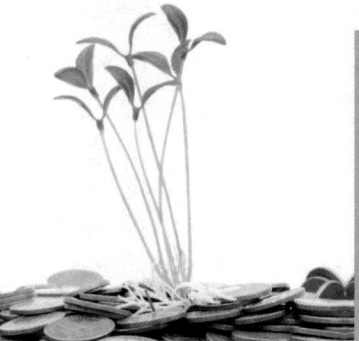
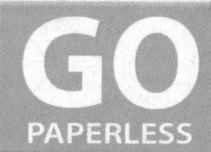
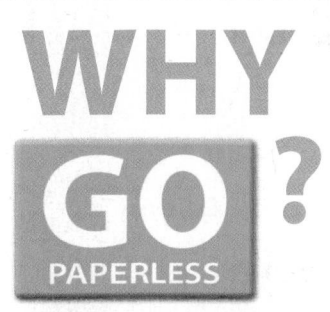
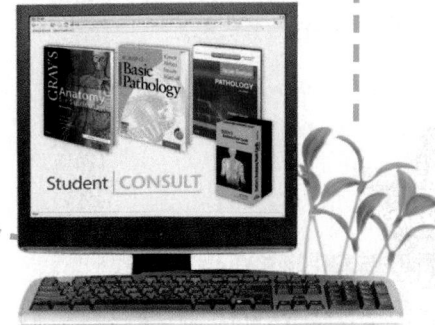
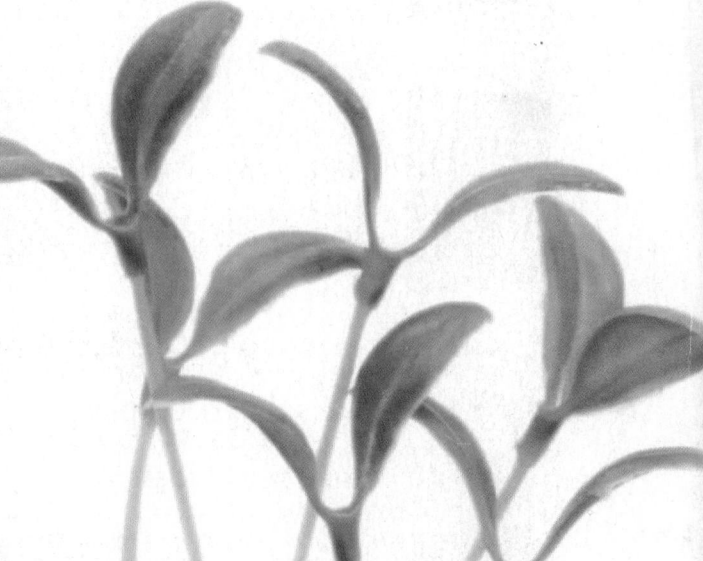

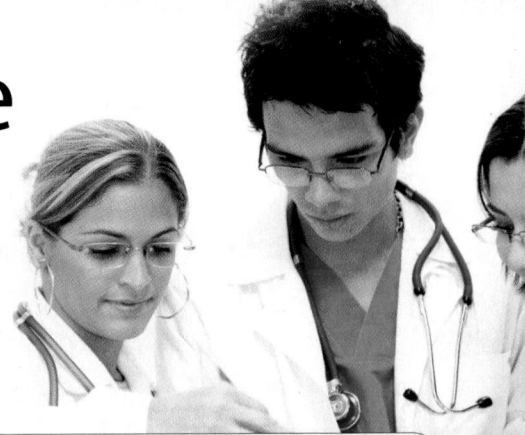
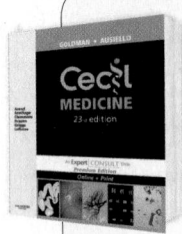
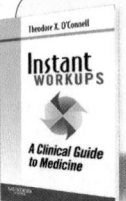
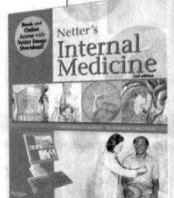
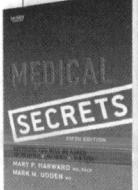
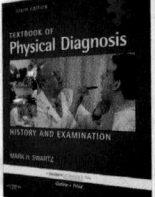
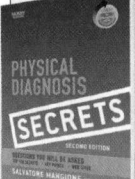
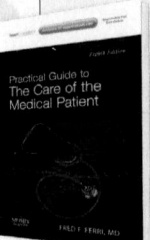
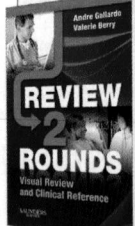
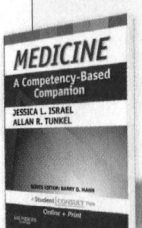
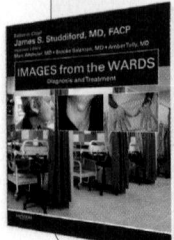

ANDREOLI and CARPENTER'S

Cecil Essentials of
MEDICINE

8th EDITION

ANDREOLI and CARPENTER'S

Cecil Essentials of
MEDICINE

8th EDITION

Editor-in-Chief

THOMAS E. ANDREOLI, MD, MACP, FRCP (Edin.), FRCP (London), ScD (hon.), Docteur (hon.), MD (hon.)[†]
Distinguished Professor
Nolan Chair Emeritus
Department of Internal Medicine
Department of Physiology and Biophysics
University of Arkansas College of Medicine
Little Rock, Arkansas
(†Deceased)

Editors

Ivor J. Benjamin, MD, FACC, FAHA
Professor of Medicine
Adjunct Professor of Biochemistry
Christi T. Smith Endowed Chair for Cardiovascular Research
Director, Center for Cardiovascular Translational Biomedicine
University of Utah School of Medicine
Salt Lake City, Utah

Robert C. Griggs, MD, FACP, FAAN
Professor of Neurology, Medicine, Pediatrics, and
Pathology and Laboratory Medicine
University of Rochester School of Medicine and Dentistry
Rochester, New York

Edward J. Wing, MD, FACP, FIDSA
Dean of Medicine and Biological Sciences
The Warren Alpert Medical School of Brown University
Providence, Rhode Island

SAUNDERS

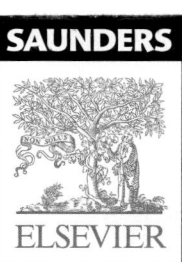

ELSEVIER

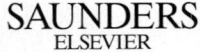

1600 John F. Kennedy Blvd.
Ste 1800
Philadelphia, PA 19103-2899

ANDREOLI AND CARPENTER'S CECIL ESSENTIALS OF MEDICINE   ISBN: 978-1-4160-6109-0

International Edition   ISBN: 978-0-8089-2428-9

Previous editions copyrighted 2007, 2004, 2001, 1997, 1993, 1990, 1986 by Saunders, an imprint of Elsevier Inc.

Library of Congress Cataloging-in-Publication Data

Andreoli and Carpenter's Cecil essentials of medicine / editor-in-chief, Thomas E. Andreoli; editors, Ivor J. Benjamin, Robert C. Griggs, Edward J. Wing.—8th ed.
   p. ; cm.
   Includes bibliographical references and index.
   ISBN 978-1-4160-6109-0
   1. Internal medicine—Textbooks.   I. Andreoli, Thomas E., 1935-2009   II. Cecil, Russell L. (Russell La Fayette), 1881-1965.   III. Title: Cecil essentials of medicine.   IV. Title: Essentials of medicine.
   [DNLM: 1. Internal Medicine. WB 115 A559 2010]
   RC46.C42 2010
   616—dc22   2009027158

Cover: Hemoglobin subunit: Phantatomix / Photo Researchers, Inc.; False-color (computer graphics) photograph of a resin cast of the human bronchial tree, the network of airways serving both lungs: Alfred Pasieka / Photo Researchers, Inc.; DNA: Dr. A. Lesk, MRC-LMB / Photo Researchers, Inc.; Osteoarthritis of foot, X-ray: DR P. MARAZZI / Photo Researchers, Inc.

Acquisitions Editor: James Merritt
Managing Editor: Rebecca Gruliow
Publishing Services Manager: Linda Van Pelt
Project Manager: Sharon Lee
Design Direction: Steven Stave

Printed in China

Last digit is the print number: 9 8 7 6 5 4 3 2 1

Dedication

Thomas E. Andreoli

When Dr. Thomas Andreoli died of a cerebral hemorrhage on April 14, 2009, he had nearly completed the editorial oversight of this, the eighth edition of the textbook he co-founded in 1986. In many ways this textbook epitomizes his career as an educator, clinical scientist, and international leader of the medical profession.

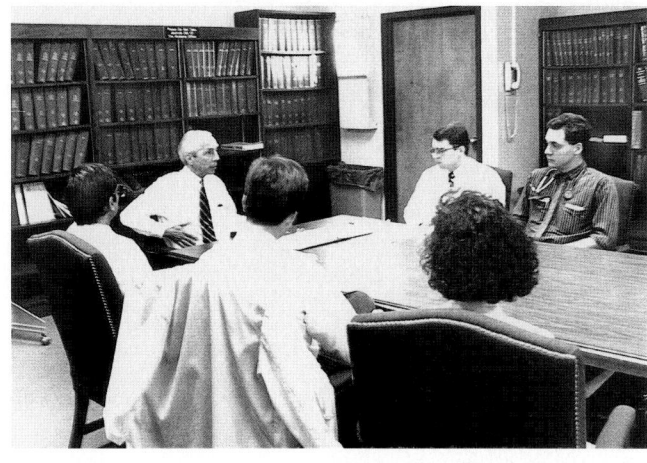

As an outstanding, life-long investigator in his chosen field of nephrology, Dr. Andreoli served as president of both national and international medical societies and was recognized by honorary doctoral degrees from both European and American universities.

As a dedicated bedside clinician and teacher, Dr. Andreoli served as an outstanding chair of medicine, and endowed chairs in his name were established at both the University of Alabama School of Medicine and the University of Arkansas College of Medicine. His superlative teaching was recognized by his receiving, inter alia, the Louis Pasteur Award from the University Louis Pasteur, Mastership of the American College of Physicians, and the Robert H. Williams Distinguished Chair of Medicine Award from the Association of Professors of Medicine.

Perhaps Dr. Andreoli's most distinguished contribution was his lifelong Oslerian devotion to translating medical science from bench to bedside. Despite his major national and international commitments, he continued throughout his career to hold morning resident teaching rounds five times weekly, maintaining a broad knowledge of all aspects of internal medicine and genuinely and gently transmitting that knowledge to two generations of medical students. He was uniquely qualified for, and committed to, imparting his wisdom and skill as a physician, which provided the basis for his serving as a founding editor of *Essentials of Medicine*, and editor-in-chief of its last three editions. We feel immensely privileged to have been his co-editors and friends, and we dedicate this text to Dr. Thomas Andreoli.

Charles C. J. Carpenter, MD, MACP
Professor of Medicine
Brown Medical School
Director, Brown University AIDS Center
Providence, Rhode Island

Clementine M. Whitman

No tribute to Dr. Andreoli's accomplishments would be complete without acknowledging the contributions of Clementine Whitman, his personal assistant of 40 years, who moved with him from Alabama to Texas and to Arkansas. Clementine was the hub of Dr. Andreoli's professional and personal life, meticulously handling every detail. Dr. Andreoli, a man as demanding of others as of himself, was indeed blessed and fortunate to have such a talented, dedicated, loyal, and hard-working person by his side.

Sudhir V. Shah, MD, FACP
Professor of Medicine
Director, Division of Nephrology
University of Arkansas College of Medicine
Little Rock, Arkansas
Chief, Renal Section, Medicine Service
John L. McClellan Memorial Veterans Hospital
Little Rock, Arkansas

Andreoli and Carpenter's Cecil Essentials of Medicine International Advisory Board

NAME	DISCIPLINE	COUNTRY
Professor J. S. Bajaj Chief Consultant and Director Department of Diabetes, Endocrine and Metabolic Medicine Batra Hospital and Medical Research Centre New Delhi, India profbajaj@hotmail.com	Endocrinology	India
Professor Massimo G. Colombo, MD Professor and Chairman Department of Gastroenterology and Endocrinology IRCCS Maggiore Hospital University of Milan Milan, Italy massimo.colombo@unimi.it	Hepatology/Gastroenterology	Italy
Professor Bertrand Fontaine, MD Professor of Neurology Faculté de Médecine Fédération des Maladies du Système Nerveux Groupe Hospitalier Pitié-Salpêtrière Paris, France bertrand.fontaine@chups.jussieu.fr	Neurology	France
Professor Arnoldo Guzmán-Sanchez Professor and Chair Department of Obstetrics and Gynecology Hospital Civil de Guadalajara Guadalajara, Jalisco, Mexico ags@cencar.udg.mx	Women's Health	Mexico
Professor Kiyoshi Kurokawa, MD President, Science Council of Japan Professor Emeritus, University of Tokyo Roppongi, Minato-ku Tokyo, Japan kurokawa@is.icc.u-tokai.ac.jp	Nephrology	Japan
Professor Umesh G. Lalloo, MD, FCCP Head, Department of Pulmonology and HIV Nelson R. Mandela School of Medicine University of Kwa-Zulu Natal Durban, South Africa lalloo@ukzn.ac.za	General Internal Medicine/HIV	South Africa
Professor Pal Magyar Head, Department of Pulmonary Medicine Semmelweis University Budapest, Hungary magyar@pulm.sote.hu	Pulmonary Medicine	Hungary
Professor John Newsom-Davis, MD *Emeritus* Professor of Clinical Neurology Radcliffe Infirmary Woodstock Road Oxford, United Kingdom John.newsomdavis@btinternet.com	Neurology	United Kingdom

NAME	DISCIPLINE	COUNTRY
Professor J. N. Pande Professor of Medicine Department of Infectious Diseases Sita Ram Bhartia Institute of Science and Research All India Institute of Medical Sciences New Delhi, India jnpande@hotmail.com	Infectious Diseases	India
Dr. Mario Paredes-Espinoza Professor and Chair Department of Internal Medicine Hospital Civil Fray Antonio Alcalde Guadalajara, Jalisco, Mexico mparedes@megared.net.mx	Men's Health/General Internal Medicine	Mexico
Professor Nestor Schor, MD, PhD Head Professor of Medicine Nephrology Division UNIFESP-Escola Paulista de Medicina São Paulo, Brazil Nschor.dmed@epm.br	Nephrology	Brazil

Lead Authors and Contributors

Section I Introduction to Molecular Medicine

Lead Author
Ivor J. Benjamin, MD, FACC, FAHA
Professor of Medicine
Adjunct Professor of Biochemistry
Christi T. Smith Endowed Chair in Cardiovascular
  Research
Director, Center for Cardiovascular Translational
  Biomedicine
University of Utah School of Medicine
Salt Lake City, Utah
Ivor.Benjamin@hsc.utah.edu

Section II Evidence-Based Medicine

Lead Authors
Sara G. Tariq, MD
Associate Professor
Department of Internal Medicine
University of Arkansas College of Medicine
Little Rock, Arkansas
TariqSaraG@uams.edu

Susan S. Beland, MD
Associate Professor
Department of Internal Medicine
University of Arkansas College of Medicine
Little Rock, Arkansas
belandsusans@uams.edu

Section III Cardiovascular Disease

Lead Author
Ivor J. Benjamin, MD, FACC, FAHA
Professor of Medicine
Adjunct Professor of Biochemistry
Christi T. Smith Endowed Chair in Cardiovascular
  Research
Director, Center for Cardiovascular Translational
  Biomedicine
University of Utah School of Medicine
Salt Lake City, Utah
Ivor.Benjamin@hsc.utah.edu

Contributors
David Bull, MD
Professor of Surgery
Director, Thoracic Surgery Residency Program
University of Utah School of Medicine
Chief of Cardiothoracic Surgery
Salt Lake City VA Medical Center
Salt Lake City, Utah
David.Bull@hsc.utah.edu

Mohamed H. Hamdan, MD
Professor and Associate Division Chief
Division of Cardiology
University of Utah School of Medicine
Section Chief, Arrhythmia
University of Utah Healthcare
Salt Lake City, Utah
Mohamed.Hamdan@hsc.utah.edu

Dean Y. Li, MD, PhD
Associate Professor
Departments of Medicine and Oncological Science
Huntsman Cancer Institute
University of Utah School of Medicine
Salt Lake City, Utah
dean@hmbg.utah.edu

Sheldon E. Litwin, MD
Amundsen Professor of Internal Medicine/Cardiology
Director of Cardiovascular Imaging
University of Utah Hospital
University of Utah School of Medicine
Salt Lake City, Utah
Sheldon.Litwin@hsc.utah.edu

Andrew D. Michaels, MD
Associate Professor of Internal Medicine
Director, Cardiac Catheterization Laboratory and
  Interventional Cardiology
University of Utah School of Medicine
Salt Lake City, Utah
andrew.michaels@hsc.utah.edu

Jack H. Morshedzadeh, MD
Instructor
Division of Cardiology
University of Utah School of Medicine
Salt Lake City, Utah
Jack.Morshedzadeh@HSC.Utah.edu

Josef Stehlik, MD
Assistant Professor of Internal Medicine
Division of Cardiology
University of Utah School of Medicine
Salt Lake City, Utah
Josef.stehlik@hsc.utah.edu

Kevin J. Whitehead, MD
Associate Professor of Cardiology
University of Utah School of Medicine
Salt Lake City, Utah
Kevin.whitehead@hsc.utah.edu

Ronald G. Victor, MD
Associate Director
Cedars-Sinai Heart Institute
Director, Cedars-Sinai Hypertension Center
Los Angeles, California
Ronald.Victor@cshs.org

Wanpen Vongpatanasin, MD
Associate Professor of Internal Medicine-Cardiology
The University of Texas Southwestern Medical School
Dallas, Texas
Wanpen.Vongpatanasin@UTSouthwestern.Edu

Section IV Pulmonary and Critical Care Medicine

Lead Author
Sharon I. Rounds, MD
Professor of Medicine and of Pathology and Laboratory
    Medicine
Brown Medical School
Chief of Pulmonary Critical Care Medicine
Providence VA Medical Center
Providence, Rhode Island
Sharon_Rounds@Brown.edu

Contributors
Jason M. Aliotta, MD
Assistant Professor of Medicine
Division of Biology and Medicine
Brown University
Providence, Rhode Island
Jason_Aliotta@brown.edu

Brian Casserly, MD
Assistant Professor of Medicine
Brown University
Providence, Rhode Island
Brian_Casserly@brown.edu

Matthew D. Jankowich, MD
Instructor in Medicine
Division of Biology and Medicine
Brown University
Providence, Rhode Island
Matthew_Jankowich@brown.edu

F. Dennis McCool, MD
Chief, Pulmonary Critical Care Medicine
Memorial Hospital of Rhode Island
Professor of Medicine
Alpert Medical School of Brown University
Pawtucket, Rhode Island
F_McCool@Brown.edu

Section V Preoperative and Postoperative Care

Lead Author
Kim A. Eagle, MD
Albion Walter Hewlett Professor of Internal Medicine
Chief, Clinical Cardiovascular Medicine
Director, Cardiovascular Center
University of Michigan Medical School
Ann Arbor, Michigan
keagle@umich.edu

Contributors
Wei C. Lau, MD
Clinical Associate Professor
Director, Adult Cardiovascular Thoracic Anesthesiology
Medical Director, Cardiovascular Center Operating Rooms
Department of Anesthesiology
University of Michigan Health System
Ann Arbor, Michigan
weiclau@umich.edu

Section VI Renal Disease

Lead Author
Raymond C. Harris, MD
Ann and Roscoe R. Robinson Professor of Medicine
Director, Division of Nephrology
Vanderbilt University School of Medicine
Nashville, Tennessee
Ray.Harris@vanderbilt.edu

Contributors
Thomas E. Andreoli, MD, MACP, FRCP (Edinburgh), FRCP (London), ScD (hon.), Docteur (hon.), MD (hon.), Doctor (hon.)
Distinguished Professor of Internal Medicine and of
    Physiology and Biophysics
Nolan Chairman Emeritus of Internal Medicine
University of Arkansas College of Medicine
Little Rock, Arkansas

Amanda W. Basford, MD
Kidney Associates, PLLC
6624 Fannin, Suite 1400
Houston, Texas
Amanda.Basford@gmail.com

Kerri L. Cavanaugh, MD
Assistant Professor of Medicine
Vanderbilt University School of Medicine
Nashville, Tennessee
kerri.cavanaugh@vanderbilt.edu

Jamie P. Dwyer, MD
Assistant Professor of Medicine, Nephrology and
    Hypertension
Vanderbilt University School of Medicine
Nashville, Tennessee
jamie.dwyer@vanderbilt.edu

Thomas A. Golper, MD
Professor of Medicine/Nephrology
Director, Medical Specialties Patient Care Center
Vanderbilt University School of Medicine
Nashville, Tennessee
Thomas.golper@vanderbilt.edu

Michelle W. Krause, MD, MPH
Assistant Professor of Medicine
Division of Nephrology
Department of Internal Medicine
University of Arkansas College of Medicine
Little Rock, Arkansas
KrauseMichelleW@uams.edu

T. Alp Ikizler, MD
Catherine McLaughlin Hakim Professor of Medicine
Director, Clinical Research in Nephrology
Director, Master of Science in Clinical Investigation
   Program
Medical Director, Vanderbilt Outpatient Dialysis Unit
Division of Nephrology
Vanderbilt University School of Medicine
Nashville, Tennessee
alp.ikizler@vanderbilt.edu

Julia B. Lewis, MD
Professor of Medicine
Director, Fellowship Training
Division of Nephrology
Vanderbilt University School of Medicine
Nashville, Tennessee
Julia.lewis@vanderbilt.edu

James M. Luther, MD, MSCI
Assistant Professor of Medicine
Division of Nephrology
Vanderbilt University School of Medicine
Nashville, Tennessee
james.luther@vanderbilt.edu

James L. Pirkle, MD
Nephrology and Hypertension Specialists, P.C.
Dalton, Georgia
JLPirkle@yahoo.com

Didier Portilla, MD
Professor of Medicine
Division of Nephrology
Department of Internal Medicine
University of Arkansas College of Medicine
Little Rock, Arkansas
PortillaDidier@uams.edu

Robert L. Safirstein, MD
Professor, Executive Vice Chair
Department of Internal Medicine
University of Arkansas College of Medicine
Chief of Medical Services
Central Arkansas Veterans Hospital
Little Rock, Arkansas
SafirsteinRobertL@uams.edu

Gerald Schulman, MD
Professor of Medicine
Division of Nephrology
Vanderbilt University School of Medicine
Nashville, Tennessee
Gerald.schulman@vanderbilt.edu

Sudhir V. Shah, MD
Professor and Director
Division of Nephrology
Department of Internal Medicine
University of Arkansas College of Medicine
Little Rock, Arkansas
ShahSudhirV@uams.edu

Roy Zent, MD
Associate Professor of Medicine, Cancer Biology, and Cell
   and Developmental Biology
Division of Nephrology
Vanderbilt University School of Medicine
Nashville, Tennessee
roy.zent@vanderbilt.edu

Section VII Gastrointestinal Disease

Lead Author
M. Michael Wolfe, MD
Professor of Medicine
Research Professor of Physiology and Biophysics
Boston University School of Medicine
Chief, Section of Gastroenterology
Boston Medical Center
Boston, Massachusetts 02118
Michael.Wolfe@bmc.org

Contributors
Wanda P. Blanton, MD
Instructor, Department of Medicine
Section of Gastroenterology
Boston University School of Medicine
Boston, Massachusetts
Wanda.Blanton@bmc.org

Charles M. Bliss Jr., MD, FACP
Assistant Professor of Medicine
Section of Gastroenterology
Boston University School of Medicine
Boston, Massachusetts
charles.bliss@bmc.org

Francis A. Farraye, MD, MSc
Clinical Director, Section of Gastroenterology
Co-Director, Center for Digestive Disorders
Professor of Medicine
Boston University School of Medicine
Boston, Massachusetts
Francis.Farraye@bmc.org

Christopher S. Huang, MD
Instructor of Medicine
Section of Gastroenterology
Boston University School of Medicine
Boston, Massachusetts
cshuang@bu.edu

Brian C. Jacobson, MD, MPH
Director of Endoscopic Ultrasonography
Associate Director of Endoscopy Services
Boston Medical Center and
Assistant Professor of Medicine
Boston University School of Medicine
Boston, Massachusetts
brian.jacobson@bmc.org

David R. Lichtenstein, MD, FACG
Director of Gastrointestinal Endoscopy
Associate Professor of Medicine
Boston University School of Medicine
Boston, Massachusetts
davidL@bu.edu

Robert Lowe, MD
Associate Professor of Medicine
Educational Director of the Section of Gastroenterology
Boston University School of Medicine
Boston, Massachusetts
RoLowe@bu.edu

Daniel S. Mishkin, MD, CM
Director, The Endoscopy Center of Brookline
Instructor of Medicine
Boston University School of Medicine
Boston, Massachusetts
damishkin@bu.edu

T. Carlton Moore, MD
Assistant Professor in Medicine
Section of Gastroenterology
Boston University School of Medicne
Boston, Massachusetts
Carlton.Moore@bmc.org

Jaime A. Oviedo, MD, FACG
Greater Boston Gastroenterology
Framingham, Massachusetts
Jaime.Oviedo@bmc.org

Marcos C. Pedrosa, MD, MPH
Chief of Endoscopy
VA Boston HealthCare System
Brigham and Women's Hospital
Boston, Massachusetts
Marcos.Pedrosa@med.va.gov

Elihu M. Schimmel, MD
Director
VA Advanced Specialty Training Program in
    Gastroenterology and Hepatology
Boston VA Hospital
Boston, Massachusetts
Elihu.Schimmel@med.va.gov

Paul C. Schroy, III, MD, MPH
Director of Clinical Research
Section of Gastroenterology
Associate Professor of Medicine
Boston University School of Medicine
Associate Professor of Epidemiology/Biostatistics
Boston University School of Public Health
Boston, Massachusetts
pschroy@bu.edu

Satish K. Singh, MD
Assistant Professor of Medicine
Boston University School of Medicine
Staff Gastroenterologist
VA Boston HealthCare System
Boston, MA 02118
singhsk@bu.edu

Chi-Chuan Tseng, MD, PhD
Associate Professor of Medicine
Department of Medicine
Boston University School of Medicine
Associate Chief
Boston Veterans Administration Health Care System
Boston, Massachusetts
ethan@bu.edu

Section VIII Diseases of the Liver and Biliary System

Lead Author
Michael B. Fallon, MD
Professor of Medicine
Director, Division of Gastroenterology, Hepatology and
    Nutrition
The University of Texas Medical School
Houston, Texas
michael.b.fallon@uth.tmc.edu

Contributors
Miguel R. Arguedas MD, MPH
Assistant Professor
Division of Gastroenterology
University of Alabama School of Medicine
MCLM 280
Birmingham, Alabama
Arguedas@uab.edu

Rudolf Garcia-Gallont, MD
Head, Department of Surgery
Amedesgua Hospital
Guatemala City, Guatemala
garciagallont@hotmail.com

Rajan Kochar, MD
Assistant Professor of Medicine
Division of Gastroenterology, Hepatology and Nutrition
The University of Texas Medical School
Houston, Texas
rajankochar@gmail.com

Brendan M. McGuire, MD, MS
Associate Professor
Medical Director, Liver Transplantation/Medicine
Liver Center, Department of Medicine
University of Alabama School of Medicine
Birmingham, Alabama
bmcguire@uab.edu

Klaus Mönkemüller, MD
Associate Professor
Chief, Endoscopy and Outpatient Clinic
Division of Gastroenterology, Hepatology and Infectious
    Diseases
Otto-von-Guericke University
Magdeburg, Germany
Klaus.Monkemuller@medizin.uni-magdeburg.de

Helmut Neumann, MD
Faculty of Medicine
Division of Gastroenterology, Hepatology and Infectious
   Diseases
Otto-von-Guericke University
Magdeburg, Germany
Helmut.Neumann@Medizin.Uni-Magdeburg.de

Aasim M. Sheikh, MD
Northwest Georgia Gastroenterology Associates
Marietta, Georgia
asheikh@uab.edu

Shyam Varadarajulu, MD
Assistant Professor, Division of Gastroenterology
Director, Interventional Endoscopy
University of Alabama at Birmingham
Birmingham, Alabama
svaradarajulu@uab.edu

Section IX Hematologic Disease

Lead Author
Nancy Berliner, MD
Professor of Medicine
Harvard Medical School
Chief, Division of Hematology
Brigham and Women's Hospital
Boston, Massachusetts
nberliner@partners.org

Contributors
Jill Lacy, MD
Associate Professor of Medical Oncology
Yale University School of Medicine
New Haven, Connecticut
Jill.Lacy@yale.edu

Christine S. Rinder, MD
Associate Professor of Anesthesiology and Laboratory
   Medicine
Yale University School of Medicine
Department of Anesthesiology
Yale-New Haven Hospital
New Haven, Connecticut
christine.rinder@yale.edu

Henry M. Rinder, MD
Professor of Laboratory Medicine and Internal Medicine
Director, Clinical Hematology Laboratory
Program Director, Clinical Pathology Residency Training
Yale University School of Medicine
New Haven, Connecticut
henry.rinder@yale.edu

Michal G. Rose, MD
Associate Professor of Medicine
Yale University School of Medicine
Chief, Cancer Center
VA Connecticut HealthCare System
New Haven, Connecticut
Michal.Rose@yale.edu

Stuart E. Seropian, MD
Associate Professor of Medicine
Yale Cancer Center
Lymphoma, Leukemia and Myeloma Program
New Haven, Connecticut
stuart.seropian@yale.edu

Christopher Tormey, MD
Instructor, Laboratory Medicine
Yale University School of Medicine
New Haven, Connecticut
christopher.tormey@yale.edu

Richard Torres, MD
Attending Hematopathologist
Yale University School of Medicine
New Haven, Connecticut
Richard.Torres@yale.edu

Eunice S. Wang, MD
Research Assistant Professor
Leukemia Service, Departments of Medicine and
   Immunology
Staff Physician
Leukemia Service
Roswell Park Cancer Institute
Buffalo, New York
Eunice.Wang@roswellpark.org

Section X Oncologic Disease

Lead Author
Jennifer J. Griggs, MD, MPH
Associate Professor
Department of Internal Medicine
Division of Hematology/Oncology
Director, Breast Cancer Survivorship Program
University of Michigan Comprehensive Cancer Center
University of Michigan Medical School
Ann Arbor, Michigan
jengriggs@med.umich.edu

Contributors
Barbara A. Burtness, MD
Medical Oncologist
Fox Chase Cancer Center
Philadelphia, Pennsylvania
Barbara.Burtness@fccc.edu

Alok A. Khorana, MD, FACP
Assistant Professor of Medicine, James P. Wilmot Cancer
   Center
University of Rochester School of Medicine and Dentistry
Rochester, New York
alok_khorana@urmc.rochester.edu

Paula M. Lantz, MD
Professor and Chair
Department of Health Management and Policy
Research Professor, Institute for Social Research
University of Michigan Health System
Ann Arbor, Michigan
plantz@umich.edu

Robert F. Todd, III, MD, PhD
Margaret M. Alkek Distinguished Chair and Professor
Department of Medicine
Baylor College of Medicine
Houston, Texas
rftodd@bcm.edu

Section XI Metabolic Disease

Lead Author
Robert J. Smith, MD
Director, Division of Endocrinology
Director, Hallett Center for Diabetes and Endocrinology
Brown University Alpert Medical School
Providence, Rhode Island
Robert_J_Smith@brown.edu

Contributors
David G. Brooks, MD, PhD
Medical Director, Global Clinical Development
Abraxis Bioscience, LLC
Burlington, Massachusetts
dbrooks@abraxisbio.com

Geetha Gopalakrishnan, MD
Assistant Professor
Division of Biology and Medicine
Brown University Alpert Medical School
Providence, Rhode Island
Geetha_Gopalakrishnan@brown.edu

Osama Hamdy, MD
Medical Director
Obesity Clinical Program
Joslin Diabetes Center
Assistant Professor of Medicine
Harvard Medical School
Boston, Massachusetts
Osama.hamdy@joslin.harvard.edu

Michelle P. Warren, MD
Wyeth-Ayerst Professor
Founder and Medical Director
Center for Menopause, Hormonal Disorders and Women's
   Health
Department of Obstetrics and Gynecology
Columbia University College of Physicians and Surgeons
New York, New York
mpw1@columbia.edu

Thomas R. Ziegler, MD
Professor of Medicine
Atlanta Clinical and Translational Science Institute
Emory University School of Medicine
Atlanta, Georgia
tzieg01@emory.edu

Section XII Endocrine Disease

Section Author
Glenn D. Braunstein, MD
Professor of Medicine
UCLA School of Medicine
Chair, Department of Medicine
Cedars-Sinai Medical Center
Los Angeles, California
Glenn.Braunstein@cshs.org

Contributors
Philip S. Barnett, MD, PhD
Director
Anna and Max Webb and Family Diabetes Outpatient
   Treatment and Education Center
Cedars Sinai Medical Center
Professor of Medicine
David Geffen School of Medicine
University of California, Los Angeles
Los Angeles, California
Philip.Barnett@cshs.org

Vivien S. Herman-Bonert, MD
Associate Professor of Medicine
David Geffen School of Medicine
Division of Endocrinology
University of California, Los Angeles
Attending Physician, Cedars Sinai Medical Center
Los Angeles, California
vivien.bonert@cshs.org

Theodore C. Friedman, MD, PhD
Associate Professor of Medicine
UCLA School of Medicine
Endocrinology Division
Cedars Sinai Medical Center
Los Angeles, California
friedmantc@csmc.edu

Section XIII Women's Health

Lead Author
Pamela A. Charney, MD
Assistant Professor of Medicine
Weill Cornell Medical College
New York, New York
pac2029@med.cornell.edu

Contributors
Patricia I. Carney, MD
Department of Obstetrics and Gynecology
Christiana Care Health Services
Newark, Delaware
pcarney@christianacare.org

Deborah B. Ehrenthal, MD, FACP
Departments of Internal Medicine and Obstetrics and
    Gynecology
Christiana Care Health Services
Newark, Delaware
Clinical Assistant Professor of Medicine
Thomas Jefferson University
Philadelphia, Pennsylvania
dehrenthal@christianacare.org

Renee K. Kottenhahn, MD
Department of Pediatrics
Christiana Care Health Services
Newark, Delaware
rkottenhahn@christianacare.org

Section XIV Men's Health

Lead Author
Joseph A. Smith, Jr., MD
Professor and Chair
Department of Urologic Surgery
Vanderbilt University School of Medicine
Nashville, Tennessee
Joseph.Smith@vanderbilt.edu

Contributors
Douglas F. Milam, MD
Associate Professor
Department of Urologic Surgery
Vanderbilt University School of Medicine
Nashville, Tennessee
doug.milam@vanderbilt.edu

Johnathan S. Starkman, MD
Clinical Instructor
Department of Urologic Surgery
Vanderbilt University School of Medicine
Nashville, Tennessee
starkman137@comcast.net

Section XV Diseases of Bone and Bone Mineral Metabolism

Lead Author
Andrew F. Stewart, MD
Professor of Medicine
Chief, Division of Endocrinology and Metabolism
University of Pittsburgh School of Medicine
Pittsburgh, Pennsylvania
stewarta@pitt.edu

Contributors
Susan L. Greenspan, MD
Professor of Medicine
Director, Osteoporosis Prevention and Treatment Center
Associate Program Director, General Clinical Research
    Center
University of Pittsburgh School of Medicine
Pittsburgh, Pennsylvania
greenspn@pitt.edu

Steven P. Hodak, MD
Clinical Assistant Professor of Medicine
Medical Director, Center for Diabetes and Endocrinology
University of Pittsburgh School of Medicine
Pittsburgh, Pennsylvania
sph12@pitt.edu

Mara J. Horwitz, MD
Assistant Professor of Medicine
Division of Endocrionology
University of Pittsburgh School of Medicine
Pittsburgh, Pennsylvania
Horwitz@pitt.edu

Shane O. LeBeau, MD
Clinical Assistant Professor of Medicine
Center for Diabetes and Endocrinology
University of Pittsburgh School of Medicine
Pittsburgh, Pennsylvania
SOL15@pitt.edu

G. David Roodman, MD, PhD
Professor of Medicine
University of Pittsburgh Hillman Cancer Center
Pittsburgh, Pennsylvania
roodmangd@msx.upmc.edu

Section XVI Musculoskeletal and Connective Tissue Disease

Lead Author
Larry W. Moreland, MD
Margaret Jane Miller Endowed Professor of Arthritis
    Research
Chief, Division of Rheumatology and Clinical Immunology
University of Pittsburgh School of Medicine
Pittsburgh, Pennsylvania
MorelandL@dom.pitt.edu

Contributors
Surabhi Agarwal, MD
Medical Resident
University of Pittsburgh School of Medicine
Pittsburgh, Pennsylvania
agarwals@upmc.edu

Dana P. Ascherman, MD
Assistant Professor of Medicine
Divison of Rheumatology and Clinical Immunology
University of Pittsburgh School of Medicine
Pittsburgh, Pennsylvania
ascher@pitt.edu

Robyn T. Domsic, MD
Assistant Professor of Medicine
Division of Rheumatology and Clinical Immunology
University of Pittsburgh School of Medicine
Pittsburgh, Pennsylvania
rtd4@pitt.edu

Jennifer Rae Elliott, MD
Division of Rheumatology and Clinical Immunology
University of Pittsburgh School of Medicine
Pittsburgh, Pennsylvania
elliottjr@upmc.edu

Amy H. Kao, MD, MPH
Assistant Professor of Medicine
Division of Rheumatology and Clinical Immunology
University of Pittsburgh School of Medicine
Pittsburgh, Pennsylvania
AHK7@pitt.edu

Fotios Koumpouras, MD
Assistant Professor of Medicine
Medical Director, Lupus Center of Excellence
Division of Rheumatology and Clinical Immunology
University of Pittsburgh School of Medicine
Pittsburgh, Pennsylvania
koumpourasf@upmc.edu

C. Kent Kwoh, MD
Professor of Medicine
Division of Rheumatology and Clinical Immunology
University of Pittsburgh School of Medicine
Pittsburgh, Pennsylvania
kwoh@pitt.edu

Douglas W. Lienesch, MD
Assistant Professor of Medicine
Division of Rheumatology and Clinical Immunology
University of Pittsburgh School of Medicine
Pittsburgh, Pennsylvania
lieneschd@upmc.edu

Kathleen McKinnon-Maksimowicz, DO
Assistant Professor of Medicine
Division of Rheumatology and Clinical Immunology
University of Pittsburgh School of Medicine
Pittsburgh, Pennsylvania
mckinnonk@dom.pitt.edu

Thomas A. Medsger, Jr., MD
Gerald P. Rodnan Professor of Medicine
Division of Rheumatology and Clinical Immunology
Director, Scleroderma Research Program
University of Pittsburgh School of Medicine
Pittsburgh, Pennsylvania
medsger@dom.pitt.edu

Niveditha Mohan, MD
Assistant Professor of Medicine
Division of Rheumatology and Clinical Immunology
University of Pittsburgh School of Medicine
Pittsburgh, Pennsylvania
mohann2@upmc.edu

Section XVII Infectious Disease

Lead Author
Edward J. Wing, MD, FACP, FIDSA
Dean of Medicine and Biological Sciences
The Warren Alpert Medical School of Brown University
Providence, Rhode Island
ewing@lifespan.org

Contributors
Keith B. Armitage, MD
Professor of Medicine
Vice Chair for Education
Department of Medicine
Co-Director, Medicine/Pediatrics Residency
Director, Internal Medicine Residency Training Program
Case Western Reserve University
Cleveland, Ohio
KBA@case.edu

Curt G. Beckwith, MD
Assistant Professor of Medicine
Division of Infectious Diseases
Brown Medical School
Providence, Rhode Island
cbeckwith@lifespan.org

David A. Bobak, MD
Associate Professor
Division of Infectious Diseases
Case Western Reserve University
University Hospitals of Cleveland
Cleveland, Ohio
David.Bobak@case.edu

Jessica K. Fairley, MD
Division of Infectious Disease and HIV Medicine
Case Western Reserve University
Division of Infectious Disease
University Hospitals
Cleveland, Ohio
jessica.fairley@case.edu

Scott A. Fulton, MD
Assistant Professor
Division of Infectious Diseases
Case Western Reserve University
University Hospitals of Cleveland
Cleveland, Ohio
Scott.Fulton@case.edu

Corrilynn O. Hileman, MD
Internal Medicine
Infectious Disease
Case Western Reserve University
Cleveland, Ohio
corrilynn.hileman@case.edu

Christoph Lange, MD, PhD
Medical Clinic
Borstel Research Center
Borstel, Germany
clange@fz-borstel.de, cgmlange@hotmail.com

Michael M. Lederman, MD
Scott R. Inkley Professor of Medicine
Case Western Reserve University
Co-Director, CWRU/University Hospitals of Cleveland
Center for AIDS Research
Cleveland, Ohio
Michael.lederman@case.edu

Tracy L. Lemonovich, MD
Instructor
Division of Infectious Diseases and HIV Medicine
Case Western Reserve University
Cleveland, Ohio
tracy.lemonovich@uhhospitals.org

Michelle V. Lisagaris, MD
Assistant Professor
Department of Medicine
University Hospitals of Cleveland
Cleveland, Ohio
MVL@case.edu

Amy J. Ray, MD
Clinical Instructor and Division Chief
University Hospitals Richmond Medical Center
Infectious Diseases Division
University Hospitals, School of Medicine
Case Western Reserve University
Cleveland, Ohio
amy.ray@uhhospitals.org

Benigno Rodriguez, MD
Assistant Professor
Department of Medicine
Case Western Reserve University
Cleveland, Ohio
rodriguez.benigno@clevelandactu.org

Robert A. Salata, MD
Division Chief
Division of Infectious Diseases and HIV Medicine
Case Western Reserve University
Cleveland, Ohio
RAS7@po.cwru.edu

Richard R. Watkins, MD, MS
Division of Infectious Diseases
Akron General Medical Center
Akron, Ohio

Section XVIII Bioterrorism

Lead Author
Robert W. Bradsher, Jr., MD
Richard V. Ebert Professor of Internal Medicine
Vice-Chair for Education, Department of Internal
  Medicine
Director, Division of Infectious Diseases
University of Arkansas College of Medicine
Little Rock, Arkansas
BradsherRobertW@uams.edu

Section XIX Neurologic Disease

Lead Author
Robert C. Griggs, MD, FACP, FAAN
Professor of Neurology, Medicine, Pathology and
  Laboratory Medicine, and Pediatrics
University of Rochester School of Medicine and Dentistry
Rochester, New York
Robert_Griggs@urmc.rochester.edu

Contributors
Michel J. Berg, MD
Associate Professor of Neurology and Medical Director,
  Strong Epilepsy Center
University of Rochester School of Medicine and Dentistry
Rochester, New York
Michel_berg@urmc.rochester.edu

Emma Ciafaloni, MD
Associate Professor
Department of Neurology (SMD)
University of Rochester School of Medicine and Dentistry
Rochester, New York
Emma_ciafaloni@urmc.rochester.edu

Timothy J. Counihan, MD, MRCPI
Department of Neurology
Galway University Hospital
Galway, Ireland
timothy.counihan@hse.ie

William P. Cheshire Jr., MD
Professor of Neurology
Mayo Clinic
Jacksonville, Florida
cheshire@mayo.edu

Emily C. de los Reyes, MD
Associate Professor of Clinical Pediatrics and Neurology
Nationwide Children's Hospital
The Ohio State University
Columbus, Ohio
emily.delosreyes@nationwidechildrens.org

Jennifer J. Griggs, MD, MPH
Associate Professor
Department of Internal Medicine
Division of Hematology/Oncology
Director, Breast Cancer Survivorship Program
University of Michigan Comprehensive Cancer Center
University of Michigan Medical School
Ann Arbor, Michigan
jengriggs@med.umich.edu

Carlayne E. Jackson, MD
Professor of Neurology
University of Texas Medical School
San Antonio, Texas
jacksonce@uthscsa.edu

Kevin A. Kerber, MD
Assistant Professor
Department of Neurology
Director, Dizziness Clinic
University of Michigan Medical School
Ann Arbor, Michigan
kakerber@umich.edu

Lynn C. Liu, MD
Chief, Strong Sleep Disorders Center
Department of Neurology
University of Rochester School of Medicine and Dentistry
Rochester, New York
Lynn_liu@urmc.rochester.edu

Geoffrey S.F. Ling, MD, PhD
Defense Advanced Research Projects Agency
Defense Sciences Office
Arlington, Virginia
geoffrey.ling@darpa.mil

Jeffery M. Lyness, MD
Professor and Associate Chair for Education
Department of Psychiatry
Director of Curriculum, Office of Curriculum and
    Assessment
University of Rochester School of Medicine and Dentistry
Rochester, New York
Jeffrey_lyness@urmc.rochester.edu

Deborah Joanne Lynn, MD
Associate Professor
The Ohio State University Department of Neurology
Director, Department of Neurology Medical Student
    Education
Staff Neurologist
The Ohio State University Medical Center and The Arthur
    James Cancer Hospital and Research Institute
Co-director, Ohio State University Multiple Sclerosis
    Center
Columbus, Ohio
Lynn.7@osu.edu

Frederick J. Marshall, MD
Associate Professor
Department of Neurology (SMD)
University of Rochester
Rochester, New York
fred.marshall@ctcc.rochester.edu

Allan McCarthy, MD, MRCPI
Department of Neurology
Galway University Hospital
Galway, Ireland
amaccarthy@gmail.com

Sinéad M. Murphy, BA, MB, BCh, MRCPI
Department of Neurology
Galway University Hospital
Galway, Ireland
smurph1@hotmail.com

Avindra Nath, MD
Professor of Neurology
Johns Hopkins University
Baltimore, Maryland
anath1@jhmi.edu

E. Steve Roach, MD
Vice Chair for Clinical Affairs
Department of Pediatrics
Director, Division of Pediatric Neurology
Professor of Child Neurology
Nationwide Children's Hospital
The Ohio State University
Columbus, Ohio
Steve.roach@nationwidechildrens.org

Lisa R. Rogers, DO
Director, Medical Neuro-Oncology
University Hospitals—Case Medical Center and
Professor of Neurology
Department of Neurology
Case Western University School of Medicine
Cleveland, Ohio
lisa.rogers@case.edu

Roger P. Simon, MD
Chair and Director
R.S. Dow Neurobiology Laboratories
Legacy Research Hospital and
Adjunct Professor
Neurology, Physiology and Pharmacology
Oregon Health and Science University
Portland, Oregon
rsimon@downeurobiology.org

Section XX The Aging Patient

Lead Author
Harvey J. Cohen, MD
Walter Kempner Professor and Chair of Medicine
Director, Center for the Study of Aging and Human
    Development
Duke University School of Medicine
Durham, North Carolina
cohen015@mc.duke.edu

Contributor
Mitchell T. Heflin, MD, MHS
Assistant Professor of Medicine and Geriatrics
Center for the Study of Aging and Human Development
Duke University School of Medicine
Durham, NC
Durham, North Carolina
heflin001@mc.duke.edu

Section XXI Palliative Care

Lead Authors
Timothy E. Quill, MD
Professor of Medicine, Psychiatry and Medical Humanities
Director, Palliative Care Program
University of Rochester School of Medicine
Rochester, New York
Timothy_Quill@urmc.rochester.edu

Robert G. Holloway, MD, MPH
Professor, Department of Neurology
Professor, Department of Community and Preventive
    Medicine (SMD)
Rochester, New York
Robert_holloway@urmc.rochester.edu

Section XXII Alcohol and Substance Abuse

Lead Authors
L. David Hillis, MD
Dan Parman Distinguished Professor
Chair, Department of Internal Medicine
University of Texas Medical School
San Antonio, Texas
HillisD@uthscsa.edu

Richard A. Lange, MD
Professor and Executive Vice-Chair
Department of Medicine
University of Texas Medical School
San Antonio, Texas
langera@uthscsa.edu

This is the eighth edition of *Andreoli and Carpenter's Cecil Essentials of Medicine*. *Essentials VIII*, like its predecessors, is intended to be comprehensive but concise. *Essentials VIII* therefore provides an exacting and thoroughly updated treatise on internal medicine, without excessive length, for students of medicine at all levels of their careers.

We welcome with enthusiasm a new editor, Edward J. Wing, MD, Frank L. Day Professor of Biology, and Dean of Medicine and Biological Sciences at Brown University Warren Alpert Medical School.

Essentials VIII has three cardinal components. First, at the beginning of each section—kidney, for example—we provide a brief but rigorous summary of the fundamental biology of the kidney and/or the cardinal signs and symptoms of diseases of the kidney. The same format has been used in all the sections of the book. Second, the main body of each section contains a detailed, but again, concise description of the diseases of the various organ systems, together with their pathophysiology and their treatment.

Finally, *Essentials* relies heavily on the Internet. *Essentials VIII* is published entirely on a Web site on the Internet. In the online version of *Essentials VIII*, we provide a substantial amount of supplemental material, indicated in the hard copy text by boldface symbols (for example, **Web Fig. 1**) and denoted by an arrow icon shown in the margin of this page. This icon is present throughout the hard copy of the book as well as in the Internet version and directs the reader to a series of illustrations, tables, or videos in the Internet version of *Essentials*. This material is clearly crucial to understanding modern medicine, but we hope that, in this manner, the supplemental material will enrich *Essentials VIII* without having enlarged the book significantly.

As in prior editions, we make abundant use of 4-color illustrations. And as in prior editions, each section has been reviewed by one or another of the editors, and finally by the editor-in-chief.

We thank James T. Merritt, Senior Acquisitions Editor, Medical Education, of Elsevier, Inc., and especially Rebecca Gruliow, Managing Editor for Global Medicine, Elsevier, Inc. Both Jim Merritt and Rebecca Gruliow contributed heartily to the preparation of this eighth edition of *Essentials*. Lastly, we thank our very able secretarial staff, Ms. Clementine M. Whitman (Little Rock); Ms. Barbara S. Bottone (Providence); Ms. Shirley E. Thomas (Rochester); Ms. Jennifer F. Schroff (Salt Lake City); and Ms. Jean M. Drinan, and Ms. Catarina A. Santos (Providence).

The Editors

Contents

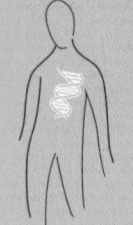

Section I

Introduction to Molecular Medicine

1   Molecular Basis of Human Disease – BENJAMIN

Chapter 1

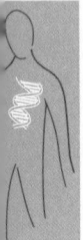

Molecular Basis of Human Disease

Ivor J. Benjamin

Medicine has evolved dramatically during the past century from a healing art in which standards of practice were established on the basis of personal experience, passed on from one practitioner to the next, to a rigorous intellectual discipline steeped in the scientific method. The scientific method, a process that tests the validity of a hypothesis or prediction through experimentation, has led to major advances in the fields of physiology, microbiology, biochemistry, and pharmacology. These advances served as the basis for the diagnostic and therapeutic approaches to illness in common use by physicians through most of the 20th century. Since the 1980s, the understanding of the molecular basis of genetics has expanded dramatically, and advances in this field have identified new and exciting dimensions for defining the basis of *conventional* genetic diseases (e.g., sickle cell disease) as well as the basis of complex genetic traits (e.g., hypertension). The molecular basis for the interaction between genes and environment has also begun to be defined. Armed with a variety of sensitive and specific molecular techniques, contemporary physicians can now begin not only to understand the molecular underpinning of complex pathobiologic processes but also to identify individuals at risk for common diseases. Understanding modern medicine, therefore, requires an understanding of molecular genetics and the molecular basis of disease. This introductory chapter offers an overview of this complex and rapidly evolving topic and attempts to summarize the principles of molecular medicine that will be highlighted in specific sections throughout this text.

Deoxyribonucleic Acid and the Genome

All organisms possess a scheme to transmit the essential information containing the genetic make-up of the species through successive generations. In human cells, 23 pairs of chromosomes are present, each pair of which contains a unique sequence and therefore unique genetic information. In the human genome, about 6×10^9 nucleotides, or 3×10^9 pairs of nucleotides, associate in the double helix. All the specificity of DNA is determined by the base sequence, and this sequence is stored in complementary form in the double-helical structure, which facilitates correction of sequence errors and provides a mechanistic basis for replication of the information during cell division. Each DNA strand serves as a template for replication, which is accomplished by the action of DNA-dependent polymerases that unwind the double-helical DNA and copy each single strand with remarkable fidelity.

All cell types except for gametocytes contain this duplicate, diploid number of genetic units, one half of which is referred to as a *haploid number*. The genetic information contained in chromosomes is separated into discrete functional elements known as *genes*. A gene is defined as a unit of base sequence that usually, but with rare exceptions, encodes a specific polypeptide sequence. New evidence suggests that small, noncoding RNAs play critical roles in expression of this essential information. An estimated 30,000 genes are present in the human haploid genome, and these are interspersed among regions of sequence that do not code for protein and whose function is as yet unknown. For example, noncoding RNAs (e.g., transfer RNA [tRNA], ribosomal RNA [rRNA], and other small RNAs) act as components of enzyme complexes such as the ribosome and spliceosome. The average chromosome contains 3000 to 5000 genes, and these range in size from about 1 kilobase (kb) to 2 megabases (Mb).

Ribonucleic Acid Synthesis

Transcription, or RNA synthesis, is the process for transferring information contained in nuclear DNA to an intermediate molecular species known as messenger RNA (mRNA).

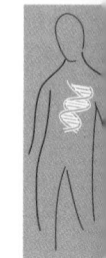

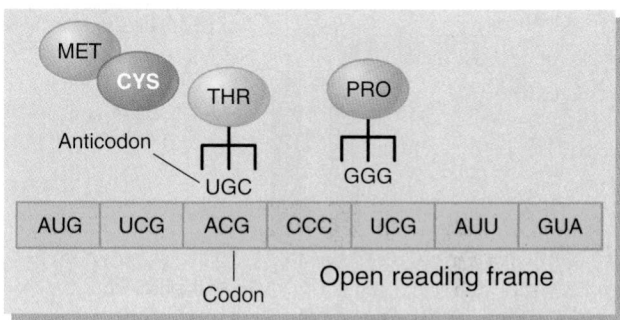

Figure 1-1 Transcription. Genomic DNA is shown with enhancer and silencer sites located 5′ upstream of the promoter region, to which RNA polymerase is bound. The transcription start site is shown downstream of the promoter region, and this site is followed by exonic sequences interrupted by intronic sequences. The former sequences are transcribed *ad seriatim* (i.e., one after another) by the RNA polymerase.

Two biochemical differences distinguish RNA from DNA: (1) the polymeric backbone is made up of ribose rather than deoxyribose sugars linked by phosphodiester bonds, and (2) the base composition is different in that uracil is substituted for thymine. RNA synthesis from a DNA template is performed by three types of DNA-dependent RNA polymerases, each a multi-subunit complex with distinct nuclear location and substrate specificity. RNA polymerase I, located in the nucleolus, directs the transcription of genes encoding the 18S, 5.8S, and 28S ribosomal RNAs, forming a molecular scaffold with both catalytic and structural functions within the ribosome. RNA polymerase II, located in the nucleoplasm instead of the nucleoli, primarily transcribes precursor mRNA transcripts and small RNA molecules. The carboxyl-terminus of RNA polymerase II is uniquely modified with a 220-kD protein domain, the site of enzymatic regulation by protein phosphorylation of critical serine and threonine residues. All tRNA precursors and other rRNA molecules are synthesized by RNA polymerase III in the nucleoplasm.

RNA polymerases are synthesized from precursor transcripts that must first be cleaved into subunits before further processing and assembling with ribosomal proteins into macromolecular complexes. Ribosomal architectural and structural integrity are derived from the secondary and tertiary structures of rRNA, which assume a series of folding patterns containing short duplex regions. Precursors of tRNA in the nucleus undergo the removal of the 5′ leader region, splicing of an internal intron sequences, and modification of terminal residues.

Precursors of mRNA are produced in the nucleus by the action of DNA-dependent RNA polymerase II, which copies the *antisense* strand of the DNA double helix to synthesize a single strand of mRNA that is identical to the *sense* strand of the DNA double helix in a process called *transcription* (Fig. 1-1). The initial, immature mRNA first undergoes modification at both the 5′ and 3′ ends. A special nucleotide structure called the *cap* is added to the 5′ end, which functions to increase binding to the ribosome and enhance translational efficiency. The 3′ end undergoes modification by nuclease cleavage of about 20 nucleotides, followed by the addition of a length of polynucleotide sequence containing a uniform stretch of adenine bases, the so-called poly A tail that stabilizes the mRNA.

In addition to these changes that uniformly occur in all mRNAs, other, more selective modifications can also occur.

Figure 1-2 Translation. The open reading frame of a mature messenger RNA is shown with its series of codons. Transfer RNA molecules are shown with their corresponding anticodons, charged with their specific amino acid. A short, growing polypeptide chain is depicted. A, adenine; C, cytosine; CYS, cysteine; G, guanine; MET, methionine; PRO, proline; THR, threonine; U, uracil.

Because each gene contains both exonic and intronic sequences and the precursor mRNA is transcribed without regard for exon-intron boundaries, this immature message must be edited in such a way that splices all exons together in appropriate sequence. The process of splicing, or removing intronic sequences to produce the mature mRNA, is an exquisitely choreographed event that involves the intermediate formation of a spliceosome, a large complex consisting of small nuclear RNAs and specific proteins, which contains a loop or lariat-like structure that includes the intron targeted for removal. Only after splicing, a catalytic process requiring adenosine triphosphate hydrolysis, has concluded is the mature mRNA able to transit from the nucleus into the cytoplasm, where the encoded information is translated into protein.

Alternative splicing is a process for efficiently generating multiple gene products often dictated by tissue specificity, developmental expression, and pathologic state. Gene splicing allows the expression of multiple isoforms by expanding the repertoire for molecular diversity. An estimated 30% of genetic diseases in humans arise from defects in splicing. The resulting mature mRNA then exits the nucleus to begin the process of *translation* or conversion of the base code to polypeptide (Fig. 1-2). Alternative splicing pathways (i.e., alternative exonic assembly pathways) for specific genes also serve at the level of transcriptional regulation. The discovery of catalytic RNA, the capacity for self-directed internal

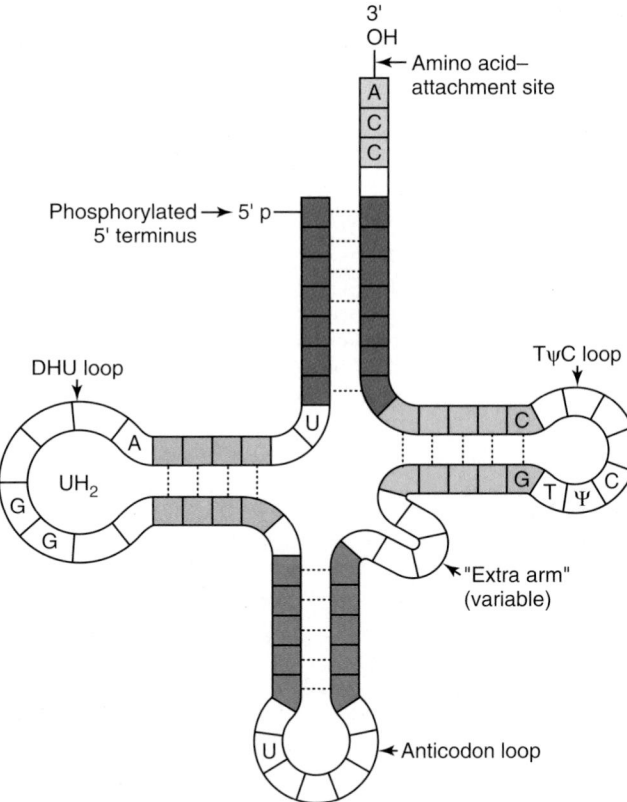

Figure 1-3 Secondary structure of transfer RNA (tRNA). The structure of each tRNA serves as an adapter molecule that recognizes a specific codon for the amino acid to be added to the polypeptide chain. About one half the hydrogen-bonded bases of the single chain of ribonucleotides are shown paired in double helices like a cloverleaf. The 5′ terminus is phosphorylated, and the 3′ terminus contains the hydroxyl group on an attached amino acid. The anticodon loop is typically located in the middle of the tRNA molecule. C, cytocide; DHU, dihydroxyuridine; G, guanine; UH_2, dihydrouridine; ψ, pseudouridine; T, ribothymidine; U, uracil. (Data from Berg JM, Tymoczko JL, Strayer JL: Berg, Tymoczko and Stryer's Biochemistry, 5th ed. New York, WH Freeman, 2006.)

excision and repair, has advanced the current view that RNA per se serves both as a template for translation of the genetic code and, simultaneously, as an enzyme (see "Transcriptional Regulation" later in this chapter).

Protein synthesis, or translation of the mRNA code, occurs on ribosomes, which are macromolecular complexes of proteins and rRNA located in the cytoplasm. Translation involves the conversion of the linear code of a triplet of bases (i.e., the codon) into the corresponding amino acid. A four-base code generates 64 possible triplet combinations (4 × 4 × 4), and these correspond to 20 different amino acids, many of which are encoded by more than one base triplet. To decode mRNA, an adapter molecule (tRNA) recognizes the codon in mRNA through complementary base pairing with a three-base anticodon that it bears; in addition, each tRNA is charged with a unique amino acid that corresponds to the anticodon (Fig. 1-3).

Translation on the mRNA template proceeds without punctuation of the non-overlapping code with the aid of rRNA on an assembly machine, termed *ribosomes*—essentially a polypeptide polymerase. At least one tRNA molecule exists for each 20 amino acids, although degeneracy in the code expands the number of available tRNA molecules, mitigates the chances of premature chain termination, and ameliorates the potential deleterious consequences of single-base mutations. The enzymatic activity of the ribosome then links amino acids through the synthesis of a peptide bond, releasing the tRNA in the process.

Consecutive linkage of amino acids in the growing polypeptide chain represents the terminal event in the conversion of information contained within the nuclear DNA sequence into mature protein (DNA → RNA → protein). Proteins are directly responsible for the form and function of an organism. Thus, abnormalities in protein structure or function brought about by changes in primary amino acid sequence are the immediate precedent cause of changes in phenotype, adverse forms of which define a disease state.

Inhibition of RNA synthesis is a well-recognized mechanism of specific toxins and antibiotics. Toxicity from the ingestion of the poisonous mushroom (*Amanita phalloides*), for example, leads to the release of the toxin α-amanitin, a cyclic octapeptide that inhibits the RNA Pol II and blocks elongation of RNA synthesis. The antibiotic actinomycin D binds with high affinity to double-helical DNA and intercolates between base pairs, precluding access of DNA-dependent RNA polymerases and the selective inhibition of transcription. Several major antibiotics function through inhibition of translation. For example, the aminoglycoside antibiotics function through the disruption of the mRNA-tRNA codon-anticodon interaction, whereas erythromycin and chloramphenicol inhibit peptide bond formation.

Control of Gene Expression

OVERVIEW

The timing, duration, localization, and magnitude of gene expression are all important elements in the complex tapestry of cell form and function governed by the genome. Gene expression represents the flow of information from the DNA template into mRNA transcripts and the process of translation into mature protein.

Four levels of organization involving transcription factors, RNAs, chromatin structure, and epigenetic factors are increasingly recognized to orchestrate gene expression in the mammalian genome. Transcriptional regulators bind to specific DNA motifs that positively or negatively control the expression of neighboring genes. The information contained in the genome must be transformed into functional units of either RNA or protein products. How DNA is packed and modified represents additional modes of gene regulation by disrupting the access of transcription factors from DNA-binding motifs. In the postgenomic era, the challenge is to understand the architecture by which the genome is organized, controlled, and modulated.

Transcription factors, chromatin architecture, and modifications of nucleosomal organization make up the major mechanisms of gene regulation in the genome.

TRANSCRIPTIONAL REGULATION

The principal regulatory step in gene expression occurs at the level of gene transcription. A specific DNA-dependent RNA polymerase performs the transcription of information contained in genomic DNA into mRNA transcripts. Transcription begins at a proximal (i.e., toward the 5′ end of the gene) transcription start site, containing nucleotide sequences that influence the rate and extent of the process (see Fig. 1-1). This region is known as the *promoter region* of the gene and often includes an element of sequence rich in adenine and thymine (the TATA box) along with other sequence motifs within about 100 bases of the start site. These regions of DNA that regulate transcription are known as *cis*-acting regulatory elements. Some of these regulatory regions of promoter sequence bind proteins known as *trans*-acting factors, or transcription factors, which are themselves encoded by other genes. The *cis*-acting regulatory sequences to which transcription factors bind are often referred to as *response elements*. Families of transcription factors have been identified and are often described by unique aspects of their predicted protein secondary structure, including helix-turn-helix motifs, zinc-finger motifs, and leucine-zipper motifs. Transcription factors make up an estimated 3% to 5% of the protein-coding products of the genome.

In addition to gene-promoter regions, enhancer sites are distinct from promoter sites in that they can exist at distances quite remote from the start site, either upstream or downstream (i.e., beyond the 3′ end of the gene), and without clear orientation requirements. *Trans*-acting factors bind to these enhancer sites and are believed to alter the tertiary structure or conformation of the DNA in a manner that facilitates the binding and assembly of the transcription-initiation complex at the promoter region, perhaps in some cases by forming a broad loop of DNA in the process. Biochemical modification of select promoter or enhancer sequences, such as methylation of CpG-rich sequences (cytosine-phosphate-guanine), can also modulate transcription; methylation typically suppresses transcription. The terms *silencer* and *suppressor* elements refer to *cis*-acting nucleotide sequences that reduce or shut off gene transcription and do so through association with *trans*-acting factors that recognize these specific sequences.

Regulation of transcription is a complex process that occurs at several levels; importantly, the expression of many genes is regulated to maintain high basal levels, which are known as *housekeeping* or *constitutively expressed* genes. They typically yield protein products that are essential for normal cell function or survival and thus must be maintained at a specific steady-state concentration under all circumstances. Many other genes, in contrast, are not expressed or are only modestly expressed under basal conditions; however, with the imposition of some stress or exposure of the cell to an agonist that elicits a cellular response distinct from that of the basal state, the expression of these genes is induced or enhanced. For example, the heat shock protein genes encoding *stress proteins* are rapidly induced in response to diverse pathophysiologic stimuli (e.g., oxidative stress, heavy metals, inflammation) in most cells and organisms. The increased heat shock protein expression is complementary to the basal level of heat shock proteins whose functions as molecular chaperones play key roles during protein synthesis to prevent protein misfolding, increase protein translocation, and accelerate protein degradation. These adaptive responses often mediate changes in phenotype that are homeostatically protective to the cell or organism.

MICRORNAS AND GENE REGULATION

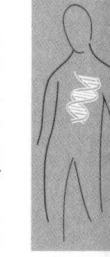

Less is currently known about the determinants of translational regulation than is known about transcriptional regulation. The recent discovery and identification of small RNAs (21 to 24 mer), termed *microRNAs* (miRNAs), adds further complexity to the regulation of gene expression within the eukaryotic genome. First discovered in worms more than 10 years ago, miRNAs are conserved noncoding strands of RNA that bind to the 3′-untranslated regions of target mRNAs, enabling gene silencing of protein expression at the translational level. Gene-encoding miRNAs exhibit tissue-specific expression and are interspersed in regions of the genome unrelated to known genes.

Transcription of miRNAs proceeds in multiple steps from sites under the control of an mRNA promoter. RNA polymerase II transcribes the precursor miRNA, termed *primary miRNA* (primiRNA), containing 5′ caps and 3′ poly (A) tails. In the nucleus, the larger primiRNAs of 70 nucleotides form an internal hairpin loop, embedding the miRNA portion that undergoes recognition and subsequent excision by double-stranded RNA-specific ribonuclease, termed *Drosha*. Gene expression is silenced by the effect of miRNA on nascent RNA molecules targeted for degradation.

Because translation occurs at a fairly invariant rate among all mRNA species, the stability or half-life of a specific mRNA also serves as another point of regulation of gene expression. The 3′-untranslated region of mRNAs contains regions of sequence that dictate the susceptibility of the message to nuclease cleavage and degradation. Stability appears to be sequence specific and, in some cases, dependent on *trans*-acting factors that bind to the mRNA. The mature mRNA contains elements of untranslated sequence at both the 5′ and 3′ ends that can regulate translation.

Beginning in the organism's early development, miRNAs may facilitate much more intricate ways for the regulation of gene expression, as have been shown for germline production, cell differentiation, proliferation, and organogenesis. Because recent studies have implicated the expression of miRNAs in brain development, cardiac organogenesis, colonic adenocarcinoma, and viral replication, this novel mechanism for gene silencing has potential therapeutic roles for congenital heart defects, viral disease, neurodegeneration, and cancer.

CHROMATIN REMODELING AND GENE REGULATION

Both the size and complexity of the human genome with 23 chromosomes, ranging in size between 50 and 250 Mb, pose formidable challenges for transcription factors to exert the specificity of DNA-binding properties in gene regulation. Control of gene expression also takes place in diverse types of cells, often with exquisite temporal and spatial specificity throughout the life span of the organism. In eukaryotic cells, the genome is highly organized into densely packed nucleic acid DNA- and RNA-protein structures, termed *chromatin*.

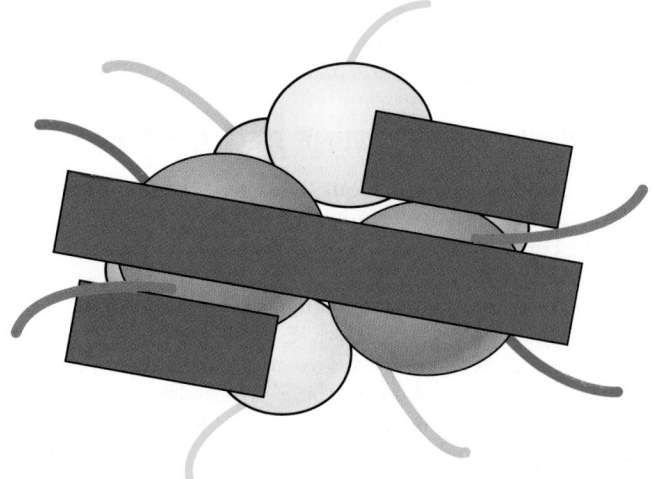

Figure 1-4 Schematic representation of a nucleosome. Rectangular blocks represent the DNA strand wrapped around the core that consists of eight histone proteins. Each histone has a protruding tail that can be modified to repress or activate transcription. (Adapted from Berg JM, Tymoczko JL, Strayer JL: Berg, Tymoczko and Stryer's Biochemistry, 5th ed. New York, WH Freeman, 2006.)

The building blocks of chromatin are called *histones,* a family of small basic proteins that occupy one half of the mass of the chromosome. Histones derive their basic properties from the high content of basic amino acids, arginine, and lysine. Five major types of histones—H1, H2A, H2B, H3, and H4—have evolved to form complexes with the DNA of the genome. Two pairs each of the four types of histones form a protein core, the histone octomer, which is wrapped by 200 base pairs of DNA to form the nucleosome (Fig. 1-4). The core proteins within the nucleosomes have protruding amino-terminal ends, exposing critical lysine and arginine residues for covalent modification. Further DNA condensation is achieved as higher-order structure is imparted on the chromosomes. The nucleosomes are further compacted in layered stacks with a left-handed superhelix resulting in negative supercoils that provide the energy for DNA strand separation during replication.

Condensation of DNA in chromatin precludes the access of regulatory molecules such as transcription factors. Reversal of chromatin condensation, on the other hand, typically occurs in response to environmental and other developmental signals in a tissue-dependent manner. Promoter sites undergoing active transcription, as well as relaxation of chromatin structure, that become susceptible to enzymatic cleavage by nonspecific DNAase I are called *hypersensitive sites.* Transcription factors on promoter sites may gain access by protein-protein interactions to enhancer elements containing tissue-specific proteins at remote sites, several thousand bases away, resulting in transcription activation or repression.

EPIGENETIC CONTROL OF GENE EXPRESSION

Complex regulatory networks revolve around transcription factors, nucleosomes, chromatin structure, and epigenetic markings. *Epigenetics* refers to heritable changes in gene expression without changes in the DNA sequence. Such examples include DNA methylation, gene silencing, chromatin remodeling, and X-chromosome inactivation. This form of inheritance involves the alterations in gene function without changes in DNA sequence. Chemical marking of DNA methylation is both cell specific and developmentally regulated. Methylation of the 5′ CpG dinucleotide by specific methyl transferases, which occurs in 70% of the mammalian genome, is another mechanism of gene regulation. Steric hindrance from the bulky methyl group of 5′ methylcytosine precludes occupancy by transcription factors that stimulate or attenuate gene expression. Most genes are found in CpG islands, reflecting sites of gene activity across the genome.

In an analogous manner, modifications of histone by phosphorylation, methylation, ubiquination, and acetylation are transmitted and reestablished in an inheritable manner. It is conceivable that other epigenetic mechanisms do not involve genomic modifications of DNA. For example, modification of the gene encoding the estrogen receptor α has been implicated in gene silencing at ^{5m}C sites of multiple downstream targets in breast cancer cells. Powerful new approaches are being developed to examine feedback and feed-forward loops in transmission of epigenetic markings.

The concept that dynamic modifications (e.g., DNA methylation and acetylation) of histones or epigenesis contribute, in part, to tumorigenic potential for progression has already been translated into current therapies. Histone acetyltransferases (HATs) and histone deacetyltransferases (HDACs) play antagonistic roles in the addition and removal of acetylation in the genome. Furthermore, genome-wide analysis of HATs and HDACs is beginning to provide important insights into complex modes of gene regulation. Several inhibitors of histone deacetylases, with a range of biochemical and biologic activities, are being developed and tested as anticancer agents in clinical trial. Phase I clinical trials have suggested these drugs are well tolerated. In general, the inhibition of deacetylase remodels chromatin assembly and reactivates transcription of the genome. Because the mechanisms of actions of HDACs extend to apoptosis, cell cycle control, and cellular differentiation, current clinical trials are seeking to determine the efficacy of these novel reagents in the drug compendium for human cancers.

Genetic Sequence Variation, Population Diversity, and Genetic Polymorphisms

A stable, heritable change in DNA is defined as a *mutation.* This strict contemporary definition does not depend on the functional relevance of the sequence alteration and implicates a change in primary DNA sequence. Considered in historical context, mutations were first defined on the basis of identifiable changes in the heritable phenotype of an organism. As biochemical phenotyping became more precise in the mid-20th century, investigators demonstrated that many proteins exist in more than one form in a population, and these forms were viewed as a consequence of variations

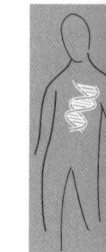

in the gene coding for that protein (i.e., allelic variation). With advances in DNA-sequencing methods, the concept of mutation evolved from one that could be appreciated only by identifying differences in phenotype to one that could precisely be defined at the level of changes in the structure of DNA. Although most mutations are stably transmitted from parents to offspring, some are genetically lethal and thus cannot be passed on. In addition, the discovery of regions of the genome that contain sequences that repeat in tandem a highly variable number of times (tandem repeats) suggests that some mutations are less stable than others. These tandem repeats are further described later in this section.

The molecular nature of mutations is varied (Table 1-1). A mutation can involve the deletion, insertion, or substitution of a single base, all of which are referred to as *point mutations.* Substitutions can be further classified as *silent* when the amino acid encoded by the mutated triplet does not change, as *missense* when the amino acid encoded by the mutated triplet changes, and as *nonsense* when the mutation leads to premature termination of translation (stop codon). On occasion, point mutations can alter the processing of precursor mRNA by producing alternate splice sites or eliminating a splice site. When a single- or double-base deletion or insertion occurs in an exon, a frameshift mutation results, usually leading to premature termination of translation at a now in-frame stop codon. The other end of the spectrum of mutations includes large deletions of an entire gene or a set of contiguous genes; deletion, duplication, and translocation of a segment of one chromosome to another; or duplication or deletion of an entire chromosome. Such chromosomal mutations play a large role in the development of many cancers.

Each individual possesses two alleles for any given gene locus, one from each parent. Identical alleles define homozy-gosity and nonidentical alleles define heterozygosity for any gene locus. The heritability of these alleles follows typical mendelian rules. With a clearer understanding of the molecular basis of mutations and of allelic variation, their distribution in populations can now be analyzed precisely by following specific DNA sequences. Differences in DNA sequences studied within the context of a population are referred to as *genetic polymorphisms,* and these polymorphisms underlie the diversity observed within a given species and among species.

Despite the high prevalence of benign polymorphisms in a population, the occurrence of harmful mutations is comparatively rare because of selective pressures that eliminate the most harmful mutations from the population (lethality) and the variability within the genomic sequence to polymorphic change. Some portions of the genome are remarkably stable and free of polymorphic variation, whereas other portions are highly polymorphic, the persistence of variation within which is a consequence of the functional benignity of the sequence change. In other words, polymorphic differences in DNA sequence between individuals can be divided into those producing no effect on phenotype, those causing benign differences in phenotype (i.e., normal genetic variation), and those producing adverse consequences in phenotype (i.e., mutations). The last group can be further subdivided into the polymorphic mutations that alone are able to produce a functionally abnormal phenotype such as monogenic disease (e.g., sickle cell anemia) and those that alone are unable to do so but in conjunction with other mutations can produce a functionally abnormal phenotype (complex disease traits [e.g., essential hypertension]).

Polymorphisms are more common in noncoding regions of the genome than they are in coding regions, and one common type of these involves the tandem repetition of short DNA sequences a variable number of times. If these tandem repeats are long, they are termed *variable number tandem repeats*; if these repeats are short, they are termed *short tandem repeats* (STRs). During mitosis, the number of tandem repeats can change, and the frequency of this kind of replication error is high enough to make alternative lengths of the tandem repeats common in a population. However, the rate of change in length of the tandem repeats is low enough to make the size of the polymorphism useful as a stable genotypic trait in families. In view of these features, polymorphic tandem repeats are useful in determining the familial heritability of specific genomic loci. Polymorphic tandem repeats are sufficiently prevalent along the entire genomic sequence, enabling them to serve as genetic markers for specific genes of interest through an analysis of their linkage to those genes during crossover and recombination events. Analyses of multiple genetic polymorphisms in the human genome reveal that a remarkable variation exists among individuals at the level of the sequence of genomic DNA (genotyping). Single-nucleotide polymorphism (SNP), the most common variant, differs by a single base between chromosomes on any given stretch of DNA sequence (Fig. 1-5). From genotyping of the world's representative population, 10 million variants (one site per 300 bases) are estimated to make up 90% of the common SNP variants in the population, with the rare variants making up the remaining 10%. With each generation of a species, the frequency of polymorphic changes in a gene is 10^{-4} to 10^{-7}.

Type	Examples
Point Mutations	
Deletion	α-Thalassemia, polycystic kidney disease
Substitution	
Silent	Cystic fibrosis
Missense	Sickle cell anemia, polycystic kidney disease, congenital long QT syndrome
Nonsense	Cystic fibrosis, polycystic kidney disease
Large Mutations (Gene or Gene Cluster)	
Deletion	Duchenne muscular dystrophy
Insertion	Factor VIII deficiency (hemophilia A)
Duplication	Duchenne muscular dystrophy
Inversion	Factor VIII deficiency
Expanding triplet	Huntington disease
Very Large Mutation (Chromosomal Segment or Chromosome)	
Deletion	Turner syndrome (45,X)
Duplication	Trisomy 21
Translocation	XX male [46,X; t(X;Y)]*

Table 1-1 Molecular Basis of Mutations

*Translocation onto an X chromosome of a segment of a Y chromosome that bears the locus for testicular differentiation.

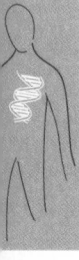

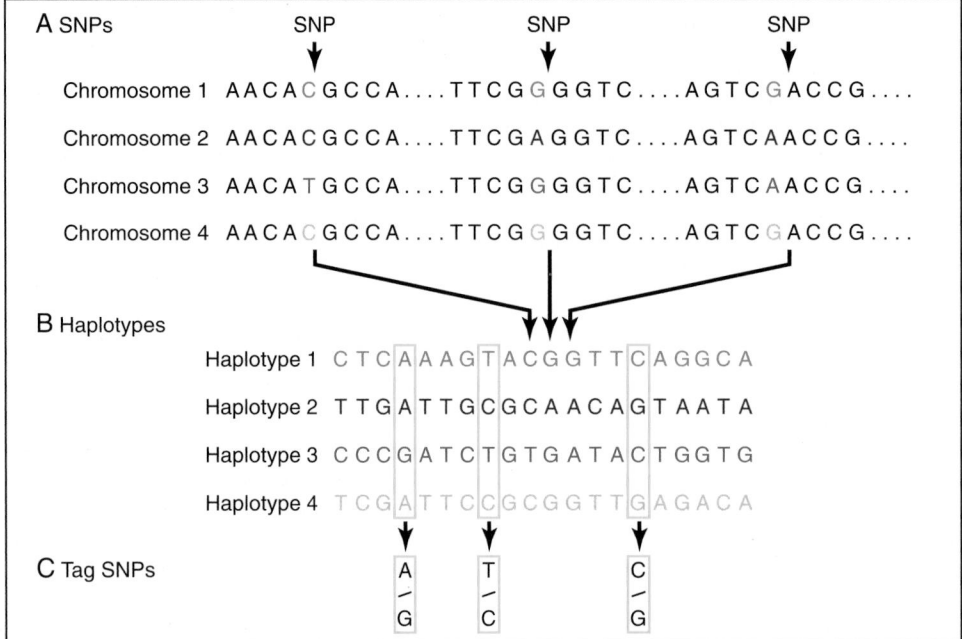

Figure 1-5 Single nucleotide polymorphisms (SNPs), haplotypes, and tag SNPs. A stretch of mostly identical DNA on the same chromosome is shown from four different individuals. SNP refers to the variation of the three bases shown in DNA region. The combination of nearby SNPs defines a haplotype. Tag SNPs are useful tools shown (**C**) for genotyping four unique haplotypes from the 20 haplotypes (**B**). (Adapted from International HapMap Consortium: The International HapMap Project. Nature 426: 789-796, 2003.)

Thus, in view of the number of genes in the human genome, between 0.5% and 1.0% of the base sequence of the human genome is polymorphic. In this context, the new variant can be traced historically to the surrounding alleles on the chromosomal background present at the time of the mutational event. A haplotype is a specific set or combination of alleles on a chromosome or part of a chromosome (see Fig. 1-5). When parental chromosomes undergo crossover, new *mosaic* haplotypes, containing additional mutations, are created from such recombinations. SNP alleles within haplotypes can be co-inherited in association with other alleles in the population, termed *linkage disequilibrium* (LD). The association between two SNPs will decline with increasing distance, enabling patterns of LD to be decided from the proximity of nearby SNPs. Conversely, a few well-selected SNPs are often sufficient to predict the location of other common variants in the region.

Haplotypes associated with a mutation are expected to become common by recombination in the general population over thousands of generations. In contrast, genetic mapping with LD departs from traditional mendelian genetics by using the entire human population as a large family tree without an established pedigree. Of the possible 10 million variants, the International HapMap Project and the Perlegen private venture have deposited more than 8 million variants comprising the public human SNP map from more than 341 people representing different population samples. The SNPs distributed across the genome of unrelated individuals provide a sufficiently robust sample set for statistical associations to be drawn between genotypes and modest phenotypes. A mutation can now be defined as a specific type of allelic polymorphism that causes a functional defect in a cell or organism.

The causal relationship between monogenic diseases with well-defined phenotypes that co-segregate with the disease requires only a small number of affected individuals compared with unaffected control individuals. In contrast, complex disorders (e.g., diabetes, hypertension, cancer) will necessitate the combinatorial effects of environmental factors and genes with subtle effects. Only through searching for variations in genetic frequency between patients and the general population can the causation of disease be discerned. In the postgenomic era, gene mapping entails the statistical association with the use of LD and high-density genetic maps that span thousands to 100,000 base pairs. To enable comprehensive association studies to become routine in clinical practice, inexpensive genotyping assays and denser maps with all common polymorphisms must be linked to all possible manifestations of the disease. Longitudinal studies of the HapMap and Perlegen cohorts will determine the effects of diet, exercise, environmental factors, and family history on future clinical events. Without similar approaches on securing adequate sample sizes and datasets, the promise of genetic population theory will not overcome the inherent limitations of linking human sequence variation with complex disease traits.

Gene Mapping and the Human Genome Project

The process of gene mapping involves identifying the relative order and distance of specific loci along the genome. Maps can be of two types: genetic and physical. Genetic maps identify the genomic location of specific genetic loci by a statistical analysis based on the frequency of recombina-

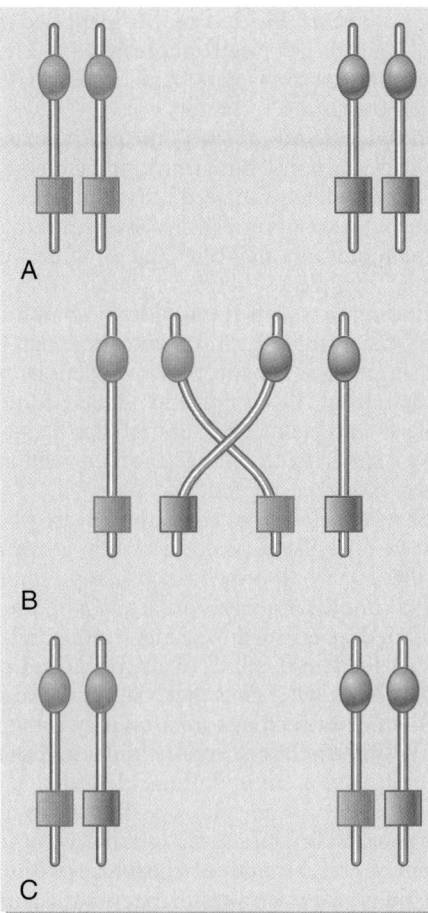

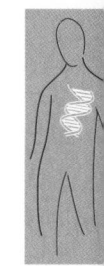

Figure 1-6 Crossing over and recombination. **A,** Two haploid chromosomes are shown, one from each parent (*red* and *blue*) with two genomic loci denoted by the circles and squares. **B,** Crossing over of one haploid chromosome from each parent. **C,** Resulting recombination of chromosomal segments now redistributes one haploid locus (*squares*) from one diploid pair to another.

for specific alleles to be inherited together indicates that the recombination distance in the human genome is about 3000 cM.

Identifying the gene or genes responsible for a specific polygenic disease phenotype requires an understanding of the topographic anatomy of the human genome, which is inextricably linked to interactions with the environment. The Human Genome Project, first proposed in 1985, represented an international effort to determine the complete nucleotide sequence of the human genome, including the construction of its detailed genetic, physical, and transcript maps, with identification and characterization of all genes. This foray into *large-scale biology* was championed by Nobel Laureate James Watson as the defining moment in his lifetime for witnessing the path from the double helix to the sequencing of 3 billion bases of the human genome, paving the way for understanding human evolution and harnessing the benefits for human health.

Among the earliest achievements of the Human Genome Project were the development of 1-cM resolution maps, each containing 3000 markers, and the identification of 52,000 sequenced tagged sites. For functional analysis on a genome-wide scale, major technologic advances were made, including as high-throughput oligonucleotide synthesis, normalized and subtracted complementary DNA (cDNA) libraries, and DNA micro-arrays. In 1998, the Celera private venture proposed a similar goal as the Human Genome Project using a revolutionary approach, termed *shotgun sequencing,* to determine the sequence of the human genome (**Web Movie 1-1**). The shotgun sequencing method was designed for random large-scale sequencing and subsequent alignment of sequenced segments using computational and mathematic modeling. In the end, the Human Genome Project, in collaboration with the Celera private venture, produced a refined map of the entire human genome in 2001.

Because of the differences in genomic sequence that arise as a consequence of normal biologic variations or sequence polymorphisms, the resulting restriction fragment length polymorphisms (RFLPs) differ among individuals and are inherited according to mendelian principles. These polymorphisms can serve as genetic markers for specific loci in the genome. One of the most useful types of RFLP for localization of genetic loci within the genome is that produced by tandem repeats of sequence. Tandem repeats arise through *slippage* or stuttering of the DNA polymerase during replication in the case of STRs; longer variations arise through unequal crossover events. STRs are distributed throughout the genome and are highly polymorphic. Of importance is that these markers have two different alleles at each locus that are derived from each parent; thus, the origins of the two chromosomes can be discerned through this analysis.

The use of highly polymorphic tandem repeats that occur throughout the genome as genomic markers has provided a basis for mapping specific gene loci through establishing the association or linkage with select markers. Linkage analysis is predicated on a simple principle: the likelihood that a crossover event will occur during meiosis decreases the closer the locus of interest is to a given marker. The extent of genetic linkage can be ascertained for any group of loci, one of which may contain a disease-producing mutation (Fig. 1-7).

tion events of the locus of interest with other known loci. Physical maps identify the genomic location of specific genetic loci by a direct measurement of the distance along the genome at which the locus of interest is located in relation to one or more defined markers. The precise location of genes on a chromosome is important for defining the likelihood that a portion of one chromosome will interchange, or cross over, with the corresponding portion of its complementary chromosome when genetic recombination occurs during meiosis (Fig. 1-6).

During meiotic recombination, genetic loci or alleles that have been acquired from one parent interchange with those acquired from the other parent to produce new combinations of alleles, and the likelihood that alleles will recombine during meiosis varies as a function of their linear distance from one another in the chromosomal sequence. This recombination probability or distance is commonly quantitated in centimorgans (cM): 1 cM is defined as the chromosomal distance over which there is a 1% chance that two alleles will undergo a crossover event during meiosis. Crossover events serve as the basis for mixing parental base sequences during development and, thereby, promoting genetic diversity among offspring. Analysis of the tendency

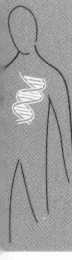

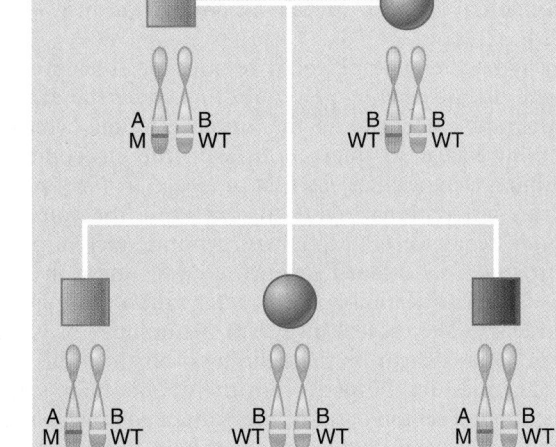

Figure 1-7 Linkage analysis. Analysis of the association (genomic contiguity) of a mutation (M) and a polymorphic allelic marker (A) shows close linkage in that the mutation segregates with the A allele, whereas the wild-type gene locus (WT) associates with the B allele.

Identifying Mutant Genes

Deducing the identity of a specific gene sequence believed to cause a specific human disease requires that mutations in the gene of interest be identified. If the gene believed to be responsible for the disease phenotype is known, its sequence can be determined by conventional cloning and sequencing strategies, and the mutation can be identified. A variety of techniques are currently available for detecting mutations. Mutations that involve insertion or deletion of large segments of DNA can be detected by Southern blot, in which the isolated DNA is annealed to a radioactively labeled fragment of cDNA sequence. Prior incubation of the DNA with a specific restriction endonuclease cleaves the DNA sequence of interest at specific sites to produce smaller fragments that can be monitored by agarose gel electrophoresis. Shifts in mobility on the gel in comparison with wild-type sequence become apparent as a function of changes in the molecular size of the fragment. Alternatively, the polymerase chain reaction (PCR) can be used to identify mutations (**Web Movie 1-2**).

In this approach, small oligonucleotides (20 to 40 bases in length), which are complementary to regions of DNA that bracket the sequence of interest and are complementary to each strand of the double-stranded DNA, are synthesized and serve as primers for the amplification of the DNA sequence of interest. These primers are added to the DNA solution. The temperature of the solution is increased to dissociate the individual DNA strands and is then reduced to permit annealing of the primers to their complementary template target sites. A thermostable DNA polymerase is included in the reaction to synthesize new DNA in the 5′-to-3′ direction from the primer annealing sites. The temperature is then increased to dissociate duplex structures, after which it is reduced, enabling another cycle of DNA synthesis to occur. Several temperature cycles (usually up to 40) are used to amplify progressively the concentration of the sequence of interest, which can be identified as a PCR product by agarose gel electrophoresis with a fluorescent dye. The product can be isolated and sequenced to identify the suggested mutation.

If the gene is large and the site of the mutation is unknown (especially if it is a point mutation), other methods can be used to identify the likely mutated site in the exonic sequence. One commonly used approach involves scanning the gene sequence for mutations that alter the structural conformation of short complexes between parent DNA and PCR products, leading to a shift in mobility on a nondenaturing agarose gel (i.e., single-strand conformational polymorphism). A single-base substitution or deletion can change the conformation of the complex in comparison with wild-type complexes and yield a shift in mobility. Sequencing this comparatively small region of the gene then facilitates precise identification of the mutation.

When the gene believed to cause the disease phenotype is unknown, when its likely position on the genome has not been identified, or when only limited mapping information is available, a candidate gene approach can be used to identify the mutated gene. In this strategy, potential candidate genes are identified on the basis of analogy to animal models or by analysis of known genes that map to the region of the genome for which limited information is available. The candidate gene is then analyzed for potential mutations. Regardless of the approach used, mutations identified in candidate genes should always be correlated with functional changes in the gene product because some mutations could be functionally silent, representing a polymorphism without phenotypic consequences. Functional changes in the gene product can be evaluated through the use of cell-culture systems to assess protein function by expressing the mutant protein through transiently transfecting the cells with a vector that carries the cDNA coding for the gene of interest and incorporating the mutation of interest. Alternatively, unique animal models can be developed in which the mutant gene is incorporated in the male pronucleus of oocytes taken from a super-ovulating impregnated female. This union produces an animal that overexpresses the mutant gene; that is, it produces a transgenic animal, an animal with more than the usual number of copies of a given gene, or an animal in which the gene of interest is disrupted and the gene product is not synthesized (i.e., a gene *knockout* animal or an animal with one half [heterozygote] or none [homozygote] of the usual number of a given gene).

MOLECULAR DIAGNOSTICS

The power of molecular techniques extends beyond their use in defining the precise molecular basis of an inherited disease. By exploiting the exquisite sensitivity of PCR to amplify rare nucleic acid sequences, it is possible to diagnose rapidly a range of infectious diseases for which unique sequences are available. In particular, infections caused by fastidious or slow-growing organisms can now be rapidly diagnosed, similar to the case for *Mycobacterium tuberculosis*. The presence of genes conferring resistance to specific antibiotics in microorganisms can also be verified by PCR techniques. The sequencing of the entire genome of organisms such as *Escherichia coli, M. tuberculosis,* and *Treponema pallidum* now offers unparalleled opportunities to monitor

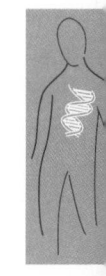

the epidemiologic structures of infections, follow the course of acquired mutations, tailor antibiotic therapies, and develop unique gene-based therapies (see later) for infectious agents for which conventional antibiotic therapies are ineffective or marginally effective.

The application of molecular methods to human genetics has clearly revolutionized the field. Through the use of approaches that incorporate linkage analysis and PCR, simple point mutations can be precisely localized and characterized. At the other end of the spectrum of genetic changes that underlie disease, chromosomal translocations, deletions, or duplications can be identified by conventional cytogenetic methods. Large deletions that can incorporate many kilobase pairs and many genes can now be visualized with fluorescent in situ hybridization (FISH), a technique in which a segment of cloned DNA is labeled with a fluorescent tag and hybridized to chromosomal DNA. With the deletion of the segment of interest from the genome, the chromosomal DNA fails to fluoresce in the corresponding chromosomal location.

Advances in molecular medicine have also revolutionized the approach to the diagnosis and treatment of neoplastic diseases, as well as the understanding of the mechanisms of carcinogenesis. According to current views, a neoplasm arises from the clonal proliferation of a single cell that is transformed from a regulated, quiescent state into an unregulated growth phase. DNA damage accumulates in the parental tumor cell as a result of either exogenous factors (e.g., radiation exposure) or heritable determinants. In early phases of carcinogenesis, certain genomic changes may impart intrinsic genetic instability that increases the likelihood of additional damage. One class of genes that becomes activated during carcinogenesis is oncogenes, which are primordial genes that normally exist in the mammalian genome in an inactive (proto-oncogene) state but, when activated, promote unregulated cell proliferation through activation of specific intracellular signaling pathways.

Molecular methods based on the acquisition of specific tumor markers and unique DNA sequences that result from oncogenetic markers of larger chromosomal abnormalities (i.e., translocations or deletions that promote oncogenesis) are now broadly applied to the diagnosis of malignancies. These methods can be used to establish the presence of specific tumor markers and oncogenes in biopsy specimens, to monitor the presence or persistence of circulating malignant cells after completion of a course of chemotherapy, and to identify the development of genetic resistance to specific chemotherapeutic agents. In addition, through the use of conventional linkage analysis and candidate gene approaches, future studies will enable the identification of individuals with a heritable predisposition to malignant transformation. Many of these specific topics are discussed in later chapters.

The advent of *gene chip* technologies or expression arrays has revolutionized molecular diagnostics and has begun to clarify the pathobiologic structures of complex diseases. These methods involve labeling the cDNA generated from the entire pool of mRNA isolated from a cell or tissue specimen with a radioactive or fluorescent marker and annealing this heterogeneous population of polynucleotides to a solid-phase substrate to which many different polynucleotides of known sequence are attached. The signals from the labeled cDNA strands bound to specific locations on the array are monitored, and the relative abundance of particular sequences is compared with that from a reference specimen. Using this approach, micro-array patterns can be used as molecular fingerprints to diagnose a particular disease (i.e., type of malignancy and its susceptibility to treatment and prognosis) as well as to identify the genes whose expression increases or decreases in a specific disease state (i.e., identification of disease-modifying genes).

Of course, many other applications of molecular medicine techniques are available, in addition to these applications in infectious diseases and oncology. Molecular methods can be used to sort out genetic differences in metabolism that may modulate pharmacologic responses in a population of individuals *(pharmacogenomics)*, address specific forensic issues such as paternity or criminal culpability, and approach epidemiologic analysis on a precise genetic basis.

GENES AND HUMAN DISEASE

Human genetic diseases can be divided into three broad categories: (1) those that are caused by a mutation in a single gene (e.g., monogenic disorders, mendelian traits); (2) those that are caused by mutations in more than one gene (e.g., polygenic disorders, complex disease traits); and (3) those that are chromosomal in nature (Table 1-2). In all three groups of disorders, environmental factors can contribute to the phenotypic expression of the disease by modulating gene expression or unmasking a biochemical abnormality that has no functional consequences in the absence of a stimulus or stress. Classic monogenic disorders include sickle cell anemia, familial hypercholesterolemia, and cystic fibrosis. Importantly, these genetic diseases can be exclusively produced by a single specific mutation (e.g., sickle cell anemia) or by any one of several mutations (e.g., familial hypercholesterolemia, cystic fibrosis) in a given family (Pauling paradigm). Interestingly, some of these disorders evolved to protect the host. For example, sickle cell anemia evolved as protection against falciparum malaria, and cystic fibrosis developed as protection against cholera. Examples of polygenic disorders or complex disease traits include type 1 (insulin-dependent) diabetes mellitus, atherosclerotic cardiovascular disease, and essential hypertension. A common

Table 1-2 **Molecular Basis of Mutations**

Type	Examples
Monogenic Disorders	
Autosomal dominant	Polycystic kidney disease 1, neurofibromatosis 1
Autosomal recessive	β-Thalassemia, Gaucher disease
X-linked	Hemophilia A, Emery-Dreifuss muscular dystrophy
One of multiple mutations	Familial hypercholesterolemia, cystic fibrosis
Polygenic Disorders	
Complex disease traits	Type 1 (insulin-dependent) diabetes, essential hypertension, atherosclerotic disease, cancer

example of a chromosomal disorder is the presence of an extra chromosome 21 (trisomy 21). The overall frequency of monogenic disorders is about 1%. About 60% of these include polygenic disorders, which includes those with a genetic substrate that develops later in life. About 0.5% of monogenic disorders include chromosomal abnormalities. Importantly, chromosomal abnormalities are frequent causes of spontaneous abortion and malformations.

Contrary to the view held by early geneticists, few phenotypes are entirely defined by a single genetic locus. Thus, monogenic disorders are comparatively uncommon; however, they are still useful as a means to understanding some basic principles of heredity. Monogenic disorders are of three types: autosomal dominant, autosomal recessive, and X-linked. *Dominance* and *recessiveness* refer to the nature of the heritability of a genetic trait and correlate with the number of alleles affected at a given locus. If a mutation in a single allele determines the phenotype, the mutation is said to be dominant; that is, the heterozygous state conveys the clinical phenotype to the individual. In contrast, if a mutation is necessary at both alleles to determine the phenotype, the mutation is said to be recessive; that is, only the homozygous state conveys the clinical phenotype to the individual. Dominant or recessive mutations can lead to either a loss or a gain of function of the gene product. If the mutation is present on the X chromosome, it is defined as X-linked (which in males can, by definition, be viewed only as dominant); otherwise, it is autosomal. The importance of identifying a potential genetic disease as inherited by one of these three mechanisms is that, if one of these patterns of inheritance is present, the disease must involve a single genomic abnormality that leads to an abnormality in a single protein. Classically identified genetic diseases are produced by mutations that affect coding (exonic) sequences. However, mutations in intronic and other untranslated regions of the genome occur that may disturb the function or expression of specific genes. Examples of diseases with these types of mutations include myotonic dystrophy and Friedreich ataxia.

An individual with a dominant monogenic disorder typically has one affected parent and a 50% chance of transmitting the mutation to his or her offspring. In addition, men and women are equally likely to be affected and equally likely to transmit the trait to their offspring. The trait cannot be transmitted to offspring by two unaffected parents. In contrast, an individual with a recessive monogenic disorder typically has parents who are clinically normal. Affected parents, each heterozygous for the mutation, have a 25% chance of transmitting the clinical phenotype to their offspring but a 50% chance of transmitting the mutation to their offspring (i.e., producing an unaffected carrier).

Notwithstanding the clear heritability of common monogenic disorders (e.g., sickle cell anemia), the clinical expression of the disease in an individual with a phenotype expected to produce the disease may vary. *Variability in clinical expression* is defined as the range of phenotypic effects observed in individuals carrying a given mutation. *Penetrance* refers to a smaller subset of individuals with variable clinical expression of a mutation and is defined as the proportion of individuals with a given genotype who exhibit any clinical phenotypic features of the disorder.

Three principal determinants of variability in clinical expression or incomplete penetrance of a given genetic disorder can occur: (1) environmental factors, (2) the effects of other genetic loci, and (3) random chance. Environmental factors can modulate disease phenotype by altering gene expression in several ways, including their action on transcription factors (e.g., transcription factors that are sensitive to cell redox state [nuclear factor κB]) or *cis*-elements in gene promoters (e.g., folate-dependent methylation of CpG-rich regions); or by post-translationally modifying proteins (e.g., lysine oxidation). That other genes can modify the effects of disease-causing mutations is a reflection of the overlay of genetic diversity on primary disease phenotype. Numerous examples exist of the effects of these so-called *disease-modifying genes* producing phenotypic variations among individuals with the identical primary disease-causing mutations *(gene-gene interactions)* and the effects of disease-modifying genes interacting with environmental determinants to alter phenotype further *(gene-environment interactions)*. These interactions are clearly important in polygenic diseases; gene-gene and gene-environment interactions can modify the phenotypic expression of the disease. Among patients with sickle cell disease, for example, some patients experience painful crises, whereas others exhibit acute chest syndrome; still other presentations include hemolytic crises.

Genetic disorders affecting a unique pool of DNA, mitochondrial DNA, have been identified. Mitochondrial DNA is unique in that it is inherited only from the mother. In addition, mutations in mitochondrial DNA can vary among mitochondria within a given cell and within a given individual (heteroplasmy). Examples of genetic disorders based in the mitochondrial genome are Kearns-Sayre syndrome and Leber hereditary optic neuropathy. The list of known mitochondrial genomic disorders is growing rapidly, and mitochondrial contributions to a large number of common polygenic disorders may also exist.

MOLECULAR MEDICINE

A principal goal of current molecular strategies is to restore normal gene function to individuals with genetic mutations. Methods to do so are currently primitive, and a number of obstacles must be surmounted for this approach to be successful.

The principal problems are that to deliver a complete gene into a cell is not easy, and persistent expression of the new gene cannot be ensured because of the variability in its incorporation in the genome and the consequent variability in its regulated expression. Many approaches have been used to date, but none has been completely successful. They include the following: (1) packaging the cDNA in a viral vector, such as an attenuated adenovirus, and using the cell's ability to take up the virus as a means for the cDNA to gain access to the cell; (2) delivering the cDNA by means of a calcium phosphate–induced perturbation of the cell membrane; and (3) encapsulating the cDNA in a liposome that can fuse with the cell membrane and thereby deliver the cDNA.

After the cDNA has been successfully delivered to the cell of interest, the magnitude and durability of expression of the gene product are important variables. The magnitude of expression is determined by the number of copies of cDNA taken up by a cell and the extent of their incorporation in the genome of the cell. The durability of expression appears to be dependent partly on the antigenicity of the sequence and protein product.

Notwithstanding these technical limitations, gene therapy has been used to treat adenosine deaminase deficiency successfully, which suggests that the principle on which the treatment is based is reasonable. Clinical trials of gene therapy have slowed considerably after unexpected deaths were widely reported in both the scientific and lay media. Efforts on other genetic disorders and as a means to induce expression of a therapeutic protein (e.g., vascular endothelial cell growth factor to promote angiogenesis in ischemic tissue) are ongoing.

Understanding the molecular basis of disease leads naturally to the identification of unique disease targets. Recent examples of this principle have led to the development of novel therapies for diseases that have been difficult to treat. Imatinib, a tyrosine kinase inhibitor that is particularly effective at blocking the action of the bcr-abl kinase, is effective for the treatment of chronic-phase chronic myelogenous leukemia. Monoclonal antibody to tumor necrosis factor-α (infliximab) and soluble tumor necrosis factor-α receptor (etanercept) are prime examples of *biologic modifiers* that are effective in the therapy of chronic inflammatory disorders, including inflammatory bowel disease and rheumatoid arthritis. This approach to molecular therapeutics is rapidly expanding and holds great promise for improving the therapeutic armamentarium for a variety of diseases.

Beyond cancer-related categories (e.g., DNA, RNA repair), gene expression arrays have provided additional interactions of regulatory pathways of clinical interest. The limitation of gene expression profile using micro-arrays, which does not account for post-transcriptional and other post-translational modifications of protein-coding products, will likely be overcome by approaches and advances in proteomics. Such processes by signaling networks tend to amplify or attenuate gene expression on time scales lasting seconds to weeks. Much work remains to improve current knowledge about the pathways that initiate and promote tumors. The basic pathways and nodal points of regulation will be identified for rational drug design and target from mechanistic insights gleaned from expression profiling of cultured cell lines, from small animal models of human disease, and from human samples. Although accounting for tissue heterogeneity and variation among different cell types, the new systems' approach for incorporating genomic and computational research appears particularly promising to decipher the pathways that promote tumorigenesis. In turn, biologists and clinicians will use information derived from these tools to understand the events that promote survival, proangiogenesis, and immune escape, all of which may confer metastatic potential and progression.

What potential diagnostic tools are available to establish genetic determinants of drug response? Genome-wide approaches from the Human Genome Project in combination with micro-arrays, proteomic analysis, and bioinformatics will identify multiple genes encoding drug targets (e.g., receptors). Similar high-throughput screening should provide insights into the predisposition to adverse effects of outcomes from treatments that are linked to genetic polymorphisms.

PHARMOCOGENETICS

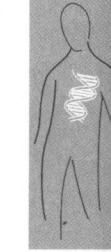

The future of pharmacogenetics is to know all the factors that influence adverse drug effects. In this way, the premature abandonment of special drug classes can be avoided in favor of rational drug design and therapy.

Many hurdles must be overcome for pharmacogenetics to become more widespread and to be integrated into medical practice. Current approaches of trial and error in medical practice are well engrained on the parts of physicians. In addition, the allure for blockbuster drugs by the pharmaceutical industry warrants a new model for approaching individualized doses. New training for physicians in molecular biology and genetics should complement clinical pharmacogenomic studies that determine efficacy in an era of evidence-based medicine. Pharmacogenetic polymorphisms, unlike other clinical variables such as renal function, need only a single test, ideally as a newborn. Polygenic models of therapeutic optimization still face hurdles that reduce the chances for abuse of genetic information and additional costs. On the other hand, SNP haplotyping has the potential to identify genetically similar subgroups of the population and to randomize therapies based on more robust genetic markers. On a population level, genomic variability is much greater within than among distinct racial and ethnic groups.

Both therapeutic efficacy and host toxicity are influenced by the patient's specific disease, age, renal function, nutritional status, and other co-morbid factors. New challenges will be posed for the selection and guide to drug therapy for patients with cancer, hypertension, and diabetes. It is conceivable that treatment of multisystem disorders (e.g., metabolic syndrome) might be derived from novel therapeutics based on individual, interacting, and complementary molecular pathways.

REGENERATIVE MEDICINE

A new era of regenerative biology has emerged with the discovery that adult mammalian cells can be reprogrammed into new cells. Regenerative medicine entails novel applications and approaches to exploit the resident population of progenitor cells for regeneration or repair of damaged tissues. After irreversible damage, transplantation of solid organs such as the heart, kidney, and lungs is a well-established medical-surgical intervention, but the limited availability of organs restricts widespread applications. Manipulation of cultured cells for transplantation heralds an alternative and complementary strategy to solid organ transplantation and offers an expanded platform for regenerative medicine. Although postmitotic, terminally differentiated organs are devoid of significant regenerative capacity, recent evidence for cellular plasticity of adult solid organs, throughout adult life, has challenged this prevailing dogma. This makeover involves approaches either to convert adult into pluripotent stem cells—retaining the ability to differentiate into new cell types—or forced reprogramming of adult cells into mature or progenitor cells.

Embryonic stem (ES) cells share common features of clonagenicity, self-renewal, and multi-potentiality, a prerequisite for differentiation into diverse cell lineages of multicellular adult organism. Both technical and ethical concerns propelled the search for new sources, including

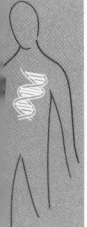

the isolation of ES cells from a single blastomere, which circumvents destruction of the embryo, and the use of post-implantation embryos as ES cell donors. Somatic cell nuclear transplantation (SCNT) or nuclear transfer (NT) is a technique for successful cloning and reprogramming of adult animal cell nuclei from healthy oocyte host cells. SCNT provides a source of stem cells tailored to the donor organism and promises to accelerate the pace for human use. Induced pluripotent stem (iPS) cells share the common features of somatic cell reprogramming but with the aid of four transcription factors by retroviral transduction. Whether symmetrical and asymmetrical cell division promotes the differentiation of pluripotent progenitor cells into distinct lineages of the mature organ awaits future studies. It is conceivable that age, gender, risk factors, and other disease status will have an impact on regenerative

plasticity, proliferation, or cellular functions. Another future hurdle will be to determine whether genetic factors enhance the cellular and molecular properties of ES cells essential for the reconstitution of a well-differentiated organ in vivo.

Might progenitor cells derived from bone marrow or circulating blood be administered safely and efficaciously? Both clinical and translational scientists are being asked to address whether stem cell therapy has efficacy for the current victims of either stroke or heart attack. Beyond the feasibility are questions related to benefits from transplantation of different cells originating from embryonic, fetal, or adult stem cell lineages. Whether priming of endogenous cell-mediated repair mechanisms using genetically engineered cell lines leads to improvement in selected endpoints and clinical outcomes awaits large-scale clinical trials.

Prospectus for the Future

The concept of personalized medicine will be realized from the functional and analytical phenotyping that aids diagnosis and treatment based on the individual's genome and disease profile. An important future challenge will be the extraction of biologically meaningful data of direct clinical relevance to diagnosis, prognosis, therapeutic response, and, ultimately, prevention.

What are the functional consequences of genome occupancy and modification in health and disease? Computational analyses will play an increasing role in understanding cancer pathogenesis and the mechanisms of disease. Information about the hierarchy of cellular functions is being coupled with powerful approaches to derive different yet complementary perspectives about molecular mechanisms. Micro-array analysis has already

provided new classes of hematologic diseases and prognostic factors in breast cancer. Experimental approaches are already underway to reduce tumorigenesis into discrete modules of regulatory networks and biologic processes. A catalog of listed genes that change with tumor type, for example, should not be equated with prognosis, therapeutic response, or adverse outcomes. How to move diagnostic tools using micro-arrays and gene expression profiles into clinical decision making will be the focus of research programs in translational and clinical outcomes.

Specific therapies for many inheritable diseases have lagged substantially behind advances in other fields, but new opportunities appear on the horizon for improving prognosis and clinical outcomes in the era of regenerative medicine.

References

Acharya MR, Sparreboom A, Venitz J, Figg WD: Rational development of histone deacetylase inhibitors as anticancer agents: A review. Mol Pharmacol 68:917-932, 2005.

Collins FS, Green ED, Guttmacher AE: A vision for the future of genomics research. Nature 422:835-847, 2003.

Evans WE, McLeod HL: Pharmacogenomics: Drug disposition, drug targets, and side effects. N Engl J Med 348:538-549, 2003.

Hinds DA, Stuve LL, Nilsen GB, et al: Whole-genome patterns of common DNA variation in three human populations. Science 307:1072-1079, 2005.

Krause DS, Van Etten RA: Tyrosine kinases as targets for cancer therapy. N Engl J Med 353:172-187, 2005.

van Steensel B: Mapping of genetic and epigenetic regulatory networks using microarrays. Nat Genet 37:S18-S24, 2005.

Willard HF, Ginsburg GS (eds): Genomic and Personalized Medicine. New York, Elsevier, 2009.

Zamore PD, Haley B: Ribo-gnome: The big world of small RNAs. Science 309:1519-1524, 2005.

Section II

Evidence-Based Medicine

Chapter **2**

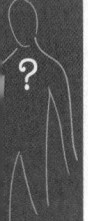

Evidence-Based Medicine, Quality of Life, and the Cost of Medicine

Sara G. Tariq and Susan S. Beland

The diagnosis and treatment of individual patients involve clinical experience and skills on the part of the physician and knowledge of scientific information obtained through clinical trials. In the past, most of the daily practice was based on informal learning and a tradition of knowledge transferred from experienced clinicians to trainees and colleagues. Increasingly, however, this informal technique is being supplanted by rigorous analysis of the scientific underpinnings of clinical logic. Electronic databases and Internet technology enable collation and dissemination of information to help identify which techniques are supported by clinical trials. *Evidence-based medicine* has evolved during the past decade and uses the best available evidence from published research as the foundation for clinical decision making. This foundation, in addition to clinical expertise and a respect for patient preference, will aid the physician in providing optimal outcomes and a quality of life for the patient. However, the development of new techniques in medicine, often at great cost, can strain the ability of a society to fund and provide such services. Critical appraisal of both new and traditional diagnostic and treatment modalities is thus needed.

Critical Appraisal of the Literature

Being cognizant of the types of evidence is crucial to practice evidence-based medicine. Research studies can be divided into two major categories: primary and secondary (Table 2-1).

Primary studies can have a number of designs. In *randomized controlled studies,* participants in the trial are ran-

domly allocated to one intervention or another. Both groups are followed for a specified period and analyzed in terms of specific outcomes defined at the outset of the study. This type of study allows rigorous assessment of a single variable in a defined patient group, has a prospective design that potentially eradicates bias by comparing two otherwise similar groups, and allows for meta-analysis. However, these studies are expensive and time-consuming. Results of randomized controlled trials can have enormous impact on the practice of medicine, as exemplified by the Women's Health Initiative randomized controlled trial. This study was designed to assess the risks and benefits for postmenopausal hormone use in healthy women. However, the trial was stopped early because of an increased incidence of breast cancer, coronary heart disease, stroke, and thromboembolic disease in the hormone-treated group. *Cohort studies* have two or more groups of participants selected on the basis of differences in their exposure to a particular agent. The participants are prospectively followed to see how many in each group develop a disease or other specific outcome. A well-known example is the Framingham Heart Study that enrolled 5200 participants in 1948 and followed them forward in time to examine the progression and risk factors for heart disease. The data provided from the Framingham Study have helped clinicians understand the development and progression of heart disease and its risk factors. As with randomized trials, cohort studies are time-consuming. *Case-control studies* involve patients with a particular disease or condition who are identified and matched with control patients. The control participants can be patients with another disease or individuals from the general population. The validity of these retrospective studies depends on careful selection of the control group. For example, the impact of risk factors for men and women was recently evaluated in the CARDIO 2000 Study. The authors

Table 2-1 **Types of Research Studies**	
Primary Studies	**Secondary Studies**
Randomized control	Meta-analyses
Case control	Clinical practice guidelines
Cohort studies	Decision analysis
Cross sectional	Cost-effectiveness analysis
Case series	
Case report	

Table 2-2 **Requirements of Screening Tests**
• Prevalence of disease must be sufficiently high.
• Disease must have significant morbidity and mortality rates.
• Effective treatment must be available.
• Improved outcomes from early diagnosis and treatment must be present.
• Test should have good sensitivity and specificity parameters.
• Test should carry acceptable risks and be cost-effective.

evaluated 848 hospitalized patients after their first episode of acute coronary syndrome and used 1078 age- and sex-matched controls. The data revealed that women experiencing their first event were significantly older than men. *Case reports* describe the medical history of a single patient. When medical histories of more than one patient with a particular condition are described together to illustrate one aspect of the disease process, the term *case series* is used.

Secondary (integrative) studies attempt to summarize and draw conclusions from primary information. Meta-analyses use statistical techniques to combine and summarize the results of primary studies. By combining the results from many trials, meta-analyses are able to estimate the magnitude of the effect of an intervention or risk factor as well as evaluate previously unanswered questions by performing subgroup analyses. The use of meta-analysis has provoked some controversy. Some investigators believe that meta-analyses may be as reliable as randomized controlled trials, whereas others believe that the technique should be used only as an alternate to randomized trials. However, in the absence of a large randomized controlled study, a meta-analysis of multiple smaller studies may be the best source of information to answer a specific question.

Clinical practice guidelines attempt to summarize diagnostic and treatment strategies for common clinical problems to assist the physician with specific circumstances. They are usually published by medical organizations, such as the American College of Physicians, and government agencies, such as the Agency for Health Care Policy and Research and the United States Preventive Services Task Force. *Decision analysis* uses the results of primary studies to generate probability trees to aid both health professionals and patients in making choices about clinical management. *Cost-effectiveness analysis* evaluates whether a particular course of action is an effective use of resources.

Testing in Medical Practice

Screening tests are performed on asymptomatic healthy people to detect occult disease and should meet the criteria listed in Table 2-2. Screening tests are most useful when a high prevalence of disease is present in the population and the test has adequate sensitivity and specificity parameters. When applied to a disease with low prevalence, a test with low specificity would have an unacceptable number of false-positive results, which would lead to further procedures that are often invasive and expensive.

Diagnostic tests are used to determine the cause of illness in symptomatic persons and can be helpful in *patient management* by evaluating the severity of disease, determining prognosis, detecting disease recurrence, or selecting appropriate medications or other therapies. When considering diagnostic tests, the physician should weigh the potential benefits against the risks and expense.

When comparing the efficacy of a new diagnostic test, the critical issues are the following: (1) Does the new test have something to offer that the currently accepted test does not? (2) Does the new test provide additional information that alters the *post-test probability*, which is the likelihood that a patient who has a positive test has the disease? Comparing the post-test probability with the *pre-test probability* before ordering the test, which is the clinical assessment of diagnostic possibilities, is also important.

Values for some pre-test probabilities have been published, but more often they are derived from the physician's clinical experience and are influenced by the practice setting. For instance, an obese African-American woman from the rural South is experiencing fatigue, blurry vision, and frequent vaginal yeast infections, and she has a strong family history of diabetes. Based on these features, she would have a high pre-test probability for type 2 diabetes mellitus. If a new diagnostic test were available for the diagnosis of diabetes, a comparison could be made on the post-test probabilities expected from the standard test (fasting blood glucose) and the new test. Ideally, the new test would offer greater diagnostic accuracy.

Sensitivity and *specificity* are important parameters to consider when evaluating a diagnostic test. Sensitivity is an index of the diagnostic test's ability to detect the disease when it is present. Specificity is the ability of the diagnostic test to identify correctly the absence of the disease. These parameters are calculated by the use of a 2 × 2 table (Table 2-3). An additional value, the *likelihood ratio,* which uses

Table 2-3 **Schematic Outcomes of a Diagnostic Test (2 × 2 Table)**		
Test Result	**Disease Present**	**Disease Absent**
Positive	True positive (*a*)	False positive (*b*)
Negative	False negative (*c*)	True negative (*d*)

Positive predictive value (true-positive rate) =$a/(a+b)$.
Negative predictive value (false-positive rate) =$d/(c+d)$.
Sensitivity =$a/(a+c)$; patients with the disease who have a positive test.
Specificity =$d/(b+d)$; patients without the disease who have a negative test.

both sensitivity and specificity, gives an even better indication of the test's performance. A high positive likelihood ratio indicates a high likelihood of the presence of disease, whereas a high negative likelihood ratio identifies the absence of disease.

Positive likelihood ratio:

$$= \frac{\text{Sensitivity (probability that test is positive in diseased patients)}}{1 - \text{Specificity (probability that test is positive in nondiseased patients)}}$$

Negative likelihood ratio:

$$= \frac{1 - \text{Sensitivity (probability that test is negative in diseased patients)}}{1 - \text{Specificity (probability that test is negative in nondiseased patients)}}$$

After determining the validity of the diagnostic test, its applicability to the patient in question and whether the test is affordable and accurate in a particular setting should be ascertained. If the diagnostic test requires special devices or skills that are not available in the practice facility, the results provided can be inaccurate. Most importantly, an assessment should be made about whether the test will change the management offered or decrease the need for the use of other tests.

Evaluating Evidence about Treatment

One of the most common problems facing physicians is the need to assess the validity of new treatments being developed as well as validity of traditional treatments that have been used for years. For example, how long after discharge from the hospital should treatment with antimicrobial agents continue for the patient who had been hospitalized for pneumonia? What is the value of plasmapheresis in thrombotic thrombocytopenic purpura? The first step in evaluating prospective treatments is to assess whether the information is derived from a properly conducted randomized controlled study. Every patient who enters the trial must be accounted for at the end of the study. The patients who are lost to follow-up often have different outcomes. If the conclusion of the trial does not change after accounting for the lost patients, then validity is added to the study. Another point to consider is whether patients were analyzed in their original randomized groups even if they did not undergo the intervention in question. This is termed an *intention-to-treat analysis*. A description of whether both groups were treated differently regarding other interventions (e.g., co-interventions) should be included.

Assessing the importance of the data provided is the next step. This includes a number of simple statistical calculations

applied to the available results. The first is *relative risk reduction* (RRR):

$$RRR = \frac{\text{Incidence of outcome in control group} - \text{Incidence of outcome in study group}}{\text{Incidence of outcome in control group}}$$

For example, the Diabetes Control and Complications Trial investigated the effect of tight control of blood glucose in patients with type 1 diabetes on the development and progression of long-term complications. The study involved more than 1400 patients, with one half randomized to intensive treatment and one half to conventional therapy. In this study, 3.4% of the patients in the conventional group and 2.2% in the intensive group developed microalbuminuria, indicating a 35% decrease in the occurrence of microalbuminuria in the primary prevention group:

$$RRR = \frac{0.034 - 0.022}{0.034} \times 100 = 35\%$$

The greater the RRR, the more effective the therapy. However, the RRR does not take into account the baseline risk of the patients entering the trial and thus does not differentiate between large and small effects.

The significance of RRR is discussed on the web site (**Web Text 2-1**).

Calculating the *absolute risk reduction* (ARR), which gives the absolute difference in rates between the two groups, is another way of assessing the outcome. The ARR is defined as the number (X) that had the ill effect in the control group minus the number (Y) in the treatment group (i.e., ARR = $X - Y$). Using the previous example, the ARR for the development of microalbuminuria is $0.034 - 0.022 = 0.012$, or 1.2%. Another valuable calculation is the *number needed to treat*, which represents the number of patients who need to be treated to prevent a single outcome event and is the inverse of the ARR (i.e., $1/[X - Y]$). The lower the number needed to treat, the more clinically relevant is the treatment. Again, using the example, to prevent 1 patient from developing microalbuminuria, 83 patients with diabetes would have to be treated with intensive therapy ($1/[X - Y] = 1/0.012 = 83$). From this example, what seems like a large RRR of 35% actually translates to a relatively small (although significant) number of patients who benefited from intensive treatment.

As before, assessment of the applicability of this information to a particular patient should be made by taking into account whether the patient in question has the same characteristics of the patients included in the study. Evidence of side effects, cause, or value of a particular clinical sign in diagnosis can be assessed along these same lines.

Internet in Clinical Practice

The use of computer systems for disseminating medical information has increased exponentially. Numerous worldwide websites offer high-quality medical news, information

Table 2-4 **Worldwide Websites**
• Cochrane Collaboration—one of the major organizations involved in evidence-based medicine (http://www.cochrane.org)
• MD Consult—comprehensive medical information service (http://www.mdconsult.com)
• Centers for Disease Control and Prevention (http://www.cdc.gov)
• National Institutes of Health (http://www.nih.gov)
• UpToDate—comprehensive clinical information website that is constantly updated (http://www.uptodate.com)
• Student Consult—provides access to full standard texts online (http://www.studentconsult.com)

about practice guidelines, online textbooks and journals, and information about evidence-based medicine. In addition, many government sites offer up-to-date information (e.g., Centers for Disease Control and Prevention, National Institutes of Health). Table 2-4 lists some of these sites.

Including the Patient in the Decision Process

Searching for the best evidence and applying it have the ultimate goal of providing better patient care. The process should also involve informing the patient of the available options and offering options based on good evidence. Effective communication, geared toward the patient's level of health literacy, is crucial to ensure that the patient makes an informed decision. Using a certain therapy or implementing a diagnostic test may be inconvenient, or the patient may develop a certain side effect that he or she is not willing to accept. Involvement of the patient in the decision-making process requires good communication and adequate resources for patient education.

Quality of Life

Health care in the millennium has changed significantly. An increasing number of patients survive illnesses that used to be fatal, and many patients have multiple co-existing illnesses. Assessing clinical improvement to a given treatment covers only one aspect of the clinician's success. For example, although survival is an important outcome for patients with cancer, overall quality of life is fundamental. A patient can have improvement in disease-free survival without having a significant change in quality of life, and vice versa. Quality of life represents a subjective concept that is defined by the subjective perception of the patient and includes physical, emotional, social, and cognitive functions and the disease symptoms and side effects of a given treatment or intervention. For example, in examining the efficacy of a drug for postchemotherapy anemia, it would not only be important to know whether the hemoglobin rises appropriately but also to know whether the patient subjectively has more energy and is able to perform the normal duties of life.

Quality of life is more commonly becoming a defined outcome measure in clinical trials. An increasing number of studies have been conducted in which health-related quality of life is either the primary or secondary endpoint. Hopefully, clinicians can then take the information gained from these data and apply it in a holistic manner to optimize patient care.

COST OF MEDICINE

The practice of medicine has significantly changed during the past 30 years. The cost of medicine has risen astronomically, and it is the duty of the physician to be cognizant of this in daily practice. Health care spending is growing much faster than the rest of the economy. Rising hospital expenses reflect many factors, including the demand for new medications and technology as well as the aging population. Physicians can contribute to the reduction of costs by being aware of medication prices and ordering tests appropriately.

The pharmaceutical industry has been accused of contributing to medical inflation. The industry spends more than $11 billion annually on promotion and marketing, and $8,000 to $13,000 per physician each year. They employ 1 drug representative for every 11 physicians in the United States. The average price of drugs rose almost 50% between 1992 and 2000. Literature suggests that the gifts and perks physicians receive from the pharmaceutical representatives have a major influence on their practices and prescribing habits. Caution is recommended when analyzing data from pharmaceutical representatives, taking into account the inherent bias that exists regarding the medication they are marketing. The medical profession is responsible for providing the best care possible for patients, and barriers to this care arise when a gift or amenity accepted from a pharmaceutical representative obscures the judgment of appropriate and cost-effective care. Generic drugs should be prescribed whenever possible. Studies have shown that if physicians substituted generic drugs for brand-name drugs, the potential national savings would be up to 5.9 billion dollars annually. In addition, all medical schools should stress the use of generic drugs to students and residents.

The use of tests is the second area in which physicians must be prudent when it comes to cost. The routine ordering of expensive and unnecessary tests has become part of the medical culture, but they can never take the place of a thorough history and physical examination. Evidence-based medicine is an important tool to use when deciding whether a certain diagnostic test is needed to help in the care of a patient. The risks and benefits of each test that is ordered must be weighed against the costs. For example, asymptomatic patients who are concerned about ovarian cancer may want their physician to order a pelvic ultrasound. The prudent physician will know that the prevalence of ovarian cancer is low in the population and thus the literature does not support the routine use of pelvic ultrasound as a screening tool. Therefore, a pelvic ultrasound is not a cost-effective test for screening ovarian cancer in all female patients.

These are two ways in which physicians can take an active role in helping reduce the cost of medical care in this nation, but the problem is clearly larger than this. Physicians will need to find a balance between being cost-conscious and maintaining high-quality patient care as the medical field continues to expand.

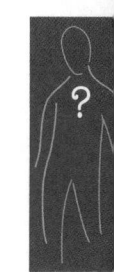

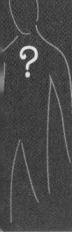

Prospectus for the Future

Challenges to be met:
- Medical schools need to expand the teaching of evidence-based medicine to students and physicians in training.
- Risks and benefits of screening tests need to be better defined (e.g., use of computed tomography in the diagnosis of early lung cancer versus risk for radiation exposure).

- To affect the cost of medicine, the overuse of technology (e.g., computed tomography for every patient with abdominal pain) needs to be addressed from the standpoint of evidence-based medicine.
- Finally, universal health care coverage for all people in the United States is desperately needed.

References

Bhat SK: The cost of medicine. Ann Intern Med 139:74-75, 2003.

Bottomley A: The cancer patient and quality of life. Oncologist 7:120-125, 2002.

Diabetes Control and Complications Trial Research Group: The effect of intensive treatment of diabetes on the development and progression of long-term complications in insulin-dependent diabetes mellitus. N Engl J Med 329:977-986, 1993.

Haas JS, Phillips KA, Gerstenberger EP: Potential savings from substituting generic drugs for brand-name drugs: Medical expenditure panel survey, 1997-2000. Ann Intern Med 142:891-897, 2005.

Hall WJ: The ethical dilemma of accepting gifts from drug makers. ACP-ASIM Observer, December, 2001.

Sacket D: Evidence-Based Medicine, 2nd ed. Oxford, Churchill Livingstone, 2000, pp 13-29.

Writing Group for the Women's Health Initiative Investigators: Risks and benefits of estrogen plus progestin in healthy postmenopausal women, JAMA 288:321-333, 2002.

Section III

Cardiovascular Disease

Chapter 3

Structure and Function of the Normal Heart and Blood Vessels

Jack Morshedzadeh, Dean Y. Li, and Ivor J. Benjamin

Gross Anatomy

The heart is composed of four chambers, two atria and two ventricles, which form two separate pumps arranged side by side and in series (Fig. 3-1). The atria are low-pressure capacitance chambers that mainly function to store blood during ventricular contraction (systole) and then fill the ventricles with blood during ventricular relaxation (diastole). The two atria are separated by a thin interatrial septum. The ventricles are high-pressure chambers responsible for pumping blood through the lungs and to the peripheral tissues. Because the pressure generated by the left ventricle is greater than that generated by the right, the left ventricular myocardium is thicker than the right. The two ventricles are separated by the interventricular septum, which is a membranous structure at its superior aspect and a thick, muscular structure at its medial and distal portions.

The atrioventricular (AV) valves separate the atria and ventricles. The mitral valve is a bileaflet valve that separates the left atrium and ventricle. The tricuspid valve is a trileaflet valve and separates the right atrium and ventricle. Strong chords (chordae tendineae) attach the ventricular aspects of these valves to the papillary muscles of their respective ventricles. These papillary muscles are extensions of normal myocardium that project into the ventricular cavities and are important for optimal valve closure. The semilunar valves separate the ventricles from the arterial chambers: the aortic valve separates the left ventricle from the aorta, and the pulmonic valve separates the right ventricle from the pulmonary artery. These valves do not have chordae. Rather, they are fibrous valves whose edges coapt closely, thus allowing for adequate valve closure. Each of the four valves is surrounded by a fibrous ring, or annulus, that forms part of the structural support of the heart. When open, the valves allow free flow of blood across them and into the adjacent chamber or vessel. When closed, the valves effectively prevent the backflow of blood into the preceding chamber.

The thin, double-layered pericardium surrounds the heart. The visceral pericardium is adherent to the heart and constitutes its outer surface, or *epicardium.* This outer surface is separated from the parietal pericardium by the pericardial space, which normally contains less than 50 mL of fluid. The parietal pericardium has attachments to the sternum, vertebral column, and diaphragm that serve to stabilize the heart in the chest. Normal pericardial fluid lubricates contact surfaces and limits direct tissue-surface contact during myocardial contraction. In addition, the normal pericardium modulates interventricular interactions during the cardiac cycle.

Circulatory Pathway

The circulatory system is composed of two distinct and parallel vascular networks, arterial and venous networks, which interconnect through capillary beds of the distal target organs (see Fig. 3-1). Deoxygenated blood drains from peripheral tissues and enters the right atrium through the superior and inferior venae cavae. Blood draining from the heart enters the right atrium through the coronary sinus. This blood mixes in the right atrium during ventricular systole and then flows across the tricuspid valve and into the right ventricle during ventricular diastole. When the right ventricle contracts, blood is ejected across the pulmonic valve and into the main pulmonary artery, which then bifurcates into the left and right pulmonary arteries as these branches enter their respective lungs. After multiple bifurcations, blood flows into the pulmonary capillaries, where

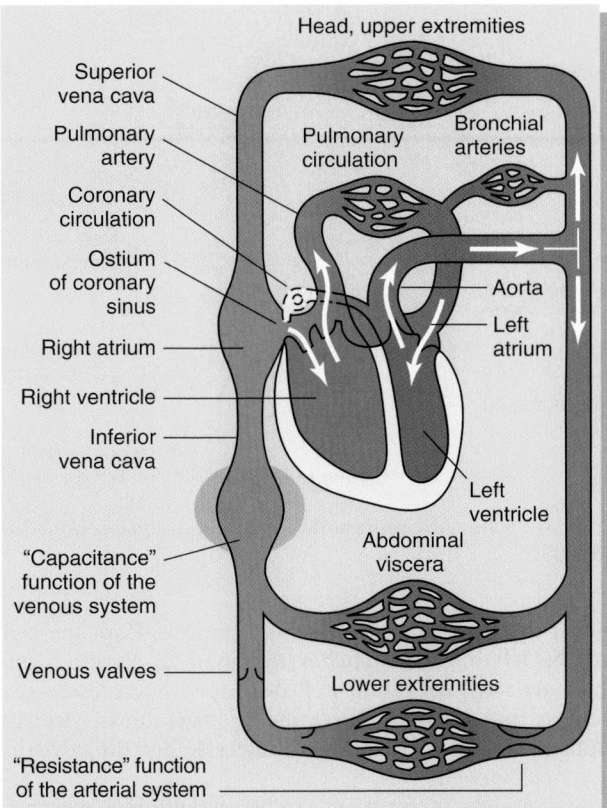

Figure 3-1 Schematic representation of the systemic and pulmonary circulatory systems. The venous system contains the greatest amount of blood at any one time and is highly distensible, accommodating a wide range of blood volumes (high capacitance). The arterial system is composed of the aorta, arteries, and arterioles. Arterioles are small muscular arteries that regulate blood pressure by changing tone (resistance).

carbon dioxide is exchanged for oxygen across the alveolar-capillary membrane. Oxygenated blood then drains from the lungs into the four pulmonary veins, which empty into the left atrium. During ventricular diastole, the blood flows across the open mitral valve and into the left ventricle. With ventricular contraction, the blood is ejected across the aortic valve and into the aorta and is subsequently delivered to the various organs, where oxygen and nutrients are exchanged for carbon dioxide and metabolic wastes.

The heart receives blood through the left and right coronary arteries (Fig. 3-2). These are the first arterial branches of the aorta and originate in outpouchings of the aortic root called the *sinuses of Valsalva*. The left main coronary artery originates in the left sinus of Valsalva and is a short vessel that bifurcates into the left anterior descending (LAD) and the left circumflex (LCx) coronary arteries. The LAD travels across the surface of the heart in the anterior interventricular groove toward the cardiac apex. It supplies blood to the anterior and anterolateral left ventricle through its diagonal branches and to the anterior two thirds of the interventricular septum through its septal branches. The LCx traverses posteriorly in the left AV groove (between the left atrium and left ventricle), supplying blood to the lateral aspect of the left ventricle through obtuse marginal branches as well as giving off branches to the left atrium. The right coronary artery (RCA) originates in the right sinus of Valsalva and courses down the right AV groove to a point where the left and right AV grooves and the inferior interventricular groove meet, the *crux* of the heart. The RCA gives off atrial branches to the right atrium and acute marginal branches to the right ventricle. The blood supply to the diaphragmatic and posterior aspects of the left ventricle varies. In 85% of individuals, the RCA bifurcates at the crux into the posterior descending coronary artery (PDA), which travels in the inferior interventricular groove to supply blood to the inferior

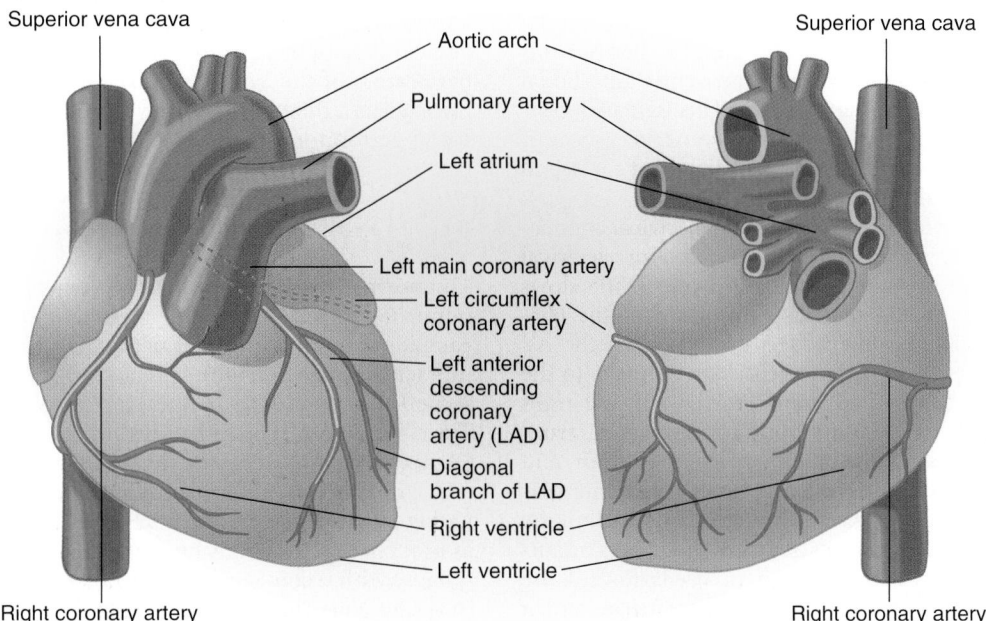

Figure 3-2 Major coronary arteries and their branches.

left ventricular wall and inferior third of the interventricular septum and to the posterior left ventricular (PLV) branches, which supply the posterior left ventricle. This course is termed a *right dominant circulation.* In 10% of individuals, the RCA terminates before reaching the crux, and the LCx supplies the PLV and PDA. This course is termed a *left dominant circulation.* In the remaining individuals, the RCA gives rise to the PDA, and the LCx gives rise to the PLV in a *co-dominant circulation.* An understanding of coronary artery anatomy and distribution of blood supply enables the clinician to define the location of coronary artery disease based on history, physical examination, and noninvasive tests such as electrocardiography (ECG), echocardiography, and radionuclide ventriculography. Small vascular channels, called *collateral vessels,* interconnect the normal coronary arteries. These vessels are nonfunctional in the normal myocardium because no pressure gradient develops across them. However, in the setting of severe stenosis or complete occlusion of a coronary artery, the pressure in the vessel distal to the stenosis decreases, and a gradient develops across the collateral vasculature, resulting in flow through the collateral vessel. The development of collateral vasculature is directly related to the severity of the coronary stenosis and may be stimulated by ischemia, hypoxia, and a variety of growth factors. Over time, these vessels may reach up to 1 mm in luminal diameter and are almost indistinguishable from similarly sized, normal coronary arteries.

Most of the venous drainage from the heart occurs through the coronary sinus, which runs in the AV groove and empties into the right atrium. A small amount of blood from the right side of the heart drains directly into the right atrium through the thebesian veins and small anterior myocardial veins.

Conduction System

The electrical impulse that initiates cardiac contraction originates in the sinoatrial (SA) node, a collection of specialized pacemaker cells measuring 1 to 2 cm in length located high in the right atrium between the superior vena cava and the right atrial appendage (Fig. 3-3). The impulse then spreads through the atrial tissue and through preferential internodal tracts, ultimately reaching the AV node. This structure consists of a meshwork of cells located at the inferior aspect of the right atrium between the coronary sinus and the septal leaflet of the tricuspid valve.

The AV node provides the only normal electrical connection between the atria and ventricles. After an electrical impulse enters the AV node, conduction transiently slows and then proceeds to the ventricles by means of the His-Purkinje system. The bundle of His extends from the AV node down the membranous interventricular septum to the muscular septum, where it divides into the left and right bundle branches. The right bundle branch is a discrete structure that extends along the interventricular septum and enters the moderator band on its way toward the anterolateral papillary muscle of the right ventricle. The left bundle branch is less distinct; it consists of an array of fibers organized into an anterior fascicle, which proceeds toward the anterolateral papillary muscle of the left ventricle, and a posterior fascicle, which proceeds posteriorly in the septum

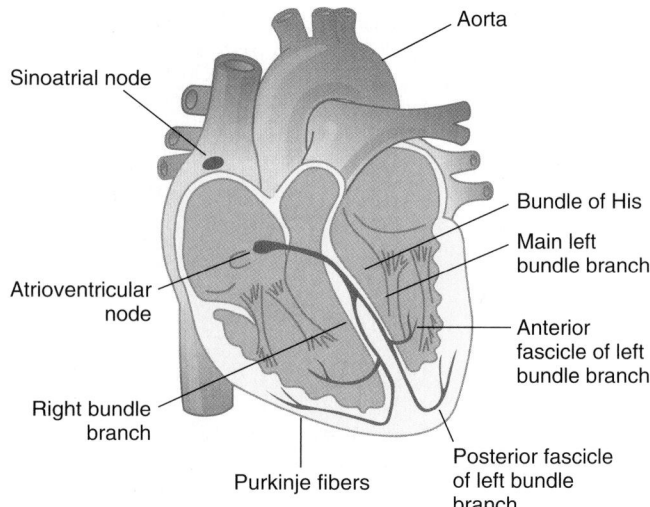

Figure 3-3 Schematic representation of the cardiac conduction system.

toward the posteromedial papillary muscle. Both the right and the left bundle branches terminate in Purkinje cells, which are large cells with well-developed intercellular connections that allow for the rapid propagation of electrical impulses. These impulse-generating cells then directly stimulate myocytes.

Heart blocks, a form of cardiac arrhythmia, may arise from intrinsic problems of the conduction system or from impaired blood supply (coronary artery disease) to the conduction system. The SA node is supplied by the SA nodal artery, which is a branch of the RCA in about 60% of the population or a branch of the LCx in 40%. The AV node is supplied by the AV nodal artery, which is a branch of the RCA in about 90% of the population or a branch of the LCx in 10%. The right bundle branch receives most of its blood supply from septal perforators that branch off of the LAD. There may also be collateral blood supply from the RCA or LCx. The left anterior fascicle is supplied by septal perforators from the LAD and is particularly susceptible to ischemia and infarction. The proximal portion of the left posterior fascicle is supplied by the AV nodal artery and by septal perforators of the LAD. The distal portion of the posterior fascicle has a dual blood supply from anterior and posterior septal perforators (i.e., the LAD and PDA).

Neural Innervation

The normal myocardium is richly innervated by the autonomic nervous system. The sympathetic supply is from preganglionic neurons located within the superior five to six thoracic segments of the spinal cord, which synapse with second-order neurons in the cervical sympathetic ganglia. Traveling within the cardiac nerves, these fibers end in the SA node, AV node, epicardial vessels, and myocardium. The parasympathetic supply is from preganglionic neurons originating in the dorsal motor nucleus of the medulla and pass as branches of the vagus nerve to the heart. Here the fibers synapse with second-order neurons located in ganglia within the heart. Nerve terminals of the parasympathetic nerves end in the SA node, AV node, epicardial vessels, and myocardium. A supply of vagal afferents from the inferior and posterior aspects of the ventricles mediate important cardiac reflexes, whereas the vagal efferent fibers to the SA and AV nodes are active in modulating impulse initiation and conduction. In general, sympathetic stimulation increases heart rate (HR) and force of myocardial contraction, and parasympathetic stimulation slows HR and reduces the force of contraction.

Myocardium

Cardiac tissue (myocardium) is composed of several cell types that together produce the organized contraction of the heart. Specialized myocardial cells make up the cardiac electrical system (conduction system) and are responsible for the generation of an electrical impulse and organized propagation of that impulse to cardiac muscle fibers (myocytes), which, in turn, respond by mechanical contraction. Atrial and ventricular myocytes are specialized, branching muscle cells connected end to end by intercalated disks. These thickened regions of the cell membrane (sarcolemma) aid in the transmission of mechanical tension between cells. The sarcolemma has functions similar to those of other cell membranes, including maintenance of ionic gradients, propagation of electrical impulses, and provision of receptors for neural and hormonal inputs. In addition, the sarcolemma is intimately involved with the coupling of myocardial excitation and contraction through small transverse tubules (T tubules) that extend from the sarcolemma into the intracellular space. The myocytes contain several other organelles: the nucleus; the multiple mitochondria responsible for generating the energy required for contraction; an extensive network of intracellular tubules called the *sarcoplasmic reticulum,* which functions as the major intracellular storage site for calcium; and the myofibrils, which are the contractile elements of the cell. Each myofibril is made up of repeating units called *sarcomeres,* which are, in turn, composed of overlapping thin actin filaments and thick myosin filaments and their regulatory proteins troponin and tropomyosin (Fig. 3-4).

Muscle Physiology and Contraction

Contraction of myocytes begins with electrical depolarization of the sarcolemma, resulting in an influx of calcium into the cell through channels in the T tubules (Fig. 3-5). This initial calcium entry stimulates the rapid release of large amounts of calcium from the sarcoplasmic reticulum into the cell cytosol. The calcium then binds to the calcium-binding troponin subunit (troponin C) on the actin filaments of the sarcomere, resulting in a conformational change in the troponin-tropomyosin complex. This change facilitates the actin-myosin interaction, which results in cellular contraction. As the wave of depolarization passes, the calcium is rapidly and actively resequestered in the sarcoplasmic reticulum, where it is stored by various proteins, including calsequestrin, until the next wave of depolarization occurs. Calcium is also extruded from the cytosol by

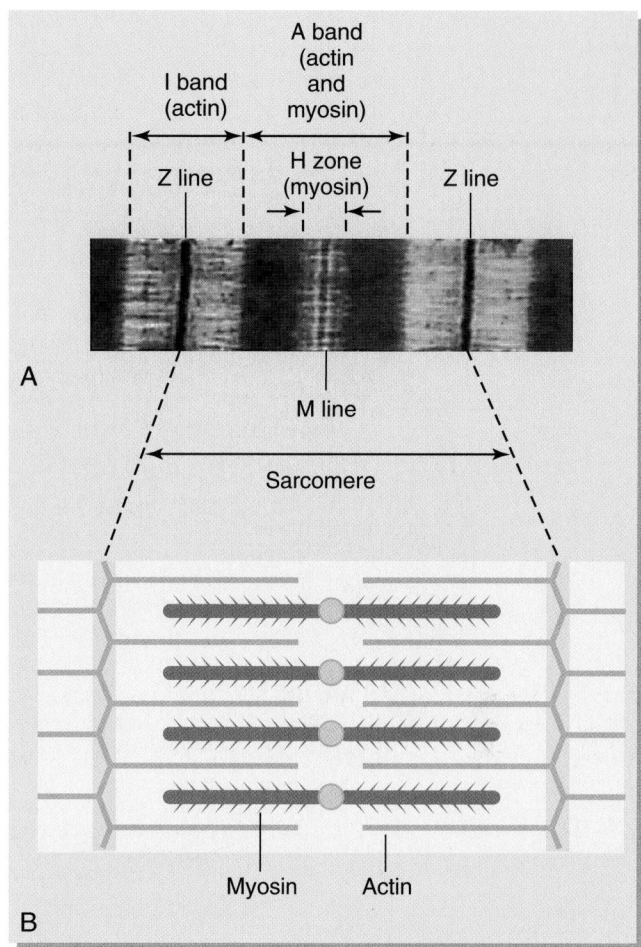

Figure 3-4 **A,** Sarcomere as it appears under the electron microscope. **B,** Schematic of the location and interaction of actin and myosin.

various calcium pumps in the sarcolemma. The force of myocyte contraction can be regulated by the amount of free calcium released into the cell by the sarcoplasmic reticulum. More calcium allows for greater actin-myosin interaction, producing a stronger contraction.

The energy for myocyte contraction is derived from adenosine triphosphate (ATP), which is generated by oxidative phosphorylation of adenosine diphosphate (ADP) in the abundant mitochondria of the cell. ATP is required both for calcium influx and for force generation by actin-myosin interaction. During contraction, ATP promotes dissociation of myosin from actin, thereby permitting the sliding of thick filaments past thin filaments as the sarcomere shortens. Under normal circumstances, fatty acids are the preferred energy source, although glucose can also be used as a substrate. These substrates must be constantly delivered to the heart through the bloodstream because minimal energy is stored in the heart. Myocardial metabolism is aerobic and thus requires a constant supply of oxygen. Under ischemic or hypoxemic conditions, glycolysis and lactate may serve as a source of ATP, although in insufficient quantities to sustain the working heart. Ischemic conditions might also promote alterations in both cytosolic and mitochondrial calcium overload, a major terminal event in muscle injury of the heart, termed *myocardial infarction.*

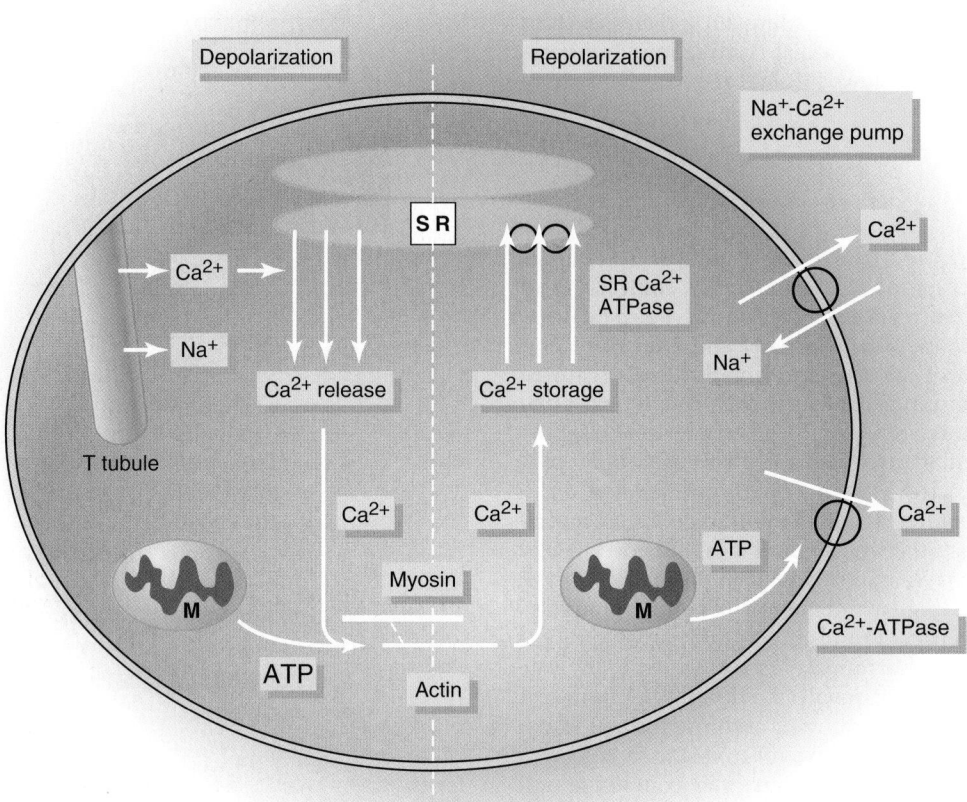

Figure 3-5 Calcium dependence of myocardial contraction. (1) Electrical depolarization of the myocyte results in an influx of Ca^{2+} into the cell through channels in the T tubules. (2) This initial phase of calcium entry stimulates the release of large amounts of Ca^{2+} from the sarcoplasmic reticulum (SR). (3) The Ca^{2+} then binds to the troponin-tropomyosin complex on the actin filaments, resulting in a conformational change that facilitates the binding interaction between actin and myosin. In the presence of adenosine triphosphate (ATP), the actin-myosin association is cyclically dissociated as the thick and thin filaments slide past each other, resulting in contraction. (4) During repolarization, the Ca^{2+} is actively pumped out of the cytosol and sequestered in the SR. M, mitochondrion.

Circulatory Physiology and the Cardiac Cycle

The cardiac cycle is a repeating series of contractile and valvular events during which the valves open and close in response to pressure gradients between different cardiac chambers (Fig. 3-6). This cycle can be divided into *systole*, the period of ventricular contraction, and *diastole*, the period of ventricular relaxation. With the onset of ventricular contraction, the pressure in the ventricles increases and exceeds that in the atria, at which time the AV valves close. Intraventricular pressure continues to rise, initially without a change in ventricular volume (isovolumic contraction), until the intraventricular pressures exceed the pressures in the aorta and pulmonary artery, at which time the semilunar valves open and ventricular ejection of blood occurs. With the onset of ventricular relaxation, the pressure in the ventricles falls until the pressure in the arterial chambers exceeds that

in the ventricles, and the semilunar valves close. Ventricular relaxation continues, initially without a change in ventricular volume (isovolumic relaxation). When the pressure in the ventricles falls below the pressure in the atria, the AV valves open, and a rapid phase of ventricular filling occurs as blood in the atria empties into the ventricles. At the end of diastole, active atrial contraction augments ventricular filling. This augmentation is particularly important in patients with poor ventricular function or stiff ventricles and is lost in patients with atrial fibrillation.

In the absence of valvular disease, no impediment to the flow of blood exists from the ventricles to the arterial beds, and the systolic arterial pressure rises sharply to a peak. During diastole, the arterial pressure gradually falls as blood flows distally, and elastic recoil of the arteries occurs. This response contrasts with the pressure response in the ventricles during diastole, in which pressure gradually increases as blood enters the ventricles from the atria. Atrial pressure can be directly measured in the right atrium, whereas occluding

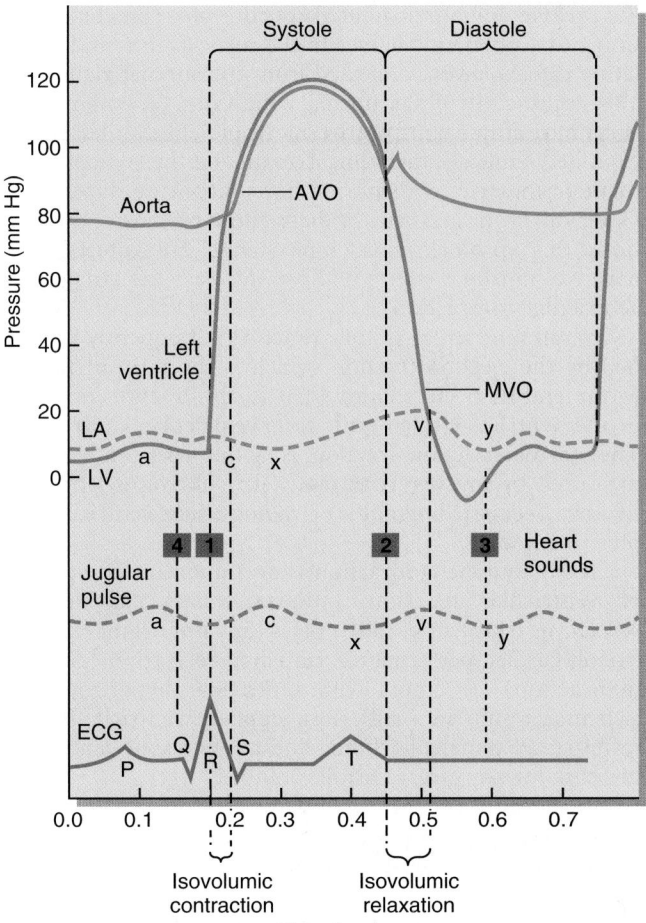

Figure 3-6 Simultaneous electrocardiogram (ECG) and pressure tracings obtained from the left atrium (LA), left ventricle (LV), and aorta, and the jugular venous pressure during the cardiac cycle. For simplification, right-sided pressures have been omitted. Normal right atrial pressure closely parallels that of the left atrium, and right ventricular and pulmonary artery pressures are timed closely with their corresponding left-sided heart counterparts; they are reduced only in magnitude. The normal mitral and aortic valve closure precedes tricuspid and pulmonic valve closure, respectively, whereas valve opening reverses this order. The jugular venous pulse lags behind the right atrial pulse.

During the course of one cardiac cycle, the electrical events (ECG) initiate and therefore precede the mechanical (pressure) events, and the latter precedes the auscultatory events (heart sounds) they themselves produce. Shortly after the P wave, the atria contract to produce the a wave. The QRS complex initiates ventricular systole, followed shortly by LV contraction and the rapid buildup of LV pressure. Almost immediately, LV pressure exceeds LA pressure, closing the mitral valve and producing the first heart sound. After a brief period of isovolumic contraction, LV pressure exceeds aortic pressure and the aortic valve opens (AVO). When the ventricular pressure once again falls below the aortic pressure, and the aortic valve closes to produce the second heart sound and terminate ventricular ejection. The LV pressure decreases during the period of isovolumic relaxation until it drops below LA pressure, and the mitral valve opens (MVO).

a small pulmonary artery branch and measuring the pressure distally (the pulmonary capillary *wedge* pressure) is often used to obtain left atrial pressure indirectly. An atrial pressure tracing is shown in Figure 3-6 and is composed of several waves. The *a wave* represents atrial contraction. As

Table 3-1 Normal Values for Common Hemodynamic Parameters

Heart Rate	60-100 Beats/Minute
Pressures	
Central venous	≤9 mm Hg
Right atrial	≤9 mm Hg
Right ventricular	
Systolic	15-30 mm Hg
End-diastolic	≤9 mm Hg
Pulmonary arterial	
Systolic	15-30 mm Hg
Diastolic	3-12 mm Hg
Pulmonary capillary wedge	≤12 mm Hg
Left atrial	≤12 mm Hg
Left ventricular	
Systolic	100-140 mm Hg
End-diastolic	3-12 mm Hg
Aortic	
Systolic	100-140 mm Hg
Diastolic	60-90 mm Hg
Resistance	
Systemic vascular resistance	800-1500 dynes-sec/cm^{-5}
Pulmonary vascular resistance	30-120 dynes-sec/cm^{-5}
Cardiac output	4-6 L/min
Cardiac index	2.5-4 L/min

the atria subsequently relax, the atrial pressure falls, and the *x descent* is noted on the pressure tracing. The x descent is interrupted by a small *c wave*, which is generated as the AV valve bulges toward the atrium during ventricular systole. As the atria fill from venous return, the *v wave* is seen, after which the *y descent* appears as the AV valves open and blood from the atria empties into the ventricles. The normal ranges of pressures in the various cardiac chambers are shown in Table 3-1.

CARDIAC PERFORMANCE

The amount of blood ejected by the heart each minute is referred to as the cardiac output (CO) and is the product of the stroke volume (SV; amount of blood ejected with each ventricular contraction) and the HR:

$$CO = SV \times HR$$

The cardiac index is the CO divided by the body surface area; it is measured in liters per minute per square meter and is a way of normalizing CO to body size. The normal CO at rest is 4 to 6 L/min, although this value can increase fourfold to sixfold during strenuous exercise as a result of increases in HR (chronotropic) and SV (inotropic).

The SV is a measure of the mechanical function of the heart and is affected by preload, afterload, and contractility (Table 3-2). *Preload* is the volume of blood in the ventricle at the end of diastole and is primarily a reflection of venous return. Within limits, as the preload increases, the ventricle stretches, and the ensuing ventricular contraction becomes more rapid and forceful. This phenomenon is known as the

Table 3-2 Factors Affecting Cardiac Performance

Preload (left ventricular diastolic volume)	Total blood volume
	Venous (sympathetic) tone
	Body position
	Intrathoracic and intrapericardial pressures
	Atrial contraction
	Pumping action of skeletal muscle
Afterload (impedance against which the left ventricle must eject blood)	Peripheral vascular resistance
	Left ventricular volume (preload, wall tension)
	Physical characteristics of the arterial tree (elasticity of vessels or presence of outflow obstruction)
Contractility (cardiac performance independent of preload or afterload)	Sympathetic nerve impulses
	Increased contractility
	Circulating catecholamines
	Digitalis, calcium, other inotropic agents
	Increased heart rate or post-extrasystolic augmentation
	Anoxia, acidosis
	Decreased contractility
	Pharmacologic depression
	Loss of myocardium
	Intrinsic depression
Heart rate	Autonomic nervous system
	Temperature, metabolic rate
	Medications, drugs

Frank-Starling relationship. Because ventricular volume is not easily measured, ventricular filling pressure (ventricular end-diastolic pressure, atrial pressure, or pulmonary capillary wedge pressure) is frequently used as a surrogate measure of preload. Two major means can manipulate the preload in a clinical setting. The first is to modulate volume status: intravenous fluids to increase preload and diuretics to decrease preload. The second is to regulate vascular tone: nitroglycerin to diminish preload.

Afterload is the force against which the ventricles must contract to eject blood. The arterial pressure is often used as a practical measure of afterload; although, in truth, the intraventricular pressure, the size of the ventricular cavity, and the thickness of the ventricular walls (Laplace's law) determine afterload. Thus, afterload is increased in the setting of systemic hypertension or stenosis of the aortic valve but may be equally increased in the setting of ventricular dilation or ventricular hypertrophy. Some antihypertensive drugs, such as angiotensin-converting enzyme (ACE) inhibitors and hydralazine, reduce blood pressure (BP) by reducing afterload.

Contractility, or inotropy, although difficult to define, represents the force of ventricular contraction independent of loading conditions. For example, an increase in contractility results in a stronger ventricular contraction even when

the preload and afterload are kept constant. Direct stimulation from adrenergic nerves in the myocardium and circulating catecholamines released from the adrenal glands can alter contractility under normal conditions. Several medications have important positive inotropic effects that can be exploited clinically, including digoxin and the sympathomimetic amines (e.g., epinephrine, norepinephrine, dopamine). Other medications, many of them antihypertensive medications, (e.g., β blockers, calcium channel antagonists) have negative inotropic effects and can decrease the strength of ventricular contraction.

Overall ventricular systolic function is frequently quantified by the ejection fraction, which is the ratio of the SV to the end-diastolic volume, that is, the fraction of blood in the ventricle ejected with each ventricular contraction. The normal ejection fraction is about 60% and can be measured by invasive (contrast ventriculography) or noninvasive (echocardiography or radionuclide ventriculography) methods.

Clearly, systolic contraction is an important component of ventricular function; however, ventricular diastolic relaxation (lusitropy) also plays an important role in overall cardiac performance. Impaired relaxation (diastolic dysfunction), as occurs with ventricular hypertrophy or ischemia, results in a stiff, noncompliant ventricle, leading to impaired ventricular filling and an increased ventricular pressure for any given diastolic volume.

PHYSIOLOGY OF THE CORONARY CIRCULATION

The heart is an aerobic organ requiring a constant supply of oxygen to maintain normal function. Under normal conditions, the supply of oxygen delivered to the heart is closely matched to the amount of oxygen required by the heart (the myocardial oxygen consumption [Mvo_2]). The main determinants of Mvo_2 are HR, contractility, and wall stress. The wall stress, as determined by Laplace's law, is directly related to the systolic pressure and the heart size and inversely proportional to wall thickness:

$$\text{Wall stress} = (\text{pressure} \times \text{radius})/(2 \times \text{wall thickness})$$

Thus, the Mvo_2 parallels changes in HR, BP, contractility, and heart size. In general, oxygen delivery to an organ can be augmented by either increasing blood flow or increasing oxygen extraction from the blood. For all practical purposes, the oxygen extraction by the heart is maximal at rest, and thus increases in coronary blood flow must meet increases in Mvo_2.

Because of the compression of intramyocardial blood vessels during systole, most coronary flow occurs during diastole. Therefore, diastolic pressure is the major pressure driving the coronary circulation. An important implication of this fact is that tachycardia, which primarily shortens the duration of diastole, results in reduced time for coronary flow, which occurs despite the increase in Mvo_2 associated with increased HR. The systolic pressure has little effect on coronary blood flow except insofar as changes in BP lead to changes in Mvo_2.

Regulation of coronary blood flow occurs primarily through changes in coronary vascular resistance. In response to a change in Mvo_2, the coronary arteries can dilate or constrict to allow for appropriate changes in coronary flow. Additionally, in the range of coronary perfusion pressures of 60 to 130 mm Hg, coronary blood flow is held constant by the process of autoregulation of the coronary arteries. This regulation of arterial resistance occurs at the level of the arterioles and is mediated by several factors. As ATP is metabolized during increased myocardial activity, adenosine is released and acts as a potent vasodilator. Decreased oxygen tension, increased carbon dioxide, acidosis, and hyperkalemia all develop during increased myocardial metabolism and may also mediate coronary vasodilation.

The coronary arteries are innervated by the autonomic nervous system, and activation of sympathetic or parasympathetic neurons alters coronary blood flow by affecting changes in vascular tone. Parasympathetic innervation through the vagus nerve and through the neurotransmitter acetylcholine results in vasodilation. Sympathetic neurons use norepinephrine as a neurotransmitter and may have opposing effects on the coronary vasculature. Stimulation of α receptors results in vasoconstriction, whereas stimulation of β receptors leads to vasodilation.

The ability of the coronary vasculature to mediate changes in blood flow through changes in vascular tone depends in large part on an intact, normally functioning endothelium. The endothelium produces several potent vasodilators, including endothelium-derived relaxing factor (EDRF) and prostacyclin. EDRF is likely to be nitric oxide or a compound containing nitric oxide and is released by the endothelium in response to acetylcholine, thrombin, ADP, serotonin, bradykinin, platelet aggregation, and an increase in shear stress. The latter stimulus accounts for the dilation of the coronary arteries in response to increases in blood flow in the setting of increases in Mvo_2 (called *flow-dependent vasodilation*).

Vasoconstricting factors, most notably endothelin, are also produced by the endothelium and are likely to play a role in regulating vascular tone. The balance of these vasodilator and vasoconstriction factors may be important in conditions such as coronary vasospasm. In addition to influencing vascular tone, the endothelium has several other functions that have important implications for blood flow and tissue perfusion. These include maintenance of a nonthrombotic surface through inhibition of platelet activity, control of thrombosis and fibrinolysis, and modulation of the inflammatory response of the vasculature. Disturbances in these normal properties of the endothelium *(endothelial dysfunction)* are likely to play an important role in the pathophysiologic conditions of coronary atherosclerosis and thrombosis.

PHYSIOLOGY OF THE SYSTEMIC CIRCULATION

The normal cardiovascular system is capable of providing appropriate blood flow to each of the organs and tissues of the body under a wide range of conditions. This is achieved by maintaining arterial BP within normal limits to meet functional needs from adjustments to the cardiac output and the resistance to blood flow in specific organs and tissues. Arterial pressure is regulated acutely and chronically through various local and systemic, humoral, and neural factors.

Poiseuille's law describes the relationship between pressure and flow. Although not exactly descriptive of blood flow through elastic tapering blood vessels, Poiseuille's law is useful in understanding blood flow. Fluid flow (F) through a tube is proportional (proportionality constant = K) to the pressure (P) difference between the ends of the tube:

$$F = K \times \Delta P$$

The reciprocal of K is the resistance to flow (R); that is $K = 1/R$. When fluid flows through a tube, the resistance to flow is determined by the properties of both the fluid and the tube. In the case of a steady, streamlined flow of fluid through a rigid tube, Poiseuille found that these factors determine resistance:

$$R = 8\eta L / \pi r^4$$

where r is the radius of the tube, L is its length, and η is the viscosity of the fluid. This equation shows that the resistance to blood flow increases proportionately with increases in fluid viscosity or tube length. In contrast, radius changes have a much greater influence because resistance is inversely proportional to the fourth power of the radius. Poiseuille's law incorporates the factors influencing flow, so that:

$$\begin{aligned} F &= \Delta P / R \\ &= \Delta P \pi r^4 / 8 \eta L \end{aligned}$$

The most important determinants of blood flow in the cardiovascular system are ΔP and r^4. Thus, small changes in arterial radius can cause large changes in flow to a tissue or organ. Systemic vascular resistance (SVR) is the total resistance of flow offered by the blood vessels of the systemic circulation. Physiologic changes in SVR are primarily caused by changes in the radius of small arteries and arterioles, the *resistance vessels* of the systemic circulation. The SVR is defined as the pressure drop across the peripheral capillary beds divided by the blood flow across the beds (e.g., SVR = BP/CO). In practice, this is calculated as the mean arterial pressure minus the right atrial pressure divided by the cardiac output and is normally in the range of 800 to 1500 dynes sec/cm^5.

As with the coronary circulation autonomic innervation alters systemic vascular tone through sympathetic and parasympathetic innervation. Local oxygen tension, carbon dioxide levels, pH, and potassium levels have direct effects on vascular tone and blood flow. And finally, a normally functioning endothelium mediates changes in blood flow through potent vasodilatory and vasoconstricting factors (see "Physiology of the Coronary Circulation").

Control of BP through neural regulation occurs by means of tonic and reflexive modulation of autonomic nervous system outflow. Acutely, changes in these outflows influence key determinants of BP, such as cardiac chronotropy, inotropy, and vascular resistance. The primary mechanism by which BP is neurally modulated is through the baroreflexes. The baroreflex loop anatomically originates at the level of the baroreceptor. The baroreceptors are highly specialized stretch-sensitive nerve endings distributed throughout various regions of the cardiovascular systems, such as the carotid artery, aorta, and the cardiopulmonary region. Baroreceptors located in the carotid artery (e.g., carotid sinus) and aorta are sometimes referred to as *high-pressure baroreceptors* and those in the cardiopulmonary areas as *low-pressure baroreceptors*. After transmission of afferent impulses to the central nervous system, signals are integrated, and the efferent arm of the reflex projects neural signals systemically through the sympathetic and parasympathetic branches of the autonomic nervous system. In general, in response to an increase in systemic BP, there is an increased firing rate of the baroreceptors, efferent sympathetic outflow is inhibited (reducing vascular tone, chronotropy, and inotropy), and parasympathetic outflow is increased (reducing cardiac chronotropy). The opposite occurs when BP decreases.

Cardiac output and systemic BP are controlled not only neurally and by local vasoactive substances through regulation of vascular tone but also by blood volume. A major physiologic control mechanism, which regulates total blood volume, is the *renin-angiotensin-aldosterone system* (RAAS). Renin is an enzyme secreted by the kidneys in response to low renal perfusion, low blood volume, low BP, or low sodium concentration. Renin converts the polypeptide angiotensinogen to angiotensin I in the liver. Angiotensin I circulates in the bloodstream and is converted to angiotensin II by the activity of ACE located primarily in the capillary beds of the lung. Angiotensin II is a powerful vasoconstrictor regulating BP through changes in vascular tone. In addition to its vasoactive properties, angiotensin II activates release of the hormone aldosterone from the adrenal cortex. Aldosterone then acts on the kidneys to retain sodium and thus water. Angiotensin II also acts directly on the posterior pituitary gland, increasing the secretion of vasopressin (e.g., antidiuretic hormone). Much like angiotensin II, vasopressin is a vasoconstrictor; it also acts on the kidney by retaining water through its action on V2 receptors in the collecting ducts. Although activity of the RAAS is to maintain blood volume, this system has adverse effects in chronic disease states, aggravating conditions such as hypertension and heart failure.

Blood leaves the arterioles and flows into the capillary systems, where oxygen and nutrients are delivered to cells and carbon dioxide and metabolic wastes are removed. The deoxygenated blood then drains into peripheral veins, which contain valves to prevent backflow. These veins have thinner walls than arteries and function as *capacitance vessels;* they are able to accommodate a significantly larger volume of blood than the arterial system. With the aid of the pumping action of skeletal muscles and the respiratory motion of the chest wall, blood returns to the right atrium. This venous return can be altered by constriction or dilation of the peripheral veins. In addition to the venous drainage, a rich system of lymphatic vessels helps drain excess interstitial fluid from the periphery. The various lymphatic vessels drain into the thoracic duct and, subsequently, into the left brachiocephalic vein.

PHYSIOLOGY OF THE PULMONARY CIRCULATION

Similar to the systemic circulation, the pulmonary circulation consists of a branching network of progressively smaller arteries, arterioles, capillaries, and veins. The pulmonary capillaries are separated from the alveoli by a thin alveolar-capillary membrane through which gas exchange occurs. Carbon dioxide thus diffuses from the capillary blood into the alveoli, and oxygen diffuses from the alveoli into the blood. The flow of blood to various lung segments is regulated by several factors, the most important being the Po_2 in the alveoli. In this manner, blood is shunted toward well-ventilated lung segments and away from poorly ventilated segments. As a result of the extensive nature of the pulmonary capillary system and the distensibility of the pulmonary vasculature, the resistance across the pulmonary system (the pulmonary vascular resistance) is about 10% that of the systemic circulation. Owing to these features, the pulmonary system is able to tolerate significant increases in blood flow with little or no rise in pulmonary pressure. Thus, intracardiac shunts (e.g., atrial septal defects) may be associated with normal pulmonary pressure.

The lung receives a dual blood supply. The pulmonary artery accounts for most pulmonary blood flow; however, the lungs also receive oxygenated blood through the bronchial arteries. These vessels supply oxygen to the lung and drain into the bronchial veins. The bronchial veins drain partly into the pulmonary veins; thus, a small amount of deoxygenated blood normally enters the systemic circulation and accounts for a physiologic right-to-left shunt. In the normal setting, this shunt is insignificant, accounting for only 1% of the total systemic blood flow.

Cardiovascular Response to Exercise

The response of the heart to exercise is multifaceted and involves many of the previously discussed mechanisms of circulatory control (Table 3-3). In anticipation of exercise, neural centers in the brain stimulate vagal withdrawal and an increase in sympathetic tone, resulting in an increase

Table 3-3 **Physiologic Responses to Exercise**	
Increased heart rate	Increased sympathetic stimulation
Increased stroke volume	Decreased parasympathetic stimulation
Increased contractility	Increased sympathetic stimulation
Increased venous return	Sympathetic-mediated venoconstriction
	Pumping action of skeletal muscles
	Decreased intrathoracic pressure with deep inspirations
	Arteriolar vasodilation in exercising muscle
Decreased afterload	Arteriolar vasodilation in exercising muscle (mediated chiefly by local metabolites)
Increased blood pressure	Increased cardiac output
	Vasoconstriction (sympathetic stimulation) on nonexercising vascular beds
Increased O_2 extraction	Shift in oxyhemoglobin dissociation curve as a result of local acidosis

in HR and contractility (thus an increase in CO) before exercise ever starts. With exercise, sympathetic venoconstriction, augmented pumping action of skeletal muscles, and increased respiratory movements of the chest wall result in an increase in venous return to the heart. Through the Frank-Starling relationship, this increase in venous return results in an increase in contractility, thus augmenting CO. Sympathetic activation may also increase contractility; however, most of the increase in CO during exercise (up to 4 to 6 times the normal rate) is a consequence of an increase in HR. The peak HR that can be achieved is dependent on age and can be estimated by the following formula: maximal HR = (220 − age) ± 15 beats/minute.

Local factors in exercising muscle cause arteriolar dilation, resulting in increased flow to the capillary beds. This vasodilation results in decreased resistance to flow, and therefore the SVR decreases with exercise. Despite this change in resistance, the systolic BP rises, owing to the augmented CO and to sympathetic vasoconstriction, which leads to the preferential shunting of blood away from nonexercising vascular beds. The diastolic BP, by contrast, generally remains constant during exercise. The pulmonary system is able to tolerate the increased flow with only small increases in pulmonary pressure. The increases in HR and contractility result in a significant increase in Mvo_2 (up to 300%), and coronary blood flow subsequently increases.

Various types of exercises have different effects on the circulatory system. The response described in this text occurs with isotonic exercises, such as running or biking. With isometric exercises, such as weight lifting, the predominant response is an increase in BP, owing to an increase in peripheral vasoconstriction.

Prospectus for the Future

Recent years have witnessed an explosion in the growth of basic knowledge governing normal heart development and function of the circulatory system. New insights about the molecular switches and factors that promote the formation of heart chambers and blood vessels are unraveling the genetic basis for unusual causes of congenital heart disease. Similarly, the recent discovery of specific growth factors and signaling pathways that guide vascular trajectory and ensure vascular stability offer new opportunities to rethink future strategies for promoting cardiac and vascular regeneration and repair. With increasing refinement in this basic knowledge, future milestones appear on the horizon for diagnosis, early treatment, and even prevention of cardiovascular diseases.

References

Berne RM, Levy MN: Physiology, Updated Edition, 5th ed., with Student Consult Access. Part IV: The Cardiovascular System. St Louis, Elsevier, 2004.

Guyton AC, Hall JE: Textbook of Medical Physiology. St. Louis, Elsevier, 2005.

Chapter 4

Evaluation of the Patient with Cardiovascular Disease

Sheldon E. Litwin and Ivor J. Benjamin

History

As with diseases of most organ systems, the ability of the physician to diagnose diseases of the cardiovascular system is in large part dependent on eliciting and interpreting the patient's clinical history. A thorough history can enable the physician to identify a patient's symptoms as characteristic of a specific cardiovascular disorder or to suggest that symptoms are unlikely to be caused by cardiovascular disease. In addition, a complete history will reveal the presence of other systemic diseases that may have cardiovascular manifestations, identify existing risk factors that may be modified to prevent the future development of cardiovascular disease (see Chapter 9), enable the selection of appropriate further diagnostic testing (see Chapter 5), and allow the assessment of functional capacity and extent of cardiovascular disability. The patient should be asked about prior medical conditions, including childhood illnesses (e.g., rheumatic fever), as well as intravenous drug use, which may lead to the development of valvular heart disease. Several cardiovascular disorders are inherited (e.g., hypertrophic cardiomyopathy, Marfan syndrome, long QT syndrome), and a thorough family history may bring this potential to the examiner's attention.

The classic symptoms of cardiac disease include precordial discomfort or pain, dyspnea, palpitations, syncope or presyncope, and edema. Although characteristic of heart disease, these symptoms are nonspecific and may also occur as a result of diseases of other organ systems (e.g., musculoskeletal, pulmonary, renal, gastrointestinal). Furthermore, some patients with established cardiovascular disease may be asymptomatic or have atypical symptoms.

Chest pain is a frequent symptom and may be a manifestation of cardiovascular or noncardiovascular disease (Tables 4-1 and 4-2). Full characterization of the pain with regard to quality, quantity, frequency, location, duration, radiation, aggravating or alleviating factors, and associated symptoms may help distinguish among various causes. Reversible myocardial ischemia caused by obstructive coronary artery disease commonly results in episodic chest pain or discomfort during exertion or stress (angina pectoris). Patients frequently deny having pain and, instead, describe a discomfort in their chest. Sometimes they will refer to the discomfort as a *squeezing, tightening, pressing,* or *burning* sensation or as a *heavy weight* on their chest, and they will sometimes clench their fist over their chest while describing the discomfort (Levine sign). Anginal discomfort is classically located substernally or over the left chest. It frequently radiates to the epigastrium, neck, jaw, or back and down the ulnar aspect of the left arm. Radiation to the right chest or arm is less common, whereas radiation above the jaw or below the epigastrium is not typical of cardiac disease. Angina is usually brought on by either physical or emotional stress, is mild to moderate in intensity, lasts 2 to 10 minutes, and resolves with rest or sublingual administration of nitroglycerin. It may occur more frequently in the morning, in cold weather, after a large meal, or after exposure to environmental factors, including cigarette smoke, and is frequently accompanied by other symptoms, such as dyspnea, diaphoresis, nausea, palpitations, or lightheadedness. Patients frequently report a stable pattern of angina that is predictably reproducible with a given amount of exertion. Unstable angina occurs when a patient reports a significant increase in the frequency or severity of angina or when angina occurs with progressively decreasing exertion or at rest. When anginal-type pain occurs mainly at rest, it may be of a noncardiac origin, or it may reflect true cardiac ischemia resulting from coronary spasm (Prinzmetal or variant angina). The pain of an acute myocardial infarction may be similar

Table 4-1 Cardiovascular Causes of Chest Pain

Condition	Location	Quality	Duration	Aggravating or Alleviating Factors	Associated Symptoms or Signs
Angina	Retrosternal region: radiates to or occasionally isolated to neck, jaw, shoulders, arms (usually left), or epigastrium	Pressure, squeezing, tightness, heaviness, burning, indigestion	<2-10 min	Precipitated by exertion, cold weather, or emotional stress; relieved by rest or nitroglycerin; variant (Prinzmetal) angina may be unrelated to exertion, often early in the morning	Dyspnea; S_3, S_4, or murmur of papillary dysfunction during pain
Myocardial infarction	Same as angina	Same as angina, although more severe	Variable; usually longer than 30 min	Unrelieved by rest or nitroglycerin	Dyspnea, nausea, vomiting, weakness, diaphoresis
Pericarditis	Left of the sternum; may radiate to neck or left shoulder, often more localized than pain of myocardial ischemia	Sharp, stabbing, knifelike	Lasts many hours to days; may wax and wane	Aggravated by deep breathing, rotating chest, or supine position; relieved by sitting up and leaning forward	Pericardial friction rub
Aortic dissection	Anterior chest; may radiate to back, interscapular region	Excruciating, tearing, knifelike	Sudden onset, unrelenting	Usually occurs in setting of hypertension or predisposition, such as Marfan syndrome	Murmur of aortic insufficiency; pulse or blood pressure asymmetry; neurologic deficit

to angina, although the former is usually more severe and prolonged (>30 minutes).

The pain of acute pericarditis is usually sharper than anginal pain, is located to the left of the sternum, and may radiate to the neck or left shoulder. In contrast to angina, the pain may last hours, typically worsens with inspiration, and improves when the patient sits up and leans forward; it may be associated with a pericardial friction rub. Acute aortic dissection produces severe, sharp, *tearing* pain that radiates to the back and may be associated with asymmetrical pulses and a murmur of aortic insufficiency. Pulmonary emboli may produce the sudden onset of sharp chest pain that is worse on inspiration, is associated with shortness of breath, and may have an associated pleural friction rub, especially if a pulmonary infarction is present. A multitude of noncardiac conditions may also produce chest pain (see Table 4-2). The clinical history and physical examination findings will often help distinguish these causes from ischemic chest pain.

Dyspnea, an uncomfortable, heightened awareness of breathing, is commonly a symptom of cardiac disease. Patients with decreased left ventricular function may exhibit significant abnormalities of the aortic or mitral valves or decreased myocardial compliance (i.e., left ventricular hypertrophy, acute ischemia), left ventricular diastolic, or left atrial pressure increases transmitted through the pulmonary veins to the pulmonary capillary system, producing vascular congestion. This congestion results in exudation of fluid into the alveolar space and impairs gas exchange across the alveolar-capillary membrane, producing the subjective

sensation of dyspnea. Dyspnea frequently occurs on exertion; however, in patients with severe cardiac disease, it may be present at rest. Patients with heart failure commonly sleep on two or more pillows because the augmented venous return that occurs on assuming the recumbent position produces an increase in dyspnea (orthopnea). In addition, these patients report awakening 2 to 4 hours after the onset of sleep with dyspnea (paroxysmal nocturnal dyspnea), which is likely caused by the central redistribution of peripheral edema in the supine position.

Dyspnea may be associated with diseases of the lungs or chest wall and is also seen in anemia, obesity, deconditioning, and anxiety disorders. In addition, the sudden onset of dyspnea, with or without chest pain, may be present with pulmonary emboli. It is frequently difficult to distinguish cardiac from pulmonary causes of dyspnea by history alone because both may produce resting or exertional dyspnea, orthopnea, or cough. Wheezing and hemoptysis are classically results of pulmonary disease, although they are also frequently present in the patient with pulmonary edema resulting from left ventricular dysfunction or mitral stenosis. True paroxysmal nocturnal dyspnea is, however, more specific for cardiac disease. In patients with coronary artery disease, dyspnea may be an *anginal equivalent*; that is, the dyspnea is the result of ischemia and occurs in a pattern consistent with angina but in the absence of chest discomfort.

Palpitation refers to the subjective sensation of the heart beating. Patients may describe a *fluttering* or *pounding* in the chest or a feeling that their heart *races* or *skips a beat*. Some

Table 4-2 Noncardiac Causes of Chest Pain

Condition	Location	Quality	Duration	Aggravating or Alleviating Factors	Associated Symptoms or Signs
Pulmonary embolism (chest pain often not present)	Substernal or over region of pulmonary infarction	Pleuritic (with pulmonary infarction) or angina-like	Sudden onset (minutes to hours)	Aggravated by deep breathing	Dyspnea, tachypnea, tachycardia; hypotension, signs of acute right ventricular heart failure, and pulmonary hypertension with large emboli; pleural rub; hemoptysis with pulmonary infarction
Pulmonary hypertension	Substernal	Pressure; oppressive	—	Aggravated by effort	Pain usually associated with dyspnea; signs of pulmonary hypertension
Pneumonia with pleurisy	Located over involved area	Pleuritic	—	Aggravated by breathing	Dyspnea, cough, fever, bronchial breath sounds, rhonchi, egophony, dullness to percussion, occasional pleural rub
Spontaneous pneumothorax	Unilateral	Sharp, well localized	Sudden onset; lasts many hours	Aggravated by breathing	Dyspnea; hyperresonance and decreased breath and voice sounds over involved lung
Musculoskeletal disorders	Variable	Aching, well localized	Variable	Aggravated by movement; history of exertion or injury	Tender to palpation or with light pressure
Herpes zoster	Dermatomal distribution	Sharp, burning	Prolonged	None	Vesicular rash appears in area of discomfort
Esophageal reflux	Substernal or epigastric; may radiate to neck	Burning, visceral discomfort	10-60 min	Aggravated by large meal, postprandial recumbency; relief with antacid	Water brash
Peptic ulcer	Epigastric, substernal	Visceral burning, aching	Prolonged	Relief with food, antacid	—
Gallbladder disease	Right upper quadrant; epigastric	Visceral	Prolonged	Spontaneous or following meals	Right upper quadrant tenderness may be present
Anxiety states	Often localized over precordium	Variable; location often moves from place to place	Varies; often fleeting	Situational	Sighing respirations; often chest wall tenderness

people feel post-extrasystolic beats as a painful or uncomfortable sensation. Common arrhythmic causes of palpitations include premature atrial or ventricular contractions, supraventricular tachycardia, ventricular tachycardia, and sinus tachycardia. Occasionally, patients report palpitations even when no rhythm disturbance is noted during monitoring, as occurs commonly in patients with anxiety disorders. The pattern of palpitations, especially when correlated to the pulse, may help narrow the differential diagnosis: rapid, regular palpitations are noted with supraventricular tachycardia or ventricular tachycardia; rapid, irregular palpita-

tions are noted with atrial fibrillation; and *skipped beats* are noted with premature atrial or ventricular contractions.

Syncope is the transient loss of consciousness resulting from inadequate cerebral blood flow and may be the result of a variety of cardiovascular diseases (see Chapter 10). True syncope must be distinguished from primary neurologic causes of loss of consciousness (i.e., seizures) and metabolic causes of loss of consciousness (e.g., hypoglycemia, hyperventilation). Cardiac syncope occurs after an abrupt decrease in cardiac output, as may occur with acute myocardial ischemia, valvular heart disease (aortic or mitral stenosis), hypertrophic obstructive cardiomyopathy, left atrial tumors, tachyarrhythmias (ventricular, or less commonly supraventricular, tachycardias), or bradyarrhythmias (e.g., sinus arrest, atrioventricular block, Stokes-Adams attacks). Reflex vasodilation or bradycardia may also result in syncope (vasovagal syncope, carotid sinus syncope, micturition syncope, cough syncope, or neurocardiogenic syncope), as may acute pulmonary embolism and hypovolemia. Because global, or at the very least bilateral, cortical ischemia is required to produce syncope, it rarely occurs as a result of unilateral carotid artery disease. However, syncope is occasionally the result of bilateral carotid artery disease and can also occur when disease of the vertebrobasilar system results in brainstem ischemia. In up to 50% of patients, the cause of a syncopal episode cannot be determined; however, in the cases in which a cause is determined, the most important factor in establishing the diagnosis is obtaining an accurate history of the event.

Edema is a nonspecific symptom that commonly accompanies cardiac disease as well as renal disease (e.g., nephrotic syndrome), hepatic disease (e.g., cirrhosis), and local venous abnormalities (e.g., thrombophlebitis, chronic venous stasis). When edema occurs as a result of cardiac disease, it reflects an increase in venous pressure. This increased pressure alters the balance between the venous hydrostatic and oncotic forces, resulting in extravasation of fluid into the extravascular space. When this process occurs as a result of elevated left-sided heart pressure, pulmonary edema results, whereas elevated right-sided heart pressure results in peripheral edema. Characteristically, the peripheral edema of heart failure is *pitting;* that is, an indentation is left in the skin after pressure is applied to the edematous region. The edema is exacerbated by long periods of standing, is worse in the evening, improves after lying down, and may first be noted when a patient has difficulty in fitting into his or her shoes. The edema may shift to the sacral region after a patient lies down for several hours. When visible edema is noted, it is usually preceded by a moderate weight gain (i.e., 5 to 10 lb), indicative of volume retention. As heart failure progresses, the edema may extend to the thighs and involve the genitalia and abdominal wall, and fluid may collect in the abdominal (ascites) or thoracic (pleural effusion) cavities. Anasarca with ascites should raise suspicion for constrictive pericarditis because this disease may progress very slowly and insidiously.

Cyanosis is an abnormal bluish discoloration of the skin resulting from an increase in the level of reduced hemoglobin in the blood and, in general, reflects an arterial oxygen saturation of 85% or less (normal arterial oxygen saturation, ≥95%). Central cyanosis exhibits as cyanosis of the lips or trunk and often reflects right-to-left shunting of blood caused by structural cardiac abnormalities (e.g., atrial or ventricular septal defects) or pulmonary parenchymal or vascular disease (e.g., chronic obstructive pulmonary disease, pulmonary embolism, pulmonary arteriovenous fistula). Peripheral cyanosis may occur because of systemic vasoconstriction in the setting of poor cardiac output or may be a localized phenomenon resulting from venous or arterial occlusive or vasospastic disease (e.g., venous or arterial thrombosis, arterial embolic disease, Raynaud disease). When cyanosis occurs in childhood, it usually reflects congenital heart disease with right-to-left shunting of blood.

Myriad *other symptoms*, many of them nonspecific, may occur with cardiac disease. Fatigue frequently occurs in the setting of poor cardiac output or may occur secondary to the medical therapy of cardiac disease from overdiuresis, aggressive blood pressure lowering, or use of β-blocking agents. Nausea and vomiting frequently occur during an acute myocardial infarction and may also reflect intestinal edema in the setting of right ventricular heart failure. Anorexia and cachexia may occur in severe heart failure. Positional fluid shifts may result in polyuria and nocturia in patients with edema. In addition, epistaxis, hoarseness, hiccups, fever, and chills may reflect underlying cardiovascular disease.

Many patients with significant cardiac disease are asymptomatic. Patients with coronary artery disease frequently have periods of asymptomatic ischemia that can be documented with ambulatory electrocardiographic monitoring. Furthermore, nearly one third of patients who suffer an acute myocardial infarction are unaware of the event. This silent ischemia appears to be more common in older adults and in patients with diabetes. Patients may also be asymptomatic despite having severely depressed ventricular function; this usually bespeaks a chronic, slowly progressive process. Reduced exercise capacity may only be seen during provocative testing. Similarly, recent findings show that a high percentage of episodes of atrial fibrillation are unrecognized by patients.

Assessment of Functional Capacity

In patients with cardiac disorders, the ability or inability to perform various activities (functional status) plays an important role in determining their extent of disability, deciding when to institute various therapies or interventions, and assessing their response to therapy as well as determining their overall prognosis. The New York Heart Association Functional Classification is a standardized method for the assessment of functional status (Table 4-3) and relates functional capacity to the presence or absence of cardiac symptoms during the performance of *usual activities*. The

Table 4-3 **Classification of Functional Status**		
Class I	Uncompromised	Ordinary activity does not cause symptoms.* Symptoms only occur with strenuous or prolonged activity.
Class II	Slightly compromised	Ordinary physical activity results in symptoms; no symptoms at rest.
Class III	Moderately compromised	Less than ordinary activity results in symptoms; no symptoms at rest.
Class IV	Severely compromised	Any activity results in symptoms; symptoms may be present at rest.

*Symptoms refer to undue fatigue, dyspnea, palpitations, or angina in the New York Heart Association classification and refer specifically to angina in the Canadian Cardiovascular Society classification.

Canadian Cardiovascular Society has provided a similar classification of functional status specifically in patients with angina pectoris. These tools are useful in that they allow a patient's symptoms to be classified and then compared with their symptoms at a different point in time.

Physical Examination

EXAMINATION OF THE JUGULAR VENOUS PULSATIONS

The examination of the neck veins allows for estimation of the right atrial pressure and for identification of the venous waveforms. The right internal jugular vein is used for this examination because it more accurately reflects right atrial pressure than the external jugular or left jugular vein. With the patient lying at a 45-degree angle (higher in patients with elevated venous pressure, lower in patients with low venous pressure) with the head turned to the left, the vertical distance from the sternal angle (angle of Louis) to the top of the venous pulsation can be determined. Because the right atrium lies about 5 cm vertically below the sternal angle, distention of the internal jugular vein 4 cm above the sternal angle reflects a right atrial pressure of 9 cm H_2O. The right atrial pressure is normally 5 to 9 cm H_2O and is increased with congestive heart failure, tricuspid insufficiency or stenosis, and restrictive or constrictive heart disease. With inspiration, negative intrathoracic pressure develops, venous blood drains into the thorax, and the normal venous pressure falls; the opposite is true with expiration. This pattern is reversed (Kussmaul sign) in the setting of right ventricular heart failure, constrictive pericarditis, or restrictive myocardial disease. With right ventricular heart failure, the elevated venous pressure results in passive congestion of the liver. Pressure applied over the liver for 1 to 3 minutes in this setting results in an increase in the jugular venous pressure (hepatojugular reflux).

The normal waveforms of the venous pulsation consist of the a, c, and v waves and the x and y descents; these waveforms are shown in Figure 4-1A and reflect events in the right side of the heart. The a wave results from atrial contraction. Subsequent atrial relaxation results in a decrease in the right atrial pressure, which is seen as the x descent. This descent is interrupted by the c wave, generated by the bulging of the tricuspid valve cusps into the right atrium during ventricular systole. As the atrial pressure increases owing to venous return, the v wave is generated. This wave is normally smaller than the a wave and is followed by the y descent as the tricuspid valve opens and blood flows from the right atrium to the right ventricle during diastole.

Abnormalities of the venous waveforms reflect underlying structural, functional, or electrical abnormalities of the heart (see Fig. 4-1B through G). The a wave increases in any condition in which greater resistance to right atrial emptying occurs (e.g., tricuspid stenosis, right ventricular hypertrophy or failure, pulmonary hypertension). *Cannon a waves* are seen when the atrium contracts against a closed tricuspid valve, as occurs with complete heart block, with junctional or ventricular rhythms, and occasionally with ventricular pacemakers. The a wave is absent in atrial fibrillation. In tricuspid regurgitation, the v wave is prominent and may merge with the c wave (c-v wave), thus diminishing or eliminating the x descent altogether. The y descent is attenuated in tricuspid stenosis, owing to the impaired atrial emptying. In pericardial constriction and restrictive cardiomyopathy, as well as in right ventricular infarction, the y descent becomes rapid and deep, and the x descent may also become prominent (w waveform). In pericardial tamponade, the x descent is prominent, but the y descent is diminished or absent.

EXAMINATION OF THE ARTERIAL PULSE

The arterial blood pressure can be measured with the use of a sphygmomanometer. The cuff is applied to the upper arm, rapidly inflated to 30 mm Hg above the anticipated systolic pressure, and then slowly deflated (= 3 mm Hg/sec) while listening for the sounds produced by blood entering the previously occluded brachial artery (Korotkoff sounds). The pressure at which the first sound is heard (usually a clear, tapping sound) represents the systolic pressure. Diastolic pressure occurs at the point at which the Korotkoff sounds disappear. Normally, the pressure in both arms is the same (about 120/70 mm Hg), and the systolic pressure in the legs is 10 to 20 mm Hg higher. Asymmetrical arm pressures can result from atherosclerotic disease of the aorta, aortic dissection, and stenosis of the innominate or subclavian arteries. Coarctation of the aorta and severe atherosclerotic disease of the aorta or the femoral or iliac arteries can result in a lower blood pressure in the legs than in the arms. Aortic insufficiency is frequently associated with a leg pressure more than 20 mm Hg higher than the arm pressure (Hill sign). Use of a cuff that is too small for a patient's arm will result in erroneously high pressure measurements. Similarly, a cuff that is too large results in erroneously low measurements.

The arterial examination should include assessments of the carotid, radial, brachial, femoral, popliteal, posterior tibial, and dorsalis pedis pulses, although the carotid artery pulse most accurately reflects the central aortic pulse. The rhythm, strength, contour, and symmetry of the pulses should be noted. The normal arterial pulse (Fig. 4-2A) rises rapidly to a peak in early systole, plateaus, and then falls. The descending pressure wave is interrupted by the dicrotic notch, related to aortic valve closure. This normal pattern is altered in a variety of cardiovascular disease states (see Fig. 4-2B *through F*). The amplitude of the pulse increases in aortic insufficiency, anemia, pregnancy, and thyrotoxicosis and decreases in conditions such as hypovolemia, tachycardia, left ventricular failure, and severe mitral stenosis. Aortic insufficiency results in a *bounding* pulse (Corrigan pulse or water-hammer pulse), owing to an increased pulse pressure (the difference between systolic and diastolic pressure), and is accompanied by a multitude of abnormalities in the peripheral pulses that reflect this increased pulse pressure. Aortic stenosis characteristically results in an attenuated carotid pulse with a delayed upstroke (pulsus parvus et tardus) and may be associated with a palpable thrill over the aortic area (the carotid shudder). A bisferious pulse is commonly felt in the presence of pure aortic regurgitation and is characterized by two systolic peaks. The first peak is the percussion wave, resulting from the rapid ejection of a large volume of blood early in systole; the second peak is the tidal

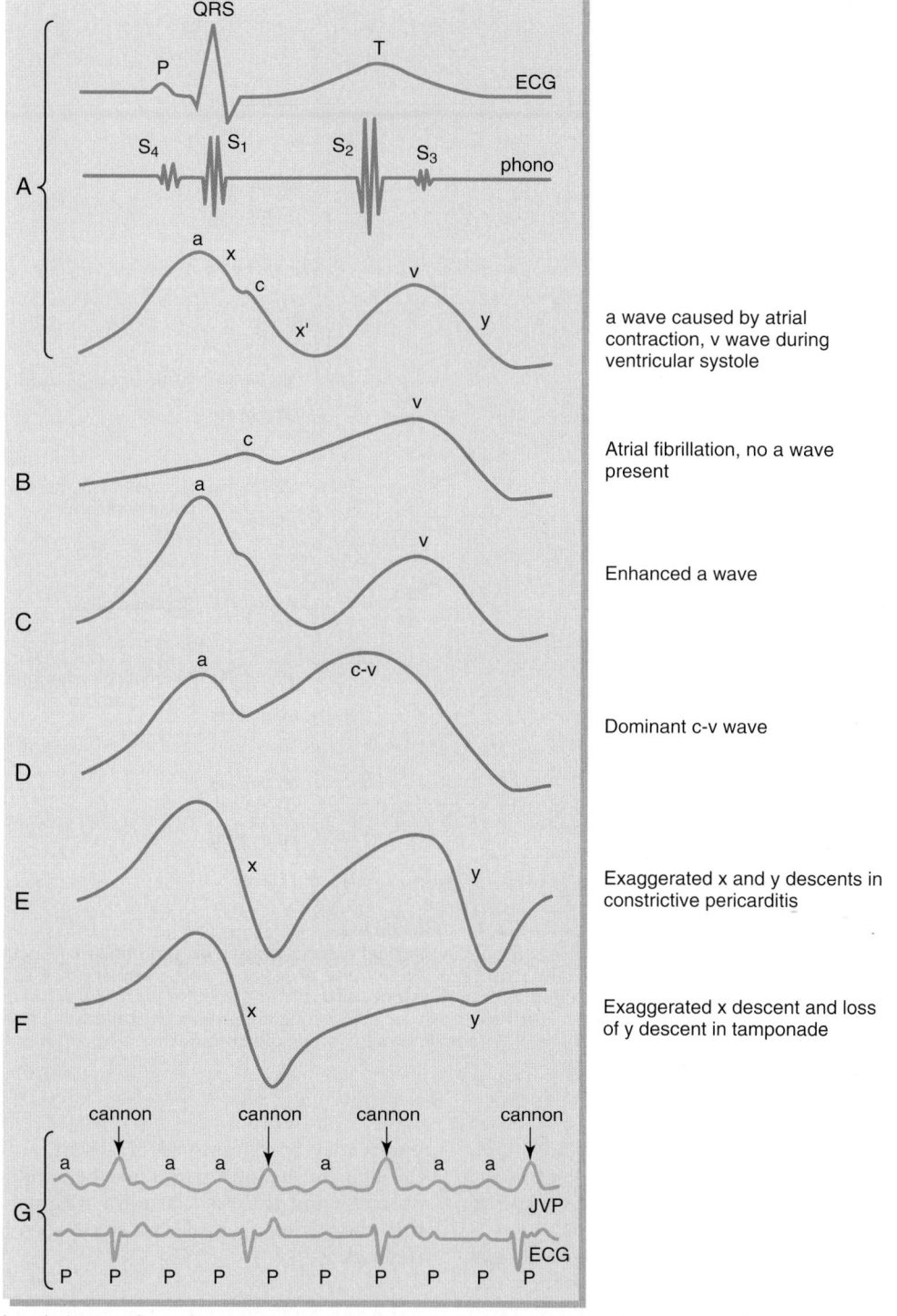

Figure 4-1 Normal and abnormal jugular venous pulse tracings. **A,** Normal jugular pulse tracing with simultaneous electrocardiogram (ECG) and phonocardiogram. **B,** Loss of the a wave in atrial fibrillation. **C,** Large a wave in tricuspid stenosis. **D,** Large c-v wave in tricuspid regurgitation. **E,** Prominent x and y descents in constrictive pericarditis. **F,** Prominent x descent and diminutive y descent in pericardial tamponade. **G,** Jugular venous pulse (JVP) tracing and simultaneous ECG during complete heart block demonstrating cannon a waves occurring when the atrium contracts against a closed tricuspid valve during ventricular systole.

wave, a reflected wave from the periphery. This bifid pulse may also be noted in hypertrophic cardiomyopathy in which the initial rapid upstroke of the pulse is cut short by the development of a left ventricular outflow tract obstruction, resulting in a fall in the pulse. The reflected wave again produces the second impulse. In severe left ventricular dysfunc-

tion, the intensity of the pulse may alternate from beat to beat (*pulsus alternans*), and in atrial fibrillation, the pulse intensity is variable. With inspiration, negative intrathoracic pressure is transmitted to the aorta, and the systolic pressure normally decreases by up to 10 mm Hg. Pulsus paradoxus is an exaggeration of this normal inspiratory fall in systolic

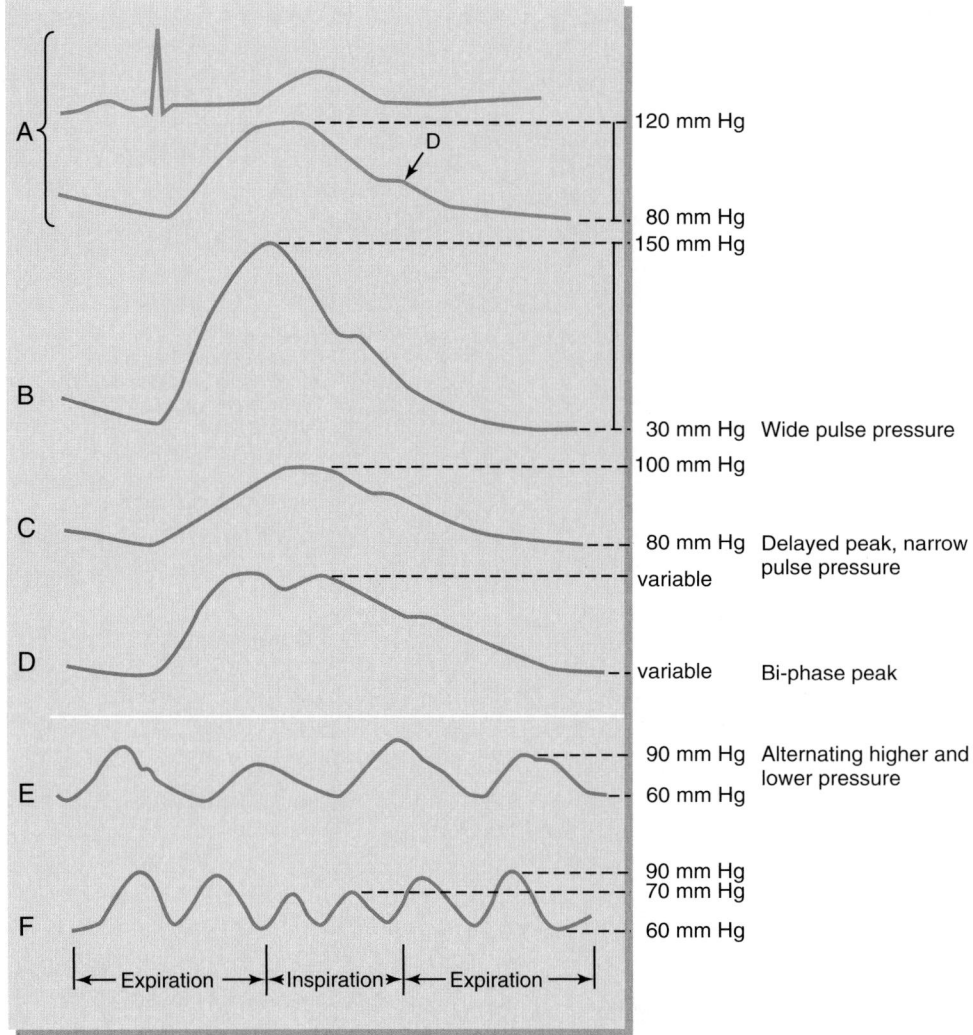

Figure 4-2 Normal and abnormal carotid arterial pulse contours. **A,** Normal arterial pulse with simultaneous electrocardiogram (ECG). The dicrotic wave (D) occurs just after aortic valve closure. **B,** Wide pulse pressure in aortic insufficiency. **C,** Pulsus parvus et tardus (small amplitude with a slow upstroke) associated with aortic stenosis. **D,** Bisferious pulse with two systolic peaks, typical of hypertrophic obstructive cardiomyopathy or aortic insufficiency, especially if concomitant aortic stenosis is present. **E,** Pulsus alternans, characteristic of severe left ventricular failure. **F,** Paradoxic pulse (systolic pressure decrease of >10 mm Hg with inspiration), most characteristic of cardiac tamponade.

pressure and is characteristically seen with pericardial tamponade, although it may also occur as a result of severe obstructive lung disease, constrictive pericarditis, hypovolemic shock, and pregnancy.

Atherosclerotic disease of the peripheral vascular system frequently accompanies coronary atherosclerosis; therefore, the presence of peripheral vascular disease warrants a search for symptoms or signs of coronary artery disease and vice versa. When atherosclerosis occurs in a peripheral artery to the lower extremity and impairs blood flow distally, the patient may complain of intermittent cramping in the buttocks, thigh, calf, or foot (claudication). Severe peripheral vascular disease may result in digital ischemia or necrosis, without or with associated erectile dysfunction (Leriche syndrome). The peripheral pulses should be palpated and the abdominal aorta assessed for enlargement in all cardiac patients; a pulsatile, expansile, periumbilical mass suggests the presence of an abdominal aortic aneurysm. With significant stenosis of the peripheral vasculature, the distal

pulses may be diminished or absent, and the blood flow through the stenotic artery may be audible (a *bruit*). With normal aging, the elastic arteries lose their compliance, and this change in physical property may obscure abnormal findings.

EXAMINATION OF THE PRECORDIUM

Inspection and palpation of the precordium may yield valuable clues as to the existence of cardiac disease. Chest wall abnormalities should be noted, such as pectus excavatum, which may be associated with Marfan syndrome or mitral valve prolapse; pectus carinatum, which may be associated with Marfan syndrome; and kyphoscoliosis, which is occasionally a cause of secondary pulmonary hypertension and right ventricular heart failure. The presence of visible pulsations in the aortic (second right intercostal space and suprasternal notch), pulmonic (third left intercostal space), right ventricular (left parasternal region), and left ventricular (fourth to fifth intercostal space and left mid-clavicular line) regions should be noted and will help direct the palpation of the heart. Retraction of the left parasternal area may be seen with severe left ventricular hypertrophy, and systolic retraction of the chest wall at the cardiac apex or left axilla (Broadbent sign) is characteristic of constrictive pericarditis.

Precordial palpation is best performed with the patient supine or in the left lateral position, with the examiner standing to the patient's right side. In this position, firm placement of the examiner's right hand over the patient's lower left chest wall places the fingertips over the region of the cardiac apex and the palm over the region of the right ventricle. The normal cardiac apical impulse is a brief, discrete impulse (about 1 cm) located in the fourth to fifth intercostal space in the left mid-clavicular line generated as the left ventricle strikes the chest wall during early systole. In a patient with a structurally normal heart, the apex is the point of maximal impulse (PMI) of the heart against the chest wall. Enlargement of the left ventricle results in lateral displacement of the apical impulse, whereas chronic obstructive pulmonary disease may result in inferior displacement of the PMI. Volume overload states, such as aortic insufficiency and mitral regurgitation, produce ventricular enlargement primarily from dilation and result in a hyperdynamic apical impulse; that is, the impulse is brisk and increased in amplitude. Pressure overload states, such as aortic stenosis and long-standing hypertension, produce ventricular enlargement primarily from hypertrophy. In this setting, the apical impulse is sustained, and atrial contraction is frequently detected (a palpable S_4). Hypertrophic cardiomyopathy characteristically produces a double or triple apical impulse. Left ventricular aneurysms produce an apical impulse that is larger than normal and dyskinetic.

The right ventricular impulse is not normally palpable. When an impulse is felt over the left parasternal region, it usually reflects right ventricular hypertrophy or dilation. Aortic aneurysms may be palpable (or visible) in the suprasternal notch or the second right intercostal space. Pulmonary hypertension may produce a palpable systolic impulse in the left third intercostal space and may also be associated with a palpable pulmonic component of the second heart sound (P_2). Harsh murmurs originating from valvular or congenital heart disease may be associated with palpable vibratory sensations (thrills), as can occur with aortic stenosis, hypertrophic cardiomyopathy, and ventricular septal defects.

Auscultation

TECHNIQUE

Auscultation of the heart should ideally be performed in a quiet room with the patient in a comfortable position and the chest fully exposed. Certain heart sounds are better heard with either the bell or diaphragm of the stethoscope. Low-frequency sounds are best heard with the bell applied to the chest wall with just enough pressure to form a seal. As more pressure is applied to the bell, low-frequency sounds are filtered out. High-frequency sounds are best heard with the diaphragm firmly applied to the chest wall. In a patient

with a normally situated heart, four major zones of cardiac auscultation are assessed. Aortic valvular events are best heard in the second right intercostal space. Pulmonary valvular events are best heard in the second left interspace. The fourth left interspace is ideal for auscultating tricuspid valvular events, and mitral valvular events are best heard at the cardiac apex or PMI. Because anatomic abnormalities, both congenital and acquired, can alter the location of the heart in the chest, the auscultatory areas may vary among patients. For instance, in patients with emphysema, the heart is shifted downward, and heart sounds may be best heard in the epigastrium. In dextrocardia, the heart lies in the right hemithorax, and the auscultatory regions are reversed. Additionally, auscultation in the axilla or supraclavicular areas or over the thoracic spine may be helpful in some settings, and having the patient lean forward, exhale, or perform various maneuvers may help accentuate particular heart sounds (Table 4-4).

NORMAL HEART SOUNDS

The two major heart sounds heard during auscultation are termed S_1 and S_2. These heart sounds are high-pitched sounds originating from valve closure (**Web Sounds, normal**). S_1 occurs at the onset of ventricular systole and corresponds to closure of the atrioventricular valves. It is usually perceived as a single sound, although occasionally its two components, M_1 and T_1, corresponding to closure of the mitral and tricuspid valves, respectively, can be heard. M_1 occurs earlier, is the louder of the two components, and is best heard at the cardiac apex. T_1 is somewhat softer and heard at the left lower sternal border. The second heart sound results from closure of the semilunar valves. The two components, A_2 and P_2, originating from aortic and pulmonic valve closure, respectively, can be easily distinguished. A_2 is usually louder than P_2 and is best heard at the right upper sternal border. P_2 is loudest over the second left intercostal space. During expiration, the normal S_2 is perceived as a single event. However, during inspiration, the augmented venous return to the right side of the heart and the increased capacitance of the pulmonary vascular bed result in a delay in pulmonic valve closure. In addition, the slightly decreased venous return to the left ventricle results in slightly earlier aortic valve closure. Thus, *physiologic splitting* of the second heart sound, with A_2 preceding P_2 during inspiration, is a normal respiratory event.

Occasionally, additional heart sounds may be heard in normal individuals. A third heart sound (see later discussion) can be heard in normal children and young adults, in whom it is referred to as a *physiologic S_3*; it is rarely heard after the age of 40 years in healthy individuals (**Web Sounds, S_3**).

A fourth heart sound (S_4) is generated by forceful atrial contraction and is rarely audible in normal young individuals but is fairly common in older individuals (**Web Sounds, S_4**).

A murmur is an auditory vibration usually generated either by abnormally increased flow across a normal valve or by normal flow across an abnormal valve or structure. *Innocent* murmurs are always systolic murmurs, are usually soft and brief, and are by definition not associated with abnormalities of the cardiovascular system. They arise from

Table 4-4 **Effects of Physiologic Maneuvers on Auscultatory Events**

Maneuver	Major Physiologic Effects	Useful Auscultatory Changes
Respiration	↑ Venous return with inspiration	↑ Right heart murmurs and gallops with inspiration; splitting of S_2 (see Fig. 4-3)
Valsalva (initial ↑ BP, phase I; followed by ↓ BP, phase II)	↓ BP, ↓ venous return, ↓ LV size (phase II)	↑ HCM ↓ AS, MR MVP click earlier in systole; murmur prolongs
Standing	↑ Venous return ↑ LV size	↑ HCM ↓ AS, MR MVP click earlier in systole; murmur prolongs
Squatting	↑ Venous return ↑ Systemic vascular resistance ↑ LV size	↑ AS, MR, AI ↓ HCM MVP click delayed; murmur shortens
Isometric exercise (e.g., handgrip)	↑ Arterial pressure ↑ Cardiac output	↑ Gallops ↑ MR, AI, MS ↓ AS, HCM
Post PVC or prolonged R-R interval	↑ Ventricular filling ↑ Contractility	↑ AS Little change in MR
Amyl nitrate	↓ Arterial pressure ↑ Cardiac output ↓ LV size	↑ HCM, AS, MS ↓ AI, MR, Austin Flint murmur MVP click earlier in systole; murmur prolongs
Phenylephrine	↑ Arterial pressure ↑ Cardiac output ↓ LV size	↑ MR, AI ↓ AS, HCM MVP click delayed; murmur shortens

↑, Increased intensity; ↓, decreased intensity; AI, aortic insufficiency; AS, aortic stenosis; BP, blood pressure; HCM, hypertrophic cardiomyopathy; LV, left ventricle; MR, mitral regurgitation; MS, mitral stenosis; MVP, mitral valve prolapse; PVC, premature ventricular contraction; R-R, interval between the R waves on an electrocardiogram.

flow across the normal aortic or pulmonic outflow tracts and are present in a large proportion of children and young adults. Murmurs associated with high-flow states (e.g., pregnancy, anemia, fever, thyrotoxicosis, exercise) are not considered innocent, although they are not usually associated with structural heart disease. These are termed *physiologic murmurs,* owing to their association with altered physiologic states. Diastolic murmurs are never *innocent* or *physiologic.*

ABNORMAL HEART SOUNDS

Abnormalities of S_1 and S_2 relate to abnormalities in their intensity (Table 4-5) or abnormalities in their respiratory splitting (Table 4-6). As noted, splitting of the S_1 is normal but not frequently noted. This splitting becomes more apparent with right bundle branch block or with Ebstein anomaly of the tricuspid valve, owing to delay in closure of the tricuspid valve in these conditions (**Web Sounds, Ebstein**). The intensity of S_1 is determined in part by the opening state of the atrioventricular valves at the onset of ventricular systole. If the valves are still widely open, as may occur with tachycardia or a short P-R interval, S_1 will be accentuated. Conversely, in the presence of a long P-R interval, the mitral valve drifts toward a closed position before the onset of ventricular systole, and the subsequent S_1 is soft. The intensity of S_1 may vary in the presence of Mobitz type I heart block, atrioventricular dissociation, and atrial fibrillation when the relationship between atrial and ventricular systole varies. In mitral stenosis with a pliable valve, the persistent pressure gradient at the end of diastole keeps the mitral valve leaflets relatively open and results in a loud S_1 at the onset of systole. In severe mitral stenosis, when the mitral valve is heavily calcified and has decreased leaflet excursion, S_1 becomes faint or absent (Figs. 4-3 and 4-4).

S_2 may be loud in systemic hypertension, owing to accentuated aortic valve closure (loud A_2), or in pulmonary hypertension, owing to accentuated pulmonic valve closure (loud P_2). When the aortic or pulmonary valves are stenotic, the force of valve closure is decreased, thus A_1 and P_2 become soft or inaudible. In this setting, S_2 may appear to be single; in the setting of aortic stenosis, prolonged left ventricular ejection narrows the normal splitting of S_2; and with severe aortic stenosis, S_2 may become absent altogether as prolonged ejection and its accompanying murmur obscure P_2. Wide splitting of the S_2 with normal respiratory variation occurs when either pulmonic valve closure is delayed (e.g., right bundle branch block, pulmonic stenosis) or aortic valve closure occurs earlier owing to more rapid ejection of left ventricular volume (e.g., mitral regurgitation, ventricular septal defect). Fixed splitting of S_2 without respiratory variation is characteristic of atrial septal defects and also occurs with right ventricular failure (**Web Sounds, ASD**). Paradoxic splitting of S_2 is a reversal of the usual closure sequence of the aortic and pulmonic valves (i.e., P_2 precedes A_2). In this setting, a single S_2 with inspiration and splitting of S_2 with expiration can be heard. This circumstance occurs most commonly when delay occurs in closure of the aortic valve resulting from either delay in electrical conduction to

Table 4-5 Abnormal Intensity of Heart Sounds

	S₁	A₂	P₂
Loud	Short PR interval Mitral stenosis with pliable valve	Systemic hypertension Aortic dilation Coarctation of the aorta	Pulmonary hypertension Thin chest wall
Soft	Long PR interval Mitral regurgitation Poor left ventricular function Mitral stenosis with rigid valve Thick chest wall	Calcific aortic stenosis Aortic regurgitation	Valvular or subvalvular pulmonic stenosis
Varying	Atrial fibrillation Heart block	—	—

Table 4-6 Abnormal Splitting of S₂

Single S₂	Widely Split S₂ with Normal Respiratory Variation	Fixed Split S₂	Paradoxically Split S₂
—	Right bundle branch block	Atrial septal defect	Left bundle branch block
Pulmonic stenosis	Left ventricular pacing	Severe right ventricular dysfunction	Right ventricular pacing
Systemic hypertension	Pulmonic stenosis	—	Angina, myocardial infarction
Coronary artery disease	Pulmonary embolism	—	Aortic stenosis
Any condition that can lead to paradoxical splitting of S₂	Idiopathic dilation of the pulmonary artery	—	Hypertrophic cardiomyopathy Aortic regurgitation
	Mitral regurgitation		
	Ventricular septal defect		

the left ventricle (e.g., left bundle branch block) or prolonged mechanical contraction of the left ventricle (e.g., aortic stenosis, hypertrophic cardiomyopathy).

The third heart sound, S₃ (also called the *ventricular diastolic gallop*), is a low-pitched sound occurring shortly after A₂ in mid-diastole and heard best at the cardiac apex with the patient in the left lateral position. A pathologic S₃ is distinguished from a physiologic S₃ by age or the presence of underlying cardiac disease. It is frequently heard with ventricular systolic dysfunction from any cause and likely results either from blood entering the ventricle during the rapid filling phase of diastole or from the impact of the ventricle against the chest wall. Maneuvers that increase venous return accentuate S₃, and maneuvers that decrease venous return make the S₃ softer. An S₃ can also be heard in hyperdynamic states, where it likely results from rapid early diastolic filling. The left ventricular S₃ is best noticed at the cardiac apex, whereas the right ventricular S₃ is heard best at the left lower sternal border and increases in intensity with inspiration. The timing of the S₃ is similar to the sound generated by atrial tumors (*tumor plop*) and constrictive pericarditis (*pericardial knock*) and can also be confused with the *opening snap* of a stenotic mitral valve.

The fourth heart sound, S₄ (also called the *atrial diastolic gallop*), is best heard at the cardiac apex with the bell of the stethoscope. It is a low-pitched sound originating from the active ejection of blood from the atrium into a noncompliant ventricle and is therefore not present in the setting of atrial fibrillation. S₄ is commonly heard in patients with left ventricular hypertrophy from any cause (e.g., hypertension, aortic stenosis, hypertrophic cardiomyopathy) or acute myocardial ischemia and in hyperkinetic states. Frequently, the S₄ is also palpable at the cardiac apex. S₃ and S₄ are occasionally present in the same patient. In the presence of tachycardia or a prolonged PR interval, the S₃ and S₄ may merge to produce a summation gallop.

The opening of normal cardiac valves is not audible. However, abnormal valves may produce opening sounds. In the presence of a bicuspid aortic valve or in aortic stenosis with pliable valve leaflets, an *ejection sound* is audible as the leaflets open to their maximal extent. A similar ejection sound may originate from a stenotic pulmonic valve, and in this case, the ejection sound decreases in intensity with inspiration. These ejection sounds are high pitched, occur early in systole, and are frequently followed by the typical ejection murmur of aortic or pulmonic stenosis. Ejection sounds are also heard with systemic or pulmonary hypertension, the exact mechanism of which is not clear.

Ejection sounds heard in mid to late systole are referred to as systolic *clicks* and are most commonly associated with mitral valve prolapse. As the redundant mitral valve prolapses and reaches its maximal superior displacement, it produces a high-pitched click. Several clicks may be heard as various parts of the redundant valve prolapse (**Web Sounds, MVP**). Frequently, the click is followed by a mitral regurgitant murmur. Maneuvers that decrease venous return cause the clicks to occur earlier in systole and the murmur to become longer (see Table 4-4).

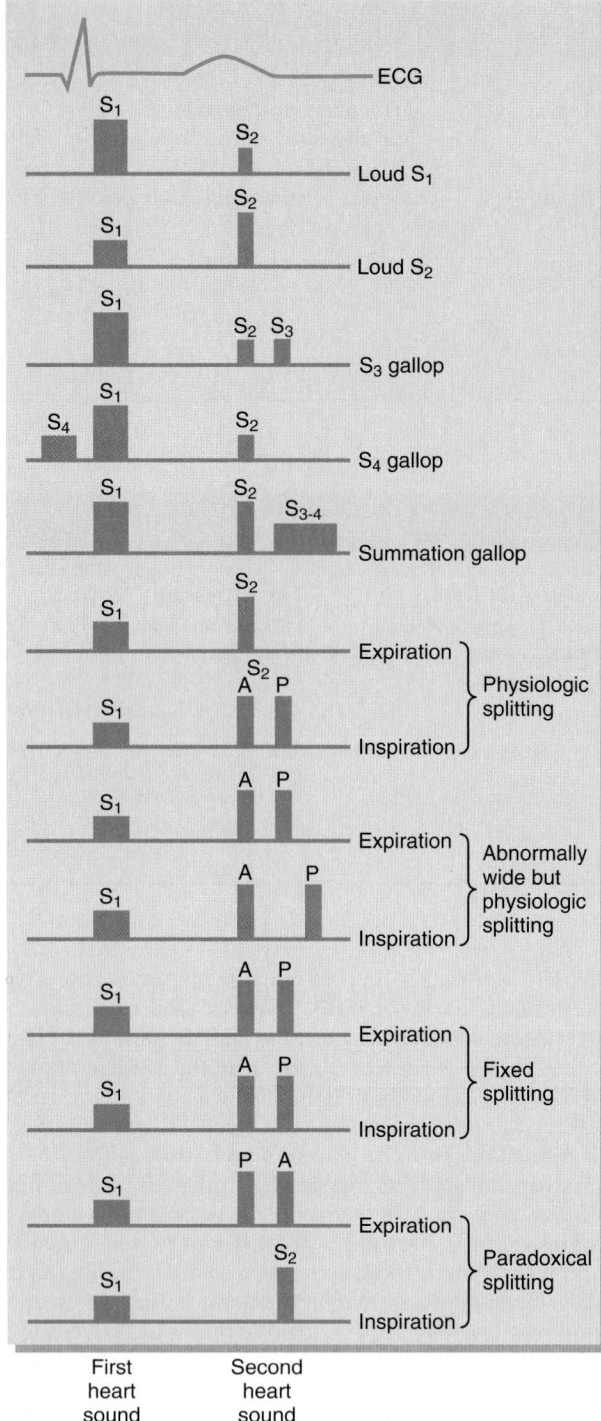

Figure 4-3 Abnormal heart sounds can be related to abnormal intensity, abnormal presence of a gallop rhythm, or abnormal splitting of S_2 with respiration. ECG, electrocardiogram.

The opening of abnormal mitral or tricuspid valves can also be heard in the presence of rheumatic valvular stenosis, when the sound is referred to as an *opening snap* (**Web Sounds, MS**). The *snap* is heard only if the valve leaflets are pliable and is generated as the leaflets abruptly dome during early diastole. The interval between S_2 and the opening snap is of diagnostic importance; as the stenosis worsens and the atrial pressure increases, the mitral valve

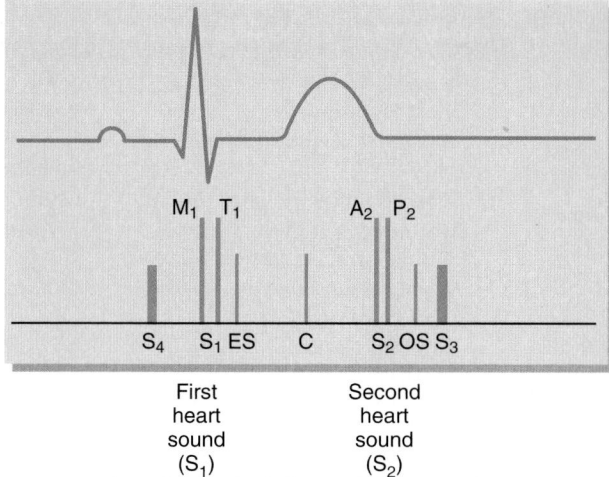

Figure 4-4 The relationship of extra heart sounds to the normal first (S_1) and second (S_2) heart sounds. S_1 is composed of the mitral (M_1) and tricuspid (T_1) closing sounds, although it is frequently perceived as a single sound. S_2 is composed of the aortic (A_2) and pulmonic (P_2) closing sounds, which are usually easily distinguished. A fourth heart sound (S_4) is soft and low pitched and precedes S_1. A pulmonic or aortic ejection sound (ES) occurs shortly after S_1. The systolic click (C) of mitral valve prolapse may be heard in mid or late systole. The opening snap (OS) of mitral stenosis is high pitched and occurs shortly after S_2. A tumor plop or pericardial knock occurs at the same time and can be confused with an OS or an S_3, which is lower in pitch and occurs slightly later.

Table 4-7	**Grading System for Intensity of Murmurs**
Grade 1	Barely audible murmur
Grade 2	Murmur of medium intensity
Grade 3	Loud murmur, no thrill
Grade 4	Loud murmur with thrill
Grade 5	Very loud murmur; stethoscope must be on the chest to hear it; may be heard posteriorly
Grade 6	Murmur audible with stethoscope off the chest

opens earlier in diastole, and the interval between the S_2 and the opening snap shortens.

MURMURS

As stated previously, murmurs are a series of auditory vibrations generated when either abnormal blood flow across a normal cardiac structure or normal flow across an abnormal cardiac structure results in turbulent flow. These sounds are longer than the individual heart sounds and can be described by their location, intensity, frequency (pitch), quality, duration, and timing in relation to systole or diastole. The intensity of a murmur is graded on a scale of 1 to 6 (Table 4-7). In general, murmurs of grade 4 or greater are associated with a palpable thrill. The loudness of a murmur does not necessarily correlate with the severity of the underlying abnormality. For instance, flow across a large atrial septal defect is essentially silent, whereas flow across a small ventricular

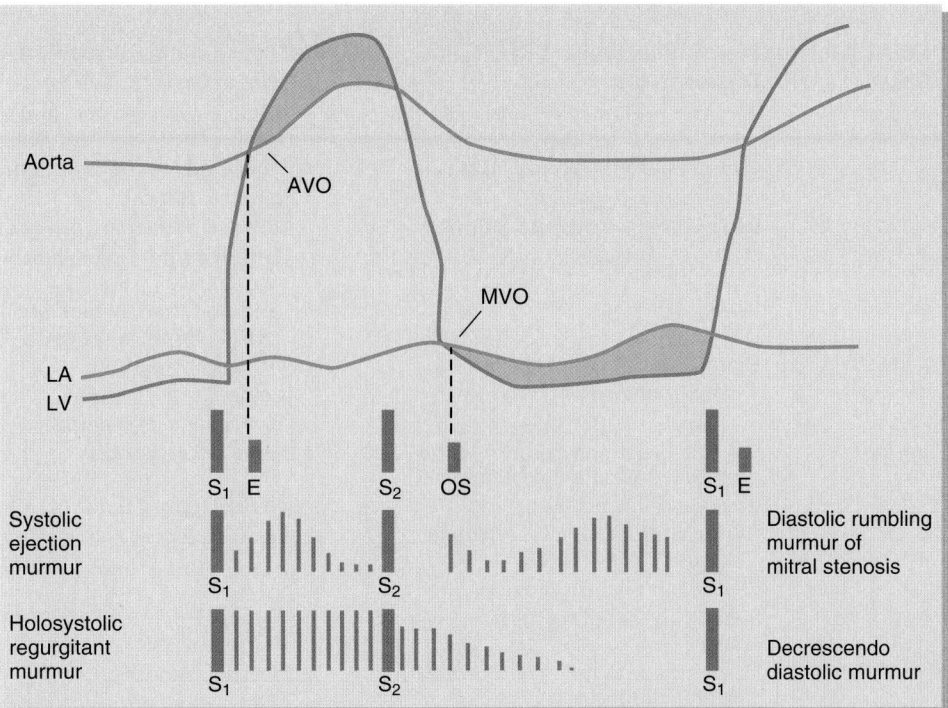

Figure 4-5 Abnormal sounds and murmurs associated with valvular dysfunction displayed simultaneously with left atrial (LA), left ventricular (LV), and aortic pressure tracings. AVO, aortic valve opening; E, ejection click of the aortic valve; MVO, mitral valve opening; OS, opening snap of the mitral valve. The *shaded areas* represent pressure gradients across the aortic valve during systole or mitral valve during diastole, characteristic of aortic stenosis and mitral stenosis, respectively.

septal defect is frequently associated with a loud murmur (**Web Sounds, VSD**). Higher-frequency murmurs correlate with a higher velocity of flow at the site of turbulence. Important to note are the pattern or configuration of the murmur (e.g., crescendo, crescendo-decrescendo, decrescendo, plateau) (Fig. 4-5) and the quality of the murmur (e.g., harsh, blowing, rumbling) as well as the location of maximal intensity and the pattern of radiation of the murmur. Various physical maneuvers may help clarify the nature of a particular murmur (see Table 4-4).

Murmurs can be divided into three categories—(1) systolic, (2) diastolic, and (3) continuous (Table 4-8)—and can result from abnormalities on the right or left side of the heart as well as the great vessels. Right-sided murmurs may become significantly louder after inspiration, owing to the resulting augmentation of venous return, whereas left-sided murmurs are relatively unaffected by respiration. Systolic murmurs can be further divided into ejection-type murmurs and regurgitant murmurs. Ejection murmurs reflect turbulent flow across the aortic or pulmonic valve (**Web Sounds, AS and PS**). They begin shortly after S_1, increase in intensity as the velocity of flow increases, and subsequently decrease in intensity as the velocity falls (crescendo-decrescendo). Examples of ejection-type murmurs include innocent murmurs and the murmurs of aortic sclerosis, aortic stenosis, pulmonic stenosis, and hypertrophic cardiomyopathy. Innocent murmurs and aortic sclerotic murmurs are short in duration and do not radiate (**Web Sounds, benign murmur**). The duration of aortic or pulmonic stenotic murmurs varies depending on the severity of the stenosis (compare **Web Sounds, AS—early** and **AS—late**). With

more severe stenosis, the murmur becomes longer, and the time to peak intensity of the murmur lengthens (i.e., early-, mid-, and late-peaking murmurs). The murmur of aortic stenosis is usually harsh, radiates to the carotid arteries, and at times may radiate to the cardiac apex (Gallavardin phenomenon). The murmur of hypertrophic cardiomyopathy may be confused with aortic stenosis, but it does not radiate to the carotids, and it is the only ejection murmur that becomes louder with decreased venous return. Mitral regurgitation associated with mitral valve prolapse may also show this response, but it is not a typical ejection murmur.

The classic regurgitant systolic murmurs of mitral (MR) and tricuspid regurgitation (TR) last throughout all of systole (holosystolic), are plateau in pattern, and terminate at S_2 (**Web Sounds, MR**). With acute MR, the murmur may be limited to early systole and may be somewhat decrescendo in pattern. When MR is secondary to mitral valve prolapse, it starts in mid to late systole and is preceded by a mitral valve click. Ventricular septal defects may also result in holosystolic murmurs, although a small muscular ventricular septal defect may have a murmur limited to early systole.

Early-diastolic murmurs result from aortic or pulmonic insufficiency and are decrescendo in pattern. The duration of the murmur reflects chronicity: a short murmur is heard in acute aortic insufficiency or mild insufficiency, whereas chronic aortic insufficiency may produce a murmur throughout diastole. A Graham Steell murmur denotes a pulmonic insufficiency murmur in the setting of pulmonary hypertension. Mid-diastolic murmurs classically result from mitral or tricuspid stenosis, are low pitched, and are referred to as

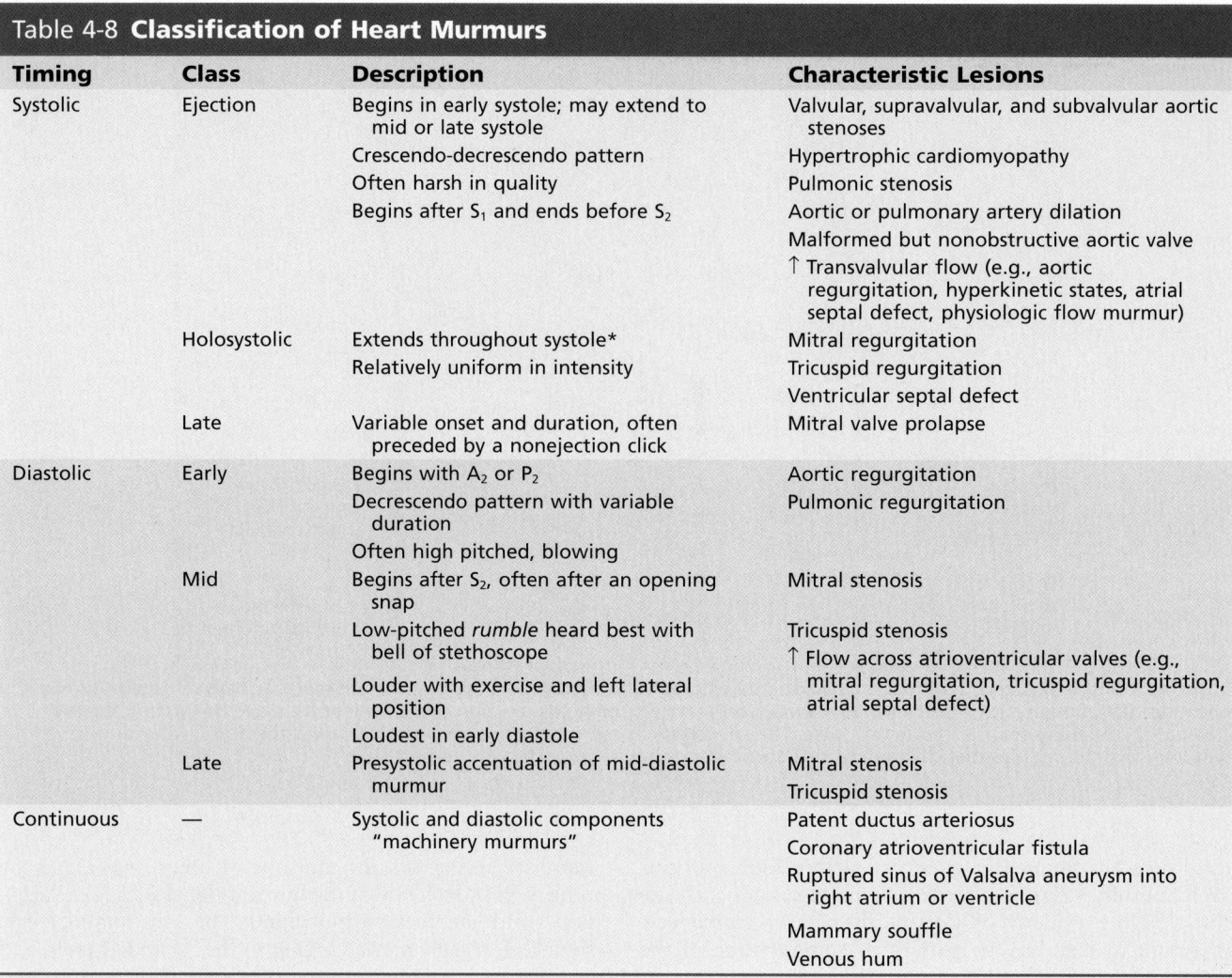

Table 4-8 **Classification of Heart Murmurs**

Timing	Class	Description	Characteristic Lesions
Systolic	Ejection	Begins in early systole; may extend to mid or late systole	Valvular, supravalvular, and subvalvular aortic stenoses
		Crescendo-decrescendo pattern	Hypertrophic cardiomyopathy
		Often harsh in quality	Pulmonic stenosis
		Begins after S_1 and ends before S_2	Aortic or pulmonary artery dilation
			Malformed but nonobstructive aortic valve
			↑ Transvalvular flow (e.g., aortic regurgitation, hyperkinetic states, atrial septal defect, physiologic flow murmur)
	Holosystolic	Extends throughout systole*	Mitral regurgitation
		Relatively uniform in intensity	Tricuspid regurgitation
			Ventricular septal defect
	Late	Variable onset and duration, often preceded by a nonejection click	Mitral valve prolapse
Diastolic	Early	Begins with A_2 or P_2	Aortic regurgitation
		Decrescendo pattern with variable duration	Pulmonic regurgitation
		Often high pitched, blowing	
	Mid	Begins after S_2, often after an opening snap	Mitral stenosis
		Low-pitched *rumble* heard best with bell of stethoscope	Tricuspid stenosis
			↑ Flow across atrioventricular valves (e.g., mitral regurgitation, tricuspid regurgitation, atrial septal defect)
		Louder with exercise and left lateral position	
		Loudest in early diastole	
	Late	Presystolic accentuation of mid-diastolic murmur	Mitral stenosis
			Tricuspid stenosis
Continuous	—	Systolic and diastolic components "machinery murmurs"	Patent ductus arteriosus
			Coronary atrioventricular fistula
			Ruptured sinus of Valsalva aneurysm into right atrium or ventricle
			Mammary souffle
			Venous hum

*Encompasses both the first and second heart sounds.

diastolic rumbles. Similar murmurs may be heard with obstructing atrial myxomas or in the presence of augmented diastolic flow across an unobstructed mitral or tricuspid valve, as occurs with an atrial or ventricular septal defect or with significant MR or TR. Severe, chronic aortic insufficiency may also produce a diastolic rumble, owing to premature closure of the mitral valve (Austin Flint murmur). Late-diastolic murmurs reflect presystolic accentuation of the mid-diastolic murmurs, owing to augmented mitral or tricuspid flow after atrial contraction.

Continuous murmurs are murmurs that last throughout all of systole and continue into at least early diastole. These murmurs are referred to as *machinery murmurs* and are generated by continuous flow from a vessel or chamber with high pressure into a vessel or chamber with low pressure. A patent ductus arteriosus produces the classic continuous murmur (**Web Sounds, PDA**).

OTHER CARDIAC SOUNDS

Pericardial rubs occur in the setting of pericarditis. These rubs produce coarse, scratching sounds heard best at the left sternal border with the patient leaning forward and holding his or her breath at end expiration. The classic rub has three components corresponding to atrial systole, ventricular systole, and ventricular diastole, although frequently only one or two of the components are audible (**Web Sounds, pericardial rubs**). Localized irritation of the surrounding pleura may result in an associated pleural friction rub (pleuropericardial rub), which varies with respiration.

Continuous venous murmurs, or venous *hums,* are almost universally present in children. They are also frequent in adults, especially during pregnancy or in the setting of thyrotoxicosis or anemia. These murmurs are best heard at the base of the neck with the patient's head turned to the opposite direction and can be eliminated by gentle pressure over the vein.

PROSTHETIC HEART SOUNDS

Prosthetic valves produce characteristic auscultatory findings. Porcine or bovine bioprosthetic valves produce heart sounds that are similar to native valve sounds; however, because these valves are smaller than the native valves that they replace, they almost always have an associated murmur (systolic ejection murmur when placed in the aortic position and diastolic rumble when placed in the mitral position). Mechanical valves result in crisp, high-pitched sounds related to valvular opening and closure. With ball-in-cage valves (e.g., Starr-Edwards valves, the opening sound is louder than the closure sound. With all other mechanical valves (e.g., Björk-Shiley valves, St. Jude valves), the closure sound is louder. These valves also produce an ejection-type murmur. Listening for all of the expected prosthetic sounds in patients with prosthetic valves is important because dysfunction of these valves may first be suggested by a change in the intensity or quality of the heart sounds or the development of a new or changing murmur.

Prospectus for the Future

Thanks to advances in chip technology, the essential art of cardiac auscultation is making a resurgence with the use of the computerized heart sound phonocardiography or acoustic cardiography. Students and experienced practitioners alike will be able to use an algorithm for predicting left ventricular dysfunction based on the characteristics of the S_3 and S_4 heart sounds and biomarkers of disease compensation and progression. Personal digital assistants, smartphones, and other technologies will make inroads for more accurate diagnosis during initial screening evaluation and bedside management of patients with cardiovascular disease.

References

Pickering TG, Hall JE, Appel LJ, et al: Recommendations for blood pressure measurement in humans and experimental animals. Part 1: Blood pressure measurement in humans: A statement for professionals from the Subcommittee of Professional and Public Education of the American Heart Association Council on High Blood Pressure Research. Circulation 111:697-716, 2005.

Goldman L, Ausiello D: Cecil Textbook of Medicine, 22nd ed. Part VIII: Cardiovascular Disease. Philadelphia, WB Saunders, 2004.

Chapter **5**

Diagnostic Tests and Procedures in the Patient with Cardiovascular Disease

Sheldon E. Litwin

Chest Radiography

The chest radiograph is an integral part of the cardiac evaluation and gives valuable information regarding structure and function of the heart, lungs, and great vessels. A routine examination includes posteroanterior and lateral projections (Fig. 5-1).

In the posteroanterior view, cardiac enlargement may be present when the transverse diameter of the cardiac silhouette is greater than one half the transverse diameter of the thorax. The heart may appear falsely enlarged when it is displaced horizontally, such as with poor inflation of the lungs, and if the film is an anteroposterior projection, which magnifies the heart shadow. Left atrial enlargement is suggested when the left-sided heart border is straightened or bulges toward the left. In addition, the main bronchi may be widely splayed, and a circular opacity or *double density* within the cardiac silhouette may be seen. Right atrial enlargement may be present when the right-sided heart border bulges toward the right. Left ventricular enlargement results in downward and lateral displacement of the apex. A rounding of the displaced apex suggests ventricular hypertrophy. Right ventricular enlargement is best assessed in the lateral view and may be present when the right ventricular border occupies more than one third of the retrosternal space between the diaphragm and thoracic apex.

The aortic arch and thoracic aorta may become dilated and tortuous in patients with severe atherosclerosis, long-standing hypertension, and aortic dissection. Dilation of the proximal pulmonary arteries may occur when pulmonary pressures are elevated and pulmonary vascular resistance is increased. Disease states associated with increased pulmonary artery flow and normal vascular resistance, such as

atrial or ventricular septal defects, may result in dilation of the proximal and distal pulmonary arteries.

Pulmonary venous congestion secondary to elevated left ventricular heart pressures results in redistribution of blood flow in the lungs and prominence of the apical vessels. Transudation of fluid into the interstitial space may result in fluid in the fissures and along the horizontal periphery of the lower lung fields (Kerley B lines). As venous pressures further increase, fluid collects within the alveolar space, which early on collects preferentially in the inner two thirds of the lung fields, resulting in a characteristic *butterfly* appearance.

Fluoroscopy or plain films may identify abnormal calcification involving the pericardium, coronary arteries, aorta, and valves. In addition, fluoroscopy can be instrumental in evaluating the function of mechanical prosthetic valves.

Specific radiographic signs of congenital and valvular diseases are discussed in their respective sections.

Electrocardiography

The electrocardiogram (ECG) represents the electrical activity of the heart recorded by skin electrodes. This wave of electrical activity is represented as a sequence of deflections on the ECG (Fig. 5-2). The horizontal scale represents time such that, at a standard paper speed of 25 mm/second, each small box (1 mm) represents 0.04 second, and each large box (5 mm) represents 0.20 second. The vertical scale represents amplitude (10 mm = 1 mV). The heart rate can be estimated by dividing the number of large boxes between complexes (R-R interval) into 300.

In the normal heart, the electrical impulse originates in the sinoatrial (SA) node and is conducted through the atria.

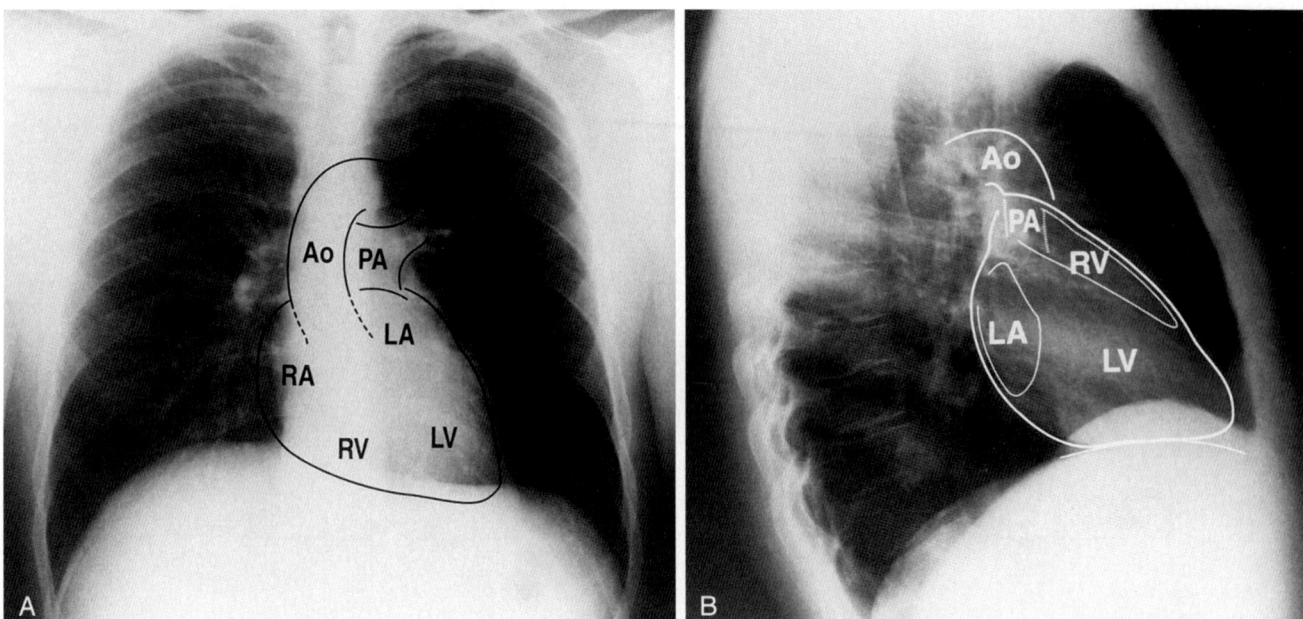

Figure 5-1 Schematic illustration of the parts of the heart, whose outlines can be identified on a routine chest radiograph. **A,** Posteroanterior chest radiograph. **B,** Lateral chest radiograph. Ao, aorta; LA, left atrium; LV, left ventricle; PA, pulmonary artery; RA, right atrium; RV, right ventricle.

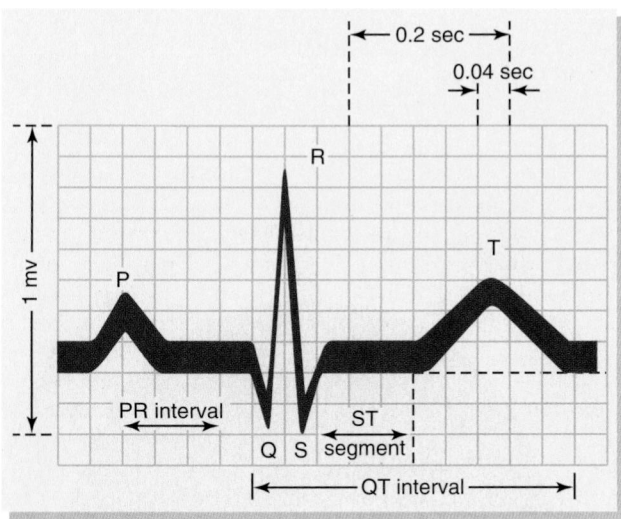

Figure 5-2 Normal electrocardiographic complex with labeling of waves and intervals.

Given that depolarization of the SA node is too weak to be detected on the surface ECG, the first, low-amplitude deflection on the surface ECG reflects atrial activation and is termed the *P wave*. The interval between the onset of the P wave and the next rapid deflection (QRS complex) is known as the PR interval and primarily represents the time taken for the impulse to travel through the atrioventricular (AV) node. The normal PR segment ranges from 0.12 to 0.20 second. A PR interval greater than 0.20 second defines AV nodal block.

After the wave of depolarization has moved through the AV node, the ventricular myocardium is depolarized in a sequence of four phases. First, the interventricular septum depolarizes from left to right. This phase is followed by depolarization of the right ventricle and inferior wall of the left ventricle, then the apex and central portions of the left ventricle, and, finally, the base and the posterior wall of the left ventricle. Ventricular depolarization results in a high-amplitude complex on the surface ECG known as the *QRS complex.* The first downward deflection of this complex is the Q wave, the first upward deflection is the R wave, and the subsequent downward deflection is the S wave. In some individuals, a second upward deflection may be present after the S wave and is termed *R prime* (R′). Normal duration of the QRS complex is less than 0.10 second. Complexes greater than 0.12 second are usually secondary to some form of interventricular conduction delay.

The isoelectric segment after the QRS complex is the ST segment and represents a brief period during which relatively little electrical activity occurs in the heart. The junction between the end of the QRS complex and the beginning of the ST segment is the J point. The upward deflection after the ST segment is the T wave and represents ventricular repolarization. The QT interval, which reflects the duration and transmural gradient of ventricular depolarization and repolarization, is measured from the onset of the QRS complex to the end of the T wave. The QT interval varies with heart rate, but for rates between 60 and 100 beats/minute, the normal QT interval ranges from 0.35 to 0.44 second. For heart rates outside this range, the QT interval can be corrected by the following formula:

$$QT_c = QT\,(sec)/\text{R-R interval}^{1/2}\,(sec)$$

In some individuals, a U wave (of varying amplitude) may be noted after the T wave, the cause of which is unknown.

The standard ECG consists of 12 leads: six limb leads (I, II, III, aVR, aVL, and aVF) and six chest or precordial leads (V_1 to V_6) (Fig. 5-3). The electrical activity recorded in each

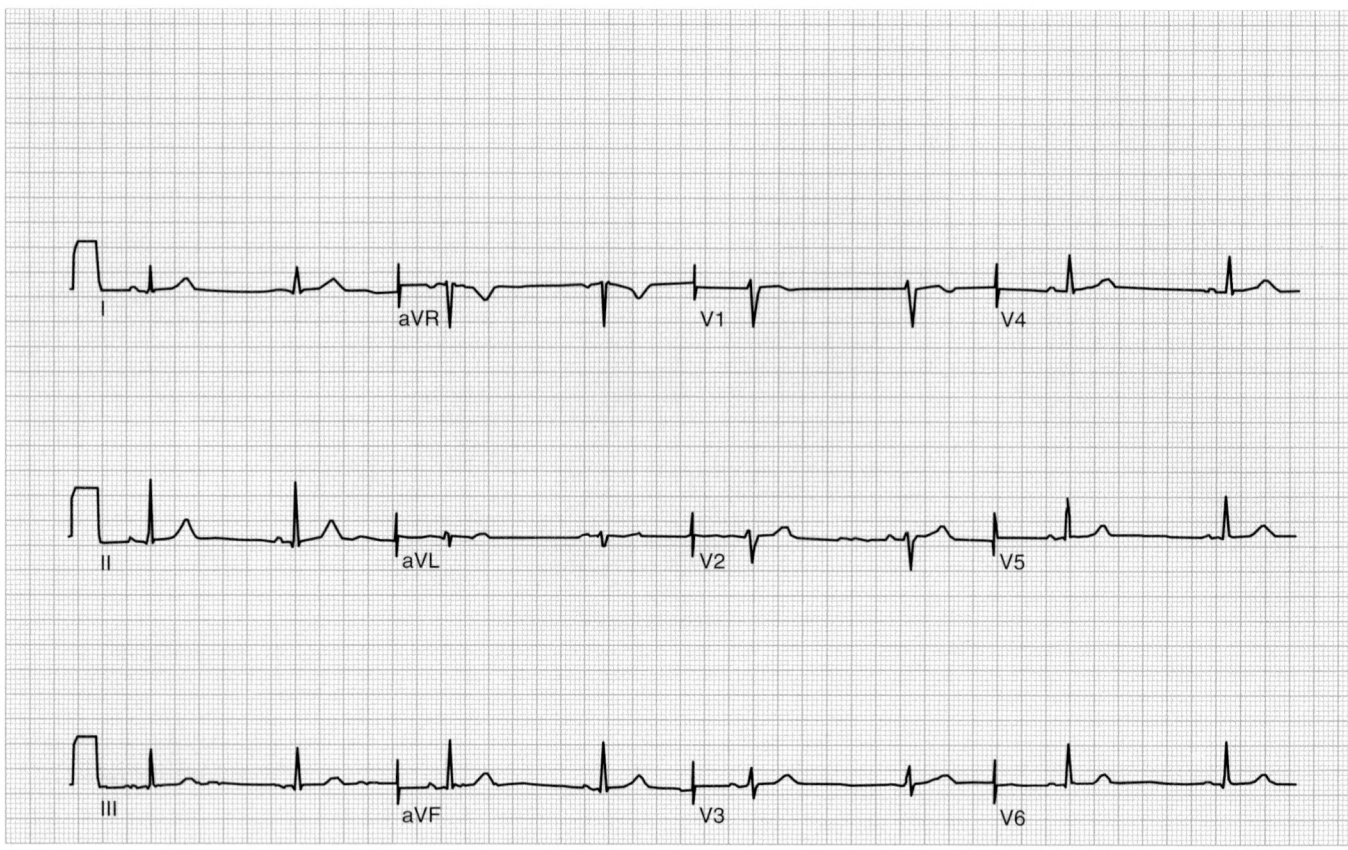

Figure 5-3 Normal 12-lead electrocardiogram.

lead represents the direction and magnitude (vector) of the electrical force as seen from that particular lead position. Electrical activity directed toward a particular lead is represented as an upward deflection, and an electrical impulse directed away from a particular lead is represented as a downward deflection. Although the overall direction of electrical activity can be determined for any of the waveforms previously described, the mean QRS axis is the most clinically useful and is determined by examining the six limb leads. Figure 5-4 illustrates Einthoven triangle and the polarity of each of the six limb leads of the standard ECG. Skin electrodes are attached to both arms and legs, with the right leg serving as the ground. Leads I, II, and III are bipolar leads and represent electrical activity between two leads: lead I represents electrical activity between the right and left arms (left arm positive), lead II between the right arm and left leg (left leg positive), and lead III between the left arm and left leg (left leg positive). Leads aVR, aVL, and aVF are designated the *augmented leads*. With these leads, the QRS will be positive or have a predominant upward deflection when the electrical forces are directed toward the right arm for aVR, left arm for aVL, and left leg for aVF. These six leads form a hexaxial frontal plane of 30-degree arc intervals. The normal QRS axis ranges from −30 to +90 degrees. An axis more negative than −30 defines left axis deviation, and an axis greater than +90 defines right axis deviation. In general, a positive QRS complex in leads I and aVF suggests a normal QRS axis between 0 and 90 degrees.

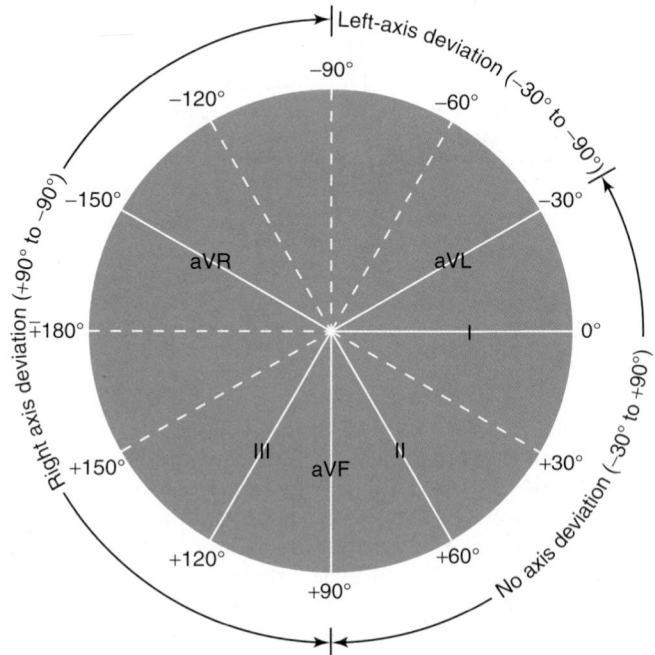

Figure 5-4 Hexaxial reference figure for frontal plane axis determination, indicating values for abnormal left and right QRS axis deviations.

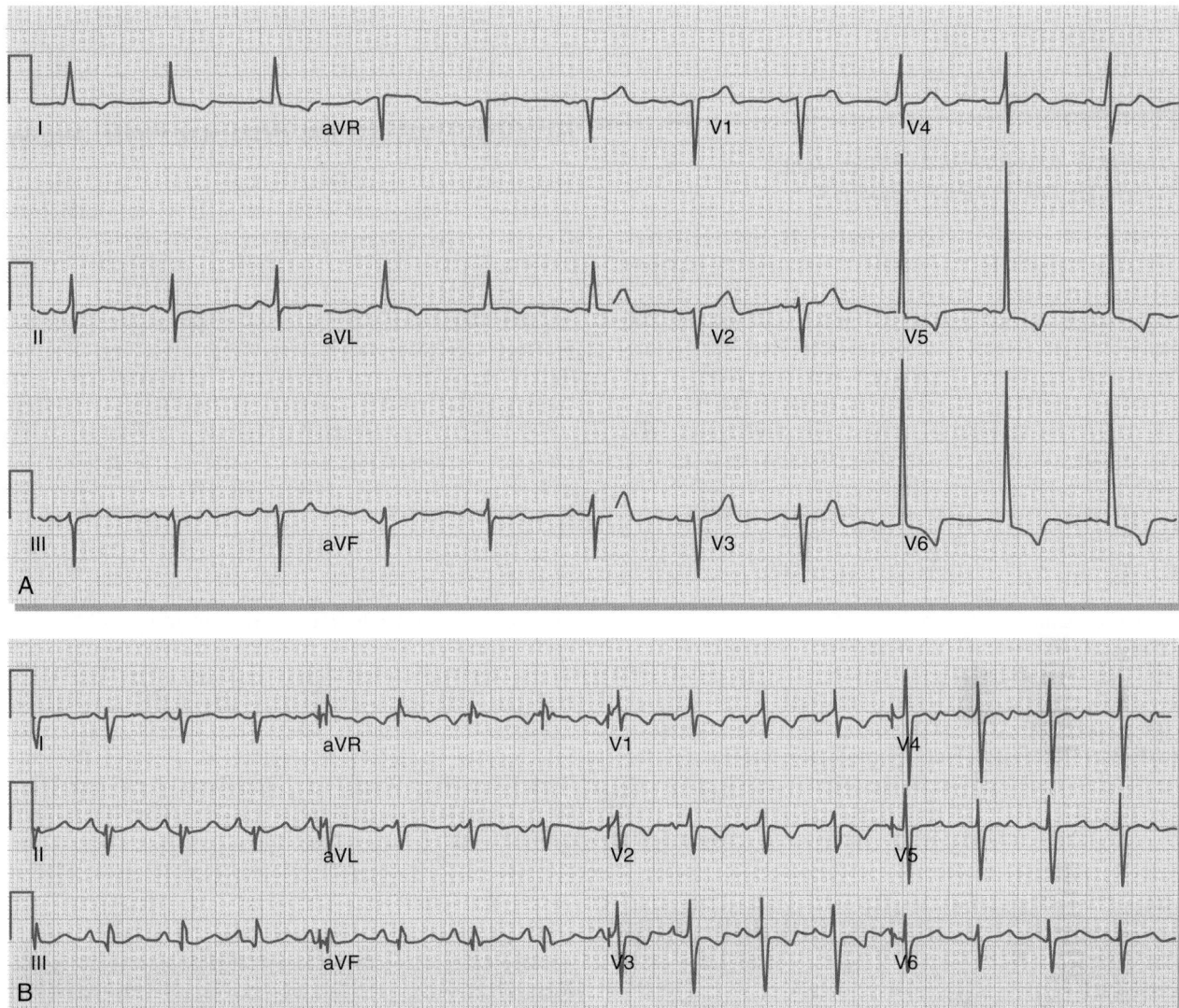

Figure 5-5 **A,** Left ventricular hypertrophy as seen on an electrocardiographic recording. Characteristic findings include increased QRS voltage in precordial leads (deep S in lead V_2 and tall R in lead V_5) and downsloping ST depression and T-wave inversion in lateral precordial leads (*strain* pattern) and leftward axis. **B,** Right ventricular hypertrophy with tall R wave in right precordial leads, downsloping ST depression in precordial leads (RV strain), right axis deviation, and evidence of right atrial enlargement.

The six standard precordial leads (V_1 to V_6) are attached to the anterior chest wall (Fig. 5-5). Lead placement should be as follows: V1—fourth intercostal space, right sternal border; V2—fourth intercostal space, left sternal border; V3—midway between V2 and V4; V4—fifth intercostal space, left mid-clavicular line; V5—level with V4, left anterior axillary line; V6—level with V4, left mid-axillary line. The chest leads should be placed under the breast. Electrical activity directed toward these leads results in a positive deflection on the ECG tracing. Leads V_1 and V_2 are closest to the right ventricle and interventricular septum, and leads V_5 and V_6 are closest to the anterior and anterolateral walls of the left ventricle. Normally, a small R wave occurs in lead V_1 reflecting septal depolarization and a deep S wave reflecting predominantly left ventricular activation. From V_1 to V_6, the R wave becomes larger (and the S wave smaller) because the predominant forces directed at these leads originate from the left ventricle. The transition from a predominant S wave to a predominant R wave usually occurs between leads V_3 and V_4. Right-sided chest leads are used to look for evidence of right ventricular infarction. ST-segment elevation in V_{4R} has the best sensitivity and specificity for making this diagnosis. For right-sided leads, standard V_1 and V_2 are switched, and V_{3R} to V_{6R} are placed mirror image to the standard left-sided chest leads. Some groups have advocated the use of posterior leads to increase the sensitivity for diagnosing lateral and posterior wall infarction or ischemia (areas that are often deemed to be *electrically silent* on traditional 12-lead ECGs). To do this, six additional leads are placed in the fifth intercostal space continuing posteriorly from the position of V_6.

Abnormal Electrocardiographic Patterns

CHAMBER ABNORMALITIES AND VENTRICULAR HYPERTROPHY

The P wave is normally upright in leads I, II, and F; inverted in aVR; and biphasic in V_1. Left atrial abnormality (defined as enlargement, hypertrophy, or increased wall stress) is characterized by a wide P wave in lead II (0.12 second) and a deeply inverted terminal component in lead V_1 (1 mm). Right atrial abnormality is present when the P waves in the limb leads are peaked and 2.5 mm or more in height.

Left ventricular hypertrophy may result in increased QRS voltage, slight widening of the QRS complex, late intrinsicoid deflection, left axis deviation, and abnormalities of the ST-T segments (see Fig. 5-5A). Multiple criteria with variable sensitivity and specificity for detecting left ventricular hypertrophy are available. The most frequently used criteria are given in Table 5-1.

Right ventricular hypertrophy is characterized by tall R waves in leads V_1 through V_3; deep S waves in leads I, aVL, V_5, and V_6; and right axis deviation (see Fig. 5-5B). In patients with chronically elevated pulmonary pressures, such as with chronic lung disease, a combination of ECG abnormalities reflecting a right-sided pathologic condition may be present and include right atrial abnormality, right ventricular hypertrophy, and right axis deviation. In patients with acute pulmonary embolus, ECG changes may suggest right ventricular strain and include right axis deviation; incomplete or complete right bundle branch block; S waves in leads I, II, and III; and T-wave inversions in leads V_1 through V_3.

INTERVENTRICULAR CONDUCTION DELAYS

The ventricular conduction system consists of two main branches, the right and left bundles. The left bundle further divides into the anterior and posterior fascicles. Conduction block can occur in either of the major branches or in the fascicles (Table 5-2).

Fascicular block results in a change in the sequence of ventricular activation but does not prolong overall conduction time (QRS duration remains < 0.10 second). Left anterior fascicular block is a relatively common ECG abnormality and is sometimes associated with right bundle branch block. This conduction abnormality is present when extreme left axis deviation occurs (more negative than −45 degrees); when the R wave is greater than the Q wave in leads I and aVL; and when the S wave is greater than the R wave in leads II, III, and aVF. Left posterior fascicular block is uncommon but is associated with right axis deviation (>90 degrees); small Q waves in leads II, III, and aVF; and small R waves in leads I and aVL. The ECG findings associated with fascicular blocks can be confused with myocardial infarction (MI). For example, with left anterior fascicular block, the prominent QS deflection in leads V_1 and V_2 can mimic an anteroseptal MI, and the rS deflection in leads II, III, and aVF can be confused with an inferior MI. Similarly, the rS deflection in leads I and aVL in left posterior fascicular block may be confused with a high lateral infarct. The presence of abnormal ST- and T-wave segments and pathologic Q waves (see

---

Table 5-1 Electrocardiographic Manifestations of Atrial Abnormalities and Ventricular Hypertrophy

Left Atrial Abnormality

P-wave duration ≥ 0.12 second
Notched, slurred P wave in leads I and II
Biphasic P wave in lead V_1 with a wide, deep, negative terminal component

Right Atrial Abnormality

P-wave duration ≤ 0.11 second
Tall, peaked P waves of ≥ 2.5 mm in leads II, III, and aVF

Left Ventricular Hypertrophy

Voltage criteria
R wave in lead aVL ≥ 12 mm
R wave in lead I ≥ 15 mm
S wave in lead V_1 or V_2 + R wave in lead V_5 or V_6 ≥ 35 mm
Depressed ST segments with inverted T waves in the lateral leads
Left axis deviation
QRS duration ≥ 0.09 second
Left atrial enlargement

Right Ventricular Hypertrophy

Tall R waves over right precordium (R:S ratio in lead V_1 > 1.0)
Right axis deviation
Depressed ST segments with inverted T waves in leads V_1 to V_3
Normal QRS duration (if no right bundle branch block)
Right atrial enlargement

Table 5-2 Electrocardiographic Manifestations of Fascicular and Bundle Branch Blocks

Left Anterior Fascicular Block

QRS duration ≤ 0.1 second
Left axis deviation (more negative than −45 degrees)
rS pattern in leads II, III, and aVF
qR pattern in leads I and aVL

Right Posterior Fascicular Block

QRS duration ≤ 0.1 second
Right axis deviation (+90 degrees or greater)
qR pattern in leads II, III, and aVF
rS pattern in leads I and aVL
Exclusion of other causes of right axis deviation (chronic obstructive pulmonary disease, right ventricular hypertrophy)

Left Bundle Branch Block

QRS duration ≥ 0.12 second
Broad, slurred, or notched R waves in lateral leads (I, aVL, V_5, and V_6)
QS or rS pattern in anterior precordium leads (V_1 and V_2)
ST-T-wave vectors opposite to terminal QRS vectors

Right Bundle Branch Block

QRS duration ≥ 0.12 second
Large R′ wave in lead V_1 (rsR′)
Deep terminal S wave in lead V_6
Normal septal Q waves
Inverted T waves in leads V_1 and V_2

"Myocardial Ischemia and Infarction" later) are helpful findings to differentiate MI from a fascicular block.

Bundle branch blocks are associated with QRS duration longer than 120 milliseconds. In left bundle branch block, depolarization proceeds down the right bundle, across the interventricular septum from right to left, and then to the left ventricle. Characteristic ECG findings include a wide QRS complex; a broad R wave in leads I, aVL, V_5, and V_6; a deep QS wave in leads V_1 and V_2; and ST depression and T-wave inversion opposite the QRS deflection (Fig. 5-6A). Given the abnormal sequence of ventricular activation with left bundle branch block, many ECG abnormalities, such as Q-wave MI and left ventricular hypertrophy, are difficult to evaluate. In some cases, acute MI is still apparent even with LBBB. Left bundle branch block almost always indicates the presence of underlying myocardial disease (most commonly fibrosis due to ischemic injury or hypertrophy). With right bundle branch block, the interventricular septum depolarizes normally from left to right, and therefore the initial QRS deflection remains unchanged. As a result, ECG abnormalities such as Q-wave MI can still be interpreted. After septal activation, the left ventricle depolarizes,

followed by the right ventricle. The ECG is characterized by a wide QRS complex; a large R' wave in lead V_1 (R-S-R'); and deep S waves in leads I, aVL, and V_6, representing delayed right ventricular activation (see Fig. 5-6B). Although right bundle branch block may be associated with underlying cardiac disease, it may also appear as a normal variant or be seen intermittently when heart rate is elevated. In the latter case, it is often referred to as *rate-related bundle branch block*.

MYOCARDIAL ISCHEMIA AND INFARCTION

Myocardial ischemia and MI may be associated with abnormalities of the ST segment, T-wave, and QRS complex. Myocardial ischemia primarily affects repolarization of the myocardium and is often associated with horizontal or down-sloping ST-segment depression and T-wave inversion. These changes may be transient, such as during an anginal episode or an exercise stress test, or may be long-lasting in the setting of unstable angina or MI. T-wave inversion without ST-segment depression is a nonspecific finding and must be correlated with the clinical setting.

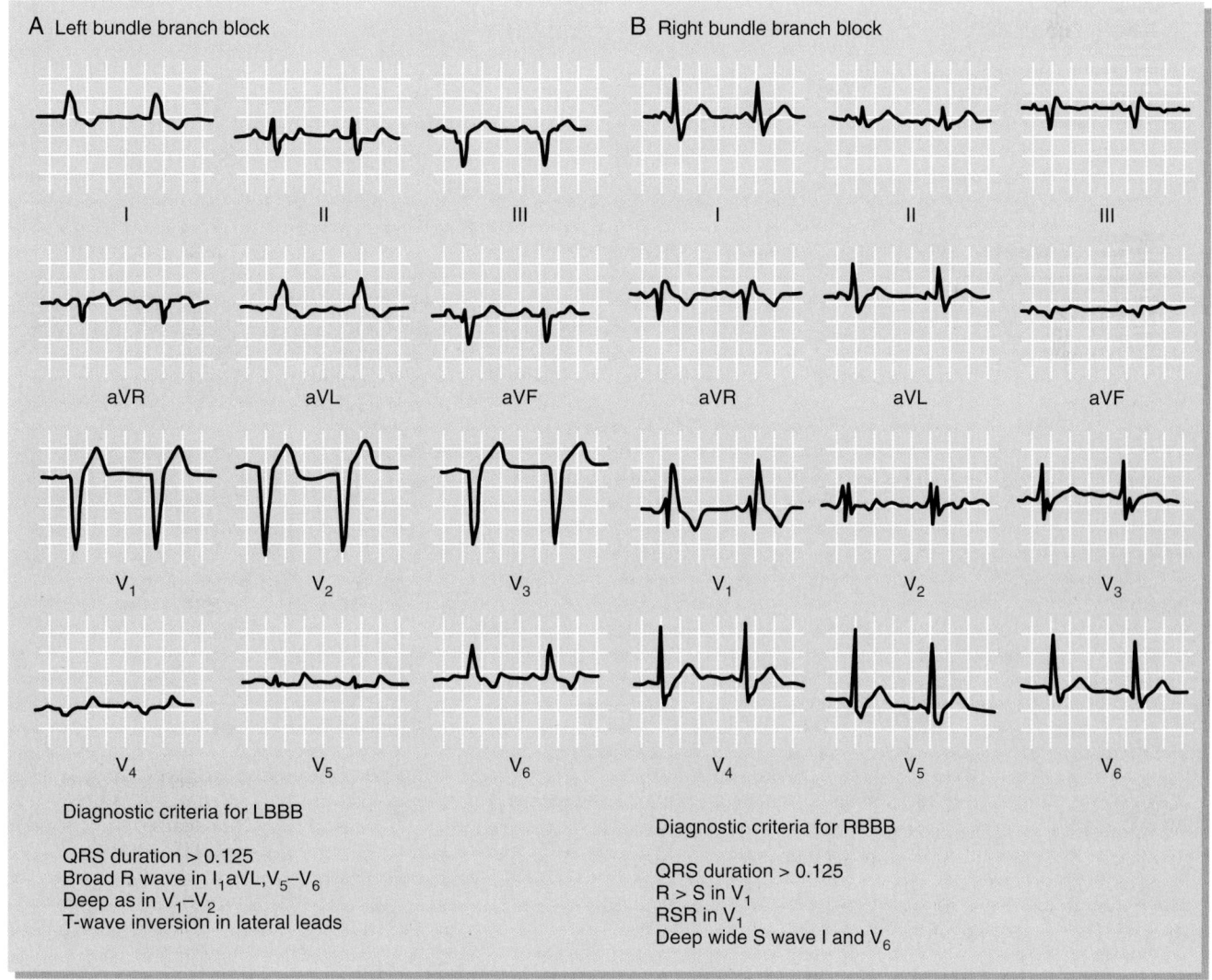

A Left bundle branch block

I II III

aVR aVL aVF

V_1 V_2 V_3

V_4 V_5 V_6

Diagnostic criteria for LBBB

QRS duration > 0.125
Broad R wave in I, aVL, V_5–V_6
Deep as in V_1–V_2
T-wave inversion in lateral leads

B Right bundle branch block

I II III

aVR aVL aVF

V_1 V_2 V_3

V_4 V_5 V_6

Diagnostic criteria for RBBB

QRS duration > 0.125
R > S in V_1
RSR in V_1
Deep wide S wave I and V_6

Figure 5-6 **A,** Left bundle branch block (LBBB). **B,** Right bundle branch block (RBBB). Criteria for bundle branch block are summarized in Table 5-2.

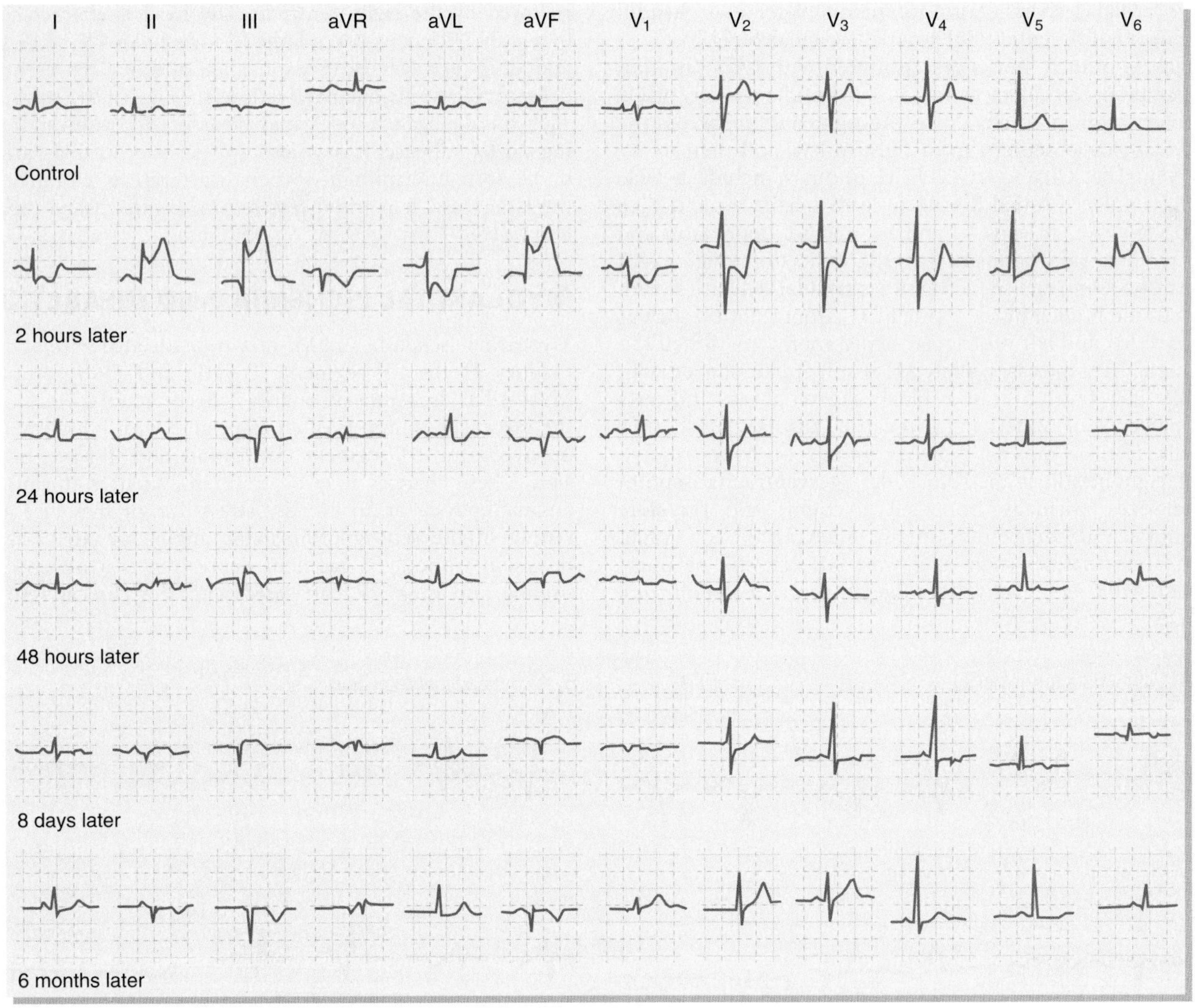

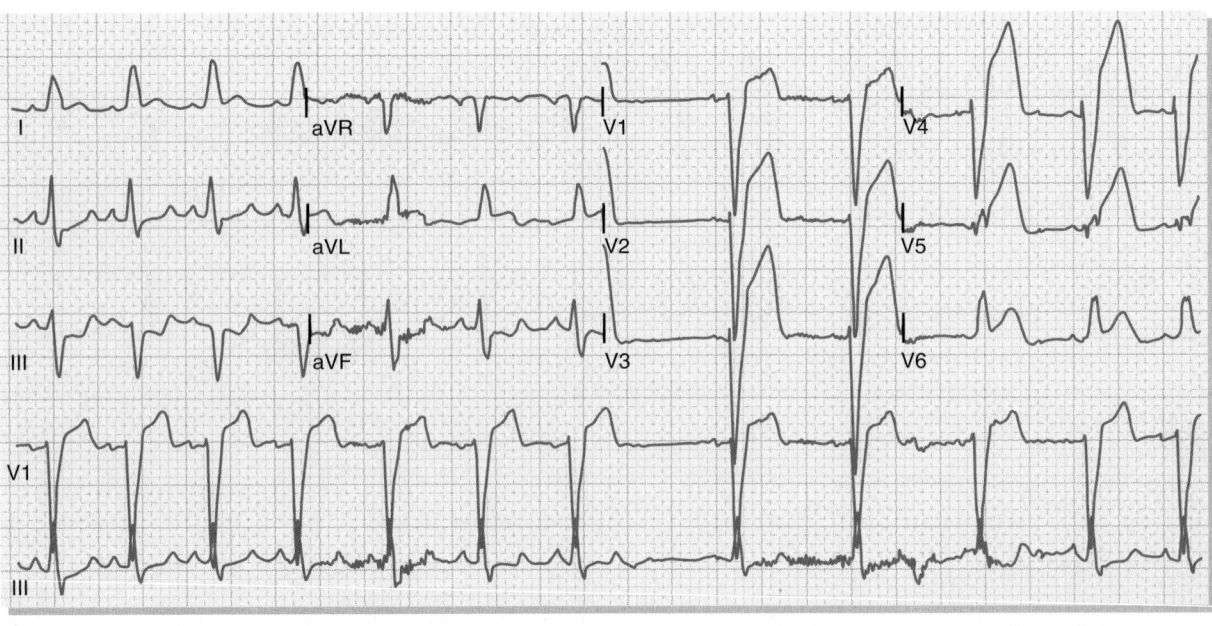

I
II
III
aVR
aVL
aVF
V_1
V_2
V_3
V_4
V_5
V_6
Control
2 hours later
24 hours later
48 hours later
8 days later
6 months later

A

I
aVR
V1
V4
II
aVL
V2
V5
III
aVF
V3
V6
V1
III

B

Figure 5-7 A, Evolutionary changes in a posteroinferior myocardial infarction. Control tracing is normal. The tracing recorded 2 hours after onset of chest pain demonstrated development of early Q waves, marked ST-segment elevation, and hyperacute T waves in leads II, III, and aVF. In addition, a larger R wave, ST-segment depression, and negative T waves have developed in leads V_1 and V_2. These are early changes indicating acute posteroinferior myocardial infarction. The 24-hour tracing demonstrates evolutionary changes. In leads II, III, and aVF, the Q wave is larger, the ST segments have almost returned to baseline, and the T wave has begun to invert. In leads V_1 to V_2, the duration of the R wave now exceeds 0.04 seconds, the ST segment is depressed, and the T wave is upright. (In this example, ECG changes of true posterior involvement extend past lead V_2; ordinarily, only leads V_1 and V_2 may be involved.) Only minor further changes occur through the 8-day tracing. Finally, 6 months later, the ECG illustrates large Q waves, isoelectric ST segments, and inverted T waves in leads II, III, and aVF and large R waves, isoelectric ST segment, and upright T waves in leads V_1 and V_2, indicative of an *old* posteroinferior myocardial infarction. **B,** Example of an ECG from a patient with an underlying LBBB who experienced an acute anterior myocardial infarction. Characteristic ST segment elevation and hyperacute T-waves are seen in leads V1-V6 and leads I and AVL despite the presence of the LBBB. Note that this is not always the case, as a patient with typical symptoms and a LBBB as well as no definite ischemic ST segment elevations should still be treated as if the individual is having an MI or acute coronary syndrome.

Localized ST-segment elevation suggests more extensive myocardial injury and is often associated with acute MI (see Fig. 5-7). Vasospastic or Prinzmetal angina may be associated with reversible ST-segment elevation without MI. ST-segment elevation may occur in other settings not related to acute ischemia or infarction. Persistent, localized ST-segment elevation in the same leads as pathologic Q waves is consistent with a ventricular aneurysm. Acute pericarditis is associated with diffuse ST-segment elevation and PR depression. Diffuse J-point elevation in association with upward-coving ST segments is a normal variant common among young men and is often referred to as *early repolarization.*

The presence of a Q wave is one of the diagnostic criteria used to verify MI. Infarcted myocardium is unable to conduct electrical activity, and therefore electrical forces will be directed away from the surface electrode overlying the infarcted region, resulting in a Q wave on the surface ECG. Knowing which region of the myocardium each lead represents enables the examiner to localize the area of infarction (Table 5-3). A pathologic Q wave has a duration of greater than or equal to 0.04 second or a depth one fourth or more the height of the corresponding R wave.

Not all MIs result in the formation of Q waves. In addition, small R waves can return many weeks to months after an MI.

Abnormal Q waves, or *pseudoinfarction,* may also be associated with nonischemic cardiac disease, such as ventricular pre-excitation, cardiac amyloidosis, sarcoidosis, idiopathic or hypertrophic cardiomyopathy, myocarditis, and chronic lung disease.

ABNORMALITIES OF THE ST SEGMENT AND T WAVE

A number of drugs and metabolic abnormalities may affect the ST segment and T wave (Fig. 5-8). Hypokalemia may result in prominent U waves in the precordial leads and prolongation of the QT interval. Hyperkalemia may result in tall, peaked T waves. Hypocalcemia typically lengthens the QT interval, whereas hypercalcemia shortens it. A commonly used cardiac medication, digoxin, often results in diffuse, scooped ST-segment depression. Minor or *nonspecific* ST-segment and T-wave abnormalities may be present in many patients and have no definable cause. In these instances, the physician must determine the significance of the abnormalities based on the clinical setting.

Several excellent websites containing examples of normal and abnormal ECGs are available.

Long-Term Ambulatory Electrocardiographic Recording

Ambulatory ECG (Holter monitoring) is a widely used, noninvasive method to evaluate cardiac arrhythmias and conduction disturbances over an extended period and to detect electrical abnormalities that may be brief or transient. With this approach, ECG data from two to three surface leads are stored on a tape recorder that the patient wears for a minimum of 24 to 48 hours. The recorders have both patient-activated event markers and time markers so that any abnormalities can be correlated with the patient's symptoms or time of day. These data can then be printed in a standard, real-time ECG format for review.

For patients with intermittent or rare symptoms, an event recorder, which can be worn for several weeks, may be helpful in identifying the arrhythmia. The simplest device is a small, hand-held monitor that is applied to the chest wall when symptoms occur. The ECG data are recorded and can be transmitted later by telephone to a monitoring center for analysis. A more sophisticated system uses a wrist recorder that allows continuous-loop storage of 4 to 5 minutes of ECG data from one lead. When the patient activates the system, ECG data preceding the event and for 1 to 2 minutes after the event are recorded and stored for further analysis. With both of these devices, the patient must be physically able to activate the recorder during the episode to store the ECG data. Implantable recording devices (subcutaneous) are sometimes used to diagnose infrequent events.

STRESS TESTING

Stress testing is an important noninvasive tool for evaluating patients with known or suggested coronary artery disease (CAD). During exercise, the increased demand for oxygen by the working skeletal muscles is met by increases in heart rate and cardiac output. In patients with significant CAD, the increase in myocardial oxygen demand cannot be met by an increase in coronary blood flow. As a result, myocardial ischemia may occur, resulting in chest pain and characteristic ECG abnormalities. These changes, combined with the hemodynamic response to exercise, can give useful diagnostic and prognostic information in the patient with cardiac abnormalities. The most frequent indications for stress testing include establishing a diagnosis of CAD in patients

Table 5-3 Electrocardiographic Localization of Myocardial Infarction

Infarct Location	Leads Depicting Primary Electrocardiographic Changes	Likely Vessel* Involved
Inferior	II, III, aVF	RCA
Septal	V_1, V_2	LAD
Anterior	V_3, V_4	LAD
Anteroseptal	V_1 to V_4	LAD
Extensive anterior	I, aVL, V_1 to V_6	LAD
Lateral	I, aVL, V_5 to V_6	CIRC
High lateral	I, aVL	CIRC
Posterior†	Prominent R in V_1	RCA or CIRC
Right ventricular‡	ST elevation in V_1 and, more specifically, V_4R in setting of inferior infarction	RCA

*This is a generalization; variations occur.
†Usually in association with inferior or lateral infarction.
‡Usually in association with inferior infarction.
CIRC, circumflex artery; LAD, left anterior descending coronary artery; RCA, right coronary artery.

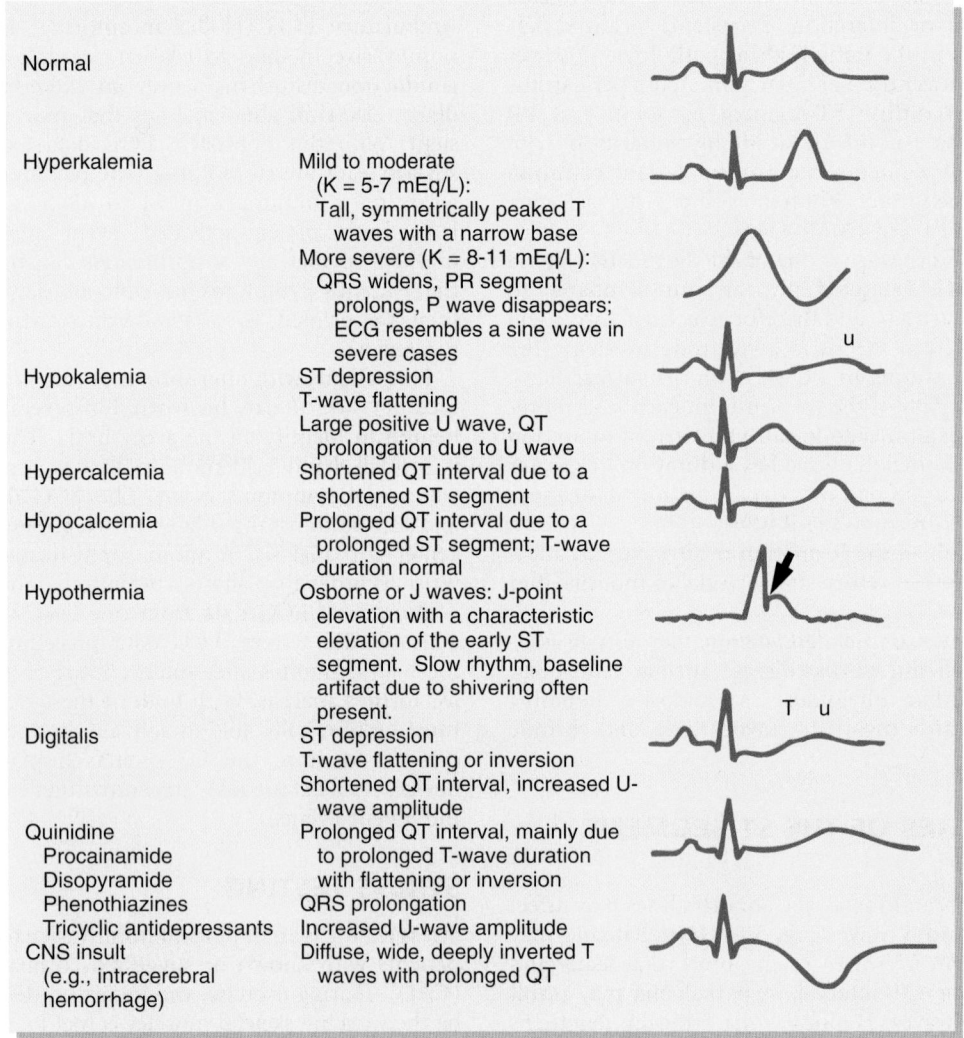

Normal		
Hyperkalemia	Mild to moderate (K = 5-7 mEq/L): Tall, symmetrically peaked T waves with a narrow base More severe (K = 8-11 mEq/L): QRS widens, PR segment prolongs, P wave disappears; ECG resembles a sine wave in severe cases	
Hypokalemia	ST depression T-wave flattening Large positive U wave, QT prolongation due to U wave	
Hypercalcemia	Shortened QT interval due to a shortened ST segment	
Hypocalcemia	Prolonged QT interval due to a prolonged ST segment; T-wave duration normal	
Hypothermia	Osborne or J waves: J-point elevation with a characteristic elevation of the early ST segment. Slow rhythm, baseline artifact due to shivering often present.	
Digitalis	ST depression T-wave flattening or inversion Shortened QT interval, increased U-wave amplitude	
Quinidine Procainamide Disopyramide Phenothiazines Tricyclic antidepressants	Prolonged QT interval, mainly due to prolonged T-wave duration with flattening or inversion QRS prolongation Increased U-wave amplitude	
CNS insult (e.g., intracerebral hemorrhage)	Diffuse, wide, deeply inverted T waves with prolonged QT	

Figure 5-8 Metabolic and drug influences on the electrocardiographic recording.

with chest pain, assessing prognosis and functional capacity in patients with chronic stable angina or after an MI, evaluating exercise-induced arrhythmias, and assessing for ischemia after a revascularization procedure.

The most common form of stress testing uses continuous ECG monitoring while the patient walks on a treadmill. With each advancing stage, the speed and incline of the belt increases, thus increasing the amount of work the patient performs. The commonly used Bruce protocol employs 3 minutes of exercise at each stage. The modified Bruce protocol incorporates two beginning stages with slower speeds and lesser inclines than are used in the standard Bruce protocol. The modified Bruce or similar protocols are generally used for older, markedly overweight, and unstable or more debilitated patients. Exercise testing may also be performed using a bicycle or arm ergometer. The stress test is generally deemed adequate if the patient achieves 90% of his or her predicted maximal heart rate, which is equal to 220 minus the patient's age. Indications for stopping the test include fatigue, severe hypertension (>220 mm Hg systolic), worsening angina during exercise, developing marked or widespread ischemic ECG changes, significant arrhythmias, or hypotension. The diagnostic accuracy of stress testing is improved with adjunctive echocardiography or radionuclide imaging. Contraindications to stress testing include unstable angina, acute MI, poorly controlled hypertension (blood pressure >220/110 mm Hg), severe aortic stenosis (valve area < 1.0 cm²), and decompensated congestive heart failure. In the era of reperfusion therapy (thrombolytic and percutaneous interventions), for acute coronary syndromes or acute MI, little role exists for the predischarge submaximal stress test that was commonly used in the past.

The diagnostic accuracy of the exercise test is dependent on the pre-test likelihood of CAD in a given patient, the sensitivity and specificity of the test results in that patient population, and the ECG criteria used to define a positive test. Clinical features that are most useful at predicting important angiographic coronary disease before exercise testing include advanced age, male sex, and the presence of typical (vs. atypical) anginal chest pain. The diagnostic accuracy and cost-effectiveness of exercise testing is best in patients with an intermediate risk for CAD (30% to 70%) and when ischemic ECG changes are accompanied by chest pain during exercise. Exercise testing is less cost-effective in diagnosing CAD in a patient with classic symptoms of angina because a positive test will not significantly increase the post-test probability of CAD, and a negative test would likely represent a false-negative result. Nonetheless, prognostic information and objective information about the efficacy of pharmacologic therapy may still be obtained. Similarly, exercise testing in young patients with atypical chest pain may not be diagnostically useful, given that an abnormal test result will likely represent a false-positive test and will not significantly increase the post-test probability of CAD.

The normal physiologic response to exercise is an increase in heart rate and systolic and diastolic blood pressures. The ECG will maintain normal T-wave polarity, and the ST segment will remain unchanged or, if depressed, will have a rapid upstroke back to baseline. An ischemic ECG response to exercise is defined as (1) 1.5 mm of up-sloping ST-segment depression measured 0.08 second past the J point, (2) at least 1 mm of horizontal ST depression, or (3) 1 mm of down-sloping ST-segment depression measured at the J point. Given the large amount of artifact on the ECG that may occur with exercise, these changes must be present in at least three consecutive depolarizations. Other findings suggestive of more extensive CAD include early onset of ST depression (6 minutes); marked, down-sloping ST depression (>2 mm), especially if present in more than five leads; ST changes persisting into recovery for more than 5 minutes; and failure to increase systolic blood pressure to 120 mm Hg or more or a sustained decrease of 10 mm Hg or more below baseline.

The ECG is not diagnostically useful in the presence of left ventricular hypertrophy, left bundle branch block, Wolff-Parkinson-White syndrome, or chronic digoxin therapy. In these instances, nuclear or echocardiographic imaging is needed to diagnose ischemia. In patients who are unable to exercise, pharmacologic stress testing with myocardial imaging has been shown to have sensitivity and specificity for detecting CAD equal to those of exercise stress imaging. Intravenous dipyridamole and adenosine and newer selective adenosine A2A receptor agonists are coronary vasodilators that result in increased blood flow in normal arteries without significantly changing flow in diseased vessels. The resulting heterogeneity in blood flow can be detected by nuclear imaging techniques and the regions of myocardium supplied by diseased vessels identified. Another commonly used technique to evaluate for ischemia is dobutamine-stress echocardiography. Dobutamine is an inotropic agent that increases myocardial oxygen demand by increasing heart rate and contractility. The echocardiogram is used to monitor for ischemia, which is defined as new or worsening wall motion abnormalities during the infusion. Demonstrating improvement in wall thickening with low-dose dobutamine suggests that there is myocardial viability of abnormal segments (i.e., segments that are hypokinetic or akinetic at baseline).

ECHOCARDIOGRAPHY

Echocardiography is a widely used, noninvasive technique in which sound waves are used to image cardiac structures and evaluate blood flow. A piezoelectric crystal housed in a transducer placed on the patient's chest wall produces ultrasound waves. As the sound waves encounter structures with different acoustic properties, some of the ultrasound waves are reflected back to the transducer and recorded. Ultrasound waves emitted from a single, stationary crystal produce an image of a thin slice of the heart (M mode), which can then be followed through time. Steering the ultrasound beam across a 90-degree arc multiple times per second creates two-dimensional imaging (Fig. 5-9). Transthoracic echocardiography is safe, simple, fast, and relatively inexpensive. Hence it is the most commonly used test to assess cardiac size, structure, and function. The development of three-dimensional echocardiographic imaging techniques offers great promise for more accurate measurements of chamber volumes and mass as well as the assessment of geometrically complex anatomy and valvular lesions (**Web Fig. 5-1** shows a three-dimensional image).

Doppler echocardiography allows assessment of both direction and velocity of blood flow within the heart and great vessels. When ultrasound waves encounter moving red blood cells, the energy reflected back to the transducer is altered. The magnitude of this change (Doppler shift) is represented as velocity on the echocardiographic display and can be used to determine whether the blood flow is normal or abnormal (Fig. 5-10). In addition, the velocity of a particular jet of blood can be converted to pressure using the modified Bernoulli equation ($\Delta P \cong 4v^2$). This process allows for the assessment of pressure gradients across valves or between chambers. Color Doppler imaging allows visualization of blood flow through the heart by assigning a color to the red blood cells based on their velocity and direction

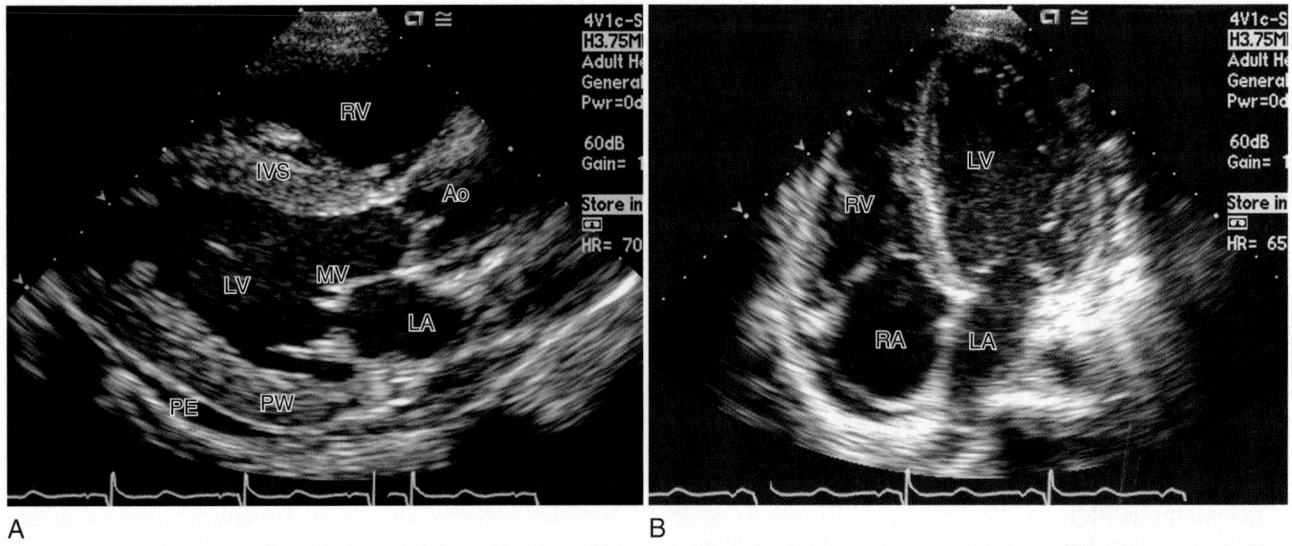

A   B

Figure 5-9 Portions of standard two-dimensional echocardiograms (**A,** parasternal long-axis view; **B,** apical four-chamber view) showing the major cardiac structures. Ao, aorta; IVS, interventricular septum; LA, left atrium; LV, left ventricle; MV, mitral valve; PE, pericardial effusion; PW, posterior LV wall; RV, right ventricle. See **Web Figure 5-3** for a moving image of a two-dimensional echocardiogram. (Image courtesy of Sheldon E. Litwin, MD, Division of Cardiology, University of Utah.)

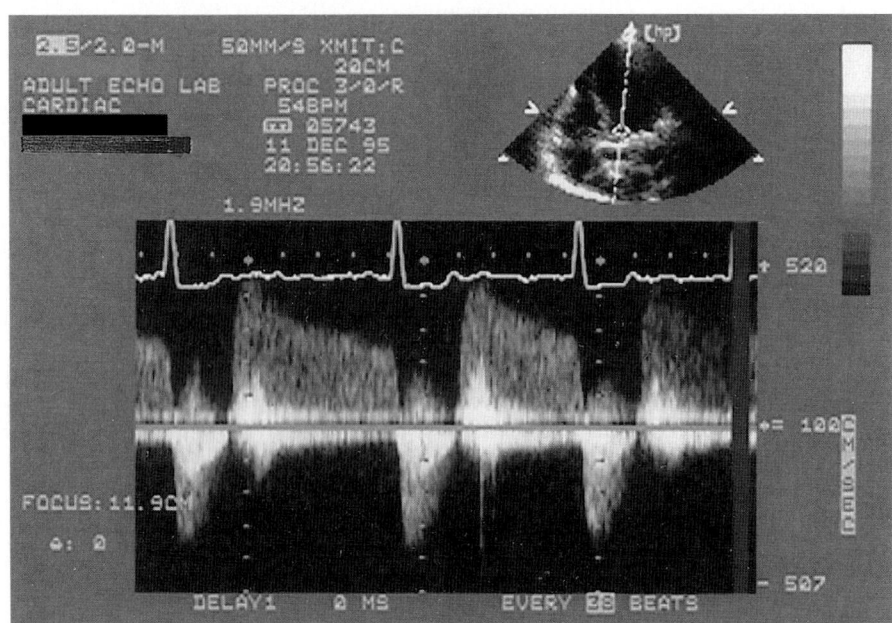

Figure 5-10 Doppler tracing in a patient with aortic stenosis and regurgitation. The velocity of systolic flow is related to the severity of obstruction.

(Fig. 5-11; **Web Fig. 5-2**). By convention, blood moving away from the transducer is represented in shades of blue, and blood moving toward the transducer is represented in red. Color Doppler imaging is particularly useful in identifying valvular insufficiency and abnormal shunt flow between chambers. Recently, the use of Doppler techniques to record myocardial velocities or strain rates has provided new insight into myocardial function and hemodynamics.

Two-dimensional echocardiography and Doppler echocardiography are often used in conjunction with exercise or pharmacologic stress testing. Although variability occurs among studies, the sensitivity of stress echocardiography is apparently slightly lower, but the specificity is slightly higher, compared with myocardial perfusion imaging with nuclear tracers. The overall cost-effectiveness of stress echocardiography is estimated to be significantly better than nuclear perfusion imaging because of the lower cost.

The development of ultrasound contrast agents composed of microbubbles that are small enough to transit through the pulmonary circulation has greatly improved the ability to use ultrasound to image obese patients, patients with lung disease, and those with otherwise difficult acoustic windows (Fig. 5-12; **Web Fig. 5-3** shows a dynamic contrast echocardiographic image). These agents are also being developed as molecular imaging agents by complexing the bubbles to compounds that can selectively bind to the target site of interest (i.e., clots, neovessels).

Transesophageal echocardiography (TEE) allows two-dimensional and Doppler imaging of the heart through the esophagus by having the patient swallow a gastroscope mounted with an ultrasound crystal within its tip. Given the close proximity of the esophagus to the heart, high-resolution images can be obtained, especially of the left atrium, mitral valve apparatus, and aorta. TEE is particularly useful in diagnosing aortic dissection, endocarditis, prosthetic valve dysfunction, and left atrial masses (Fig. 5-13; **Web Fig. 5-4**).

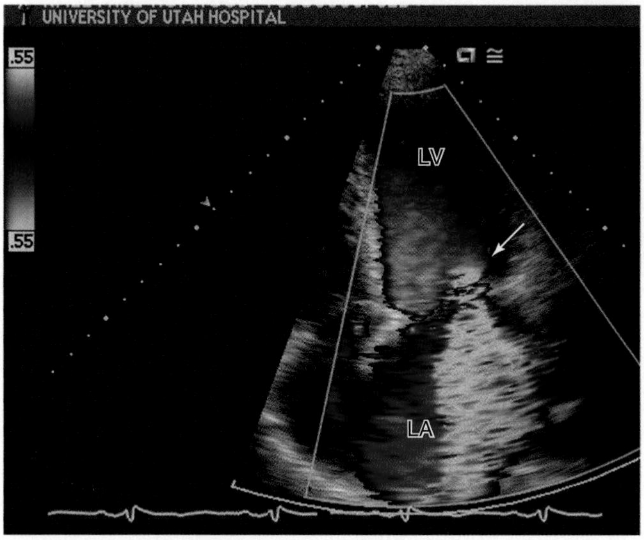

NUCLEAR CARDIOLOGY

Radionuclide imaging of the heart allows quantification of left ventricular size and systolic function as well as myocardial perfusion. With radionuclide ventriculography, the patient's red blood cells are labeled with a small amount of a radioactive tracer (usually technetium-99m). Left ventricular function can then be assessed by one of two methods. With the first-pass technique, radiation emitted by the tagged red blood cells as they initially flow though the heart is detected by a gamma camera positioned over the patient's chest. With the gated equilibrium method, or multigated acquisition (MUGA) method, the tracer is allowed to achieve an equilibrium distribution throughout the blood pool before count acquisition begins. This second method improves the resolution of the ventriculogram. For both techniques, the gamma camera can be gated to the ECG, allowing for determination of the total emitted end-diastole counts (EDC) and end-systole counts (ESC). Left ventricular ejection fraction (LVEF) can then be calculated as follows:

$$LVEF = (EDC - ESC)/EDC$$

If scintigraphic information is collected throughout the cardiac cycle, a computer-generated image of the heart can be displayed in a cinematic fashion, allowing for the assessment of wall motion.

Myocardial perfusion imaging is usually performed in conjunction with exercise or pharmacologic (vasodilator) stress testing. Persantine, or more commonly adenosine, is

Figure 5-11 Color Doppler recording demonstrating severe mitral regurgitation. The regurgitant jet seen in the left atrium (LA) is represented in blue because blood flow is directed away from the transducer. The yellow components are the mosaic pattern traditionally assigned to turbulent or high-velocity flow. The *arrow* points to the hemisphere of blood accelerating proximal to the regurgitant orifice (proximal isovelocity surface area [PISA]). The size of the PISA can be used to help grade the severity of regurgitation. LA, left atrium; LV, left ventricle. See **Web Figure 5-2** for a dynamic echocardiographic image in a patient with mitral regurgitation. (Image courtesy of Sheldon E. Litwin, MD, Division of Cardiology, University of Utah.)

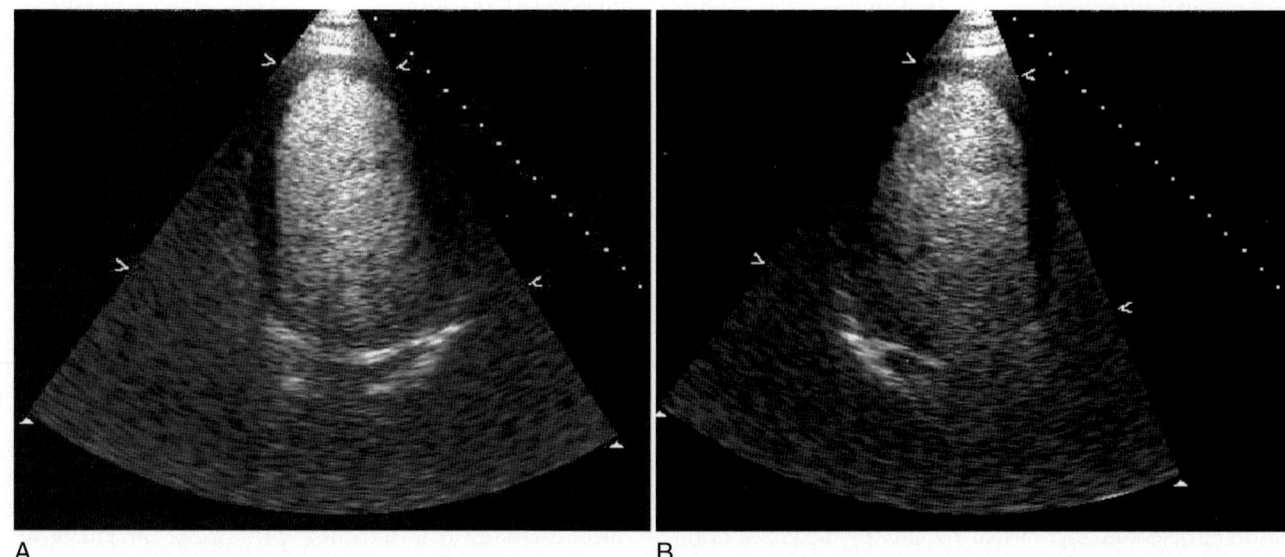

A   B

Figure 5-12 Echocardiogram enhanced with intravenous ultrasound contrast agent (**A**, apical four-chamber view; **B**, apical long-axis view). Highly echo-reflectant microbubbles make the left ventricular cavity appear white, whereas the myocardium appears dark. See **Web Figure 5-3** for a dynamic image of echocardiographic contrast. (Image courtesy of Sheldon E. Litwin, MD, Division of Cardiology, University of Utah.)

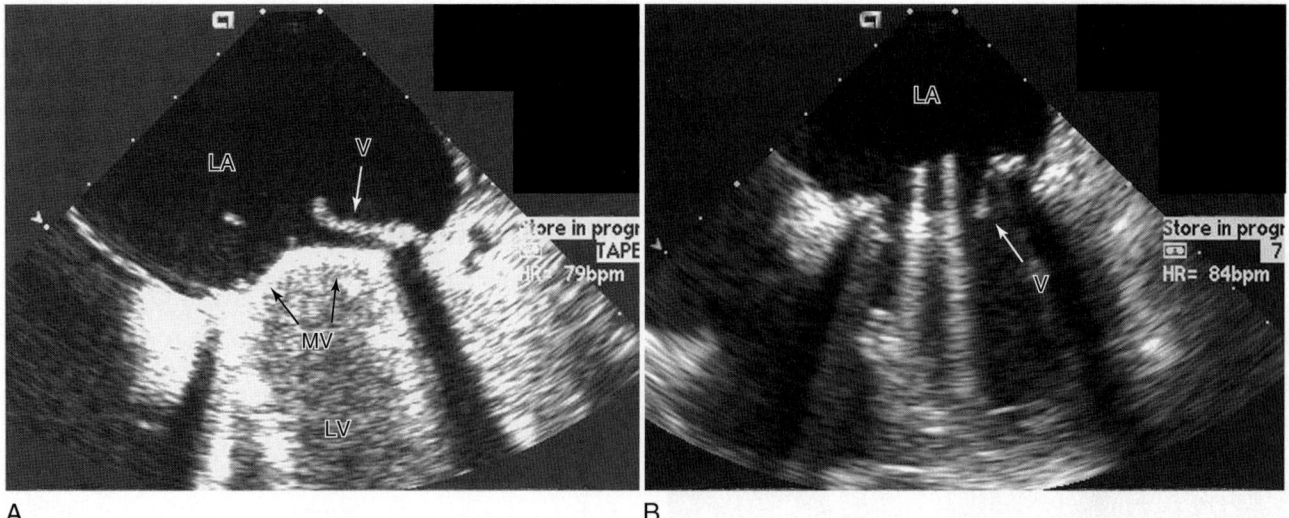

A   B

Figure 5-13 Transesophageal echocardiogram demonstrating the presence of a vegetation adherent to the ring of a bi-leaflet tilting-disk mitral valve prostheses (**A,** systole, leaflets closed with vegetation seen in left atrium; **B,** diastole, leaflets open, vegetation prolapsing into left ventricle). Transesophageal echocardiography is the diagnostic test of choice for assessing prosthetic mitral valves because the esophageal window allows unimpeded views of the atrial surface of the valve. LA, left atrium; LV, left ventricle; MV, prosthetic mitral valve disks; V, vegetation. See **Web Figure 5-4** for a dynamic transesophageal echocardiographic image. (Image courtesy of Sheldon E. Litwin, MD, Division of Cardiology, University of Utah.)

used as the coronary vasodilator. Each agent can increase myocardial blood flow by fourfold to fivefold. Adenosine is more expensive, but has the advantage over Persantine of a very short half-life. Newer adenosine-like agents with reduced side-effect profiles are starting to be used clinically. Technetium-99m sestamibi is the most frequently used radionuclide and is usually injected just before completion of the stress test. Tomographic (single-photon emission computed tomography [SPECT]) images of the heart are obtained for qualitative and quantitative analyses at rest and after stress. In the normal heart, radioisotope is relatively equally distributed throughout the myocardium. In patients with ischemia, a localized area of decreased uptake will occur after exercise but partially or completely fill in at rest (redistribution). A persistent defect at peak exercise and rest (fixed defect) is consistent with MI or scarring. However, in some patients with apparently fixed defects, repeat rest imaging at 24 hours or after reinjection of a smaller quantity of isotope will demonstrate improved uptake, indicating the presence of viable, but severely ischemic, myocardium. The use of new approaches such as combined low-level exercise and vasodilators, prone imaging, attenuation correction, and computerized data analysis has improved the quality and reproducibility of the data from these studies.

Myocardial perfusion imaging may also be combined with ECG-gated image acquisition to allow for simultaneous assessment of ventricular function and perfusion. Not only can LVEF be quantitated with this technique, but also regional wall motion can be assessed to help rule out artifactual perfusion defects (**Web Fig. 5-5**).

Positron-emission tomography (PET) is a noninvasive method of detecting myocardial viability by the use of both perfusion and metabolic tracers. In patients with left ventricular dysfunction, the presence of metabolic activity in a region of myocardium supplied by a severely stenotic coronary artery suggests viable tissue that may regain more

normal function after revascularization (Fig. 5-14). PET is less widely available than conventional SPECT imaging; however, PET offers improved spatial resolution because of the higher energy of the isotopes used for this type of imaging.

CARDIAC CATHETERIZATION

Cardiac catheterization is an invasive technique in which fluid-filled catheters are introduced percutaneously into the arterial and venous circulation. This method allows for the direct measurement of intracardiac pressures and oxygen saturation and, with the injection of a contrast agent, visualization of the coronary arteries, cardiac chambers, and great vessels. Cardiac catheterization is generally indicated when a clinically suggested cardiac abnormality requires confirmation and its anatomic and physiologic importance needs to be quantified. In the current era, coronary angiography for the diagnosis of CAD is the most common indication for this test. Noninvasive testing, compared with catheterization, is safer, cheaper, and equally effective in the evaluation of most valvular and hemodynamic questions. Most often, catheterization will precede some type of beneficial intervention, such as coronary artery angioplasty, coronary bypass surgery, or valvular surgery. Although cardiac catheterization is generally safe (0.1% to 0.2% overall mortality rate), procedure-related complications such as vascular injury, renal failure, stroke, and MI can occur.

An important objective during the cardiac catheterization is to document the filling pressures within the heart and great vessels. This task is accomplished through use of fluid-filled catheters that transmit intracardiac pressures to a transducer that displays the pressure waveform on an oscilloscope. During a right ventricular heart catheterization, pressures within the right atrium, right ventricle, and pulmonary artery are routinely measured in this manner. The

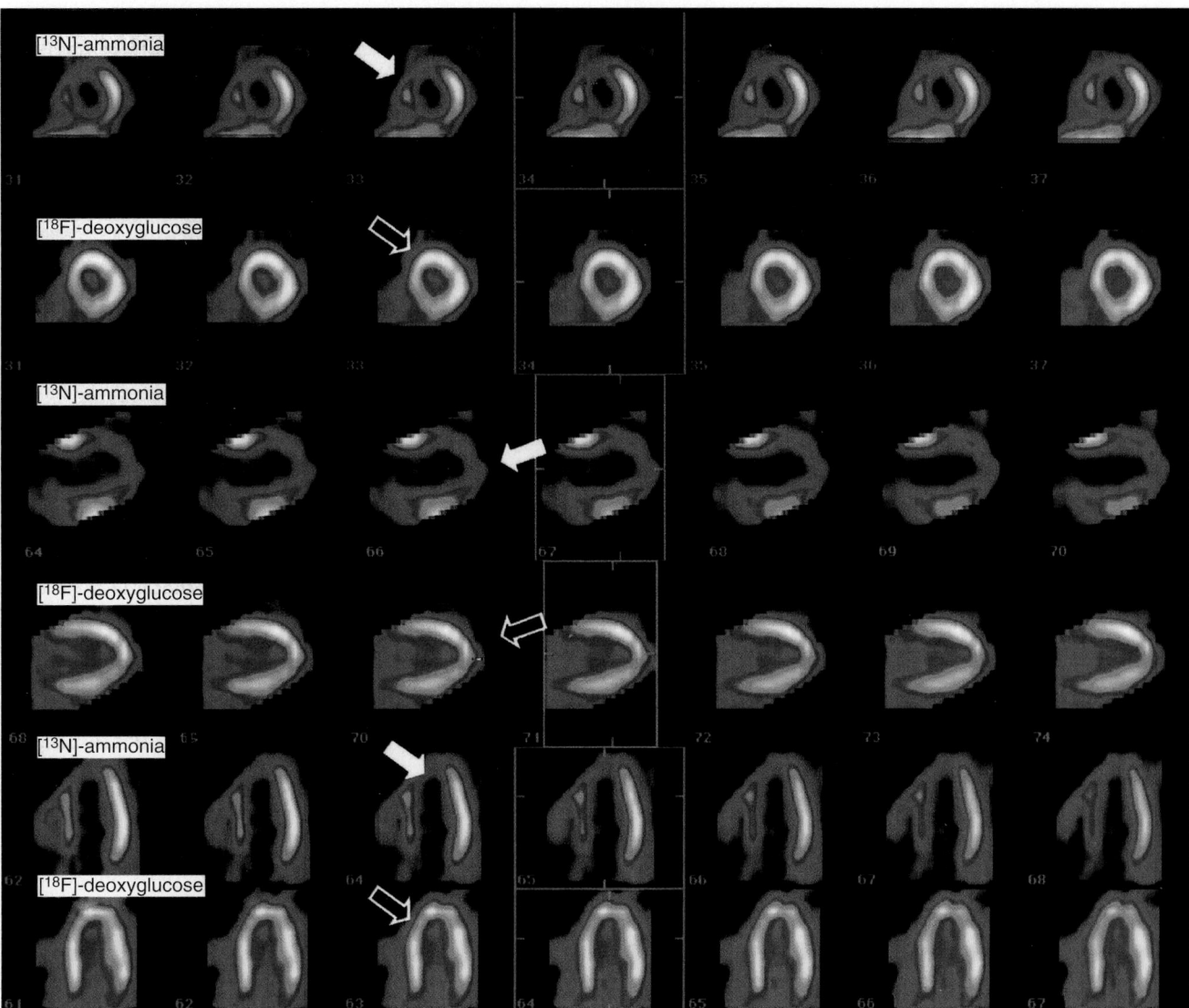

Figure 5-14 Resting myocardial perfusion (obtained with [^{13}N]-ammonia) and metabolism (obtained with [^{18}F]-deoxyglucose) Positron-emission tomography images of a patient with ischemic cardiomyopathy. The study demonstrates a perfusion-metabolic mismatch (reflecting hibernating myocardium) in which large areas of hypoperfused *(solid arrows)* but metabolically viable *(open arrows)* myocardium are involving the anterior, septal, and inferior walls and the left ventricular apex. See **Web Figure 5-5** for a dynamic image obtained with cardiac single-photon emission computed tomography imaging. (Courtesy of Marcelo F. Di Carli, MD, Brigham and Women's Hospital, Boston.)

catheter can then be advanced further until it *wedges* in the distal pulmonary artery. The transmitted pressure measured in this location originates from the pulmonary venous system and is known as the *pulmonary capillary wedge pressure.* In the absence of pulmonary venous disease, the pulmonary capillary wedge pressure reflects left atrial pressure and, similarly, if no significant mitral valve pathologic condition exists, reflects left ventricular diastolic pressure. A more direct method of obtaining left ventricular filling pressures is to advance an arterial catheter into the left ventricular cavity. With these two methods of obtaining intracardiac pressures, each chamber of the heart can be assessed and the gradients across any of the valves determined (Fig. 5-15).

Cardiac output can be determined by one of two widely accepted methods: the Fick oxygen method and the indicator dilution technique. The basis of the Fick method

is that total uptake or release of a substance by an organ is equal to the product of blood flow to that organ and the concentration difference of that substance between the arterial and venous circulation of that organ. If this method is applied to the lungs, the substance released into the blood is oxygen; if no intrapulmonary shunts exist, pulmonary blood flow is equal to systemic blood flow or cardiac output. Thus the cardiac output can be determined by the following equation:

$$\text{Cardiac output} = \text{oxygen consumption}/(\text{arterial oxygen content} - \text{venous oxygen content})$$

Oxygen consumption is measured in milliliters per minute by collecting the patient's expired air over a known period while simultaneously measuring oxygen saturation in a

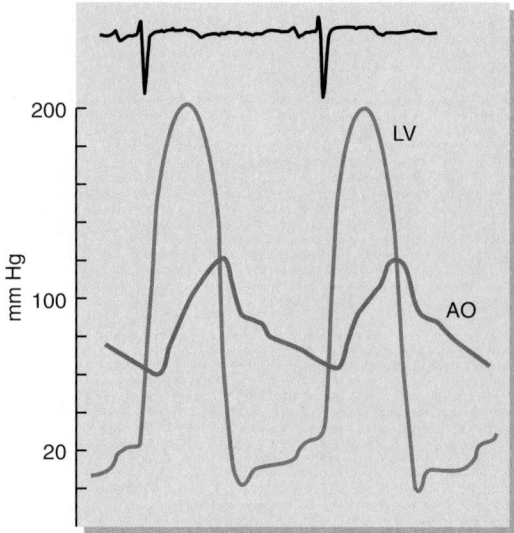

Figure 5-15 Electrocardiographic and left ventricular (LV) and aortic (AO) pressure curves in a patient with aortic stenosis. A pressure gradient occurs across the aortic valve during systole.

sample of arterial and mixed venous blood (arterial and venous oxygen content, respectively, measured in milliliters per liter). The cardiac output is expressed in liters per minute and then corrected for body surface area (cardiac index). The normal range of cardiac index is 2.6 to 4.2 L/min/m². Cardiac output can also be determined by the indicator dilution technique, which most commonly uses cold saline as the indicator. With this method, cold saline is injected into the blood, and the resulting temperature change *downstream* is monitored. This action generates a curve in which temperature change is plotted over time, and the area under the curve represents cardiac output.

Detection and localization of intracardiac shunts can be performed by sequential measurement of oxygen saturation in the venous system, right side of the heart, and two main pulmonary arteries. In patients with left-to-right shunt flow, an increase in the oxygen saturation, or *step-up*, will occur as one sample from the chamber where arterial blood is mixing with venous blood. By using the Fick method for calculating blood flow in the pulmonary and systemic systems, the shunt ratio can be calculated. Noninvasive approaches have large supplanted catheterization laboratory assessment of shunts.

Left ventricular size, wall motion, and ejection fraction can be accurately assessed by injecting contrast into the left ventricle (left ventriculography). Aortic and mitral valve insufficiency can be qualitatively assessed during angiography by observing the reflux of contrast medium into the left ventricle and left atrium, respectively. The degree of valvular stenosis can be determined by measuring pressure gradients across the valve and determining cardiac output (Gorlin formula).

The coronary anatomy can be defined by injecting contrast medium into the coronary tree. Atherosclerotic lesions appear as narrowing of the internal diameter (lumen) of the vessel. A hemodynamically important stenosis is defined as 70% or more narrowing of the luminal diameter. However, the hemodynamic significance of a lesion can be underesti-

mated by coronary angiography, particularly in settings in which the atherosclerotic plaque is eccentric or elongated. Use of intravascular ultrasound, Doppler flow wires, or miniaturized pressure sensors can be used during invasive procedures to help evaluate the severity or estimate the physiologic significance of intermediate lesions.

Biopsy of the ventricular endomyocardium can be performed during cardiac catheterization. With this technique, a bioptome is introduced into the venous system through the right internal jugular vein and guided into the right ventricle by fluoroscopy. Small samples of the endocardium are then taken for histologic evaluation. The primary indication for endomyocardial biopsy is the diagnosis of rejection after cardiac transplantation and documentation of cardiac amyloidosis; however, endomyocardial biopsy may have some use in diagnosing specific etiologic agents responsible for myocarditis.

RIGHT VENTRICULAR HEART CATHETERIZATION

A right ventricular heart catheterization can be performed at the bedside with a balloon-tipped pulmonary artery (Swan-Ganz) catheter. This technique allows for serial measurements of right atrial, pulmonary artery, and pulmonary capillary wedge pressures as well as cardiac output by thermodilution (Fig. 5-16). Such measurements may be useful in monitoring the response to various treatments, such as diuretic therapy, inotropic agents, and vasopressors (Table 5-4). The pulmonary artery catheter is most useful in the critically ill patient for assessing volume status and differentiating cardiogenic from noncardiogenic pulmonary edema. Notably, however, several papers have suggested no improvements in outcomes of critically ill patients in whom pulmonary artery catheterization was performed. Improvements in noninvasive imaging techniques have made the pulmonary artery catheter much less important in diagnosing cardiac conditions, such as pericardial tamponade, constrictive pericarditis, right ventricular infarction, and ventricular septal defect.

MAGNETIC RESONANCE IMAGING

Magnetic resonance angiography or imaging (MRI) is an increasingly used noninvasive method for studying the heart and vasculature, especially in patients who have contraindications to standard contrast angiography. MRI offers high-resolution dynamic and static images of the heart that can be obtained in any plane. Good-quality images can be obtained in a higher number of subjects than is typically possible with echocardiography. Obesity, claustrophobia, inability to perform multiple breath-holds of 10 to 20 seconds, and arrhythmias are all causes of reduced image quality. Currently, the presence of cardiac pacemakers or implantable defibrillators is considered a contraindication for MRI. Magnetic resonance angiography is useful in the evaluation of cerebral, renovascular, and lower extremity arterial disease. MRI offers significant advantages over other imaging techniques for the characterization of different tissues (e.g., muscle, fat, scar). MRI is useful in the evaluation of ischemic heart disease because stress-rest myocardial perfusion (Fig. 5-17A) and areas of prior infarction

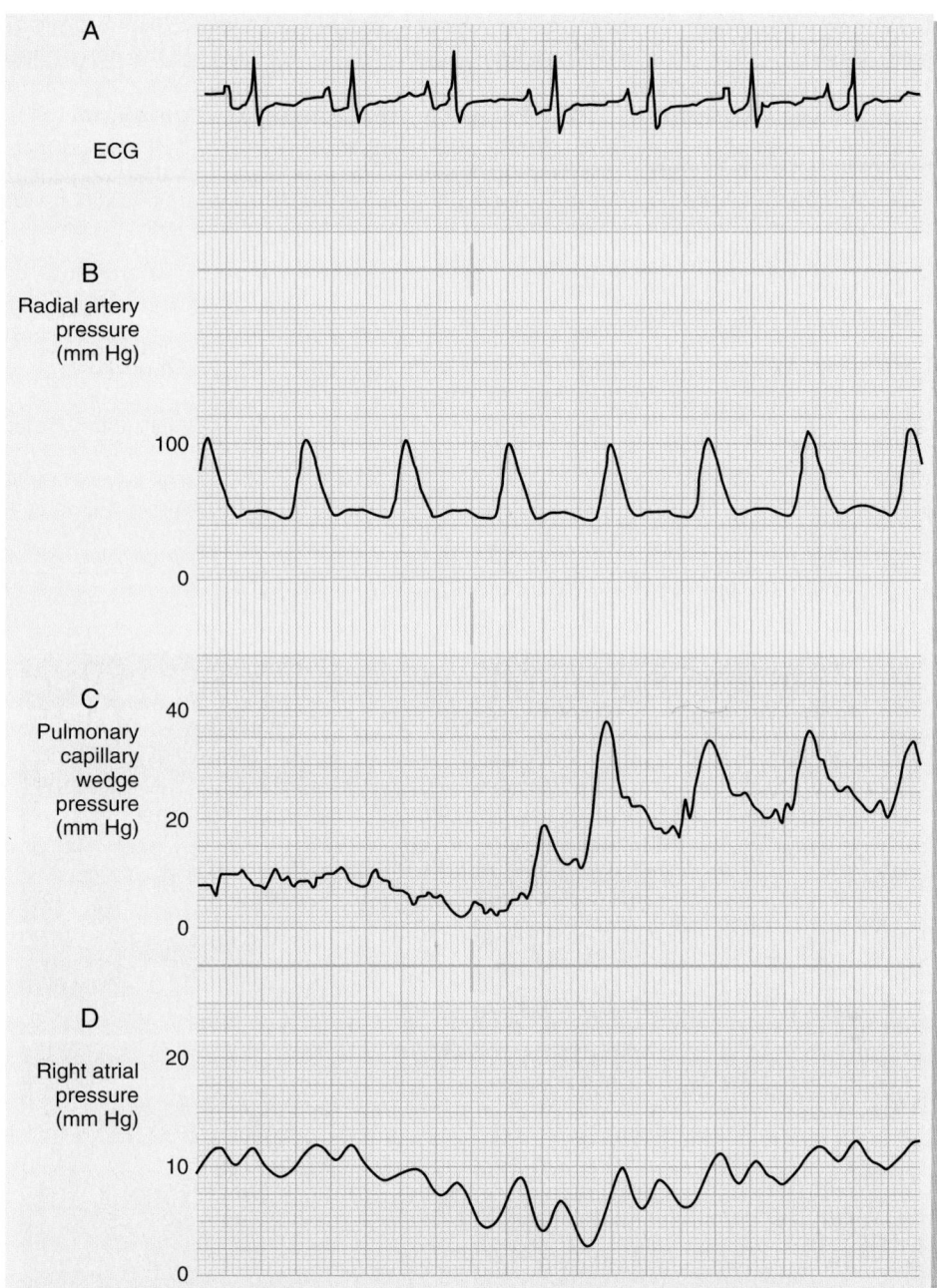

Figure 5-16 Electrocardiographic (ECG) and Swan-Ganz flotation catheter recordings are shown in tracings A and C, respectively. The left portion of tracing C was obtained with the balloon inflated, yielding the pulmonary arterial wedge pressure. The right portion of tracing C was recorded with the balloon deflated, depicting the pulmonary arterial pressure. In this patient, the pulmonary arterial wedge pressure (left ventricular filling pressure) is normal, and the pulmonary artery pressure is elevated because of lung disease.

(see Fig. 5-17B to D) can be visualized with excellent special resolution. The presence of delayed gadolinium contrast enhancement within the myocardium is characteristic of scar or permanently damaged tissue (**Web Fig. 5-6**). The greater the transmural extent of delayed enhancement in a given segment, the lower is the likelihood of improved function in that segment after revascularization. Because of the better spatial resolution, delayed enhancement imaging can depict localized or subendocardial scars that are not detectable with nuclear imaging techniques. The combined use of stress-rest perfusion and delayed enhancement imaging

has performance characteristics for diagnosing CAD that are at least as good as, and probably superior to, those of conventional stress tests using nuclear scintigraphy or echocardiography. MRI is excellent for evaluating a variety of cardiomyopathies (Fig. 5-18). In addition to morphology and function, characteristic patterns of delayed enhancement have been reported in myocarditis, hypertrophic cardiomyopathy, and cardiac amyloidosis. MRI has also been used to help assess right ventricular morphology and function in patients with suspected arrhythmogenic right ventricular cardiomyopathy.

Table 5-4 **Differential Diagnosis Using a Bedside Balloon Flow-Directed (Swan-Ganz) Catheter**

Disease State	Thermodilution Cardiac Output	PCW Pressure	RA Pressure	Comments
Cardiogenic shock	↓	↑	nl or ↓	↑ Systemic vascular resistance
Septic shock (early)	↑	↓	↓	↑ Systemic vascular resistance; myocardial dysfunction can occur late
Volume overload	nl or ↑	↑	↑	—
Volume depletion	↓	↓	↓	—
Noncardiac pulmonary edema	nl	nl	nl	—
Pulmonary heart disease	nl or ↑	nl	↑	↑ PA pressure
RV infarction	↓	↓ or nl	↑	—
Pericardial tamponade	↓	nl or ↑	↑	Equalization of diastolic RA, RV, PA, and PCW pressure
Papillary muscle rupture	↓	↑	nl or ↑	Large v waves in PCW tracing
Ventricular septal rupture	↑	↑	nl or ↑	Artifact caused by RA → PA sampling higher in PA than RA; may have large v waves in PCW tracing

↑, Increased; ↓, decreased; nl, normal; PA, pulmonary artery; PCW, pulmonary capillary wedge; RA, right atrium; RV, right ventricle.

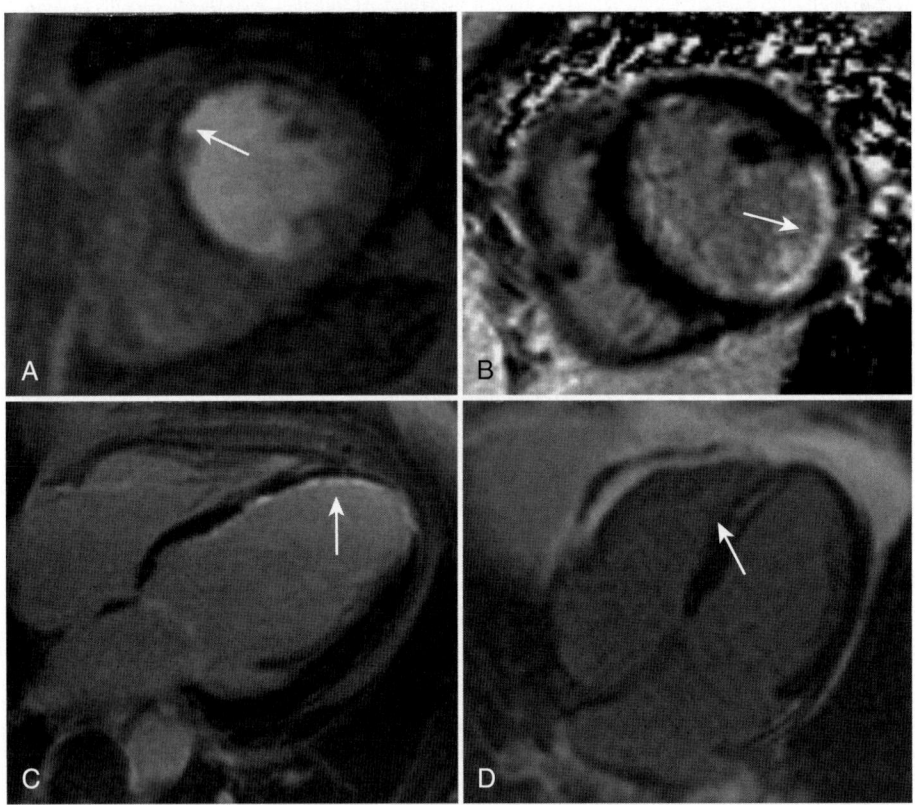

Figure 5-17 Cardiac magnetic resonance imaging (MRI) showing use of cardiac MRI in evaluation of cardiomyopathies. **A,** Severe left ventricular hypertrophy in a patient with hypertrophic cardiomyopathy. Diastolic frame shows open mitral valve. **B,** Systolic frame showing systolic anterior motion of mitral valve with flow disturbance in left ventricular outflow tract. **C,** Patient with left ventricular noncompaction as evidenced by deep trabeculations in the left ventricular apex. **D,** Patient with ischemic cardiomyopathy who has transmural apical infarction and adjacent mural thrombus. See **Web Figure 5-6** for a dynamic cardiac MRI image. (Images courtesy of Sheldon E. Litwin, MD, Division of Cardiology, University of Utah.)

COMPUTED TOMOGRAPHY OF THE HEART

New applications of computed tomography (CT) have greatly advanced our ability to diagnose cardiovascular disease noninvasively. The development of fast gantry rotation speeds and the addition of multiple rows of detectors (multidetector CT) has allowed unprecedented visualization of the great vessels, heart, and coronary arteries with images acquired during a single breath-hold (10 to 15 seconds). Until recently, CT has been used most frequently to diagnose aortic aneurysm and acute aortic dissection and pulmonary embolism. CT is also useful for defining con-

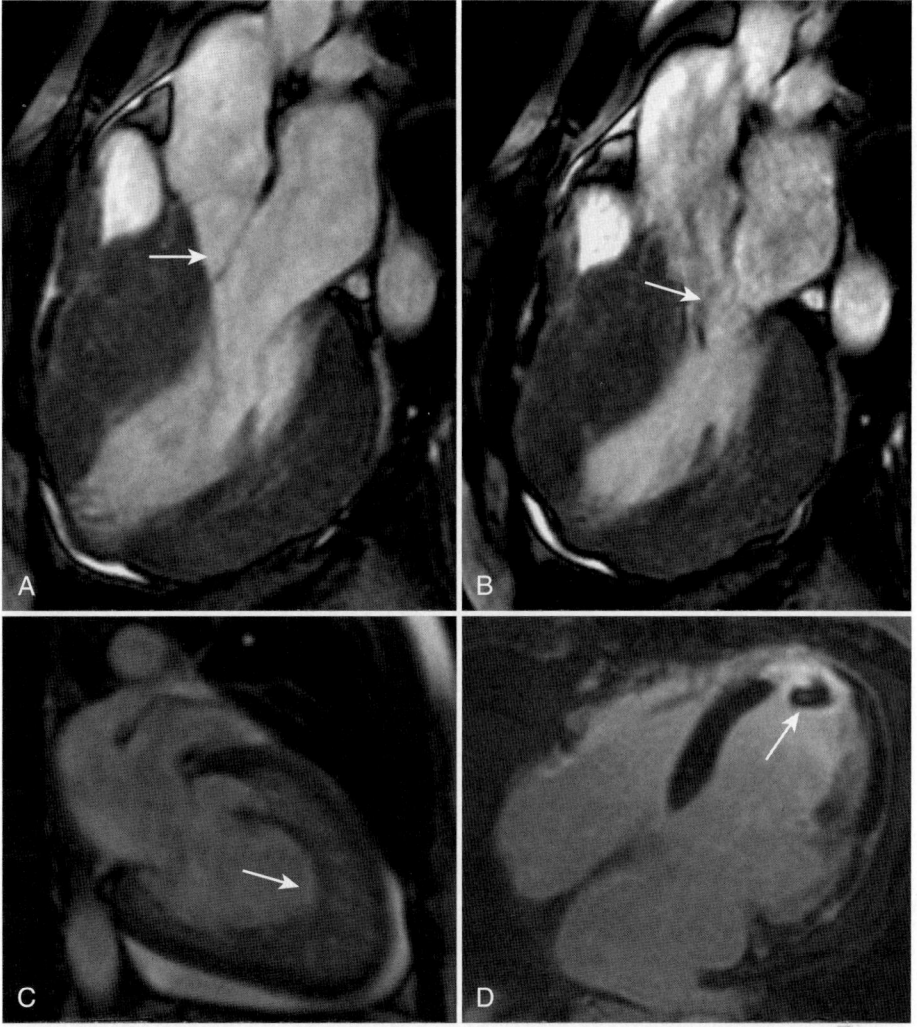

Figure 5-18 Use of cardiac magnetic resonance imaging in the evaluation of chest pain or ischemic heart disease. **A,** First-pass perfusion study during vasodilator stress showing large septal perfusion defect. The hypoperfused area appears dark compared with the myocardium with normal perfusion. **B,** Example of delayed enhancement imaging with nearly transmural infarction of the mid-inferolateral wall, including the posterior papillary muscle. Infarcted myocardium appears white, whereas normal myocardium is black. **C,** Nontransmural (subendocardial) infarction of the septum and apex. **D,** Patient with acute myocarditis mimicking an acute coronary syndrome. Mid-myocardial, rather than subendocardial, delayed enhancement is characteristic of myocarditis.

genital abnormalities and detecting pericardial thickening or calcification associated with constrictive pericarditis. More recently, ECG-gated dynamic CT images have been used to quantify ventricular size, function, and regional wall motion (**Web Fig. 5-7**), and in contrast to echocardiography, CT is not limited by the presence of lung disease or chest wall deformity. However, obesity and the presence of prosthetic materials (i.e., mechanical valves or pacing wires) may affect image quality.

The greatest excitement and controversy over cardiac CT relates to the evaluation of coronary atherosclerosis. Electron-beam and multidetector CT scans can be used to quickly and reliably visualize and quantitate the extent of coronary artery calcification (Fig. 5-19). The presence of coronary calcium is pathognomonic of atherosclerosis, and the extent of coronary calcium (usually reported as an Agatston score) is a powerful marker of future cardiac events. The coronary calcium score adds substantial, independent

improvement in risk prediction to the commonly employed clinical risk scores (e.g., the Framingham risk score). Although the extent of coronary artery calcification does not reliably predict the severity of stenoses, the calcium score is a good marker of the overall atherosclerotic burden. Contrast-enhanced coronary computed tomographic angiography (CTA) has improved dramatically in recent years. Coronary CTA has been reported to have a sensitivity of more than 95% in diagnosing significant coronary artery obstruction. This is superior to the sensitivity of stress echo or nuclear myocardial perfusion scanning. Given the speed and accuracy of this test, it is likely to assume a major role in the evaluation of patients with acute chest pain syndromes. Some advocates of cardiac CT have proposed the use of this test for the *triple rule-out* in patients with acute chest pain—namely, the ability to diagnose pulmonary embolism, aortic dissection, and coronary artery disease with one imaging study. Formal evaluation of this hypoth-

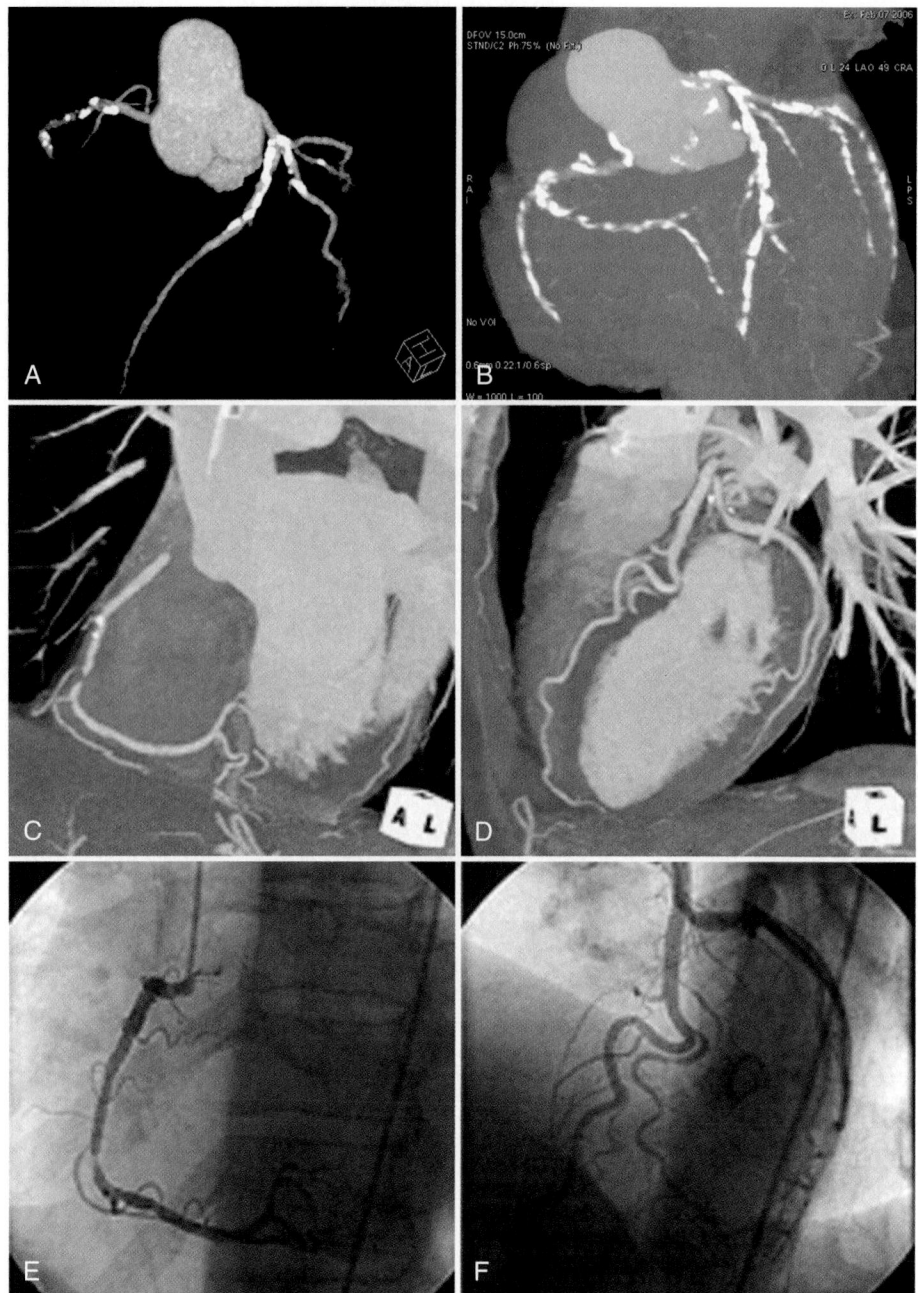

Figure 5-19 Computed tomographic coronary angiography compared with conventional radiographic contrast angiography. **A** and **B,** Volume-rendering technique demonstrating stenosis of the right coronary artery and normal left coronary artery. **C** and **D,** Maximal intensity projection of the same arteries demonstrating severe noncalcified plaque in the right coronary artery with superficial calcified plaque. **E** and **F,** Invasive angiography of the same arteries. (From Raff GL, Gallagher MJ, O'Neill WW, et al: Diagnostic accuracy of noninvasive coronary angiography using 64-slice spiral computed tomography. J Am Coll Cardiol 46:552, 2005.)

esis still needs to be undertaken. Detractors of cardiac CT most frequently cite the risks of radiation and contrast exposure as well as a lack of prospective studies showing improvement in outcome with this testing modality. Of note, the calculated radiation exposure of a cardiac CTA is about double that of a diagnostic invasive coronary angiogram, but is similar to that of a typical nuclear myocardial perfusion scan. As of this writing, the future role of cardiac CTA in routine clinical practice remains uncertain.

NONINVASIVE VASCULAR TESTING

Assessment for the presence and severity of peripheral vascular disease is an important component of the cardiovascular evaluation. Comparison of the systolic blood pressure in the upper and lower extremities is one of the simplest tests to detect the presence of hemodynamically important arterial disease. Normally, the systolic pressure in the thigh is similar to that in the brachial artery. An ankle-to-brachial pressure ratio (ankle-brachial index) of less than or equal to 0.9 is abnormal. Patients with claudication usually have an index ranging from 0.5 to 0.8, and patients with rest pain have an index less than 0.5. In some patients, measuring the ankle-brachial index after treadmill exercise may be helpful in identifying the importance of borderline lesions. During normal exercise, blood flow increases to the upper and lower extremities and decreases in peripheral vascular resistance, whereas the ankle-brachial index remains unchanged. In the presence of a hemodynamically significant lesion, the increase in systolic blood pressure in the arm is not matched by an increase in blood pressure in the leg. As a result, the ankle-brachial index will decrease, the magnitude of which is proportional to the severity of the stenosis.

After significant vascular disease in the extremities has been identified, plethysmography can be used to determine the location and severity of the disease. With this method, a pneumatic cuff is positioned on the leg or thigh and, when inflated, temporarily obstructs venous return. Volume changes in the limb segment below the cuff are converted to a pressure waveform, which can then be analyzed. The degree of amplitude reduction in the pressure waveform corresponds to the severity of arterial disease at that level.

Doppler ultrasound uses reflected sound waves to identify and localize stenotic lesions in the peripheral arteries. This test is particularly useful in patients with severely calcified arteries, in whom pneumatic compression is not possible and ankle-brachial indices are inaccurate. In combination with real-time imaging (duplex imaging), this technique is useful in assessing specific arterial segments and bypass grafts for stenotic or occlusive lesions.

Both magnetic resonance angiography and CTA allow high-quality and comprehensive imaging of the entire peripheral arterial circulation in a single study. The three-dimensional nature of these studies and their ability to perform extensive postprocessing views (including cross-sectional views) of any vessel, even those that are very tortuous, are attractive features of these modalities.

Prospectus for the Future

Multidisciplinary teams consisting of cardiologists, cardiac surgeons, vascular surgeons, and radiologists will replace existing and traditional approaches for the evaluation and management of patients with cardiac disease. Such collaboration will foster efficiency and rapid advances for improvements in patient care, education, and research within a seamless, integrated environment. Career opportunities within organizations with the supporting infrastructure for cardiac imaging will likely realize the promise for patient-oriented, team-based cardiovascular medicine. Tissue enhancement using MRI of either the atria or ventricles will assist practitioners with classification and forecasting of outcomes after interventions such as ablation for atrial fibrillation.

References

Cheitlin MD, Armstrong WF, Aurigemma GP, et al: ACC/AHA/ASE 2003 guideline update for the clinical application of echocardiography—summary article: A report of the American College of Cardiology/American Heart Association Task Force on Practice Guidelines (ACC/AHA/ASE Committee to Update the 1997 Guidelines for the Clinical Application of Echocardiography). J Am Soc Echocardiogr 16:1091-1110, 2003.

Eagle KA, Berger PB, Calkins H, et al: ACC/AHA guideline update for perioperative cardiovascular evaluation for noncardiac surgery—executive summary: A report of the American College of Cardiology/American Heart Association Task Force on Practice Guidelines (Committee to Update the 1996 Guidelines on Perioperative Cardiovascular Evaluation of Noncardiac Surgery). Circulation 105:1257-1267, 2002.

Gibbons RJ, Abrams J, Chatterjee K, et al: ACC/AHA 2002 guideline update for the management of patients with chronic stable angina—summary article: A report of the American College of Cardiology/American Heart Association Task Force on Practice Guidelines (Committee on the Management of Patients with Chronic Stable Angina). Circulation 107:149-158, 2003.

Gibbons RJ, Balady GJ, Bricker JT, et al: ACC/AHA 2002 guideline update for exercise testing—summary article: A report of the American College of Cardiology/American Heart Association Task Force on Practice Guidelines (Committee to Update the 1997 Exercise Testing Guidelines). J Am Coll Cardiol 40:1531-1540, 2002.

Klein C, Nekolla SG: Assessment of myocardial viability with contrast-enhanced magnetic resonance imaging: Comparison with positron emission tomography. Circulation 105:162-167, 2002.

Morey SS: ACC and AHA update guidelines for coronary angiography. American College of Cardiology. American Heart Association. Am Fam Physician 60:1017-1020, 1999.

Raff GL, Goldstein JA: Coronary angiography by computed tomography. J Am Coll Cardiol 49:1830-1833, 2007.

Sandham JD, Hull RD, Brant RF, et al: A randomized, controlled trial of the use of pulmonary artery catheters in high-risk surgical patients. N Engl J Med 348:5-14, 2003.

Chapter **6**

Heart Failure and Cardiomyopathy

Sheldon E. Litwin and Ivor J. Benjamin

The syndrome of heart failure occurs when an abnormality of cardiac function results in failure to provide adequate blood flow to meet the metabolic needs of the body's tissues and organs or in an excessive rise in cardiac filling pressures. In most cases, myocardial dysfunction causes impaired ventricular filling, as well as emptying. Heart failure can result from a large number of heterogeneous disorders (Table 6-1). Idiopathic cardiomyopathy is defined as a primary abnormality of myocardial tissue in the absence of coronary occlusive, valvular, or systemic disease. However, in the clinical setting, the term *cardiomyopathy* is often used to refer to myocardial dysfunction that is the result of a known genetic, cardiac, or systemic disease. These *secondary* cardiomyopathies may be related to a significant number of disorders, but in the United States, they are most often the result of ischemic heart disease. Ventricular dysfunction can also result from excessive pressure overload, such as with long-standing hypertension or aortic stenosis, or volume overload, such as aortic insufficiency or mitral regurgitation. Diseases that result in infiltration and replacement of normal myocardial tissue, such as amyloidosis, are rare causes of heart failure. Hemochromatosis can cause a dilated cardiomyopathy that is believed to result from iron-mediated mitochondrial damage. Diseases of the pericardium, such as chronic pericarditis or pericardial tamponade, can impair cardiac function without directly affecting the myocardial tissue. Long-standing tachyarrhythmias have been associated with myocardial dysfunction that is often reversible. In addition, an individual with underlying myocardial or valvular disease may develop heart failure with the acute onset of an arrhythmia. Finally, multiple metabolic abnormalities (e.g., thiamine deficiency, thyrotoxicosis), drugs (e.g., alcohol, doxorubicin), and toxic chemicals (e.g., lead, cobalt) can damage the myocardium.

Forms of Heart Failure

Heart failure can be classified as predominantly left or right sided, high output or low output, and acute or chronic. High-output failure is an uncommon disorder that can occur with severe anemia, vascular shunting, or thyrotoxicosis. This failure results when the heart is unable to meet the abnormally elevated metabolic demands of the peripheral tissues even though cardiac output is elevated. Fluid retention is a common component of this syndrome. Low-output failure is much more common than high-output failure and is characterized by insufficient forward output, particularly during times of increased metabolic demand. Cardiac dysfunction may predominantly affect the left ventricle, as with a large myocardial infarction, or the right ventricle, as with an acute pulmonary embolus; however, in many disease states, both ventricles will be impaired (biventricular heart failure). *Acute heart failure* usually refers to the situation in which an individual who was previously asymptomatic develops heart failure signs or symptoms following an acute injury to the heart, such as myocardial infarction, myocarditis, or rupture of a heart valve. *Chronic heart failure* refers to the situation in which an individual whose symptoms have developed over a long period, most often when preexisting cardiac disease is present. However, a patient with myocardial dysfunction from any cause may be well compensated for long periods and then develop acute heart failure symptoms in the setting of arrhythmia, anemia, hypertension, ischemia or infection.

The severity of heart failure symptoms does not correlate closely with the usual clinical measures of cardiac function (i.e., left ventricular ejection fraction [LVEF]), although the LVEF is a good prognostic marker. This situation likely reflects the fact that ventricular filling pressures are a more important determinant of symptoms than myocardial

Table 6-1 **Causes of Congestive Heart Failure and Cardiomyopathy**

Coronary Artery Disease

Acute ischemia
Myocardial infarction
Ischemic cardiomyopathy with hibernating myocardium

Idiopathic

Idiopathic dilated cardiomyopathy*
Idiopathic restrictive cardiomyopathy
Peripartum

Pressure Overload

Hypertension
Aortic stenosis

Volume Overload

Mitral regurgitation
Aortic insufficiency
Anemia
Atrioventricular fistula

Toxins

Ethanol
Cocaine
Doxorubicin (Adriamycin)
Methamphetamine

Metabolic-Endocrine

Thiamine deficiency
Diabetes
Hemochromatosis
Thyrotoxicosis
Obesity
Hemochromatosis

Infiltrative

Amyloidosis

Inflammatory

Viral myocarditis

Hereditary

Hypertrophic
Dilated

*Genetic bases for these cardiomyopathies have been identified in a large number of individual patients and families. Most of the mutations have been found in cardiac contractile or structural proteins.

function per se. Heart failure may occur in the setting of a reduced or preserved ejection fraction (EF). Recent data suggest that when sensitive methods for assessing myocardial function (i.e., tissue velocity or strain rate imaging) are used, changes are usually detected in both systolic and diastolic function in patients with heart failure (even when the EF is normal or near normal). Importantly, the predisposing conditions for heart failure (e.g., hypertension, advanced age, coronary artery disease, renal dysfunction) are similar, the prognosis is similar irrespective of whether the LVEF is preserved or reduced. Despite many similarities, medical treatments that have been proved beneficial in heart failure with reduced EF have not shown similar efficacy in heart failure with preserved ejection fraction.

ACUTE PULMONARY EDEMA

In patients with the acute onset of pulmonary edema, initial management should be directed at improving oxygenation and providing hemodynamic stability. These patients commonly have marked elevation of blood pressure, cardiac ischemia, and worsening mitral regurgitation as contributing factors to the pulmonary edema. Standard therapy includes supplemental oxygen and an intravenous loop diuretic. Sublingual or intravenous nitroglycerin helps reduce preload through venodilation and may provide symptomatic relief in patients with ischemic and nonischemic ventricular dysfunction. Intravenous morphine acts in a similar manner but must be used with caution, given its depressive effects on respiratory drive. In patients with hypertensive urgency, severe hypertension, or congestive heart failure related to aortic or mitral regurgitation, an arterial vasodilator, such as nitroprusside, may be helpful in reducing afterload.

Evaluation of the patient's response to treatment requires frequent assessments of blood pressure, heart rate, end-organ perfusion, and oxygen saturation. In patients with persistent hypoxia or respiratory acidosis, mechanical ventilation or external ventilatory support may be necessary. Pulmonary artery catheterization may be helpful in documenting filling pressures, cardiac output, and peripheral vascular resistance and in monitoring the response to therapy, although invasive monitoring has not been associated with improved patient outcomes. In patients with refractory pulmonary edema or systemic hypotension, an inotropic agent, an intra-aortic balloon pump, or a ventricular assist device may be necessary.

HEART FAILURE WITH PRESERVED EJECTION FRACTION

Slowed relaxation of the left ventricle and increased chamber stiffness impair ventricular filling and may contribute to elevated left ventricular, left atrial, and pulmonary venous pressures. Diastolic filling abnormalities contribute to heart failure symptoms in most patients with reduced left ventricular function. However, some patients with a diagnosis of heart failure have normal or *nearly normal* EF. These patients have been commonly labeled as having *diastolic heart failure*. As described earlier in this chapter, newer imaging techniques have revealed that most of these patients also have a component of systolic dysfunction as well. Thus, the term *heart failure with preserved EF* is now the preferred terminology to describe this condition.

Relaxation abnormalities are present in most people older than 65 years and are almost universal after age 75 years; however, most of these individuals do not have heart failure. Thus, isolated abnormalities of left ventricular relaxation are apparently not sufficient to directly cause heart failure in the absence of other predisposing conditions.

In patients with a variety of cardiovascular diseases, relaxation abnormalities appear at earlier ages than would otherwise be expected. As of this writing, no therapeutic agents that specifically target impaired relaxation have been developed. β–Receptor agonists (dobutamine) and phosphodiesterase inhibitors (milrinone) have potent lusitropic effects (improve relaxation); however, they also directly increase contractility and enhance myocyte calcium cycling. Chronic β-blocker therapy is associated with parallel improvements in systolic and diastolic function, even though both of these may actually deteriorate during the early phases of treatment. Although calcium channel blockers have been proposed as therapy for diastolic abnormalities, little evidence supports their use for this purpose. Moreover, calcium entry into cardiac myocytes through L-type calcium channels occurs almost exclusively during systole; thus, the theoretical basis for their use is also not firm. In general, all therapies that result in improved systolic function also tend to improve diastolic function, or at least diastolic filling pressures. The use of diuretics to control volume overload and the vigorous treatment of hypertension are the mainstay of therapy for this condition.

RESYNCHRONIZATION THERAPY

Interventricular conduction delays, demonstrated as a prolonged QRS duration, are a common complication in patients with heart failure and have been associated with reduced exercise capacity and a poor long-term prognosis. Biventricular pacing or resynchronization therapy results in more normal ventricular contraction and has been associated with an improvement in cardiac output and LVEF. Biventricular pacing may have a beneficial effect on left ventricular remodeling by reducing left ventricular volume, left ventricular mass, and severity of mitral regurgitation. Clinically, these hemodynamic and structural changes have translated into an improvement in exercise duration, functional capacity, and quality of life. Biventricular pacing has also been shown to reduce mortality. Unfortunately, up to 30% of patients undergoing biventricular pacemaker placements do not respond favorably to the treatment. At present, this therapy is generally reserved for patients with severe heart failure and a widened QRS complex who remain symptomatic despite optimal pharmacologic therapy. Intense research efforts are underway to identify with increased accuracy the patients who are likely to derive the greatest benefit. Efforts are currently focused on the quantification of mechanical asynchrony using newer imaging techniques including tissue Doppler imaging and strain imaging (echocardiography or magnetic resonance imaging), wall thickening analysis by computed tomography, and phase imaging with nuclear scintigraphy. Resynchronization therapy is indicated for ambulatory patients with sinus rhythm and class III or IV symptoms. This therapy has not been well studied in patients with atrial fibrillation. Because of the significant expense of this treatment, it is not currently recommended for patients with short life expectancy, including those with refractory, decompensated heart failure.

Adaptive Mechanisms in Heart Failure

A large number of compensatory changes occur in the cardiovascular and renal systems to maintain adequate blood flow to the vital organs of the body in the setting of myocardial dysfunction. These changes include increases in left ventricular volume and pressure through the Frank-Starling mechanism, ventricular remodeling, and neurohormonal activation.

In the normal heart, increasing the stroke volume or heart rate can augment cardiac output. Stroke volume is dependent on the contractile state of the myocardium, left

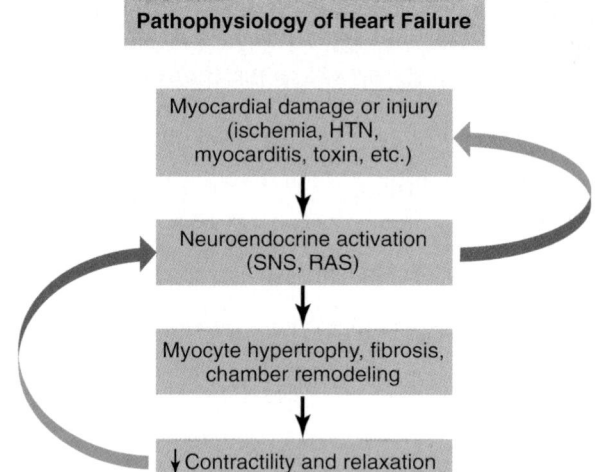

Pathophysiology of Heart Failure

Figure 6-1 Schematic diagram illustrating the progressive nature of left ventricular dysfunction that can follow an initial cardiac insult. Attenuation of the neurohumoral activation (or blockade of the downstream effects) may interrupt the positive feedback and slow or reverse the progression of heart failure. HTN, hypertension; RAS, renin-angiotensin system; SNS, sympathetic nervous system.

ventricular filling (preload), and resistance to left ventricular emptying (afterload). According to the Frank-Starling law (Fig. 6-1), stroke volume can be increased with minimal elevation in left ventricular pressure as long as contractility is normal and outflow is not impeded. In the failing heart with depressed intrinsic contractility (Fig. 6-2, curve A), larger increases in filling pressures are required to produce similar increases in stroke volume. When left ventricular diastolic pressure approaches 20 to 25 mm Hg, the hydrostatic pressure in the pulmonary capillaries exceeds the oncotic pressure, and pulmonary edema may ensue. Both depressed myocardial contractility and increased chamber stiffness can lead to pulmonary congestion through similar mechanisms.

The failing heart may also undergo changes in left ventricular size, shape, and mass to maintain adequate forward flow. This process is known as *remodeling* and occurs in response to myocyte loss, such as after a myocardial infarction, or to hemodynamic overload, such as aortic or mitral valve insufficiency. The initial response to increased cardiac stress or load is usually hypertrophy of the viable myocytes. If the increase occurs mainly in cell length, then ventricular dilation is the predominant form of remodeling (usually seen in volume overload or myocardial infarction). The eccentric pattern of remodeling helps maintain cardiac output but occurs at the expense of increased ventricular wall stress. If the myocytes predominantly increase in width (as in the setting of pressure overload), the heart will tend to thicken with maintenance of cavity volume. This form of remodeling, usually referred to as *concentric hypertrophy,* will tend to reduce wall stress but may do so at the expense of increased filling pressures. If the extent of hypertrophy is inadequate to normalize wall stress, a vicious cycle is established. Overstretching of the myocytes can lead to an increase in myocyte death, ventricular dilation, development of a spherical left ventricular cavity, and further elevation in wall stress.

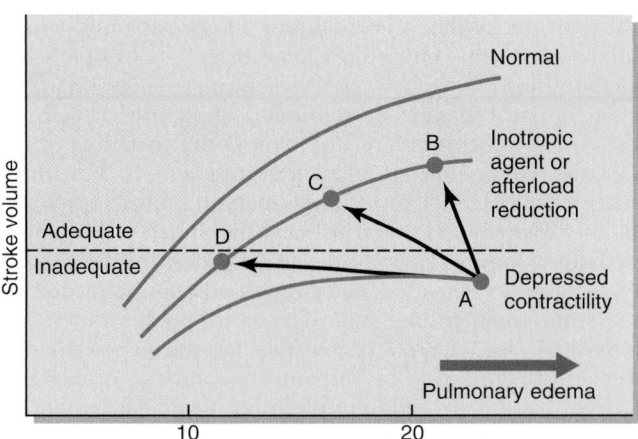

Figure 6-2 Normal and abnormal ventricular function curves. When the left ventricular end-diastolic pressure acutely rises above 20 mm Hg (A), pulmonary edema often occurs. The effect of diuresis or venodilation is to move leftward along the same curve, with a resultant improvement in pulmonary congestion and with minimal decrease in cardiac output. The stroke volume is poor at any point along this depressed contractility curve; thus, therapeutic maneuvers that would raise it more toward the normal curve would be necessary to improve cardiac output significantly. Unlike the effect of diuretics, the effect of digitalis or arterial vasodilator therapy in a patient with heart failure is to move the patient into another ventricular function curve intermediately between the normal and depressed curves. When the patient's ventricular function moves from A to B by the administration of one of these agents, the left ventricular end-diastolic pressure may also decrease because of improved cardiac function; further administration of diuretics or venodilators may shift the patient further to the left along the same curve from B to C and eliminate the risk for pulmonary edema. A vasodilating agent that has both arteriolar and venous dilating properties (e.g., nitroprusside) would shift this patient directly from A to C. If this agent shifts the patient from A to D because of excessive venodilation or administration of diuretics, then the cardiac output may fall too low, even though the left ventricular end-diastolic pressure would be normal (10 mm Hg) for a normal heart. Thus, left ventricular end-diastolic pressures between 15 and 18 mm Hg are usually optimal in the failing heart to maximize cardiac output but avoid pulmonary edema.

The mechanical changes are triggered, in part, by activation of several neurohormonal systems. The renin-angiotensin-aldosterone system helps maintain cardiac output through expansion of intravascular volume by promoting retention of sodium and water. Stimulating arterial vasoconstriction through the actions of angiotensin II enhances tissue perfusion. In addition, release of vasopressin will promote free water absorption by the kidney. The sympathetic nervous system helps maintain tissue perfusion by increasing arterial tone as well as increasing heart rate and ventricular contractility.

Although adaptive in the short term, activation of these systems is associated with several deleterious effects, including elevation in ventricular filling pressures, depression of stroke volume secondary to an increase in peripheral vascular resistance, and stimulation of myocardial hypertrophy and left ventricular remodeling. These maladaptive changes are ultimately responsible for many of the signs and symptoms associated with congestive heart failure and provide the rationale for treatment.

Table 6-2 **New York Heart Association Functional Classification for Heart Failure**	
Class	**Patient Symptoms**
I (Mild)	No limitation of physical activity. Ordinary physical activity does not cause undue fatigue, palpitation, or dyspnea (shortness of breath).
II (Mild)	Slight limitation of physical activity. Comfortable at rest, but ordinary physical activity results in fatigue, palpitation, or dyspnea.
III (Moderate)	Marked limitation of physical activity. Comfortable at rest, but less than ordinary activity causes fatigue, palpitation, or dyspnea.
IV (Severe)	Unable to carry out any physical activity without discomfort. Symptoms of cardiac insufficiency at rest. If any physical activity is undertaken, discomfort is increased.

From the Heart Failure Society of America © 2002 HFSA, Inc. Available at: http://www.abouthf.org/questions_stages.htm.

Countering these effects, and in response to the increase in ventricular filling pressures, the myocardial cells secrete atrial natriuretic peptide and brain natriuretic peptide (BNP). The plasma concentration of both of these hormones has been shown to increase in patients with heart failure. The measurement of serum BNP or its precursors has proved to be clinically useful in the diagnosis of heart failure. Although endogenous natriuretic peptides promote salt and water excretion by the kidneys and result in arterial vasodilation, they are relatively ineffective at reversing the maladaptive changes associated with the powerful renin-angiotensin and sympathetic nervous systems.

Evaluation of Patients with Heart Failure

The history and physical examination are integral parts of the diagnosis of heart failure and the determination of its underlying or precipitating cause. One of the cardinal manifestations of left ventricular heart failure is dyspnea, which is related to elevation in pulmonary venous pressure. In patients with chronic heart failure, shortness of breath initially occurs only with exertion but may progress to occur at rest. Cardiac dyspnea is often worsened by the recumbent position (orthopnea) when increased venous return further elevates pulmonary venous pressure. Paroxysmal nocturnal dyspnea occurs after several hours of sleep and is probably caused by central redistribution of edema. If cardiac output is low but left ventricular filling pressures are normal, the patient may complain primarily of fatigue resulting from diminished blood flow to the exercising muscles. In some instances, heart failure is slow to progress, and the patient may unknowingly restrict his or her activities. Thus, the history should include an assessment not only of the patient's symptoms but also of his or her level of activity (functional capacity; Table 6-2). Many patients complain of peripheral edema, usually involving the lower extremities. The edema commonly worsens during the day and decreases overnight with elevation of the legs. In patients with severe, long-standing heart failure, the edema can involve the thighs and abdomen, and ascites may develop. Importantly, peripheral edema often does not have a cardiac cause.

Many of the physical findings of heart failure are related to the neurohormonal changes that help compensate for the reduced cardiac output. An increased heart rate may be present as a result of increased sympathetic tone. The pulse pressure may be narrowed secondary to peripheral vasoconstriction and low stroke volume. If left ventricular filling pressures are elevated, then crackles may be heard on auscultation of the lung fields. Elevation in right-sided filling pressures will result in distended neck veins. If the liver is also congested, firm pressure applied to the right upper quadrant will cause the jugular veins to become further engorged (hepatojugular reflux). Palpation of the precordium may reveal left ventricular enlargement. An early-diastolic third heart sound (S_3) or gallop suggests elevated atrial pressure and increased ventricular chamber stiffness. The sound results from rapid deceleration of the passive component of blood flow from the atrium into the noncompliant ventricle. An S_3 can be generated from the left or right ventricle. A fourth heart sound (S_4) suggests an increased atrial contribution to left ventricular filling but is not specific for heart failure. The murmurs of both mitral and tricuspid regurgitation are common in patients with congestive heart failure and may become accentuated during an acute decompensation. As stated earlier, peripheral edema is a common finding on physical examination and may be related to elevation in venous pressure or increased sodium and water retention. In bedridden patients, the edema may predominantly be in the presacral region.

The electrocardiogram in patients with congestive heart failure is not specific, but it may provide insight into the cause of the cardiac dysfunction, such as prior myocardial infarction, left ventricular hypertrophy, or significant arrhythmias. The chest radiograph may show chamber enlargement and signs of pulmonary congestion (Fig. 6-3). Treatment of heart failure will result in improvement of the vascular congestion on the chest radiograph, but these changes may lag 24 to 48 hours behind clinical improvement. Certain blood chemistries may be altered in the patient with heart failure. The serum sodium concentration may be low, owing to increased water retention with activation of the renin-angiotensin system. The use of potent diuretics is almost always partially responsible for the hyponatremia. Renal function may be impaired secondary to intrinsic kidney disease or reduced perfusion secondary to renal artery vasoconstriction and low cardiac output. Hepatic congestion is common with right ventricular heart failure and may result in elevated liver enzyme levels.

Because many of the signs and symptoms of heart failure may also occur with pulmonary disease, differentiating between these two disease processes may be difficult. Initial therapy will often be directed at both potential pulmonary and cardiac causes until further testing can be performed. Echocardiography is arguably the central means for diagnostic testing in patients with suspected heart failure. This test is fast, safe, and portable and allows for noninvasive assessments of chamber sizes, systolic function, valvular function, both right and left ventricular filling pressures, and quantification of stroke volume or cardiac output. Documentation of heart size, wall thickness, and ventricular function will have important therapeutic implications in most patients (Fig. 6-4). Rapid measurement of the plasma concentration of BNP provides objective and complementary data to aid in the diagnosis of heart failure in the patient with dyspnea. Clinical studies have shown that plasma levels of BNP are elevated in patients with symptomatic left or right ventricular dysfunction but are usually normal in patients with

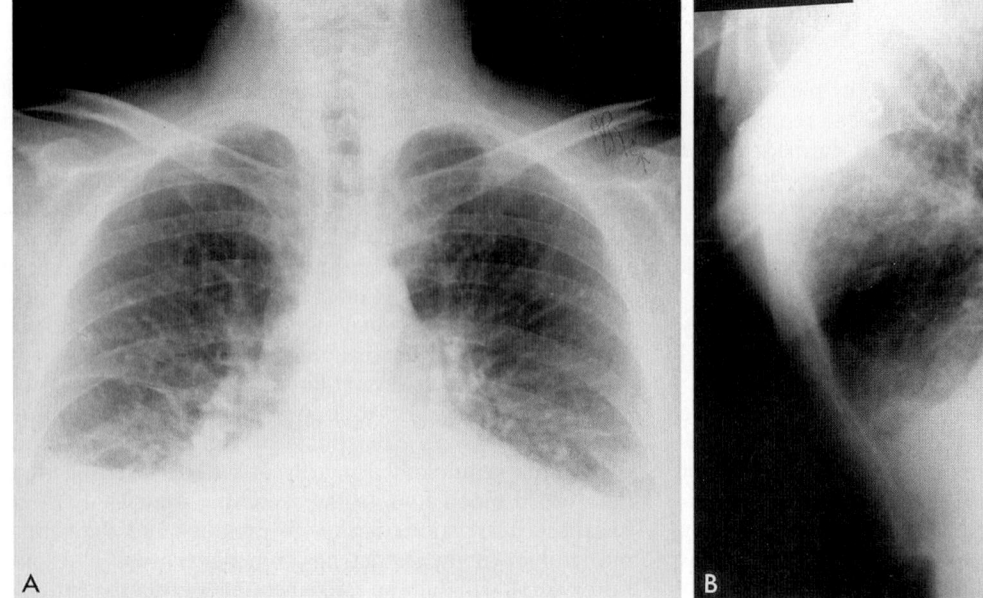
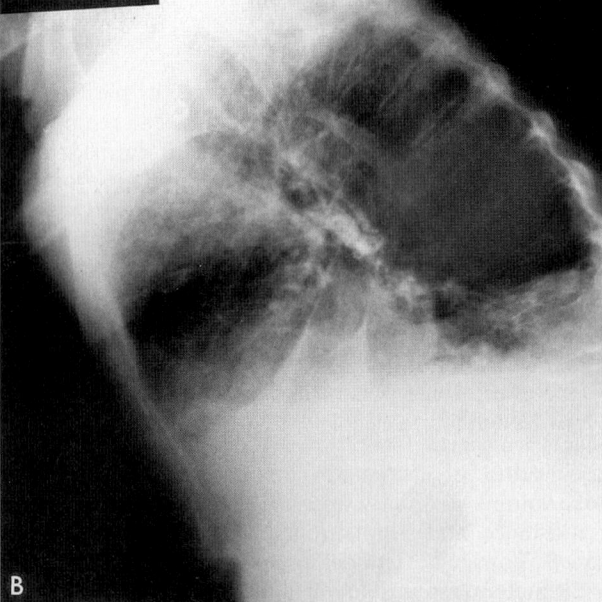

Figure 6-3 A, Posteroanterior chest radiograph showing cardiomegaly. **B,** Lateral chest radiograph showing pulmonary vascular congestion typical of pulmonary edema.

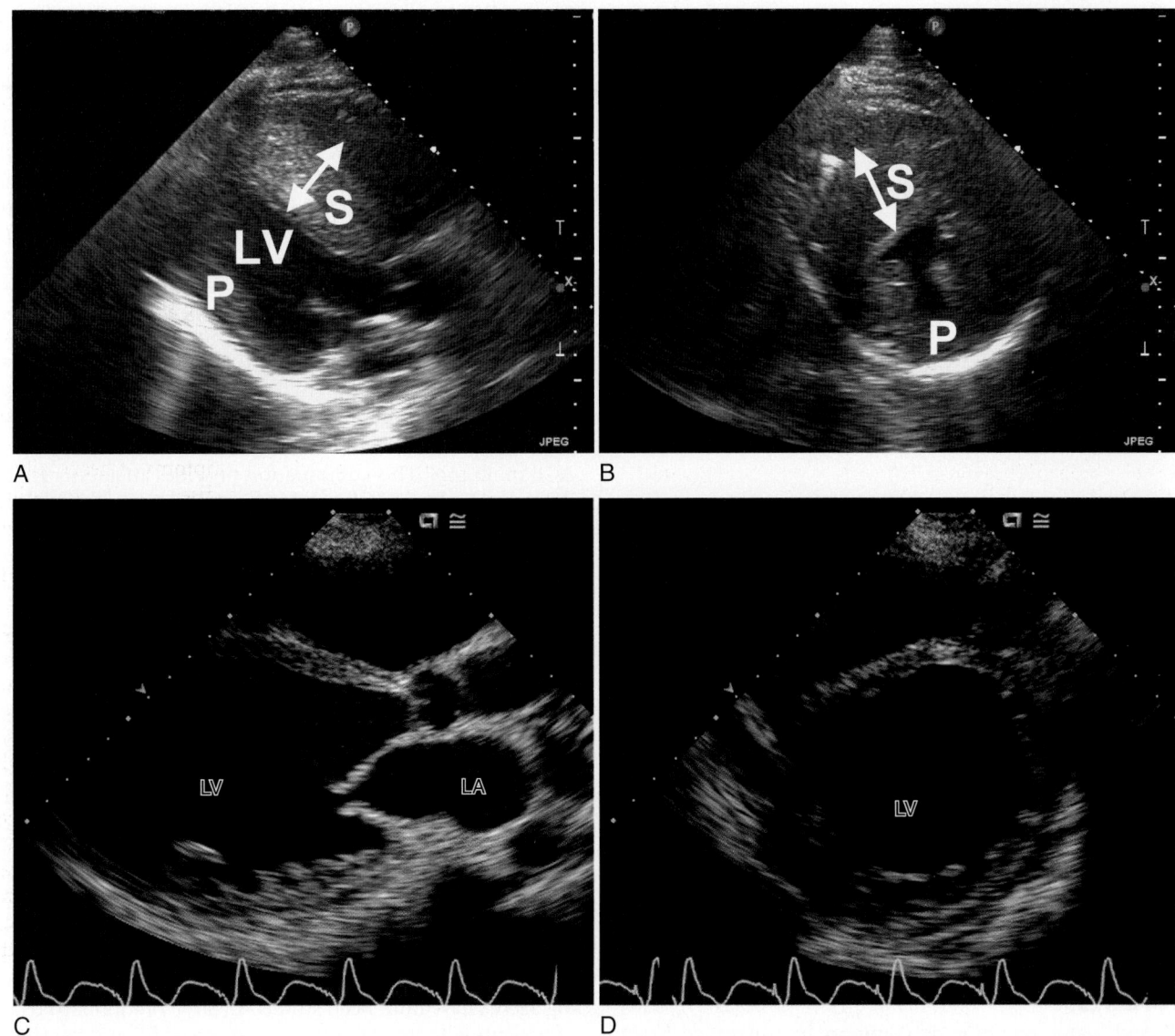

Figure 6-4 Echocardiographic examples of hypertrophic cardiomyopathy seen in long axis (**A**) and short axis (**B**) views. Note normal size of left ventricular (LV) cavity and marked thickening of interventricular septum (S) compared with posterior wall (P). In contrast, similar views in a patient with dilated cardiomyopathy (**C** and **D**) reveal a markedly enlarged left ventricular cavity with diffuse wall thinning.

dyspnea secondary to noncardiac causes. Unfortunately, a relatively large indeterminate range exists in which the test is not helpful. Advanced age and renal dysfunction also reduce the utility of the test, particularly if the BNP concentration is mildly elevated.

An important point to note is that pulmonary edema may also be secondary to noncardiac causes, such as sepsis, certain pulmonary infections, drug toxicity, or neurologic injury. This syndrome, termed *adult respiratory distress syndrome,* can be differentiated from cardiogenic pulmonary edema by the presence of a low or normal pulmonary capillary wedge pressure. The wedge pressure can be estimated noninvasively using left ventricular filling velocities and mitral annular velocities assessed by conventional and tissue Doppler techniques. Peripheral edema may also occur in disease states other than congestive heart failure. Renal disease, especially nephrotic syndrome, cirrhosis, and severe venous stasis disease, may be associated with peripheral edema.

Treatment

Treatment of congestive heart failure should be directed not only at relieving the patient's symptoms but also at treating the underlying or precipitating causes (Table 6-3) and preventing progression. Patients should be educated about the importance of compliance with medical therapy as well as dietary salt and fluid restriction. Rhythm disturbances, such as atrial fibrillation, may precipitate congestive heart failure and may require specific therapy. Treatment of active coronary artery disease, hypertension, or valvular disease may

---

Table 6-3 **Precipitants of Heart Failure**

Dietary (sodium and fluid) indiscretion
Noncompliance with medications
Development of cardiac arrhythmia
Anemia
Uncontrolled hypertension
Superimposed medical illness (pneumonia, renal dysfunction)
New cardiac abnormality (acute ischemia, acute valvular insufficiency)

---

relieve heart failure symptoms. In addition, correction of concomitant medical problems may help stabilize heart function.

NONPHARMACOLOGIC TREATMENT

All patients with heart failure should be instructed to restrict sodium intake to about 2 g/day. Fluid intake should also be limited to avoid hyponatremia. Weight reduction in the obese patient helps reduce the workload of the failing heart. Although a growing body of data suggests that a higher body mass index may paradoxically have protective effects in patients with heart failure, each condition is an independent risk factor for increased morbidity and mortality of cardiac disease. A supervised exercise cardiac rehabilitation program can help reduce heart failure symptoms and improve functional capacity in select patients. Although briefly popular, external enhanced counterpulsation (EECP) has fallen out of favor.

PHARMACOLOGIC TREATMENT

Diuretics

Salt and water retention is common in congestive heart failure secondary to activation of the renin-angiotensin-aldosterone system. Diuretics help promote renal excretion of sodium and water and provide rapid relief of pulmonary congestion and peripheral edema. Loop diuretics, such as furosemide, are the preferred agents in the treatment of symptomatic heart failure. In patients who are refractory to high doses of these agents, diuretics that block sodium absorption at different sites within the nephron may be beneficial (i.e., thiazide-type diuretics). Diuretic therapy is currently considered a mainstay in the treatment of patients with heart failure and preserved EF who have elevated left ventricular filling pressures or peripheral edema. Spironolactone is an aldosterone antagonist with weak diuretic effects that has been shown to reduce hospitalizations for heart failure and cardiac mortality in patients with reduced LVEF and New York Heart Association class III or IV symptoms of heart failure.

Notably, diuretic therapy will lower intracardiac filling pressures and thus cardiac output through the Frank-Starling mechanism. In most patients, this change is well tolerated. However, in some patients, the reduced cardiac output will result in decreased renal perfusion and a rise in the blood urea nitrogen and creatinine levels.

Vasodilators

A large number of vasodilators have been shown to reverse the peripheral vasoconstriction that occurs in congestive heart failure. The most important group of vasodilator agents is the angiotensin-converting enzyme (ACE) inhibitors. These agents help relieve heart failure symptoms, in part, by blocking production of angiotensin II and reducing afterload. In addition, ACE inhibitors have been shown to reduce mortality in patients with both symptomatic and asymptomatic left ventricular dysfunction. The major side effects of ACE inhibitors include hypotension, hyperkalemia, and azotemia. Cough may occur in about 10% of patients and is related to increased bradykinin levels associated with ACE inhibitor use.

Hydralazine in combination with oral nitrates has also been shown to reduce mortality in patients with symptomatic congestive heart failure, although not to the degree of ACE inhibitors. This combination provides an alternative to the patient who is ACE inhibitor intolerant or may require additional therapy for blood pressure control. In addition, recent prospective studies reveal that the combination of hydralazine and nitrates was more beneficial than ACE inhibitors in the African American population.

A newer class of agents, the angiotensin II receptor antagonists, prevents the binding of angiotensin II to its receptor. This action has the theoretical advantage of blocking the effects of angiotensin II produced in the bloodstream as well as at the tissue level. In addition, the angiotensin II receptor blockers do not interfere with bradykinin metabolism and therefore are not associated with cough. Several studies comparing ACE inhibitors to angiotensin II blockers suggest that these two classes of agents are equally effective in reducing morbidity and mortality in patients with heart failure. The current guidelines for the management of chronic heart failure, however, recommend that angiotensin II receptor blockers be reserved for patients who are intolerant of ACE inhibitors. ACE inhibitors and angiotensin II receptor blocking agents have both been studied in large randomized trials of patients with heart failure and preserved EF, and they have been found to be ineffective in this large patient group.

The negative inotropic effects of the calcium channel blockers and their activation of the sympathetic nervous system make these agents less attractive in the treatment of patients with congestive heart failure. In particular, several studies have shown worsening of heart failure symptoms in patients treated with nifedipine. Other calcium channel blockers, such as diltiazem, have been shown to relieve symptoms and increase functional capacity without a deleterious effect on survival in patients with idiopathic dilated cardiomyopathy. Amlodipine has been studied in patients with both ischemic and nonischemic cardiomyopathy and also has not been associated with an increased cardiac morbidity and mortality. In addition, patients with nonischemic cardiomyopathy treated with amlodipine may have a modest survival benefit. Further studies with these agents are necessary before general recommendations regarding their use in patients with heart failure can be made.

Inotropic Agents

Inotropic agents help relieve heart failure symptoms by increasing ventricular contractility. The oldest and most commonly used agent in this class is digoxin, which has been associated with symptomatic improvement in heart failure in patients with systolic dysfunction. However, a recent trial found no significant improvement in survival among patients randomized to digoxin compared with patients treated with placebo. A small reduction in hospitalizations and in death secondary to heart failure was observed, but this was counterbalanced by a slight increase in death secondary to arrhythmias. In general, digoxin therapy should be considered in the patient with left ventricular systolic dysfunction who remains symptomatic after treatment with an ACE inhibitor and a diuretic. No evidence has been found that digoxin should be administered to the patient with asymptomatic left ventricular dysfunction. In addition, digoxin may be harmful in patients with infiltrative cardiomyopathies, such as amyloidosis. Digoxin toxicity results in gastrointestinal, neurologic, and generalized systemic side effects as well as causing a number of tachyarrhythmias and bradyarrhythmias.

Several other classes of oral inotropic agents have been evaluated for treatment of congestive heart failure, such as flosequinan, milrinone, vesnarinone, and xamoterol. All these agents have been associated with increased mortality with long-term use. More recently, promising data have emerged involving the calcium-sensitizing agent levosimendan. This class of agents has the theoretical advantage of not increasing calcium fluxes into the myocyte; therefore, these agents should be less arrhythmogenic and have a more favorable energetic effect.

β Blockers

As previously discussed, many of the symptoms associated with heart failure are related to activation of several neurohormonal systems, including the sympathetic nervous system. Release of catecholamines may initially help maintain blood pressure and cardiac output but, in the long term, may induce further myocardial injury. To date, long-term use of three different β blockers—metoprolol, bisoprolol, and carvedilol—has been shown in clinical trials to improve LVEF and survival in patients with symptomatic left ventricular dysfunction. Of these agents, carvedilol is unique in that it is also an antioxidant and an α blocker, additional properties that may be beneficial in patients with heart failure. Data from clinical trials comparing the efficacy of metoprolol to carvedilol in patients with heart failure have recently been reported. These data suggest superior effects of carvedilol; however, controversy about the experimental design has limited widespread adoption of a single agent. Therapy with one of the aforementioned β blockers should be strongly considered in all patients who have been stabilized on an ACE inhibitor, digoxin, and a diuretic but remain symptomatic (New York Heart Association classes II to IV). β blockers also appear to be effective in patients who are not taking ACE inhibitors. β-blocker therapy is generally withheld from patients with acutely decompensated heart failure or significant volume overload. Gradual up-titration of the dose improves the ability to tolerate these drugs, which are intrinsically negatively inotropic.

Anticoagulation

Thrombosis and thromboemboli occur in patients with left ventricular remodeling and congestive heart failure secondary to stasis of blood, intracardiac thrombi, and atrial arrhythmias. Although long-term warfarin therapy remains controversial, certain patients may benefit from its use, including patients with chronic atrial fibrillation or flutter, patients with definite mural thrombi noted by echocardiography or ventriculography, and patients in sinus rhythm with LVEF less than 20%. In the general heart failure population, prevention of thromboembolism is roughly balanced by increased bleeding risks. Thus, the routine use of anticoagulation is only recommended in heart failure patients with atrial fibrillation, prior arterial embolic events, or mechanical heart valves and in patients who have had an anterior myocardial infarction in the past 3 months.

Refractory Heart Failure

Despite adequate medical therapy, many patients with congestive heart failure fail to have significant reduction in their symptoms. In these instances, therapy with intravenous inotropic agents for 24 to 96 hours, sometimes with hemodynamic monitoring (Swan-Ganz catheter), may be necessary to stabilize the patient. One commonly used agent is dobutamine, which enhances contractility of the heart and reduces peripheral vasoconstriction through stimulation of β_2 receptors. Milrinone is an intravenous phosphodiesterase inhibitor that has similar effects on contractility and afterload. Administration of these agents often promotes diuresis, especially when given concomitantly with intravenous loop diuretics. In patients with markedly elevated systemic vascular resistance, the use of intravenous vasodilators, such as sodium nitroprusside, can significantly reduce afterload and improve cardiac output. A newly available agent, nesiritide, is a recombinant form of human BNP that has been shown to reduce systemic and pulmonary vascular resistance, increase cardiac output, and promote diuresis comparable to standard inotropic agents and vasodilators. Although nesiritide is less likely to provoke serious dysrhythmias compared with dobutamine, recent data have questioned the safety profile and efficacy of nesiritide. Until further studies document safety, nesiritide is not a first-line agent.

If the previously mentioned measures fail to produce a satisfactory diuretic response, dopamine given in doses ranging from 2 to 5 mcg/kg per minute may facilitate sodium and water excretion by stimulating renal dopaminergic receptors. If heart failure is accompanied by hypotension, higher doses of dopamine may be necessary. With doses higher than 5 mcg/kg per minute, dopamine can increase heart rate and peripheral vascular resistance through stimulation of β_1 and α receptors. Although this dose range of dopamine may help stabilize blood pressure, the increase in afterload may have further deleterious effects on the failing heart. In addition, dopamine may provoke arrhythmias that may lead to further hemodynamic instability. If hypotension persists despite dopamine doses greater than 15 mcg/kg per minute, mechanical assist devices, such as the intra-aortic balloon pump, should be considered as a means to stabilize the patient.

In patients who cannot be weaned from pharmacologic or mechanical support and in ambulatory patients with severe functional impairment refractory to medical therapy, cardiac transplantation should be considered a means to improve symptoms and prolong survival (see Chapter 12). Currently, the use of cardiac resynchronization therapy is not a routine consideration in this group of patients who have markedly reduced long-term survival.

Cardiovascular Assist Devices

The most commonly used mechanical support device is the intra-aortic balloon pump. This device can be inserted percutaneously through the femoral artery and advanced into the descending thoracic aorta. Inflation of the balloon occurs during diastole such that perfusion pressure in the proximal aorta and coronary arteries is enhanced. Deflation, which occurs just before the onset of systole, greatly reduces aortic impedance and thus significantly reduces afterload. This device is particularly useful in stabilizing patients with severe coronary disease before percutaneous or after surgical revascularization. In addition, this device may provide hemodynamic support in patients with severe mitral regurgitation or acquired ventricular septal defect before surgical repair. In patients with refractory congestive heart failure, the intra-aortic balloon pump may serve as a temporizing measure until cardiac transplantation can be performed.

In addition to the intra-aortic balloon pump, several ventricular assist devices are available that provide hemodynamic support. These devices can be placed percutaneously but most commonly are implanted through a sternotomy incision. They can be used to support either ventricle. Blood is collected from the right atrium, left atrium, or the left ventricular apex into an extracorporeal reservoir and then actively pumped back into the pulmonary or systemic circulation by the assist device. These units were initially intended to provide hemodynamic support for several days to weeks (most often a *bridge* to transplantation in the patient who is critically ill). Because of the success with these devices and the limited availability of donor hearts, assist devices are now being implanted as *destination* therapy. The pump is placed within the peritoneum, and portable battery packs allow the patient to ambulate. Newer left ventricular assist devices, as well as total artificial hearts, are undergoing clinical investigation as permanent cardiac replacement therapy.

Prospectus for the Future

External Containment Devices

In patients with left ventricular dysfunction, cardiac remodeling characterized by progressive ventricular chamber dilation and wall thinning can lead to elevation in wall stress and activation of neurohormonal mechanisms that further impair myocardial function. Experimental devices that passively contain the heart have been shown, in animal models, to reduce ventricular cavity size and improve myocardial responsiveness to β-adrenergic stimulation without impairing left ventricular filling or interfering with coronary blood flow. Randomized trials evaluating the efficacy of these devices in patients with end-stage cardiomyopathy are underway.

Mitral Valve Repair

Mitral regurgitation contributes to the progression of heart failure in a large number of patients. However, most patients with severe heart failure are deemed poor surgical candidates. Several new and exciting percutaneous approaches to mitral and aortic valve repair are being explored as ways to treat some of these patients.

Cell-Based Therapies

Permanent loss of myocytes is the final common pathway in most forms of heart failure. Presently, some experimental data support the notion that implantation of cells into the failing heart might effectively regenerate new cardiac muscle. Skeletal myoblasts, bone marrow–derived progenitor cells, and embryonic stem cells are all undergoing testing in both animals and humans. Although many types of transplanted cells are able to contract, ineffective formation of gap junctions and hence ineffective electrical continuity between the transplanted cells and the existing myocardial syncytium continue to be obstacles.

References

Burkhoff D, Maurer MS, Packer M, et al: Heart failure with a normal ejection fraction: Is it really a disorder of diastolic function? Circulation 107:656-658, 2003.

Cleland JG, Daubert JD, Erdmann E, et al: The effect of cardiac resynchronization on morbidity and mortality in heart failure. N Engl J Med 352:1539-1549, 2005.

Dokainish H, Zoghbi WA, Lakkis NM, et al: Optimal noninvasive assessment of left ventricular filling pressures: A comparison of tissue Doppler echocardiography and B-type natriuretic peptide in patients with pulmonary artery catheters. Circulation 109:2432-2439, 2004.

Poole-Wilson PA, Swedberg K, Cleland JG, et al: Comparison of carvedilol and metoprolol on clinical outcomes in patients with chronic heart failure in the Carvedilol or Metoprolol European Trial (COMET): Randomised controlled trial. Lancet 362:7-13, 2003.

Rose EA, Gelijns AC, Moskowitz AJ, et al: Long-term mechanical left ventricular assistance for end-stage heart failure. N Engl J Med 345:1435-1443, 2001.

Taylor AL, Ziesche S, Yancy C, et al: Combination of isosorbide dinitrate and hydralazine in blacks with heart failure. N Engl J Med 351:2049-2057, 2004.

Young JB, Abraham WT, Smith AL, et al: Combined cardiac resynchronization and implantable cardioversion defibrillation in advanced chronic heart failure: The MIRACLE ICD trial. JAMA 289:2685-2694, 2003.

Congenital Heart Disease

Kevin J. Whitehead

About 0.8% of all live births are complicated by congenital cardiac abnormalities, not including infants with bicuspid aortic valve and mitral valve prolapse (see Chapter 8), which are more prevalent (2% and 2.4%, respectively). Congenital heart disease is a major cause of infant morbidity and mortality. As a result of advances in pediatric cardiology and cardiothoracic surgery, about 85% of infants born with congenital heart disease can be expected to survive into adulthood. In turn, adults with congenital heart disease represent a large and growing population that is encountered more frequently in clinical practice. An equal number of adults and children live with congenital heart disease, with an estimated 800,000 adult patients in the United States alone.

Most cases of congenital heart disease occur sporadically, without a known specific cause. Genetic abnormalities are responsible for a proportion of cases and may contribute to cases occurring sporadically as well. Environmental factors are also known to cause congenital heart disease. An increased incidence is found in children of patients with congenital heart disease, with a higher risk in mothers than in fathers. In most cases, the nature of the parent's defect does not predict the lesion in affected offspring.

The size and nature of the congenital defect often determine the onset of symptoms. Normal physiologic changes in cardiovascular hemodynamics at birth can prompt presentation. Symptoms can develop shortly after birth when transition from fetal to adult circulation represents a new dependence on biventricular circulation with a pulmonary circuit. The isolated pulmonary and systemic circulations of D-transposition of the great arteries become apparent on closure of the last fetal connections between circuits, the ductus arteriosus and the foramen ovale. In other conditions, the primary lesion results in changes that delay presentation until such compensatory mechanisms fail. Hypertrophy of the morphologic right ventricle in L-transposition of the great arteries is sufficient to compensate for systemic vascular resistance and maintain normal perfusion for years, with symptoms often developing when the systemic ventricle fails. Still other lesions may develop in adulthood when degenerative changes, such as stenosis

of a previously well-functioning bicuspid aortic valve, are superimposed on an initial lesion. Some congenital defects may go undetected throughout life (e.g., small atrial septal defects [ASDs], whereas some may resolve spontaneously (small muscular ventricular septal defects [VSDs]). Many adult patients with congenital heart disease will have already undergone palliative or reparative surgical procedures and will have subsequent care directed at residual defects and sequelae of such procedures. This chapter focuses on the most common congenital abnormalities observed in adults, including those that develop in adulthood and those for which surgical correction during infancy and childhood permits survival into adulthood.

Septal Defects

ATRIAL SEPTAL DEFECTS

ASDs are some of the most common congenital defects, representing 10% to 17% of cases, with a higher prevalence in women (60%). Defects are classified according to their location in the interatrial septum. The most common ASD (60%), the ostium secundum defect, involves the fossa ovalis. Ostium primum defects (20%) involve the atrioventricular junction and are at one end of the spectrum of atrioventricular septal defects (or endocardial cushion defects). Primum ASDs are usually associated with a cleft mitral valve and mitral regurgitation. In rare cases, primum ASD can be associated with a large VSD and a single atrioventricular (AV) valve, forming an AV septal defect. Sinus venosus defects are located in the superior septum and may be associated with partially anomalous pulmonary venous drainage into the superior vena cava or right atrium.

In patients with uncomplicated ASDs (e.g., with normal pulmonary vascular resistance), oxygenated blood shunts from the left to the right atrium. The magnitude of the shunting is determined by the size of the defect and the compliance of the left and right ventricles. Small ASDs accommodate the increased blood flow in the right atrium without sequelae and no significant hemodynamic compromise of the right heart. If the defect is large, the right atrium and right ventricle dilate to accommodate the increased volume of shunted blood (Fig. 7-1). Pressure in the pulmonary artery increases secondary to the increased volume of blood; however, with the exception of extremely large, long-standing defects, pulmonary vascular resistance usually remains normal.

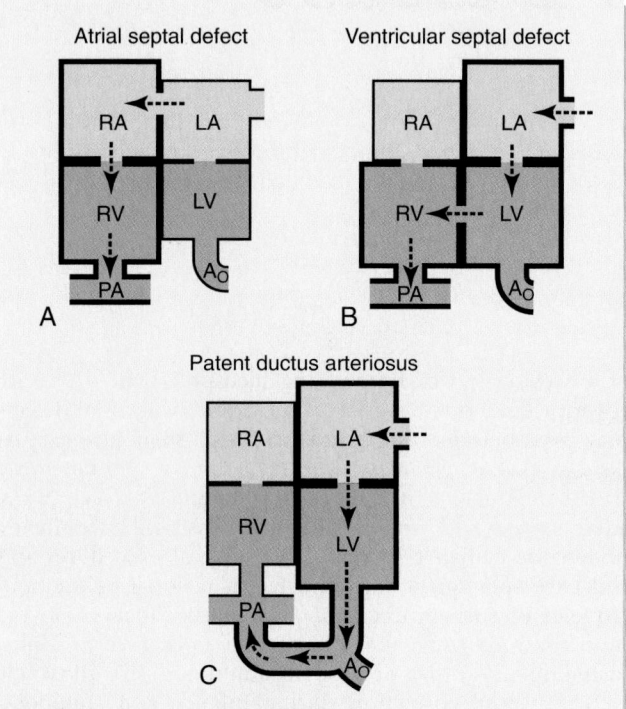

Figure 7-1 Diagram illustrates the three types of shunt lesions that commonly survive until adulthood and their effects on chamber size. **A,** Uncomplicated atrial septal defect demonstrating left-to-right shunt flow across the interatrial septum and resulting in dilation of the right atrium (RA), right ventricle (RV), and pulmonary artery (PA). **B,** Uncomplicated ventricular septal defect, resulting in dilation of the RV, left atrium (LA), and left ventricle (LV). **C,** Uncomplicated patent ductus arteriosus, resulting in dilation of the LA, LV, and PA. Ao, aorta. (From Liberthson RR, Waldman H: Congenital heart disease in the adult. In Kloner RA [ed]: The Guide to Cardiology, 3rd ed. Greenwich, Conn, Le Jacq Communications, 1991, pp 24-47. Copyright ©1991 by Le Jacq Communications, Inc.)

Most patients with ASD are asymptomatic until adulthood, when symptoms such as fatigue, dyspnea, and poor exercise tolerance develop, secondary to right ventricular dysfunction. Older patients may decompensate when acquired heart disease leads to a rise in left ventricular filling pressures and more blood is shunted from the left atrium to the already volume-overloaded right heart. Patients with ASD are prone to atrial fibrillation, especially after 50 years of age. Irreversible pulmonary vascular obstruction resulting in right-to-left shunting and cyanosis (Eisenmenger syndrome) is uncommon and occurs infrequently (<5% of patients with ASDs). The presence of an ASD may be heralded by a paradoxical embolus traversing the defect, resulting in stroke or transient ischemic attack.

A prominent right ventricular pulsation may be observed on physical examination, along the left sternal border secondary to a dilated, hyperdynamic right ventricle (Table 7-1). The S_2 sound is widely split and fixed. Wide splitting occurs because right ventricular volume overload results in a prolonged ejection period and delayed closure of the pulmonic valve. Fixed splitting results from a lack of respiratory variation in right ventricular filling with variation in the left-to-right shunt, compensating for varying venous return. An ejection-quality murmur that increases with inspiration is commonly heard at the left sternal border and is secondary to increased blood flow across the pulmonic valve. If severe pulmonary vascular obstruction develops, the P_2 sound becomes loud, the splitting of S_2 narrows, and a right ventricular gallop may be heard.

The diagnosis of ASD is usually made with two-dimensional and color Doppler echocardiography. In particular, transesophageal imaging allows for excellent visualization of the interatrial septum as well as associated congenital defects such as anomalous pulmonary veins, VSDs, and abnormalities of the mitral leaflets. This technique provides additional information pertaining to right ventricular size and function and the degree of shunt flow. Cardiac magnetic resonance imaging (MRI) is another noninvasive imaging modality that provides excellent visualization of the interatrial septum and pulmonary veins and can provide diagnostic information in cases of uncertainty after echo imaging. MRI is particularly well suited for analysis of right ventricular size and function. Cardiac catheterization is useful to assess and define the shunt fraction (Qp/Qs ratio) to measure pulmonary arterial pressures and to estimate pulmonary vascular

Table 7-1 **Findings in Uncomplicated Shunt Lesions**			
Type	**Physical Findings**	**Electrocardiogram**	**Chest Radiograph**
Atrial septal defect	Parasternal RV impulse Widely and fixed split S_2 Ejection murmur across pulmonic valve	Right bundle branch block Left axis deviation with ostium primum defect	Large pulmonary artery Increased pulmonary markings
Ventricular septal defect	Hyperdynamic precordium Holosystolic left parasternal murmur, with or without thrill	LV and RV hypertrophy	Cardiomegaly Prominent pulmonary vasculature
Patent ductus arteriosus	Hyperdynamic apical impulse Continuous machinery-like murmur	LV hypertrophy	Prominent pulmonary artery Enlarged LA and LV

LA, left atrium; LV, left ventricle; RV, right ventricle.

resistance, but is rarely necessary after noninvasive imaging. The most common indication for catheterization is now the identification of concomitant coronary artery disease in adults older than 40 years who are contemplating surgical repair.

Once diagnosed, ASDs should be closed without delay. The presence of right ventricular enlargement should prompt referral for closure, even in the absence of symptoms. Paradoxical embolism, elevation of pulmonary artery pressure, or a net left-to-right shunt should also prompt consideration of closure. Defects less than 8 mm in diameter are rarely significant. Significant pulmonary hypertension is a contraindication to ASD closure. When pulmonary arterial pressures exceed two thirds of systemic pressure, evidence of ongoing significant left-to-right shunt must also be present, or the reversibility of pulmonary hypertension with the administration of vasodilators or oxygen must be administered to justify the increased risk for closure.

Percutaneous device closure of a secundum ASD is an acceptable alternative to surgical closure and is becoming the preferred intervention for this condition. A sufficient rim of tissue is required for successful device deployment. Short- and intermediate-term results with the Amplatzer closure device have been excellent. The long-term results remain unknown, and patients who have received such devices should continue to receive close follow-up care. Primum and sinus venosus defects should be surgically closed.

Closure of a hemodynamically significant ASD before the age of 25 years is expected to convey a mortality benefit. Closure before the age of 40 years of age is expected to decrease the long-term risk for atrial arrhythmias. After the fourth decade, symptoms are usually significantly improved after surgical repair; however, some degree of right ventricular dysfunction may persist. Antibiotic prophylaxis for infective endocarditis is not required for small ASDs or patent foramen ovale or after ASD closure.

VENTRICULAR SEPTAL DEFECT

VSD is a common congenital abnormality in newborns and is present in about 1 in 500 normal births. Because nearly 50% of VSDs close spontaneously during childhood and most large defects are surgically corrected at an early age, this defect is rarely encountered in adults. VSDs are classified according to their location within the interventricular septum. Type I VSDs (also known as supracristal VSD) are located beneath the aortic annulus and often lead to aortic valvular incompetence. Type II VSDs (or perimembranous VSD) are the most common (about 80%) and are located in the membranous portion of the septum between the left ventricular outflow tract and the right ventricle near the septal leaflet of the tricuspid valve. Type III defects involve the atrioventricular canal, which is often associated with ostium primum ASDs, along with mitral and tricuspid leaflet abnormalities. Such congenital defects are common in patients with Down syndrome. Type IV defects (or muscular VSDs) make up 5% to 20% of VSDs and involve the muscular portion of the interventricular septum and often close spontaneously during childhood if small.

In patients with uncomplicated VSDs, oxygenated blood from the left ventricle is shunted across the defect into the right ventricle. If the defect is small, then right ventricular size and function are normal, and pulmonary vascular resistance does not increase. If the defect is large, however, the right ventricle dilates to accommodate the increased volume, and pulmonary blood flow increases (see Fig. 7-1). If the condition is uncorrected, pulmonary vascular obstruction may develop and may lead to pulmonary artery hypertension, reversal of the interventricular shunt, and systemic desaturation and cyanosis (Eisenmenger syndrome).

The clinical course of a patient with VSD depends on the size of the defect. Most small defects spontaneously close, or if still present in adulthood, they are usually not associated with any significant hemodynamic complications. Large defects are usually detected and repaired during infancy. Affected individuals with uncorrected defects who survive to adulthood may have signs and symptoms of right-sided ventricular heart failure. If pulmonary vascular obstruction with reversed central shunt (so-called Eisenmenger physiology) develops, cyanosis and clubbing of the fingers may be present. All patients with VSD (or repaired VSD with residual shunt flow) are at risk for bacterial endocarditis that usually involves the right ventricular outflow tract.

On physical examination, the patient with an uncomplicated VSD has a hyperdynamic precordium and a palpable thrill along the left sternal border (see Table 7-1). The murmur is usually holosystolic and is best heard at the left sternal border. In general, small defects are associated with loud murmurs because of the significant pressure gradient between the left and the right ventricles. As pulmonary hypertension develops and left-to-right shunt flow decreases, the murmur may soften, and a loud P_2 sound may be present.

Two-dimensional and Doppler echocardiography are useful in diagnosing VSDs as well as in assessing right ventricular size and function and associated cardiac abnormalities. The evaluation of VSD can be complemented by cardiac MRI or computed tomography (CT) studies in cases of uncertainty with echo imaging. Cardiac catheterization may be necessary before surgical repair to document the severity of shunt flow and to determine pulmonary artery pressure and pulmonary vascular resistance, especially in cases with suspected pulmonary arterial hypertension. Documentation involves identifying a rise in oxygen content in blood that is sampled from the right ventricle and pulmonary artery compared with blood from the right atrium. Patients with Eisenmenger syndrome and net right-to-left shunt flow are not surgical candidates. Surgical closure of the VSD with sutures or a prosthetic patch is recommended for patients with left-to-right shunt flow greater than 1.5 : 1 without evidence of irreversible pulmonary hypertension. Percutaneous device closure is an attractive option for muscular VSDs.

Valvular Defects

CONGENITAL AORTIC STENOSIS AND BICUSPID AORTIC VALVE

Congenital left ventricular outflow obstruction may occur at the valvular, subvalvular, or supravalvular level. Valvular stenosis is most often secondary to a bicuspid aortic valve, which is present in about 2% of the population and occurs more frequently in men than in women. Associated cardiovascular abnormalities can occur in less than or equal to 20% of affected persons and include coarctation of the aorta and patent ductus arteriosus (PDA). Bicuspid aortic valves rarely cause significant obstruction during infancy and early childhood. However, their abnormal structure results in turbulent flow that leads to leaflet injury and thickening, calcification, and, ultimately, narrowing of the orifice.

Although a few patients with bicuspid aortic stenosis remain asymptomatic throughout life, most affected individuals develop symptoms during the fifth and sixth decades of life. As with acquired aortic stenosis, chest pain, syncope, and congestive heart failure are the most frequent symptoms. Bicuspid aortic valves may be complicated by aneurismal enlargement of the thoracic aorta and aortic dissection. Other complications include sudden death, particularly in the setting of significant outflow obstruction, and infective endocarditis, which can lead to significant aortic regurgitation. Less commonly, aortic regurgitation is the predominant abnormality associated with a bicuspid aortic valve.

The physical examination of a patient with a stenotic bicuspid aortic valve is similar to that of the patient with acquired aortic stenosis and is usually characterized by an ejection-quality murmur at the left sternal border (Table 7-2). If the leaflets are still pliable, an early systolic ejection click may be appreciated as the leaflets open. The decrescendo diastolic murmur of aortic insufficiency may also be present, as may typical signs of significant aortic regurgitation.

The diagnosis of bicuspid aortic valve and the determination of degree of stenosis and regurgitation are usually made by two-dimensional and Doppler echocardiography. (Treatment of patients with significant obstruction or insufficiency is outlined in Chapter 8.) Children and young adults with significant stenosis may have improvement with percutaneous valvuloplasty, especially when calcification of the valve cusps is minimal. In older adults or those patients with significant leaflet calcification, aortic valve replacement remains the treatment of choice. Although aortic root enlargement may be identified by echocardiography, cardiac MRI and CT provide more accurate measurements for serial follow-up and should be performed if enlargement is suspected. Although endocarditis is always a concern with bicuspid aortic valves, antibiotic prophylaxis is unlikely to prevent most cases, and the risks are now thought to outweigh the benefits. Meticulous oral hygiene is the recommended practice to prevent endocarditis in these patients.

Other causes of congenital left ventricular outflow tract obstruction are much less common. *Subaortic stenosis* is often first diagnosed in adulthood and is characterized by the presence of a discrete, fibrous diaphragm that encircles the left ventricular outflow tract between the mitral annulus and the basal interventricular septum. Patients with this defect have a characteristic outflow murmur but not the systolic ejection click appreciated in patients with bicuspid

Table 7-2 **Findings in Select Uncomplicated, Unrepaired Cardiac Defects**			
Type	**Physical Findings**	**Electrocardiogram**	**Chest Radiogram**
Congenital aortic stenosis	Decreased carotid upstroke	LV hypertrophy	Post-stenotic aortic dilation
	Sustained apical impulse		Prominent LV
	Single S₂, S₄		
	Systolic ejection murmur		
Coarctation of aorta	Delayed femoral pulses	LV hypertrophy	Post-stenotic aortic dilation
	Reduced blood pressure in lower extremities		Prominent ascending aorta
	Findings associated with bicuspid aortic valve		LV enlargement
Pulmonic valve stenosis	RV lift	RV hypertrophy	Post-stenotic dilation of the main or left pulmonary artery
	Pulmonic ejection sound	RA abnormality	
	Systolic ejection murmur at left sternal border		RA and RV enlargement
	RV S₄, widely split S₂, soft P₂		
Tetralogy of Fallot	Usually cyanotic	RV hypertrophy	Boot-shaped heart
	Possible clubbing	RA abnormality	Small pulmonary artery
	Prominent ejection murmur at left sternal border		Normal pulmonary vasculature
	Soft or absent P₂		
Ebstein anomaly	Acyanotic or cyanotic	RA abnormality	Enlarged RA
	Increased jugular venous pressure	Right bundle branch block	Normal pulmonary vasculature
	Prominent v wave	PR prolongation	
	Systolic murmur at sternal border, increases with inspiration	Ventricular pre-excitation	

LV, left ventricle; PR, pulse rate; RA, right atrium; RV, right ventricle.

aortic valves. *Supravalvar aortic stenosis* (SVAS) is a rare form of outflow obstruction characterized by varying degrees of ascending aortic root stricture. Loss-of-function mutations in the extracellular matrix protein, elastin, are responsible for smooth muscle hypertrophy in SVAS, which is a generalized arteriopathy most commonly affecting the sinotubular junction of the ascending aorta but also affecting the pulmonary and other systemic arteries. This abnormality is usually diagnosed in childhood and is often part of a syndrome with hypercalcemia and multiple skeletal, vascular, and developmental abnormalities. Nonsyndromic cases also occur in both sporadic and familial forms.

PULMONIC VALVE STENOSIS

Pulmonic valve stenosis is the most common cause of obstruction to right ventricular outflow and usually occurs as an isolated congenital lesion. Fusion of the pulmonary leaflets creates the pressure-overloaded state and results in right ventricular hypertrophy. Some patients develop discrete hypertrophy of the infundibulum beneath the pulmonic valve, further contributing to outflow obstruction.

Unless the valve is severely stenotic at birth, most affected persons live a normal life until adolescence or young adulthood. The development of symptoms depends on the severity of the stenosis and right ventricular function. Patients with mild-to-moderate stenosis are usually asymptomatic and rarely have complications associated with the defect. Patients with moderate-to-severe obstruction often exhibit progressive fatigue and dyspnea. If right ventricular dysfunction occurs, symptoms and signs of right-sided ventricular heart failure may be present.

On physical examination, the patient with severe stenosis has a right ventricular lift on palpation of the precordium (see Table 7-2). The S_1 sound is usually normal and is followed by an opening click that becomes louder with expiration. The P_2 sound becomes softer and is delayed as the severity of the stenosis increases. The characteristic murmur of pulmonic stenosis is a systolic ejection murmur heard best at the left upper sternal border, which increases with inspiration. As with aortic stenosis, a late-peaking murmur indicates more severe stenosis. A prominent jugular venous a wave and right-sided S_4 sound may also be present in patients with severe obstruction to right ventricular outflow.

For asymptomatic patients with mild pulmonic stenosis (<30 mm Hg peak gradient), symptoms are unlikely, and obstruction is unlikely to progress. Patients with moderate stenosis (peak gradient > 50 mm Hg) are likely to develop symptoms and require closer observation. In children and adults with isolated pulmonic stenosis, percutaneous balloon valvuloplasty is a suitable therapeutic option that offers results comparable with those achieved with surgery. Valvuloplasty should be offered to symptomatic patients (who will often have peak gradients higher than 50 mm Hg. Asymptomatic patients with peak gradients higher than 60 mm Hg should also be treated. Balloon valvuloplasty is unlikely to relieve obstruction from significant infundibular stenosis or in cases with moderate or worse pulmonary regurgitation, in which case surgical repair is preferred. Repair of the valve involves separation of the fused commissures and resection of the infundibulum if significant hypertrophy is present. Valve replacement is rarely necessary.

OTHER VALVULAR DEFECTS

Ebstein anomaly is a rare condition (0.5% of patients with congenital heart disease) characterized by apical displacement of the tricuspid valve into the right ventricle. As a result, the basal portion of the right ventricle forms part of the right atrium and leaves a small functional right ventricle. The tricuspid leaflets are often dysplastic and may partially adhere to the interventricular septum or right ventricular free wall, often with significant tricuspid regurgitation. The degree of right ventricular dysfunction depends on the size of the *functioning* right ventricle and the severity of the tricuspid regurgitation. Ebstein anomaly frequently presents in adulthood. A patent foramen ovale or ostium secundum ASD is present in more than 50% of patients and may result in right-to-left shunt flow as right atrial pressure increases. Supraventricular arrhythmias are common in those with Ebstein anomaly, as is ventricular pre-excitation associated with Wolff-Parkinson-White syndrome.

Diseases of the Aorta
COARCTATION OF THE AORTA

Coarctation of the aorta is a fibrotic narrowing of the aortic lumen usually located distal to the left subclavian artery in the region of the ligamentum (ductus) arteriosus. The defect is more common in men than in women (2:1) and represents 5% to 8% of all congenital heart defects. About 25% to 50% of patients have an associated bicuspid aortic valve. The most common extracardiac abnormality is an aneurysm of the circle of Willis (present in 3% to 5% of patients).

Coarctation produces obstruction to left ventricular outflow and results in a rise in blood pressure in the proximal aorta and great vessels relative to the distal aorta and lower extremities. The development of left ventricular hypertrophy helps maintain normal stroke volume in the presence of increased afterload. Most cases of coarctation are diagnosed in infancy or childhood, during which a high mortality rate is observed for severe coarctation that has not been repaired. Occasional cases of mild coarctation will remain undiagnosed until adulthood, when a work-up for secondary causes of hypertension may reveal the abnormality. A coarctation should be excluded in all young patients with hypertension. If the condition is left untreated, more than two thirds of patients will develop left ventricular dysfunction and congestive heart failure by the fourth decade of life. Other complications include aortic dissection or rupture, stroke secondary to chronic hypertension, or spontaneous rupture of cerebral aneurysms. As such, patients with coarctation can be considered to have a generalized arteriopathy. Endocarditis involving the coarctation or the associated bicuspid aortic valve is a dangerous complication.

Clinically, most patients with coarctation have upper extremity hypertension with forceful carotid and upper extremity pulses (Fig. 7-2; see also Table 7-2). The pulses in the lower extremities are typically weak and delayed relative to the carotid upstroke. An ejection-quality murmur may be

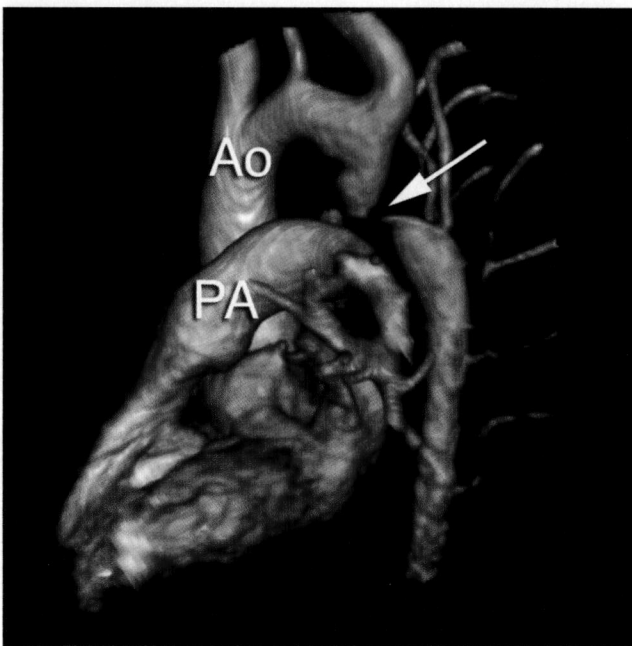

Figure 7-2 Three-dimensional reconstruction of cardiac magnetic resonance image from a patient with uncorrected coarctation of the aorta. The coarctation *(arrow)* of the descending thoracic aorta (Ao) occurs in close proximity to the pulmonary artery (PA) in the expected location of the ligamentum arteriosus. Prominent intercostal arterial collaterals are observed.

heard if a bicuspid aortic valve is present. A systolic murmur originating from the coarctation is typically heard over the left upper back. Older adults may have findings of heart failure.

The diagnosis of coarctation may be made by two-dimensional and Doppler echocardiography. Echocardiography may be the only study required for diagnosis in infants and children. However, in adults, MRI and cardiac catheterization are the preferred methods for defining the location of the coarctation and the anatomy of the arch vessels. Repair in adults is recommended at the time of diagnosis, although only about 50% of patients become normotensive after the procedure. Surgical repair is standard in many centers, although primary percutaneous treatment with balloon angioplasty and stenting of discrete coarctation is preferred in others. Restenosis of the aorta may occur postoperatively, although in many instances, this recurrent stenosis may be dilated using percutaneous techniques. A new or unusual headache in a patient with coarctation should prompt an evaluation for intracranial aneurysms. Progressive enlargement of the thoracic aorta with dissection is a concern in patients with coarctation. Hypertension is common after repair of coarctation and may be manifest primarily with exercise.

PATENT DUCTUS ARTERIOSUS

The ductus arteriosus functionally closes several hours after birth and anatomically closes within 4 to 8 weeks thereafter. PDA is more common in infants who are premature or who are born at a high altitude. PDA is also more common in women than in men, and it may be associated with other cardiac abnormalities such as coarctation and VSD.

A persistent communication between the aorta and pulmonary artery is the result of the failure of the ductus arteriosus to close. The hemodynamic consequences of this communication depend on the size of the ductus. If the defect is small, pulmonary artery resistance remains normal, and blood flows from left to right from the aorta to the pulmonary circulation. Most patients with small PDAs are asymptomatic and survive into adulthood without developing significant hemodynamic complications. When the ductus is large, blood flow through the pulmonary circulation and returning to the left side of the heart is significantly increased, resulting in left ventricular volume overload and pulmonary congestion (see Fig. 7-1). Persistence of a large PDA may result in elevated pulmonary vascular resistance with Eisenmenger physiology. When pulmonary vascular resistance exceeds systemic vascular resistance, shunt flow reverses and passes from right to left. Such patients have cyanosis of the lower extremities with clubbing of the toes, whereas the upper extremities are usually normal in color without evidence of clubbing of the fingers. This differential cyanosis is secondary to shunting of poorly oxygenated blood from the pulmonary artery to the aorta distal to the left subclavian artery, whereas well-oxygenated blood from the left ventricle is supplied to the head and upper limbs. The increased volume and pressure load on the right ventricle can precipitate right-sided ventricular failure.

The characteristic physical examination finding of uncomplicated PDA is a loud, continuous, machinery-like murmur best heard in the left infraclavicular region (see Table 7-2). If the PDA is small, the peripheral pulses remain normal. A hemodynamically significant PDA also has a continuous murmur, but it is typically associated with bounding pulses and a wide pulse pressure. The left ventricle may be enlarged, and signs of pulmonary congestion may be present. An Eisenmenger PDA is characterized by the loss of the continuous murmur, signs of pulmonary hypertension, and differential cyanosis and clubbing.

The diagnosis of PDA is usually confirmed with two-dimensional and Doppler echocardiography, at which time the size of the shunt and the pulmonary pressures can be estimated. Oximetry should be performed on both fingers and toes. Cardiac catheterization is usually performed at the same time as percutaneous closure for further confirmation. Evidence for reversibility of pulmonary hypertension at cardiac catheterization is reassuring. Closure of the PDA is indicated in all cases except in those patients with silent PDAs, found only by a screening examination and without audible murmur, and in those with large PDAs associated with severe, irreversible pulmonary vascular disease.

Percutaneous device closure is the preferred intervention in most centers, particularly if calcification of the duct is present. Surgery is reserved for the PDA that is too large for percutaneous closure or with distorted anatomy such as a ductal aneurysm or after endarteritis. Surgical complications include recurrent laryngeal or phrenic nerve injury and thoracic duct damage. As with most congenital heart lesions, infective endocarditis is a concern and should be managed primarily by optimal oral hygiene. Antibiotic prophylaxis is reserved for patients with previous endocarditis.

Cyanotic and Other Complex Conditions

TETRALOGY OF FALLOT

Tetralogy of Fallot is the most common cyanotic congenital heart lesion in adults and represents 10% of all congenital heart defects. It may be exhibited to the physician before or, more commonly, after corrective or palliative surgery (see Table 7-2). Tetralogy is the result of a malalignment of the aorticopulmonary septum that divides the truncus arteriosus into the aorta and pulmonary artery during development, resulting in deviation of the aorta anteriorly toward the pulmonary artery. The four components of tetralogy are the following: (1) overriding of the aorta in relation to the ventricular septum; (2) right ventricular outflow obstruction, which may be valvular, subvalvular, supravalvular, or a combination of all three; (3) membranous VSD; and (4) right ventricular hypertrophy. The VSD is usually large and allows free communication between the right and left ventricles. The presence of right ventricular outflow obstruction is protective, preventing volume and pressure overload of the pulmonary circulation, which would result in fixed pulmonary hypertension. The degree of right-to-left shunt flow depends on the degree of right ventricular outflow obstruction. If pulmonic stenosis is mild, right-to-left shunt flow is minimal, and the patient remains acyanotic (pink tetralogy). More commonly, the pulmonic stenosis is severe, and a large volume of poorly oxygenated blood is shunted into the systemic circulation with resulting cyanosis. The degree of cyanosis is worsened with exercise, when the fall in systemic vascular resistance increases the degree of right-to-left shunt flow. Tetralogy may also be associated with ASD, muscular VSD, right aortic arch, and other coronary anomalies. A chromosomal deletion (22q11) is found in 15% of cases, particularly in those with associated anomalies. Such a deletion implies a higher risk for transmission of congenital heart disease to offspring.

Surgical correction of tetralogy is usually performed during infancy or childhood and involves relief of right ventricular obstruction and patch closure of the VSD. After reparative surgery, patients are at risk for residual pulmonary stenosis or regurgitation, which may lead to right ventricular enlargement and dysfunction and tricuspid regurgitation. Aortic insufficiency is common after repair and may become clinically significant. Residual VSDs, aneurysms of the right ventricular outflow tract, and sustained arrhythmias are also recognized complications. Arrhythmias may be supraventricular or ventricular, may signify hemodynamic impairment, and may contribute to an increased risk for sudden death. Prolongation of the QRS duration (to >180 milliseconds) on the surface electrocardiographic study is a marker for increased risk for ventricular tachycardia and sudden death.

Palliative surgery may have been performed in childhood to improve pulmonary blood flow. Occasionally, patients may elect not to undergo complete repair. Such palliation involves the creation of a shunt between the systemic and pulmonary circulation (e.g., subclavian artery to ipsilateral pulmonary artery [Blalock-Taussig shunt]), which results in increased pulmonary blood flow and improved oxygenation of the systemic blood. A variety of palliative shunts have been used for this purpose. Although such procedures often result in long-term palliation of hypoxia, several complications can occur. Patients may outgrow their shunts, or the shunts may spontaneously close and may lead to progressive cyanosis. If the shunt is too large, the increased volume of blood into the pulmonary circulation and left heart may result in pulmonary congestion and progress to irreversible pulmonary vascular obstruction. In patients surviving to adulthood, corrective surgery should still be undertaken, but the operative risk is higher secondary to the presence of right ventricular dysfunction.

COMPLETE TRANSPOSITION OF THE GREAT ARTERIES

Complete transposition (also known as D-transposition) represents 5% to 7% of congenital heart disease and is the most common cyanotic congenital heart disease in the newborn. It is characterized by abnormal ventriculoarterial connections with the aorta arising from the right ventricle and the pulmonary artery arising from the left. The circulation is thus two circuits in parallel. This anatomy can support fetal development, but serious consequences result on closure of the foramen ovale and ductus arteriosus shortly after birth, at which point the systemic and pulmonary circuits are separated and oxygenated blood no longer mixes with the systemic circulation. Uncorrected D-transposition has a 90% mortality rate in the first year of life. Associated defects include VSD, left ventricular outflow tract (subpulmonic) stenosis, and coarctation of the aorta.

The first successful palliative procedure for D-transposition was the atrial switch procedure (e.g., Mustard or Senning procedures) in which the venous return is baffled to the contralateral ventricle to achieve two circuits in series. These procedures result in excellent short- and mid-term outcomes. Complications include failure of the systemic right ventricle, tricuspid regurgitation, sinus node dysfunction, tachyarrhythmias, and baffle leaks or obstruction. Progressive ventricular failure should prompt consideration of heart transplantation.

In the 1980s, the arterial switch procedure supplanted the Mustard and Senning procedures. This technically challenging procedure restores normal anatomy by attaching the aorta to the left ventricle and the pulmonary artery to the right ventricle with reimplantation of the coronary arteries into the new aorta. Less long-term follow-up data are available for patients following arterial switch, but similar favorable mid-term outcomes have been noted, relative to the Mustard and Senning procedures. Late complications include obstruction of the reimplanted coronary arteries with associated myocardial ischemia, and progressive enlargement of the new aortic root with associated valvular regurgitation. It is recommended that all adults be evaluated at least once for coronary artery patency following arterial switch.

CORRECTED TRANSPOSITION OF THE GREAT ARTERIES

Inversion of the ventricles and abnormal positioning of the great arteries characterize congenital-corrected transposition of the great arteries (L-transposition). In this anomaly, the anatomic right ventricle lies on the left and receives oxygenated blood from the left atrium. Blood is ejected into an anteriorly displaced aorta. The anatomic left ventricle lies on the right and receives venous blood from the right atrium and ejects it into the posteriorly displaced pulmonary artery. This condition is not generally cyanotic and is uncommon, representing 0.5% of cases in patients with congenital heart disease.

The clinical course of patients with corrected transposition depends on the severity of other intracardiac anomalies. When the abnormality is an isolated lesion, many individuals survive into adulthood without symptoms. In some patients, the systemic ventricle (anatomic right ventricle) may fail, and pulmonary congestion may result. Associated anomalies include atrioventricular nodal block, VSD, and Ebstein anomaly.

SINGLE VENTRICLE AND FONTAN OPERATION

A variety of anatomic defects can functionally result in a single ventricle supporting both the pulmonary and systemic circulation. As such, tricuspid atresia, double-inlet left ventricle with VSD, and large atrioventricular septal defect (among others) may all have similar consequences for the patient. The cardiac output is directed in common to both the aorta and the pulmonary artery, with the balance between the two circulatory beds determined by the degree of outflow tract obstruction. If outflow obstruction is equal, the lower pulmonary vascular resistance will tend to favor pulmonary flow; thus, the ideal single ventricle will have some degree of pulmonary outflow obstruction to prevent the development of fixed pulmonary hypertension. Patients with univentricular hearts who are not repaired have a poor prognosis, with a median survival of 14 years of age. Most patients have cyanosis and functional limitations and would benefit from palliative surgery.

The goal with palliation is to optimize pulmonary blood flow without volume loading the ventricle. In suitable patients, the Fontan procedure can offer improved functional status and relieve cyanosis. The Fontan procedure and its modifications connect all systemic venous return to the pulmonary artery without an intervening ventricular pump. This can be accomplished by anastomosis of the right atrium to the pulmonary arteries, separate connections between the superior vena cava and the adjacent right pulmonary artery, and the inferior vena cava through a graft to the left pulmonary artery or a tunnel connecting the vena cava and anastomosed to the pulmonary artery. The Fontan procedure separates the two circulations and provides relief of cyanosis without providing a volume load on the left ventricle or a pressure load on the pulmonary arteries. Complications include thrombosis, obstruction, or leaks in the Fontan circuit, ventricular dysfunction, arrhythmias, hepatic dysfunction, and protein-losing enteropathy. Patients with poor ventricular function or intractable protein-losing enteropathy after the Fontan procedure should be considered for transplantation.

EISENMENGER SYNDROME

In 1897, Victor Eisenmenger first described the clinical and pathologic features of a patient with fixed pulmonary hypertension resulting from a large VSD. In 1958, Paul Wood used the term *Eisenmenger complex* to describe the combination of a large VSD with systemic pulmonary pressures and a reversed or bidirectional shunt. The same pulmonary pathologic changes can result from a large shunt at any level, and the term *Eisenmenger syndrome* was suggested to describe pulmonary hypertension with reversed or bidirectional shunting at any level. Thus a VSD, a PDA, or an ASD could all result in Eisenmenger physiologic characteristics. The defect size generally exceeds 1.5 cm in diameter for VSD, with about half that diameter for PDA and twice that diameter for ASD. Large surgical shunts can also lead to Eisenmenger syndrome.

Most patients with Eisenmenger syndrome survive to adulthood, with complications generally occurring from the third decade onward. The prognosis is better than that for patients with other causes of pulmonary hypertension such as primary pulmonary hypertension.

Complications include hyperviscosity syndrome, hemorrhage or thrombosis, arrhythmias and sudden death, endocarditis and cerebral abscess, ventricular dysfunction, hyperuricemia and gout, and renal impairment, among others. Hyperviscosity syndrome results from excessive erythrocytosis driven by increased erythropoietin in response to chronic hypoxia. Symptoms include headache, myalgias, and altered mentation. Many patients can tolerate a high hematocrit level with mild or no symptoms, and phlebotomy should not be undertaken simply in response to the hematocrit level. Excessive phlebotomy can lead to iron deficiency. Iron-deficient erythrocytes are less distensible and result in higher blood viscosity for any given hematocrit level, with microcytosis being the strongest independent predictor for cerebrovascular events.

Patients with Eisenmenger syndrome have achieved a delicate balance, and management of such patients should respect that balance. Prevention of complications is the preferred strategy. Influenza inoculations, endocarditis prophylaxis, and an avoidance of inappropriate phlebotomy are the mainstays of management. Extreme caution should be exercised with noncardiac surgery to avoid precipitous changes in vascular resistance that may lead to cardiovascular collapse. Pregnancy is strongly discouraged, considering the high risk to both the mother and the fetus. Sterilization is preferred because oral contraceptives can aggravate the risk for thrombosis. Pulmonary vasodilator therapy may improve quality of life, but carries recognized risks and should be supervised by expert care.

Other Conditions

Congenital anomalies of the coronary arteries are not uncommon and may be asymptomatic or associated with myocardial ischemia. The left circumflex or left anterior descending artery may arise from the right sinus of Valsalva and is usually not associated with abnormalities of myocardial perfusion. Either coronary artery may arise from the right sinus and may pass between the pulmonary trunk and aorta. This abnormality may result in myocardial ischemia, infarction, or sudden death in young adults, especially during exertion. Coronary artery fistulas with drainage into the right ventricle, vena cava, or pulmonary vein may be associated with myocardial ischemia if a significant amount of coronary blood flow is shunted into the venous system. Diagnosis of these abnormalities is made by coronary angiography.

Prospectus for the Future

The growing population of patients with successful outcomes after intervention for congenital heart disease is posing new challenges during adulthood. The increasing prevalence of genetic studies must be linked to genetic counseling. Early prenatal diagnoses that are linked to specific molecular defects will engender therapeutic strategies in utero. Genetic epidemiologic studies will provide important insights about the influences of the in utero environment on the subsequent susceptibility and risk factors for heart disease during adulthood.

References

Deanfield J, Thaulow E, Warnes C, et al: Management of grown up congenital heart disease. Eur Heart J 24:1035, 2003.

Gatzoulis MA, Webb GD, Daubeney PEF: Diagnosis and Management of Adult Congenital Heart Disease. Philadelphia, Elsevier, 2003.

Therrien J, Dore A, Gersony W, et al: Canadian Cardiovascular Society Consensus Conference 2001 update: Recommendations for the management of adults with congenital heart disease—Part I. Can J Cardiol 17:940, 2001.

Therrien J, Gatzoulis M, Graham T, et al: Canadian Cardiovascular Society Consensus Conference 2001 update: Recommendations for the management of adults with congenital heart disease—Part II. Can J Cardiol 17:1029, 2001.

Therrien J, Warnes C, Daliento L, et al: Canadian Cardiovascular Society Consensus Conference 2001 update: Recommendations for the management of adults with congenital heart disease—Part III. Can J Cardiol 17:1135, 2001.

Warnes CA, Williams RG, Bashore TM, et al: ACC/AHA 2008 guidelines for the management of adults with congenital heart disease. Circulation 118:e714-e833, 2008.

Webb GD, Williams RG: Care of the adult with congenital heart disease. J Am Coll Cardiol 37:1166, 2001.

Wilson W, Taubert KA, Gewitz M, et al: Prevention of endocarditis: Guidelines from the American Heart Association. Circulation 116:1736-1754, 2007.

Chapter **8**

Acquired Valvular Heart Disease

Sheldon E. Litwin

Aortic Stenosis

Aortic stenosis can be congenital or acquired in origin (Table 8-1). The most common congenital cardiac abnormality affects the bicuspid aortic valve. Significant narrowing of the orifice usually occurs during middle age after years of turbulent flow through the valve results in leaflet injury, thickening, and calcification. Rheumatic aortic stenosis results from fusion of the leaflet commissures and is usually associated with mitral valve disease. The most common cause of aortic stenosis in adults is degenerative or senile aortic stenosis, which usually occurs in patients older than 65 years. Aortic stenosis is more common in men than it is in women.

In patients with aortic stenosis, the outflow obstruction gradually increases over many years, resulting in left ventricular hypertrophy. This response allows the left ventricle to generate and maintain a large pressure gradient across the valve without a reduction in stroke volume. However, left ventricular hypertrophy often results in increased diastolic chamber stiffness because greater intracavitary pressure is required to maintain left ventricular filling. Systolic dysfunction may also occur as a result of changes in expression of myocyte contractile and calcium-cycling proteins.

Patients with severe aortic stenosis may be asymptomatic for many years despite the presence of severe obstruction. The cardinal symptoms associated with aortic stenosis are angina, syncope, and congestive heart failure. Angina can occur in the absence of epicardial coronary artery disease because of the increased oxygen demand of the hypertrophied ventricle and decreased coronary blood flow secondary to elevated left ventricular diastolic pressure. Syncope may result from transient arrhythmias but more commonly occurs with exertion when cardiac output is insufficient to maintain arterial pressure in the presence of exercise-induced peripheral vasodilation. Dyspnea may result from increased filling pressures associated with the noncompliant, hypertrophied left ventricle or may signal the onset of systolic

dysfunction. Once patients with severe aortic stenosis develop symptoms, the prognosis is poor unless surgical correction is undertaken. Previous studies have shown that the mean survival rate after the onset of symptoms is about 2 years in patients with heart failure, 3 years in patients with syncope, and 5 years in patients with angina (Fig. 8-1).

On physical examination, the patient with aortic stenosis may have a laterally displaced, sustained apical impulse secondary to left ventricular hypertrophy (Table 8-2). An audible or palpable S_4 may also be present if the patient is in sinus rhythm. Decreased mobility of the aortic cusps may cause the A_2 component of S_2 to be soft or absent. The murmur of aortic stenosis is a harsh, crescendo-decrescendo murmur that is best heard over the right upper sternal border and often radiates to the neck. As the obstruction increases, the *peak* of the murmur occurs later in systole. If left ventricular dysfunction develops, the murmur may decrease in intensity secondary to a reduction in stroke volume. The carotid impulse is often diminished in intensity and delayed (i.e., pulsus parvus et tardus) (see Chapter 4), although in older adults, these changes may be present secondary to intrinsic vascular disease in the absence of significant aortic stenosis.

The principal electrocardiographic finding in aortic stenosis is left ventricular hypertrophy. Heart block may develop as a result of calcification from the aortic valve extending into the conducting system. Echocardiography is the most important diagnostic test and is useful to determine the cause of the aortic stenosis and to quantitate the degree of obstruction. The mean transvalvular gradient and valve area can be measured and calculated using Doppler techniques. Patients with severe stenosis will often undergo cardiac catheterization both to confirm the presence of severe aortic stenosis and to determine whether concomitant coronary artery disease is present. A valve area less than or equal to 0.7 cm^2 defines critical aortic stenosis (normal valve area is 3 cm^2) and is usually associated with a mean transvalvular gradient of more than 50 mm Hg when normal left

Table 8-1 **Major Causes of Valvular Heart Disease in Adults**

Aortic Stenosis

Bicuspid aortic valve
Rheumatic fever
Degenerative stenosis

Aortic Regurgitation

Bicuspid aortic valve
Aortic dissection
Endocarditis
Rheumatic fever
Aortic root dilation

Mitral Stenosis

Rheumatic fever

Mitral Regurgitation

Chronic

Mitral valve prolapse
Left ventricular dilation
Posterior wall myocardial infarction
Rheumatic fever
Endocarditis

Acute

Posterior wall or papillary muscle ischemia
Papillary muscle or chordal rupture
Endocarditis
Prosthetic valve dysfunction
Systolic anterior motion of mitral valve

Tricuspid Regurgitation

Functional (annular) dilation
Tricuspid valve prolapse
Endocarditis
Carcinoid heart disease

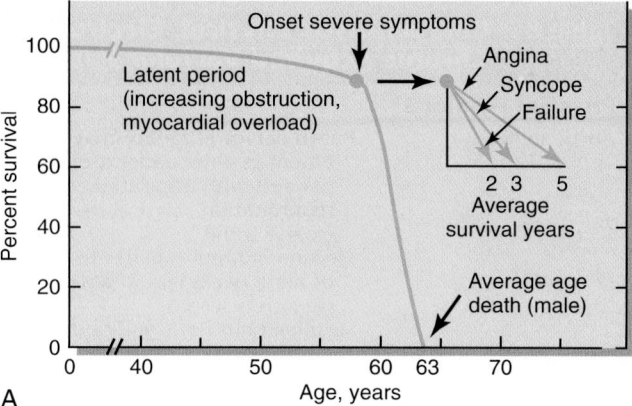

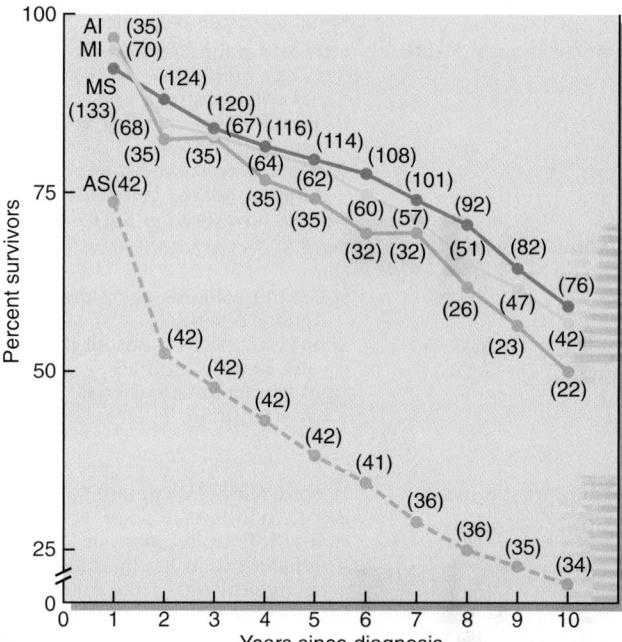

Figure 8-1 A, Natural history of aortic stenosis without surgical therapy. **B,** Natural history of mitral and aortic valve disease in an era when surgical therapy was not widely available. Survival rates in 42 patients with aortic stenosis (AS, *orange circles with dotted line*), 35 patients with aortic insufficiency (AI, *orange circles with solid line*), and 133 patients with mitral insufficiency (MI, *yellow circles with solid line*). Clinical course in AI, MS *(red circles with dotted line),* and MI is similar with a 5-year survival rate of about 80% and a 10-year survival rate of about 60%. Patients with AS have a worse prognosis, with 5- and 10-year survival rates of about 40% and 20%, respectively. (**A** from Ross J Jr, Braunwald E: Aortic stenosis. Circulation 38[Suppl V]:61, 1968. Copyright © 1968 American Heart Association. **B** from Rapaport E: Natural history of aortic and mitral valve disease, Am J Cardiol 35:221-227, 1975.)

ventricular function is present. It should be noted that in patients with reduced systolic function, the mean gradient might be low despite the presence of severe aortic stenosis. Moreover, symptoms are often present with valve areas of 0.7 to 1 cm^2.

Treatment in most adults with symptomatic aortic stenosis is surgical replacement of the valve. The operative risk and prognosis are best in patients with preserved left ventricular systolic function. However, surgery should still be considered in patients with left ventricular dysfunction because relief of the obstruction can result in significant clinical and hemodynamic improvement. A more nuanced approach is required for patients with asymptomatic aortic stenosis in whom a recommendation for surgical intervention might be based on the functional assessment by exercise stress testing. Advanced age is associated with higher operative morbidity but is not a contraindication to surgical therapy. Balloon aortic valvuloplasty is a percutaneous technique in which a balloon catheter is positioned across the aortic valve. Inflation results in fracture or separation of the fused and calcified cusps. This procedure is most effective in young patients with noncalcified congenital aortic stenosis and is rarely used in adult patients with calcific aortic stenosis because of significant complications and a high restenosis rate (about 30% at 6 months). Medical interventions with cholesterol-lowering therapies to slow the progression of mild to moderate aortic stenosis are still under clinical inves-

tigation. Routine antibiotic prophylaxis is no longer recommended unless there is prior history of endocarditis.

Aortic Regurgitation

Aortic regurgitation (AR) may be secondary to primary disease of the aortic leaflets, aortic root, or both (see Table 8-1). Abnormalities of the aortic leaflets may be secondary

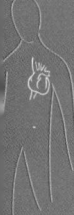

Table 8-2 Characteristic Physical, Electrocardiographic, and Chest Radiographic Findings in Chronic Acquired Valvular Heart Disease

Physical Findings*		Electrocardiogram	Radiograph
Aortic stenosis	Pulsus parvus et tardus (may be absent in older patients or in patients with associated aortic regurgitation); carotid *shudder* (coarse thrill) Ejection murmur radiates to base of neck; peaks late in systole if stenosis is severe Sustained but not significantly displaced LV impulse A_2 decreased, S_2 single or paradoxically split S_4 gallop, often palpable	LV hypertrophy Left bundle branch block is also common Rare heart block from calcific involvement of conduction system	LV prominence without dilation Post-stenotic aortic root dilation Aortic valve calcification
Aortic regurgitation	Increased pulse pressure Bifid carotid pulses Rapid pulse upstroke and collapse LV impulse hyperdynamic and displaced laterally Diastolic decrescendo murmur; duration related to severity Systolic flow murmur S_{3G} common	LV hypertrophy, often with narrow deep Q waves	LV and aortic dilation
Mitral stenosis	Loud S_1 OS S_2-OS interval inversely related to stenosis severity S_1 not loud, and OS absent if valve heavily calcified Signs of pulmonary arterial hypertension	Left atrial abnormality Atrial fibrillation common RV hypertrophy pattern may develop if associated pulmonary arterial hypertension is present	Large LA: double-density, posterior displacement of esophagus, elevation of left main stem bronchus Straightening of left heart border as a result of enlarged left appendage Small or normal-sized LV Large pulmonary artery Pulmonary venous congestion
Mitral regurgitation	Hyperdynamic LV impulse S_3 Widely split S_2 may occur Holosystolic apical murmur radiating to axilla (murmur may be atypical with acute mitral regurgitation, papillary muscle dysfunction, or mitral valve prolapse)	LA abnormality LV hypertrophy Atrial fibrillation	Enlarged LA and LV Pulmonary venous congestion
Mitral valve prolapse	One or more systolic clicks, often mid-systolic, followed by late systolic murmur Auscultatory findings dynamic Symptoms may include tall thin habitus, pectus excavatum, straight back syndrome	Often normal Occasionally ST-segment depression and/or T-wave changes in inferior leads	Depends on degree of valve regurgitation and presence or absence of those abnormalities
Tricuspid stenosis	Jugular venous distention with prominent α wave if sinus rhythm Tricuspid OS and diastolic rumble at left sternal border; may be overshadowed by concomitant mitral stenosis Tricuspid OS and rumble increased during inspiration	Right atrial abnormality Atrial fibrillation common	Large RA
Tricuspid regurgitation	Jugular venous distention with large regurgitant (systolic) wave Systolic murmur at left sternal border, increased with inspiration Diastolic flow rumble RV S_3 increased with inspiration Hepatomegaly with systolic pulsation	RA abnormality; findings are often related to cause of the tricuspid regurgitation	RA and RV are enlarged; findings are often related to cause of the tricuspid regurgitation

*Findings are influenced by the severity and chronicity of the valve disorder.
LA, left atrium; LV, left ventricle; OS, opening snap; RA, right atrium; RV, right ventricle.

to rheumatic disease, congenital abnormalities, endocarditis, or use of certain anorexigenic drugs. In addition, AR is commonly a consequence of degenerative and bicuspid aortic stenosis. An aortic root pathologic condition associated with annular and root dilation may result in separation or prolapse of the leaflets.

With chronic AR, the left ventricle must accommodate the normal inflow from the left atrium in addition to the aortic regurgitant volume. As a result, the left ventricle dilates and hypertrophies to maintain normal effective forward flow and to minimize wall stress. As the AR progresses, these changes in left ventricular size and wall thickness may be insufficient to maintain normal left ventricular filling pressures, and irreversible myocyte damage may occur. As a result, the left ventricle will dilate further, and systolic function and effective stroke volume will decrease.

Clinically, patients with chronic, severe AR may be asymptomatic for long periods secondary to the compensatory changes in the left ventricle. When symptoms do develop, they are primarily related to an elevation in left ventricular filling pressures and include dyspnea on exertion, orthopnea, and paroxysmal nocturnal dyspnea. Many patients will describe chest or head pounding secondary to the hyperdynamic circulation. If effective cardiac output is reduced, the patient may complain primarily of fatigue and weakness. As with aortic stenosis, angina may occur in patients with AR even in the absence of epicardial coronary artery disease secondary to elevated left ventricular filling pressures and reduced coronary perfusion pressure.

On physical examination, patients with severe AR have a widened pulse pressure (difference between the systolic and diastolic pressures) as a result of the runoff of blood back into the left ventricle (see Table 8-2). The arterial pulse is usually bounding, with a rapid upstroke and quick collapse (Corrigan disease or water-hammer pulse) (see Chapter 4). The cardiac impulse is hyperdynamic and is displaced laterally and inferiorly. The murmur of AR is a high-pitched, decrescendo diastolic murmur best heard at the lower left sternal border with the patient sitting up and leaning forward. Asking the patient to hold his or her breath at end expiration while the hands are held behind the head may also improve the ability to auscultate the murmur of AR. A systolic ejection murmur is often heard secondary to increased forward flow across the aortic valve. An S_3 gallop may be present, especially if the patient has developed symptoms of heart failure. A low-pitched, diastolic murmur (Austin Flint murmur) may be heard at the apex and confused with the murmur of mitral stenosis (MS). This sound is thought to be secondary to the incomplete opening of the mitral leaflets (functional MS) secondary to elevated left ventricular filling pressures or impingement of the AR jet on the anterior mitral leaflet.

The natural history of chronic AR is varied. Many patients with moderate to severe AR will remain asymptomatic for many years and generally have a favorable prognosis. Other patients may have progression of AR severity and develop left ventricular dysfunction and symptoms of congestive heart failure. Echocardiography is the primary tool to monitor the progression of disease and optimize the timing of surgery. Prior studies have shown that patients at high risk are those with left ventricular end-systolic diameters greater than 50 mm or an ejection fraction of less than 50%. Surgery is usually recommended before developing this degree of left ventricular enlargement or dysfunction. Therefore patients with known moderate to severe AR should be monitored regularly with noninvasive testing to detect early signs of cardiac (i.e., left ventricular) decompensation.

Treatment of patients with moderate to severe AR theoretically should include vasodilator therapy, such as nifedipine or angiotensin-converting enzyme (ACE) inhibitors, because these agents unload the left ventricle. Although some published data suggest that these agents may slow the progression of myocardial dysfunction and delay the need for surgery, more recent data do not support that contention.

Valve replacement surgery should be considered in symptomatic patients and those with evidence of significant left ventricular enlargement or left ventricular systolic dysfunction. In patients with reduced left ventricular ejection fraction of short duration (14 months), valve replacement usually results in significant improvement in ventricular function. If left ventricular dysfunction has been present for a prolonged period, then permanent myocardial damage may occur. Although such patients should not be excluded from surgery, their long-term prognosis remains poor.

As compared with chronic AR, acute AR is a medical emergency that often requires immediate surgical intervention. The causes of acute AR include infective endocarditis, traumatic rupture of the aortic leaflets, aortic root dissection, and acute dysfunction of a prosthetic valve. Acute AR is the result of hemodynamic instability because the left ventricle is unable to dilate to accommodate the increased diastolic volume, resulting in decreased effective forward flow. Left ventricular and left atrial pressures rise quickly, leading to pulmonary congestion.

Patients with acute AR often exhibit symptoms and signs of cardiogenic shock. The patient is usually pale with cool extremities as a result of peripheral vasoconstriction. The pulse is weak and rapid, and the pulse pressure is normal or decreased. The murmur of acute AR is low pitched and short because of rapid equilibration of aortic and left ventricular pressures during diastole. An S_3 gallop is often present. Echocardiography is useful to assess AR severity and to determine its cause and can be quickly performed at the bedside in the patient who is acutely ill.

The medical treatment of acute AR includes vasodilator therapy and diuretics if the blood pressure is stable. In patients who are hemodynamically compromised, inotropic support and vasopressors may be necessary. For most patients with acute AR, urgent valve replacement remains the treatment of choice. Intra-aortic balloon counterpulsation is relatively contraindicated because it may worsen AR severity.

Mitral Stenosis

MS occurs when thickening and immobility of the mitral leaflets impede flow from the left atrium to the left ventricle. Rheumatic fever is by far the most common cause of MS. Rarely, congenital abnormalities, connective tissue disorders, left atrial tumors, and overly aggressive surgical repair

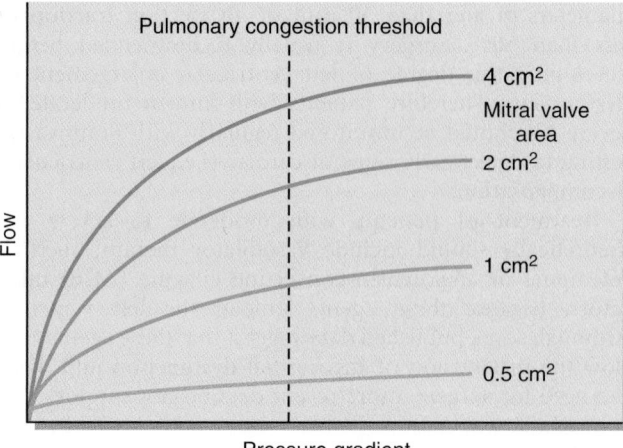

Figure 8-2 Graphic illustration of the relationship between the diastolic gradient across the mitral valve and the flow through the mitral valve. As the mitral valve becomes more stenotic, the pressure gradient across the mitral valve must increase to maintain flow into the left ventricle. When the mitral valve area is 1 cm^2 or less, the flow rate into the left ventricle cannot be significantly increased, despite a significantly elevated pressure gradient across the mitral valve. (Adapted from Wallace AG: Pathophysiology of cardiovascular disease. In Smith LH Jr, Thier SO [eds]: The International Textbook of Medicine, vol 1. Philadelphia, WB Saunders, 1981, p 1192.)

of a regurgitant valve may lead to obstruction of the mitral valve. Two thirds of patients with MS are women. The pathologic changes that occur with rheumatic MS include fusion of the leaflet commissures and thickening, fibrosis, and calcification of the mitral leaflets and chordae. These changes occur over many years before dysfunction becomes hemodynamically important.

The initial hemodynamic change that occurs with MS is an elevated left atrial pressure created by obstruction to left ventricular inflow (Fig. 8-2). This pressure change is transmitted back to the pulmonary venous system and may result in pulmonary congestion. Initially, this change may only occur at more rapid heart rates, such as with exercise or atrial arrhythmias, when higher left atrial pressures develop during the shortened diastolic period. As the MS becomes more severe, left atrial pressure remains elevated even at normal heart rates, and symptoms related to elevated pulmonary venous pressures may be present at rest. Chronic elevations in pulmonary venous pressures may lead to an increase in pulmonary vascular resistance and pulmonary arterial pressures. If the MS is not corrected, irreversible changes in the pulmonary vasculature may occur, and signs and symptoms of right ventricular heart failure may develop. In contrast, left ventricular filling pressures are usually normal or low with mild to moderate MS. As the stenosis becomes severe, filling of the left ventricle is impaired, and stroke volume and cardiac output are reduced.

Patients with MS of rheumatic origins usually develop symptoms during the third or fourth decade of life. Dyspnea, orthopnea, and atrial fibrillation are the most common symptoms. Some patients may have sudden hemoptysis secondary to rupture of the dilated bronchial veins (pulmonary apoplexy) or blood-tinged sputum associated with pulmonary edema. Peripheral embolism from left atrial thrombus

may also occur, even in the absence of atrial fibrillation. In long-standing, severe MS, patients may develop peripheral edema secondary to elevated right ventricular pressures and right ventricular dysfunction. Compression of the left recurrent laryngeal nerve from a severely dilated left atrium may result in hoarseness (Ortner syndrome).

On physical examination, S$_1$ is loud early in the course of MS because the leaflets remain fully open throughout diastole and then quickly close (see Table 8-2). As the leaflets become more calcified and immobile, S$_1$ will become softer or completely absent. The opening snap is a high-pitched sound after the S$_2$ and reflects the abrupt mitral valve opening. As the MS becomes more severe, the interval between the S$_2$ and opening snap becomes shorter because left atrial pressure exceeds left ventricular pressure earlier in diastole. The characteristic low-pitched rumbling murmur of MS is best heard at the left ventricular apex with the patient in the left lateral decubitus position. The murmur is loudest in early diastole when rapid ventricular filling occurs. If sinus rhythm is present, the murmur may increase in intensity after atrial contraction (presystolic accentuation). In some patients, the murmur may only be heard at times of increased blood flow through the mitral valve, such as after exercise. If pulmonary artery pressures are elevated, a palpable P$_2$ may be detected at the upper left sternal border. On auscultation, the pulmonic component of S$_2$ is prominent and a right ventricular gallop may be present.

Echocardiography is the most useful tool for pathologic assessment of the mitral apparatus as well as the severity of the stenosis. The characteristic rheumatic deformity observed with two-dimensional imaging is doming (i.e., hockey stick deformity) of the anterior mitral valve leaflet, which is secondary to fusion of the commissures and tethering of the leaflet tips (Fig. 8-3). In addition, the mobility of the leaflets

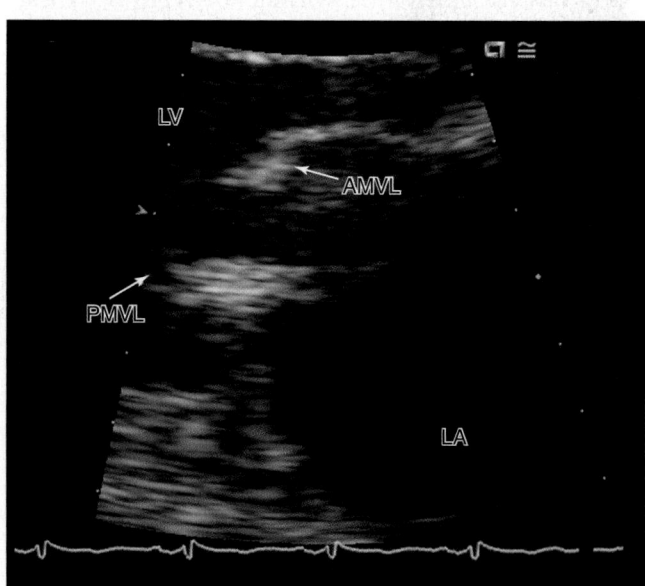

Figure 8-3 Example of hockey stick deformity of mitral valve in chronic rheumatic heart disease as visualized by echocardiography. Tips of anterior mitral valve leaflet (AMVL) are tethered, thus restricting opening of the valve. Posterior mitral valve leaflet (PMVL) is thickened and has reduced mobility. Left atrium (LA) is characteristically enlarged.

and the extent of valvular calcification can be assessed and used to determine treatment options. Doppler techniques allow calculation of the mitral valve area and the transvalvular gradient. Transesophageal echocardiography is a useful tool for studying the mitral apparatus and examining the left atrium for thrombus before percutaneous valvuloplasty.

The severity of MS and associated hemodynamic changes can also be evaluated with cardiac catheterization. Measurements of the cardiac output and transvalvular gradient can be used to calculate the valve area by means of the Gorlin formula. A normal mitral valve area is 4 to 6 cm^2, and critical MS is defined as a valve area less than 1 cm^2.

Patients with mild to moderate MS can usually be managed medically. Heart rate control is imperative in these patients because more rapid rates reduce the length of the diastolic filling period. This is especially true in patients with atrial fibrillation, in whom loss of atrial contraction may further reduce left ventricular filling. Anticoagulant therapy is indicated for patients with atrial fibrillation and for those with sinus rhythm who have had prior embolic events or who have moderate to severe MS. Diuretics are useful in relieving pulmonary congestion and signs of right ventricular heart failure. All patients should be instructed on the importance of endocarditis prophylaxis. Prophylaxis against recurrent bouts of rheumatic fever may be used in patients younger than 30 years.

Patients with severe symptoms (New York Heart Association classes III through IV) and moderate to severe MS should be considered for a percutaneous or surgical intervention. Percutaneous balloon valvuloplasty is a new technique in which a balloon catheter positioned across the mitral valve is quickly inflated, resulting in separation of the fused cusps. Optimal short- and long-term results are obtained in patients with pliable, noncalcified leaflets and chords, minimal mitral regurgitation (MR), and no evidence of left atrial thrombus. A surgical option in this same group of patients is open mitral valve commissurotomy. With direct visualization of the mitral valve, the surgeon is able to débride the valve, separate the fused cusps, and remove left atrial thrombi. Although the valve remains abnormal, this procedure is associated with a low operative mortality and a good hemodynamic result and may spare the patient from a valve replacement for many years. If mitral commissurotomy is not an option, valve replacement with a bioprosthetic or mechanical prosthesis can be performed.

Mitral Regurgitation

MR can result from abnormalities of the mitral leaflets, annulus, chordae, or papillary muscles (see Table 8-1). The most common leaflet abnormality resulting in chronic MR is myxomatous degeneration of the mitral valves. This condition results in mitral valve prolapse (MVP), which progresses as the chordae become elongated or rupture (Fig. 8-4). Both acute and chronic rheumatic fever may also cause MR.

With chronic MR, the left ventricle dilates to compensate for the increased regurgitant volume. However, in contrast to aortic insufficiency, the increased volume is ejected into the low-pressure left atrium. Thus, left ventricular wall stress and pressure remain normal for a significant period. If the left atrium dilates sufficiently to accommodate the increased

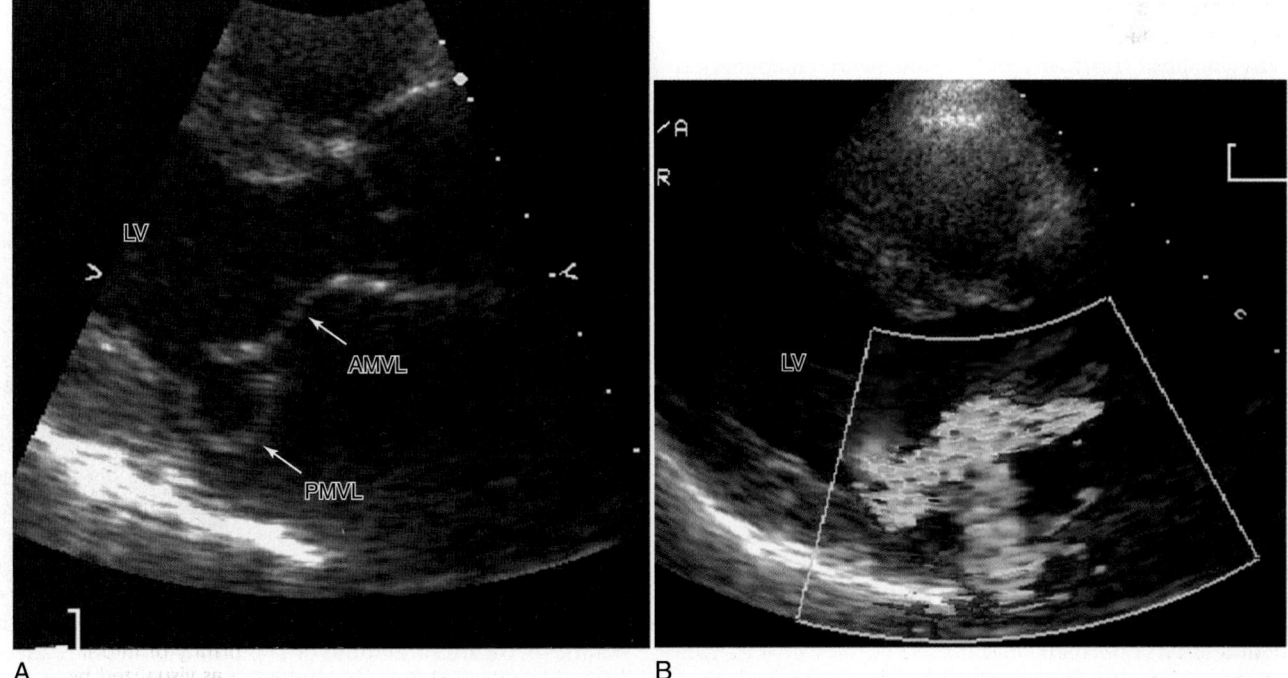

A   B

Figure 8-4 Typical example of mitral valve prolapse is visualized with transthoracic echocardiography. **A,** Prolapse of the posterior mitral valve leaflet (PMVL) behind the mitral valve annular plane results from lengthening and rupture of chordae tendineae. In this patient, a highly eccentric *(blue)* jet of moderate-to-severe mitral regurgitation is observed **(B).** AMVL, anterior mitral valve leaflet; LV, left ventricle.

volume, left atrial and pulmonary venous pressures will remain normal. As the MR progresses, myocyte damage may occur, resulting in further left ventricular dilation, an elevation in diastolic filling pressures, and a reduction in left ventricular systolic function. As left atrial and pulmonary venous pressures increase, pulmonary congestion may occur.

Patients with chronic compensated MR are usually asymptomatic and have normal functional capacity. When symptoms do occur, left ventricular systolic function is sometimes depressed. Patients may initially complain of fatigue and dyspnea with exertion secondary to reduced cardiac output and elevation in pulmonary venous pressures. If the MR remains untreated, pulmonary hypertension and right ventricular heart failure may occur.

MR characteristically produces a holosystolic murmur best heard at the apex and radiating to the axilla and back (see Table 8-2). If an eccentric, anteriorly directed jet of MR is present, an ejection-quality murmur may be present and confused with an aortic outflow murmur. If the MR is secondary to MVP, a mid-systolic click may be present, followed by a late systolic murmur. MR associated with rheumatic mitral disease may be accompanied by heart sounds typical of MS.

Echocardiography is the primary noninvasive method for defining mitral valve pathologic evaluation and assessing left ventricular size and function. Doppler techniques are useful in grading the severity of MR. Quantitative echocardiographic measures of MR severity are predictive of long-term survival, even in patients who are asymptomatic. Mitral valve repair appears to normalize the survival curves in this group of patients. MR can also be assessed during cardiac catheterization by estimating the amount of contrast medium that is ejected into the left atrium during left ventriculography. In addition, left ventricular size and systolic function can be quantitated, filling pressures can be measured, and the coronary anatomy can be defined.

The medical treatment of patients with compensated chronic MR is afterload reduction with vasodilator therapy, such as ACE inhibitors or hydralazine. The timing of surgery is difficult because the development of symptoms often indicates the presence of left ventricular dysfunction and irreversible myocardial damage. In addition, mitral valve replacement with disruption of the chordal apparatus often results in further left ventricular dilation and decline in systolic function.

Echocardiographic parameters that identify patients at risk for a poor response to mitral valve replacement are a left ventricular end-diastolic diameter greater than 70 mm, an end-systolic diameter greater than 45 mm, and a low-normal or reduced left ventricular ejection fraction. Patients with known MR should be followed with yearly studies to monitor left ventricular function and size so that surgery can be performed *before* irreversible myocyte damage and left ventricular remodeling occur. The development of either atrial fibrillation or pulmonary hypertension may be an indication for earlier surgical intervention, even if left ventricle size and function are still normal.

In many patients, the mitral valve may be repaired, thus avoiding many of the potential complications associated with valve replacement. With this surgery, sections of redundant leaflet can be excised, leaflets débrided, and chordae

shortened. A prosthetic ring (annuloplasty) can be sewn into the mitral annulus to reduce the size of the orifice and increase the degree of leaflet coaptation. The advantage of this procedure is that preservation of the mitral apparatus helps maintain normal left ventricular geometry and function. In addition, long-term anticoagulation is not necessary in most patients in sinus rhythm. Valve repair is generally not indicated if the mitral valve is heavily calcified or disrupted secondary to papillary muscle disease or endocarditis. In these instances, valve replacement is the procedure of choice.

Based on excellent surgical outcomes and long-term durability, mitral valve repair is the procedure of choice in all patients in whom it is technically feasible. Severe MR, even in the absence of symptoms or left ventricular dysfunction, may be an appropriate reason for surgical intervention. A variety of percutaneous mitral valve repair techniques are in development.

Acute severe MR is often a life-threatening condition that can result from a variety of papillary muscle, chordal, and leaflet abnormalities (see Table 8-1). Patients with acute MR usually become severely ill because the left atrium does not dilate to accommodate the regurgitant volume. As a result, left atrial and pulmonary venous pressures abruptly increase, resulting in pulmonary congestion. In addition, the decreases in stroke volume and cardiac output result in an increase in systemic vascular resistance and, as a consequence, an increase in the severity of MR. Patients usually exhibit pulmonary edema and signs of cardiogenic shock. On auscultation, the MR murmur is often a soft, low-pitched sound in early systole, resulting from rapid equilibration of left ventricular and left atrial pressures. Afterload reduction with either an intravenous vasodilator, such as nitroprusside, or an intra-aortic balloon pump may help stabilize the patient before urgent valve replacement surgery. Ischemia of the posterior wall or papillary muscles may cause acute but transient MR.

Mitral Valve Prolapse

MVP is reported to be present in about 1% to 3% of the population. Although MVP can be observed in all ages and in both sexes, epidemiologic studies suggest that the prevalence is greater in women than it is in men. In some patients, MVP is inherited as an autosomal dominant trait with variable penetrance.

MVP is present when superior displacement in ventricular systole of one or both mitral valve leaflets exists across the plane of the mitral annulus toward the left atrium (see Fig. 8-4). Primary or classic MVP occurs when myxomatous degeneration of the mitral valve occurs without evidence of systemic disease. Secondary MVP is also characterized by myxomatous degeneration of the mitral apparatus but in the presence of a recognizable systemic or connective tissue disease, such as Marfan syndrome or systemic lupus erythematosus. Functional MVP results from structural abnormalities of the mitral annulus or papillary muscles or reduced left ventricular volume, but the mitral leaflets are anatomically normal.

Most patients with MVP are asymptomatic. Although a variety of nonspecific symptoms have been associated with

MVP (e.g., chest pain, palpitations, dizziness, anxiety [MVP syndrome]), the frequency of these symptoms is no different from that in the general population. MVP may be associated with varying degrees of MR. MR severity is probably the main determinant of long-term complications. The characteristic physical examination finding in MVP is the mid-systolic click, followed by a late systolic murmur (see Table 8-2). The auscultatory findings of MVP are subtle and are greatly affected by changes in left ventricular volume. Maneuvers that reduce left ventricular volume will result in prolapse of the redundant leaflets early in systole; as a result, the click will occur early in systole, and the MR murmur will sound more holosystolic. If left ventricular volume is increased, the click will be heard late in systole, followed by a short systolic murmur. The diagnosis of MVP is usually confirmed by echocardiography, which allows examination of the mitral apparatus and determination of the MR severity.

Most patients with mild prolapse and insignificant MR are asymptomatic and require no specific intervention. Endocarditis prophylaxis is generally recommended only if mild or greater MR exists. However, in some individuals, the MR may progress to such a degree that serial examinations and echocardiograms are necessary to monitor MR severity and left ventricular function. Middle-aged and older men and patients with asymmetrical prolapse are at highest risk for developing complications from MVP, such as severe MR and endocarditis. MR that acutely worsens may be related to rupture of the chordae tendineae. Sudden death in the absence of hemodynamically significant MR is rare.

Patients with MVP and evidence of structural leaflet abnormalities or significant MR should receive endocarditis prophylaxis. Symptomatic arrhythmias should be treated as discussed in Chapter 10. For patients with severe MR, mitral valve repair or replacement may be indicated as discussed earlier (see "Mitral Regurgitation").

Tricuspid Stenosis

Tricuspid stenosis is most often rheumatic in origin and is usually associated with mitral or aortic disease. Other rare causes include carcinoid syndrome, congenital valve abnormalities, and leaflet tumors or vegetations.

Similar to MS, tricuspid stenosis is more common in women than it is in men and tends to be a slowly progressive disease. Patients generally exhibit symptoms and signs of right ventricular heart failure, such as fatigue, abdominal bloating, and peripheral edema. On physical examination, a prominent jugular venous a wave may be present if the patient is in sinus rhythm and may be confused with an arterial pulsation. In addition, a palpable presystolic pulsation coinciding with atrial contraction may be felt on palpation of the liver. On auscultation, the findings of tricuspid stenosis may not be detected secondary to the presence of mitral and aortic valve disease. However, an opening snap may be audible at the left sternal border, followed by a soft, high-pitched diastolic murmur. In contrast to MS, the murmur of tricuspid stenosis is shorter in duration and accentuated with inspiration.

Tricuspid stenosis can be diagnosed by echocardiography or right ventricular catheterization. Because the right heart is a low-pressure system, the mean gradient across the tricuspid valve may be quite small (5 mm Hg) yet still clinically important.

Tricuspid Regurgitation

Tricuspid regurgitation (TR) is most often secondary to dilation of the right ventricle and tricuspid annulus that may occur with right ventricular heart failure of any cause. Other causes include endocarditis, carcinoid syndrome, congenital abnormalities, and chest wall trauma.

In the absence of pulmonary hypertension, TR is usually well tolerated. However, if right ventricular dysfunction is present, patients usually have symptoms of right ventricular heart failure. On physical examination, the jugular veins are distended, and a prominent v wave is usually present. Hepatic congestion is common and often associated with a palpable systolic pulsation. The murmur of TR is high pitched and pansystolic and is best heard along the sternal border. Maneuvers that increase venous return, such as inspiration or leg raising, accentuate the murmur and are helpful in differentiating TR from MR or aortic outflow tract murmurs. If the TR is acute, the murmur is usually soft and present only during early systole.

TR related to pulmonary hypertension and right ventricular dysfunction will usually significantly improve with treatment of the underlying cause. Repair of the tricuspid annulus (annuloplasty) may restore tricuspid valve competence in patients with persistent symptoms despite treatment. In individuals with a primary leaflet pathologic condition, tricuspid valve replacement may be necessary.

Pulmonic Stenosis and Regurgitation

Pulmonic stenosis is most often congenital in origin and is discussed further in Chapter 7. Rheumatic deformity of the pulmonic valve is rare and not usually associated with hemodynamically important obstruction.

Pulmonic regurgitation is most often the result of dilation of the annulus secondary to pulmonary hypertension of any cause. Symptoms are usually related to the primary disease and in most cases are secondary to right ventricular heart failure. In this setting, the murmur of pulmonic regurgitation is a high-pitched, blowing murmur best heard at the second left intercostal space (Graham Steell murmur). In the absence of pulmonary hypertension, the murmur is usually low pitched and occurs late in diastole. Treatment is usually directed at the underlying cause of the pulmonary hypertension. Rarely and usually in the setting of congenital or previously repaired pulmonic valve disease, the valve will need to be replaced because of intractable right ventricular heart failure.

Multivalvular Disease

Multivalvular disease is common, especially in patients with rheumatic heart disease and in the older adult population.

Often, regurgitant lesions, such as TR and pulmonic regurgitation, are the result of another valve lesion, such as MS in association with pulmonary hypertension. In general, symptoms are most often related to the most proximal valve lesion. However, the severity of each individual lesion may be difficult to assess clinically, and, therefore, careful evaluation with echocardiography and right and left ventricular heart catheterization is necessary to assess valve function before any planned surgery. Failure to correct all significant valvular lesions may result in a poor clinical outcome. Double valve replacement is associated with a higher operative and long-term mortality than single valve replacement.

Rheumatic Heart Disease

Acute rheumatic fever (ARF) is the sequelae of group A β-hemolytic streptococcal infection. The disease is thought to be secondary to an abnormal immunologic response to the streptococcal infection. ARF usually occurs in children 4 to 9 years of age, with boys and girls being equally affected. Although the prevalence of this disease has significantly decreased in the United States over the past several decades, it still poses a major health care problem in many developing nations, and endemic outbreaks have been identified even in the United States.

ARF is characterized by a diffuse inflammation of the heart (pancarditis). An exudative pericarditis is common and often results in fibrosis and obliteration of the pericardial sac. Constrictive pericarditis is rare. The myocardium is often infiltrated with lymphocytes, and areas of necrosis may occur. The characteristic histologic finding in the myocardium is the Aschoff body, which is a confluence of monocytes and macrophages surrounded by fibrous tissue. Valvulitis is characterized by verrucous lesions on the leaflet edge, which are composed of cellular infiltrates and fibrin. The mitral valve is most frequently involved, followed by the aortic valve. Involvement of the tricuspid or pulmonic valve is rare. Valvulitis can be recognized by the presence of a new insufficiency murmur. Aortic stenosis and MS do not occur for many years, when progression of the fibrosis results in restricted leaflet mobility.

The presentation of ARF is usually an acute, febrile illness 2 to 4 weeks after a streptococcal pharyngitis infection. Because the diagnosis of ARF cannot be made by laboratory tests alone, guidelines based on the symptoms and a physical examination have been established (modified Jones criteria) (Table 8-3). A diagnosis of ARF can be made if two major, or one major and two minor, criteria are present after a recent, documented streptococcal pharyngitis infection. Major criteria include evidence of carditis (e.g., pleuritic chest pain, friction rub, heart failure, MR), polyarthritis, chorea, erythema marginatum, and subcutaneous nodules. Minor criteria include fever, arthralgia, and a history of rheumatic fever or known rheumatic heart disease.

Once the diagnosis is established, a course of therapy with penicillin is indicated to eradicate the streptococcal infection. Salicylates are effective for the treatment of fever and arthritis. Corticosteroids and immunosuppressive therapy have not been proved beneficial in the management of the carditis. Heart failure should be treated with standard therapy.

Recurrent attacks of rheumatic fever are common, especially during the first 5 to 10 years after the primary illness. Rheumatic fever prophylaxis should be continued during this period, and for 10 years in patients with a high exposure rate to streptococcal infection (e.g., health care professionals, child care workers, military recruits). Patients with significant rheumatic heart disease should receive prophylaxis indefinitely, considering the high rate of recurrence in these individuals. The recommended therapy for prophylaxis is an intramuscular injection of 1.2 million units of benzathine penicillin monthly. Alternatively, oral penicillin or erythromycin may be used. Noncompliance with these agents reduces the effectiveness of this mode of therapy.

Prosthetic Heart Valves

Two types of artificial heart valves are available: mechanical valves (tilting disk and bi-leaflet) and tissue valves (bioprostheses) (Fig. 8-5). The mechanical valves have a favorable

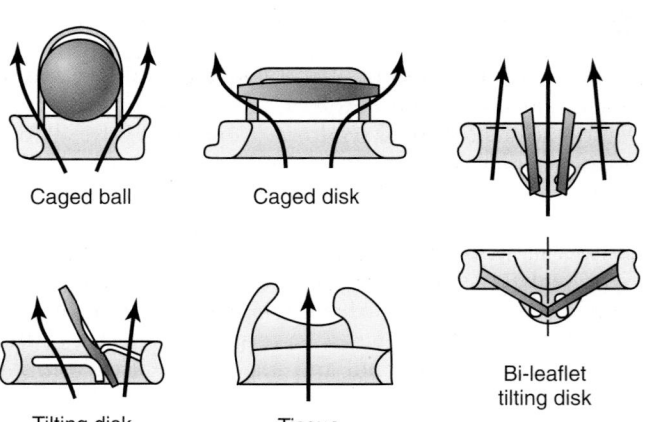

Caged ball   Caged disk

Tilting disk   Tissue   Bi-leaflet tilting disk

Figure 8-5 Designs and flow patterns of major categories of prosthetic heart valves: caged ball, caged disk, tilting disk, bi-leaflet tilting disk, and bioprosthetic (tissue) valves. Whereas flow in mechanical valves must course along both sides of the occluder, bioprostheses have a central flow pattern. (From Schoen FJ, Titus JL, Lawrie GM: Bioengineering aspects of heart valve replacement. Ann Biomed Eng 10:97-128, 1982; Schoen FJ: Pathology of cardiac valve replacement. In Morse D, Steiner RM, Fernandez J [eds]: Guide to Prosthetic Cardiac Valves. New York, Springer-Verlag, 1985, p 208.Copyright © 1985 Springer-Verlag.)

Table 8-3 **Revised Jones Criteria**

Major Criteria

Carditis (pleuritic chest pain, friction rub, heart failure)
Polyarthritis
Chorea
Erythema marginatum
Subcutaneous nodules

Minor Criteria

Fever
Arthralgia
Previous rheumatic fever or known rheumatic heart disease

hemodynamic profile and are extremely durable. However, mechanical valves carry a high thromboembolic risk and require long-term anticoagulation. Bioprosthetic use is less likely to be complicated by thromboembolic disease, but the durability of the valve is significantly less than with mechanical valves, especially in young patients. The type of prosthesis used in a particular patient is dependent on multiple factors, including the patient's age, suitability for long-term anticoagulation, and valve position. The American College of Cardiology/American Heart Association guidelines are available for anticoagulation therapy in patients with prosthetic heart valves. All patients with mechanical valves require warfarin therapy. Aspirin (75 to 100 mg/day) is recommended as sole long-term therapy in patients with biologic prosthetic valves and in combination with warfarin in patients with mechanical valves. Warfarin is recommended during the first 3 months after surgery in patients receiving biologic prostheses. The INR should be maintained at 2.3 to 3 in low-risk patients with mechanical aortic valves. High-risk features (e.g., atrial fibrillation, left ventricular dysfunction, previous thromboembolism, and hypercoagulable state) should lead to an INR goal of 2.5 to 3.5 in patients with mechanical AVR. The INR should be maintained at 2.5 to 3.5 in all patients with mechanical mitral valves.

Replacement of a diseased valve with an artificial valve results in a new set of potential risks and complications with the prosthesis. All valve prostheses result in some degree of stenosis because the effective valve orifice is smaller than that of the native valve. Thrombosis or calcification of the prosthetic valve can result in prosthetic dysfunction and hemodynamically important stenosis. Prosthetic valve insufficiency can result from perivalvular leaks in the area of the sewing ring. With bioprosthetic valves, deterioration of the prosthetic valve leaflets can lead to valve insufficiency and stenosis. Hemolysis is a frequent complication of the older mechanical valves (e.g., ball cage, disk cage) and can occur with present-day prostheses if turbulent flow associated with prosthetic valve dysfunction exists, especially regurgitation. Endocarditis remains a potential complication in all patients with prosthetic valves. The guidelines for endocarditis prophylaxis are provided later (see "Endocarditis Prophylaxis").

Evaluation of prosthetic valve function is best performed with two-dimensional and Doppler echocardiographic techniques. Transesophageal echocardiography is particularly useful in studying prosthetic valves when thrombosis or endocarditis is suggested. Mechanical valves can be assessed with fluoroscopy to determine whether leaflet excursion is normal. Gated cardiac computed tomography may also be helpful (Fig 8-6; **Web Fig 8-1**).

Endocarditis Prophylaxis

Patients with valvular heart disease and prosthetic heart valves are at increased risk for developing endocarditis (Table 8-4) (see Chapter 100). In the past, endocarditis prophylaxis was widely recommended for abnormal valves. However, recently updated guidelines reflect the fact that only an extremely small number of cases of infective endocarditis may be prevented by antibiotic prophylaxis, even if it were 100% effective. Infective endocarditis is more likely

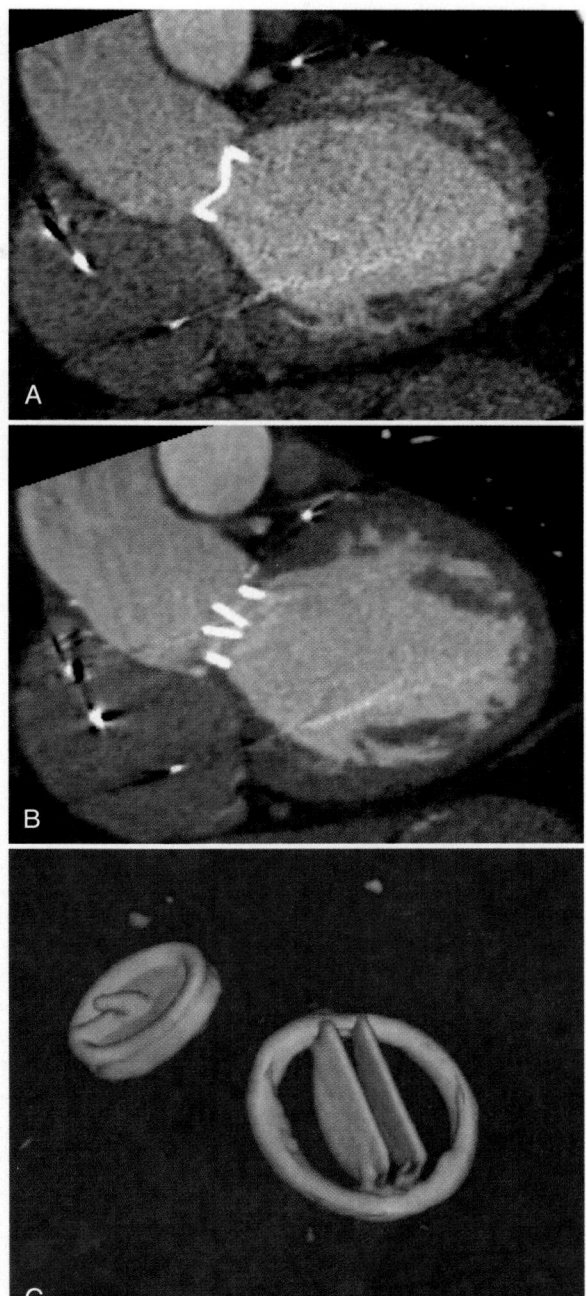

Figure 8-6 Images of mechanical heart valves obtained with gated cardiac CT. Maximum intensity projection of bileaflet tilting disk mechanical aortic prosthesis in closed (**A**) and open (**B**) positions. Dynamic images of this valve can be seen on **Web Figure 8-1**. (**C**) Volume-rendered image showing closed, single-leaflet aortic valve and open bi-leaflet tilting disk mitral valve in diastole. Both valves were clearly seen to open and close normally on the dynamic line images. This patient had suspected prosthetic valve dysfunction that was incompletely evaluated by both fluoroscopy and transesophageal echocardiography.

Table 8-4 Cardiac Conditions in which Antibiotic Prophylaxis Is Recommended

Prosthetic heart valves
Previous bacterial endocarditis
Congenital cardiac malformations (class IIa)
Unrepaired cyanotic
Repaired with residual shunt
First 6 months after repair with prosthetic material
Cardiac transplant recipients with valve regurgitation due to structurally abnormal valve

Table 8-5 Dental and Surgical Procedures in which Endocarditis Prophylaxis Is Recommended

For patients with the underlying cardiac conditions shown in Table 8-4, prophylaxis is reasonable for all dental procedures that involve manipulation of either gingival tissue or the periapical region of teeth or perforation of oral mucosa.
Prophylaxis is not recommended solely on the basis of an increased lifetime risk for acquisition of infective endocarditis.
Administration of antibiotics solely to prevent endocarditis is not recommended for patients who undergo a genitourinary or gastrointestinal tract procedure.

to result from frequent exposure to random bacteremia associated with daily activities than from bacteremia caused by a dental, gastrointestinal tract, or genitourinary procedure. Lastly, the risk for antibiotic-associated adverse events exceeds the benefit (if any) of prophylactic therapy. The role of antibiotic prophylaxis is to prevent infection of the abnormal valve during procedures that are associated with transient bacteremia (Table 8-5). The flora commonly found in the part of the body being instrumented determines the choice of antibiotics. All patients with known valve disease or prosthetic heart valves should carry a card indicating the nature of their valve lesion and the type of endocarditis prophylaxis recommended.

The Committee on Rheumatic Fever, Endocarditis, and Kawasaki Disease of the American Heart Association does not recommend routine antibiotic prophylaxis in patients with valvular heart disease undergoing uncomplicated vaginal delivery or caesarean section unless infection is suspected. Antibiotics are optional for high-risk patients with prosthetic heart valves, a previous history of endocarditis, complex congenital heart disease, or a surgically constructed systemic-pulmonary conduit.

Prospectus for the Future

Infectious disease such as ARF as the principal cause of acquired valvular heart disease will continue to decline worldwide. For isolated mitral valvular stenosis, for example, percutaneous approaches by a skilled operator will become the standard and the preferred treatment modality over a surgical procedure. Aortic and mitral regurgitation caused by degenerative and other acquired diseases will create the major morbidity and mortality rates with advancing age. In the next decade, rapid advances in percutaneous approaches to address mitral regurgitation and aortic stenosis may radically change our practice and strategies for treating these conditions.

References

American College of Cardiology/American Heart Association Task Force on Practice Guidelines: 2008 Focused update incorporated into the ACC/AHA 2006 guidelines for the management of patients with valvular heart disease. J Am Coll Cardiol 32:el-e142, 2008.

Freed LA, Levy D, Levine RA, et al: Prevalence and clinical outcome of mitral-valve prolapse. N Engl J Med 341:1-7, 1999.

Enriquez-Sarano M, Avierinos JF, Messika-Zeitoun D, et al: Quantitative determinants of the outcome of asymptomatic mitral regurgitation. N Engl J Med 352:875-883, 2005.

Freeman RV, Otto CM: Spectrum of calcific aortic valve disease: Pathogenesis, disease progression, and treatment strategies. Circulation 111:3316-3326, 2005.

Zoghbi WA, Enriquez-Sarano M, Foster E, et al: Recommendations for evaluation of the severity of native valvular regurgitation with two-dimensional and Doppler echocardiography. J Am Soc Echocardiogr 16:777-802, 2003.

ACC/AHA guidelines update on valvular heart disease: focused update on infective endocarditis. J Am Coll Cardiol 52:676-685, 2008.

Coronary Heart Disease

Andrew D. Michaels

Epidemiology

Coronary heart disease (CHD) is the leading cause of death in the industrialized world. Apart from its influence on mortality, it causes substantial morbidity, disability, and loss of productivity. With improvements in diagnosis, prevention, and treatment, the mortality rate from CHD has declined gradually over the past several decades. Nonetheless, 1.2 million people have a myocardial infarction (MI) or fatal cardiac event each year in the United States alone. Nearly half of all deaths in industrialized nations and 25% of those in developing countries are due to CHD. By the year 2020, CHD is predicted to surpass infectious disease as the world's leading cause of death and disability.

Pathophysiology of Atherosclerosis

In the industrialized world, atherosclerosis often begins in the early decades of life. One in six American teenagers dying accidentally has pathologic evidence of coronary atherosclerosis. Several processes contribute to the initiation and progression of atherosclerosis, including accumulation of lipoproteins, endothelial injury, and inflammation.

In the early phase of atherosclerosis, small lipoprotein particles penetrate the vascular endothelium, where they are oxidized and coalesce into aggregates in the intimal layer. This process is accelerated at sites of endothelial injury, which may be caused or accelerated by systemic hypertension, hypercholesterolemia, cigarette smoking, or excessive sheer forces. The accumulation of intimal lipid aggregates stimulates the expression of adhesion molecules (e.g., intracellular adhesion molecule-1, vascular cell adhesion molecule-1, selectins) on the luminal surface of the endothelial cells, thereby enabling them to bind circulating monocytes (e.g., macrophages). The adherent monocytes intercalate between the endothelial cells into the intimal layer in response to chemokines and cytokines produced by endothelial and medial smooth muscle cells. The intimal monocytes ingest the lipoprotein aggregates to become lipid-filled monocytes, or *foam cells*. Aggregates of these foam cells make up the earliest visible evidence of atherosclerosis, or the *fatty streak*.

Foam cells replicate and release proinflammatory mediators, thereby perpetuating the local inflammatory process with resultant lesion progression. In addition, they release enzymes that cause endothelial denudation. Because the endothelium is involved in the control of vascular tone through its production of vasodilating substances such as prostacyclin and nitric oxide (e.g., endothelium-derived relaxing factor) and thrombosis, injury to these cells impairs vasodilation and creates a local prothrombotic state. Circulating platelets adhere to sites of endothelial injury and release growth factors, which stimulate the migration and proliferation of smooth muscle cells and fibroblasts from the media. This leads to formation of a fibrous cap over the lipid-rich core (**Web video 1—Coronary Atherosclerosis,** http://www.heartsite.com/html/cad.html).

As lipids continue to accumulate in the foam cells, they undergo necrosis and leave a remnant lipid pool in the core of the plaque. Metalloproteinase enzymes (e.g., collagenase, gelatinase) released by macrophages and mast cells in the plaque degrade collagen and extracellular matrix proteins adjacent to the lipid pool, whereas cytokines (e.g., interferon-α) released by T lymphocytes inhibit the formation of collagen by vascular smooth muscle cells. This combination of increased collagen degradation and decreased collagen production creates a vulnerable plaque, which is predisposed to fissure or rupture. Such vulnerable plaques have a lipid-laden core and a thin, weakened fibrous cap. When the thin fibrous cap fissures or ruptures, highly thrombogenic collagen and lipid are exposed to circulating blood with resultant adhesion of platelets and formation of an intraluminal thrombus. Activated platelets release substances (e.g., thromboxane, serotonin) that promote vasoconstriction and thrombus propagation. When the extent of platelet aggregation and thrombosis is sufficient to impair blood flow (partially or completely), an acute coronary event (unstable angina, non–ST-segment elevation myocardial infarction [NSTEMI] or ST-segment elevation myocardial infarction [STEMI]) occurs.

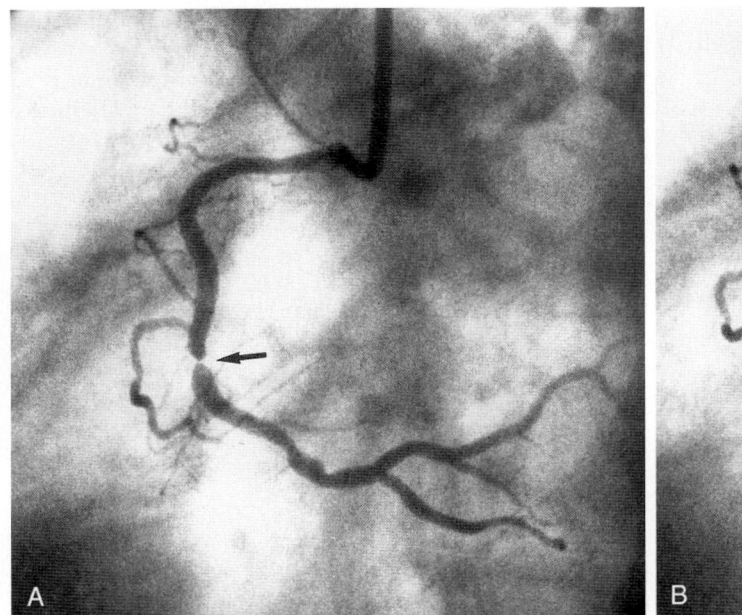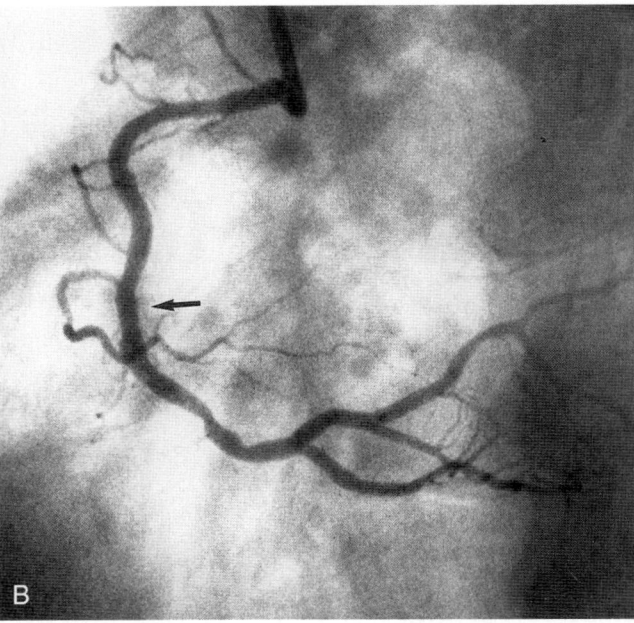

Figure 9-1 Angiograms of the right coronary artery. **A,** Discrete stenosis is observed in the middle segment of the artery *(arrow).* **B,** Same artery is shown after successful balloon angioplasty of the stenosis and placement of an intracoronary stent.

When the atherosclerotic plaque is covered with a thick fibrous cap, rupture is less likely, but the plaque may gradually increase in size. As plaque volume increases, the coronary arterial lumen is compromised, and blood flow is impaired (Fig. 9-1). The hemodynamic significance of plaque is determined by the length and severity of the luminal narrowing; in general, a 70% decrease in the luminal diameter of a coronary artery limits blood flow in the presence of increased myocardial oxygen demands (e.g., exercise, emotional excitement), leading to the clinical condition of exertional angina. A 90% decrease in luminal diameter is sufficient to limit flow even when myocardial oxygen demands are normal. For intermediate-severity lesions with a diameter stenosis between 40% and 70%, assessing the hemodynamic significance of the stenosis with either fractional flow reserve (FFR; ratio of the mean coronary pressure distal to the stenosis [acquired by a micromanometer pressure transducer on a coronary angioplasty guidewire] divided by the mean arterial pressure proximal to the stenosis) or stress testing may help determine the requirement for coronary revascularization.

Risk Factors

Several risk factors for the development of atherosclerosis have been identified (Table 9-1). Nonmodifiable risk factors include (1) advanced age, (2) male sex, and (3) family history of premature atherosclerosis. The prevalence of coronary artery disease (CAD) increases with age. At any given age, the prevalence is higher in men than in women. On average, the clinical manifestations of CAD become evident about 10 years later in women than in men. A family history of premature atherosclerosis (occurring in men before age 55 years and in women before age 65 years) increases the risk for atherosclerosis in an individual, likely as a result of environ-

mental factors (e.g., dietary habits, cigarette smoking) and a genetic predisposition to the disease.

Other risk factors are modifiable, and their treatment may decrease the risk for atherosclerosis. These modifiable risk factors include hyperlipidemia, hypertension, diabetes mellitus, metabolic syndrome, cigarette smoking, obesity, sedentary lifestyle, and excessive alcohol intake. Although several definitions of the metabolic syndrome have been endorsed, the definition adopted by the National Cholesterol Education Program Adult Treatment Panel requires at least three of the following five criteria: waist circumference

Table 9-1 **Risk Factors and Markers for Coronary Artery Disease**
Nonmodifiable Risk Factors
Age
Male sex
Family history of premature coronary artery disease
Modifiable Independent Risk Factors
Hyperlipidemia
Hypertension
Diabetes mellitus
Metabolic syndrome
Cigarette smoking
Obesity
Sedentary lifestyle
Heavy alcohol intake
Markers
Elevated lipoprotein(a)
Hyperhomocysteinemia
Elevated high-sensitivity C-reactive protein (hsCRP)
Coronary arterial calcification detected by electron-beam computed tomography (EBCT) or multidetector computed tomography (MDCT)

more than 102 cm in men and more than 88 cm in women; triglyceride level 150 mg/dL or higher; high-density lipoprotein (HDL) cholesterol level lower than 40 mg/dL in men and lower than 50 mg/dL in women; blood pressure 130/85 mm Hg or higher; and serum glucose 110 mg/dL or higher. Using these criteria, nearly 25% of the U.S. population has metabolic syndrome. Finally, markers associated with an increased incidence of CAD include lipoprotein(a), hyperhomocysteinemia, high-sensitivity C-reactive protein (hsCRP), and coronary arterial calcification.

Lipids play a central role in the atherosclerotic process, and elevated levels of cholesterol, primarily low-density lipoprotein (LDL) cholesterol, are associated with accelerated atherosclerosis (**Web video 1—Coronary Atherosclerosis,** http://www.heartsite.com/html/cad.html). HDL cholesterol, by contrast, functions as a protective agent, and its serum level is inversely related to the risk of CAD. Elevated triglycerides are often associated with reduced levels of HDL cholesterol and are an independent risk factor for CAD. Large trials of lipid-lowering therapy have demonstrated the effectiveness of cholesterol reduction in the primary and secondary prevention of CAD.

Systemic hypertension, defined as a systolic arterial pressure greater than 140 mm Hg or a diastolic pressure greater than 90 mm Hg, increases the risk for CAD. The risk increases proportionally with the extent of blood pressure elevation, and proper treatment of hypertension reduces the risk.

Diabetes mellitus increases both the risk for developing CAD and the mortality associated with it. Although CAD is the leading cause of death in adult patients with diabetes, tight glycemic control has not been shown to reduce the risk. Diabetes mellitus often co-exists with other risk factors, including dyslipidemia (elevated triglyceride level, low HDL level), hypertension, and obesity. This grouping of risk factors has been termed the *metabolic syndrome*, and its presence identifies a person at increased risk for having or developing atherosclerotic disease.

Cigarette smoking has adverse effects on the lipid profile, clotting factors, and platelet function and is associated with a twofold to threefold increase in the risk for CAD. Cessation of smoking reduces the excess risk for a coronary event by 50% within the first 1 to 2 years of quitting.

Obesity, defined as a body mass index greater than 30 kg/m^2, is often associated with other risk factors (e.g., hypertension, dyslipidemia, glucose intolerance); in addition, obesity appears to be an independent risk factor for CAD. The distribution of body fat is important, with abdominal adiposity posing a substantially greater risk for CAD in both men and women.

Multiple observational studies have demonstrated an inverse relationship between the amount of physical activity and the risk for CAD. Although the ideal duration, frequency, and intensity of such physical activity have not been determined, numerous studies have shown that exercise is beneficial in healthy patients and those with or at risk for CAD.

Moderate alcohol intake (1 to 2 drinks daily) is associated with a reduction in the risk for cardiovascular events; in contrast, heavy alcohol intake increases cardiovascular mortality.

Lipoprotein(a) consists of LDL cholesterol linked to an apo(a) molecule. It has a homologic structure with plasminogen and interferes with the generation of plasmin, thereby creating a predisposition to thrombosis.

Elevated levels of homocysteine are associated with an increased risk for coronary, cerebral, and peripheral vascular disease. Hyperhomocysteinemia can be treated effectively with dietary folate supplementation. However, such treatments have not been shown to reduce the incidence of stroke or cardiovascular events in patients with elevated serum homocysteine levels.

CRP, a marker of inflammation, may indicate or contribute to an increased propensity for plaque rupture and thrombosis. Elevated serum CRP levels—when measured with the new high-sensitivity assays (i.e., hsCRP)—strongly correlate with the risks for MI, stroke, peripheral arterial disease, and sudden cardiac death. Levels of hsCRP lower than 1 mg/L are associated with a low risk for vascular events; levels of 1 to 3 mg/L pose an intermediate risk; levels greater than 3 mg/L create a high risk. In healthy patients without hyperlipidemia but with an hsCRP greater than 2 mg/L, statin therapy has been shown to reduce the risk for myocardial infarction, stroke, revascularization for unstable angina, and death from cardiovascular causes.

Coronary arterial calcification is a prominent feature of coronary atherosclerosis, and it correlates with the presence and severity of CAD. Electron-beam computed tomography (EBCT) or multidetector computed tomography (MDCT) can accurately quantify coronary calcification, thereby serving as screening tests for CAD in asymptomatic patients. Currently, the usefulness of EBCT or MDCT and hsCRP in the clinical setting is poorly defined. However, the finding of coronary calcification in patients without known CAD or risk factors for CAD may identify those who warrant aggressive risk factor modification.

Nonatherosclerotic Causes of Cardiac Ischemia

Although atherosclerosis is the most common disease affecting the coronary arteries, several nonatherosclerotic processes may produce myocardial ischemia or MI. Embolization from infective endocarditis, mural thrombi in the left atrium or ventricle, prosthetic valves, intracardiac tumors, or paradoxical emboli from the venous system across an atrial or a ventricular septal defect or pulmonary arteriovenous malformation may compromise coronary blood flow, leading to myocardial ischemia or MI. Chest wall trauma may result in coronary arterial dissection or thrombosis. Aortic dissection can propagate to the aortic root and occlude a coronary artery at its origin. Coronary arterial dissection may occur spontaneously during pregnancy or with connective tissue disorders such as Marfan syndrome or Ehlers-Danlos syndrome.

Several forms of arteritis may involve the coronary arteries, including syphilis, Takayasu arteritis, polyarteritis nodosa, systemic lupus erythematosus, and giant cell arteritis. These syndromes may result in obstruction, occlusion, or thrombosis of the coronary arteries. Kawasaki disease, a mucocutaneous lymph node syndrome, is a systemic disease of children that causes coronary vasculitis with resultant coronary aneurysms. Spontaneous in situ coronary thrombosis may occur in the setting of hematologic disorders (e.g., polycythemia vera, essential thrombocytosis, disseminated intravascular coagulation, sickle cell anemia, paroxysmal nocturnal hemoglobinuria). Congenital coronary anomalies may cause myocardial ischemia. Spontaneous coronary spasm (e.g., Prinzmetal vasospastic angina) with or without underlying CAD may cause myocardial ischemia or, rarely, MI. Cocaine use may result in myocardial ischemia or MI through several mechanisms, including coronary vasospasm, thrombosis, and accelerated atherosclerosis. An occasional patient treated with sumatriptan for migraine headaches or paclitaxel for cancer may experience MI in the absence of CAD.

In 10% to 20% of patients with suggested angina, coronary angiography reveals normal epicardial coronary arteries. In some of these individuals, microvascular or small vessel disease, the *syndrome X*, has been implicated. Studies have suggested that women have a higher prevalence of syndrome X compared with men presenting with possible acute coronary syndrome. The small resistance vessels in these patients, which are not visualized angiographically, have reduced vasodilatory capability. This dysfunction may lead to myocardial ischemia, as evidenced by exercise-related abnormalities on echocardiographic or nuclear scintigraphic studies. Some patients respond to treatment with common anti-anginal medications; although, in general, these drugs are less effective in patients with syndrome X than in those with atherosclerotic CAD.

Finally, myocardial ischemia may result when significant increases in the demand for myocardial oxygen exceed oxygen supply. Such an oxygen supply-demand imbalance may occur in individuals with thyrotoxicosis, aortic stenosis, aortic insufficiency, tachyarrhythmia, or sepsis. Diminished oxygen supply may occur as a result of acute blood loss, hypotension, severe anemia, or carbon monoxide poisoning.

Pathophysiology and Consequences of Myocardial Ischemia

In the normal myocardium, a balance between myocardial oxygen supply and demand is present at rest and during physical exertion or emotional excitement. In response to an increase in oxygen demand, an appropriate increase in oxygen supply maintains adequate tissue oxygenation. When oxygen demand increases in the setting of limited oxygen supply, myocardial ischemia results. At rest, the myocardium extracts most of the oxygen that is delivered to it through the coronary arteries. As a result, any increase in myocardial oxygen demand, as a result of an increase in heart rate, wall stress, or contractility, must be accompanied by a concomitant proportional increase in myocardial blood flow. Regulation of coronary blood flow occurs at the level of the arterioles and is dependent on autonomic tone and an intact, functioning endothelium.

Endothelial dysfunction secondary to atherosclerosis impairs the ability of the coronary arterioles to dilate when oxygen demands increase. In addition, when a flow-limiting stenosis is present in an epicardial coronary artery, the arterioles distal to the stenosis may already be maximally or nearly maximally dilated in the resting state. The inability of the arterioles to dilate and increase coronary arterial flow during periods of increased demand (e.g., decreased coronary vasodilator reserve) results in a supply-demand mismatch, with resultant ischemia and the clinical pattern of stable angina.

When myocardial oxygen supply cannot meet oxygen demand, myocardial ischemia occurs. This ischemia, in turn, initiates a series of pathophysiologic events. Regional myocardial hypoxia causes anaerobic glycolysis, lactate production, intracellular acidosis, and disordered calcium homeostasis. These intracellular changes induce abnormalities in myocardial relaxation, leading to reduced compliance and contraction, which cause regional wall motion abnormalities. Finally, electrocardiographic (ECG) evidence of ischemia (i.e., ST-segment depression or elevation) occurs, and angina pectoris ensues.

If myocardial ischemia is transient, the duration of the resultant mechanical dysfunction may be short. In contrast, more prolonged ischemia may produce myocardial stunning, hibernation, or even an MI. *Myocardial stunning* refers to a prolonged period (e.g., hours, days) of reversible myocardial dysfunction after an ischemic event. Hibernation occurs in the setting of chronic ischemia when oxygen delivery is adequate to maintain myocardial viability but inadequate to maintain normal function. The clinical importance of the hibernating state is that restoration of blood flow to the involved myocardium results in improved mechanical function.

Because of limited energy expenditure, conduction tissue is more resistant to ischemia than contractile tissue. Nevertheless, ischemia may result in altered ionic transport, altered autonomic tone, and injury to the conduction system, resulting in a variety of ischemia-induced arrhythmias and conduction abnormalities.

Angina Pectoris

For many years, patients with chronic, stable angina pectoris were believed to develop myocardial ischemia because of a transient increase in myocardial oxygen demand as a result of physical exertion or emotional excitement in the setting of limited oxygen supply caused by fixed atherosclerotic CAD. Effort-induced angina was thought to be a problem of excessive oxygen demand with limited oxygen supply. However, some patients with chronic, stable angina may develop myocardial ischemia because of dynamic coronary vasoconstriction in the setting of fixed atherosclerotic CAD. Such *inappropriate coronary vasoconstriction* has been shown to occur during exposure to cold, while under mental stress, and during isometric or isotonic exercise as well as during exposure to cigarette smoking. In short, chronic, stable angina is a syndrome of both increased myocardial oxygen demands in the setting of limited supply and dynamic reductions in myocardial oxygen supply, most of which are induced by common, everyday events.

Table 9-2 Angina Pectoris

Type	Pattern	ECG	Abnormality	Medical Therapy
Stable	Stable pattern, induced by physical exertion, exposure to cold, eating, emotional stress	Baseline often normal or nonspecific ST-T changes	≥70% Luminal narrowing of one or more coronary arteries from atherosclerosis	Aspirin Sublingual nitroglycerin
	Lasts 5-10 min Relieved by rest or nitroglycerin	Signs of previous MI ST-segment depression during angina		Anti-ischemic medications Statin
Unstable	Increase in anginal frequency, severity, or duration	Same as stable angina, although changes during discomfort may be more pronounced	Plaque rupture with platelet and fibrin thrombus, causing worsening coronary obstruction	Aspirin and clopidogrel Anti-ischemic medications
	Angina of new onset or now occurring at low level of activity or at rest	Occasional ST-segment elevation during discomfort		Heparin or LMWH Glycoprotein IIb/IIIa inhibitors
	May be less responsive to sublingual nitroglycerin			Statin
Prinzmetal or variant angina	Angina without provocation, typically occurring at rest	Transient ST-segment elevation during pain Often with associated AV block or ventricular arrhythmias	Coronary artery spasm	Calcium channel blockers Nitrates

AV, atrioventricular; ECG, electrocardiography; LMWH, low-molecular-weight heparin; MI, myocardial infarction.

The patient with exertional angina pectoris (Table 9-2) usually complains of a retrosternal pressure or dull ache during physical exertion, while eating, during exposure to cold, or with emotional excitement. Other adjectives that the patient may use to describe the chest discomfort include "viselike," "constricting," "crushing," "heavy," and "squeezing." In many patients, the retrosternal pain radiates to the jaw, neck, and left shoulder and arm. Dyspnea often accompanies exertional angina pectoris and may be associated with diaphoresis and nausea. Although its duration varies considerably from one patient to another, the episode usually lasts 3 to 10 minutes. On occasion, however, it may linger for as long as 20 to 30 minutes. It is typically relieved by sublingual nitroglycerin within 1 to 3 minutes.

At a time when the patient is not experiencing angina, the physical examination is usually normal. During an episode of chest discomfort, the patient may become somewhat pale and diaphoretic, and the respiratory rate and effort may increase. The heart rate and systemic arterial pressure are usually greater than at rest. Pulmonary congestion (e.g., rales at both bases posteriorly) may be evident. On auscultation of the heart, an S_4 is usually audible as a result of decreased left ventricular compliance, and a transient S_3 may be present if left ventricular systolic dysfunction occurs. In an occasional patient, ischemia-induced papillary muscle dysfunction will cause a murmur of mitral regurgitation to be audible at the cardiac apex. As the episode of angina resolves, the pulmonary rales, diastolic heart sounds, and systolic murmur may quickly disappear.

Three noninvasive techniques have been used to demonstrate transient episodes of myocardial ischemia in the patient with exertional angina pectoris: (1) During exercise-induced or spontaneous chest pain, the ECG usually shows ST-segment depression that is reflective of subendocardial

ischemia, which resolves within minutes of the pain's disappearance (Fig. 9-2). (2) During episodes of angina, global left ventricular systolic function may decline, and segmental wall motion abnormalities may develop. These abnormalities can be observed with two-dimensional echocardiography, magnetic resonance imaging, or gated blood pool scintigraphy. The assessment of regional abnormalities and systolic function using two-dimensional echocardiography performed during exercise or intravenous dobutamine infusion is a particularly useful technique for detecting myocardial ischemia. As with the ECG alterations, these segmental wall motion abnormalities may resolve within minutes after relief of pain, or they may linger for hours. (3) Myocardial perfusion may be assessed during exercise-induced angina by the intravenous injection of a radioactive tracer, such as thallium-201 or technetium sestamibi, followed by imaging with the appropriate equipment.

EVALUATION OF THE PATIENT WITH ANGINA

For the patient in whom the cause of chest pain is unclear, stress testing may help clarify the diagnosis by reproducing the patient's symptoms and demonstrating objective evidence of ischemia. Submitting the patient to exercise or pharmacologic stress provides an opportunity to assess the evidence of ischemia through the evaluation of ECG abnormalities (e.g., routine stress testing), perfusion defects (e.g., radionuclide imaging), or segmental wall motion abnormalities (e.g., echocardiography). As with all diagnostic tests, the predictive value of exercise testing is influenced by the pre-test probability that the patient has CAD. For example, in the patient with a high pre-test probability of having CAD, a positive test is highly predictive, whereas a test with

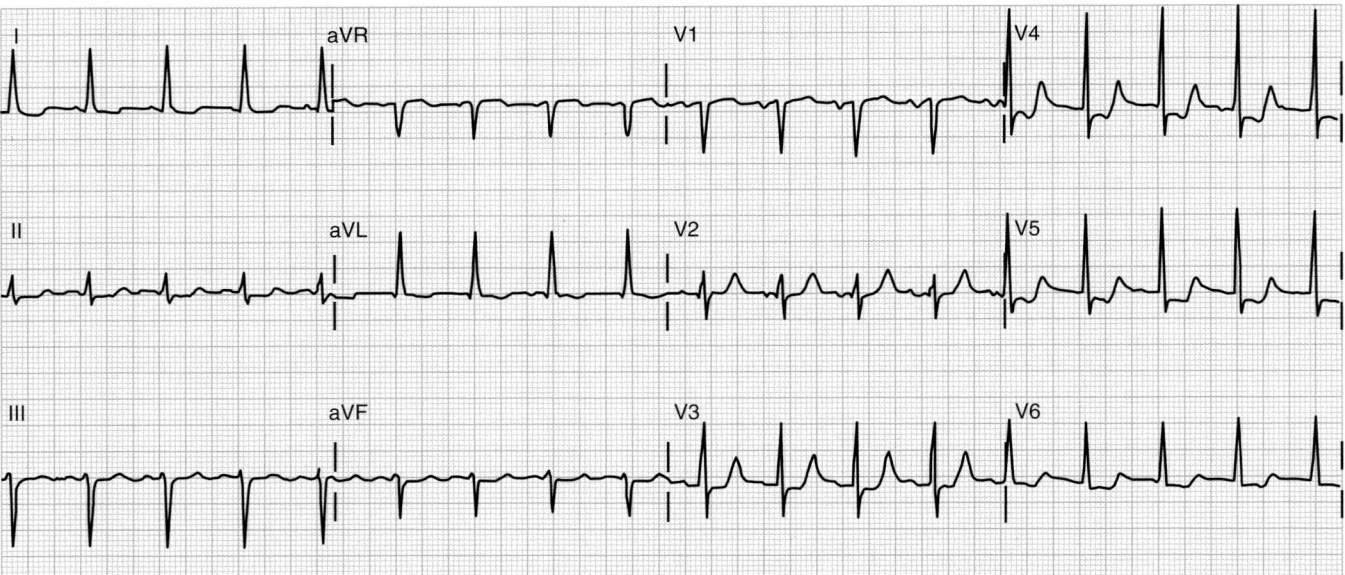

A

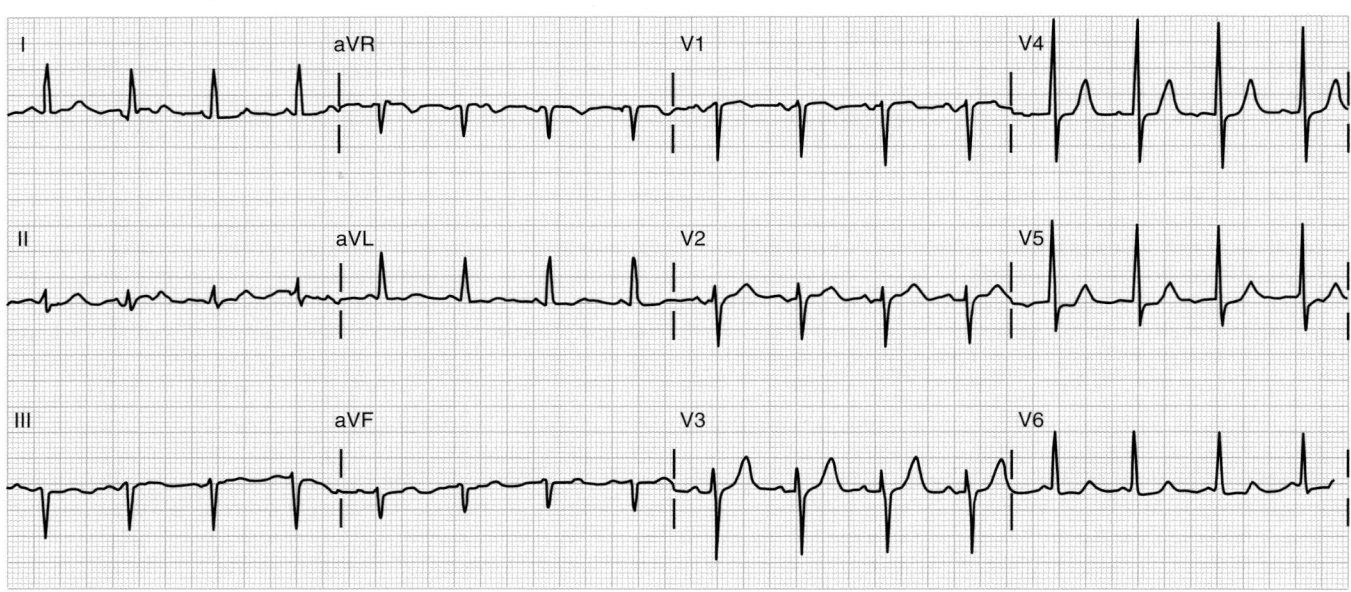

B

Figure 9-2 Electrocardiogram obtained during angina (**A**) and after the administration of sublingual nitroglycerin and subsequent resolution of angina (**B**). During angina, transient ST-segment depression and T-wave abnormalities are present.

negative results has a high likelihood of being falsely negative. Conversely, in the individual with a low likelihood of having CAD, a negative test is highly predictive, but a positive test result has a high likelihood of being falsely positive.

Stress testing may also be useful in the patient with chronic stable angina for the determination of exercise capacity, documentation of the effectiveness of medications, and risk stratification (i.e., identifying patients at risk for CAD in whom more aggressive therapies may be warranted) (Fig. 9-3). The Clinical Outcomes Utilizing Revascularization and Aggressive Drug Evaluation (COURAGE) trial has demonstrated that patients with a large degree of ischemic myocardium during stress testing are most likely to benefit with coronary revascularization.

In a patient with a normal resting ECG, routine stress testing with ECG monitoring is usually sufficient. However, in patients with baseline ECG abnormalities (e.g., nonspecific ST-segment abnormalities, left ventricular hypertrophy, left bundle branch block [LBBB], or ventricular pre-excitation) and in patients taking digoxin, the specificity of exercise-induced ST-T-wave changes is diminished. In these

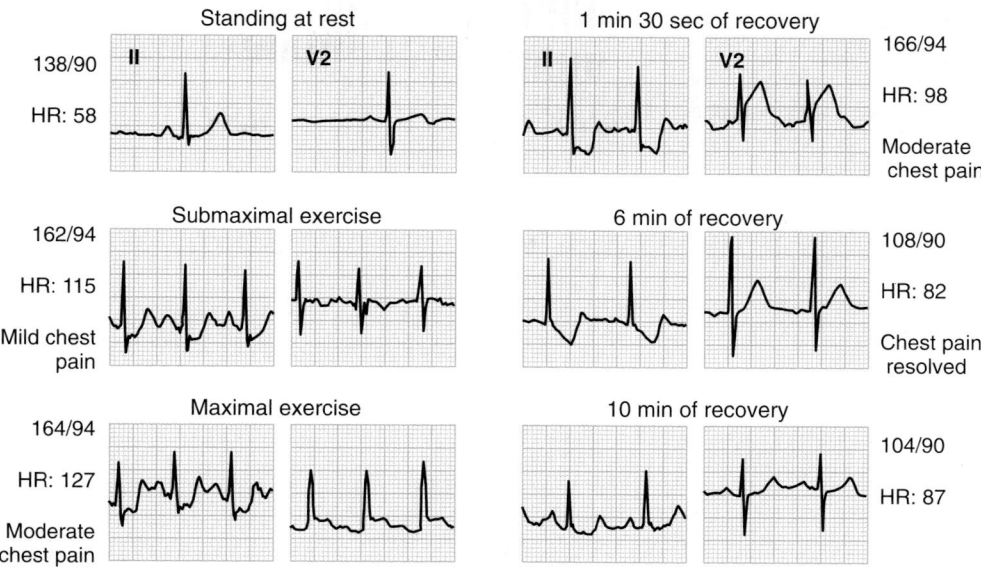

Figure 9-3 Treadmill exercise test demonstrates a markedly ischemic electrocardiogram (ECG) response. The resting ECG is normal. The test was stopped when the patient developed angina at a relatively low workload, accompanied by ST-segment depression in lead II and ST-segment elevation in lead V_2. These changes worsened early in recovery and resolved after administration of sublingual nitroglycerin. Only leads II and V_2 are shown; however, ischemic changes were seen in 10 of the 12 recorded leads. Severe atherosclerotic disease of all three coronary arteries was documented at subsequent cardiac catheterization.

individuals, echocardiographic, nuclear scintigraphic, or magnetic resonance imaging improves both the sensitivity and the specificity of stress testing, albeit at substantially increased cost. Nuclear imaging is preferred over echocardiography in patients with LBBB. Exercise-induced ECG changes in women are less specific than in men; for this reason, many physicians perform exercise testing with imaging in all women. Several prognostic markers associated with a poor clinical outcome have been identified in the patient undergoing routine stress testing; these include (1) ischemic ECG changes (ST-segment depression) that occur early in exercise, in multiple leads, or persist for several minutes after the completion of exercise; (2) an associated decrease (rather than the normal increase) in blood pressure levels; and (3) poor exercise tolerance (e.g., less than 6 minutes exercise duration on the standard Bruce protocol).

In patients whose baseline ECG is sufficiently abnormal to preclude an adequate interpretation during exercise, the standard exercise test may be combined with radionuclide perfusion imaging, ECG assessment of left ventricular global and segmental function, or magnetic resonance imaging of left ventricular function. When stress testing is combined with imaging, the sensitivity for detecting CAD is about 90%, which is greater than that achieved with standard ECG-guided exercise testing. The specificity is about 80%, and the predictive value is about 90%.

When a radionuclide stress perfusion imaging study is performed, a radioactive tracer, such as thallium-201, technetium-99m sestamibi, or technetium-99 tetrofosmin, is immediately administered intravenously before exercise is terminated. Because the radioactive tracer is distributed to the myocardium in proportion to coronary arterial blood flow, segments of myocardium that become ischemic during exercise have decreased uptake of the radioactive tracer relative to normally perfused areas of myocardium. Within 4

hours of the injection of thallium, about 50% is redistributed throughout viable myocardium, which results in a *filling in* of areas that were hypoperfused at peak exercise. Unlike thallium, technetium sestamibi and tetrofosmin do not redistribute to areas that were ischemic. The presence and extent of exercise-induced perfusion abnormalities provide prognostic information. Patients with a normal stress perfusion study—with or without CAD—have an extremely low risk for future cardiac events (<1% per year), whereas those with an abnormal stress perfusion study have an event rate of about 7% annually, the risk in correlation with the magnitude of the perfusion defects.

When exercise induces ischemia, global left ventricular systolic function may decline, and regional wall motion abnormalities may develop. These changes can be observed with two-dimensional echocardiography, magnetic resonance imaging, or gated equilibrium blood pool scintigraphy (e.g., radionuclide ventriculography, multigated acquisition [MUGA] scanning). The extent of wall motion abnormalities correlates with the extent of CAD and the risk for future cardiac events.

For patients who are able to ambulate, exercise stress is preferable to pharmacologic stress because it provides more physiologic information. In patients who are nonambulatory or have limited exercise capacity, pharmacologic stress may provide similar diagnostic information, but it cannot yield information regarding exercise capacity or the hemodynamic response to exercise. A vasodilator (dipyridamole or adenosine) or an intravenous inotropic agent (dobutamine) is typically administered to perform a pharmacologic stress test. With the former, blood flow in unobstructed coronary arteries increases to a greater extent than in obstructed arteries, and this can be detected with perfusion imaging. In contrast, dobutamine infusion increases myocardial contractility—and hence myocardial oxygen demand—and is combined with radionuclide perfusion,

Table 9-3 **Indications for Coronary Angiography in Patients with Stable Angina Pectoris**
• Unacceptable angina despite medical therapy (for consideration of revascularization) • Noninvasive testing results with high-risk features • Angina or risk factors for coronary artery disease in the setting of depressed left ventricular systolic function • For diagnostic purposes in the individual in whom the results of noninvasive testing are unclear

Table 9-4 **Goals of Risk Factor Modification**	
Risk Factor	**Goal**
Dyslipidemia Elevated LDL cholesterol level Patients with CAD or CAD equivalent*	LDL < 70 mg/dL
Without CAD, at least two risk factors†	LDL < 130 mg/dL (or <100 mg/dL‡)
Without CAD, zero or one risk factor†	LDL < 160 mg/dL
Elevated TG	TG < 200 mg/dL
Reduced HDL cholesterol level	HDL > 40 mg/dL
Hypertension	Systolic blood pressure < 140 mm Hg Diastolic blood pressure < 90 mm Hg
Smoking	Complete cessation
Obesity	<120% of ideal body weight for height
Sedentary lifestyle	30-60 min moderate intensity activity (e.g., walking, jogging, cycling, rowing) 5 times per week

*CAD equivalents include diabetes mellitus, noncoronary atherosclerotic vascular disease, or >20% 10-year risk for a cardiovascular event as predicted by the Framingham risk score.
†Risk factors include cigarette smoking, blood pressure ≥ 140/90 mm Hg or on antihypertensive medication, HDL cholesterol level < 40 mg/dL, family history of premature coronary atherosclerosis (e.g., male, ≤45 years; female, ≤55 years).
‡Target of 100 mg/dL should be strongly considered for men ≥ 60 years of age and individuals with a high burden of subclinical atherosclerosis (>75th percentile of patient's age and sex for coronary calcification), hsCRP > 3 mg/dL, or metabolic syndrome.
CAD, coronary artery disease; CRP, C-reactive protein; HDL, high-density lipoprotein; hsCRP, high-sensitivity C-reactive protein; LDL, low-density lipoprotein; TG, triglycerides.

magnetic resonance imaging, or echocardiographic imaging to assess the presence of perfusion defects or regional wall motion abnormalities.

As previously noted, EBCT has been used for the detection of CAD. The absence of calcification on computed tomography (CT) strongly correlates with the absence of hemodynamically significant coronary atherosclerosis. Moreover, the extent of coronary calcification is predictive of the risk for myocardial infarction. The presence of coronary calcification is diagnostic of coronary atherosclerosis, although the extent of luminal diameter narrowing cannot be predicted by the extent of calcification. With the addition of intravenous contrast administration, MDCT machines may perform a noninvasive CT coronary angiogram (CTA) to visualize coronary arterial stenoses in addition to detecting coronary calcification. Their roles in the detection and management of CAD are evolving.

Invasive cardiac catheterization with coronary angiography allows visual assessment of the extent and severity of CAD. The anatomic information obtained must be interpreted in light of functional information (e.g., stress testing) because the anatomic severity of a given coronary stenosis does not necessarily correlate with its physiologic significance. FFR measurements may be performed in the cardiac catheterization laboratory to demonstrate the functional significance of intermediate-severity coronary stenoses. Coronary angiography is invasive and is associated with a small risk. Nonetheless, the risk-benefit analysis of catheterization favors the procedure in many patients with angina (Table 9-3).

MEDICAL MANAGEMENT OF STABLE ANGINA

The approach to the management of the patient with angina involves (1) risk factor modification and lifestyle changes to slow or to arrest the progression of CAD and thrombosis, (2) pharmacotherapy to prevent or to relieve angina, and (3) revascularization to improve symptoms, prognosis, or both. In addition, concurrent medical conditions (e.g., anemia, congestive heart failure, chronic obstructive pulmonary disease, obstructive sleep apnea, hyperthyroidism) that may precipitate or worsen angina should be corrected, if possible.

Control of hypertension, diabetes mellitus, hyperlipidemia, and smoking cessation are important in controlling the progression of disease in patients with coronary atherosclerosis. Guidelines for aggressive risk factor reduction have

been established (Table 9-4). Patients should be instructed on dietary changes; an evaluation by a nutritionist may be helpful. Patients with CAD generally should be treated aggressively for hyperlipidemia management. Statin medications are most commonly prescribed for a goal LDL lower than 100 mg/dL. Recent studies suggest that further LDL reductions below 70 mg/dL provide further risk reduction. For those CAD patients with normal cholesterol levels, statin therapy may be helpful in stabilizing atherosclerotic plaque, resulting in a reduced risk for MI and stroke. For those with low HDL, niacin or fibrate agents may be helpful, in addition to aerobic exercise, to achieve a goal HDL of greater than 40 mg/dL.

All patients with known or suggested CAD should be placed on antiplatelet therapy (e.g., aspirin, 75 to 325 mg daily; clopidogrel, 75 mg daily for patients allergic to aspirin) unless a contraindication to antiplatelet therapy is present. These agents decrease the rates of MI and death in patients with angina or previous MI. In addition, they may decrease the risk for MI in individuals without suggested CAD but with multiple risk factors. Angiotensin-converting enzyme (ACE) inhibitors should be prescribed to patients with CAD who have diabetes mellitus or left ventricular systolic dysfunction unless contraindicated. Angiotensin receptor blockers may be used in patients who develop an ACE inhibitor–induced dry cough. Although exercise is often limited by angina, regular activity at a level that is tolerated should be encouraged. Isometric exercise, such as weight lifting and high-intensity activities, especially in the cold (e.g., skiing, shoveling snow), are not advisable. However, many patients with stable angina may perform vigorous activities, including moderate physical exertion at work. For obese patients and those with a sedentary lifestyle, regular aerobic activity is recommended.

As previously noted, the pathophysiologic characteristics of angina are one of supply-demand mismatch. Therefore, its therapy is directed at correcting the mismatch by decreasing myocardial oxygen demands, augmenting myocardial oxygen supply, or both. Nitrates, β blockers, and calcium channel blockers are among the pharmacologic options most commonly used for the control of symptoms in patients with chronic stable angina (Table 9-5). They appear to be of similar efficacy in controlling anginal symptoms. When a single agent fails to control angina, combination therapy is usually effective. Ranolazine, a selective inhibitor of late sodium influx, is an effective antianginal agent that has no effect on heart rate or systemic blood pressure. Ranolazine may be used as either a first- or second-line agent for patients with angina. Unlike aspirin and lipid-lowering therapy, none of these agents has been convincingly shown to decrease mortality in patients with CAD.

Nitrate preparations have been used in the medical management of exertional angina for many years. The effect of nitrates is mediated through relaxation of vascular smooth muscle. Dilation of arterioles reduces systemic vascular resistance and therefore afterload. Nitrates have a more pronounced effect on the venous system; venodilation results in venous pooling, decreased venous return, and therefore decreased preload. The arteriolar and venodilatory effects substantially reduce myocardial oxygen demands, thereby decreasing angina. In addition, nitrates augment coronary blood flow by dilating epicardial coronary arteries (although this effect is minimal in extensively diseased arteries) and increasing blood flow through collateral vessels. Several formulations are available. Sublingual nitroglycerin tablets or oral spray is effective for the acute treatment of anginal episodes and as prophylactic therapy before an activity that is likely to provoke angina. Topical nitroglycerin ointment and oral preparations are effective for the chronic management of stable angina, whereas intravenous nitroglycerin is appropriate for patients with unstable angina and acute MI. The chronic use of nitrates may result in tolerance, an effect that can be minimized by allowing for a daily nitrate-free period; for example, removing topical nitrate preparations during sleeping hours or prescribing oral nitrates that avoid around-the-clock administration.

β-adrenergic blocking drugs are competitive inhibitors of catecholamine β receptors. They decrease myocardial oxygen

Table 9-5 Medications for Angina Pectoris

Drug Class	Examples	Anti-anginal Effect	Physiologic Side Effects	Comments
Nitroglycerin	Sublingual Topical Intravenous Oral	Decreased preload and afterload Coronary vasodilation Increased collateral blood flow	Headache Flushing Orthostasis	Tolerance develops with continuous use
β-adrenergic blocking agents	Metoprolol Atenolol Propranolol Nadolol	Decreased heart rate Decreased blood pressure Decreased contractility	Bradycardia Hypotension Bronchospasm Depression	May worsen heart failure and AV conduction block; avoid in vasospastic angina
Calcium channel blocking agents	Phenylalkylamine (verapamil) Benzothiazepine (diltiazem)	Decreased heart rate Decreased blood pressure Decreased contractility Coronary vasodilation	Bradycardia Hypotension Constipation with verapamil	May worsen heart failure and AV conduction
Calcium channel blocking agents	Dihydropyridine (nifedipine, amlodipine)	Decreased blood pressure Coronary vasodilation	Hypotension, reflex tachycardia Peripheral edema	Short-acting nifedipine associated with increased risk for cardiovascular events
Late sodium current blocking agents	Ranolazine	Inhibits cardiac late I_{Na} Prevents calcium overload	Dizziness Headache Constipation Nausea	No effects on blood pressure or heart rate Modest QTc prolongation

AV, atrioventricular; I_{Na}, sodium current.

demands by reducing heart rate, blood pressure, and contractility. These agents are effective in controlling anginal symptoms (especially exercise-induced symptoms), and they decrease mortality and reinfarction in survivors of MI. β blockers differ in their lipid solubility, duration of action, and β-receptor selectivity. β_1 receptors predominate in the heart, where they mediate increases in heart rate, contractility, and atrioventricular (AV) conduction. β_2 receptors predominate in the vascular and bronchial smooth muscle. Blockade of β_1 receptors produces several beneficial cardiac effects, whereas β_2-receptor blockade may induce bronchospasm and peripheral vasoconstriction. Atenolol and metoprolol are β_1 selective at low doses; however, at the moderate to high doses often used in clinical practice, all β blockers lose their selectivity. Because β blockers may worsen underlying conduction system abnormalities, they should be used with caution in patients with conduction system dysfunction. In addition, these agents may result in a mild increase in the triglyceride level and a mild decrease in the HDL cholesterol level.

Calcium ions play a critical role in myocardial and vascular smooth muscle contraction and in the genesis of the cardiac action potential (see Chapter 10). Blocking these effects with a calcium antagonist results in a decrease in heart rate, myocardial contractility, and peripheral arterial vasodilation, all of which decrease myocardial oxygen demand. In addition, coronary vasodilation occurs, resulting in augmented oxygen supply. Three major classes of calcium antagonists are available, and the specific agent of choice should be individualized for the particular patient. The dihydropyridine medications (e.g., nifedipine, amlodipine) predominantly cause vasodilation with little or no effect on heart rate, contractility, or AV conduction. In fact, the vasodilation may lead to a reflex tachycardia. The phenylalkylamine medications (e.g., verapamil) reduce heart rate, slow AV conduction, depress contractility, and have less of an effect on peripheral vascular tone than the dihydropyridine medications. They may not be tolerated in patients with depressed ventricular systolic function or underlying conduction system disease. The benzothiazepine medications (e.g., diltiazem) have less vasodilatory action than the dihydropyridine medications and less myocardial suppressant action than the phenylalkylamine medications.

REVASCULARIZATION IN PATIENTS WITH ANGINA

In patients for whom medical therapy does not effectively control anginal symptoms and in patients considered to be at increased risk clinically (e.g., unstable angina, angina associated with heart failure, angina associated with arrhythmia, poor exercise capacity) or by noninvasive testing (e.g., large amount of ischemic myocardium, depressed left ventricular systolic function), coronary revascularization plays an important therapeutic role. Several modalities for coronary revascularization exist, including surgical revascularization (e.g., coronary artery bypass grafting [CABG]) and catheter-based percutaneous techniques (e.g., percutaneous coronary intervention [PCI]).

With advances in equipment, adjunctive pharmacologic agents, and increasing operator experience, PCI can now be achieved with high success rates and at relatively low risk.

More than 1 million PCI procedures are performed each year in the United States alone. (**Web video 9-1—Angioplasty**, http://www.heartsite.com/html/ptca.html). With percutaneous transluminal coronary angioplasty (PTCA), a high-pressure inflation of a distensible balloon is performed at the site of coronary arterial narrowing with resultant enlargement of the lumen. Balloon inflation causes denudation of the endothelial surface, fracture of the atherosclerotic plaque, and disruption of the vessel intima. The vessel lumen can be successfully dilated in greater than 90% of cases. In 2% to 5% of patients undergoing PTCA, the coronary arterial injury is severe, and, as a result, the artery occludes abruptly. Such patients are usually treated with intracoronary stenting or rarely urgent CABG to prevent acute MI. In patients in whom PTCA is initially successful, up to 50% develop restenosis at the site of balloon dilation within 1 to 6 months of the angioplasty. Of the patients who develop restenosis, about 50% experience recurrent angina. Restenosis is a complex process involving elastic recoil of the artery, vascular remodeling, and hyperplasia of the vascular intima. It is not prevented by the administration of antiplatelet, anticoagulant, anti-anginal, or hypolipidemic medications.

During the past decade, intracoronary stenting now has become the technique of choice for PCI (**Web video 9-2—Intracoronary Stenting**, http://www.heartsite.com/html/stent.html). The coronary stent—a cylindric, expandable metal structure available in varying diameters and lengths—is premounted on an angioplasty balloon. When the balloon is positioned at the site of the stenosis and inflated to expand the stent, the stent becomes permanently embedded in the arterial wall. Subsequently, the balloon is deflated and removed, but the stent maintains its expanded cylindric configuration, thereby acting as a scaffold to maintain vessel patency. In this way, stenting results in a greater increase in luminal size than can be achieved with balloon angioplasty alone (see Fig. 9-1B). Stents can be used to treat PTCA-related coronary arterial dissections, thereby avoiding the need for urgent CABG. In comparison with balloon angioplasty, stenting is associated with a reduced incidence of abrupt closure (about 1% to 2%) and restenosis (about 20% to 25%), thereby explaining why it is the procedure of choice in more than 90% of PCIs. At the same time, stenting may not be the procedure of choice in small coronary arteries (luminal diameter < 2.0 mm) because these vessels are too small for the smallest available stents. The person in whom intracoronary bare metal stenting (BMS) has been performed should receive aspirin indefinitely and clopidogrel for 2 to 4 weeks to prevent thrombosis. During the weeks after stent deployment, the stent becomes endothelialized, at which time it is no longer thrombogenic or subject to abrupt closure. Studies have demonstrated that a 1-year course of clopidogrel is superior compared with a 4-week course after bare metal stenting, with a reduction in adverse ischemic events.

Beginning in 2003, drug-eluting stents (DES) have been coated with antiproliferative drugs (e.g., sirolimus [Rapamycin], paclitaxel [Taxol]), which are extremely effective in preventing restenosis. There are five FDA-approved DES in the United States, listed in order of their approval with the year of approval: Cordis Cypher (sirolimus; 2003), Boston Scientific Taxus (paclitaxel; 2004), Medtronic Endeavor (zotarolimus; 2007), Abbott Xience V (everolimus;

2008), and Boston Scientific Promus (everolimus; 2008). The incidence of restenosis with DES is 5% to 10%. Randomized trials have demonstrated a roughly 70% reduction in stent restenosis with DES compared with BMS. In stenting procedures in the United States, roughly 65% involve DES, and 35% involve BMS. The person who receives a DES should take aspirin indefinitely and clopidogrel for at least 12 months. The antiproliferative agent that coats the stent delays the process of endothelialization; as a result, these stents are subject to thrombosis and abrupt closure for months after their placement.

Other percutaneous interventional techniques that have a limited role in coronary revascularization include rotational and directional atherectomy; thrombectomy; brachytherapy, which is the application of local radiation therapy to treat restenosis after stenting; and coronary laser therapy. Of these, thrombectomy has the most promising role in PCI procedures for STEMI patients.

Studies performed in the 1970s and 1980s established the effectiveness of CABG for the control of anginal symptoms and, in some patients, offered an improvement in survival when compared with anti-anginal medical therapy. Harvesting a segment of saphenous vein or radial artery and anastomosing it to the ascending aorta (proximally) and the distal portion of the diseased coronary artery (distally) is performed with CABG. The internal mammary artery can be dissected free from the pleural surface and its distal end anastomosed to a diseased coronary artery. These procedures effectively bypass the sites of atherosclerotic narrowing, thereby allowing blood to flow freely to the myocardium perfused by the diseased artery. The left internal mammary artery is most commonly used to bypass the left anterior descending coronary artery, and has 10-year patency rates of roughly 90%. In comparison, the patency rate for saphenous vein grafts is 50% at 10 years. Whenever possible, the mammary artery is used because its long-term patency is superior to that of venous or radial arterial conduits. Experienced surgeons perform CABG with a peri-operative mortality rate of 1% to 2%, a stroke rate of 1% to 2%, and a peri-operative MI rate of 5% to 10%.

CABG improves survival (when compared with medical therapy) in patients with greater than 50% luminal diameter narrowing of the left main coronary artery or narrowing of all three major epicardial coronary arteries in conjunction with mildly or moderately depressed left ventricular systolic function (e.g., ejection fraction, 35% to 50%). In addition, CABG improves long-term survival in patients with a narrowing of two or three epicardial coronary arteries and normal left ventricular systolic performance, provided that the proximal portion of the left anterior descending coronary artery is significantly narrowed.

In the short term (within 1 to 2 years of the procedure), those having PCI are more likely than those undergoing CABG to require anti-anginal medications or a subsequent revascularization procedure largely because of the incidence of symptomatic restenosis after successful percutaneous coronary revascularization. Because of the progressive decline of graft patency between 5 and 10 years postoperatively, the benefits of surgery over percutaneous revascularization are less apparent in the long term. Small, randomized studies comparing the two approaches to revascularization in patients with multivessel CAD and preserved left ven-

tricular systolic function (e.g., ejection fraction > 50%) demonstrate no difference in mortality after 1 to 5 years of follow-up, except in patients with diabetes, who fare better with CABG. Recently, however, larger observational studies showed that CABG is associated with higher long-term survival than stenting in patients with multivessel CAD. A recently completed trial showed no difference between CABG and DES for left main or multivessel CAD in mortality or myocardial infarction. DES did have higher rates of repeat revascularization because of restenosis, but lower rates of stroke. There are ongoing randomized trials in diabetic patients with multivessel CAD randomized to CABG or DES.

Unfortunately, neither percutaneous nor surgical revascularization techniques halt the underlying atherosclerotic process, and new stenoses may develop at previously uninvolved sites in native coronary arteries and in the bypass grafts. Aspirin should be administered immediately after CABG and continued thereafter because it improves graft patency. If a stenosis develops in a bypass graft, percutaneous revascularization is often effective. In addition, repeat CABG is possible, although the surgical risks are higher than with the first procedure.

For patients with severe angina refractory to maximal medical therapy and coronary revascularization, treatment options include external counterpulsation and spinal cord stimulation. External counterpulsation involves inflation of three lower extremity cuffs during diastole and deflation during systole. This treatment is performed in 1-hour sessions for a total of 35 treatments. Roughly 75% of patients report an improvement in angina severity, and the treatment is generally well-tolerated. The likely mechanism of action involves improved endothelial function. Spinal cord stimulation provides analgesia for patients with severe angina by placing a stimulating electrode in the dorsal epidural space at the C7-T1 level. Although preliminary data appear promising, there is a paucity of data on intermediate- or long-term outcomes. Transmyocardial laser revascularization is no longer recommended for refractory angina.

VARIANT ANGINA

In 1959, Prinzmetal and colleagues described a group of patients with *variant* angina. These patients usually experienced chest pain at rest rather than with physical exertion or emotional excitement, and the ECG recorded during chest pain showed ST-segment elevation rather than depression, which resolved as the pain subsided (Fig. 9-4). On occasion, episodes of chest discomfort were accompanied by varying degrees of AV block or ventricular ectopy, but MI was uncommon. Patients with variant angina did not often have the usual risk factors for coronary atherosclerosis, although cigarette smoking was frequent. Subsequent angiographic studies demonstrated that variant angina is the result of epicardial coronary arterial spasm, which may occur either at the site of an atherosclerotic plaque or in the setting of angiographically normal coronary arteries.

During coronary angiography, coronary vasospasm may be provoked by the intracoronary infusion of acetylcholine or ergonovine. In addition, methacholine, a parasympathomimetic agent, has been used to induce coronary arterial spasm, similar to the arterial spasm in response to exposure

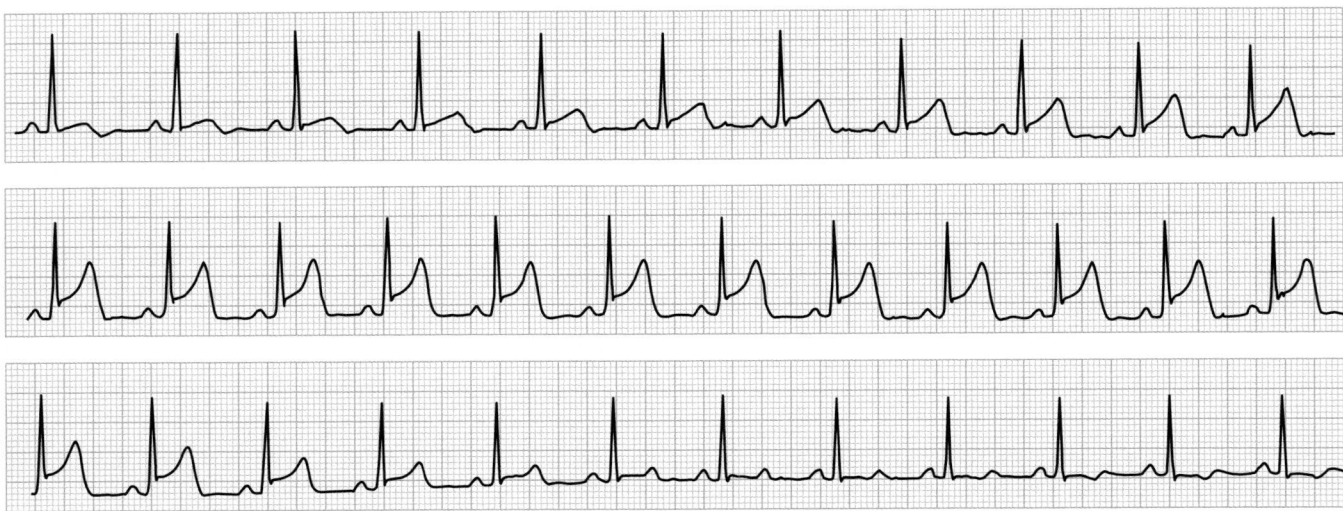

Figure 9-4 Continuous electrocardiogram recording in a patient with Prinzmetal (variant) angina. The spontaneous onset of chest discomfort began during the *top strip*, accompanied by transient ST-segment elevation. By the *bottom strip*, several minutes later, both discomfort and ST-segment elevation had resolved.

to cold (e.g., cold pressor test), the production of a significant alkalosis (e.g., vigorous hyperventilation during the intravenous infusion of an alkalotic buffer solution), and histamine administration.

Calcium channel blockers, alone or in combination with long-acting nitrate preparations, are highly effective in patients with coronary arterial spasm. They are the treatment of choice for patients with variant angina. β blockers are contraindicated in patients with vasospastic angina because blockade of the vasodilatory effects of β₂-receptor stimulation may result in unopposed α-adrenergic vasoconstriction. For the rare patient who has continued episodes of coronary arterial spasm despite maximal medical therapy, intracoronary stenting may be performed.

Acute Coronary Syndromes

The term *acute coronary syndrome* encompasses the clinical syndromes of unstable angina, NSTEMI, and STEMI. Patients with unstable angina or NSTEMI are usually indistinguishable by history, physical examination, and ECG findings. The distinction between these two groups is made only after the results of the serum cardiac enzyme analyses are available.

The patient with unstable angina or NSTEMI may develop myocardial ischemia or MI through several mechanisms. Most commonly, these individuals have subendocardial ischemia or necrosis as a result of decreased coronary blood flow, which is due to platelet aggregation or a partially occlusive intracoronary thrombus at the site of an ulcerated atherosclerotic plaque. In addition, concomitant platelet-mediated coronary arterial vasoconstriction at the site of plaque ulceration may occur. Alternatively, the patient may develop myocardial ischemia or MI because of an increase in myocardial oxygen demand that cannot be met by an appropriate increase in coronary blood flow. In some indi-

viduals, the coronary blood flow cannot appropriately increase because of severe CAD. In those without CAD, subendocardial ischemia or infarction may occur solely as a result of significantly augmented myocardial oxygen demands in the setting of a normal supply (e.g., uncontrolled hypertension, thyrotoxicosis) or a decrease in myocardial oxygen delivery (e.g., profound anemia, hypoxemia). Patients with left ventricular hypertrophy (due to hypertension or aortic stenosis) are at increased risk for subendocardial ischemia.

The patient with unstable angina pectoris usually complains of retrosternal chest pain similar in character and consistency to that of the patient with stable, exertional chest pain. In contrast to the patient whose angina is stable, however, these individuals usually report that their anginal frequency, severity, or duration has worsened, and they may report pain at rest. Furthermore, the patient may note that nitroglycerin is ineffective or less effective in relieving the chest pain.

On physical examination, the patient may exhibit no visible or audible abnormalities at a time when he or she is pain free. During an episode of chest pain, however, the patient may become anxious, diaphoretic, and dyspneic. The heart rate often increases, although bradycardia may occur secondary to enhanced vagal tone or transient AV block and most commonly with inferior wall ischemia or infarction. On cardiac auscultation, an S₄ may be audible as a result of decreased left ventricular compliance. An S₃ may be present if left ventricular systolic dysfunction occurs, and a systolic murmur of mitral valve papillary muscle dysfunction may be appreciated. Evidence of pulmonary congestion is often present and may reflect an elevated left ventricular filling pressure as a result of decreased left ventricular compliance or systolic dysfunction. If a large area of myocardium is involved and left ventricular systolic dysfunction ensues, then frank pulmonary edema may occur.

For the patient who is experiencing chest pain, a 12-lead ECG should be immediately obtained because it is frequently diagnostic of myocardial ischemia or MI and is important

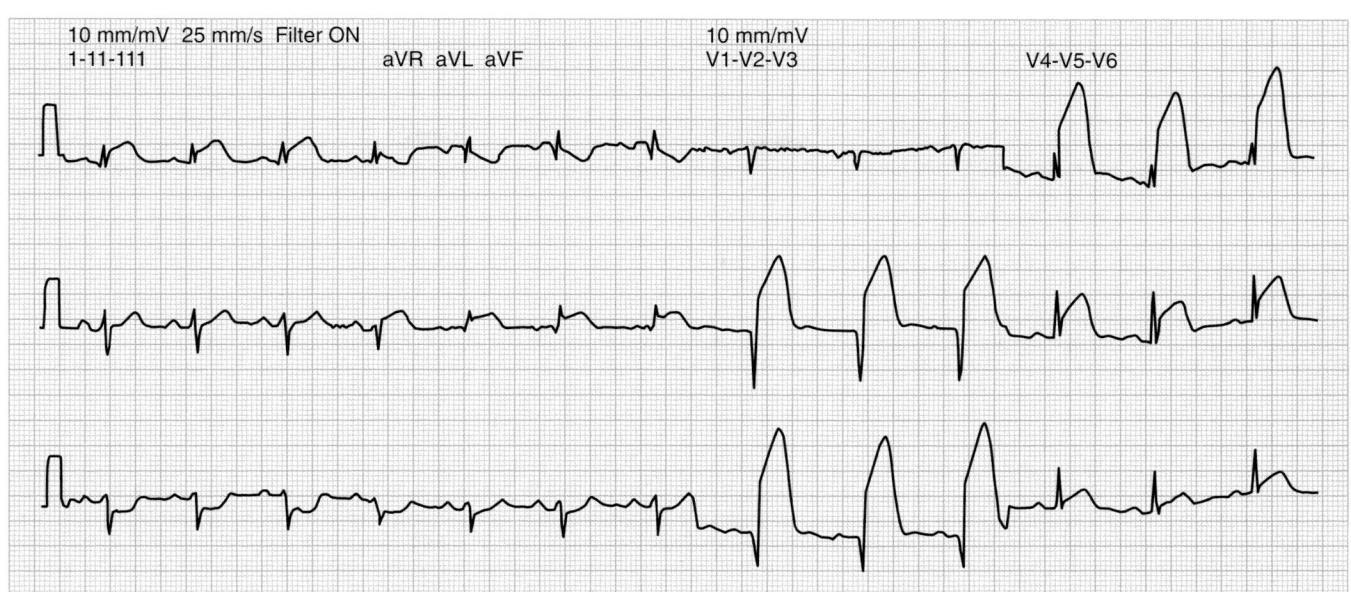

Figure 9-5 Acute anterolateral myocardial infarction. Leads I, aVL, and V_2 to V_6 demonstrate ST-segment elevation. Reciprocal ST-segment depression is seen in leads II, III, and aVF. Deep Q waves have developed in leads V_2 and V_3.

in determining the appropriate treatment plan. STEMI, previously referred to by the pathologically inaccurate term, *transmural infarction* or *Q-wave myocardial infarction*, refers to an acute coronary syndrome in which ST-segment elevation (e.g., ST-segment elevation at the J point in two contiguous leads at least 0.2 mV in men or at least 0.15 mV in women in leads V_2 to V_3 or at least 0.1 mV in other leads) is present on the surface ECG. These infarctions typically are the result of complete thrombotic occlusion of a coronary artery and may first be exhibited on the ECG by symmetrically peaked or hyperacute T waves. These peaked T waves resolve after several minutes as the characteristic ST-segment elevation develops (Fig. 9-5). The distribution of leads with ST-segment elevation can identify the myocardial location and the culprit coronary artery: anterior MI, V_2 to V_5, left anterior descending coronary artery; inferior MI, II, III, aVF, right coronary artery; lateral MI, I, aVL, V_6, left circumflex or diagonal; posterior, V_7 to V_9, left circumflex coronary artery; right ventricular RV_4, right coronary artery.

NSTEMI, previously termed *subendocardial infarction* or *non–Q-wave myocardial infarction*, and unstable angina occur as a result of a subtotally occlusive thrombus or a thrombus that was initially totally occlusive but not sustained, enabling partial or complete lysis to occur within minutes to hours of its formation. They are associated with ST-segment depression and T-wave inversions on the surface ECG (Fig. 9-6).

In one fourth to one half of patients with acute MI, the first ECG does not demonstrate typical ST-segment changes. In this situation, serial ECGs should be obtained to increase the diagnostic yield. If a patient has ongoing chest pain without ST-segment changes, posterior lead ECG recording of leads V_7 to V_9 should be performed. A posterior lead ECG is used to assess for posterior wall injury, usually the result of left circumflex coronary artery occlusion, which is not readily apparent on a standard 12-lead ECG. If acute MI is

suggestive but the initial ECG does not confirm the diagnosis, demonstration of new regional wall motion abnormalities with echocardiography may be helpful in confirming the diagnosis.

Myocardial necrosis results in the release of certain intracellular enzymes into the blood. Their appearance in the blood allows the identification of myocardial necrosis, and their quantitation over a number of hours allows for the estimate of its amount. Because 20% of patients with acute MI have atypical or no symptoms (i.e., *silent* MI) and the initial ECG is nondiagnostic in up to 50% of patients, serologic identification of myocyte necrosis has become an important diagnostic tool. Several serum markers have been identified (Fig. 9-7).

Creatine kinase (CK) and its myocardial-specific isoenzyme, creatine kinase muscle band (CK-MB) are detectable in the blood within 3 to 6 hours of the onset of MI. They reach their peak concentration at 24 hours and return to normal within 48 hours. Although CK-MB is relatively specific for cardiac injury, it may be elevated in subjects with extensive skeletal muscle injury or disease, chronic renal disease, or hypothyroidism.

Troponins I and T are regulatory proteins involved in the interaction of cardiac actin and myosin. Because they are not present to any extent in other organs and are not detectable in blood under normal circumstances, an increase in their serum concentration is more specific and sensitive for myocyte necrosis than an increase in the concentration of other enzymes. After cardiac injury, the serum troponin concentration begins to rise within 4 to 6 hours and remains elevated for 7 to 10 days. False-positive elevations of troponin T, but not troponin I, have been observed in patients with renal failure. The presence of heterophilic antibodies or fibrin may interfere with the assay for troponin I and give false-positive results. The former is found in 3% of the general population and a high percentage of patients with autoimmune disease; the latter may be found in blood that

Boston University Hospital

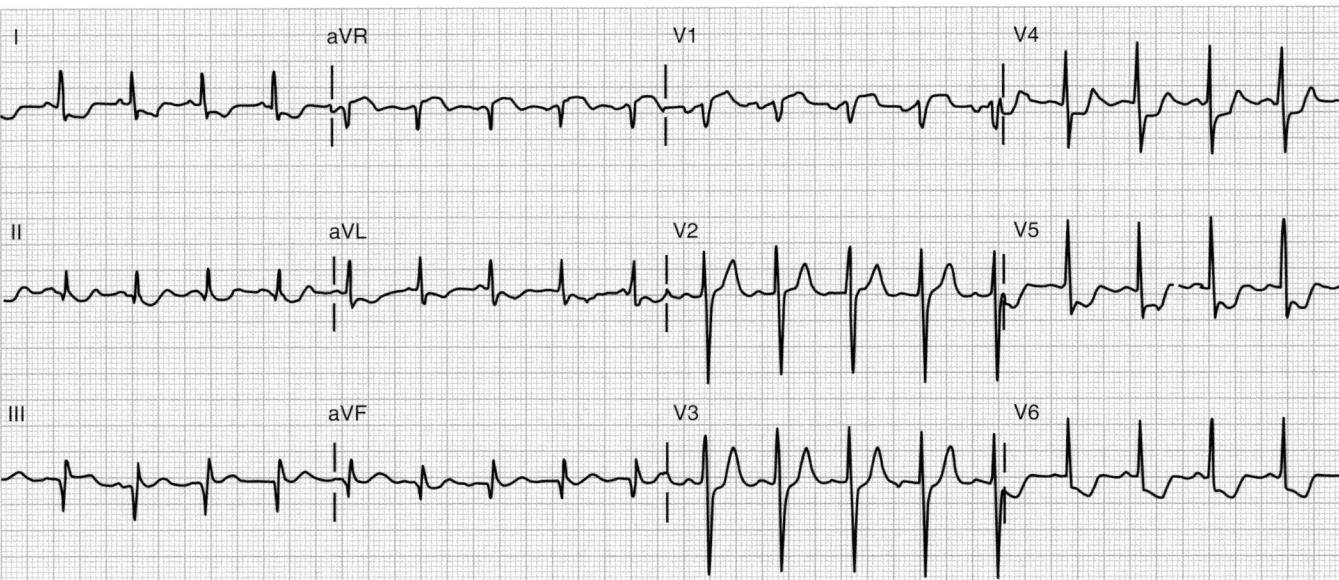

Figure 9-6 Marked ST-segment depression in a patient with prolonged chest pain is the result of an acute non–ST-segment elevation myocardial infarction (NSTEMI). Between 1 and 3 mm of ST-segment depression is seen in leads I, aVL, and V₄ to V₆. The patient is known to have had a previous inferior myocardial infarction.

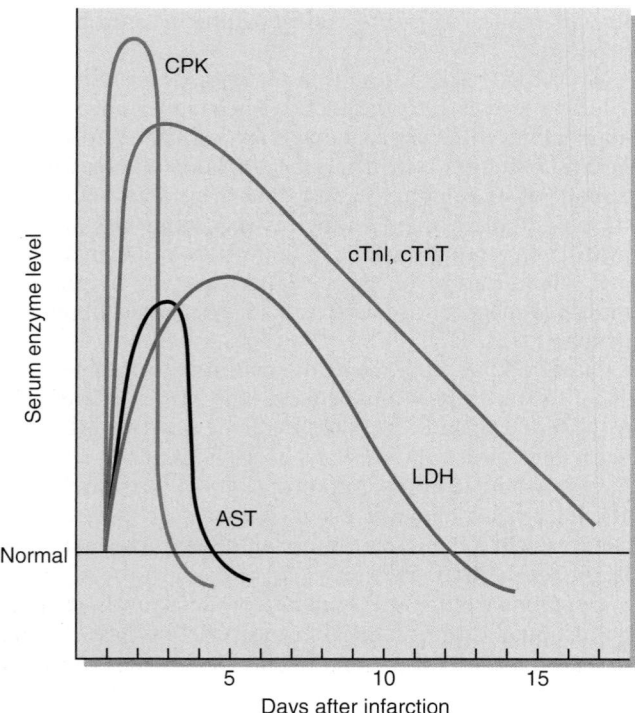

Figure 9-7 Typical time course for the detection of enzymes released after myocardial infarction. AST, serum aspartate aminotransferase; CPK, creatine kinase; cTnI, cardiac troponin I; cTnT, cardiac troponin T; LDH, lactate dehydrogenase.

has been heparinized. Because serum troponin concentration is an extremely sensitive measure of myocardial necrosis, such elevations are sometimes observed in patients with myocardial necrosis as a result of increased myocardial oxygen demand (i.e., subjects with a significantly elevated heart rate or blood pressure, pulmonary embolism, hypoxemia) or reduced supply (i.e., hypotension) in the absence of epicardial CAD.

TREATMENT OF UNSTABLE ANGINA AND NON–ST-SEGMENT ELEVATION MYOCARDIAL INFARCTION

Unstable angina and NSTEMI may be clinically indistinguishable with ECG studies. They are differentiated only by the presence of serologic evidence of myocardial necrosis. Accordingly, the initial treatment of these patients is similar and includes (1) hospital admission with serial assessment of ECGs and sequential measurements of cardiac enzymes; (2) aggressive anti-anginal, antiplatelet, and antithrombotic therapy; and (3) identification of the patient at increased risk for recurrent ischemia, MI, or death who may benefit from revascularization. With optimal medical therapy, the 1-year mortality rate of patients with unstable angina or NSTEMI is 3% to 5% (Fig. 9-8).

Rest for 24 to 48 hours with continuous ECG monitoring, analgesics, and supplemental oxygen therapy are frequently prescribed. Sublingual nitroglycerin should be given initially, followed by oral or topical nitroglycerin. Intravenous nitroglycerin should be administered if recurrent chest pain occurs. In the absence of a contraindication, β blockers should be promptly instituted because they decrease heart rate and blood pressure levels and left ventricular contractility, thereby reducing myocardial oxygen demand. The calcium antagonists, verapamil and diltiazem, may be useful for the patient who fails to respond to nitrates and β blockers as well as for the patient with a contraindication to β blockers. However, calcium antagonists should not be used in the patient with known depressed left ventricular systolic function or with evidence of pulmonary vascular congestion on

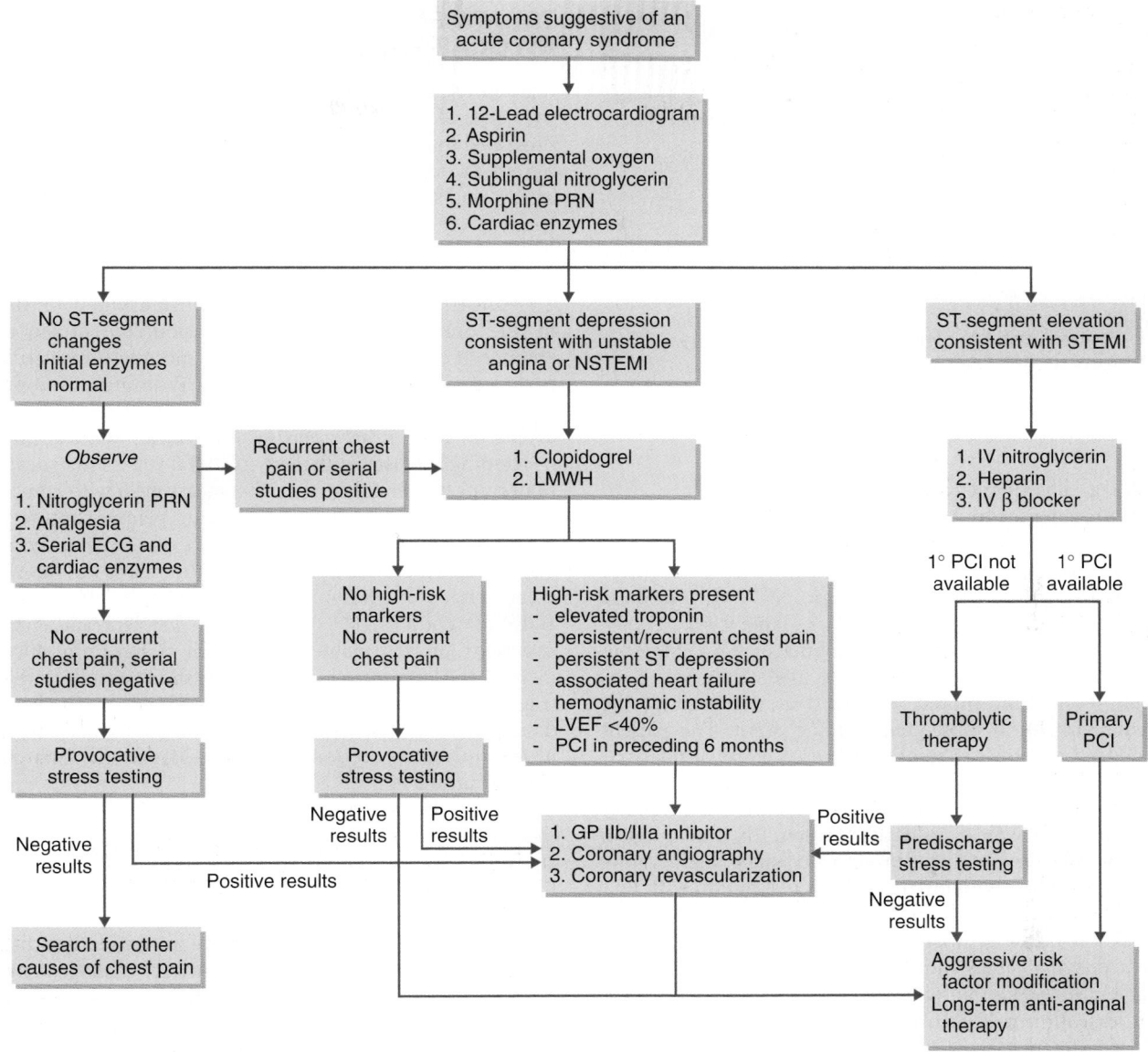

Figure 9-8 Treatment algorithm for patients with symptoms suggestive of an acute coronary syndrome. ECG, electrocardiogram; LMWH, low-molecular-weight heparin; NSTEMI, non–ST-segment elevation myocardial infarction; PCI, percutaneous coronary intervention; STEMI, ST-segment elevation myocardial infarction.

physical examination or chest radiograph. Because dihydropyridine calcium antagonists (e.g., nifedipine, amlodipine) may cause a reflex tachycardia with a resultant worsening of angina, they should be avoided unless they can be used in combination with a β blocker.

As noted, enhanced platelet aggregation and partial coronary arterial occlusion by platelet-rich thrombus play important pathophysiologic roles in most patients with unstable angina or NSTEMI. Aspirin has been shown to decrease mortality and rates of recurrent MI in these patients. Accordingly, the patient without a contraindication should receive oral aspirin, an initial 325-mg dose followed by 75 to 325 mg daily. The addition of oral clopidogrel or an intravenous glycoprotein IIb/IIIa inhibitor (e.g., tirofiban, eptifibatide) provides more effective platelet inhibition, thereby reducing the risk for recurrent ischemia or infarction. If

clopidogrel is administered, it is continued for 9 to 12 months. If a glycoprotein IIb/IIIa inhibitor is used, it is infused for 48 to 96 hours. Glycoprotein IIb/IIIa inhibitors are typically used in patients who have high-risk features predictive of a subsequent cardiac event, such as ST-segment depressions, T-wave inversions, or positive biomarkers, or those in whom percutaneous revascularization is planned.

Heparin, unfractionated or low-molecular-weight, is given concomitantly with antiplatelet therapy. If unfractionated heparin is used, it is usually infused for 48 hours. Enoxaparin, a low-molecular-weight heparin, may be used instead of unfractionated heparin. It is administered subcutaneously twice daily and continued until hospital discharge. Unlike unfractionated heparin, it does not require monitoring of its anticoagulant effects by serially measuring the activated partial thromboplastin time. In patients considered at

Table 9-6 Selection Criteria for Thrombolytic Therapy in Acute Myocardial Infarction

- Chest pain consistent with acute myocardial infarction
- Electrocardiographic changes:
  - ST-segment elevation at the J point in two or more contiguous leads with ≥0.2 mV in men or ≥0.15 mV in women in leads V_2-V_3 and/or ≥0.1 mV in other leads
  - New or presumed new left bundle branch block
  - ST-segment depression with prominent R wave in leads V_2 and V_3 if believed to represent posterior infarction
- Time from onset of symptoms: <12 hr
- Age:
  - <75 years: definite benefit
  - ≥75 years: benefit less clear

risk for a subsequent cardiac event, low-molecular-weight heparin is superior to unfractionated heparin in preventing recurrent ischemia. Thrombolytic therapy or abciximab have not been shown to be beneficial for the treatment of individuals with unstable angina or NSTEMI. In these patients, in fact, it may be detrimental (Table 9-6).

For the patient with unstable angina or NSTEMI who promptly and completely responds to medical therapy, subsequent evaluation should be aimed at determining the patient's risk for a subsequent cardiac event. The patient deemed to be at low risk might undergo exercise or pharmacologic stress testing. The patient considered to be at high risk for subsequent events should receive maximal antiplatelet therapy with aspirin and a glycoprotein IIb/IIIa inhibitor, low-molecular-weight heparin, and coronary angiography within 4 to 48 hours, followed by revascularization with PCI or CABG, if indicated. Patients most likely to benefit from this early invasive approach are those with elevated serum cardiac enzyme values and those with three or more at-risk variables, including the following: (1) age 65 years or older, (2) at least three risk factors for atherosclerosis, (3) a previously documented coronary arterial stenosis of 50% or greater, (4) ECG ST-segment deviation at the time of hospital arrival, (5) at least two anginal episodes in the 24 hours before hospitalization, or (6) use of aspirin during the 7 days before hospitalization. This risk stratification system is termed the *TIMI risk score*.

Urgent coronary angiography should be performed in the patient with continued or recurrent chest pain despite optimal medical therapy or hypotension or severe heart failure during medical therapy. (**Web video 9-3, Cardiac Cath,** http://www.heartsite.com/html/cardiac_cath.html). Coronary angiography should be considered for the patient with an acute coronary syndrome and any of the following risk factors: (1) previous PCI or CABG, (2) congestive heart failure or depressed left ventricular systolic function, (3) life-threatening ventricular arrhythmias, (4) recurrent low-threshold ischemia, or (5) exercise or pharmacologic stress testing that indicates a high likelihood of severe CAD. Based on coronary anatomy, the experience of the medical personnel, the presence of co-existing medical conditions, and the preferences of the patient, a recommendation for percutaneous or surgical revascularization can be made.

TREATMENT OF ST-SEGMENT ELEVATION MYOCARDIAL INFARCTION

Numerous studies have shown that coronary thrombosis is the cause of most STEMIs. Postmortem studies have demonstrated that 85% to 95% of patients dying of STEMI have a fresh thrombotic occlusion of a large epicardial coronary artery, and angiographic studies performed within several hours of the onset of STEMI have shown a similar incidence of total occlusion. After as little as 15 minutes of coronary occlusion, irreversible cellular injury and necrosis ensue. The subsequent extent of myocardial injury is determined by the duration of coronary occlusion, the presence or absence of collateral vessels, and the amount of myocardium perfused by the infarct-related artery. Prompt restoration of antegrade flow in the infarct-related artery minimizes the extent of myocardial necrosis. In arteries with gradually developing stenoses, sufficient collateral vessels may develop to prevent irreversible myocardial injury even with complete arterial occlusion. In contrast, if acute plaque rupture and thrombotic occlusion occur at the site of a previously nonobstructive stenosis, collateral circulation does not have sufficient time to develop, and extensive infarction ensues. With infarction of 20% to 25% of the left ventricle, congestive heart failure usually ensues. With infarction of 40% or more of the left ventricle, cardiogenic shock usually develops (Fig. 9-9). Cardiogenic shock is defined as inadequate tissue perfusion due to cardiac dysfunction and is discussed in the upcoming section (see "Post–Myocardial Infarction Complications").

In the patient with suggested acute MI, a 12-lead ECG should be performed within 5 minutes of the patient's arrival, and serum cardiac enzyme levels should be assessed. If ST-segment elevation in contiguous ECG leads or LBBB is present, subsequent care should be focused on sedation and pain relief, prompt restoration of antegrade flow in the occluded infarct-related coronary artery, management of ventricular dysfunction or arrhythmias, and prevention or treatment of immediate and late complications.

A large-bore intravenous line should be introduced for the administration of fluids and medications, and supplemental oxygen should be initiated. Intravenous morphine sulfate should be used to relieve chest pain and to decrease sympathetic stimulation. However, it should be given cautiously because it may cause hypotension, respiratory depression, or bradycardia. The usual dose is 2 to 5 mg every 5 to 10 minutes until chest pain is relieved; systemic arterial pressure should be monitored carefully during its administration. The patient should be kept on bed rest for the first 24 hours of hospitalization. Intravenous nitroglycerin should be administered to patients with continued chest pain, congestive heart failure, or systemic arterial hypertension. The nitroglycerin infusion should be initiated at 5 to 10 mcg/minute and gradually increased up to 200 mcg/minute until a 10% reduction in systolic arterial pressure in normotensive patients or a 25% to 30% reduction in systolic arterial pressure in hypertensive patients is realized. Morphine and nitroglycerin should be avoided in the patient suggested as having right ventricular infarction because a medication-induced reduction in preload may cause profound systemic arterial hypotension. The patient with acute MI should receive oral or rectal aspirin, 325 mg immediately and then

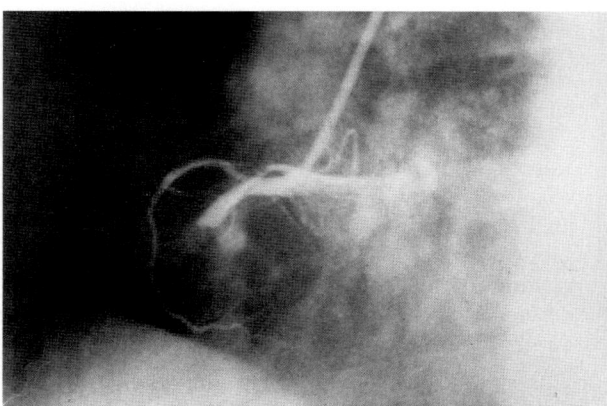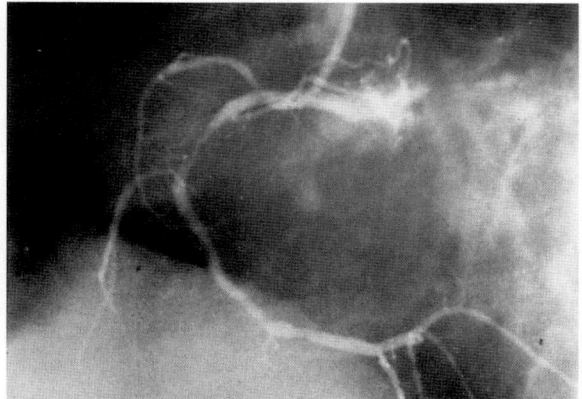

Figure 9-9 Right coronary artery angiogram in a patient with acute inferior myocardial infarction. The *left panel* demonstrates total occlusion of the right coronary artery. The *right panel* depicts restoration of flow 90 minutes after the intravenous administration of tissue-type plasminogen activator.

daily (75 to 325 mg) thereafter, because of its effectiveness in reducing mortality. In addition to aspirin, clopidogrel should be initiated with a 300- to 600-mg oral loading dose followed by a 75 mg daily maintenance dose. In patients older than 75 years treated with thrombolytics, there is a higher risk for bleeding complications with the addition of clopidogrel.

Restoration of antegrade flow in the occluded infarct-related artery within 12 hours of pain onset reduces morbidity and mortality. This reduction can be accomplished mechanically with a primary PCI or with a pharmacologic intervention using a thrombolytic agent. Randomized trials have established the superiority of PCI over thrombolytics in patients who can receive PCI expeditiously, generally within 90 minutes of presentation to medical attention. Thrombolytic therapy should be reserved for patients in whom PCI cannot be completed within 2 hours of medical attention. A delay in immediate reperfusion therapy increases the extent of myocardial damage and mortality.

An intravenous β blocker may be administered cautiously for those without a contraindication (i.e., heart rate < 60 beats/minute, systolic arterial pressure < 100 mm Hg, any congestive heart failure or peripheral hypoperfusion, first-degree AV block with a PR interval > 0.24 second, second- or third-degree AV block, severe obstructive lung disease, asthma). In the STEMI patient treated with intravenous β blocker, the beneficial effects of a reduction in arrhythmia, recurrent ischemia, and reinfarction are offset by an increased risk for cardiogenic shock. Therefore, intravenous β blockade is contraindicated in STEMI patients with any signs of heart failure or evidence of a low cardiac output state. Intravenous β blockade is reserved for hypertensive patients without any evidence of ventricular dysfunction, risk factors for cardiogenic shock, or contraindications to therapy. The β blocker most often used in this setting is metoprolol. Metoprolol is administered as three 5-mg boluses at 2- to 5-minute intervals to achieve a resting heart rate less than 70 beats/minute. Oral β blockade, initiated within 1 day and continued indefinitely, reduces the risk for nonfatal reinfarction and cardiovascular mortality by 20% to 25% when compared with placebo. The specific oral β blockers shown to exert this beneficial effect are propranolol, timolol, metoprolol, and atenolol. Although the mechanisms by which β

blockers exert their beneficial effect are not completely understood, they appear to have an anti-arrhythmic and anti-ischemic influence. For the patient in whom β blockers are contraindicated, verapamil may decrease the incidence of reinfarction and mortality; however, verapamil should be avoided in patients with ventricular systolic dysfunction, clinical heart failure, or any evidence of a low cardiac output state. The other calcium antagonists are not beneficial, and the dihydropyridine agents actually increase mortality.

In the patient with congestive heart failure or depressed left ventricular systolic function (ejection fraction < 0.40%) without systemic arterial hypotension, the administration of an oral ACE inhibitor improves outcome. Randomized, placebo-controlled trials have demonstrated that ACE inhibitor therapy with captopril, enalapril, ramipril, trandolapril, or zofenopril begun 24 hours to 16 days after MI limits left ventricular dilation, improves left ventricular ejection fraction, reduces the incidence of reinfarction and heart failure, and improves short- and long-term survival. In two large trials, the administration of ACE inhibitors within 1 day of hospitalization reduced short-term mortality. The recommended initial regimens include captopril (initial dose, 6.25 mg, increased every 6 to 8 hours to a maximum of 50 mg 3 times daily as long as the systolic arterial pressure is > 90 to 100 mm Hg); enalapril (initial dose, 2.5 mg/day, gradually increased to 20 mg twice daily), or lisinopril (initial dose, 2.5 mg/daily, increased to a maximum of 40 mg/day). ACE inhibitors should not be administered to patients with systemic arterial hypotension (systolic pressure < 90 to 100 mm Hg), an allergy to ACE inhibitors, hyperkalemia, a history of bilateral renal arterial stenosis, previous worsening of renal failure with ACE inhibitors, or pregnancy. Intravenous ACE inhibitors are not recommended for acute STEMI management because of the risk for hypotension.

During the hours after the initiation of the therapies previously described, the patient should be closely observed for the development of early complications related to the MI. Systemic arterial hypotension during the early hours of infarction may be due to intravascular volume depletion, right ventricular infarction, severe left ventricular systolic dysfunction, medications (most notably morphine or nitroglycerin), bradycardia, or tachyarrhythmia. Less commonly, a mechanical complication (e.g., left ventricular free-wall rupture, ventricular septal defect, papillary muscle rupture with resultant mitral regurgitation) can occur within hours of the onset of MI.

Immediate Reperfusion Therapy

In patients with STEMI, early restoration of blood flow to the jeopardized myocardium can limit necrosis, improve left ventricular function, and reduce mortality. This can be mechanically accomplished with primary PCI or pharmacologically with a thrombolytic agent. If a cardiac catheterization facility is accessible and experienced physicians and personnel can quickly perform primary PCI (i.e., within 90 minutes of the patient's first contact with medical personnel), it is the preferred method of restoring antegrade flow in most patients. On the other hand, if primary PCI is not immediately available or the delay in transporting the patient to a catheterization facility would be inordinately long, thrombolytic therapy should be given. Primary PCI is particularly preferable in patients with a contraindication to thrombolytic therapy, with prior CABG, in cardiogenic shock, or older than 70 years.

Thrombolytic therapy is effective in restoring infarct-related artery patency. In 50% to 60% of patients, normal coronary flow is reestablished within 90 minutes of thrombolytic administration. It should be administered to the STEMI patient who seeks medical attention at a center without catheterization facilities or appropriately experienced personnel as well as to the patient with a condition that would make catheterization inappropriate (i.e., allergy to radiographic contrast material, severe renal insufficiency, severe peripheral vascular disease). In the United States, five thrombolytic agents are currently approved for use in patients with STEMI (Table 9-7): (1) streptokinase, (2) anistreplase (anisoylated plasminogen streptokinase activator complex [APSAC]), (3) alteplase (tissue plasminogen activator [t-PA]), (4) reteplase plasminogen activator (r-PA), and (5) tenecteplase tissue plasminogen activator (TNK-tPA). Currently, r-PA and TNK-tPA are the most commonly used thrombolytics. Although slight differences in their effectiveness and bleeding complications have been reported, the choice of agent is less important than the timely decision to administer it.

Streptokinase (1.5 million units) is given as a 1-hour infusion. Rarely, the recipient may experience an acute allergic reaction. Although its administration is frequently associated with mild hypotension, the drop in systemic arterial pressure is rarely of sufficient magnitude to warrant interruption of the infusion. Because antibodies to streptokinase develop within days of its administration, it should not be given to patients who have previously received it or who have had a recent streptococcal infection. APSAC is derived from and has the same limitations as streptokinase, but it is significantly more costly. These agents are seldom used in the United States.

t-PA and its derivatives r-PA and TNK-tPA are much more expensive than streptokinase and are associated with a slightly higher rate of intracranial hemorrhage (0.7% versus 0.5%, respectively). However, they are also more *clot specific* in that they do not cause a generalized fibrinolytic state, and they are more effective at lysing older thrombi (e.g., those associated with an MI of >4 hours' duration). t-PA and its derivatives do not elicit an antibody response or hypotension. t-PA is given as an initial bolus or *front loaded*, followed by a 90-minute infusion (15 mg as a bolus, another 50 mg infused over 30 minutes, and the remaining 35 mg infused over the next 60 minutes). r-PA is administered as a double bolus (two 10-unit boluses delivered 30 minutes apart), and TNK-tPA is administered as a single bolus (0.5 mg/kg to a maximum of 50 mg). Although r-PA and TNK-tPA are somewhat more likely than t-PA to restore early patency of the infarct-related artery, the mortality rate with these three agents is similar.

Overall, thrombolytic therapy decreases short-term mortality in subjects with STEMI by about 20%. Angiographic studies comparing thrombolytic regimens demonstrate that restoration of blood flow in the infarct-related artery is faster and more complete with t-PA than with streptokinase, and this translates into a modestly decreased mortality rate with t-PA, especially when it is given in a front-loaded fashion. Specifically, in the Global Utilization of Streptokinase and Tissue Plasminogen Activator for Occluded Coronary Arteries (GUSTO) trial, t-PA was associated with a statistically significant 1% absolute reduction in mortality when compared with streptokinase. Most of this benefit occurred in patients younger than 70 years within 4 hours of the onset of an anterior STEMI. In older patients, in patients more than 4 hours after symptom onset, and in those with an MI in a territory other than the anterior wall, the mortality difference between these two agents was negligible.

The contraindications to thrombolytic therapy are listed in Table 9-8; they identify those with an unacceptably high risk for bleeding complications. The most catastrophic potential complication of thrombolytic therapy is intracranial hemorrhage. This risk is substantially increased in patients with a history of hemorrhagic stroke, uncontrolled hypertension, body weight less than 70 kg, and age more than 65 years.

Aspirin is an obligatory adjunct to thrombolysis; its use is associated with an additive benefit on mortality and a decrease in recurrent ischemic events. Clopidogrel therapy

Table 9-7 **Dosing Regimens of Commonly Used Thrombolytic Agents**	
Thrombolytic Agent	**Dosing Regimen**
t-PA (alteplase)	15 mg bolus IV, followed by 0.75 mg/kg body weight (not to exceed 50 mg) over 30 min, followed by 0.5 mg/kg (not to exceed 35 mg) over 60 min
r-PA (reteplase)	Two 10U IV boluses, given 30 min apart
TNK-tPA (tenecteplase)	Single bolus IV 0.5 mg/kg (dose rounded to the nearest 5 mg, ranging from 30 to 50 mg)
Streptokinase	1.5 million U IV over 60 min

IV, intravenous; PA, plasminogen activator; r-PA, reteplase plasminogen activator; TNK-tPA, tenecteplase tissue plasminogen activator; U, units.

Table 9-8 Contraindications to Thrombolytic Therapy in Acute Myocardial Infarction

Absolute

Suspected aortic dissection
Active bleeding*
Any prior cerebral hemorrhage
Intracranial neoplasm
Cerebral aneurysm or arteriovenous malformation
Ischemic cerebrovascular accident within 3 months

Relative

Bleeding diathesis, coagulopathy, or anticoagulant use
Major surgery within 3 weeks
Puncture of a noncompressible vessel, internal bleeding, or head or major body trauma within previous 2 weeks
Nonhemorrhagic stroke or gastrointestinal hemorrhage within 6 months
Proliferative retinopathy
Active peptic ulcer disease
History of chronic, severe, poorly controlled hypertension
Severe uncontrolled hypertension on presentation (systolic blood pressure > 180 mm Hg or diastolic blood pressure >110 mm Hg)
Traumatic or prolonged (>10 min) cardiopulmonary resuscitation
Pregnancy

*Does not include menstrual bleeding.

Table 9-9 Complications of Acute Myocardial Infarction

Functional

Left ventricular failure
Right ventricular failure
Cardiogenic shock

Mechanical

Free-wall rupture
Ventricular septal defect
Papillary muscle rupture with acute mitral regurgitation

Electrical

Bradyarrhythmias (first-, second-, and third-degree atrioventricular blocks)
Tachyarrhythmias (supraventricular, ventricular)
Conduction abnormalities (bundle branch and fascicular blocks)

with a 300-mg load followed by a daily maintenance dose of 75 mg improves mortality compared with placebo in STEMI patients 75 years and older. Intravenous heparin administered for 48 hours is necessary to maintain patency of the infarct-related artery after successful thrombolysis when a t-PA is administered, but not with streptokinase. Low-molecular-weight heparin may be slightly more effective than unfractionated heparin as adjunctive therapy after successful thrombolysis. Its use is associated with a higher rate of vessel patency and a lower rate of reocclusion, leading to fewer episodes of recurrent ischemia and infarction, albeit with a somewhat increased risk for hemorrhagic complications. For patients who do not reperfuse within 90 minutes of receiving thrombolytics (as evidenced by continued chest pain or continued ST-segment elevation), rescue PCI is generally recommended. Even with successful thrombolysis, there is a 30% chance of culprit vessel reocclusion within 3 months. Risk stratification with a submaximal, symptom-limited stress test or coronary angiography is required during the STEMI hospitalization for thrombolyzed patients.

POST–MYOCARDIAL INFARCTION COMPLICATIONS

The complications of MI may be categorized as electrical or mechanical (Table 9-9).

Arrhythmias and Conduction Abnormalities

Cardiac arrhythmias may occur in patients with acute coronary syndromes. Those that cause symptoms or hemodynamic compromise almost always warrant treatment, whereas those that do not often can be managed expectantly.

Although most of these arrhythmias are a direct result of the ischemic process, other reversible aggravating factors, such as electrolyte disturbances, hypoxemia, and medication toxicity, must be excluded.

Premature ventricular complexes, ventricular couplets, and nonsustained ventricular tachycardia (VT) occur frequently in the peri-infarction period. Although such ectopy can be effectively suppressed with anti-arrhythmic agents, treatment is not warranted in the absence of symptoms or hemodynamic compromise. The presence of frequent ventricular ectopy does not predict the development of more malignant arrhythmias, and empiric therapy of such ectopy is associated with an increased mortality rate. Accelerated idioventricular rhythm, or *slow VT*, often occurs shortly after successful reperfusion, is self-limited, and does not require treatment.

During the past several decades, mortality in hospitalized patients with acute MI has substantially declined in large part because of the early recognition and treatment of lethal arrhythmias. Because most deaths from acute MI occur as a result of sustained VT or ventricular fibrillation (VF), these rhythm disturbances should be treated with immediate electrical defibrillation, after which administering intravenous anti-arrhythmic medications (e.g., lidocaine, amiodarone) is reasonable for 24 to 48 hours. Sustained but hemodynamically stable VT can be treated initially with anti-arrhythmic agents with electrical cardioversion held in reserve. In the absence of electrolyte abnormalities, polymorphic VT is usually a marker of recurrent or persistent ischemia, and aggressive anti-ischemic treatment is warranted. When sustained VT or VF occurs in the first 48 hours after MI, it does not portend the same poor prognosis as it does when it occurs later.

Transient supraventricular tachyarrhythmias may occur in patients with acute MI, with sinus tachycardia and atrial fibrillation being the most common. The cause of sinus tachycardia (e.g., anxiety, pain, fever, anemia, hypoxemia, hypovolemia, pulmonary vascular congestion, thyrotoxicosis) should be promptly identified and corrected. If atrial fibrillation is accompanied by a rapid ventricular response, with resultant ongoing ischemia or hemodynamic compromise, electrical shock cardioversion should be considered. In the patient with atrial fibrillation and a rapid ventricular response, intravenous β blockers or amiodarone is usually effective for controlling the ventricular response, provided no contraindications to their use exist. Calcium channel blocking agents are also effective but should be avoided in the patient with heart failure. (These arrhythmias are discussed at length in Chapter 10.)

Bradyarrhythmias may complicate acute MI. The most common bradyarrhythmia is sinus bradycardia, which is observed in 20% to 25% of patients with acute MI and is more common in those with inferior than anterior MI. In patients with inferior MI, sinus bradycardia is often associated with hypotension caused by increased vagal tone as a result of stimulation of vagal afferent fibers in the inferoposterior portion of the left ventricle (Bezold-Jarisch reflex). Unless accompanied by hemodynamic instability, sinus bradycardia should be simply observed. If treatment is necessary, intravenous atropine (0.5 to 2 mg) should be administered, aiming for a heart rate of 60 beats/minute and a resolution of symptoms. Temporary pacing is rarely required.

Ischemia and infarction can result in transient or permanent injury to the conduction system. Varying degrees of AV block may occur in patients with acute MI. Ischemia of the AV node can result in first-degree or Mobitz type I second-degree (Wenckebach phenomenon) AV block. These rhythms are most often associated with inferior MI; they are transient, do not adversely affect survival, and do not require treatment unless the ventricular rate is sufficiently slow to produce syncope, congestive heart failure, or angina. Mobitz type II second-degree AV block is a rare complication of acute MI (1% of cases) and usually results from injury to the His-Purkinje system in the setting of an extensive anterior MI. It often is associated with progression to complete or third-degree AV block and is an indication for temporary transvenous or transcutaneous pacing in anticipation of implantation of a permanent pacemaker. Complete or third-degree AV block may occur with inferior or anterior MI. When it occurs in the setting of an inferior MI, the block is usually at the level of the AV node. It is associated with a stable escape rhythm and tends to be transient, although it may take up to 1 to 2 weeks to resolve. As a result, treatment with only a temporary and not a permanent pacemaker is usually required. In contrast, when complete AV block occurs in the setting of an anterior MI, the His-Purkinje system is usually involved. The block is usually permanent, and a permanent pacemaker should be implanted.

Block in one or more branches of the conduction system may occur with acute MI and is more common with anterior than with inferior infarction. Patients with isolated left anterior or left posterior fascicular block or right bundle branch block (RBBB) do not require specific therapy. Conversely, temporary pacing is suggested in patients with new bifascicular blocks (e.g., LBBB or RBBB with left anterior or left posterior fascicular block) because progression to complete heart block is common. If bifascicular block persists after an MI, a permanent pacemaker should be placed.

Congestive Heart Failure and Cardiogenic Shock

Patients who die of cardiac failure after acute MI have extensive myocardial necrosis with loss of at least 40% of the functioning left ventricular muscle mass, as either a consequence of new infarction or a combination of old and new infarctions.

The patient with an acute MI and no evidence on physical examination or chest radiographic studies of left ventricular failure has an excellent prognosis, with only a 2% to 5% in-hospital mortality rate (Killip class I). The individual with some evidence of pulmonary vascular congestion (e.g., basilar rales, S_3, radiographic evidence of pulmonary venous congestion) is classified as Killip class II and has a short-term mortality rate of 10% to 15%. In the patient with overt pulmonary edema evidenced on physical examination or chest radiographic studies, mortality rate is 20% to 30% (Killip class III). Finally, the patient with cardiogenic shock is said to be Killip class IV and has a mortality rate of 50% to 60% even with maximal therapy. In these individuals, infarction is associated with systemic arterial hypotension and diminished peripheral perfusion, as manifested by mental confusion, cold and clammy skin, peripheral cyanosis, and oliguria. Hemodynamically, the systemic arterial systolic pressure is less than 90 mm Hg, the cardiac index is less than 1.8 L/m² per minute, the systemic arteriolar resistance is greatly increased (>2000 dynes/cm⁵ per second), and the left ventricular filling pressure is elevated (more than 20 mm Hg) for more than 30 minutes. The reduced systemic arterial pressure further diminishes coronary arterial perfusion pressure, thereby increasing myocardial ischemia. The low cardiac output and systemic arterial pressure induce an intense sympathetic discharge that produces peripheral vasoconstriction, further decreasing tissue perfusion and causing a systemic lactic acidosis, which depresses myocardial function. In response to a reduced cardiac output, the heart rate increases, thereby increasing myocardial oxygen demand. As left ventricular filling pressure rises, subendocardial perfusion is further compromised. In short, the hemodynamic and metabolic consequences of cardiogenic shock cause worsening myocardial ischemic injury, which, in turn, leads to worsening left ventricular dysfunction. A cycle of severe hemodynamic impairment and deteriorating myocardial oxygenation is established.

The therapy of the patient with an acute MI and resultant left ventricular dysfunction depends on the extent of such dysfunction. The normotensive individual with symptoms and signs of Killip class II congestive heart failure (i.e., mild orthopnea, basilar rales, S_3) usually responds to bed rest, salt restriction, a loop diuretic, and low-dose vasodilator therapy with an ACE inhibitor. Additional therapy with digitalis or other inotropic agents is not usually necessary, nor is invasive hemodynamic monitoring. The management of the patient with more severe heart failure (Killip class III or IV) should be based on a careful assessment of hemodynamic variables obtained with a balloon-tipped flotation catheter in the pulmonary artery and an intra-arterial cannula. Adequate oxygenation should be ensured by continuous pulse oximetry with supplemental oxygen or ventilator support as needed. Placement of a urinary catheter enables the urine output to be assessed accurately, and endotracheal intubation and assisted ventilation may reduce the work of breathing and improve tissue oxygenation. Intravenous furosemide should be administered in an attempt to reduce the pulmonary capillary wedge pressure in the range of 18 to 20 mm Hg; this appears to be the optimal preload in the setting of acute MI. In the normotensive individual, vasodilator therapy with nitroglycerin and oral ACE inhibitors should be instituted to reduce afterload, increase cardiac output, and lower left ventricular filling pressure. The resultant decrease in left ventricular wall stress reduces myocardial oxygen requirements, improves subendocardial perfusion, and helps relieve ischemia. Nitroglycerin should be administered to avoid an excessive reduction in systemic arterial pressure, which may compromise myocardial perfusion, while keeping pulmonary capillary wedge pressure in the range of 18 to 20 mm Hg. The patient with heart failure and hypotension or an inadequate response to diuretics and vasodilators (i.e., cardiac output < 1.8 L/m² per minute pulmonary capillary wedge pressure > 20 mm Hg) should be treated with intravenous inotropic agents (e.g., dopamine or dobutamine, depending on the systemic arterial pressure). If the patient is only mildly hypotensive, dobutamine is the preferred inotropic agent. Dopamine should be reserved for the patient with more severe hypotension because it may increase pulmonary capillary wedge pressure.

In the patient with severe heart failure or cardiogenic shock, a careful search for a potentially correctable cause should be undertaken. Two-dimensional and color Doppler echocardiography, which can rapidly be performed at the bedside, will allow the clinician to determine whether the shock is due to extensive left ventricular dysfunction or a mechanical problem, such as acute mitral regurgitation, acute ventricular septal defect, extensive right ventricular infarction, or a contained rupture of the left ventricular free wall (see "Mechanical Complications").

Patients with shock who are examined within the first few hours of the onset of MI should be considered for immediate reperfusion therapy. Thrombolytic agents are less effective in opening the occluded infarct-related artery in the patient with cardiogenic shock, and these agents have not convincingly exerted a beneficial effect in such patients. Conversely, early coronary revascularization within 12 hours of the onset of cardiogenic shock, accomplished percutaneously or surgically, has been shown to improve in-hospital and 1-year survival.

By reducing afterload and increasing myocardial perfusion pressure, intra-aortic balloon counterpulsation may be effective in stabilizing the patient with cardiogenic shock. Although initial hemodynamic improvement in this setting may be dramatic, balloon counterpulsation alone probably does not improve the poor prognosis associated with cardiogenic shock. Rather, counterpulsation should be considered a supportive measure in patients with potentially reversible abnormalities before cardiac catheterization, cardiac surgery, or, in some cases, cardiac transplantation. In patients who remain hemodynamically unstable despite pressors and intra-aortic balloon counterpulsation, percutaneous left ventricular support device implantation should be considered. If these therapies do not improve hemodynamics, a surgical ventricular assist device could be considered.

Right Ventricular Infarction

Right ventricular infarction usually occurs in association with inferior MI because the blood supply to both these areas usually comes from the right coronary artery. The presence of a concomitant right ventricular infarction substantially increases the mortality of an inferior MI. Right ventricular

MI results in the clinical triad of hypotension, clear lungs (i.e., normal pulmonary capillary wedge pressure), and prominent jugular venous distention. In the absence of hemodynamic measurements, right ventricular infarction may be confused with hypovolemia, pulmonary embolism, or cardiac tamponade. In fact, the patient with acute right ventricular failure may have a prominent y descent in the atrial pressure tracing (Fig. 9-10), Kussmaul sign, and pulsus paradoxus, all of which mimic pericardial tamponade. Demonstrating ST-segment elevation in the right precordial leads (e.g., >0.1 mV elevation in V₄R) confirms the diagnosis of right ventricular infarction. For this reason, a right-sided precordial ECG should be obtained in all patients with inferior MI. The treatment of hypotension in the patient with right ventricular infarction often requires rapid intravascular volume repletion (with a goal right atrial pressure of 12 to 15 mm Hg) and inotropic agents (e.g., dobutamine). A balloon-tipped flotation catheter in the pulmonary artery and an intra-arterial cannula should be used for hemodynamic monitoring. Diuretic and vasodilator (e.g., nitroglycerin) therapy should be avoided because they may provoke hypotension in this setting. If the patient can be supported during the first few days of hemodynamic instability, considerable improvement in right ventricular function often occurs.

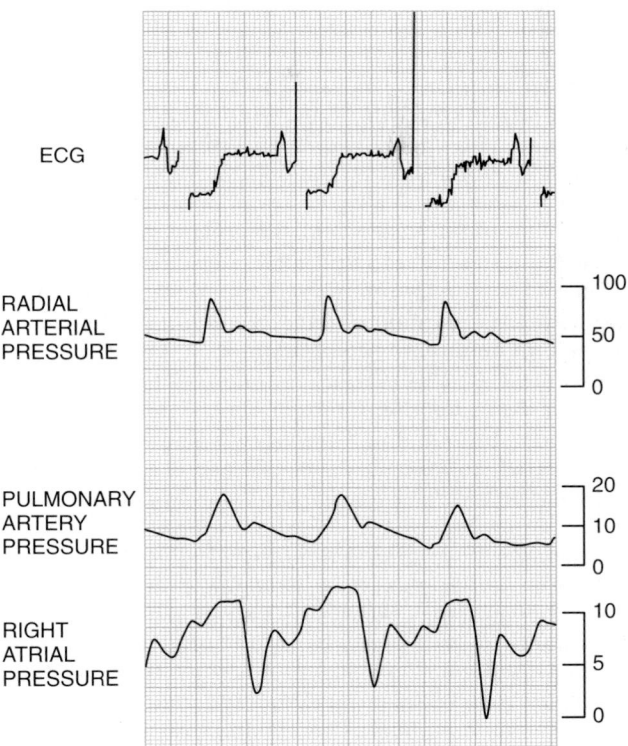

Figure 9-10 Electrocardiographic (ECG), arterial, and Swan-Ganz bedside catheter recordings in a patient with right ventricular infarction. Hypotension is present, and cardiac output, estimated by thermodilution (not shown), is reduced. The pulmonary arterial pressures are normal, whereas the right atrial pressure is elevated, and it demonstrates a prominent y descent.

Mechanical Complications

Mechanical complications of acute MI include papillary muscle rupture, ventricular septal defect, and ventricular free-wall rupture. Patients with these complications frequently experience hemodynamic collapse 3 to 5 days after acute MI. These complications are associated with high mortality rates; they account for about 15% of the mortality from acute MI. Successful immediate reperfusion therapy has reduced the appearance of these complications. Patients with late or unsuccessful reperfusion therapy are at higher risk for these mechanical complications.

Papillary muscle rupture results in acute mitral regurgitation. The resultant sudden increase in left atrial volume causes a significantly elevated left atrial pressure, with resultant pulmonary edema. Papillary muscle rupture occurs most commonly with inferior MI because the posteromedial papillary muscle usually has a single source of blood supply from the right coronary artery. Conversely, the anterolateral papillary muscle has a dual blood supply. A loud, apical holosystolic murmur is usually audible, although an occasional patient with severe mitral regurgitation has no audible murmur. The diagnosis may be rapidly confirmed with transthoracic echocardiography or right-heart ventricular catheterization, with the latter demonstrating large v waves in the pulmonary capillary wedge tracing in the absence of an oxygen *step-up* in the right ventricle.

An acute ventricular septal defect may occur after anterior or inferior MI. On physical examination, a harsh holosystolic murmur is audible at the left lower sternal border, which may be difficult to differentiate from acute mitral regurgitation; this murmur is often accompanied by a palpable thrill. The diagnosis can be confirmed by obtaining blood samples from each of the cardiac chambers during right heart ventricular catheterization and by demonstrating a higher oxygen saturation in the samples obtained from the right ventricle or pulmonary artery compared with those obtained from the right atrium (e.g., oxygen step-up). Specifically, an increase in oxygen saturation of more than 6% between the right atrium and pulmonary artery strongly suggests the presence of a ventricular septal defect with concomitant left-to-right shunting. Doppler echocardiography also allows visualization of left-to-right shunting of blood through the ventricular septal defect.

Treatment of acute papillary muscle rupture or ventricular septal defect includes inotropic agents, vasodilators, and intra-aortic balloon counterpulsation. These temporizing measures help prepare the patient for urgent cardiac surgery to repair the ventricular septal defect or replace the mitral valve.

Free-wall rupture of the left ventricle almost always results in hemopericardium, cardiac tamponade, and electromechanical dissociation. Survival is uncommon and depends on prompt recognition and emergent surgical repair. In an occasional patient, a pseudoaneurysm or false aneurysm develops when free-wall rupture occurs, so that the rupture is confined by the adherent pericardium, organized thrombus, and hematoma. Because the wall of the pseudoaneurysm contains no myocardium, it may rupture at a later date. The pseudoaneurysm maintains continuity with the left ventricular cavity through a narrow connecting orifice (e.g., neck). In contrast, a true aneurysm represents an area of infarcted myocardium that has become thinned and dilated through a process of ventricular remodeling. True aneurysms have a wide orifice or neck, their walls always contain some myocardial elements, and they rarely rupture. Pseudoaneurysms should undergo prompt surgical resection because of the risk for rupture. Conversely, a true aneurysm does not require urgent surgical resection. Medical treatment of post-MI aneurysms includes aggressive heart failure management with ACE inhibitors, β blockers, aldosterone inhibitors for those with class III or IV heart failure, and consideration of anticoagulant therapy. Those undergoing subsequent CABG and those with aneurysm-related chest pain may be considered for aneurysmectomy.

SECONDARY PREVENTION OF ACUTE CORONARY SYNDROME

Secondary prevention therapies are a critical component of the management of all patients with acute coronary syndrome. About 70% of coronary heart disease deaths and 50% of MIs occur in patients with a prior history of coronary artery disease. Secondary prevention therapies in patients recovering from acute coronary syndrome represent a major opportunity to reduce cardiovascular morbidity and mortality.

Before hospital discharge, patients should be educated regarding adherence to the recommended lifestyle changes and pharmacologic therapies. Patients and their families should receive discharge instructions about recognizing acute cardiac symptoms and appropriate actions to take in order to ensure early evaluation and treatment should symptoms recur. Family members should be advised about cardiopulmonary resuscitation and automatic external defibrillator (AED) training programs.

Lipid management involves dietary therapy that is low in saturated fat and cholesterol (<7% of total calories as saturated fat and <200 mg/day cholesterol). Consumption of fruits, vegetables, fiber, whole grains, and foods enriched with omega-3 fatty acids are encouraged. Antioxidants are not recommended for the secondary prevention of MI. Statins are recommended for patients following an acute coronary syndrome for a goal LDL of less than 70 mg/dL. Weight reduction is recommended to achieve a desirable body mass index range between 18.5 and 24.9 kg/m². Patients should be advised regarding strategies for weight management and regular aerobic physical activity, usually prescribed initially with cardiac rehabilitation. Patients are encouraged to exercise for at least 30 minutes, preferably daily. Cardiac rehabilitation is recommended for patients with heart failure and after MI or coronary revascularization. Patients with a history of cigarette smoking should be encouraged to stop smoking and avoid secondhand smoke. In addition to smoking cessation counseling, pharmacologic therapy (nicotine replacement, varenicline, bupropion) should be considered. For those with systemic hypertension, a low-sodium diet and antihypertensive medication should be prescribed. Typically, ACE inhibitors and β blockers are recommended. An angiotensin receptor blocker may be used in patients who develop a cough attributed to the ACE inhibitor. For those with systolic dysfunction, diuretics may be prescribed to promote euvolemia. In addition to ACE inhibitors and β blockers (most commonly carvedilol or metoprolol succinate), aldosterone inhibitors are recommended for patients with class III or IV heart failure symptoms. Antiplatelet therapy with both aspirin (75 to 162 mg daily indefinitely) and clopidogrel (75 mg daily for 1 year) is recommended. Warfarin may be used for patients with persistent or paroxysmal atrial fibrillation or flutter and those with a left ventricular thrombus. For patients with an indication for anticoagulation who received a stent, aspirin (75 to 162 mg), clopidogrel (75 mg), and warfarin (goal INR 2 to 3) may be given to those younger than 75 years with a low bleeding risk. Diabetic patients should have hypoglycemic therapy for a goal hemoglobin A1c of less than 7%. Hormone replacement therapy with estrogen plus progestin should not be started for postmenopausal women recovering from an acute coronary syndrome. Women already taking hormone therapy at the time of an acute coronary syndrome should not continue hormone therapy.

Prospectus for the Future

- New methods are needed to identify patients at risk for CAD using genomics and proteomics.
- New treatments are required for treating components of ischemic heart disease (e.g., raising HDL level, lowering hsCRP level, targeting antiplatelet therapy) to reduce cardiac events.
- Evaluation is needed to compare the efficacy and safety of drug-eluting stents with CABG for patients needing coronary revascularization.
- Development of regional cardiac centers is necessary to provide reperfusion therapy for patients with acute MI who enter a hospital that does not have a catheterization laboratory.

References

Anderson JL, Adams CD, Antman EM, et al: ACC/AHA 2007 guidelines for the management of patients with unstable angina/non-ST-elevation myocardial infarction: A report of the American College of Cardiology/American Heart Association Task Force on Practice Guidelines (Writing Committee to Revise the 2002 Guidelines for the Management of Patients With Unstable Angina/Non-ST-Elevation Myocardial Infarction). Developed in collaboration with the American College of Emergency Physicians, American College of Physicians, Society for Academic Emergency Medicine, Society for Cardiovascular Angiography and Interventions, and Society of Thoracic Surgeons. J Am Coll Cardiol 50:e1-e157, 2007.

Antman EM, Hand M, Armstrong PW, et al: 2007 Focused update of the ACC/AHA 2004 Guidelines for the Management of Patients with ST-Elevation Myocardial Infarction: A report of the American College of Cardiology/American Heart Association Task Force on Practice Guidelines (Writing Group to Review New Evidence and Update the ACC/AHA 2004 Guidelines for the Management of Patients With ST-Elevation Myocardial Infarction). J Am Coll Cardiol 51:210-247, 2008.

Eagle KA, Guyton RA, Davidoff R, et al: ACC/AHA 2004 guideline update for coronary artery bypass graft surgery. Circulation 110:e340-e437, 2004.

Fraker TD Jr, Fihn SD, writing on behalf of the 2002 Chronic Stable Angina Writing Committee: 2007 Chronic angina focused update of the ACC/AHA 2002 Guidelines for the Management of Patients with Chronic Stable Angina: A report of the American College of Cardiology/American Heart Association Task Force on Practice Guidelines Writing Group to Develop the Focused Update of the 2002 Guidelines for the Management of Patients with Chronic Stable Angina. J Am Coll Cardiol 50:2064-2074, 2007.

Gibler WB, Cannon CP, Blomkalns AL, et al: Practical implementation of the guidelines for unstable angina/non-ST-segment elevation myocardial infarction in the emergency department. Circulation 111:2699-2710, 2005.

King SB III, Smith SC Jr, Hirshfeld JW Jr, et al: 2007 Focused update of the ACC/AHA/SCAI 2005 Guideline Update for Percutaneous Coronary Intervention: A report of the American College of Cardiology/American Heart Association Task Force on Practice Guidelines (2007 Writing Group to Review New Evidence and Update the 2005 ACC/AHA/SCAI Guideline Update for Percutaneous Coronary Intervention). J Am Coll Cardiol 51:172-209, 2008.

Klocke FJ, Baird MG, Lorell BH, et al: ACC/AHA/ASNC guidelines for the clinical use of cardiac radionuclide imaging. Circulation 108:1404-1418, 2003.

Lauer M, Froelicher ES, Williams M, et al: Exercise testing in asymptomatic adults: A statement for professionals from the American Heart Association Council on Clinical Cardiology. Circulation 112:771-776, 2005.

Scanlon PJ, Faxon DP, Audet AM, et al: ACC/AHA guidelines for coronary angiography. J Am Coll Cardiol 33:1756-1824, 1999.

Shaw LJ, Berman DS, Maron DJ, et al: Optimal medical therapy with or without percutaneous coronary intervention to reduce ischemic burden: Results from the Clinical Outcomes Utilizing Revascularization and Aggressive Drug Evaluation (COURAGE) trial nuclear substudy. Circulation 117:1283-1291, 2008.

Thygesen K, Alpert JS, White HD; Joint ESC/ACCF/AHA/WHF Task Force for the Redefinition of Myocardial Infarction. Universal definition of myocardial infarction. J Am Coll Cardiol 50:2173-2195, 2007.

Chapter 10

Cardiac Arrhythmias

Mohamed H. Hamdan

Cardiac Action Potential and Normal Conduction

The electrical activity of a single cardiac cell can be recorded with the aid of a microelectrode and demonstrates that the resting potential of a myocyte is −80 to −90 mV. This resting potential is maintained by the accumulation of potassium inside the cell and the removal of sodium from the cell by the energy-requiring sodium-potassium adenosine triphosphatase (Na^+,K^+-ATPase). When a cardiac myocyte is depolarized to below threshold level (threshold potential), an action potential is produced by a complex series of ionic shifts (Fig. 10-1A). The action potential can be divided into five phases. Phase 0 is the rapid initial depolarization and is mediated by an increased permeability of the sarcolemma to sodium ions. This phase is followed by phase 1, an early, rapid, repolarization resulting from the movement of potassium out of the cell. The plateau phase (phase 2) of the action potential is mainly determined by the inward movement of calcium ions but also by the movement of sodium, chloride, and potassium ions. Phase 3 constitutes the repolarization phase of the action potential and is the result of the movement of potassium ions out of the cell. Phase 4 of the action potential represents the outward flow of potassium and the inward flow of sodium and results in the gradual depolarization of the cell from resting to threshold potential (see Fig. 10-1B). During the action potential and shortly thereafter, a period occurs during which an adequate depolarizing stimulus fails to elicit an action potential. This period is termed the *absolute refractory period* and is most closely related to the duration of phase 3 of the action potential.

The appearance of the action potential of sinus and atrioventricular (AV) nodal cells is different from that of the typical myocyte. The normal resting potential of these cells is higher (−60 mV), the initial upstroke of depolarization is slower and calcium dependent, and the phase 4 depolariza-

tion is highly pronounced (see Fig. 10-1B). The slope of the phase 4 depolarization determines the rate at which a cell will spontaneously depolarize (automaticity) until it reaches threshold potential, thus generating an action potential that is then propagated to surrounding cells. The sinus node usually has the fastest phase 4 depolarization and thus functions as the normal pacemaker of the heart, producing a rate of contraction (heart rate) of 60 to 100 beats/min. If the sinus node fails, the AV node has the next fastest pacemaker rate (about 50 beats/minute). The ventricular myocytes have slow phase 4 depolarization and produce a heart rate of 30 to 40 beats/minute if higher pacemakers fail. When a lower pacemaker focus appropriately fires in the setting of slowing of the higher focus, the firing is termed an *escape beat* (if single) or an *escape rhythm* (if sustained).

The autonomic nervous system has important effects on the generation and propagation of cardiac impulses. The sinus and AV nodes are the most richly innervated regions of the heart and are most affected by changes in autonomic tone. Sympathetic stimulation, either directly from sympathetic nerve endings in the heart or indirectly by means of circulating catecholamines, increases the heart rate by increasing the rate of phase 4 depolarization and also increases intercellular conduction velocity. Parasympathetic stimulation has the opposite effects. Vagal tone is, in part, controlled by the baroreceptors of the carotid sinus and aortic arch and responds to increases in blood pressure by increasing vagal output, with a resulting decrease in heart rate and AV nodal conduction velocity.

The normal cardiac impulse starts at the sinoatrial node, passes through the atria to the AV node, where it slows, and then continues down the His-Purkinje system to the ventricular myocardium, where the wave of depolarization terminates because no further tissue exists to depolarize. Further conduction occurs only after a new impulse is formed in the sinoatrial node.

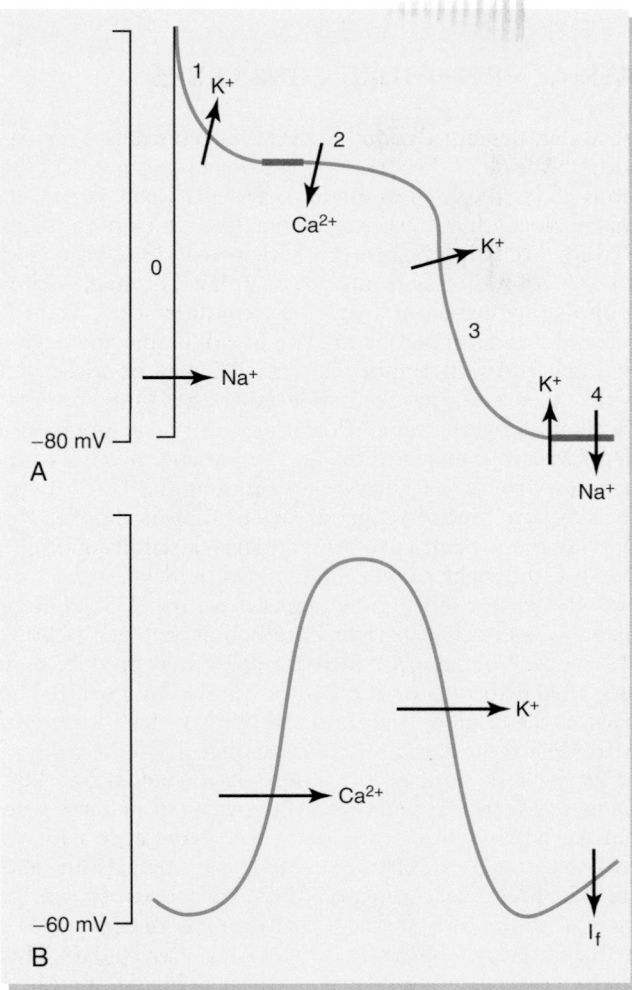

Figure 10-1 Genesis of the cardiac action potential. **A,** Ventricular action potential with predominant ionic currents. **B,** Sinus node action potential with predominant ionic currents. See text for details. 1_f, Hyperpolarization-activated current.

Cardiac Arrhythmias

Cardiac arrhythmias result from disorders of (1) *impulse formation* and (2) *impulse conduction*. Disorders of impulse formation include enhanced or abnormal automaticity and triggered activity. Disorders of impulse conduction include conduction block with or without re-entry (defined later). One or more of the previously described electrophysiologic (EP) mechanisms can explain most cardiac arrhythmias.

DISORDERS OF IMPULSE FORMATION

Cardiac depolarization is driven by the sinus node (normal pacemaker), which is located in the high right atrium along the cristae terminalis. This waveform propagates down the AV node and His-Purkinje system, resulting in synchronized activation of both ventricles. Subsidiary pacemakers with a lower discharge rate are mainly present in the AV junction and the His-Purkinje system. These pacemakers do not reach threshold because of overdrive suppression by the sinus node. However, under certain conditions, such as sinus node slowing or conduction block, these pacemaker sites may become active and discharge at their normal rate.

Enhanced automaticity refers to pacemaker cells discharging at a rate faster than their normal rate. By definition, these cells have intrinsic automaticity (slow response type of action potential; see Fig. 10-1B), but under certain conditions (partial depolarization, decrease in threshold, or increase in the slope of phase 4), the automaticity rate is enhanced. *Abnormal automaticity* refers to spontaneous depolarization resulting in impulse formation in cardiac tissues that lack intrinsic automaticity (fast response type of action potential; see Fig. 10-1A). Under certain conditions, these cells may show spontaneous automaticity, resulting in premature depolarizations, which, if repetitive, can lead to tachycardia. Singular premature atrial or ventricular depolarizations may arise by this mechanism. Some sustained rhythms, including ectopic atrial tachycardia, accelerated junctional or idioventricular rhythms, and some forms of ventricular tachycardia (VT), may also result from increased automaticity. Ischemia, digoxin, methylxanthine toxicity, electrolyte abnormalities, and high catecholamine states are well-known causes of abnormal and enhanced automaticity.

Triggered activity means impulse initiation caused by afterdepolarizations. Afterdepolarizations are oscillations in membrane potentials that occur after the upstroke of the action potential. If the amplitude is large enough to reach threshold, afterdepolarizations can generate a subsequent action potential. By definition, afterdepolarizations must be preceded by at least one action potential, thus the term triggered activity. They do not occur spontaneously but, rather, are triggered by prior activation of the heart. When afterdepolarizations occur during repolarization, they are called *early afterdepolarizations* (EADs). EADs are usually exacerbated by hypokalemia or potassium channel blockade or drugs and may be catecholamine driven or provoked by a critical heart rate. EADs may also occur spontaneously in patients with congenital long QT syndrome (LQTS). When afterdepolarizations occur after full repolarization, they are called *delayed afterdepolarizations* (DADs). DADs are more pronounced at fast heart rates, are facilitated by intracellular calcium overload, and account for the mechanism underlying most digoxin-toxic rhythms. They are usually caused by ischemia, catecholamines, and digitalis.

DISORDERS OF IMPULSE CONDUCTION

Disorders of impulse conduction include conduction block with or without *reentry*. Reentry is the most common mechanism of arrhythmogenesis. During reentry, a depolarization propagates in one direction while blocking in adjacent tissue, returns to depolarize the area not initially excited, and, if successful, will travel around repeating its course. Therefore, three criteria are needed for reentry to be present: (1) two available pathways, (2) unidirectional block in one, and (3) conduction delay in the other with return excitation. Based on these general concepts, three types of reentry have been described: (1) anatomic, (2) functional (leading circle or reentry), and (3) reentry by reflection. Describing these mechanisms in detail is not the purpose of this chapter; however, it should be emphasized that the presence of a discrete anatomic obstacle (such as a scar) is not always needed for reentry, given that conduction delay and block can be caused by many factors, including differences in refractoriness, ischemia, fibrosis, electrolyte abnormalities, and drug toxicity. An example of reentry in which two distinct pathways are present is provided in Figure 10-2. Pathway A conducts rapidly but has a relatively long refractory period. Pathway B conducts slowly but has a relatively short refractory period. In the usual state (see Fig. 10-2A), an impulse enters the two pathways by means of a proximal common pathway. Conduction occurs rapidly down pathway A and, after reaching the distal common pathway, continues distally and proceeds retrograde up pathway B until it intercepts the slow antegrade impulse traveling down this pathway and is extinguished. The surface electrocardiogram (ECG) may appear normal, without evidence of the dual pathways. If a premature depolarization occurs, it also enters the two pathways through the proximal common pathway. If it occurs early enough, it is unable to conduct down pathway A because of the long refractory period of this path (see Fig. 10-2B). The impulse therefore travels down pathway B, which has the short refractory period, and reaches the distal common pathway, where it continues distally. However, because pathway B conducts relatively slowly, by the time the impulse reaches the distal aspect of pathway A, this path is no longer refractory, and the impulse rapidly conducts in a retrograde direction up pathway A, reenters the loop by means of pathway B, and conducts retrograde up the proximal common pathway. If the reentrant circuit is in the AV node, the resulting surface ECG demonstrates a premature complex, initiating a tachycardia, and retrograde P waves may be seen.

Reentry can occur at any point along the normal conduction system, including the sinoatrial node, the AV node, and atrial or ventricular myocardium. It may occur in a small focus of cardiac tissue such as the AV node (a micro-reentrant circuit) or involve anatomically distinct pathways such as bypass tracts (a macro-reentrant circuit).

As stated previously, cardiac arrhythmias are the result of disorders in impulse formation or impulse conduction, with reentry being the most common underlying mechanism. Clinically, cardiac arrhythmias can be divided into three categories: (1) premature beats, (2) bradyarrhythmias (slow heart rates), and (3) tachyarrhythmias (fast heart rates).

Premature Beats
ATRIAL PREMATURE COMPLEXES

An atrial premature complex (APC) is defined as a premature activation of the atria arising from a site other than the sinus node. APCs appear on the surface ECG as P waves with morphologic characteristics different from those of the sinus P wave occurring before the anticipated sinus beat (Fig. 10-3A). An APC may conduct with a short, normal, or prolonged PR interval, or it may not conduct at all. The PR interval is determined by the site of origin and the degree of prematurity. If conducted, an APC may be associated with either a normal or a wide (aberrant) QRS complex. Distinguishing aberrant APCs from ventricular premature depolarizations may be difficult. The presence of a full compensatory pause (RR interval surrounding the APC = twice the sinus cycle length) suggests lack of sinus node resetting, thus favoring a ventricular rather than an atrial site of origin. Because the right bundle branch has a longer refractory period than the left bundle branch, an early APC is more likely to conduct with right bundle branch block (RBBB) aberrancy. When nonconducted, an APC may produce only as a small deformity on the T wave followed by a pause. The pause is the result of sinus node resetting, which is common with APCs regardless of whether conducted.

Twenty-four-hour Holter studies have shown that APC frequency increases with age. APCs occur in patients with normal hearts but appear to be more frequent in patients with structural heart disease such as chronic renal failure and chronic pulmonary disease. APCs have been shown to increase in the early stages of a myocardial infarction (MI), with a subsequent decrease in frequency after 10 days. This characteristic may be related to atrial ischemia, increased filling pressures, or the increased catecholamine state often seen during MI. APCs also appear to be frequent in the setting of pericarditis.

The most common symptoms include palpitations, or the sensation of skipped beats. Dizziness and heart failure–like

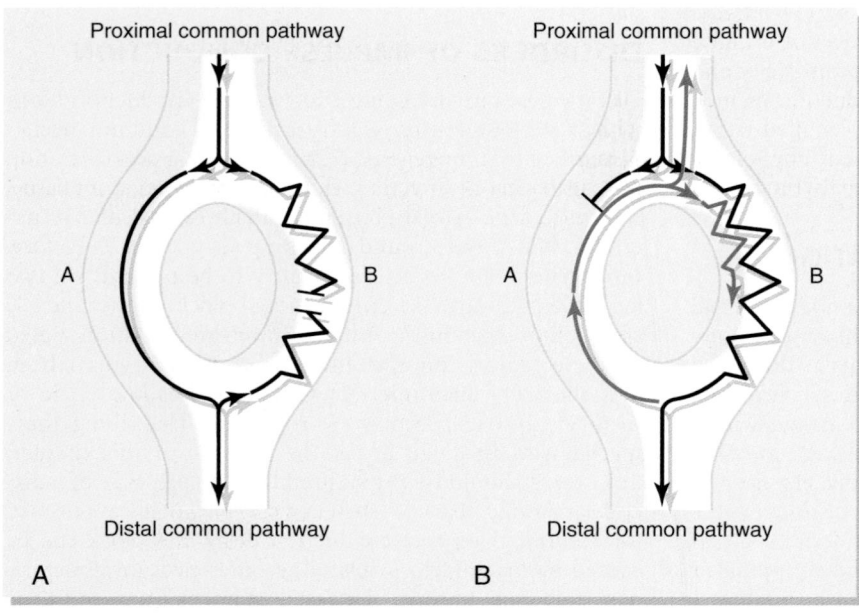

Proximal common pathway   Proximal common pathway

A   B   A   B

Distal common pathway   Distal common pathway

A   B

Figure 10-2 Mechanism of reentry. Reentry requires two distinct pathways with disparate conductive and repolarizing properties. **A,** An impulse enters the two pathways and conducts rapidly down pathway A and slowly down pathway B. When the impulse reaches the distal common pathway, it proceeds distally, as well as traveling retrograde up pathway B, where it is extinguished, owing to collision with the antegrade depolarization in this pathway. **B,** A premature depolarization enters the pathways but is blocked in pathway A, owing to the long refractory period of this pathway. The impulse travels down pathway B (slowly conducting and rapidly repolarizing) to the distal common pathway, where it proceeds distally, as well as traveling up pathway A, which by then is fully repolarized and able to conduct in a retrograde fashion, allowing the impulse to reenter the loop and produce the reciprocating rhythm.

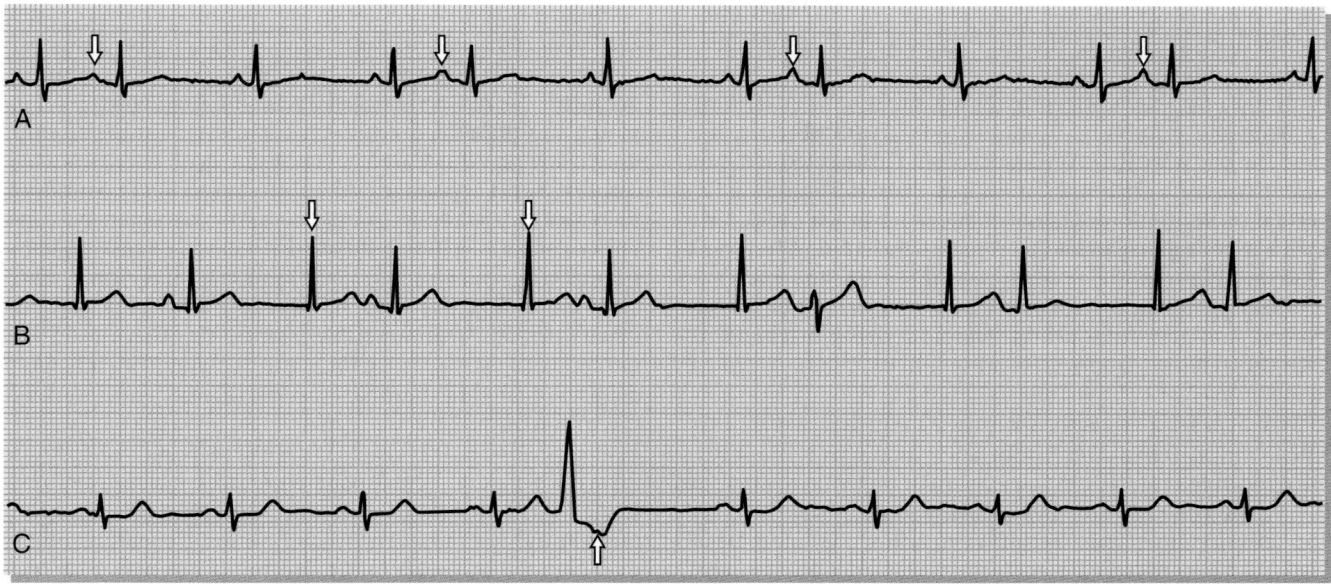

Figure 10-3 Premature complexes. **A,** Atrial premature complexes (APCs) with a trigeminal rhythm. An atrial premature beat occurs after every two sinus beats. Note the presence of a P wave *(arrows)* preceding the QRS complex with a long PR interval caused by decremental conduction in the AV node. The QRS complex is narrow because the origin of the impulse is supraventricular. **B,** Junctional premature complexes (JPCs) *(arrows).* JPCs often conduct in a retrograde fashion, resulting in a P wave that is buried in the QRS complex. Similar to APCs, the QRS complex is narrow because the origin of the impulse is supraventricular. **C,** Ventricular premature complexes (VPCs). Note the wide QRS morphology and the presence of a retrograde P wave *(arrow).* PVCs might conduct retrograde, resulting in a P wave that follows the QRS.

symptoms might occur in the setting of atrial bigeminy with nonconducted atrial premature beats. Therapy is aimed at treating the underlying disease and eliminating factors that are known to cause ectopic beats such as alcohol and caffeine intake. In patients with symptoms, β blockers should be the first line of therapy, followed by calcium channel blockers and class IC agents such as flecainide and propafenone. Class III agents such as sotalol and amiodarone should be avoided because of pro-arrhythmia risks.

JUNCTIONAL PREMATURE COMPLEXES

A junctional premature complex (JPC) refers to a premature beat originating from the AV junction area, which includes the AV node, the peri-nodal area, and the His bundle. After impulse formation, propagation occurs both in the antegrade direction down the His bundles and in the retrograde direction up to the atria. The result is nearly simultaneous atrial and ventricular depolarization with a surface P wave buried in the QRS complex (see Fig. 10-3B). At times, retrograde atrial activation precedes ventricular activation, resulting in a PR interval as long as 90 minutes. This action is more common when the impulse originates from a peri-nodal site. When the impulse originates from the His bundle, retrograde atrial activation always follows ventricular depolarization, resulting in a retrograde P wave that follows the QRS complex. On some occasions, the impulse fails to propagate in the antegrade direction, resulting in a retrograde P wave that mimics an APC. When a JPC fails to conduct in the retrograde direction, the result is a QRS complex without a P wave. Finally, the impulse might not conduct in either direction but may affect the conduction of subsequent impulses (concealed JPCs), resulting in AV block. In such

instances, the diagnosis is based on the presence of manifest JPC in a patient with otherwise normal QRS duration and evidence of intermittent AV block. The mechanism of JPC is believed to be abnormal automaticity, although triggered activity may also be a potential mechanism. They can occur in both normal and abnormal hearts. JPCs are more common in the setting of digitalis toxicity, high-catecholamine states, hypokalemia, and MI.

Most patients with JPCs are asymptomatic. When symptoms occur, skipped beats and palpitations are the most common complaints. More severe symptoms such as dizziness, near syncope, and syncope might occur if the patient has AV block caused by concealed JPCs. Management of JPCs should be focused on correcting the underlying problems. In symptomatic patients with no underlying cause, β blockers are often helpful in suppressing JPCs. Classes I and III antiarrhythmic drugs should only be used in patients with symptoms refractory to β-blocker therapy. In patients with AV block secondary to concealed JPCs, therapy should be aimed at suppressing the junctional beats rather than implanting a pacemaker.

VENTRICULAR PREMATURE COMPLEXES

A ventricular premature complex (VPC) refers to a premature depolarization originating from the ventricles. The impulse often does not conduct to the atria and thus does not reset the sinus node. The result is a wide QRS complex with a compensatory pause (see Fig. 10-3C). When retrograde conduction occurs and the sinus node is reset, a noncompensatory pause will be inscribed. A VPC that occurs early and fails to affect both the next ventricular depolarization and sinus node activity is referred to as *interpolated*

VPC. With an interpolated VPC, the RR interval surrounding the VPC is equal to the sinus RR interval. A supraventricular premature beat may conduct with aberrancy, resulting in a wide QRS complex similar to a VPC. Criteria in favor of a ventricular origin include (1) the absence of a preceding P wave, (2) AV dissociation, (3) marked left axis deviation, (4) a QRS interval longer than 160 minutes, (5) certain configurational characteristics such as Rsr′ in lead V_1, QS or rS in lead V_6, and concordance (upright or downward QRS in all precordial leads), and finally (6) the presence of a full compensatory pause. VPCs occur in patients with normal and abnormal hearts. The underlying mechanisms include reentry, abnormal automaticity, and triggered activity.

When associated with symptoms, patients with VPCs often complain of *skipped* beats and palpitations. The presence of frequent VPCs such as in a bigeminal rhythm (VPCs alternating with sinus beats) can significantly lower the effective heart rate, resulting in a low cardiac output state. In such instances, symptoms might include dizziness, near syncope, and syncope. In addition to the presence of symptoms, VPCs can have an impact on prognosis and risk for sudden death. Although VPCs have no prognostic significance in patients with a normal heart, their presence in patients with heart disease is often associated with poor outcome. In patients with a history of MI, the presence of VPCs increases mortality. Suppression of VPCs with antiarrhythmic drugs, however, has not been shown to reduce mortality. In the Cardiac Arrhythmia Suppression Trial (CAST), randomization of patients with a history of MI, ventricular arrhythmias, and documented arrhythmia suppression with flecainide or encainide showed increased mortality. The largest trial that assessed the effect of amiodarone on the risk for arrhythmic death among MI survivors with frequent VPCs was the Canadian Amiodarone Myocardial Infraction Arrhythmia Trial (CAMIAT). The consensus from this trial was that, unlike other antiarrhythmic drugs, amiodarone was not associated with excess risk for death. At present, the first drug of choice for the treatment of symptomatic VPCs should be a β blocker. If β-blocker therapy fails, amiodarone or catheter ablation should be considered. With catheter ablation, the VPC site of origin is identified, and radiofrequency energy is applied to eliminate the ectopy. Both amiodarone therapy and catheter ablation should only be considered in patients who continue to have symptomatic VPCs despite β-blocker therapy. In the asymptomatic patient, no drug therapy is needed.

Bradyarrhythmias

Bradyarrhythmias are usually the result of either *sinus node dysfunction* or *atrioventricular block*.

SINUS NODE DYSFUNCTION

Sinus node dysfunction may be exhibited as sinus bradycardia, sinus pauses or arrest, or sinoatrial exit block. Patients with sinus node disease may have lightheadedness, dizziness, near syncope, or syncope, or may not have any symptoms at all.

Sinus bradycardia indicates, by definition, a sinus rate less than 60 beats/minute (Fig. 10-4A). The diagnosis of sinus node disease requires that secondary causes be excluded. Increases in vagal tone are frequently seen in young healthy athletes and are a common cause of sinus node slowing. Increased vagal tone also occurs during carotid sinus massage, Valsalva maneuvers, vomiting, increased intracranial pressure, and vasovagal syncope. Other causes of sinus bradycardia include drugs (digitalis, β blockers, calcium channel blockers, and some antiarrhythmic agents such as sotalol and amiodarone), hyperkalemia, hypothyroidism, and hypothermia. Sinus bradycardia also occurs in the setting of many organic heart diseases, including coronary artery disease, cardiomyopathy, and myocarditis.

Sinus pause is the result of transient failure of impulse formation in the sinus node. When this inactivity is prolonged, it is called *sinus arrest.* Both conditions are visualized on the ECG as a flat line with no P waves. Depending on the duration of sinus node inactivity, the pause may be terminated by a junctional or ventricular escape beat. Sinus pause or arrest should be differentiated from (1) nonconducted atrial premature beats and (2) sinoatrial exit block (see later discussion). A nonconducted APC usually shows as a small deformity on the T wave (see Fig. 10-4B). Causes of sinus pauses and sinus arrest are similar to those of sinus bradycardia.

Sinoatrial exit block is the result of abnormal transmission between the sinus node and the atrium. Several types of sinoatrial conduction block exist (see later discussion). Because sinoatrial electrograms are not routinely available, only second-degree sinoatrial block might be diagnosed from the surface ECG. Second-degree (type II) sinoatrial exit block is usually inferred by the presence of a pause equal to a multiple of the basic PP interval (see Fig. 10-4C). In some instances, the Wenckebach phenomenon (second-degree [type I]) is observed, resulting in progressive shortening of the PP interval before seeing the absence of a P wave (see Fig. 10-4D). Patients with sinoatrial exit block often have other arrhythmias, including atrial fibrillation, atrial tachycardia (tachycardia-bradycardine syndrome) (see Fig. 10-4E), sinus bradycardia, and AV block.

ATRIOVENTRICULAR BLOCK

The sinus impulse has to traverse the atrium, the AV node, and the His-Purkinje system before reaching the ventricles. This interval is reflected on the ECG as the PR interval. Conduction delay or block can occur at any level, resulting in various types of AV block. AV block is classified into (1) first-degree AV block, (2) second-degree AV block (types I and II), and (3) third-degree AV block.

First-degree AV block occurs when enough prolongation in AV conduction occurs, resulting in a PR interval longer than 200 minutes (Fig. 10-5A). Despite the prolonged PR interval, each P wave is followed by a QRS interval. In patients with first-degree AV block and a narrow QRS complex, the site of block is usually in the AV node. In the setting of a wide QRS complex, the site of block can be at any level but remains most commonly at the level of the AV node. A PR interval longer than 290 milliseconds is almost always associated with AV nodal disease.

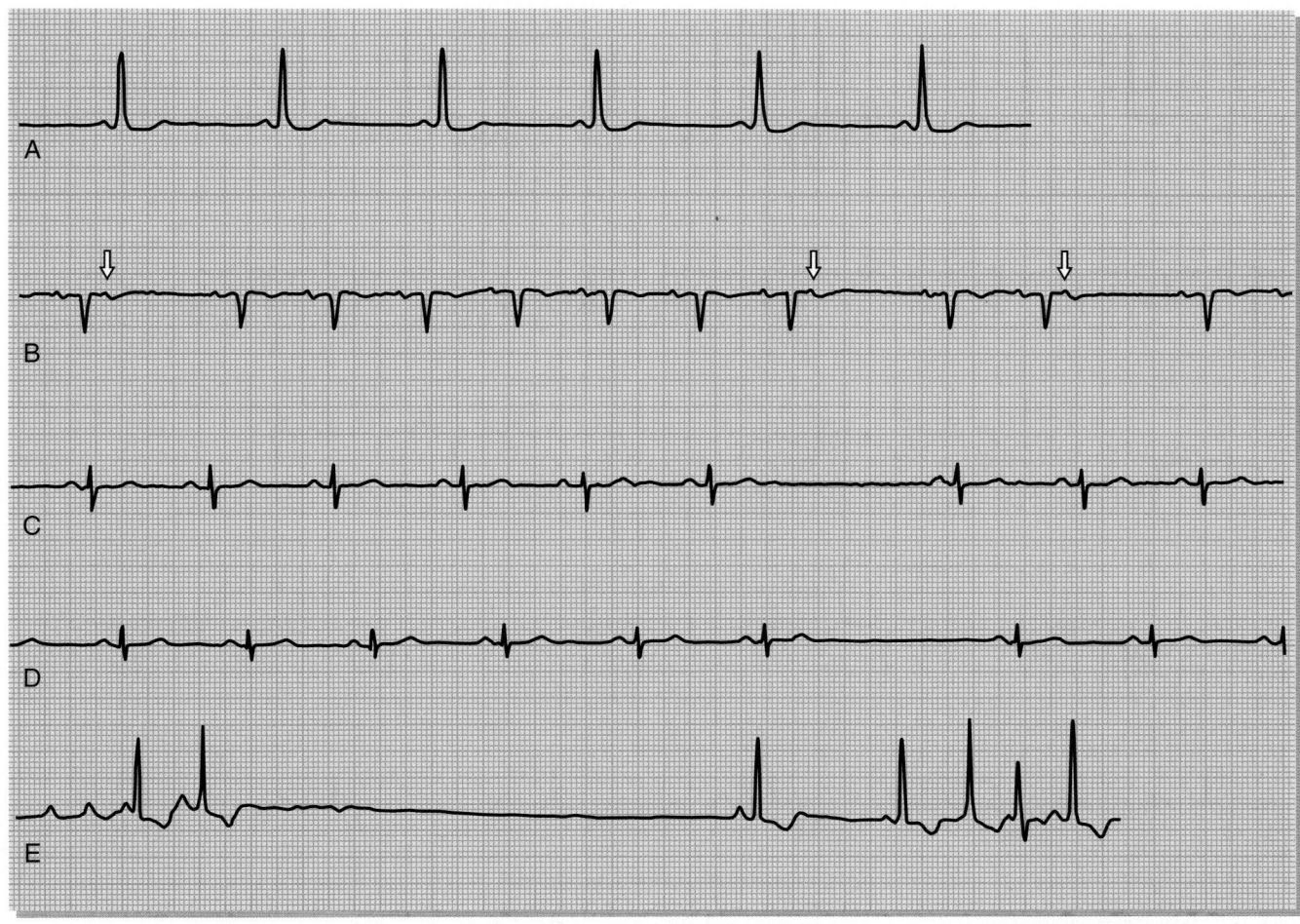

Figure 10-4 Sinus node disturbances. **A,** Sinus bradycardia at a rate of 49 beats/minute in a patient receiving metoprolol. **B,** Nonconducted atrial premature complexes (APCs). Note the small deformity on the T wave *(arrows)* caused by the APCs. The following pause is caused by resetting of the sinus node. **C,** Sinoatrial exit (second-degree type II) block. Note that the pause is equal to a multiple of the basic PP interval (twice). **D,** Sinoatrial exit (Wenckebach) block. Note the progressive shortening of the PP interval before seeing the absence of a P wave. **E,** Sick sinus syndrome. Coarse atrial fibrillation was followed by a prolonged spontaneous period of asystole before restoration of sinus rhythm (tachy-brady syndrome).

Second-degree AV block is associated with intermittent failure of the P wave to be conducted to the ventricles. The ratio of P waves to QRS complexes may vary in the same patient. Two types of second-degree AV block have been classified: *type I,* also called Mobitz type I or Wenckebach phenomenon, and *type II,* or Mobitz type II. *Type I* second-degree AV block is characterized by (1) progressive length-ening of the PR interval until a P wave is blocked, (2) progressive shortening of the RR interval until a P wave is blocked, and (3) the RR interval surrounding the blocked P wave is shorter than two PP intervals (see Fig. 10-5B). In the presence of narrow QRS complex, the site of AV block is in the AV node. In patients with a wide QRS complex, the site of AV block can be infranodal in up to 25% of instances. *Type II* AV block is characterized by intermittent blocked P waves with no change in the PR interval (see Fig. 10-5C). The sinus cycle length is usually constant with the RR interval surrounding the nonconducted P wave equal to twice the sinus cycle length. In the presence of a wide QRS complex, the site of AV block is usually infranodal. In the setting of a narrow QRS complex, the site of block is

usually in the His bundle above the bifurcation but may occasionally be in the AV node. In 2:1 AV block (see Fig. 10-5D), the site of block is unknown. Findings that favor infranodal block include (1) a history of near syncope or syncope, (2) a QRS duration above 120 minutes, (3) the presence of type II second-degree AV block or third-degree AV block during continuous ECG monitoring, (4) improved AV conduction with carotid sinus massage, and (5) worsening AV conduction with atropine and exercise. Identifying the site of block is important in the asymptomatic patient with 2:1 AV block because infranodal block is associated with worse prognosis and mandates the implantation of a pacemaker.

Third-degree AV block or complete AV block is defined by the presence of atrioventricular dissociation *and* an atrial rate that is faster than the ventricular rate. By definition, the sinus P waves are not conducted, and the QRS complexes are from a subsidiary pacemaker, which usually has a slower rate. The RR and PP intervals are usually constant but bear no relation to each other. The PR interval will vary because the P is independent of the QRS (see Fig. 10-5E).

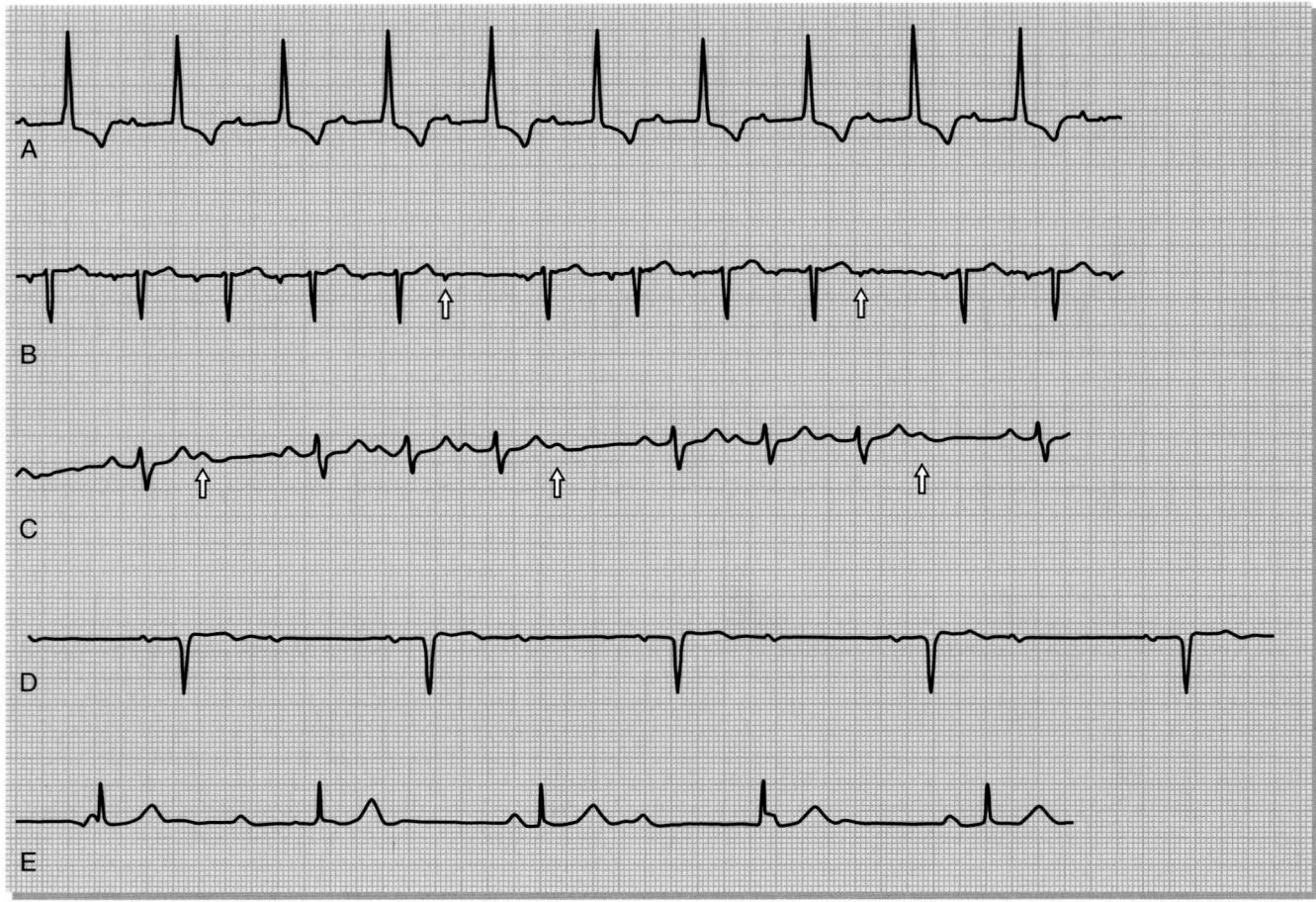

Figure 10-5 Heart block. **A,** First-degree atrioventricular (AV) block; the PR interval is prolonged (>200 minutes). **B,** Second-degree AV block, type 1 (Wenckebach). Progressive PR prolongation preceding a nonconducted P wave *(arrows)* occurs. **C,** Second-degree AV block, type II. Nonconducted P waves are seen *(arrows)* in the absence of progressive PR prolongation. **D,** 2:1 AV block in which every other P wave is conducted. **E,** Third-degree (complete) AV block with AV dissociation and a narrow-complex (AV nodal) escape rhythm.

Tachyarrhythmias

Tachyarrhythmias are divided into *supraventricular, ventricular,* and *preexcited tachycardias.* During supraventricular tachycardia (SVT), the ventricles are depolarized through the normal His-Purkinje system, with or without aberrancy, resulting in a narrow or wide complex tachycardia. During VT, the impulse originates from the ventricle and depolarizes the ventricles in an asynchronized fashion, resulting in a wide QRS complex. With preexcited tachycardias, some or all ventricular activation is caused by antegrade conduction down an accessory pathway, resulting in a wide complex tachycardia. A summary of the most common tachyarrhythmias follows.

ATRIAL TACHYARRHYTHMIAS

Atrial Tachycardia

Atrial tachycardia results from an ectopic atrial focus discharging at a rate faster than the sinus rate. The rate is usually 100 to 250 beats/minute, and the P-wave morphology is different from the sinus P wave (Fig. 10-6A) unless the tachycardia focus site is close to the sinus node. The PR

interval is usually normal or longer than the PR interval during sinus rhythm. The rhythm is usually regular, although episodes of AV block may result in some irregularities. Most commonly, AV conduction is 1:1; however, variable AV block might be seen. When atrial tachycardia occurs with AV block, digoxin toxicity is suggested. Atrial tachycardias are more likely to occur in patients with concomitant heart disease, including coronary artery disease, valvular disease, cardiomyopathies, cor pulmonale, and congenital heart disease. The mechanism of atrial tachycardia can be automaticity, reentry, or triggered activity. In a young patient, automaticity is the most likely mechanism, and, as the age increases, reentry becomes more common. Triggered activity has been suggested, but its role remains poorly defined. In patients with cardiac surgery resulting in atrial scars, reentry around the existing scar can result in atrial tachycardia, called *incisional tachycardia.* The ECG manifestation of the latter is similar to focal atrial tachycardia, except that the P-wave duration is usually longer. The P-wave morphology and axis are determined by the exit site. Vagal maneuvers usually do not terminate atrial tachycardias but can result in transient AV block, thus unmasking the P waves. When the arrhythmia is not a result of digoxin toxicity, β blockers and calcium channel blockers are the mainstays of therapy, with

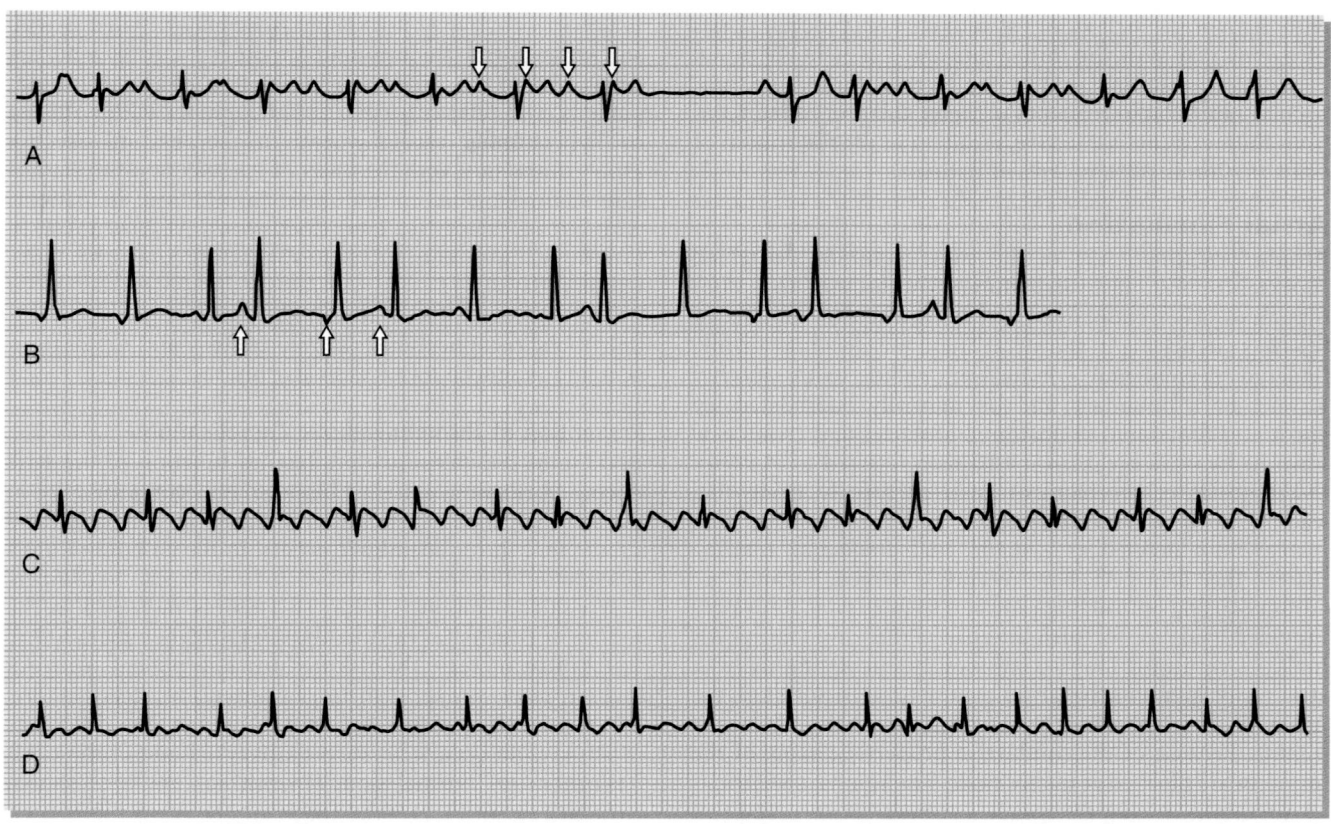

Figure 10-6 Atrial tachyarrhythmias. **A,** Atrial tachycardia with 2:1 and variable AV conduction. Note the presence of more P waves *(arrows)* than QRS complexes. **B,** Multifocal atrial tachycardia demonstrating an irregularly irregular rhythm at a rate of about 110 beats/minute, with at least three different P-wave morphologies *(arrows)* and without a dominant underlying rhythm. **C,** Atrial flutter. Flutter waves are seen as the discrete undulations of the baseline (sawtooth pattern). The conduction rate is variable. **D,** Atrial fibrillation. The rhythm is irregularly irregular without evidence of organized atrial electrical activity.

class I or class III anti-arrhythmic agents reserved for refractory patients. Catheter ablation can eliminate this arrhythmia in 75% to 90% of patients. When atrial tachycardia is the result of digoxin therapy, withholding the agent should be the first step, followed by the administration of digoxin-specific antibodies if the patient is symptomatic.

Multifocal atrial tachycardia (MAT) is an irregular rhythm defined by the presence of three or more P-wave morphologies and a rate greater than 100 beats/minute (see Fig. 10-6B). It occurs most commonly in patients with underlying lung disease; it is also seen in the setting of an acute MI, hypokalemia, or hypomagnesemia; and it may be a precursor of atrial fibrillation. Aminophylline use may also be a contributing factor. Treatment is directed at the underlying disease. Rate control of this arrhythmia may be difficult, although verapamil is frequently effective.

Atrial Flutter

Atrial flutter (AFL) is a reentrant tachycardia localized to the right atrium with passive activation of the left atrium. The reentrant circuit is limited anteriorly by the tricuspid valve and posteriorly by the cristae terminalis and the eustachian ridge. The direction of impulse propagation around the tricuspid annulus determines the P-wave morphology. If propagation is in the counterclockwise direction, the impulse propagates up the septum and down the lateral wall, resulting in a negative P wave in the inferior leads with a typical

sawtooth pattern (see Fig. 10-6C), called *typical AFL*. If propagation is in the clockwise direction, the P wave is upright in the inferior leads, and the tachycardia is called *atypical AFL*. The atrial rate during AFL is usually about 250 to 350 beats/minute, with an average rate of 300 beats/minute. The ventricular rate depends on the conduction down the AV node. Usually, conduction is 2:1, resulting in a ventricular rate of about 150 beats/minute. In young patients with enhanced AV nodal conduction, the ventricular rate can be as high as the atrial rate, reaching 300 beats/minute. Similarly, in the presence of an accessory pathway, the ventricular rate can be rapid, resulting in hemodynamic compromise and ventricular fibrillation.

AFL may occur in patients with or without structural heart disease and may be precipitated by thyrotoxicosis, pericarditis, and alcohol ingestion. When AFL is associated with hemodynamic compromise or angina, immediate cardioversion should be performed. Relatively low-energy shocks are frequently effective because of the stable nature of the circuit. When the patient is hemodynamically stable, the focus should be on rate control to reduce the risk for tachycardia-induced cardiomyopathy and anticoagulation to reduce the risk for stroke. If patients remain symptomatic despite rate control, rhythm control either pharmacologically or with catheter ablation should be attempted. When class IA anti-arrhythmic agents are used to convert AFL to sinus rhythm, the ventricular rate must first be controlled with digoxin, β blockers, or calcium channel blockers. Class IA agents may slow the flutter rate and augment AV nodal conduction, resulting in 1:1 conduction with rapid ventricular rates. Radiofrequency catheter ablation of the reentrant flutter circuit is effective, resulting in the restoration of sinus rhythm in 90% to 95% of patients.

Atrial Fibrillation

Atrial fibrillation (AF) is the most common sustained supraventricular tachyarrhythmia. According to *Moe's hypothesis*, AF is maintained by having a critical number of wavelets circulating in the atria. These wavelets may shrink, undergo decremental conduction, collide with another wavelet or a boundary and be mutually annihilated, or encounter functional or anatomic obstacles and create new wavelets by wave breaks, a mechanism referred to as *vortex shedding*. Other mechanisms such as rapidly firing foci leading to *fibrillatory conduction,* and the presence of a *mother rotor* defined as a stable, high-frequency rotating pattern that drives AF, have recently emerged. Technologic advances using optical mapping and frequency analysis have provided evidence for such alternative theories. During AF, multiple reentrant loops continuously circulating in both atria result in ineffective atrial contraction. In addition, the AV node is bombarded at rates greater than 400 beats/minute. Because of the conductive properties, many of the impulses are blocked at the AV node. The resultant ventricular rhythm is irregularly irregular at rates between 120 and 170 beats/minute. At rapid ventricular rates, the rhythm may appear to be regular, although careful measurements will disclose the irregularity. A truly regular ventricular rate in the setting of AF suggests the development of a junctional or ventricular rhythm, both of which may be a reflection of digoxin toxicity. AF may be paroxysmal or chronic and may be the only arrhythmia present or be part of a more generalized rhythm disturbance (sick sinus syndrome). The surface ECG demonstrates an irregular ventricular pattern and the absence of organized atrial activity; that is, no P waves are present (see Fig. 10-6D). Physical examination of a patient in AF reveals variation in the intensity of S_1, an irregular cardiac rhythm, and absence of a waves in the jugular venous pulsations. At the very short RR intervals that occur intermittently during rapid heart rates, the minimal diastolic filling time and subsequent low stroke volume fail to produce a palpable pulse. A discrepancy may therefore exist between the auscultated heart rate and the palpable pulse rate, with the auscultated rate being a more accurate reflection of the true ventricular rate.

A clear association of AF with age exists, and a sharp increase in incidence is noted after the seventh decade of life. AF may occur without any identifiable cardiac abnormality but is common in the setting of underlying cardiac disease, including valvular heart disease (especially rheumatic), heart failure, and ischemic cardiac disease. The most frequent predisposing cardiovascular condition for the development of AF is hypertension. AF may also be precipitated by pericarditis, thyrotoxicosis, pulmonary emboli, pneumonia, and acute alcohol ingestion and occurs postoperatively in about one third of patients who undergo cardiac surgery. AF is frequently asymptomatic or associated with only minor symptoms, such as palpitations. In patients with obstructive coronary artery disease, the rapid heart rate associated with the onset of AF may precipitate ischemia. In patients with aortic or mitral stenosis and in other patients who are dependent on the atrial contribution to cardiac output (e.g., patients with left ventricular hypertrophy or with a dilated or hypertrophic cardiomyopathy), the loss of effective atrial contraction with the onset of AF may result in significant hemodynamic compromise. In addition, in patients with bypass tracts (see later discussion), AF may result in extremely rapid ventricular rates with subsequent hemodynamic collapse.

The treatment of AF is threefold: (1) prevention of thromboembolic complications, (2) rate control, and (3) restoration and maintenance of sinus rhythm.

Prevention of Thromboembolic Complications

Because of the ineffective mechanical function of the atria during fibrillation, stasis of blood may occur, especially in the atrial appendages, and result in thrombus formation and subsequent thromboembolic events. In the absence of anticoagulation therapy, AF is associated with a 5%- to 6%-per-year risk for embolic stroke. This risk is increased in the setting of rheumatic valvular disease (>10%). Other clinical factors that increase the risk for stroke in patients with AF include prior stroke, diabetes, hypertension, heart failure, left atrial enlargement, and increasing age. No difference in stroke rate occurs between paroxysmal and chronic AF. Restoration of normal sinus rhythm has not been shown to reduce the risk for stroke. In fact, in the Atrial Fibrillation Follow-up Investigation of Rhythm Management (AFFIRM) trial, a trend toward a higher incidence of stroke in patients randomized to rhythm control was found when compared with rate control, albeit not statistically significant. This trend was most likely caused by the decreased use of warfarin in the rhythm control group. Therefore, any patient with paroxysmal, persistent, or permanent AF who does not have a contraindication to anticoagulation should be treated with warfarin therapy with a target international normalized ratio between 2 and 3.

Rate Control

Rate control in AF is important for several reasons. It has been shown to improve symptoms and quality of life. Symptoms and hemodynamic compromise are increased at faster ventricular rates, and the tachycardic response may induce ischemia in patients with coronary artery disease. In addition, the poorly controlled heart rate may result in the development of progressive ventricular dysfunction. The heart rate can usually be controlled with digoxin, β blockers, or calcium channel blockers. In rare instances, the ventricular rate cannot be controlled by pharmacologic means, and catheter ablation of the AV node and permanent pacemaker implantation are necessary for adequate heart rate control. Occasionally, patients exhibit AF and a relatively slow ventricular rate in the absence of rate-lowering medications. This circumstance usually reflects significant underlying conduction system disease that also often involves the sinus node.

Rhythm Control

Rhythm control has several advantages, including (1) abolition of symptoms, (2) halting atrial enlargement (an independent predictor of stroke), and (3) improvement of left ventricular function and exercise capacity. The main disadvantage is subjecting patients to a drug therapy or procedure that might be associated with complications. As stated before, rhythm control has not been shown to reduce the risk for stroke or to have an impact on mortality when compared with rate control. Therefore, rhythm control should be attempted in patients who are symptomatic despite rate control and in those who have left ventricular dysfunction. When AF is associated with hemodynamic compromise, electrical cardioversion (with 100 to 360 joules) is the treatment of choice. In hemodynamically stable patients with less than 48 hours of AF, the risk for thromboembolism is low, and pharmacologic or electrical cardioversion can be attempted without the need for 3 weeks of anticoagulation (see later discussion). Patients with more than 48 hours of AF, or in whom the duration of the arrhythmia is unknown, are at increased risk for atrial thrombi and should be treated with anticoagulation for at least 3 weeks before an attempt at cardioversion. An alternative approach is to perform a transesophageal echocardiogram; if atrial thrombi are not present, cardioversion can be safely performed. Anticoagulation should be continued for at least 4 weeks after successful cardioversion because effective atrial contraction may be slow to return. The options for maintaining rhythm control include (1) pharmacologic therapy, (2) catheter ablation, and (3) surgical Maze procedure. The class IA (quinidine, procainamide, and disopyramide), class IC (propafenone and flecainide), and class III (sotalol and amiodarone) agents are effective in restoring sinus rhythm and for long-term maintenance therapy. However, the benefits of such therapy must be weighed against the risks for toxicity with these agents, and the probability of maintaining sinus rhythm must be taken into account. The preferred choice of drug therapy for the maintenance of sinus rhythm in patients with paroxysmal and persistent AF, based on the most recent American College of Cardiology/American Heart Association guidelines, is provided in Figure 10-7. Radiofrequency ablation of the ostia of the pulmonary veins or electrical isolation of the pulmonary veins from the left atrium is a procedure that should be reserved to symptomatic patients who have failed drug therapy. Ablation therapy frequently abolishes the arrhythmia, improving symptoms and, at times, left ventricular function in patients with baseline congestive heart failure. The surgical maze procedure involves making surgical lesions in the atria that interrupt reentrant circuits and may restore sinus rhythm in more than 90% of patients. This procedure is usually performed in conjunction with mitral valve surgery.

ATRIOVENTRICULAR NODAL (JUNCTIONAL) RHYTHM DISTURBANCES

Atrioventricular Nodal Reentrant Tachycardia

Atrioventricular nodal reentrant tachycardia (AVNRT) is the most common type of paroxysmal SVT and is characterized by the sudden onset and termination of a regular narrow QRS complex tachycardia at rates of 150 to 250 beats/minute (Fig. 10-8A). A wide QRS complex may occur if aberrant conduction occurs in the His-Purkinje system. These rhythms may occur at any age, are somewhat more common in women than men, may occur in the absence of organic heart disease, may be short lived or sustained, and may produce palpitations, chest pain, dyspnea, and presyncope. The substrate for this tachycardia is dual AV node pathways with different effective refractory period (ERP): a fast pathway with a longer ERP and a slow pathway with a shorter ERP. Whether these pathways are exclusively intranodal or not remains controversial, but catheter ablation studies of these pathways have revealed distinct atrial insertion sites, with the fast pathway inserting anteriorly near the His bundle and the slow pathway posteriorly near the coronary sinus ostium.

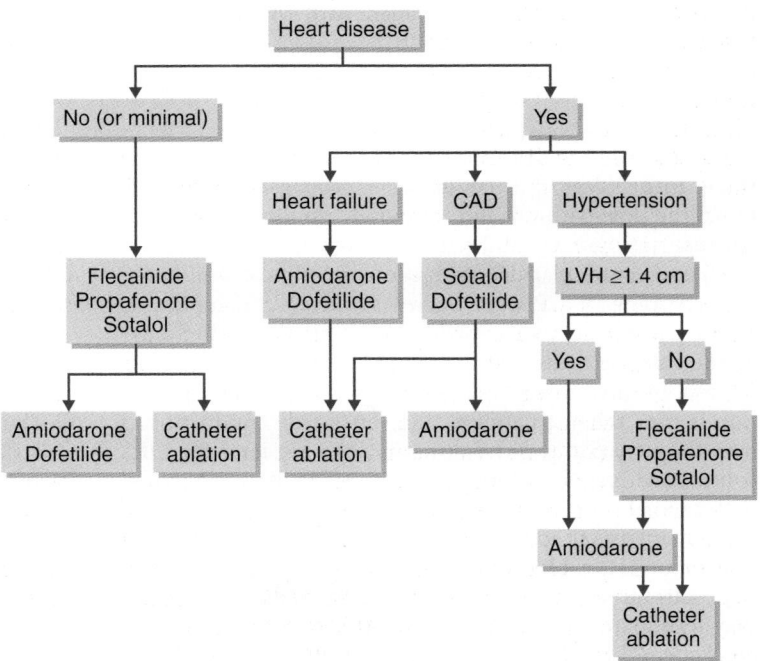

Figure 10-7 Drug therapy to maintain sinus rhythm in patients with recurrent paroxysmal or persistent atrial fibrillation. CAD, coronary artery disease; LVH, left ventricular hypertrophy.

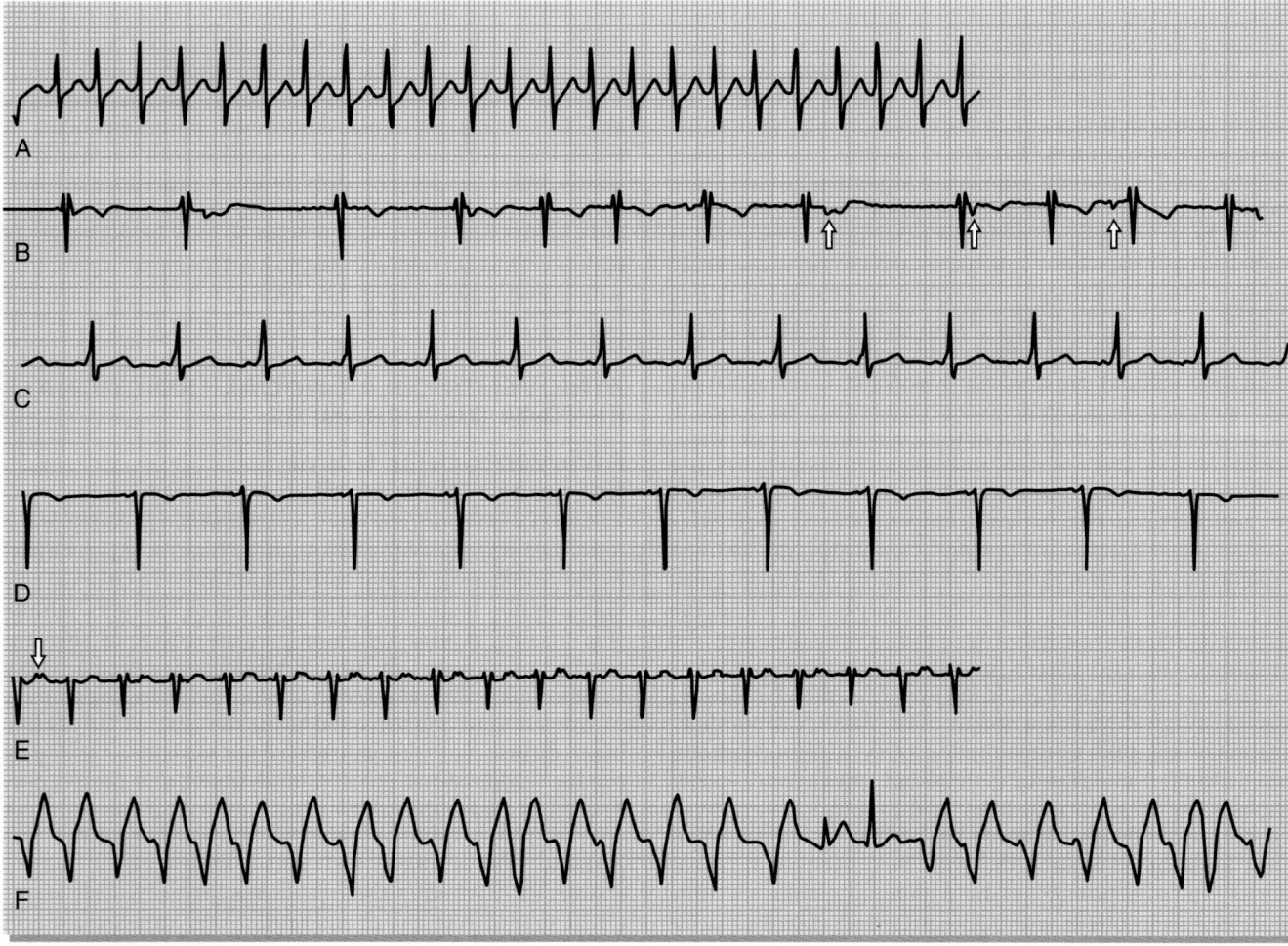

Figure 10-8 Atrioventricular (AV) nodal (junctional) rhythm disturbances. **A,** AV nodal reentrant tachycardia at a rate of 185 beats/minute. The retrograde P waves are hidden in the QRS complexes. **B,** Automatic junctional tachycardia. Note the presence of AV dissociation during tachycardia. The P waves *(arrows)* are dissociated from the QRS complexes. **C,** Normal sinus rhythm in a patient with Wolff-Parkinson-White (WPW) syndrome. Note the short PR interval (<120 minutes), the *slurring* of the initial portion of the QRS (delta wave), and the wide QRS complex. **D,** Normal sinus rhythm in a patient with Lown-Ganong-Levine pattern. Note the short PR interval without the presence of a delta wave or wide QRS complex. **E,** Orthodromic AV reentrant tachycardia at a rate of 146 beats/minute in a patient with WPW syndrome. The retrograde P waves are clearly seen altering the normal T-wave contour *(arrow).* **F,** Atrial fibrillation in a patient with WPW syndrome. Note the rapid and irregular ventricular response with widening of the QRS secondary to preexcitation.

At least two types of AVNRT have been identified. In the usual form (typical), the impulse propagates antegrade down the slow pathway and retrograde up the fast pathway. Because retrograde conduction is over the fast pathway, atrial and ventricular depolarizations are almost simultaneous, resulting in a P wave buried in the QRS complex, or appearing at its terminal portion, resulting in pseudo S wave in the inferior leads and a pseudo R′ in lead V_1 (see Fig. 10-8A). In the unusual form of AVNRT, antegrade conduction is over the fast pathway, and retrograde conduction is over the slow pathway, resulting in a P wave after the QRS complex with a long RP interval. AVNRT is usually initiated with premature stimuli and terminated by premature beats, vagal maneuvers, adenosine, or other cardiac medications known to cause block in the AV node. Vagal maneuvers (e.g., carotid sinus massage, Valsalva maneuver, coughing) may terminate an episode by causing a transient AV nodal blockade. Adenosine (6 to 12 mg intravenously) terminates

episodes in more than 95% of patients and is the treatment of choice if vagal maneuvers fail. In rare instances, direct current cardioversion is necessary. Intravenous β blockers, digoxin, or calcium channel blockers are also an extremely effective acute therapy, and their oral formulations are effective chronically. Classes IC and III anti-arrhythmic agents are useful in resistant patients. In rare instances, direct current cardioversion is necessary. Radiofrequency catheter ablation of one limb of the reentrant circuit (slow pathway) can cure AVNRT in more than 90% of patients, with a low risk for inducing complete heart block (<2%) that might require the placement of a permanent pacemaker.

Automatic Junctional Tachycardia

Automatic junctional tachycardia (AJT) is characterized as a rapid irregular SVT with episodes of AV dissociation (see Fig. 10-8B). The rate ranges between 110 and 250 beats/minute, and the QRS interval is usually narrow but may be wide secondary to bundle branch block. AJT was first described in infants and children but has also been reported in adults in which the prognosis is more benign. Abnormal automaticity is believed to be the mechanism responsible for AJT. This tachycardia is usually sensitive to catecholamines but can sometimes be terminated with carotid sinus massage and adenosine. β blockers, calcium channel blockers, and classes IC and III anti-arrhythmic drugs should be the first line of therapy. When drug therapy fails, radiofrequency can result in cure; however, it is associated with a significant risk for AV block (20%), requiring the implantation of a permanent pacemaker. AJT must be differentiated from the more common nonparoxysmal junctional tachycardia. The latter is regular, has a slower rate (70 to 120 beats/minute) and occurs in the setting of digitalis toxicity, inferior MI, metabolic derangements, chronic lung disease, or after cardiac surgery. The mechanism of nonparoxysmal junctional tachycardia is believed to be triggered activity secondary to DADs. Digoxin toxicity must always be excluded as a cause. Specific therapy for nonparoxysmal junctional tachycardia is usually not necessary.

WOLFF-PARKINSON-WHITE SYNDROME AND ATRIOVENTRICULAR RECIPROCATING ARRHYTHMIAS

Normally, the AV node is the only pathway that allows the wave of depolarization to conduct from the atria to the ventricles. However, anomalous bands of tissue (accessory pathways or bypass tracts) may exist and form an additional conduction pathway. The conductive properties of these bypass tracts differ from those of the AV node in that they do not produce the decremental conduction property of normal conduction tissue. In other words, they do not conduct slower at rapid rates. Conduction through the bypass tracts may be unidirectional or bidirectional. These properties provide the substrate for macro-reentrant arrhythmias (see previous discussion) using the bypass tract as one limb of the reentrant circuit and the AV node as the other. Other, less frequent pathways have been reported, such as AV nodal bypass tract, a direct communication between the atria and the His-Purkinje system, nodoventricular fibers connecting the AV node to the ventricular myocardium, and fasciculoventricular connections from the His-Purkinje system to the ventricles. Most patients with bypass tracts have otherwise anatomically normal hearts, although the incidence of right-sided accessory pathways is increased in patients with Ebstein anomaly of the tricuspid valve. Similarly, an association with left-sided accessory pathways and mitral valve prolapse and hypertrophic cardiomyopathy has been noted.

Wolff-Parkinson-White Syndrome during Normal Sinus Rhythm

During normal sinus rhythm, when the AV bypass tract conducts in an antegrade fashion, the ventricular muscle will be activated by the atrial impulse sooner than would be expected if the impulse reached the ventricles only by way of the normal AV conduction. This activity is referred to as *preexcitation*. The result is a short PR interval (<120 minutes) and a wide QRS complex with *slurring* of the initial portion

of the QRS, referred to also as a *delta wave*. The QRS is wide because it is a fusion complex created by ventricular activation through two separate pathways, the AV node and the accessory pathway (see Fig. 10-8C). The extent of preexcitation is determined by the conductive properties of the pathway and the AV node in addition to the accessory pathway location. Wolff-Parkinson-White (WPW) syndrome refers to the presence of preexcitation and a history of paroxysmal tachycardia. When preexcitation is present alone without paroxysmal tachycardia, the patient is referred to as having WPW pattern. Occasionally, the accessory pathway conducts only in the retrograde direction, that is, from the ventricle to the atrium without any antegrade conduction and thus ventricular preexcitation. This circumstance is referred to as a *concealed* accessory pathway because its presence is not evident on the surface ECG when the patient is in normal sinus rhythm. As stated before, some accessory pathways connect the atria to the His-Purkinje system. The result is a short PR interval because the atrial impulse will be bypassing the AV node, but a normal QRS complex is seen because the ventricles are activated through the normal His-Purkinje system (see Fig. 10-8D). This circumstance is referred to as *Lown-Ganong-Levine pattern*; when it is associated with a history of tachycardias, it is referred to as the *Lown-Ganong-Levine syndrome*.

Arrhythmias in Patients with Wolff-Parkinson-White Syndrome

The most common arrhythmia in WPW syndrome is *orthodromic* AV reentrant tachycardia (AVRT) in which the AV node is used as the antegrade limb of the circuit and the bypass tract as the retrograde limb. This circumstance results in a narrow-complex QRS tachycardia on the surface ECG (see Fig. 10-8E), unless aberrant conduction is present. A retrograde P wave may be noted, usually with a short RP interval. Less commonly, *antidromic* AVRT may occur that uses the accessory pathway as the antegrade limb and the AV node as the retrograde limb. This circumstance results in complete preexcitation of the ventricles with a wide, bizarre QRS complex on the ECG. Because the AV node is an intrinsic component of both forms of AVRT, transient blockade of the AV node by vagal maneuvers or medications will interrupt the circuit and terminate the tachyarrhythmia. The incidence of *atrial tachyarrhythmias*, such as AF or AFL, is increased in patients with bypass tracts. When these arrhythmias occur, rapid ventricular rates often occur and may precipitate hemodynamic collapse and sudden death (see Fig. 10-8F).

Treatment of Patients with Wolff-Parkinson-White Syndrome

In a patient with a delta wave noted on the ECG but without any symptoms, no specific therapy is required. In patients with frequent episodes of AVRT, *transient* blockade of the AV node by vagal maneuvers or medications will interrupt the circuit and terminate the tachyarrhythmia. Chronic pharmacologic therapy with drugs that prolong the refractory period of the accessory pathway (class IA, IC, or III anti-arrhythmic agents) is effective. Drugs that slow conduction in the AV node (digoxin, β blockers, or calcium channel blockers) should be avoided in patients with WPW because they may enhance conduction down the accessory pathway and increase the ventricular rate during AF and AFL. Indeed, when atrial tachyarrhythmias occur in patients with WPW, AV nodal-blocking drugs are contraindicated; in this setting, digoxin, β blockers, or calcium channel blockers may result in slowing of conduction through the AV node with resultant preferential excitation of the ventricles through the accessory AV connection. Intravenous procainamide is the drug of choice for acutely controlling the rate of AF or AFL in patients with bypass tracts. Electrical cardioversion should be considered early in these patients. Radiofrequency catheter ablation of the accessory pathway has become the therapy of choice for symptomatic patients and has a success rate in excess of 95%.

VENTRICULAR RHYTHM DISTURBANCES

Ventricular Tachycardia

VT is defined as three or more consecutive ventricular depolarizations occurring at a rate greater than 100 beats/minute. The resulting QRS complexes on the surface ECG are aberrant, as described earlier for VPCs, and may be monomorphic or polymorphic (Fig. 10-9A). Evidence of independent atrial activity may be present (AV dissociation); however, when retrograde conduction to the atria is present, AV dissociation is not seen. Occasionally, a normal sinus depolarization may be conducted to the ventricles before the pathologic ventricular depolarization occurs and results in a normal-appearing QRS complex, called a *capture* beat. If the atrial depolarization reaches the ventricles simultaneously with the spontaneous ventricular depolarization, a *fusion* complex will result. These abnormalities are pathognomonic for VT. VT that lasts for more than 30 seconds or requires termination because of hemodynamic instability is considered *sustained;* VT that lasts less than 30 seconds and is hemodynamically stable is considered *nonsustained.*

VT occurs most frequently in patients with underlying heart disease, including acute ischemia, prior infarction with scar formation, congestive cardiomyopathy, right ventricular dysplasia, and hypertrophic heart disease. The mechanism is usually reentry in the ventricular myocardium, although it may also arise in a diseased portion of the conduction system (e.g., bundle branch reentry). Metabolic abnormalities, such as hyperkalemia and hypoxia, and medications, such as digoxin and antiarrhythmic agents, may also precipitate VT, likely as a result of triggered activity. On the other hand, VT can occur in the absence of structural heart disease. This type of VT accounts for only 6% of all clinical VTs and is called idiopathic VT. Idiopathic VT is best classified according to its site of origin. Right ventricular outflow tract VT (RVOT-VT) is the most common type of idiopathic VT originating from the right ventricular outflow tract with left bundle branch block–inferior axis morphology. The mechanism of this tachycardia is believed to be triggered activity. This tachycardia occurs in otherwise healthy individuals, is very sensitive to catecholamines, and terminates with adenosine, thus the term *adenosine-sensitive VT.* The other type of idiopathic VT originates from the septum near the apex of the left ventricle resulting in RBBB–superior axis morphology. The mechanism of idiopathic left VT has been shown to be reentry with involvement of the distal His-Purkinje system. Idiopathic left VT is known to be verapamil sensitive, thus the term *verapamil-sensitive VT.*

Nonsustained VT requires no treatment unless the patient is symptomatic. In most instances, nonsustained VT is associated with left ventricular dysfunction, which independently, if moderate to severe, is an indication for the implantation of an implantable cardioverter-defibrillator (ICD). When patients are symptomatic, the choice of medical therapy is dictated by the presence or absence of structural heart disease. In patients with normal left ventricular function, β blockers, calcium channel blockers, and class IC and class III agents should be used, in that order. In patients with left ventricular dysfunction, β blockers followed by

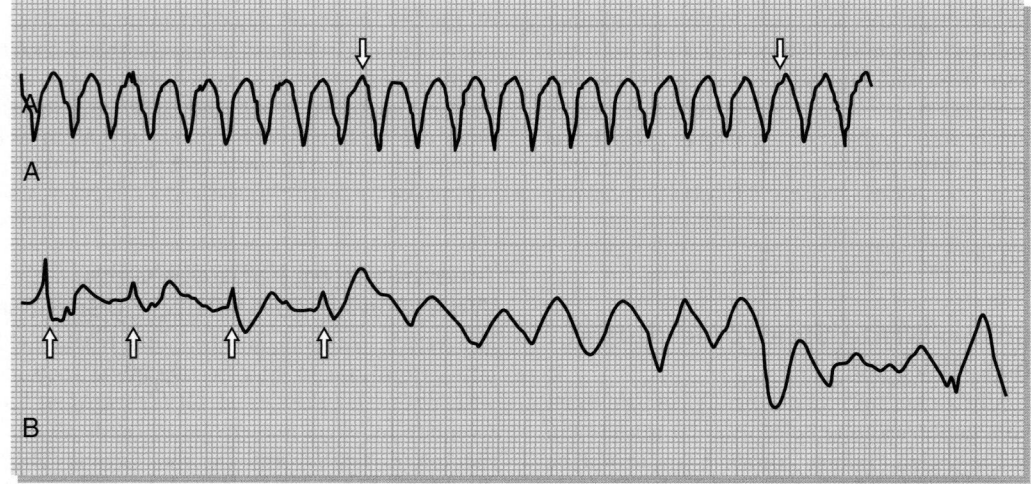

Figure 10-9 Ventricular rhythm disturbances. **A,** Monomorphic ventricular tachycardia at a rate of 200 beats/minute. The QRS complex is wide, and P waves are seen to occasionally alter the QRS morphology *(arrows),* reflecting AV dissociation. **B,** Ventricular fibrillation. An *agonal* rhythm is initially present *(arrows)* but deteriorates into ventricular fibrillation. The baseline is irregular without evidence of organized ventricular electrical activity.

amiodarone are usually the drugs of choice. An important point to note is that, although this arrhythmia is often a marker for increased cardiac mortality in some patients with structural or ischemic heart disease, suppression of this arrhythmia with pharmacologic treatment has not been shown to decrease mortality in most settings. Patients with *sustained VT* that is associated with hemodynamic compromise, angina, or heart failure should undergo synchronized cardioversion. When stable, sustained VT should be managed with intravenous drug therapy such as amiodarone or lidocaine. If left ventricular function is normal, procainamide and sotalol may also be used. If drug therapy fails, synchronized cardioversion should be performed. Following the acute treatment, most patients receive an ICD unless a reversible cause has been identified (e.g., ischemia, metabolic abnormalities, drug toxicity). Ventricular tachyarrhythmias that occur in the setting of acute MI respond to treatment of the ischemia and do not necessarily require prolonged anti-arrhythmic therapy. In the rare instances of idiopathic VT, catheter ablation may provide a permanent cure, with a success rate of 90%. Catheter ablation is also used as an adjunctive therapy in patients with ICDs who have recurrent or incessant VT. With improvements in interventional techniques, localization of the abnormal ventricular foci and subsequent radiofrequency ablation may be curative in many forms of VT, including those associated with previous MI.

Ventricular Flutter

Ventricular flutter (VFL) is a form of monomorphic VT occurring at a rate of 280 to 300 beats/minute and is a hemodynamically unstable rhythm. *Ventricular fibrillation* (VF) is a disorganized, chaotic, ventricular rhythm that results in ineffective ventricular contraction, rapid hemodynamic collapse, and death if not immediately terminated (see Fig. 10-9B). VF is recognized on ECG by coarse undulations of the baseline without identifiable QRS complexes, ST segments, or T waves. It may occur in the setting of ischemia, metabolic abnormalities, and drug toxicity, or it may degenerate from VT, either spontaneously or after attempted cardioversion. Treatment with immediate nonsynchronized direct current shock at 360 joules (or equivalent biphasic) is required in all instances. Several shocks may be required for termination of this arrhythmia, and concurrent treatment of precipitating causes is essential. Once the rhythm has been successfully terminated, an intravenous anti-arrhythmic agent such as amiodarone or lidocaine should be started to prevent recurrences. If VF is the result of an acute reversible cause, no chronic therapy is required. However, if VF occurs as a result of fixed underlying cardiac disease, implantation of an ICD is indicated.

Approach to the Patient with Suspected Arrhythmias

HISTORY

Many, if not most, arrhythmias occur intermittently, and patients are often asymptomatic at the time of evaluation. Therefore, with the suggestion of an arrhythmic problem, the necessity and urgency for further evaluation must frequently be determined by the history alone. Palpitations, syncope, presyncope, dizziness, chest pain, and symptoms of heart failure are the most common complaints of patients with arrhythmic disorders. Palpitations give a sensation of a rapid or irregular heartbeat. Characterizing the pattern (regular or irregular, intermittent or continuous) and rate of palpitations by having patients tap their fingers on a table to the rhythm of the palpitations may help determine their cause. For instance, occasional *skipped beats* are likely the result of premature atrial or ventricular beats, whereas periods of rapid, irregular heartbeats may be reflective of paroxysmal AF. The perception of palpitations does not invariably correlate with arrhythmias; some patients have tachyarrhythmias without palpitations, whereas other patients have palpitations without tachyarrhythmias. Only simultaneously recording the ECG and documenting the symptoms can confirm the correlation between the symptoms and an arrhythmia. Syncope is the sudden, transient loss of consciousness. Obtaining a complete history of the events immediately preceding and after a syncopal episode will suggest the diagnosis in most patients for whom a diagnosis is eventually determined. Chest pain may be a manifestation of palpitations or may represent arrhythmia-induced cardiac ischemia. Similarly, cardiac arrhythmias may also precipitate or exacerbate congestive heart failure. A prior history of cardiac disease is important to elicit. Patients with palpitations or syncope and a history of cardiomyopathy or prior MI frequently have ventricular tachyarrhythmias, whereas patients with valvular heart disease or hypertension frequently develop AF. A family history of cardiac disease (e.g., dilated or hypertrophic cardiomyopathy, bypass tracts, sudden cardiac death, LQTS) is important to note.

PHYSICAL EXAMINATION

In addition to noting the pulse rate and rhythm, a thorough examination is useful for identifying evidence of underlying cardiac disease. When patients are examined during an arrhythmic episode, several clues to the nature of the arrhythmia may be present. Evidence of AV dissociation suggests a ventricular arrhythmia and includes variable intensity of S_1 (because of variations in the PR interval), intermittent cannon a waves in the jugular venous pulsation, and a cacophony of sounds (as a result of atrial systole occurring during various parts of the cardiac cycle, generating intermittent S_3 and S_4). The S_2 may become widely or paradoxically split if a bundle branch block develops during an arrhythmia. Nonetheless, these findings are not diagnostic of a ventricular source of the arrhythmia because bundle branch blocks and, rarely, AV dissociation may occur during supraventricular tachyarrhythmias as well.

USEFUL TESTS

Electrocardiogram

The ECG taken during the arrhythmia is usually diagnostic. If P waves are not obvious, moving the arm leads to a parasternal position (Lewis leads) or using an esophageal electrode (placed 40 cm into the esophagus by means of a

CSM

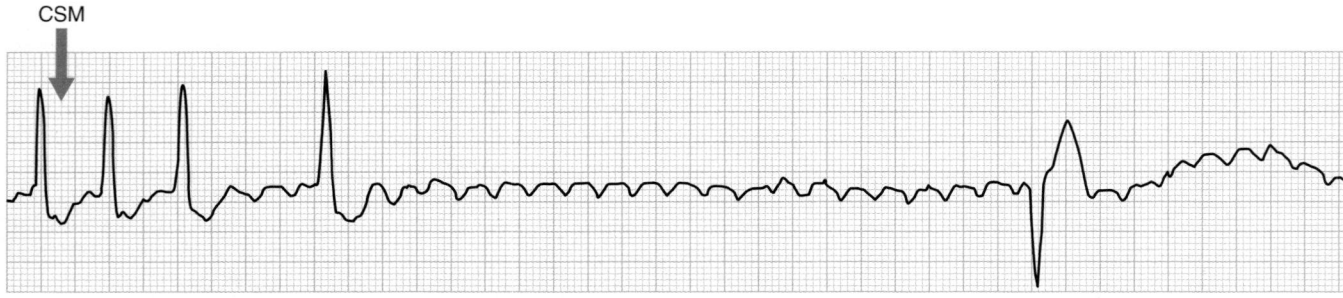

Figure 10-10 Carotid sinus massage during atrial flutter with resultant unmasking of the underlying flutter waves.

nasogastric tube) may help discern atrial activity. In patients who exhibit a hemodynamically stable supraventricular tachyarrhythmia, carotid sinus massage or pharmacologic therapy with adenosine or verapamil may slow or block conduction in the AV node, resulting in either tachycardia termination or the identification of the underlying rhythm. Carotid sinus massage is performed with the patient in the supine position by applying light pressure for 5 to 10 seconds over the carotid impulse at the angle of the jaw. A successful test should result in slowing of the ventricular rate (Fig. 10-10). If no effect is noted, massage can be performed over the contralateral carotid impulse. This test should not be performed if carotid bruits are present. Unfortunately, many patients are examined after the arrhythmia has resolved. Nonetheless, clues may be present on the resting ECG. A delta wave is diagnostic of WPW syndrome, which is associated with AV reentrant arrhythmias and AF. Evidence of prior MI raises the suspicion of ventricular tachyarrhythmias.

When a *wide-complex tachycardia* is present, determining whether it is VT or SVT with aberrancy is important because the therapeutic and prognostic implications differ significantly. When an SVT is associated with a narrow-complex QRS, the diagnosis is straightforward. However, when an SVT occurs in the setting of a preexisting bundle branch block or conducts aberrantly as a result of rate-related block in the His-Purkinje system, the resulting QRS complex is wide and may be difficult to distinguish from VT. Several features may be helpful in making this distinction. The presence of AV dissociation, capture beats, or fusion complexes is diagnostic of VT. However, the absence of these findings is not helpful because they are present in less than 50% of instances. A wide-complex tachycardia occurring in the presence of ischemia or in a patient with known ischemic heart disease is VT in more than 90% of instances. The heart rate, blood pressure, and presence or absence of symptoms do not differentiate these arrhythmias, whereas intermittent cannon a waves in the jugular venous pulsations suggest VT. If an abnormal QRS complex is present when the patient is in normal sinus rhythm and the QRS complex during the tachycardia is identical to the one in normal sinus rhythm, the rhythm is likely SVT. Adenosine may be useful in determining the cause; with SVT, adenosine-induced blockade of the AV node will terminate the tachycardia in most instances, given that 90% of SVT involve the AV node (60% AVNRT, 30% AVRT). In the remainder of patients, adenosine-induced AV block will unmask the atrial activity and thus help make the diagnosis. In rare instances, adenosine may terminate a VT when the tachycardia originates from the right ventricular outflow tract. Verapamil should never be used as a diagnostic test because it may precipitate ventricular fibrillation if the initial rhythm is VT. Table 10-1 lists the features that may help differentiate these arrhythmias from one another.

Recording Devices

Because of the intermittent nature of arrhythmias, prolonged recording devices are more effective than a single ECG in electrocardiographically capturing an arrhythmia. Ambulatory ECG (Holter) monitors continuously record the rhythm and are useful in patients who have frequent episodes of presumed arrhythmic symptoms. Patient-activated event monitors, or loop recorders, can be worn for weeks at a time and continuously monitor the patient's heart rhythm. If symptoms occur, the patient activates the device, which then permanently records the rhythm for several minutes before and after the event and transmits the recorded rhythm by telephone to a central monitoring

Table 10-1 **Features that May Differentiate Ventricular Tachycardia from Supraventricular Tachycardia with Aberrancy**	
Helpful Features	**Implications**
Positive QRS concordance	Diagnostic of VT
Presence of AV dissociation, capture beats, or fusion beats	Diagnostic of VT
Atypical RBBB (monophasic R, QR, RS, or triphasic QRS in V₁; R:S ratio < 1, QS or QR, monophasic R in V₆)	Suggests VT
Atypical LBBB (R >30 min or R to S [nadir or notch] > 60 min in V₁ or V₂; R:S ratio < 1, QS or QR in V₆)	Suggests VT
Shift of axis from baseline	Suggests VT
History of CAD	Suggests VT
QRS during tachycardia identical to QRS during sinus rhythm	Suggests SVT
Termination with adenosine	Suggests SVT

AV, atrioventricular; CAD, coronary artery disease; LBBB, left bundle branch block; RBBB, right bundle branch block; SVT, supraventricular tachycardia; VT, ventricular tachycardia.

facility. This type of monitor is useful if the patient has infrequent symptoms. For patients with very infrequent symptoms, an implantable event monitor can be placed under the skin of the chest wall and can remain in place for up to 1 year. All these devices are useful in diagnosing arrhythmias, determining the relationship (if any) of the patient's symptoms to an arrhythmia, monitoring the efficacy of anti-arrhythmic therapy, and evaluating artificial pacemaker function. If a patient's symptoms are exertion related, formal exercise testing may be useful.

Head-Up Tilt-Table Testing

In patients with suggested neurocardiogenic syncope, *head-up tilt-table* testing may reproduce their symptoms. This procedure is performed by strapping a patient to the tilt table, then tilting the table 60 to 80 degrees vertically for 15 to 60 minutes. The presumed mechanism of tilt-induced syncope involves a postural decrease in ventricular filling, resulting in increased sympathetic activity and ventricular contraction. This increased contraction is believed to result in the activation of cardiac mechanoreceptors (C fibers), leading to reflex increase in vagal tone and withdrawal of peripheral sympathetic tone. The result is bradycardia-induced low cardiac output in addition to vasodilation leading to hypotension. The sensitivity of the test in detecting neurocardiogenic syncope can be up to 85% depending on the tilt protocol used, with a relatively low false-positive rate (<15%). The administration of intravenous isoproterenol or sublingual nitroglycerin increases the diagnostic yield of the test while decreasing its specificity.

Electrophysiologic Study

Invasive EP studies are performed by recording the electrical activity of the heart through catheters strategically positioned in the right atrial and ventricular chambers. This test may be useful in a group of patients in whom conduction disorders of the sinus or AV node are suggested. The results may help determine the mechanism of heart block and the need for permanent pacemaker implantation. More commonly, EP studies are used to evaluate patients with documented tachyarrhythmias or with syncope for which a tachyarrhythmia is suggested as the cause. Both supraventricular and ventricular tachyarrhythmias may be reproduced by programmed electrical stimulation. If a tachyarrhythmia is induced, the application of radiofrequency energy at the arrhythmia site of origin or targeting a critical component of the arrhythmia circuit often leads to tachycardia termination.

Syncope

Syncope is defined as sudden, transient loss of consciousness and may be the result of a variety of cardiac and noncardiac conditions (Table 10-2). Presyncope is a feeling of impending syncope without true loss of consciousness. Cardiovascular causes are responsible for most syncope episodes and produce loss of consciousness by means of a drop in blood pressure, with resultant bilateral cortical or brainstem hypoperfusion. Cerebrovascular disease is an uncommon cause of syncope, unless bilateral carotid artery disease or vertebrobasilar disease is present.

Table 10-2 **Causes of Syncope**

Cause	Features
Peripheral Vascular or Circulatory	
Vasovagal syncope (neurally mediated)	Prodrome of pallor, yawning, nausea, diaphoresis; precipitated by stress or pain; occurs when patient is upright, aborted by recumbency; fall in blood pressure with or without a decrease in heart rate
Micturition syncope	Syncope with urination (probably vagal)
Post-tussive syncope	Syncope after paroxysm of coughing
Hypersensitive carotid sinus syndrome	Vasodepressor and/or cardioinhibitory responses with light carotid sinus massage (see text)
Drugs	Orthostasis
	Occurs with antihypertensive drugs, tricyclic antidepressants, phenothiazines
Volume depletion	Orthostasis
	Occurs with hemorrhage, excessive vomiting or diarrhea, Addison disease
Autonomic dysfunction	Orthostasis
	Occurs in diabetes, alcoholism, Parkinson disease, deconditioning after a prolonged illness
Central Nervous System	
Cerebrovascular	Transient ischemic attacks and strokes are unusual causes of syncope; associated neurologic abnormalities are usually present
Seizures	Warning aura sometimes present, jerking of extremities, tongue biting, urinary incontinence, postictal confusion
Metabolic	
Hypoglycemia	Confusion, tachycardia, jitteriness before syncope; patient may be taking insulin
Cardiac	
Obstructive	Syncope is often exertional; physical findings consistent with aortic stenosis, hypertrophic obstructive cardiomyopathy, cardiac tamponade, atrial myxoma, prosthetic valve malfunction, Eisenmenger syndrome, tetralogy of Fallot, primary pulmonary hypertension, pulmonic stenosis, massive pulmonary embolism
Arrhythmias	Syncope may be sudden and occurs in any position; episodes of dizziness or palpitations; may be a history of heart disease; bradyarrhythmias or tachyarrhythmias may be responsible—check for hypersensitive carotid sinus

The most important aspect of the approach to the patient with syncope is obtaining a thorough history, both from the patient and from any witnesses to the episode. The conditions during which a syncopal episode occurs may suggest the cause. For instance, syncope that occurs on arising from a lying or sitting position suggests orthostasis. Exercise-induced syncope suggests obstructive cardiac disease, such as aortic or mitral valve stenosis or hypertrophic cardiomyopathy. Syncope during straining, coughing, or micturition is the result of Valsalva-induced decrease in venous return. A history of palpitations preceding the event suggests an arrhythmic cause. Syncope that occurs during emotional stress suggests a vasovagal episode. Certain features may suggest a noncardiac cause, including incontinence or tonic-clonic movements, which suggest seizure. Patients who suffer a cardiac syncopal episode usually regain consciousness rapidly (<5 minutes). Longer episodes of unresponsiveness suggest a noncardiac cause. Review of the patient's medications is important and may suggest drug-induced hypotension or arrhythmias as the cause of a syncopal episode.

The physical examination of a patient with syncope should include evaluation of orthostatic changes in the heart rate and blood pressure, a thorough cardiac examination to exclude significant murmurs, a neurologic examination, and carotid sinus massage when the history suggests carotid sinus sensitivity as the diagnosis. A 12-lead ECG should be obtained and may be diagnostic of the cause of syncope (e.g., complete heart block) or reveal abnormalities that warrant further evaluation (e.g., prior myocardial infarction, conduction system disease, nonsustained VT, a delta wave of WPW syndrome).

Further cardiac testing is useful in select patients. An echocardiogram is helpful in patients in whom structural heart disease or an arrhythmic cause is suspected. A 24-hour Holter monitor or an event monitor may be helpful in evaluating for possible arrhythmias. In patients with recurrent syncope without evidence of a structural or arrhythmic cause and in patients in whom the history suggests vasovagal or neurocardiogenic syncope, tilt-table testing may be useful (see earlier discussion). In patients in whom the history, ECG, or Holter monitoring suggest a tachyarrhythmia or bradyarrhythmia as the cause of syncope, EP testing is indicated (see earlier discussion). However, in patients with a normal resting ECG and no structural heart disease, the diagnostic yield of EP testing is so low that it is rarely useful. Figure 10-11 offers a diagnostic approach to the patient with syncope. Despite all these diagnostic modalities, in more than 30% of all patients with syncope, the cause remains unknown. Fortunately, these patients can be reassured of a good prognosis.

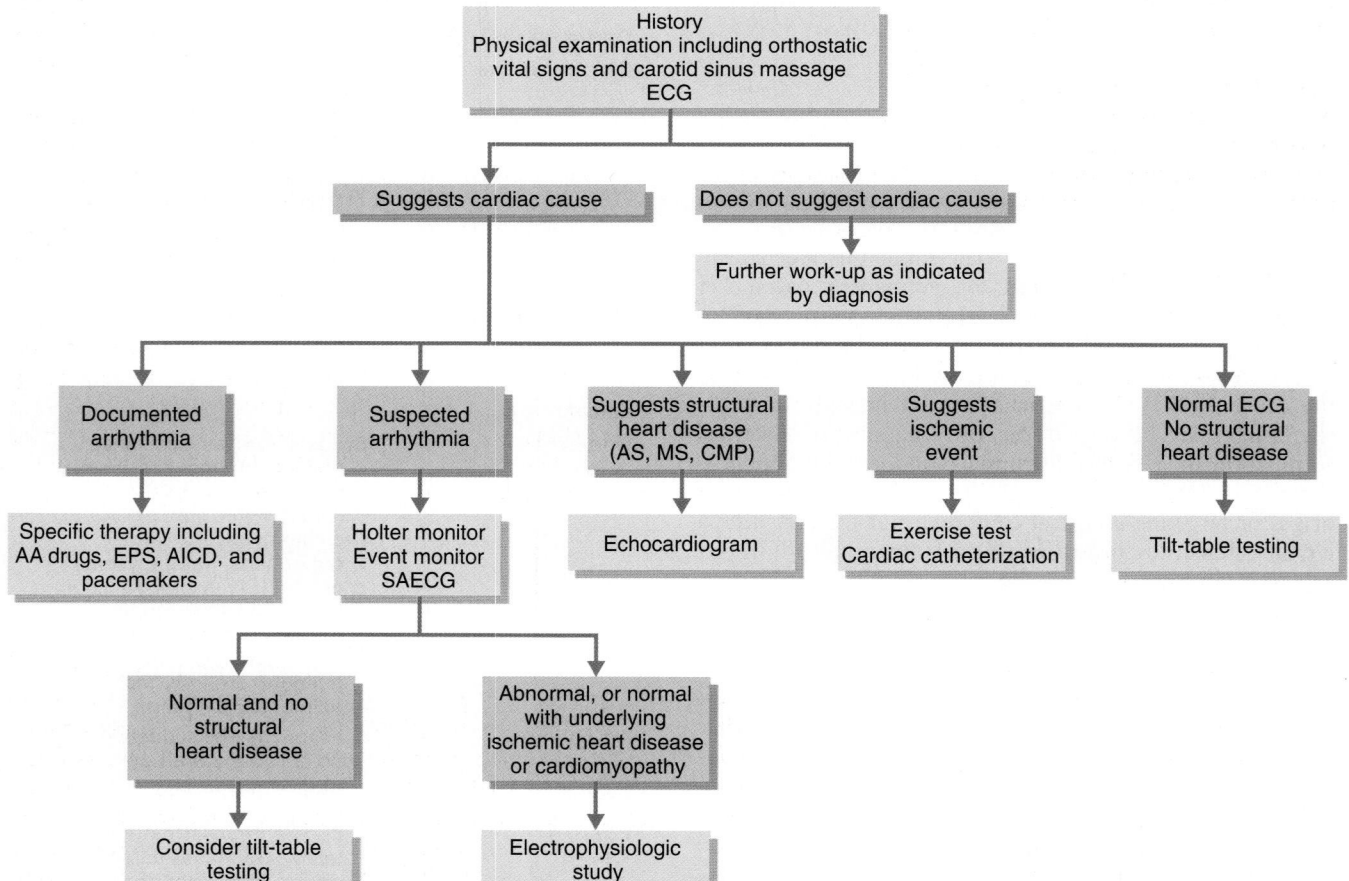

Figure 10-11 Diagnostic approach to the patient with syncope. AA, anti-arrhythmic; AICD, automatic implantable cardioverter-defibrillator; AS, aortic stenosis; CMP, cardiomyopathy; ECG, electrocardiogram; EPS, electrophysiologic study; MS, mitral stenosis; SAECG, signal-averaged ECG.

Sudden Cardiac Death

Sudden cardiac death (SCD) is commonly defined as a natural, unexpected death occurring within 1 hour of the onset of symptoms. Sudden death may be the result of a variety of cardiac and noncardiac diseases (Table 10-3), although cardiac causes are by far the most common. SCD accounts for an estimated 300,000 deaths per year—more than 50% of all deaths from cardiac causes—and is the leading cause of death among men 20 to 60 years old. Ventricular tachyarrhythmias (VT and VF) occurring in the setting of ischemic heart disease account for the mechanism of death in most of these patients. Polymorphic VT occurring in the setting of LTQS (see later discussion), short QT syndrome (see later discussion), Brugada syndrome (see later discussion), and hypertrophic cardiomyopathy are also common causes of SCD, particularly in young patients. VT in the absence of underlying heart disease and rapid conduction of AF or AFL over an accessory bypass tract precipitating VT or VF account for other tachyarrhythmic causes of SCD. Bradyarrhythmias and pulseless electrical activity, a condition during which the electrical activity of the heart continues in the absence of mechanical contraction, account for only a small proportion of SCD.

Ischemic heart disease is present in at least 80% of patients who die suddenly of a cardiac cause, and as many as 75% of these patients have a prior history of a MI (Table 10-4). In the remainder, SCD is their first manifestation of ischemic heart disease. Nonetheless, only 20% of patients resuscitated from an episode of SCD have evidence of having had an acute transmural MI at the time of the event. This circumstance is of prognostic importance; survivors of SCD that occurred in the setting of an acute MI have a recurrence rate of less than 5% in the following year, compared with a 30% recurrence rate in survivors in whom SCD occurred in the absence of an acute infarction.

Table 10-3 Causes of Sudden Cardiac Death

Noncardiac

Central nervous system hemorrhage
Massive pulmonary embolus
Drug overdose
Hypoxia secondary to lung disease
Aortic dissection or rupture

Cardiac

Ventricular fibrillation
Myocardial ischemia/injury
Long QT syndrome
Short QT syndrome
Brugada syndrome
Arrhythmogenic right ventricular dysplasia
Ventricular tachycardia
Bradyarrhythmias, sick sinus syndrome
Aortic stenosis
Tetralogy of Fallot
Pericardial tamponade
Cardiac tumors
Complications of infective endocarditis
Hypertrophic cardiomyopathy (arrhythmia or obstruction)
Myocardial ischemia
Atherosclerosis
Prinzmetal angina
Kawasaki arteritis

Table 10-4 Predictors of Sudden Cardiac Death after Myocardial Infarction

Decreased left ventricular ejection fraction
Residual ischemia
Complex ventricular ectopy (nonsustained ventricular tachycardia) on ambulatory ECG monitoring
Late potentials on signal-averaged ECG
Decreased heart rate variability
Prolonged QT on ECG
Induction of sustained monomorphic ventricular tachycardia with programmed electrical stimulation

ECG, electrocardiogram.

The only effective treatment of an acute episode of SCD is immediate circulatory support with cardiopulmonary resuscitation and establishment of an effective cardiac rhythm with electrical defibrillation. Once a stable rhythm has been restored, intravenous anti-arrhythmic therapy, usually with amiodarone, should be instituted for the first 24 hours while determination of the precipitating cause is made. That VT or VF was the mechanism of SCD cannot be assumed, unless these rhythms were documented at the time of arrest. A thorough search for other possible causes is mandatory. In SCD survivors, a full cardiac evaluation should be performed to define cardiac function, identify the presence of reversible heart disease, and assess the risk for recurrent arrhythmias. Echocardiography can identify possible structural cardiac causes of SCD (e.g., aortic stenosis, hypertrophic cardiomyopathy) and allows assessment of left ventricular function. This identification is important prognostically; patients with depressed ventricular function have a higher likelihood of recurrent SCD, a poorer response to anti-arrhythmic drug therapy, and a higher mortality rate than do those with normal ventricular function. Ambulatory ECG monitoring and stress testing are useful in documenting the frequency and severity of recurrent ventricular arrhythmias and in assessing for residual ischemia.

Patients in whom acute MI precipitates SCD do not require anti-arrhythmic therapy. Cardiac catheterization and revascularization should be performed if possible. In SCD survivors in whom the event occurred in the absence of an acute MI, and in patients with recurrent ventricular tachyarrhythmias, the implantation of an ICD has been the mainstay of treatment.

Management of Cardiac Arrhythmias

When initiating treatment of an arrhythmia, several clinical factors should be considered, including the nature of the specific arrhythmia, the setting in which the arrhythmia occurred, the consequences of the arrhythmia, and the potential risks of therapy. Certain arrhythmias (e.g., VT) can cause hemodynamic instability or SCD and warrant aggressive treatment to prevent recurrences. Other arrhythmias are hemodynamically stable but produce intolerable symptoms (e.g., palpitations, dizziness) and should be similarly suppressed. Certain arrhythmias may not be a problem acutely but warrant treatment to prevent long-term complications (e.g., stroke prevention in AF). The situation in which an arrhythmia occurs may dictate the need for therapy. For example, VF occurring in the setting of an acute MI is unlikely to recur if the underlying ischemic process is treated and warrants no specific therapy for the arrhythmia itself. Conversely, VF occurring in the absence of acute ischemia is likely to recur and requires aggressive therapy. Arrhythmias that are tolerated well and require no therapy in patients with structurally normal hearts may not be tolerated at all in patients with depressed left ventricular systolic function or valvular heart disease and may require aggressive therapy in these settings. Some arrhythmias are secondary to an underlying disease process. Metabolic abnormalities (e.g., hypokalemia, hypomagnesemia, hypoxia, hyperthyroidism) and acute illness (e.g., congestive heart failure, sepsis, anemia) may precipitate arrhythmias, as may emotional upset, certain foods or beverages (e.g., caffeine-containing products, alcohol), and both prescription (e.g., digoxin, theophylline, anti-arrhythmic agents) and nonprescription (e.g., decongestants, certain antibiotics, cocaine) drugs. Although treatment of arrhythmias associated with these factors may be warranted acutely, long-term therapy is not required, provided that the inciting factor is removed or controlled.

Asymptomatic arrhythmias are difficult clinical problems. Ventricular premature contractions and nonsustained VT may be markers of underlying heart disease and, although benign themselves, may progress to more malignant arrhythmias. Treatment with anti-arrhythmic medications in these instances has not been shown to decrease mortality, and, in fact, some agents are associated with increased mortality because of their pro-arrhythmic side effects. The presence of symptoms is clearly important in deciding whether to treat an arrhythmia. In patients who are asymptomatic, the risks of the arrhythmia must be compared with the risks of therapy before instituting an anti-arrhythmic agent.

Pharmacologic Therapy

Anti-arrhythmic medications work by interfering with various aspects of myocardial depolarization or repolarization and can be classified based on their particular mechanism of action. The most frequently used classification system is the Vaughn Williams classification, which categorizes these drugs based on their in vitro EP effects on normal Purkinje fibers (Table 10-5). This classification is a helpful construct; however, several limitations to its interpretation and use exist. First, whether the in vivo effects of a drug in a specific class are the same as those seen in vitro is unclear. Second, a given drug may have properties of more than one class. Third, drugs in the same class may differ somewhat in their modes of action, side-effect profile, and clinical effectiveness for treating a given arrhythmia. Nonetheless, the classification remains a useful communication tool.

Several general points are worth noting in the management with anti-arrhythmic agents. Many drugs are given as a standard dose, whereas others are titrated, depending on clinical effect. Therapeutic blood levels of many drugs have been established; however, the absolute concentration of the agent in the patient's blood is a much less useful guide to therapy than is the clinical effectiveness of the drug and the

Table 10-5 **Vaughn Williams Classification of Anti-arrhythmic Drugs**		
Class	**Physiologic Effect***	**Examples**
I	Blocks sodium channels; predominantly reduces the maximum velocity of the upstroke of the action potential (phase 0)	—
IA	Intermediate potency blockade	Quinidine, procainamide, disopyramide
IB	Least potent blockade	Lidocaine, tocainide, mexiletine, phenytoin
IC	Most potent blockade	Flecainide, propafenone, moricizine
II	β-Adrenergic receptor blockade	Propranolol, metoprolol, atenolol
III	Potassium channel blockade: predominantly prolongs action potential duration	Amiodarone, sotalol, bretylium, ibutilide, dofetilide
IV	Calcium channel blockade	Verapamil, diltiazem

*Several agents have physiologic effects characteristic of more than one class.

presence or absence of side effects. The therapeutic-to-toxic ratio of most anti-arrhythmic agents is small such that, at therapeutically effective doses, toxic side effects are common. Knowledge of the metabolism of these agents is important. Either the kidney or the liver metabolizes most anti-arrhythmic drugs (Table 10-6), and doses must be decreased in patients with renal or hepatic dysfunction to avoid toxicity. Many of these agents have negative inotropic effects, and, even at nontoxic levels, noncardiac side effects are common. These drugs frequently interact with other medications and may interfere with nonpharmacologic modes of therapy. For example, quinidine and amiodarone increase the serum digoxin level and augment the anticoagulant effect of warfarin. Flecainide and propafenone increase the amount of energy required for an artificial pacemaker to pace the heart effectively (pacing threshold), whereas amiodarone increases the amount of energy required to defibrillate the heart effectively (defibrillation threshold). For this reason, artificial pacemakers and ICDs need to be checked after instituting anti-arrhythmic agents.

Table 10-6 and Table 10-7 summarize the important characteristics of the most commonly used anti-arrhythmic agents. An in-depth discussion of each agent is beyond the scope of this chapter; however, several points warrant specific mention.

CLASS I ANTIARRHYTHMIC AGENTS

Class IA agents block sodium channels to a moderate degree and are useful for the long-term oral treatment of both supraventricular and ventricular arrhythmias. Procainamide is also available in an intravenous preparation and is useful for the acute management of these arrhythmias. These agents prolong the conduction time and the ERP of most cardiac tissues, including accessory pathways, and may be

Table 10-6 Select Characteristics of Anti-arrhythmic Drugs

Drug	Effect on Surface ECG	Effect on LV Function	Important Drug Interactions	Effect on Pacing and Defibrillation Thresholds	Major Route of Elimination
Quinidine	Prolongs QRS and QT	Negative inotropic effect	Increases digoxin level and warfarin effect Cimetidine increases quinidine level Phenobarbital, phenytoin, and rifampin decrease quinidine level	Increases PT and DT at high doses	Liver and kidney
Procainamide	Prolongs PR, QRS, and QT	Negative inotrope	Cimetidine, alcohol, and amiodarone increase procainamide level	Increases PT at high doses	Liver and kidney
Disopyramide	Prolongs QRS and QT	Negative inotrope	Phenobarbital, phenytoin, and rifampin all decrease disopyramide level	Increases PT at high doses	Liver and kidney
Lidocaine	Shortens QT	None	Propranolol, metoprolol, and cimetidine all increase lidocaine level	Increases DT	Liver
Mexiletine	Shortens QT	None	Increases theophylline level Phenobarbital, phenytoin, and rifampin all decrease mexiletine level	Variable effects	Liver
Flecainide	Prolongs PR and QRS	Negative inotrope	Increases digoxin level	Increases PT; variable effect on DT	Liver and kidney
Propafenone	Prolongs PR and QRS	Negative inotrope	Increases digoxin, theophylline, and cyclosporine levels; increases warfarin effect Phenobarbital, phenytoin, and rifampin decrease propafenone level Cimetidine and quinidine increase propafenone level	Increases PT; variable effect on DT	Liver
Moricizine	Prolongs PR and QRS	Negative inotrope	Decreases theophylline level Cimetidine increases moricizine level	—	Liver
Amiodarone	Prolongs PR and QT; slows sinus rate	None	Increases digoxin and cyclosporine levels; increases warfarin effect	Increases DT	Liver
Sotalol	Prolongs PR and QT; slows sinus rate	Negative inotrope	Additive effects with other β blockers	Decreases DT	Kidney
Bretylium	Prolongs PR and QT	None	—	—	Kidney
Ibutilide	Prolongs PR and QT	None	—	Decreases DT	Liver
Dofetilide	Prolongs QT	None	Verapamil, diltiazem, cimetidine, and ketoconazole all increase dofetilide level	Decreases DT	Liver and kidney

DT, defibrillation threshold; ECG, electrocardiogram; LV, left ventricle; PT, pacing threshold.

effective therapy for patients with AVNRT or AVRT. Because these agents slow the spontaneous sinoatrial rate and can enhance conduction through the AV node through vagolytic effects, they can induce more rapid ventricular rates in patients with AF and AFL. Therefore, care must be taken to ensure that the ventricular rate is controlled with a β blocker, calcium channel blocker, or digoxin before instituting a class IA agent in patients with atrial arrhythmias. Owing to its α-adrenergic blocking effects, quinidine may cause significant hypotension and may also produce syncope in 0.5% to 2% of patients as a result of QT prolongation and subse-

quent polymorphic VT. This pro-arrhythmic effect may also be seen with the other agents in this class. Between 60% and 70% of patients who receive procainamide develop antinuclear antibodies (specifically antihistone antibodies), whereas a clinical lupus-like syndrome occurs in only 20% to 30%; this rate is reversible on stopping the drug. Disopyramide has significant negative inotropic effects and should be used with extreme caution (if at all) in patients with left ventricular dysfunction.

Class IB agents are weak sodium channel blockers. They are useful for treating ventricular tachyarrhythmias, but,

Table 10-7　Common Side Effects of Select Anti-arrhythmic Drugs

Drug	Major Side Effects
Quinidine	Nausea, diarrhea, abdominal cramping
	Cinchonism: decreased hearing, tinnitus, blurred vision, delirium
	Rash, thrombocytopenia, hemolytic anemia
	Hypotension, torsades de pointes, quinidine syncope
Procainamide	Drug-induced lupus syndrome
	Nausea, vomiting
	Rash, fever, hypotension, psychosis, agranulocytosis
	Torsades de pointes
Disopyramide	Anticholinergic: dry mouth, blurred vision, constipation, urinary retention, closed-angle glaucoma
	Hypotension, worsening heart failure
Lidocaine	CNS: dizziness, peri-oral numbness, paresthesias, altered consciousness, coma, seizures
Mexiletine	Nausea, vomiting
	CNS: dizziness, tremor, paresthesias, ataxia, confusion
Flecainide	CNS: blurred vision, headache, ataxia
	Congestive heart failure, ventricular pro-arrhythmia
Propafenone	Nausea, vomiting, constipation, metallic taste to food
	Dizziness, headache, exacerbation of asthma, ventricular pro-arrhythmia
Moricizine	Nausea, dizziness, headache
β Blockers	Bronchospasm, bradycardia, fatigue, depression, impotence
	Congestive heart failure
Calcium channel blockers	Congestive heart failure, bradycardia, heart block, constipation
Amiodarone	Agranulocytosis, pulmonary fibrosis, hepatopathy, hyperthyroidism or hypothyroidism, corneal micro-deposits, bluish discoloration of the skin, nausea, constipation, bradycardia
Sotalol	Same as β blockers, torsades de pointes
Bretylium	Orthostatic hypotension
	Transient hypertension, tachycardia, and worsening of arrhythmia (initial catecholamine release)
Ibutilide	Torsades de pointes
Dofetilide	Torsades de pointes, headache, dizziness, diarrhea

CNS, central nervous system.

because they have minimal effects on the sinus or AV nodes, they are not effective for supraventricular arrhythmias. Lidocaine is the most clinically useful drug in this class and is the initial intravenous drug of choice in patients with ventricular tachyarrhythmias. Lidocaine appears particularly effective in ischemia-related arrhythmias; however, its prophylactic use during an acute infarction is not indicated and may increase mortality. Phenytoin is a potent anti-epileptic that also has

class IB anti-arrhythmic properties. It is particularly effective in treating atrial and ventricular arrhythmias caused by digoxin toxicity. These agents have relatively little effect on hemodynamics, and clinically important pro-arrhythmia is rare.

Class IC agents are potent blockers of sodium channels. They are effective therapy for both ventricular and supraventricular arrhythmias; however, the use of flecainide and moricizine to treat asymptomatic ventricular arrhythmias after MI has been proved to increase mortality, especially in patients with left ventricular dysfunction. Flecainide remains an effective and relatively safe therapy for supraventricular arrhythmias (especially paroxysmal AF) in patients with structurally normal hearts. Propafenone is similar to flecainide but with β-blocking effects and therefore may exacerbate bradycardia, heart block, heart failure, and bronchospasm. Both drugs can convert AF to AFL (class IC AFL), which usually conducts at faster rates. Therefore, similar to class IA agents, class IC agents should only be used after the initiation of an AV-nodal agent (β blockers, calcium channel blockers, digoxin) when treating patients with atrial arrhythmias.

CLASS II AND IV ANTIARRHYTHMIC AGENTS

The β blockers and *nondihydropyridine calcium channel blockers* constitute *class II* and *class IV* anti-arrhythmic agents, respectively. The anti-arrhythmic effectiveness of these drugs relates mainly to their ability to slow the rate of the sinus node and decrease conduction through the AV node. They are effective for controlling the rate of AF and AFL, although they are not effective for converting these arrhythmias to normal sinus rhythm. Intravenous administration of these agents may acutely terminate some supraventricular tachyarrhythmias, especially reentrant rhythms that use the AV node as one limb of the reentrant circuit (i.e., AVNRT, AVRT). By virtue of their ability to slow conduction in the AV node selectively, these agents may facilitate conduction down a bypass tract and are contraindicated in patients with WPW syndrome and atrial tachyarrhythmias. These agents also have a negative inotropic effect and thus must be used with caution in patients with left ventricular dysfunction or overt heart failure.

CLASS III ANTIARRHYTHMIC AGENTS

Amiodarone

Amiodarone is mainly a class III agent but has physiologic effects of all four classes. Similar to other class III anti-arrhythmic drugs, it prolongs the action potential duration. It is an effective therapy for a wide range of both supraventricular and ventricular arrhythmias and is safe to use in patients with left ventricular dysfunction. Amiodarone is the drug of choice for the treatment of AF in patients with heart failure and may decrease arrhythmic death after MI and in patients with nonischemic cardiomyopathy. It is more effective than other antiarrhythmic agents in preventing recurrences of VT or VF and is the drug of choice for treating these arrhythmias in the setting of cardiac arrest. In addition, amiodarone may be administered intravenously for the acute treatment of refractory ventricular tachyarrhythmias. Its use has been somewhat limited by the fear of significant side effects; however, with maintenance doses of less than 300 mg/day, adverse effects are less common.

Drug Interactions

Before using amiodarone, it is important to make sure the patient is not taking other medicines that may interact with this drug. The effect of warfarin is increased with amiodarone, necessitating a reduction in the dosage. Similarly, the side effects of β blockers and calcium channel blockers are increased, often leading to bradycardia and AV block. The concomitant use of most antiarrhythmic agents is prohibited because of the risk for serious side effects, including malignant ventricular arrhythmias and bradycardia. Amiodarone stays in the body for weeks or months after drug discontinuation. Therefore, drug interactions should be monitored even after stopping the medication for at least few weeks.

Side Effects

Adverse effects are common, with prevalence as high as 15% in the first year and 50% during long-term use. Fortunately, many of these adverse effects are manageable, and the need to discontinue amiodarone therapy is relatively low, occurring in less than 20% of patients. The most serious side effect is pulmonary fibrosis, which shows as an interstitial pattern on chest radiographs and a restrictive pattern on pulmonary function tests. When this occurs, immediate discontinuation of the drug is recommended. Cases of optic neuropathy and optic neuritis, usually resulting in visual impairment, have been reported in patients treated with amiodarone. In some cases, visual impairment has progressed to permanent blindness. Optic neuropathy or neuritis may occur at any time following initiation of therapy. Although a causal relationship to the drug has not been clearly established, the presence of any visual impairment warrants prompt ophthalmic examination. Appearance of optic neuropathy or neuritis calls for re-evaluation of amiodarone therapy and frequently drug discontinuation. Elevations of hepatic enzyme levels are seen frequently in patients exposed to amiodarone and in most cases are asymptomatic. If the increase exceeds 3 times normal, or doubles in a patient with an elevated baseline, discontinuation of amiodarone or dosage reduction should be considered. Excess sinus bradycardia and AV block are also serious cardiovascular adverse effects, particularly when combined with class II and IV agents. Thyroid function abnormalities are relatively common; however, they are rarely a cause for drug discontinuation. Finally, long-term exposure may cause blue-gray discoloration of the skin, particularly the face and hands. This effect is not harmful and usually reverses after the medicine is stopped. Avoiding prolonged exposure to the sun may help to prevent this effect. A more comprehensive list of the potential side effects is available in Table 10-7.

Monitoring and Follow-Up

Initial assessment of patients started on amiodarone therapy should occur every 3 to 6 months for the first year and every 6 months thereafter. Patients receiving amiodarone therapy should have liver and thyroid function tests performed at baseline and every 6 months. They also need to have a chest radiograph and pulmonary function tests at baseline and every year. High-resolution CT scan is indicated if there is a clinical suspicion of pulmonary toxicity. Similarly, ophthalmologic evaluation is indicated if visual symptoms develop.

Sotalol, Ibutilide, Dofetilide, and Bretylium

Sotalol has both class III and β-blocking effects. It is particularly effective for treating ventricular tachyarrhythmias, but it is also effective for a large number of supraventricular arrhythmias, including AF. *Ibutilide* is a parenteral class III agent that is effective for the acute termination of AF and AFL of recent onset (<90 days), and it enhances the success of electrical cardioversion of this arrhythmia. *Dofetilide* is a pure class III agent that is effective for the treatment of atrial arrhythmias; it is especially effective for the termination and prevention of AF and AFL. Dofetilide has no demonstrable negative inotropic effect, is more effective than sotalol for the acute conversion of AF, and is not associated with the risk for pulmonary and hepatic toxicity that is seen with amiodarone. At initiation, patients are routinely monitored for prolongation of the QT intervals and the increased risk for torsades de pointes. The incidence of this arrhythmia is low in patients given amiodarone but is as high as 2% and 5% in patients with impaired ventricular function who are given dofetilide or ibutilide, respectively. *Bretylium* causes an initial release of norepinephrine from nerve terminals and may result in transient hypertension and aggravation of arrhythmias. It subsequently prevents norepinephrine release and thus prevents arrhythmia recurrence. Bretylium is administered intravenously and is indicated for treating life-threatening ventricular tachyarrhythmias when other agents have failed.

Other Antiarrhythmic Agents

Several other anti-arrhythmic agents that do not fit into the Vaughn Williams classification are worthy of mention. *Adenosine* is an endogenous nucleoside that, when given intravenously in pharmacologic doses, results in profound, albeit transient, slowing of AV conduction and sinus node discharge rate. Flushing, chest pain, and dyspnea commonly occur after adenosine injection but are short lived because of the short half-life of this agent (about 6 seconds). The main use of adenosine is in the treatment of SVT; it terminates more than 95% of AVNRTs and AVRTs. During rapid atrial tachyarrhythmias, transient adenosine-induced heart block may help unmask the underlying rhythm. Theophylline blocks the effects of adenosine, and dipyridamole potentiates its effects. *Atropine* blocks the effects of the vagus nerve on the heart and results in an increased sinus rate and increased conduction through the AV node. It is indicated for the treatment of symptomatic bradycardia. *Digoxin* enhances vagal tone and results in slowing of the sinus node rate and conduction through the AV node. It is useful for controlling the ventricular response to a SVT when combined with a β blocker or a calcium channel blocker.

Nonpharmacologic Therapy of Bradyarrhythmias

CARDIAC PACEMAKERS

Artificial cardiac pacemakers are devices that deliver a small electrical impulse to a localized region of the heart, causing the affected myocytes to depolarize to the threshold potential, thus initiating an action potential that then spreads to the remainder of the heart. These devices can be used temporarily to treat a transient bradyarrhythmia resulting from a reversible cause, or they can be implanted permanently to treat irreversible disorders of impulse formation or conduction that result in recurrent or persistent bradyarrhythmias. Temporary pacemakers can deliver the electrical impulse indirectly through the chest wall (transcutaneous pacing), or they can be placed intravenously into the right side of the heart to deliver the impulse locally (transvenous pacing). Transcutaneous pacing requires higher energy to *capture* the heart electrically and therefore can be somewhat uncomfortable. In addition, some patients, especially obese individuals, cannot be effectively paced transcutaneously. Nonetheless, this type of pacemaker can be an effective mode of pacing in most patients, may help stabilize a patient who has an unstable bradyarrhythmia until a transvenous or permanent pacemaker can be inserted, and is useful to have as prophylaxis for acutely ill patients who are at high risk for developing significant bradyarrhythmias. Permanent pacemakers are usually inserted intravenously. The pulse generator is buried in a *pocket* created in the pectoral region of the chest wall, and the leads pass from the generator through the cephalic, axillary, or subclavian vein and into the right atrium or ventricle where they are anchored in place. Indications for permanent pacemaker insertion are listed in Table 10-8.

Current pacemakers allow for the tailoring of the pacemaker function to the specific needs of the patient. A code has been developed that describes these various functions. The first letter reflects the cardiac chamber being paced (V, ventricle; A, atrium; D, dual chamber—atrium and ventricle). The second letter reflects the chamber in which electrical activity is being sensed (V, ventricle; A, atrium; D, dual chamber—atrium and ventricle; O, none). The third letter reflects the response mode of the pacemaker. If the pacemaker senses the patient's own native beat, it may respond by being inhibited (I), triggered to fire (T), or triggered to fire after a sensed atrial event but inhibited by a sensed ventricular event (D). Newer pacemakers are also capable of sensing a patient's activity level (through temperature, vibration, or respiratory sensors) and changing their paced rate in response to a sensed increase in metabolic need. This mode is termed a *rate-responsive* mode and is indicated by an *R* after the first three letters. Examples of common pacing modes are listed in Table 10-9.

The choice of pacing mode depends on the needs of the individual patient. Dual-chamber pacing maintains AV synchrony, which is an advantage because the timing of atrial contraction is important for maximizing cardiac output. Therefore, AV synchronous pacing is useful for patients with left ventricular dysfunction in whom loss of AV synchrony may result in the precipitation of heart

Table 10-8 **Indications for Pacemaker Insertion**	
Pacing is definitely indicated.	Acquired third-degree AVB with or without symptoms* Congenital third-degree AVB with symptoms Mobitz I (Wenckebach) second-degree AVB with symptomatic bradycardia Mobitz II second-degree AVB with or without symptomatic bradycardia Sinus bradycardia (heart rate < 40 beats/minute) with symptoms Alternating bundle branch block
Pacing is probably indicated.	Congenital AVB with moderate bradycardia Bifascicular block (RBBB + LAFB or RBBB + LPFB) with a history of syncope after ruling out other causes Incidental finding of significant His-Purkinje disease during invasive cardiac electrophysiologic evaluation Transient third-degree AVB or Mobitz II second-degree heart block after an AMI Neurocardiogenic syncope with a positive tilt-table test
Pacing is not indicated.	Asymptomatic sinus bradycardia Asymptomatic sinus node dysfunction Bradycardia during sleep First-degree AVB Asymptomatic Mobitz I (Wenckebach) second-degree AVB Transient asymptomatic pause during atrial fibrillation Asymptomatic, >3-second pause with CSM Recurrent syncope of undetermined cause

AMI, acute myocardial infarction; AVB, atrioventricular block; CSM, carotid sinus massage; LAFB, left anterior fascicular block; LBBB, left bundle branch block; LPFB, left posterior fascicular block; RBBB, right bundle branch block.
*Symptoms include syncope, dizziness, confusion, congestive heart failure, and decreased exercise tolerance.

failure. For patients who have structurally normal hearts or who have a pacemaker implanted for only occasional symptomatic bradyarrhythmias, maintaining AV synchrony is not as important, and a single ventricular pacing electrode is sufficient. In patients with chronic AF, AV synchrony is not possible, and a single ventricular pacing electrode is also adequate.

Safeguards have been programmed into the pacemakers that limit the upper pacing rate, thus preventing rapid ventricular pacing in response to a supraventricular tachyarrhythmia. Newer pacemakers can detect the onset of an atrial tachyarrhythmia and switch to an appropriate pacing mode (mode switching). Pacemaker malfunction may be demonstrated as failure of a pacemaker impulse to depolarize the heart (failure to capture), abnormalities of sensing (oversensing or undersensing), or pacing at an abnormal rate. Many pacemakers decrease their pacing rate or change their pacing mode as the battery life is depleted.

Table 10-9 Common Pacemaker Modes

Pacemaker Type	Code	Chamber Paced	Chamber Sensed	Mode
Ventricular asynchronous	VOO	V	None	Continuous ventricular pacing regardless of the presence of intrinsic QRS complexes
Ventricular demand	VVI	V	V	Ventricular pacing inhibited by spontaneous QRS complexes
Atrial demand	AAI	A	A	Atrial pacing inhibited by spontaneous P waves
Atrial synchronous, ventricular inhibited	VDD	V	AV	Ventricular pacing follows a sensed P wave after a preset AV delay; ventricular pacing inhibited by spontaneous QRS complexes; no atrial pacing
AV sequential	DVI	AV	V	Ventricular pacing follows atrial pacing after a preset AV delay; ventricular and atrial pacing inhibited by spontaneous QRS; no P-wave sensing
Optimal sequential	DDD	AV	AV	Ventricular pacing follows sensed P waves or atrial pacing after a preset AV delay; ventricular pacing inhibited by spontaneous QRS complexes; atrial pacing inhibited by spontaneous P waves
Rate responsive	VVIR	V	V	Same as VVI or DDD, but pacing rate increases with physiologic demand
	DDDR	AV	AV	

A, atrial; AV, atrioventricular; V, ventricular.

Nonpharmacologic Therapy of Tachyarrhythmias

DIRECT CURRENT CARDIOVERSION AND DEFIBRILLATION

Direct current cardioversion and electrical defibrillation are effective methods for treating atrial or ventricular tachyarrhythmias and are the methods of choice for terminating hemodynamically unstable tachyarrhythmias, as well as stable tachyarrhythmias that are refractory to pharmacologic therapy. Cardioversion refers to the synchronized application of an electrical shock to the heart in an attempt to terminate a tachyarrhythmia. Synchronization of the shock to the QRS complex is a critical feature because the inadvertent administration of an electrical shock during ventricular repolarization (i.e., during the T wave) may precipitate VF. Defibrillation refers to the asynchronous delivery of an electrical shock to terminate VF. Synchronization in this setting is not possible because no organized ventricular activity (QRS) occurs during VF.

Small, although real, risks are inherent with electrical cardioversion. For this reason, several factors need to be addressed before elective procedures. Hyperkalemia should be excluded, as should a supratherapeutic digoxin level; cardioversion in the setting of digoxin toxicity may precipitate refractory ventricular arrhythmias. Adequate sedation is important and can usually be accomplished by the intravenous administration of benzodiazepines (e.g., midazolam) or short-acting anesthetic agents (e.g., propofol). Aspiration of gastric contents can occur because patients are unable to protect their airways during this type of sedation; therefore, patients should have fasted for at least 6 hours before the procedure. Minor cutaneous burns at the site of application of the electrical current are common, especially if multiple shocks are delivered. Even with appropriate synchronization, electrical cardioversion may precipitate VF, in which case immediate defibrillation is required. In patients with AF, systemic embolization of atrial thrombus may occur after conversion to normal sinus rhythm. Therefore, patients who are undergoing elective cardioversion of AF must be adequately anticoagulated with warfarin for at least 3 weeks before and 4 weeks after electrical cardioversion.

The electrical shock is delivered through paddles applied to the patient's chest. These shocks can be arranged either with both paddles placed on the anterior chest (one paddle at the upper sternal border and the other at the cardiac apex) or with one paddle anteriorly located over the right upper sternal border and the other posteriorly over the left interscapular region. Lubrication with electrolyte gel or the use of electrolyte pads improves contact and decreases burns. AFL can frequently be converted to normal sinus rhythm with low-energy shocks (<50 joules), whereas AF frequently requires higher energy (100 to 360 joules). VT can be cardioverted with low-energy shocks (<50 joules), but VF should always be defibrillated with high-energy shocks (200 to 360 joules). If the initial shock is not successful, the energy should be titrated up and several paddle positions tried before accepting failure. Traditional defibrillators deliver monophasic electrical impulses, whereas newer devices deliver biphasic impulses. These biphasic defibrillators require significantly reduced energy for successful arrhythmia termination and are more effective than monophasic systems. Many tachyarrhythmias recur after initially successful cardioversion. Administering an antiarrhythmic agent may help maintain sinus rhythm in these patients.

RADIOFREQUENCY CATHETER ABLATION, AUTOMATIC IMPLANTABLE CARDIOVERTER-DEFIBRILLATORS, AND SURGICAL THERAPY

Radiofrequency Catheter Ablation

Because of the frequent recurrence of tachyarrhythmias despite pharmacologic therapy and the risk for pro-arrhythmia with most anti-arrhythmic agents, several non-pharmacologic approaches to the chronic management of tachyarrhythmias have been developed. Radiofrequency catheter ablation involves the application of alternating current electrical energy in the radiofrequency range to a strategically chosen area of the endocardium. An arrhythmogenic focus or the pathway by which the arrhythmia is perpetuated can be identified (mapped), and a radiofrequency-induced lesion can be created at that site, thereby eliminating (i.e., ablating) the arrhythmia. Ablation is effective in eliminating AFL and supraventricular tachyarrhythmias caused by accessory pathways (e.g., WPW syndrome) and dual pathways in the AV node such as AVNRT. The success rate of this procedure in curing these arrhythmias is greater than 95%. In addition, radiofrequency ablation is effective in treating AF, although the success rate is less with this arrhythmia. Ablation is associated with a relatively low risk for complications that include tamponade, stroke, and inadvertent complete AV block in up to 2% of patients, depending on the site of ablation. In patients with AF or AFL that is refractory to pharmacologic rate control, production of iatrogenic complete heart block by ablation of the AV node and subsequent placement of a permanent ventricular pacemaker offers a definitive method of controlling the ventricular rate. Catheter ablation of VT is more difficult than it is for SVT but can be effective in select patients. Patients with monomorphic VT in the absence of structural heart disease (e.g., RVOT-VT and idiopathic left VT) and patients with bundle branch reentry VT are good candidates, and success can be expected in about 90% of these instances. VT related to prior MI is difficult to treat with ablation, and such therapy should be attempted only if affected patients have incessant or recurrent VT despite anti-arrhythmic therapy.

Automatic Implantable Cardioverter-Defibrillators

ICD therapy is the anti-tachycardic equivalent of a pacemaker and is used for treating ventricular tachyarrhythmias. Similar to the pacemaker, the ICD has a generator that is buried in the pectoral region and is connected to an electrode that is placed transvenously and anchored to the endocardium. The device monitors heart rate and identifies a tachyarrhythmia as any rhythm that is faster than the rate programmed into the device. Most ICDs have several possible therapeutic responses to a sensed tachyarrhythmic event. Pacing the ventricle at a faster rate (antitachycardia pacing) may successfully terminate a relatively slow VT. If this level is not successful, the device may then deliver a 20- to 36-joule electrical discharge, which may be repeated several times at escalating energy levels in an attempt to terminate the tachyarrhythmia. Fast VT and VF are usually treated with high-energy shock, although painless antitachycardia pacing has been used with some success in treating fast VT. All current devices also have pacemaker capabilities in the event of a bradyarrhythmia.

Implantable Cardioverter-Defibrillator Indications for Secondary Prevention

ICDs have been shown to decrease mortality compared with anti-arrhythmic therapy in survivors of VF or hemodynamically unstable VT. Trials during the 1990s suggested that sotalol and amiodarone are effective anti-arrhythmic drugs in the treatment of patients with SCD or recurrent VT. Several secondary prevention trials including the Antiarrhythmics Versus Implantable Defibrillators (AVID) trial significantly changed the therapeutic approach to SCD survivors. This study was a randomized trial of anti-arrhythmic therapy (primarily amiodarone) versus ICD implantation in patients with depressed ventricular function who had survived an episode of life-threatening ventricular tachyarrhythmia, and it demonstrated a mortality benefit with ICD therapy. Therefore, in SCD survivors in whom the event occurred in the absence of an acute MI or a reversible cause, and in patients with hemodynamically unstable VT, the implantation of an ICD is indicated.

Implantable Cardioverter-Defibrillator Indications for Primary Prevention

Perhaps the most effective method of treating SCD is by identifying patients at highest risk and instituting therapy aimed at preventing its occurrence. In the patient who has had an MI, several factors have been shown to be associated with an increased risk for SCD (see Table 10-4). The occurrence of frequent complex ventricular ectopy in patients after an acute MI is associated with a near tripling of the risk for subsequent SCD; however, attempts at suppression of these arrhythmias with anti-arrhythmic agents have resulted in an increased mortality. Several studies have, however, demonstrated a decrease in overall mortality, as well as in SCD, in patients treated with β-blocking agents after a MI. Therefore, these agents should be instituted in these patients unless a contraindication to their use exists. Patients who have had an MI with moderate left ventricular dysfunction, nonsustained VT on ambulatory ECG monitoring, and inducible monomorphic VT during EP testing have been shown to have an improved survival with ICD implantation (according to the Multicenter Unsustained Tachycardia Trial [MUSTT] and Multicenter Automatic Defibrillator Implantation Trial [MADIT]). Recently, the MADIT-II and Sudden Cardiac Death in Heart Failure Trial (SCD-HeFT) demonstrated improved survival with ICD therapy regardless of the presence of spontaneous or inducible ventricular arrhythmias. The MADIT-II trial was designed to evaluate the effect of prophylactic ICD therapy on survival in patients with prior MI and left ventricular ejection fraction of 30% or less. The trial was stopped in November 2001 because ICD therapy was shown to save lives. The SCD-HeFT trial compared ICD therapy with amiodarone and placebo in patients with ischemic or nonischemic dilated cardiomyopathy with a left ventricular ejection fraction of 35% or less, New York Heart Association Functional Classification II-III, and no history or suspicion of sustained VT or VF. Similar to the MADIT-II, ICD therapy was shown to improve all-cause mortality in this patient population. As a result of these multicenter trials, patients with moderate to severe left ventricular dysfunction should be referred for an ICD implant for primary prevention of SCD.

Surgical Therapy

Given the effectiveness of radiofrequency ablation and ICDs, surgical therapy of tachyarrhythmias is rarely necessary. Surgery is occasionally used after failed ablation in patients with accessory bypass tracts and those with recurrent or incessant VT that failed medical therapy and ablation. In addition, in patients with refractory VT in the setting of a ventricular aneurysm, surgical aneurysmectomy may eliminate the arrhythmia, with a success rate of about 70%, and improves pharmacologic control of the arrhythmia in an additional 20% of patients.

Clinical Syndromes

LONG QT SYNDROME

LQTS refers to specific congenital and acquired abnormalities of repolarization that result in prolongation of the QT interval on the surface ECG (Table 10-10). This circumstance is defined as a QTc longer than 440 minutes (QTc equals the QT interval divided by the square root of the RR interval). Acquired forms are the result of various drugs or metabolic abnormalities. At least four separate genetic mutations account for the congenital forms of this disorder and do so by alterations in potassium or sodium channels. Congenital forms may be associated with deafness (Jervell and Lange-Nielsen syndrome) or occur in isolation (Romano-Ward syndrome). The significance of the LQTS is its association with the development of a specific type of VT called *torsades de pointes*. This arrhythmia occurs in the setting of a prolonged QT interval, is usually initiated with a VPC, occurs during the susceptible period of repolarization (i.e., at the peak of the T wave), and is characterized by

Table 10-10	**Conditions Associated with Prolongation of the QT Interval**
Condition	**Examples**
Congenital	Romano-Ward syndrome (without deafness)
	Jervell and Lange-Nielsen syndrome (with deafness)
Acquired: drugs	Class IA and class III anti-arrhythmic agents
	Tricyclic antidepressants
	Phenothiazines
	Antibiotics (macrolides, pentamidine, trimethoprim-sulfamethoxazole)
	Terfenadine (especially when combined with macrolides or antifungal agents)
Metabolic	Hypokalemia
	Hypocalcemia
	Hypomagnesemia
Other	Liquid protein diets

a wide-complex tachyarrhythmia with QRS complexes of varying axis and morphology that appear to rotate around the isoelectric baseline. Frequently, these episodes are self-limited, although syncope and sudden death may occur.

The treatment of torsades de pointes differs from that of other forms of VT. Many anti-arrhythmic agents prolong the QT interval and exacerbate the arrhythmia. Intravenous magnesium (2 to 3 g) is effective in terminating this arrhythmia even in the presence of normal serum magnesium levels. Treatment with isoproterenol or temporary transvenous pacing at rates of 100 to 120 beats/minute can effectively help prevent the arrhythmia, presumably through tachycardia-induced shortening of the QT interval. Removing the inciting agent is of paramount importance in acquired cases. Chronic treatment in patients with the congenital syndromes is with β-blocker therapy at the highest doses tolerated. Chronic pacemaker or ICD implantation, or both, is indicated in patients with recurrent arrhythmia despite β-blocker therapy. Screening family members of these patients is also important to identify those at risk for this arrhythmia.

SHORT QT SYNDROME

Short QT syndrome is a new clinical entity that is associated with a high incidence SCD, AF, or both. The diagnosis is made when a patient exhibits syncope and a corrected QT interval shorter than 320 minutes. Missense mutations in *KCNH2 (HERG)* linked to a gain of function of the rapidly activating delayed-rectifier current *I(Kr)* have been identified in the first two reported families with familial SCD. In addition, two more gain-of-function mutations in the *KCNJ2* gene encoding the strong inwardly rectifying channel protein *Kir2.1* and in the *KCNQ1* gene encoding the α subunit of the *KvLQT1 (I[Ks])* channel confirmed a genetically heterogeneous disease. The treatment of choice for syncope or SCD is the implantation of an ICD. In the asymptomatic patient, the treatment remains unclear.

BRUGADA SYNDROME

Brugada syndrome is characterized by the presence of an ST-segment elevation in V_1 to V_3 that is unrelated to ischemia, structural heart disease, or electrolyte abnormalities. This syndrome has been linked to mutations in *SCN5A*, the gene encoding for the α subunit of the sodium channel. Brugada syndrome is a familial disease with an autosomal dominant mode of transmission and incomplete penetrance and is found in 5 to 66 per 10,000 persons. Unfortunately, syncope and SCD caused by rapid polymorphic VT are often the first symptoms in patients with this disease. Unlike ischemia-induced polymorphic VT, the arrhythmia in patients with Brugada syndrome often occurs during sleep. Elevated parasympathetic activity and sodium channel blockers such as procainamide and flecainide exacerbate the occurrence of ventricular arrhythmias in patients with Brugada syndrome. On the other hand, high catecholamine states, isoproterenol (Isuprel), and potassium I_{to} blockers such as quinidine are effective in suppressing ventricular arrhythmias in patients with this syndrome. Similar to other clinical syndromes associated with SCD, ICD implantation is the preferred therapy in patients with Brugada syndrome and a history of near syncope, syncope, or SCD. In the asymptomatic patient, the performance of a diagnostic EP study for further risk stratification has been suggested. In patients with inducible sustained ventricular arrhythmias, the implantation of an ICD has been shown to improve long-term outcome. In the asymptomatic patient with a negative EP study, close follow-up is usually sufficient.

Prospectus for the Future

- Identification of specific populations of patients with paroxysmal AF who benefit from pulmonary vein isolation and ablation for maintenance of sinus rhythm
- Evaluation of atrial pacing as a modality to prevent recurrences of AF
- Further clarification of which patient populations benefit from implantation of a cardioverter-defibrillator

- Programming of cardioverter-defibrillators to provide therapy before arrhythmia onset by identifying electrical characteristics that may predict impending arrhythmias (e.g., long RR intervals, R-on-T phenomenon, T-wave alternans)
- Progress on the development of genetically engineered biologic pacemakers as alternatives to mechanical pacemakers

References

American College of Cardiology/American Heart Association Task Force on Practice Guidelines: ACC/AHA/NASPE 2002 guideline update for implantation of cardiac pacemakers and antiarrhythmia devices: Summary article. Circulation 106:2145-2161, 2002.

American College of Cardiology/American Heart Association Task Force on Practice Guidelines and the European Society of Cardiology Committee for Practice Guidelines and Policy Conferences: ACC/AHA/ESC guidelines for the management of patients with atrial fibrillation: Executive summary. J Am Coll Cardiol 38:1231-1265, 2001.

Bardy GH, Lee KL, Mark DB, et al: Amiodarone or an implantable cardioverter-defibrillator for congestive heart failure. N Engl J Med 352:225-237, 2005.

Wyse DG, Waldo AL, DiMarco JP, et al: The Atrial Fibrillation Follow-up Investigation of Rhythm Management (AFFIRM) investigators: A comparison of rate control and rhythm control in patients with atrial fibrillation. N Engl J Med 347:1825-1833, 2002.

Pericardial and Myocardial Disease

Josef Stehlik and Ivor J. Benjamin

Pericardial Disease

The pericardium is a protective sac around the heart composed of two distinct layers: the *visceral* pericardium, an inner layer tightly attached to the heart muscle, and the parietal pericardium, a fibrous outer layer. The space between the two layers is called *pericardial space* and is lubricated by 5 to 15 mL of clear pericardial fluid produced by the visceral pericardium.

ACUTE PERICARDITIS

Acute pericarditis, inflammation of the visceral and parietal pericardium, can result from a number of different causes. Although a definitive cause is often not determined (and the condition is then called *idiopathic pericarditis*), viral infection is probably the most common cause. *Viral pericarditis* is usually self-limiting, although occasionally the symptoms may recur once or more before complete resolution. Although less common, pericarditis caused by bacterial infection or tuberculosis can be life-threatening. Pericardial inflammation can also result from direct pericardial injury (trauma, injury early after myocardial infarction or pericardiotomy) due to autoimmune mechanisms (late after myocardial infarction—Dressler syndrome, in connective tissue disease) or to uremia. A comprehensive list of conditions that can affect the pericardium is shown in Table 11-1.

The classic clinical presentation of pericarditis is chest pain, typically abrupt in onset, sharp, worse in supine position, and relieved by sitting upright and leaning forward. On heart auscultation, the presence of a *pericardial rub* indicates contact between two inflamed layers of the pericardium. Pericardial rub usually has a characteristic high-pitched, leathery quality, with three components that correspond to movement of the heart during the cardiac cycle (ventricular systole, early ventricular diastole, and atrial contraction; not all three components are always audible). Serial auscultation is advised because the rub may be intermittent and vary in intensity. The absence of an audible rub does not exclude the diagnosis of pericarditis. Chest pain from myocardial ischemia or pulmonary embolism may mimic pericarditis, and these conditions should be considered in the differential diagnosis.

Electrocardiogram (ECG) changes are common. During the acute phase, depression of the PR segments and diffuse ST-segment elevations are typical and result from inflammation of the myocardium adjacent to visceral pericardium. Flattening and inversion of T waves may also be present. Most of the ECG abnormalities resolve over several days to weeks, but T-wave abnormalities may persist longer. ST-segment elevations in pericarditis may be mistaken for the current of injury seen in ST-elevation myocardial infarction. In pericarditis, however, multiple leads are affected, reciprocal ST-segment depressions are not seen, and ECG changes evolve much slower than in acute myocardial infarction.

Laboratory testing in pericarditis often shows elevated erythrocyte sedimentation rate, C-reactive protein, and white blood cell count. Testing directed at excluding specific causes of pericarditis may include tuberculin skin test, evaluation of thyroid and renal function, antinuclear antibody, complement levels, rheumatoid factor, and human immunodeficiency virus (HIV) serologic testing. Viral serologic studies have been insensitive and generally do not alter the therapeutic decision. Cardiac enzymes (serum levels of creatine kinase muscle band [CK-MB], troponin) may be elevated as a result of concomitant involvement of the myocardium. Chest radiographic and echocardiographic findings are normal unless pericardial effusion is also present.

The treatment of acute pericarditis is directed at managing the underlying cause and providing pain relief. For most patients, nonsteroidal anti-inflammatory drugs are effective in relieving the chest discomfort and facilitating the resolution of inflammation; colchicine can be an effective alternative. Glucocorticoids are used if the former therapy is not sufficiently effective. Although most cases of idiopathic and

Table 11-1 **Causes of Pericarditis**
Idiopathic
Infectious
Viral (echovirus, coxsackievirus, adenovirus, cytomegalovirus, hepatitis B virus, Ebstein-Barr virus, human immunodeficiency virus)
Bacterial (*Staphylococcus, Streptococcus*, and *Mycoplasma* species; *Borrelia burgdorferi, Haemophilus influenzae, Neisseria meningitidis*)
Mycobacterial (*Mycobacterium tuberculosis, Mycobacterium avium-intracellulare*)
Fungal (*Histoplasma* and *Coccidioides* species)
Protozoal
Immune or Inflammatory
Connective tissue disease (systemic lupus erythematosus, rheumatoid arthritis, scleroderma)
Arteritis (polyarteritis nodosa, temporal arteritis)
Late after myocardial infarction (Dressler syndrome), late postcardiotomy or thoracotomy,
Drug Induced
Procainamide, hydralazine, isoniazid, cyclosporine
Trauma or Damage to Adjacent Structures
Penetrating trauma
Acute myocardial infarction, cardiac surgery, coronary angioplasty, implantable defibrillators, pacemakers
Pneumonia
Neoplastic Disease
Primary: mesothelioma, fibrosarcoma, lipoma
Secondary (metastatic or direct extension): breast, lung, thyroid carcinoma, lymphoma, leukemia, melanoma
Radiation Induced
Miscellaneous
Uremia
Hypothyroidism
Gout

viral pericarditis are self-limited, complications include recurrences, large pericardial effusion, cardiac tamponade, and pericardial constriction. These conditions are discussed later in more detail.

PERICARDIAL EFFUSION

Pericardial effusion is an abnormal accumulation of fluid within the pericardial space. Most causes of pericarditis can result in pericardial effusion (see Table 11-1). Additional causes include hypothyroidism, *chylopericardium* (accumulation of chylous from an injured thoracic duct) and *hemopericardium* (accumulation of blood in the pericardial space). *Hemopericardium* most often results from direct trauma (thoracic injury, pacemaker placement, coronary intervention, endomyocardial biopsy), cardiac rupture after myocardial infarction, or aortic dissection communicating with the pericardial space.

Symptoms of pericardial effusion depend on its size and rate of accumulation. Effusions that accumulate slowly are initially asymptomatic; significant accumulation of pericardial fluid may result in chest pressure as well as symptoms related to compression of adjacent structures. Pressure on the phrenic nerve, recurrent laryngeal nerve, lungs, or esophagus will cause cough, hoarseness, dyspnea and dysphagia. Maybe more importantly, pericardial effusion can result in hemodynamic compromise. When accumulation is

slow, the pericardial space can accommodate up to 2 liters of fluid without a significant increase in pericardial pressure. However, a rapidly accumulating effusion, such as in hemopericardium caused by trauma, may result in severe hemodynamic compromise with the collection of as little as 100 to 200 mL of fluid (see "Cardiac Tamponade").

The physical examination in a patient with a small pericardial effusion is often normal. If the effusion is large, the apical impulse may be difficult to palpate, and the heart sounds may be muffled. On chest radiographic examination, the cardiac silhouette may be enlarged. On ECG, a large pericardial effusion will result in low voltage of QRS complexes; the amplitude of the QRS complexes may vary from beat to beat, an abnormality thought to be secondary to changes in the electrical axis resulting from the heart's swinging motion within the pericardial sac (*QRS alternans*). Echocardiography is a sensitive test for detection of pericardial effusion and provides an accurate assessment of its size, location, and hemodynamic significance. Computed tomography (CT) and magnetic resonance imaging (MRI) also detect the presence of pericardial effusion with high accuracy and may determine the cause of the pericardial effusion through evaluation of surrounding structures and enhanced myocardial tissue characterization.

Drainage of the pericardial fluid by percutaneous fine-needle aspiration (*pericardiocentesis*) can be performed for diagnostic and therapeutic reasons. In general, diagnostic pericardiocentesis is usually of low yield and should be reserved for patients with persistent (>2 weeks) pericardial effusion or suspected purulent or tuberculous pericarditis. Pericardiocentesis is usually performed in the cardiac catheterization laboratory under fluoroscopic or echocardiographic guidance. Laboratory analysis of the fluid includes hematocrit and cell count determination; glucose, protein, cholesterol and triglyceride levels; Gram stain; and cultures. Examination for acid-fast bacilli is done when tuberculous disease is suspected. Tuberculous pericarditis is also associated with elevated levels of adenosine deaminase in the fluid. When appropriate, cytologic examination to rule out malignancy is done. Elevated triglyceride level suggests a chylous effusion seen in thoracic duct injury, and a high level of cholesterol suggests hypothyroidism as the cause. When the diagnosis remains unclear after fluid analysis, a sample of the pericardium can be obtained by surgical excision. Tissue examination is especially important when an effusion results from a chronic infectious process, such as tuberculosis, because pericardial fluid alone identifies the organism only in a minority of patients. Therapeutic pericardiocentesis is performed to remove pericardial fluid in patients with effusions resulting in significant symptoms or when there is evidence of hemodynamic compromise. For patients with recurrent effusions, pericardiotomy (pericardial window) may provide a longer-term continuous drainage into the pleural or peritoneal cavity.

The treatment for asymptomatic pericardial effusions is directed at the underlying illness, and, in turn, the prognosis depends on the underlying disease.

CARDIAC TAMPONADE

Cardiac tamponade occurs when pericardial effusion causes an increase in pericardial pressure that impairs proper cardiac function. Hemodynamic compromise is a result of impaired filling of the cardiac chambers. The right atrium and right ventricle are first to be affected, and compression of left-sided chambers follows with further pericardial pressure increase. As a result, the cardiac stroke volume declines, and systemic blood pressure drops. Compensatory activation of the adrenergic system results in tachycardia and an increase in systemic vascular resistance. The amount of pericardial fluid necessary to cause tamponade depends on the rate of its accumulation. In addition, the state of intravascular volume will affect symptoms—decreased preload (e.g., in dehydration) exacerbates the hemodynamic changes, and high preload counteracts the effects of high pericardial pressures.

Fatigue, dyspnea, and lightheadedness are the main symptoms when pericardial fluid accumulates slowly. Rapid fluid accumulation leading to acute tamponade results in loss of consciousness and shock.

The classic diagnostic triad seen on physical examination includes hypotension, jugular venous distention (with absent y descent), and muffled heart sounds. Tachypnea, tachycardia, and hypotension are also present. *Pulsus paradoxus*, a decrease in the systemic systolic blood pressure of more than 10 mm Hg with inspiration, is an additional characteristic finding. Under normal conditions, intrathoracic pressures decrease during inspiration, which leads to an increase in venous blood return from the periphery and an increase of right ventricular filling. As a result, the right ventricle increases in size to accommodate the extra volume. In cardiac tamponade, the compressive effect of the pericardial fluid limits expansion of the right ventricle into the intrathoracic cavity, and instead the interventricular septum is displaced toward the left ventricle, impairing left ventricular filling. This results in lower left ventricular stroke volume and lower systemic blood pressure. In expiration, the intraventricular septum returns to midline, and systemic pressure recovers. Pulsus paradoxus is not specific for cardiac tamponade. It may occur in chronic obstructive pulmonary disease, asthma, severe congestive heart failure, pulmonary embolism, and, in some instances, constrictive pericarditis.

If the effusion is large, the chest radiographic examination may reveal an enlarged globular (flask-shaped) cardiac silhouette. The ECG may show reduced voltage and electrical alternans (see explanation under "Effusive Constrictive Pericarditis"). Echocardiography is the gold standard for noninvasive assessment and demonstrates the pericardial effusion and its hemodynamic effects: compression of the right atrium, compression of the right ventricle in diastole, increased flow into the right ventricle, leftward bulging of the interventricular septum, and decreased left ventricular filling during inspiration. The inferior vena cava is typically distended. Right-sided heart catheterization can also be used to determine the hemodynamic significance of pericardial effusion. Typically, the pressure in the atria and diastolic pressure in the ventricles are elevated and equalized in all four chambers. This pressure is equal to the elevated pericardial pressure, which can be measured with a pericardial catheter.

Cardiac tamponade is a medical emergency and requires immediate treatment. Temporizing measures include immediate initiation of intravenous hydration, which increases preload and aids in filling of the cardiac chambers. The effect of this therapy will only be temporary, however. Vasopressors may be necessary to support systemic blood pressure. The definitive treatment is pericardiocentesis, which usually leads to quick improvement of hemodynamics. If the effusion is recurrent or loculated, surgical drainage might be necessary. Treatment of the condition that leads to formation of the pericardial effusion is also necessary.

CONSTRICTIVE PERICARDITIS

Constrictive pericarditis results from scarring of the pericardium in response to various inflammatory conditions. It is characterized by a thickened, fibrotic (or calcified) pericardium that restricts diastolic filling of the heart. The disease process is often diffuse and symmetrical and results in elevated and equalized diastolic pressures in all four cardiac chambers. In contrast to pericardial tamponade, in which ventricular filling is impaired throughout diastole, early diastolic filling in constrictive pericarditis is not impaired but is slowed in mid and late diastole as the ventricles meet the resistance of the thickened pericardium.

Historically, the most common cause of pericardial constriction was tuberculous pericarditis that often leads to thickening and calcification of the pericardium. Currently, pericardial constriction is most often a sequel of nontuberculous pericarditis caused by viral infection, radiation exposure, connective tissue disorders, and thoracotomy, for example. Frequently, the exact cause will not be identified.

Symptoms of pericardial constriction are typically symptoms of right heart failure, and the onset is often insidious. Patients present with fatigue and dyspnea, abdominal pain, hepatic distension, ascites, and lower extremity swelling. On physical examination, the jugular veins are distended. Changes in intrathoracic pressure are not transmitted to the heart encased in thickened pericardium, and as a result, the jugular pressure during inspiration stays the same or increases (*Kussmaul sign*), rather than falling. There are prominent x and y descents in the jugular venous tracing. In contrast to pericardial tamponade, pulsus paradoxus is not typically present. On cardiac examination, an early diastolic sound (*pericardial knock*) that follows the aortic component of the second heart sound may be heard at the left sternal border. The pericardial knock corresponds to abrupt cessation of early, rapid diastolic filling.

Diagnosis of pericardial constriction may be difficult. Chest radiography may reveal pericardial calcification and pleural effusions. Echocardiographic examination may show thickened pericardium with reduced mobility, abnormalities of ventricular septal wall motion, and dilation of the inferior vena cava. Doppler echocardiography demonstrates abnormal flow velocities in the pulmonary and hepatic veins and an abnormal pattern of ventricular diastolic filling. CT and MRI can be used to measure pericardial thickness. MRI can also assess mobility of the pericardium and hemodynamic changes associated with constrictive pericarditis. Right-sided heart catheterization is used to confirm the diagnosis. Typical findings include prominent x and y descents in atrial tracings and elevation and equalization of atrial and ventricular diastolic pressures. The early diastolic pressure in the ventricles is normal; the early diastolic ventricular filling is rapid

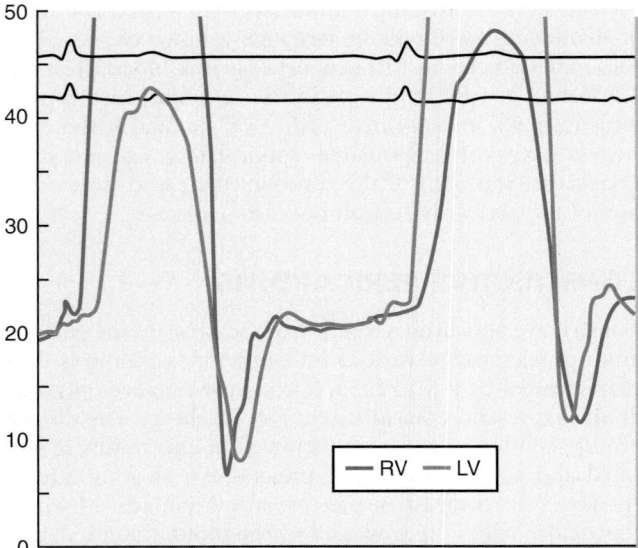

Figure 11-1 Pressure recordings in a patient with constrictive pericarditis: simultaneous right ventricular and left ventricular pressure tracings with equalization of diastolic pressure, as well as *dip-and-plateau* morphology.

owing to elevated atrial pressure, and it slows abruptly in mid and late diastole as the ventricular volume reaches the limit set by the nondistensible pericardium. This characteristic appearance of the diastolic ventricular pressure curve— low early diastolic pressure that rises quickly and plateaus in late diastole, has been called the *dip-and-plateau sign* or the *square-root sign* (Fig. 11-1). Although many of the hemodynamic findings are similar to those seen in restrictive pericarditis, in pericardial constriction, the left and right ventricular diastolic pressure tracings are nearly superimposable and do not change with volume loading or exercise.

The treatment of constrictive pericarditis consists of salt restriction and use of diuretics to control the excess volume. If symptoms cannot be controlled by medical therapy, surgical removal of the pericardium (*pericardiectomy)* is recommended. In pure pericardial constriction, pericardiectomy is effective and leads to resolution of symptoms. Some patients, especially those with radiation heart injury, may have a combination of pericardial constriction and myocardial restriction. In these patients, pericardiectomy might lead only to partial improvement.

EFFUSIVE CONSTRICTIVE PERICARDITIS

Effusive constrictive pericarditis refers to a syndrome in which there is pericardial effusion as well as abnormally tense noncompliant visceral pericardium. It may represent an intermediate stage in the development of constrictive pericarditis. The clinical features resemble those of both tamponade and constriction. Drainage of the pericardial fluid leads to drop of the intrapericardial pressure; however, features of constrictive physiology remain. Effusive constrictive pericarditis can result from pericarditis of any cause but is more commonly seen with radiation-induced pericarditis.

The diagnosis of effusive constrictive pericarditis is generally made after successful pericardiocentesis does not lead to resolution of symptoms and hemodynamic abnormalities. If constriction is confirmed, pericardectomy is the treatment of choice.

Diseases of the Myocardium

MYOCARDITIS

Myocarditis is an inflammatory process that affects the myocardium. Most cases of myocarditis are attributed to viral infection (*viral myocarditis*), but other infectious and noninfectious triggers also lead to myocardial inflammation.

Viruses most commonly associated with viral myocarditis are enteroviruses, specifically Coxsackie group B serotypes, adenoviruses, parvovirus B19, hepatitis C virus, cytomegalovirus, and HIV. The pathogenesis of viral myocarditis is believed to evolve in several phases. Initially, during the active viremia, the viruses infect the myocytes, and this is followed by cellular and antibody-mediated immune response. Although normal immune response will lead to viral clearing and myocardial healing, abnormal immune response can cause myocardial damage. This abnormal immune response leads to inflammatory cellular infiltration of the myocardium with T lymphocytes and macrophages, production of a wide range of pro-inflammatory cytokines (interleukins, tumor necrosis factor) that have negative inotropic effects, and production of autoantibodies directed against myocardial proteins. Although viral replication in the myocytes contributes to myocardial dysfunction, it is the immune response of the organism that is believed to result in the potentially permanent myocardial damage. In this last stage, which happens only in some patients, dilated cardiomyopathy and heart failure develop. The exact mechanisms of this process are not known, but it is believed that the cytokines, autoantibodies, and possibly other processes associated with persistent low-level viral replication in myocytes lead to myocyte atrophy, myocyte apoptosis, and adverse remodeling of the ventricles. It is believed that viral myocarditis accounts for more than one fifth of cases of nonischemic cardiomyopathy.

Many nonviral infectious agents also cause myocarditis. The most common bacterial infections in which myocarditis is seen are diphtheria, brucellosis, clostridial infections, legionnaires disease, meningococcal infections, streptococcal infection, and *Mycoplasma pneumoniae* infections. In many of these, the damage is attributed to the bacterial toxins, and myocardial function is expected to recover with treatment of the underlying infection. Rickettsial infections (Q fever, Rocky Mountain spotted fever), spirochetal infections (leptospirosis, Lyme disease), and fungal infections can also be complicated by myocarditis. In Central and South America, myocarditis caused by infection with protozoa *Trypanosoma cruzi* results in dilated cardiomyopathy (Chagas disease). Treatment with antiprotozoal therapy, if initiated early in the course of infection, may be beneficial; however, the myocardial damage seen in this parasitic infection is largely immune mediated.

Numerous noninfectious causes of myocarditis have also been described. Multiple chemicals and drugs can lead to myocardial inflammation by direct effect or as part of a hypersensitivity reaction. Some of the common causes include cocaine, chemotherapeutics (daunorubicin, doxorubicin), and antibiotics, among many others.

A distinct entity is *giant cell myocarditis*, which is usually associated with ventricular arrhythmias and progressive severe heart failure. The cause of this disease is not known, but it is believed to result from an autoimmune process. Multinucleated giant cells seen on myocardial biopsy are pathognomonic.

The clinical features of inflammatory myocarditis vary from asymptomatic to life-threatening presentations. The acute stage of viral myocarditis usually presents with symptoms of acute viral illness—fevers, muscle aches, fatigue. Patients usually seek medical attention once symptoms of heart failure develop, including exertion intolerance, shortness of breath, fluid retention, and persistent fatigue. In most cases, these symptoms develop several weeks after the acute viral illness has resolved. Presentation in patients with nonviral infectious myocarditis includes a combination of the primary infectious process and heart failure symptoms.

On physical examination, the patients are often tachycardic and hypotensive. Findings of heart failure—elevated jugular venous pressure, S_3 gallop, crackles, and peripheral edema, may be seen.

Elevated levels of serum cardiac enzymes (troponin, CK-MB) support the suspicion of myocardial injury in myocarditis. Testing aimed at determining the possible infectious etiology should be performed. Rising viral titers are often seen in viral myocarditis. Sinus tachycardia and nonspecific ST- and T-wave abnormalities are common ECG findings. When pericardium is also involved by the inflammatory process, diffuse ST-segment elevations typical for acute pericarditis are also seen. Ventricular ectopy is frequent, and atrioventricular conduction defects are seen in myocarditis associated with Lyme disease. Echocardiography will determine the presence of ventricular remodeling, including increasing chamber size and presence of ventricular systolic dysfunction. Increasingly, MRI has been used because it can detect focal changes in myocardial tissue that are highly suggestive of an inflammatory process. The role of transvenous endomyocardial biopsy in diagnosing acute myocarditis is evolving. The biopsy can detect the presence of infiltrating white cells (macrophages, lymphocytes, eosinophils), evidence of myocardial damage, and interstitial fibrosis. Although the presence of these histopathologic abnormalities is used to determine whether acute myocarditis is present, there is significant intraobserver and interobserver variability in evaluating these changes, and maybe more importantly, the biopsy findings often do not provide a conclusive diagnosis. A descriptive term of *acute lymphocytic myocarditis* is used when there is clear evidence of inflammation and the presence of infiltrating lymphocytes. There are some situations, however, in which endomyocardial biopsy will prove helpful, such as in giant cell myocarditis (multinucleated giant cells are seen) or hypersensitivity myocarditis (eosinophilic infiltrate is seen). Polymerase chain reaction to detect specific viral genomes in the myocardium can also be performed.

To date, no effective therapy for viral myocarditis has been established. Empiric trials in which specific antiviral agents are administered based on genomic diagnosis have for the most part enrolled only a small number of patients and lack long-term follow-up. Clinical trials of various forms of immunosuppressive therapy (prednisone, cyclosporine, azathioprine, intravenous immunoglobulin, interferon, immunoadsorption) have so far not resulted in conclusive evidence of benefit. The treatment of cardiomyopathy believed to have resulted from viral myocarditis is similar to that of nonischemic cardiomyopathy of other etiologies. β-adrenergic blockers, angiotensin-converting enzyme inhibitors, aldosterone receptor blockers, and diuretics are the mainstay of medical therapy; mechanical circulatory support and heart transplantation are considered for those who do not stabilize with medical therapy. The natural history of acute viral myocarditis is hard to determine because of the difficulties associated with establishing the diagnosis. It is believed, however, that roughly one third of the patients will recover fully, one third of the patients will have some sequelae in the form of left ventricular systolic dysfunction but be stable on medical therapy, and one third of patients may progress to advanced heart failure.

Treatment of nonviral infectious myocarditis is aimed at eradication of the specific infection. Hypersensitivity myocarditis and myocarditis associated with toxins responds to withdrawal of the offending agent. Immunosuppressive therapy has shown to be effective in giant cell myocarditis.

Patients with myocarditis should not participate in competitive sports for at least 6 months after the onset of clinical manifestations. Athletes may return to training and competition after this period if cardiac size and function return to normal, clinically relevant arrhythmias are absent, and serum markers of inflammation have normalized.

CARDIOMYOPATHIES

Cardiomyopathies are a heterogeneous group of diseases of the myocardium associated with structural and functional abnormalities. Different classifications of cardiomyopathies abound, and there are frequent changes to the classifications as a result of our better understanding of mechanisms of disease. The four main cardiomyopathic groups identified based on structural and functional characteristics are dilated, hypertrophic, restrictive, and arrhythmogenic right ventricular cardiomyopathy. Both familial (genetic) and nonfamilial (acquired) forms of the diseases have been described.

DILATED CARDIOMYOPATHY

Dilated cardiomyopathy (DCM) is characterized by enlargement and impaired systolic function of the left ventricle or both the left and right ventricles. Although abnormal loading conditions such as hypertension or valvular disease, as well as coronary artery disease, can lead to similar structural and functional changes (i.e., *hypertensive, valvular,* or *ischemic cardiomyopathy*), these conditions are not considered to be part of the DCM group and are discussed elsewhere. DCM can be familial (genetic) or acquired (Table 11-2).

Table 11-2 **Cardiomyopathies**

Disorder	Description, Cause
Dilated cardiomyopathy	Dilation and impaired systolic function of the left or both ventricles
Familial (genetic)	Known or unknown genetic mutations
Nonfamilial	Viral myocarditis, nonviral infective myocarditis, idiopathic (immune) myocarditis
	Toxins (drugs, alcohol)
	Pregnancy (peripartum cardiomyopathy)
	Nutritional (thiamine deficiency—beriberi, vitamine C deficiency—scurvy, selenium deficiency)
	Endocrine (diabetes mellitus, hyperthyroidism, hypothyroidism, hyperparathyroidism, pheochromocytoma, acromegaly)
	Autoimmune (rheumatoid arthritis, systemic lupus erythematosus, dermatomyositis)
	Tachycardia induced
Hypertrophic cardiomyopathy	Left and/or right ventricular hypertrophy, often asymmetrical (usually more prominent hypertrophy of interventricular septum)
Familial (genetic)	Mutations of sarcoplasmic proteins (several hundred described so far)
	Metabolic storage diseases of the myocyte
Restrictive cardiomyopathy	Restrictive filling of the ventricles; ventricles are usually small, atria are markedly enlarged
Familial (genetic)	Mutations of sarcomeric proteins
	Familial amyloidosis (transthyretin, apolipoprotein)
	Hemochromatosis
	Desminopathy, pseudoxanthoma elasticum, glycogen storage diseases
	Unknown genetic mutations
Nonfamilial	Amyloidosis, sarcoidosis, carcinoid, scleroderma
	Endomyocardial fibrosis (hypereosinophilic syndrome, idiopathic, chromosomal cause, drugs)
	Radiation, metastatic cancer, anthracycline toxicity
Arrhythmogenic right ventricular	Progressive fibrofatty replacement of the right and, to lesser degree, left ventricular cardiomyopathy; familial, unknown gene
Familial	Unknown mutation
	Mutations of intercalated disk protein, cardiac ryanodine receptor, transforming growth factor-$\beta3$
Unclassified Cardiomyopathies	
Takotsubo (stress-induced) cardiomyopathy	Transient dilation and dysfunction of the distal parts of the left ventricle (apical ballooning) seen in the setting of a stressful situation; usually resolves within weeks
Left ventricular noncompaction	Characterized by prominent left ventricular trabeculae and deep intertrabecular recesses; familial in most cases, caused by arrest in the normal embryogenesis of the heart; apex and periapical regions of the left ventricle most affected; some patients remain asymptomatic, others develop left ventricular dilation and systolic dysfunction
Cardiomyopathies associated with muscular dystrophies and neuromuscular disorders	Duchenne-Becker muscular dystrophy, Emery-Dreifuss muscular dystrophy, myotonic dystrophy, Friedreich ataxia, neurofibromatosis, tuberous sclerosis
Ion channelopathies	Disorders caused by mutations in genes encoding ionic channel proteins; not typically considered cardiomyopathies because they are not associated with typical structural changes of the heart but rather present with electrical dysfunction; some classifications now include these disorders as cardiomyopathies; long-QT syndrome, short-QT syndrome, Brugada syndrome, catecholaminergic polymorphic ventricular tachycardia

About one fourth of cases of DCM are familial, caused by genetic mutations. Some of the specific mutations that have been described involve genes that encode proteins of the sarcomere, cytoskeleton, nuclear membrane, and mitochondria; many mutations remain unknown. The mode of inheritance is typically autosomal dominant.

Nonfamilial DCM has different causes. Most cases are believed to be a result of acute viral myocarditis, a process described in detail earlier in this chapter. Exposure to cardiac toxins can also lead to DCM. Anthracyclines, such as doxorubicin (Adriamycin), daunorubicin, and chemotherapeutic agents frequently used to treat hematologic malignancies, cause a dose-dependent cardiac toxicity. Despite the use of routine echocardiographic screening and discontinuation of anthracycline therapy when signs of ventricular dysfunction develop, this is still a frequent cause of DCM.

Long-term exposure to alcohol is an important preventable cause of DCM. The risk is seen when more than 90 g of alcohol (about seven standard alcoholic drinks) is consumed daily for more than 5 years; lower exposure may lead to cardiomyopathy in women. Abstinence from alcohol may lead to sustained improvements in ventricular function.

Deficiency of certain nutrients—thiamine (beriberi), vitamin C (scurvy), carnitine, selenium, phosphate, and calcium—can also lead to DCM.

Peripartum cardiomyopathy is a form of idiopathic DCM that develops during the last month of pregnancy or within several months of delivery. The pathogenesis of this often life-threatening disease is not completely understood; autoimmunity, concurrent viral myocarditis, and hemodynamic stress of pregnancy have all been suggested as possible causes.

Prolonged periods of supraventricular or ventricular tachycardia can lead to idiopathic DCM (tachycardia-induced cardiomyopathy). The structural and functional changes usually reverse after the rapid heart rhythm is controlled.

The development of the structural and functional changes of DCM can be gradual, and many patients are asymptomatic for a significant amount of time. The first presentation of DCM is usually due to symptoms of heart failure, including fatigue, weakness, dyspnea, and edema. In some patients, the presenting episode is related to arrhythmia or an embolic event.

On physical examination, tachycardia is often present, with a narrow pulse pressure, as well as tachypnea and jugular venous distention. The cardiac examination reveals a laterally displaced apex. S_3 gallop is common; murmurs of mitral and tricuspid regurgitation are frequently heard because of dilation of the mitral and tricuspid annuli caused by ventricular enlargement. Crackles indicating pulmonary edema may be present over the lung fields, and breath sounds may be diminished if pleural effusions are present. In some patients, the clinical features of right ventricular heart failure may predominate, with hepatomegaly, ascites, lower extremity edema, and anasarca.

Diagnostic testing will show cardiomegaly, pulmonary venous congestion, and pleural effusions on chest radiography. Serum B-type natriuretic peptide (BNP) levels are elevated. ECG will determine the cardiac rhythm and will usually show only nonspecific ST- and T-wave abnormalities. Echocardiography provides a comprehensive evaluation of ventricular size and function, detects abnormalities of valvular function, and can also show the presence of a ventricular thrombus. Similar information can be now obtained with MRI. Complete work-up should rule out ischemic, valvular, and hypertensive heart disease as the etiology of myocardial dysfunction and should also include evaluation for potentially reversible causes of DCM (e.g., alcohol, nutritional deficiencies). Myocardial biopsy may be considered if the etiology of DCM is in question. In patients with a strong family history, a referral for genetic testing should be considered.

Management of patients with DCM will entail long-term therapy. First, potential reversible causes of DCM should be addressed (e.g., alcohol cessation, correction of nutritional deficiencies, removal of cardiotoxic agents). Loop diuretics are used to decongest patients who show signs of fluid overload. Although this therapy is clearly associated with symptom improvement, especially dyspnea, the effect of diuretic on survival has not been well studied. A number of medication classes have been extensively studied in heart failure in respect to long-term morbidity and mortality. Vasodilators, such as angiotensin-converting enzyme inhibitors, angiotensin receptor blockers, and hydralazine, in combination with nitrates, have been shown to reduce both morbidity (hospital readmissions) and mortality of patients with systolic dysfunction of the left ventricle. Their effect is through decrease of left ventricular afterload. Angiotensin-converting enzyme inhibitors and angiotensin receptor blockers have additional beneficial effects associated with the blockade of the rennin-angiotensin-aldosterone axis. Blockade of the adrenergic system, which contributes to the detrimental remodeling of the left ventricle, has also been shown to decrease morbidity and mortality. The compounds studied in heart failure include carvedilol, metoprolol succinate, bisoprolol, and, in a subgroup of patients, bucindolol. β-adrenergic blockers should be avoided in cardiogenic shock and in patients with marked fluid overload. Aldosterone receptor blockade with spironolactone or eplerenone has also been shown to reduce long-term morbidity and mortality. Digitalis is used in patients with symptoms despite the use of therapies with proven mortality benefit. Although digitalis does not reduce mortality, it has been shown to reduce hospitalization for heart failure.

Patients with idiopathic DCM and persistent moderate to severe symptoms of heart failure, who also have a QRS duration longer than 120 milliseconds (evidence of dyssynchrony of left ventricular contraction), may benefit from cardiac resynchronization therapy with a biventricular pacemaker. The concurrent pacing of both left and right ventricle leads to a more efficient contraction, improvement of symptoms, and probably a survival benefit. Patients with idiopathic DCM are at an increased risk for possibly fatal ventricular tachycardia and ventricular fibrillation. Survival of patients with a left ventricular ejection fraction less than 35% despite maximal medical management has been shown to be improved with the use of implantable cardioverter-defibrillators (ICDs).

Patients with limiting heart failure symptoms despite the use of the previously described therapies may be considered for heart transplantation or support with a left ventricular assist device.

The prognosis of patients with DCM depends on the response to medical therapy. Although some patients will see a significant improvement in symptoms and cardiac function, in others, the disease will be progressive and associated with a high mortality rate.

HYPERTROPHIC CARDIOMYOPATHY

Hypertrophic cardiomyopathy (HCM) is characterized by left ventricular hypertrophy with nondilated or even small left ventricular cavity size and absence of an apparent cause for hypertrophy (e.g., hypertensive disease or aortic stenosis). This is a relatively common genetic disease (1 in 500 in the general population) with autosomal dominant inheritance. More than 400 individual mutations on 11 different genes encoding proteins of the cardiac sarcomere have been described, with mutations of the β-myosin heavy chain being the most frequent. Sporadic forms of the disease are believed to be a result of spontaneous mutations. The microscopic phenotype includes cardiomyocyte hypertrophy, myofibrillar disarray, and interstitial fibrosis.

An additional group of diseases have recently been added to the category of HCM. These are metabolic storage diseases that result in changes in myocardial appearance that resemble changes caused by the classic sarcomeric mutations. These include glycogen storage diseases, lysosomal storage diseases, disorders of fatty acid metabolism, and mitochondrial cytopathies—all caused by mutations of nonsarcomeric proteins.

The phenotypical expression of the disease varies not only based on the specific mutation but also within families. This is probably due to different penetrance as a result of various largely unknown environmental factors.

The main pathophysiologic abnormalities seen in HCM are left ventricular outflow obstruction, diastolic dysfunction, mitral regurgitation, and arrhythmias. Obstruction of left ventricular outflow occurs in roughly half of the patients (hence the old terms *hypertrophic obstructive cardiomyopathy* and *idiopathic hypertrophic subaortic stenosis*). During systole, the hypertrophied septum bulges into the left ventricular outflow tract, creating a gradient between the lower part of the left ventricular cavity and the left ventricular outflow. This causes high-velocity turbulent flow through the narrowed path, which results in a suction force (Venturi effect) that pulls the anterior leaflet of the mitral valve into the outflow tract. This not only further worsens the obstruction but also causes mitral regurgitation. The relaxation properties of the abnormal myocardium are impaired, sufficient filling of the left ventricle requires higher than normal pressures, and the stroke volume is limited. This is called diastolic dysfunction. Patients with HCM are also predisposed to supraventricular and ventricular arrhythmias.

The symptomatic presentation of HCM varies as a result of the wide phenotypical spectrum. Some patients are asymptomatic, and HCM is diagnosed incidentally. Others present with symptoms resulting from the dynamic obstruction to left ventricular outflow and diastolic dysfunction. The most frequent symptom is dyspnea on exertion, which causes marked elevation of left ventricular filling pressures and pulmonary venous pressures, pulmonary congestion, and limitation in cardiac output. Ischemic chest pain can occur in the absence of epicardial coronary artery disease and is caused by increased oxygen demand by the hypertrophied ventricle and elevated wall tension that reduces blood flow to the subendocardium. Abnormalities of the structure of small myocardial arteries in HCM can also contribute to myocardial ischemia. Presyncope or syncope can be a result of outflow tract obstruction and inability to increase cardiac output during exertion, or a result of arrhythmias that can be triggered by exertion. In some, sudden death caused by ventricular arrhythmia is the initial manifestation of the disease.

A number of important findings can be found on physical examination. Patients with obstruction to flow have *pulsus bisferiens*—brisk initial upstroke in pulse followed by a midsystolic dip corresponding to the development of left ventricular outflow tract obstruction, followed by another rise in late systole. Precordial examination shows a forceful and sustained apical impulse. Decreased compliance of the left ventricle during atrial contraction may lead to an audible S_4 gallop. Turbulent flow through the outflow tract causes a harsh crescendo-decrescendo systolic murmur best heard along the left sternal border with radiation to the base of the heart. Patients may also have an apical holosystolic murmur of mitral regurgitation. The intensity of the murmur of HCM will change with changing degrees of obstruction. This can be observed with physiologic or pharmacologic maneuvers that change preload (left ventricular filling) or contractility. The intensity of the murmur will increase with Valsalva maneuver, with assuming a standing position, and after administration of nitroglycerin or inotropic drugs. The intensity of the murmur will decrease with squatting, volume loading, and administration of β-adrenergic blockers.

The ECG in HCM typically shows increased QRS voltage suggestive of left ventricular hypertrophy. Secondary ST depressions and deep T-wave inversions are also seen. In some patients, a pseudoinfarct pattern with Q waves in the inferior, lateral, or anterior leads is seen and reflects depolarization of the abnormally hypertrophic myocardium. Echocardiography and MRI are helpful in confirming the diagnosis and allow for evaluation of the degree and location of the hypertrophy, the presence and degree of outflow obstruction, and the presence of systolic anterior motion of the anterior mitral leaflet. Doppler echocardiography can be used to monitor for changes in the gradient during provocative maneuvers or for assessment of treatment effect. Echocardiography is also used for screening of family members of patients newly diagnosed with HCM. Cardiac catheterization can be used when echocardiography is inadequate in defining the severity of obstruction. It can confirm the presence of the intracavitary gradient and evaluate for changes in the gradient to the maneuvers described previously.

Management of HCM is aimed at reducing the left ventricular outflow obstruction, improving diastolic dysfunction, and reducing the risk for sudden cardiac death. β blockers and calcium channel blockers improve symptoms in many patients. The benefits are derived from a decrease in heart rate (which prolongs diastole and allows for improved ventricular filling) and decreased contractility (which relieves the severity of left ventricular outflow tract obstruction). Disopyramide, a medication with potent negative inotropic effects, has also been used. In some patients, significant symptoms due to persistent obstruction persist despite medical therapy, and in this situation, nonpharmacologic therapies should be considered. A dual-chamber pacemaker with intentional pacing of the right ventricle may decrease the obstruction by altering the sequence of ventricular contraction. A more predictable response is seen with surgical myectomy, in which resection of the basal anterior septum typically results in dramatic relief of the obstruction and improvement of symptoms (Fig. 11-2). Long-term follow-up studies after septal myectomy show lasting improvements in symptoms and exercise capacity without recurrence of outflow tract obstruction.

A less invasive alternative to septal myectomy is alcohol-induced septal ablation performed percutaneously in the cardiac catheterization laboratory. Alcohol is selectively injected into the septal perforator (a branch of the left anterior descending coronary artery), which provides blood supply to the proximal septum. This produces a controlled myocardial infarction and eventual thinning of the septum,

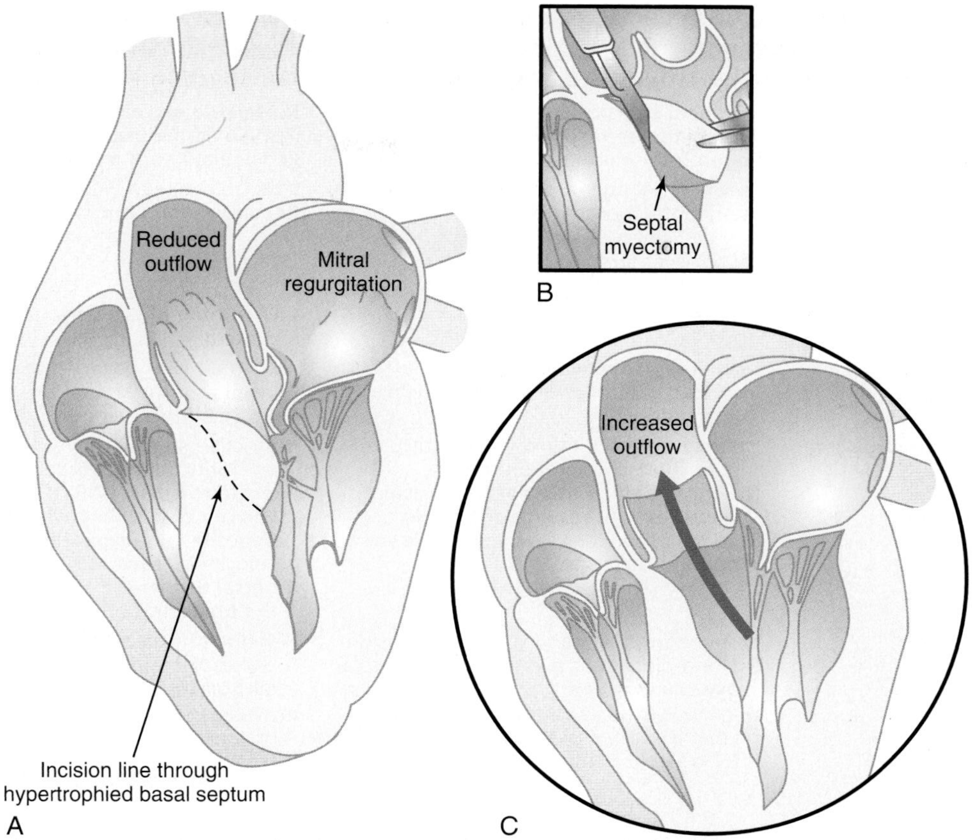

Figure 11-2 Schematic diagram of a patient undergoing surgical septal myectomy. (From Nishimura RA, Holmes DR Jr: Clinical practice: Hypertrophic obstructive cardiomyopathy. N Engl J Med 350:1320-1327, 2004.)

which widens the left ventricular outflow and decreases the outflow gradient. Both surgical septal myectomy and alcohol septal ablation are used in the management of HCM.

Supraventricular arrhythmias, such as atrial fibrillation, are seen frequently and are poorly tolerated. The loss of atrial contribution and shortening of the diastole due to tachycardia result in impaired ventricular filing and raise the outflow gradient. Thus, prompt restoration of sinus rhythm with cardioversion and antiarrhythmic therapy is recommended. Ventricular tachycardia and ventricular fibrillation are the primary mechanism of sudden death in patients with HCM. This can be prevented with ICD therapy. Use of ICD therapy is guided by the perceived risk for ventricular arrhythmias in individual patients. Some of the characteristics that have been associated with this risk are (1) prior cardiac arrest or sustained ventricular tachycardia, (2) high (>30 mm) ventricular wall thickness, (3) syncope, especially if exertional or recurrent, and (4) first-degree relative with sudden cardiac death. Certain genotypes also appear to convey an increased risk for sudden cardiac death.

Patients with HCM should be excluded from most competitive sports and avoid strenuous exercise.

The clinical course of HCM is varied. Sudden death is the leading cause of mortality. Heart failure symptoms may gradually progress, and some patients unresponsive to conventional therapy may require heart transplantation. Relatives of patients with HCM should have serial screening echocardiograms performed yearly during adolescence and less frequently throughout adulthood. Genetic testing can be helpful in determining the presence of the HCM mutation in first-degree relatives of patients with HCM.

RESTRICTIVE CARDIOMYOPATHIES

Restrictive cardiomyopathy (RCM) is a relatively rare form of cardiomyopathy characterized by impaired ventricular filling with normal or decreased diastolic volume of either or both ventricles. Increased myocardial stiffness causes left ventricular pressure to rise significantly with only small changes in volume. Systolic function is usually preserved. Restrictive cardiomyopathies are familial (genetic) or acquired, and the exact causes for some idiopathic forms have not yet been established.

One of the more common genetic forms of RCM is familial amyloidosis, a result of known genetic mutations of transthyretin and apolipoprotein. Familial hemochromatosis is also associated with RCM. Certain sarcomeric protein mutations or mutations of the desmin gene can equally result in RCM.

Acquired forms of RCM result from different systemic disorders. Amyloidosis, sarcoidosis, carcinoid heart disease, and scleroderma have all been associated with RCM. Endocardial pathology that impairs ventricular filling also presents as RCM; examples are hypereosinophilic syndromes and endomyocardial fibrosis. The exact pathogenesis of these disorders is not well known, but parasitic infections and certain drugs (serotonin, methysergide, ergotamine) have been implicated. It is also likely that some nutritional factors

Table 11-3 Differentiation between Restrictive Cardiomyopathy and Constrictive Pericarditis

Type of Evaluation	Restrictive Cardiomyopathy	Constrictive Pericarditis
Physical examination	Kussmaul sign present Apical impulse may be prominent Regurgitant murmurs are common	Kussmaul sign may be present Apical impulse usually not palpable Pericardial knock may be present
Electrocardiography	Low QRS voltage (especially in amyloidosis) Pseudoinfarction pattern Bundle branch blocks AV conduction disturbances Atrial fibrillation	Low QRS voltage Repolarization abnormalities
Chest radiography		Calcification of the pericardium may be present
Echocardiography	Marked enlargement of the atria Increased wall thickness (especially in amyloidosis)	Atria usually of normal size Normal wall thickness Pericardial thickening may be seen
Doppler echocardiography	Restrictive mitral inflow (dominant E wave with short deceleration time) No significant variation of transvalvular velocities with respiration (<10%) Reversal of forward flow in hepatic veins during inspiration	Restrictive mitral inflow (dominant E wave with short deceleration time) Increased velocity of RV filling and decreased velocity of LV filling with inspiration; opposite with expiration; variation in velocity exceeds 15% Reversal of forward flow in hepatic veins during expiration
Cardiac catheterization	Prominent atrial x and y descents (w sign) Dip-and-plateau appearance of ventricular diastolic pressure Diastolic pressures increased but not equalized (LV diastolic pressure higher than RV diastolic pressure)	Prominent atrial x and y descents (w sign) Dip-and-plateau appearance of ventricular diastolic pressure Increase and equalization of diastolic pressures Discordance of RV and LV peak systolic pressures (with inspiration, RV systolic pressure increases and LV systolic pressure decreases)
Endomyocardial biopsy	May reveal specific cause of restrictive cardiomyopathy	No specific findings on endomyocardial biopsy Pericardial biopsy may reveal abnormality
Computed tomography, magnetic resonance imaging		Pericardial thickening

AV, atrioventricular, LV, left ventricular; RV, right ventricular.

play a role because there are significant geographic variations in the prevalence of the disease.

The diagnosis of restrictive cardiomyopathy should be considered in patients with predominantly right ventricular heart failure without evidence of either cardiomegaly or systolic dysfunction. Often, the correct diagnosis is not made until months or even years after symptom onset. Constrictive pericarditis can present similarly to RCM, and establishing the correct diagnosis can be challenging. Distinctive features of the two disorders are described in Table 11-3.

Treatment of restrictive cardiomyopathies is focused on alleviating the symptoms of heart failure and on the underlying disorder when treatment is available. Diuretics are used for decongestion, but intravascular depletion may compromise ventricular filling and lead to reduced cardiac output and hypotension. Supraventricular tachyarrhythmias are poorly tolerated. In patients with conduction system disease such as advanced atrioventricular block, a permanent pacemaker may be indicated. Some specific therapies include chemotherapy in amyloidosis, phlebotomy and iron chelation therapy in hemochromatosis, and steroids in sarcoidosis and endomyocardial fibrosis.

ARRHYTHMOGENIC RIGHT VENTRICULAR CARDIOMYOPATHY

Arrhythmogenic right ventricular cardiomyopathy (ARVC), or arrhythmogenic right ventricular dysplasia, is an autosomal dominant disease with male predominance characterized by progressive replacement of right ventricular myocardium by fibrous and adipose tissue. This results in morphologic and functional changes in the right ventricle. In some patients, the fibrous and adipose infiltration also involves the left ventricle, and in these patients, the presentation may resemble DCM. The prevalence of ARVC is estimated at about 1 in 1000 to 5000, with significant regional variation.

The disease typically presents in young adults, and the presenting symptom is usually arrhythmia—palpitations, syncope, or sudden cardiac death (ARVC is a frequent cause of sudden death in young adults). Symptoms of right ventricular failure are rare, despite evidence of right ventricular dysfunction on imaging studies.

The clinical diagnosis of ARVC is suggested by integration of the information from clinical presentation (arrhythmias), resting ECG, family history, and imaging studies. Histologic examination of the right ventricle, when available, confirms the diagnosis. Resting ECG may be normal, but some frequent abnormalities include incomplete or complete right bundle branch block, the so-called epsilon waves that follow the QRS complex, and inverted T waves in the precordial leads. Typical arrhythmia is a monomorphic sustained ventricular tachycardia originating in the right ventricle (left bundle branch block morphology). However, nonsustained ventricular tachycardias, frequent ventricular premature beats, and supraventricular tachycardias are also common. Right ventricular dilation and systolic dysfunction can be seen with echocardiography and MRI. The latter modality can also show presence of myocardial fat. Histologic examination of the right ventricular wall will demonstrate transmural fibrous and adipose infiltration.

Treatment consists of ICD therapy for patients with history of ventricular tachycardia and possibly even for primary prevention of sudden cardiac death. Antiarrhythmics and radiofrequency ablation of ventricular tachycardia are used in patients with frequent arrhythmias.

Patients with probable or definite diagnosis of ARVC should be excluded from competitive sports.

Unclassified Cardiomyopathies

Some cardiomyopathies, which do not fit into the current categories, are included and briefly described in Table 11-2.

Prospectus for the Future

Genetically engineered animal models have emerged as powerful tools for molecular and genetic studies of human diseases. Genetic testing for disease-causing genes of inherited cardiac disorders are available, but advances about the underlying pathogenesis are still needed to identify effective therapeutic targets. Emerging technologies such as proteomics and genomics might lend important insights into the pathogenesis of human viral myocarditis. Molecular aids using PCR and other serologic methods are likely to speed diagnosis with greater accuracy and specificity. In parallel, medical providers must be alert to epidemiologic shifts in the prevalence of cardiotropic agents such as hepatitis C that can contribute to new cases of viral myocarditis worldwide. Most importantly, future efforts are needed to forge consensus for the treatment of inflammatory phases and prevention of viral sequelae. Lastly, the global effort in basic and clinical research on AIDS is anticipated to yield spin-offs in pathogenesis, vaccine development, and other unforeseen benefits for the treatment and prevention of virus-mediated diseases in humans.

References

American College of Cardiology/American Heart Association Task Force on Practice Guidelines (Writing Committee): ACC/AHA 2005 guideline update for the diagnosis and management of chronic heart failure in the adult—summary article. Circulation 112:1825-1852, 2005.

American College of Cardiology/European Society of Cardiology: Clinical expert consensus document on hypertrophic cardiomyopathy. J Am Coll Cardiol 42:1687-1713, 2003.

Maron BJ, Ackerman MJ, Nishimura RA, et al: Task Force 4: HCM and other cardiomyopathies, mitral valve prolapse, myocarditis, and Marfan syndrome. J Am Coll Cardiol 45:1340-1345, 2005.

Elliott P, Andersson B, Arbustini E, et al: Classification of the cardiomyopathies: A position statement from the European Society of Cardiology Working Group on Myocardial and Pericardial Diseases. Eur Heart J 29:270-276, 2008.

Magnani JW, Dec GW: Myocarditis: Current trends in diagnosis and treatment. Circulation 113:876-890, 2006.

Maron BJ, Towbin JA, Thiene G, et al: Contemporary definitions and classification of the cardiomyopathies: An American Heart Association Scientific Statement from the Council on Clinical Cardiology, Heart Failure and Transplantation Committee; Quality of Care and Outcomes Research and Functional Genomics and Translational Biology Interdisciplinary Working Groups; and Council on Epidemiology and Prevention. Circulation 113:1807-1816, 2006.

Chapter 12

Other Cardiac Topics

David A. Bull and Ivor J. Benjamin

Cardiac Tumors

Primary cardiac tumors are extremely rare, with a prevalence of less than 0.3% in most pathologic series (Table 12-1). Myxoma is the most common primary tumor of the heart and is usually benign. These tumors are frequently isolated lesions, arising most often in the left atrium in the region of the fossa ovalis. Less commonly, myxomas may be detected in the right atrium, in the right or left ventricle, or in multiple sites within the heart. A familial pattern of myxomas can occur and is transmitted in an autosomal dominant manner. In these patients, multiple cardiac myxomas may be present in association with a constellation of extracardiac abnormalities, including pigmented nevi, cutaneous myxomas, breast fibroadenomas, and pituitary and adrenal gland disease. In addition, patients with familial myxoma may have recurrence of the tumor or tumors after surgical excision. Whether sporadic or familial, less than 10% of myxomas are malignant.

Symptoms associated with myxoma are usually related to embolization of tumor fragments and obstruction of the mitral valve. In addition, patients may exhibit a constellation of nonspecific symptoms and laboratory abnormalities, including fever, malaise, weight loss, anemia, and elevated erythrocyte sedimentation rate. The diagnosis is usually made with echocardiography; the transesophageal approach is the most sensitive method for detecting small left atrial tumors. Considering the propensity for embolization, most myxomas are surgically removed when diagnosed. Because tumors may recur, follow-up echocardiograms should be performed.

Other, less common benign tumors include papillary fibroelastomas, fibromas, and rhabdomyomas. Fibroelastomas are pedunculated tumors with frondlike attachments that usually arise from the surface of the mitral and aortic valve leaflets. These tumors do not result in valve dysfunction but may be a source of systemic embolization. Fibromas most often arise within the interventricular septum and may be associated with arrhythmias or conduction disturbances. Rhabdomyomas are the most common cardiac tumors found in children and are often associated with tuberous sclerosis.

Cardiac lipomas may occur throughout the heart and pericardium. Pericardial lipomas can be large, whereas intramyocardial lipomas are small and often encapsulated. Surgical excision is the treatment of choice. Lipomatous hypertrophy of the interatrial septum should be considered in the differential of atrial masses. This lesion is a consequence of nonencapsulated adipose tissue hyperplasia and, although occasionally found incidentally at autopsy, may be associated with supraventricular arrhythmias, conduction disturbances, and, in rare cases, sudden cardiac death.

About one fourth of all primary cardiac tumors are malignant, and most are sarcomas. These tumors grow rapidly and often result in chamber obliteration and obstruction of blood flow. If there is involvement of the pericardium, a hemorrhagic effusion with pericardial tamponade may develop. The prognosis in affected individuals is poor; surgical excision is possible in rare cases. Irradiation and chemotherapy may provide palliative relief.

In contrast with primary cardiac tumors, metastatic disease involving the heart is common, occurring in up to one in five patients dying with malignancy. The most common tumors to metastasize to the heart are carcinomas of the lung, breast, and kidney; melanoma and lymphoma may also have cardiac involvement. Metastasis to the pericardium is common and often complicated by a hemorrhagic effusion and pericardial tamponade. Infiltration of the myocardium may result in conduction disturbances and arrhythmias. Intracavitary masses are unusual but may result from local tumor invasion or direct extension of the malignancy through the venous system (i.e., renal cell carcinoma may metastasize to the heart through the inferior vena cava). Treatment is directed at the underlying malignancy. If pericardial tamponade is present, immediate drainage will help stabilize the patient. A pericardotomy is often necessary to prevent reaccumulation of fluid within the pericardial sac. Surgical excision of an obstructing tumor mass is usually palliative.

Table 12-1 Examples of Tumors of the Heart and Pericardium

Primary

Benign

Myxoma
Lipoma
Papillary fibroelastoma
Rhabdomyoma
Fibroma

Malignant

Angiosarcoma
Rhabdomyosarcoma
Mesothelioma
Fibrosarcoma

Metastatic

Melanoma
Lung
Breast
Lymphoma
Renal cell

Table 12-2 Cardiac Lesions from Nonpenetrating Trauma

Pericardium

Hematoma
Hemopericardium
Rupture
Pericarditis
Constriction (late complication)

Myocardium

Contusion
Intracavitary thrombus
Aneurysms and pseudoaneurysms
Rupture (e.g., free wall, septum)
Acute rupture (e.g., atrium, ventricle, septa)

Valves

Rupture (e.g., leaflets, chordae, papillary muscle)

Coronary Arteries

Laceration

Great Vessels

Aortic rupture

Data from Schick EC: Nonpenetrating cardiac trauma. Cardiol Clin 13:241-247, 1995.

Traumatic Heart Disease

NONPENETRATING CARDIAC INJURIES

Blunt cardiac trauma accounts for about 10% of all traumatic heart disease (Table 12-2). Motion-related injuries secondary to abrupt body deceleration (motor vehicle accidents) and chest wall compression (e.g., steering wheel impact, athletic blow, cardiac resuscitative maneuvers) are the most common causes of blunt injury to the heart. Changes in the myocardium range from small ecchymotic areas in the subepicardium to transmural injury with myocardial hemorrhage and necrosis. Pericarditis is present in most patients and may be complicated by a tear or rupture of the pericardium or cardiac tamponade. Less common complications include rupture of a papillary muscle or chordae tendineae and coronary artery laceration.

Patients most often experience precordial pain that is similar to that associated with myocardial infarction. However, musculoskeletal pain secondary to chest wall injury may confuse the clinical presentation. Congestive heart failure is unusual unless myocardial injury has been extensive or valve dysfunction has occurred. Life-threatening ventricular arrhythmias may occur with severe trauma and are a frequent cause of death in such patients. The electrocardiogram most often demonstrates nonspecific repolarization abnormalities or ST-segment and T-wave changes consistent with acute pericarditis. If myocardial injury is extensive, localized ST-segment elevation and pathologic Q waves may be present. Elevation of the myocardial component of the creatine kinase muscle band (CK-MB) is supportive of a diagnosis of cardiac contusion but is of limited diagnostic use in patients with massive chest wall trauma because the CK-MB fraction may be elevated as a result of severe skeletal muscle injury. Newer markers of myocardial injury, such as troponins T and I, may be more specific for establishing a diagnosis of myocardial contusion. Echocardiography is a useful, noninvasive tool to assess for wall motion abnormalities, valve dysfunction, and the presence of hemodynamically significant pericardial effusion.

Treatment of patients with cardiac contusion is similar to that for myocardial infarction, with initial observation and monitoring, followed by a gradual increase in physical activity. Anticoagulants and thrombolytic agents are contraindicated given the risk for hemorrhage into the myocardium and pericardial sac. Most patients who survive the initial injury will have partial or complete recovery of myocardial function. However, patients should be monitored for late complications that include aneurysm formation, free-wall or papillary muscle rupture, and significant arrhythmias.

GREAT VESSEL INJURY

Rupture of the aorta is one of the most common cardiovascular injuries resulting from blunt chest wall trauma. In more than 90% of cases, rupture occurs in the descending thoracic aorta just distal to the origin of the subclavian artery. Most individuals die immediately of exsanguination. However, up to 20% of patients may survive the initial injury if the blood is confined within the aortic adventitia and surrounding mediastinal tissues (pseudoaneurysm). Characteristic symptoms and findings on presentation include chest and interscapular back pain, increased arterial pressure and pulse amplitude in the upper extremities, decreased pressure and pulse amplitude in the lower extremities, and mediastinal widening on the chest radiograph. Previously, aortography had been the standard for diagnosing blunt aortic injury. Aortography, however, is a relatively invasive, time-consuming procedure with the potential for additional morbidity in this critically ill group of patients. Although conventional chest computed tomography (CT) could not match the diagnostic accuracy of aortography, helical thin-cut CT angiography has emerged as a superior alternative to aortography for diagnosing blunt aortic injury. Helical CT scanning is an ideal diagnostic method for aortic injury because of its relatively low cost compared with aortography, its nearly universal availability in emergency departments, and its lack of operator dependence. In addition, at most trauma centers, CT scanning is already an integral part of the diagnosis and management of serious blunt injury, with patients typically undergoing simultaneous CT scanning of other areas of the body to evaluate potential injuries.

The overall diagnostic accuracy for helical CT scanning in the setting of blunt aortic injury exceeds 99%, with the positive and negative predictive values for helical CT scanning meeting or exceeding the same values for aortography. Patients without direct helical CT scan evidence of blunt aortic injury require no further evaluation. Aortography should be reserved for indeterminate helical CT scans. Such a strategy helps substantially reduce the morbidity and cost of unnecessary aortograms for blunt aortic injury.

The force from rapid deceleration necessary to tear the aorta often leads to injuries of other organs. Associated injuries may be present in more than 90% of patients with aortic transection, and 24% of these patients require a major surgical procedure before aortic repair. The extremely high death rate of acute blunt rupture of the thoracic aorta has led surgeons in the past to repair the tear as quickly as possible. This form of management, however, has resulted in high rates of death and complications, often because of associated injuries in other organs. Patients with traumatic rupture of the aorta fall into two broad categories: (1) About 5% are hemodynamically unstable or deteriorate within 6 hours of admission. These patients require emergent surgical correction because mortality without intervention exceeds 90%. (2) The other 95% of patients are hemodynamically stable at the time of presentation, allowing time for a work-up and staging of any intervention. Mortality in this group is as low as 25% and is rarely the result of free rupture if the blood pressure is controlled. In the past decade, the philosophy of managing traumatic rupture of the aorta in this subgroup of patients has changed to emphasizing blood pressure control and assessing the need for emergent repair against the risks of operation. Recent prospective studies have demonstrated the value of initial antihypertensive therapy to allow delayed repair of blunt aortic injury in patients with severe co-existent injuries to other organ systems. In a substantial number of cases, associated injuries or co-morbidities make the risks of immediate surgical repair prohibitive. The current indications for considering delayed aortic repair include trauma to the central nervous system, contaminated wounds, respiratory insufficiency from lung contusion or other causes, body surface burns, blunt cardiac injury, tears of solid organs that will undergo nonoperative management, and retroperitoneal hematoma, as well as patients 50 years or older and those with medical co-morbidities. Patients with significant neurologic, pulmonary, or cardiac injuries have better outcomes if their confounding pathologic condition can be ameliorated before thoracotomy.

PENETRATING CARDIAC INJURIES

Penetrating cardiac injuries are frequently the result of physical violence secondary to bullet and knife wounds. Similar wounds may result from the inward displacement of bone fragments or fractured ribs secondary to blunt chest wall injury. Iatrogenic injuries may occur during placement of central venous catheters and wires.

With traumatic perforations, the right ventricle is the most frequently involved chamber, considering its anterior location in the chest, and is often associated with pericardial laceration. Symptoms are related to the size of the wound and the nature of the concomitant pericardial injury. If the pericardium remains open, extravasated blood drains freely into the mediastinum and pleural cavity, and symptoms are related to the resulting hemothorax. If the pericardial sac limits blood loss, pericardial tamponade results. In this situation, treatment includes emergent pericardiocentesis followed by emergent surgical closure of the wound. Small penetrating wounds to the ventricles that are not associated with extensive cardiac damage have the highest rate of survival. Late complications include chronic pericarditis, arrhythmias, aneurysm formation, and ventricular septal defects.

Cardiac Surgery
CORONARY ARTERY BYPASS GRAFTING

Despite the effectiveness of current medical therapy for the treatment of coronary artery disease, many patients may require revascularization. Coronary artery bypass grafting (CABG) is an effective means of reducing or eliminating symptoms of angina pectoris. In addition, previous studies have shown that CABG may improve survival in certain subgroups of patients, including patients with angina refractory to medical therapy, patients with greater than 50% stenosis of the left main coronary artery, and patients with severe three-vessel coronary artery disease associated with left ventricular dysfunction. In addition, patients with two-vessel coronary artery disease in which a severe stenosis (>75%) is present in the proximal left anterior descending artery appear to benefit from CABG even if left ventricular function is normal.

Standard CABG is performed through a median sternotomy incision with cardiopulmonary bypass and cardioplegic arrest. Operative mortality is 1% or less in stable patients with normal left ventricular function; the incidences of perioperative myocardial infarction and stroke range from 1% to 4%. An increase in adverse events is associated with advancing age, female gender, short stature, diabetes, unstable angina or recent myocardial infarction, and severely reduced left ventricular function. Overall survival at 10 years is about 80%, with recurrent or progressive angina occurring in about 50% of patients.

Long-term success of surgery is dependent on the type of conduit used during surgery (saphenous vein grafts versus internal mammary artery) and the progression of atherosclerotic disease in the native and graft vessels. The internal mammary artery is particularly resistant to atherosclerotic disease and has a patency rate of about 90% at 10 years. In comparison, venous grafts are subject to closure both during the immediate postoperative period (usually secondary to technical factors) and months to years after surgery, secondary to intimal hyperplasia and progression of atherosclerosis. As a result, only 50% of venous grafts are patent 7 to 10 years after CABG. The major predictor of the subsequent development of atherosclerotic disease in the surgically placed bypass grafts is the ability of patients to control their risk factors for the development of atherosclerotic disease generally after surgery, particularly cigarette smoking, hypertension, diabetes, hypercholesterolemia, and obesity. Aggressive lowering of low-density lipoprotein levels after CABG and the administration of a daily aspirin have been shown to reduce the incidence of venous graft occlusion. Most cases of recurrent angina can be managed successfully with medication (see Chapter 9). In many cases, percutaneous revascularization of a native vessel or graft will provide symptomatic relief and is the initial procedure of choice in this setting. In patients with refractory symptoms not amenable to percutaneous revascularization, repeat CABG is an option; however, in this setting, repeat CABG is associated with increased peri-operative mortality and less satisfactory long-term control of angina.

MINIMALLY INVASIVE CARDIAC SURGERY

Minimally invasive approaches for cardiac surgery can be broadly grouped into two categories: (1) those approaches that avoid the performance of a sternotomy, and (2) those approaches that avoid the use of cardiopulmonary bypass. During the past 15 years, progressive experience incorporating these approaches has led to the application of minimally invasive techniques to select patients undergoing cardiac surgery. Many of the approaches have significant limitations, however, and the development of minimally invasive techniques for the performance of cardiac surgery continues to evolve.

In highly select patients, minimally invasive direct coronary artery bypass (MIDCAB) can be performed through a limited thoracotomy, sparing the patient the peri-operative morbidity associated with a median sternotomy. This technique also avoids the use of cardiopulmonary bypass. The most common approach is through a small left anterior thoracotomy incision and allows for the harvesting of the left internal mammary artery under direct visualization. Therefore, this technique is most suitable for patients with proximal disease in the distribution of the left anterior descending coronary artery, although other coronary arteries can be bypassed using different thoracotomy approaches. The major limitation to this approach has been the lower patency rates in the left internal mammary grafts placed using this technique and a higher incidence of recurrent ischemia compared with conventional CABG. The MIDCAB procedure therefore is only applicable to highly select patients with disease in the distribution of the left anterior descending coronary artery and significant co-morbidities, which preclude the performance of a median sternotomy and use of cardiopulmonary bypass.

The initial experience with the MIDCAB approach and the subsequent demonstration of its limitations prompted the development of port-access cardiac surgery. This technique incorporates the MIDCAB approach of a limited lateral thoracotomy, thereby avoiding a median sternotomy, but uses cardiopulmonary bypass to facilitate performance of intracardiac procedures, including mitral valve repair or replacement, as well as the potential for access to other coronary artery distributions beyond the left anterior descending coronary artery for CABG. The port-access approach uses an endoaortic balloon through cannulas placed in the femoral vessels for cardiopulmonary bypass.

A few centers have successfully used the port-access platform for performance of select cardiac surgical procedures, particularly mitral valve repair or replacement. The widespread adoption of this platform has been limited by persistent difficulties with access to all areas of the heart for coronary revascularization and the potentially catastrophic complication of aortic dissection in a small number of patients.

The limitations encountered with both the MIDCAB and port-access platforms have spurred the development of performing coronary bypass surgery through a median sternotomy but without cardiopulmonary bypass (e.g., off-pump coronary artery bypass [OPCAB]), allowing for surgery on the beating heart. The advantages of OPCAB over other platforms for minimally invasive coronary surgery are that complete revascularization can be performed and both internal mammary arteries can be harvested. Compared with conventional CABG, OPCAB is associated with decreased blood loss, decreased need for transfusion, decreased myocardial enzyme release up to 24 hours after surgery, decreased renal dysfunction, and, typically, decreased number of grafts placed per patient. Also compared with conventional CABG, however, OPCAB is not associated with a decreased length of hospital stay, a decreased mortality rate, or improved long-term neurologic function. Although the OPCAB platform has become the most widely adopted approach for minimally invasive cardiac surgery, major questions remain regarding the intermediate and long-term patencies of the bypass grafts placed using this technique and whether the decreased number of grafts placed per patient compromises the long-term cardiac outcomes of patients undergoing this procedure, compared with conventional CABG. Large-scale prospective clinical trials need to be conducted to answer these questions definitively.

VALVULAR SURGERY

Surgical repair or replacement of a diseased valve is dependent on multiple factors, including the type and severity of the valve lesion, the presence of symptoms, and the functional status of the left and in some cases the right ventricle (see Chapter 8). In most adults, the diseased valve is usually replaced with a prosthesis, although some forms of valve disease, such as mitral valve regurgitation or mitral stenosis without significant valvular or chordal calcification, may be amenable to repair. Because prosthetic heart valves are associated with a number of complications, including thrombosis, endocarditis, and hemolysis, the decision to proceed with valve surgery should only be made after the risks of valve replacement are weighed against the potential benefits of symptom relief and improved survival.

Valve surgery is performed in a manner similar to CABG, with most cases requiring a median sternotomy, cardiopulmonary bypass, and cardioplegic arrest. Minimally invasive surgery through a modified sternotomy or thoracotomy incision may be possible in select patients with isolated aortic or mitral valve disease. Operative mortality for all techniques ranges from 1% to 8% for most patients with preserved left ventricular function and good exercise capacity. The risk of surgery increases further with advancing age, depressed left ventricular ejection fraction, presence of severe coronary artery disease, and replacement of multiple valves. Symptomatic patients usually have significant clinical improvement after valve surgery; however, long-term survival is strongly dependent on the patient's preoperative functional status and ventricular function.

CARDIAC TRANSPLANTATION

During the past two decades, cardiac transplantation has become a life-saving treatment choice in patients with end-stage congestive heart failure. With advances in surgical techniques and immunosuppressive therapy, 1- and 5-year survival rates are about 90% and 75%, respectively. These rates are far superior to the 1-year survival rate in patients with advanced heart failure, which can be as low as 50%. Unfortunately, many patients suitable for cardiac transplantation die before surgery as a result of the limited number of donor hearts available each year. The development and widespread application of left ventricular assist devices has allowed many of these patients who would otherwise die awaiting transplantation to survive until a donor heart becomes available. In many cardiac transplant centers today, more than half of patients undergoing cardiac transplantation have previously undergone placement of a left ventricular assist device.

The major indications for cardiac transplantation are to prolong survival and improve the quality of life. Determining which patients are suitable for cardiac transplantation can be difficult because many patients may have clinical and hemodynamic improvement with intensification of medical therapy. In general, functional capacity, as assessed by exercise stress testing with measurement of maximal oxygen consumption at peak exercise, is the best predictor of which patients should be selected for cardiac transplantation. Individuals with severely impaired exercise capacity (e.g., peak oxygen consumption less than 10 to 12 mL/kg per minute, with the lower limit of normal 20 mL/kg per minute) are most likely to experience a survival benefit from transplantation. Exclusion criteria include irreversible pulmonary vascular hypertension, malignancy, active infection, diabetes mellitus with end-organ damage, and advanced liver or kidney disease. Although advanced age is associated with higher surgical and 1-year mortality rates, an age limit for cardiac transplantation is no longer strictly enforced at most centers, with patients instead being listed for transplantation based on an overall assessment of their physiologic status and potential for long-term survival after transplantation.

The procedure is performed through a median sternotomy incision. The posterior walls of the left and right atria with their venous connections are left in place and used to suture to the donor heart. The aorta and pulmonary artery are directly anastomosed to the recipient's great vessels. Immunosuppressive therapy is begun immediately after surgery and continued throughout the patient's life. Although new immunosuppressive agents are available, most regimens still include combinations of cyclosporine, azathioprine, and prednisone. Frequent complications during the first year include infection and rejection of the donor heart. In addition, hyperlipidemia and hypertension are common medical problems that may require treatment.

The major long-term complication is the development of coronary vasculopathy in the transplanted heart. In contrast to coronary artery atherosclerosis, which tends to be a focal process affecting primarily the proximal vessels, this disease is characterized by diffuse myointimal proliferation involving primarily the medial and distal segments of the coronary arteries. Although the cause of this disease is not entirely known, coronary vasculopathy is thought to be secondary to an immune-mediated response directed against the donor vessels. Monitoring for this complication can be difficult because angina is not provoked in the denervated heart and standard exercise stress testing has a low sensitivity for detecting this disease. Coronary angiography is performed after transplantation and yearly thereafter to monitor for significant narrowing of the coronary arteries. Unfortunately, the diffuse nature of the vasculopathy makes coronary angiography less accurate for the detection of this disease. Intracoronary ultrasound, with measurements of the intimal layer and coronary artery lumen size, is a new technique that appears to be more sensitive than coronary angiography for the detection of this complication. Treatment options are limited, but aggressive management of hypercholesterolemia and the use of calcium channel blockers, specifically diltiazem, have been associated with a slowing of disease progression and a higher survival rate. Retransplantation is reserved for patients with severe, three-vessel coronary artery disease with reduced left ventricular function and symptoms of congestive heart failure.

NONCARDIAC SURGERY IN THE PATIENT WITH CARDIOVASCULAR DISEASE

Noncardiac surgery in patients with known cardiovascular disease may be associated with an increased risk for death or cardiac complications, such as myocardial infarction, congestive heart failure, and arrhythmias. To determine an individual patient's risk for a procedure, the consulting physician must have knowledge of the type and severity of the patient's cardiac disease, his or her co-morbid risk factors, and the type and urgency of surgery. In general, the preoperative evaluation and management of patients with cardiovascular disease are similar to those in the nonoperative setting, with additional noninvasive and invasive testing targeted toward those at-risk patients in whom the results would affect treatment or outcome.

Usually, estimation of a patient's peri-operative risk can be determined by a careful clinical evaluation, including a history, physical examination, and review of the electrocardiogram. Patients at highest risk for a peri-operative cardiac event are those with a recent myocardial infarction (defined as more than 7 days but less than 1 month earlier), unstable or severe angina, decompensated congestive heart failure, significant arrhythmias, or severe valvular disease (Table 12-3). Predictors of moderate or intermediate cardiac risk include a history of stable angina, compensated heart failure, prior myocardial infarction, or diabetes mellitus. Advanced age, an abnormal electrocardiogram, low-functional capacity, and poorly controlled hypertension are associated with cardiovascular disease but are not independent predictors of a peri-operative cardiac event.

Risks associated with the type of surgery are highest in patients undergoing major emergency procedures, especially when performed in the older adult population (Table 12-4). Cardiac complications are also common after vascular

Table 12-3 Clinical Predictors of Increased Perioperative Cardiovascular Risk (Myocardial Infarction, Congestive Heart Failure, Death)

Major

Unstable coronary syndromes
Recent myocardial infarction (e.g., >1 wk and ≤1 mo)
Unstable or severe angina (Canadian Cardiovascular Society angina class III or IV)
Decompensated heart failure
Significant arrhythmias
High-grade atrioventricular block
Symptomatic ventricular arrhythmias
Supraventricular arrhythmias with uncontrolled ventricular response
Severe valvular disease

Intermediate

Mild angina (Canadian Cardiovascular Society angina class I or II)
Prior myocardial infarction
Compensated or prior congestive heart failure
Diabetes mellitus

Minor

Advanced age
Abnormal electrocardiogram (e.g., left ventricular hypertrophy, left bundle branch block)
Rhythm other than sinus
Low functional capacity (i.e., unable to climb one flight of stairs with a bag of groceries)
History of a stroke
Uncontrolled systemic hypertension

Table 12-4 Cardiac Risk Stratification for Noncardiac Surgical Procedures

High (Reported Cardiac Risk > 5%)

Emergent major operations, particularly in the older adult population
Major vascular surgery, aortic aneurysm repair
Peripheral vascular surgery
Prolonged procedures associated with large fluid shifts or blood loss or both

Intermediate (Reported Cardiac Risk < 5%)

Carotid endarterectomy
Head and neck
Intraperitoneal and intrathoracic
Orthopedic
Prostate

Low (Reported Cardiac Risk < 1%)

Endoscopic procedures
Cataract extraction
Breast biopsy

Data from Eagle KA, Brundage BH, Chaitman BR, et al: Guidelines for perioperative cardiovascular evaluation for noncardiac surgery: Report of the ACC/AHA Task Force on Practice Guidelines. J Am Coll Cardiol 27:910-948, 1996.

surgery, considering that the prevalence of underlying coronary artery disease is high in this patient population. In addition, any surgery associated with large volume shifts or blood loss may place increased demands on an already diseased heart. Procedures associated with the lowest risk in the patient with cardiac disease are cataract extraction and endoscopy.

Once the clinical evaluation is complete and the type of surgery is known, the need for additional testing and treatment can be determined. If emergency surgery is contemplated, little in the way of cardiac assessment can be performed, and recommendations may be directed at perioperative medical management and surveillance. If surgery is not urgent, additional evaluation is based on the clinical assessments of the risk and type of surgery. Patients with major risk factors for cardiac complications should have surgery delayed until the cardiac condition is treated and stabilized. Patients with intermediate predictors of cardiac risk scheduled for high-risk surgery should undergo noninvasive testing, such as exercise or pharmacologic stress testing or echocardiography. The results of these tests will help determine future management, such as cardiac catheterization or intensification of medical therapy. Patients scheduled for low- or intermediate-risk surgery, especially if the patient has good exercise capacity, should proceed with surgery with appropriate medical management and postoperative surveillance. Noncardiac surgery is generally safe for patients with minor or no clinical risk factors for cardiac complications, although some patients with poor functional capacity scheduled for high-risk operations may benefit from additional cardiac evaluation.

Disease-Specific Approaches

CORONARY ARTERY DISEASE AND MYOCARDIAL INFARCTION

About 70% of postoperative myocardial infarctions occur within the first 6 days, with the peak incidence between 24 and 72 hours. Mortality associated with noncardiac surgery has been reported as high as 30% to 40%, especially if associated with congestive heart failure or significant arrhythmias. Multiple stresses associated with surgery can provoke ischemia. Physiologic tachycardia and hypertension secondary to volume shifts, anemia, infection, and the stress of wound healing increase myocardial oxygen demand and may provoke ischemia. In addition, increased platelet reactivity during the postoperative period may increase the risk for coronary thrombosis and subsequent infarction.

Despite the high mortality associated with peri-operative myocardial infarction, few studies have examined the effects of anti-ischemic therapy on the prevention of this complication. Several small, uncontrolled trials have suggested that β blockers may reduce intraoperative ischemia. More recently, the use of atenolol before and after surgery was associated with a reduction in myocardial infarction and cardiac death, especially during the first 6 to 12 months after surgery. Although the data are limited, the use of a peri-operative β blocker should be considered in all patients with suggested or known coronary artery disease unless a specific contraindication to its use is present. The data available on the usefulness of calcium channel blockers and nitrates are even more limited, but this approach may be appropriate for the treatment of symptomatic coronary disease in individuals who are not candidates for revascularization. Coronary angiography and revascularization should be reserved for individuals in whom this treatment would otherwise result in significant improvement in symptoms or long-term survival. In rare cases, revascularization may be indicated in high-risk patients undergoing major noncardiac surgery.

All patients with suggested or known cardiac disease should have routine electrocardiograms the first 3 days after surgery to monitor for ischemia. When the electrocardiogram is inconclusive, measurement of troponin levels may be helpful to document an ischemic event. Treatment of a myocardial infarction in this setting is similar to that for the nonsurgical patient (see Chapter 9), although the use of anticoagulants and thrombolytic agents may be contraindicated in the immediate postoperative period. Special attention should be paid to correcting abnormalities that may provoke additional ischemia (e.g., hypoxia, anemia).

CONGESTIVE HEART FAILURE

Several studies have shown that decompensated heart failure is associated with increased peri-operative cardiac complications. In these patients, surgery should be postponed until appropriate treatment is instituted and symptoms have been stabilized. If planned surgery is associated with large blood loss or fluid shifts, a pulmonary artery catheter may be helpful in managing the patient.

During the postoperative period, congestive heart failure most commonly occurs during the first 24 to 48 hours when fluid administered during surgery is mobilized from the extravascular space. However, heart failure may also result from myocardial ischemia and new arrhythmias. Initial management includes identification and treatment of the underlying cause. In addition, intravenous diuretics usually provide rapid relief of pulmonary congestion. If heart failure is complicated by hypotension or poor urine output, insertion of a pulmonary artery catheter may be helpful to guide additional therapy (see Chapter 6).

VALVULAR HEART DISEASE

Aortic and mitral stenosis are associated with the greatest risk for complications after noncardiac surgery. Patients with symptomatic, severe aortic stenosis should have valve replacement before noncardiac surgery. In patients with mild to moderate mitral stenosis, careful attention to volume status and heart rate control are necessary to optimize left ventricular filling and to avoid pulmonary congestion. Patients with severe mitral stenosis should be considered for percutaneous valvuloplasty or mitral valve replacement before high-risk surgery. In patients with valve disease or prosthetic heart valves, prophylactic antibiotics are recommended when appropriate.

ARRHYTHMIAS AND CONDUCTION DEFECTS

Patients with symptomatic, high-grade conduction disturbances, such as third-degree atrioventricular (AV) block, have an increased peri-operative risk for cardiac complications and should have a temporary pacemaker inserted before surgery. Patients with first-degree AV block, Mobitz type I AV block, or bifascicular block (right bundle branch block and left anterior fascicular block) do not require prophylactic pacemaker insertion.

Atrial arrhythmias, such as atrial fibrillation, are common after surgery and are usually not associated with significant complications if the ventricular rate is well controlled. Ventricular premature beats and nonsustained ventricular tachycardia are also common after noncardiac surgery and do not require specific therapy unless associated with myocardial ischemia or heart failure. In most instances, treatment of the underlying cause (e.g., hypoxia, metabolic abnormalities, ischemia, volume overload) will result in significant improvement or resolution of the rhythm disturbance without specific anti-arrhythmic therapy.

CARDIAC DISEASE IN PREGNANCY

Pregnancy is associated with dramatic changes in the cardiovascular system that may result in significant hemodynamic stress to the patient with underlying heart disease. During a normal pregnancy, plasma volume increases an average of 50%, beginning in the first trimester and peaking between the 20th and 24th weeks of pregnancy. This change is accompanied by an increase in stroke volume, heart rate, and, accordingly, cardiac output. In addition, a concomitant fall in systemic vascular resistance and mean arterial pressure occurs because of the effects of gestational hormones on the vasculature and the creation of a low-resistance circulation in the pregnant uterus and placenta. During labor, uterine contractions result in a transient increase of up to 500 mL of blood in the central circulation, resulting in further increases in stroke volume and cardiac output. After delivery, intravascular volume and cardiac output increase further as compression of the inferior vena cava by the gravid uterus is relieved and extravascular fluid is mobilized. Symptoms and signs that may mimic cardiac disease often accompany these hemodynamic changes and include fatigue, reduced exercise tolerance, lower extremity edema, distention of the neck veins, S_3 gallop, and new systolic murmurs. Differentiating symptoms produced by cardiac disease versus those attributable to a normal pregnancy can be difficult. Under such circumstances, echocardiography can be a safe and helpful noninvasive test to assess cardiac structure and function in the pregnant patient.

Many pregnant patients with known cardiac disease can complete a normal pregnancy and delivery without significant harm to the mother or fetus. However, certain cardiac conditions, including irreversible pulmonary hypertension, cardiomyopathy associated with severe heart failure, and Marfan syndrome with a dilated aortic root, are associated with a high risk for cardiovascular complications and death. Under these circumstances, patients should be advised against having children. If pregnancy occurs, a first-trimester therapeutic abortion should be strongly recommended.

Specific Cardiac Conditions

MITRAL STENOSIS

Mitral stenosis secondary to rheumatic heart disease frequently occurs in young women of childbearing age. The physiologic increases in heart rate and cardiac output during pregnancy result in a significant increase in the gradient across the mitral valve and a rise in left atrial and pulmonary venous pressures. Congestive heart failure may develop as the pregnancy progresses through the second and third trimesters or may occur more acutely with the onset of atrial fibrillation. The management of the patient with mitral stenosis depends on her prepregnant functional capacity and the severity of the valve obstruction. In general, patients with severely symptomatic mitral valve stenosis should have percutaneous or surgical correction of the valve before conception. Women with minimal symptoms (New York Heart Association functional classes I to II) usually tolerate pregnancy and vaginal delivery well even if moderate to severe stenosis is present. Management includes salt restriction, diuretic therapy, and aggressive treatment of pulmonary infections. Patients who develop atrial fibrillation with a rapid ventricular response should be treated with AV nodal blocking agents and cardioversion if possible. Patients who develop refractory heart failure during pregnancy should be considered for mitral balloon valvuloplasty because surgical commissurotomy or valve replacement may be associated with fetal demise.

AORTIC STENOSIS

Aortic stenosis in a pregnant woman is usually congenital in origin. Patients with significant outflow obstruction may develop angina or heart failure during the later portion of the pregnancy as cardiac output increases. Supportive therapy includes bed rest and prevention of hypovolemia. If these measures fail to control symptoms and the fetus is not near term, balloon valvuloplasty or aortic valve surgery should be considered to reduce the risk for maternal death.

MARFAN SYNDROME

Pregnant women with Marfan syndrome are at an increased risk for aortic dissection and rupture, especially during the third trimester and first postpartum month. Patients with an aortic root diameter greater than 40 mm are at greatest risk for this complication and should strongly consider therapeutic abortion during the first trimester. Women with an aortic root diameter less than 40 mm should have serial echocardiograms to monitor the size of the aortic root during pregnancy. In addition, restriction in physical activity and treatment with a β blocker may help prevent further dilation of the aorta.

CONGENITAL HEART DISEASE

Survival to reproductive age is common in patients with corrected congenital defects. The risk for pregnancy in these patients is related to the completeness of the repair and the mother's functional capacity. Uncomplicated atrial or ventricular septal defects not associated with symptoms or pulmonary hypertension are usually well tolerated during pregnancy. Intracardiac shunts associated with pulmonary vascular hypertension are associated with a high maternal mortality rate during pregnancy as a result of an increase in right-to-left shunting and worsening oxygen desaturation of the blood. In these women, pregnancy is contraindicated. If pregnancy occurs, a therapeutic abortion during the first trimester should be recommended. Women with uncor-

rected tetralogy of Fallot should undergo palliative or definitive repair before conception to improve maternal and fetal outcomes with pregnancy. Women with residual obstruction of the right ventricular outflow tract remain at high risk for right ventricular heart failure during pregnancy.

PROSTHETIC HEART VALVES

Most patients with a normal-functioning prosthetic valve tolerate pregnancy without complications. However, in patients with mechanical valves, special attention to the choice and dose of anticoagulant therapy is necessary to avoid thromboembolic complications in the mother and teratogenic effects in the fetus. Women should start subcutaneous heparin before conception to avoid the potential teratogenic effects of warfarin during the first several months of critical fetal organ development. This therapy can be continued throughout pregnancy, or, alternatively, warfarin can be reinstituted late in the second trimester or during the third trimester. Heparin therapy, although reducing the risk for teratogenicity associated with warfarin use, is associated with a high risk for maternal bleeding complications. Low-molecular-weight heparin may be an acceptable alternative; however, no firm data are available to support these recommendations. At the time of delivery, anticoagulation therapy is interrupted to avoid bleeding complications. Antibiotic prophylaxis is generally not recommended at the time of delivery.

HEART DISEASE ARISING DURING PREGNANCY

Cardiovascular disease can develop during pregnancy and may pose a significant risk to the mother and fetus. Hypertension is not an uncommon problem during pregnancy and is defined as a consistent increase in blood pressure of 30/15 mm Hg or as an absolute blood pressure greater than 140/90 mm Hg. The three major forms of hypertension that may develop during pregnancy include chronic hypertension, gestational hypertension, and toxemia. Toxemia is a form of hypertension that develops during the second half of pregnancy and is associated with proteinuria, edema, and, in severe forms, seizures. This problem is primarily managed by the obstetrician and is not discussed in this text. Gestational hypertension is an elevation in blood pressure that occurs late in the pregnancy, during delivery, or in the first postpartum days. This disease entity is not associated with proteinuria or edema and resolves within 2 weeks of delivery. Chronic hypertension is presumed to be present if an elevation in blood pressure is detected before the 20th week of pregnancy. No matter what the cause, fetal mortality correlates with the severity of the hypertension and begins to rise when the diastolic pressure exceeds 75 mm Hg during the second trimester and 85 mm Hg during the third trimester. Initial treatments include a reduction in physical activity and salt restriction. If the blood pressure remains greater than 150/90 mm Hg, then antihypertensive treatment should be instituted. Agents that have been safely used in pregnancy include hydralazine, α-methyldopa, clonidine, β blockers, and labetalol. Diuretics should be used with caution because of the increased risk for placental hypoperfusion.

Peripartum cardiomyopathy (PCM) is a form of dilated cardiomyopathy that may begin during the last trimester of pregnancy or within the first 6 months after delivery in a woman without prior heart disease or other definable causes for cardiac dysfunction. The true incidence of the disease is unknown, but estimates conclude that one woman in 3000 to 4000 pregnancies is affected. Although the cause of PCM is unknown, myocardial injury is thought to be immunologically mediated. Women usually exhibit symptoms and signs of congestive heart failure. Echocardiography is useful to assess chamber size and degree of ventricular dysfunction. The outcome with PCM is variable, with death or progressive heart failure occurring in about one third of affected women. The prognosis is particularly poor if symptoms develop before delivery. Despite this risk, many patients will have complete recovery of ventricular function, although recurrence is possible, especially with subsequent pregnancies. Treatment is similar to that for congestive heart failure (see Chapter 6) and usually includes vasodilators, such as hydralazine, digoxin, and diuretics. Angiotensin-converting enzyme inhibitors have been associated with increased fetal wastage in pregnant animals and should be avoided. A thorough evaluation of cardiac function should be performed before subsequent pregnancies. If a woman decides to proceed with another pregnancy, she should be monitored regularly for signs of cardiac decompensation.

About 50% of aortic dissections that occur in women younger than 40 years are associated with pregnancy. Although the cause of aortic dissection during pregnancy is unknown, it has been postulated that hemodynamic and hormonal changes associated with pregnancy may weaken the aortic wall. The highest incidence of dissection is during the third trimester, although it may occur at any time during the pregnancy and during the early postpartum period. The presenting symptoms and diagnostic work-up are similar to those for the nonpregnant patient (see Chapter 13). Transesophageal echocardiography is highly sensitive and specific for the detection of aortic dissection and offers the advantage of not exposing the fetus to ionizing radiation. Management includes aggressive blood pressure control and β-blocker therapy to reduce shear forces of the ejected blood. Recommendations for corrective surgery are similar to those for the nonpregnant patient and are discussed in Chapter 13.

Prospectus for the Future

CABG remains an important but less commonly used mode for revascularization of symptomatic coronary artery disease. Technical advances of percutaneous coronary angioplasty (PTCA), however, have emboldened such attempts for revascularization of unprotected left main disease, the established domain for CABG, even in octogenarians. Prospective studies are needed to evaluate the efficacy, health outcomes, and cost benefits for combined approaches of CABG and PTCA with drug-eluting stents. Percutaneous and minimally invasive surgical options will gain greater widespread application in the management of heart disease. With the limited donor pool for cardiac transplantation, advanced heart failure will be managed with resynchronization therapy, left ventricular assist devices, and stem- and cell-based therapies.

References

Butany J, Nair V, Naseemuddin A, et al: Cardiac tumours: Diagnosis and management. Lancet Oncol 6:219-228, 2005.

Elkayam U, Bitar F: Valvular heart disease and pregnancy. Part I: Native valves. J Am Coll Cardiol 46:223-230, 2005.

Elkayam U, Bitar F: Valvular heart disease and pregnancy. Part II: Prosthetic valves. J Am Coll Cardiol 46:403-410, 2005.

Froehlich JB, Karavite D, Russman PL, et al: ACC/AHA preoperative assessment guidelines reduce resource utilization before aortic surgery. J Vasc Surg 36:758-763, 2002.

Gray DT, Veenstra DL: Comparative economic analyses of minimally invasive direct coronary artery bypass surgery. J Thorac Cardiovasc Surg 125:618-624, 2003.

Rodés-Cabau J, DeBlois J, Bertrand OF, et al: Nonrandomized comparison of coronary artery bypass surgery and percutaneous coronary intervention for the treatment of unprotected left main coronary artery disease in octogenarians. Circulation 118:2374-2381, 2008.

Vascular Diseases and Hypertension

Wanpen Vongpatanasin and Ronald G. Victor

Diseases of the systemic and pulmonary vasculature are among the most common clinical problems encountered in internal medicine. Yet these important diseases are not often given the emphasis they deserve; they fall between the cracks of traditional medical subspecialties. Early clinical recognition is important because in many cases effective therapy can prevent or at least delay needless suffering and death. This chapter reviews the causes, clinical manifestations, diagnostic evaluations, and therapeutic approaches to the major forms of systemic and pulmonary vascular diseases, as well as arterial hypertension. New qualifying examinations are now available in both vascular medicine and hypertension, highlighting the increasing need for expertise in these fields.

Systemic Vascular Disease

PERIPHERAL ARTERIAL DISEASE

Peripheral arterial disease (PAD) refers to atherosclerotic vascular disease of mainly the lower extremities. Similar to other atherosclerotic vascular diseases, PAD is more prevalent in men than in women, particularly before the age of menopause. The prevalence increases with age, ranging from 2% to 6% for adults younger than 60 years to 20% to 30% for those older than 70 years. As with coronary atherosclerosis, the major reversible risk factors are cigarette smoking, diabetes mellitus, hyperlipidemia, and hypertension. Only 30% to 50% of patients with PAD become symptomatic. The classic syndrome of intermittent claudication refers to ischemic muscle pain or weakness that is brought on by exertion and promptly relieved by rest. Claudication is associated with a significant 10-year risk for morbidity and mortality. About 25% of patients develop worsening claudication, 5% require amputation, 10% to 20% require revascularization (e.g., surgery, angioplasty), and 30% die of a cardiovascular event (e.g., heart attack, stroke) as a result of

concomitant coronary or cerebrovascular atherosclerosis. To minimize the progression of PAD and avoid complications, risk factor modification is absolutely essential. This modification includes tight control of blood pressure (BP), plasma lipids, and blood glucose. Complete cessation of tobacco use is a must.

The diagnosis of PAD begins with a careful history and physical examination and is confirmed with noninvasive laboratory testing. Ischemic pain occurs in the leg muscles supplied by arterial segments that are distal to the site of stenosis. Thus, calf claudication is the hallmark of femoral-popliteal disease, whereas discomfort in the thigh, hip, or buttock associated with impotence indicates aortoiliac disease (Leriche syndrome). Depending on the severity of the stenosis, the pain is experienced at a predictable walking distance and is promptly relieved by rest. Claudication must be differentiated from the pseudoclaudication of lumbar degenerative spinal canal stenosis. In the latter condition, walking can also aggravate leg pain, but it is not relieved simply by the cessation of exercise. Rather, assuming positions that minimize lumbar extension such as stooping forward or sitting alleviates the pain. The characteristic physical findings of PAD are absent or diminished pulses distal to the stenosis, bruits over the diseased artery, hair loss, thin shiny skin, and muscle atrophy. Severe ischemia causes pallor, cyanosis, decreased skin temperature, ulceration, and gangrene.

Noninvasive techniques are effective. The *ankle-brachial index* (ABI) is the ratio of the highest systolic BP measured from either the dorsalis pedis or posterior tibialis artery to the highest systolic BP obtained from the brachial artery using a Doppler stethoscope. The normal ABI range is 0.9 to 1.3. An ABI of less than 0.9 indicates PAD. This simple noninvasive test has a sensitivity and a specificity of 95% and 99%, respectively. In some patients with diabetes mellitus or renal failure, the media of the affected leg vessels become so heavily calcified that they resist compression except during very high levels of cuff inflation. The result is a falsely elevated ankle BP and an artificially normal or supernormal ABI (Table 13-1).

Duplex ultrasonography is an important adjunct to the ABI, with a similar sensitivity and specificity. This test is particularly useful to diagnose PAD in patients with non-compressible vessels from medial wall calcification. The Doppler velocity waveform remains abnormal, despite a spuriously normal or elevated ABI. Magnetic resonance (MR) angiography and computed tomographic (CT) angiography are newer techniques that now permit excellent visualization of vascular stenosis and identification of runoff vessels. With these noninvasive imaging modalities, spatial resolution is comparable with that of traditional invasive angiography. Catheter-based angiography, the gold standard, now is reserved for patients undergoing revascularization.

The medical management of patients with PAD includes lifestyle and risk factor modification as well as antiplatelet therapy. Smoking cessation reduces the risk for limb loss, myocardial infarction, and death. Lipid-lowering therapy with a statin hydroxymethylglutaryl–coenzyme A (HMG-CoA) reductase inhibitor should be initiated and intensified if low-density lipoprotein (LDL) cholesterol is greater than 100 mg/dL. Hypertension should be treated with appropriate medication, which should be intensified until BP is less than 140/90 mm Hg. The target BP is even lower (<130/80 mm Hg) in PAD patients with diabetes or chronic kidney disease and in patients who have had a prior cardiovascular event or who have left ventricular hypertrophy (LVH) visualized by electrocardiography (ECG) or echocardiography. In contrast to traditional teaching, β-adrenergic blockers do not reduce walking capacity or worsen intermittent claudication in patients with PAD. Aspirin reduces the risk for myocardial infarction, death, and stroke. However, clopidogrel has proved more effective than aspirin in this setting. Each patient needs an exercise prescription because exercise training improves walking capacity and quality of life. Pentoxifylline is a methylxanthine derivative that may improve maximal walking distance, but the data are inconclusive. Better data is available with cilostazol, a phosphodiesterase III inhibitor, whereas sildenafil is a phosphodiesterase V inhibitor. In several studies of patients with symptomatic PAD, cilostazol consistently improved walking capacity and quality of life. It is one of the most effective agents for intermittent claudication. However, cilostazol must be avoided in patients with congestive heart failure because its use may increase mortality.

Revascularization (percutaneous or surgical) is indicated for patients with severe claudication that is resistant to medical therapy, limb-threatening ischemia, or vasculogenic impotence. Percutaneous revascularization offers a comparable patency rate with less morbidity and mortality than does surgery in patients with short focal stenoses in large arteries such as the distal aorta or iliac arteries (Fig. 13-1). Surgical revascularization is more suitable for longer areas of stenosis or obstructive lesions distal to the origin of the iliac arteries.

Acute limb ischemia (ALI) constitutes a vascular emergency. Sudden occlusion of a peripheral artery is caused by either arterial embolism or thrombosis in situ. Arterial emboli usually originate in the cardiac chambers in the

Table 13-1 **Interpretation of Ankle-Brachial Index**	
Ankle-Brachial Index	**Interpretation**
0.90-1.30	Normal
0.70-0.89	Mild PAD
0.40-069	Moderate PAD
<0.40	Severe PAD
>1.30	Noncompressible vessels

PAD, peripheral arterial disease.

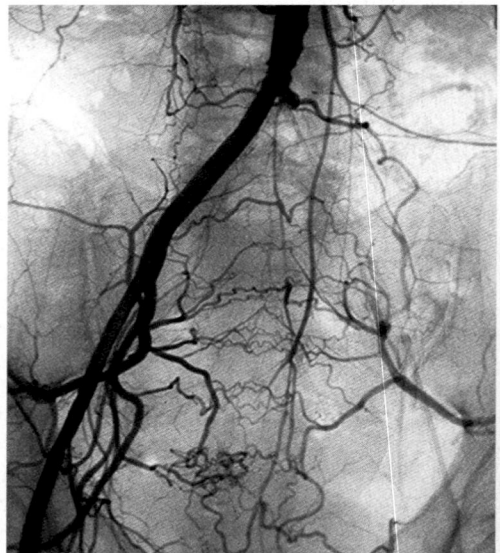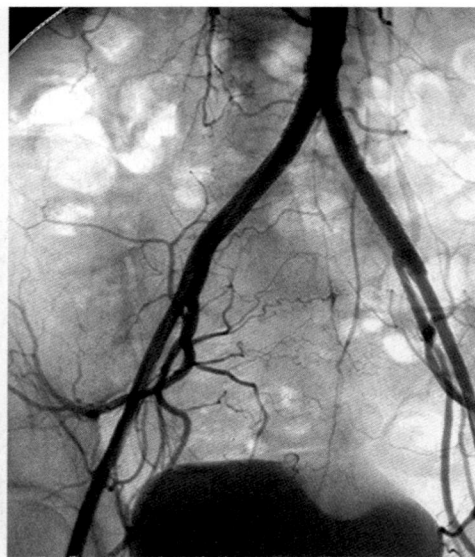

Figure 13-1 Angiogram of the distal abdominal aorta and iliac arteries demonstrates an occluded left common iliac artery with extensive collateral circulation from the contralateral internal iliac artery *(left panel)*, which resolved after successful stent implantation *(right panel)*. (Images courtesy of Bart Domatch, MD, Radiology Department, University of Texas Southwestern Medical Center, Dallas, Texas.)

setting of preexisting cardiac disease such as myocardial infarction (e.g., left ventricular mural thrombus), congestive heart failure, or atrial arrhythmias (e.g., left atrial thrombus in a patient with atrial fibrillation). Thrombosis in situ usually occurs in arteries with a preexisting severe stenosis in the setting of longstanding PAD with or without previous vascular surgery. Patients with arterial embolism usually experience sudden onset of symptoms without a history of claudication, whereas those with thrombosis in situ typically have a history of claudication that has previously been stable and then suddenly assumes a crescendo pattern over a period of days. In either case, the physical examination reveals a cold, cyanotic (bluish) extremity with absent pulses distal to the site of arterial occlusion and diminished motor or sensory function. A hand-held Doppler device is used to assess signals at different arterial segments and confirms the diagnosis of acute vascular occlusion. Anticoagulation should be initiated immediately with intravenous heparin titrated to maintain the activated partial thromboplastin time equal to 2.0 to 2.5 times control. Patients with ALI who developed symptoms for more than 14 days or occlusion in the suprainguinal sites generally require surgical thromboembolectomy or bypass surgery. In contrast, patients with more recent onset of symptoms or infrainguinal occlusion should be treated with catheter-directed infusion of thrombolytic therapy or percutaneous thrombus extraction. Patients with irreversible tissue necrosis, regardless of the cause, should be treated with emergent amputation rather than revascularization to reduce the risk for kidney failure (myoglobinemia), sepsis, and multiple-organ failure.

AORTIC ANEURYSM

Abdominal aortic aneurysm (AAA) is a common vascular disease in older adults, affecting 4% to 8% of men and 0.5% to 1.5% of women older than 65 years. Thoracic aortic aneurysm is much less prevalent (0.4% to 0.5%). Besides age, the major risk factors for AAA are cigarette smoking, hypertension, and a family history of aortic aneurysms. Atherosclerosis is responsible for most cases of AAA, but other causes include cystic medial necrosis (Marfan syndrome, Ehlers-Danlos syndrome), vasculitis with connective tissue disease (Takayasu arteritis, giant cell arteritis), chronic infection (syphilitic aortitis), and trauma. Abdominal aortic aneurysms gradually grow in size over time at an average rate of 1 to 4 mm per year. The risk for rupture is low until the diameter reaches 5 cm, and then it increases exponentially. The risk for aortic rupture is 1% per year for aneurysms between 3.5 and 4.9 cm in diameter and 5% per year for aneurysms larger than 5 cm.

Most patients with AAA are asymptomatic, but some develop vascular complications such as aneurysm expansion with compression of adjacent structures. Occasionally, mural thrombi form within the aneurysm embolize, causing acute occlusion of distal arterial segments. Patients with iliac aneurysm may develop hydronephrosis or recurrent urinary tract infection from ureteral compression. Others develop neurologic symptoms from compression of sciatic or femoral nerves. The classic physical finding is a pulsatile nontender mass below the umbilicus (distal to the origin of the renal arteries). In thin patients, normal aortic pulsations are often

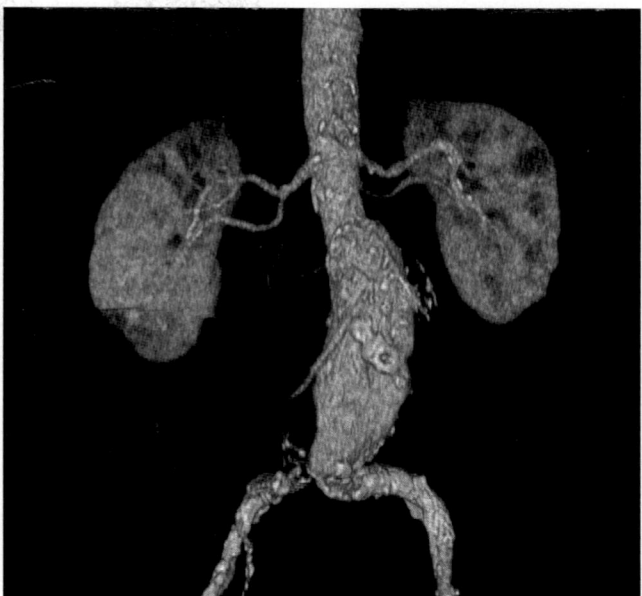

Figure 13-2 Computed tomographic angiogram of the distal abdominal aorta shows an abdominal aortic aneurysm with the largest diameter of 6.2 cm and severe stenosis at the origin of the right common iliac artery. (Image courtesy of Bart Domatch, MD, Radiology Department, University of Texas Southwestern Medical Center, Dallas, Texas.)

Table 13-2 Indications for Surgical Treatment of Arterial Aneurysms

Symptoms from expansion of aneurysm or compression of adjacent structure
Rupture of aneurysm
Rapid aortic aneurysm expansion of ≥1 cm per year
Large aneurysm
Ascending aorta >4.5 cm for patients with Marfan syndrome and >5 cm for all others
Aortic arch >5.5 cm
Descending thoracic aorta >5 cm
Abdominal aorta >5.5 cm
Iliac aneurysm >3 cm

palpable but above the umbilicus. Hypotension and acute abdominal pain should prompt consideration of aneurysm rupture, which requires emergent operative repair. Duplex ultrasonography is an accurate and reliable diagnostic tool for abdominal aortic and iliac aneurysms. Routine screening for AAA with ultrasonography is recommended for all men between the ages of 65 and 75 years or men above the age of 60 with family history of AAA among first-degree relatives. Such screening has a proven mortality benefit. CT and MR angiography allow visualization of the thoracic and abdominal aorta as well as the iliac arteries and its branches (Fig. 13-2). Medical treatment for aortic aneurysm includes smoking cessation, tight BP control, and cholesterol reduction. β-Adrenergic blockade reduces the rate of aortic root enlargement in patients with Marfan syndrome but has not proved beneficial in patients with AAA from other causes. Patients with large aneurysms or rapid aneurysm expansion regardless of the size should undergo aneurysm repair (Table 13-2). Elective AAA repair carries a peri-operative mortality rate of 2% to 6%. Furthermore, a large randomized study failed to demonstrate any benefit of surgery in patients with aneurysms 4 to 5.5 cm in diameter. For these reasons, patients with small aortic aneurysms should be treated medically with close monitoring of aneurysm size with periodic imaging studies every 6 to 12 months (see Table 13-2).

Percutaneous endovascular aneurysm repair (EVAR) is an alternative method to open surgical repair for treatment of AAA. EVAR offers lower perioperative death than surgical repair, but long-term survival rates are not different from surgery. EVAR has not been shown to improve mortality in patients with multiple co-morbidities, who are considered to be unfit for surgery, when compared with conservative management. Therefore, it should be offered only to selected patients with symptoms from compression of adjacent organs or vascular complications.

Aortic Dissection

In aortic dissection, the intimal layer is torn from the aortic wall, leading to the formation of a false lumen in parallel with the true lumen. Risk factors include hypertension, cocaine use, trauma, hereditary connective tissue disease (e.g., Marfan syndrome, Ehlers-Danlos syndrome), vasculitis (e.g., Takayasu arteritis, giant cell arteritis), Behçet disease, bicuspid aortic valve, and aortic coarctation. Aortic dissection can be classified as types A and B (Stanford system). Type A dissection involves the ascending aorta, whereas type B dissection involves the distal aorta. The DeBakey system subdivides aortic dissection into three subtypes: types I, II, and III. Type I dissection involves the entire aorta, whereas type II involves only the ascending aorta, and type III involves only the descending aorta. Aortic dissection involving the ascending aorta carries a high mortality rate of 1% to 2% per hour during the first 24 to 48 hours. Patients usually develop acute onset of severe chest or back pain. Abdominal pain, syncope, and stroke are common. Retrograde propagation of the dissection can cause pericardial tamponade or coronary artery dissection with acute myocardial infarction. Dissection involving the aortic valve causes acute severe aortic insufficiency with acute pulmonary edema. The dissection plane may propagate in an antegrade direction to compromise flow in the carotid and subclavian arteries, producing a stroke or acute upper limb ischemia. Patients with distal (type B) aortic dissection exhibit acute onset of back pain or chest pain often accompanied by lower extremity ischemia and ischemic neuropathy. The physical findings include pulse deficits, neurologic deficits, or a diastolic murmur of aortic regurgitation. However, acute aortic regurgitation into an unprepared ventricle produces only a short, soft diastolic murmur that is often missed. The widened pulse pressure and associated physical findings of chronic aortic regurgitation are absent, and the clinical picture is that of an acutely ill patient with tachypnea, tachycardia, and a narrow pulse pressure. Hypotension, jugular venous distention, and pulsus paradoxus should prompt the diagnosis of pericardial tamponade. Transesophageal echocardiography, MR angiography, or CT angiography confirms the diagnosis by demonstrating an intimal flap that separates the true lumen from the false lumen (Fig. 13-3). Type A aortic dissection is uniformly fatal without emergent surgical repair. With surgery, mortality is reduced to 10% at

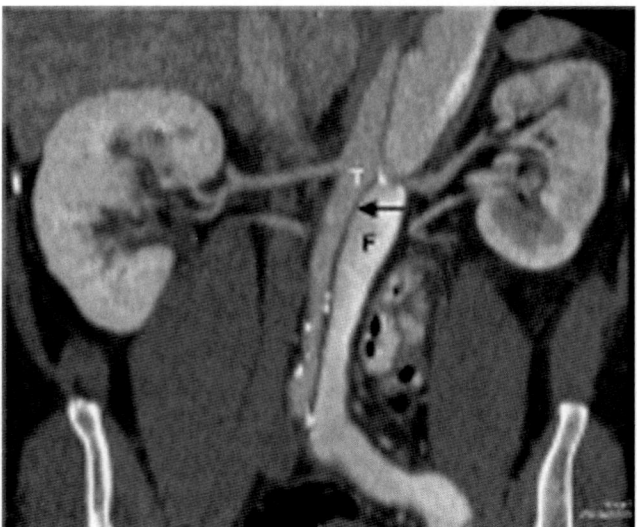

Figure 13-3 Computed tomographic angiogram of the aorta shows type B aortic dissection. The intimal flap *(arrow)* separates the true lumen *(T)* from the false lumen *(F)* and compromises blood flow to the right kidney, causing renal atrophy and cortical thinning. (Image courtesy of Bart Domatch, MD, Radiology Department, University of Texas Southwestern Medical Center, Dallas, Texas.)

24 hours and 20% at 30 days. Patients with type B aortic dissection should be treated medically because 1-year survival is higher with medical therapy than it is with surgery (75% versus 50%). However, surgery is indicated if type B dissection compromises blood flow to the legs, kidneys, or other viscera. Tight control of BP is essential because aortic aneurysm develops in 30% to 50% of patients with type B aortic dissection studied for 4 years.

Penetrating Aortic Ulcers and Intramural Hematoma

Penetrating aortic ulcers and intramural hematomas exhibit chest pain that is indistinguishable from that of aortic dissection. In contrast to aortic dissection, however, the pathologic condition is localized. No identifiable intimal flap and thus no branch vessel occlusion are produced. Disruption of the internal elastic lamina produces aortic ulcers that erode into the medial wall and protrude into the surrounding structures. Rupture of the vasa vasorum causes formation of localized hematoma underneath the adventitia with resultant asymmetrical thickening of the aortic wall. Patients with either condition typically are older than those with aortic dissection, have a larger aortic size, and have a higher prevalence of AAA. Aortic rupture is the major complication of both penetrating ulcers and intramural hematomas, particularly with those aneurysms located in the ascending aorta. The diagnosis is made with invasive angiography, CT angiography, or MR angiography (Fig. 13-4). Surgical intervention should be considered for ulcers and hematomas of the ascending aorta, deeply penetrating ulcers, or severely bulging hematomas, irrespective of their location. Ulcers and hematomas of the descending aorta may be managed successfully with β-adrenergic blockade and tight control of BP.

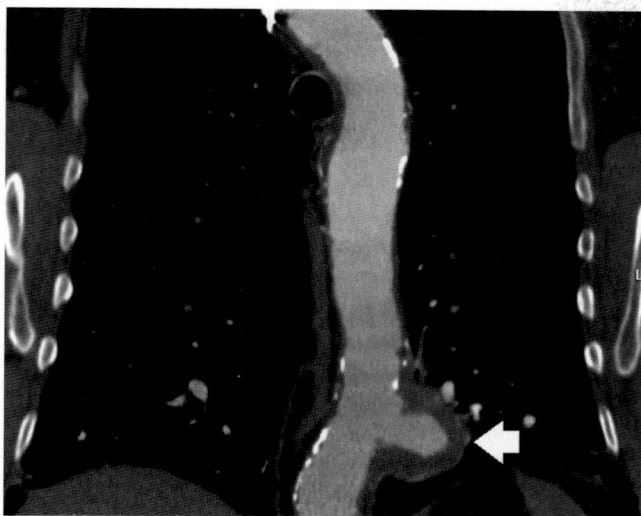

Figure 13-4 Computed tomographic angiogram of the descending thoracic aorta shows a large penetrating aortic ulcer above the diaphragm *(arrow)*. (Image courtesy of Bart Domatch, MD, Radiology Department, University of Texas Southwestern Medical Center, Dallas, Texas.)

Other Arterial Diseases

Buerger disease is a nonatherosclerotic disease of the arteries, veins, and nerves of the arms and legs affecting mostly young men before the age of 45 years. The cause is unknown, but all patients have a history of heavy tobacco addiction. The presenting symptom is claudication of the feet, legs, hands, or arms. Multiple-limb involvement and superficial thrombophlebitis are common. The C-reactive protein and Westergren sedimentation rate typically are normal, and a search for serologic markers for connective tissue disease (e.g., antinuclear antibody or rheumatoid factor, antiphospholipid antibody) is negative. The diagnosis is usually based on the typical clinical presentation. If the presentation is atypical, biopsy may be needed to make the diagnosis. The histologic hallmark is inflammatory intramural thrombi within the arteries and veins with sparing of internal elastic lamina and other arterial wall structures. The most effective treatment of Buerger disease is complete tobacco abstinence. The prostacyclin analogue iloprost constitutes adjunctive therapy to reduce limb ischemia and improve wound healing.

Raynaud phenomenon is a vasospastic disease of the small arteries of mainly the fingers and toes. Primary (idiopathic) Raynaud phenomenon occurs in the absence of underlying disorders. Secondary Raynaud phenomenon occurs in association with connective tissue diseases (e.g., scleroderma, polymyositis, rheumatoid arthritis, systemic lupus erythematosus) as well as with repeated mild physical trauma (e.g., use of jack hammers), certain drugs (e.g., antineoplastic chemotherapeutic agents, interferon, monoamine-reuptake inhibitors such as tricyclic antidepressants, serotonin agonists), and Buerger disease. Patients usually complain of recurrent episodes of digital ischemia, with a characteristic white-blue-red color sequence. Pallor is followed by cyanosis if ischemia is prolonged and then by erythema (reactive hyperemia) when the episode resolves. Episodes are precipitated by cold temperature or emotional stress. Physical examination can be entirely normal between

attacks with normal radial, ulnar, and pedal pulses. Some patients may have digital ulcers or thickening of fat pad (sclerodactyly). Patients should be instructed to avoid cold temperatures and dress warmly. Calcium channel blockers (CCBs) reduce the frequency and severity of vasospastic episodes.

Giant cell arteritis is an immune-mediated vasculitis predominantly involving medium-sized and large arteries such as the subclavian artery, axillary artery, and aorta of the older adult with a strong male predominance. About 40% of patients with giant cell arteritis also have polymyalgia rheumatica, a syndrome characterized by severe stiffness and pain originating in the muscles of the shoulders and pelvic girdle. Patients may exhibit headache from temporal arteritis, jaw claudication from ischemia of the masseter muscles, or visual loss from involvement of ophthalmic artery. Chest pain suggests the co-existence of aortic aneurysm or dissection. Physical findings include low-grade fever, scalp tenderness in the temporal area, pale and edematous fundi, or a diastolic murmur of aortic regurgitation. BP difference of more than 15 mm Hg between arms suggests subclavian artery stenosis. Laboratory findings include significantly elevated C-reactive protein and Westergren sedimentation rate plus anemia. The diagnosis is confirmed by histologic examination of the arterial tissue (frequently from temporal artery biopsy), showing infiltration of lymphocytes and macrophages (i.e., giant cells) in all layers of the vascular wall. High-dose corticosteroids are highly effective. To minimize complications from long-term corticosteroid administration, the steroid dose should be tapered to find the lowest dose needed to suppress symptoms, which often wane. Every attempt should be made to discontinue corticosteroids over time.

Takayasu arteritis is an idiopathic granulomatous vasculitis of the aorta, its main branches, and the pulmonary artery. This condition is particularly common in young women of Asian descent, but it also occurs in occidental women and men. The inflammatory process in the vascular wall can lead to stenosis and aneurysm formation. Hypertension, as a result of renal artery stenosis or aortic coarctation, is the most common manifestation and is present in as many as 80% of affected individuals. Because the vascular involvement is so widespread, patients may have symptoms and signs of coronary ischemia, congestive heart failure, stroke, vertebrobasilar insufficiency, or intermittent claudication. Physical findings include bruits over the subclavian arteries or aorta as well as diminished brachial pulses and thus a low brachial artery BP. The diagnosis is based primarily on this clinical presentation. First-line treatment is with corticosteroids. Other immunosuppressive agents such as methotrexate or cyclophosphamide are often added to prevent disease progression and relapse. Immunosuppressive therapy does not cause regression of preexisting vascular stenoses or aneurysms. For this reason, percutaneous or surgical revascularization is usually required.

Arteriovenous (AV) fistulas are abnormal vascular communications that shunt blood flow from the arterial system directly into the venous system, bypassing the capillary beds that normally ensure optimal tissue perfusion and nutrient exchange. AV fistulas may be congenital, as in AV malformation (AVM), or acquired. The main causes of acquired AV fistula are penetrating trauma (e.g., gunshot, knife wound) and surgically created shunts for hemodialysis access. Patients may exhibit a pulsatile mass, symptoms related to compression of an adjacent organ, or bleeding from spontaneous rupture of an AVM. Systolic and diastolic bruits or thrills may be detectable over the fistula or AVM. An AVM in skeletal muscle may lead to bone malformation or a pathologic fracture, whereas AVM in the brain may result in neurologic deficits or seizures. High-output heart failure is another complication from a large AVM or fistula. MR angiography, CT angiography, or conventional angiography confirms the diagnosis. Depending on the size and location of the AVM, treatment options include surgical resection, transcatheter embolization, or pulse laser irradiation. Patients with acquired AV fistulas from trauma usually need surgical closure.

Pulmonary Vascular Disease

Pulmonary hypertension is characterized by elevated mean pulmonary pressure of greater than 25 mm Hg at rest or greater than 30 mm Hg during exercise. The many causes of pulmonary hypertension are summarized in Table 13-3.

Patients with pulmonary hypertension have not only an elevated pulmonary arterial pressure but also a low cardiac output, causing symptoms of exertional dyspnea, fatigue, and syncope. Pulmonary capillary wedge pressure is usually normal except in patients with pulmonary venous hypertension and congenital heart disease.

PULMONARY ARTERIAL HYPERTENSION

Pulmonary arterial hypertension (PAH) is caused by a combination of pulmonary vasoconstriction, endothelial cell or smooth muscle proliferation, intimal fibrosis, and thrombosis in the pulmonary capillaries and arterioles. PAH is either idiopathic (primary pulmonary hypertension [PPH]) or secondary to connective tissue disease, congenital heart disease, portal hypertension, or human immunodeficiency virus (HIV) infection as well as anorexigenic drugs or toxins. Connective tissue diseases, particularly scleroderma, are the most common secondary causes of PAH.

Patients with mild PAH can be asymptomatic, but patients with more advanced disease complain of dyspnea, chest pain, syncope, or presyncope. Physical findings include a left parasternal lift, loud pulmonary component of the second heart sound, murmur of tricuspid or pulmonic regurgitation, hepatomegaly, peripheral edema, or ascites. Associated ECG abnormalities indicate right ventricular hypertrophy, right atrial enlargement, or right axis deviation. Echocardiography provides important information about the severity of the pulmonary hypertension (i.e., estimated pulmonary artery pressure, right ventricular dimensions and function) and its potential causes (e.g., left ventricular failure, valvular lesions, congenital heart disease with left-to-right shunts). Pulmonary function tests, ventilation-perfusion $(\dot{V}/\dot{Q})$ lung scans, polysomnography or overnight oximetry, autoantibody tests, HIV serology, and liver function tests also should be performed to determine other potential causes. Right ventricular catheterization should be performed in all patients with suggested PAH. Under basal conditions in the catheterization laboratory, an elevated mean pulmonary artery pressure exceeding 25 mm Hg, a pulmonary capillary wedge pressure below 15 mm Hg, and a pulmonary vascular resistance exceeding 3 units confirm the diagnosis. Acute vasodilator drug challenge should be performed during right ventricular catheterization to guide appropriate treatment.

Without treatment, the prognosis of PAH is poor, with a median survival of less than 3 years. Patients with severe symptoms should be treated with prostacyclin or epoprostenol (an intravenous prostacyclin analogue) because of their proven efficacy in improving exercise capacity, quality of life, and survival. Other prostacyclin analogues, such as treprostinil and iloprost, are also effective in reducing pulmonary artery pressure and improving exercise capacity. Other classes of drugs approved for treatment of PAH include endothelin receptor blockers and phosphodiesterase-5 inhibitors. Oral CCBs are indicated for the small subset of patients with mild to moderate symptoms who demonstrate significant reduction in pulmonary pressure with acute CCB challenge. Supplemental home oxygen is indicated for all patients with hypoxemia. Higher elevations exacerbate hypoxemia, and relocation to sea level improves symptoms. Oral anticoagulation is recommended for all patients with PAH. Diuretics should be prescribed for patients with peripheral edema or hepatic congestion. Lung transplantation is recommended only for patients in whom severe symptoms occur despite intensive medical therapy.

Table 13-3 Classification of Pulmonary Hypertension

Category 1: Pulmonary Arterial Hypertension

Primary pulmonary hypertension or idiopathic pulmonary hypertension:
- Sporadic
- Familial

PPH associated with:
- Connective tissue disease
- Congenital heart disease
- Portal hypertension
- Human immunodeficiency viral infection

Drugs and toxins:
- Anorexigens
- Cocaine

Category 2: Pulmonary Venous Hypertension

Left ventricular heart failure
Left ventricular valvular heart disease

Category 3: Pulmonary Hypertension associated with Chronic Respiratory Disease or Hypoxemia

Chronic obstructive pulmonary disease
Obstructive sleep apnea

Category 4: Pulmonary Hypertension associated with Chronic Venous Thromboembolism

Left ventricular valvular heart disease

Category 5: Pulmonary Hypertension Due to Miscellaneous Disorders Directly Affecting the Pulmonary Vasculature

Sarcoidosis
Histiocytosis X
Compression of pulmonary vessels (adenopathy, tumor, fibrosing mediastinitis)

Venous Thromboembolic Disease

Venous thromboembolism (VTE) encompasses both deep vein thrombosis (DVT) and pulmonary embolism (PE). Among the adult U.S. population, the overall combined annual incidence is as high as 1 new case per 1000 persons. The incidence of VTE is higher in men than in women and higher in African Americans and whites than in Asians and Hispanics. More than 150 years ago, Dr. Rudolf Virchow recognized three predisposing factors: (1) endothelial damage, (2) venous stasis, and (3) hypercoagulation (Virchow triad). Endothelial damage is common with surgery or trauma, venous stasis is common with prolonged bed rest or immobilization (leg cast), and hypercoagulation is common with cancer. Trousseau syndrome consists of migratory thrombophlebitis with noninfectious vegetations on the heart valves (marantic endocarditis) typically in the setting of mucin-secreting adenocarcinoma. Dr. Trousseau, a pathologist, diagnosed his own pancreatic carcinoma on the basis of the association that now bears his name. Hypercoagulable states include hereditary diseases such as deficiencies in antithrombin III, protein C, or protein S; mutation in factor V gene (factor V Leiden) or factor II gene (prothrombin G20210A); and hyperhomocysteinemia. However, a thorough search for identifiable risk factors will come up negative in 25% to 50% of patients with VTE.

DEEP VEIN THROMBOSIS

Most DVT starts in the calf veins. Without treatment, 15% to 30% of these clots propagate to the proximal calf veins. The risk for a subsequent PE is much higher with proximal DVT than those confined to the distal calf vessels (40% to 50% versus 5% to 10%, respectively). Involvement of the upper extremities is much less common, but subclavian and axillary vein thrombosis also can lead to PE in as many as 30% of affected individuals. The same risk factors that cause lower extremity DVT also cause upper extremity DVT. In addition, other specific causes of upper extremity DVT include traumatic damage of the vessel intima from heavy exertion such as rowing, wrestling, or weight lifting (Paget-Schroetter syndrome); from extrinsic compression at the level of thoracic inlet (thoracic outlet obstruction); or from insertion of central venous catheters or pacemakers. Pain and swelling are the major complaints from patients with DVT; however, a large number of patients with DVT are asymptomatic, particularly if the DVT is restricted to the calf. Patients with upper extremity DVT can develop the superior vena caval syndrome of facial swelling, blurred vision, and dyspnea. Thoracic outlet obstruction can compress the brachial plexus leading to unilateral arm pain associated with hand weakness. Physical examination frequently reveals tenderness, erythema, warmth, and swelling below the site of thrombosis. Pain with dorsiflexion of the foot (Homan sign) may be present, but the low sensitivity and the low specificity limit its usefulness in the diagnosis of lower extremity DVT. A palpable tender cord, dilated superficial veins, and low-grade fever occur in some patients. Upper extremity DVT can cause brachial plexus tenderness in the supraclavicular fossa and atrophic hand muscles. For patients with probable thoracic outlet obstruction, several provocative tests should be performed. Adson test is positive if the radial pulses weaken during inspiration and during extension of the arm of the affected side while rotating the head to the same side. Wright test is positive if the radial pulses become weaker and painful symptoms are reproduced while abducting the shoulder of the affected side with the humerus externally rotated.

The laboratory diagnosis of DVT includes measurement of D-dimers, which are fibrin degradation products. D-dimer elevation is a highly sensitive indicator of DVT that can be performed rapidly in the emergency department. In a patient in whom the index of probability is low, a negative D-dimer test effectively excludes the diagnosis of DVT. However, the test is not specific and can be elevated in many other conditions frequently encountered in hospitalized patients (e.g., inflammation, recent surgery, malignancy). Duplex ultrasonography can be used to demonstrate the presence of a blood clot or noncompressibility of the affected veins proximal to the site of occlusion. Duplex ultrasonography has greater sensitivity in detecting proximal DVT (90% to 100%) than distal DVT (40% to 90%) of the lower extremities. With upper extremity DVT, acoustic shadowing of the clavicle may obscure detection of thrombosis in subclavian vein segments. MR angiography is particularly helpful in making the diagnosis of upper extremity DVT and pelvic vein thrombosis. Contrast venography is the conventional gold standard test, but it is invasive and technically difficult in patients with edematous extremities. Therefore, invasive venography should be reserved for patients in whom the clinical suggestion is high, despite negative or inconclusive results from noninvasive imaging.

Patients with proximal lower extremity DVT and those with upper extremity DVT should be treated initially with subcutaneous low-molecular-weight heparin (LMWH), intravenous or subcutaneous unfractionated heparin (UFH), or subcutaneous selective factor Xa inhibitor fondaparinux to prevent thrombus propagation and to maintain the patency of venous collaterals. Intravenous UFH should be given as a bolus, followed by continuous infusion to maintain an activated partial thromboplastin time of at least 1.5 times the control value. LMWH and fondaparinux has a longer half-life than UFH and can be given once or twice daily with similar efficacy. Oral warfarin should be initiated together with LMWH, UFH, or fondaparinux without delay and titrated until the international normalized ratio (INR) reaches a value between 2 and 3. When DVT is confined to the calf, the risk for PE is low, and the risk-to-benefit ratio of anticoagulation remains controversial.

When upper extremity DVT occurs in young patients who are otherwise healthy, two invasive approaches to thrombus removal should be considered: (1) infusion of a fibrinolytic drug through a catheter inserted directly into the affected vein, or (2) mechanical fragmentation of the thrombus through catheter-based technology. The purpose of these invasive procedures is to prevent or minimize the postthrombotic syndrome, which includes chronic arm pain, swelling, hyperpigmentation, and ulceration from residual venous obstruction.

Catheter-based placement of a filter in the inferior vena cava should be considered for patients with proximal DVT who either have an absolute contraindication to anticoagulation or develop recurrent PE despite an adequate trial of anticoagulation. Vena cava filters are effective in reducing the incidence of PE, but they increase the risk for recurrent DVT. Some proximal or distal migration of the filter occurs in up to 50% of cases; however, clinically evident filter embolization is limited to case reports.

PULMONARY EMBOLISM

PE occurs when a thrombus dislodges from the deep veins of the upper or lower extremities. Pulmonary vascular resistance and pulmonary arterial pressure increase from two mechanisms: (1) anatomic reduction in cross-sectional area of the pulmonary vascular bed, and (2) functional hypoxia-induced pulmonary vasoconstriction. The pressure overload on the right ventricle can lead to dilation, hypokinesis, and tricuspid regurgitation. When severe, elevated right ventricular end-diastolic pressure can compress the right coronary artery, causing subendocardial ischemia. In acute PE, areas of lung tissue are ventilated but underperfused. This $\dot{V}/\dot{Q}$ mismatch and the resultant redistribution of pulmonary blood flow from obstructed pulmonary artery to other lung regions with lower $\dot{V}/\dot{Q}$ cause arterial hypoxemia. In patients with a patent foramen ovale, hypoxemia worsens when the sudden elevation in right atrial pressure causes right-to-left shunting across the foramen.

The classic symptoms of acute PE are the sudden onset of dyspnea and pleuritic chest pain. Additional symptoms include anginal chest pain from right ventricular ischemia, hemoptysis from pulmonary infarction, and syncope or presyncope from massive PE with acute right ventricular failure (cor pulmonale). The most common physical findings are tachypnea and tachycardia. Additional physical findings include a right ventricular lift, inspiratory crackles, a loud pulmonary component of the second sound, expiratory wheezing, and a pleural rub. Symptoms and signs of proximal DVT are present in 10% to 20% of patients. Arterial blood gas analysis often reveals hypoxemia, respiratory alkalosis, and a high alveolar-to-arterial oxygen tension gradient. However, normal arterial blood gas values do not exclude the diagnosis. The most common finding with ECG analysis is sinus tachycardia. Atrial fibrillation, premature atrial contraction, and supraventricular tachycardia are less common. Other ECG changes suggest acute right ventricular strain. These include the S_1-Q_3-T_3 pattern, a new right bundle branch block or right axis deviation, and P-wave pulmonale. However, these findings are present in only 30% of patients with even massive PE. Common but nonspecific abnormalities with chest radiographic studies include atelectasis, pleural effusion, and pulmonary infiltrates. Less common but more specific radiographic findings include Hampton hump (i.e., wedge-shaped infiltrate in the peripheral lung field), which is indicative of pulmonary infarction, and Westermark sign (decreased vascularity). The plasma D-dimer test is elevated in most patients with PE as a result of activation of the endogenous fibrinolytic system, which is not sufficient to dissolve the clot. Commercially available D-dimer assays have a high sensitivity and negative predictive value but low specificity. Therefore, a normal D-dimer test effectively excludes the diagnosis of PE in patients in whom the clinical suggestion is low or intermediate. However, it should not be used to screen patients with a high

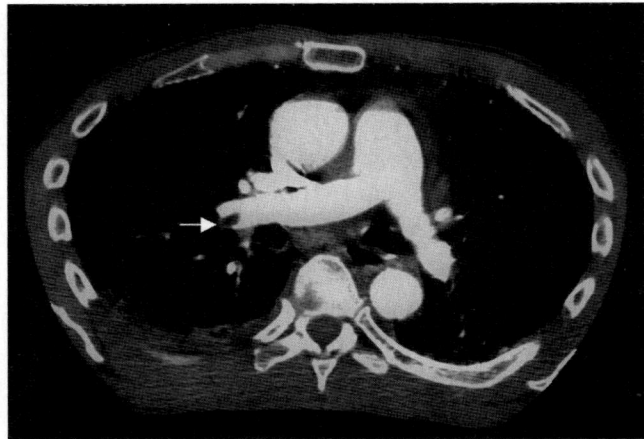

Figure 13-5 Spiral chest computed tomographic angiogram shows a large thrombus in the right main pulmonary artery *(arrow)*. (Image provided by Michael Landay, MD, Department of Radiology, University of Texas Southwestern Medical Center, Dallas, Texas.)

index of suspicion because of low negative predictive value. Elevated levels of cardiac troponin I and troponin T and other markers of myocardial injury can be found in patients with PE and are indicative of right ventricular dysfunction and a poor prognosis.

In patients with suggested PE, a completely normal $\dot{V}/\dot{Q}$ scan effectively excludes the diagnosis without further testing. However, less than 10% of $\dot{V}/\dot{Q}$ scans are interpreted as definitively normal. In patients in whom a moderate or high level of clinical probability of PE exists, a high-probability $\dot{V}/\dot{Q}$ scan has a diagnostic accuracy of 90% to 100%; however, a low or intermediate probability scan is no more helpful than a coin flip. More recently, multidetector CT angiography has become the imaging modality of choice in patients with acute PE because of its excellent visualization of the pulmonary artery (Fig. 13-5). The resolution of 1 mm or less rivals that of conventional invasive angiography. The speed of the newer-generation scanners allows acquisition of all images within a single breath-hold, avoiding respiratory motion artifacts. The overall negative predictive value of multidetector CT angiography exceeds 99%. A negative CT scan excludes the diagnosis of PE and eliminates the need for further diagnostic testing. CT also permits detection of other pathologic conditions involving the lung parenchyma, pleura, and mediastinal structures. Such pathologic findings may mimic PE and constitute alternative causes of chest pain and dyspnea. Multidetector CT angiography is not yet available at all centers. The requirement for intravenous injection of iodinated contrast material restricts applicability to those without a history of kidney disease or an allergic reaction to contrast dye. Figure 13-6 presents an algorithm for the work-up of PE based on current evidence. Echocardiography may directly detect thrombi in the right atrium, right ventricle, or pulmonary artery or indirectly demonstrate right ventricular dysfunction, signifying presence of hemodynamically significant emboli. Therefore, it is helpful in diagnosis of PE in patients with hypotension or shock, particularly when multidetector CT are not immediately available. Invasive pulmonary angiography should

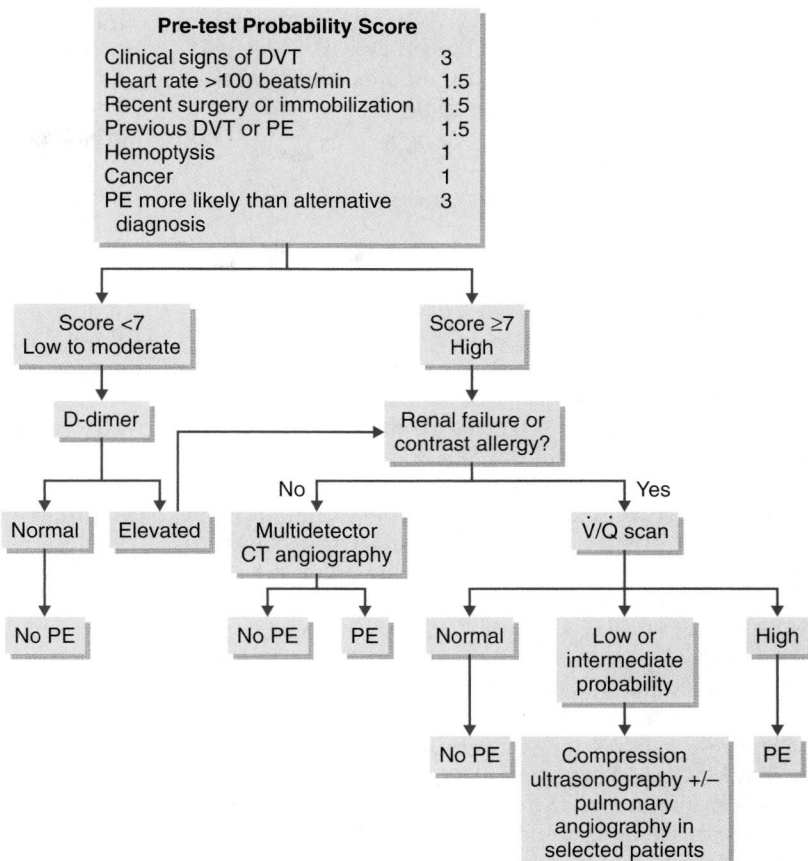

Figure 13-6 Diagnostic algorithm for patients with suggested pulmonary embolism (PE). DVT, deep vein thrombosis.

be reserved for patients in whom noninvasive testing is inconclusive.

Treatment of acute PE includes immediate anticoagulation with UFH, LMWH, or fondaparinux. LMWH and fondaparinux are preferred agents in patients with normal renal function due to the ease of subcutaneous administration and lower rates of thrombocytopenia. Because these drugs are excreted renally, they should be avoided in patients with renal failure and intravenous UFH should be used. Thrombolytic therapy with recombinant tissue plasminogen activator (rt-PA) is indicated for patients with hypotension or shock from massive PE. Surgical or percutaneous removal of emboli should be considered in patients with massive PE who have contraindications for thrombolytic therapy. Thrombolytic therapy should also be considered in patients with right ventricular enlargement or dysfunction, particularly when they have limited cardiovascular reserve or other predictors of poor outcomes such as elevated cardiac troponins. After initiation of heparins or fondaparinux, warfarin should be administered. Infusion of heparins or fondaparinux needs to be continued for at least the first 5 days of warfarin therapy until a therapeutic INR of 2 to 3 is reached.

The time necessary to continue anticoagulation after an acute PE or DVT episode depends on the presence or absence of reversible risk factors for recurrent VTE. Patients with a history of trauma or surgery generally have a low rate of recurrent VTE; therefore, warfarin can be discontinued after 3 to 6 months of administration. Patients with cancer and

VTE should be treated initially with subcutaneous fixed-dose LMWH for 3 to 6 months because of its greater efficacy than warfarin in preventing recurrent thromboembolism in this setting. After this period, treatment with LMWH or warfarin should be continued indefinitely unless the cancer is cured. Patients with idiopathic VTE with low risk for bleeding should be treated with warfarin indefinitely, whereas those with high bleeding risk should be treated for at least 3 months.

VENOUS THROMBOEMBOLISM PROPHYLAXIS

Patients who are at high risk for VTE should receive prophylaxis with subcutaneous UFH or LMWH. Patients at high risk include those who are hospitalized with acute medical illness, particularly congestive heart failure, acute respiratory illness, acute inflammatory diseases, those who are expected to be immobilized for 3 days or longer, or patients with previous VTE. Major surgery, either elective or emergent, is an important indication for VTE prophylaxis. Subcutaneous UFH is equally effective to LMWH and fondaparinux in preventing symptomatic DVT in patients undergoing general surgery, gynecologic surgery, or neurosurgery. However, LMWH, fondaparinux, or adjusted-dose warfarin to INR between 2 and 3 are preferred to UFH for prevention of DVT in orthopedic surgery such as hip surgery or total knee replacement because of superior efficacy. Patients undergoing major cancer surgery should receive continued prophylaxis after discharge up to 28 days. Mechanical prophylaxis with intermittent pneumatic compression provides additional protection from VTE and should be administered in all surgical patients whenever possible.

Arterial Hypertension

Affecting nearly one third of the adult population (65 million in the United States and 1 billion people worldwide), arterial hypertension is the leading cause of death in the world, the most common cause for an outpatient visit to a physician, and the most easily recognized treatable risk factor for stroke, myocardial infarction, heart failure, peripheral vascular disease, aortic dissection, atrial fibrillation, and end-stage kidney disease. Despite this knowledge and unequivocal scientific proof that treating hypertension with medication dramatically reduces its attendant morbidity and mortality, hypertension remains untreated or undertreated in most affected individuals in all countries, including those with the most advanced systems of medical care (Fig. 13-7). Thus, hypertension remains one of the world's great public health problems. The asymptomatic nature of the condition impedes early detection, which requires regular BP measurement. Because most cases of hypertension cannot be cured, BP control requires lifelong treatment with prescription medications, which are costly and may cause more symptoms than the underlying disease process. Effective hypertension management requires continuity of care by a regular and knowledgeable medical provider as well as sustained active participation by an educated patient. This section reviews the most important principles in the early detection and effective treatment of hypertension.

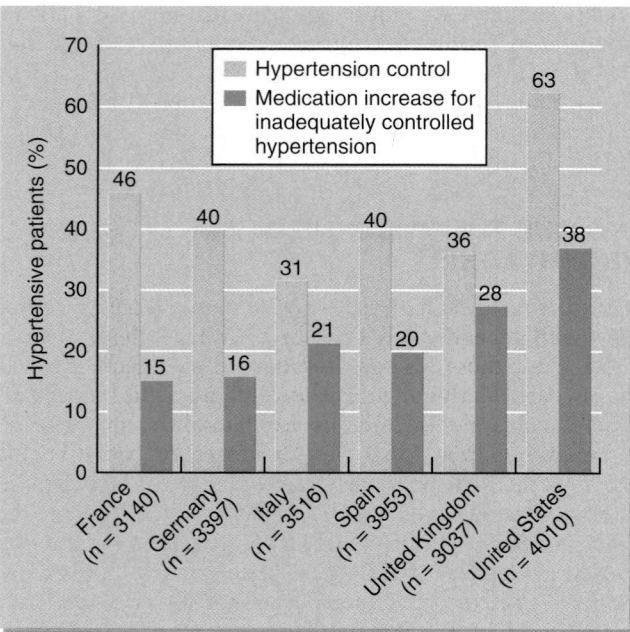

Figure 13-7 Hypertension control rates in North America and Europe. (From Wang YR, Alexander GC, Stafford RS: Outpatient hypertension treatment, treatment intensification, and control in Western Europe and the United States. Arch Intern Med 141-147, 2007.)

INITIAL EVALUATION FOR HYPERTENSION

The initial evaluation for hypertension needs to accomplish three goals: (1) staging of BP, (2) assessing the patient's overall cardiovascular risk, and (3) detecting clues of secondary hypertension. The initial clinical data needed to accomplish these goals are obtained through a thorough history and physical examination, routine blood tests, a spot (preferably first morning) urine specimen, and a resting 12-lead ECG. In some patients, ambulatory BP monitoring and an echocardiogram provide helpful additional data about the time-integral burden of BP on the cardiovascular system.

GOAL 1: ACCURATE ASSESSMENT OF BLOOD PRESSURE

Across populations, the risks for heart disease and stroke increase continuously and logarithmically with increasing levels of systolic and diastolic BP at or above 115/75 mm Hg (Fig. 13-8). Thus, the dichotomous separation of *normal* from *high* BP is artificial. BP is currently staged as normal, prehypertension, or hypertension based on the average of two or more readings taken at two or more office visits. When a patient's average systolic and diastolic pressures fall into different stages, the higher stage applies (Table 13-4).

Prehypertension is designated as BPs in the 120 to 139 mm Hg systolic, 80 to 89 mm Hg diastolic ranges. Prehypertensive individuals are twice as likely to progress to hypertension as are those with lower values.

BP normally varies dramatically throughout a 24-hour period. To minimize variability in readings, BP should be measured at least twice after 5 minutes of rest with the patient seated, the back supported, and the arm bare and at heart level. The most common mistake in measuring BP is using a standard-issue cuff that is too small for a large arm, producing spuriously elevated readings. Most overweight adults require a large adult cuff. Tobacco and caffeine should be avoided for at least 30 minutes. To avoid underestimation of systolic pressure in older adults who may have an *auscultatory gap* as a result of arteriosclerosis, radial artery palpation should be performed to estimate systolic pressure; the cuff should then be inflated to a value 20 mm Hg higher than the level that obliterates the radial pulse and deflated at a rate of 3 to 5 mm Hg per second. BP should be measured in both arms and after 5 minutes of standing, the latter to exclude a significant postural fall in BP, particularly in older persons and in those with diabetes or other conditions (e.g., Parkinson disease) that predispose the patient to autonomic insufficiency.

Because of the anxiety of going to the physician, BPs often are higher in the physician's office than when measured at home or during normal daily life outside the home. Self-monitoring of BP outside of the physician's office actively engages a patient in his or her own health care and provides a better estimate of a person's usual BP for medical decision making. BP should be measured in early morning and evening times. Three BP readings should be obtained during each measurement, separated by at least 1 minute. Because the first BP tends to be the highest, average BP should be used to assess home BP. Many *electronic home monitors* are available, but only a handful of models have been rigorously

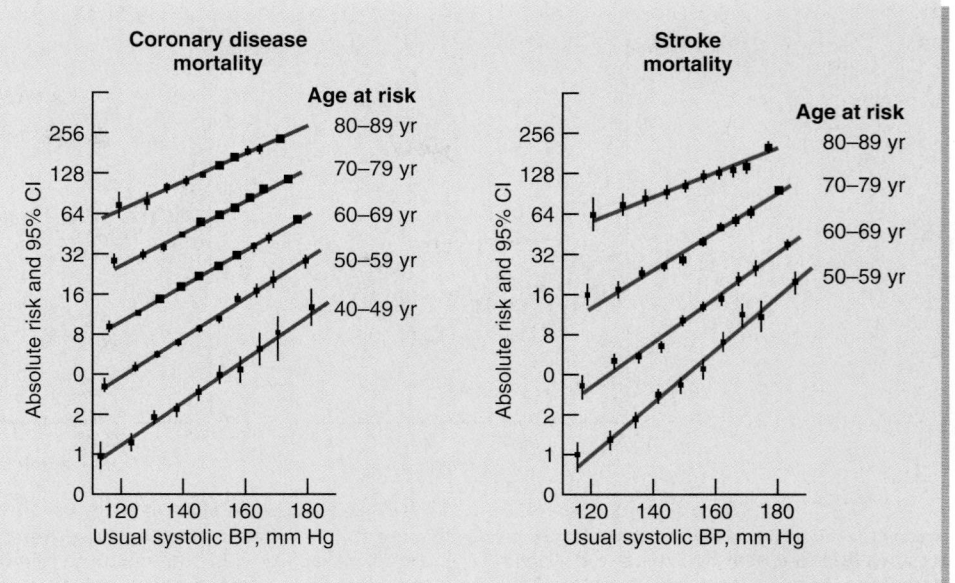

Figure 13-8 Absolute risk for coronary artery disease and stroke mortality by usual systolic blood pressure (BP) levels. (From Prospective Studies Collaboration: Age-specific relevance of usual BP to vascular mortality: A meta-analysis of individual data for one million adults in 61 prospective studies. Lancet 360:1903-1913, 2002.)

Blood Pressure Stage	Systolic Blood Pressure (mm Hg)	Diastolic Blood Pressure (mm Hg)
Normal	<120	<80
Prehypertension	120-139	80-89
Stage 1 hypertension	140-159	90-99
Stage 2 hypertension	≥160	≥100

Table 13-4 Staging of Office Blood Pressure*

*Calculation of seated blood pressure is based on the mean of two or more readings on two separate office visits.
    From Chobanian A, Bakris G, Black H, et al: The seventh report of the Joint National Committee on Prevention, Detection, Evaluation, and Treatment of High Blood Pressure. The JNC 7 report. JAMA 289:2560-2572, 2003.

validated against mercury sphygmomanometry and can be recommended.

Ambulatory monitoring provides automated measurements of BP over a 24-hour period while patients are engaged in their usual activities, including sleep (Fig. 13-9). With ambulatory monitoring, current recommendations for *upper limits of normal* are a mean daytime BP of 135/85 mm Hg, mean nighttime BP of 120/70 mm Hg, and a mean 24-hour BP of 130/80 mm Hg. However, an *optimal* mean daytime ambulatory BP is less than 130/80 mm Hg. To avoid undertreating hypertension, these lower treatment thresholds must be used when incorporating ambulatory monitoring in medical decision making. With self-monitoring of BP at home, an average value of 130/80 mm Hg should be considered the upper limit of normal; BP should be lower in the patient's own home than with daily activities outside the home.

Up to one third of patients with elevated office BPs have normal home or ambulatory BPs. If the 24-hour BP profile is completely normal and no target organ damage has occurred despite consistently elevated office readings, the patient has *office-only*, or *white-coat*, hypertension, presumably the result of a transient adrenergic response to the measurement of BP in the physician's office (see Fig. 13-9). In other patients, office readings underestimate ambulatory BPs, presumably because of sympathetic overactivity in daily life owing to job or home stress, tobacco abuse, or other adrenergic stimulation that dissipates when coming to the office (Fig. 13-10). Such documentation prevents underdiagnosing and undertreating this *masked hypertension*, which is also associated with high cardiovascular risks and identified in 10% of hypertensive patients in general and 60% to 70% of African American patients with hypertensive kidney disease.

GOAL 2: CARDIOVASCULAR RISK STRATIFICATION

Most patients with BPs in the prehypertensive or hypertensive range will have one or more additional modifiable risk factors for atherosclerosis (e.g., hypercholesterolemia, cigarette smoking, diabetes). Many patients already have evidence of target organ involvement at the time of the initial office evaluation for newly diagnosed hypertension. In addition to hypertensive stage, the other two components to cardiovascular risk are (1) co-morbidity, and (2) target organ damage (Table 13-5).

The current U.S. treatment guidelines recommend a usual BP of 140/90 mm Hg as the threshold for initiating a lifetime of antihypertensive medication in most patients and a lower threshold of 130/80 mm Hg for high-risk patients. The definition of *high-risk* patients has been expanded to include those with any of the following conditions: (1) diabetes mellitus; (2) chronic kidney disease (estimated glomerular filtration rate [GFR] < 60 mL/1.73 m² per minute or estimated urinary albumin excretion > 300 mg per 24 hours); (3) high Framingham risk score with estimated cardiovascular 10-year risk of 10% or greater; (4) unstable or stable angina;

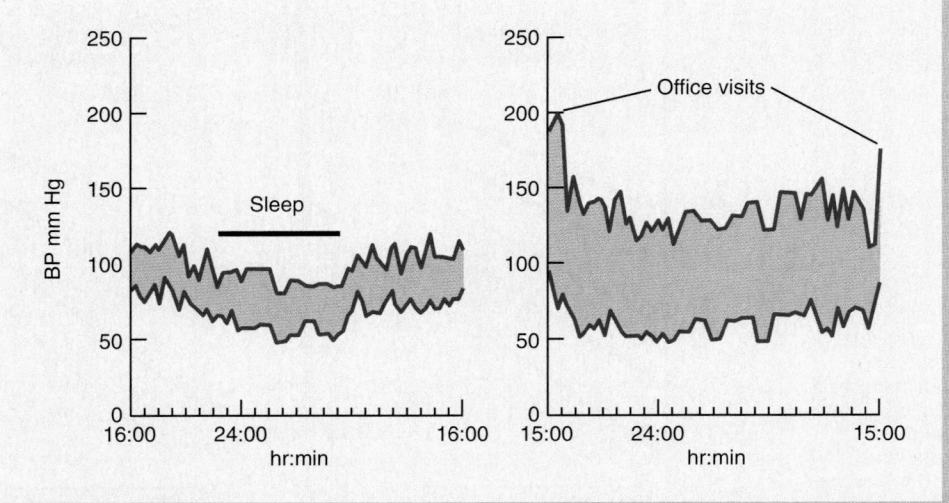

Figure 13-9 Twenty-four-hour ambulatory blood pressure (BP) monitor tracings in two different patients. **A,** Optimal blood pressure (BP) in a healthy 37-year-old woman. The normal variability in BP, the nocturnal dip in BP during sleep, and the sharp increase in BP on awakening are noted. **B,** Pronounced white-coat effect in an 80-year-old woman referred for evaluation of medically refractory hypertension. Documentation of the white-coat effect prevented overtreatment of the patient's isolated systolic hypertension. (**A,** Courtesy of Meryem Tuncel, MD, Hypertension Division, Department of Internal Medicine, University of Texas Southwestern Medical Center, Dallas, Texas. **B,** Tracing provided by Wanpen Vongpatanasin, MD, Hypertension Division, Department of Internal Medicine, University of Texas Southwestern Medical Center, Dallas, Texas.)

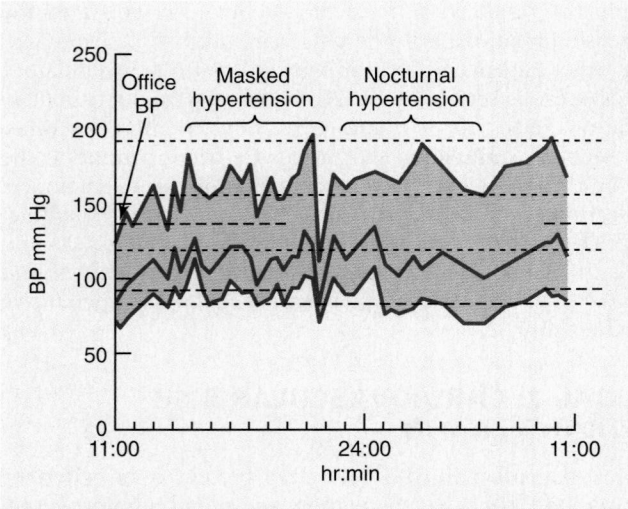

Figure 13-10 Twenty-four-hour ambulatory blood pressure (BP) monitor tracing shows both masked hypertension and nocturnal hypertension in a 55-year-old man with stage 3 chronic kidney disease. Treatment with three different antihypertensive medications in this patient produced an office BP of 125/75 mm Hg, which seems to be at goal. However, progressive hypertensive heart disease and deterioration of renal function suggested masked hypertension. Ambulatory monitoring revealed that the patient's treated BP was much higher out of the office, documenting both masked hypertension (ambulatory BP of 175/95 mm Hg and sustained nocturnal hypertension (BP of 175/90 mm Hg). Additional medication was added. (Tracing provided by Ronald G. Victor, MD, Hypertension Division, Department of Internal Medicine, University of Texas Southwestern Medical Center, Dallas, Texas.)

Table 13-5 **Components of Cardiovascular Risk Stratification in Patients with Hypertension or Prehypertension**
Indications for BP < 130/80 mm Hg
Diabetes mellitus
Chronic kidney disease
GFR < 60 mL/1.73 m²/min
Urine albumin: Cr > 300 mg/24 hr
Ten-year Framingham cardiovascular risk score ≥10%
Stable or unstable angina
ST-elevation or non–ST-elevation myocardial infarction
Congestive heart failure or left ventricular ejection fraction < 40%
Peripheral arterial disease, carotid disease, aortic aneurysm

BP, blood pressure; Cr, serum creatinine; GFR, glomerular filtration rate.

Data from Executive Summary of the Third Report of the National Cholesterol Education Program (NCEP) Expert Panel on Detection, Evaluation, and Treatment of High Cholesterol in Adults (Adult Treatment Panel III). JAMA 285:2486-2497, 2001; and Scientific statement from the American Heart Association Council for High Blood Pressure Research and the Councils on Clinical Cardiology and Epidemiology and Prevention. Circulation 115:2761-2788, 2007.

(5) acute myocardial infarction (with or without ST elevation); (6) carotid artery disease, peripheral arterial disease, or AAA; and (7) congestive heart failure or left ventricular ejection fraction of less than 40%.

GOAL 3: IDENTIFICATION OF SECONDARY (IDENTIFIABLE) CAUSES OF HYPERTENSION

A thorough search for secondary causes is not cost-effective in most patients with hypertension, but it becomes critically important in two circumstances: (1) when a com-

Table 13-6 Guide to Evaluation of Secondary Hypertension

Probable Diagnosis	Clinical Clues	Diagnostic Testing
Renal parenchymal hypertension	Estimated GFR < 60 mL/1.73 m²/min Urine albumin-to-creatinine ratio > 30 mg/g	Renal ultrasound
Renovascular disease	New elevation in serum creatinine, significant elevation in serum creatinine with initiation of ACEI or ARBs, refractory hypertension, flash pulmonary edema, abdominal bruit	MR or CT angiography, invasive angiogram
Coarctation of the aorta	Arm pulses > leg pulses, arm BP > leg BP, chest bruits, rib notching on chest radiograph	Chest MRI or CT, aortogram
Primary aldosteronism	Hypokalemia, refractory hypertension	Plasma renin and aldosterone, 24-hr urine potassium, 24-hr urine aldosterone and potassium after salt loading, adrenal CT, adrenal vein sampling
Cushing syndrome	Truncal obesity, wide and blanching purple striae, muscle weakness	24-hr urine cortisol, dexamethasone suppression test, adrenal CT
Pheochromocytoma	Spells of paroxysmal hypertension, palpitations, perspiration, pallor, pain in the head Diabetes	Plasma and 24-hr urine metanephrines and catecholamines, adrenal CT
Obstructive sleep apnea	Loud snoring, daytime somnolence, obesity, large neck	Sleep study

ACEI, angiotensin-converting enzyme inhibitor; ARB, angiotensin receptor blocker; BP, blood pressure; CT, computed tomography; GFR, glomerular filtration rate; MR, magnetic resonance; MRI, magnetic resonance imaging.
Data from Kaplan NM: Clinical Hypertension, 8th ed. Philadelphia, Williams & Wilkins, 2002.

pelling cause is found on the initial evaluation, or (2) when the hypertensive process is so severe that it either is refractory to intensive multiple-drug therapy or requires hospitalization. Table 13-6 summarizes the major causes of secondary hypertension that should be suggested on the basis of a good history, physical examination, and routine laboratory tests.

Renal Parenchymal Hypertension

Chronic kidney disease is the most common cause of secondary hypertension. Hypertension is present in more than 85% of patients with chronic kidney disease and is a major factor causing their increased cardiovascular morbidity and mortality. The mechanisms causing the hypertension include an expanded plasma volume and peripheral vasoconstriction, with the latter caused by both activation of vasoconstrictor pathways (renin-angiotensin and sympathetic nervous systems) and inhibition of vasodilator pathways (nitric oxide). Renal insufficiency should be considered when proteinuria is found by dipstick or when the serum creatinine level is greater than 1.2 mg/dL in women with hypertension or greater than 1.4 mg/dL in men with hypertension.

Renovascular Hypertension

Unilateral or bilateral renal artery stenosis is present in less than 2% of patients with hypertension in a general medical practice but in up to 30% in patients with medically refractory hypertension. The main causes of renal artery stenosis are atherosclerosis (85% of patients), typically in older adults with other clinical manifestations of systemic atherosclerosis, and fibromuscular dysplasia (15% of patients), typically in women between the ages of 15 and 50 years. Unilateral renal artery stenosis leads to underperfusion of the juxta-

glomerular cells, thereby producing renin-dependent hypertension even though the contralateral kidney is able to maintain normal blood volume. In contrast, bilateral renal artery stenosis (or unilateral stenosis with a solitary kidney) constitutes a potentially reversible cause of progressive renal failure and volume-dependent hypertension. The following clinical clues increase the suggestion of renovascular hypertension: any hospitalization for urgent or emergent hypertension; recurrent *flash* pulmonary edema; recent worsening of longstanding, previously well-controlled hypertension; severe hypertension in a young adult or in an adult after 50 years of age; precipitously and progressively worsening of renal function in response to angiotensin-converting enzyme (ACE) inhibition or angiotensin receptor blockade (ARB); unilateral small kidney by any radiographic study; extensive peripheral arteriosclerosis; or a flank bruit. The diagnosis is confirmed by noninvasive testing with MR or spiral CT angiography (Fig. 13-11). Renal artery angioplasty often cures fibromuscular dysplasia. Atherosclerotic renal artery stenosis should be treated with intensive medical management of atherosclerotic risk factors (hypertension, lipids, smoking cessation). Revascularization should be considered for the following indications: (1) medically refractory hypertension, (2) progressive renal failure on medical therapy, and (3) bilateral renal artery stenosis or stenosis of a solitary functioning kidney.

Primary Aldosteronism

The most common causes of primary aldosteronism are (1) a unilateral aldosterone-producing adenoma and (2) bilateral adrenal hyperplasia. Because aldosterone is the principal ligand for the mineralocorticoid receptor in the distal nephron, excessive aldosterone production causes excessive renal Na⁺-K⁻ exchange, often resulting in hypokalemia. The

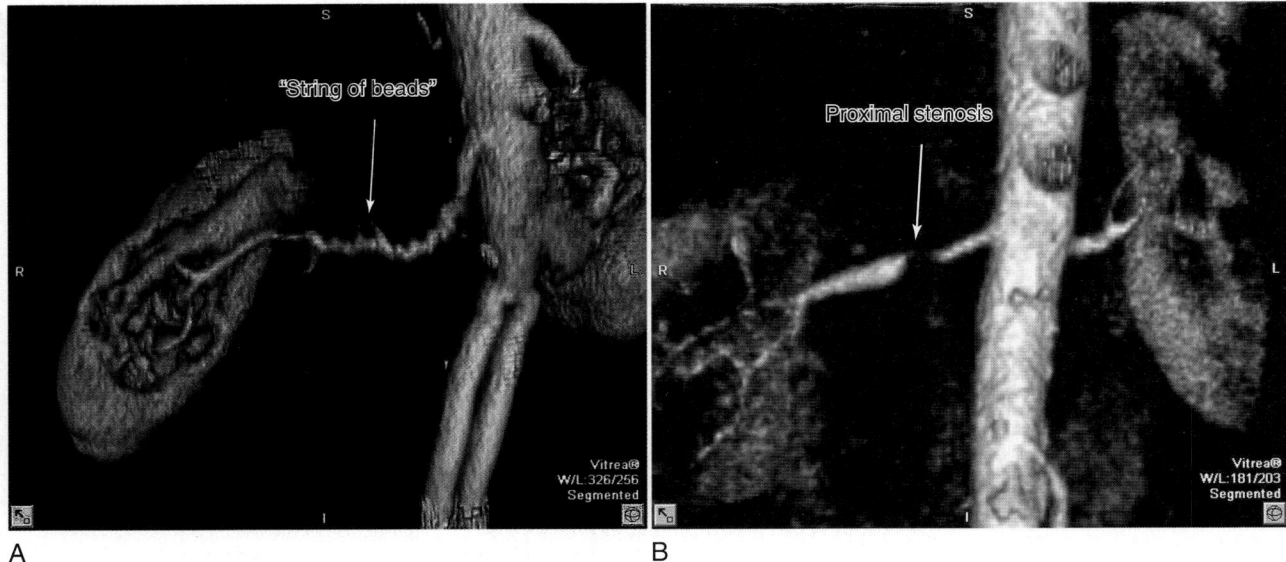

Figure 13-11 Computed tomographic angiogram with three-dimensional reconstruction. **A,** Classic *string-of-beads* lesion of fibromuscular dysplasia. **B,** Severe proximal atherosclerotic stenosis of the right renal artery. (Images courtesy of Bart Domatch, MD, Radiology Department, University of Texas Southwestern Medical Center, Dallas, Texas.)

diagnosis should always be suggested when hypertension is accompanied by either unprovoked hypokalemia (serum K^+ < 3.5 mmol/L in the absence of diuretic therapy) or a tendency to develop excessive hypokalemia during diuretic therapy (serum K^+ < 3 mmol/L). However, more than one third of patients do not have hypokalemia on initial presentation, and the diagnosis should be considered in any patient with refractory hypertension. The diagnosis is confirmed by the demonstration of nonsuppressible hyperaldosteronism during salt loading, followed by adrenal vein sampling to distinguish between a unilateral adenoma and bilateral hyperplasia. Laparoscopic adrenalectomy is the treatment of choice for unilateral aldosterone-producing adenoma, whereas pharmacologic mineralocorticoid receptor blockade with eplerenone is the treatment for bilateral adrenal hyperplasia.

Mendelian Forms of Hypertension

Nine rare forms of severe early-onset hypertension are inherited as mendelian traits. In each case, the hypertension is mineralocorticoid induced and involves excessive activation of the epithelial sodium channel (*ENaC*), the final common pathway for reabsorption of sodium from the distal nephron. The resultant salt-dependent hypertension can be caused by gain-of-function mutations of *ENaC* (Liddle syndrome) or the mineralocorticoid receptor (i.e., a rare form of pregnancy-induced hypertension) and by increased production or decreased clearance of mineralocorticoids. These include aldosterone (glucocorticoid-remediable aldosteronism), deoxycorticosterone (17-hydroxylase deficiency), and cortisol (syndrome of apparent mineralocorticoid excess).

Pheochromocytoma

Pheochromocytomas are rare catecholamine-producing tumors of the adrenal (or sometimes extra-adrenal) chromaffin cells. The diagnosis should be suggested when hypertension is accompanied by paroxysms of headaches, palpitations, pallor, or diaphoresis. In some patients, pheochromocytoma is misdiagnosed as panic disorder. A family history of early-onset hypertension may suggest pheochromocytoma as part of the multiple endocrine neoplasia syndromes. If the diagnosis is missed, outpouring of catecholamines from the tumor can cause an unsuspected hypertensive crisis during unrelated radiologic or surgical procedures; the perioperative mortality rate exceeds 80% in such patients.

Laboratory confirmation of pheochromocytoma is made by demonstrating elevated levels of plasma or urinary metanephrines, catecholamines, or other metabolites such as vanillylmandelic acid. These are typically large tumors that can usually be localized by CT or magnetic resonance imaging (MRI), although nuclear scanning with specific isotopes that localize to chromaffin tissue is occasionally needed to identify smaller tumors.

Treatment of these tumors is surgical resection. Patients must receive adequate α blockade (phentolamine), β blockade, and volume expansion before surgery to prevent the hemodynamic swings that can occur during manual manipulation of the tumor peri-operatively. For unresectable tumors, chronic therapy with the α-adrenergic blocker phenoxybenzamine is usually effective.

The differential diagnosis includes other causes of neurogenic hypertension such as sympathomimetic agents (cocaine, methamphetamine), baroreflex failure, and obstructive sleep apnea. A history of surgery and radiation therapy for head-and-neck tumors suggests the possibility of baroreceptor damage. Loud snoring, obesity, and somnolence suggest obstructive sleep apnea. Weight loss, continuous positive airway pressure, and corrective surgery improve BP control in some patients with sleep apnea.

Other causes of secondary hypertension include hypothyroidism, hyperthyroidism coarctation of the aorta, and immunosuppressive drugs, especially cyclosporine and tacrolimus.

TREATMENT OF HYPERTENSION

Prescription medication is the cornerstone of treating hypertension. Lifestyle modification should be used as an adjunct but not as an alternative to life-saving BP medication. Most dietary sodium comes from processed foods, and daily salt consumption can be reduced from 10 to 6 g by teaching patients to read food labels (6 g of NaCl = 2.4 g of Na$^+$ = 100 mmol of Na$^+$. The *Dietary Approaches to Stop Hypertension* (DASH) guidelines, which are rich in fresh fruits and vegetables (for high potassium content) and low-fat dairy products, has been shown to lower BP in feeding trials. Other lifestyle modifications that can lower BP include weight loss in overweight patients with hypertension, regular aerobic exercise, smoking cessation, and moderation in alcohol intake.

Currently, 92 prescription medications and many fixed-dose combinations are marketed for the treatment of hypertension in the United States (see Table 13-4).

WHICH DRUGS FOR WHICH PATIENTS?

Patients with Uncomplicated Hypertension

Choosing the best drugs to treat hypertension in a given patient comes down to two considerations: (1) effectively lowering BP and preventing hypertensive complications with minimal side effects and cost, and (2) concomitant treatment of co-morbid cardiovascular diseases (e.g., angina, heart failure). The seventh report of the U.S. Joint National Committee (JNC 7) recommends a thiazide-type diuretic as cost-effective first-line therapy for most patients with hypertension. It also recommends initiating therapy with two drugs—one being a thiazide—for stage 2 hypertension. In contrast, the European Society of Hypertension makes no specific drug class recommendation, arguing that the most effective drugs are those that the patient will tolerate and take. The British Hypertension Society advocates a treatment strategy that is based on the patient's age and ethnicity. It recommends initiating therapy with an ACE inhibitor or ARB or a β blocker (*A* or *B* drug) for young white patients (<55 years of age) who often have high-renin hypertension but a CCB or diuretic (*C* or *D* drug) for older and black patients who often have low-renin hypertension (Tables 13-7 and 13-8).

A growing body of evidence from clinical trials emphasizes the overriding importance of lowering BP with combinations of drugs rather than belaboring the choice of a single, best agent to begin therapy. Primary hypertension is multifactorial, and typically several medications (usually three or more) with different mechanisms of action (see Table 13-4) are required simultaneously to reach currently recommended BP levels (<140/90 mm Hg for most patients, <130/80 mm Hg for high-risk patients). In most patients with hypertension, low-dose combination drug therapy is the only way to control BP adequately and to minimize side effects. With many classes of antihypertensive medication, the dose-response relationship for BP is rather flat. Most of the BP lowering occurs at the lower end of the dose range. However, many of the side effects are steeply dose dependent, becoming problematic mainly at the high end of the

Table 13-7 **Oral Antihypertensive Agents**

Drug*	Dose Range, Total Doses per Day (mg/day)
Diuretics	
Thiazide Diuretics	
HCTZ	6.25-50 (1)
Chlorthalidone	6.25-50 (1)
Indapamide	1.25-5 (1)
Metolazone	2.5-5 (1)
Loop Diuretics	
Furosemide	20-160 (2)
Torsemide	2.5-20 (1-2)
Bumetanide	0.5-2 (2)
Ethacrynic acid	25-100 (2)
Potassium sparing	
Amiloride	5-20 (1)
Triamterene	25-100 (1)
Spironolactone	12.5-400 (1-2)
Eplerenone	25-100 (1-2)
β Blockers	
Acebutolol	200-800 (2)
Atenolol	25-100 (1)
Betaxolol	5-20 (1)
Bisoprolol	2.5-20 (1)
Carteolol	2.5-10 (1)
Metoprolol	50-450 (2)
Metoprolol XL	50-200 (1-2)
Nadolol	20-320 (1)
Nebivolol	5-40 (1)
Penbutolol	10-80 (1)
Pindolol	10-60 (2)
Propranolol	40-180 (2)
Propranolol LA	60-180 (1-2)
Timolol	20-60 (2)
β/α Blockers	
Labetalol	200-2400 (2)
Carvedilol	6.25-50 (2)
Calcium Channel Blockers	
Dihydropyridines	
Amlodipine	2.5-10 (1)
Felodipine	2.5-20 (1-2)
Isradipine CR	2.5-20 (2)
Nicardipine SR	30-120 (2)
Nifedipine XL	30-120 (1)
Nisoldipine	10-40 (1-2)
Nondihydropyridines	
Diltiazem CD	120-540 (1)
Verapamil HS	120-480 (1)
Angiotensin-Converting Enzyme Inhibitors	
Benazepril	10-80 (1-2)
Captopril	25-150 (2)
Enalapril	2.5-40 (2)
Fosinopril	10-80 (1-2)
Lisinopril	5-80 (1-2)
Moexipril	7.5-30 (1)
Perindopril	4-16 (1)
Quinapril	5-80 (1-2)
Ramipril	2.5-20 (1)
Trandolapril	1-8 (1)

*The major contraindications and side effects of these drugs are summarized in Table 13-8.

Continued

Table 13-7 Oral Antihypertensive Agents—cont'd

Drug	Dose Range, Total Doses per Day (mg/day)
Angiotensin Receptor Blockers	
Candesartan	8-32 (1)
Eprosartan	400-800 (1-2)
Irbesartan	150-300 (1)
Losartan	25-100 (2)
Olmesartin	5-40 (1)
Telmisartan	20-80 (1)
Valsartan	80-320 (1-2)
Direct Renin Inhibitors	
Aliskiren	75-300 (1)
α Blockers	
Doxazosin	1-16 (1)
Prazosin	1-40 (2-3)
Terazosin	1-20 (1)
Phenoxybenzamine	20-120 (2) for pheochromocytoma
Central Sympatholytics	
Clonidine	0.2-1.2 (2-3)
Clonidine patch	0.1-0.6 (weekly)
Guanabenz	2-32 (2)
Guanfacine	1-3 (1) (q hr)
Methyldopa	250-1000 (2)
Reserpine	0.05-0.25 (1)
Direct Vasodilators	
Hydralazine	10-200 (2)
Minoxidil	2.5-100 (1)
Fixed-Dose Combinations	
Aliskiren/HCTZ	75-300/12.5-25 (1)
Amiloride/HCTZ	5/50 (1)
Amlodipine/benazepril	2.5-5/10-20 (1)
Amlodipine/valsartan	5-10/160-320 (1)
Amlodipine/olmesartan 5-10/20-40 (1)	
Atenolol/chlorthalidone	50-100/25 (1)
Benazepril/HCTZ	5-20/6.25-25 (1)
Bisoprolol/HCTZ	2.5-10/6.25 (1)
Candesartan/HCTZ	16-32/12.5-25 (1)
Enalapril/HCTZ	5-10/25 (1-2)
Eprosartan/HCTZ	600/12.5-25 (1)
Fosinopril/HCTZ	10-20/12.5 (1)
Irbesartan/HCTZ	15-30/12.5-25 (1)
Losartan/HCTZ	50-100/12.5-25 (1)
Olmesartan/HCTZ	20-40/12.5 (1)
Spironolactone/HCTZ	25/25 (½-1)
Telmisartan/HCTZ	40-80/12.5-25 (1)
Trandolapril/verapamil	2-4/180-240 (1)
Triamterene/HCTZ	37.5/25 (½-1)
Valsartan/HCTZ	80-160/12.5-25 (1)

HCTZ, hydrochlorothiazide.

clinical dose range. Thus, low-dose combinations achieve therapeutic synergy and minimize side effects. Fixed-dose combinations reduce pill burden and cost. Additional ways to facilitate patient adherence include (1) titrating medical therapy based on home readings, which engages the patient's active participation; (2) teaching the patient to know his or her goal BP values; and (3) prescribing long-acting preparations with once-daily dosing.

Along with antihypertensive medication and lifestyle modification, additional cardiovascular risk reduction with low-dose aspirin (81 mg per day) and lipid-lowering medication should be strongly considered as an integral part of most antihypertensive regimens. In patients who are treated for hypertension, low-dose aspirin has been shown to reduce the risk for myocardial infarction by 36% without increasing the risk for intracerebral hemorrhage. A sizeable cardiovascular benefit of adding 10 mg of the HMG-CoA reductase inhibitor atorvastatin to antihypertensive therapy has been demonstrated in patients older than 60 years with moderate hypertension and an average LDL cholesterol of only 130 mg/dL.

Patients with High Cardiovascular Risks

Aggressive BP reduction to reach target goal of less than 130/80 mm Hg is warranted in patients at high risk for cardiovascular events (see Table 13-5). In patients with very high cardiovascular risk profiles but without known left ventricular dysfunction, the ACE inhibitor ramipril (10 mg/day) reduces cardiovascular events, an effect that may or may not be beyond what can be explained by BP reduction alone. The ARB telmisartan similarly offers cardiovascular protection in these high-risk individuals with less side effects such as angioedema. In contrast, a combination of ARB and ACE inhibitor results in deterioration of renal function and increases risk for hypotension without added cardiovascular benefit. A recent clinical trial demonstrated a large benefit of combination therapy with dihydropyridine CCB and ACE inhibitor over the combination of thiazide diuretics and ACE inhibitor in reducing cardiovascular events. Thus, the former combination should be considered in high-risk patients who have an elevated BP of more than 20 mm Hg above target goal.

Hypertension in African Americans

Hypertension disproportionately affects African Americans. The explanation is unknown, but the dominant importance of environmental factors is indicated by a significant geographic variation in hypertension prevalence among African-origin and European-origin populations. Hypertension is rare in Africans living in Africa and is more prevalent in several European countries than it is in the United States. As monotherapy, an ACE inhibitor or ARB or a β blocker generally yields a smaller decrease in BP in an African American than it does in a white person with hypertension and thus affords less protection against stroke. However, when high doses of an ACE inhibitor or ARB are used in combination with a diuretic, antihypertensive efficacy is amplified, and ethnic differences seem to disappear. When used as part of an appropriate multidrug regimen, ACE inhibitor–based treatment can achieve excellent control of hypertension in African American patients with hypertensive nephrosclerosis, and it slows the deterioration in renal function.

Table 13-8 Major Contraindications and Side Effects of Antihypertensive Drugs

Drug Class	Major Contraindications	Side Effects
Diuretics		
Thiazides	Gout	Insulin resistance, new-onset type 2 diabetes (especially in combination with β blockers)
		Hypokalemia, hyponatremia
		Hypertriglyceridemia
		Hyperuricemia, precipitation of gout
		Erectile dysfunction (more than other drug classes)
		Potentiate nondepolarizing muscle relaxants
		Photosensitive dermatitis
Loop diuretics	Hepatic coma	Interstitial nephritis
		Hypokalemia
		Potentiate succinylcholine
		Potentiate aminoglycoside ototoxicity
Potassium-sparing diuretics	Serum K >5.5 mEq/L GFR <30 mg/mL/1.73 m^2	Fatal hyperkalemia if used with salt substitutes, ACE inhibitors, ARBs, high-potassium foods, NSAIDs
β blockers	Heart block	Insulin resistance, new-onset type 2 diabetes (especially in combination with thiazides)
	Asthma	Heart block, acute decompensated CHF
	Depression	Bronchospasm
	Cocaine and/or methamphetamine abuse	Depression, nightmares, fatigue
		Cold extremities, claudication (β$_2$ effect)
		Stevens-Johnson syndrome
		Agranulocytosis
ACE inhibitors	Pregnancy	Cough
	Bilateral renal artery stenosis	Hyperkalemia
	Hyperkalemia	Angioedema
		Leukopenia
		Fetal toxicity
		Cholestatic jaundice (rare fulminant hepatic necrosis if the drug is not discontinued)
ARBs	Pregnancy	Hyperkalemia
	Bilateral renal artery stenosis	Angioedema (very rare)
	Hyperkalemia	Fetal toxicity
Direct renin inhibitors	Pregnancy	Hyperkalemia
	Bilateral renal artery stenosis	diarrhea
	Hyperkalemia	Fetal toxicity
Dihydropyridine CCBs	As monotherapy in chronic kidney disease with proteinuria	Headaches
		Flushing
		Ankle edema
		CHF
		Gingival hyperplasia
		Esophageal reflux
Nondihydropyridine CCBs	Heart block	Bradycardia, AV block (especially with verapamil)
	Systolic heart failure	Constipation (often severe with verapamil)
		Worsening of systolic function, CHF
		Gingival edema and/or hypertrophy
		Increase cyclosporine blood levels
		Esophageal reflux
α blockers	Monotherapy for hypertension	Orthostatic hypotension
	Orthostatic hypotension	Drug tolerance (in the absence of diuretic therapy)
	Systolic heart failure	Ankle edema
	Left ventricular dysfunction	CHF
		First-dose effect (acute hypotension)
		Potentiate hypotension with PDE-5 inhibitors (e.g., sildenafil)

Continued

Table 13-8 Major Contraindications and Side Effects of Antihypertensive Drugs—cont'd

Drug Class	Major Contraindications	Side Effects
Central sympatholytics	Orthostatic hypotension	Depression, dry mouth, lethargy Erectile dysfunction (dose dependent) Rebound hypertension with clonidine withdrawal Coombs-positive hemolytic anemia and elevated LFTs with α-methyldopa
Direct vasodilators	Orthostatic hypotension	Reflex tachycardia Fluid retention Hirsutism, pericardial effusion with minoxidil Lupus with hydralazine

ACE, angiotensin-converting enzyme; ARB, angiotensin receptor blocker; AV, arteriovenous; CCB, calcium channel blocker, CHF, congestive heart failure; GFR, glomerular filtration rate; LFT, liver function test; NSAID, nonsteroidal anti-inflammatory drug; PDE-5, phosphodiesterase type 5.

Hypertensive Nephrosclerosis

Hypertension is the second most common cause of chronic kidney disease, accounting for more than 25% of cases. Hypertensive nephrosclerosis is the result of persistently uncontrolled hypertension, causing chronic glomerular ischemia. Typically, proteinuria is mild (<0.5 g per 24 hours). Nondiabetic chronic kidney disease is a compelling indication for ACE inhibitor–based or ARB-based antihypertensive therapy. ACE inhibitors cause greater dilation of the efferent renal arterioles, thereby minimizing intraglomerular hypertension. In contrast, arterial vasodilators such as dihydropyridine CCBs, when used without an ACE inhibitor or ARB, preferentially dilate the afferent arteriole and impair renal autoregulation. Glomerular hypertension can result if systemic BP is not sufficiently lowered. The ACE inhibitor should be withdrawn only if the rise in serum creatinine exceeds 30% of the baseline value or the serum K⁻ increases to greater than 5.6 mmol/L.

Hypertensive Patients with Diabetes

Compared with its 25% prevalence in the general adult population, hypertension is present in 75% of patients with diabetes and is a major factor contributing to excessive risk for myocardial infarction, stroke, heart failure, microvascular complications, and diabetic nephropathy progressing to end-stage renal disease. To reduce these risks, BPs should be lowered to less than 130/80 mm Hg. The cardiovascular benefits of tight BP control in patients with diabetes cannot be overemphasized because they exceed and are additive to those of tight glucose control. To achieve such stringent BP goals typically requires three to five drugs. An ACE inhibitor or ARB should be the drug of first choice for the hypertensive patient with diabetes because of mounting evidence that these agents provide special renoprotective effects. However, an ACE inhibitor or ARB alone rarely achieves the stringent BP goals in patients with diabetic nephropathy. A loop diuretic is usually needed to shrink the expanded plasma volume. A dihydropyridine CCB is usually needed for antihypertensive synergy. The dihydropyridine CCB should not be started until antihypertensive therapy has been initiated with an ACE inhibitor or ARB. A β blocker should be added if the patient has coronary disease, which is prevalent in diabetes or heart failure. The α,β blocker carvedilol has a better metabolic profile than standard β blockers.

Hypertensive Patients with Coronary Artery Disease

To lower myocardial oxygen demands in patients with coronary disease, the antihypertensive regimen should reduce BP without causing reflex tachycardia. For this reason, a β blocker is often prescribed in conjunction with a dihydropyridine CCB. β blockers are indicated for patients with hypertension who have sustained a myocardial infarction and for most patients with chronic heart failure. ACE inhibitors are indicated for almost all patients with left ventricular systolic dysfunction and may be considered for patients after myocardial infarction even in the absence of ventricular dysfunction. In patients with stable coronary artery disease, a cardioprotective effect of ACE inhibition has also been demonstrated in patients with moderate cardiovascular risk profiles but not in those with lower risk profiles.

Isolated Systolic Hypertension in Older Adults

In developed countries, systolic pressure rises progressively with age; if individuals live long enough, almost all (>90%) develop hypertension. Diastolic pressure rises until the age of 50 years and decreases thereafter, producing a progressive rise in pulse pressure (i.e., systolic pressure minus diastolic pressure) (Fig. 13-12).

Different hemodynamic faults underlie hypertension in young and old persons. Patients who develop hypertension before 50 years of age typically have *combined systolic and diastolic hypertension*: systolic pressure greater than 140 mm Hg *and* diastolic pressure greater than 90 mm Hg. The main hemodynamic fault is vasoconstriction at the level of the resistance arterioles. In contrast, most patients who develop hypertension after 50 years of age have *isolated systolic hypertension*: systolic pressure greater than 140 mm Hg but diastolic pressure less than 90 mm Hg (often <80 mm Hg). In isolated systolic hypertension, the primary hemodynamic fault is decreased distensibility of the large conduit arteries (see Fig. 13-12). Collagen replaces elastin in the elastic lamina of the aorta, an age-dependent process that is accelerated by atherosclerosis and hypertension. The cardiovascular risk associated with isolated systolic hypertension is related to pulsatility, the repetitive pounding of the blood vessels with each cardiac cycle and a more rapid return of the arterial pulse wave from the periphery, both begetting more

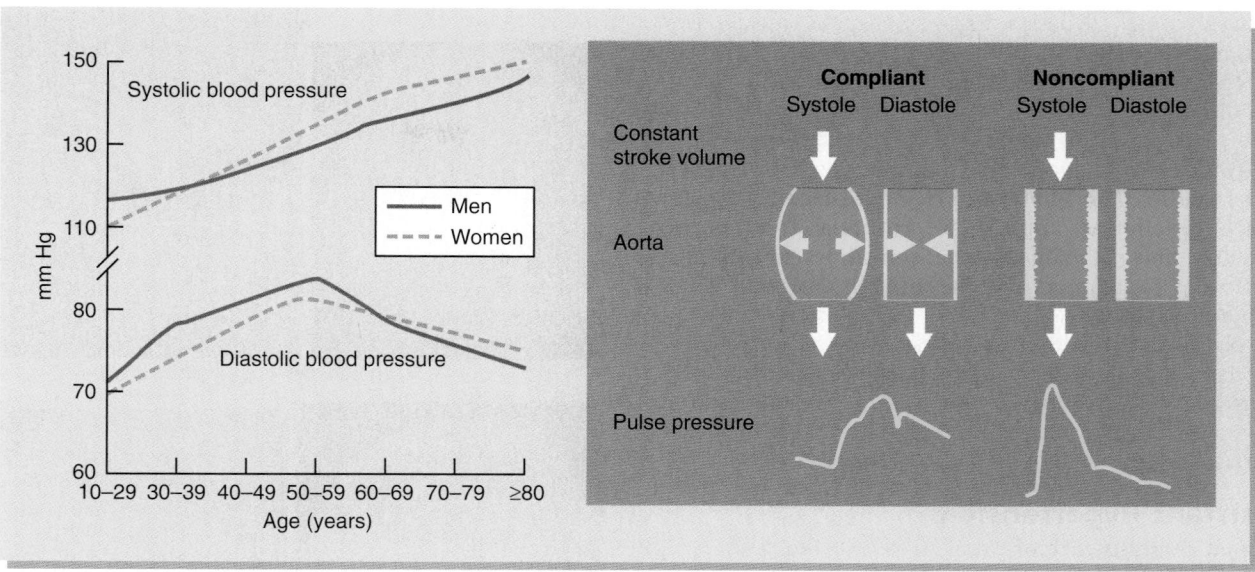

Figure 13-12 Age-dependent changes in systolic and diastolic blood pressure (BP) in the United States *(left panel)*. Schematic diagram explains the relation between aortic compliance and pulse pressure *(right panel)*. *(Left panel,* From Burt V, Whelton P, Rocella EJ, et al: Prevalence of hypertension in the U.S. adult population: Results from the Third National Health and Nutrition Examination Survey, 1988-1991. Hypertension 25:305-313, 1995. *Right panel,* From Dr. Stanley Franklin University of California at Irvine.)

systolic hypertension. In the United States and Europe, most uncontrolled hypertension occurs in older patients with isolated systolic hypertension. A BP of 160/60 mm Hg (pulse pressure of 100 mm Hg) carries twice the risk for fatal coronary heart disease as 140/110 mm Hg (pulse pressure of 30 mm Hg) (Fig. 13-13)!

In older persons with isolated systolic hypertension, lowering systolic pressure from higher than 160 to lower than 150 mm Hg reduces the risks for stroke, myocardial infarction, and overall cardiovascular mortality; it also reduces heart failure admissions and slows the progression of dementia. Trial data do not yet exist in older persons to determine whether the treatment of isolated elevations in systolic pressure between 140 and 160 mm Hg is beneficial; however, in the absence of such data, most authorities recommend treatment to prevent progression of systolic hypertension. No studies have specifically tested for a mortality benefit of treating systolic hypertension in patients older than 80 years; however, post hoc analyses strongly suggest a large reduction in strokes and heart failure admissions.

Based on data from several large randomized trials, low-dose thiazide diuretics and dihydropyridine CCBs are the drugs of choice for isolated systolic hypertension. For many older patients with hypertension, especially those with diabetes, the addition of an ACE inhibitor or ARB will be necessary to achieve recommended BP goals. To prevent the development of orthostatic hypotension, medication should be titrated to standing BP.

Blood Pressure Lowering for Secondary Prevention of Stroke

Most neurologists do not recommend BP reduction during an acute stroke. After the acute phase, BP should be lowered with a thiazide diuretic, adding an ACE inhibitor or additional drugs as needed to achieve BP goals.

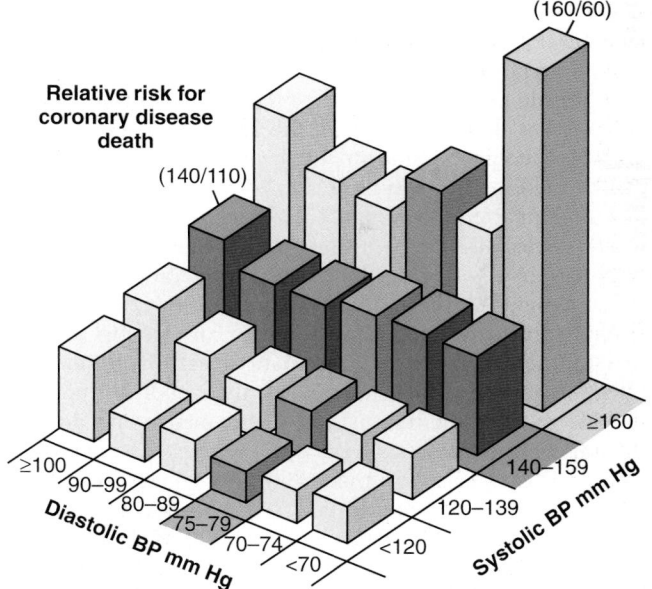

Figure 13-13 Joint influences of systolic blood pressure (SBP) and diastolic BP on coronary heart disease (CHD) risk in the Multiple Risk Factor Intervention Trial. (From Neaton JD, Wentworth D: Serum cholesterol, blood pressure, cigarette smoking, and death from coronary heart disease: Overall findings and differences by age for 316,099 white men. Arch Intern Med 152:56-64, 1992.)

Hypertensive Disorders of Women

Oral contraceptives cause a small increase in BP in most women but rarely cause a large increase into the hypertensive range. If hypertension develops, oral contraceptive therapy should be discontinued in favor of other methods of contraception. Oral estrogen replacement therapy appears to cause a small increase in BP. In contrast, transdermal estrogen (which bypasses first-pass hepatic metabolism) appears to cause a small but consistent decrease in BP.

Hypertension, the most common nonobstetric complication of pregnancy, is present in 10% of all pregnancies. Of these cases, one third are caused by chronic hypertension, and two thirds are due to preeclampsia, which is defined as an increase in BP to 140/90 mm Hg or greater after the 20th week of gestation accompanied by proteinuria (>300 mg per 24 hours) and pathologic edema, sometimes accompanied by seizures (eclampsia) and the multisystem HELLP syndrome of hemolysis (H), elevated liver enzymes (EL), and low platelets (LP). Although the cause remains an enigma, preeclampsia is the most common cause of maternal mortality and perinatal mortality. α-Methyldopa remains the drug of choice for chronic hypertension in pregnancy, and hydralazine (plus bed rest) for preeclampsia.

Resistant Hypertension

Defined as persistence of usual BP above 140/90 mm Hg despite treatment with full doses of three or more different classes of medications in rational combination and including a diuretic, *resistant hypertension* is the most common reason for referral to a hypertension specialist. In practice, the problem usually falls into one of four categories: (1) pseudoresistance, (2) inadequate medical regimen, (3) nonadherence or ingestion of pressor substances, or (4) secondary hypertension. Pseudoresistant hypertension is caused by *white-coat aggravation,* a white-coat effect superimposed on chronic hypertension that is well-controlled with medication outside the physician's office. The most common cause of apparent drug resistance is the absence of appropriate diuretic therapy. Significant impairment in renal function can be present with serum creatinine in the 1.2 to 1.4 mg/dL range or even lower, particularly in older patients with little muscle mass. To avoid this pitfall, calculation of GFR by equations based on serum creatinine, age, and weight and measurement of the urinary albumin-to-creatinine ratio from a spot-urine specimen should be an essential part of the routine evaluation of every patient with hypertension. Other common shortcomings of the medical regimen include reliance on monotherapy and inadequate dosing. Several common causes of resistant hypertension are related to the patient's behavior: medication nonadherence, recidivism with lifestyle modification (e.g., obesity, a high-salt diet, excessive alcohol intake), or habitual use of pressor substances such as sympathomimetics (e.g., tobacco, cocaine, methamphetamine, phenylephrine-containing cold or herbal remedies) or nonsteroidal anti-inflammatory drugs, with the latter causing renal sodium retention. After these behavioral factors have been excluded, the search should begin for secondary hypertension. The most common unrecognized factors are chronic kidney disease and primary aldosteronism. An increasing body of evidence suggests addition of spironolactone as a highly effective treatment in patients with resistant hypertension even in the absence of aldosteronism. Therefore, it should be part of antihypertensive regimen unless contraindicated.

Acute Severe Hypertension

Of all the patients in the emergency department, 25% have an elevated BP. *Hypertensive emergencies* are acute, often severe elevations in BP that are accompanied by acute or

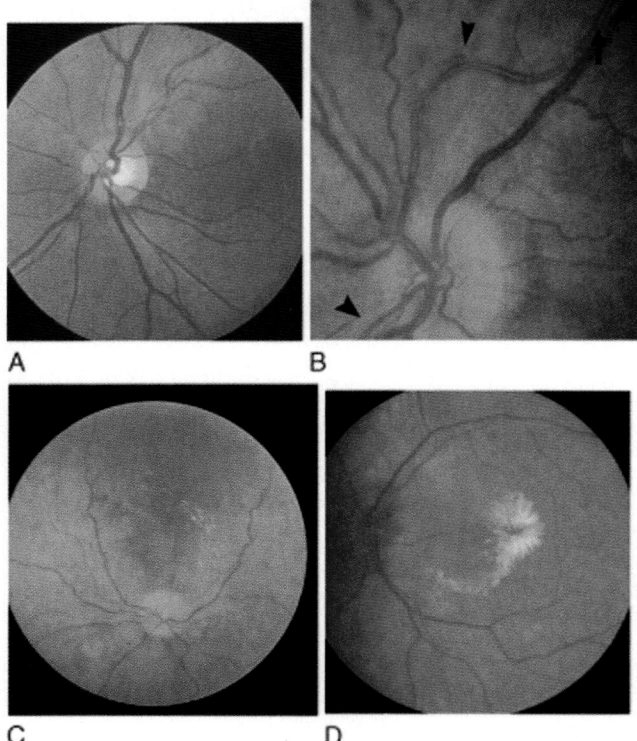

Figure 13-14 Hypertensive retinopathy is traditionally divided into four grades. **A,** Grade 1 shows very early and minor changes in a young patient; increased tortuosity of a retinal vessel and increased reflectiveness (silver wiring) of a retinal artery are seen at the 1-o'clock position in this view. Otherwise, the fundus is completely normal. **B,** Grade 2 also shows increased tortuosity and silver wiring *(arrowheads).* In addition, *nipping* of the venules at arteriovenous (AV) crossings is visualized *(arrow).* **C,** Grade 3 shows the same changes as grade 2 plus flame-shaped retinal hemorrhages and soft *cotton-wool* exudates. **D,** In grade 4, swelling of the optic disc (papilledema) is observed, retinal edema is present, and hard exudates may collect around the fovea, producing a typical *macular star.* (From Forbes CD, Jackson WF: Color Atlas and Text of Clinical Medicine, 3rd ed. London, Mosby, 2003.)

rapidly progressive target organ dysfunction such as myocardial or cerebral ischemia or infarction, pulmonary edema, or renal failure. *Hypertensive urgencies* are severe elevations in BP without severe symptoms and without evidence of acute or progressive target organ dysfunction. Thus the key distinction and approach to the patient depends on the state of the patient and the assessment of target organ damage, not simply the absolute level of BP. The full-blown clinical picture of a hypertensive emergency is a critically ill patient with a BP greater than 220/140 mm Hg, headaches, confusion, blurred vision, nausea and vomiting, seizures, heart failure, oliguria, and grade III or IV hypertensive retinopathy (Fig. 13-14). Hypertensive emergencies require immediate admission in an intensive care unit (ICU) for intravenous therapy and continuous BP monitoring, whereas hypertensive urgencies can often be managed with oral medications and appropriate outpatient follow-up in 24 to 72 hours. The most common hypertensive cardiac emergencies include acute aortic dissection, hypertension after coronary artery bypass graft surgery, acute myocardial infarction, and unstable angina. Other hypertensive emergencies include eclampsia, head trauma, severe body burns, postoperative bleeding from vascular suture lines, and epistaxis that cannot be controlled with anterior and posterior nasal packing. Neurologic emergencies, which include acute ischemic stroke, hemorrhagic stroke, subarachnoid hemorrhage, and hypertensive encephalopathy, can be difficult to distinguish from one another. Hypertensive encephalopathy is characterized by severe hypertensive retinopathy (i.e., retinal hemorrhages and exudates, with or without papilledema) and a posterior leukoencephalopathy affecting mainly the white matter of the parieto-occipital regions as seen on cerebral MRI or CT. A new focal neurologic deficit suggests a stroke in evolution, which demands a much more conservative approach to correcting the elevated BP.

In most other hypertensive emergencies, the goal of parenteral therapy is to achieve a controlled and gradual lowering of BP. A good rule of thumb is to lower the initially elevated arterial pressure by 10% in the first hour and by an additional 15% over the next 3 to 12 hours to a BP of no less than 160/110 mm Hg. BP can be reduced further over the next 48 hours. Unnecessarily rapid correction of the elevated BP to completely normal values places the patient at high risk for worsening cerebral, cardiac, and renal ischemia. In chronic hypertension, cerebral autoregulation is reset to higher than normal BP. This compensatory adjustment prevents tissue overperfusion (i.e., increased intracranial pressure) at very high BP, but it also predisposes the patient to tissue underperfusion (i.e., cerebral ischemia) when an elevated BP is lowered too quickly. In patients with coronary disease, overly rapid or excessive reduction in diastolic BP in the ICU can precipitate an acute myocardial ischemia or infarction. Secondary causes of hypertension should be considered in every patient admitted to the ICU with hypertensive crisis.

Parenteral agents for the treatment of hypertensive emergency are summarized in Table 13-9. Sodium nitroprusside, a nitric oxide donor, is the most popular agent because it can be titrated rapidly to control BP. Intravenous nitroglycerin, another nitric oxide donor, is indicated mainly for hypertension in the setting of acute coronary syndrome or decompensated heart failure. Nicardipine is a parenteral dihydropyridine CCB that is particularly useful in postoperative cardiac patients and in patients with renal failure to avoid the thiocyanate toxicity with nitroprusside. Fenoldopam is a selective dopamine-1 receptor agonist that causes both systemic and renal vasodilation as well as increased glomerular filtration, natriuresis, and diuresis. Intravenous labetalol is an effective treatment for hypertensive crisis, particularly in the setting of myocardial ischemia with preserved ventricular function.

Most patients in the emergency department with hypertensive urgencies are either nonadherent with their medical regimen or are being treated with an inadequate regimen. To expedite the necessary changes in medications, outpatient follow-up should be arranged within 72 hours. To manage the patient during the short interim period, effective oral medication includes labetalol, clonidine, or captopril, which is a short-acting ACE inhibitor.

BPs greater than 160/110 mm Hg are a common incidental finding among patients in emergency departments and other acute care settings for urgent medical or surgical care of symptoms that are unrelated to BP (e.g., musculoskeletal pain, orthopedic injury). In these settings, the elevated BP is more often the first indication of chronic hypertension than a simple physiologic stress reaction, providing an important opportunity to initiate primary care referral for formal evaluation and treatment of chronic hypertension. Home and ambulatory BP monitoring is indicated to determine whether the patient's BP normalizes completely once the acute illness has resolved.

Table 13-9 Parenteral Agents for Management of Hypertensive Emergencies

Agent	Dose	Onset of Action	Precautions
Parenteral Vasodilators			
Sodium nitroprusside	0.25-10 mcg/kg/min IV infusion	Immediate	Thiocyanate toxicity with prolonged use
Nitroglycerin	5-100 mcg/min IV infusion	2-5 min	Headache, tachycardia, tolerance
Nicardipine	5-15 mg/hr IV infusion	1-5 min	Protracted hypotension after prolonged use
Fenoldopam mesylate	0.1-0.3 mcg/kg/min IV infusion	1-5 min	Headache, tachycardia, increased intraocular pressure
Hydralazine	5-10 mg as IV bolus or 10-40 mg IM; repeat every 4-6 hr	10 min IV 20 min IM	Unpredictable and excessive falls in blood pressure; tachycardia; angina exacerbation
Enalaprilat	0.625-1.25 mg every 6 hr IV bolus	15-60 min blood pressure	Unpredictable and excessive falls in acute renal failure in patients with bilateral renal artery stenosis
Parenteral Adrenergic Inhibitors			
Labetalol	20-80 mg as slow IV injection every 10 min, or 0.5-2.0 mg/min IV as infusion	5-10 min	Bronchospasm, heart block, orthostatic hypotension
Metoprolol	5 mg IV every 10 min for three doses	5-10 min	Bronchospasm, heart block, heart failure, exacerbation of cocaine-induced myocardial ischemia
Esmolol	500 mcg/kg IV over 3 min; then 25-100 mg/kg/min as IV infusion	1-5 min	Bronchospasm, heart block, heart failure
Phentolamine	5-10 mg IV bolus every 5-15 min	1-2 min	Tachycardia, orthostatic hypotension

IM, intramuscular; IV, intravenous.

PROGNOSIS

One of the most important prognostic factors in hypertension is ECG or echocardiographic LVH, with the latter already present in as many as 25% of patients with newly diagnosed hypertension. LVH predisposes the patient to heart failure, atrial fibrillation, and sudden cardiac death. For these reasons, BP should be lowered to below 130/80 mm Hg in hypertensive patients with LVH.

Because of their relatively short duration (typically, <5 years), randomized trials underestimate the lifetime protection against premature disability and death afforded by several decades of antihypertensive therapy in clinical practice. In the Framingham Heart Study, treating hypertension for 20 years in middle-aged adults reduced total cardiovascular mortality by 60%, which is considerably greater than the results of most randomized trials despite the less intense treatment guidelines when therapy was initiated in the 1950s through the 1970s.

Prospectus for the Future

- Further delineation of genetic causes of hypertension and application of this research to the treatment and prevention of hypertension, including development of pharmacologic and nonpharmacologic therapy that target the various signaling pathways in hypertension and prehypertension
- Improvement of endovascular techniques (stent grafts) for the treatment of aortic aneurysms, aortic dissection, and peripheral vascular diseases and evaluation of the role of these techniques in patients who are unfit for surgery

- Evaluation of drug-eluting stents for the prevention of restenosis after percutaneous revascularization of infrainguinal vascular disease
- Further assessment of safety and efficacy of emerging antithrombotic therapy in patients with atrial fibrillation, venous thromboembolism, and vascular disease
- Improvements in noninvasive imaging techniques of the vasculature, including three-dimensional reconstruction using CT angiography, MR angiography, and duplex ultrasonography

---

References

American Heart Association: Proceedings: Atherosclerotic Vascular Disease Conference. Circulation 118:2811-2878, 2008.

Chobanian A, Bakris G, Black H, et al: The seventh report of the Joint National Committee on Prevention, Detection, Evaluation, and Treatment of High Blood Pressure. The JNC 7 report. JAMA 289:2560-2572, 2003. (The latest United States consensus guidelines.)

Kearon C, Kahn SR, Agnelli G, et al: American College of Chest Physicians. Antithrombotic therapy for venous thromboembolic disease: American College of Chest Physicians Evidence-Based Clinical Practice Guidelines, 8th ed. Chest 133:454S-545S, 2008.

Jamerson K, Weber MA, Bakris GL, et al, for the ACCOMPLISH Trial Investigators: Benazepril plus amlodipine or hydrochlorothiazide for hypertension in high-risk patients. N Engl J Med 359:2417-2428, 2008.

Julius S, Nesbitt SD, Egan BM, et al, for the Trial of Preventing Hypertension (TROPHY) Study Investigators: Feasibility of treating prehypertension with an angiotensin-receptor blocker. N Engl J Med 354:1685-1697, 2006.

Rosendorff C, Black HR, Cannon CP, et al: Treatment of hypertension in the prevention and management of ischemic heart disease: A scientific statement from the American Heart Association Council for High Blood Pressure Research and the Councils on Clinical Cardiology and Epidemiology and Prevention. Circulation 115:2761-2788, 2007.

Sakalihasan N, Limet R, Defawe OD: Abdominal aortic aneurysm. Lancet 365:1577-1589, 2005.

Task Force for the Management of Arterial Hypertension of the European Society of Hypertension (ESH) and of the European Society of Cardiology (ESC). 2007 Guidelines for the management of arterial hypertension. Eur Heart J 28:1462-1536, 2007.

Torbicki A, Perrier A, Konstantinides S, et al: Task Force for the Diagnosis and Management of Acute Pulmonary Embolism of the European Society of Cardiology. Guidelines on the diagnosis and management of acute pulmonary embolism: The Task Force for the Diagnosis and Management of Acute Pulmonary Embolism of the European Society of Cardiology (ESC). Eur Heart J 29:2276-2315, 2008.

Yusuf S, Teo KK, Pogue J, et al, for the ONTARGET Investigators: Telmisartan, ramipril, or both in patients at high risk for vascular events. N Engl J Med 358:1547-1559, 2008.

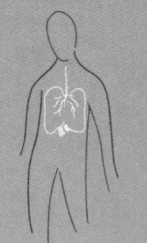

Section IV

Pulmonary and Critical Care Medicine

Chapter 14

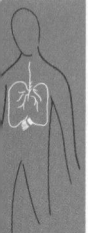

The Lung in Health and Disease

Sharon Rounds and Matthew D. Jankowich

The lung is part of the respiratory system. The respiratory system includes the centers for respiratory control in the brain cortex and medulla, the spinal cord, and peripheral nerves that innervate the skeletal muscles of respiration and the airways and vessels. The upper airway, including the nose, pharynx, and larynx, are where inspired air is humidified and particulate matter is filtered. The chest wall bony structure serves to maintain the lungs in an inflated state. The skeletal muscles of respiration include the diaphragm and the accessory muscles; the latter are important when disease states result in diaphragm fatigue. The lung consists of conducting airways and blood vessels and the gas exchange unit with alveolar gas space and capillaries. The lung is a complex organ with an extensive array of airways and vessels arranged to efficiently transfer the gases necessary for sustaining life. This organ has an immense capacity for gas exchange; therefore, it is not a limiting factor in exercise tolerance in healthy individuals. However, gas exchange becomes compromised in lung disease, rendering the host unable to function properly. The most dramatic consequence of acute and chronic abnormalities in lung function is systemic hypoxemia, leading to tissue hypoxia. Thus, the sequelae of lung dysfunction involve detrimental effects to other organs.

In addition to gas exchange, it is increasingly recognized that the lungs have other functions, such as defense against inhaled infectious agents or environmental toxins. Also, the entire cardiac output passes through the pulmonary circulation that serves as a filter for blood-borne clots or infections. The massive surface area of endothelial cells lining the pulmonary circulation serves metabolic functions, such as conversion of angiotensin I to angiotensin II.

Lung disorders are common and range from well-known conditions such as asthma and chronic obstructive pulmonary disease (COPD) to rarely encountered disorders such as lymphangioleiomyomatosis. This section discusses the diagnosis, evaluation, and treatment of disorders that develop in direct response to lung injury as well as disorders that develop indirectly through injuries to other organs. This chapter begins with a brief discussion of how the basic structural-functional relationships of the lung are established during lung development, followed by a description of the classification of pulmonary disorders discussed in the chapters in this section.

Lung Development

The lung begins to develop during the first trimester of pregnancy through complex and overlapping processes that transform the embryonic lung bud into a functioning organ with an extensive airway network, two complete circulatory systems, and millions of alveoli responsible for the transfer of gases to and from the body. Lung development can be described in five consecutive stages: *embryonic, pseudoglandular, canalicular* or *vascular, saccular,* and *alveolar postnatal* (Table 14-1). During the embryonic stage, between 21 days and 7 weeks of gestation, the rudimentary lung emerges from the foregut as a single epithelial bud surrounded by mesenchymal tissue. This stage is followed by the pseudoglandular stage (between 5 and 17 weeks of gestation), during which repeated monochotomous and dichotomous branching forms rudimentary airways—a process termed *branching morphogenesis* (Fig. 14-1). Coinciding with airway formation, new bronchial arteries arise from the aorta. The canalicular stage is next (between 17 and 24 weeks of gestation) and is characterized by the formation of the acinus, the differentiation of the acinar epithelium, and the development of the distal pulmonary circulation. Through the process of *vasculogenesis,* capillary networks derived from endothelial cell precursors are formed, extend from and around the distal air spaces, and connect with the developing pulmonary arteries and veins. By the end of this stage, the thickness of the alveolar capillary membrane is similar to that in the adult. During the saccular or prenatal alveolar stage (between 24 and 38 weeks of gestation), vascularized crests emerging from the parenchyma divide the terminal airway structures termed *saccules.* Thinning of the interstitium continues, bringing capillaries from adjacent alveolar structures into close apposition, leading to a double capillary

Table 14-1 **Stages of Lung Development**		
Stage	**Period**	**Comments**
Embryonic	3-7 wk	Embryonic lung bud emerges from the foregut.
Pseudoglandular	5-17 wk	Airway tree is formed through a process of monochotomous and dichotomous branching accompanied by growth.
Canalicular	17-24 wk	Angiogenesis and vasculogenesis occur to form the developing vascular network.
Saccular	24-38 wk	Alveoli begin to form through thinning of the mesenchyme and apposition of vascular structures with the air spaces and maturation.
Alveolar (postnatal)	36 wk-2 yr	Further development of alveoli and maturation occurs.

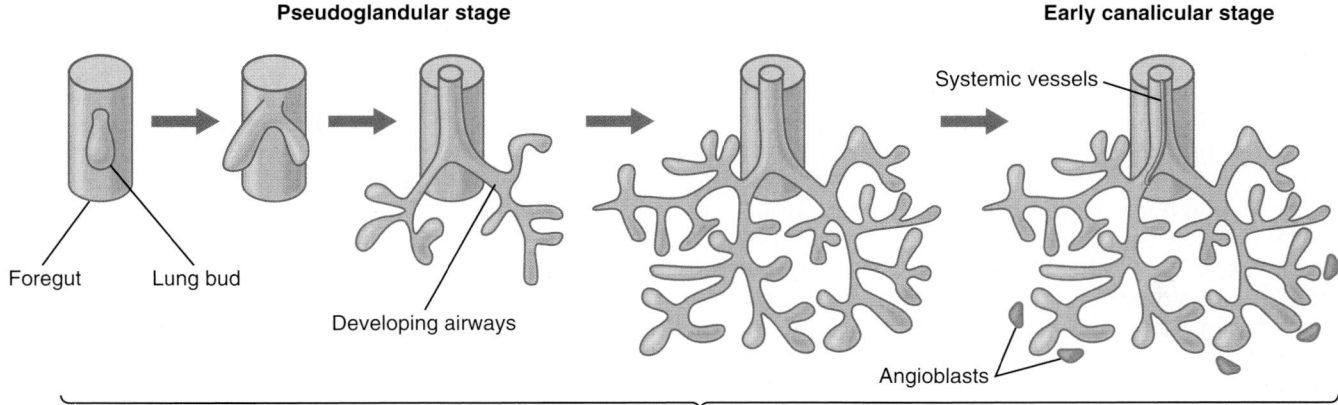

Figure 14-1 Lung branching morphogenesis. Branching morphogenesis occurs during the pseudoglandular stage of lung development and is the process by which the embryonic lung develops the primitive airway system through monochotomous and dichotomous branching.

network. Near birth, capillaries from opposing networks fuse to form a single network, and capillary volume increases with continuing lung growth and expansion. After birth, the lung continues to grow through the first few years of childhood with the creation of more alveoli through the septation of the air sacs. By age 2 years, the lung contains double arterial supplies and venous drainage systems, a complex airway system designed to generate progressive decreases in resistance to airflow as the air travels distally, and a vast alveolar network that efficiently transfers gases to and from the blood.

The processes that drive lung development are tightly controlled, but mishaps do happen, leading to congenital lung disorders such as cystic adenomatoid malformation of the lung, lung hypoplasia or agenesis, bullous changes in the lung parenchyma, and abnormalities in the vasculature, including aberrant connections between systemic vessels and lung compartments (e.g., lung sequestration) and congenital absence of one or both pulmonary arteries. However, these conditions are rare when compared with the number of infants born annually with abnormal lung function as a result of prematurity. In premature infants, the type II pneumatocytes of the lung are underdeveloped and produce insufficient quantities of surfactant, a surface-active substance produced by specific alveolar epithelial cells that helps decrease surface tension, thereby preventing alveolar collapse. This disorder is known as the *infant respiratory distress syndrome* (IRDS). The treatment of IRDS is administration

of exogenous surfactant and corticosteroids to enhance lung maturation. To sustain life while allowing maturation, mechanical ventilation and oxygen supplementation are required but may promote the development of bronchopulmonary dysplasia. In children without congenital abnormalities, lung disorders are relatively rare, except those caused by infection and accidents.

Pulmonary Disease

Diseases of the respiratory system in the adult are some of the most common clinical entities confronted by physicians. At least 4 of the top 10 causes of death by medical illnesses in the United States are related to pulmonary dysfunction in one way or another: cancer (of which lung cancer is the most common), COPD, pneumonia, and sepsis. COPDs, such as emphysema and chronic bronchitis, are the fourth leading cause of death and the second leading cause of disability in the United States. At a time when a decrease in the age-adjusted death rate by other common disorders such as coronary artery disease and stroke is occurring, death by COPD continues to increase and is projected to become the third leading cause of death in the United States by 2020. More than 16 million Americans are estimated to have COPD, but because COPD takes years to develop and the incidence of cigarette smoking (the most common etiologic factor for COPD) is staggering (in 2005, more than 44.5

million Americans were daily smokers), the true disease burden of COPD is much greater.

Asthma is also a common illness, affecting 6% to 8% of the population in the United States. Between the decades of 1960 and 1990, the prevalence, hospitalization rate, and mortality rate related to asthma increased dramatically. Sleep-disordered breathing is estimated to affect 7 to 18 million people in the United States, with 1.8 to 4 million of these having severe sleep apnea. Interstitial lung diseases are being increasingly recognized, and their true incidence appears to have been underestimated. For example, idiopathic pulmonary fibrosis, the most common of the idiopathic interstitial pneumonias, affects 85,000 to 100,000 Americans annually. Another interstitial lung disease, sarcoidosis, affects about 45,000 Americans each year. Acute respiratory conditions are also common. Viral upper respiratory infections account for 40% of all acute respiratory conditions. Pneumonia occurs in 6 million people per year and is one of the top leading causes of death in the United States.

These conditions affect individuals of all ages, races, and sex. However, a disproportionate increase in the incidence, morbidity, and mortality related to lung diseases exists in minority populations. This finding is true for COPD, asthma, and certain interstitial lung disorders, among others. Although these differences point to genetic differences among these populations, they also point to differences in culture, socioeconomic status, exposure to pollutants (e.g., inner-city living), and access to health care.

This section reviews the epidemiologic factors, pathophysiologic conditions, clinical presentation, evaluation, and management of the most common lung diseases. Lung diseases are often classified on the basis of the affected anatomic areas of the lung (e.g., interstitial lung diseases, pleural diseases, airways diseases) and the physiologic abnormalities detected by pulmonary function testing (e.g., obstructive lung diseases, restrictive lung diseases). In general, classification schemes based exclusively on physiologic factors are inaccurate because distinctly different disorders with different causes, consequences, and responses to therapy show similar physiologic abnormalities (Fig. 14-2).

The *obstructive lung diseases* share a common physiologic characterization of airflow limitation, as determined by pulmonary function testing (referred to as an *obstructive pattern*). Obstructive lung diseases include emphysema, chronic bronchitis, asthma, and bronchiectasis, among others. The *interstitial lung diseases* are less common disorders but are more difficult to subclassify because this category includes more than 120 distinct entities, some that are inherited and most without an obvious cause. In general, a restrictive physiologic condition that is due to decreased lung compliance and small lung volumes characterizes these disorders, and this characterization is the reason they are often referred to as *restrictive lung disorders* (e.g., idiopathic pulmonary fibrosis). However, not all interstitial lung diseases exhibit a restrictive pattern on pulmonary function testing. They may have airflow limitation as a result of small airway involvement (e.g., sarcoidosis, bronchiolitis obliterans). The *pulmonary vascular diseases* are disorders in which involvement of the pulmonary vasculature causes increased intraluminal pressure or pulmonary hypertension. These range from disorders caused by obstruction to blood flow as a result of blood clots (e.g., pulmonary embolus) to disorders characterized by tissue remodeling and obliteration or compression of the vascular structures by connective tissue (e.g., primary pulmonary hypertension). The *disorders of respiratory control* include conditions in which extrapulmonary abnormalities are responsible for dysfunction of the respiratory system, causing abnormal ventilation. These include disorders of sleep such as obstructive sleep apnea. These also include disorders of the neuromuscular system in which ventilatory abnormalities are due to poor excursion of the respiratory muscles, as observed in myasthenia gravis and polymyositis. *Disorders of the pleura, chest wall, and mediastinum* are classified as such because they affect these specific structures. Infectious agents, of which viral and bacterial infections are the most frequent, cause conditions that include *infectious diseases of the lung.* *Neoplastic disorders* of the lung include both benign (e.g., hamartomas) and malignant (e.g., lung carcinoma) disorders, which can affect the lung parenchyma or its surrounding pleura (e.g., mesothelioma). This section also discusses illnesses requiring critical care such as acute lung injury and sepsis, which are often triggered by injuries to the lung and are frequently managed by pulmonologists and critical care specialists.

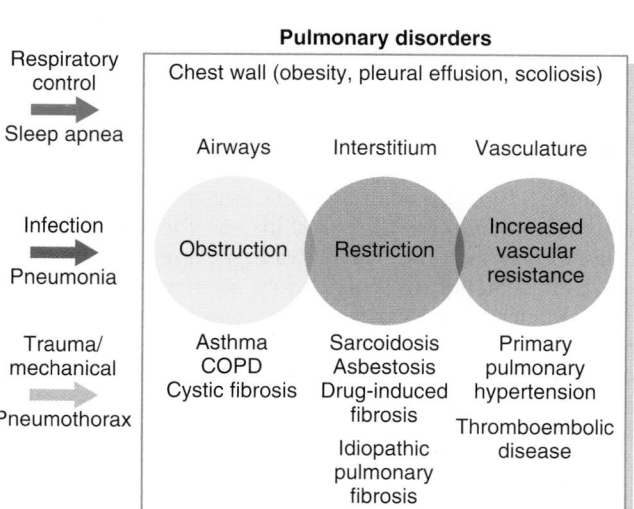

Figure 14-2 Lung diseases. Lung diseases are caused by abnormalities in the lung structure (e.g., airways, interstitium, vasculature), the chest wall, or external forces (e.g., infection). Disorders affecting the lung structure cause physiologic derangements (e.g., obstruction to airflow, restricted lung volumes, pulmonary hypertension, and hypoxia), but these derangements are not necessarily specific to any particular lung disease caused by the extensive overlap among the mechanisms responsible for their manifestation.

Prospectus for the Future

Important questions remain in lung development. What are the primary stimuli for branching morphogenesis? How does gene regulation alter lung development? How do lung airway and blood vessel development remain coordinated? What are the environment-gene interactions that cause abnormal lung development?

In addition, there are important fundamental questions in the epidemiology of lung diseases. For example, it is not clear whether or how childhood asthma and adult COPD are related. In addition, the role of fine particulate matter air pollution in the pathogenesis of lung diseases is unclear.

Finally, the causes and pathogenesis of many lung diseases, such as sarcoidosis, are unclear.

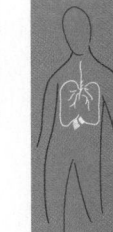

References

Mannino DM: Epidemiology and global impact of chronic obstructive pulmonary disease. Semin Respir Crit Care Med 26:204-210, 2005.

Whitsett JA, Wert SE, Trapnell BC: Genetic disorders influencing lung formation and function at birth. Hum Mol Genet 13:R207-R215, 2004.

Chapter 15

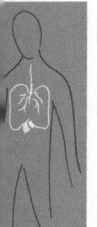

General Approach to Patients with Respiratory Disorders

Brian Casserly and Sharon Rounds

History

A detailed history is necessary to assess effectively a patient who may have pulmonary disease. Patients with lung disorders often complain of one or more of the following symptoms: dyspnea or shortness of breath, fatigue, exercise intolerance, chest tightness, cough, sputum production, and chest pain, among others. Although individually these symptoms are not specific, the presence of certain symptoms coinciding in the same individual may point to a specific diagnosis.

Important to note, common symptoms of respiratory disease, such as dyspnea and cough, are frequently seen in diseases of other organ systems (Table 15-1). For example, dyspnea is also a cardinal symptom of heart disease, and cough may be caused by gastroesophageal reflux or chronic sinusitis. An organized approach to the patient, starting with a careful history and a detailed physical examination, will focus further investigation to determine the cause of the symptom.

Common Presenting Complaints

Dyspnea (shortness of breath) is a common complaint of patients with pulmonary disease (Table 15-2). Timing and acuity of onset, exacerbating and alleviating factors, and degree of functional impairment are key elements of the history. Associated symptoms such as cough, hemoptysis, chest pain, wheezing, orthopnea, and paroxysmal nocturnal dyspnea, as well as environmental triggers, should be elicited and are helpful in developing a differential diagnosis. If dyspnea is recent, of sudden onset, and accompanied by chest pain, then diseases such as pneumothorax, pulmonary

embolism, and pulmonary edema should come to mind. If the dyspnea is long-standing and is slowly progressive, then chronic conditions such as chronic obstructive pulmonary disease (COPD), pulmonary fibrosis, pulmonary arterial hypertension, and neuromuscular disorders are in the differential diagnosis. The progression of chronic dyspnea may be insidious. Asking specific questions to quantify changes in functional status over time is important. Dyspnea may occur during exertion or at rest and may be episodic or continuous. Episodic dyspnea associated with exertion suggests parenchymal lung disease or cardiac dysfunction. Dyspnea that is seasonal or triggered by environmental exposure suggests diseases such as asthma and hypersensitivity pneumonitis. Positional dyspnea can occur in patients with severe obstructive lung disease, diaphragmatic paralysis, or neuromuscular weakness.

Orthopnea is defined as dyspnea that occurs in the supine position. This condition may occur as a result of a decrease in vital capacity caused by abdominal contents exerting force against the diaphragm. *Paroxysmal nocturnal dyspnea* is dyspnea that occurs 1 to several hours after lying down and is associated with congestive heart failure. Increased venous return to the heart causes this condition, resulting in mild interstitial edema. Asthma can also be associated with nocturnal dyspnea and is thought to be due to decreased vital capacity, decreased production of endogenous agents with bronchodilator functions, and increased exposure to allergens present in beddings. Exercise-induced asthma causes dyspnea out of proportion to the degree of exertion, with dyspnea often being most severe in the 15 to 30 minutes after the cessation of exercise.

Wheezing, although associated with asthma, has many causes. The absence of wheezing does not rule out asthma in any setting, and the presence of wheezing does not establish the diagnosis. Other conditions that cause wheezing are congestive heart failure; endobronchial obstruction by

Table 15-1 **Major Symptoms of Respiratory Disease**
Cough
Sputum
Hemoptysis
Dyspnea (acute, progressive, or paroxysmal)
Wheezing
Chest pain
Fever
Hoarseness
Night sweats

Table 15-2 **Some Causes of Dyspnea**	
Airways disease	Chronic obstructive lung diseases Laryngeal disorders Tracheal obstruction or stenosis Tracheomalacia
Parenchymal lung disease	Pneumonia Interstitial lung diseases Obliterative bronchiolitis Pulmonary edema due to increased vascular permeability (acute respiratory distress syndrome) Infiltrative and metastatic malignancies
Pulmonary circulation	Pulmonary thromboembolism Pulmonary arterial hypertension Pulmonary arteriovenous malformation
Chest wall and pleura	Pneumothorax Pleural effusion or massive ascites Pleural tumor Fractured ribs Chest wall deformities Neuromuscular diseases Bilateral diaphragmatic paresis
Cardiac	Pulmonary edema due to left heart failure Pericardial effusion or constrictive pericarditis Intracardiac shunt
Hematologic	Anemia
Noncardiorespiratory	Psychogenic Acidosis (with compensatory respiratory alkalosis) Midbrain lesion

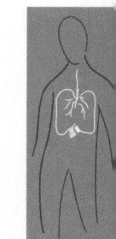

tumor, foreign body, or mucus; vocal cord abnormalities; and acute bronchitis.

Cough is a frustrating symptom for both the patient and the physician. The three most common causes of chronic cough are postnasal drip, asthma, and gastroesophageal reflux disease. Cough may be mild and infrequent, or it may be severe enough to induce emesis or syncope. Cough may be dry or may produce sputum or blood (*hemoptysis*). The symptom may begin months after initiation of a drug (e.g., angiotensin-converting enzyme [ACE] inhibitors) leading to a dry, hacking cough. *Bordetella pertussis* infection (whooping cough) and viral lower respiratory infections can produce a cough that may last for 3 months or longer. Patients with asthma often have a cough. On occasion, cough is their only symptom, a condition sometimes referred to as *cough-variant asthma*. Nocturnal cough should raise the suggestion of asthma, heart failure, or gastroesophageal reflux disease.

More than occasional production of *sputum* is abnormal and should be characterized with regard to quantity, color, presence or absence of blood, and timing. The physician should ask the patient to estimate the frequency and volume of sputum produced in 24 hours as well as any diurnal variation. *Chronic bronchitis* is defined as a persistent cough resulting in sputum production for more than 3 months in each of the last 3 years. Patients with asthma often have a productive cough resulting from excess mucus production. Colored sputum does not always signify a bacterial infection because the concentration of cellular debris, predominantly white cells present in any inflammatory process, influences sputum color. Patients with difficult to control asthma who report brown plugs or casts of the small bronchi in their sputum may have *allergic bronchopulmonary aspergillosis*.

Hemoptysis is a frightening symptom. The volume of blood may be scant or large enough to cause asphyxiation or exsanguination. The most common cause of hemoptysis in the United States is bronchitis, whereas the most common cause worldwide is pulmonary tuberculosis. Most cases of hemoptysis are small in volume and self-limited and resolve with the treatment of the underlying process. Massive hemoptysis, defined as more than 500 mL of blood in 24 hours, is rare and considered a medical emergency when it occurs. Causes of massive hemoptysis include lung cancer, lung cavities containing mycetomas, cavitary tuberculosis, pulmonary hemorrhage syndromes, pulmonary arteriovenous malformations, and bronchiectasis. The physician should distinguish among hemoptysis, epistaxis, and hematemesis. Because many patients have trouble identify-

ing the source of the bleeding, a careful upper airway physical examination is essential.

Chest pain attributable to the lungs usually results from pleural disease, pulmonary vascular disease, or musculoskeletal pain precipitated by coughing because no pain receptors exist in the lung parenchyma. Lung cancer, for example, does not cause pain until it invades the pleura, chest wall, vertebral bodies, or mediastinal structures. Disease or inflammation of the pleura causes pleuritic chest pain characterized as a sharp or stabbing pain with deep inspiration. Pain caused by pulmonary emboli, infection, pneumothorax, and collagen vascular disease is also usually pleuritic. Pulmonary hypertension may produce dull anterior chest pain unrelated to respiration caused by right ventricular strain and demand ischemia. Other examples of noncardiac causes of chest pain include esophageal disease, herpetic neuralgia, musculoskeletal pain, and trauma. Older patients or those with a history of chronic systemic steroid use may have thoracic pain resulting from vertebral compression or rib fractures. Adequate analgesia, including narcotics, is essential in the treatment of chest pain in patients with underlying lung disease to prevent the reduction in vital capacity caused by splinting of the chest in reaction to the pain. Musculoskeletal chest pain should be a diagnosis of exclusion after serious causes have been ruled out. This pain is usually reproducible with movement or palpation over the affected area.

Past History

One should always ask about previous respiratory illness including pneumonia, tuberculosis, or chronic bronchitis, or abnormalities of the chest radiograph that have been previously reported to the patient. Patients with the acquired immunodeficiency syndrome (AIDS) have a high risk for developing *Pneumocystis jiroveci* pneumonia and other chest infections including tuberculosis. Immunosuppression from long-standing steroid use may predispose to tuberculosis and other lung infections. Almost every class of drug can be associated with lung toxicity. Examples include pulmonary embolism from use of the oral contraceptive pill, interstitial lung disease from cytotoxic agents (e.g., methotrexate, cyclophosphamide, bleomycin), bronchospasm from β blockers or nonsteroidal anti-inflammatory drugs and cough from ACE inhibitors. Some medications known to cause lung disease may not be mentioned by the patient because they are illegal (e.g., cocaine, heroin).

An accurate history of tobacco use, as well as other *toxic* and *environmental exposures*, is essential in patients with respiratory complaints. Tobacco smoke is the most prevalent environmental toxin causing lung disease. Patients may be anxious about other inhaled toxins or irritants and yet may continue to smoke without concern. Asking about tobacco use and attempting to motivate patients to quit smoking is the physician's duty. The risk for lung disease from smoking is directly related to individual genetic susceptibility and the total pack-years of exposure, and it is inversely related to the age at onset of smoking and, in the case of lung cancer, the interval since smoking cessation.

A history of exposure to other inhaled toxins, irritants, or allergens should be elicited. A careful occupational history often uncovers exposure to inorganic dust or fibers such as asbestos, silica, or coal dust. Organic dusts may cause hypersensitivity pneumonitis and other interstitial lung diseases. Solvents and corrosive gases are also causes of pulmonary disease. The presence of household pets should be documented. Cats are the most allergenic for asthma, and birds may cause hypersensitivity or fungal lung disease. A travel history is important in evaluating infectious causes of pulmonary disease. For example, histoplasmosis is common in the Ohio and Mississippi River valleys, and coccidioidomycosis is found in the desert Southwest. Travel to developing countries increases the risk for exposure to tuberculosis. A family history is important in assessing the risk for genetic lung diseases such as cystic fibrosis and α_1-antitrypsin deficiency as well as susceptibility to asthma, emphysema, or lung cancer.

Physical Examination

The physical examination should be complete, with emphasis on areas highlighted by the history. The first steps in the physical examination of the patient with pulmonary disease are observation and inspection, which must be done when the patient's chest is bare (Table 15-3). The physician should start by evaluating the general appearance of the patient. In particular, attention should be given to the presence or absence of respiratory distress. This observation will

Table 15-3 **Physical Examination of the Chest**
Inspection
Observation for anxiety, distress, malnutrition, somnolence
Chest wall shape, deformity
Respiratory rate, depth, pattern
Paradoxic respiratory motion of chest and abdomen
Retractions
Use of accessory muscles
Pursed-lip breathing
Cyanosis
Palpation
Tracheal deviation
Chest expansion
Vocal fremitus
Lymphadenopathy
Subcutaneous emphysema
Percussion
Normal, dull, or hyperresonant
Auscultation
Breath sounds: normal vesicular over periphery and bronchial centrally
Pleural rub
Added sounds: wheezes, crackles
Stridor

not only help in diagnosis but also point to the urgency of the case.

Body habitus is important because morbid obesity in a patient with exercise intolerance and sleepiness might point to a diagnosis of sleep-disordered breathing, whereas dyspnea in a thin middle-aged man with pursed lips might suggest emphysema. Race and sex should also be noted because certain conditions are more frequently encountered in specific populations. For example, sarcoidosis is most common in African Americans in the Southeast, whereas lymphangioleiomyomatosis is a rare disorder that essentially affects young women of childbearing age. *Tachycardia and pulsus paradoxus* are important signs of severe asthma.

The physician should watch the patient breathe and note the effort required for breathing. Increased respiratory rate, use of accessory muscles of respiration, pursed-lip breathing, and paradoxic abdominal movement all indicate increased work of breathing. The patient's inability to speak in full sentences indicates severe airway obstruction or neuromuscular weakness. The physician should listen for cough during the history and physical examination and should note the strength of the cough because this may signal respiratory muscle weakness or severe obstructive lung disease. The patient's rib cage should expand symmetrically with inspiration. The shape of the thoracic cage should also be noted. Increased anteroposterior diameter is observed in those with lung hyperinflation due to obstructive lung disease. Severe kyphoscoliosis, pectus excavatum, ankylosing spondylitis, and morbid obesity can produce restrictive ventilatory disease as a consequence of distortion and restriction of the volume of the thoracic cavity.

The hands may reveal important signs of lung diseases. Look for *clubbing*, which is commonly associated with respiratory disease. An uncommon association with clubbing is hypertrophic pulmonary osteoarthropathy (HPO). HPO is characterized by the presence of periosteal inflammation at the distal ends of long bones, the wrists, the ankles, and the metacarpal and metatarsal bones. There is swelling and tenderness over the wrists and other involved areas. Rarely HPO may occur without clubbing. The causes of HPO include primary lung carcinoma and pleural mesothelioma. Look for *staining* of the fingers (actually caused by tar because nicotine is colorless), a sign of cigarette smoking. The density of staining does not indicate the number of cigarettes smoked, but depends rather on the way the cigarette is held in the hand. Ask the patient to dorsiflex the wrists with the arms outstretched and to spread out the fingers. A flapping tremor *(asterixis)* may be seen with severe carbon dioxide retention. *Wasting and weakness* are signs of cachexia due to malignancy. In addition, compression and infiltration by a peripheral lung tumor of a lower trunk of the brachial plexus results in wasting of the small muscles of the hand and weakness of finger abduction.

Examination of the head and neck are also important. Inspect the eyes for evidence of *Horner syndrome* (a constricted pupil, partial ptosis, and loss of sweating), which can be due to an apical lung tumor compressing the sympathetic nerves in the neck. Listen to the voice for *hoarseness,* which may indicate recurrent laryngeal nerve palsy associated with carcinoma of the lung (usually left sided), or laryngeal carcinoma. However, the most common cause is laryngitis. Look for nasal polyps (associated with asthma), engorged turbinates (various allergic conditions), and a deviated septum (nasal obstruction). Look at the tongue for central cyanosis. The mouth may hold evidence of an upper respiratory tract infection (a reddened pharynx and tonsillar enlargement with or without a coating of pus). A broken tooth or gingivitis may predispose to lung abscess or pneumonia. Sinusitis is indicated by tenderness over the sinuses on palpation. There may be facial plethora or cyanosis if superior vena caval obstruction is present. Some patients with obstructive sleep apnea will be obese with a receding chin, a small pharynx, and a short, thick neck.

Palpation of the chest is performed by first palpating the accessory muscles of respiration in the patient's neck—the scalene and sternocleidomastoid muscles. Hypertrophy and contraction indicate increased respiratory effort. The trachea should be palpated and should lie in the midline of the neck. Deviation of the trachea may suggest lung collapse or a mass. Neck masses should be noted. The physician should place both hands on the lower half of the patient's posterior thorax with thumbs touching and fingers spread; the hands should be kept in place while the patient takes several deep inspirations. The physician's thumbs should separate slightly and the hands should move symmetrically apart during the patient's inspiration.

Fremitus is a faint vibration felt best with the edge of the hand against the patient's chest wall while the patient speaks. Fremitus is increased in areas with underlying lung consolidation, and it is decreased over a pleural effusion. Next, the patient's chest should be percussed. The level of the diaphragms on each side should be noted. The percussion note should be compared on the two sides starting at the apex and moving down, including the posterior, anterior, and lateral aspects. A pleural effusion, consolidation, mass, or elevated diaphragm can cause dullness to percussion; a pneumothorax or hyperinflation can cause hyperresonance.

Auscultation of the lungs is performed to evaluate the quality of the breath sounds and to detect the presence of extra (adventitious) sounds not heard in normal lungs. Normal breath sounds have two qualities, vesicular and bronchial. Bronchial breath sounds are heard over the central airways and are louder and coarser than vesicular breath sounds, which are heard at the periphery and base of the lungs. Bronchovesicular sounds are a combination of the two and are heard over medium-sized airways. Bronchial sounds have a longer inhaled component, whereas vesicular sounds have a much longer expiratory component and are much softer. Bronchial breath sounds and bronchovesicular breath sounds at the periphery of the lungs are abnormal and may be caused by underlying consolidation. In the presence of consolidation, increased transmission of vocal sounds, called *whispered pectoriloquy,* occurs; *egophony,* in which the spoken letter *e* sounds like an *a* over the area of consolidation, is heard and sometimes compared with the bleating of a goat.

Abnormal or extrapulmonary sounds are crackles, wheezes, and rubs. *Crackles* can be coarse rattles or fine, *Velcro-like* sounds. Mucus in the airways or the opening of large- and medium-sized airways often causes coarse crackles. Fine crackles, produced with inspiration by the opening of collapsed alveoli, are most common at the bases and are heard in pulmonary edema and interstitial fibrosis as well as in healthy older patients during deep inspiration. *Wheezing* is a higher-pitched sound and, when heard locally, suggests large airway obstruction. The wheezing of patients with asthma or congestive heart failure is lower in pitch and heard diffusely over all lung fields. Localized wheezing can be heard in conditions such as pulmonary embolism, obstruction of a bronchus by a tumor, and foreign-body aspiration. A *rub* is a pleural sound caused by inflamed pleural surfaces rubbing together. A rub has been described as the sound of pieces of leather rubbing against each other. Rubs are often evanescent and depend on the amount of fluid in the pleural space. Often, pleuritic chest pain and a rub develop after large-volume thoracentesis. A crunching sound timed with the cardiac cycle, called *Hamman crunch,* is heard in patients with a pneumomediastinum. The complete absence of breath sounds on one side should cause the examiner to think of pneumothorax, hydrothorax, or hemothorax; obstruction of a main stem bronchus; or surgical or congenital absence of the lung. The physical findings associated with various pulmonary disorders are outlined in Table 15-4.

Evaluation

The clinician should be able to develop a differential diagnosis based on a detailed history and a thorough physical examination. This preliminary differential diagnosis is the basis on which a battery of tests is ordered, recognizing that these tests might unveil disorders not considered in the initial assessment. The objective of this extended evaluation is twofold: (1) to confirm a diagnosis or discard other disorders, and (2) to assess the severity of the lung derangement. In general, patients with a suggested lung disorder should undergo pulmonary function testing. *Spirometry* evaluates airflows and helps distinguish between an obstructive pattern characteristic of COPD, asthma, and related

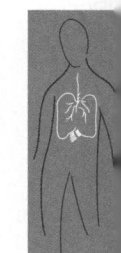

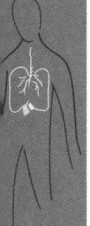

Table 15-4   Physical Findings in Common Pulmonary Disorders

Disorder	Mediastinal Displacement	Chest Wall Movement	Vocal Fremitus	Percussion Note	Breath Sounds	Added Sounds	Voice Sounds
Pleural effusion	Heart displaced to opposite side	Reduced over affected area	Absent or markedly decreased	Dull	Absent over fluid; bronchial breath at upper border	Absent; pleural rub may be found above effusion	Absent over effusion; increased with egophony at upper border
Consolidation	None	Reduced over affected area	Normal or increased	Dull	Bronchial	Crackles	Increased with egobronchophony and whispered pectoriloquy
Pneumothorax	Tracheal deviation to opposite side if under tension	Decreased over affected area	Absent	Resonant	Absent or decreased	Absent	Absent
Atelectasis	Ipsilateral shift	Decreased over affected area	Variable	Dull	Absent or diminished	Crackles may be heard	Absent
Bronchospasm	None	Decreased symmetrically	Normal or decreased	Normal or decreased	Bronchovesicular	Wheezing	Normal or decreased
Interstitial fibrosis	None	Decreased symmetrically	Normal or increased	Normal	Bronchovesicular	End-inspiratory crackles unaffected by cough or posture	Normal

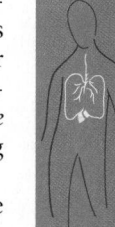

disorders, as well as a restrictive pattern observed in fibrosing lung disease. Spirometry will also provide information regarding the severity of the physiologic derangement. *Lung volume measurements* are helpful in assessing hyperinflation or confirming a restrictive process. Measuring diffusion capacity for carbon monoxide (D_LCO) will provide information about alterations in gas-exchanging capability. Further assessment of gas exchange can be obtained through the determination of oxygen saturation using pulse oximetry. Information regarding both oxygenation and acid-base status is obtained from *arterial blood gas* determination. A *6-minute walk test* will evaluate oxygenation during exertion; through this test, patients are often found to require supplemental oxygen for the first time. Other, more specialized tests (e.g., bronchoprovocation, cardiopulmonary stress testing, polysomnography) might be required, depending on the circumstances.

Imaging studies of the chest are extremely useful in evaluating lung structure. The *chest radiograph* will provide information about the lung parenchyma and pleura, the cardiac silhouette, mediastinal structures, and even body habitus. Frequently, examining old chest radiographic images is useful to assess progression of disease. *Computed tomography* will provide more accurate information about the pulmonary and mediastinal structures, and it is essential in the assessment of interstitial lung disease and lung masses, among other disorders. Together with *ventilation-perfusion scanning* and *pulmonary angiography,* the computed tomogram is one of the many tools available to evaluate the lung vasculature. *Magnetic resonance imaging, positron-emission tomography,* and related tests are becoming more frequently used in the evaluation of patients with lung masses and other lung disorders. Standard blood tests such as the *blood counts* and *blood chemistry* point to specific disorders or may provide information about the severity of a lung disorder (e.g., polycythemia in chronic hypoxemia, leukocytosis in lung infection). Some specialized tests should be reserved when specific diagnoses such as *serologic conditions* (e.g., rheumatoid factor, antinuclear antibodies) are suggested in patients who may have connective tissue–related lung disease or *hypersensitivity profile* when the diagnosis of hypersensitivity pneumonitis is being entertained.

Together with the history and physical examination, these tests are useful at narrowing a diagnosis to establish a specific plan of treatment. This plan can often be created in a single visit. However, patients will frequently require several visits to a clinician. These follow-up visits serve to assess progression of disease, patient compliance with therapy, and response to management. If these noninvasive tests do not allow for diagnosing the problem, more invasive tests might be necessary. *Fiberoptic* or *rigid bronchoscopy* allows for direct visualization of the airways and for obtaining valuable clinical samples for study. *Transthoracic percutaneous needle aspiration* is useful in evaluating peripheral lung lesions. Ultimately, surgery might be required to obtain tissue through *open* or *video-assisted thoracoscopic-guided lung biopsy.*

Prospectus for the Future

The predictive values of various aspects of history and physical examination need to be clarified. The role of quantitative computed tomography analysis in diagnosis and assessment of disability of lung diseases needs to be clarified. The role of interventional pulmonary procedures must be ascertained for both diagnosis and treatment of lung diseases.

Reference

Fitzgerald FT, Murray JF: History and physical examinations. In Mason RJ, Murray JF, Broaddus VC, Nadel JA (eds): Murray and Nadel's Textbook of Respiratory Medicine, 4th ed. Philadelphia, Elsevier, 2005.

Chapter 16

Evaluating Lung Structure and Function

F. Dennis McCool

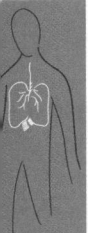

The satisfactory functioning of all organ systems depends on their capacity to consume oxygen and eliminate carbon dioxide. The primary function of the lung is to deliver oxygen to the pulmonary capillary blood and to excrete carbon dioxide. To accomplish this, a volume of air must be delivered through numerous branching airways to small alveolar sacs. Oxygen can then diffuse across the thin alveolar membrane into the capillary blood, where it is bound to hemoglobin. As oxygen is removed from the alveolus, carbon dioxide diffuses from the pulmonary vasculature into the alveolar sacs. It is excreted from the body when air is exhaled from the lungs and airways. The remarkable matching of oxygen consumption and carbon dioxide production allows the human to maintain optimal oxygenation and acid-base balance over a wide range of activities that require enormous differences in ventilation. This chapter provides an overview of the anatomy and physiology that enable the respiratory system to perform its life-sustaining functions as well as a discussion of tests available to evaluate lung structure and function.

Anatomy

AIRWAY

Inspired air travels through the nose and mouth and then passes into the pharynx, larynx, and trachea. In the nose and nasopharynx, the air is heated, humidified, and filtered of airborne particles greater than 10 μm in diameter. Air then quickly enters the trachea and the left and right main stem bronchi. The bronchi separate into segmental and subsegmental airways. Cartilaginous rings help to maintain the patency of these large airways. In the main stem bronchi, the rings are circumferential, whereas in the trachea, the cartilaginous rings are U-shaped, with the posterior membrane of the trachea sharing a wall with the esophagus. The region of the lung that includes the first 18 branches of the airways is referred to as the *conducting zone*. This region consists of the trachea, bronchi, bronchioles, and alveolar ducts (Fig. 16-1). After about 18 subdivisions, the airways branch another 3 to 5 times until they become alveolar sacs. This area of the lung is referred to as the *respiratory zone* and consists of the terminal bronchioles and alveolar ducts. Gas exchange commences in the terminal bronchioles but primarily occurs in the alveoli. All totaled, there are about 27 subdivisions of the airway from the trachea to the alveolar ducts. The total cross-sectional area of this zone is far greater than the cross-sectional area of the more proximal airways. Thus, for a given airflow rate (Δ volume/time), air travels at a lower velocity (Δ distance/time) in the distal airways than in the larger proximal airways. This difference in velocity in concert with the difference in overall cross-sectional area results in low resistance to flow in the distal airways and greater resistance to airflow in the proximal airways.

ALVEOLI

The alveoli are the grapelike clusters of air sacs that interface with the pulmonary capillaries. There are about 300 million individual alveolar sacs. The alveoli are thin-walled structures with a total surface area of about 100 m². This is roughly half the size of a tennis court. The surface of the alveoli is lined by two types of cells. The flat type I pneumocyte constitutes 95% of the cells. Type II pneumocytes account for about 5% of the alveolar lining cells and secrete surfactant; a complex lipoprotein whose role in lowering surface tension in the alveolar space is critical to reducing the forces needed to expand the lung. Surfactant is also important in preventing alveolar collapse at low lung volumes and thereby promoting normal gas exchange. The epithelial lining of the alveoli, the endothelial lining of the capillaries, and the intervening basement membrane present a barrier to gas exchange. Normally this barrier is less than 1 μm thick and does not significantly interfere with gas exchange.

BLOOD VESSELS

The pulmonary artery arises from the right ventricle and branches until it terminates in a meshwork of capillaries that

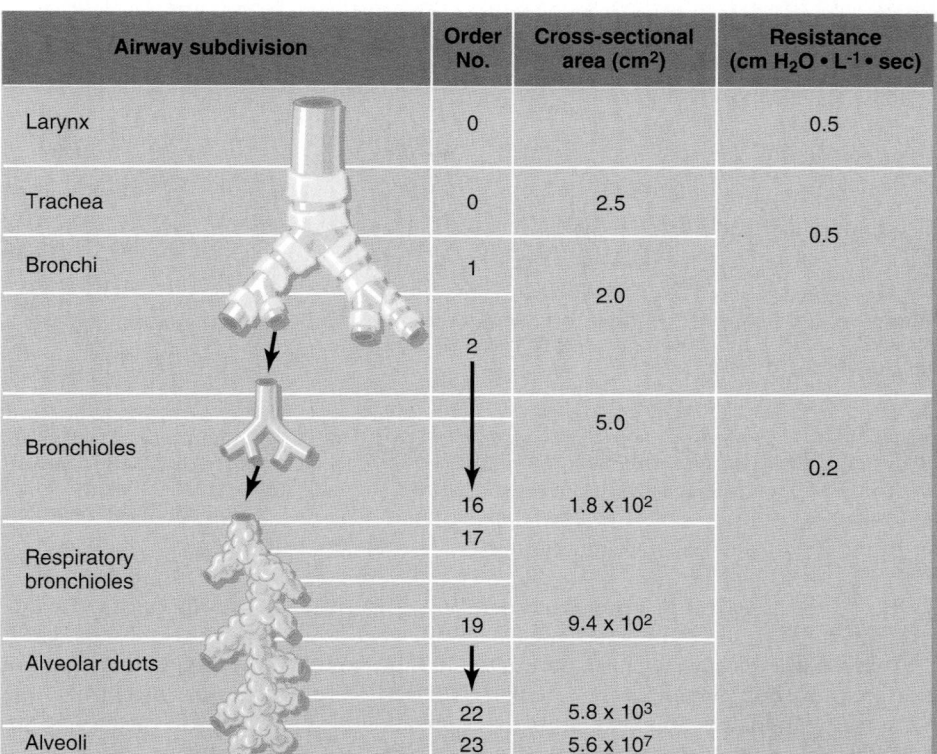

Airway subdivision	Order No.	Cross-sectional area (cm²)	Resistance (cm H₂O • L⁻¹ • sec)
Larynx	0		0.5
Trachea	0	2.5	0.5
Bronchi	1	2.0	
	2		
Bronchioles		5.0	0.2
	16	1.8 × 10²	
Respiratory bronchioles	17		
	19	9.4 × 10²	
Alveolar ducts			
	22	5.8 × 10³	
Alveoli	23	5.6 × 10⁷	

Figure 16-1 The subdivision of the airways and their nomenclature. The cross-sectional area increases dramatically toward the peripheral, small airways. (Adapted from Weibel ER: Morphometry of the Human Lung. Berlin, Springer, 1963.)

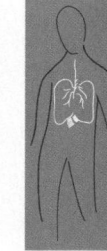

surround the alveoli. This creates a large surface area that facilitates gas exchange. Blood returns to the heart through pulmonary veins that course through the lungs, coalesce into four main pulmonary veins, and empty into the left atrium. The pulmonary circulation is a low-resistance circuit with pulmonary vascular resistance about $\frac{1}{10}$ of the resistance in the systemic circulation. Pulmonary vessels can be easily recruited to accommodate increases in blood flow while maintaining low pressures and resistance. Accordingly, during exercise, any increase in cardiac output can be distributed through the lung without significantly increasing pulmonary arterial pressures. A separate vascular system, the bronchial system, also supplies the lung. The bronchial arteries originate from the aorta and, in contrast to the pulmonary arteries, are under systemic pressure. These vessels provide nutrients to lung structures proximal to the alveoli. Two thirds of the bronchial circulation drains into the pulmonary veins and then empties into the left atrium. This blood, which has low oxygen content, mixes with the freshly oxygenated blood from the pulmonary veins to lower the oxygen content of the blood that enters the systemic circulation.

Physiology

VENTILATION

Overall, gas exchange consists of a series of four steps. First is ventilation, second is diffusion of oxygen and carbon dioxide between alveolar sacs and alveolar capillaries, third is circulation, and the fourth is diffusion of oxygen

and carbon dioxide between systemic capillaries and cells. Ventilation refers to the bulk transport of air from the atmosphere to the alveolus. The product of tidal volume (V_T) and breathing frequency (f) represents the total volume of air delivered to the lung (minute ventilation, V_E). However, not all air entering the lung is in contact with gas-exchanging units. The portion of the inhaled breath that fills the respiratory zone is the alveolar volume (V_A), and the portion remaining in the conducting airways is the dead space volume (V_D) (Fig. 16-2). The fraction of the tidal breath that is dead space varies with the size of the breath. With larger breaths, the dead space is a smaller fraction of the total tidal volume. Thus, for a given tidal volume, slow, deep breathing results in greater V_A and improved gas exchange when compared with rapid, shallow breathing. The fraction of the tidal breath that is dead space can be calculated as follows:

$$V_D/V_T = (Pa_{CO_2} - Pe_{CO_2})/Pa_{CO_2},$$

where Pa_{CO_2} is arterial P_{CO_2} and Pe_{CO_2} is the P_{CO_2} of mixed expired gas.

Normally, one third of a breath is dead space ($V_D / V_T = \frac{1}{3}$). At end-expiration, the V_D contains exhaled alveolar gas that had been in equilibrium with pulmonary capillary blood. The amount of fresh air reaching the alveoli on the next breath is the $V_A - V_D$.

Because every breath includes a portion that is dead space, minute ventilation (V_E) includes a portion of ventilation that is dead space and a portion that is alveolar ventilation. As the metabolic rate and CO_2 production increase, alveolar ventilation must increase to maintain an arterial P_{CO_2}

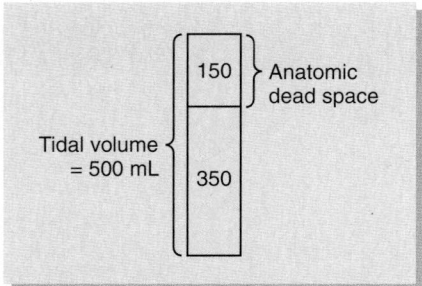

Figure 16-2 Schematic of the inspired air that participates in gas exchange (350 mL) and the anatomic dead space (150 mL) for a tidal breath of 500 mL.

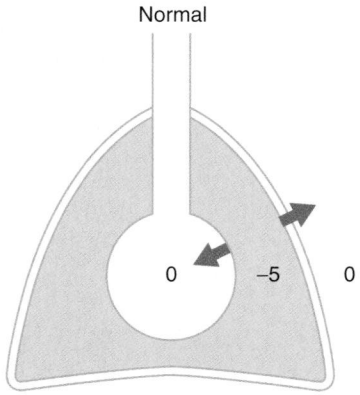

Figure 16-3 Schematic of the lung and chest wall at functional residual capacity. The *arrows* show that the expanding elastic force of the chest wall equals the collapsing elastic force of the lung. The intrapleural pressure is –5 because of both forces tugging on the pleural space in opposite directions.

of 40 mm Hg. The relationship among these variables is described by the alveolar carbon dioxide equation.

$$P_{ACO_2} = CO_2 \text{ production}/V_A,$$

where P_{ACO_2} is alveolar ventilation and V_A is alveolar ventilation.

From the above equation, one appreciates that the partial pressure of carbon dioxide in the alveolus is indirectly proportional to alveolar ventilation. Similarly, as metabolic rate increases and O_2 consumption increases, alveolar ventilation must increase to maintain a normal arterial P_{O_2}. The relationship among these variables is described by the alveolar oxygen equation.

$$P_{AO_2} = \text{Oxygen consumption}/V_A$$

This relationship is somewhat more complicated because P_{AO_2} also is proportional to the fraction of inspired oxygen, water vapor pressure, and the partial pressure of CO_2 in the alveolus. The implications of these two relationships are that (1) the maintenance of a constant alveolar gas composition depends on a constant ratio of ventilation to metabolic rate; (2) if ventilation is too high (hyperventilation), alveolar P_{CO_2} will be low, and alveolar P_{O_2} will be high; and (3) if ventilation is too low (hypoventilation), alveolar P_{CO_2} will be high, and alveolar P_{O_2} will be low.

MECHANICS OF BREATHING

Respiratory mechanics is the study of forces needed to deliver air to the lung and how these forces govern the volume and flow of gases. Mechanically, the respiratory system consists of two structures: the lungs and the chest wall. The lungs are elastic (springlike) structures that are situated within another elastic structure, the chest wall. At end-expiration, with absent respiratory muscle activity, the inward recoil of the lung is exactly balanced by the outward recoil of the chest wall. Normally, the recoil of the lung is always inward (favoring lung deflation), and the recoil of the chest wall is outward (favoring inflation), except at high lung volumes, where the chest wall also recoils inward (Fig. 16-3). The inspiratory and expiratory muscles can disturb this balance and cause gas to flow in and out of the lung. The energy required to stretch the respiratory system above its equilibrium state (end-expiration during quiet breathing) is provided by the inspiratory muscles. With normal quiet breathing, gas flow out of the lung is usually accomplished by the passive recoil of the respiratory system.

During a typical breath, inspiratory muscle contraction lowers intrapleural pressure, which in turn lowers intraalveolar pressure. Once alveolar pressure becomes subatmospheric, air can flow from the mouth through the airways to the alveoli. At the end of inspiration, the inspiratory muscles are turned off, and the lungs and chest wall recoil passively back to their equilibrium states. This passive respiratory system recoil causes alveolar pressure to become positive throughout expiration until the resting position of the lung and chest wall are reestablished and alveolar pressure once again equals atmospheric pressure. During quiet breathing, pleural pressure is always subatmospheric, whereas alveolar pressure oscillates above and below zero (atmospheric) pressure (Fig. 16-4). The major inspiratory muscle is the diaphragm. Others include the sternocleidomastoid muscles, the scalenus muscles, and the external intercostal muscles. Diaphragm contraction results in expansion of the lower rib cage and compression of the intraabdominal contents. The latter action results in expansion of the abdominal wall. The expiratory muscles consist of the internal intercostal muscles and the abdominal muscles. Expiratory flows can be enhanced by recruiting the expiratory muscles, which occur during exercise or cough.

To inflate the respiratory system, the inspiratory muscles must overcome two types of forces; the elastic forces imposed by the lung and the chest wall (elastic loads) and resistive forces related to airflow (resistive loads). The elastic loads on the inspiratory muscles are due to the respiratory system's tendency to resist stretch. The elastic forces are volume dependent such that the respiratory system becomes more difficult to stretch at volumes above functional residual capacity (FRC) and more difficult to compress as volumes below FRC. The elastic forces can be characterized by examining the relationship between lung volume and recoil pressure (Fig. 16-5). When either deflated or inflated, the lung and chest wall have characteristic recoil pressures. The slope of the relationship between lung volume and recoil pressure of the chest wall or lung represents the compliance of each structure. The sum of the chest wall and lung recoil pressures represents the recoil pressure of the total respiratory system.

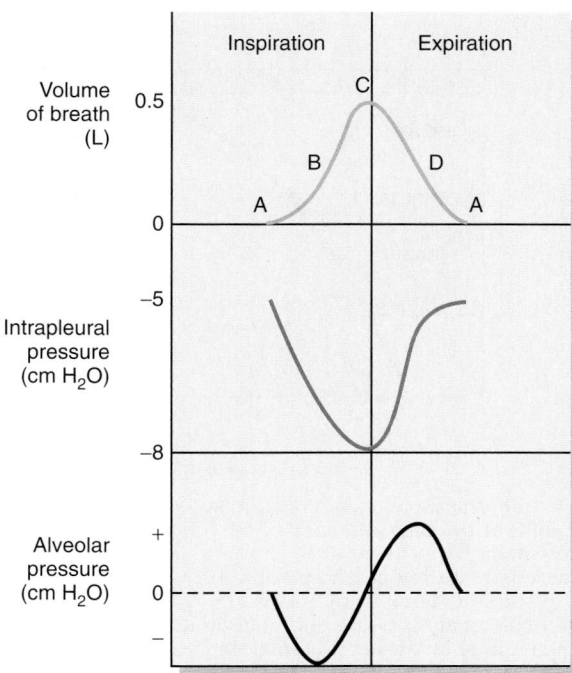

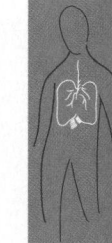

Figure 16-4 Volume, intrapleural pressure, and alveolar pressure during a normal breathing cycle. The letters A to D correspond to different phases of the cycle. Alveolar pressure is biphasic with zero crossings at times of no flow (end-expiration [A] and end-inspiration [C]). Intrapleural pressure remains subatmospheric throughout.

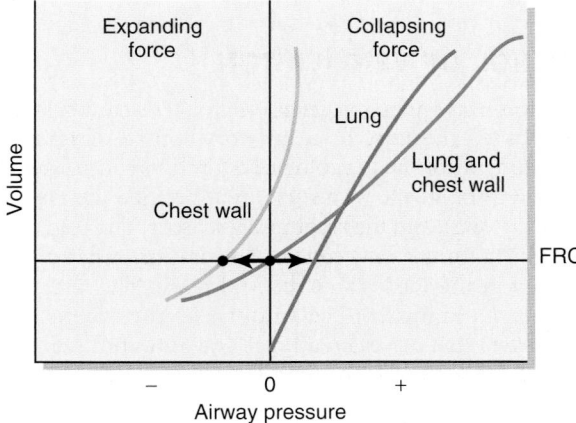

Figure 16-5 Volume-pressure (V-P) relationship of the respiratory system and its components: the lung and chest wall. Respiratory system recoil pressure at any volume is the sum of the lung and chest wall recoil pressures. The slope of the V-P curve represents the compliance of each structure. FRC, functional residual capacity.

The elastic properties of the lung are related to two factors: (1) the elastic behavior of fibrin and elastin in the lung parenchyma, and (2) the surface tension in the alveolus due to the air-liquid interface. Both factors contribute equally to lung elastic recoil. A surface active substance called *surfactant* is produced by type II alveolar cells and lines alveolar fluid. This substance consists of primarily phospholipids and lowers surface tension, making it easier to inflate the lung. The lungs are stiff and difficult to inflate in diseases charac-

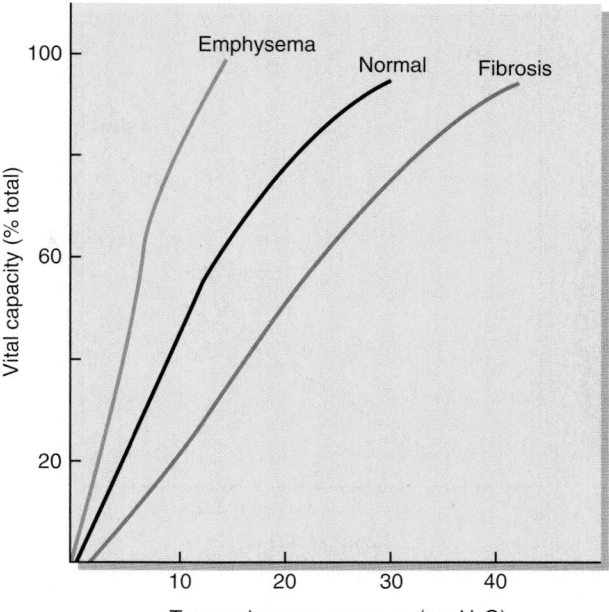

Figure 16-6 Compliance curves for normal individuals and for patients with emphysema and pulmonary fibrosis. An elevation in the transpulmonary pressure required to achieve a given lung volume increases the work of breathing.

terized by a loss of surfactant such as infant respiratory distress syndrome. Diseases such as pulmonary fibrosis, which are characterized by excessive collagen in the lung, can make the lung stiff and difficult to inflate, whereas diseases such as emphysema, characterized by a loss of elastin and collagen, will decrease lung compliance (Fig. 16-6). Normally, at FRC, it takes about 1 cm of water pressure (cm H_2O) to inflate the lungs 200 mL and to inflate the chest wall 200 mL. Since the lung and chest wall both need to be inflated to the same volume during inspiration, it would take 2 cm H_2O of pressure to inflate both. Thus, normal respiratory system compliance is roughly 100 mL/cm H_2O, and lung and chest wall compliance 200 mL/cm H_2O, at volumes near FRC.

The second set of forces that the inspiratory muscles must overcome to inflate the lungs are flow-dependent forces; namely, tissue viscosity and airway flow resistance; the latter constituting the major component of the flow-dependent forces. Airway resistance during inspiration can be calculated by measuring inspiratory flow and the difference in pressure between the alveolus and the airway opening (ΔP_{A-ao}).

$$R = \Delta P_{A-ao}/flow$$

Airflow velocity, the type of airflow (laminar or turbulent), and the physical attributes of the airway (radius and length) are the key determinants of airway resistance. Of the physical properties, the radius of the airways is the major factor. Resistance increases to the fourth power as diameter decreases under conditions of laminar flow (streamline flow profile) and to the fifth power under conditions of turbulent flow (chaotic flow profile). Because airway diameter increases as lung volume increases, airway resistance decreases as lung

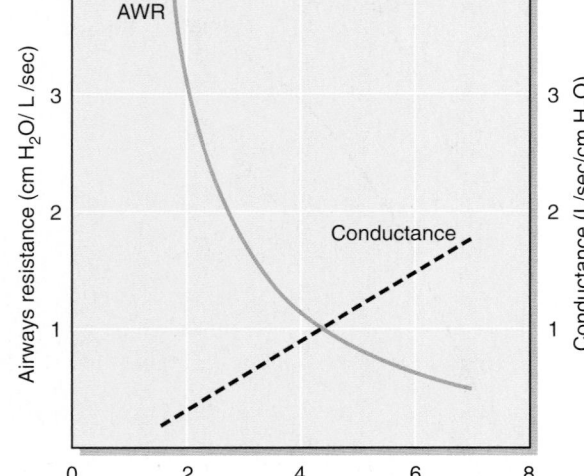

Figure 16-7 As lung volume increases, the airways are dilated, and resistance decreases. The reciprocal of resistance (conductance) increases as lung volume increases. AWR, airway resistance.

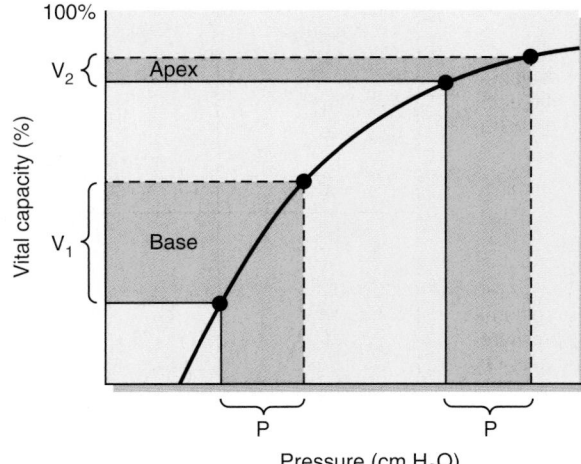

Figure 16-8 Transpulmonary pressure (Ppl-Pal) and volume for lung units at the base and apex of the lung. Pleural pressure is more negative at the apex of the lung, thereby stretching the alveoli in this region and placing them on a less compliant part of the volume-pressure (V-P) curve. For a given change in transpulmonary pressure during inspiration, the more compliant base inflates to a greater degree than the apex.

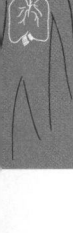

volume increases (Fig. 16-7). Airway diameter also contributes to regional differences in airway resistance. Although the peripheral airways are narrower than the central airways, their total cross-sectional area is much greater than that of the central airways. Consequently, resistance to airflow of the peripheral airways is low relative to the central airways (see Fig. 16-1). The velocity of airflow is another key determinant of airway resistance. Resistance is directly proportional to flow rate when flow is laminar and proportional to the square of flow rate when it is turbulent. In addition, the velocity of airflow determines, in part, whether the flow pattern is laminar or turbulent (higher resistance than laminar flow). Clinically, increased airway resistance can be seen in diseases associated with airway obstruction caused by an intrinsic mass, mucus within the airway, airway smooth muscle contraction, or dynamic compression of the airways. Lung elastic recoil also influences airflow. Decreased elastic recoil decreases airflow (**Web Fig. 16-1**). Normal resistance when breathing at FRC at low flow rates is in the range of 1 to 2 cm H_2O/L per second.

DISTRIBUTION OF VENTILATION

The distribution of inhaled volume throughout the lung is unequal. Generally more of the inhaled volume goes to the bases of the lung than to the apex when inhaling in the upright body position. This pattern of volume distribution leads to greater ventilation of the bases than the apices. This inhomogeneity of ventilation is due largely to regional differences in lung compliance. At the lung apex, the alveoli are relatively more inflated at FRC than at the lung base. The difference in alveolar distention from apex to base is related to pleural pressure differences from apex to base. The weight of the lung causes pleural pressure to be more negative at the apex and less negative at the base. The normal difference in pleural pressure from apex to base is about 8 cm H_2O (Fig.

16-8). Because the apical alveoli are more stretched at FRC, they are operating on a stiffer, less compliant region of their volume-pressure curve than the alveoli at the bases. Thus, at the beginning of inspiration, more volume is directed toward the base than to the apex of the lung.

CONTROL OF VENTILATION

Maintaining adequate oxygenation and acid-base balance is accomplished through the respiratory control system. This system consists of the neurologic respiratory control centers, the respiratory effectors (muscles that provide the power to inflate the lung), and the respiratory sensors. The respiratory center that automatically controls inspiration and expiration is located in the medulla of the brainstem. The respiratory center in the brainstem has an intrinsic rhythm generator (pacemaker) that drives breathing. The output of this center is modulated by inputs from peripheral and central chemoreceptors, mechanoreceptors in the lung, and higher centers in the brain, including conscious control from the cerebral cortex. The respiratory center in the medulla is primarily responsible for determining the level of ventilation.

Carbon dioxide is the primary factor controlling ventilation. CO_2 in the arterial blood diffuses across the blood-brain barrier, thereby reducing cerebral spinal fluid pH and stimulating the central chemoreceptors. A change in $PaCO_2$ above or below normal will increase or decrease ventilation, respectively. During quiet, restful breathing, the level of $PaCO_2$ is thought to be the major factor controlling breathing. Only when PaO_2 (partial pressure of oxygen dissolved in the blood and not bound to hemoglobin) falls substantially does ventilation respond significantly. Typically, PaO_2 needs to fall below 50 mm Hg before ventilation dramatically increases (Fig. 16-9). Low oxygen levels in the blood are not sensed by the respiratory center in the brain but are sensed by receptors located in the carotid body. This is a vascular

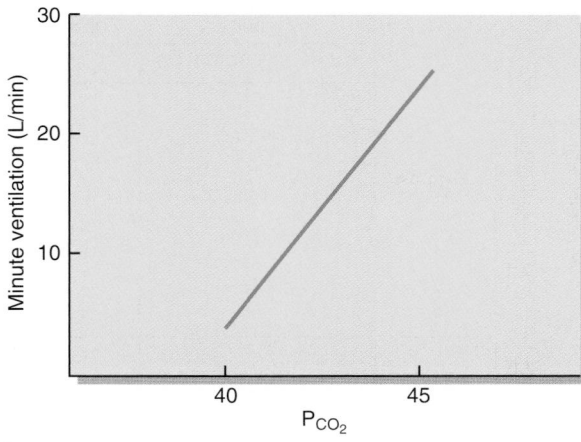

A

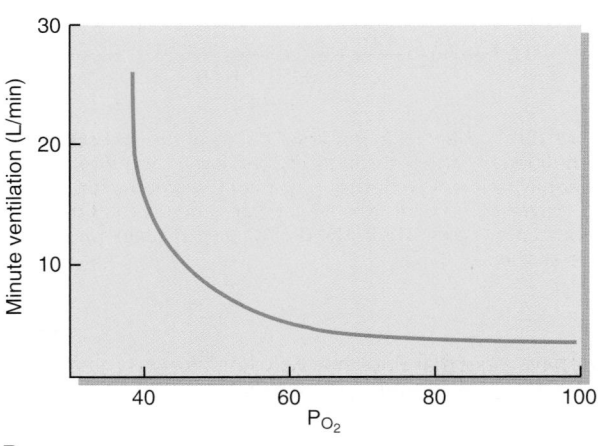

B

Figure 16-9 A rising P_{CO_2} leads to a linear increase in minute ventilation (**A**). The ventilatory response to hypoxemia (**B**) is less sensitive and is clinically relevant only when the P_{O_2} has dropped significantly.

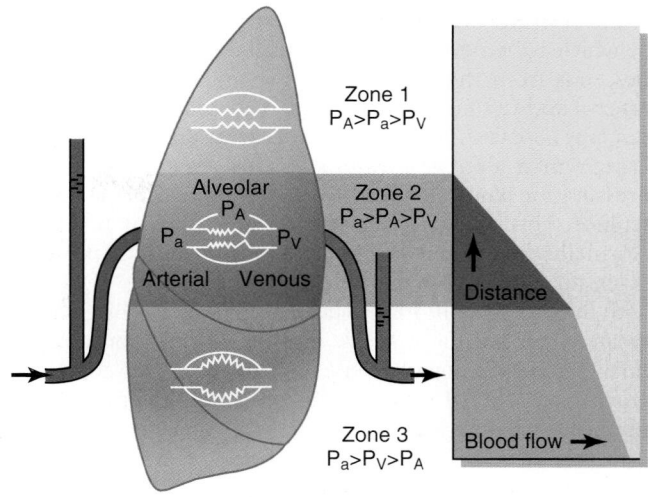

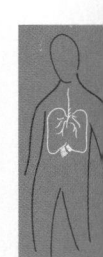

Figure 16-10 Zonal model of blood flow in the lung. Because of the inter-relationship of vascular and alveolar pressures, the lung base receives the most flow (see text for explanation). (From West JB, Dollery CT, Naimark A: Distribution of blood flow in isolated lung: Relation to vascular and alveolar pressures. J Appl Physiol 19:713-724, 1964.)

receptor located between the internal and external branches of carotid artery. Changes in Pa_{O_2} are sensed by the carotid sinus nerve. Neural traffic projects to the respiratory center through the glossopharyngeal nerve, which serves to modulate ventilation. The carotid body also senses changes in Pa_{CO_2} and pH. Nonvolatile acids (i.e., ketoacids) stimulate ventilation through their effects on the carotid body.

The outcome of this complex respiratory control system is that variables such as Pa_{O_2}, Pa_{CO_2}, and pH are held within narrow limits under most circumstances. The respiratory control center also can adjust V_T and f to minimize the energetic cost of breathing and can adapt to special circumstances such as speaking, swimming, eating, and exercise. Breathing can be stimulated when P_{CO_2}, P_{O_2}, and pH are artificially manipulated. For example, rebreathing carbon dioxide, inhaling a concentration of low oxygen, or infusion of acid into the bloodstream will increase ventilation.

PERFUSION

The pulmonary vascular bed differs from the system circulation in several respects. The pulmonary vascular bed receives the entire cardiac output of the right ventricle, whereas the cardiac output from the left ventricle is dispersed among several organ systems. Despite receiving the entire cardiac output, the pulmonary system is a low-resistance, low-pressure circuit. The normal mean systemic arterial pressure is about 100 mm Hg, whereas the normal mean pulmonary artery pressure is in the range of 15 mm Hg. The vasculature bed can passively accommodate an increase in blood flow without raising arterial pressure by recruiting more vessels in the lung. Thus, during exercise, there is little increase in pulmonary artery resistance despite a large increase in pulmonary blood flow. Hypoxic vasoconstriction also is a feature unique to the pulmonary vascular system and regulates regional blood flow. This regulation aids in matching blood flow to ventilation by reducing flow to poorly ventilated regions of the lung.

In the upright individual, there is greater perfusion of the lung bases than apices (Fig. 16-10). In a low-pressure system such as the pulmonary circulation, the effects of gravity on blood flow need to be considered. Usually the arterial-venous pressure difference provides the "driving" pressure for blood flow. Although this is true for the systemic circulation, it is true only for certain regions of the lung. With the respiratory system, pulmonary blood flow also needs to be considered in the context of alveolar pressure. Venous and arterial pressures are importantly affected by gravity, whereas alveolar pressure remains constant throughout the lung, assuming the airways are open. Thus, as one descends from the apex to the base of the lung, arterial and venous pressures increase because of gravity, but alveolar pressure remains constant. At the apex of the lung, alveolar pressure may be greater than arterial pressure. This region of the lung is referred to as *zone 1* and, in theory, receives no blood flow. Alveolar pressure may exceed arterial pressure under special circumstances such as hypovolemic shock, in which pulmonary arterial pressure may fall below alveolar pressure, and with very high levels of positive end-expiratory pressure

(PEEP), which may increase alveolar pressure to the extent at which it becomes greater than arterial pressure. As one descends from the apex toward the midzone of the lung, arterial and venous pressures increase, and alveolar pressure remains constant. At some point, arterial pressure becomes greater than alveolar pressure. In this region, the driving pressure for blood flow is the arterial-alveolar pressure difference. This region is referred to as *zone 2* of the lung. Normally, there is very little zone 2 because alveolar pressure is less than venous pressure in most of the lung. However, with high levels of PEEP, alveolar pressure will become greater than venous pressure in more lung regions. When further approaching the base of the lung, the effects of gravity on arterial and venous pressures are more pronounced, venous pressure becomes greater than alveolar pressure, and the arterial-venous pressure difference provides the driving pressure for blood flow. This region is referred to as *zone 3* of the lung. Normally, most of the lung is in zone 3, and most of the perfusion is to the lung base. This inequality in perfusion from apex to base is qualitatively similar to the inequality of ventilation from apex to base, thereby optimizing the matching of ventilation and perfusion.

GAS TRANSFER

Oxygen and carbon dioxide are easily dissolved in plasma. Nitrogen is much less soluble and is not significantly exchanged across the alveolar-capillary interface. The pressure gradient for oxygen between the alveolus and capillary promotes diffusion of oxygen from the alveolus to the capillary (P_{AO_2} of 150 mm Hg versus P_{AO_2} of 40 mm Hg). This pressure difference is greater than that driving carbon dioxide from the mixed venous blood to the alveolus (P_{MVCO_2} of 45 mm Hg versus P_{ACO_2} of 40 mm Hg). Despite the lower driving pressure, the greater solubility of carbon dioxide allows complete equilibration between the alveolus and plasma during each respiratory cycle (Fig. 16-11).

Most of the oxygen contained in the blood is bound to hemoglobin, with a small fraction dissolved and measured as the P_{AO_2}. The amount of oxygen dissolved is about 3 mL/L in arterial blood, whereas the amount of oxygen bound to hemoglobin is about 197 mL/L in arterial blood, assuming a normal hematocrit. Each molecule of hemoglobin is capable of carrying four molecules of oxygen. The shape of the oxyhemoglobin association curve reflects the cooperative binding of oxygen to hemoglobin (Fig. 16-12). In general, the percent hemoglobin saturation is between 80% and 100% with P_{AO_2} above 60 mm Hg and drops dramatically when the P_{AO_2} is less than 60 mm Hg. Factors that decrease the affinity of hemoglobin for oxygen include a reduction in blood pH, an increase in temperature, an increase in P_{CO_2}, and an increase in 2,3-diphosphoglyceric acid (2,3-DPG). These factors facilitate unloading of oxygen into tissues. This is seen as a shift of the oxyhemoglobin dissociation curve to the right. The oxygen carrying capacity of hemoglobin is also affected by competitive inhibitors for binding sites such as carbon monoxide. Carbon monoxide has an affinity for hemoglobin that is 240 times greater than oxygen. Thus, it will preferentially bind to hemoglobin. However, it does not affect the amount of oxygen dissolved in the blood. Someone with carbon monoxide poisoning

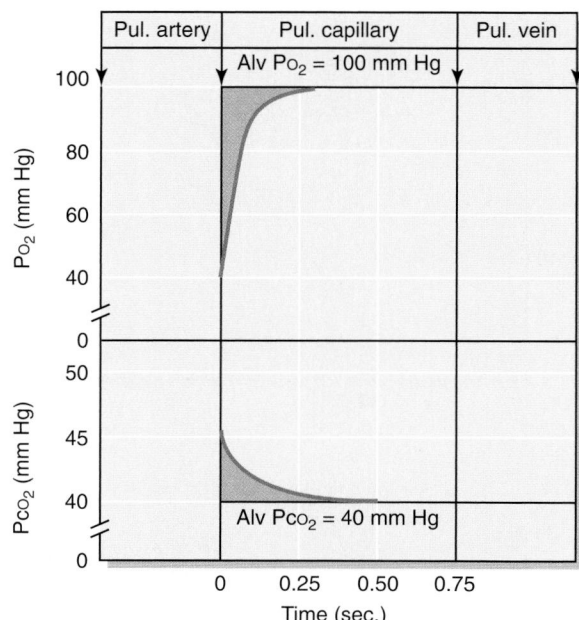

Figure 16-11 Changes in P_{O_2} and P_{CO_2} as blood courses from the pulmonary artery through the capillaries and into the pulmonary veins. The diffusion gradient is greater for O_2 than CO_2. However, equilibration of capillary and alveolar gas occurs for both molecules within the 0.75 second it takes for blood to traverse the capillaries.

may have a normal P_{AO_2} but very low blood oxygen content due to the desaturated hemoglobin.

About 5% of carbon dioxide is dissolved in plasma, and the remainder is transported in other forms. A small amount of carbon dioxide also binds to hemoglobin. However, carbon dioxide does not exhibit cooperative binding; therefore, the shape of the carbon dioxide–hemoglobin dissociation curve is linear (see Fig. 16-12). Carbon dioxide binds to the protein component of the hemoglobin molecule and to the amino groups of the polypeptide chains of plasma proteins to form carbamino compounds. About 10% of carbon dioxide is transported in this fashion. Most of the carbon dioxide is transported as bicarbonate ion. As carbon dioxide diffuses from metabolically active tissue into the blood, it reacts with water to form carbonic acid. This reaction primarily occurs in the red blood cell because it is catalyzed by the enzyme carbonic anhydrase, which resides in the red blood cell. Carbonic acid then dissociates to bicarbonate and hydrogen ion. Although there is more carbon dioxide dissolved in blood than oxygen, it is still a small fraction of the total carbon dioxide transported by blood.

ABNORMALITIES OF PULMONARY GAS EXCHANGE

The P_{AO_2} and P_{ACO_2} are determined by the degree of equilibration between the alveolar gas and capillary blood. The degree of equilibration depends on four major factors: (1) ventilation, (2) matching of ventilation with perfusion, (3) shunt, and (4) diffusion. A fifth cause of hypoxemia is a low inspired P_{O_2}. *Hypoxemia* refers to a reduction in the oxygen content in the blood. Specifically, hypoxemia is determined by measuring the P_{O_2} of arterial blood. In contrast, *hypoxia*

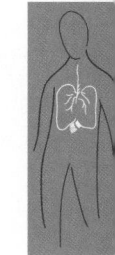

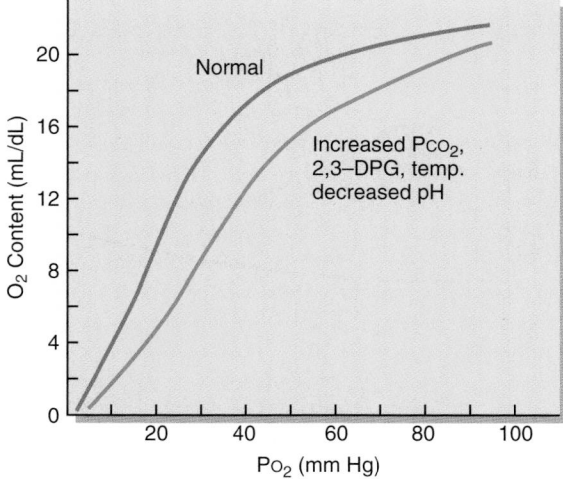

A

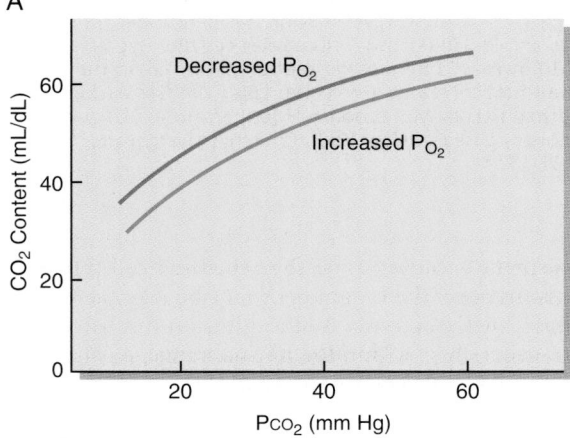

B

Figure 16-12 **A,** The oxyhemoglobin dissociation curve. The bulk of the oxygen is combined with hemoglobin. The various factors that decrease the hemoglobin oxygen affinity are shown. Opposite changes increase hemoglobin oxygen affinity, shifting the curve to the left. **B,** The carbon dioxide dissociation curve is more linear than the oxyhemoglobin curve throughout the physiologic range. Increased PaO_2 shifts the curve to the right, which decreases carbon dioxide content for any given $PaCO_2$ and thus facilitates carbon dioxide off-loading in the lungs. The shift to the left at a lower PaO_2 facilitates carbon dioxide on-loading at the tissues. DPG, diphosphoglycerate.

refers to a decrease in oxygen content of an organ, for example, myocardial hypoxemia.

Hypoventilation is defined as ventilation inadequate to keep PCO_2 from increasing above normal. In this situation, hypoxemia may occur when increased carbon dioxide in alveoli displaces alveolar oxygen. The reciprocal relationship between alveolar carbon dioxide and alveolar oxygen is described by the alveolar gas equation.

$$PAO_2 = [(PB - PH_2O) \times FIO_2] - (PaCO_2/R),$$

where PAO_2 is the partial pressure of oxygen in the alveolus; PB is barometric pressure; PH_2O is water vapor pressure; FIO_2 is the fraction of inspired oxygen; and R is the respiratory exchange ratio.

From this equation, it is apparent that as alveolar ventilation falls and $PaCO_2$ rises, PAO_2 will have to fall. Administering supplemental oxygen (increasing the FIO_2) can reverse hypoventilation-induced hypoxemia. When breathing room air, the difference between alveolar oxygen and arterial oxygen ($PA–a$ gradient) is normally about 20 mm Hg. Generally, this difference increases when hypoxemia is present. However, when hypoxemia is due to hypoventilation, the O_2 gradient is within normal limits. Causes of hypoventilation are varied and range from diseases or drugs that depress the respiratory control center to disorders of the chest wall or respiratory muscles that impair respiratory pump function. Disorders associated with hypoventilation include inflammation trauma or hemorrhage in the brainstem, spinal cord pathology, anterior horn cell disease, peripheral neuropathies, myopathies, abnormalities of the chest wall such as kyphoscoliosis, and upper airway obstruction. Administering a higher FIO_2 will alleviate the hypoxemia but will do little to improve the elevated $PaCO_2$.

A second cause of hypoxemia is ventilation-perfusion ratio $(\dot{V}/\dot{Q})$ mismatch. This is the most common cause of hypoxemia in disease states. In the ideal lung, ventilation and perfusion would be perfectly matched. Although both ventilation and perfusion are greater at the base relative to the apex of the lung, the $\dot{V}/\dot{Q}$ is lower at the base than at the apex of the lung. In the normal lung, the $\dot{V}/\dot{Q}$ ranges from 0.5 at the base to 3 at the apex. The overall $\dot{V}/\dot{Q}$ for the normal lung is 0.8. If lung disease develops, $\dot{V}/\dot{Q}$ inequality may develop. If the $\dot{V}/\dot{Q}$ is less than 0.8, the $PA–a$ gradient is increased, and hypoxia ensues. The $PaCO_2$ is usually within the normal range but will increase slightly at extremely low ratios (Fig. 16-13). Typically, hypoxemia seen in diseases that affect the airways, such as chronic obstructive pulmonary disease (COPD), is due to $\dot{V}/\dot{Q}$ mismatch. As with hypoxemia due to hypoventilation, administering a higher FIO_2 improves hypoxemia due to $\dot{V}/\dot{Q}$ mismatch.

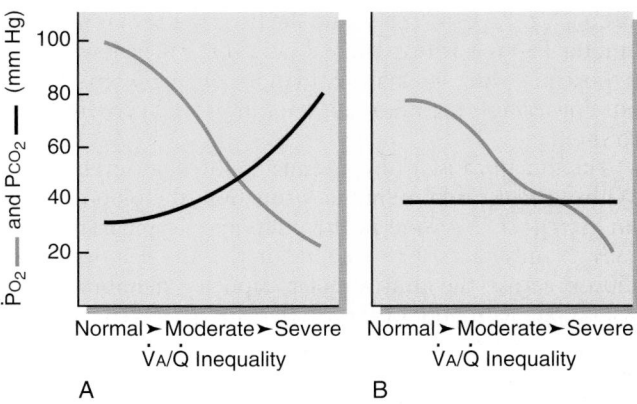

A   **B**

Figure 16-13 **A,** The effect of increasing ventilation-perfusion $(\dot{V}/\dot{Q})$ inequality on PaO_2 and $PaCO_2$ when cardiac output and minute ventilation are held constant. **B,** The gas tensions change when ventilation is allowed to increase. Increased ventilation can maintain a normal $PaCO_2$ but can only partially correct the hypoxemia. (Adapted from Dantzker DR: Gas exchange abnormalities. In Montenegro H [ed]: Chronic Obstructive Pulmonary Disease. New York, Churchill Livingstone, 1984, pp 141-160.)

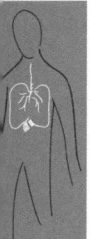

The third cause of hypoxemia is shunt. A right-to-left shunt occurs when a portion of blood travels from the right side to the left side of the heart without the opportunity to exchange oxygen and carbon dioxide in the lung. Right to left shunts can be classified as anatomic or physiologic. With an anatomic shunt, a portion of the blood bypasses the lung by traversing through an anatomic canal. In all healthy individuals, there is a small fraction of blood in the bronchial circulation that passes to the pulmonary veins and empties into the left atrium, thereby reducing Pa_{O_2} of the systemic circulation. A smaller portion of the normal shunt is related to the coronary circulation draining through the thebesian veins into the left ventricle. Anatomic shunts found in disease states can be classified as intracardiac or intrapulmonary shunts. Intracardiac shunts occur when right atrial pressures are elevated and deoxygenated blood travels from the right atrium to the left atrium through an atrial septal defect or patent foramen ovale. Intrapulmonary anatomic shunts consist primarily of arteriovenous malformations or telangiectasias. A physiologic right-to-left shunt consists of a portion of the pulmonary arterial blood passing through normal vasculature but not coming into contact with alveolar air. This is an extreme example of ventilation-perfusion mismatch ($\dot{V}/\dot{Q} = 0$). Physiologic shunt can be due to diffuse flooding of the alveoli with fluid, as seen with congestive heart failure or acute respiratory distress syndrome. Alveolar flooding with inflammatory exudates as seen in lobar pneumonia also causes a shunt. The fraction of blood shunted can be calculated when the F_{IO_2} is 100% by using the following equation.

$$QS/Qt = (Cc_{O_2} - Ca_{O_2})/(Cc_{O_2} - Cv_{O_2}),$$

where QS is the shunted blood flow, Qt is the total blood flow, Cc_{O_2} is the end pulmonary capillary oxygen content; Ca_{O_2} is the arterial oxygen content; and Cv_{O_2} is the mixed venous oxygen content.

If the shunt is severe enough, patients will require mechanical ventilation and the application of positive end expiratory pressure to improve arterial oxygenation. At values less than 50% of the cardiac output, a shunt has very little effect on Pa_{CO_2} (Fig. 16-14). With shunt, the P_A–a gradient is elevated, and the Pa_{CO_2} is within normal range or may be low. Unlike hypoxemia due to hypoventilation or $\dot{V}/\dot{Q}$ mismatch, administering a high F_{IO_2} does not improve hypoxemia due to shunt.

The fourth cause of hypoxemia is diffusion impairment. With normal cardiopulmonary function, the blood spends on average 0.75 second in the pulmonary capillaries. Typically, it only takes 0.25 second for the alveolar oxygen to diffuse across the thin alveolar capillary membrane and equilibrate with pulmonary arterial blood. However, if there is impairment to diffusion across this membrane (thickening of the alveolar capillary membrane by fluid, fibrous tissue, cellular debris, or inflammatory cells), it will take longer for the oxygen in the alveoli to equilibrate with pulmonary arterial blood. If the impediment to diffusion is such that it takes longer than 0.75 second for oxygen to diffuse, hypoxemia ensues. Alternatively, if the time the red cell spends traversing the pulmonary capillary decreases to 0.25 second or less, hypoxemia may develop. Hypoxemia may only be evident during exercise in individuals with diffusion

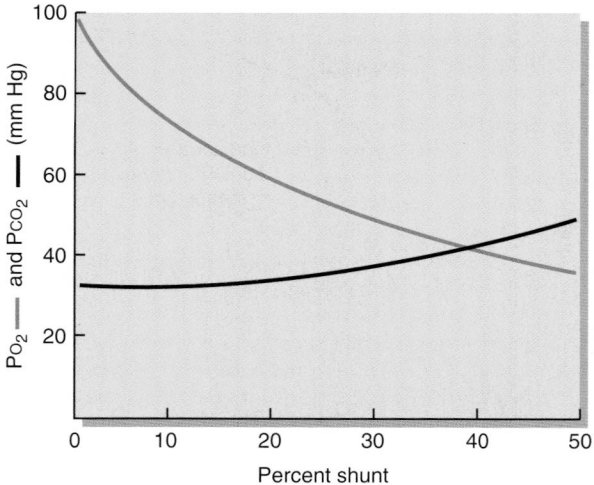

Figure 16-14 The effect of increasing shunt on the arterial Pa_{O_2} and Pa_{CO_2}. The minute ventilation has been held constant in this example. Under usual circumstances, the hypoxemia would lead to increased minute ventilation and a fall in the Pa_{CO_2} as the shunt increases. (From Dantzker DR: Gas exchange abnormalities. In Montenegro H [ed]: Chronic Obstructive Pulmonary Disease. New York, Churchill Livingstone, 1984, pp 141-160.)

impairment because of the shortened red cell transit time. In this instance, the O_2 gradient may be normal at rest but increases with exercise. With diffusion impairment, the Pa_{CO_2} generally is within the normal range. As with hypoxemia due to hypoventilation and $\dot{V}/\dot{Q}$ mismatch, administering a higher F_{IO_2} improves hypoxemia due to impaired diffusion.

A fifth cause of hypoxemia is due to low inspired oxygen. This is seen at an altitude at which the fraction of inspired oxygen is normal, but the partial pressure of oxygen is low because barometric pressure is low (P_{atm}). Rarely, circumstances occur in which the F_{IO_2} is low (e.g., rebreathing air). Hypoxemia due to low inspired oxygen is associated with a normal O_2 gradient and is usually accompanied by a low Pa_{CO_2}. Providing supplemental oxygen will correct this form of hypoxemia. Finally, a low mixed venous P_{O_2} will predispose individuals to hypoxia (Fig. 16-15).

Evaluation of Lung Function

Pulmonary function tests evaluate one or more major aspects of the respiratory systems. Accurate measurements of lung volumes, airway function, and gas exchange require a pulmonary function testing laboratory. Pulmonary function tests are commonly used to aid in the diagnosis of disease and assess disease severity. In addition, they are helpful in monitoring the course of the disease, assessing risk for surgical procedures, and measuring the effects of varied environmental exposures. Assessment of bronchodilator response or other forms of treatment also can be evaluated with serial pulmonary function tests (Table 16-1). Accurate interpretation of pulmonary function tests requires the appropriate reference standards. Variables that affect the predicted

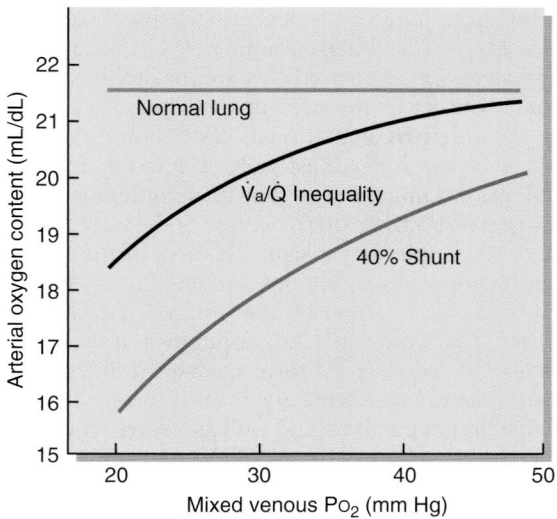

Figure 16-15 The effect of altering mixed venous PV_{O_2} on the arterial oxygen content under three assumed conditions: a normal lung, severe ventilation-perfusion ($\dot{V}/\dot{Q}$) inequality, and the presence of a 40% shunt. For each situation, the patient is breathing 50% oxygen and the PV_{O_2} or mixed venous P_{O_2} is altered, keeping all other variables constant. (From Dantzker DR: Gas exchange in the adult respiratory distress syndrome. Clin Chest Med 3:57-67, 1982.)

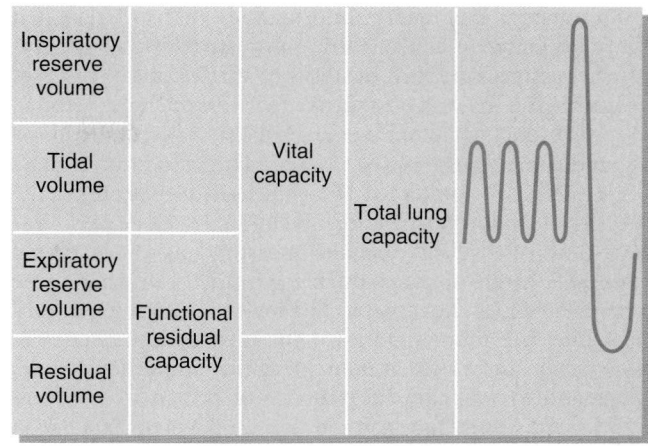

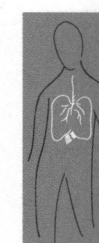

Figure 16-16 Lung volumes and capacities. Although spirometry can measure vital capacity and its subdivisions, calculation of residual volume requires measurement of functional residual capacity by body plethysmography, helium dilution technique, or nitrogen washout.

Table 16-1 **Indications for Pulmonary Function Testing**
• Evaluation of signs and symptoms
• Shortness of breath, exertional dyspnea, chronic cough
• Screening at-risk populations
• Monitoring pulmonary drug toxicity
• Follow-up abnormal study
• Chest radiograph, electrocardiogram, arterial blood gases, hemoglobin
• Preoperative assessment
• Assess severity
• Follow response to therapy
• Determine further treatment goals
• Assess disability

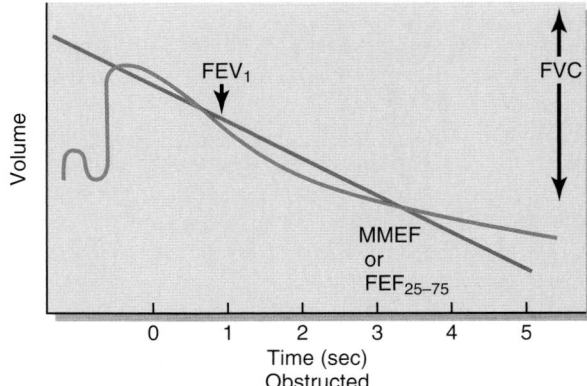

Figure 16-17 Spirometry in a normal individual and in a patient with obstructive lung disease. FEV_1 represents the forced expired volume in 1 second, and FVC represents the forced vital capacity. The slope of the line connecting the points at 25% and 75% of the FVC represents the forced expired flow (FEF at 25% to 75%) or maximum mid-expiratory flow (MMEF). The FEF at 25% to 75% is less reproducible and less specific than the FEV_1.

standards for pulmonary function tests include age, height, gender, race, and hemoglobin concentration.

Spirometry is the simplest means of measuring lung function and can be performed in an office practice. A spirometer is an apparatus that measures inspiratory and expiratory volumes. Flow rates can be calculated from tracings of volume versus time. Typically, vital capacity (VC) is measured as the difference between a full inspiration to total lung capacity (TLC) and a full exhalation to residual volume (RV) (Fig. 16-16). Flow rates are measured after instructing someone to forcefully exhale from TLC to RV. Such a forced expiratory maneuver allows one to calculate the forced expired volume in 1 second (FEV_1) and the forced vital capacity (FVC) (Fig. 16-17). A value of 80% to 120% predicted is considered normal for FVC. Normally, people can exhale more than 75% to 80% of their FVC in the first second, and the majority of FVC can be exhaled in 3 seconds. The ratio of these two variables is normally more than 0.8.

Spirometry can reveal abnormalities that are classified into two patterns—obstructive and restrictive. Obstructive impairments are defined by a low FEV_1/FVC ratio. Diseases characterized by an obstructive pattern include asthma, chronic bronchitis, emphysema, bronchiectasis, cystic fibrosis, and some central airway lesions. The reduction in FEV_1 (expressed as % predicted FEV_1) is used to determine the severity of airflow obstruction (**Web Fig. 16-2**). Peak expiratory flow rate (PEFR) can be measured as the maximal expired flow rate obtained during spirometry or when using a hand-held peak flow meter. The lower the peak expiratory flow rate, the more significant the obstruction. The peak flow meter can be used at home or in the emergency department and to evaluate the presence of obstruction. Severe attacks of asthma, for example, are usually associated with peak expiratory flow rates of less than 200 L per minute (normal is 500 to 600 L per minute). A restrictive pattern is characterized by loss of lung volume. With spirometry, both the FVC and FEV_1 are reduced with a normal FEV_1/FVC ratio. The restrictive pattern must be confirmed by measurements of lung volumes.

Lung volumes are measured using body plethysmography or by dilution of an inert gas such as helium. Lung volumes that can be measured with these techniques include FRC, TLC, and RV (see Fig. 16-16). As mentioned previously, FRC is the lung volume at which the inward elastic recoil of the lung equals the outward elastic recoil of the chest wall. Changes in FRC reflect abnormalities in lung elastic recoil. Diseases associated with increased elastic recoil such as pulmonary fibrosis are associated with a reduction in FRC, whereas those with decreased recoil such as emphysema are associated with an increase in FRC. TLC is the amount of air in the thorax after a maximal inspiration and is determined by the balance of the forces generated by the respiratory muscles to expand the respiratory system and the elastic

recoil of the respiratory system. Restrictive lung disease is defined as a TLC less than 80% predicted, whereas values of TLC greater than 120% predicted are consistent with hyperinflation. The lower the percent predicted TLC, the more severe the restrictive impairment. Restriction may be due to disorders of the lung, chest wall, respiratory muscles, or pleural space. Lung diseases that cause pulmonary fibrosis will cause a restrictive pattern because of the increased elastic recoil of the respiratory system. Diseases of the chest wall, such as kyphoscoliosis, obesity, and ankylosing spondylitis can also cause restriction by reducing the elasticity of the chest wall. Weakness of the respiratory muscles causes restriction by reducing the force available to inflate the respiratory system. Myasthenia gravis, amyotrophic lateral sclerosis, diaphragm paralysis, and Guillain-Barré syndrome can be associated with weakness sufficient to cause restrictive lung disease. Finally, space-occupying lesions involving the pleural space such as pleural effusions, pneumothorax, or pleural tumors can cause restriction. Occasionally, RV and FRC may be elevated with no increase in total lung capacity. This pattern is referred to as *air trapping* and can be seen with COPD or asthma.

The forced expiratory maneuver can be analyzed in terms of flow and volume, that is, a flow-volume loop (Fig. 16-18). Flow-volume loops are useful when identifying obstructive and restrictive patterns. The characteristic appearance of obstructive impairment is concavity ("scooping") of the expiratory loop (**Web Fig. 16-3**). With restrictive impairments, the loops are similar in appearance to normal but reduced in size. In addition, flow-volume loops are the primary means of identifying upper airway obstruction. Upper airway obstruction is characterized by a truncated (clipped) inspiratory or expiratory loop. A fixed obstruction has clipping of both inspiratory and expiratory loops. Variable intrathoracic upper airway obstruction exhibits

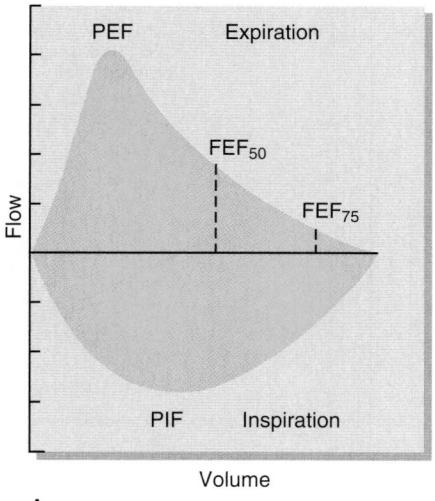

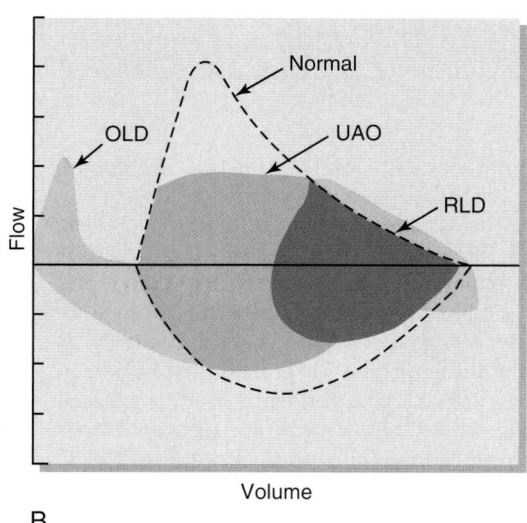

A   B

Figure 16-18 **A,** The maximum expired flow and volume curve in a normal individual. The peak expiratory flow (PEF) and forced expiratory flows at 50% and 75% of the exhaled vital capacity (FEF at 50% and 75%) are indicated. PIF, peak inspiratory flow. **B,** In obstructive lung disease (OLD), hyperinflation pushes the position of the curve to the left, and characteristic scalloping on expiration develops. In restrictive lung disease (RLD), lung volumes are reduced, but flow for any point in volume is normal. The flow-volume curve displays different patterns with various forms of upper airway obstruction (UAO), with reduction in respiratory flow if the obstruction is outside the thoracic cavity and, in addition, in expiratory flow if the obstruction is caused by a fixed deformity.

clipping of the expiratory loop, whereas variable extrathoracic obstruction exhibits clipping of the inspiratory loop (see Fig. 16-18).

BRONCHOPROVOCATION TESTING

Bronchoprovocation testing is typically used to determine the presence or absence of hyperreactive airways disease. Some individuals in whom there is a clinical suspicion of asthma may have normal expiratory flow rates and lung volumes. Bronchoprovocation testing in these individuals can be important in identifying hyperreactive airways disease and supporting the diagnosis of asthma. Methacholine is a cholinergic agonist that causes bronchoconstriction. Individuals with hyperreactive airways exhibit airflow limitation after inhaling low concentrations of methacholine. During the bronchoprovocation test, the subject inhales increasing concentrations of methacholine. Measurements of FEV_1 and FVC, as well as specific airways conductance, are obtained after the inhalation of each concentration. If the FEV_1 is reduced by 20% or more or the specific airways conductance is reduced by 40% or more, a diagnosis of hyperreactive airways disease can be ascertained. Patients with asthma demonstrate a fall in FEV_1 of 20% from baseline at doses considerably smaller than normal individuals (Fig. 16-19).

LUNG DIFFUSION CAPACITY

The diffusion of oxygen from the alveolus into the capillary can be assessed by measuring the diffusion capacity for carbon monoxide. To calculate diffusion capacity for oxygen, one needs to know the alveolar volume and the partial pressure of oxygen in the alveolus and in the pulmonary capil-

lary. Because it is not practical to measure the oxygen tension of pulmonary capillary blood, carbon monoxide is used rather than oxygen to assess diffusion capacity. Carbon monoxide diffuses across the alveolar capillary membranes much as oxygen does. However, carbon monoxide has the advantage of completely binding to hemoglobin. Therefore, the partial pressure of carbon monoxide in the pulmonary venous blood is negligible. Diffusion capacity for carbon monoxide (D_{LCO}) is then measured as the rate of disappearance of carbon monoxide from the alveolus and is used as a surrogate for oxygen diffusion capacity. This measurement provides an overall assessment of gas exchange and depends on factors including the surface area of the lung, the physical properties of the gas, perfusion of ventilated areas, hemoglobin concentration, and the thickness of the alveolar-capillary membrane. Thus, an abnormal D_{LCO} may not only signify disruption of the alveolar-capillary membrane but may also be related to a reduction in surface area of the lung (pneumonectomy), poor perfusion (pulmonary embolus), or poor ventilation of alveolar units. An increased D_{LCO} may be associated with engorgement of the pulmonary circulation with red blood cells or polycythemia. A low D_{LCO} may be seen in interstitial lung diseases that alter the alveolar-capillary membrane or diseases such as emphysema that destroy both alveolar septa and capillaries (**Web Fig. 16-4**). Anemia lowers the D_{LCO}. Most laboratories provide a hemoglobin correction for diffusion capacity.

ARTERIAL BLOOD GASES

The measurement of Pa_{O_2} and Pa_{CO_2} provides information about the adequacy of oxygenation and ventilation. This requires arterial blood sampling through arterial puncture or indwelling cannula (Table 16-2). Oxygenation can also be measured through noninvasive devices including the pulse oximeter, which measures hemoglobin oxygen saturation, and through transcutaneous devices that measure Pa_{O_2} and Pa_{CO_2}. These devices are particularly useful for measuring oxygenation during exertion in the office setting. Often, alterations in oxygenation are not detected at rest, but they are unveiled during exertion. The 6-minute walk test is a standardized test in which the patient walks for 6 minutes while the oxygen hemoglobin saturation is measured. A decrease in the oxygen hemoglobin saturation is abnormal and suggests impaired gas exchange capabilities.

In summary, pulmonary function tests, in conjunction with history and physical examination, can be used to diagnose pulmonary disorders and assess severity and response to therapy, as illustrated in the flow diagram (**Web Fig. 16-5**).

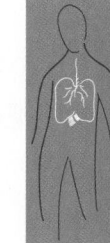

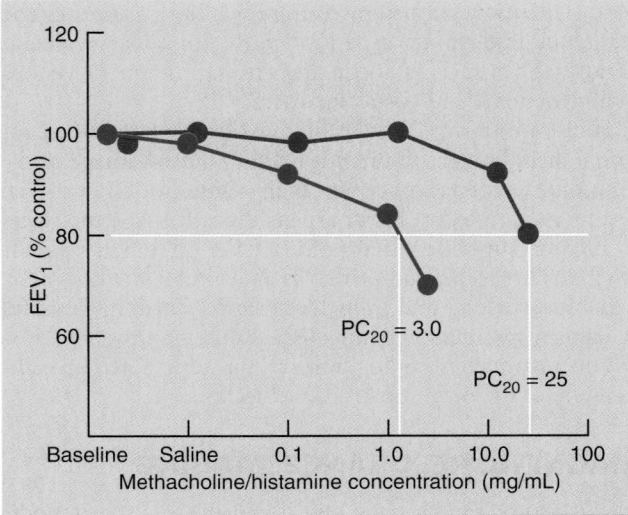

Figure 16-19 Bronchoprovocation challenge. Patients are exposed to increasing concentrations of an inhaled challenge (e.g., methacholine, histamine) followed by evaluation of FEV_1 (percent control, PC). The FEV_1 falls at lower concentrations of the challenge drug in a patient with asthma *(blue circles)* when compared with an individual without asthma *(red circles)*.

Table 16-2 **Normal Values for Arterial Blood Gases**
P_{O_2}: 104 − (0.27 × age)
P_{CO_2}: 36-44
pH: 7.35-7.45
Alveolar-arterial O_2 difference = 2.5 + 0.21 × age

Evaluation of Lung Structure

CHEST RADIOGRAPH

Generally, the evaluation of a patient with lung disease begins with routine chest radiography and then proceeds to more specialized techniques such as computed tomography (CT) or magnetic resonance imaging (MRI). Ideally, the chest radiograph consists of two different films, a postero-anterior (PA) radiograph and a lateral radiograph (**Web Fig. 16-6**). Many pathologic processes can be identified on a PA chest radiograph; however, the lateral view adds valuable information about areas that are not well seen on the PA projection. In particular, the retrocardiac region, the posterior bases of the lung, and the bony structure of the thorax such as the vertebral column are visualized better on the lateral radiograph. The PA chest radiograph is obtained with the patient standing with his or her back to the x-ray beam and the anterior chest wall placed against the film cassette. The chest radiograph should be obtained while the patient takes the deepest breath possible. When the patient is too weak to stand or too sick to travel to the radiology department, the cassette is placed behind the patient's back, and the x-ray beam travels from anterior to posterior (AP film). The quality of a portable film is not that of a standard PA film, but it still provides valuable information.

The approach to examining a chest radiograph should be systematic so that subtle abnormalities are not missed. An examination of a chest radiograph includes evaluating the lungs and pulmonary vasculature, the bony thorax, the heart and great vessels, the diaphragm and pleura, the mediastinum, the soft tissues, and the subdiaphragmatic areas. Abnormalities seen on a chest radiograph include pulmonary infiltrates, nodules, interstitial disease, vascular disease, masses, pleural effusions and thickening, cavitary lung disease, cardiac enlargement, some airway diseases, and vertebral or rib fractures. In addition to the PA and lateral chest radiographs, the lateral decubitus projection is often used to identify the presence or absence of pleural effusion. The decubitus view is particularly useful in determining whether blunting of the costal phrenic sulcus is due to freely flowing pleural fluid or related to pleural thickening. The chest radiograph in concert with a good history and physical examination allows the clinician to diagnose chest disease in many circumstances.

FLUOROSCOPY

Fluoroscopic examination of the chest is useful in evaluating motion of the diaphragm. This technique is particularly helpful in diagnosing unilateral diaphragm paralysis. A paralyzed hemidiaphragm moves paradoxically when the patient is instructed to inhale or forcefully sniff. However, fluoroscopy is limited when evaluating for bilateral diaphragm paralysis. Because of compensatory respiratory strategies in the setting of bilateral diaphragm paralysis, apparent normal descent of the diaphragm may be seen during inspiration, leading to a false-negative result by fluoroscopy. Furthermore, paradoxical hemidiaphragm motion is seen in as many as 6% of normal subjects during the sniff maneuver. This observation leads to a false-positive interpretation.

Alternatively, two-dimensional B-mode ultrasound of the diaphragm can be used to visualize diaphragm contraction during inspiration. With this technique, the diaphragm muscle is visualized in the zone of apposition of the diaphragm to the rib cage. Absence of contraction correlates with the absence of active transdiaphragmatic pressure and indicates diaphragm paralysis. This technique can be used to diagnose bilateral and unilateral diaphragm paralysis.

COMPUTED TOMOGRAPHY

CT has many applications in pulmonary medicine and provides more detailed information about lung structure than chest radiography. Using this technique, cross sections of the entire thorax can be obtained, usually at 1-cm intervals. Image contrast can be adjusted to optimize visualization of the lung parenchyma or pleural and mediastinal structures. The use of intravenous contrast material as part of the examination permits separation of vascular from nonvascular mediastinal structures. CT of the chest adds tremendous anatomic detail when compared with chest radiography. Its increased resolution permits elucidation of many findings. It helps to characterize pulmonary nodules and masses, distinguish between pleural thickening and pleural fluid, estimate the size of the heart and presence of pericardial fluid, identify patterns of involvement of interstitial lung disease, detect cavities, identify intracavitary processes such as mycetomas, quantify the extent and distribution of emphysema, detect and measure mediastinal adenopathy for staging of lung cancer, and identify vascular invasion by neoplasm. Newer generations of CT scanners are able to use multiple x-ray beams so that 4 to 64 images are created simultaneously at a much faster rate than the older models, which used only a single x-ray beam and detector.

CT angiography allows for construction of three-dimensional images of the pulmonary vascular system. This imaging technique has emerged as the procedure of choice for identifying pulmonary embolism supplanting pulmonary ventilation-perfusion scintigraphic lung scanning. The technique also can be used to identify pulmonary vascular abnormalities such as aortic dissection, pulmonary venous malformations, and aortic aneurism.

High-resolution CT is a technique that generates thin anatomic slices (1 mm) to provide a high-contrast image of the pulmonary parenchyma. With high-resolution CT, a special reconstruction algorithm sharpens the soft tissue interfaces to provide superior visualization of the pulmonary parenchyma. This technique primarily is used to identify interstitial lung disease and bronchiectasis. It is extremely useful in identifying interstitial lung disease that may not be apparent on a plain chest radiograph and has supplanted bronchography in the diagnosis of bronchiectasis.

MAGNETIC RESONANCE IMAGING

MRI is a tomographic technique that uses radio waves modified by a strong magnetic field to produce an image. It provides images that are similar to those produced with CT but with better definition of vascular structures. MRIs can be constructed in one of several anatomic planes. Although the standard image is usually an axial view, sagittal and coronal images can be easily created from the information obtained

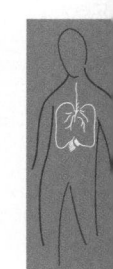

at the time of the study. Intravenous administration of gadolinium acts as a contrast agent and allows better visualization of vascular structures. MRI can be used to study aortic dissection and may have a role in the evaluation of pulmonary emboli.

PULMONARY ANGIOGRAPHY

Pulmonary angiography entails placement of a catheter in the pulmonary artery followed by rapid injection of contrast. Angiography was the gold-standard for diagnosing pulmonary thromboembolic disease. Pulmonary angiography can be useful in detecting congenital abnormalities of the pulmonary vascular tree, but CT and MRI have largely supplanted pulmonary angiography.

POSITRON-EMISSION TOMOGRAPHY

Positron-emission tomography (PET) detects metabolically active masses greater than 1 cm in diameter. It is helpful in assessing whether a pulmonary nodule is benign or malignant. However, it does not distinguish between inflammation and malignancy. Thus, assessment of multiple pulmonary nodules using PET scanning is limited because of false-positive findings due to active granulomatous disease such as tuberculosis, sarcoidosis, or fungal infections. Dual-modality integrated PET-CT combines morphologic and functional imaging. The combination of PET and CT is helpful in localizing solitary metastatic lymph nodes in the hilum, which allows better staging of lung cancer. In addition, PET-CT is helpful in planning radiation therapy for patients with lung cancer associated with atelectasis.

BRONCHOSCOPY

Fiberoptic bronchoscopy is used for diagnostic or therapeutic indications. It is most commonly performed to directly visualize the nasopharynx, larynx, vocal cords, and proximal tracheobronchial tree for diagnostic purposes. The procedure is performed by sedating the patient and providing local anesthesia with inhaled and bronchoscopically instilled lidocaine. The bronchial mucosa is assessed for endobronchial masses, mucosal integrity, extrinsic compression, dynamic compression, and hemorrhage. The bronchoscope is equipped with a channel for passage of biopsy forceps, bronchial brushes, or needles for aspiration and tissue biopsy. Saline also can be instilled through the channel for bronchial washings or bronchoalveolar lavage. Bronchial washings can be analyzed for cytology, culture, and special stains. A bronchial brush is used to scrape the bronchial mucosa and harvest cells for cytology. Bronchoscopes can also be adapted to provide ultrasound images of the airways and neighboring tissues. Endobronchial ultrasound (EBUS) uses high acoustic frequencies, in the range of 20 MHz, which provide high-resolution images of proximal tissue. EBUS can provide guidance for needle aspiration of mediastinal lymph nodes.

Common therapeutic indications for bronchoscopy include the retrieval of foreign bodies, suctioning of secretions, re-expansion of atelectatic lung, and assistance with difficult endotracheal intubations. In special centers, bronchoscopy is used to perform YAG laser therapy of endobronchial lesions, guide placements of catheters for brachytherapy of lung cancer, or guide placement of stents. Lasers produce a beam of light that can induce tissue vaporization, coagulation, and necrosis. Cryotherapy probes induce tissue necrosis through hypothermic cellular crystallization and microthrombosis. Cryotherapy and electrocautery have been used to treat and relieve airway obstruction caused by benign tracheal bronchial tumors, polyps, and granulation tissue. The goal of endobronchial brachytherapy is to relieve airway obstruction from central tumors. This is generally used as an adjunct to conventional external-beam irradiation. Tracheobronchial stenting can be performed to manage airway compression associated with malignant tumors, tracheoesophageal fistulas, and tracheobronchomalacia. Bronchoscopy is generally a safe procedure, with major complications, including significant bleeding, pneumothorax, and respiratory failure, occurring in 0.1% to 1.7% of patients.

Prospectus for the Future

Continued refinement and evolution of techniques and methods currently used to assess pulmonary structure and function will enhance our ability to diagnose and treat individuals with lung disease. Although pulmonary function testing has been performed for decades, advances in equipment design and better standardization of methods will improve accuracy and reproducibility. Further development of noninvasive techniques used to measure changes in lung volume from body surface displacements may allow for assessment of pulmonary function in settings outside of the pulmonary function laboratory. Great strides in assessing lung structure will evolve from advances in CT, PET, and MRI technology. CT volume-rendering techniques will provide images of the central airways enabling "virtual bronchoscopy." This technique may be useful to guide biopsy location for conventional bronchoscopy and allow visualization of airways distal to an endobronchial obstruction. Volumetric measurements of pulmonary nodules using CT segmentation techniques will allow more accurate calculation of nodule volume and better assessment of tumor doubling times. This, in concert with PET-CT, may provide more accurate means of determining malignant potential of solitary pulmonary nodules. MRI may evolve into the preferred method for evaluating pulmonary emboli and mediastinal disease. Velocity-encoded MRI is a promising modality for assessing pulmonary vascular blood flow and pressures, which may prove to be more accurate than current noninvasive methods. Lymph node specific magnetic resonance contrast agents and the development of PET molecular tracers targeting tumor proteins and receptors may better differentiate enlarged lymph nodes due to hyperplasia from those due to neoplasia. Finally, new insights into function of the respiratory control centers in the cortex and brainstem may be attained from studies using functional MRI of the brain.

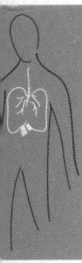

References

McCool FD, Hoppin FG Jr: Respiratory mechanics. In Baum GL (Ed-in-Chief): Textbook of Pulmonary Diseases. Philadelphia, Lippincott-Raven Publishers, 1998, pp 117-130.

Miller WT: Radiographic evaluation of the chest. In Fishman AP (Ed-in-Chief): Fishman's Pulmonary Diseases and Disorders. New York, McGraw-Hill, 2007, pp 455-510.

Wagner PD: Ventilation, pulmonary blood flow, and ventilation-perfusion relationships. In Fishman AP (Ed-in-Chief): Fishman's Pulmonary Diseases and Disorders. New York, McGraw-Hill, 2007, pp 147-160.

West JB: Respiratory Physiology: The Essentials, 5th ed. Baltimore, Williams & Wilkins, 1995.

West JB, Wagner PD: Pulmonary gas exchange. Am J Respir Crit Care Med 157:S82-S87, 1988.

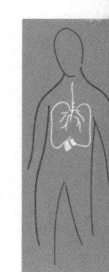

Obstructive Lung Diseases

Matthew D. Jankowich

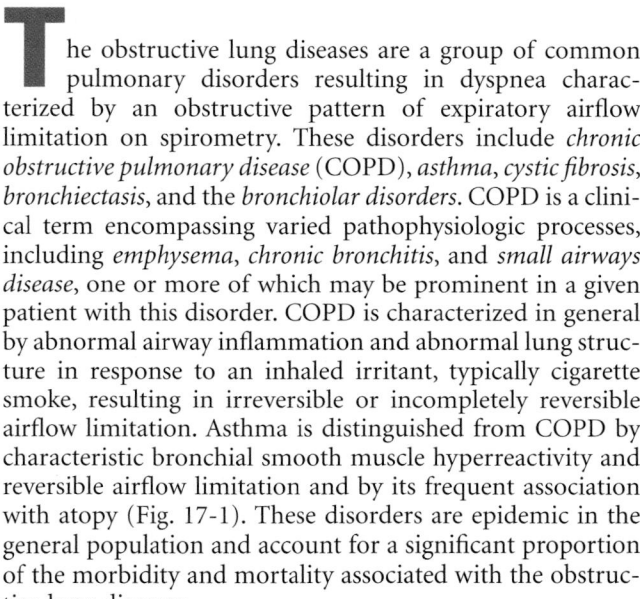

The obstructive lung diseases are a group of common pulmonary disorders resulting in dyspnea characterized by an obstructive pattern of expiratory airflow limitation on spirometry. These disorders include *chronic obstructive pulmonary disease* (COPD), *asthma*, *cystic fibrosis*, *bronchiectasis*, and the *bronchiolar disorders*. COPD is a clinical term encompassing varied pathophysiologic processes, including *emphysema*, *chronic bronchitis*, and *small airways disease*, one or more of which may be prominent in a given patient with this disorder. COPD is characterized in general by abnormal airway inflammation and abnormal lung structure in response to an inhaled irritant, typically cigarette smoke, resulting in irreversible or incompletely reversible airflow limitation. Asthma is distinguished from COPD by characteristic bronchial smooth muscle hyperreactivity and reversible airflow limitation and by its frequent association with atopy (Fig. 17-1). These disorders are epidemic in the general population and account for a significant proportion of the morbidity and mortality associated with the obstructive lung diseases.

All the obstructive lung disorders cause an obstructive pattern of expiratory airflow limitation, although the basis for airflow obstruction varies among disorders. The flow of air through the bronchial tree is directly proportional to the driving pressure and is inversely proportional to the resistance. In obstructive lung disease, alterations in one or both of these processes might be present. For example, in emphysema, airflow limitation is caused by decreased elastic recoil resulting in decreased driving pressure. By contrast, in asthma, airflow limitation is due to bronchoconstriction that increases airway resistance. Airway obstruction to flow causes characteristic changes in lung volumes. The residual volume and functional residual capacity are increased, whereas the total lung capacity remains normal or is increased. Vital capacity is reduced by the increase in residual volume. Several factors may contribute to the increase in functional residual capacity and residual volume in obstructive lung disease. Decreased lung elastic recoil in emphysema increases the functional residual capacity because of reduced opposition to the outward force exerted by the chest wall. Loss of airway tone and decreased tethering by surrounding lung in COPD, as well as bronchoconstriction and mucus plugging in acute asthma, allow airways to collapse at higher lung volumes and trap excessive air. Finally, under demands for increased minute ventilation such as during exercise, the increased resistance to airflow may not allow the lungs to empty completely during the time available for expiration, leading to so-called dynamic hyperinflation of the lungs as the volume of trapped air progressively increases while the inspiratory capacity is progressively limited.

The three major consequences of the changes in lung volume seen with obstructive lung disease are as follows: (1) Breathing at higher lung volumes requires a higher change in pressure for the same change in lung volume, and this requirement increases the work of breathing. (2) Larger lung volumes place the inspiratory muscles at a mechanical disadvantage. The diaphragm is flattened, thereby decreasing its ability to change intrathoracic volume, and all the inspiratory muscle fibers are shortened, decreasing the tension they are able to exert to effect changes in lung volume. (3) Lung volumes are larger, resulting in tethering of the narrowed and collapsing airways by the surrounding lung parenchyma, tending to retain airway patency and reduce airway resistance and air trapping; this consequence is beneficial. These three physiologic derangements explain many of the clinical features of obstructive lung diseases (Table 17-1).

Although the consequences to lung function are relatively similar in the obstructive lung diseases, their pathogenesis, treatment, and prognosis are different. Therefore, a careful evaluation is needed to reach a definitive diagnosis that will guide targeted therapy.

Chronic Obstructive Pulmonary Disease

COPD results in slowly progressive dyspnea and is characterized by abnormalities of airway and lung structure occurring in response to noxious inhaled substances, especially cigarette smoke. The abnormalities of airway and lung structure in COPD result in irreversible airflow limitation, the physiologic hallmark of COPD. The term COPD encompasses emphysema, chronic bronchitis, and small airways disease, pulmonary disorders that have common clinical manifestations and often co-exist in the same patient. The term excludes other causes of airflow obstruction, such as asthma, although in practice these diseases may at times overlap.

COPD is one of the most common disorders seen by physicians, and it is the fourth leading cause of death in the United States. There are an estimated 1,500,000 emergency department visits related to COPD annually, and about 700,000 patients with COPD are hospitalized each year. From 1997 to 2001, about 90,000 deaths per year attributable to COPD occurred in the United States. Although COPD has historically been more prevalent in males than females, the prevalence of COPD in females has been increasing, and annual death rates for COPD have been steadily rising in both white and black women. Prevalence rates for COPD are correlated with increasing age, lower socioeconomic status, and smoking.

Cigarette smoking is by far the most common cause of COPD; however, other factors such as inhalation of cooking fire smoke, air pollution, occupational exposures to dust and fumes, and infections contribute to the occurrence, severity, and progression of the disease. Although cigarette smoking is the most common cause, it is important to note that only 20% of smokers are thought to develop clinically significant COPD (although many more may experience some loss of lung function). This finding suggests that COPD results from a susceptibility to environmental factors (e.g., tobacco) as a result of a genetic predisposition. A genetic predisposition is also implied by the documentation of familial clusters of COPD.

Several longitudinal studies have defined patterns of age-related decline in lung function and have documented the concept of susceptibility to COPD. These studies show that most adult nonsmoking men exhibit a decline in forced expiratory volume in 1 second (FEV_1) of 35 to 40 mL per year. This rate is increased to 45 to 60 mL per year in most cigarette smokers. However, the susceptible smoker may demonstrate losses of 70 to 120 mL per year (Fig. 17-2). This information allows the physician to project the rate of decrease of lung function in patients with COPD and assess the effects of therapeutic interventions.

Although COPD results in chronic, progressive dyspnea, periodic acute exacerbations are characteristic of COPD. Exacerbations are characterized by a rapidly developing worsening of pulmonary function respiratory symptoms such as cough and sputum production. Acute exacerbations are associated with various triggers, including viral or bacterial respiratory infections, air pollution, and cardiac failure. Exacerbations vary widely in severity, but severe exacerbations may lead to hospitalization, acute respiratory failure, and death. Following an exacerbation, a patient may take weeks to return to a baseline level of function. Patients with

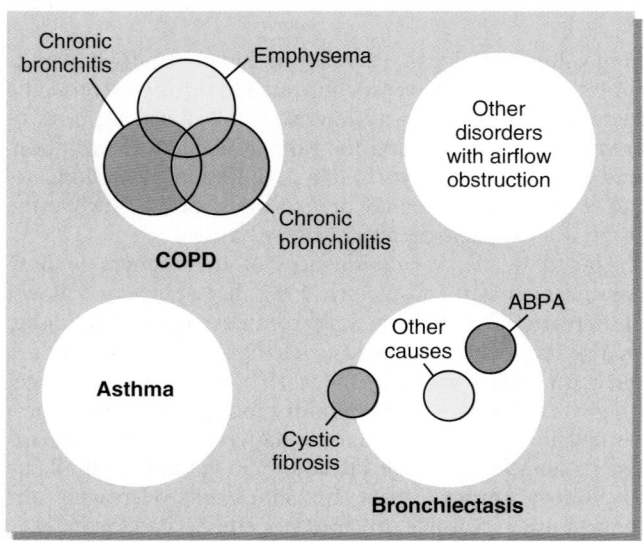

Figure 17-1 Classification of obstructive lung diseases. COPD, chronic obstructive lung disease.

Table 17-1 Features of Obstructive Lung Diseases

Disorder	Clinical Features	Laboratory Findings
Chronic obstructive pulmonary disease	Chronic progressive dyspnea	Decreased expiratory flow rates, hypoxia and hypercapnia in end-stage disease
Emphysema	Little or no sputum, end-stage cachexia	Hyperinflation, increased compliance, low D_LCO, rarely α_1-antitrypsin deficiency
Chronic bronchitis	Sputum, history of smoking, industrial exposure	Nonspecific; rarely occurs in isolation without varying degrees of emphysema
Asthma	Episodic dyspnea, cough, wheezing, with or without environmental triggers	Airway hyperreactivity, response to bronchodilators
Bronchiectasis	Usually large volume of sputum	Chest radiograph: dilated bronchi, thick-walled, tram track shadows, obstruction with or without restriction on pulmonary function tests
Immotile cilia syndrome	Situs inversus, dextrocardia, sinusitis, infertility	Abnormal dynein in ciliated cells
Hypogammaglobulinemia		Decrease in one or more immunoglobulins
Cystic fibrosis	Sinusitis, bronchiectasis, meconium ileus, malabsorption, infertility	Increased sweat chloride, mutation in CFTR chloride channel, elevated fecal fat, abnormal nasal mucosal potential difference

CFTR, cystic fibrosis transmembrane conductance regulator; D_LCO, diffusion capacity for carbon monoxide.

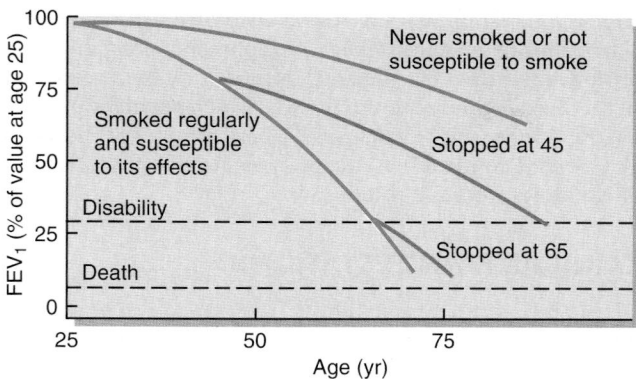

Figure 17-2 Pattern of decline in forced expiratory volume in 1 second (FEV$_1$) with risks for morbidity and mortality from respiration disease in a susceptible smoker in comparison with a normal patient and with a nonsusceptible smoker. Although cessation of smoking does not replenish the lung function already lost in a susceptible smoker, it decreases the rate of further decline. (Data from Fletcher C, Peto R: The natural history of chronic airflow obstruction. BMJ 1:1645-1648, 1977.)

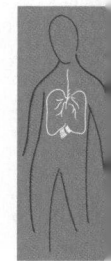

frequent exacerbations of COPD appear to experience an accelerated rate of decline in FEV$_1$.

The only genetic disorder thus far definitively linked to COPD is α_1-antitrypsin deficiency, which accounts for less than 1% of all cases. The deficient enzyme, α_1-antitrypsin, an acute-phase reactant, is produced primarily in the liver, from which it travels to the lung, where it deactivates elastases released by inflammatory cells that are capable of degrading connective tissue matrices. In doing so, α_1-antitrypsin prevents the uncontrolled degradation of elastin in the lung parenchyma and protects against the development of emphysema. Individuals with the ZZ genotype of α_1-antitrypsin deficiency produce mutant forms of α_1-antitrypsin that have a tendency to inappropriately polymerize within the hepatocyte, leading to a deficiency in secreted α_1-antitrypsin and in some cases to collateral damage to the liver caused by accumulation of intracellular misfolded, mutant α_1-antitrypsin. Patients who develop emphysema at a young age (<40 years) should be evaluated for this condition whether or not they smoke. Polymorphisms in various other candidate genes that may be relevant to susceptibility to COPD are under investigation.

As noted previously, the main pathophysiologic abnormalities potentially present in COPD are emphysema, chronic bronchitis, and small airways disease. These disorders are individually discussed next.

Emphysema

Emphysema is defined as a permanent enlargement of the air spaces distal to the terminal bronchiole (**Web Fig. 17-1**). This occurs as a result of destruction of lung parenchyma, but in the absence of significant fibrosis. These changes result in an abnormal acinus with limited capabilities for gas exchange. Based on thin gross lung sections, emphysema can be classified into *centrilobular* and *panlobular* types (**Web Figs. 17-2 and 17-3**). In centrilobular emphysema, the proximal part of the lobule (the respiratory bronchiole) is affected, which represents the most common

histologic feature observed in emphysema related to smoking, whereas panlobular emphysema is typically seen in α_1-antitrypsin deficiency.

The observation that α_1-antitrypsin deficiency was associated with emphysema, and that emphysema could be reproduced in experimental models by the instillation of papain, a protease, into the lungs, led to the hypothesis that emphysema is caused by an imbalance between protease and antiprotease systems in the lung. This theorized imbalance would favor proteolytic destruction of lung connective tissue, resulting in emphysema (the *protease-antiprotease hypothesis*). Research has focused on neutrophil elastase and its role in the destruction of lung elastin. Neutrophil elastase is the main target for inactivation by α_1-antitrypsin and has relatively unopposed effects. However, evidence of a primary role of this enzyme in cigarette smoke-induced emphysema is less clear, so the focus has since broadened to include examination of the role of the matrix metalloproteinases (MMPs), produced by macrophages and other cells, in emphysema. Transgenic mice deficient in the *MMP-12* gene are resistant to the development of emphysema, supporting a role for this enzyme in mediating lung connective tissue loss leading to emphysema.

The *inflammation* induced by cigarette smoke is a trigger of the cycle of protease release and lung destruction resulting in emphysema (**Web Fig. 17-4**). Macrophages are activated by cigarette smoke and recruit neutrophils and other inflammatory cells to the lung, leading to the release of elastase and MMPs. The destruction of elastin and other connective tissue elements in the lungs over time by these proteases leads in turn to the loss of elastic recoil and the destruction of alveolar structures characteristic of emphysema.

Cigarette smoke contains many oxidant molecules, capable of inducing *oxidative stress* in the lung. Oxidative stress has diverse effects, including the oxidative inactivation of antiproteases in the lung as well as acetylation of specific histones in the chromatin of lung cells and macrophages, allowing the expression of various pro-inflammatory genes. Histone deacetylase activity is reduced in COPD, which in turn may result in an inability to control the pro-inflammatory response in this condition. Pro-inflammatory gene expression promotes cytokine production and release, contributing to further inflammatory cell recruitment and activation. Systemic inflammation, triggered by ongoing pulmonary inflammation, may lead to nonpulmonary abnormalities associated with emphysema, including cachexia and skeletal muscle alterations. Finally, increased *apoptosis* of pneumocytes and endothelial cells has been observed in lungs with emphysema and could contribute to the loss of alveoli.

Understanding of emphysema pathogenesis has improved, with the recognition that inflammation, oxidative stress, protease-antiprotease balance, and apoptosis are linked in a complex interaction induced by cigarette smoke. This improved understanding has broadened the range of therapeutic possibilities that may be effective in ameliorating the destructive process. To date, however, specific therapies targeted at molecular pathways involved in emphysema pathogenesis have not been successful at altering disease progression, with the possible exception of α_1-antitrypsin replacement therapy in α_1-antitrypsin deficiency.

Chronic Bronchitis

Chronic bronchitis often coincides with emphysema in the patient with COPD, and it is defined in clinical terms as a persistent cough resulting in sputum production for more than 3 months in each of the past 2 years. Cigarette smoking is the major cause, although exposure to pollutants such as dusts may also play a role. Pathologic findings are goblet cell hyperplasia, mucus hypersecretion and plugging, and airway inflammation and fibrosis.

The disease mechanisms involved in the development of emphysema are also important in the pathogenesis of chronic bronchitis. However, in contrast to emphysema, chronic bronchitis is a disease of the large airways and not the lung parenchyma. Therefore, the relationship of chronic bronchitis to airflow obstruction is less robust than for emphysema, and airflow limitation in a patient with chronic bronchitis may be more reflective of concomitant emphysema and small airways disease. Inflammation in chronic bronchitis leads to effects on the airway epithelium, including *excess mucus production* and *impairment in mucociliary clearance*. *Neurogenic stimuli* are also important in the pathogenesis of airway obstruction in chronic bronchitis. The conducting airways are surrounded by smooth muscle, which contains adrenergic and cholinergic receptors. Stimulation of β_2-adrenergic receptors by circulating catecholamines dilates airways, whereas stimulation of airway irritant receptors constricts airways through a cholinergic mechanism by means of the vagus nerve. The irritant bronchoconstrictive pathways are normally present to protect against inhalation of noxious agents, but in pathologic states, these pathways may contribute to airway hyperreactivity. A host of endogenous chemical mediators such as proteases, growth factors, and cytokines can also affect airway tone.

By definition, the predominant symptom in chronic bronchitis is sputum production. Bronchospasm may also be prominent. Recurrent bacterial airway infections are typical. As with all patients with COPD, the evaluation of patients with chronic bronchitis should include pulmonary function tests and a chest radiograph in addition to standard laboratory testing.

Small Airways Disease

The role of small airways (<2 mm in diameter) in the pathogenesis of COPD continues to be elucidated. The small airways are thought to be a major site of resistance to airflow in COPD. *Respiratory bronchiolitis,* with an accumulation of pigmented macrophages in and around the bronchioles (**Web Fig. 17-5**), may be an incidental finding in asymptomatic smokers without COPD. However, as COPD develops, other inflammatory cells are recruited to the small conducting airways, presumably in reaction to ongoing irritation from cigarette smoke or inhaled particles. With inflammation, the small airways in COPD can be affected by remodeling, leading to airway wall thickening and fibrosis, smooth muscle hypertrophy, and airway luminal narrowing, contributing to airflow obstruction. Small airways can be occluded by mucus plugs and inflammatory exudates, leading to an overall loss of cross-sectional area and increased resistance to airflow. Lymphoid follicles may form around the airways in response to ongoing antigenic stimulation and

bacterial infection, with a prominence of B cells and CD8[+] cells in more advanced COPD. Emphysema contributes to airflow obstruction at the small airway level by destruction of the alveoli tethered to the airways, which normally provide a force opposing airway closure. These changes at the small airway level contribute to the physiologic abnormalities and altered local immune response in COPD.

CLINICAL MANIFESTATIONS

COPD related to chronic tobacco exposure is characterized by slowly progressive dyspnea that is first noted during exertion but that progresses over years until it is evident at rest. Affected individuals complain of exercise intolerance and fatigue, and the disease eventually leads to weight loss, depression, and anxiety as a result of increased work of breathing. Chronic cough can be present and is productive or dry, depending on the degree of airway involvement (e.g., chronic bronchitis). In general, emphysema caused by chronic cigarette smoking is almost never observed in patients before 40 years of age. If it is, consideration should be given to genetic disorders, such as α_1-antitrypsin deficiency.

During the early stages of COPD, the physical examination may be normal. A normal examination and the absence of symptoms often delay diagnosis. Inspection of the thorax and palpation may fail to reveal findings. As the disease progresses, the lungs may be hyperresonant to percussion, and auscultation may show diminished breath sounds with rhonchi, wheezes, or faint crackles. The chest wall may begin to remodel, giving the patient the appearance of a "barrel chest." During the late stages of COPD, patients show evidence of increased work of breathing with use of accessory muscles, pursed-lip breathing, and weight loss. Skeletal muscle wasting may also become evident. Despite their respiratory insufficiency, some patients are able to sustain relatively normal oxygen levels in blood until very late in the disease, leading to the classic clinical presentation of the "pink puffer." Other patients tend to retain CO_2 and diminish their work of breathing, resulting in chronic respiratory acidosis and, in extreme cases, polycythemia and cyanosis; this is the prototypical "blue bloater" phenotype.

As the disease progresses, the lung volumes increase (hyperinflation) and the diaphragms flatten, which renders inspiratory excursions inefficient. Tidal volume decreases and respiratory rate increases in an effort to decrease work of breathing. In advanced disease, the cardiovascular system becomes affected as a result of loss of vasculature in destroyed alveolar walls and vascular remodeling due to chronic hypoxia. With limited area for blood flow, pulmonary vascular resistance is increased, leading to increased right ventricular afterload and development of pulmonary hypertension. This accelerates the development of right ventricular failure, which is referred to as *cor pulmonale* in the setting of lung disease. Right heart gallop, distended neck veins, hepatojugular reflux, and leg edema characterize cor pulmonale.

EVALUATION

Airway narrowing, which increases resistance to airflow, and a loss of elastic recoil of the lung, which decreases driving pressure, decrease airflow in the lungs. Both these physiologic abnormalities are often present in COPD. They can be detected by pulmonary function tests, which are essential for the diagnosis of obstructive pulmonary disease, for assessing its severity, and for evaluating response to therapy. COPD is characterized by airflow obstruction, with decreased FEV_1. The decrease in FEV_1 predominates when compared with that of the forced vital capacity (FVC), leading to reduction of the FEV_1/FVC ratio; a reduced FEV_1 and FEV_1/FVC ratio is pathognomonic of airflow obstruction.

Although some degree of reversibility can be detected with bronchodilators, and hyper-reactivity can be unveiled by bronchoprovocation challenge, the obstructive defect is not entirely reversible in COPD. This characteristic and the progressive nature of the obstruction represent key features that help distinguish COPD from asthma. The severity of disease and prognosis can be estimated by the FEV_1; an FEV_1 of about 1 L (usually 50% of predicted levels) suggests severe obstruction and, in the case of COPD, predicts a mean survival of 50% at 5 years. FEV_1 can be incorporated into a validated prognostic scoring system, the BODE index, that is a better predictor of mortality than FEV_1 alone. The BODE index includes the assessment of body mass index (B); degree of obstruction (O) as assessed by FEV_1, modified Medical Research Council dyspnea (D) score, and exercise (E) capacity as denoted by 6-minute walk distance.

Lung volumes should be measured with pulmonary function testing because the limitation to expired airflow and decreased elastic recoil lead to lung hyperinflation, evidenced by increased residual volume, functional residual capacity, and, ultimately, total lung capacity. Increased lung volume causes flattening of the diaphragm, which causes shortening of its muscle fibers, thereby reducing contractile efficiency.

Destruction of alveoli decreases the surface area for gas exchange in emphysema. This loss of surface area, coupled with bronchial obstruction and altered distribution of ventilated air, results in ventilation-perfusion ratio $(\dot{V}/\dot{Q})$ inequality or mismatch, a cause of hypoxemia. Hyperinflation of the lungs increases zone 1 conditions, in which alveolar pressure exceeds pulmonary arterial pressure, a process that decreases perfusion and increases physiologic dead space. Hypercarbia, but not hypoxemia, can be avoided by hyperventilation, even with substantial $\dot{V}/\dot{Q}$ mismatching. However, eventually, the metabolic costs of breathing become excessive, and respiratory muscles fatigue. Over time, chemoreceptors *reset,* allowing the level of partial pressure of carbon dioxide in arterial blood ($Paco_2$) to rise, which increases the efficiency of ventilation by eliminating a higher concentration of carbon dioxide per breath, and thereby lowering the metabolic cost of breathing. Significant individual variation is observed in the degree of mechanical impairment and in the magnitude of increase in $Paco_2$. Derangements in gas exchange can be detected by performing arterial blood gases. They can also be detected by showing a decrease in lung *diffusion capacity for carbon monoxide* (D_Lco) or by evaluating hemoglobin oxygen desaturation during exertion. The degree of decrease in D_Lco correlates well with the radiologic extent of emphysema in COPD.

Chest radiographs may fail to reveal abnormalities during the early stages of COPD, but in later stages, radiographic studies show hyperinflation, hyperlucency, flattening of the diaphragms, and bullous changes in lung parenchyma (**Web Fig. 17-6**). Pleural abnormalities, lymphadenopathy, and mediastinal widening are not characteristic of emphysema and should point to other diagnoses, such as lung cancer. *Computed tomography* (CT) is more sensitive than plain radiographs because CT allows for a more detailed evaluation of the lung parenchyma and surrounding structures. CT is useful in assessing the distribution of emphysema (**Web Fig. 17-7**) in patients for whom operative interventions such as lung volume reduction surgery are being contemplated. High-resolution computed tomography (HRCT) is highly sensitive for the detection of occult emphysema and can reveal the pattern of emphysematous changes. The *electrocardiogram* might show evidence of right ventricular strain. *Echocardiography* can reveal evidence of right ventricular hypertrophy or dilation and can often provide an estimate of pulmonary arterial pressures in patients with advanced COPD. Blood hemoglobin might reveal erythrocytosis in the setting of chronic hypoxemia, whereas increased white blood cell counts might suggest infection. The *arterial blood gas* may show hypoxemia, hypercarbia, or both, whereas acidemia due to acute hypercarbia may be present during an exacerbation.

MANAGEMENT

Because a cure for COPD does not exist, the best approach to this condition resides in its prevention. Most cases of COPD in the United States are due to cigarette smoking. Thus, an appropriate major emphasis has been placed on the development of community education programs that emphasize smoking prevention and promote smoking cessation. Legislative measures banning smoking in various public settings and levying increased taxes on cigarettes have been used to diminish the effects of environmental or second-hand tobacco smoke exposure and to discourage smoking. Although smoking cessation interventions are only effective in a minority of patients, smoking cessation will decrease mortality in patients with COPD who do succeed at quitting. Most patients who are successful at smoking cessation have had at least one prior failed attempt, so physicians should encourage smoking cessation with at least brief interventions at every opportunity, even in patients who have tried but failed to quit in the past. Long-term physician and group support increases the success of cessation attempts, and pharmacologic smoking cessation aides, including nicotine replacement with gum or transdermal patches, bupropion, and varencycline, may provide additional benefit.

After COPD is established, therapy is directed at avoiding complications such as exacerbations, relieving airflow obstruction through use of bronchodilators, and providing supplemental oxygen to patients with hypoxemia. Commonly used inhaled bronchodilators include sympathomimetic agents (β_2-adrenoreceptor agonists) and anticholinergic agents. Ipratropium bromide, a short-acting anticholinergic agent, is efficacious at decreasing dyspnea and improving FEV_1 in COPD. Albuterol is the most commonly used β_2 agonist; its bronchodilator effect is rapid in onset and is also relatively short lived. In practice, a combination of albuterol and ipratropium is frequently prescribed because these agents produce greater benefits when used in combination than individually. Short-acting agents are typically initiated in patients with mild disease or intermittent symptoms on an as-needed basis. Long-acting bronchodilators are effective for maintenance therapy in patients with persistent symptoms and may improve compliance. The long-acting β_2 agonists formoterol and salmeterol can be administered twice daily. Tiotropium is a long-acting anticholinergic that has been found to improve symptoms and lung function and to reduce the frequency of exacerbations in patients with COPD.

Short-acting bronchodilators can be delivered either by a metered-dose inhaler (MDI) or nebulizer. The MDI offers advantages of portability and ease of administration and convenience. When used correctly with a spacer, MDIs are as effective as nebulizers in delivering the drug. Nebulization has no advantage over the use of MDIs in the long-term management of obstructive lung disease except in patients unable to use an MDI properly.

Theophylline, a methylxanthine, is a weak systemic sympathomimetic agent with a narrow therapeutic window. It is not a first-line drug in the treatment of obstructive lung disease, although long-acting derivatives with improved safety profiles have been developed. Theophylline preparations have some anti-inflammatory activity and may provide additional bronchodilation in patients with COPD who do not respond adequately to inhaled β agonists. When these preparations are used, blood concentrations should be maintained in the lower end of the therapeutic range (between 8 and 12 mcg/mL). Toxicity is common at concentrations higher than 20 mcg/mL. The metabolism of theophylline is decreased by many commonly used drugs (e.g., erythromycin), and toxic serum concentrations of theophylline can be reached quickly when these other drugs are administered unless the theophylline dose is adjusted appropriately. Toxic effects of theophylline may be observed in the gastrointestinal, cardiac, and neurologic systems. Severe theophylline toxicity could be fatal and may require treatment with charcoal hemoperfusion.

Current data suggest that the chronic use of inhaled corticosteroids improves symptoms and decreases the frequency of exacerbations. For this reason, inhaled long-acting corticosteroids (e.g., fluticasone propionate, budesonide) are frequently used in the treatment of COPD. Inhaled corticosteroids are less clearly effective in COPD than in asthma, and pneumonia may occur more frequently in patients with COPD treated with inhaled corticosteroids. Inhaled corticosteroids can be combined with long-acting β agonists. Combination of a long-acting β agonist, salmeterol, with an inhaled corticosteroid, fluticasone, in patients with moderate to severe COPD improved health-related quality of life and reduced exacerbations to a greater extent than either component alone. Systemic use of corticosteroids is indicated during acute exacerbations, and intravenous corticosteroids have been proved useful in the acute setting. Intravenous corticosteroids have also proved effective for the management of acute exacerbations of most obstructive lung diseases, including cases of asthma (Fig. 17-3). Patients with acute exacerbations are generally transitioned from intravenous to oral steroids within 72 hours, with a subsequent tapering of the oral steroid dose over 2 weeks. Other agents with anti-inflammatory capabilities, such

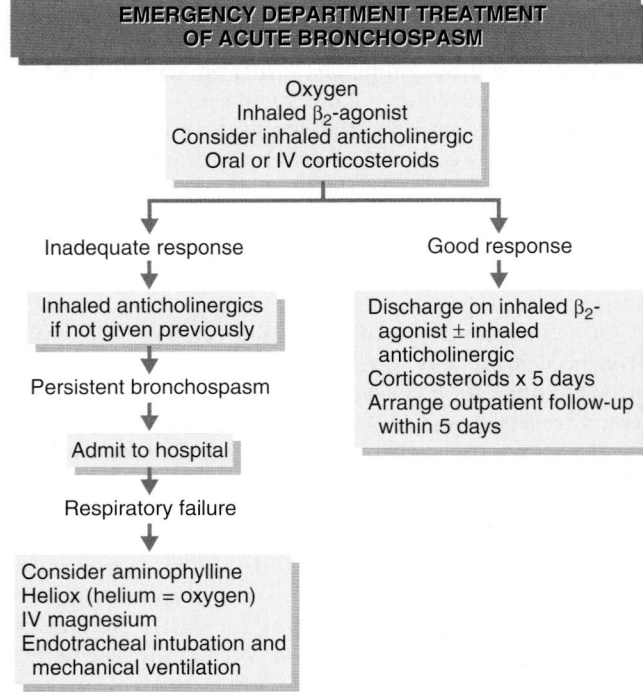

EMERGENCY DEPARTMENT TREATMENT OF ACUTE BRONCHOSPASM

A

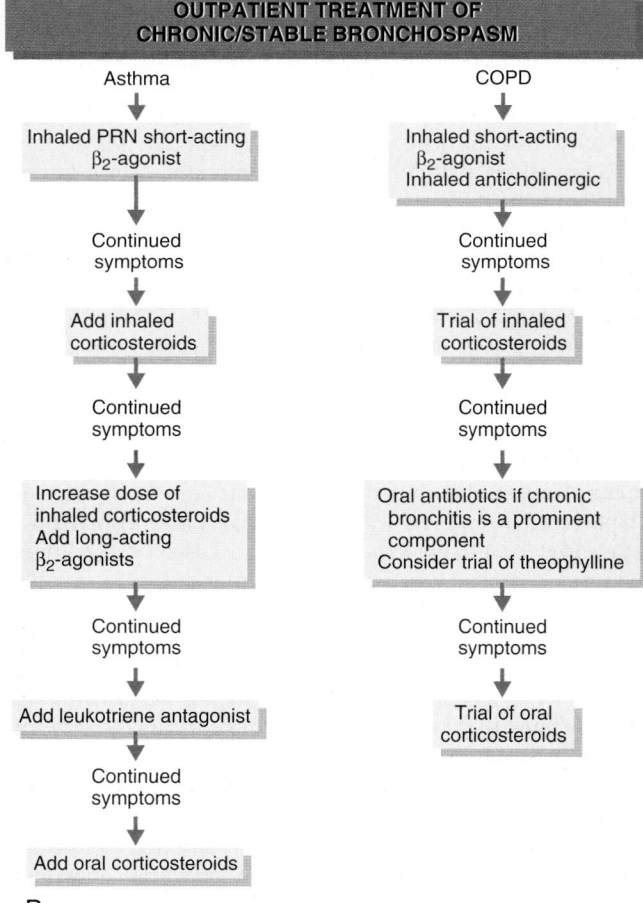

OUTPATIENT TREATMENT OF CHRONIC/STABLE BRONCHOSPASM

B

Figure 17-3 Algorithms for the treatment of bronchospasm in the emergency department (**A**) and in outpatients with stable disease (**B**).

as leukotriene inhibitors, are not indicated for treatment of COPD.

Continuous oxygen therapy has been shown to improve survival in patients with COPD and hypoxemia. Oxygen supplementation is recommended once the partial pressure of oxygen in arterial blood (Pa_{O_2}) drops below 55 mm Hg or the hemoglobin oxygen saturation decreases to 88%. Oxygen supplementation is indicated at higher levels of Pa_{O_2} if end-organ damage is present.

Oxygen therapy is frequently necessary for treatment of acute exacerbations of obstructive lung disease. In patients who hypoventilate chronically and therefore have an elevated Pa_{CO_2}, elevating the inspired oxygen content may acutely worsen hypercarbia by inhibiting the hypoxic ventilatory drive and by promoting the dissociation of carbon dioxide from oxygenated hemoglobin (the *Haldane effect*). Nonetheless, arterial oxygen must be maintained in a range compatible with life even at the expense of precipitating respiratory failure requiring mechanical ventilation. During exacerbations of COPD leading to hypercarbic respiratory failure, noninvasive positive airway pressure ventilation has proved useful in reducing the work of breathing, alleviating diaphragm fatigue, and reducing the need for endotracheal intubation and mechanical ventilation.

Exacerbations of airway obstruction may result from viral or bacterial infection. The most common bacterial pathogens in COPD are *Streptococcus pneumoniae*, *Haemophilus influenzae*, and *Moraxella catarrhalis*. Management of acute exacerbations should include empiric antibiotics. Immunization with influenza vaccines directed at specific epidemic strains reduces exacerbations of COPD. Pneumococcal vaccination is also recommended in patients with COPD.

Multiple airway clearance techniques aid in clearing of airway secretions, but their effectiveness in the management of emphysema and other obstructive lung diseases in adults is questionable. If needed, chest physiotherapy and postural drainage might be useful in patients with chronic bronchitis and increased sputum production. Few data support the use of specific mucolytics or expectorant agents for patients with COPD.

Patients with pulmonary disease of sufficient severity to compromise normal activities of daily living commonly demonstrate improved quality of life and less subjective dyspnea when enrolled in a comprehensive, high-quality *pulmonary rehabilitation program*. Pulmonary rehabilitation has not been shown to improve objective measures of pulmonary function, to affect the rate of decline in lung function, or to improve survival. However, it has been shown to improve the quality of life in motivated patients. An important part of pulmonary rehabilitation is nutritional assessment and careful attention to maintaining adequate nutrition. Malnutrition and cachexia are common in later stages of obstructive lung disease and result in decreased respiratory muscle strength and compromised immune function.

In certain patients with advanced emphysema, surgical interventions might prove beneficial. Of these, bullectomy, lung volume reduction surgery (LVRS), and lung transplantation are all potentially effective surgical options for select patients. Resection of nonfunctional areas of lung (e.g., bullectomy) may allow for compressed functional areas to expand and may improve symptoms, airflow, and oxygena-

tion by improving $\dot{V}/\dot{Q}$ matching in a subgroup of patients. In addition, resection of bullae can decrease lung volumes, resulting in enhanced diaphragmatic function and decreased work of breathing. The best candidates for LVRS are those with predominantly upper lobe disease with a low exercise tolerance despite rehabilitation and without other major co-morbidities. In general, a high surgical mortality risk exists in patients with an FEV_1 or $D_{L}CO$ of less than 20% predicted and in those with more homogeneous distribution of emphysema. Endoscopic placement of one-way endobronchial valves to deflate regions of lung with emphysema is under active investigation.

Single or bilateral lung transplantation is an option for patients with end-stage airflow obstruction. In general, the average survival after lung transplantation is 4 to 5 years. Chronic rejection, viral infections, transplant-associated lymphoproliferative disease, and late occurrence of obliterative bronchiolitis remain significant problems of lung transplantation, but the procedure can clearly improve the quality of life and can extend productive life in properly selected patients.

Although the disease course can be unpredictable, discussion of end-of-life issues with the patient is an important component of longitudinal care as COPD progresses to an advanced stage. Developing advance directives regarding use of intensive care measures at the end of life may be desirable. Opioid narcotics can be highly effective at relieving dyspnea in patients with terminal complications of COPD.

Bronchiolar Disorders

The bronchiolar disorders are known for patchy inflammation and epithelial injury, fibrosis, or obliteration of the noncartilaginous small airways, the bronchioles (**Web Fig. 17-8**). This results in airflow limitation that is due to increased airway resistance. Bronchiolitis contributes to the syndrome of COPD, as discussed previously under "Small Airways Disease," but isolated bronchiolar disorders with different etiologies than cigarette smoking also exist. These disorders may be self-limited, as in *acute bronchiolitis* caused by viral infections including respiratory syncytial virus (RSV), or relentlessly progressive, as in the *bronchiolitis obliterans syndrome* occurring after lung transplantation. Acute bronchiolitis is most common in infants, occurring in epidemic form during wintertime in association with RSV, and can complicate adult viral respiratory infections or can result from aspiration injury. Wheezing and dyspnea are typical symptoms of acute bronchiolitis. *Diffuse panbronchiolitis* is an idiopathic disorder most common in Japan and is characterized by cough with purulent sputum, sinusitis, and dyspnea. Recurrent respiratory infections with bacterial organisms such as *Pseudomonas aeruginosa* complicate the course of diffuse panbronchiolitis. *Bronchiolitis obliterans* is seen with connective tissue diseases, the bronchiolitis obliterans syndrome of chronic allograft rejection after lung transplantation, as well as after occupational toxin exposures. For example, occupational clusters of bronchiolitis obliterans have recently been described following exposure to diacetyl, a flavoring chemical used in the manufacture of microwave popcorn.

In general, the bronchiolar disorders cause an obstructive pattern of expiratory airflow limitation on pulmonary function testing without evidence of reversibility. The bronchiolitis obliterans syndrome is diagnosed clinically by a decline in FEV_1 of 20% from a stable baseline value on serial testing after lung transplantation. HRCT is valuable in the diagnosis and assessment of the bronchiolar disorders. Characteristic findings on HRCT include centrilobular nodules or *tree-in-bud opacities*, reflecting impacted inflammatory exudates or sloughed epithelial cells in the bronchioles. A "mosaic" pattern, with decreased attenuation in geographic regions of lung reflecting areas of air trapping distal to obstructed bronchioles, is often seen, and CT scanning during the expiratory phase can confirm that this finding is caused by air trapping as opposed to decreased perfusion from pulmonary vascular disease. Lung biopsy is often of limited value because of the scattered, patchy nature of the abnormalities present in the bronchiolar disorders.

Treatment of the bronchiolar disorders is challenging. Acute bronchiolitis typically resolves without treatment; bronchodilators and steroids are not clearly beneficial, although they are often prescribed. The bronchiolitis obliterans syndrome responds poorly to increased immunosuppression and is a frequent cause of death after transplantation. Azithromycin, a macrolide antibiotic, has been reported to increase FEV_1 in the bronchiolitis obliterans syndrome. Macrolide antibiotics have also been reported to positively affect the clinical course of diffuse panbronchiolitis, possibly reflecting immunomodulatory or antifibrotic effects of these medications. Lung transplantation may be necessary in progressive bronchiolitis obliterans, and retransplantation has sometimes been performed in patients affected by the bronchiolitis obliterans syndrome after transplant rejection.

Bronchiectasis

Bronchiectasis is abnormal dilation of the bronchi (**Web Fig. 17-9**) resulting from inflammation and permanent destructive changes in the elastic and muscular layers of the bronchial walls. Bronchiectasis may be localized to a certain bronchus or may be diffuse. This disorder is usually caused by recurrent or chronic severe infections such as necrotizing pneumonias (e.g., *Staphylococcus aureus* pneumonia), tuberculosis, or infection with atypical mycobacteria (e.g., *Mycobacterium avium-intracellulare*). Viral (e.g., *measles*) and fungal (e.g., *histoplasmosis* and *coccidioidomycosis*) infections may cause bronchiectasis as well. *Allergic bronchopulmonary aspergillosis* is a condition associated with hypersensitivity to aspergillus fungi that is usually exhibited as severe intractable asthma, central bronchiectasis, high levels of immunoglobulin E (IgE), and precipitins for *Aspergillus* species.

Localized bronchiectasis may result from anatomic obstruction, either by an endobronchial foreign body, tumor, or broncholith, or as a result of extrinsic compression by lymphadenopathy. The *right middle lobe syndrome* results from narrowing of the right middle lobe bronchial orifice, often by lymph nodes, leading to localized bronchiectasis distal to the site of obstruction. Anatomic obstruction results in chronic or recurrent infection and inflammation leading to bronchial distortion and destruction over time.

Bronchiectasis is more frequent in middle-aged to older individuals. In addition to infections and anatomic obstruction, bronchiectasis may be related to connective tissue diseases including rheumatoid arthritis. Bronchiectasis may occur in younger patients when associated with congenital defects like *cystic fibrosis* or *primary ciliary dyskinesia*, a rare inherited abnormality of the ciliary microtubules that impairs airway clearance and is associated with recurrent infections. The classic triad of sinusitis, *situs inversus,* and infertility is diagnostic of *Kartagener syndrome*, a form of primary ciliary dyskinesia. Other congenital syndromes associated with bronchiectasis include α_1-antitrypsin deficiency and immunodeficiency states related to hypogammaglobulinemia.

Patients with bronchiectasis exhibit chronic cough and foul-smelling sputum, shortness of breath, abnormal chest sounds, and fatigue. Blood-streaked sputum is common, and massive hemoptysis may occur. Clubbing may be present. Periodic exacerbations due to infection with bacterial pathogens, including *P. aeruginosa, S. pneumoniae,* and *H. influenzae,* are common. Pulmonary function tests may show varying degrees of obstruction. Evidence of bronchial hyperresponsiveness is not infrequent. Chest radiographs may be normal or may show increased interstitial markings. The classic finding is parallel lines in peripheral lung fields described as *tram tracks,* which represent thickened bronchial walls that do not taper from proximal to distal sites. HRCT is more sensitive for the detection of dilated airways and is the test of choice in the diagnosis of suspected bronchiectasis. Bronchiectasis on HRCT is suggested by lack of airway tapering at the lung periphery and by airways that are larger in diameter than their accompanying blood vessel. Bronchoscopy may be indicated in localized bronchiectasis to assess for endobronchial abnormalities. Sputum can be cultured to assess for fungal or mycobacterial organisms that may be causative of the bronchiectasis, or for identification of specific bacterial pathogens during exacerbations.

Treatment of the underlying cause of the bronchiectasis should be undertaken if possible. An anatomic obstruction, such as from a foreign body or benign tumor, should be relieved. Atypical mycobacterial infection should be treated with an appropriate multidrug regimen in symptomatic patients following confirmation of the diagnosis with multiple smears and cultures. Allergic bronchopulmonary aspergillosis is typically treated with corticosteroids; addition of azole antifungals may also be beneficial. Bacterial exacerbations of bronchiectasis should be treated with a broad-spectrum antibiotic effective against the likely pathogens, such as a quinolone. Aerosolized antibiotics are of benefit in the suppression of bacterial growth in bronchiectasis associated with cystic fibrosis but are less clearly beneficial in noncystic fibrosis bronchiectasis. Immunoglobulin supplementation may aid in the host defense against bacterial infection in individuals with hypogammaglobulinemia. Airway clearance and postural drainage are frequently employed in bronchiectasis but are of uncertain benefit. Bronchodilators may provide symptomatic relief. Massive hemoptysis should be managed with airway protection and identification of the bleeding site; bronchial artery angiography with embolization of the causative bleeding vessels may be life-saving. The role of surgery is mainly in the removal of a badly damaged isolated segment of bronchiectatic lung, for the resection of obstructing lesions causing distal bronchiectasis, and on occasion as a salvage therapy in resection of a site with uncontrolled hemorrhage.

Cystic Fibrosis

Cystic fibrosis is an autosomal recessive genetic disorder that affects about 30,000 children and adults in the United States. This disorder affects many organs, including the lungs, pancreas, and reproductive organs, although most mortality related to cystic fibrosis is due to lung disease. It is the most common lethal genetic disorder in the white population, with a carrier frequency of about 1 in 29, affecting 1 in 3300 live births. About 1000 new patients with cystic fibrosis are diagnosed each year. Cystic fibrosis results from a mutation in a single gene that encodes the cystic fibrosis transmembrane conductance regulator (CFTR), which is a cyclic adenosine monophosphate-regulated chloride channel present on the apical surface of epithelial cells (**Web Fig. 17-10**). The most common mutation is the ΔF508 mutation, a 3 base-pair deletion that results in absence of the phenylalanine residue at the 508 position of the protein. However, more than 1600 mutations have been identified to date. The abnormal CFTR protein results in defective chloride transport and increased sodium reabsorption in airway and ductal epithelia, creating abnormally thick and viscous secretions in the respiratory, hepatobiliary, gastrointestinal, and reproductive tracts. The thick secretions do not easily clear from the airways, resulting in respiratory symptoms, and cause luminal obstruction and destruction of exocrine ducts in other organs, leading to exocrine organ dysfunction.

Infants with cystic fibrosis may present with meconium ileus or failure to thrive with steatorrhea. Salty-tasting skin may be noted by caregivers. Patients with cystic fibrosis typically have chronic cough with thick sputum production, wheezing, and dyspnea. Pancreatic insufficiency and diabetes are common, and male patients have azoospermia (Table 17-2). Nasal polyps are often present, and clubbing is typical. Cystic fibrosis should be considered in the differential diagnosis of patients with unexplained chronic sinus disease, bronchiectasis, male infertility associated with absence of the vas deferens, pancreatitis, or malabsorption. Pulmonary function tests demonstrate hyperinflation and obstruction; a bronchodilator response may be present. Chest imaging studies show hyperinflation, bronchial wall thickening, and bronchiectasis.

In patients with cystic fibrosis, the airways become colonized initially with S. aureus or H. influenzae, followed by P. aeruginosa in ensuing years. Persistent inflammation and infection cause bronchial wall destruction and bronchiectasis. Mucus plugging of small airways results in postobstructive cystic dilations and parenchymal destruction, and progressive airflow obstruction and eventually hypoxemia ensue. The course of cystic fibrosis may additionally be complicated by the development of allergic bronchopulmonary aspergillosis and by nontuberculous mycobacterial infection. Colonization and infection with multidrug resistant *Burkholderia cepacia* complex may occur in advanced cystic

Table 17-2 **Organ Involvement in Cystic Fibrosis**
Pulmonary
Cough and sputum production
Recurrent pneumonias
Bronchial hyperreactivity
Hemoptysis
Pneumothorax
Significant digital clubbing
Cor pulmonale
Upper Respiratory Tract
Nasal polyps
Chronic sinusitis
Gastrointestinal
Meconium ileus in the neonate
Distal intestinal obstruction
Rectal prolapse
Hernias
Exocrine pancreatic dysfunction causing steatorrhea, malnutrition, and vitamin deficiency
Acute pancreatitis (rare)
Diabetes mellitus
Cirrhosis and portal hypertension
Salivary gland inflammation
Cholelithiasis
Genitourinary
Azoospermia
Decreased fertility rate in women
Nephrolithiasis

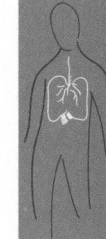

fibrosis, creating challenging management issues. Most patients die of respiratory failure.

The diagnosis of cystic fibrosis is made by measuring the concentration of chloride in sweat (*sweat test*). The diagnosis is considered definitive if the clinical picture is consistent with cystic fibrosis and if the chloride concentration performed in a certified laboratory is greater than 60 mEq/L on at least two occasions. Genotyping can also confirm the diagnosis if known mutations are identified in both gene alleles and can be used if sweat testing is equivocal.

Although most patients are diagnosed in childhood, some patients are not diagnosed until adulthood. About 45% of the population with cystic fibrosis in the United States is older than 18 years. Before 1940, infants with cystic fibrosis rarely lived to their first birthday. Currently, the median predicted life span for a person with cystic fibrosis is about 37 years of age.

The treatment of cystic fibrosis relies on aggressive airway hygiene, nutritional support including pancreatic enzyme replacement, antibiotics, and bronchodilators. Aerosolized recombinant human DNase (dornase alfa) decreases sputum viscosity, improves lung function, and reduces exacerbations in cystic fibrosis. Inhaled hypertonic saline helps to hydrate secretions, allowing them to be coughed out more easily, and also improves pulmonary function, although likely to a lesser extent than dornase alfa. Inhaled tobramycin provided twice daily every other month is indicated in moderate to severe cystic fibrosis patients with pseudomonal infections. Anti-inflammatory therapy with ibuprofen and azithromycin may be helpful in certain patients with cystic fibrosis. However, inhaled corticosteroids are not clearly beneficial. As is the case for other obstructive lung diseases, the ultimate therapy for patients with cystic fibrosis with end-stage lung disease is lung transplantation; bilateral lung transplantation is preferred in this condition.

Asthma

Asthma is a common pulmonary disorder characterized by airway inflammation, airway hyper-reactivity, and reversible airflow obstruction. The incidence of asthma is highest in children, but it affects all ages and occurs worldwide, with a preponderance of the disease in developed industrialized countries. Asthma results in a large burden of morbidity as well as economic cost in the United States. From 2001 to 2003, about 20 million persons per year reported having asthma in the United States. The prevalence of asthma has increased markedly over a period of decades. Asthma prevalence more than doubled among children from 1980 to 1995 alone, and the overall prevalence of asthma increased from 3.1% to 5.6% of the population during that time. Although asthma prevalence continued to increase up to 2001, it has recently appeared to plateau, and about 7% of the United States population is estimated to have asthma. Disturbingly, despite modern therapies and improved understanding of asthma, the number of deaths caused by asthma in the United States increased from 2891 in 1980 to 5637 deaths in 1995. Since then, the number of asthma deaths has appeared to decline, although about 4000 deaths per year still occur as a result of asthma. The reasons for the increase in asthma-related deaths in the late 20th century remain uncertain.

The cause of asthma is unknown, but it is likely to be a polygenic disease influenced by environmental factors. Atopy is strongly linked to asthma. Asthma is generally associated with an allergic-type activation of the immune system typified by a helper T-cell subtype 2 (T_H2)-predominant T-cell response to inhaled antigens, with consequent IgE production and allergic airway inflammation. Exposure to indoor allergens like dust mites, cockroaches, furry pets, and fungi is a significant factor, as are outdoor pollution and other irritants, including cigarette smoke. Current concepts of asthma pathogenesis include a focus on impairment of the shift from T_H2-predominant immunity to a T_H1 immune response early in life. Paradoxically, the perpetuation of T_H2 immune responses and the development of inappropriate allergic responses may be related to the relative lack of exposure of the immune system to appropriate infectious antigenic stimuli in childhood in the developed world, the so-called *hygiene hypothesis*. Farming, for example, appears to be protective against the development of asthma and allergic disease, possibly in part because of the increased exposure to microbial antigens eliciting a T_H1 response. Increased exposure to other children, as in daycare settings, and less frequent use of antibiotics may also decrease asthma risk, supporting this hypothesis. On the other hand, asthma is common in poor urban settings in which there is heavy exposure to allergic antigens from dust mites and cockroaches. The timing and role of particular environmental exposures in utero and in early life in the pathogenesis of asthma and allergic diseases remains to be fully elucidated, and there is no current theory that completely explains asthma pathogenesis or the recent increased incidence of asthma. The interplay of other aspects of modern life, such

as diet, with regards to asthma propensity continues to be explored.

Several genetic polymorphisms have been associated with asthma, including variations in the β-adrenergic receptor leading to diminished responsiveness to β agonists. Identifying other genetic polymorphisms important in asthma is a subject of ongoing research. Although asthma is more common in male children than female children, the prevalence of asthma changes following puberty, and asthma is more common in adult women than men, suggesting possible hormonal influences on asthma pathogenesis. Asthma can also be induced by workplace exposures in persons having no previous history of asthma (*occupational asthma*). Certain substances, like isocyanates, used in spray paints, and Western red cedar wood dust, are strongly provocative agents for the development of occupational asthma. Obesity has been linked to a higher incidence of asthma, a disturbing observation in view of the increasing prevalence of obesity. The mechanisms by which obesity may influence asthma development are unclear. Certain infectious agents and other conditions can cause acute bronchospasm even in patients without the diagnosis of asthma. Such is the case for viral infections, gastroesophageal reflux disease, and exposure to gases or fumes, and these disorders may play a role in the development or control of some cases of asthma.

The hallmark of asthma is *airway hyperresponsiveness*, a tendency of the airway smooth muscle to constrict in response to levels of inhaled allergens or irritants that would not typically elicit such a response in normal hosts. Inhaled allergens provoke airway mast cell degranulation by binding to and cross-linking IgE on the mast cell surface. Mast cell degranulation leads to the release of chemical mediators, which cause acute bronchoconstriction and thus increased airway resistance and wheezing, as well as mucus hypersecretion (**Web Fig. 17-11**). In addition, disruption of the continuity of the ciliated columnar epithelium and increased vascularity and edema of the airway wall follow antigen exposure. In addition to allergens, factors such as stimulation of irritant receptors, respiratory tract infections, and airway cooling can provoke bronchoconstriction in asthmatic individuals. Airway cooling appears to be responsible for exercise-induced bronchoconstriction as well as some wintertime asthma attacks. Underlying chronic *airway inflammation* is considered a major pathogenetic mechanism responsible for asthma. Patients with asthma have higher numbers of activated inflammatory cells within the airway wall, and the epithelium is typically infiltrated with eosinophils, mast cells, macrophages, and T lymphocytes, which produce multiple soluble mediators (e.g., cytokines, leukotrienes, bradykinins). However, although airway inflammation in asthma is generally typified by a T_H2-type response with predominantly eosinophilic inflammation, some patients with severe asthma exhibit neutrophilic airway inflammation and cytokine production more characteristic of T_H1 inflammation, suggesting asthma may be a common clinical phenotype resulting from heterogeneous forms of airway inflammation.

Asthma is associated with *airway wall remodeling*, which is characterized by hyperplasia and hypertrophy of smooth muscle cells (**Web Fig. 17-12**), edema, inflammatory infiltration, angiogenesis, and increased deposition of connective tissue components such as types I and III collagens. The latter leads to not only a thickening of the subepithelial lamina reticularis (**Web Fig. 17-13**) but also an expansion of the entire airway wall. Airway remodeling may begin fairly early in the course of the disease. Whether inflammation leads to remodeling or these processes represent two independent manifestations of the disease is unknown. Pulmonary function does seem to decline at an accelerated rate over time in patients with asthma, and airway wall remodeling may play a role in this functional loss. Over time, airway wall remodeling may lead to irreversible airflow limitation, which can worsen the disease by rendering bronchodilator drugs less effective; airway wall remodeling may make the distinction between asthma and COPD difficult.

CLINICAL MANIFESTATIONS

The classic triad of symptoms is wheezing, chronic episodic dyspnea, and chronic cough. However, the clinical manifestations of asthma may vary widely from mild intermittent symptoms to catastrophic attacks resulting in asphyxiation and death. Although wheezing is not a pathognomonic feature of asthma, in the setting of a compatible clinical picture, asthma is the most common diagnosis. Asthma can develop at any age as episodic cough, shortness of breath, and chest tightness. Often these symptoms worsen at night or during the early hours of the morning. Other associated symptoms are sputum production and chest pain or tightness. Patients may exhibit only one or a combination of the foregoing symptoms. Physical examination may be normal or may show evidence of wheezing. Rhinitis or nasal polyps may be present. In the case of an acute exacerbation, the clinician may find that the patient has difficulty talking, is using accessory muscles of inspiration, has *pulsus paradoxus*, is diaphoretic, and has mental status changes ranging from agitation to somnolence. In patients with these findings, treatment should be immediate and aggressive.

EVALUATION

A diagnosis of asthma requires documentation of hyperactivity and reversible airway obstruction to flow. The history might be sufficient to assess this because most patients complain of repeated but reversible episodes of wheezing. Airflow limitation is easily detected by spirometry when present. However, because asthma is episodic, patients might exhibit symptoms at a time when this cannot be documented. Depending on the circumstances, it might be necessary to test for airway hyperactivity by bronchoprovocation challenge (Table 17-3). The patient is given an airway application of a stimulant with bronchoconstrictor activity; histamine, methacholine, and cold air are among the most commonly used stimulants. Methacholine, a synthetic form of acetylcholine, is generally preferred to histamine because there are less systemic side effects. Exercise can also be used to trigger an attack. Although most patients with or without asthma may develop some degree of airflow limitation during bronchoprovocation testing, the diagnosis depends on the dose of the stimulus needed to elicit an effect; those with asthma develop airflow limitation at much lower doses than patients without. For methacholine challenges, the concentration of methacholine required to produce a 20% decline in FEV_1 from baseline is reported. Although a positive bronchoprovocation challenge is not by itself diagnostic of asthma, a negative bronchoprovocation challenge is generally helpful in ruling out asthma as a diagnosis.

Lung volume measurements may show hyperinflation during active disease, but D_LCO is typically normal because asthma is an airways disease and does not cause destruction of the acinus. Decreased D_LCO may be due to artifacts created by the measurement, which is highly sensitive to distribution of the gas (as is the case in mucus plugging). In this setting, the D_LCO value normalizes when corrected for gas volume distribution. During acute exacerbations of asthma, arterial blood gases are useful to determine gas-exchange status. A chest radiograph should be obtained if a concern for pulmonary infection exists. Fleeting or migratory infiltrates on chest radiograph in a patient with difficult asthma should suggest the possibility of allergic bronchopulmonary aspergillosis. Blood tests in asthma might reveal eosinophilia and increased levels of IgE. Skin tests might be useful to identify household and other antigens that may precipitate asthma attacks in a particular patient (see Table 17-3).

MANAGEMENT

The management of asthma requires education and cooperation on the part of the patient. Simple, inexpensive peak expiratory flow meters can be used at home to monitor airflow obstruction. A diary should be maintained, and a clear written plan should be in place for using symptoms and peak flow information to intervene early in exacerbations and to alter long-term therapy for optimal control of symptoms. Short-acting β agonists are used for the acute relief of symptoms such as wheezing. However, the cornerstone of maintenance therapy in all but mild intermittent asthma is scheduled administration of inhaled corticosteroids. Long-acting β agonists may be added for additional

Table 17-3 **Diagnostic Studies in Asthma**	
Routine pulmonary function test	Decreased FEV_1; hyperinflation; improvement with bronchodilator
Special pulmonary function test	
Methacholine or cold-air challenge	Indicates the presence of nonspecific bronchial hyperreactivity; bronchoconstriction occurs at lower doses in asthma
Challenge with specific agents: occupational, drugs	Occasionally performed
Chest radiograph	Fleeting infiltrates and central bronchiectasis in ABPA
Skin tests	Demonstrate atopy; little value except prick test to *Aspergillus fumigatus* positive in ABPA
Blood tests	Eosinophils and IgE are usually increased in atopy; levels may be very high in ABPA; *Aspergillus precipitins* increased in many, but not all, patients with ABPA

ABPA, allergic bronchopulmonary aspergillosis; FEV_1, forced expiratory volume in 1 second; IgE, immunoglobulin E.

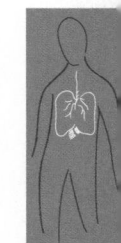

symptomatic control as needed. Long-acting β agonists should not be employed as a monotherapy for asthma control, especially in African American patients, because there has been an increased mortality demonstrated in this patient population using this therapeutic approach. Leukotriene inhibitors can be used as adjuncts in maintenance therapy, although they generally appear to be less effective than inhaled corticosteroids. Theophylline preparations may have additional beneficial effects in some patients, but the narrow therapeutic window and modest efficacy of these preparations limit their value. Oral or intravenous corticosteroids are used during acute asthma exacerbations, although long-term use of oral corticosteroids should be avoided if possible given the various side effects associated with chronic glucocorticoid administration.

Allergen avoidance is a reasonable measure in asthma, although the effects of specific interventions, such as mattress barrier protection to reduce dust mite exposure, appear limited. Treatment of associated conditions that may exacerbate asthma, such as allergic rhinitis and gastroesophageal reflux disease, may be clinically beneficial and aid in achieving asthma control. Use of recombinant human anti-IgE monoclonal antibody may be effective at reducing exacerbations in patients with allergic asthma.

Acute severe asthma, or *status asthmaticus*, is an attack of severe bronchospasm that is unresponsive to routine therapy. Such attacks may be sudden (*hyperacute asthma*) and may be rapidly fatal, often before medical care can be obtained. In most cases, however, patients have a history of progressive dyspnea over hours to days, with increasing bronchodilator use. Treatment of status asthmaticus should be aggressive, with the administration of nebulized bronchodilators and intravenous steroids and with continuous monitoring of blood oxygen saturation by pulse oximetry, often supplemented by arterial blood gas analysis to evaluate for hypercarbia. A rising $Paco_2$ in a patient with asthma is an ominous sign and may portend a need for ventilatory support. Noninvasive ventilation has been used successfully to decrease the work of breathing and avoid the need for endotracheal intubation in patients with exacerbations of asthma. However, in some cases, intubation and mechanical ventilation is necessary for the management of respiratory failure in status asthmaticus. Mechanical ventilation of the patient with status asthmaticus can be extremely challenging and may require the use of paralytic agents to control the breathing pattern and even use of inhaled general anesthesia to relieve bronchospasm.

Prospectus for the Future

The obstructive lung diseases are common and account for a tremendous burden of morbidity and mortality in the general population. Public health strategies to discourage smoking, the major cause of COPD, have shown promise in developed countries, but more attention to strategies aimed at discouraging smoking in developing countries is needed. In addition, more effective treatments for tobacco addiction are needed. Our understanding of the causes of the asthma epidemic remain limited, a crucial hindrance to developing effective methods to prevent the development of this disease. Improved understanding of the genetic and environmental risk factors for asthma development may allow the implementation of novel forms of immune modulation in susceptible individuals early in life. Therapies that are effective at altering the natural course of COPD or asthma once disease is established using disease-modifying agents are currently lacking, despite improved understanding of the molecular pathogenesis of these disorders. New approaches to counter histone acetylation-deacetyla-tion balance may generate more effective anti-inflammatory agents for use in COPD, whereas an understanding of the role of chitinases in asthma may result in novel treatments for this chronic condition. Clinicians caring for patients with cystic fibrosis now have an effective array of tools capable of allowing the supportive care of patients for decades of life. Molecular approaches to the treatment of cystic fibrosis aimed at improving the intracellular trafficking and function of the cystic fibrosis transmembrane receptor, attacking the disease at its root cause, are also underway. Finally, the increasing recognition of the pathogenetic heterogeneity of individuals with obstructive lung disease displaying asthma or COPD phenotypes means that current one-size-fits-all approaches to therapy using agents such as inhaled steroids or β agonists will be abandoned in favor of sophisticated personalized therapeutic regimens and perhaps regenerative medical approaches. The significant economic costs of such personalized medicine, however, demand a greater focus on disease prevention.

References

American Thoracic Society/European Respiratory Society Task Force: Standards for the diagnosis and management of patients with COPD [Internet]. Version 1.2. New York, American Thoracic Society, 2004 [updated September 8, 2005]. Available from: http://www.thoracic.org/go/copd.

Barker AF: Bronchiectasis. N Engl J Med 346:1383-1393, 2002.

Celli BR: Update on the management of COPD. Chest 133:1451-1462, 2008.

Expert Panel Report 3: Guidelines for the Diagnosis and Management of Asthma. National Asthma Education and Prevention Program, National Heart, Lung and Blood Institute. Available online at http://www.nhlbi.nih.gov/guidelines/asthma/asthgdln.pdf. Accessed October 2008.

Flume PA, O'Sullivan BP, Robinson KA, et al: Cystic fibrosis pulmonary guidelines: Chronic medications for maintenance of lung health. Am J Respir Crit Care Med 176:957-969. 2007.

Moorman JE, Rudd RA, Johnson CA, et al: National Surveillance for Asthma—United States 1980-2004. MMWR Morb Mortal Wkly Rep 56:1, 2007.

Ryu JH, Myers JL, Swensen SJ: Bronchiolar disorders. Am J Respir Crit Care Med 168:1277-1292, 2003.

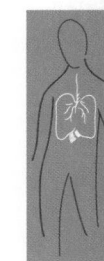

Interstitial Lung Diseases

Jason M. Aliotta and Matthew D. Jankowich

The interstitial lung diseases (ILDs) form a complex group of dozens of disorders with heterogeneous clinical courses and prognoses that are characterized by diffuse, typically chronic, lung injury, occurring in the setting of variable amounts of inflammation, which often leads to lung fibrosis. These diseases are daunting for the clinician because the differential diagnosis may be broad, and the work-up required to make the appropriate diagnosis may be extensive. Understanding of these disorders has been hampered in the past by use of confusing and nonspecific terminology, especially with regard to the idiopathic interstitial pneumonias. Current classifications use histopathology and clinical syndromes to divide these disorders into more understandable groupings. This text uses a classification that divides ILDs into the following categories: *idiopathic interstitial pneumonitides, granulomatous disorders, connective tissue–related ILDs, drug-induced ILDs, pulmonary vasculitic disorders,* and *distinct entities of unknown origin that exhibit well-defined syndromes* such as *pulmonary Langerhans cell histiocytosis* and *lymphangioleiomyomatosis.*

The presentation of ILD is often nonspecific, with common clinical symptoms including dyspnea on exertion, dry cough, and sometimes constitutional symptoms. Pulmonary function tests generally show restriction and gas-exchange abnormalities. Imaging demonstrating *diffuse lung disease* often leads to the consideration of ILD as a diagnosis. However, early radiographic changes may be subtle, and other clinical entities such as congestive heart failure or lymphangitic carcinomatosis may cause similar clinical, physiologic, and radiographic findings. Therefore, diagnosis may be delayed in some circumstances until other clinical entities are excluded and biopsy is undertaken. High-resolution computed tomography (HRCT) has contributed greatly to the diagnostic work-up of patients with suspected ILD because typical HRCT patterns in appropriate clinical settings may be sufficient for diagnosis.

Most ILDs, including more common entities like idiopathic pulmonary fibrosis (IPF), often present with chronic progressive symptoms. However, some ILDs can present in an acute fashion. Such entities include acute pneumonitis due to systemic lupus erythematosus, acute hypersensitivity pneumonitis, some drug reactions, and acute interstitial pneumonia. In such cases, infection often needs to be ruled out, and diagnosis may be challenging in critically ill individuals.

When ILD is suspected in a patient with typical symptoms and diffuse lung disease on imaging, the epidemiologic background, including the age, race, and sex of the patient, is helpful in formulating the diagnostic possibilities. For example, IPF typically occurs in middle-aged or elderly individuals, whereas sarcoidosis often presents in young individuals and is most common in those of African American background in the United States. Sex is also a consideration because lymphangioleiomyomatosis presents almost exclusively in women of childbearing age, whereas pulmonary Langerhans cell histiocytosis most often occurs in young male smokers. This background data can help to focus the initial differential diagnosis.

History can further narrow the differential in the setting of suspected ILD. Important factors to elicit are a history of rash, dysphagia, arthritis, or Raynaud phenomenon that may suggest an underlying connective tissue disorder. If the patient carries a diagnosis of connective tissue disease, this may be helpful in limiting the work-up if imaging findings typical of the usual pulmonary manifestations of the particular connective tissue disease are present. Other past medical history is informative; a history of severe or poorly controlled asthma in a patient with radiographic infiltrates and constitutional symptoms should lead to consideration of *Churg-Strauss syndrome,* whereas a history of severe sinus disease should raise the possibility of *Wegener granulomatosis.* Drug-induced ILD should be considered in all patients presenting with diffuse lung disease on imaging, and a careful medication usage history is critical. The smoking history is also important because a number of ILDs are associated with cigarette smoking, including *respiratory bronchiolitis interstitial lung disease, desquamative interstitial pneumonitis,* and pulmonary Langerhans cell histiocytosis.

Environmental exposures should be elicited because a typical exposure to, for example, pet birds or hot tubs may be suggestive of *hypersensitivity pneumonitis.* Home visits can be very informative. The occupational history is also important. Although the pneumoconioses due to asbestos and silica exposure are becoming much less common with modern safeguards and restrictions, these diseases continue to present long after exposure. High-technology manufacturing has particular hazards, for example, with beryllium exposure leading to berylliosis in susceptible individuals. Nonindustrial professions still carry occupational risks; for example, outbreaks of granulomatous pneumonitis have been described in indoor lifeguards exposed to molds.

The physical examination may reveal only oxygen desaturation with exertion in early ILD. Patients may show evidence of decreased chest expansion during inspection. Auscultation of the lungs typically reveals Velcro-like crackles at the lung bases. Clubbing may be present. Skin rashes, arthritis and joint deformities, Raynaud phenomenon, and dysphagia may point to a connective tissue–related ILD such as *dermatomyositis* or *polymyositis, progressive systemic sclerosis,* or *mixed connective tissue disorder.* Evidence of right ventricular heart failure with jugular vein distention, a cardiac gallop, loud P_2 sound, and leg edema suggests pulmonary hypertension; right ventricular heart failure is usually the result of chronic hypoxemia and is often related to end-stage lung disease. Laboratory studies may be of benefit; for example, eosinophilia will suggest the particular group of disorders associated with pulmonary infiltrates and peripheral blood eosinophilia.

A chest radiograph can narrow the possible diagnosis based on the distribution of the typical reticulonodular changes found in ILD. For example, sarcoidosis, lymphangioleiomyomatosis, silicosis, hypersensitivity pneumonitis, eosinophilic granuloma, and ankylosing spondylitis most often affect the upper- and mid-level lung fields, whereas IPF, asbestosis, and many connective tissue-related ILDs typically involve the lower-level lung fields. These patterns are best analyzed through the use of HRCT of the chest, a test considered essential in the evaluation of patients suggested as having ILD. HRCT can reveal patterns of disease that allow the diagnostic considerations to be significantly narrowed. For example, upper lobe–predominant cystic lung disease on HRCT suggests a group of entities including Langerhans cell histiocytosis, sarcoidosis, and lymphangioleiomyomatosis. Lower lobe and peripheral reticular opacities with associated traction bronchiectasis and honeycombing suggest idiopathic pulmonary fibrosis, asbestosis, or certain connective tissue disease–related ILDs. Visualization of abnormalities of the mediastinum or pleura occurring in association with parenchymal lung disease is also helpful. Sarcoidosis, for example, typically exhibits hilar and mediastinal lymphadenopathy in association with beadlike septal nodules, whereas pleural plaques in association with lower lobe fibrosis is consistent with asbestosis. Incorporation of HRCT imaging data with clinical history may in some circumstances be sufficient for diagnosis.

Pulmonary function tests in ILD typically reveal a restrictive pattern characterized by proportionately decreased airflows with preserved forced expiratory volume in 1 second–to–forced vital capacity (FEV_1/FVC) ratio (no obstruction to airflow) and decreased lung volumes as highlighted by decreased total lung capacity and functional residual capacity. The diffusion capacity for carbon dioxide (D_{LCO}) of the lung is often decreased and may be the earliest change present in drug-induced ILD or connective tissue disease-related ILD. The restrictive abnormality found in most forms of ILD is due to the decreased compliance of the lung in the setting of fibrosis. Histologically, ILD affects the interstitium of the lung, the space located between the base-

ment membrane of the vascular structures within the distal air spaces and the basement membranes of the epithelial cells that line the alveoli (Fig. 18-1). This space also extends proximally toward the alveolar ducts and respiratory bronchioles. Normally, the interstitium of the lung contains a few fibroblasts and connective tissue components within a very thin wall that allows for the efficient diffusion of gases. In ILD, however, this space expands with the accumulation of fibroblasts or other cells and the deposition of an aberrant matrix that increases the distance between the alveolar space and vascular structures, thereby delaying and sometimes preventing gas exchange. This thickened interstitium accounts for the poor oxygenation and increased lung stiffness exhibited as decreased compliance, small lung volumes, and increased work of breathing. Because lung involvement by ILD may be sporadic, with areas of normal lung adjacent to areas of fibrosis, local differences in compliance may result in abnormal $\dot{V}/\dot{Q}$ matching, contributing to hypoxemia. The processes outlined above account for the physiologic manifestations seen in disorders like *idiopathic pulmonary fibrosis* (IPF) and *asbestosis.*

In some ILDs, an obstructive rather than restrictive abnormality or mixed findings are present on pulmonary function testing, and lung volumes are relatively preserved on physiologic testing and imaging (Fig. 18-2). In such diseases as lymphangioleiomyomatosis, pulmonary Langerhans cell histiocytosis, and hypersensitivity pneumonitis, as well as in some cases of sarcoidosis, obstructive or mixed patterns on pulmonary function testing with preservation of lung volumes are typical. This pattern of disease is due to proximal extension of the interstitial disease in the lung parenchyma with consequent involvement of the small airways. For example, in lymphangioleiomyomatosis, the small airways are narrowed by the proliferation of surrounding abnormal smooth muscle–like cells. This leads to increased airways resistance and airflow obstruction. Endobronchial disease with direct narrowing of the airways can occur in sarcoidosis, leading to similar effects. Therefore, the presence of airflow obstruction does not rule out a diagnosis of interstitial lung disease but may help to focus the differential diagnosis on particular entities.

As outlined earlier, in ILD, a synthesis of clinical, functional, and imaging data, often in the context of a multidisciplinary approach, is crucial to arriving at an appropriate diagnosis. In many circumstances, however, clinical and imaging data are insufficiently specific, and lung biopsy must be undertaken. In general, surgical lung biopsy, typically through a thoracoscopic approach, is the preferred method of obtaining tissue for examination. Transbronchial lung biopsy through the bronchoscope yields small fragments of tissue, typically too small to allow for appropriate examination of the lung architecture, and is not recommended for the assessment of suspected IPF. However, transbronchial biopsies may be useful in the setting of certain ILDs, including sarcoidosis, cryptogenic organizing pneumonia, and hypersensitivity pneumonitis. In general, the lung's response to injury is relatively stereotyped, with particular biopsy patterns of injury such as usual interstitial pneumonitis or granulomatous inflammation, being seen in a variety of disorders. Interpretation of lung biopsy results must therefore be done in the appropriate context, with incorporation of clinical and imaging data, because a biopsy

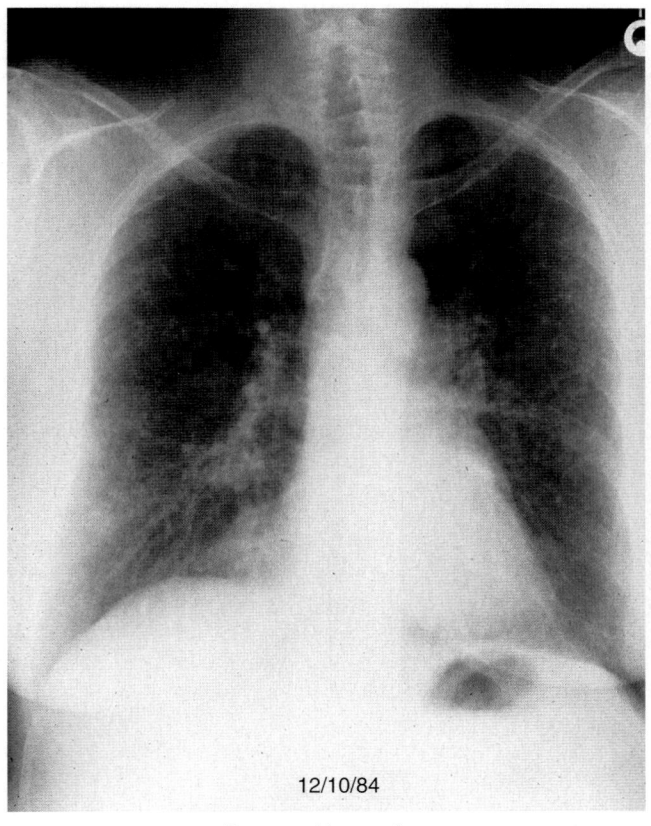

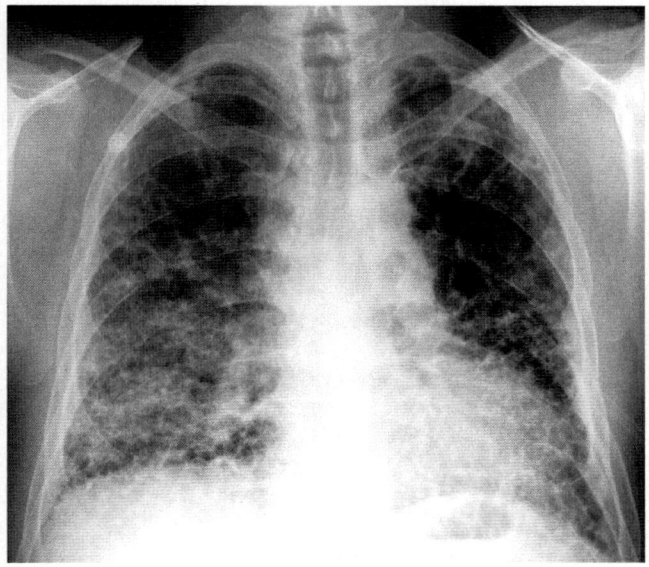

Small lung volumes

Idiopathic pulmonary fibrosis
Asbestosis

12/10/84

Preserved lung volumes

Sarcoidosis
Hypersensitivity pneumonitis

Figure 18-1 Radiographic manifestations of interstitial lung diseases. *Left image* shows well-preserved lung volumes with bilateral interstitial reticulonodular infiltrates as seen in diseases similar to sarcoidosis and hypersensitivity pneumonitis. *Right image* shows reduced lung volumes with bilateral basilar infiltrates as seen in idiopathic pulmonary fibrosis.

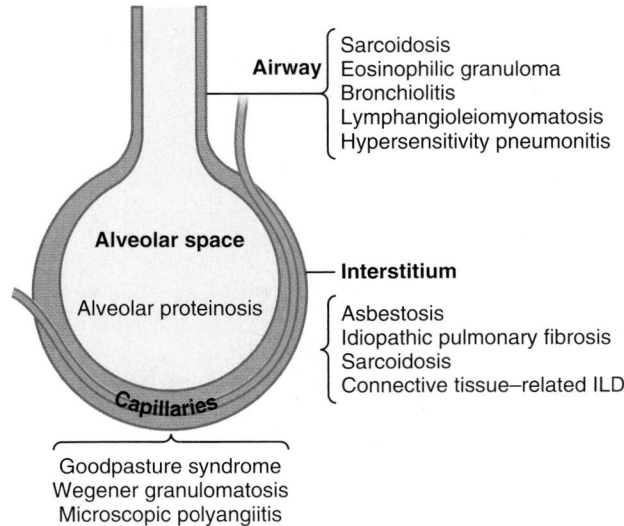

Figure 18-2 Interstitial lung disease (ILD) affects the interstitium of the lung at different locations. Depending on the site of disease activity, its consequences may vary. Specifically, diseases that affect the interstitium that surrounds the distal part of the alveoli lead to physiologic restrictions with reduced lung volumes. In contrast, diseases that preferentially affect the interstitium located near the more proximal parts of the acinus near the distal bronchioles may exhibit predominantly with well-preserved lung volumes and physiologic obstruction.

result of, for example, usual interstitial pneumonitis may carry a different prognosis in the setting of rheumatoid arthritis–associated ILD than in the setting of IPF. The summary of the typical manifestations of several ILDs is included in Table 18-1.

The management of ILD varies depending on the underlying cause, and treatments appropriate to specific entities are discussed later. Exposure avoidance is critical in the setting of hypersensitivity pneumonitis, smoking-related ILD, and drug-induced ILD. Immunosuppressants are employed in a variety of the ILDs with variable results depending on the specific entity. Supplemental oxygen and pulmonary rehabilitation may be helpful in advanced disease. Lung transplantation is performed in patients with limited life expectancy; early referral is suggested for patients with poor prognosis, as in IPF.

Idiopathic Interstitial Pneumonias

The idiopathic interstitial pneumonias (IIPs) are a group of ILDs of unknown origins. In the 1970s, these conditions were generally considered different variations of *IPF.* However, the distinct clinical presentations, natural courses,

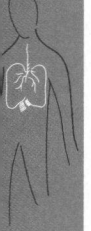

Table 18-1 Manifestations of Interstitial Lung Disease

Disease	Physical Examination	Radiographs	Laboratory Findings	Histologic Findings
Pneumoconioses Coal worker's pneumoconiosis	Variable findings Normal Crackles	Diffuse reticulonodular infiltrates	Nonspecific except beryllium: lymphocyte transformation test	Fibrosis Coal: anthracotic pigment
Asbestosis Silica-induced ILD Beryllium exposure	Clubbing	Large nodules Eggshell calcification of hilar nodes Pleural plaques	Obstructive and/or restrictive PFTs	Silica: inflammation, bi-refringent crystals, alveolar proteinosis Asbestos: mesothelioma
Hypersensitivity pneumonitis	Fever Cough Crackles	Waxing and waning reticulonodular infiltrates Fibrosis	Serum precipitins to specific proteins Obstructive and/or restrictive PFTs	Obliterative bronchiolitis without granulomas Desquamative interstitial pneumonitis and diffuse alveolar damage Diffuse or patchy, intra-alveolar
IPF DIP and/or RB-ILD	Variable findings Normal Crackles Clubbing	Normal to end-stage honeycombing Abnormalities usually diffuse	Nonspecific Restrictive PFTs	Macrophages
UIP AIP NSIP				Patchy, fibroblasts, fibrosis Uniform, fibroblasts, no fibrosis Patchy or diffuse, prominent interstitial inflammation, fibrosis
Collagen vascular	Collagen vascular disease Crackles Pleural rub	Pleural effusions Diffuse interstitial infiltrates Nodular infiltrates Occasional cavities	Serologic findings for specific disease Occasionally obstructive, usually restrictive PFTs	Interstitial inflammation Vasculitis Bronchiolar obstruction Organizing pneumonia Fibrosis
Drug-induced ILD	Fever Crackles Pleural rub	Fibrosis Migratory infiltrates Diffuse interstitial infiltrates Pulmonary edema	Restrictive PFTs Anti-RNP antibodies	Alveolar macrophages with lamellar bodies in amiodarone Interstitial inflammation Fibrosis Eosinophilic infiltration

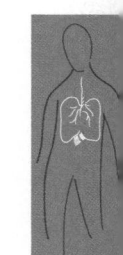

Sarcoidosis	Fever Malaise Weight loss Erythema nodosum Lupus pernio and skin plaques Salivary and lacrimal gland enlargement Iritis, uveitis, chorioretinitis; keratoconjunctivitis Cranial nerve palsies Arthritis Occasional rales or wheezes	Reticulonodular infiltrates Nodules Hilar adenopathy Mediastinal adenopathy Fibrosis	Lymphocytic bronchoalveolar lavage, T4 > T8 subsets Obstructive and/or restrictive PFTs Elevated transaminases with liver involvement Occasional hypercalcemia	Noncaseating granuloma with giant cells and negative acid-fast bacilli and fungal stains Fibrosis
Radiation exposure	Crackles Fever	Focal interstitial infiltrates corresponding to radiation port Occasional diffuse infiltrates Fibrosis	None	*Acute:* endothelial and alveolar lining cell damage *Chronic:* fibrosis
Pulmonary Langerhans cell histiocytosis	None to cough Dyspnea Chest pain Fatigue Weight loss Occasional fever	Spontaneous pneumothorax Nodules Reticulonodular infiltrates Middle and upper lobe predominance Honeycombing Sparing of costophrenic angle Cysts and nodules on HRCT	Normal lung volumes with decreased D$_{LCO}$	OKT-6 (CD1) and S100-positive immunostaining Few eosinophils Peribronchiolar inflammation Macrophages filling lumen of bronchioles and intraluminal fibrosis
Lymphangioleiomyomatosis	Dyspnea Cough Chest pain Decreased breath sounds or rales Hemoptysis Ascites	Spontaneous pneumothorax Pleural effusions Reticulonodular infiltrate Miliary pattern Honeycombing Hyperinflation Diffuse, small, thin-walled cysts on HRCT	Obstructive and/or restrictive PFTs Chylous pleural effusions Chylous ascites	HMB-45-positive immunostaining Atypical smooth muscle cell proliferation around bronchovascular bundles
COP	Fever Chills Malaise Fatigue Cough Dyspnea on exertion Weight loss	Peripheral patchy infiltrates, occasionally migratory CT scan: patchy consolidation, ground glass opacities, small nodules	Restrictive and occasionally obstructive PFTs in smokers	Patchy peri-bronchiolar distribution Foamy macrophages in alveolar spaces Intraluminal buds of granulation tissue

AIP, acute interstitial pneumonia; BOOP, bronchiolitis obliterans and organizing pneumonia; COP, cryptogenic organizing pneumonia; CT, computed tomography; DIP, desquamative interstitial pneumonia; HRCT, high-resolution computed tomography; ILD, interstitial lung disease; IPF, idiopathic pulmonary fibrosis; NSIP, nonspecific interstitial pneumonia; PFT, pulmonary function test; RB, respiratory bronchiolitis; RNP, antiribonucleoprotein antibodies; UIP, usual interstitial.

and responses to treatment observed in these patients led to their reclassification into a group of idiopathic interstitial disorders. The latest classification scheme was suggested in a 2002 consensus statement by the American Thoracic and the European Respiratory Societies. These disorders are recognized as distinct clinicopathologic entities and can be classified based on their *histologic pattern* as well as their *clinical course*. Those with an *acute* clinical course include *acute interstitial pneumonia (AIP);* a *subacute* clinical course include *nonspecific interstitial pneumonia (NSIP), cryptogenic organizing pneumonia (COP), respiratory bronchiolitis–associated interstitial lung disease (RB-ILD), desquamative interstitial pneumonia (DIP),* and *lymphoid interstitial pneumonia (LIP);* or a *chronic* clinical course as seen in *usual interstitial pneumonia (UIP).*

Of the IIPs, IPF, also known as *cryptogenic fibrosing alveolitis,* is the most common, affecting 85,000 to 100,000 individuals in the United States. Although initially thought to be a relatively rare disease, IPF is now considered to be one of the most common ILDs with prevalence in some populations of 29 cases per 100,000; the prevalence is much higher in patients older than 70 years. In most patients with IPF, the disease is sporadic; however, IPF has been found in members of certain families (termed *familial IPF*), indicating that genetic alterations might predispose patients to this illness. The disease is idiopathic, but gamma herpesviruses have been detected in the lungs of a large proportion of patients with IPF, and an animal model resembling this condition has been reported. Many environmental, occupational, and infectious agents can cause lung fibrosis, including asbestos, silica, and tuberculosis. Therefore, distinguishing IPF from these other lung disorders is important because of the implications for prognosis and therapy.

IPF is characterized by progressive fibrosis of the lungs resulting in nonproductive cough and shortness of breath that worsens with exertion and, ultimately, causes hypoxemic respiratory failure. A typical patient with IPF is between 50 and 70 years of age, and the symptoms frequently develop 1 to 2 years before a diagnosis is confirmed. Physical examination often reveals crackles in the bases of both lungs, indicating the predominant site of scarring. With increased connective tissue deposition, the lung becomes stiff as evidenced by decreased compliance. Pulmonary function tests show decreased lung volumes consistent with a restrictive process. Poor oxygenation in IPF often requires long-term oxygen supplementation. The chest radiograph shows infiltrates that are most predominant at the bases and periphery of the lungs. HRCT allows for better visualization of the lung and is useful in evaluating the extent of disease. It delineates the areas of fibrosis and provides information about other structures in the chest. The classic HRCT findings of IPF are bilateral reticulonodular infiltrates with peripheral distribution and the presence of honeycombing and traction bronchiectasis in the absence of ground-glass opacification, lymphadenopathy, and pleural disease (Fig. 18-3; **Web Fig. 18-1**). In the setting of a typical clinical presentation and classic HRCT findings, a lung biopsy may not be necessary. Unfortunately, a lung biopsy is required for confirmation in many patients.

The histologic patterns of IPF show areas of scar tissue interspersed with normal alveolar structures. An interesting pathologic feature is the presence of *fibroblastic foci,* which

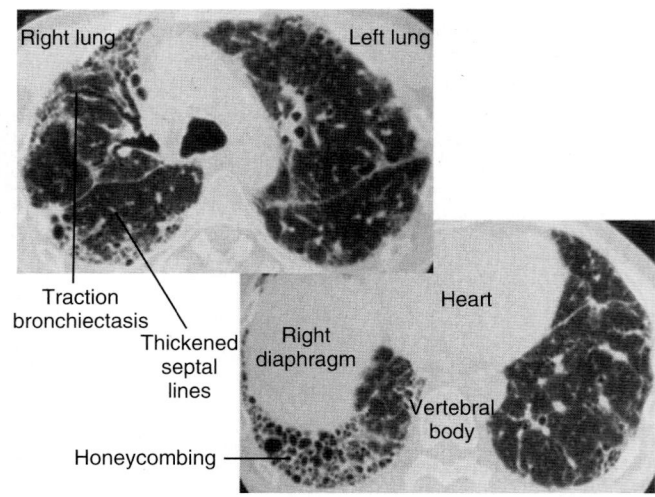

Figure 18-3 Computer tomography of the chest in a patient with idiopathic pulmonary fibrosis.

are areas in which fibroblasts accumulate and are believed to be the site of disease activity. This overall pattern of tissue organization is UIP, which can accompany other disorders (e.g., connective tissue-related ILD); thus, the diagnosis of IPF depends on a clinical, radiographic, and histologic picture that includes the syndrome of ILD in the absence of an obvious cause and a histologic manifestation consistent with UIP.

There is insufficient clinical evidence to suggest that any pharmacologic treatment improves survival or the quality of life for patients with IPF. As a result, clinicians typically consider offering treatment on a case-by-case basis after carefully weighing the benefits against the risks of treatment. Younger patients (<50 years of age) with significant ground-glass opacification, little fibrosis by HRCT, and minimal loss of lung function who have no contraindications to therapy are reasonable candidates for offering pharmacologic treatment. Combination therapy, using corticosteroids along with azathioprine, is generally recommended. The addition of *N*-acetylcysteine may offer additional benefit when added to this regimen. Other medications, including cyclophosphamide, cyclosporine, colchicine, penicillamine, and interferon-γ do little to stop the progression of IPF and may be more harmful than beneficial. More recently, it has been recognized that some patients with IPF experience acute respiratory deterioration in the absence of any clinically apparent cause (heart failure, pulmonary embolism, pneumonia). These episodes of idiopathic acute deterioration have been termed *acute exacerbations of IPF* and are associated with a poor prognosis. HRCT findings include new ground-glass opacities and consolidation superimposed on a background reticular or honeycomb pattern consistent with UIP. Histologically, evidence of acute lung injury (diffuse alveolar damage) can be found on the background of UIP. Acute exacerbations of IPF are typically treated with high doses of corticosteroids. Because survival on the lung transplantation waiting list for patients with IPF is worse than for patients with other indications for lung transplantation, early referral for transplantation evaluation should be initiated. Unfortunately, the 5-year survival rate for lung transplantation in patients with IPF is only 40% to 50%.

The second most common IIP is *NSIP*. As the term suggests, this condition exhibits a histologic picture that is nonspecific and characterized by diffuse interstitial inflammation. It is often associated with other conditions such as connective tissue disorders (e.g., systemic lupus erythematosus, rheumatoid arthritis, polymyositis) or hypersensitivity pneumonitis. The association with these disorders is so strong that histologic confirmation of NSIP should prompt a search for these conditions. As in IPF, patients with NSIP exhibit slowly progressive dyspnea and bilateral interstitial infiltrates. Ground-glass opacification is often noted by HRCT. NSIP is more responsive to immunosuppressants than is IPF, and a 3-month trial period with these agents should be considered. However, occasionally, NSIP is associated with significant fibrosis (*fibrosing NSIP*), and lung transplantation should be considered in these patients, if possible.

DIP is usually seen in young individuals and is associated with a history of cigarette smoking. Patients exhibit a progressive shortness of breath and bilateral infiltrates on chest radiograph. The HRCT pattern is nonspecific, and a biopsy may be required for diagnosis. Tissue histologic findings show the accumulation of activated macrophages in the alveolar spaces. Treatment relies on immunosuppressant therapy and the avoidance of tobacco exposure. DIP is often confused with (and is considered by some experts to be identical to) *RB-ILD*, which has a similar clinical presentation and is associated with tobacco exposure.

AIP is another IIP that is not commonly seen. There is no sex predominance in AIP and no association with smoking. Its presentation differs from other IIPs in that it is more acute, with dyspnea progressing from days to a few weeks, invariably leading to respiratory failure. Patients often have a prior illness suggestive of a viral upper respiratory infection with constitutional symptoms such as myalgias, arthralgias, fever, chills, and malaise. The histologic pattern shows diffuse alveolar damage. Although a trial with immunosuppressants is recommended, this condition is often fatal, independent of treatment.

COP is often considered within the group of IIPs because it mimics these disorders clinically. Patients with COP exhibit subacute or chronic dyspnea first noted on exertion and sometimes triggered after an acute illness like an upper respiratory viral infection. Connective tissue disorders, inhaled irritants, and drugs (e.g., methotrexate) can cause COP. Histologically, COP is characterized by distal airway and interstitial inflammation and obliteration of distal air spaces with fibroblasts and fibrosis. Similar to NSIP and DIP, this condition is likely to respond to immunosuppressant therapy.

LIP is still classified by many groups as being one of the pulmonary lymphoproliferative disorders because many cases were thought to develop into lymphoma. However, with recent advances in immunohistochemistry and molecular analysis techniques, it would appear that only a small number of cases of LIP are found to actually undergo malignant transformation. LIP is an uncommon disease that is seen predominantly in women. Patients present with gradual-onset dyspnea and cough and occasionally fever, weight loss, chest pain, and arthralgias. Clinically, cases of LIP must be investigated for any known cause or associations, such as collagen vascular diseases (i.e., Sjögren syn-

drome), rheumatologic diseases (i.e., rheumatoid arthritis), and immunodeficiency diseases (i.e., AIDS). Histologically, infiltration of cells, including lymphocytes, plasma cells, and histiocytes, can be seen within alveolar septae. In addition, type II pneumocyte hyperplasia and an increase in the number of alveolar macrophages can be seen in LIP. Lymphoid follicles are often present, usually in the distribution of pulmonary lymphatics. Corticosteroids are used to treat LIP with variable success; however, more than one third of patients progress to develop diffuse fibrosis. It is unclear whether treatment influences the course of the disease or has a significant effect on lung physiology.

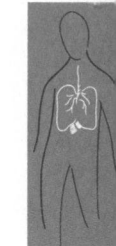

Granulomatous Disorders

A variety of noninfectious ILDs are characterized by granuloma formation within the lungs, including Wegener granulomatosis, hypersensitivity pneumonitis, and chronic beryllium disease. These disorders are discussed elsewhere in this chapter. Of the ILDs characterized by granulomatous lung inflammation, *sarcoidosis* is the most common. Sarcoidosis is a multisystem illness with frequent lung involvement with a prevalence of 1 to 40 cases per 100,000 worldwide. A higher incidence of sarcoidosis is reported among Scandinavian, German, and Irish individuals residing in northern Europe. In the United States, the prevalence rates of sarcoidosis are 10.9 per 100,000 for whites and 35.5 per 100,000 for African Americans, with women being more frequently affected. Sarcoidosis typically occurs in young individuals between 10 and 40 years of age, with women being affected more often than men.

Sarcoidosis is characterized by the formation in tissues of noncaseating granulomas that organize in an inner core of epithelioid cells, macrophages, and giant cells, surrounded by a rim of lymphocytes, fibroblasts, and connective tissue. Granulomas are present in the airways or lung parenchyma in more than 90% of patients with sarcoidosis. Granulomatous angiitis may also be found in the lungs. The upper respiratory system, lymph nodes, skin, and eyes are commonly involved. Virtually any other organ may be affected, including the liver, bone marrow, spleen, musculoskeletal system, heart, salivary glands, and nervous system (Table 18-2). The granulomas may be clinically silent, or, if extensive, may result in a disruption of normal organ structure and function. The cause of these lesions is unknown, but given the frequency of lung involvement, inhaled antigens, ranging from bacteria to environmental substances, have been hypothesized to trigger the onset of granulomatous inflammation. This inflammation may be self-limited or may be propagated, possibly by repeated exposure to the unknown antigen or because of the development of an autoimmune cross-reaction. Familial susceptibility to sarcoidosis seems to exist. To date, however, neither genetic factors nor specific environmental triggers have been firmly established. A single causative antigen may not exist, and sarcoidosis instead may represent a stereotypical inflammatory reaction to various possible antigens in a genetically susceptible host.

Sarcoidosis is associated with abnormal immune function as evidenced by cutaneous anergy and as exhibited in lung by an increased ratio of CD4$^+$ to CD8$^+$ T lymphocytes and

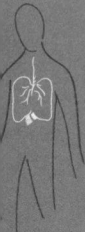

Table 18-2	**Clinical Manifestations of Sarcoidosis**
Organ Systems	
Pulmonary	Dyspnea, cough, wheezing, hemoptysis, endobronchial lesions
Dermatologic	Erythema nodosum, papules, plaques
Otolaryngologic	Saddle nose deformity, sinusitis, laryngeal lesions, parotitis
Ocular	Uveitis, chorioretinitis, keratoconjunctivitis, lacrimal gland enlargement, chronic tearing, optic neuritis
Neurologic	Cranial nerve palsy, headache, diabetes insipidus, mass lesions, seizures, meningitis, encephalitis
Rheumatologic	Arthralgias, arthropathy, myopathy
Gastrointestinal	Elevated transaminases, abdominal pain, jaundice
Cardiologic	Arrhythmias, conduction abnormalities, sudden cardiac death, pulmonary hypertension, congestive heart failure
Hematologic	Lymphadenopathy (especially hilar), hypersplenism
Endocrine	Hypercalcemia, hypercalciuria, epididymitis
Renal	Renal calculi, interstitial nephritis, renal failure
Syndromes	
Löfgren syndrome	Fever, arthralgias, bilateral hilar adenopathy, erythema nodosum
Heerfordt syndrome (uveoparotid fever)	Fever, swelling of parotid gland and uveal tracts, cranial nerve VII palsy

Table 18-3	**Radiographic Staging of Sarcoidosis**	
Stage	**Radiographic Findings**	
0	Normal radiograph	
I	Adenopathy without parenchymal abnormality	
II	Adenopathy and parenchymal disease	
III	Parenchymal disease without lymphadenopathy	
IV	End-stage fibrosis	

Skin manifestations include erythema nodosum; plaques; nodules; and lupus pernio, a violaceous, often disfiguring, nodular lesion of the nose and cheeks. Ocular symptoms are also common, and the onset of uveitis may eventually lead to the diagnosis of sarcoidosis when granulomatous extraocular organ involvement is uncovered. Neurosarcoidosis may present with cranial nerve palsies or with headache in the setting of lymphocytic meningitis. Sarcoidosis can involve the heart, resulting in a cardiomyopathy. Arrhythmias and sudden cardiac death can occur as a result of the disruption of the conducting system by granulomatous infiltration. Pulmonary hypertension may result from pulmonary fibrosis or directly from granulomatous vasculitis.

In 90% of patients, the chest radiograph shows abnormalities that include bilateral hilar adenopathy (**Web Fig. 18-2**), infiltrates (**Web Fig. 18-3**), and fibrosis. The radiographic changes characteristic of sarcoidosis have been classified in stages 0 through IV (Table 18-3), but this staging system does not imply a typical chronologic progression. As in other ILDs, computed tomography (CT) is more sensitive for the detection of parenchymal abnormalities, and also more clearly demonstrates the extent of mediastinal adenopathy. Parenchymal HRCT findings include nodularity along the bronchovascular bundles emanating from the hila (**Web Fig. 18-4**). Positron-emission tomography (PET) scans may reveal other sites of organ involvement. Pulmonary function tests typically show restriction or obstruction. Liver involvement may cause mild elevation of transaminases, and cirrhosis and liver failure have been reported, although they are rare. Hypercalcemia and hypercalciuria may be detected and are due to increased intestinal absorption of calcium as a result of increased conversion of vitamin D to its active form in sarcoid granulomas. Kidney stones may result from the abnormal calcium metabolism. Elevated levels of angiotensin-converting enzyme (ACE) are common but are not specific. The use of ACE levels in the diagnosis or management of sarcoidosis is controversial.

The diagnosis of sarcoidosis is dependent on a typical clinical, radiographic, and histologic picture and is a diagnosis of exclusion. Tissue samples will show noncaseating granulomas, but because this finding is nonspecific, careful attention should be given to ruling out infectious causes of granulomatous inflammation, such as mycobacterial infection, through stains and cultures. Necrotizing granulomas have rarely been reported in sarcoidosis, but this finding should prompt an intense search for infection. In contrast to most ILDs, in which tissue diagnosis requires open-lung biopsy, the granulomas in sarcoidosis can be identified in skin nodules or in lymph nodes. A transbronchial lung biopsy is positive in 50% to 60% of patients with normal

increased concentrations of pro-inflammatory cytokines such as interferon-γ, interleukin-12, and tumor necrosis factor-α (TNF-α). These derangements can be detected in the bronchoalveolar lavage fluid and are consistent with an imbalance in the production of T_h1 versus T_h2 cytokines, favoring the production of the former and promoting persistent inflammation. Sarcoidosis may occur in the setting of immunomodulatory therapy, especially with interferon alfa, highlighting the role of immune imbalances in the disorder.

The clinical presentation of sarcoidosis is variable. The disease is frequently detected incidentally on routine chest radiograph in asymptomatic individuals. Others may present with diverse acute or chronic symptoms. Patients may develop well-described acute syndromes such as *Löfgren syndrome*, which includes erythema nodosum, arthritis, and hilar adenopathy, or *uveoparotid fever*, also known as Heerfordt syndrome, which exhibits the triad of uveitis, parotitis, and facial nerve palsy. Both syndromes are associated with better outcomes when compared with other clinical presentations of sarcoidosis. In many cases, symptoms are vague and chronic and may include systemic symptoms such as low-grade fevers, night sweats, or joint pains. Respiratory manifestations, including shortness of breath, dry cough, and chest pain, occur in one third to one half of patients.

parenchyma and close to 90% of patients with parenchymal abnormalities detected by chest radiograph. Because airway involvement is common, endobronchial biopsies may also demonstrate granulomas. After the diagnosis is made, all patients should have an ophthalmologic evaluation as well as a 24-hour collection of urine to evaluate for hypercalciuria. Electrocardiographic (ECG) examination and sometimes Holter monitoring should be performed to assess for conduction system abnormalities or arrhythmias resulting from involvement of the heart by sarcoidosis.

The course of sarcoidosis is variable. Spontaneous remission is common, and death and disability are relatively rare, making decisions regarding treatment initiation difficult. The acute sarcoidosis syndromes tend to remit and not recur. However, about one third of all patients with sarcoidosis will have chronic progressive disease, and some patients will develop pulmonary fibrosis or other end-organ damage. Corticosteroids are the standard therapy but should not be used indiscriminately in all patients with the diagnosis of sarcoidosis. Whether corticosteroids alter the disease course is uncertain. However, corticosteroid therapy should be considered in patients with extrapulmonary organ involvement or progressive pulmonary dysfunction. Patients with erythema nodosum in the setting of Löfgren syndrome may be managed with nonsteroidal anti-inflammatory medications alone. Other skin involvement may respond to hydroxychloroquine or corticosteroids, although the treatment of lupus pernio is challenging. Anterior uveitis may be treated with topical steroids, but other eye involvement may require systemic corticosteroids. Systemic corticosteroids are also generally used for the treatment of cardiac sarcoidosis. Conduction system disease and arrhythmias may necessitate placement of pacemakers or automatic implantable cardioverter-defibrillators. Neurosarcoidosis and hypercalcemia, as well as progressive pulmonary disease, are among the other indications for systemic steroid treatment (Table 18-4). Methotrexate has been used as a steroid-sparing agent. Anti–tumor necrosis factor-α agents, minocycline, hydroxychloroquine (Plaquenil), and thalidomide have been tested, although efficacy data are relatively sparse.

Interstitial Lung Diseases Related to Connective Tissue Disorders

In patients with ILD, a thorough history and physical examination may reveal abnormalities, such as arthritis and hand deformities, rashes, esophageal dysmotility, Raynaud syndrome, or skin changes suggestive of an underlying connective tissue disease. Connective tissue disorders, such as *systemic lupus erythematosus, rheumatoid arthritis (RA), mixed connective tissue disorder, systemic sclerosis (scleroderma), polymyositis* or *dermatomyositis,* and *Sjögren syndrome,* can cause ILD as well as a wide variety of other pulmonary manifestations (Table 18-5). Lung disease is a major cause of morbidity and mortality in some of these conditions, especially systemic sclerosis. Although not typical, an ILD related to connective tissue disorders (CTD-ILD) can even develop before other symptoms such as arthritis manifest, making the diagnosis more difficult.

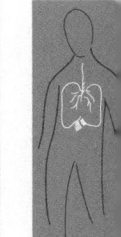

Table 18-4 **Indications for Use of Corticosteroids in Sarcoidosis**	
Disorder	**Treatment**
Iridocyclitis	Corticosteroid eye drops
	Local subconjunctival deposit of cortisone
Posterior uveitis	Oral prednisone
Pulmonary involvement	Steroids rarely recommended for stage 1; usually used if infiltrate remains static or worsens over 3-month period or if patient is symptomatic
Upper airway obstruction	Rare indication for intravenous steroids
Lupus pernio	Oral prednisone shrinks the disfiguring lesions
Hypercalcemia	Responds well to corticosteroids
Cardiac involvement	Corticosteroids usually recommended if patient has arrhythmias or conduction disturbances
Central nervous system involvement	Response is best in patients with acute symptoms
Lacrimal and salivary gland involvement	Corticosteroids recommended for disordered function, *not* gland swelling
Bone cysts	Corticosteroids recommended if symptomatic

Clinical manifestations of CTD-ILD are nonspecific and include exertional dyspnea and dry cough. Exertional dyspnea may be obscured by disabilities caused by the underlying CTD. CTD-ILD may also be relatively asymptomatic, manifesting as an incidental finding on imaging. Lung examination in patients with CTD-ILD may reveal bibasilar crackles, and pulmonary function tests often show a restrictive pattern with decreased diffusion capacity. If obstruction is present on pulmonary function testing, airway manifestations of the CTD, such as obliterative bronchiolitis in the setting of RA, must be considered. Chest imaging studies are useful because they may reveal typical patterns associated with the underlying CTD, often obviating the need for biopsy. Such patterns include apical fibrocavitary disease in ankylosing spondylitis and basilar fibrotic changes in RA, polymyositis, and systemic sclerosis. Imaging may also reveal pulmonary nodules in RA, or pleural disease in the setting of RA or systemic lupus erythematosus. Pulmonary hypertension in the absence of fibrosis can occur in these patients, especially with limited scleroderma (CREST syndrome) and systemic lupus erythematosus, so echocardiography may be helpful in patients with these disorders and otherwise unexplained dyspnea. Drug-induced lung disorders related to immunosuppressant therapy should always be considered in patients with CTD. Although CTD-ILD typically is chronic in nature, acute or fulminant pneumonitis that may be difficult to distinguish from opportunistic infection can be seen in systemic lupus erythematosus, Sjögren syndrome, polymyositis, and dermatomyositis.

Bronchoscopy with bronchoalveolar lavage is often used to rule out infection in acute presentations or if imaging reveals areas of consolidation as may occur with organizing

Table 18-5 Pulmonary Involvement in Connective Tissue Disorders

Syndrome	RA	Lupus	SS	PM/DM	Sjögren Syndrome
Pleural effusion	+ (5%-40%)	+ (30%-40%)			
Necrobiotic nodules	+				
Fibrosis	+ (20%-60%)	+ (3%)	+ (15%-90%)	+ (10%-40%)	+ (33%)
Bronchiolitis	+	+			+
Pulmonary arthropathy	+	+	+	+	
Atelectasis		+			
Pulmonary edema		+			
Pneumonitis, hemorrhage		+			
Diaphragm dysfunction		+			
Aspiration			+	+ (14%)	
Secondary carcinoma			+		

DM, dermatomyositis; PM, polymyositis; RA, rheumatoid arthritis; SS, Sjögren syndrome.

pneumonia in RA. Lung biopsy may be necessary if the clinical presentation or imaging findings are atypical. Biopsies of areas of typical basilar fibrosis in CTD frequently reveal patterns consistent with NSIP or UIP. In Sjögren syndrome with ILD, lymphocytic interstitial pneumonia or even lymphoma may be found on biopsy. Diffuse alveolar damage is found in the setting of acute lupus pneumonitis. Immunosuppressants are the mainstay of treatment for CTD-ILD, and, in general, these disorders are more responsive to this therapy than is IPF.

Drug-Induced Lung Disorders

A large number and variety of drugs can induce adverse reactions in the lung, often in the form of an ILD (Table 18-6). These reactions can vary in severity from self-limited hypersensitivity reactions (**Web Fig. 18-5**) to diffuse alveolar damage resulting in respiratory failure and death. In general, a high index of suspicion is needed to make the association between a drug and a pulmonary reaction, and a careful review of medications and other pharmacologic substances used by a patient is necessary in the setting of diffuse lung disease. Other pharmacologic substances that commonly produce adverse pulmonary reactions include illicit drugs such as heroin and cocaine. Substances like talc may also be injected inadvertently during the use of illicit drugs, resulting in pulmonary vascular or interstitial disease.

The clinical presentation of drug-induced ILD is often nonspecific, with fever, cough, and dyspnea accompanied by radiographic infiltrates. Eosinophilia may sometimes be present. Antinuclear antibodies are positive, but anti–double-stranded DNA antibodies are negative, in the setting of *drug-induced lupus.* Pulmonary function tests, if performed, generally reveal decreases in diffusion capacity and often a restrictive pattern. ILD caused by medications generally does not produce a unique radiographic or histologic pattern of lung injury but may result in a variety of nonspecific reactions, including pulmonary infiltrates with peripheral eosinophilia, a hypersensitivity pneumonitis pattern, and interstitial fibrosis. Alveolar filling may also occur in the

setting of drug-induced organizing pneumonia and acute lung injury or diffuse alveolar damage. Pleural and pericardial effusions may be present in lupus-like drug reactions. Because the presentation of drug-induced ILDs lacks specificity, ILDs are typically diagnoses of exclusion.

There are particular settings in which drug-induced lung disease may be especially relevant and should be strongly considered in the differential diagnosis. These settings include the use of chemotherapeutic agents, the use of illicit drugs, patients presenting with lupus-like illness, and patients using particular agents well-known to produce pulmonary toxicity such as *amiodarone* or *nitrofurantoin.* Many chemotherapeutic agents, ranging from the newer tyrosine kinase inhibitors to older agents such as *bleomycin* and *methotrexate,* may produce lung injury and ILD. Diagnosis of a drug-induced ILD may be challenging in patients treated with chemotherapy because atypical infections and chemotherapy-induced heart failure may result in similar symptoms and radiographic findings.

Heroin use typically results in pulmonary edema or aspiration injury and not ILD per se. Cocaine use can produce a variety of pulmonary effects, including organizing pneumonia, alveolar hemorrhage, and diffuse alveolar damage. "Crack lung" is a clinical diagnosis typified by dyspnea, hemoptysis, and pulmonary infiltrates occurring in the setting of crack cocaine use. Drug-induced lupus occurs with particular drugs, such as *procainamide* or *hydralazine.* Amiodarone lung toxicity is a classic drug-induced lung disorder that results in alveolar or interstitial infiltrates accompanied by dyspnea on exertion; foamy macrophages can be detected by bronchoalveolar lavage, but only indicate amiodarone use, not toxicity. Nitrofurantoin may cause an acute pulmonary syndrome with fever, dyspnea, and cough soon after initiation of the drug, or a chronic pulmonary fibrosis with long-standing use. Amiodarone and nitrofurantoin reactions necessitate drug withdrawal and often corticosteroids for resolution.

Pulmonary toxicity from drugs may be dose-dependent, as with bleomycin, in which the risk of lung toxicity increases with cumulative doses exceeding 450 U. Amiodarone lung disease typically occurs with doses over 400 mg/day. Synergistic lung toxicities may occur. For example, exposure to

Table 18-6 Common Drug-Induced Lung Diseases

Drug	Dose Relation	Manifestation
Chemotherapeutic		
Bevacizumab	Acute	Hemoptysis, pulmonary hemorrhage
Bleomycin	Acute or delayed, >450 U increased risk	Pneumonitis, fibrosis, BOOP, lung nodules
Busulfan	Chronic	Fibrosis, alveolar proteinosis
Cyclophosphamide	Chronic	Fibrosis, BOOP
Cytosine arabinoside	Acute	Pulmonary edema, ARDS
Gefitinib	Acute	Pulmonary fibrosis, interstitial pneumonitis, diffuse alveolar damage
Gemcitabine	Acute	Dyspnea, bronchospasm, capillary leak syndrome with pulmonary edema, ARDS, alveolar hemorrhage
Imatinib	Acute, chronic	Pulmonary edema, pneumonitis
Interferon alfa	Chronic	Sarcoidosis
Irinotecan	Acute	Pneumonitis
Methotrexate	Acute or chronic	Hypersensitivity pneumonitis, resolves with discontinuation, BOOP
Mitomycin C	Acute or delayed	Pneumonitis, ARDS, BOOP, hemolytic uremic syndrome
Paclitaxel and docetaxel	Acute	Interstitial and hypersensitivity pneumonitis
Antimicrobial		
Nitrofurantoin	Acute or chronic	Acute pneumonitis, chronic fibrosis
Sulfasalazine	Acute or chronic	Pulmonary infiltrates with eosinophilia, BOOP
Cardiovascular		
Amiodarone	Acute or chronic, >400 mg/day	Pneumonitis, fibrosis
Flecainide	Acute	ARDS, LIP
Tocainide	Weeks or months	Pneumonitis
Procainamide	Subacute or chronic	Drug-induced systemic lupus erythematosus, pleural effusions, pulmonary infiltrates
Anti-inflammatory		
Aspirin	Acute	Pulmonary edema, bronchospasm
Illicit		
Opiates	Acute	Pulmonary edema
Cocaine	Acute	Pulmonary edema, diffuse alveolar damage, pulmonary hemorrhage, BOOP
Talc (in intravenous and inhaled illicit drugs)	Acute or chronic	Granulomatous interstitial fibrosis, granulomatous pulmonary artery occlusion, particulate embolization
Tocolytics		
Terbutaline, albuterol, ritodrine	Acute	Pulmonary edema

ARDS, acute respiratory distress syndrome; BOOP, bronchiolitis obliterans and organizing pneumonia; LIP, lymphoid interstitial pneumonia.

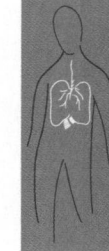

high levels of inspired oxygen may precipitate bleomycin lung injury and should be avoided if possible in exposed patients.

The website http://www.pneumotox.com is an online reference site tabulating the reported pulmonary toxicities of various drugs that is searchable by drug name as well as by pattern of lung involvement.

Pulmonary Vasculitis and Diffuse Alveolar Hemorrhage

Diffuse alveolar hemorrhage (DAH) syndromes encompass diverse group of specific entities that are all characterized by the disruption of the alveolar-capillary membrane, resulting in bleeding into the alveolar spaces. Unfortunately, patients with DAH do not always present with signs, symptoms, and laboratory and radiographic findings that support a specific underlying diagnosis. Often, DAH is found without features that identify a specific etiology.

All DAH syndromes are characterized by the abrupt onset of cough, fever, and dyspnea. Hemoptysis is common but not universal because it may be absent in up to one third of patients with DAH. Physical findings are generally nonspecific, although ocular, nasopharyngeal, or cutaneous abnormalities may suggest systemic vasculitis or collagen vascular disease as an etiology. The cardiopulmonary examination is often normal but may reveal inspiratory crackles, a systolic murmur suggestive of mitral stenosis or evidence of pulmonary hypertension. Falling hemoglobin levels, the presence of increasingly hemorrhagic fluid on sequential bronchoalveolar lavage and new patchy alveolar infiltrates (**Web Fig 18-6**) by chest imaging favor the diagnosis of DAH. Other laboratory abnormalities may include the presence of azotemia, suggesting a pulmonary-renal syndrome. In this setting, an abnormal urinalysis with proteinuria, hematuria, and red blood cell casts is usually seen. The erythrocyte sedimentation rate (ESR) may be increased, particularly in those with an underlying systemic disease. Some lung disorders characterized by DAH are associated with the production of antineutrophil cytoplasmic antibodies (ANCA) directed against neutrophil cytoplasmic antigens or antibodies directed at the glomerular basement membrane. ANCA testing, in particular, can play an important role in the workup of DAH because it is used in the diagnosis and classification of various pulmonary vasculitides that cause DAH. Two major immunofluorescent patterns can be seen in ANCA testing: diffuse staining throughout the cytoplasm (c-ANCA) or staining around the nucleus (p-ANCA). Specific antigens that ANCAs are directed against include proteinase-3 (PR-3), typically causing the c-ANCA pattern, and myeloperoxidase (MPO), which typically causes the p-ANCA pattern.

All DAH syndromes are characterized by three distinct histologic patterns. *Bland pulmonary hemorrhage* is due to alveolar hemorrhage without inflammation or destruction of the alveolar structures. This pattern is seen in conditions where there is elevated pulmonary capillary hydrostatic pressure, such as congestive heart failure or mitral stenosis, or with the use of certain anticoagulation medications. *Diffuse alveolar damage* (DAD) is caused by a variety of pulmonary infections, connective tissue diseases, and medications. DAD is also seen in acute respiratory distress syndrome (ARDS) from any etiology. Histologically, alveolar walls appear edematous and are lined with hyaline membranes. The most common histologic pattern seen on lung biopsy obtained from patients with DAH is *pulmonary capillaritis*, which is characterized by neutrophilic infiltration of the alveolar septa. This sequentially leads to necrosis, loss of capillary structural integrity, and extravasation of red blood cells into the interstitium and alveolar spaces. This finding is seen in a variety of connective tissue diseases and is the most common histologic pattern of the pulmonary vasculitides.

The pulmonary vasculitides represent a group of specific entities, many of which are associated with elevated serum ANCA levels. These entities include *Wegener granulomatosis, microscopic polyangiitis, Churg-Strauss syndrome,* and certain drug-induced vasculitis syndromes. *Pauci-immune glomerulonephritis without evidence of extrarenal disease* is a disorder that is considered to be on the spectrum of Wegener granulomatosis and microscopic polyangiitis because its histologic features are indistinguishable from these disorders and some patients eventually develop extrarenal (pulmonary) manifestations. *Wegener granulomatosis* is a systemic necrotizing granulomatous vasculitis that often involves the small and medium-sized vessels of the upper airway, the lower respiratory tract, and the kidney. Although this triad is not always seen at initial presentation, as only 40% of those affected have renal disease at that time, 80% to 90% of patients eventually develop glomerulonephritis. The most frequent manifestations of this illness are pulmonary, as highlighted by cough, chest pain, hemoptysis, and dyspnea. Constitutional symptoms, such as fever and weight loss, as well as symptoms due to involvement of the skin, eye, heart, nervous system, and musculoskeletal system, are also common. The diagnosis of Wegener granulomatosis is supported by clinical findings and by the presence of circulating ANCAs, which are seen in 90% of all patients. The remaining 10% are ANCA negative. In ANCA-positive patients, antibodies are

usually directed against PR-3; however, 10% to 20% may have anti-MPO antibodies. Chest imaging may show bilateral disease and infiltrates that evolve over the course of the illness. Lung nodules are common and may cavitate. Effusions and adenopathy are not common. Sinus films or CT scans serve to diagnose upper airway involvement. Tissue biopsy at a site of active disease is generally needed to confirm Wegener's granulomatosis. The presence of granulomatous inflammation is common, but actual vasculitis is seen in only 35% of patients. A renal biopsy is preferred because it is easier to perform and more often diagnostic. In the absence of renal involvement, a lung biopsy should be considered. Pathologically, Wegener granulomatosis is characterized by small and medium vessel necrotizing vasculitis and granulomatous inflammation. Special stains and cultures should be performed to exclude the presence of infections that can produce similar findings.

Microscopic polyangiitis is a form of systemic necrotizing small vessel vasculitis that universally affects the kidneys, whereas pulmonary involvement occurs in only a minority of patients (10% to 30%). This rare condition has a prevalence of 1 to 3 cases per 100,000, but it is the most common cause of pulmonary-renal syndrome. It is often heralded by a long prodromal phase, characterized by constitutional symptoms followed by the development of rapidly progressive glomerulonephritis (RPGN). In those patients who do develop lung involvement, DAH secondary to capillaritis is the most common manifestation. Joint, skin, peripheral nervous system, and gastrointestinal involvement can be seen as well. Seventy percent of patients with microscopic polyangiitis are ANCA positive, most of whom have anti-MPO antibodies. Because anti-MPO and anti-PR3 antibodies can be present in both microscopic polyangiitis and Wegener granulomatosis, these diseases cannot be distinguished based on their ANCA pattern. However, the two diseases can be distinguished pathologically because microscopic polyangiitis is characterized by a focal, segmental necrotizing vasculitis affecting venules, capillaries, arterioles, and small arteries *without* clinical or pathologic evidence of necrotizing granulomatous inflammation. The absence or paucity of immunoglobulin localization in vessel walls distinguishes microscopic polyangiitis from immune complex–mediated small vessel vasculitis such as *Henoch-Schönlein purpura* and *cryoglobulinemic vasculitis*.

Treatments of Wegener granulomatosis and microscopic polyangiitis are similar. Combination therapy with corticosteroids and cyclophosphamide is the standard of care. Azathioprine can be substituted for cyclophosphamide if remission is achieved. Intravenous immunoglobulin may be effective for those with persistent disease. Novel therapies, including trimethoprim-sulfamethoxazole, antilymphocyte monoclonal antibodies, and tumor necrosis factor inhibitors, have been tried with some success.

Allergic granulomatosis or *Churg-Strauss syndrome* is characterized by the triad of asthma, hypereosinophilia, and necrotizing vasculitis. Many other organ systems, including the nervous system, skin, heart, and gastrointestinal tract, may be involved as well. The vasculitis can be associated with skin nodules and purpura. Although DAH and glomerulonephritis may occur, they are much less common than in the other small vessel vasculitides. Morbidity and mortality are often due to cardiac or gastrointestinal complications or to status asthmaticus and respiratory failure. ANCAs are less helpful in Churg-Strauss syndrome because only 50% of patients are ANCA positive. Anti-MPO antibodies are more commonly seen in these patients. Pathologically, both a necrotizing, small vessel vasculitis and an eosinophil-rich inflammatory infiltrate with necrotizing granulomas are seen. Most patients respond well to corticosteroids, but other immunosuppressants similar to cyclophosphamide may be required in patients with refractory disorders.

Other well-known causes of pulmonary capillaritis include the systemic vasculitides, collagen vascular disorders, antiglomerular membrane antibody syndrome (*Goodpasture syndrome*), and *Henoch-Schönlein purpura*. Goodpasture syndrome causes DAH associated with glomerulonephritis caused by antiglomerular basement membrane antibodies to the α_3 chain of type IV collagen that is also found in the lung basement membrane. More than 90% of patients with Goodpasture syndrome have antiglomerular basement membrane antibodies detectable in the serum. In those without circulating antibodies, the diagnosis may be confirmed by lung biopsy, although the kidney is the preferred site. Up to 40% may also be ANCA positive, primarily with anti-MPO antibodies. Pathologically, linear deposition of antibody along the alveolar or glomerular basement membrane that is visible by direct immunofluorescence occurs. The treatment of Goodpasture syndrome is plasmapheresis and immunosuppression. The disease is fatal if left untreated.

Idiopathic pulmonary hemorrhage or *hemosiderosis* is a diagnosis of exclusion. Patients with this syndrome have recurrent DAH without associated renal or systemic disease. Histologically, the lung shows hemorrhage and hemosiderin accumulation without inflammation. Treatment includes supportive care, immunosuppression, and occasionally plasmapheresis, but response to therapy is varied. This syndrome is most common in children, who have a worse prognosis than adults.

Environmental and Occupational Interstitial Lung Diseases

Several environmental and occupational exposures may cause ILDs. These include the *pneumoconioses, drug-induced ILD* (discussed earlier), and *hypersensitivity pneumonitis.* Pneumoconiosis and hypersensitivity pneumonitis are discussed later. The pneumoconioses are lung diseases resulting from the inhalation of mineral dusts, including silica, coal dust, or asbestos. Hypersensitivity pneumonitis is caused by the inhalation of organic dusts.

PNEUMOCONIOSIS

The pneumoconioses result from the effects of accumulation of mineral dusts in the lungs, with the typical reaction being fibrosis. In general, the risk and extent of these diseases are related to the intensity and cumulative amount of exposure over time. Prevention of the pneumoconioses through occupational safeguards or, in the case of asbestos, legislative bans on use, is most important because there are not effective treatments for these diseases once established.

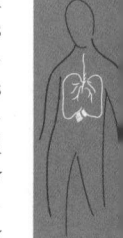

Silicosis is a lung disease caused by exposure to crystalline-free silica, which results in an inflammatory and fibrotic reaction resulting in the characteristic silicotic nodule. Certain occupations that have a higher propensity for exposure to silica include mining, stone cutting, carving, polishing, foundry work, and abrasive clearing (sandblasting). Although exposure is usually chronic (over years), accelerated and acute disease manifestations have been described in the setting of heavier short-term exposures. Acute silicosis causes a pulmonary alveolar proteinosis, with an accumulation of surfactant in the alveolar spaces. Chronic silicosis results in *simple nodular silicosis,* which is usually asymptomatic unless the patient is also exposed to tobacco, and *progressive massive fibrosis* (PMF), which is characterized by extensive bilateral apical fibrosis resulting from the confluence of many silicotic nodules. Patients with silicosis may present with dyspnea or may be relatively asymptomatic but present for evaluation of an abnormal chest radiograph. Chest radiographs in uncomplicated silicosis show upper lobe nodular opacities, which may be subtle, whereas PMF results in marked architectural distortion of the upper lobes (**Web Fig 18-7**). Hilar node enlargement may be seen accompanied by *eggshell* nodal calcification (**Web Fig 18-8**). Pulmonary function tests in simple nodular silicosis may be normal or show a mixed obstructive or restrictive pattern, whereas PMF is typically associated with severe restriction and hypoxemia. Patients with silicosis are at elevated risk for tuberculosis and should be screened for latent tuberculosis infection; there is also an association between silicosis and rheumatoid arthritis.

Coal worker's pneumoconiosis is an uncommon cause of pulmonary fibrosis, occurring in workers exposed to coal dust and graphite. Usually, the patients are exposed while working in underground mines. Coal worker's pneumoconiosis results in the formation of pigmented lesions in the lung, surrounded by emphysema, known as *coal macules.* PMF may subsequently occur. Most patients show chronic cough, which is usually productive, because of bronchitis related to coal exposure or to tobacco. The chest radiograph shows diffuse small rounded opacities. As with silicosis, there is an association with rheumatoid arthritis; Caplan syndrome is the occurrence of multiple large, sometimes cavitary, lung nodules in association with rheumatoid arthritis following coal dust exposure.

Asbestosis is due to chronic exposure to asbestos, which is a fibrous silicate used for insulation, for friction-bearing surfaces, and to strengthen materials. The inhaled asbestos fibers are deposited in the lungs, where small fibers may be phagocytosed and cleared through lymphatics to the pleural space, but longer fibers are often retained. Typically, asbestos exposure may lead to pleural disease characterized by pleural plaques, effusion, and fibrosis, but it does not necessarily affect the lung parenchyma. If it does, it is called *asbestosis* and is associated with interstitial lung fibrosis. Asbestosis is characterized by a gradual onset of dyspnea. As with other pneumoconioses, the risk and severity of disease are related to the extent and duration of cumulative exposure. Asbestosis is often diagnosed after exposure has ceased, and disease progression may continue to occur in the absence of ongoing exposure, owing to the reaction to retained asbestos fibers in the lung. The clinical presentation, pulmonary function tests, and imaging studies are similar to those

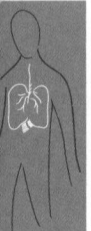

found in restrictive lung diseases like IPF. However, the detection of significant pleural disease is useful in distinguishing this illness from other ILDs. The diagnosis is made from the history and demonstration of concomitant pleural plaques and lower lobe–predominant fibrotic changes on chest radiographs or CT scan. In uncertain cases, the demonstration of asbestos in tissue specimens may be necessary; asbestos bodies are the characteristic finding and consist of asbestos fibers coated by iron-containing (ferruginous) material. Asbestos exposure results in an elevated incidence of malignancy, including lung carcinoma and mesothelioma, especially in persons who also smoke. Whether the presence of asbestosis itself confers a heightened risk for malignancy, independent of the effects of asbestos exposure alone, is uncertain. No specific treatment for asbestosis exists.

Berylliosis results from exposure to beryllium, a rare metal useful in modern, high-technology industries. Exposure to beryllium can lead to an acute chemical bronchitis and pneumonitis or chronic beryllium disease. Chronic beryllium disease is characterized by a multisystemic granulomatosis that is difficult to distinguish from sarcoidosis. The diagnosis is made by history of exposure, histologic examination, and laboratory confirmation through the beryllium lymphocyte proliferation test that is available at specialized centers. Corticosteroids may be useful in the treatment of berylliosis, but patients should avoid further exposure to beryllium.

HYPERSENSITIVITY PNEUMONITIS

Hypersensitivity pneumonitis (also termed *extrinsic allergic alveolitis*) is a relatively common ILD resulting from an exaggerated immune reaction to various inhaled organic antigens in sensitized individuals. Potential sensitizing antigens are diverse, ranging from bacterial, fungal, and animal proteins to low–molecular-weight chemicals (Table 18-7). Although evocative descriptions have been given to occupational forms of this disease ("paprika splitter's lung" resulting from sensitivity to *Mucor stolonifer*), more prosaic exposures may occur in everyday life, for example, to contaminated hot tub water or to pet birds. The disease may present in an acute fashion several hours after intense exposure to a provocative antigen, with fever, chills, cough, dyspnea, and malaise that last for up to 24 hours. Subacute or chronic disease may occur with repeated or prolonged antigen exposure and may result in chronic dyspnea and cough, with eventual progression to pulmonary fibrosis.

Diffuse crackles and wheezes are common physical findings. Hypoxemia may be present. In general, hypersensitivity pneumonitis is characterized by nonspecific infiltrates in the mid and upper lung fields on chest radiographs. CT scanning is more sensitive than chest radiography, revealing ground-glass opacities, centrilobular nodules, and mosaic attenuation patterns resulting from airway obstruction. In chronic hypersensitivity pneumonitis, emphysema and lower lobe honeycombing may be present. Restrictive or mixed obstructive-restrictive patterns may be seen on pulmonary function testing, along with abnormalities of gas exchange. Bronchoalveolar lavage may demonstrate a lymphocytic alveolitis, with CD8 T-lymphocyte predominance. Patients with hypersensitivity pneumonitis may have pre-

Table 18-7 **Hypersensitivity Pneumonitis**		
Antigen	**Source**	**Disease Examples**
Thermophilic bacteria	Moldy hay, sugar cane, compost	Farmer's lung, bagassosis, mushroom worker's disease
Other bacteria	Contaminated water, wood dust, fertilizer, paprika dust	Humidifier, detergent worker's disease, and familial hypersensitivity pneumonitis
Fungi	Moldy cork, contaminated wood dust, barley, maple logs	Suberosis, sequoiosis, and maple bark stripper's disease, malt worker's disease, and paprika splitter's lung
Animal protein	Bird droppings, animal urine, bovine and porcine pituitary powder	Pigeon breeder's lung, duck fever, turkey handler's disease, pituitary snuff taker's disease, laboratory worker's hypersensitivity pneumonitis
Chemically altered human proteins (albumin and others)	Toluene diisocyanate Trimellitic anhydride Diphenylmethane diisocyanate	Hypersensitivity pneumonitis
Phthalic anhydride	Heated epoxy resin	Epoxy resin lung

cipitating antibodies to the offending antigen, but serum precipitins are not sufficiently sensitive or specific for diagnosis, and the specific antigen may not be known or may not be tested for with standard test panels.

An appropriate exposure, clinical history, and imaging findings can suggest the diagnosis, but lung biopsy may be necessary for confirmation. Transbronchial biopsy is often sufficient. Typical biopsy findings include poorly formed granulomas containing foreign body giant cells and interstitial chronic inflammation with a bronchiolocentric component. Clinical improvement often occurs in the hospital setting when patients are isolated from the offending antigen, and relapse may occur after discharge. Corticosteroids can relieve symptoms in the acute phase, but their efficacy in chronic forms of the disease is less clear. Identification of the cause of hypersensitivity pneumonitis is important because chronic disease management requires avoidance of exposure to the antigen, which can be financially or psychologically challenging for patients in the setting of occupational, pet, or residential exposures.

Specific Entities

PULMONARY LANGERHANS CELL HISTIOCYTOSIS (EOSINOPHILIC GRANULOMA)

Pulmonary Langerhans cell histiocytosis (LCH), also called *eosinophilic granuloma*, is a disease of young- to middle-aged adults. Nearly all cases occur in white men who smoke. The disorder results from the infiltration of Langerhans cells, which are dendritic cells, into the lung parenchyma. Smoking may alter local immune signaling, attracting the Langerhans cells to the lungs. Patients typically exhibit constitutional symptoms, dyspnea on exertion, and cough, possibly with hemoptysis. Pneumothorax may also occur. Imaging shows micronodular lesions and cysts that predominate in the mid and upper lung zones. Pulmonary function tests show an obstructive pattern and impaired diffusion capacity. Specific diagnosis can be made with open lung biopsy, which demonstrates multiple stellate lung nodules that may be cellular or fibrotic, containing Langerhans cells that stain for Cd1a and S100. Electron microscopy may reveal Birbeck granules, distinctive racquet-shaped structures within the cells. In the right clinical setting and with a typical HRCT, a biopsy might not be needed for diagnosis. In contrast to systemic LCH, pulmonary LCH is not a neoplastic disorder, and spontaneous regression may occur. The main treatment is tobacco cessation. Corticosteroids and other immunosuppressants are sometimes employed as adjunctive therapy.

LYMPHANGIOLEIOMYOMATOSIS

Lymphangioleiomyomatosis (LAM) is a rare disorder that may occur in association with the tuberous sclerosis complex or sporadically in women of childbearing age. The disease is characterized by extensive nodular infiltration of the lungs and lymphatics with growths of smooth muscle–like cells. Mutations in the *TSC-1* or *TSC-2* gene, encoding for tumor suppressor proteins that normally act as inhibitors of protein synthesis and cell growth, may result in tuberous sclerosis or LAM, with mutations in *TSC-2* being associated with greater disease severity. Dyspnea and pneumothorax are the most common presentations, with chylous pleural effusions and hemoptysis also occurring. These clinical presentations result from the lung parenchymal destruction, airway narrowing, and lymphatic obstruction caused by the abnormal proliferation of the smooth muscle–like cells. Imaging studies show an interstitial pattern with mid and upper lung predominance, multiple thin-walled cystic lesions, and characteristically preserved lung volumes. Pleural effusion or pneumothorax may also be present on imaging. CT of the abdomen may reveal fat-containing kidney lesions consistent with angiomyolipomas. Pulmonary function tests typically show a progressive obstructive pattern, although mixed obstruction and restriction may also be seen.

Although the clinical features coupled with characteristic imaging are often diagnostic, lung biopsy might be necessary in some cases. This demonstrates interstitial nodules composed centrally of spindle-shaped cells that stain for smooth muscle cell actin as well as with HMB-45, an antibody to the melanocytic glycoprotein gp-100, involving the alveolar walls, lobular septa, venules, small airways, and pleura. Treatment involves management of pleural complications, including use of pleurodesis to prevent recurrent pneumothorax or effusion; bronchodilator and oxygen therapy; and avoidance of pharmacologic estrogens, which may exacerbate the disease. Progesterones have been used in an attempt to modulate disease progression, although efficacy data are limited. Because the products of the *TSC-1* and *TSC-2* genes normally act as inhibitors of the mammalian target of rapamycin (m-TOR), use of inhibitors of m-TOR activity like sirolimus is under investigation in LAM, with sirolimus being shown in one small study to improve lung function in LAM. Lung transplantation can be performed in patients with severe pulmonary dysfunction.

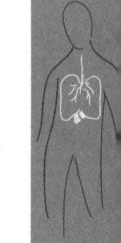

EOSINOPHILIC LUNG DISEASE

Eosinophilic lung diseases are characterized by the presence of pulmonary infiltrates and eosinophilia of the peripheral blood or lung. Because eosinophilia is a feature of many diseases, it is important to distinguish primary pulmonary eosinophilic lung disorders from lung disorders in which eosinophilia is secondary to a specific cause. Eosinophilic lung diseases can be categorized as follows: *primary pulmonary eosinophilic disorders* (including *acute* and *chronic eosinophilic pneumonia, hypereosinophilic syndrome*), *pulmonary disorders of known cause associated with eosinophilia* (including *asthma, allergic bronchopulmonary aspergillosis, drug reactions, parasitic infections*), *lung diseases associated with eosinophilia* (including *hypersensitivity pneumonitis, COP, IPF*), *malignancies associated with eosinophilia* (including *lung cancer, leukemia, lymphoma*), and *systemic disease associated with eosinophilia* (including *rheumatoid arthritis, sarcoidosis*, and *Sjögren syndrome*).

Acute eosinophilic pneumonia is characterized by fever, a nonproductive cough, and dyspnea of less than 7 days' duration, often leading to respiratory failure. This disease typically affects men between the ages of 20 and 40 years who are otherwise healthy. Chest imaging reveals diffuse bilateral pulmonary infiltrates. Eosinophilia is not present in the peripheral blood initially but may occur 7 to 30 days after onset. However, abundant eosinophils can be found in bronchoalveolar lavage fluid, and a level of greater than 25% of all nucleated cells is helpful in making the correct diagnosis. Although lung biopsy is typically not required to make the diagnosis, it can show eosinophilic infiltration with acute and organizing diffuse alveolar damage. Treatment with corticosteroids typically offers complete clinical and radiographic resolution without recurrence or residual sequelae.

Chronic eosinophilic pneumonia is an idiopathic disease predominantly of middle-aged women. Also termed *prolonged pulmonary eosinophilia*, this illness is characterized by a productive cough, dyspnea, malaise, weight loss, night sweats, and fever associated with progressive peripheral lung infiltrates that, on chest radiography, have been described as resembling the "photographic negative of pulmonary edema" (**Web Fig 18-9**). On presentation, most patients have a peripheral eosinophilia of greater than 30% and bronchoalveolar lavage fluid eosinophilia as well. Histologic examination shows eosinophils and histiocytes in the lung parenchyma and interstitium, areas of COP, but minimal fibrosis. Spontaneous remissions have been reported, but respiratory failure can also develop. Typically, treatment with corticosteroids is rapidly effective. Prolonged therapy is recommended because unlike with acute eosinophilic pneumonia, relapses are common.

Simple pulmonary eosinophilia, also known as *Löffler syndrome*, is characterized by transient migratory infiltrates that last less than 1 month. In some cases, no symptoms are present, but dyspnea and dry cough may occur. Pathologic examination of tissues reveals interstitial and intra-alveolar

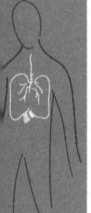

accumulation of eosinophils, macrophages, and edema. The syndrome might be idiopathic or caused by parasitic infections (e.g., *Ascaris* species, *Strongyloides* species, hookworms) or drugs (e.g., nitrofurantoin, minocycline, sulfonamides, penicillin, nonsteroidal anti-inflammatory drugs). Treatment requires removal of the offending agent or treatment of the parasitic infection. In idiopathic cases, corticosteroids may be used.

Allergic bronchopulmonary aspergillosis (ABPA) is a hypersensitivity reaction that occurs when *Aspergillus* species colonizes the airways in patients with asthma or cystic fibrosis. Patients may present with fever, malaise, a cough productive of thick brown mucus plugs, and occasionally hemoptysis. On chest radiograph, pulmonary infiltrates, which are often transient and migratory, and central bronchiectasis may be seen. Peripheral eosinophilia of greater than 10%, elevated IgE levels (as well as the presence of aspergillus-specific IgE), and precipitating antibodies to aspergillus are among the laboratory abnormalities seen in ABPA. Response to corticosteroids is good. Itraconazole can be added to the treatment regimen as well.

PULMONARY ALVEOLAR PROTEINOSIS

Pulmonary alveolar proteinosis (PAP) is a rare disorder in which lipoproteinaceous material, similar to surfactant, accumulates within the alveoli. PAP has a congenital form, characterized by mutations of the genes encoding surfactant protein B or C or for the receptor for granulocyte-macrophage colony-stimulating factor (GM-CSF). Secondary PAP occurs in conditions in which there is a functional impairment or decrease in the number of alveolar macrophages, as seen in various hematologic malignancies (leukemia), infections (pneumocystis pneumonia), and inhalation of toxic dusts (silica, aluminum) or following allogeneic bone marrow transplantation. Acquired or idiopathic forms of PAP may represent an autoimmune disease, with neutralizing antibodies directly targeting GM-CSF playing a role in its pathogenesis. Patients with PAP present with progressive dyspnea on exertion, malaise, low-grade fever, and cough. Chest radiograph typically reveals bilateral perihilar opacities. CT scan may show thickening of the intralobular and interlobular septae, creating a pattern referred to as *crazy paving*, which is a nonspecific finding because it is seen in many other diseases of the lung. Bronchoalveolar lavage fluid can establish the diagnosis because the lavage fluid has a milky, opaque appearance that contains large "foamy" alveolar macrophages with few inflammatory cells. Asymptomatic patients and those with mild symptoms require no immediate treatment. Whole-lung lavage is indicated for patients with hypoxemia or severe dyspnea and, in up to 40% of patients, may be required only one time. GM-CSF administration in patients with acquired PAP may be beneficial, but less so than whole-lung lavage.

Prospectus for the Future

Sensitive and specific noninvasive methods are needed for the early identification of ILDs when attempts at preventing progression of lung fibrosis are likely to be more effective. IPF, the most common of the IIPs, is almost invariably fatal, and current treatment strategies are ineffective. Several clinical trials are examining the effectiveness of novel drugs in its treatment, including anti–TNF-α agents, endothelin receptor antagonists, and antioxidants. The National Institutes of Health have established the *Idiopathic Pulmonary Fibrosis Clinical Research Network* to accelerate discovery. However, much confusion about this disease remains in the community, and educational strategies will be needed to accelerate diagnosis. Sarcoidosis is another enigmatic disease that, when progressive, is largely unresponsive to current treatment strategies. Small studies suggest agents capable of immunomodulation might be useful, but further work is needed in this area. The advent of new technology able to evaluate genetic abnormalities related to disease has unveiled gene polymorphisms associated with IPF and sarcoidosis, among other ILDs. However, the true role of these abnormalities in causing the disease remains unclear, and the ability to exploit this information for early detection of disease is still limited. Interesting research is ongoing related to less common ILDs such as lymphangioleiomyomatosis, which affects women of childbearing age, and is focusing on the intracellular pathways that lead to cellular dysfunction in these disorders. Further work in this area and in the detection of the environmental hazards responsible for ILD is desperately needed. Until new and effective treatment strategies are generated, lung transplantation represents the only hope for an increasing number of patients with fibrosing ILDs. Therefore, efforts to extend life in lung transplant recipients are underway, particularly those targeting chronic rejection and bronchiolitis obliterans, the main cause of death in this population.

References

Allen TC: Pulmonary Langerhans cell histiocytosis and other pulmonary histiocytic diseases: A review. Arch Pathol Lab Med 132:1171-1181, 2008.

Collard HR, Schwarz MI: Diffuse alveolar hemorrhage. Clin Chest Med 25;583-592, 2004.

Frankel SK, Cosgrove GP, Fischer A, et al: Update in the diagnosis and management of pulmonary vasculitis. Chest 129;452-465, 2006.

Ianuzzi MC, Rybicki BA, Teirstein AS: Sarcoidosis. N Engl J Med 357:2153-2165, 2007.

Joint statement of the American Thoracic Society (ATS) and the European Respiratory Society (ERS): American Thoracic Society/European Respiratory Society international multidisciplinary consensus classification of the idiopathic interstitial pneumonias. Am J Respir Crit Care Med 165:277-304, 2002.

Leslie KO: Historical perspective: A pathologic approach to the classification of idiopathic interstitial pneumonias. Chest 128(5 Suppl 1):513S-519S, 2005.

Limper AH: Drug-induced pulmonary disease. In Mason R, Broaddus VC, Murray JF, Nadel JA (eds): Murray and Nadel's Textbook of Respiratory Medicine, 4th ed. Philadelphia, Elsevier Saunders, 2005, pp 1888-1908.

Krymakaya VP: Smooth muscle-like cells in pulmonary lymphangioleiomyomatosis. Proc Am Thorac Soc 5:119-126, 2008.

Noth I, Martinez FJ: Recent advances in idiopathic pulmonary fibrosis. Chest 132;637-650, 2007.

Trapnell BC, Whitsett JA, Nakata K: Pulmonary alveolar proteinosis. N Engl J Med. 349:2527-2539, 2003.

Wechsler ME: Pulmonary eosinophilic syndromes. Immunol Allergy Clin North Am 27:477-492, 2007.

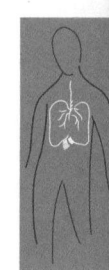

Pulmonary Vascular Disease

Sharon Rounds

Pulmonary vascular diseases are a heterogenous group of disorders with multiple causes. Pulmonary vascular disorders are caused by conditions that directly affect the pulmonary vessels, as in idiopathic pulmonary arterial hypertension (IPAH), or by disorders outside of the lung, as in pulmonary hypertension associated with lung disease and hypoxemia. The World Health Organization classification of pulmonary hypertensive disorders is presented in Table 19-1. The main complication of these disorders is the development of pulmonary hypertension, which is defined as mean pulmonary artery pressure over 25 mm Hg at rest or over 30 mm Hg with exercise. Factors that increase pulmonary arterial pressure include cardiac output, left atrial pressure, blood viscosity, and (most importantly) loss of cross-sectional area of the vascular bed, which increases vascular resistance. The loss of a cross-sectional area may be the result of mechanical occlusion, loss of vessels, vascular remodeling, or vasoconstriction. Clinical manifestations of the disease may not be exhibited until late in the course of the disease. This delayed onset occurs because the pulmonary vasculature is a high-flow, low-resistance, highly compliant system with very high capacitance such that it can accept the entire output of the right ventricle with only slight increases in pressure—even when one half of the pulmonary vasculature is removed.

Pulmonary Thromboembolic Disease

Pulmonary thromboembolic disease is a relatively common entity with an incidence ranging from 400,000 to 650,000 patients per year in the United States. Pulmonary thromboembolic disease is usually a complication of venous thrombosis. The deep veins of the femoral and popliteal systems of the lower extremities are most often affected, but right atrial, right ventricular, and upper extremity thromboses can also embolize to the lung. In view of this, predisposing factors for pulmonary embolism are the same as those for venous thrombosis and include venous stasis, hypercoagulability, and endothelial injury. Congenital or acquired procoagulant disorders (e.g., activated protein C deficiency) are also considered predisposing factors.

After a clot dislodges from the lower extremity circulation, it travels to the pulmonary circulation, where it can obstruct a branch of the pulmonary artery. The affected lung segment develops an increased ventilation-perfusion ratio $(\dot{V}/\dot{Q})$. This increases overall dead space ventilation, which leads to an inefficient excretion of partial pressure of carbon dioxide in arterial blood ($Paco_2$). In addition, blood flow is shifted from the obstructed site to other areas, which may include areas of low $\dot{V}/\dot{Q}$, thereby leading to shunting and hypoxemia. Pulmonary infarction of the area distal to the occlusion is rare because of the redundancy of the pulmonary circulation and because of oxygenation of lung parenchyma by bronchial arteries and by alveolar oxygen.

CLINICAL PRESENTATION

The classic presentation of acute pulmonary embolism includes acute shortness of breath accompanied by chest pain, hemoptysis, severe hypoxemia, and circulatory collapse as a result of shock. However, more often than not, the presentation is subtle, and the diagnosis might be difficult to make without a high level of suspicion, particularly in young individuals with otherwise healthy lungs. Dyspnea on exertion and atypical chest pain might be the only symptoms on initial presentation. Therefore, a careful history is paramount when evaluating patients for thromboembolic disease, especially those at high risk for this disorder as a result of stasis, malignancy, and previous history of venous thrombosis as well as other risk factors. The physical examination might reveal abnormalities in lung auscultation ranging from isolated crackles to diffuse wheezing. Pleural effusions might be underlying areas of dullness to percussion during the physical examination. Edema of the extremities, especially if the edema is asymmetrical, might point to venous thrombosis. In deep vein thrombosis, dorsiflexion of

Table 19-1 World Health Organization Classification of Pulmonary Hypertension

Group I. Pulmonary Arterial Hypertension

- Idiopathic (primary)
- Familial
- Related conditions, e.g., collagen vascular disease, portal hypertension, systemic-to-pulmonary shunts, HIV infection
- Associated with significant venous or capillary involvement: pulmonary veno-occlusive disease and pulmonary-capillary hemangiomatosis
- Persistent pulmonary hypertension of the newborn

Group II. Pulmonary Venous Hypertension

- Left-sided atrial or ventricular heart disease
- Left-sided valvular heart disease

Group III. Pulmonary Hypertension associated with Hypoxemia

- Chronic obstructive pulmonary disease
- Interstitial lung disease
- Sleep-disordered breathing
- Alveolar hypoventilation disorders
- Chronic exposure to high altitude
- Developmental abnormalities

Group IV. Pulmonary Hypertension Due to Chronic Thrombotic Disease, Embolic Disease, or Both

- Thromboembolic obstruction of proximal pulmonary arteries
- Thromboembolic obstruction of distal pulmonary arteries
- Pulmonary embolism (tumor, parasites, foreign material)

Group V. Miscellaneous

- Sarcoidosis, pulmonary Langerhans cell histiocytosis, lymphangiomatosis, compression of pulmonary vessels (adenopathy, tumor, fibrosing mediastinitis)

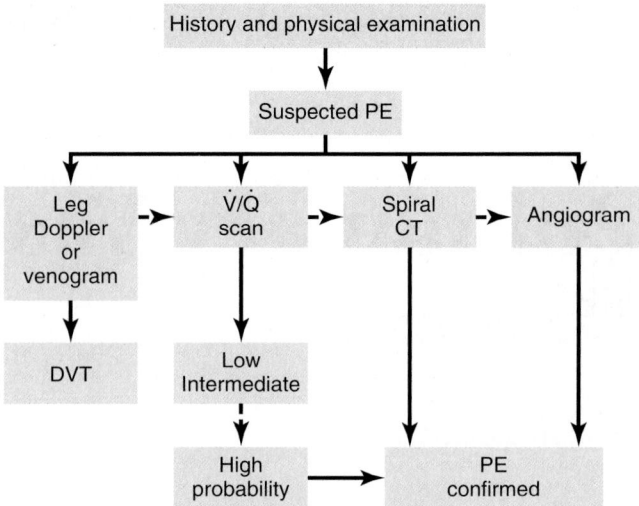

Figure 19-1 Tests commonly used in the evaluation of patients who may have pulmonary embolism (PE). Doppler ultrasound or venogram of the leg is useful to evaluate deep vein thrombosis (DVT). Ventilation-perfusion ($\dot{V}/\dot{Q}$) scans are most useful when they are normal or show lesions highly suggestive of intravascular clot. Unfortunately, these findings are not the case in many patients, requiring further investigation. Spiral computed tomography (CT) has high sensitivity and specificity and allows for the evaluation of thoracic structures in addition to assessing the vasculature. Angiography is considered the gold standard, but it is often not needed if other noninvasive tests are used alone or in combination.

the foot may cause calf pain as a result of stretching the calf muscles and deep veins (Homan sign). Signs of pulmonary hypertension and right ventricular strain, such as increased pulmonary component of the second heart sound or right ventricular heave, are not usually appreciated unless there is a massive pulmonary embolus or preexisting heart or lung disease.

EVALUATION

In severe cases, arterial blood gas measurement may show acidemia, hypoxemia, and hypercapnia, but subtle changes such as mild alkalosis might be the only abnormalities. A normal $Paco_2$ in a patient with tachypnea and presumably hyperventilation suggests increased dead space and, in the appropriate setting, might point to the diagnosis. However, a normal alveolar-arterial oxygen-tension gradient (A-aDo$_2$) does not exclude acute pulmonary embolism. An elevated level of lactic dehydrogenase (LDH) might be the result of tissue infarction, but this test is also insensitive and nonspecific. Some have advocated the use of plasma D-dimer levels in patients who might have pulmonary thromboembolism, but these are not specific either because they are elevated in patients with several unrelated medical conditions such as congestive heart failure, chronic illness, and connective tissue disorders. The main usefulness of plasma D-dimer levels is its negative predictive value.

The electrocardiogram may show atrial tachyarrhythmias or evidence of right heart strain as evidenced by a new right bundle branch block, right ventricular strain pattern, and the $S_IQ_{III}T_{III}$ pattern that mimics inferior myocardial infarction. The chest radiograph is often normal but may show atelectasis, isolated infiltrates, or a small pleural effusion. Oligemia (Westermark sign), an abrupt cutoff of pulmonary vessels or enlarged central pulmonary arteries (Fleischer sign), and pleural-based area of increased opacity (Hampton hump) might also be noted. Independent of these findings, chest radiographs are not sensitive enough to diagnose pulmonary embolism. Three diagnostic methods are used for the diagnosis of pulmonary embolism: the $\dot{V}/\dot{Q}$ scan, chest computed tomography (CT), and pulmonary arteriography (Fig. 19-1). The $\dot{V}/\dot{Q}$ scan compares lung ventilation by radiolabeled tracer gas with lung perfusion by radiolabeled micro-occlusive particles. The usefulness of the $\dot{V}/\dot{Q}$ scan depends greatly on the pre-test probability of the disease, which, in turn, is dependent on the expertise of the clinician and his or her level of certainty. A *high-probability* $\dot{V}/\dot{Q}$ scan is characterized by lobar or multilobar perfusion defects that coincide with areas of normal or relatively normal ventilation and is more than 90% accurate in diagnosing pulmonary embolism. A *normal* $\dot{V}/\dot{Q}$ scan shows no perfusion or ventilation defects and can exclude pulmonary embolism in essentially all cases. However, the test is less reliable when interpreted as *low, intermediate,* or *indeterminate* probability. Under such circumstances, pulmonary embolism is likely in between 4% and 66% of patients (Table 19-2), and further testing is necessary for an accurate diagnosis of pulmonary embolism.

Table 19-2 **Pulmonary Embolism Likelihood Using Clinical Suggestion and Ventilation-Perfusion Scan**				
Scan Result	*Clinical Probability*			
	80%-100%	**20%-79%**	**0%-19%**	**All**
High	96	88	56	87
Intermediate	66	28	16	30
Low	40	16	4	14
Normal	0	6	2	4
All scans	68	30	9	28

Data from The PIOPED Investigators: Value of ventilation/perfusion scan in acute pulmonary embolism: Results of the Prospective Investigation of Pulmonary Embolism Diagnosis (PIOPED). JAMA;263:2753-2759, 1990.

Spiral CT angiography provides a noninvasive and sensitive way to evaluate for pulmonary emboli (**Web Fig. 19-1**). Pulmonary arteriography is the gold standard and should be considered in patients without contraindications to the procedure when other tests are inconclusive and a high likelihood of pulmonary embolism exists. Although complication rates related to this procedure are low, the complications are significant if developed, ranging from pulmonary hypertension and sudden death to idiosyncratic hypersensitivity reactions to dye. For this reason, many clinicians rely on a combination of interventions to arrive at the diagnosis, particularly when pulmonary tests are combined with tests that evaluate the deep veins of the lower extremities such as venography and Doppler ultrasound.

MANAGEMENT

Pulmonary embolism is treated with supportive measures directed at sustaining organ function (e.g., fluid replacement for hypotension, mechanical ventilation for respiratory failure). To date, the only mechanical way to dislodge reliably a pulmonary artery clot is with surgical thromboembolectomy, a procedure with high mortality that requires a high level of expertise. Thromboembolectomy is only used for proximal clots that are long-standing (*chronic thromboembolism syndrome*). Consequently, medical treatments are preferred, and these are directed to prevent further clotting or to dissolve an existing clot. Anticoagulation with regular or low–molecular-weight heparin is recommended in patients without major contraindications to anticoagulation (e.g., upper gastrointestinal bleeding, hemorrhagic stroke). Their administration through subcutaneous injection appears to be as efficient as intravascular administration. The use of thrombolytic medications (e.g., tissue plasminogen activator) is usually reserved for patients with increased risk for mortality as a result of circulatory collapse caused by obstruction to the flow in large or multiple pulmonary vessels.

Idiopathic Pulmonary Arterial Hypertension

IPAH is an uncommon disorder that is progressive and usually fatal without treatment. The median survival after

the diagnosis of the disease is about 3 years without treatment. Variables associated with poor survival include heart failure, Raynaud phenomenon, elevated right atrial pressure, significantly elevated mean pulmonary arterial pressure, and decreased cardiac index. The peak incidence of IPAH is between the ages of 20 and 45 years, and it affects women more frequently than men. The cause of IPAH is unknown. However, some cases occur in families, termed *familial pulmonary arterial hypertension* (FPAH). The genetic cause of FPAH has been determined and is due to mutations in bone morphogenetic protein receptor type 2 and related receptors in the transforming growth factor-β family. Some cases of pulmonary arterial hypertension are associated with other disorders, such as HIV infection, scleroderma, hepatic cirrhosis, and anorectic drug use (see Table 19-1).

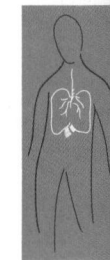

The histologic characteristics of IPAH are changes in both the arterial and venous systems. The arteries are more commonly affected, with changes in intima, media, and adventitia. There is medial vascular smooth muscle hypertrophy, adventitial thickening, and in situ thromboses of small pulmonary arteries. Plexogenic pulmonary arteriopathy is the classic pathologic finding in pulmonary arterial hypertension, consisting of medial hypertrophy, intimal proliferation and fibroelastosis, and necrotizing arteritis. The plexiform lesion is an abnormal proliferation of pulmonary endothelial cells with slitlike channels (**Web Fig. 19-2**).

Like pulmonary thromboembolism, the clinical presentation of IPAH can be subtle. The usual symptoms are dyspnea on exertion or chest pains, not typical of angina pectoris. In more severe cases, patients may present with syncope on exertion caused by inability of the restricted pulmonary circulation to accommodate increased cardiac output with exercise. Chest radiographs may reveal prominent pulmonary arteries or right ventricular enlargement (**Web Fig. 19-3**). Pulmonary function tests are usually normal, with the exception of decreased diffusing capacity, reflecting the restricted circulation and decreased surface area available for gas exchange. Indeed, the diagnosis of IPAH is dependent on exclusion of other underlying heart or lung diseases that might result in pulmonary hypertension. Echocardiogram is useful to exclude heart diseases that increase pulmonary venous pressures (e.g., mitral valve stenosis). In addition, echocardiogram may reveal enlarged right atrial and right ventricular cavity size and encroachment of the interventricular septum on the left ventricle (**Web Fig. 19-4**). Furthermore, echocardiogram may be used to estimate the level of pulmonary artery systolic pressure. The definitive diagnosis of IPAH requires right heart catheterization with measurement of pulmonary artery pressures and resistance.

Modern treatment of IPAH improves survival and includes drugs with vasodilator activity such as calcium channel blockers and prostacyclin. Because of the potential adverse effects of calcium channel blockers (decreased preload leading to acute hypotension), continuous intravenous prostacyclin is considered the most effective medical treatment. Other vasodilator drugs now available include endothelin receptor antagonists (e.g., bosentan) and drugs increasing cyclic guanosine monophosphate because of phosphodiesterase inhibition (e.g. sildenafil). These oral agents, plus inhaled or subcutaneous prostacyclin preparations, have dramatically enhanced treatment options for patients with IPAH. In addition to effects on relaxing vascular smooth muscle constriction, vasodilator drugs also appear to stabilize or reverse vascular remodeling in IPAH. Other interventions include supplemental oxygen, anticoagulation, and judicious use of diuretic medications. Heart-lung, double-lung, or single-lung transplantations have been performed in these patients with some success, but the overall 5-year survival rate in all patients undergoing lung transplantation is only 50%.

Secondary Pulmonary Hypertension

As shown in Table 19-1, pulmonary hypertension is also associated with other disorders that increase pulmonary venous pressure (e.g., mitral valve stenosis) and diseases of the lungs associated with hypoxemia (e.g., sleep apnea and chronic obstructive pulmonary disease). These conditions are frequently termed *secondary pulmonary hypertension*. Both vasoconstriction and vascular remodeling contribute to increased pulmonary vascular resistance in secondary pulmonary hypertension. For example, alveolar hypoxia causes intense pulmonary vasoconstriction. Long-standing hypoxia causes vascular remodeling that is similar to plexogenic pulmonary arteriopathy, but does not include in situ thromboses or formation of plexiform lesions (**Web Fig. 19-5**). Treatment of secondary pulmonary hypertension is directed at the underlying heart or lung disease. If hypoxia is present, home oxygen therapy should be used.

Cor Pulmonale

It is now recognized that the most frequent cause of death in patients with IPAH is right ventricular failure, also termed *cor pulmonale*. Prolonged increased afterload causes the right ventricle to hypertrophy and then dilate. The interventricular septum shifts to the left, and filling of the left ventricle is decreased, with subsequent decreased cardiac output. Dilation of the right atrium causes atrial tachyarrhythmias and further decreased cardiac output. Treatment of cor pulmonale is directed at treatment of the underlying cause of pulmonary hypertension.

Prospectus for the Future

Translational research has markedly enhanced understanding of the pathogenesis of pulmonary hypertensive disorders, and this has resulted in development of therapies that increase quality of life and improve mortality. There is increased appreciation of the role of increased vascular cell proliferation in the development of pulmonary vascular remodeling. In particular, abnormal proliferation of pulmonary endothelial cells and development of plexiform lesions have raised the suggestion that IPAH might be a disease of hyperproliferative pulmonary endothelium. In addition, little is understood regarding the adaptive changes of the right ventricle to chronically increased afterload. Future investigations are needed to understand and better treat cor pulmonale. In contrast, less new information is available about pulmonary thromboembolic disease. Although new inhibitors of the coagulation cascade are currently under investigation, understanding of the mechanisms that lead to this illness has not dramatically changed during the past decade. Studies are needed in the area of genetic predisposition for thromboembolic disease as well as in vascular dysfunction leading to thrombus formation.

References

Farber HW, Loscalzo J: Pulmonary arterial hypertension. N Engl J Med 351:1655-1665, 2004.

Humbert M, Sitbon O, Simonneau G: Treatment of pulmonary arterial hypertension. N Engl J Med 351:1425-1436, 2004.

Newman JH, Phillips JA III, Loyd JE: Narrative review: The enigma of pulmonary arterial hypertension: New insights from genetic studies. Ann Intern Med 148:278-283, 2008.

Tapson VF: Acute pulmonary embolism. N Engl J Med 358:1037-1052, 2008.

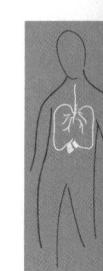

Chapter 20

Disorders of Respiratory Control

Sharon Rounds and Matthew D. Jankowich

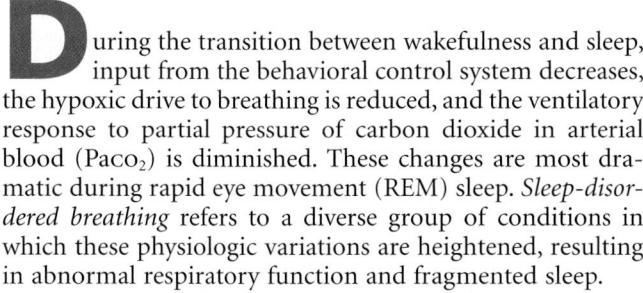

During the transition between wakefulness and sleep, input from the behavioral control system decreases, the hypoxic drive to breathing is reduced, and the ventilatory response to partial pressure of carbon dioxide in arterial blood ($Paco_2$) is diminished. These changes are most dramatic during rapid eye movement (REM) sleep. *Sleep-disordered breathing* refers to a diverse group of conditions in which these physiologic variations are heightened, resulting in abnormal respiratory function and fragmented sleep.

Of the sleep-related disorders, sleep apnea has received the most attention. *Apnea* is defined as the complete cessation of airflow for 10 seconds or longer. *Hypopnea* is a significant decrease in airflow. Occasional episodes of apnea and hypopnea are expected during normal sleep, and their frequency increases with age. However, in patients with sleep apnea, the frequency and duration of the episodes are increased, leading to sleep fragmentation and to hypoxemia and hypercapnia. Upper airway obstruction (i.e., obstructive sleep apnea [OSA]) or decreased central respiratory drive (i.e., central sleep apnea) may be the cause of sleep apnea. In some patients, both disorders are present.

Some studies suggest that the prevalence of sleep-disordered breathing may be as high as 9% in women and 24% in men, but prevalence levels depend on the definition used. Sleep-disordered breathing is usually defined as a respiratory disturbance index or frequency of abnormal respiratory events that number at least five episodes per hour of sleep. Higher prevalence estimates occur in the older adult population, with some studies showing more than 80% prevalence in older patients. Children are also affected, although less frequently (about 2%).

Obstructive Sleep Apnea

OSA is the most common of the sleep apnea syndromes and is considered to affect close to 6% of middle-aged and older men; it is less common in women. In these patients, the upper airway relaxation that occurs during sleep is such that complete occlusion of the airway results, and, consequently,

cessation of airflow occurs. After variable periods of airway occlusion, the patient arouses, re-establishes muscle tone, and opens the airway. This vicious cycle is repeated many times during the night, resulting in recurring episodes of hypoxemia. During airway occlusion, sympathetic tone is increased, resulting in vasoconstriction and hypertension, which persists during the waking hours. Indeed, OSA is the most common identifiable cause of systemic hypertension. With airway occlusion, intrathoracic pressure becomes more negative with inspiration. Episodes of hypoxemia can be associated with bradycardia and cardiac arrhythmias. These events are believed to be linked mechanistically to the increased incidence of stroke and coronary artery disease in patients with OSA. An important physiologic consequence of airway occlusion is arousal from sleep, resulting in fragmented sleep. Because apneas are more frequent during REM sleep, patients complain of lack of refreshing sleep. Patients with OSA have an increased incidence of motor vehicle crashes, presumably related to somnolence while driving. Interestingly, patients with OSA display an increased incidence of diabetes mellitus and other manifestations of the metabolic syndrome. The cardiovascular complications of OSA appear to be at least partially reversible with treatment of OSA.

CLINICAL MANIFESTATIONS

The diagnosis of OSA is suggested when patients complain of morning headaches, recurrent awakenings, and daytime somnolence that affects daytime activities, including driving. Complaints of snoring and gasping episodes may be elicited from sleeping partners. Difficulties in maintaining sleep as a result of frequent awakenings may lead to mood effects and decreased quality of life. Recent weight gain, sedatives and sleeping pills, or alcohol intake may heighten these symptoms.

The primary risk factors for OSA are obesity (although variable) and abnormal upper airway anatomy caused by macroglossia, long soft palate and uvula, enlarged tonsils, or micrognathia. Increased neck diameter (>17 cm in men and

>16 cm in women) may also be noted. A narrow oropharynx as a result of a small pharyngeal opening or redundant soft tissue is often observed. Patients may be hypertensive and, in extreme cases, may show right-sided heart failure, which results as a consequence of prolonged episodes of hypoxemia and pulmonary vasoconstriction leading to pulmonary hypertension.

EVALUATION

Chest radiographic images and pulmonary function testing are usually not helpful in the evaluation of patients with sleep apnea. In some cases, OSA is associated with the obesity-hypoventilation syndrome, which is characterized by significant obesity associated with chronic hypoventilation and hypoxemia (*pickwickian syndrome*). In such cases, arterial blood gases show hypoxemia and hypercapnia, and blood cell counts might suggest polycythemia. Although rare, hypothyroidism, acromegaly, and amyloidosis can cause or enhance OSA, and these conditions should be considered.

A formal diagnosis requires overnight polysomnography during which continuous recordings of electrocardiographic and electroencephalographic tracings are made while the patient sleeps. In addition, airflow, oxygen saturation, and respiratory, eye, chin, and limb muscle movements are monitored and recorded. OSA is diagnosed in sleeping patients (confirmed by the electroencephalographic tracings) who develop cessation of airflow despite repeated muscular efforts to breathe (**Web Fig. 20-1**). These episodes may be accompanied by transient hypoxemia and cardiac arrhythmias. A score is derived from these data that defines clinically significant sleep apnea.

Polysomnography will distinguish OSA from central sleep apnea, during which cessation of airflow is associated with halted respiratory movements. Polysomnography is also important to rule out other sleep disturbances, such as insomnia, narcolepsy, and parasomnias, as well as restless leg syndrome.

Treatment of sleep apnea includes behavioral and medical approaches. When associated with obesity, weight loss should be enthusiastically encouraged. Avoidance of sedatives and alcohol is also important. Airway obstruction can be prevented with the use of continuous positive airway pressure (CPAP) provided through a tightly fitted mask. CPAP maintains positive airway pressure throughout expiration, thereby preventing collapse of the upper airway. The amount of pressure needed can be titrated, and oxygen can be added to further prevent hypoxemic episodes. CPAP is effective in most patients, but compliance with this technique is variable. Surgical removal of obstructing tonsils, adenoids, and polyps or uvulopalatopharyngoplasty may be useful in patients with specific anatomic abnormalities. A permanent tracheostomy may be necessary in severe cases when other approaches fail. However, in general, the surgical approach to this disorder is limited to select patients only after CPAP has failed.

Other Disorders Related to Respiratory Control

Central sleep apnea is a rare disorder. It predominates in men and is generally associated with normal body habitus. Patients may complain of daytime sleepiness and insomnia with frequent awakenings. This disorder is due to apnea or hypopnea, resulting from decreased central respiratory drive, and may be a consequence of central nervous system injury (i.e., central apnea may be the result of a structural abnormality of the brainstem) or idiopathic. Affected individuals may hypoventilate even while awake, although they are capable of normal voluntary breaths. During sleep, frequent apnea is common.

In patients with obstructive lung disease, increased work of breathing eventually makes it difficult to maintain sufficient ventilation to maintain normal levels of $Paco_2$. When ventilatory capacity declines, hypoventilation causes $Paco_2$ to increase; the kidneys respond by retaining bicarbonate to keep arterial blood pH at normal levels. These patients appear to have normal ventilatory drive, but they lack the ability to increase minute ventilation to meet increased metabolic demand. This characteristic is observed in certain patients with chronic bronchitis who exhibit the classic description of the "blue bloater."

Lower brainstem and upper pontine lesions may cause *central hyperventilation*. However, this disorder rarely occurs in the absence of other physiologic or chemical abnormalities. Hepatic cirrhosis and extreme anxiety are all causes of central hyperventilation. Pregnancy can also cause hyperventilation and is thought to be caused by elevated levels of progesterone and other hormones that increase central actions. *Apneustic breathing* consists of sustained inspiratory pauses, resulting from damage to the mid-pons, most commonly caused by basilar artery infarction. *Biot respiration* or *ataxic breathing* is a haphazardly random pattern of sleep and is characterized by shallow breaths; a disruption of the respiratory rhythm generator in the medulla causes this sign.

The regular cycling of crescendo-decrescendo tidal volumes, separated by apneic or hypopneic pauses, characterizes *Cheyne-Stokes respiration*. Patients with this disorder usually have generalized central nervous system disease or congestive heart failure. Heart failure prolongs circulatory times, causing a delay between changes in blood gases at the tissue level and the arrival of those changes at the brainstem chemoreceptors. This delay sets up a cycle of gradual increase to hyperventilation, followed by gradually decreasing ventilation to apnea, and then a repetition of the cycle. Recent studies suggest that OSA and Cheyne-Stokes respiration not only are consequences of congestive heart failure but also contribute to progression of CHF.

Prospectus for the Future

With more than 5% of the population in the United States suffering from sleep-disordered breathing, and with the recognition that these disorders may contribute to systemic illnesses such as hypertension and cardiovascular disorders, interest in early diagnosis and treatment of disorders of respiratory control is growing. In view of the high incidence and potential health consequences of sleep-disordered breathing, physicians must be on the lookout for this condition. The increased inci-

dence of OSA parallels that of obesity in the United States, a public health problem that has been associated with asthma and increased risk for death. It is highly likely that genetic predisposition to OSA accounts for increased incidence in some families. Sleep medicine is an emerging clinical and research area that will continue to receive great attention in the coming decade.

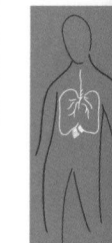

References

Arzt M, Bradley TD: Treatment of sleep apnea in heart failure. Am J Resp Crit Care Med 173:1300, 2006.

Caples SM, Gami AS, Somers VK: Obstructive sleep apnea. Ann Intern Med 142:187-197, 2005.

Somers VK, White DP, Amin R, et al: Sleep apnea and cardiovascular disease. J Am Coll Cardiol 52:686, 2008.

Stephen GA, Eichling PS, Quan SF: Treatment of sleep disordered breathing and obstructive sleep apnea. Minerva Med 95:323-336, 2004.

White DP: Pathogenesis of obstructive and central sleep apnea. Am J Resp Crit Care Med. 172:1363, 2005.

Young T, Skatrud J, Peppard PE: Risk factors for obstructive sleep apnea in adults. JAMA. 201:2013, 2004.

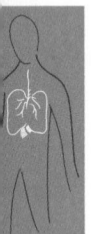

Disorders of the Pleura, Mediastinum, and Chest Wall

F. Dennis McCool

Pleural Disease

The pleura is a thin membrane that covers the entire surface of the lung as well as the inner surface of the rib cage, diaphragm, and mediastinum. There are two pleural membranes: the visceral pleura, which covers the lung; and the parietal pleura, which lines the rib cage, diaphragm, and mediastinum. A layer of mesothelial cells lines both pleural surfaces. The closed space in between the surface of the lung and the chest cavity is referred to as the *pleural space*. A small amount of fluid normally resides in this space and forms a thin layer between the pleural surfaces. Pleural fluid serves as a lubricant for the visceral and parietal pleura as they move against each other during inspiration and expiration.

The blood vessels in the visceral pleura are supplied from the pulmonary circulation and have greater hydrostatic pressure than the blood vessels in the parietal pleura, which are supplied by the systemic circulation. The pressure within the pleural space is subatmospheric during quiet breathing. Fluid is filtered from the higher-pressure vascular structures into the pleural space. The normal fluid turnover is about 10 to 20 mL per day with 0.2 to 1 mL remaining in the pleural space. Pleural fluid usually contains a small amount of protein and a small number of cells that are mostly mononuclear cells. Although both the parietal and visceral pleura contribute to pleural fluid formation, most of the fluid results from filtration of the higher-pressure vessels supplying the parietal pleura. After the fluid enters the pleural space, it is drained from the pleural space by a network of pleural lymphatics located beneath the mesothelial monolayer. The lymphatics originate in stomas on the parietal pleural surface. Under abnormal circumstances, fluid can accumulate in the pleural space. Factors that promote the entry of fluid into the pleural space include an increase in systemic venous pressure, an increase in pulmonary venous pressure, an increase in permeability of pleural vessels, or a reduction in pleural pressure. Conditions that increase hydrostatic pressure can be seen with congestive heart failure; changes in pleural membrane permeability can be seen in varied inflammatory states; and a reduction in pleural pressure can be seen with atelectasis. Occasionally, microvascular oncotic pressure may be sufficiently reduced to promote fluid entry into the pleural space in patients with hypoalbuminemia. Factors that block lymphatic drainage and interfere with the egress of fluid from the pleural space include central lymphatic obstruction or obstruction of lymphatic channels at the pleural surface by tumor.

PLEURAL EFFUSION

Pleural effusion is the accumulation of fluid in the pleural space. Pleural effusions are generally detected by chest radiography; however, the volume of fluid in the pleural space needs to exceed 250 mL to be visualized on a chest radiograph. When an effusion is present, there is blunting of the costophrenic angle on a posteroanterior chest film; this is a fluid meniscus that can be detected posteriorly also on the lateral chest radiograph, and occasionally fluid can be demonstrated in either the minor or major fissures (**Web Figs. 21-1 and 21-2**). Changes in the contour of the diaphragm may signify a subpulmonic effusion. A decubitus chest radiograph can be obtained to determine whether the fluid is free-flowing or loculated. A computed tomography (CT) scan of the chest provides better definition of the pleural space than plain radiography. Chest CT is particularly useful in differentiating pulmonary parenchymal abnormalities from pleural abnormalities, defining loculated effusions, distinguishing between atelectasis and effusion, and distinguishing loculated effusion from lung abscess (**Web Fig. 21-3**). The edge of a lung abscess usually touches the chest wall and forms an acute angle whereas that of an empyema is usually an obtuse angle.

Table 21-1 **Pleural Effusions**

Transudates		Exudates	
Congestive heart failure	Infection	Systemic lupus erythematosus	Trauma
Hypoalbuminemia	Empyema	Rheumatoid arthritis	Hemothorax
Nephrotic syndrome Malnutrition	Parapneumonic Malignancy	Intra-abdominal pathologic abnormalities	Chylothorax Ruptured esophagus
Cirrhosis	Primary lung cancer	Pancreatitis	Miscellaneous
Intra-abdominal fluid	Lymphoma	Subphrenic abscess	Myxedema
Ascites	Metastatic cancer	Complications of abdominal surgery	Uremia
Peritoneal dialysis	Pulmonary embolism and infarction Collagen vascular disease	Meigs syndrome Urinothorax	Asbestosis Lymphedema Drug-induced lupus Dressler syndrome

From Light RW, Macgregor MI, Luchsinger PC, et al: Pleural effusions: The diagnostic separation of transudates and exudates. Ann Intern Med 77:507-513, 1972.

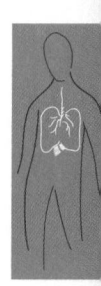

Thoracentesis is a procedure in which fluid is aspirated from the pleural space. Ultrasound or a CT scan can be used to help direct the thoracentesis catheter into collections of fluid that are otherwise difficult to drain. Analysis of pleural fluid may provide a definitive diagnosis; however, even without a definitive diagnosis, pleural fluid analysis can be useful in excluding other possible causes of disease such as infection. Classifying pleural effusions as transudates or exudates greatly assists with the differential diagnosis. The general approach to pleural effusions is outlined in **Web Figure 21-4**.

TRANSUDATES

Effusions that accumulate due to changes in osmotic and hydrostatic forces usually have low protein states and are considered transudates (Table 21-1). Congestive heart failure is the most common cause of a transudate. With heart failure, the effusions are typically bilateral. If the effusion is unilateral, it involves the right hemithorax in most instances. Effusions due to heart failure are related to dysfunction of the left side of the heart, not the right side of the heart. Transudative effusions also may be seen in cirrhosis, nephrotic syndrome, myxedema, pulmonary embolism, superior vena cava obstruction, and peritoneal dialysis. In patients with cirrhosis, the effusions are often right sided, and the mechanism may be related to flow from the peritoneal space across diaphragmatic defects into the pleural space. Transudative effusions are typically small and rarely require drainage to improve symptoms.

EXUDATES

Exudative effusions occur when there is an alteration in vascular permeability and can be observed in inflammatory states, with infection, or with neoplasm. To distinguish an exudate from a transudate, one of three criteria must be fulfilled: (1) pleural fluid–to–serum protein ratio is greater than 0.5; (2) pleural fluid–to–serum lactate dehydrogenase (LDH) ratio is greater than 0.6; and (3) pleural fluid LDH is greater than two thirds the upper limit of normal (Table 21-2). When all three criteria are met, the sensitivity, specificity, and predicted value exceed 98% for an exudative effusion. Measuring pleural fluid cholesterol may also help

Table 21-2 **Differentiation of Exudative and Transudative Pleural Effusions**

	Exudate	Transudate
Protein	>3 g/dL	<3 g/dL
Pleural and serum protein	>0.5	<0.5
LDH	Two thirds the upper limit of normal	Two thirds the upper limit of normal
Pleural and serum LDH	>0.6	<0.6

LDH, lactate dehydrogenase.
Adapted from Light RW, Macgregor MI, Luchsinger PC, et al: Pleural effusions: The diagnostic separation of transudates and exudates. Ann Intern Med 77:507-513, 1972.

distinguish an exudate from a transudate. Pleural fluid cholesterol is derived from degenerating cells within the pleural space and from vascular leakage due to increased permeability. A cholesterol level greater than 45 mg/dL is consistent with an exudative effusion.

Exudative effusions are commonly due to infection. Parapneumonic effusion occurs in patients with bacterial pneumonia and can be further classified as uncomplicated or complicated effusions. Uncomplicated parapneumonic effusions are those that do not require drainage and will respond to antibiotic therapy alone for the underlying pneumonia. By contrast, complicated parapneumonic effusions are those that will not respond to antibiotic therapy alone and will require drainage to prevent the formation of empyema. The transition from uncomplicated to complicated can occur extremely rapidly and in some cases within a 24-hour period. Typically, an uncomplicated parapneumonic effusion will have a pH greater than 7.3, a glucose greater than 60 mg/dL, and an LDH less than 1000 IU/L. A pH level of less than 7.2 usually identifies a complicated effusion. However, this finding is not specific for infection and may be due to malignancy, rheumatoid arthritis, or trauma with esophageal disruption causing an associated reduction in pH level. Complicated exudative effusions due to infections need drainage to avoid sepsis and prevent development of loculation, cutaneous fistulas, lung abscess, bronchopleural fistulas, or fibrothorax. The injection of fibrolytic agents into

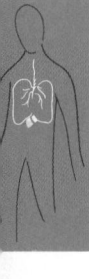

the pleural space may prevent the occurrence of fibrothorax; however, treatment of complicated pleural effusions may require thoracotomy and decortication. If pus is aspirated from the pleural space, this defines an empyema, which requires immediate drainage.

Pleural effusions secondary to primary tuberculosis may be seen in up to 30% of patients in endemic areas. The effusion is secondary to increased vascular permeability of the pleural membrane because of a hypersensitivity reaction and not due to direct infection. Typically, the pleural fluid is lymphocyte predominant and culture negative for acid-fast bacilli. Adenosine deaminase levels greater than 50 U/L may be helpful in identifying tuberculous pleural effusions. Tuberculous empyema is distinct from tuberculous pleural effusions and can occur when there is an extension of infection from the thoracic lymph nodes into the pleural space or hematogenesis spread of tuberculosis to the pleural space.

Malignant effusions are the second most common cause of exudative pleural effusions and imply a poor prognosis. Seeding of the parietal or visceral pleura with malignant cells can change vascular permeability, resulting in effusion formation. However, the finding of a pleural effusion in an individual with malignancy does not necessarily imply that there is a malignant process in the pleural space. Effusions in these individuals may be due to atelectasis, postobstructive pneumonia, hypoalbuminemia, pulmonary emboli, or complications from radiation or chemotherapy. The most common cause of malignant effusion is lung cancer, followed by breast cancer and lymphoma. An effusion that is bloody suggests a malignant process; however, other causes of bloody pleural effusions include trauma, tuberculosis, collagen vascular disease, or thromboembolic disease. To confirm the diagnosis of malignancy, cytologic examination of the fluid is needed. Malignant cells can be seen in 60% of malignant effusions on the first thoracentesis. Sensitivity rises to 80% if three separate samples are obtained. If needed, a biopsy of the pleura may be useful in identifying the presence of malignancy. Biopsies may be obtained with video-assisted thoracoscopy or, less optimally, in a blinded fashion (through a Cope or Abrams needle). A low pleural fluid pH has prognostic and therapeutic implications for patients with malignant effusions. Patients with low pleural fluid pH due to malignancy tend to have shorter survival and poorer response to chemical pleurodesis. Recurrent malignant pleural effusions may improve with chemical pleurodesis with talc or tetracycline derivatives, but effectiveness is variable, achieving a complete response in little more than 50% of patients.

Systemic inflammatory disorders such as rheumatoid arthritis and lupus erythematosus can be associated with exudative effusions. Rheumatoid pleural effusions are a common intrathoracic manifestation of rheumatoid disease and may be seen in as many as 5% of patients. Pleural fluid rheumatoid factor is often greater than 1:320, and pleural fluid glucose is less than 60 mg/dL, or the pleural fluid–to–serum glucose ratio is less than 0.5. However, a low glucose may be present in complicated parapneumonic effusions or empyema, malignant effusion, tuberculosis pleurisy, lupus pleuritis, and esophageal rupture. In systemic lupus erythematosus, 15% to 50% of patients will have pleural effusions. The pleural fluid antinuclear antibody titer is greater than 1:160.

Measuring pleural fluid amylase may further refine the differential diagnosis of an exudative effusion. Finding amylase greater than the upper limits of normal for serum amylase is consistent with acute pancreatitis, chronic pancreatic pleural effusion, esophageal rupture, or malignancy. Pancreatic disease is associated with pancreatic isoenzymes amylase, whereas malignancy and esophageal rupture are characterized by a predominance of salivary isoenzymes.

PNEUMOTHORAX

Pneumothorax is the accumulation of air in the pleural space. In this instance, pleural pressure becomes positive, and there is compression of underlying lung. Patients with pneumothorax typically present with acute onset of dyspnea. Findings include tachycardia, decreased breath sounds, decreased tactile fremitus, a pleural friction rub, subcutaneous emphysema, hyperresonance, and a tracheal shift to the opposite side. Diagnosis can be made by obtaining an upright chest radiograph. Typically, the visceral pleura separates from the parietal pleura, and air can be seen between the visceral pleural lining and the rib cage. An end-expiratory radiograph will increase the density of lung while reducing its volume, thus highlighting the difference between the lung parenchyma and the pleural gas. Management usually requires insertion of a thoracostomy tube and suction followed by water-seal drainage. However, if the pneumothorax is small and the patient is not in distress, observation alone may be indicated. If there is not a continuing air leak, as from a bronchopleural fistula, the pleural air is reabsorbed into the blood with resolution of the pneumothorax. A tension pneumothorax is a medical emergency that requires immediate decompression by placement of a chest catheter. A tension pneumothorax occurs when pleural pressure reaches levels sufficient to cause mediastinal shift, compression of the vena cava and heart, and hemodynamic compromise. Such physiology implies an ongoing leak of air into the pleural space.

Pneumothorax is often associated with blunt or penetrating trauma. With penetrating trauma, air may leak into the pleural space through the chest wall or the lung. Mechanical ventilation has also been associated with pneumothorax. Patients with underlying lung disease receiving mechanical ventilation may acutely develop a pneumothorax. A sudden rise in peak airway pressures with a reduction in breath sounds can alert the clinician to this complication. Pneumothorax also may occur spontaneously or be secondary to underlying lung disease. Typically, spontaneous pneumothorax occurs in tall, young, thin men, presumably a result of rupture of apical blebs. Underlying lung diseases that can be complicated by pneumothorax include emphysema, cystic fibrosis, granulomatosis inflammation, necrotizing pneumonia, pulmonary fibrosis, and lung abscess. Catamenial pneumothorax occurs in patients who have subpleural and diaphragmatic endometriosis; rupture of the endometrial nodules at the time of menstruation causes pneumothorax.

MESOTHELIOMA

Malignant mesotheliomas are neoplasms arising from the serosal membranes of the body cavities. Eighty percent of mesotheliomas originate in the pleural space. Generally, individuals are older than 55 years, and there is an association with asbestos exposure in the distant past. Symptoms include shortness of breath, chest pain, and weight loss. The most common radiologic presentation is a large unilateral pleural effusion that may completely opacify the hemithorax. There may be circumferential pleural thickening, usually associated with various amounts of calcified pleural plaque and effusions. CT of the chest is the most accurate noninvasive method for assessing stage and progression of mesothelioma. The diagnosis requires a biopsy; the most efficient way of obtaining tissue is by thoracoscopy. The overall prognosis for patients with malignant mesothelioma is poor. No particular therapy has emerged as superior to supportive therapy alone in terms of survival.

Mediastinal Disease

The mediastinum is the central part of the thoracic cavity between the lungs that contains the heart and aorta, esophagus, trachea, lymph nodes, and thymus. The mediastinum is bordered by the two pleural cavities laterally, the diaphragm inferiorly, and the thoracic inlet superiorly. The mediastinal space can be divided into three compartments: anterior, middle, and posterior. The localization of mediastinal masses into one of these compartments assists in the differential diagnosis (Fig. 21-1).

The anterior mediastinal compartment is anterior to the pericardium and includes lymphatic tissue, thymus, and the great veins. Lesions most commonly found in the anterior mediastinum are thymomas, germ cell tumors, lymphomas, intrathoracic thyroid tissue, and parathyroid lesions. Thymomas consist of 20% of mediastinal neoplasms in adults, and they are the most common anterior mediastinal primary neoplasm in adults. Symptoms due to myasthenia gravis may be present in one third of patients with thymoma. Patients with systemic lymphoma often have involvement of the mediastinum. However, 5% to 10% of patients with lymphoma present with primary mediastinal lesions. Posterior mediastinal masses include neurogenic tumors and cysts, meningocele, lymphoma, aneurysm of the aorta, and esophageal disorders such as diverticula and neoplasm. Cysts found in the mediastinum include pericardial cysts, bronchogenic cysts, enteric cysts, thymic cysts, and thoracic duct cysts. All these are benign but can produce compressive symptoms. Lung cancer can present with mediastinal adenopathy, a sign of unresectable disease (**Web Fig. 21-3**). The treatment of a mediastinal mass depends on the underlying pathology. For example, some require surgical resection, others radiation or chemotherapy, and some can be monitored over time.

MEDIASTINITIS

Inflammation of the mediastinal structures can be acute or chronic. Acute mediastinitis is a rapidly progressive condition secondary to infection and can be iatrogenic secondary to invasive procedures resulting in esophageal or tracheobronchial rupture or occur as a result of trauma and tissue necrosis. Chest imagining studies may show a widening of the mediastinum, pneumothorax, or hydrothorax. Treat-

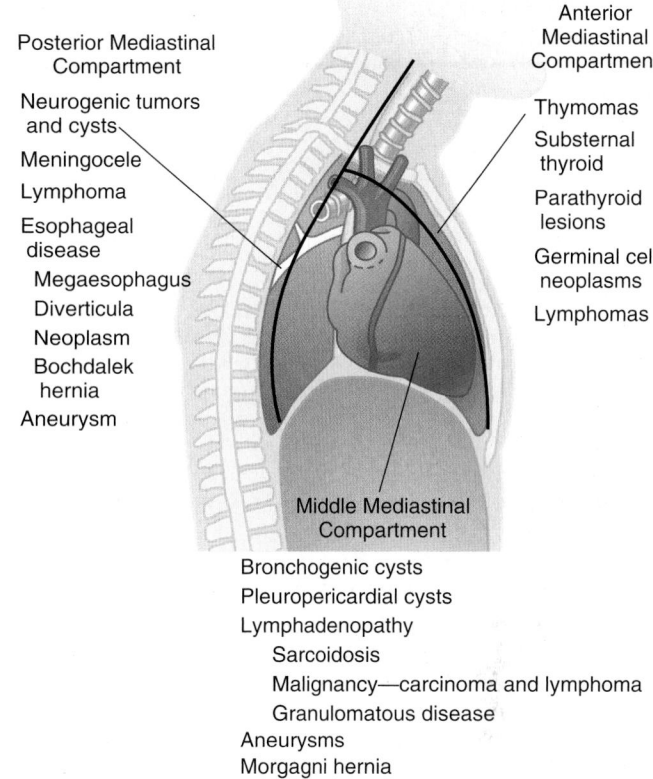

Figure 21-1 Masses of the mediastinum and their anatomic location.

ment requires antibiotics, pleural drainage, and mediastinal evacuation. Chronic mediastinitis (fibrosing mediastinitis) is a progressive illness that is due to granulomatous infections, neoplasm, radiotherapy, or occasionally drugs such as methysergide, or is idiopathic. Patients usually remain asymptomatic until vascular or neurologic structures are affected. Superior vena cava syndrome may be a consequence of chronic mediastinitis. Diagnosis and treatment often require surgical exploration.

Chest Wall Disease

The chest wall is composed of the bony structures of the rib cage, the articulations between the ribs and the vertebrae, the diaphragm, and other respiratory muscles. Normal function of this "ventilatory pump" is needed to bring oxygen from the atmosphere into the body. A wide variety of chest wall and neuromuscular disorders can result in dysfunction of the ventilatory pump. These disorders typically result in a restrictive dysfunction characterized by a reduction in total lung capacity and vital capacity with a normal residual volume. Hypoventilation may ensue resulting in hypercapnia, atelectasis, and hypoxemia.

SKELETAL DISEASE

Kyphoscoliosis and ankylosing spondylitis are disorders that involve the spine and its articulations; pectus excavatum involves the sternum, flail chest affects the ribs, and obesity

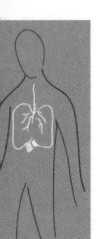

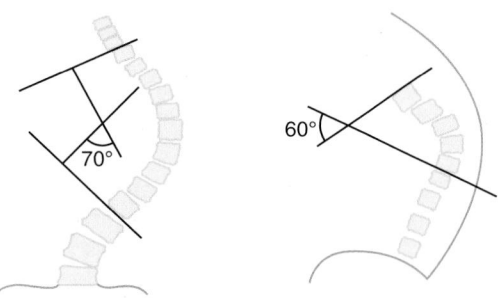

A Posteroanterior B Lateral

Figure 21-2 Schematic depicting the lines constructed to measure the Cobb angle of scoliosis (**A**) and kyphosis (**B**).

adds to the soft tissue mass of the ribcage and abdomen. These disorders primarily affect the respiratory system by stiffening the chest wall. Of these disorders, kyphoscoliosis produces the most severe restrictive impairment. Kyphoscoliosis refers to a group of disorders characterized by excessive spinal curvature in the lateral plane (scoliosis) and sagittal plane (kyphosis). The degree of curvature can be assessed by measuring the Cobb angle (Fig. 21-2). Greater degrees of spinal curvature are associated with greater restriction and an increased risk for respiratory failure. Kyphoscoliosis may be due to neuromuscular disease, associated with congenital vertebral malformations, or idiopathic. Idiopathic kyphoscoliosis is the most common form, usually manifesting in late childhood or early adolescence and affecting females more than males (ratio of 4 : 1). It is thought to be a multigene condition with autosomal or sex-linked inheritance and variable phenotypic expression. A defect in the chromatin-remodeling gene family (*CHD-7*) has been associated with idiopathic kyphoscoliosis.

Factors that contribute to respiratory failure in these patients are inspiratory muscle weakness, underlying neuromuscular disease, sleep disordered breathing, and airway compression due to distortion of lung parenchyma and twisting or airways. Treatment consists of general supportive measures such as immunizations against influenza and pneumococci, smoking cessation, maintenance of a normal body weight, supplemental oxygen, and treatment of respiratory infections. Nocturnal hypoventilation can be treated with noninvasive positive-pressure ventilation, which is typically delivered through a nasal or full facemask. Indications for instituting noninvasive ventilation include symptoms suggestive of nocturnal hypoventilations, signs of cor pulmonale, nocturnal oxyhemoglobin desaturation, or an elevated daytime $Paco_2$.

OBESITY

Obesity is a major health problem throughout the world affecting both children and adults. Body fat usually constitutes 15% to 20% of body mass in healthy men and 25% to 30% of body mass in healthy women. In obesity, the body fat content may increase by as much as 500% in women and 800% in men. The degree of obesity can be assessed by the body mass index, which is the ratio of body weight (BW) in kilograms to the square of the height (Ht) in meters (BW/

Ht^2). Individuals with a BMI between 18.5 and 24.9 kg/m^2 are normal, and those with a BMI greater than 40 kg/m^2 are considered severely or morbidly obese. Reductions in functional residual capacity and expiratory reserve volume are the most common pulmonary function abnormalities in obesity. When obesity is associated with hypoventilation, it is termed the *obesity-hypoventilation syndrome* (pickwickian syndrome). The most important consequence of this is chronic hypoventilation and pulmonary hypertension. Nocturnal noninvasive positive-pressure ventilation can be helpful in reversing these abnormalities. Weight loss is the optimal therapy but is not always attainable, and long-term weight loss maintenance is even more difficult. Pharmacotherapy or bariatric surgery should be considered in obese individuals who do not achieve weight control with conventional therapy (diet, enhanced physical activity, and behavioral therapy).

DIAPHRAGM PARALYSIS

The diaphragm separates the thorax from the abdomen and is the major muscle of inspiration. Diaphragm weakness or paralysis can involve either one or both hemidiaphragms. Unilateral diaphragm paralysis is more common than bilateral diaphragm paralysis. The most frequent causes of unilateral paralysis include traumatic phrenic nerve injury, herpes zoster, cervical spinal disease, and compressive tumors. Patients may be asymptomatic, or the abnormality may be discovered as an incidental finding of an elevated hemidiaphragm on chest radiograph. Diagnosis is confirmed by noting paradoxical upward motion of the affected diaphragm during a vigorous sniff maneuver with fluoroscopy. There is no specific treatment for this disorder, but recovery following the initial injury is occasionally seen. When disabling symptoms are present and there is significant elevation on chest radiograph, surgical plication of the diaphragm has been attempted with some success.

Bilateral diaphragm paralysis is most often seen in the setting of a disease producing generalized muscle weakness or motor neuron disease such as amyotrophic lateral sclerosis. Orthopnea is an especially prominent symptom, and patients often have difficulty sleeping in the supine position. Pulmonary function tests are associated with severe restrictive impairments. When assuming the supine position, there may be a further reduction in vital capacity by as much as 50%. Bilateral diaphragm paralysis can be difficult to diagnosis. Finding low lung volumes is often attributed to a poor inspiratory effort, and fluoroscopic sniff testing can yield false-negative results as well as false-positive results. Measurement of transdiaphragmatic pressure is reliable; however, this is somewhat invasive requiring placement of catheters in the esophagus and stomach. Alternatively, B-mode ultrasound of the diaphragm in the zone of apposition is a noninvasive means of diagnosing diaphragm paralysis. Bilateral diaphragm paralysis may not be reversible unless the underlying disease is treatable; however, recovery has been noted in more than 50% of individuals with idiopathic diaphragm paralysis or paralysis due to neuralgic amyotrophy (brachial plexus neuritis) in small series. Nocturnal hypoventilation can be treated with noninvasive positive pressure ventilation.

Prospectus for the Future

Numerous advances can be expected in treating individuals with pleural, mediastinal, and chest wall diseases. Recent progress in pleural fluid analysis using novel biomarkers and nucleic acid amplification tests may lead to more rapid and accurate diagnosis of tuberculous pleural effusions. Assays of pleural fluid tumor markers and chromosome analysis are promising developments in attempts to differentiate malignant and nonmalignant effusions. Mesothelioma remains resistant to traditional therapeutic approaches; however, evolving technology centered on gene therapy may constitute a new treatment modality. Better visualization of mediastinal structures will be achieved as magnetic resonance imaging (MRI) evolves and becomes more routinely applied to examine the chest. Molecular tracers targeting tumor receptors or proteins may be used with MRI and positron-emission tomography imaging techniques to better differentiate between malignant and benign mediastinal masses. Noninvasive nocturnal ventilation remains a cornerstone of therapy in patents with chest wall and neuromuscular diseases, but compliance can be problematic. Continued evolution of techniques to deliver nocturnal noninvasive ventilation may improve compliance with treatment, and application of this technique to patients with obesity-hypoventilation syndrome may reduce morbidity and mortality in these individuals. Patients with diaphragm paralysis due to high cervical spinal cord lesions may benefit from recent advances in intramuscular diaphragm pacing. This technique may provide an alternate means of treating respiratory failure in these individuals and others with diaphragm paralysis.

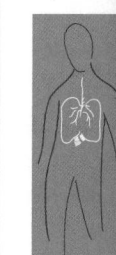

References

Colice GE, Curtis A, Deslauriers J, Heffner J, et al: Medical and surgical treatment of parapneumonic effusions: An evidence-based guideline. Chest 18:1158-1171, 2000.

Gottesman E, McCool FD: Ultrasound evaluation of the paralyzed diaphragm. Am J Respir Crit Care Med 155:1570-1574, 1997.

Heffner JE, Klein JS: Recent advances in the diagnosis and management of malignant pleural effusions. Mayo Clin Proc 83:235-250, 2008.

Light RW: The undiagnosed pleural effusion. Clin Chest Med 27:309-319, 2006.

Summerhill EM, Abu el-Sameed Y, Glidden TJ, McCool FD: Monitoring recovery from diaphragm paralysis with ultrasound. Chest 133:737-743, 2008.

Tzelepis GE, McCool FD: Non-muscular diseases of the chest wall. In Fishman AP (Ed-in-Chief): Fishman's Pulmonary Diseases and Disorders. New York, McGraw-Hill, 2007, pp 1617-1635.

Yusen RD: Medical and surgical treatment of parapneumonic effusions: An evidence-based guideline. Chest 118:1158-1171, 2000.

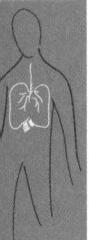

Infectious Diseases of the Lung

Brian Casserly and Sharon Rounds

Pneumonia is defined as infection of the lower respiratory tract parenchyma by agents such as bacteria, viruses, fungi, or even parasites. It should be distinguished from pneumonitis, which is an inflammation of the lungs from a variety of noninfectious causes, including chemicals, blood, radiation, and autoimmune processes. Pneumonia, the sixth leading cause of death in the United States, is responsible for 4 to 10 million respiratory infections each year.

Microbial agents can be introduced to the lungs through several routes. The most common route is by aspiration of oropharyngeal secretions. *Legionella* species, mycobacteria, endemic fungi, *Mycoplasma pneumoniae*, *Chlamydia pneumoniae*, and most viral infections are examples of pneumonia caused by direct inhalation of organisms, resulting in geographic and seasonal clustering of cases. Much less commonly, pneumonia can arise from hematogenous or embolic spread of infection from infected heart valves or venous clot. The small vessels of the pulmonary circulation act as filters for venous blood carrying small clusters of bacteria from the source. Hematogenous pneumonias, therefore, are often multifocal with peripheral lesions susceptible to rapid cavitation.

Diagnosis and therapy are dependent on clinical, imaging, and laboratory data. Patients usually exhibit respiratory symptoms, including productive cough, dyspnea, chest pain, and occasionally hemoptysis. Other, less specific symptoms include fever, general malaise, myalgias, and weight loss. The presentation may be acute (days to weeks), as observed in bacterial pneumonia, or subacute or chronic (weeks to years), as observed with tuberculosis (TB). Immunocompromised patients (e.g., those with human immunodeficiency virus [HIV] infection), may be predisposed to specific illnesses, and knowledge of the specific impairment in host defense mechanisms may help determine the cause of the infection.

The chest radiograph plays an important role. A parenchymal opacity is observed in the patient with pneumonia (**Web Fig. 22-1**); however, noninfectious disorders that mimic pneumonia exist, and no radiographic finding is entirely specific for infection.

The initial antibiotic choice may be guided by Gram stain of respiratory secretions. This requires the demonstration of a satisfactory sputum sample (defined as >25 polymorphonuclear leukocytes and <10 epithelial cells in each low-power field) and the presence of a predominant organism (>8 to 10 organisms per high-power field), particularly if the same bacteria are found within white blood cells. However, despite extensive laboratory testing, a causative organism can be identified in only about 50% of all pneumonia cases. See Table 22-1 for the most common causative agents of pulmonary infections.

Clinical guidelines have been developed to provide a systematic approach to the diagnosis and management of pneumonia. A key question that should be asked in the initial evaluation of pneumonia is whether the pneumonia is community acquired or health care associated.

Community-Acquired Pneumonia

Community-acquired pneumonia occurs twice as frequently during winter, and those at the extremes of age (<5 years and >65 years) are at increased risk. *Streptococcus pneumoniae* is the most common causative agent. *S. pneumoniae* is a gram-positive, diplococcal bacterium whose encapsulated structure protects it from host defense. Patients may have an antecedent upper respiratory tract infection, followed by the sudden onset of fever, shaking chills, dyspnea, and pleurisy. Cough productive of purulent, rust-colored sputum is common. Imaging studies show alveolar consolidation. Sputum Gram stain is positive in only 45% of bacteremic cases. Therefore, the diagnosis is confirmed by culture of the organism from a usually sterile site, such as blood, pleural fluid, or cerebrospinal fluid. In many cases, the diagnosis is presumptive, and recommended antibiotic coverage for

Table 22-1 **Organisms Causing Pulmonary Infections**		
Pathogen	**Community Acquired**	**Nosocomial**
Bacterial	**70%-80%**	**90%**
Streptococcus pneumoniae	60%-75%	3%-9%
Haemophilus influenzae	4%-5%	
Legionella sp.	2%-5%	Up to 25%
Staphylococcus aureus	1%-5%	10%-20%
Gram-negative bacilli	Rare	50%
Atypical	**10%-20%**	**Rare**
Mycoplasma pneumoniae	5%-18%	—
Chlamydia psittaci	2%-3%	—
Coxiella burnetii	1%	—
Virus	**10%-20%**	**Rare**
Influenza virus	—	8%
Hantavirus	—	Rare

Adapted from Modai J: Empiric therapy of severe infections in adults. Am J Med 88:12S-17S, 1990.

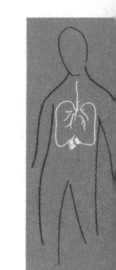

An important decision in the care of community-acquired pneumonia is whether the patient requires hospital admission. This decision should take into consideration the known risk factors for increased mortality from pneumonia. These include age 65 years or older; the presence of co-morbidities such as diabetes mellitus, renal, or congestive heart failure; altered mental status; tachycardia (>125 beats per minute); tachypnea (>30 breaths per minute); high fever (>38.3° to 40° C); hypotension (systolic blood pressure < 90 mm Hg); hypoxia (Sao_2 < 90% or Pao_2 < 60 mm Hg); multilobar involvement on chest radiograph; and identification of high-risk pathogens such as gram-negative organisms and S. aureus. For hospitalized patients, initial therapy for community-acquired pneumonia usually includes a cephalosporin such as ceftriaxone or cefuroxime, with or without a macrolide. Antibiotic treatment should be given as soon as possible because mortality can increase even after a short delay (>8 hours) in receiving appropriate antibiotics. Sputum and blood cultures should be obtained before instituting antibiotic therapy.

community-acquired pneumonia is designed to cover this organism (see later).

M. pneumoniae is a slow-growing, facultative anaerobic organism that accounts for 25% to 60% of all atypical pneumonias. M. pneumoniae is a common cause of pneumonia in patients between the ages of 5 and 35 years who may initially exhibit upper respiratory tract symptoms, pharyngitis, and bullous myringitis. Dry cough, fever, gastrointestinal symptoms, headache, and myalgias are common. Uncommon complications include cold agglutinin–induced hemolysis, hepatitis, erythema multiforme, the syndrome of inappropriate antidiuretic hormone, pericarditis, myocarditis, and neurologic abnormalities. The chest radiograph may show fine interstitial reticulonodular infiltrates in patients, which are often relatively asymptomatic. The diagnosis is based on clinical and epidemiologic features. Acute and convalescent serologic findings are required to confirm the diagnosis, but are not helpful during the acute illness.

Other common causes of community-acquired pneumonia are C. pneumoniae and Haemophilus influenzae. Patients with co-morbid conditions and those older than 65 years are also at risk for pneumonia from Legionella species, Staphylococcus aureus, and gram-negative organisms. Anaerobic infection should be considered when large amounts of oropharyngeal secretions are aspirated and in patients with chronic infections in the gingivodental crevice.

Diagnostic tests for community-acquired pneumonia should include a chest radiograph and complete blood count. The role of routine sputum and blood cultures in this setting is controversial. The recommended treatment for community-acquired pneumonia is a course (7 to 10 days) of a macrolide antibiotic (erythromycin, clarithromycin, or azithromycin). If there are co-morbidities such as chronic heart or lung disease, an extended spectrum fluoroquinolone (e.g., levofloxacin, moxifloxacin, or gemifloxacin) or a β lactam (amoxicillin) plus a macrolide should be used. The choice of treatment should also be influenced by local antibiotic resistance patterns.

Nosocomial Pneumonia

Nosocomial pneumonia is pneumonia that occurs after hospitalization. Nosocomial pneumonia is subdivided into three categories: hospital-acquired pneumonia (HAP); ventilator-associated pneumonia (VAP); and health care–associated pneumonia (HCAP). HAP is defined as pneumonia that occurs 48 hours or more after admission and that did not appear to be incubating at the time of admission. VAP is a type of HAP that develops more than 48 to 72 hours after endotracheal intubation. HCAP is defined as pneumonia that occurs in a nonhospitalized patient with extensive health care contact. This includes recent hospitalization, residence in a nursing home or other long-term care facility, and recent intravenous therapy. These patients should be considered at high risk for resistant organisms and therefore inappropriate for routine, empirical therapy for community-acquired pneumonia.

Nosocomial pneumonia is the second most common infection in hospitalized patients and the most common infection in the intensive care unit. The pathogenesis of nosocomial pneumonia is based on colonization of the oropharynx and stomach with virulent pathogens and the subsequent aspiration of these organisms into the lower respiratory tract. Gastric colonization by gram-negative organisms is enhanced by neutralization of gastric acidity. In the first 5 days of hospitalization, H. influenzae, S. pneumoniae, and S. aureus are often isolated. After this time, pneumonia is often caused by Pseudomonas aeruginosa, S. aureus, anaerobic microbes, Acinetobacter species, and various gram-negative enteric bacilli. This finding has important therapeutic implications because these organisms are more commonly associated with multidrug antibiotic resistance. Treatment is dependent on combined chemotherapy with β lactam antipseudomonal penicillin or cephalosporin, together with an aminoglycoside or a quinolone. Vancomycin is added if methicillin-resistant S. aureus is suspected. A more definitive identification of organisms and their sensitivity to antibiotics is often sought in these patients using more invasive measures, including endotracheal aspirate in intubated patients or flexible fiberoptic bronchoscopy. However, the best predictor of patient outcome with nosocomial pneumonia appears to be adequacy of the initial empirical antibiotic regimen.

Complications of Pneumonia

Parapneumonic effusion is a neutrophilic exudative effusion adjacent to a lung with pneumonia (**Web Fig. 22-2**). It can resolve with antibiotics alone or can require drainage in addition to antibiotics. As a pneumonia progresses, inflammatory pulmonary liquid leaks into the pleural space, first appearing as an uncomplicated effusion. At this point, the effusion will resolve with antibiotic therapy alone. As bacteria and inflammatory cells follow, the inflammatory process is marked by anaerobic metabolism, cytokine production, fibrin deposition in the pleural space, and thickening of the pleura. There is no universally accepted definition of *empyema*. However, most clinicians include in the term empyema all pleural effusions that are grossly purulent or contain microorganisms identified by a positive Gram stain or culture. Empyema must always be treated with pleural drainage, usually by a chest thoracostomy tube. Highly inflammatory parapneumonic effusions may behave as if they are infected, although microorganisms are never identified. There have been effusions described as "complicated" parapneumonic effusions, and these are identified clinically by a pH of less than 7.1 and a glucose level of less than 40 mg/dL. It is important to recognize that complicated effusions generally require drainage in addition to antibiotic therapy.

The major risk factor for the development of *lung abscess* is aspiration resulting in a more indolent, polymicrobial infection, usually involving both aerobes and anaerobes. Conditions predisposing patients to aspiration, such as alcoholism, seizures, or stroke, are associated with an increased incidence of lung abscess. The presence of poor dentition increases the anaerobic bacterial load in the mouth and thus the likelihood of infection after an aspiration event. For aspiration-related infection, the antibiotic chosen should reflect the predominance of anaerobes. In trials of empirical therapy for lung abscess, clindamycin showed superiority over penicillin, probably because the incidence of penicillin-resistant anaerobes in lung abscesses is 15% to 20%. Antibiotics should be continued for 6 weeks, and drainage should be reserved for very large abscesses or failure to resolve with antibiotics.

Mycobacterium Tuberculosis Infection

Infection with *Mycobacterium tuberculosis,* an aerobic, nonmotile, acid-fast rod with niacin production, causes TB. In 1997, the World Health Organization Global Surveillance and Monitoring Project estimated 8 million new cases per year of TB, including 3.5 million cases of infectious pulmonary disease. In addition, 16.2 million cases of the disease existed. An estimated 1.87 million individuals die from TB each year, and the global case-fatality rate was 23%, with 50% in some African countries with high HIV rates. In the United States, TB increased at an alarming rate in the early 1990s as a result of the surge of HIV infection, drug abuse, inner-city poverty, and homelessness.

TB infection occurs when aerosolized, contaminated droplets (expectorated by a diseased person) are inhaled by another individual and the droplet or droplet nuclei reaches an alveolus. This is almost always a latent infection, called *latent tuberculosis infection* (LTBI). If the innate immune system of the host fails to eliminate the latent infection, the bacilli proliferate inside alveolar macrophages and kill the cells. The infected macrophages produce cytokines and chemokines that attract other phagocytic cells, including monocytes, other alveolar macrophages, and neutrophils, which eventually form a nodular granulomatous structure called the *tubercle*. If the bacterial replication is not controlled, the tubercle enlarges, and the bacilli enter the local draining lymph nodes. This leads to lymphadenopathy, a characteristic manifestation of primary TB. The lesion produced by the expansion of the tubercle into the lung parenchyma and lymph node involvement is called the *Ghon complex*. The bacilli continue to proliferate until an effective cell-mediated immune (CMI) response develops, usually 2 to 6 weeks after infection. Failure by the host to mount an effective CMI response and tissue repair leads to progressive destruction of the lung. Bacterial products, tumor necrosis factor-α, macrophage antimicrobial effector molecules such as reactive oxygen intermediates (ROI) and reactive nitrogen intermediates (RNI), and the contents of cytotoxic cells (granzymes, perforin) all can contribute to the development of caseating necrosis that characterizes a tuberculous granuloma (Fig. 22-1).

If mycobacterial growth is unchecked, the bacilli may spread hematogenously to produce disseminated TB. Miliary

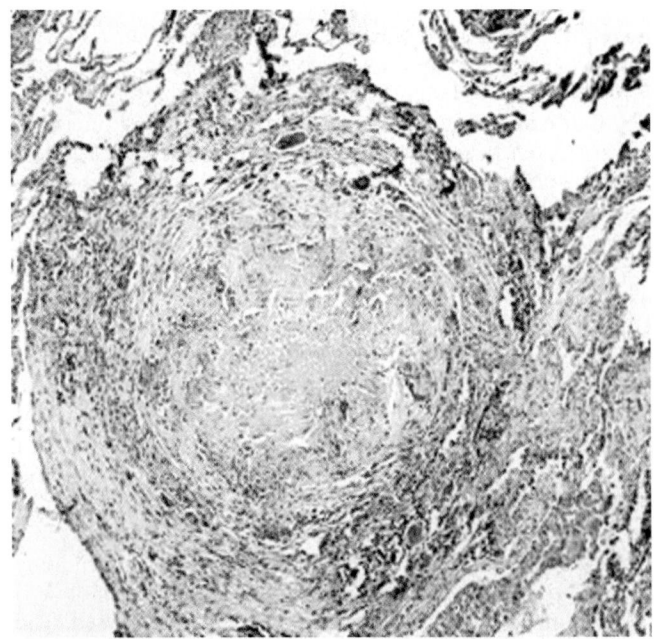

Figure 22-1 Necrotizing granuloma in lung infected with *Mycobacterium tuberculosis.*

TB is a disseminated form with lesions resembling millet seeds. Bacilli can also spread mechanically by erosion of the caseating lesions into the lung airways. It is at this point that the host becomes infectious to others. If untreated, 80% of patients will die. Others will develop chronic disease or recover spontaneously. The chronic disease is characterized by repeated episodes of spontaneous healing with fibrotic changes around the lesions and tissue breakdown. Healing by complete spontaneous eradication of the bacilli is rare.

Reactivation TB results when the persistent bacteria in a host suddenly proliferate. Only 5% to 10% of patients with no underlying medical problems who become infected develop reactivation disease in their lifetime. Although immunosuppression is clearly associated with reactivation TB, it is not clear what host factors specifically maintain the infection in a latent state for many years and what triggers the latent infection to become overt.

The diagnosis of latent TB infection is dependent on a positive tuberculin test, which does not necessarily indicate active disease, but only previous infection. The standard Mantoux test is an intradermal injection of 0.1 mL (5 tuberculin units) of purified protein derivative (PPD) tuberculin in the skin of the forearm. The injection site is evaluated 48 to 72 hours later. The reading is based on the diameter of the indurated or swollen area. Patients are at high risk for developing active TB early after tuberculin conversion, and thus treatment is recommended for LTBI. The risk for active disease is 5% within 2 years of exposure and another 5% per year thereafter. HIV patients are an exception and have a 40% risk for active disease within several months of conversion. The current recommendations as to what constitutes a positive PPD test take into account the degree of clinical suspicion of LTBI (Table 22-2).

Treatment of patients suspected of having active disease includes at least four drugs—isoniazid, 5 mg/kg per day; rifampin, 10 mg/kg per day; ethambutol, 5 to 25 mg/kg per day; pyrazinamide, 15 to 30 mg/kg per day—and should be considered before a formal diagnosis is made. Factors suggesting active disease include exposure to active TB, pulmonary symptoms, and cavitary disease on imaging studies. If the diagnosis of TB is confirmed, the drugs are continued for 2 months, barring adverse reactions to drug therapy. After 2 months, the regimen can be tailored, depending on drug-sensitivity studies, and continued for another 4 months with at least two active drugs. Rates of drug-resistant TB are increased in certain populations (e.g., recent immigrants from high TB areas, homeless people).

Resistance is detected in 9% of patients who have not received previous therapy and in 22.8% of those with prior treatment. In patients with drug-resistant TB, treatment should include at least three drugs that have not been administered before and to which the organism is susceptible in vitro. Treatment should continue for at least 18 to 24 months. Direct observation of therapy is recommended to ensure compliance.

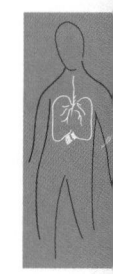

Pneumocystis Pneumonia

Pneumocystis jiroveci, formerly called *pneumocystis carinii* (PCP), is an opportunistic fungus that occurred mainly in malnourished premature infants and in adults with hematologic malignancy undergoing chemotherapy in the pre–acquired immunodeficiency syndrome (AIDS) era. However, its incidence rose significantly in the late 1980s and 1990s in patients with AIDS with low CD4$^+$ lymphocyte counts (<250 cells/m^2). Patients may complain of nonproductive cough, fever, dyspnea, and weight loss. The symptoms are slowly progressive over weeks in the patient infected with HIV. Oral candidiasis, increased serum lactic dehydrogenase (LDH), increased Aa-oxygen gradient, and a decreased CD4$^+$ count are independent predictors of HIV-related pneumocystis pneumonia.

Chest radiographic images may show diffuse, bilateral interstitial infiltrates, but they may be clear in up to 15% of patients (**Web Fig. 22-3**). Other findings include isolated infiltrates, cavitary lesions, nodular masses, pneumothorax, and a military pattern. Hilar and mediastinal adenopathy are rare. Identifying the organism in sputum, which is effective in 60% to 85% of patients, will help with diagnosis. Bronchoscopy with bronchoalveolar lavage can increase the yield (86%), especially if a transbronchial biopsy is included (98% to 100%).

Prophylaxis can be provided by oral trimethoprim-sulfamethoxazole or aerosolized pentamidine. When pneumonia is present, the therapy of choice is trimethoprim-sulfamethoxazole. However, significant adverse effects, including leukopenia, nausea, vomiting, and elevation of liver transaminases, are associated with this therapy. Intravenous pentamidine is a reasonable alternative to trimethoprim-sulfamethoxazole, but this therapy could be complicated by hypoglycemia. Less toxic drug regimens are available (e.g., trimethoprim and dapsone, clindamycin and primaquine), but these are recommended only after failure of other medications. Corticosteroids should be considered in patients with severe disease as demonstrated by significant hypoxemia (e.g., Pao$_2$ < 70 mm Hg). Corticosteroids decrease the likelihood of progression to respiratory failure.

PPD	Prophylaxis Indicated Regardless of Age	Prophylaxis Indicated if <35 Years Old
5 mm	Close contacts recently diagnosed with TB HIV positive or HIV risk factors Fibrotic changes on chest radiograph	
10 mm	Diabetes mellitus Immunosuppression Hematologic malignancy Injection drug use Renal failure Malnutrition	PPD increased >10 mm within 2 yr Native of high-prevalence country High-risk ethnic minorities Residents and staff of long-term care facilities
15 mm	PPD increased >15 mm within 2 yr	No risk factors

Table 22-2 Prophylaxis against Tuberculosis in Adults

HIV, human immunodeficiency virus; PPD, purified protein derivative of tuberculin; TB, tuberculosis.

Prospectus for the Future

Lung infection continues to represent a source of high morbidity and mortality rates, both in the community and in health care settings. A significant portion of these infections affect the extremes of age—children and older adults. Although industry continues to search for new antibiotics with higher safety and effectiveness profiles, the judicious use of agents currently available will help prevent or delay drug resistance while newer agents are being developed.

Continued efforts are needed to reinforce vaccination against infectious agents including influenza and *Streptococcus pneumoniae*. HIV infection and tuberculosis continue to be public health problems in the United States, but are particularly a problem in Africa, where effective HIV therapy is less available. This was highlighted by the identification of extensively drug-resistant tuberculosis (XDR-Tb), which is caused by a strain of *M. tuberculosis* that is resistant to many available anti-mycobacterial agents and is difficult to cure. Emerging organisms present new challenges.

On March 15, 2003, worldwide attention was drawn to Severe Acute Respiratory Syndrome (SARS) by the World Health Organization (WHO), with descriptions of cases of a rapidly progressive respiratory illness in the Guangdong province of China, Hong Kong, Vietnam, Singapore, and Canada.

There have been four influenza pandemics during the past century, and each has been caused by the emergence of a novel influenza virus. In the 1957 and 1968 pandemics, the new viruses contained components of previous human and avian influenza viruses. Sporadic transmission of avian influenza H5N1 to more than 350 humans since 2004 has prompted concerns that conditions are suitable for emergence of the next pandemic. Estimates of potential global mortality related to pandemic avian influenza are as high as 62 million deaths, and presently there is no specific treatment available. In 2009 the H1N1 ("swine") influenza virus emerged in Mexico, has spread world-wide, and is officially termed a pandemic by the WHO. At least initially, H1N1 has been complicated by relatively low mortality, but it is possible that this influenza virus may mutate to produce more severe disease in humans.

References

Blumberg HM, Burman WJ, Chaisson RE, et al: American Thoracic Society/Centers for Disease Control and Prevention/Infectious Diseases Society of America: Treatment of tuberculosis. Am J Respir Crit Care Med 167: 603, 2003.

Guidelines for the management of adults with hospital acquired, ventilator-associated, and healthcare-associated pneumonia. Am J Respir Crit Care Med 171:388, 2005.

Kollef MH, Morrow LE, Baughman RP, et al: Health-care associated pneumonia (HCAP): A critical appraisal to improve identification, management, and outcomes. Proceedings of the HCAP summit. Clin Infect Dis 46:S295, 2008.

Kovacs JA, Gill VJ, Meshnick S, Masur H: New insights into transmission, diagnosis, and drug treatment of *Pneumocystis carinii* pneumonia. JAMA 286:2450, 2001.

Maher D, Raviglione M: Global epidemiology of tuberculosis. Clin Chest Med 26:167, 2005.

Mandell LA, Wunderink RG, Anzueto A, et al: Infectious Diseases Society of America/American Thoracic Society consensus guidelines on the management of community-acquired pneumonia in adults. Clin Infect Dis 44S:S27, 2007.

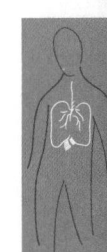

Essentials in Critical Care Medicine

Brian Casserly and Sharon Rounds

Critical care medicine has evolved dramatically during the past decades because of the development of new technologies as well as clinical trials that have established standards for the management of patients in the critical care setting. Since the epidemic of poliomyelitis in the 1950s, intensive care units have clearly proved beneficial in treating acute reversible disorders. However, because of the innovative nature of the technology used and the need for close monitoring and intensive management, the delivery of critical care medicine is expensive, accounting for up to 30% of total hospital costs.

Patients in intensive care units (ICUs) are a heterogeneous population treated for diverse conditions ranging from septic shock and respiratory failure to diabetic ketoacidosis and upper gastrointestinal bleeding. This chapter discusses a few of the most common conditions encountered in the ICU setting that are often managed by pulmonologists. These topics include acute respiratory failure and mechanical ventilation, acute lung injury, and shock.

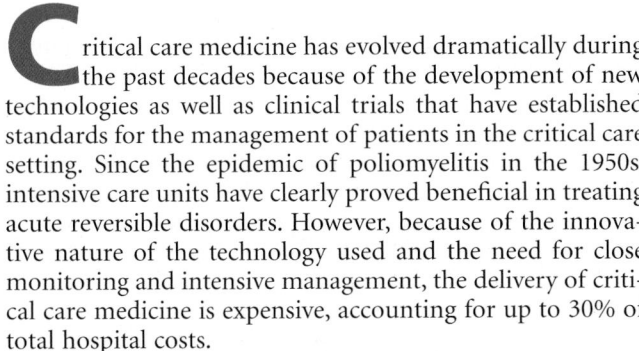

Acute Respiratory Failure and Mechanical Ventilation

Acute respiratory failure results when the lung can no longer accomplish adequate gas exchange, a condition that is fatal if left untreated. Hypoxemic respiratory failure refers to respiratory failure associated with failure to oxygenate, whereas hypercarbic respiratory failure is the failure to ventilate. These disorders are manifested by alterations in arterial partial pressure of oxygen (Pao_2) and carbon dioxide ($Paco_2$), respectively. The values of Pao_2 and $Paco_2$ that define respiratory failure are somewhat arbitrary, but respiratory compromise is evident when the Pao_2 is less than 60 mm Hg while the patient breathes room air or the $Paco_2$ is higher than 45 mm Hg. It is important to recognize that these values are not synonymous with the need for mechani-

cal ventilation, nor do they preclude the need for mechanical ventilation.

The management of respiratory failure depends on the clinical presentation. Patients with respiratory failure who are awake, cooperative, and hemodynamically stable may tolerate aggressive respiratory therapy, without intubation and mechanical ventilation, as long as gas exchange and overall status are continually monitored. This setting often describes patients with chronic obstructive pulmonary disease (COPD) who can sometimes tolerate a $Paco_2$ level as high as 85 mm Hg, which can occur in the absence of severe respiratory acidosis. In contrast, patients in respiratory failure with evidence of severe respiratory distress (e.g., respiratory rate >30 breaths per minute), mental deterioration (e.g., impaired judgment, confusion, hallucinations, somnolence), or hemodynamic instability (e.g., bradydysrhythmias or tachydysrhythmias, hypotension) usually require intubation and mechanical ventilation. In the latter circumstances, waiting for arterial blood gas determinations is not necessary and could dangerously delay therapy. Although arterial blood gas evaluation is crucial when determining the need for mechanical ventilation in the patient with respiratory failure, the patient's clinical status will ultimately dictate the course of action.

Mechanical Ventilation

Mechanical ventilation primarily uses the principals of positive pressure ventilation. Air is forced into the central airways, increasing central airway pressure. Air follows the pressure gradient from the central airways to the alveoli, which inflates the lungs. As the lungs inflate and the device stops forcing air into the central airways, the intra-alveolar pressure increases and central airway pressure decreases. Exhalation occurs when the air follows the newly reversed pressure gradient from the alveoli to the central airways.

The principal benefits of mechanical ventilation during respiratory failure are improved gas exchange and decreased work of breathing. Mechanical ventilation improves gas exchange by improving ventilation-perfusion ratio ($\dot{V}/\dot{Q}$) matching. The improved $\dot{V}/\dot{Q}$ matching is primarily a consequence of decreased physiologic shunting. Altered lung mechanics (e.g., increased airways resistance, decreased compliance) and increased respiratory demand (e.g., metabolic acidosis) increase the work of breathing. The ventilatory muscles and diaphragm can tire while trying to maintain the elevated work of breathing, resulting in respiratory failure. Mechanical ventilation can assume some or all of the increased work of breathing, allowing the ventilatory muscles to recover from their fatigue. Deteriorating gas exchange, unresponsive to conservative measures, and respiratory distress are the most common reasons for mechanical ventilation in patients with acute respiratory failure.

NONINVASIVE MECHANICAL VENTILATION

Although intubation and mechanical ventilation are usually the preferred options in respiratory failure that is considered reversible, noninvasive positive-pressure ventilation (NPPV) has proved useful in selected patients. NPPV refers to positive-pressure ventilation delivered through a noninvasive interface (nasal mask, facemask, or nasal plugs), rather than an invasive interface (endotracheal tube, tracheostomy). Its use has become more common as benefits are increasingly recognized. Selecting patients for NPPV requires careful consideration of its indications and contraindications. Generally speaking, a trial of NPPV is worthwhile in patients with acute cardiogenic pulmonary edema or hypercapnic respiratory failure due to COPD who do not require emergent intubation and do not have contraindications to NPPV. Contraindications to NPPV include cardiac or respiratory arrest; inability to cooperate, protect the airway, or clear secretions; severely impaired consciousness; facial surgery, trauma, or deformity; anticipated prolonged duration of mechanical ventilation; and recent esophageal anastomosis.

INVASIVE MECHANICAL VENTILATION

Once a decision to intubate is made, an experienced operator should expeditiously perform intubation. Complications of intubation are usually related to prolonged hypoxemia as a result of delays in the procedure, but they also include vomiting and aspiration of gastric contents, trauma to the vocal cords, bleeding, pneumothorax, cardiac arrhythmias, and cardiac arrest. Once inserted, the endotracheal tube should be secured and its position assessed by examining for breath sounds, followed by chest radiography for confirmation. Direct visualization through a bronchoscope is occasionally needed for successful intubation. A ventilator should be available before the procedure is begun so that mechanical ventilation can start as soon as the endotracheal tube is secured.

Initial ventilator settings may vary, but typically they include a ventilator mode, fraction of inspired oxygen (FIO_2) of 1 (or 100%), respiratory rate set at 10 to 12 breaths per minute, and tidal volume of 400 to 600 mL. The adequacy of the ventilator settings needs to be determined with repeated arterial blood gas levels and the clinical evaluation of the patient. Persistent cyanosis, pallor, diaphoresis, and restlessness may suggest that the tube is misplaced or that

the ventilator settings are insufficient to ventilate the patient appropriately. Positive end-expiratory pressure (PEEP) might be required in patients with refractory hypoxemia. PEEP prevents the premature collapse of the alveoli during expiration and improves $\dot{V}/\dot{Q}$ matching, leading to improved oxygenation. Once the settings are adjusted to maintain relatively normal levels of arterial blood gases (pH, 7.3 to 7.45; $Pao_2 > 60$ mm Hg; Pco_2, 30 to 45 mm Hg), attention should be given to developing a *maintenance* plan that will secure adequate oxygenation and ventilation until the cause of the respiratory failure is treated and the failure is reversed. This plan should include assessment of the need for sedation, appropriate strategy of mechanical ventilation, supportive measures to achieve hemodynamic stability, nutritional assessment, and therapies targeting the initial injurious process that triggered the respiratory failure (e.g., pneumonia, pulmonary embolism, asthma, shock). Most patients require sedation to diminish discomfort and to decrease the work of breathing, but it should be administered carefully because sedation is often accompanied by a decrease in blood pressure.

Commonly used modes of ventilation are determined by the duration of inspiration, which can be limited by volume, pressure, flow, or time. During volume-limited ventilation, inspiration ends after delivery of a preset tidal volume. Airway pressure is variable during volume-limited ventilation and is related to respiratory system compliance, airway resistance, and tubing resistance. *Assist control* (AC), *continuous mandatory ventilation* (CMV), and *synchronized intermittent mandatory ventilation* (SIMV) are examples of modes of ventilation that can be volume limited. CMV has a set rate and set tidal volume which does not allow spontaneous breathing by the patient. Patient-ventilator asynchrony is a big problem, and therefore CMV is rarely used. The assist-control mode of ventilation is similar to CMV in that there is a set rate and tidal volume, but this mode allows the patient to initiate additional spontaneous breaths. When the machine senses that the patient is attempting to take a breath, it delivers the selected tidal volume. SIMV is similar to assist-control in that a set rate and tidal volume are selected. The patient is also able to generate a spontaneous breath. However, this spontaneous breath may have a very small tidal volume, yet entail significant work of breathing. Consequently, this mode of mechanical ventilation is seldom used except when weaning patients from mechanical ventilation.

The pressure control mode of ventilation uses machine breaths that are pressure cycled, not volume cycled. With pressure control ventilation, the pressure to be used for each breath is ordered. If the patient attempts a spontaneous breath, a machine breath at the designated pressure is delivered. This may be helpful in limiting airway pressures in patients with bronchospasm or stiff lungs because it limits the risk for pneumothorax (barotrauma). Because tidal volumes may vary, the pressure control mode must be titrated carefully at the bedside to determine the proper pressure settings.

Pressure support ventilation is used only for spontaneously breathing patients. The inspiratory and expiratory pressures are selected, and there are no mandatory machine breaths. Patients find this to be a more comfortable mode of mechanical ventilation. However, pressure support ventilation should only be used for patients with a stable respiratory drive (not sedated heavily) and stable lung compliance. Pressure support ventilation is typically used for patients who are weaning from mechanical ventilator support.

Pressure-regulated volume control, airway pressure release ventilation, and high-frequency ventilation are newer modalities that are increasingly used in clinical practice.

SETTINGS

Numerous settings need to be considered when mechanical ventilation is initiated. These include tidal volume, respiratory rate, trigger mode and sensitivity, fraction of inspired oxygen, PEEP, flow rate, and flow pattern.

The appropriate initial *tidal volume* depends on numerous factors, most notably the disease for which the patient requires mechanical ventilation. The tidal volume can then be increased or decreased incrementally to achieve the desired pH and arterial carbon dioxide tension ($Paco_2$). Generally speaking, large tidal volumes can cause barotrauma or volutrauma, which increases the risk for ventilator-associated lung injury. Therefore, tidal volume should not be increased without considering effects on airway pressure or the likelihood of ventilator-induced lung injury.

An optimal method for setting the *respiratory rate* has not been established. Once the tidal volume has been established, the respiratory rate can be incrementally increased or decreased to achieve the desired pH and $Paco_2$, while monitoring auto-PEEP. Patients who are breathing spontaneously will set their own respiratory rates in all modes of ventilation except CMV.

The lowest possible *fraction of inspired oxygen* (Fio_2) necessary to meet oxygenation goals should be used. This will decrease the likelihood that adverse consequences of supplemental oxygen will develop, such as absorption atelectasis, accentuation of hypercapnia, airway injury, and parenchymal lung injury.

PEEP is generally added to prevent end-expiratory alveolar collapse. This generally improves $\dot{V}/\dot{Q}$ matching and arterial oxygenation and allows reduction in Fio_2, thereby reducing the risk for oxygen toxicity. However, elevated levels of applied PEEP can have adverse consequences, such as reduced preload (decreases cardiac output), elevated plateau airway pressure (increases risk for barotrauma), and impaired cerebral venous outflow (increases intracranial pressure). The optimal PEEP is that which enhances oxygenation without lung hyperinflation and decreased blood pressure.

Respiratory therapists typically also adjust the inspiratory flow rate, flow pattern, and amount of negative pressure required to "trigger" a mechanical ventilator breath. If these ventilator settings are not adjusted with due consideration of the patient's respiratory mechanics, two common problems can occur: *asynchrony* and *auto-PEEP*. Patient-ventilator asynchrony occurs if the phases of breaths delivered by the ventilator do not match the breathing pattern of the patient. Patient-ventilator asynchrony can cause dyspnea, increase the work of breathing, and prolong the duration of mechanical ventilation. It is detected by careful observation of the patient and examination of the ventilator waveforms. Generally, the abnormality that is most readily apparent is failure of the ventilator to trigger a breath when the patient makes an inspiratory effort. Auto-PEEP is usually seen when patients are not fully emptying their lungs during expiration before the initiation of the next breath. This is known as *stacking breaths* or generating auto-PEEP. This is particularly worrisome in patients who have exacerbations of COPD or status asthmaticus requiring mechanical ventilation. In ventilated patients, auto-PEEP may cause barotrauma or hemodynamic collapse owing to high intrathoracic pressures preventing blood return to the right ventricle.

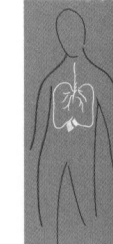

Weaning from Mechanical Ventilation

The complications of endotracheal intubation and mechanical ventilation are many; trauma to the lung from high ventilator pressures (barotrauma), volutrauma and ventilator-induced lung injury, and pneumonia are the most significant. Therefore, the patient who is mechanically ventilated must be treated aggressively and monitored carefully. Weaning from mechanical ventilation should be considered when the original insult that caused respiratory failure has cleared, especially if the patient is awake and cooperative and shows no signs of respiratory or hemodynamic instability. Weaning is usually not attempted if requirements for oxygen supplementation remain high ($Fio_2 > 0.5$). Conventional parameters that determine whether weaning is possible include negative inspiratory force, vital capacity, tidal volume, respiratory rate, and minute ventilation (Table 23-1). Unfortunately, the strength of these parameters lies in the ability to predict failure to wean rather than in the ability to predict successful spontaneous breathing. A better way to assess weaning capability is to engage the patient in a short *weaning trial* during which support from the ventilator is diminished. This trial can be achieved by allowing the patient to breathe oxygen for 1 hour without providing supporting pressure. Another strategy is to decrease the pressure generated by the ventilator during a trial of continuous positive airway pressure (CPAP). The patient is monitored for any signs of distress or hemodynamic instability, and arterial blood gas levels are measured to determine the effectiveness of spontaneous ventilation. If the patient tolerates the trial, extubation may be indicated, depending on the patient's clinical status and his or her underlying condition. In general,

Table 23-1 Conventional Weaning Parameters

Parameters	Weanable Values	Normal Ranges
NIF (cm of water)	<−20	<−50
VC (mL/kg)	>10	>65-75
V_T (mL/kg)	<5	>5-7
RR (breaths/min)	<32	12-20
V_E (L/min)	>10	>10
Rapid shallow breathing index (RSBI) (RR/V_T)	<105	<40

NIF, negative inspiratory force; RR, respiratory rate; VC, vital capacity; V_E, minute ventilation; V_T, tidal volume.

only 10% to 15% of patients who are extubated on the basis of the results of these trials require reintubation.

If the patient fails the weaning trial, attempts should be made to identify the factors responsible for the failure to wean. In very sick patients, all obvious contributory factors may have been identified and corrected, but the patient still requires a more prolonged weaning trial before extubation. Two weaning strategies are recommended in this setting. The first is to engage the patient in spontaneous ventilation trials without positive pressure for 1 hour once or twice each day with total ventilatory support between trials, usually through assisted-control ventilation. The length of the spontaneous breathing trials can be progressively increased until the patient no longer requires mechanical support. The other strategy uses pressure support ventilation. The inspiratory pressure is progressively decreased until the patient can breathe spontaneously without ventilatory support. Both strategies appear to be equally effective, although weaning through pressure support ventilation might be preferred in patients with chronic lung disease who have been mechanically ventilated for prolonged periods.

Acute Lung Injury

Acute lung injury in its most severe form is called *acute respiratory distress syndrome* (ARDS). Acute lung injury is characterized by increased permeability of the alveolar-capillary membrane leading to flooding of the alveolar spaces with proteinaceous material. ARDS is defined by clinical measures of the severity of lung dysfunction (e.g., Pao_2/Fio_2). This process is triggered by direct injury to the lung, as observed in aspiration pneumonia, smoke inhalation, and a near-drowning event, or systemic injury such as trauma, surgery, sepsis, burns, long-bone fractures, pancreatitis, uremia, transfusion therapy, shock, drug intoxication, or cardiopulmonary bypass. About 150,000 cases of ARDS are reported each year in the United States, and aspiration pneumonia and sepsis are the most common associated conditions. The morbidity rate associated with ARDS is high, and about 30% to 50% of patients die.

ARDS is the pulmonary manifestation of a systemic disorder that appears to trigger a dysregulated inflammatory response to injury. Uncontrolled inflammation causes injury to the pulmonary vascular endothelium and epithelium, which results in increased permeability of both physiologic barriers, allowing the extravasation of proteinaceous edema fluid from the intravascular space and its accumulation into the lung interstitium and alveolar spaces (**Web Fig. 23-1**). Injury to the lung epithelium results in decreased absorption of water from the alveolar space. This condition is often referred to as *noncardiogenic* or *increased permeability pulmonary edema*. In the lung, these processes cause right-to-left intrapulmonary shunting of blood, resulting in refractory hypoxemia, and decreased lung compliance that increases the work of breathing. The chest radiograph reveals diffuse bilateral alveolar infiltrates (**Web Fig. 23-2**). Failure of other organs is frequent; consequently, multiorgan failure is common, especially in the setting of sepsis.

Histologically, ARDS is characterized by diffuse alveolar damage with hyaline membranes (**Web Fig. 23-3**). The damage is further exaggerated by reductions in the quantity and quality of the synthesized surfactant leading to atelectasis. After a few days, the tissue shows hyperplasia of type II pneumocytes (**Web Fig. 23-4**) and deposition of connective tissue resulting in fibrosis. These events can be worsened by mechanical ventilation through positive pressure, hyperdistention, and hyperoxia.

A diagnosis of ARDS should be considered in patients with a predisposing condition (e.g., sepsis), bilateral pulmonary infiltrates on chest radiograph, and refractory hypoxemia (i.e., usually a Pao_2/Fio_2 of 200 mm Hg or less), in the absence of significant cardiac dysfunction. Currently, the treatment of ARDS relies on supportive measures directed at eradicating the injurious agent, sustaining the cardiovascular system, providing nutrition, and avoiding fluid overload. Recently, a ventilatory management strategy designed to deliver low-tidal volumes (about 6 mL/kg body weight) has proved beneficial, resulting in increased survival. Corticosteroids, surfactant replacement, and extracorporeal oxygenation have not proved beneficial and are not recommended. Oxygenation can be improved by PEEP and prone ventilation, but these interventions do not appear to affect the natural course of the disease. Because there is no available therapy that lessens acute lung injury or hastens repair, the key to care of patients with ARDS is meticulous supportive care and avoidance of complications, such as ventilator-associated pneumonia or catheter-related sepsis.

Shock

Shock is defined as systemic organ hypoperfusion, usually associated with hypotension, which leads to cell injury and death. Four classifications are provided: (1) cardiogenic shock (i.e., decreased cardiac output as a result of dysfunction), (2) hypovolemic shock (i.e., decreased intravascular volume), (3) septic or redistributive shock (i.e., decreased systemic vascular resistance), and (4) obstructive shock (i.e., decreased cardiac output as a result of obstruction to flow). (Anaphylactic shock caused by an allergic reaction to a drug or a related insult is not discussed in this text.)

When encountering a patient in shock, the strategy is to gain vascular access quickly and to replace volume aggressively while making a careful assessment of the situation. This strategy is particularly appropriate when shock is thought to be the result of hypovolemia or sepsis. In the case of cardiogenic shock, strategies designed to improve cardiac function should be implemented, including administration of inotropic drugs or, in severe unresponsive cases, cardiac bypass or cardiac-assist devices. In the case of severe hypovolemia, administration of saline is usually sufficient. With sepsis, fluid replacement, antibiotic therapy, and drainage of any infected space are paramount. In select patients in whom severe sepsis is diagnosed early, intravascular administration of a recombinant version of activated protein C (drotrecogin alfa [activated]) has been shown to improve survival. Obstructive shock is the result of obstruction to blood flow, as observed in massive pulmonary embolism or *saddle embolus* lodged at the bifurcation of the right and left pulmonary arteries. In this setting, relieving the obstruction mechanically or through other methods (e.g., thrombolysis) or supporting the patient's circulation until the obstruction subsides is important.

Table 23-2 Useful Resting Hemodynamic Parameters (Pulmonary Artery Catheter)

Parameters	Normal Ranges
Right atrial pressure or central venous pressure	0-5 mm Hg
Right ventricular pressure (systolic/diastolic)	25/0-5 mm Hg
Pulmonary artery pressure (systolic/diastolic)	25/8-12 mm Hg
Pulmonary capillary wedge pressure	8-12 mm Hg
Cardiac output	3.5-7 L/min
Cardiac index	2.5-4.5 L/min/m^2
Oxygen consumption	200-250 mL/min
Arteriovenous oxygen content	3.5-5.5 mL/100 mL
Mixed venous oxygen content	18 mL/100 mL
Mixed venous oxygen saturation	75%
Stroke volume	70-130 mL/beat
Stroke volume index	40-50 mL/beat/m^2
Left ventricular stroke work index	45-60 g/beat/m^2
Systemic vascular resistance	800-1200 dyne/sec/cm^{-5}
Pulmonary vascular resistance	150-250 dyne/sec/cm^{-5}

Table 23-3 Equations to Calculate Derived Parameters

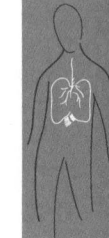

$$CO = \frac{VA}{(CaO_2 - CvO_2)}$$

$$CI = \frac{CO}{\text{Body surface area (BSA)}(m^2)}$$

Oxygen content (CxO_2) = % saturation × Hgb (g/dL) × 1.39 + $(PxO_2 × 0.003)$

Oxygen delivery (DO_2) (mL/min/m^2) = CI × CaO_2

$$SV = \frac{CO}{\text{Heart rate (beats/min)}}$$

$$SVI = \frac{SV}{BSA}$$

$$LVSWI = \frac{1.36 X (MAP - PCWP) \times SI}{100}$$

$$\text{Mean arterial pressure (MAP)} = \frac{(2 \times \text{diastolic}) + \text{systolic}}{3}$$
$$= \frac{\text{diastolic} + \text{systolic} - \text{diastolic}}{3}$$
$$= \frac{\text{diastolic} + \text{pulse pressure}}{3}$$

$$SVR = \frac{MAP - CVP}{CO} \times 80$$

$$PVR = \frac{\text{Mean PA pressure} - PCWP}{CO} \times 80$$

In the management of shock, monitoring blood pressure and organ perfusion is of utmost importance. A central venous line will facilitate the delivery of fluids, and an arterial line will allow for accurate monitoring of blood pressure. In cases in which aggressive fluid replacement is not effective and the exact cause of shock remains unknown, the placement of a pulmonary artery catheter (Swan-Ganz catheter) may be useful. This catheter allows for the direct assessment of pressures in the right atrium, right ventricle, and pulmonary artery, as well as measurement of the pulmonary capillary wedge pressure, and it allows for the assessment of the cardiac output. These values can then be used in equations that allow for calculating derived parameters such as cardiac index, systemic and pulmonary vascular resistance, and oxygen content. Information generated by the use of this catheter and the equations needed to calculate derived parameters are described in Tables 23-2 and 23-3. These values are useful in distinguishing the different types of shock (Table 23-4). Concerns have been raised about the true usefulness and benefit-risk ratio associated with this procedure. Significant expertise is required for the insertion of these catheters and for the adequate interpretation of the data generated.

Table 23-4 Hemodynamic Variables in the Four Types of Shock

Type of Shock	Pulmonary Capillary Wedge Pressure	Cardiac Index	Systemic Vascular Resistance Index
Hypovolemic	Low	Low	High
Cardiogenic	High	Low	High
Extracardiac obstructive	Normal or low (high in tamponade)	Low	High
Distributive	Normal or low	High (rarely low)	Low

Adapted from Parrillo JE, Ayres SM (eds): Major Issues in Critical Care Medicine. Baltimore, Williams & Wilkins, 1984.

Systemic Inflammatory Response Syndrome

The systemic inflammatory response syndrome (SIRS) is a constellation of clinical signs and symptoms triggered by the host response to diverse insults. The most common cause of SIRS is infection, which is called *sepsis*. However, not infrequently, SIRS can be triggered by noninfectious disorders such as pancreatitis and drug intoxication. The diagnosis of

SIRS requires at least two of the following criteria: (1) temperature higher than 38° C or less than 36° C; (2) tachycardia greater than 90 beats per minute; (3) tachypnea greater than 20 breaths per minute; or (4) Paco$_2$ less than 32 mm Hg; and (5) white blood cell count greater than 12,000/μL or less than 4000/μL. This systemic response may result in dysfunction of many organs, including the lung, liver, kidneys, heart, and central nervous system, which is referred to as multiple-organ dysfunction syndrome or multiple-organ system failure. The prognosis worsens as more organs become involved with mortality ranging from 30% in less severe cases to more than 90% with five or more failing organs.

Noxious Gases, Fumes, and Smoke Inhalation

The inhalation of certain gases and fumes may cause asphyxia or cellular and metabolic injury (Table 23-5). Carbon monoxide poisoning is a common and frequently unsuspected cause of inhalational injury and results in tissue hypoxia by competitively displacing oxygen from hemoglobin. Affinity of carbon monoxide for hemoglobin is about 250 times greater than that of oxygen. The correlation between carbon monoxide levels and symptoms is weak, but generally patients with levels greater than 30% are symptomatic. Symptoms may range from confusion or fatigue to nausea, headache, and profound coma. The diagnosis is based on clinical grounds and supported by laboratory data. Carbon monoxide intoxication might occur in closed automobiles and by exposure to kerosene heaters or charcoal fires in closed spaces. In suggested cases, arterial blood gas levels should be obtained with measured (not calculated) hemoglobin-oxygen saturation. A carbon monoxide level should be measured in patients with a measured systemic arterial oxygen saturation (Sao_2) lower than the calculated Sao_2 obtained from the arterial oxygen tension. Treatment includes 100% inspired oxygen. Hyperbaric oxygen might be useful, but the clinical use of this therapy is unclear.

Inhalation of caustic substances such as ammonia, chlorine, and hydrogen fluoride causes acute symptoms of eye and upper airway inflammation. Pain, lacrimation, rhinorrhea, and upper airway symptoms usually prompt the individual to flee the environment. Inhalation of nitrogen dioxide (silo filler's disease) occurs in farmers who work in silos where fermentation of grain produces large quantities of the gas. Most patients recover without sequelae, but a small minority of patients may develop bronchiolitis obliterans.

Table 23-5 Toxic Gases and Fumes

Injuries	Agents	Occupational Exposures
Simple asphyxia	Carbon dioxide	Mining, foundries
	Nitrogen	Mining, diving
	Methane	Mining
Cellular hypoxia and oxygen transport	Carbon monoxide	Mining, combustion in closed spaces
		Smoke inhalation
	Cyanide	Petroleum refining
	Hydrogen sulfide	
Direct tissue injury	Ammonia	Fertilizer, cleaning agents
	Chlorine	Bleaches, swimming pools
	Nitrogen dioxide	Farming, fertilizer, combustion in closed spaces
	Phosgene	Welding, paint removal
	Cadmium, mercury	Welding

Table 23-6 Common Drug Overdoses

Drug Overdose	Clinical Syndrome	Basic Treatment
Acetaminophen (paracetamol)	0.5-24 hr: nausea, vomiting 24-72 hr: nausea, vomiting, right upper quadrant pain, abnormal liver function tests and prothrombin time 72-96 hr: liver necrosis, coagulation, defects, jaundice, renal failure, hepatic encephalopathy 4 days-2 wk: resolution of liver dysfunction	Elimination: gastric lavage (if <1 hr after ingestion) Activated charcoal (if <4 hr after ingestion) (both longer if sustained-release product) Treatment: N-acetylcysteine for toxic ingestion
Amphetamines	Hypertension, tachycardia, arrhythmias, myocardial infarction, vasospasm, seizures, paranoid psychosis, diaphoresis, tachypnea	Elimination: Activated charcoal for oral ingestion Agitation/seizures: benzodiazepines Hypertension: control agitation, α-antagonists (phentolamine), vasodilators (nitroglycerin, nitroprusside, nifedipine) Hyperthermia: control agitation, external cooling
Iron	0.5-6 hr: nausea, vomiting, gastrointestinal discomfort, gastrointestinal bleed, drowsiness, hypoglycemia, hypotension 6-24 hr: latency, quiescence (may not occur in severe ingestions) 6-48 hr: shock, coma, seizures, coagulopathy, acidosis, cardiac failure 2-7 days: hepatotoxicity, coagulopathy, metabolic acidosis, renal insufficiency 1-8 wk: gastrointestinal disorders, achlorhydria	Elimination: gastric lavage and/or whole-bowel irrigation with polyethylene glycol electrolyte solution, especially when radio-opaque tablets on kidney-ureter-bladder radiograph Shock: intravenous fluids and blood (if hemorrhage present); vasopressors if needed Antidote: deferoxamine to chelate iron, when iron levels >500 mcg/dL or severe ingestion suspected
Tricyclic antidepressants	Wide-complex tachyarrhythmias, hypotension, seizures	Tachyarrhythmias: alkalizing blood (pH 7.5-7.55) with intravenous bicarbonate Seizures: benzodiazepines Hypotension: fluid resuscitation, vasopressors
Salicylate	Respiratory alkalosis (initially), metabolic acidosis (after substantial absorption), pulmonary edema, platelet dysfunction, nausea, vomiting, hearing loss, agitation, delirium	Elimination: activated charcoal, hemodialysis (for severe poisoning), alkalinization of urine Agitation/delirium: alkalinize blood with intravenous bicarbonate

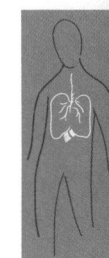

Metal fume fever causes influenza-like symptoms as a result of the inhalation of metal oxides generated by welding. Inhalation of platinum, formalin, and isocyanates may precipitate asthma. Pneumonitis can be induced by high-intensity inhalation of cadmium and mercury vapors.

Smoke inhalation may cause direct thermal injury that is usually confined to the upper airways, but it may also produce injury to the lower airways if exposure to sufficient steam occurs as a result of the high thermal content of water. Laryngeal edema, airway inflammation, and mucus can lead to airway obstruction, which requires intubation. Anoxia occurs from consumption of oxygen by fire, as well as from cytotoxic injury from gases such as carbon monoxide, cyanide, and oxidants liberated during combustion. Cyanide poisoning uncouples oxygen from energy production and requires prompt treatment with 100% oxygen and sodium thiosulfate. The combustion of natural and synthetic polymers often produces aldehydes, acetaldehyde, and acrolein, which have a high irritant potential. The treatment of patients with inhalation injuries is supportive with close attention to the airway. Oxygen should be provided, and continuous monitoring of cardiac and hemodynamic status is necessary. Sometimes intubation and mechanical ventilation are needed to overcome airway obstruction and the development of respiratory failure.

Drug Overdoses

Drug overdoses are common causes of admission to the ICU. The presenting complaints and management of the more common overdoses that result in medical emergencies are summarized in Table 23-6.

Prospectus for the Future

It is anticipated that in the very near future there will be an explosion of demand for intensive care hospital resources. First, an aging society with multiple co-morbidities is poised to require intensive care when hospitalized. The oldest baby boomers are 62 years old, and they are quickly coming to an age at which their need for critical care services markedly rises. This will have significant implications for allocation of health care resources. The administration of critical care medicine units and the delivery of care in those units are changing at a rapid pace with the standardization of care through the development of critical care pathways. Over the past few years, studies have assessed the value of early assessment and aggressive treatment of shock through *goal-directed therapy,* the use of low-volume ventilation in patients with ARDS, the development of new strategies designed to accelerate weaning from mechanical ventilation, and the development of biomarkers for the early detection of ventilator-associated pneumonia. Although more information about critical illnesses is generated each year, the main obstacle to improving the outcomes in the critical care setting is the limited use of these relatively new strategies in critical care units inside and outside academic institutions. Of note, compliance with proved new therapies is being fostered, among other mechanisms, through 24-hour coverage of critical care units by trained experts, the use of electronic records, and assessment of compliance with treatment protocols. Randomized, controlled studies designed to test new drugs and other strategies in the critical care setting are underway and are likely to improve care of the critically ill patient. Research into mechanisms of acute lung injury and repair will hopefully result in more specific therapies for ARDS.

References

Acute Respiratory Distress Syndrome Network: Ventilation with lower tidal volumes as compared with traditional tidal volumes for acute lung injury and the acute respiratory distress syndrome. N Engl J Med 342:1301, 2000.
Bernard GR: Acute respiratory distress syndrome: A historical perspective. Am J Respir Crit Care Med 172:798, 2005.
Hill NS: Noninvasive ventilation for chronic obstructive pulmonary disease. Respir Care 49:87-89, 2004.

Levy, MM, Fink, MP, Marshall, JC, et al: 2001 SCCM/ESICM/ACCP/ATS/SIS International Sepsis Definitions Conference. Crit Care Med 31:1250, 2003.
Rivers, E, Nguyen, B, Havstad, S, et al: Early goal-directed therapy in the treatment of severe sepsis and septic shock. N Engl J Med 345:1368, 2001.
Sehti JM, Siegel MD: Mechanical ventilation in chronic obstructive pulmonary disease. Clin Chest Med 21:799-818, 2000.
Ware LB, Matthay MA: The acute respiratory distress syndrome. N Engl J Med 342:1334-1349, 2000.

Chapter **24**

Neoplastic Disorders of the Lung

Matthew D. Jankowich and Jason M. Aliotta

Lung Cancer

Lung cancer is the leading cause of cancer death in both men and women in the United States, and an estimated 1 million people die worldwide of lung cancer each year. Despite recent advances in the understanding of the biology of lung cancer and the introduction of new chemotherapeutic agents for its treatment, the 5-year survival rate for patients with lung cancer is 15%. A major reason for this poor rate of survival relates to the fact that most patients with lung cancer are diagnosed during the advanced stages of the disease when surgical resection is less likely to be curative. Most bronchogenic carcinomas are classified as two major types: (1) *small cell* carcinoma (SCLC) (**Web Fig. 24-1**) and (2) *non–small cell* carcinoma (NSCLC). NSCLCs are the most common and include squamous cell carcinoma (30%) (**Web Fig. 24-2**), adenocarcinoma (32%) (**Web Fig. 24-3**), and large cell carcinoma (10%) (**Web Fig. 24-4**), whereas SCLCs account for less than 20% of all bronchogenic carcinomas.

Smoking is the leading cause of lung cancer, a cause-and-effect relationship that was recognized as early as the 1940s. The risk for lung cancer is proportionate to cigarette pack-years smoked (packs per day × years smoked) with a peak incidence in the sixth and seventh decades. Exsmokers show a persistent risk for lung cancer throughout life. Passive smoking is thought to be the cause of lung cancer in a significant percentage of nonsmokers who develop the disease. Nonsmokers who live with smokers have more than a 30% increased risk for developing lung cancer. However, nonsmokers do develop lung cancer that is thought to be unrelated to environmental tobacco exposure; the cause of this phenomenon is poorly understood. Other risk factors for lung cancer include environmental hazards such as asbestos exposure. Tobacco smoking is an important cofactor of lung cancer in the setting of asbestos exposure. Radon increases the risk for lung cancer; this risk is most common in miners. Radon exposure in the home is less significant, but in view of the increased risk, home radon testing is recommended.

The exact mechanisms by which these factors promote lung cancer remain unclear, but they are likely to cause genetic abnormalities that, when unopposed, promote the oncogenic transformation of lung epithelial cells. Because of the redundant repair mechanisms available to the lung, many individual genetic *hits* appear necessary. These *hits* affect the expression of proto-oncogenes, suppressor genes, and growth factors. Proto-oncogenes, similar to members of the *ras* family (e.g., *k-ras*), control cell cycling, growth, and differentiation. Mutations in *ras* genes have been detected in more than 50% of squamous cell cancers and in 68% of adenocarcinoma cells. Other proto-oncogenes implicated in the pathogenesis of lung cancer are *c-erb*, *rb*, *p53*, *c-myc*, and *c-src*. Mutations in tumor suppressor genes (e.g., *p21*) might also promote the development of lung cancer. Growth factors, such as gastrin-releasing peptide, insulin-like growth factor, and epidermal growth factor, promote tumor cell proliferation through the activation of protein kinase pathways (e.g., protein kinase B, mammalian target of rapamycin [mTOR]) that stimulate cellular proliferation. Epidermal growth factor receptor mutations are prominent in nonsmokers who develop lung cancer and may indicate a unique molecular basis for lung cancer in these patients.

There is growing evidence that different lung cancers arise not only as a result of certain permissive oncogenic mutations but also because the cancer cell's local environment, or *niche*, supports its growth. Data generated from animal models support the concept that the lung has specific anatomic regions that contain populations of cells responsible for replacing damaged cells during routine maintenance and injury. These *resident stem cells* are not only capable of self-renewal but also can give rise to specialized and fully differentiated cells of the lung, including tracheal and alveolar epithelium. It has been suggested that resident stem cell signaling and differentiation pathways are maintained within distinct cancer types and that destabilization of this signaling machinery may participate in the pathogenesis of certain lung cancers. Animal models support a direct relationship between tracheal epithelial progenitor cells and tumor cells in human squamous cell carcinoma. These cells are basal epithelial cells located in submucosal gland duct junctions or intracartilaginous boundaries of the trachea and express cytokeratins 5 and 14. Neuroendocrine body (NEB) microenvironments maintain putative stem cell populations for the bronchiolar epithelium. Cells within this niche include variant Clara cell–specific protein (CCSP)-expressing cells, linked to nonsquamous NSCLC, and pulmonary neuroendocrine cells (PNEC), linked to SCLC. PNEC-derived SCLC tumors are believed to be capable of circumventing existing control mechanisms that regulate normal NEB-associated proliferation, in part by undergoing genetic mutations that result in autonomous sonic hedgehog (Shh) signaling. In addition, alveolar epithelial stem cells located in the bronchoalveolar duct junction (BADJ) have been linked to the pathogenesis of various adenocarcinomas because both cell types co-express CCSP and surfactant protein C (Sp-C).

CLINICAL PRESENTATION

Patients may complain of mild cough, dyspnea, increased sputum production, hemoptysis, chest pain, and weight loss. Localized pleuritic chest pain suggests chest wall invasion (**Web Fig. 24-5**). Hoarseness is caused by involvement (or compression) of the left recurrent laryngeal nerve and suggests mediastinal or hilar involvement. A pleural effusion is observed in 9% of patients and can be related to direct tumor involvement of the pleura or obstruction of lymph flow from the mediastinal nodes (**Web Fig. 24-6**). The presence of a malignant pleural effusion precludes resection. The superior vena cava is involved in less than 5% of patients, but obstruction may result in *superior vena cava syndrome,* characterized by edema of the face and upper extremities due to impaired venous return. Despite its implications, its involvement typically does not represent a medical emergency. Dysphagia suggests esophageal involvement.

The physical examination may be normal or may reveal changes in the lung examination, such as crackles (e.g., postobstructive pneumonia (**Web Fig. 24-7**); inspiratory wheeze, suggestive of airway obstruction; or dullness to percussion as a result of underlying pleural effusion. Lymph node enlargement in the neck (**Web Fig. 24-8**) or axillary areas is suggestive of metastatic disease. The most common sites of metastases are the lymph nodes, liver (**Web Fig. 24-9**), brain, adrenal glands, kidneys, and lungs.

Lung cancers that occur in the apex of the chest and invade apical chest wall structures are known as *superior sulcus* or *Pancoast tumors* (**Web Fig. 24-10**). These tumors often result in symptoms and physical findings caused by direct extension to adjacent structures. The classic description involves a syndrome of pain radiating down the arm due to tumor erosion into the brachial plexus. Tumor erosion into the cervical sympathetic chain can result in *Horner syndrome,* which is characterized by the following triad of physical findings: ptosis, miosis, and anhidrosis over the face and forehead.

NON–SMALL CELL CARCINOMAS

Most cases of lung cancer are due to NSCLCs. Of these, *adenocarcinomas* and *squamous cell carcinomas* are the most common.

Squamous cell carcinomas arise from the epithelial layer of the bronchial wall as normal columnar epithelial cells undergo metaplasia, eventually being replaced by increasingly atypical squamous epithelial cells. A localized carcinoma (*carcinoma in situ*) forms and later extends beyond the bronchial mucosa as it becomes invasive. Because most squamous cell carcinomas (60% to 80%) tend to be located within central airways (**Web Fig. 24-11**), the airway lumen may become obstructed, leading to collapse of the lung (atelectasis) or postobstructive pneumonia. Although necrosis and cavity formation may occur in any lung tumor, this feature is more common with squamous cell carcinomas (see **Web Fig. 24-5**). Because of their slow rate of growth, these tumors have the lowest propensity for metastasis of all types of lung cancer. Pathologically, squamous cell carcinomas can be distinguished from other NSCLCs by the presence of keratinization, pearl formation, and intercellular bridging.

Adenocarcinomas represent the most common type of lung cancer as well the most common type in nonsmokers (nearly 20% of all cases). In contrast to squamous cell carcinomas, adenocarcinomas are most often found in the periphery of the lung (75%) (**Web Fig. 24-12**). This tumor is frequently associated with malignant pleural effusions (60%) and has a high propensity for distant metastasis. Pathologically, adenocarcinomas can form glandlike structures and produce mucus. The tumor cells stain positive for carcinoembryonic antigen (CEA), mucin, and surfactant apoprotein. Adenocarcinomas respond poorly to therapy and carry a very poor prognosis. Alveolar or *bronchoalveolar cell carcinomas* represent a subset of adenocarcinomas and are the most common form of lung cancer found in nonsmokers and young patients. They can develop as a lung infiltrate or as a solitary nodule and can be accompanied by bronchorrhea. Pathologically, malignant cells can appear to grow and spread along preexisting alveolar walls.

Large cell carcinomas also frequently develop as a peripheral lesion and may be associated with pneumonitis and hilar adenopathy. Two subtypes can exist: *giant cell,* an anaplastic tumor that has a median survival for patients younger than 1 year; and *clear cell,* a tumor that resembles renal cell carcinoma and has fewer malignant features. Pathologically, large cell carcinomas lack the glandular and squamous features typical of other NSCLCs and cytologic features typical of SCLCs. In this respect, it is considered a diagnosis by exclusion.

SMALL CELL LUNG CARCINOMA

Small cell carcinoma is strongly associated with cigarette smoking. Tumor cells are of pulmonary neuroendocrine cell origin and are often associated with paraneoplastic syndromes (Table 24-1). SCLCs typically are perihilar in location, not infrequently originating in the main bronchi, and often have associated lymphadenopathy (**Web Fig. 24-13**). These tumors metastasize rapidly, most commonly to the thoracic lymph nodes, bones, liver, adrenal glands, and brain. Most patients have metastatic disease at the time of presentation. SCLC has traditionally been staged as *limited disease* (confined to one hemithorax) or *extensive disease* (distant metastases), although a TNM staging system has recently been suggested. SCLC is an aggressive lung tumor,

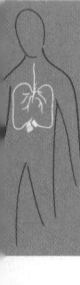

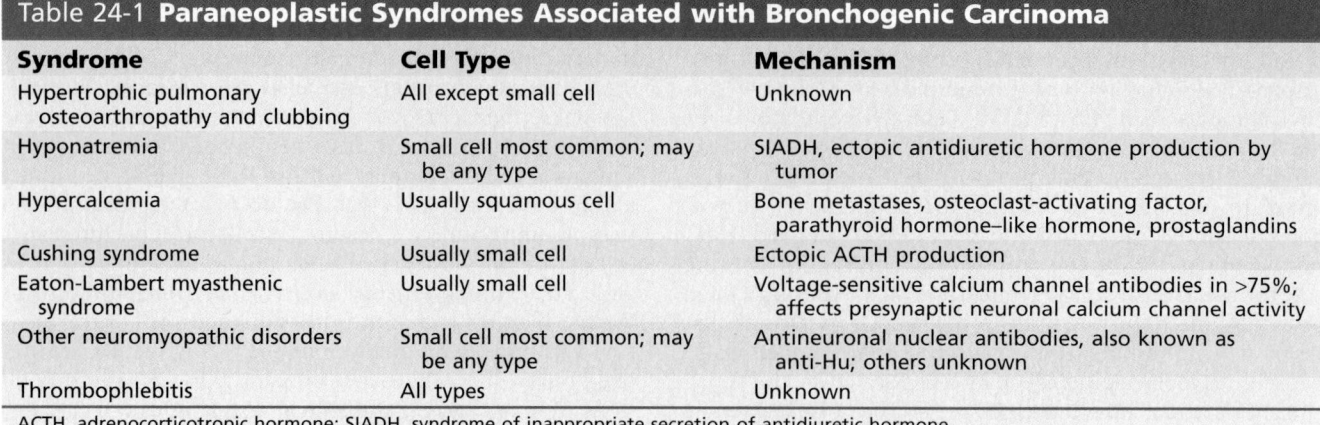

Syndrome	Cell Type	Mechanism
Hypertrophic pulmonary osteoarthropathy and clubbing	All except small cell	Unknown
Hyponatremia	Small cell most common; may be any type	SIADH, ectopic antidiuretic hormone production by tumor
Hypercalcemia	Usually squamous cell	Bone metastases, osteoclast-activating factor, parathyroid hormone–like hormone, prostaglandins
Cushing syndrome	Usually small cell	Ectopic ACTH production
Eaton-Lambert myasthenic syndrome	Usually small cell	Voltage-sensitive calcium channel antibodies in >75%; affects presynaptic neuronal calcium channel activity
Other neuromyopathic disorders	Small cell most common; may be any type	Antineuronal nuclear antibodies, also known as anti-Hu; others unknown
Thrombophlebitis	All types	Unknown

ACTH, adrenocorticotropic hormone; SIADH, syndrome of inappropriate secretion of antidiuretic hormone.

and, without treatment, the median survival of patients with this cancer is less than 5 months. The overall survival at 5 years is 5% and has not improved significantly over the past several decades.

MANAGEMENT

The management of lung cancer includes strategies targeting prevention, early detection, and treatment. Of these, the most effective approach is prevention. Because tobacco abuse is the main causal agent known to promote the development of lung cancer, strategies designed to prevent people from smoking or to promote smoking cessation should be encouraged. Individuals who are successful at quitting smoking have a lower long-term rate of lung cancer death than individuals who continue to smoke. A diet rich in fruits and vegetables may protect against the development of lung cancer in smokers. However, high-dose supplemental β carotene has been shown to increase the relative risk for lung cancer in two randomized controlled trials, and should not be recommended. There is no evidence that other supplemental vitamins reduce lung cancer risk.

Because lung cancer typically presents at an advanced stage, when cure is not possible, an effective strategy for early detection of lung cancer at a curative stage would be desirable. Therefore, there has long been interest in lung cancer screening. Unfortunately, randomized trials of screening with chest radiographic studies or sputum cytologic testing did not demonstrate a decrease in lung cancer mortality. Current trials focus on the use of low dose computed tomography (CT). The National Lung Screening Trial, sponsored by the National Cancer Institute, is a randomized trial of whether CT or chest radiography can reduce lung cancer mortality in smokers and has recently completed enrollment. Until results from this trial are available, there is no current recommended screening modality for the early detection of lung cancer in at risk patients.

When a suspected lung cancer is identified, either incidentally or because of clinical symptoms, a tissue diagnosis is essential in most patients, unless they are too debilitated to undergo treatment. If imaging reveals sites of suspected metastasis, the site of biopsy should be chosen to determine the greatest extent of spread, or highest stage, of the tumor if this is feasible. If the apparent tumor is confined to the chest, bronchoscopy is appropriate for central masses, whereas transthoracic needle aspiration of more peripheral lesions can be performed. If present, pleural effusion should be sampled to assess for malignant cells. In some cases, if the pretest probability is very high that the lung lesion is a primary lung cancer, and there is no imaging evidence of disease spread, direct referral for surgical resection may be appropriate.

Once a lung cancer is diagnosed, staging is necessary to determine the treatment and prognosis. For NSCLC, staging is critical to determine whether the patient would benefit from surgical resection for curative intent, or from other treatment modalities such as chemotherapy. Chest CT, including images of the upper abdomen, is useful to delineate the location and size of the primary tumor and to examine for mediastinal lymph nodes, pleural disease, and adrenal or liver metastases. However, CT has limited ability to distinguish benign versus malignant lymphadenopathy in the mediastinum. Positron-emission tomography (PET) using 18-fluorodeoxyglucose (FDG) is more sensitive and specific than CT in the detection of mediastinal lymph node metastases and may also detect unexpected metastases elsewhere in the body. In general, suspected mediastinal or extrathoracic metastases demonstrated by imaging should be confirmed with tissue sampling before determining that a patient is not an operative candidate. Techniques for invasive staging of the mediastinal lymph nodes include endoscopic transbronchial needle aspiration, endoscopic ultrasound-guided needle aspiration, and mediastinoscopy. Mediastinoscopy is also frequently performed to rule out mediastinal spread of disease in patients without definite imaging evidence of lymph node involvement before definitive resection of the lung cancer. PET scanning is limited in its ability to detect brain lesions, and head CT with intravenous contrast or magnetic resonance imaging (MRI) should be performed if the clinical history or examination suggests brain metastasis. Bone scans are useful for the investigation of suspected bony metastases if there are corresponding symptoms.

The treatment of lung carcinoma depends on the stage. See Table 24-2 for the International Staging System for Lung Cancer. Occasionally, SCLCs can be resected if no evidence of metastasis is found, but most SCLCs are treated with chemotherapy, with thoracic external-beam radiation if

Table 24-2 TNM Staging System for Lung Cancer

Primary Tumor (T)

T1—Tumor ≤3 cm diameter without invasion more proximal than lobar bronchus

T2—Tumor >3 cm diameter *or* tumor of any size with any of the following characteristics:
  Invasion of visceral pleura
  Atelectasis of less than entire lung
  Proximal extent at least 2 cm from carina

T3—Tumor of any size with any of the following characteristics:
  Invasion of chest wall
  Involvement of diaphragm, mediastinal pleura, or pericardium
  Atelectasis involving entire lung
  Proximal extent within 2 cm of carina

T4—Tumor of any size with any of the following:
  Invasion of mediastinum
  Invasion of heart or great vessels
  Invasion of trachea or esophagus
  Invasion of vertebral body or carina
  Presence of malignant pleural or pericardial effusion
  Satellite tumor nodule(s) within same lobe as primary tumor

Nodal Involvement (N)

N0—No regional node involvement

N1—Metastasis to ipsilateral hilar and/or ipsilateral peribronchial nodes

N2—Metastasis to ipsilateral mediastinal and/or subcarinal nodes

N3—Metastasis to contralateral mediastinal or hilar nodes *or* ipsilateral or contralateral scalene or supraclavicular nodes

Metastasis (M)

M0—Distant metastasis absent

M1—Distant metastasis present (includes metastatic tumor nodules in a different lobe from the primary tumor)

Stage Groupings of TNM Subsets

Stage IA	T1 N0 M0	Stage IIIA	T3 N1 M0
Stage IB	T2 N0 M0		T1-3 N2 M0
Stage IIA	T1 N1 M0	Stage IIIB	Any T N3 M0
Stage IIB	T2 N1 M0		T4 Any N M0
	T3 N0 M0	Stage IV	Any T Any N M1

Adapted from Greene FL, Page DL, Fleming ID: AJCC Cancer Staging Manual, 6th ed. New York, Springer, 2002.

disease is limited. Combinations of cisplatin and etoposide are the standard chemotherapeutic regimen. Although chemotherapy and radiation often produce a dramatic response and sometimes are curative for limited disease, relapse is typical, and subsequent treatments are less effective. Prophylactic cranial radiation may be performed. Surgery is the only curative therapy for NSCLC and is indicated for patients with stage I or II NSCLC who are operative candidates. Lobectomy (or greater) extent of resection is considered superior to more limited resection such as a wedge resection. Adjuvant chemotherapy is appropriate for patients with stage II disease. For patients with stage IIIA lung cancer, the optimal treatment strategy remains unclear, in part because of the heterogeneity of patients in this group. In general, these patients are not candidates for surgery alone, if at all, and a treatment plan should be developed for each patient in a multidisciplinary setting. In stage IIIB,

surgery may rarely be indicated for some T4 N0-1 M0 tumors. However, most patients with stage IIIB NSCLC are not surgical candidates, and 5-year survival is poor for this group. Combined, ideally concurrent, chemotherapy and radiotherapy are preferable to radiotherapy alone in patients with stage IIIB NSCLC. In stage IV, chemotherapy is recommended because it improves survival and provides palliation for symptoms.

Targeted molecular therapies are an area of active interest in lung cancer treatment. Highlighting the challenges of these new targeted therapies, bevacizumab, a humanized monoclonal antibody against vascular endothelial growth factor, was associated with hemoptysis, which was sometimes fatal, in patients with squamous cell carcinoma in an early-stage trial. However, bevacizumab improved survival when added to a standard platinum-based chemotherapeutic regimen in patients with nonsquamous NSCLC. Erlotinib, a tyrosine kinase inhibitor targeting the activity of the epidermal growth factor receptor, is approved for the second-line treatment of metastatic NSCLC. Targeting the epidermal growth factor receptor appears to have benefit in particular patient groups, such as women, never-smokers, and Asians, harboring particular receptor mutations.

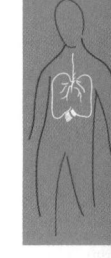

Special Circumstances

SOLITARY PULMONARY NODULE

A *solitary pulmonary nodule* (SPN) is a single, rounded lesion in the lung that is 3 cm or less in diameter. Although these lesions are commonly lung cancers in certain patient populations, the differential diagnosis of this radiographic finding is broad and includes many malignant and benign etiologies. In addition to primary lung cancer (with adenocarcinoma the most common type to present as an SPN (see **Web Fig. 24-12**), other malignant etiologies include bronchial carcinoid tumors and metastatic foci from extrapulmonary malignancies (most common sources include malignant melanoma, sarcoma, colon, kidney, breast, and testicle). Benign etiologies include benign tumors of the lung (hamartomas (**Web Fig. 24-14**), infectious granulomas (from fungal diseases including histoplasmosis and coccidioidomycosis as well as mycobacterial disease), lung abscess, vascular abnormalities (arteriovenous malformation), rounded atelectasis, and pseudotumor (pleural fluid trapped within a fissure).

When confronted with a patient with a solitary pulmonary nodule, determining the likelihood of malignancy is critically important because early resection of malignant nodules is usually curative, whereas resection of benign nodules exposes the patient to an unnecessary risk for surgery. Diagnostic evaluation includes consideration of certain *clinical features*, including patient **age** and **risk factors**. The probability of an SPN being malignant increases with patient age. However, even in younger individuals (<35 years), SPNs may still be malignant, so a benign etiology should not be assumed. The probability of lung cancer is greater when an SPN is detected in an individual with a heavy smoking history. Certain *radiographic features* can also be helpful in predicting whether an SPN is benign or malignant. **Size** of the SPN is important because larger lesions are more likely to be malignant. Lesions 4 to 7 mm in size in individuals without a history of cancer have been described to have a 0.9% chance of being malignant, whereas this likelihood increases to 18% for lesions 8 mm to 2 cm and 50% for those above 2 cm. SPNs with smooth and discrete **borders** are more likely to be benign, whereas those with irregular and spiculated boarders are more likely to be malignant. Patterns of **calcification** suggestive of a benign SPN include diffuse, central, laminated (or onion-skin), and popcorn patterns. Lesions with peripheral or eccentric (asymmetrical) calcifications are more likely to be malignant. Imaging studies should be compared with previous studies if available because the presence of an SPN without a **change in size** for more than 2 years dramatically reduces the likelihood of it being malignant.

Further characterization of SPNs typically includes the use of imaging modalities including **chest CT** because it is able to provide more specific information about the location, pattern of calcification, and edge characteristics of nodules as well as identifying unsuspected lymphadenopathy, synchronous parenchymal lesions, or invasion of the chest wall or mediastinum. More recently, metabolic imaging with **PET** has been used by clinicians to distinguish benign and malignant SPNs as those that are malignant typically take up FDG avidly. A negative PET will exclude malignancy in most cases because the negative predictive value for the test is quite high (90% to 95%). However, false-negative results can occur with certain tumors, including bronchioloalveolar cell carcinomas and carcinoids. In addition, PET is less sensitive for small lesions and should not be used routinely to evaluate SPNs smaller than 8 to 10 mm. A positive PET can be less helpful because the positive predictive value of the test is lower (80%) as certain benign lesions (infectious, inflammatory, granulomatous) take up FDG.

The initial management of an SPN uses *clinical* and *radiographic features* to help the clinician to estimate a *pretest probability* of malignancy. Several validated prediction models exist and may aid in this process, but these are generally as accurate as estimates made based on the clinical judgment of experienced clinicians. Although many reasonable approaches exist, guidelines published by the American College of Chest Physicians in 2007 describe a diagnostic algorithm for SPNs 8 mm to 3 cm in size. These guidelines recommend that SPNs with a **low** pretest probability of malignancy can be followed with serial CT scans at 3, 6, 12, and 24 months. SPNs with a **high** pretest probability of malignancy should be removed surgically (provided that the patient is a candidate for surgery), either by thoracotomy or by a less invasive thoracoscopic approach for more peripherally located lesions (video-assisted thoracic surgery [VATS]). A more definitive resection (lobectomy) would then be offered if the SPN is found to be malignant. Management of the most common type of SPN, those with an **intermediate** pretest probability, may include the use of **FDG-PET** to further characterize the lesion, or nonsurgical biopsies, either CT-guided (for peripheral lesions) or bronchoscopic (for central lesions). Those with a negative work-up may be followed by serial CT scans with the low probability group. For those with positive tests or for patients who desire a more aggressive diagnostic approach, surgical options may be pursued. Management recommendations for SPNs smaller than 8 mm were published by the Fleischner Society in 2005. Serial CT scans at various intervals, as determined by SPN size and whether the patient is considered to be high risk (history of smoking or of other risk factors) or low risk (minimal or absent history of smoking and of other risk factors) have been suggested.

PARANEOPLASTIC SYNDROMES

Paraneoplastic syndromes are usually neurologic syndromes that are rare and are elicited by a patient's immune response to tumors of the lung, ovaries, breast, and lymphatic system (see Table 24-2). Neurologic symptoms develop over weeks and may include difficulties in walking or swallowing, loss of muscle tone, loss of fine-motor coordination, slurred speech, memory loss, vision problems, dementia, sleep disturbances, seizures, and vertigo. Neurologic paraneoplastic syndromes include stiff person syndrome, encephalomyelitis, cerebellar degeneration, neuromyotonia, and sensory neuropathy. Neuromuscular junction disorders can occur, as observed in the Lambert-Eaton myasthenic syndrome and in myasthenia gravis. Myopathies are observed and can exhibit symptoms reminiscent of polymyositis. Retinopathies, certain visual loss syndromes, hyponatremia, hypercalcemia, and Cushing syndrome can also be manifestations of a paraneoplastic syndrome.

Evaluation of Surgery for the Patient with Lung Cancer

A multidisciplinary approach, using the expertise of a thoracic surgeon specializing in lung cancer, a medical oncologist, a radiation oncologist, and a pulmonologist, is often used to evaluate patients with lung cancer for surgical resection. The presurgical evaluation of patients with lung cancer involves staging of the tumor (see Table 24-2), the determination of surgical resectability, and the evaluation of lung function to determine whether the patient is a good candidate for surgery. Staging of a tumor begins with a careful history and physical examination, followed by a CT scan of the chest. Mediastinoscopy is often needed to evaluate mediastinal nodes. Other tests (e.g., PET scans, CT scans of the head) are necessary if specific symptoms or findings from the physical examination or laboratory results are suggestive of extrapulmonary involvement. Once it is determined that surgery is the most appropriate approach based on staging, evaluation of the patient's general status and ability to tolerate the procedure is necessary. Because many patients with lung cancer have co-morbid conditions that increase the likelihood of an adverse perioperative cardiovascular event, a preoperative cardiologic evaluation may be warranted.

A comprehensive preoperative physiologic assessment is important to estimate the preoperative risk from underlying pulmonary disease. Because lung cancer is more common in smokers, many patients have chronic lung disease (e.g., chronic obstructive pulmonary disease [COPD]), and lung function testing is necessary as an initial step in the presurgical evaluation. Forced expiratory volume in 1 second (FEV_1) measured by spirometry is commonly used to assess the suitability of patients with lung cancer for surgery. Patients

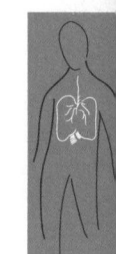

with an FEV_1 higher than 2 L (for pneumonectomy), higher than 1.5 L (for lobectomy), or more than 80% of predicted are considered to have an average preoperative risk. For patients with an acceptable FEV_1 but with unexplained dyspnea on exertion or evidence of interstitial lung disease on chest imaging, further work-up, including the measurement of carbon monoxide diffusion capacity (D_{LCO}), is necessary. In this situation, if the measured D_{LCO} is more than 80% of predicted, the patient is still considered to have an average preoperative risk. For patients with a low D_{LCO} or FEV_1, a radionucleotide perfusion scan may be performed to estimate the predicted postoperative values for both of these tests. If the predicted postoperative D_{LCO} or FEV_1 is more than 40%, it is thought that these patients also have an average preoperative risk. For all others, cardiopulmonary exercise testing (CPET) may be done to determine the maximum capacity of an individual's body to transport and utilize oxygen during *incremental exercise*, or Vo_2max. If the measured Vo_2max is less than 10 to 15 mL O_2/kg body weight per minute (roughly equivalent to being unable to climb one flight of stairs), the patient would be considered to have increased preoperative risk.

Prospectus for the Future

Lung cancer is the number one cause of cancer death in both women and men in the United States, with tobacco exposure representing the main predisposing factor. Despite the widespread use of aggressive treatment, including chemotherapy, the 5-year survival rate for lung cancer was 15% in the United States for the period from 1996 to 2004. The focus of efforts should remain prevention through smoking cessation programs, continued public education on the hazards of smoking, and discouraging young individuals from using cigarettes. Screening for lung cancer in at-risk individuals may ultimately become a part of the routine assessment, although whether imaging strategies or novel techniques for identifying signature DNA modifications in the respiratory epithelium or blood of a smoker will ultimately be the modality of choice remains to be seen. Chemoprevention remains elusive, with trials of vitamin and antioxidant strategies proving disappointing or even hazardous. The focus in chemopreventive strategies has shifted to anti-inflammatory drugs, and the outcomes of trials of these agents will be of interest. Improvements in the care of patients with a diagnosis of lung cancer are needed. Novel approaches to SCLC are emerging from the research on this tumor's molecular pathogenesis, and targeting of specific pathways, like the sonic hedgehog signaling pathway, may provide the breakthrough needed to improve survival in this condition after a decades-long plateau. Defining the best adjuvant strategies to decrease recurrence rates after surgery; individualizing care by identifying optimal candidates for targeted molecular therapies to maximize treatment effects; identifying and targeting cancer stem cells and overcoming cancer stem cell drug resistance; and examination of nonsurgical tumor ablative strategies for the marginal surgical candidate are among the many areas of necessary and ongoing research in NSCLC.

References

Diagnosis and Management of Lung Cancer: ACCP Evidence-Based Clinical Practice Guidelines, 2nd ed. Chest 132:1S, 2007.

Giangreco A, Groot KR, Janes SM: Lung cancer and lung stem cells: Strange bedfellows? Am J Respir Crit Care Med 175:547-553, 2007.

Gustafsson BI, Kidd M, Chan A, et al: Bronchopulmonary neuroendocrine tumors. Cancer 113:5-21, 2008.

MacMahon H, Austin JHM, Gamsu G, et al: Guidelines for management of small pulmonary nodules detected on CT Scans: A statement from the Fleischner Society. Radiology 237:395-400, 2005.

Mulshine JL, Sullivan DC: Clinical practice: Lung cancer screening. N Engl J Med 352:2714-2720, 2005.

Surveillance Epidemiology and End Results (SEER) Program website. Accessed October, 2008, from: http://seer.cancer.gov.

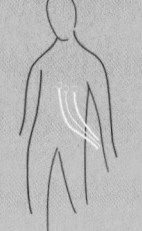

Section V

Preoperative and Postoperative Care

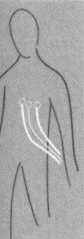

Preoperative and Postoperative Care

Wei C. Lau and Kim A. Eagle

More than 40 million people undergo noncardiac surgical procedures in the United States annually. It is estimated that the incidence of cardiac complications after noncardiac surgical procedures is between 0.5% and 1%. Consequently, about 200,000 to 400,000 people will suffer from perioperative cardiac complications. Moreover, one out of four or more of these patients will die. Patients who survive a postoperative myocardial infarction (MI) are twice as likely to die in the following 2 years as patients with uneventful surgical procedures. Emerging evidence-based practices dictate that the practicing physician should thoughtfully perform an individualized evaluation of the surgical patient to provide an accurate preoperative risk assessment, risk stratification, and modification of risk parameters that can then guide the framework for optimal perioperative risk reduction strategies. This chapter reviews preoperative and postoperative cardiovascular risk assessment, targeting intermediate-risk to high-risk patients to strategically guide perioperative preventive therapies that may favor optimal outcome.

Evaluation of Intermediate-Risk to High-Risk Patients

Mortality is extremely low with safe delivery of modern-day anesthesia in low-risk patients undergoing low-risk surgery (Table 25-1). Simple standardized preoperative screening questionnaires have been developed for the purpose of identifying patients at intermediate to high risk that may benefit from a more detailed clinical evaluation (Table 25-2). Evaluation of such surgical patients should always begin with a thorough history and physical examination with 12-lead resting echocardiogram (ECG) in accordance with the American College of Cardiology/American Heart Association (ACC/AHA) guideline recommendations. Determining the urgency of the surgery should be included in the history

because true emergent procedures are associated with an unavoidably higher morbidity and mortality. Preoperative testing should only be done for specific clinical conditions based on the history. Thus, healthy patients of any age undergoing elective surgical procedures without coexisting medical conditions should not require any testing unless the degree of surgical stress may result in unusual changes from the baseline state. The history should focus on symptoms of occult cardiac disease.

Preoperative Cardiac Risk Assessment

Assessment of exercise tolerance in preoperative risk stratification and precise prediction of in-hospital perioperative risk is most applicable in patients who self-report worsening exercise-induced cardiopulmonary symptoms, patients who may benefit from noninvasive or invasive cardiac testing regardless of scheduled surgical procedure, and patients with known coronary artery disease (CAD) or with multiple risk factors and the ability to exercise. For predicting perioperative events, "poor" exercise tolerance has been defined as the inability to walk four blocks and climb two flights of stairs or as the inability to meet a metabolic equivalent (MET) level of 4 (Table 25-3). Further clinical risk assessment often uses risk indices derived from empirical multivariable predictive models based on available clinical information that identified risk factors to identify patients at elevated perioperative cardiac risk. Previous studies have prospectively compared several cardiac risk indices with one another, and the revised cardiac risk index (RCRI) is favored by many given its accuracy and simplicity (Table 25-4). The RCRI relies on the presence or absence of six identifiable predictive factors, which include high-risk surgery, ischemic heart disease, congestive heart failure, cerebrovascular disease, diabetes mellitus, and renal failure. Each of the RCRI predictors is assigned one point, when present. The risk for cardiac events (including MI, pulmonary edema, ventricular

Table 25-1 Surgery-Specific Risk

Higher Risk

- Emergent major operations, especially in elderly patients
- Aortic and other major vascular (endovascular and nonendovascular) surgery
- Noncarotid peripheral vascular surgery
- Prolonged surgery associated with large fluid shift and/or blood loss

Intermediate Risk

- Major thoracic surgery
- Major abdominal surgery
- Carotid endarterectomy
- Head/neck surgery
- Orthopedic surgery
- Prostate surgery

Lower Risk

- Eye, skin, and superficial surgery
- Endoscopic procedures

From Eagle KA, Berger PB, Calkins H, et al: ACC/AHA guideline update for perioperative cardiovascular evaluation for noncardiac surgery—executive summary: A report of the American College of Cardiology/American Heart Association Task Force on Practice Guidelines (Committee to Update the 1996 Guidelines on Perioperative Cardiovascular Evaluation for Noncardiac Surgery). J Am Coll Cardiol 39:542-553, 2002.

Table 25-3 Functional Status

Excellent (activities requiring >7 METs)

Carry 24 lb up eight steps

Carry objects that weigh 80 lb

Outdoor work (shovel snow, spade soil)

Recreation (ski, basketball, squash, handball, jog or walk 5 mph)

Moderate (activities requiring >4 but <7 METs)

Have sexual intercourse without stopping

Walk at 4 mph on level ground

Outdoor work (garden, rake, weed)

Recreation (roller-skate, dance, foxtrot)

Poor (activities requiring <4 METs)

Shower/dress without stopping, strip and make bed, dust, wash dishes

Walk at 2.5 mph on level ground

Outdoor work (clean windows)

Recreation (golf, bowl)

MET, metabolic equivalent.
   Adapted from Hlatky MA, Boineau RE, Higginbotham MB, et al: A brief self-administered questionnaire to determine functional capacity (the Duke Activity Status Index). Am J Cardiol 64:651-654, 1989.

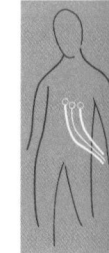

Table 25-2 Standardized Preoperative Questionnaires*

1. Age, Weight, Height
2. Are you:
   a. Female and 55 years of age or older or male and 45 years of age or older?
   b. If yes, are you also 70 years of age or older?
3. Do you take anticoagulant medications ("blood thinners")?
4. Do you have or have you had any of the following heart related conditions?
   a. Heart disease
   b. Heart attack within the last 6 months
   c. Angina (chest pain)
   d. Irregular heartbeat
   e. Heart failure
5. Do you have or have you ever had any of the following?
   a. Rheumatoid arthritis
   b. Kidney disease
   c. Liver disease
   d. Diabetes
6. Do you get short of breath when you lie flat?
7. Are you currently on oxygen treatment?
8. Do you have a chronic cough that produces any discharge or fluid?
9. Do you have lung problems or diseases?
10. Have you or any blood member of your family ever had a problem with any anesthesia other than nausea?
    a. If yes, describe
11. If female, is it possible that you could be pregnant?
    a. Pregnancy test
    b. Please list date of last menstrual period

*University of Michigan Health System patient information report. Patients who answer yes to any of questions 2 through 9 should receive a more detailed clinical evaluation.
   From Tremper KK, Benedict P: Paper "preoperative computer." Anesthesiology 92:1212-1213, 2000.

Table 25-4 Revised Cardiac Risk Index Clinical Markers*

1. High-risk surgical procedures
2. Ischemic heart disease
   a. History of myocardial infarction
   b. Current angina considered to be ischemic
   c. Requiring sublingual nitroglycerin
   d. Positive exercise test
   e. Pathologic Q waves on ECG
   f. History of PTCA and/or CABG with current angina considered to be ischemic
3. Congestive heart failure
   a. Left ventricular failure by physical examination
   b. History of paroxysmal nocturnal dyspnea
   c. History of pulmonary edema
   d. S_3 gallop on cardiac auscultation
   e. Bilateral rales on pulmonary auscultation
   f. Pulmonary edema on chest radiograph
4. Cerebrovascular disease
   a. History of transient ischemic attack
   b. History of cerebrovascular accident
5. Diabetes mellitus
   a. Treatment with insulin
6. Chronic renal insufficiency
   a. Serum creatinine > 2 mg/dL

*See Table 25-1.
   CABG, coronary artery bypass grafting; ECG, electrocardiogram; PTCA, percutaneous transluminal coronary angioplasty.
   Adapted from Lee TH, Marcantonio ER, Mangione CM et al. Derivation and prospective validation of a simple index for prediction of cardiac risk of major noncardiac surgery. Circulation 100:1043-1049, 1999.

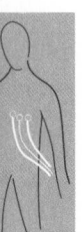

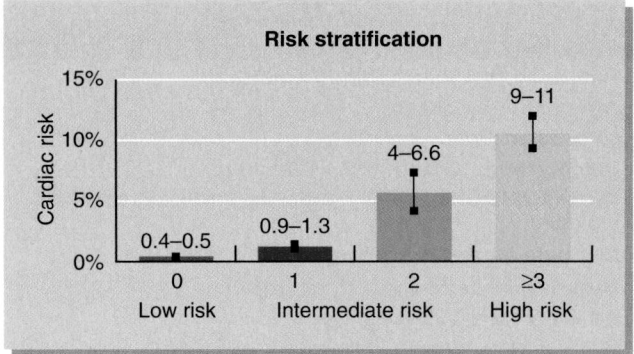

Figure 25-1 Revised cardiac risk index score.

fibrillation or primary cardiac arrest, and complete heart block) (see Table 25-4) can then be predicted. Based on the presence of 0, 1, 2, 3, or more of these clinical predictors, the rates of major cardiac complications are estimated to be 0.4% to 0.5%, 0.9% to 1.3%, 4% to 6.6%, and 9% to 11%, respectively (Fig. 25-1). Cardiac risk particularly increases with two or more predictors, and is greatest with three predictors or more. The clinical utility of the RCRI is to identify patients at higher risk for cardiac complications and to determine whether they may benefit from further risk stratification with noninvasive cardiac testing or initiation of preoperative preventive medical management.

PREOPERATIVE NONINVASIVE CARDIAC TESTING FOR RISK STRATIFICATION

Evidence discourages widespread application of preoperative noninvasive cardiac testing for all patients. Rather, a selective approach based on clinical risk categorization appears to be both effective and cost-effective. The selection of noninvasive cardiac stress tests for the occasional patient should anticipate that the patient will meet guidelines for coronary revascularization after coronary angiography or an adjustment in medical therapy, and no testing is recommended when it might delay surgical intervention for urgent or emergent conditions. There is potential benefit of coronary revascularization through identification of asymptomatic but high-risk patients (patients with left main disease, left main equivalent disease, or triple coronary vessel disease with poor left ventricular function). However, evidence does not support aggressive attempts to identifying intermediate-risk patients with asymptomatic but advanced CAD when coronary revascularization appears to offer little advantage over excellent medical therapy. An RCRI score of ≥3 in patients with severe myocardial ischemia suggestive of left main or three-vessel disease should lead to consideration of coronary revascularization before noncardiac surgery for appropriate patients. Noninvasive cardiac testing is most appropriate if it is anticipated that a patient will meet guidelines for initiation of additional medical therapy or coronary angiography and coronary revascularization in the event of a positive test. Pharmacologic stress tests, instead of exercise tests, are typically reserved for patients with functional limitations. Dobutamine echocardiography and nuclear perfusion testing for purposes of identifying patients at risk for perioperative MI or death have excellent negative predictive values (near 100%) but poor positive predictive values (<20%). Thus, a negative study is reassuring, but a positive study is still only a weak predictor of a "hard" perioperative cardiac event. Which higher risk patients are most likely to benefit from preoperative noninvasive cardiac testing and treatment strategies to improve outcomes is not well defined.

CHOICES OF NONINVASIVE CARDIAC TESTING

The choices among noninvasive tests should be based on the need to assess valvular or ventricular function and on which test is most reliable and available locally. Dobutamine stress echocardiography is often used because it has excellent overall predictive performance, as well as providing additional information about valvular and left ventricular dysfunction. A rapidly developing diagnostic modality is dobutamine stress magnetic resonance imaging (MRI), although sensitivity and specificity data are still pending at this time.

Exercise Testing

In general, poor functional capacity associated with exercise-induced ischemia indicates a higher risk for perioperative cardiac events, and achieving an excellent workload indicates a lower risk. The ability to attain 75% to 85% of maximal age-predicted heart rate is predictive of a lower rate of perioperative cardiac events. In patients with baseline ECG abnormalities and an inability to exercise secondary to comorbid conditions, pharmacologic stress echocardiography or nuclear imaging is preferred.

Dipyridamole-Thallium Imaging Stress Test

Preoperative dipyridamole-thallium imaging has excellent negative predictive value (between 90% and 100%), and low positive predictive value (6% and 67%), making it more useful for reducing risk estimates when negative than for identifying very–high-risk patients when positive. The presence of thallium redistribution, especially in increasing numbers of myocardial segments, identifies patients at greater risk for perioperative cardiac complications, whereas the presence of fixed defects identifies patients at intermediate risk, particularly for late cardiac events.

Dobutamine Stress Echocardiography

The number of myocardial segments demonstrating wall motion abnormalities or wall motion changes at low infusion rates of dobutamine identifies patients at higher risk for perioperative cardiac events. The predictive value of dobutamine and dipyridamole stress echocardiography and of dipyridamole-thallium myocardial perfusion scintigraphy in patients undergoing major vascular surgery demonstrated a trend favoring dobutamine stress echocardiography.

Ambulatory Electrocardiographic Monitoring

Studies using preoperative ambulatory ECG monitoring have demonstrated a predictive value similar to that of dipyridamole thallium. However, current evidence does not support its sole use for identifying patients to be referred for coronary angiography.

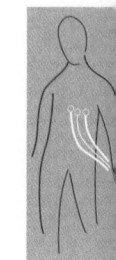

PREOPERATIVE INVASIVE CARDIAC TESTING FOR RISK STRATIFICATION

Recommendations for perioperative coronary angiography are similar to those for patients with suspected or known CAD in general and should conform to the ACC/AHA guidelines for coronary angiography. This procedure should be considered for patients who have evidence of being at high risk for adverse outcome based on noninvasive test results, unstable angina, angina refractory to medical treatment, high-risk results on noninvasive testing, or a nondiagnostic test in patients at high risk undergoing high-risk noncardiac surgery. It should be considered on an individual basis for limited to extensive ischemia during noninvasive testing, for patients at intermediate risk undergoing high-risk surgery with nondiagnostic test results, for patients convalescing from MI who need urgent noncardiac surgery, and for patients with perioperative MI. In patients who have a high clinical risk (RCRI > 3) and who have high-risk features on noninvasive cardiac testing should be considered for diagnostic cardiac catheterization (see Fig. 25-1).

PREOPERATIVE RISK MODIFICATION TO REDUCE PERIOPERATIVE CARDIAC RISK

Coronary Revascularization

Retrospective analyses of the Coronary Artery Surgery Study (CASS) registry and Bypass Angioplasty Revascularization Investigation (BARI) and prospective study of patients enrolled in the Coronary Artery Revascularization Prophylaxis (CARP) trial have shown that prophylactic coronary revascularization with either coronary artery bypass grafting (CABG) or percutaneous coronary intervention (PCI) provides no short-term or mid-term benefit for patients without left main disease or multivessel CAD in the presence of poor left ventricular systolic function. High-risk patients who have successfully undergone PCI or CABG before elective noncardiac surgeries experience fewer adverse perioperative cardiovascular events compared with similar patients treated with medications alone. However, the mortality and morbidity associated with PCI or CABG appears to offset the potential benefit of coronary revascularization before any high-risk cardiac surgery like major vascular surgery. Thus, evidence is lacking in support for elective coronary revascularization as a primary strategy in perioperative risk reduction in intermediate-risk patients undergoing major noncardiac surgery. Recommendations for PCI are similar to those for patients with suspected or known CAD in general and should conform to the ACC/AHA guidelines. Although catheter-based PCI in the perioperative setting is associated with lower procedural risk than CABG, studies have shown that the placement of a stent in a coronary artery shortly before plastic surgery may increase perioperative risk for MI and cardiac death due to in-stent thrombosis. Recommendations by the AHA/ACC Society for Cardiovascular Angiography and Intervention, American College of Surgeons, and American Dental Association Science Advisory Committee are for a 30- to 45-day delay of surgery in patients taking administration of thienopyridine dual-antiplatelet therapy after bare-metal coronary stent placement, and a 365-day wait for a drug-eluting stent. For patients who need to undergo noncardiac surgery imminently (2 to 6 weeks), drug-eluted stents should not be implanted, and balloon angioplasty appears to be a reasonable alternative. If noncardiac surgery is urgent or emergent, CABG combined with the noncardiac surgery could be considered; however, cardiac risks, the risk for bleeding, and the long-term benefit of coronary revascularization must be weighed.

Currently, studies suggest that optimal medical therapy is the preferred strategy for the intermediate- to high-risk patient population with RCRI score greater than or equal to 2 and without documented severe myocardial ischemia. As noted previously, the CARP trial demonstrated that preoperative coronary revascularization strategies to reduce perioperative cardiovascular risk did not offer significant benefit above and beyond excellent medical treatment in intermediate- to high-risk patients undergoing vascular surgery. However, high-risk patients with left main coronary stenosis, severe aortic stenosis, left ventricular ejection fraction less than or equal to 20%, or unstable coronary symptoms were excluded from the trial. In many of these patients, coronary or valve surgery is indicated on its own merit, without factoring in the noncardiac surgery. Thus, coronary revascularization may be appropriate if diagnostic catheterization reveals left main disease or multivessel disease with depressed ejection fraction. Using the information obtained from the composite algorithm (Fig. 25-2), a key decision is whether the risk for perioperative cardiac events is sufficiently low to proceed with surgery. For patients identified at high cardiac risk who are not candidates for coronary revascularization, this may result in a decision to perform a less extensive or limiting major plastic reconstruction, consider laparoscopic versus open procedures or alternative palliative procedures, or attempt to modify cardiac risk by additional intraoperative and perioperative therapies.

β-adrenergic Antagonists

Two previous clinical trials and a recent retrospective analysis of a large national database supported the use of β blockers for perioperative cardiac risk reduction in intermediate- to high-risk patients undergoing major noncardiac surgery, and particularly for major vascular surgery. However, prescribing perioperative β blockers should be based on a thorough assessment of a patient's perioperative cardiac risk (RCRI = 2) and not broad inclusion criteria, to yield a favorable risk-to-benefit ratio in patients who are at increased cardiac risk. For patients with or without mild to moderate reactive airway disease, it is advised to use the cardioselective β blocker of choice, and titrate to a target resting heart rate of 60 to 65 beats per minute. In intermediate- to high-risk patients without a long-term indication for β blockers, the medications can be administered intravenously as a preoperative medication on the day of surgery, with a targeted heart rate of 60 to 65 beats per minute, and continued for more than 7 days, preferably 30 days, after surgery. This targeted heart rate of 60 to 65 beats per minute should be titrated to avoid intraoperative and postoperative heart rate of less than 50 beats per minute and systolic blood pressure of less than 100 mm Hg. Intravenous preparations should be substituted for oral medication if patients are unable to take or absorb pills in the perioperative period.

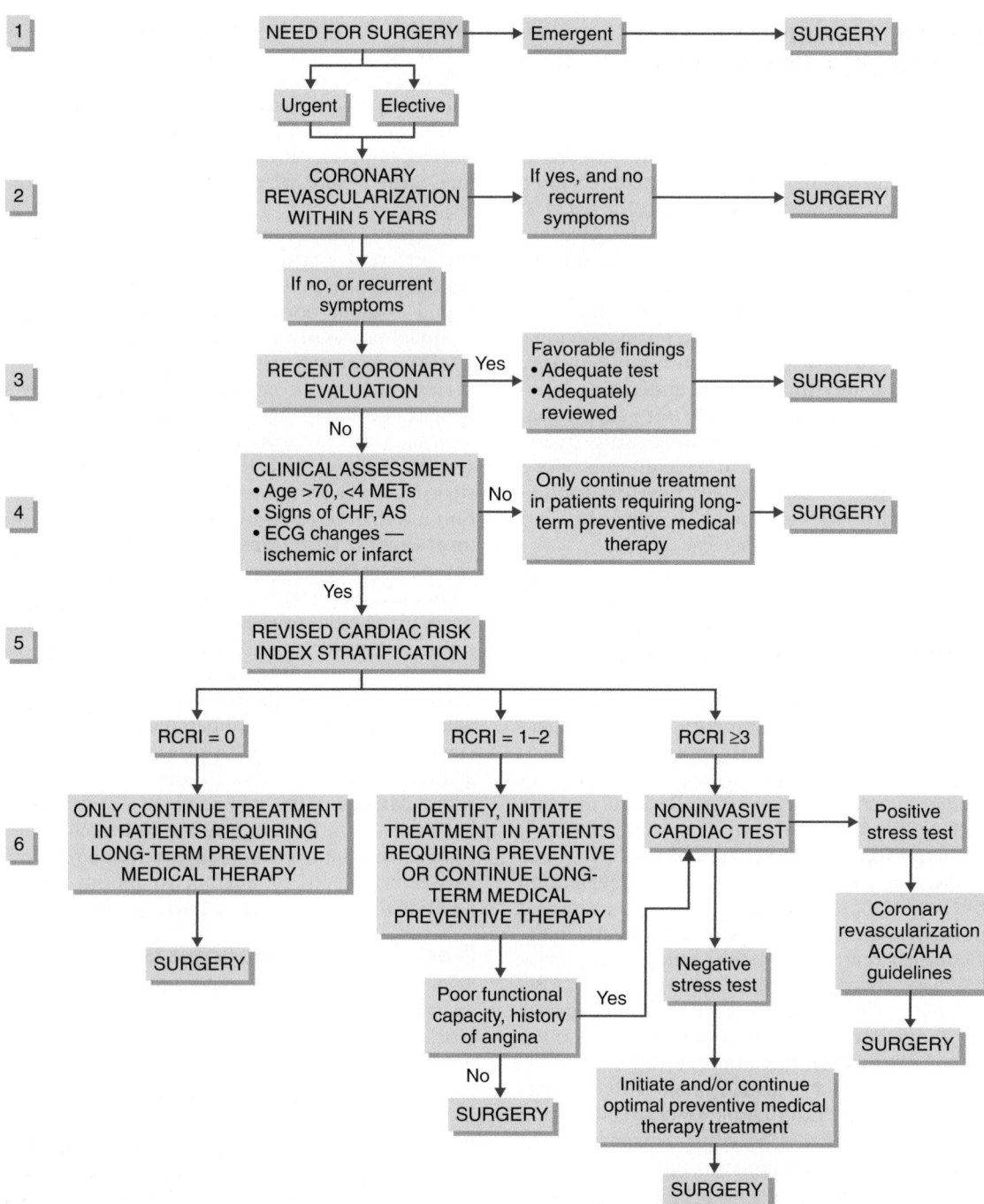

Figure 25-2 Stepwise clinical evaluation for diagnostic cardiac catheterization: (1) emergency surgery; (2) prior coronary revascularization; (3) prior coronary evaluation; (4) clinical assessment; (5) revised cardiac risk index; (6) risk modification strategies. Preventive medical therapy included β-blocker and statin therapy. ACC, American College of Cardiology; AHA, American Heart Association; CHF, congestive heart failure; ECG, electrocardiogram; MET, metabolic equivalent; RCRI, reverse cardiac risk index.

The ACC/AHA guideline focusing on recommendations for perioperative β-blocker therapy suggested using β blockers for the following situations: (1) β blockers should be continued in all high-risk patients previously receiving β-blocker therapy undergoing vascular surgery; (2) β blockers should be administered to all high-risk patients identified by myocardial ischemia on preoperative assessment undergoing vascular surgery; (3) β blockers are probably recommended for high-risk patients defined by multiple clinical predictors undergoing intermediate- or high-risk procedures; (4) β blockers may also be considered for intermediate-risk patients defined by a single clinical predictor undergoing intermediate- or high-risk procedures; (5) β blockers may be considered in low-risk patients defined by clinical predictors not receiving β-blocker therapy undergoing vascular surgery; and (6) β blockers should not be administered in preoperative patients with absolute contraindications to β blockers. As noted, the data favoring a benefit of β blockers for perioperative risk reduction are most robust in patients undergoing vascular surgery, in whom concomitant CAD is particularly common.

The recent results from the Perioperative Ischemic Evaluation (POISE) trial have addressed the limitation of the ACC/AHA recommendations for perioperative β blockers due to few randomized control trials, in regard to the beneficial effects, the method of titration, the optimal dosing regimen, the route of administration, and the risks of perioperative β blockers. The POISE trial randomized 8351 intermediate- to high-risk patients older than 45 years to either a long-acting oral metoprolol succinate (metoprolol CR) or placebo. A high starting dose of metoprolol CR was administered: 100 mg was started orally 2 to 4 hours before surgery and was continued 0 to 6 hours after surgery (or slow intravenous infusion of 15 mg every 6 hours was administered until patients were able to receive the drug orally), and was continued daily for 30 days. The medication was withheld if systolic blood pressure fell below 100 mm Hg or heart rate was below 50 beats per minute. The results showed that cardiac death, nonfatal MI, or cardiac arrest was reduced in the metoprolol group compared with placebo (5.8% versus 6.9%; hazard ratio, 0.84; 95% confidence interval [CI], 0.70 to 0.99; $P = .04$). However, there was an increased incidence of mortality and stroke in the metoprolol group compared with the placebo group (3.1% versus 2.3%, $P = .03$; and 1% versus 0.5%, $P = .005$, respectively,). Thus, for every 1000 patients treated, metoprolol CR would prevent 11 MIs in intermediate- to high-risk patients undergoing major noncardiac surgery, at a cost, however, of eight deaths and five disabling strokes. Stroke was associated with perioperative hypotension, bleeding, atrial fibrillation, and a history of stroke or transient ischemic attack. The POISE trialists highlighted the importance of a clear risk and benefit assessment for the initiation of preoperative β blockers (see Fig. 25-2). β blockers should also be carefully titrated and not abruptly initiated on a high-dose regimen to achieve the desired heart rate in the intermediate- and high-risk patients undergoing noncardiac surgery.

α₂-adrenergic Agonists

For intermediate- to high-risk patients undergoing major noncardiac surgery who do not tolerate β blockers, evidence supports alternative prophylactic use of α₂-adrenergic agonists for perioperative cardiac risk reduction. These should only be initiated in stable patients and titrated carefully to prevent significant hypotension and bradycardia.

HMG-CoA Reductase Inhibitors (Statins)

Prospective and retrospective evidence support the perioperative prophylactic use of statins for reduction of perioperative cardiac complications in patients with established atherosclerosis. Although the future role of statin prophylaxis in the reduction of perioperative cardiac risk reduction awaits definitive clarification by the ongoing European (DECREASE IV) trial, perioperative statin therapy should currently be considered in intermediate- to high-risk patients with known atherosclerosis undergoing major noncardiac surgery to reduce perioperative and long-term cardiac risk.

Calcium Channel Blockers

Evidence is lacking to support the use of calcium channel blockers as a prophylaxis strategy to decrease perioperative risk for major noncardiac surgery.

Angiotensin-Converting Enzyme Inhibitors

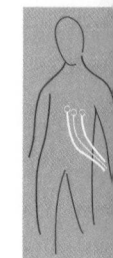

Angiotensin-converting enzyme (ACE) inhibitors and angiotensin II receptor antagonists are frequently prescribed for the management of hypertension, congestive heart failure, chronic renal failure, and ischemic heart disease. Evidence supports the discontinuation of ACE inhibitors and angiotensin receptor antagonists for 24 hours before noncardiac surgery because of adverse circulatory effects after induction of anesthesia in patients on a chronic ACE inhibitor regimen, and use of vasopressin agonists for refractory hypotension after induction of anesthesia.

Oral Antithrombotic Agents

Evidence-based recommendations regarding perioperative use of aspirin, clopidogrel, or both to reduce cardiac risk currently lacks clarity. A substantial increase in perioperative bleeding and transfusion requirement in patients receiving dual antiplatelet therapy has been observed. The discontinuation of clopidogrel 5 days before and the decision to hold aspirin 5 to 7 days before major surgery to minimize the risk for perioperative bleeding and transfusion must be balanced with the potential increased risk for an acute coronary syndrome, especially in high-risk patients with recent coronary stent implantation. If clinicians elect to withhold aspirin before surgery, it should be restarted as soon as possible postoperatively, especially after vascular graft procedures.

Intraoperative Strategies for Reducing Perioperative Risk

ANESTHETIC MANAGEMENT

Epidural anesthesia and analgesia may improve the outcome of major noncardiac surgery by better suppression of surgical stress, a positive effect on postoperative nitrogen balance, more stable cardiovascular hemodynamic response, reduced blood loss, better peripheral vascular circulation, and better postoperative pain control. Conflicting results from several meta-analyses have been published that examined the safety of general and neuraxial (epidural or spinal) anesthesia on cardiac complications. Rodgers and colleagues reviewed 141 trials, including 9559 patients, and found that overall mortality was reduced by about one third (odds ratio, 0.70; 95% CI, 0.54 to 0.90) in patients randomized to receive neuraxial anesthesia compared with patients who received general anesthesia. Lower rates of venous thrombosis, pulmonary embolism, pneumonia, and respiratory depression were also observed in patients who were provided neuraxial anesthesia. However, there are no existing data to support significant differences in cardiovascular events between the two techniques. A combined neuraxial blockade and general

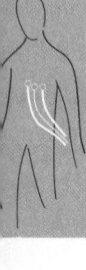

anesthesia technique has its merits when indicated to reduce the intraoperative general anesthesia requirements. Evidence from a meta-analysis of randomized controlled trials supported postoperative epidural analgesia for the purposes of pain relief for more than 24 hours to help reduce the rate of postoperative MI (rate difference, −3.8%; 95% CI, −7.4%, −0.2%; $P = .049$), with subgroup analysis favoring thoracic epidural analgesia compared with systemic analgesia. Neuraxial anesthesia, especially when used for postoperative analgesia, confers reduced postoperative cardiopulmonary complications better or equal to general anesthesia; however, conflicting evidence limits the support for its broad recommendation as the technique of choice for major surgery. Studies have demonstrated that pain management in the perioperative period is crucial for reducing cardiac risk. Adequate pain control reduces catecholamine surges, which are probably responsible for increasing myocardial oxygen demand, induction of coronary vasospasm, increasing the tendency for plaque rupture, and development of a hypercoagulable state. A hematocrit of more than 10 mg/dL and an oxygen tension higher than 60 facilitate tissue oxygenation and help decrease myocardial necrosis.

INTRAOPERATIVE PULMONARY ARTERY CATHETER

The current evidence on whether the use of pulmonary artery catheters (PACs) or a central venous catheter is beneficial for high-risk patients undergoing major noncardiac surgery is controversial. Recommendations from the practice guidelines for PAC in an updated report by the American Society of Anesthesiologist Task Force on PAC does not support the routine use of PAC when there is a low risk for hemodynamic complications in low- or intermediate-risk patients. In a large multicenter randomized trial, Sandham and associates found no benefit to therapy directed by a PAC over standard care in elderly, high-risk surgical patients. PAC may be considered for patients with signs and symptoms of heart failure preoperatively who have a very high postoperative incidence of heart failure, or for high-risk patients with limited ventricular reserve who are undergoing procedures that are likely to cause major hemodynamic shifts.

INTRAOPERATIVE TRANSESOPHAGEAL ECHOCARDIOGRAPHY

Because ischemia-induced myocardial wall motion abnormalities appear earlier than ischemia-induced electric abnormalities, intraoperative transesophageal echocardiography (TEE) was proposed to be a more sensitive monitor of ischemia than conventional intraoperative 2-lead ECG. Similarly, 12-lead ECG monitoring was also proposed to have greater sensitivity than conventional intraoperative ECG. However, when compared with intraoperative monitoring using 2-lead ECG, routine monitoring for myocardial ischemia with TEE or 12-lead ECG during noncardiac surgery lacked robust evidence for incremental value in identifying patients at high risk for perioperative ischemic outcomes. Thus, the routine use of intraoperative TEE is not recommended for monitoring and guiding therapy during noncardiac surgery, except in emergent scenarios in which

the etiology of an acute persistent and life-threatening hemodynamic instability needs to be determined.

MAINTENANCE OF BODY TEMPERATURE DURING NONCARDIAC SURGERY

Current ACC/AHA guidelines recommend the maintenance of body temperature in a normothermic range for procedures other than using hypothermia to provide organ protection. A retrospective analysis of a prospective randomized controlled trial demonstrated that hypothermia (core temperature < 35° C) was associated with an increased risk for myocardial ischemia compared with a core temperature greater than or equal to 35° C. A randomized controlled trial in 300 high-risk patients undergoing noncardiac surgery in which patients were randomized to active warming or routine care demonstrated that adverse cardiac events (unstable angina, myocardial ischemia, cardiac arrest, and MI) occurred less frequently in the normothermic group than in the hypothermic group (1.4% versus 6.3%; $P = .02$). Furthermore, hypothermia was an independent predictor of adverse cardiac events by multivariable analysis (relative risk, 2.2; 95% CI, 1.1 to 4.7; $P = .04$), indicating a 55% reduction in risk when normothermia was maintained.

Postoperative Cardiac Risk Assessment

MONITORING FOR MYOCARDIAL INFARCTION

A protocol involving an ECG immediately after surgery and on the first and second postoperative days has the highest sensitivity for detection of postoperative MI, whereas routine measurements of serial creatine kinase and CK-MB had high false-positive rates and do not increase the sensitivity. The myocardium-specific biomarkers such as troponin I and troponin T have emerged as the most sensitive and specific biochemical markers of myocardial injury and infarction and have been associated with an increased risk for cardiac events if their levels are found elevated in the postoperative period. Current recommendations favor monitoring for signs of cardiac dysfunction in patients with evidence of CAD. In such patients undergoing surgical procedures associated with high cardiac risk, ECG at baseline, immediately after surgery, and on the first 2 days postoperatively is recommended. Measurement of cardiac biomarkers should be reserved for patients at high risk and for those who demonstrate ECG changes, angina typical of acute coronary syndrome, or hemodynamic evidence of cardiovascular dysfunction.

POSTOPERATIVE RISK STRATIFICATION AND MANAGEMENT STRATEGIES

Postoperative patient care involves assessment and treatment of modifiable cardiac risk factors, including hypertension, hyperlipidemia, smoking, obesity, hyperglycemia, and physical inactivity. Patients who sustain a perioperative MI or develop evidence of myocardial ischemia should be carefully investigated because they are at substantial cardiac risk over the subsequent 5 to 10 years. Noninvasive testing to assess left ventricular function and inducible ischemia should be undertaken to identify patients who may benefit from revascularization or optimization of medical therapy. Postoperative heart failure and pulmonary edema should be treated similar to pulmonary edema in the nonoperative setting. An emergency ECG and serial troponin assays are helpful in the event of acute myocardial ischemia.

Noncardiac Surgery in Patients with Specific Cardiovascular Conditions

VALVULAR HEART DISEASE

Special consideration has to be given in preoperative risk assessment for patients with valvular heart disease. All patients undergoing noncardiac surgery should be assessed especially for aortic stenosis by physical examination and two-dimensional echocardiography for any suspicious murmur. One recent study has demonstrated that patients with aortic stenosis have a fivefold increased risk for perioperative mortality and nonfatal MI compared with patients without aortic stenosis. The adjusted relative risks for adverse events is 5.2 for asymptomatic aortic valve gradients between 25 and 50 mm Hg (moderate aortic stenosis) and 6.8 for gradients above 50 mm Hg (severe aortic stenosis). Patients with severe symptomatic aortic stenosis should undergo aortic valve replacement before plastic surgery, if they are thought to be acceptable surgical candidates. In rare instances, balloon aortic valvuloplasty may be justified before elective plastic surgery. A retrospective study suggested that selected patients with asymptomatic severe aortic stenosis could safely undergo noncardiac surgery with careful hemodynamic monitoring. Thus, all patients undergoing noncardiac surgery should be assessed diligently for systolic murmurs accompanied by chest radiography with or without ECG and echocardiographic confirmation as a stepwise diagnostic approach.

There is less known about the perioperative risks associated with mitral stenosis and mitral regurgitation in patients undergoing noncardiac surgery. Clearly, a preoperative history and physical examination, chest radiograph, or ECG will usually provide clues to the diagnosis, which can be confirmed by echocardiography. Accurate diagnosis may help optimize intraoperative anesthetic strategies, choice of pharmacologic intervention and invasive monitoring, and postoperative medical management. Heart rate should be controlled to ensure a sufficient diastolic filling period and avoid pulmonary congestion in patients with mild to moderate mitral stenosis. Patients with severe mitral stenosis are likely to benefit from balloon mitral valvuloplasty or surgical repair before high-risk surgery.

Patients with aortic or mitral valvular regurgitation benefit from volume control and afterload reduction. In aortic insufficiency, it is thought that faster heart rates are better tolerated in this particular condition than slow heart rates because slow heart rates lead to increased diastolic filling and can exacerbate left ventricular volume overload.

Except for perioperative antibiotic prophylaxis to prevent bacterial endocarditis and the need for effective anticoagulation strategies, perioperative complications in patients with prosthetic heart valves are probably similar to those in patients with comparable degrees of native valvular heart disease. In patients with a mechanical valve prosthesis, recommendation for anticoagulation are as follows: in patients requiring minimally invasive procedures (dental, superficial plastic surgery, and biopsies), the international normalized ratio should be reduced briefly to the low or subtherapeutic range, the normal dose of oral anticoagulation resumed promptly after the procedure; and perioperative unfractionated heparin is recommended for patients in whom the risk for bleeding with oral anticoagulation is high and the risk for thromboembolic without anticoagulation is also high (e.g., mechanical mitral valve). Patients between these two extremes should undergo individual assessment for the risk and benefit of reduced anticoagulation with warfarin versus perioperative heparin initiation and brief interruption surrounding surgery.

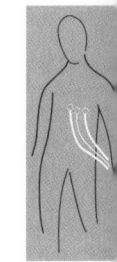

ARRHYTHMIAS AND CONDUCTION DEFECT

Ventricular and atrial arrhythmias historically are identified as predictors of perioperative cardiac complications. As such, identification of a preoperative arrhythmia warrants a careful evaluation for the presence and severity of underlying ischemic heart disease, cardiomyopathy, or other conditions that may contribute to perioperative complications. Generally, asymptomatic arrhythmias or conduction defects warrant observation only and maintenance of an optimal metabolic state. However, third-degree atrioventricular block can increase operative risk and may necessitate pacing.

CONGESTIVE HEART FAILURE AND LEFT VENTRICULAR DYSFUNCTION

Congestive heart failure (CHF) has been identified as a significant marker of cardiac risk for noncardiac surgery. Every effort should be made to identify the etiology of CHF and optimally control it preoperatively because it is a known risk factor for postoperative cardiac complications. However, there are no evidence-based recommendations for optimal perioperative strategy in patients with heart failure undergoing intermediate- to high-risk noncardiac surgery other than making sure that such patients are taking medications known to improve patients with heart failure in the long-term. Because proper treatment of heart failure depends greatly on its underlying etiology (especially systolic dysfunction versus diastolic dysfunction), characterizing this before elective noncardiac surgery can help in tailoring therapy to each patient. Close monitoring of the volume status is needed to avoid perioperative decompensation. Use of intravenous inotropic agents, vasodilators, or both for a short duration in the perioperative period may be useful to prevent or treat CHF depending on the situation.

HYPERTROPHIC CARDIOMYOPATHY

Patients with echocardiographically documented hypertrophic cardiomyopathy (HCM) are at risk for exacerbation of dynamic left ventricular outflow tract (LVOT) obstruction during periods of tachycardia, hypotension, or increased inotropy. General anesthesia or neuraxial block can lead to peripheral vasodilation and sympathetic autonomic blockade that may decrease venous return and further exacerbate LVOT obstruction. Observational studies of patients with HCM undergoing noncardiac surgery suggest that for most operations, patients with compensated HCM tolerate the perioperative period well. Perioperative cardiac risk reduction strategies should include avoidance of hypovolemia, vasodilators, phosphodiesterase inhibitors, β-adrenergic agonists, and diligent attention to volume repletion and selected use of α-adrenergic agonists. Patients with hypertrophic cardiomyopathy are at significant risk for developing perioperative hypotension, CHF, and arrhythmias and should be monitored closely.

CONGENITAL HEART DISEASE

Studies have demonstrated that patients with left-to-right cardiac shunts with residual hemodynamic abnormalities after surgical repair experience decreased cardiac output in response to stress. Vigorous treatment of ongoing CHF is required for such patients before noncardiac surgery. Patients with a large left-to-right shunt but only a slight increase in pulmonary artery resistance should undergo cardiac repair before noncardiac surgery. Patients with irreversible pulmonary artery hypertension have an extremely high risk associated with nonsurgical procedures and should not undergo elective procedures unless there is absolutely no alternative. Patients with prior repair of coarctation of the aorta have a significant risk for sudden death during follow-up, caused by residual cardiac defects with CHF, rupture of a major vessel, dissecting aneurysm, or complications arising from severe atherosclerosis. Such patients also have a high incidence of residual hypertension. Therefore, these patients require careful preoperative assessment and close hemodynamic monitoring during the intraoperative and postoperative periods. Patients with tetralogy of Fallot are also prone to sudden cardiac death. Monitoring and aggressive prevention and treatment of life-threatening arrhythmias such as ventricular tachycardia, or atrioventricular block, are needed for such patients in the perioperative period.

Surgery in patients with cyanotic congenital heart disease with right-to-left shunts poses several unique problems. Most cyanotic patients are polycythemic and therefore are prone to thrombotic complications. Use of diuretics should generally be avoided in such patients because dehydration may increase the blood viscosity and, in turn, increase the tendency for thrombosis, particularly cerebral thrombosis. Patients with a hematocrit greater than 70% should be considered for plasmapheresis before noncardiac surgery. Phlebotomy is not advisable in this circumstance because this can decrease intravascular blood volume and thus increase cyanosis. Patients with a hematocrit between 55% and 65% should receive intravenous fluids starting the night before the surgery. Patients with congenital heart disease should also receive appropriate prophylaxis for bacterial endocarditis. One retrospective report suggested that, with careful monitoring and precautions as outlined previously, patients with right-to-left shunts could undergo noncardiac surgery with relatively few complications, with careful attention not to introduce air into the vascular system.

Prospectus for the Future

CAD accounts for most deaths in patients undergoing noncardiac surgery, in whom perioperative MI is associated with high mortality rates. The success of standardized evidence-based preoperative and postoperative cardiac risk reduction strategies in patients undergoing noncardiac surgery pivots around collaborative teamwork and sound communication among surgeons, anesthesiologist, the patient's primary care physician, and the consultant. The risk for a perioperative cardiac complication varies with the severity of the surgical procedure and with RCRI stratification. A systematic stepwise approach for preoperative cardiac risk assessment for noncardiac surgery facilitates a decision as to whether the risk for perioperative cardiac events is sufficiently low to proceed with surgery. Preoperative noninvasive cardiac testing should be based on a discrete clinical risk categorization, and the choices among noninvasive tests should be based on the need for coronary, valvular, or ventricular function assessment, and which test is most reliable and available locally. In patients with strong suspicion of having or being at risk for CAD, β blockers should be given in the perioperative period, starting at least 24 hours and preferably days before the procedure and titrated to a heart rate of 60 beats per minute and continued postoperatively. Optimal postoperative patient care involves assessment and treatment of modifiable cardiac risk factors, including pain management, hypertension, hyperlipidemia, smoking, obesity, hyperglycemia, and physical inactivity. Finally, patients who sustain a nonfatal perioperative MI or develop evidence of ischemia should be carefully investigated because they are at substantial cardiac risk over the subsequent months and years.

References

Auerbach A, Goldman L: Assessing and reducing the cardiac risk of noncardiac surgery. Circulation 113:1361-1376, 2006.

Boersma E, Kertai MD, Schouten O, et al: Perioperative cardiovascular mortality in noncardiac surgery: Validation of the Lee cardiac risk index. Am J Med 118:1134-1141, 2005.

Eagle KA, Berger PB, Calkins H, et al: ACC/AHA guideline update for perioperative cardiovascular evaluation for noncardiac surgery—executive summary: A report of the American College of Cardiology/American Heart Association Task Force on Practice Guidelines (Committee to Update the 1996 Guidelines on Perioperative Cardiovascular Evaluation for Noncardiac Surgery). J Am Coll Cardiol 39:542-553, 2002.

Fleisher LA, Beckman JA, Brown KA, et al: ACC/AHA 2006 guideline update on perioperative cardiovascular evaluation for noncardiac surgery: Focused update on perioperative beta-blocker therapy. A report of the American College of Cardiology/American Heart Association Task Force on Practice Guidelines (Writing Committee to Update the 2002 Guidelines on Perioperative Cardiovascular Evaluation for Noncardiac Surgery), developed in collaboration with the American Society of Echocardiography, American Society of Nuclear Cardiology, Heart Rhythm Society, Society of Cardiovascular Anesthesiologists, Society for Cardiovascular Angiography and Interventions, and Society for Vascular Medicine and Biology. Circulation 113:2662-2674, 2006.

Hassan SA, Hlatky MA, Boothroyd DB, et al: Outcomes of noncardiac surgery after coronary bypass surgery or coronary angioplasty in the Bypass Angioplasty Revascularization Investigation (BARI). Am J Med 110:260-266, 2001.

Lindenauer PK, Pekow P, Wang K, et al: Perioperative beta-blocker therapy and mortality after major noncardiac surgery. N Engl J Med 353:349-361, 2005.

POISE Study Group: Effects of extended-release metoprolol succinate in patients undergoing non-cardiac surgery (POISE trial): A randomised controlled trial. Lancet 371:1839-1847, 2008.

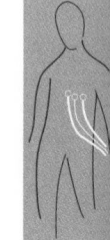

Section VI

Renal Disease

Chapter **26**

Elements of Renal Structure and Function

Robert L. Safirstein

Elements of Renal Structure

GROSS ANATOMY

The human kidneys are a pair of bean-shaped organs situated in the retroperitoneal space, positioned on either side of the vertebral column at the level of the lower thoracic and upper lumbar vertebrae. The right kidney is slightly lower than the left kidney because of the location of the liver. Each adult kidney weighs about 120 to 170 g and measures about 12 × 6 × 3 cm. A coronal section of the kidney shows two distinct regions (Fig. 26-1A). The pale outer region, or *cortex*, is about 1 cm thick. The dark inner region is the medulla and contains 6 to 15 (average, 8) conical structures called *pyramids*. The base of each pyramid is situated at the corticomedullary junction, and the apex extends into the hilum of the kidney as the papilla. The medulla is subdivided further into an outer zone containing the outer and inner stripe of the outer medulla, and an inner zone containing the papilla. This distinction, which is apparent grossly, is important because of the specific tubular and vascular components distinct to each region, all of which are important in the function of the kidney, to be described in subsequent sections.

The concave medial aspect of the kidney is the site of the renal hilum through which pass the branches of the renal artery and vein, lymphatics, nerves, and the expanding upper region of the ureter called the *renal pelvis*. The renal pelvis communicates with a flattened space within the kidney called the *renal sinus*, in which the renal pelvis branches into major and minor calyces to collect the urine emerging through the merged collecting ducts within the renal pyramids.

RENAL BLOOD SUPPLY

Blood is delivered to each kidney from a main renal artery branching from the aorta at the level of the first lumbar vertebra (see Fig. 26-1B). The renal artery enters the hilum and usually divides into two main segmental branches, which are further subdivided into several lobar arteries supplying the upper, middle, and lower regions of the kidney. These vessels branch further as they enter the renal parenchyma and create interlobar arteries that course toward the renal cortex along the lateral margin of the medullary pyramids. At the corticomedullary junction, these smaller arteries provide perpendicular branches that continue in an archlike manner, appropriately named the *arcuate arteries.* Interlobular arteries arise from the arcuate arteries and branch radially within the cortex. The glomerular capillaries receive blood through afferent arterioles that originate from these terminal interlobular arteries. The efferent arteriole leaves the glomerular capillary bed and supplies a network of vessels that surround the tubular structures. The efferent arterioles of the juxtamedullary glomeruli form hairpin loops called *vasa recta* that extend deep into the medulla.

INNERVATION OF THE KIDNEY

Kidneys are richly innervated by the autonomic nervous system. Sympathetic nerve endings are present in all segments of renal vasculature, tubules, and the juxtaglomerular apparatus. Stimulation of the renal sympathetic nerves enhances the release of renin from the juxtaglomerular cells, thereby increasing angiotensin and aldosterone production.

NEPHRON

The basic structural and functional unit of the kidney is the nephron (Fig. 26-2). Each human kidney contains about 1 million nephrons, and each nephron is composed of two major components: a filtering element that consists of an enclosed capillary network (the renal corpuscle) and its attached tubule. Most of the components of the renal corpuscle are contained within the glomerulus, which consists of Bowman capsule, which in turn encloses the glomerular tuft. The tubule components that emerge from Bowman capsule include in succession the proximal tubule, a

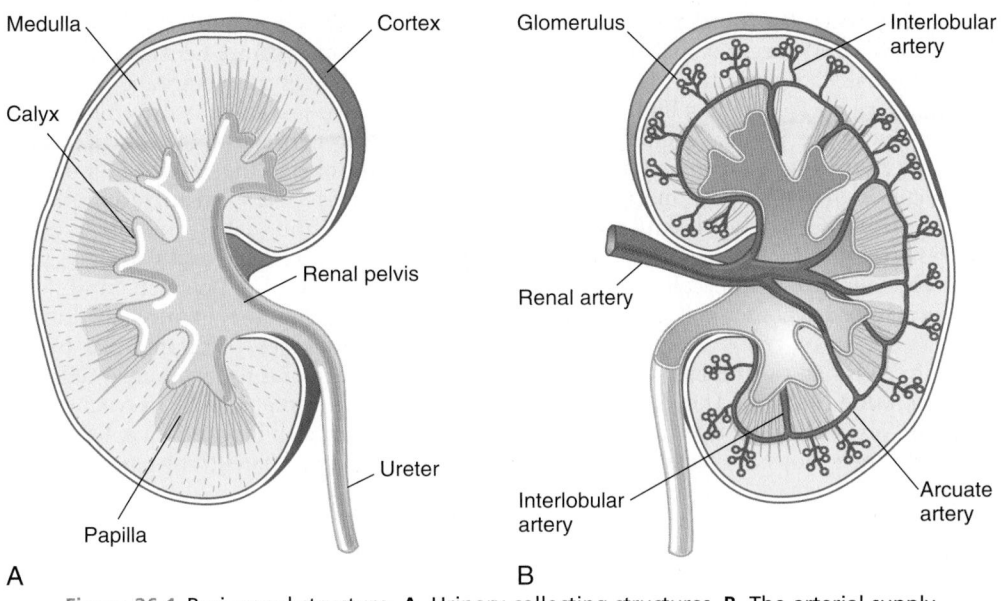

Figure 26-1 Basic renal structure. **A,** Urinary collecting structures. **B,** The arterial supply.

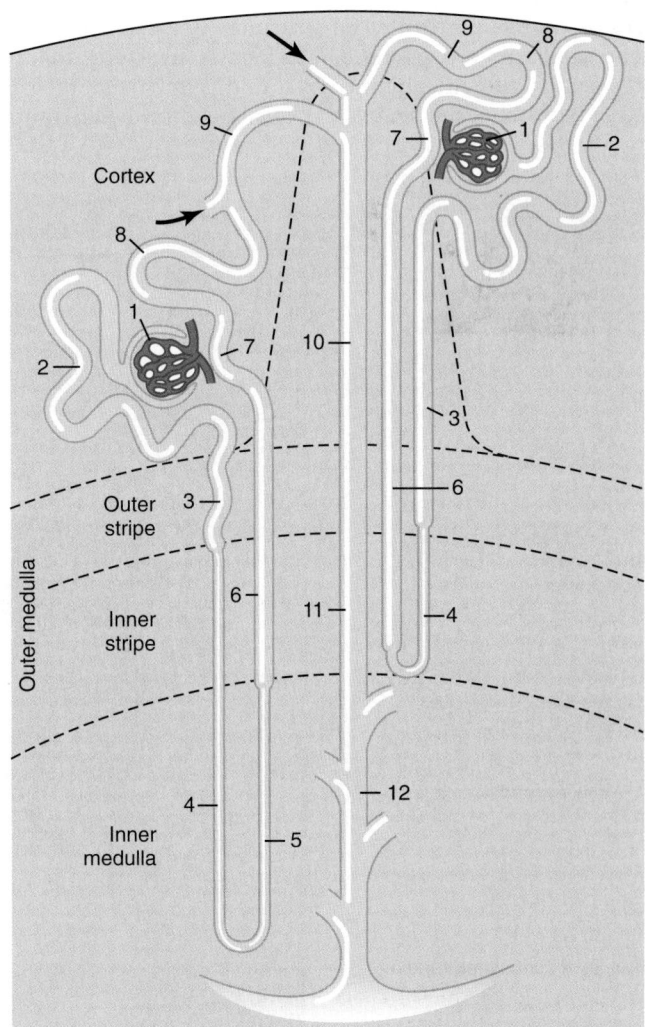

Figure 26-2 Organization of two nephrons. Each nephron consists of a glomerulus (1), proximal convoluted tubule (2), proximal straight tubule (3), thin descending limb of the loop of Henle (4), thin ascending limb (5), thick ascending limb (6), macula densa (7), distal convoluted tubule (8), and connecting tubule (9). Several nephrons coalesce to empty into a collecting duct (10), the outer medullary collecting duct (11), and the inner medullary collecting duct (12). The deeper glomerulus gives rise to nephron along with loop of Henle, which descend to the papillary tip, whereas the more superficial glomerulus has a loop of Henle that bends at the junction between the inner and outer medulla. (Modified from Briggs JP, Kriz W, Schnermann JB: Overview of kidney function and structure. In: Primer on Kidney Diseases, 4th ed. Philadelphia, Saunders, 2005).

convoluted and straight portion; the loop of Henle (composed of the straight portion of the proximal tubule, the thin descending limb, thin ascending limbs of long-looped nephrons, and the medullary thick ascending limb); and the distal tubule, which includes the cortical segment of the thick ascending limb that courses close to its glomerular pole and includes the macula densa, the post macula densa segment, and the convoluted portion of the distal tubule. The collecting duct system follows and is composed first of the connecting segment followed by the collecting ducts, which have both cortical as well as outer and inner medullary segments.

Nephrons are mainly classified on the basis of whether they possess a short or a long loop of Henle. The short-looped nephrons usually originate from the superficial and mid-cortical regions, and their loops of Henle bend within the outer medulla. By contrast, the long-looped nephrons originate from the juxtamedullary (corticomedullary) region, and their loops of Henle extend into the inner medulla. A minority of these juxtamedullary nephrons have loops that penetrate deeply in the inner medulla to reach the papilla before turning upward.

RENAL CORPUSCLE (GLOMERULUS)

The glomerulus (Fig. 26-3) is a unique network of capillaries suspended between the afferent and efferent arterioles enclosed within an epithelial structure (Bowman capsule). The capillaries are arranged into lobular structures called *glomerular tufts* and are lined by a thin layer of endothelial cells. The core of the glomerulus consists of the mesangium,

which consists of mesangial cells and a surrounding mesangial matrix. Other components of the glomerulus include the glomerular basement membrane and visceral and parietal epithelial cells. The afferent and efferent arterioles enter and leave the glomerulus at the vascular pole, and Bowman capsule continues as the proximal tubule at the urinary pole. The efferent arteriole splits up into another capillary network that surrounds the adjacent tubules to form the peritubular capillary network. The renal corpuscle thus consists of the parietal epithelium of Bowman capsule, a visceral epithelium surrounding the glomerular tuft, endothelial cells lining the capillaries, the glomerular basement membrane, and the intraglomerular mesangial cells within a mesangial matrix. These elements work in synchrony to maintain high hydraulic permeability and establish the charge and size permselectivity of the ultrafiltration process.

Epithelial Cells

The visceral epithelial cells, or podocytes, are highly specialized pericytes with a complex cytoarchitecture and prominent surface features best exemplified by interdigitating projections onto the surface of the glomerular endothelium called *foot processes*. Between these projections is the slit diaphragm, which is the most important barrier to transglomerular passage of macromolecules into the glomerular ultrafiltrate (Fig. 26-4). Hereditary forms of nephrotic syndrome are associated with mutations in genes whose products establish the slit diaphragm structure, and which are derived from the podocyte. Included in this group are mutations in nephrin, podocin, α-actinin 4, and CD2-associated

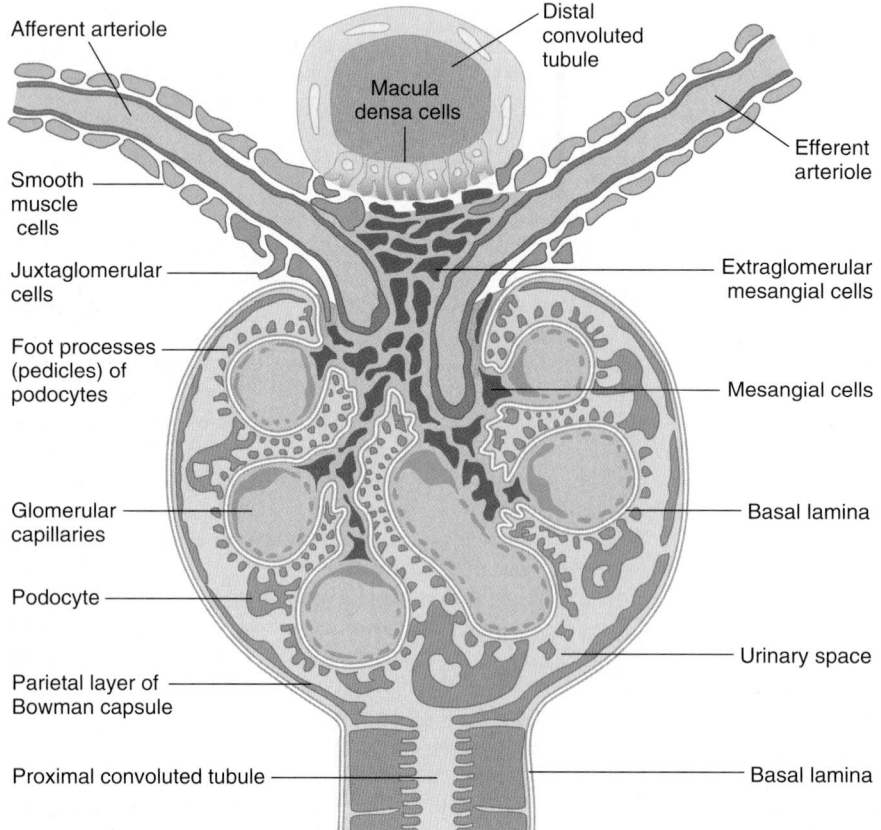

Afferent arteriole

Distal convoluted tubule

Macula densa cells

Efferent arteriole

Smooth muscle cells

Juxtaglomerular cells

Extraglomerular mesangial cells

Foot processes (pedicles) of podocytes

Mesangial cells

Glomerular capillaries

Basal lamina

Podocyte

Urinary space

Parietal layer of Bowman capsule

Proximal convoluted tubule

Basal lamina

Figure 26-3 Schematic diagram of a renal glomerulus and the structures associated at the vascular pole (*top*) and urinary pole (*bottom*) (not drawn to scale). Mesangial cells are associated with the capillary endothelium and the glomerular basement membrane. The macula densa cells of the distal tubule are shown intimately associated with the juxtaglomerular cells of the afferent arteriole and the extraglomerular mesangial cells. (Modified from Kriz W, Sakai T: Morphological aspects of glomerular function. In Davison AM [ed]: Nephrology: Proceedings of the Tenth International Congress of Nephrology. London, Baillière-Tindall, 1987.)

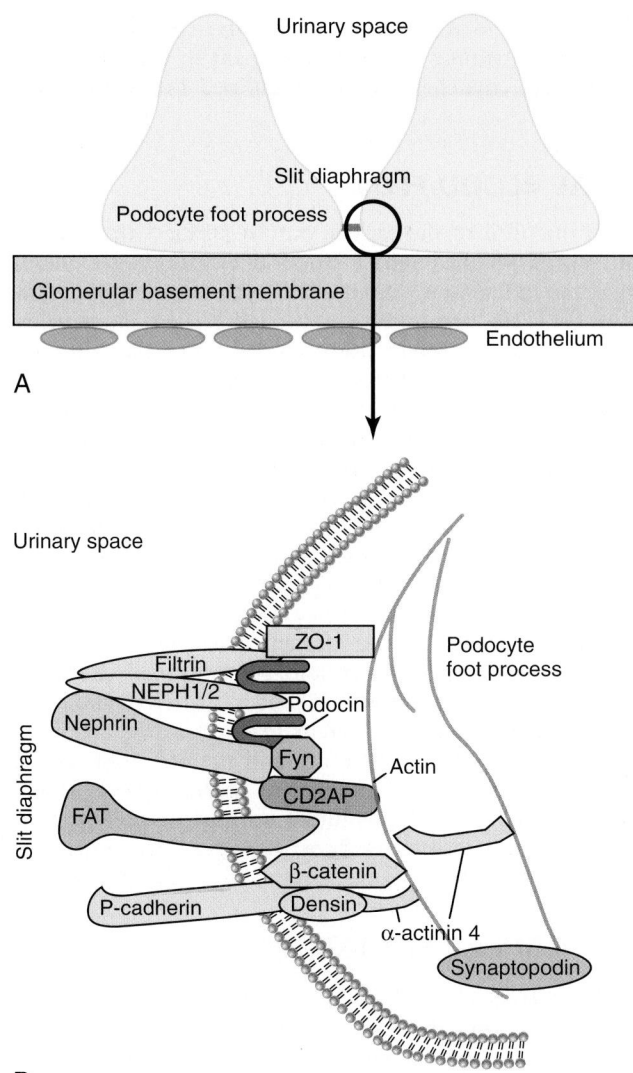

Figure 26-4 A, Schematic picture of podocyte architecture. **B,** Key slit area molecules and their interlinkages. (From Holthofer, H. Molecular architecture of the glomerular slit diaphragm. Nephrol Dial Transplant 2007;22:2124-2128.)

protein. An activating mutation in the transient receptor potential cation channel 6, another podocyte protein, causes a congenital form of focal glomerular sclerosis with onset of disease during the third and fourth decade of life. Injury to the podocytes leads to proteinuria and disturbances of podocyte architecture and results in the retraction, or effacement, of these foot processes and proteinuria. These changes are characteristic of all progressive renal disease syndromes.

Endothelial Cells

A thin layer of fenestrated endothelial cells lines the glomerular capillary lumen. These fenestrae are larger than most in the body and are in part responsible for the high ultrafiltration coefficient of the human glomerulus. A cell coat that is rich in polyanionic glycoproteins covers the endothelial surface and accounts for the lower permeability of negatively charged proteins, like albumen, of the glomerular filtration barrier. As elsewhere in the body, these endothelial cells regulate coagulation, inflammation, and vasomotor tone. They express surface antigens of the class 2 histocompatibility complex, express adhesion molecules for leukocytes, bind

factors IXa and Xa, release and bind von Willebrand factor, and synthesize and release endothelin-1 and nitric oxide. Diminished vascular epidermal growth factor action at the glomerular endothelial cell is responsible for the syndrome of preeclampsia.

Glomerular Basement Membrane

The glomerular basement membrane is a layer of hydrated gel composed of glycoproteins containing interwoven collagen fibers (type IV and V collagen). Heparinases that digest heparin-rich glycoproteins lead to dramatic increases in the permeability of the basement membrane to anionic proteins, indicating that the basement membrane is an important determinant of the glomerular protein filtration barrier. These components are made by both podocytes and endothelial cells. The lack of type IV collagen as a result of mutation of the collagen type IV α_5 subunit gene on the X chromosome leads to Alport syndrome.

Mesangium

Glomerular capillaries course along a structure called the *mesangium*, which is composed of mesangial cells embedded in a mesangial matrix (see Fig. 26-3). Mesangial cells have structural characteristics of smooth muscle cells and contain actin, myosin, and α-actin. The cells are attached through cytoplasmic projections that tether them to the basement membrane through microfibrils, which associate with fibronectin, the most abundant protein of the mesangial matrix. This arrangement affects the contractile force of the mesangial cells. A minority of the mesangial cells also participate in the phagocytosis of macromolecules, including immune complexes. These cells possess receptors for growth factors, such as platelet-derived growth factor; constrictor peptides, such as endothelin and arginine vasopressin; and cytokines. They can produce extracellular matrix when stimulated by these factors and may participate in the abnormal matrix production in many forms of glomerular disease.

Juxtaglomerular Apparatus

Tightly adherent to every glomerulus at a site between the entry and the exit of the arterioles is a plaque of distal tubule cells called the *macula densa*. These specialized cells, together with the intervening matrix of the mesangium and the specialized granular cells of the contacting arterioles, form the juxtaglomerular apparatus. Under conditions of varying salt delivery, this region has been shown to regulate glomerular filtration, whereby the flow of NaCl past this region is kept constant by a process termed *tubuloglomerular feedback*. Modulation of tubuloglomerular feedback by the reninangiotensin system, nitric oxide, and adenosine can be demonstrated in genetic ablation of these systems. Ablation of the juxtaglomerular apparatus renin-producing cells causes severe developmental abnormalities of the kidney demonstrating that these cells play a role in normal kidney development. The structure is also the site of renin formation, which is sensitive to salt concentration. These cells are richly innervated by sympathetic neurons.

TUBULE

The glomerular corpuscle funnels ultrafiltrate into the renal tubules. The proximal tubule begins at the urinary pole of the glomerulus and consists of two segments. The initial segment, the proximal convoluted tubule, is located in the cortex. The second segment, the straight portion of the proximal tubule, is located in the medullary ray and enters the medulla to form part of the loop of Henle. The thin descending limb of the loop of Henle forms a hairpin turn in the medulla and returns toward the cortex, forming the distal tubule. The distal tubule consists of two segments: the thick ascending limb of the loop of Henle and the distal convoluted tubule. The distal tubule leads to the connecting segment, which marks the transition between distal tubule and the collecting segment. The collecting segment comprises the cortical collecting duct and the outer and inner medullary collecting ducts. These segments of the collecting duct differ not only in regional distribution but also in the mix of cells found within each segment, the distribution of transporters specific to each segment, and responsiveness to hormones that regulate transport. The collecting ducts terminate as the papillary collecting ducts, or the ducts of Bellini, which empty into the renal pelvis at the tips of the renal papillae.

Elements of Renal Physiology

The main functions of the kidney are to maintain and regulate body fluid composition, including its red blood cell mass, excrete waste products of metabolism and xenobiotics, and regulate calcium and phosphate balance (Table 26-1). Although filtration, reabsorption, and secretion are fundamental to the regulation of body fluid composition, less obvious is how the kidney's capacity to synthesize, metabolize, and secrete hormones and lipids contributes to its regulation of electrolyte metabolism and blood pressure. The first step in this complex process is the formation of an ultrafiltrate of plasma at the glomerulus. This fluid, which is free of cellular elements and most of the plasma proteins, flows through the various tubular segments, where it is modified by the processes of reabsorption and secretion to restore the fluid and ionic composition of the body perturbed by

metabolism and diet. How each of the structures of the nephron contributes to the achievement of this balance in which intake matches output is outlined in the following sections.

RENAL BLOOD FLOW

About one fifth of the cardiac output perfuses the kidneys and represents the highest blood flow rate by weight of any organ in the body. About one fourth of the blood reaching the kidney per minute is filtered by the glomerulus. Blood cells and protein are excluded from the filtration barrier, and this blood passes to the peritubular capillary network, where its high oncotic pressure helps return the fluid reabsorbed from the filtrate to the blood. The medulla, which receives its blood from the postglomerular blood through the specialized capillaries of the vasa recta, receives only 15% of the renal blood flow (RBF). The normal kidney possesses the ability to autoregulate RBF, during which it is held constant over a wide range of arterial pressures. When arterial pressure increases, the operation of the system increases resistance in the afferent arteriole and reduces resistance in the efferent arteriole, whereas a fall in arterial pressure results in the opposite changes in afferent and efferent resistance. Both the inherent reaction of the arterioles to changes in perfusion pressure and the operation of the tubuloglomerular feedback system participate in these autoregulatory adjustments under normal physiologic conditions. In the diseased kidney, however, this process is severely restricted.

GLOMERULAR FILTRATION RATE

An ultrafiltrate of the blood is formed in the glomerulus driven by Starling forces as in other capillary beds. The glomerular circulation is ideally suited for high rates of filtration because the high ultrafiltration pressure generated by the afferent and efferent arterioles, the unusually high hydraulic permeability of the filtration barrier, and the tortuous course of the capillaries in the glomerular stalk, which increases the surface area available for filtration, all contribute to the large volume of fluids entering the tubule com-

Table 26-1 **Renal Homeostatic Functions**		
Function	**Mechanism**	**Affected Elements**
Waste excretion	Glomerular filtration	Urea, creatinine
	Tubular secretion	Urate, lactate, drugs (diuretics)
	Tubular catabolism	Pituitary hormones, insulin
Electrolyte balance	Tubular NaCl absorption	Volume status, osmolar balance
	Tubular K^+ secretion	K^+ concentration
	Tubular H^+ secretion	Acid-base balance
	Tubular water absorption	Osmolar balance
	Tubular Ca^+, phosphate, Mg^+ transport	Ca^+, phosphate, Mg^+ homeostasis
Hormonal regulation	Erythropoietin production	Red blood cell mass
	Vitamin D activation	Ca^+ homeostasis
Blood pressure regulation	Altered Na^+ excretion	Extracellular volume
	Renin production	Vascular resistance
Glucose homeostasis	Gluconeogenesis	Glucose supply (maintained) in prolonged starvation

partment. Normal glomerular filtration rate (GFR), which depends on body size, age, diet, and physiologic state, is typically given as 100 mL per minute for women and 120 mL per minute for men. Normal pregnancy raises GFR. Although the most accurate means by which GFR is measured is the clearance of inulin, its measurement is labor intensive and thus not clinically useful for screening purposes. Instead, serum creatinine and endogenous creatinine clearance are used most frequently to estimate changes in GFR. Reductions in GFR, the hallmark of renal disease, can be caused by multiple changes in glomerular function. They include reductions in numbers of nephrons, as occurs in chronic renal disease, reduced glomerular perfusion, from circulatory collapse or specific elevation in the resistance in the afferent arteriole, or obstruction to the flow of urine by urinary bladder outflow obstruction. Reductions in blood flow, without reduced hydrostatic pressure, as occurs in severe heart failure, also reduce GFR by reducing effective net ultrafiltration pressure. Renal disease, whether primary or secondary, impairs the generation of filtrate by different combinations of these mechanisms and will be highlighted in subsequent chapters.

TUBULAR FUNCTION

The glomerular filtrate is modified as it courses down the nephron to become the urine. Net absorption of the filtrate and its constituents best characterize Na^+, Cl^-, H_2O, HCO_3^-, glucose, amino acids, phosphates, Ca^{2+}, Mg^{2+}, uric acid, and others, whereas H^+, NH^{4+}, and a number of organic acids and bases are added to the filtrate. Urea and K^+ undergo both processes, and the net result depends primarily on the underlying physiologic state and diet. One of the most striking characteristics of the renal tubule is its cellular heterogeneity, and these differences underlie its unique transport characteristics. This heterogeneity is best exemplified by the transport proteins that are unique to each segment and the responsiveness to drugs that inhibit transport. Each segment's role in modifying the final urine will be discussed separately.

PROXIMAL TUBULE

The proximal tubule reclaims at least 60% of the filtered load of Na^+, Cl^-, H_2O, urea, and K^+ and fully 90% of the filtered HCO_3^- (Fig. 26-5). It achieves these high rates of absorption without detectable differences in osmotic gradients between blood and filtrate. Almost all the filtered glucose and amino acids are reclaimed from the filtrate during passage along the proximal tubule. Phosphates are reabsorbed at this site, and the activity of this transport route is significantly affected by parathyroid hormone (PTH). The primary mechanisms of transport of these solutes across the proximal tubule are linked to sodium by coupling primary active transport through the Na^+,K^+-ATPase at the basolateral membrane, with secondary active transport mechanisms primarily distributed in the luminal brush border membranes of the proximal tubule (see Fig. 26-5). The structural feature of the proximal tubule that enables large transepithelial mass flow is the large brush border of the luminal membrane, which enlarges membrane area greatly. This polarity of the renal epithelium is basic to achieving vectorial transport throughout the nephron.

The other structural attribute that defines a transporting epithelium is the presence of highly specialized regions where cells are joined, called *junctional complexes*. These complexes are found at the apical surface and not only bind the cells together and maintain polarity but also establish a potential space by which solute and water may pass through a paracellular transport route. The electrical classification of the proximal tubule as a "leaky epithelium" is determined by the specific characteristics of the constituents of the junctional complex. Water movement through these channels and the differing selectivity for solutes establish the solvent drag effect, in which significant movement of salt and water may be accomplished. Protein constituents of the junctional complex may be defective and lead to transport defects such as the congenital hypercalciuria noted in the syndrome of hypomagnesemic hypercalciuria, in which a mutation of paracellin appears to be responsible for the urinary calcium and magnesium loss.

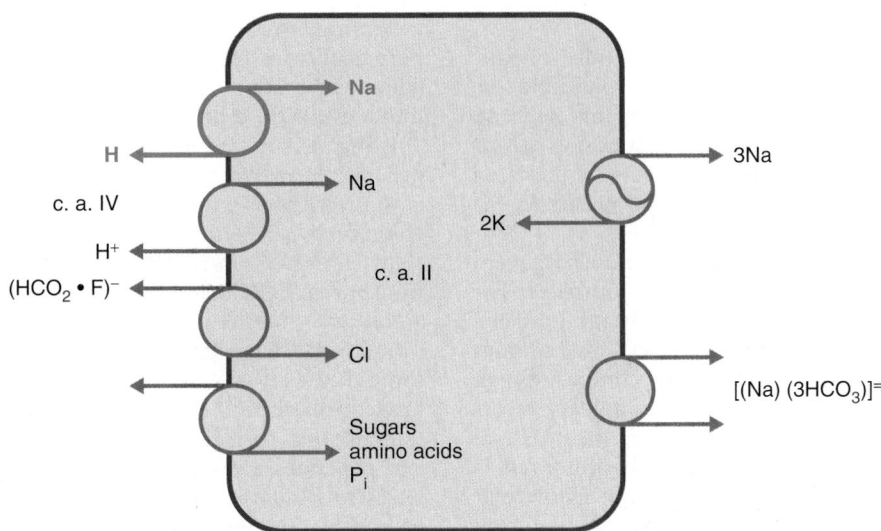

Figure 26-5 The major transport processes of the proximal tubular cells. See text for explanation.

The reabsorption of bicarbonate in the proximal tubule perhaps best illustrates the exquisite efficiency of the structural-functional relationships illustrated in Figure 26-5. Protons are secreted into the lumen through the operation of the Na^+-H^+ exchanger (NHE) located in the brush border. The transporter is regulated by cAMP, whose action depends on specific structural associations with the NHE-related factor (NHERF) and the cytoskeleton (**Web Fig. 26-1**). The potential energy stored in the Na^+ gradient established by the operation of the Na^+,K^+-ATPase drives this exchange. The HCO_3^- thus generated is extruded across the basolateral membrane accompanied by Na through the Na^+-HCO_3^- co-transporter. The efficient operation of the system is facilitated by two isozymes of carbonic anhydrase: one at the luminal membrane to dehydrate the carbonic acid formed by H excretion into the lumen, and another intracellularly to form HCO_3^- from the hydroxyl ions formed by H exit from the cell. When the operation of the NHE is coupled to a formate/chloride exchanger present on the apical membrane of the proximal tubule, the net result is NaCl reabsorption. Thus, the polarity of these transport processes and their coupling achieves efficient proton secretion and NaCl and Na^+ HCO_3^- reabsorption at low expenditure of energy.

Phosphate transport is achieved by sodium-dependent phosphate co-transporters in the proximal tubule and is regulated by hormones. PTH, secreted by the parathyroid glands, is phosphaturic and inhibits phosphate transport through a G-protein–coupled receptor that reduces cyclic adenosine monophosphate (cAMP) generation in the proximal tubule cell. Genetic studies of a familial disorder of phosphate metabolism have revealed mutations in genes that regulate phosphate reabsorption. Fibroblast growth factor 23 (*FGF-23*) is perhaps most important in this regards and the most important regulator of renal phosphate reabsorption as well as the synthesis of 1,25-dihydroxyvitamin D. Activating mutations in *FGF-23* is responsible for autosomal dominant hypophosphatemic rickets and for tumor-associated osteomalacia. *FGF-23* inhibits phosphate reabsorption by reducing expression of Na^+-dependent phosphate transporters. The predominant source of *FGF-23* is bone osteocytes and osteoblasts. Extremely high levels of *FGF-23* characterize chronic renal failure and may be responsible for the defective 1,25-dihydroxyvitamin D synthesis in this disease.

In the straight portion of the proximal tubule, organic acids such as uric acid and drugs such as penicillin are secreted. Most diuretics are also secreted in this nephron segment and inhibit luminal solute transport at sites downstream in the nephron. Furthermore, ammonia synthesis, an important step in renal acid excretion, also occurs in the proximal tubule.

The physical forces surrounding the tubule also govern solute and water reabsorption in proximal tubules. For example, a high peritubular capillary hydrostatic pressure, as occurs in volume infusion, impairs water and sodium reabsorption from the proximal tubule. By contrast, a high colloid oncotic pressure in the peritubular capillary favors the absorption of water and electrolytes from the proximal tubule. The primary determinant of these physical forces is the filtration fraction, or that portion of the glomerular plasma that is filtered. It is low during volume expansion and high during heart failure.

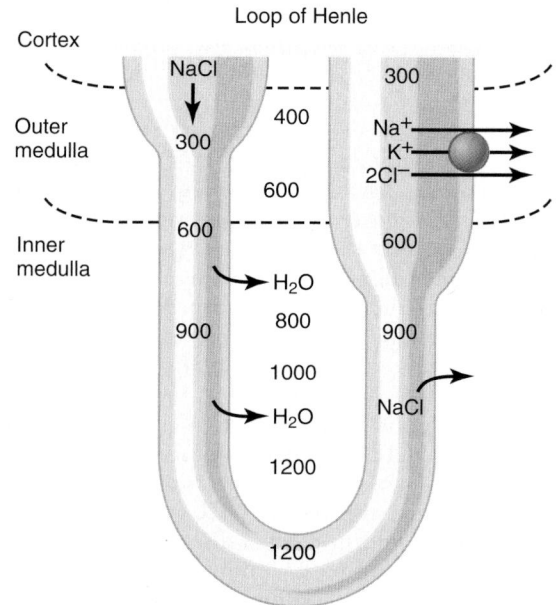

Figure 26-6 The loop of Henle is responsible for additional absorption of filtrate. Water is absorbed in the solute-impermeable descending limb. The concentrated medullary interstitium, established by solute transport at the water-impermeable ascending limb, drives water absorption from the descending limb. The hyperosmolar interstitium also provides the driving force for urinary concentration at the collecting duct. The relative osmolarity of the tubular fluid and interstitium is demonstrated by the numerals.

LOOP OF HENLE

The loop of Henle begins at the corticomedullary junction as the thin descending limb and then makes a hairpin turn and continues as the thin ascending limb (Fig. 26-6). It becomes the medullary thick ascending limb (MTAL) at the level of the outer medulla and ends in the macula densa at the level of the glomerulus from which it originated. Each segment of the loop has a different permeability for sodium chloride and water, so that about 15% of the volume of the isosmotic ultrafiltrate is absorbed and about 25% of the sodium chloride is absorbed. Passive water absorption in the thin descending limb and salt absorption in the thin ascending limb of the loop occur as a result of the selective permeability of these segments. This differential absorption converts the isotonic fluid entering from the proximal tubule into a dilute fluid delivered to the distal tubule.

A major participant in both diluting the tubule fluid and generating high medullary interstitial solute concentration is the MTAL (Fig. 26-7). The MTAL limb absorbs sodium chloride by an active, energy-dependent process. Specifically, luminal transport involves a Na^+/K^+/2 Cl^- co-transporter (NKCC2). Chloride exit from the cell is through a chloride channel whose activity is augmented by raising intracellular chloride concentration. K^+ entering the cell through the co-transporter is recycled at the luminal membrane through a K^+ channel and supports several functions. It maintains co-transporter activity, enables K^+ secretion, and generates a positive transcellular potential that drives Na^+, Ca^{2+}, and Mg^{2+} absorption through the cation selective paracellular pathway. This cation selectivity is determined by the specific paracellular protein paracellin. Genetic defects

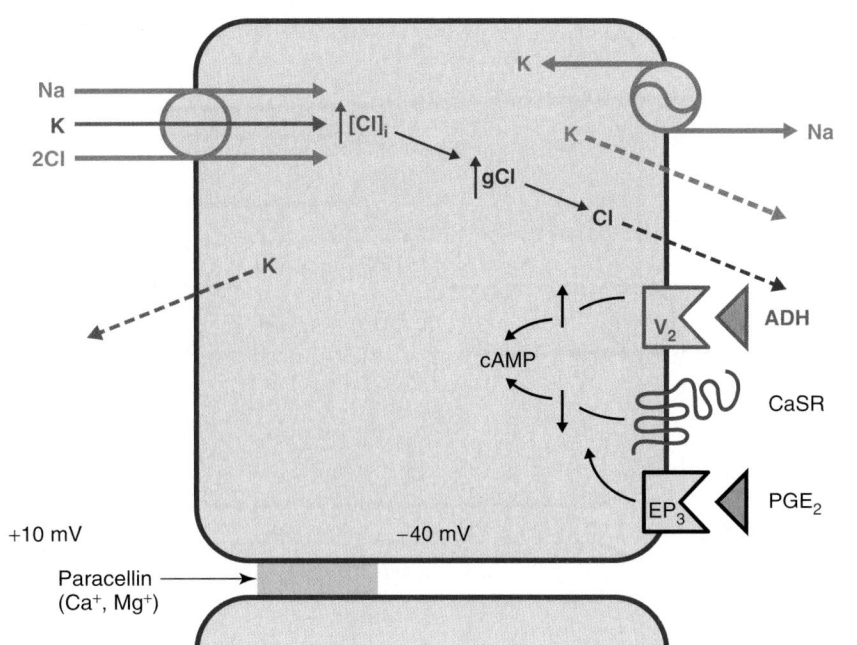

Figure 26-7 Major transport process of the medullary thick ascending limb (MTAL). See text.

in each of these proteins have been found in patients with phenotypes typical of Bartter syndrome (see Chapter 28). Because this segment is impermeable to water, the luminal fluid leaving the thick ascending limb is made hypotonic with regard to plasma by active salt absorption, a critical step in urinary dilution. The addition of sodium chloride to the medullary interstitium is the primary step that allows a multiplicative process to build and maintain the interstitial hypertonicity necessary to absorb water from thin descending limbs and from collecting ducts during antidiuresis. Furosemide is a potent inhibitor of the co-transporter. Antidiuretic hormone (ADH) increases thick ascending limb NaCl transport by raising cAMP within the cell, whereas prostaglandin inhibits ADH-induced increased intracellular cAMP content and NaCl transport. A newly recognized regulatory role occurs through the activation of the calcium-sensing receptor (CaSR) (**Web Fig. 26-2**), which inhibits NaCl transport by reducing K^+ recycling and reduces the concentration of urine. This latter function is important to prevent urinary stone formation in periods of high calcium intake.

The hairpin arrangement and countercurrent flow of the loop helps maintain high interstitial osmolality compared with the isotonic nature of the cortex. A similar organization of the vasa recta allows the sodium chloride absorbed from the loop of Henle and urea absorbed from the papillary collecting duct to be trapped within the interstitium and increases interstitial osmolality further. The integrity of these anatomic relationships is essential to the concentrating ability of the kidney.

A significant portion of calcium reabsorption occurs within the loop of Henle. Calcium absorption in the medullary portion of the thick ascending limb varies with the magnitude of the positive luminal transepithelial voltage generated by active salt absorption and occurs through the Ca^{2+}-selective paracellular pathway. The thick ascending limb of the loop of Henle is also the major site of magnesium reabsorption and most probably occurs by a similar mechanism.

DISTAL NEPHRON

The distal nephron may be divided into three segments: the distal convoluted tubule (DCT), the connecting tubule (CNT), which is a transitional epithelial, and the collecting duct. The collecting duct in the cortex consists of both intercalated cells and principal cells, whereas the collecting ducts in the medulla are exclusively composed of principal cells.

The DCT (Fig. 26-8) is a water-impermeable segment of the nephron that continues the dilution of luminal fluid initiated by the thick ascending limb. Sodium absorption in the distal convoluted tubule occurs primarily by a thiazide diuretic–sensitive (TSC), chloride-coupled co-transporter similar to the one found in the thick ascending limb but that does not depend on K^+. Genetic defects in the NaCl co-transporter are responsible for Gitelman syndrome (discussed in Chapter 28). A series of newly described kinases, the WNKs (*with no lysine*), regulate this co-transporter, and mutations in this group of genes cause a syndrome that is the mirror image of Gitelman syndrome by activating TSC function. This segment is also important in the regulation of calcium balance because PTH and vitamin D increase calcium transport here. Luminal calcium uptake proceeds through channels in the luminal membrane driven by the large electrochemical gradient for calcium entry and is regulated by the *KLOTHO* gene, originally identified as an anti-aging gene, but later shown to increase calcium reabsorption at this site as well. Calcium exit, which is active, proceeds predominantly through an Na-Ca exchanger and to a minor degree through a calcium adenosine triphosphatase (ATPase). The exit step is the major site by which PTH regulation occurs. Sodium transport in this segment is

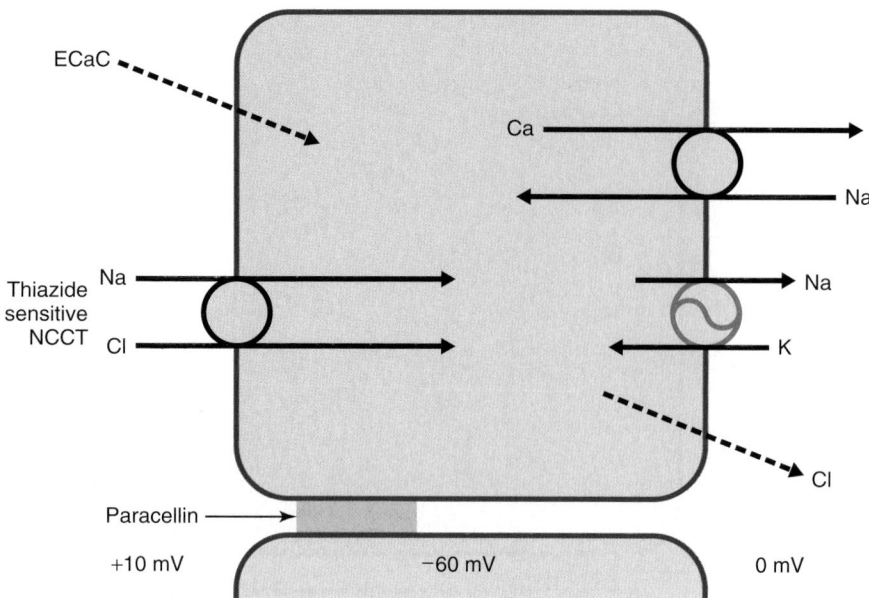

Figure 26-8 Major transport processes of the distal convoluted tubule (DCT) See text.

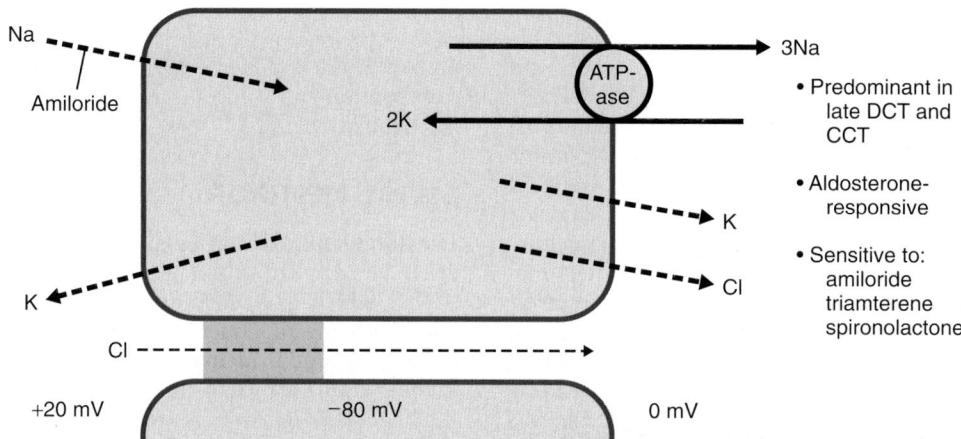

Figure 26-9 Major transport processes of the cortical collecting duct (CCD). See text. CCT, cortical collecting duct; DCT, distal convoluted tubule.

not affected by ADH or aldosterone. Inhibition of the NaCl co-transporter, by thiazides for example, augments calcium reabsorption by increasing calcium entry and promoting calcium exit as a consequence of reduced NaCl entry.

The collecting duct begins with the connecting tubule, which possesses a mixture of distal tubule and cortical collecting duct transport characteristics. The functional aspects of the collecting duct epithelium are crucial to achieving salt and water homeostasis (Fig. 26-9). In states of volume depletion and maximal aldosterone production, the urine can be rendered virtually free of sodium. The first or cortical regions of the collecting duct are lined by a mixture of principal cells and intercalated cells (Fig. 26-10). The number of the intercalated cells decreases as the collecting descend into the medulla, so they are absent in collecting ducts below the first portion of the inner medulla. Transepithelial sodium reabsorption is accomplished by the operation of the epithelial sodium channel (ENaC) (**Web Fig. 26-3**) at the luminal

membrane and the basolateral Na+,K+-ATPase. The principal mode of regulation of ENaC is by regulating its expression at the luminal surface of the cell. Aldosterone increases the rate of Na+ transport in this segment, as does ADH, whereas prostaglandins and the natriuretic peptides reduce it. Aldosterone also hyperpolarizes the basolateral membrane, provoking net K+ secretion through K+ channels in each membrane.

The intercalated cells do not participate in Na+ reabsorption or K+ secretion but instead participate in acid-base homeostasis and K+ secretion. Two types of intercalated cells exist; the first secrete acid, while the second secrete base, depending on the polarity of the transport proteins. The type A cell (see Fig. 26-10) reclaims the last amount of filtered bicarbonate and achieves final titration of urinary buffers, including ammonia, by proton secretion. There is evidence for the existence of both an H− and an H+,K+-ATPase. Basolateral HCO_3^- exit is accomplished in exchange for Cl−

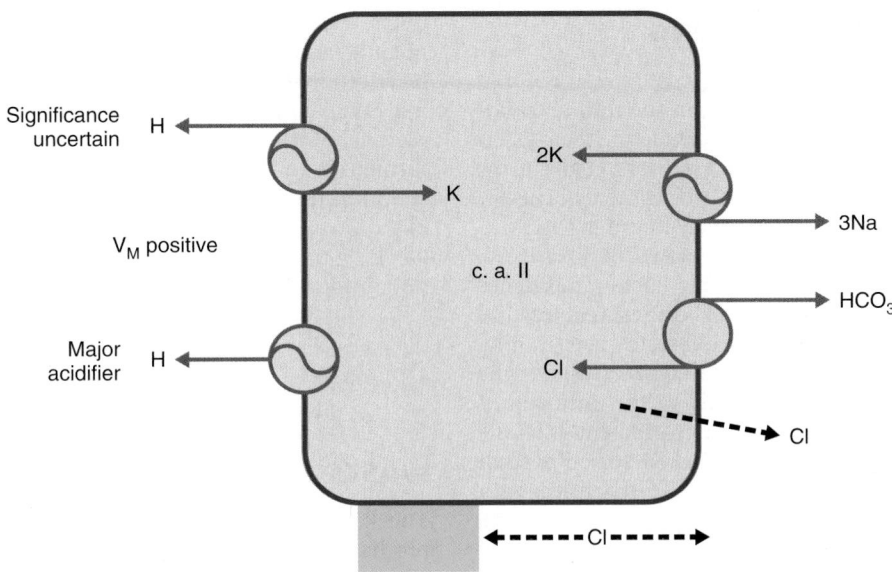

Figure 26-10 Major transport processes of the type A intercalated cell of the outer medullary collecting duct. See text for information.

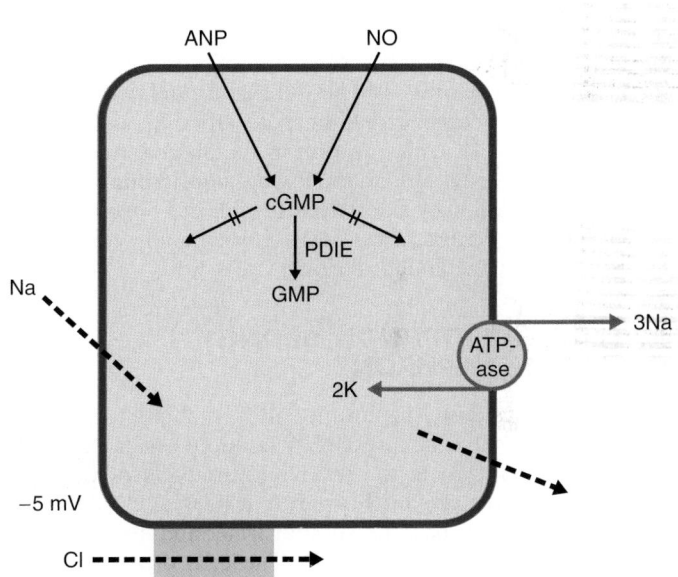

Figure 26-11 The inner medullary collecting duct (IMCD) cell and the effect of intracellular cGMP elevation in its inhibition. The failure of this inhibitory system to repress salt transport during congestive heart failure suggests that it is an important therapeutic site for its treatment. Cl, chloride; PDIE, phosphodiesterase.

through an anion exchanger (pendrin), and the Cl^- that enters the cell is extruded through a Cl^- channel. Reversal of this polarity of the proton pumps and anion exchanger leads to HCO_3^- secretion in the type B intercalated cell, but these cells disappear at the inner stripe of the outer medulla. Aldosterone stimulates urinary acidification principally by promoting Na^+ reabsorption and increasing luminal electronegativity. Increased sodium delivery to these sites, as occurs during volume expansion and diuretic use, stimulates proton excretion by stimulation of sodium transport at this site as well. The role of the intercalated cell in K^+ secretion is discussed in the next section.

The epithelial cells of the inner medullary collecting duct (IMCD) (Fig. 26-11) are taller and have less mitochondria than those of the outer medullary collecting duct

(OMCD). There is also a richly featured lateral intercellular space that probably facilitates the transfer of fluid and urea that is provoked by ADH here. This site demonstrates the presence of inhibitory cyclic guanosine monophosphate (cGMP)-responsive ENaC proteins that are activated by natriuretic peptides, like atrial natriuretic peptide (ANP). This is the site for the operation of the "escape phenomenon," in which atrial stretch due to volume expansion leads to the release of ANP and suppression of collecting duct sodium transport and natriuresis. Another key regulator is nitric oxide (NO), which also inhibits ENaC through a cGMP pathway. Failure of these systems to operate during congestive heart failure (CHF) is an important determinant of edema production and suggests that it would be a fruitful therapeutic target.

POTASSIUM SECRETION ALONG THE DISTAL NEPHRON

Potassium secretion, which may begin in the thin descending limb of the loop of Henle, is significant along the collecting ducts because the potassium that appears in the urine is mostly a result of secretion by these segments. The SK channel, which has a low conductance, is found in the principal cells, whereas the maxi-K^+ channel is found in both principal and intercalated cells. Many factors influence potassium secretion, and these can be classified as apical and peritubular factors. The principal apical factor determining K^+ secretion is tubule flow rate. In addition to reducing the luminal K^+ concentration and stimulating the diffusion of intracellular K^+ down its concentration gradient into the tubular lumen, tubule flow rate increases K^+ secretion itself by activating the maxi-K^+ channel. Volume expansion with NaCl also raises sodium delivery to the collecting ducts, which stimulates sodium reabsorption and increases luminal electronegativity. Increased luminal weak acids and decreased Cl concentration increase K^+ secretion, whereas intraluminal acidity inhibits K^+ secretion. The latter effect has been shown to be due to a decrease in luminal membrane K^+ conductance. Inhibitors of K^+ secretion are either inhibitors of Na^+ channels, like triamterene and amiloride, which depolarize the luminal membrane potential, or inhibitors of the K^+ channel itself like barium. The peritubular factors that affect K^+ transport are potassium, hydrogen, bicarbonate, and hormones. Increased K^+ concentration in the plasma increases K^+ secretion directly and by provoking aldosterone secretion. This stimulation by aldosterone is inhibited by spironolactone. Distal K^+ secretion is decreased by metabolic acidosis and increased by metabolic alkalosis.

WATER REABSORPTION ALONG THE DISTAL NEPHRON

The ability of the distal nephron to alter its ability to reabsorb water and urea in response to reduced water intake is in striking contrast to the relative invariability of water reabsorption in the proximal nephron, it does so by changing its permeability characteristics for water and urea along the nephron in response to ADH. The cells of the distal nephron are minimally permeable to water and urea in the absence of ADH and, in that circumstance, can deliver the hypotonic (50 to 100 mOsm/kg of H_2O) fluid issuing from the distal convoluted tubule unchanged into the urine. When ADH is present, water passes across the collecting duct tubule wall readily, and the luminal fluid tonicity approaches that of the interstitium. It does so by inserting preformed water channels in the luminal membrane of principal cells. Maximal urinary concentrating ability thus depends on the availability of ADH and its receptor, plus the hypertonicity of the medullary interstitium generated from thick ascending limb sodium chloride absorption and trapping of salt and urea through the countercurrent system. Urea plays a special role because its permeability is increased only in the most terminal portions of the collecting duct. The movement of urea is mediated by specific urea transporters responsive to ADH along a steep gradient for urea diffusion established by the continued water reabsorption that takes place at sites proximal to these terminal collecting

ducts. The urea moving into the interstitium deep in the medulla is trapped by the countercurrent system and exerts an additional osmotic force to draw water out of the collecting ducts and thin descending limbs that extend to these regions. Prostaglandins impair distal water reabsorption through several mechanisms, including blockade of ADH action in the collecting duct as well as increasing medullary blood flow. Thus, nonsteroidal anti-inflammatory drugs, by blocking prostaglandins, may impair renal free water excretion. Endothelin also inhibits water reabsorption at this site.

Other Renal Homeostatic Functions

WASTE EXCRETION

The kidney is responsible for elimination of nitrogenous products of protein catabolism. This is accomplished primarily by filtration at the glomerulus. Because homeostatic requirements necessitate the maintenance of low concentrations of these compounds, large volumes of ultrafiltrate formation are necessary for excretion of the absolute quantity of material. The normal daily GFR of 180 L makes such mass elimination possible.

Tubule secretion, especially at the straight portion of the proximal tubule is another route by which xenobiotics and toxins are cleared from the blood. Organic acids (e.g., hippurate, urate, and lactate), organic bases (e.g., morphine), and many xenobiotics are excreted by carrier-mediated processes served by two families of proteins; the adenosine triphosphate (ATP)-binding cassette proteins and the solute carrier proteins. The secretory process is the major route of elimination for substances that are protein bound. A large number of drugs, including antibiotics and diuretics, are excreted through this mechanism. Mutations and polymorphisms in these proteins have been shown to be responsible for potentially nephrotoxic retention of drugs, and changes in the levels of these proteins correlate with response to chemotherapy. These carrier proteins have ushered in the era of pharmacogenomic research, by which specific targeting of therapy will be individualized to the particular genomic structure of these carriers.

REGULATION OF BLOOD PRESSURE

The kidney plays a major role in the genesis of hypertension, as confirmed by genetic disorders of salt transport. Regulation of the abundance of each of the major salt transport proteins has been documented to regulate blood pressure. Activating mutations in the TSC transporter causes a syndrome of hypertension and hyperkalemia, or familial hyperkalemic hypertension. Perhaps most important among them is the gain-in-function mutation discovered in patients with Liddle syndrome in which the ENaC is activated. These patients have severe hypertension and die from early-onset cardiovascular and cerebrovascular disease. Inactivating mutations in ENaC cause pseudohypoaldosteronism type I, a disorder of severe sodium wasting and hypotension. It appears likely that genomic variations in transport proteins and their regulatory pathways may underlie the syndrome of essential hypertension.

RENAL HORMONAL REGULATION

The kidney contributes to the metabolic degradation of a number of peptide hormones, including most pituitary hormones, glucagon, and insulin, by tubular cells. Decreased renal catabolism of insulin in diabetic patients with renal insufficiency may cause hypoglycemic episodes.

The kidney is also the major site of *erythropoietin* production. This hormone is a highly glycosylated, 39,000-Da protein. It is produced in the renal cortex, but the cell has not been identified with certainty. Erythropoietin stimulates red blood cell production by its effect on the bone marrow. Erythropoietin production increases in states of decreased tissue oxygen delivery. This may occur as a result of chronic hypoxemia, as seen in persons living at high altitudes or in patients with lung disease, or as a result of decreased oxygen-carrying capacity of blood, as seen in anemic individuals.

The kidney contributes to calcium homeostasis not only by directly regulating the excretion of Ca^+, phosphate, and acid but also by affecting hormonal production. *Vitamin D* requires two enzymatic hydroxylations to become a potent hormone that regulates intestinal calcium absorption. After hydroxylation in the liver at the 25 position of the molecule, renal proximal tubular cells add a second hydroxyl ion at the 1 or 26 position. This hydroxylation step is controlled and stimulated by several hormones, including PTH and *KLOTHO*, as well as by low serum phosphate. As noted previously, the juxtaglomerular cells produce and secrete *renin*. Renin promotes the formation of angiotensin II, a potent vasoconstrictor that is a stimulus to aldosterone secretion. Aldosterone stimulates renal sodium absorption and excretion of potassium and hydrogen ions. Overproduction of elements of the renin-angiotensin system, including aldosterone, cause clinical syndromes of hypertension.

GLUCOSE HOMEOSTASIS

The kidney participates in the regulation of plasma glucose by its ability to synthesize glucose by the gluconeogenetic pathway. Lactate, pyruvate, and amino acids are used by the kidney for gluconeogenesis. This function becomes important in prolonged starvation states, in which up to 40% of plasma glucose is contributed by the kidney. Absence of this gluconeogenetic pathway in patients with severe renal dysfunction may contribute to hypoglycemia in diabetics.

Prospectus for the Future

- The role of podocyte injury in renal disease progression will be elucidated further.
- The detailed three-dimensional molecular structure of the major salt and water transporters not only will reveal the mechanism by which they accomplish transfer of molecules across biologic membranes but also will reveal how they interact with regulatory proteins, how disease causing mutations work. Such detailed information may help in the design of newer therapeutic agents for such disorders.
- More detailed understanding of the operation of the tubuloglomerular feedback system will have important therapeutic implications for the treatment of acute and chronic renal disease.
- Molecular biology and molecular genetics will continue to inform the pathophysiology of human renal disease.

References

Alpern RJ, Hebert SC (eds): Seldin and Giebisch's The Kidney: Physiology and Pathophysiology, 4th ed. Sections I, II, and III. Burlington, Academic Press, 2008.

Ellison DH: Divalent cation transport by the distal nephron: Insights from Bartter's and Gitelman's syndromes. Am J Physiol 279:F616-F625, 2000.

Strom TM, Jüppner H: PHEX, FGF23, DMP1 and beyond. Curr Opin Nephrol Hypertens 17:357-362, 2008.

Chapter **27**

Approach to the Patient with Renal Disease

Michelle W. Krause, Thomas A. Golper, Raymond C. Harris, and Sudhir V. Shah

Assessment of the Patient with Kidney Disease

HISTORY AND PHYSICAL EXAMINATION

It is estimated that kidney disease affects about 10% of the adult population in the United States and worldwide. Given these numbers, it is disturbing that there is still inadequate physician awareness of how to identify these patients with chronic kidney disease. The recognition that both acute and chronic forms of kidney disease are common should prompt physicians to pay particular attention to the detection of kidney disease. Individuals with insidious chronic kidney disease may exhibit either few or vague symptoms, such as fatigue, malaise, or anorexia, or more easily detected signs and symptoms in acute renal failure with hypertension, edema, changes in urine production, hematuria, or dark-colored (*cola-colored*) urine. A history of diabetes and hypertension, along with duration and other concomitant organ complications such as retinopathy or neuropathy, are important in determining the association to the cause of kidney disease. Similarly, a history of recurrent urinary tract infections with reflux nephropathy, chronic obstruction with recurrent renal calculi, or a family history of kidney disease in Alport syndrome is helpful in determining the cause of kidney disease. With an aging population, it is important to inquire about the quality of the urinary stream in males, including hesitancy and frequent nocturia, and these symptoms must not be dismissed as merely a sign of aging. Incomplete bladder emptying can occur with neuropathy as well as prostatism and can contribute to subclinical obstruction with significant long-term consequences to kidney function. Other pertinent historical information required when assessing kidney disease includes inquiry into other systemic disorders that affect kidney function such as arthralgias and skin rash in autoimmune diseases, fever and pharyngitis in postinfectious glomeru-

lonephritis, and medications—including prescription drugs, over-the-counter medications, illicit drugs, and herbs—in acute and chronic interstitial nephritis. One of the most important factors in determining whether kidney disease is acute or chronic in nature is to review previous medical records to obtain a baseline assessment of kidney function.

The physical examination may show signs of a systemic illness that is responsible for the patient's kidney disease. A careful examination of the retina may suggest the presence of diabetes, hypertension, bacterial endocarditis, and cholesterol emboli (**Web Fig. 27-1**). In addition, examination of skin for the presence of edema, rash, and purpura and joint examination for signs of arthritis are important (**Web Fig. 27-2**). A rectal examination in men or a pelvic examination in women is crucial to exclude a process that might cause urinary obstruction.

RENAL FUNCTION TESTS

An approximate assessment of glomerular filtration rate (GFR) is most easily obtained by measuring the concentration of creatinine and urea nitrogen in the serum. Creatinine is a metabolite of creatine, a major muscle constituent. In a specific individual, the daily rate of production of creatinine is constant and is determined by the mass of skeletal muscle. Glomerular filtration eliminates nearly all creatinine, and the concentration of creatinine in the serum has been used as a marker of renal function. The normal range for serum creatinine concentration is 0.8 to 1.3 mg/dL in men and 0.6 to 1.1 mg/dL in women. The serum creatinine value is lower in women and elderly people because of less muscle mass, which leads to a lower rate of creatinine production. However, a value in this range does not necessarily imply normal renal function. For example, in a patient whose creatinine increases from 0.6 to 1.2 mg/dL, a 50% decrease in GFR has occurred, despite creatinine remaining in the normal range. Certain drugs such as cimetidine, trimethoprim, triamterene, and amiloride may interfere with creati-

Table 27-1 **Factors Affecting Blood Urea Nitrogen Level Independent of Renal Function**
Disproportionate Increase in Blood Urea Nitrogen
Volume depletion
Gastrointestinal hemorrhage
Corticosteroid or cytotoxic agents
High-protein diet
Obstructive uropathy
Sepsis
Catabolic states
Tissue breakdown
Disproportionate Decrease in Blood Urea Nitrogen
Low-protein diet
Liver disease

Table 27-2 **Calculation of the Creatinine Clearance**
24-Hour Urine Collection
$C_{cr} = U_{cr} \times V/P_{cr}$
where C_{cr} = clearance of creatinine (mL/min)
U_{cr} = urine creatinine (mg/dL)
V = volume of urine (mL/min) (for 24-hr volume: divide by 1440)
P_{cr} = plasma creatinine (mg/dL)
Cockroft-Gault Formula
C_{cr} = (140 − age in years) × (lean body weight in kg)
Scr = serum creatinine in mg/dL × 72
For women, multiply final value by 0.85
Modification of Diet in Renal Disease Formula
GFR = 186 × (Cr) − 1.154 × age − 0.203 × 1.212 (if African American) × 0.742 (if woman)
Normal range: 95-105 mL/1.75 m² per minute

nine excretion and cause a false elevation in the serum creatinine value.

The blood urea nitrogen (BUN) concentration is often used in conjunction with the serum creatinine concentration as a measure of renal function. Urea is the major end product of protein metabolism, and its production reflects both the dietary intake of protein and the protein catabolic rate. Glomerular filtration excretes urea, but a significant amount of urea is reabsorbed along the tubule, particularly in sodium-avid states such as volume depletion. Consequently, the BUN value may vary in relation to the extracellular fluid volume, whereas the serum creatinine concentration is less dependent on volume status, although serum creatinine will also increase somewhat in sodium-avid states (so-called prerenal azotemia). The usual ratio of urea nitrogen to creatinine concentration in the serum is 10:1. This ratio is increased in a large number of clinical settings (Table 27-1).

Based on the limitations of creatinine and BUN alone in estimating kidney function, the National Kidney Foundation (NKF) and the Kidney Disease Outcomes Quality Initiative (K/DOQI) developed clinical practice guidelines that recommend measuring the creatinine clearance (C_{cr}) to estimate the GFR (see http://www.kdoqi.org). The C_{cr} may be measured by 24-hour urine collection or mathematically by the Cockroft-Gault formula or Modification of Diet in Renal Disease (MDRD) formula (Table 27-2). Two major errors limit the accuracy of C_{cr} in 24-hour urine collections: (1) increasing creatinine secretion and (2) incomplete urine collection. About 10% of creatinine is secreted by proximal tubular cells into the urine in individuals with normal kidney function, and this percentage may be increased in individuals with kidney disease, thus leading to an overestimation of the true GFR. Therefore, the NKF K/DOQI clinical practice guidelines recommend using mathematical equations rather than 24-hour urine collections for C_{cr} to estimate the GFR.

Recently, cystatin C has been described as another valid marker in estimating kidney function. Cystatin C is a cysteine protease that is produced by all nucleated cells, released into the bloodstream, and then completely filtered by the glomerulus. Cystatin C is not affected by conditions that alter muscle mass such as sex, age, and chronic diseases (e.g., cancer, liver disease), and it may be more reliable than cre-

atinine is in estimating the GFR. The widespread use of cystatin C, however, has not been uniformly adopted, and its future use in assessing kidney function is not clear.

Tests that examine the ability of the kidney to maintain salt and water balance, as well as acid-base homeostasis, are used to evaluate renal tubular function. The water deprivation test can assess the maximal urinary concentrating ability. In the patient with polyuria who may have a defect in urinary concentrating ability, the administration of 5 units of aqueous vasopressin, once the urinary osmolality reaches a steady state, distinguishes between patients with central and those with nephrogenic diabetes insipidus. Patients with central diabetes insipidus develop a doubling of the urinary osmolality with aqueous vasopressin. In contrast, individuals with nephrogenic diabetes insipidus do not respond with further increase in urinary concentration.

The fractional excretion of various solutes in the urine provides useful information about the tubular handling of a solute relative to its GFR. The fractional excretion of sodium (Fe_{Na}) or chloride (Fe_{Cl}) is the fraction of sodium (or chloride) filtered at the glomerulus that is ultimately excreted in the urine (Table 27-3). Determinations of the Fe_{Na} and Fe_{Cl} are most useful in the differential diagnosis of acute oliguric renal failure. Notably, they can be calculated on a spot specimen because the volume terms in the numerator and denominator cancel each other. A value for Fe_{Na} less than 1% suggests a prerenal condition, such as volume depletion, whereas a value greater than 3% is consistent with parenchymal renal disease, such as acute tubular necrosis or interstitial nephritis. The Fe_{Na} may, however, be less than 1% in patients with acute glomerular disease or radiocontrast-induced acute renal failure. In patients with persistent vomiting, the urinary chloride concentration is typically low and is an accurate index of volume depletion.

Acidification of the urine is an important tubular function that can be assessed by the measurement of the urine pH. In the presence of systemic acidosis (arterial pH < 7.3), the urine pH should be less than 5.3. Failure to acidify urine in the presence of systemic acidosis suggests distal renal tubular acidosis. In patients with a hyperchloremic metabolic acidosis, the urinary anion gap ($U_{Na} + U_K − U_{Cl}$) can be used to

Table 27-3 **Calculation of the Fractional Excretion of Sodium**
Fractional Excretion of Sodium (Fe$_{Na}$) = Fraction of Sodium Filtered at the Glomerulus that Is Ultimately Excreted in the Urine
Fe$_{Na}$ = clearance of sodium/clearance of creatinine
Fe$_{Na}$ = $(U_{Na}/P_{Na})/(U_{Cr}/P_{Cr})$
where P$_{Na}$ = plasma sodium (mEq/L)
P$_{cr}$ = plasma creatinine (mg/dL)
U$_{Na}$ = urine sodium (mEq/L)
U$_{cr}$ = urine creatinine (mg/dL)

distinguish extrarenal versus renal causes of the acidosis. A negative urinary anion gap is seen with extrarenal causes, such as loss of bicarbonate with diarrhea.

A normal individual excretes less than 150 mg per day of protein. The glomerular basement membrane serves as an effective barrier to the passage of high–molecular-weight proteins such as albumin, and the renal tubules have the capacity to reabsorb the small amount of protein that is filtered. An increase in proteinuria may occur as a transient phenomenon in individuals with febrile illnesses or after vigorous exercise. Postural or orthostatic proteinuria is a benign condition that is confirmed by the absence of proteinuria in overnight urine collection while the patient is supine. Persistent proteinuria almost always indicates renal disease. There are settings with markedly elevated central venous pressures in which some proteinuria is frequently seen in the absence of significant glomerular pathology, such as severe heart failure and possibly morbid obesity; however, in patients with underlying renal disease, such conditions will frequently exacerbate the amount of proteinuria. Proteinuria may be quantified with either a 24-hour urine collection or a random urine protein–to–urine creatinine (U pro/Cr) ratio. For example, a random U pro/Cr ratio of 1 correlates to 1 g per day of proteinuria. Because of the limitations of 24-hour urine collections previously discussed, the NKF K/DOQI clinical practice guidelines recommend that a U pro/Cr ratio assessment be performed to quantify proteinuria. Individuals who excrete more than 3.5 g per day of protein have, with rare exceptions, glomerular disease. Less than 3.5 g per day of urinary protein can be found in patients with both glomerular and tubular diseases. For individuals without overt proteinuria on urinalysis but with conditions that are associated with kidney disease such as diabetes mellitus, early identification of underlying kidney damage can be assessed by measuring microalbuminuria. Microalbuminuria is defined as the excretion of 30 to 300 mg per day of albumin and is associated with progression of renal disease and with higher cardiovascular morbidity and mortality in patients with diabetes mellitus and hypertension.

URINALYSIS

Urinalysis is a simple, noninvasive, and inexpensive means of detecting renal disease. A clean-catch voided urine specimen should be examined promptly using both chemical and microscopic means. Normal urine ranges from almost colorless to deep yellow, depending on the concentration of the urochrome pigment. Abnormal urine colors may be a sign of disease or may indicate the presence of an infection, pigment, drug, or dye. The presence of red blood cells or myoglobin often results in red or smoke-colored urine. Cloudiness of the urine may occur when a high concentration of white blood cells is present (pyuria) or when amorphous phosphates precipitate in alkaline urine.

A chemical assessment of the urine is performed with the *dipstick,* a plastic strip impregnated with various reagents that detect the pH, protein, hemoglobin, glucose, ketones, leukocyte esterase, and nitrite in the urine. These assays are semiquantitative and are graded on the basis of color changes in the various reagent strips. The dipstick method for detecting urinary protein is more sensitive for albumin, although it does not detect albumin in the microalbuminuria range (discussed earlier) and does not detect immunoglobulins or tubular proteins (Tamm-Horsfall mucoprotein). The major disadvantage of the dipstick method is its failure to detect immunoglobulin light chains or Bence Jones proteins secreted in multiple myeloma. The urine sulfosalicylic acid test is an alternate test that detects all urinary proteins by a process of precipitation. Highly concentrated urine may show trace to 1+ protein (10 to 30 mg/dL) in a normal individual. The finding of blood in the urine is abnormal and generally indicates the presence of intact red blood cells. Blood detected by a dipstick that cannot be accounted for by red blood cells in the urine sediment is the result of either hemoglobin or myoglobin, often in association with rhabdomyolysis. Leukocyte esterase and nitrites are usually positive in the presence of infection. A negative test, however, does not rule out infection.

Microscopic examination of the urine sediment is used to detect cellular elements, casts, crystals, and micro-organisms (Table 27-4) (**Web Fig. 27-3**). *Microscopic hematuria* is defined as more than two red blood cells per high-power field on a centrifuged urine specimen. Red cells of glomerular origin tend to be dysmorphic, whereas nonglomerular red cells are uniform in size and shape. *Pyuria* is defined as the presence of more than four white blood cells per high-power field. The presence of pyuria suggests urinary tract infection or inflammation. Sterile pyuria (negative culture in the presence of pyuria) suggests the diagnosis of prostatitis, chronic urethritis, renal tuberculosis, renal stones, papillary necrosis, or interstitial nephritis. A more specific test for interstitial nephritis involves documenting eosinophiluria by Wright stain or Hansel stain. However, certain infections can also cause eosinophiluria. Furthermore, the absence of urinary eosinophils does not rule out a diagnosis of interstitial nephritis. Renal tubular epithelial cells are large, with prominent nuclei, and are often seen in acute tubular necrosis, glomerulonephritis, or pyelonephritis. Epithelial cells in the urinary sediment may derive from any site along the urinary tract from the renal pelvis to the urethra. Renal tubular cells that contain absorbed lipids are termed *oval fat bodies.* Free fat droplets in the urine are usually observed in association with heavy proteinuria.

Urinary casts are cylindric structures derived from the intratubular precipitation of Tamm-Horsfall protein. The presence of red or white blood cells in the casts provides presumptive evidence of inflammatory parenchymal renal disease. *Red blood cell casts* most frequently indicate the presence of a proliferative glomerular lesion but may also be seen in patients with acute interstitial nephritis. *Renal tubular cell casts* in a patient with acute renal failure help confirm the diagnosis of acute tubular necrosis. The presence of *leukocyte casts* in a patient with urinary tract infection indicates a diagnosis of pyelonephritis rather than a lower urinary tract infection. Leukocyte casts may also be observed in patients with interstitial nephritis and, less commonly, in those with glomerulonephritis. Mixed cellular casts are noted when casts contain both red and white blood cells and are more frequently seen with acute interstitial nephritis.

In the absence of specific symptoms, crystals of calcium oxalate (envelope shaped) and uric acid (rhomboid shaped) identified in acidic urine are of little clinical significance. The presence of cystine crystals (benzene-ring shaped) in the urine indicates the rare disease cystinuria. Triple phosphate crystals (coffin-lid shaped) may be identified in alkaline urine. The presence of bacteria in an unspun urine specimen is significant and provides presumptive evidence for a urinary tract infection.

Table 27-4 Microscopic Examination of the Urine

Finding	Associations
Casts	
Red blood cells	Glomerulonephritis, vasculitis, interstitial nephritis
White blood cells	Interstitial nephritis, pyelonephritis
Epithelial cells	Acute tubular necrosis, interstitial nephritis, glomerulonephritis
Granular	Renal parenchymal disease (nonspecific)
Waxy, broad	Advanced renal failure
Hyaline	Normal finding in concentrated urine
Fatty	Heavy proteinuria
Cells	
Red blood cells	Urinary tract infection, urinary tract inflammation
White blood cells	Urinary tract infection, urinary tract inflammation
Eosinophils	Acute interstitial nephritis, atheroembolic disease, some infections
(Squamous) epithelial cells	Contaminants
Crystals	
Uric acid	Acid urine, acute uric acid nephropathy, hyperuricosuria
Calcium phosphate	Alkaline urine
Calcium oxalate	Acid urine, hyperoxaluria, ethylene glycol poisoning
Cystine	Cystinuria
Sulfur	Sulfa-containing antibiotics

Major Renal Syndromes

A patient with renal disease may be classified into separate clinical syndromes based on type and manifestation of renal injury as described in Table 27-5.

Acute nephritic syndrome is a clinical syndrome characterized by the relatively abrupt onset of kidney dysfunction accompanied by the presence of red blood cell casts and dysmorphic erythrocytes in the urine sediment, as well as varying degrees of proteinuria, which are highly suggestive of glomerular origin. Sodium avidity in the acute nephritic syndrome is considerably greater than what would be expected from decreased GFR. Plasma albumin is generally normal; consequently, a significant fraction of the retained sodium remains intravascularly and may explain the presence of hypertension, plasma volume dilution, circulatory overload, and congestive heart failure. Although acute poststreptococcal glomerulonephritis is the prototype for the acute nephritic syndrome, other infections may also lead to

Table 27-5 Major Renal Syndromes

Syndrome	Definition	Example
Acute nephritic syndrome	Abrupt onset of renal insufficiency accompanied by edema and hematuria that is glomerular or tubular in origin	Poststreptococcal glomerulonephritis
Nephrotic syndrome	Increased glomerular permeability manifested by massive proteinuria (>3.5 g/1.73 m² per day), edema, and hypoalbuminuria	
With *bland* urine sediment (pure nephrotic)	Oval fat bodies, coarse granular casts	Minimal change disease
Asymptomatic urinary abnormalities	Isolated proteinuria (<2.0 g/1.73 m² per day) or hematuria (with or without proteinuria)	Immunoglobulin A nephropathy
Tubulointerstitial nephropathy	Renal insufficiency associated with non-nephrotic–range proteinuria and functional tubular defects	Sarcoidosis
Acute renal failure	An abrupt decline in renal function sufficient to result in retention of nitrogenous waste (e.g., blood urea nitrogen and creatinine)	Acute tubular necrosis
Rapidly progressive renal failure	Rapid deterioration of renal function over a period of weeks to months	Rapidly progressive glomerulonephritis
Tubular defects	Isolated or multiple tubular transport defects	Renal tubular acidosis

this syndrome. Acute nephritic syndrome may also be caused by primary glomerular diseases, such as mesangioproliferative glomerulonephritis, and multisystem diseases that include systemic lupus erythematosus, Henoch-Schönlein purpura, vasculitis, and essential mixed cryoglobulinemia (**Web Fig. 27-4**).

Nephrotic syndrome is characterized by increased glomerular permeability exhibited by proteinuria in excess of 3.5 g/1.73 m² body surface area per day. A variable tendency exists toward edema, hypoalbuminemia, and hyperlipidemia. Patients with the nephrotic syndrome, in addition to proteinuria, may demonstrate oval fat bodies, coarse granular casts, and occasional cellular elements, but the lack of *active* sediment with dysmorphic red blood cells, and red blood cell casts is characteristic. The differential diagnosis includes glomerular diseases such as minimal change disease, membranous nephropathy, focal segmental glomerulosclerosis (FSGS), diabetic nephropathy, and amyloidosis. In patients with a mixed clinical picture (nephrotic-nephritic syndrome), membrane proliferative nephritis, systemic lupus erythematosus, postinfectious glomerulonephritis, and mixed essential cryoglobulinemia are the most likely diagnostic considerations.

The term *rapidly progressive renal failure* is applied to patients who have more than a 50% loss in kidney function over weeks to months. This condition is in contrast to patients with *acute renal failure,* who have an abrupt decline in renal function over several days, and to patients with *chronic renal failure,* who have a decline in renal function over months to years. The differential diagnosis of a patient who presents with rapidly progressive renal failure is shown in Table 27-6. One of the important but uncommon causes of rapidly progressive renal failure is rapidly progressive glomerulonephritis. This condition is a clinical syndrome that is typically associated with extensive glomerular crescent formation (**Web Fig. 27-5**) as the principal histologic finding on renal biopsy. Dysmorphic erythrocytes, red blood cell casts, and moderate proteinuria are characteristic in rapidly progressive glomerulonephritis.

Acute renal failure is a syndrome that can be broadly defined as an abrupt decline in renal function sufficient to result in kidney impairment over days to a few weeks. Acute renal failure can result from a decrease in renal blood flow (prerenal azotemia), intrinsic parenchymal disease (intrare-

nal azotemia), or obstruction to urine flow (postrenal azotemia). The general approach for evaluating acute renal failure is detailed in Chapter 33.

Tubulointerstitial nephropathy represents a group of clinical disorders that principally affect the renal tubules and interstitium, with relative sparing of the glomeruli and renal vasculature. In most patients, the disease can possibly be classified into acute interstitial nephritis or chronic interstitial nephropathy based on the rate of progression of renal dysfunction. Chronic tubulointerstitial nephropathy is characterized by renal insufficiency, non-nephrotic–range proteinuria, and tubular damage disproportionately severe relative to the degree of kidney impairment. Thus, patients with chronic tubulointerstitial disease often have modest degrees of sodium wasting, hyperkalemia, and a normal anion gap metabolic acidosis even when renal dysfunction is modest. Acute interstitial nephritis, often caused by a medication, is characterized by the sudden onset of clinical signs of renal dysfunction associated with a prominent inflammatory cell infiltrate within the renal interstitium and is often important in the differential diagnosis of patients with acute renal failure.

Imaging of the Urinary Tract

One of the most common imaging studies of the urinary tract is the renal ultrasound. Renal ultrasonography is a noninvasive method of obtaining an anatomic image of the kidney and the collecting system. This technique is particularly useful for determining kidney size; for detecting renal masses, cysts, and dilation of the collecting system; and for identifying hydronephrosis. At the time of the sonogram, the bladder should be imaged, especially in the immediate postvoiding state, because an accurate determination of bladder emptying is easy to obtain. The absence of hydronephrosis on a sonogram does not rule out obstructive uropathy, particularly in the presence of acute obstruction, volume depletion, or retroperitoneal fibrosis. In a patient with advanced renal failure, the presence of bilateral kidneys typically smaller than 8 cm implies a chronic, irreversible process, whereas the presence of normal-sized kidneys of 11 to 13 cm indicates acute renal failure or chronic renal failure caused by diseases such as diabetes, amyloidosis, or multiple myeloma. In addition to size, the echogenicity of the parenchyma is assessed. Scarred kidneys are far more echogenic. Duplex ultrasonography, in which B-mode ultrasonography has been combined with pulsed Doppler imaging, may be useful in detecting disease of the major renal arteries or veins. Ultrasound can easily identify simple cysts. However, complex cysts or solid lesions require further investigation by computed tomography (CT) or magnetic resonance imaging (MRI). Discrepancy in kidney size by more than 1.5 cm may suggest ischemic damage to the kidney such as renovascular disease, reflux nephropathy with scarring of the kidney, or congenital abnormalities. Ultrasonography is routinely used to guide kidney biopsy, to introduce nephrostomy tubes, or to drain fluid collection around the kidney.

Table 27-6 **Causes of Rapidly Progressive Renal Failure**
Obstructive uropathy
Malignant hypertension
Rapidly progressive glomerulonephritis
Thrombotic thrombocytopenic purpura, hemolytic uremic syndrome
Atheromatous embolic disease
Bilateral renal artery stenosis
Scleroderma crisis
Multiple myeloma
Systemic lupus erythematosus

Intravenous pyelography (IVP) involves the intravenous administration of iodinated radiographic contrast medium that is excreted through the kidney by glomerular filtration. The contrast medium concentrates in the renal tubules and produces a nephrogram image within the first few minutes after injection. As the medium passes into the collecting system, the calyces, renal pelvis, ureters, and bladder are visualized. The use of IVP over ultrasonography is required when a more detailed imaging study of anatomic structures is required or when evaluating obstruction and acute nephrolithiasis. The disadvantage of IVP is the requirement for radiocontrast, which can induce nephrotoxicity, particularly in patients with renal insufficiency as defined by an estimated GFR of less than 60 mL/1.73 m² per minute, volume depletion, diabetes, or congestive heart failure. For most institutions, contrast CT has taken the place of classic IVP.

Retrograde pyelography is performed by injecting radiocontrast material directly into the ureters at the time of cystoscopy. This technique is useful in defining obstructing lesions within the ureter or renal pelvis, particularly in the setting of a nonvisualizing kidney on IVP. Ureteric stones can be removed during this procedure using a special basket.

CT of the kidney is usually done by instilling a contrast medium, except when investigating renal calculi or hemorrhage. CT is most helpful in evaluating renal masses, complex cysts, and perinephric and vascular pathologic conditions such as renal vein thrombosis. In select cases, CT is used to guide kidney biopsy or fluid collection, such as that from a perinephric abscess. As in other imaging studies of the urinary tract, CT often uses radiocontrast agents and is contraindicated in individuals with impaired kidney function.

MRI uses high magnetic fields and radiofrequencies to construct images. MRI is most helpful in delineating complex renal masses, staging renal tumors, detecting invasion of renal veins, and diagnosing renovascular disease; it is also used as an alternative to CT in patients with kidney failure to avoid using radiocontrast agents because as gadolinium is non-nephrotoxic, although gadolinium should be avoided if possible when the GFR is less than 40 mL per minute because of its possible role in inducing nephrogenic systemic fibrosis. Technical improvement in magnetic resonance angiography has enhanced the detection of renal artery stenosis and may grade the severity of the disease. MRI should be avoided in patients with implanted ferromagnetic devices such as pacemakers.

Radionuclide imaging provides important noninvasive information about kidneys. The test involves the intravenous administration of radiolabeled compounds, after which images are taken with a gamma camera. Pregnancy is the only contraindication for renal radionuclide imaging. The uses of renal radionuclide imaging are listed in Table 27-7.

Renal arteriography involves the direct injection of radiographic contrast medium into the aorta and renal arteries and is used to assess renal vasculature. It is particularly useful in evaluating patients with suggested renal artery stenosis or thrombosis and those with a renal mass. Patients with unexplained hematuria or with a suggested vascular malforma-

Table 27-7 **Common Uses of Radionuclide Renal Imaging**
Renal perfusion
Renovascular hypertension
Glomerular filtration rate estimation for each kidney
Pyelonephritis, renal abscess
Interstitial nephritis
Renal cortical scarring
Obstruction
Renal pseudotumor

Table 27-8 **Indications for Kidney Biopsy**
Nephrotic syndrome
Persistent proteinuria, particularly with abnormal sediment or abnormal renal function
Hematuria associated with abnormal urine sediment or proteinuria
Unexplained hematuria after exclusion of lower urinary tract causes
Systemic disorders with kidney involvement (e.g., systemic lupus erythematosus, Henoch-Schönlein purpura)
Acute renal failure with atypical features or failure to recover renal function in 8 weeks
Rapidly progressive renal failure
Renal allograft dysfunction
Unexplained reduction in kidney function

tion should have a renal arteriogram. Individuals with polyarteritis nodosa may require selective renal arteriography to detect microaneurysms. Renal vein catheterization is used to confirm the diagnosis of renal vein thrombosis or to obtain blood samples from the renal vein. Although CT or MRI is used to confirm the diagnosis of renal vein thrombosis, renal venography may be required when the diagnosis is in doubt or when the initial diagnostic suspicion is high. CT angiogram and magnetic resonance angiography have been used in screening, but these involve venous injections without direct access to the renal arteries, so that interventions require a separate procedure.

Renal Biopsy

Most renal biopsies are performed when a glomerular lesion is suggested and less commonly in patients with unexplained acute or chronic renal failure. Table 27-8 lists the indications for kidney biopsy. The percutaneous biopsy is the most commonly used technique and is a relatively safe procedure. Potential complications of a closed renal biopsy include hematuria, renal hematoma, vascular laceration with the development of arteriovenous fistula, and the inadvertent biopsy of liver, spleen, or bowel. Percutaneous kidney biopsy is contraindicated in solitary or ectopic kidneys (except kidney transplants), horseshoe kidney, uncontrolled bleeding disorders, uncontrolled hypertension, renal infection, renal neoplasm, and uncooperative patients.

Prospectus for the Future

The early identification of kidney disease needs to be determined well before changes in serum parameters that are elevated after significant kidney impairment has occurred. Novel urinary biomarkers are emerging as diagnostic tools that will help identify individuals at risk for kidney disease and will allow for the development of novel therapeutic interventions that prevent the development of kidney failure or limit progressive loss of kidney function.

Additionally, genetic analysis of individuals with kidney disease may allow for directed therapeutic regimens that decrease the risk for progressive kidney disease and the ultimate need for dialysis therapies or renal transplantation in the future.

References

National Kidney Foundation: K/DOQI clinical practice guidelines for chronic kidney disease: Evaluation, classification, and stratification. Am J Kidney Dis 39:S1-S62, 2002.

Stevens LA, Fares G, Fleming J, et al: Low rates of testing and diagnostic codes usage in a commercial clinical laboratory: Evidence for lack of physician awareness of chronic kidney disease. J Am Soc Nephrol 16:2439-2448, 2005.

Fluid and Electrolyte Disorders

Thomas E. Andreoli* and Robert L. Safirstein

The content of fluid and electrolytes in the cells and fluid compartments of the body are remarkably constant under normal conditions despite a widely varying intake. This constancy is maintained by fluid and solute shifts across the cells of the body and by the capacity of the kidney to adjust the urinary excretion of water, electrolytes, and solutes to match intake and the needs of the body. In health, the solute content of body water is maintained between 285 and 295 mOsm/kg of water. Tight regulation of body water and solute concentrations is made possible by the remarkable ability of the kidney to regulate urine volume from 500 mL to 24 L per 24-hour period. The ability of the kidney to carry out its functions is intrinsically tied to the thirst-neurohypophyseal-renal axis.

Volume Disorders

Water constitutes about 60% of total-body weight in humans (Fig. 28-1). Total-body water is inversely proportional to the amount of body fat, which varies with age, gender, and nutritional status. About two thirds of the total-body water is in the intracellular compartment. Three fourths of the extracellular water is in the interstitial space, and one fourth is in the plasma. Potassium and magnesium constitute the major cations of the intracellular space, whereas sodium is the major cation of the extracellular space. Phosphate and protein are the major anions of the intracellular space, whereas chloride and bicarbonate are the major anions of extracellular space. The cell membrane represents the barrier between the intracellular and extracellular fluid compartments. Because membranes are relatively permeable to water, the osmotic gradient determines the movement of fluid across the cell membrane. Thus, except for transient changes, the intracellular and extracellular fluid compartments are in *osmotic equilibrium*. The transfer of fluid between the vascular and interstitial compartments occurs across the capillary wall and is governed by the balance between hydrostatic pressure gradients and plasma oncotic pressure gradients, as related in the *Starling equation*:

*Deceased.

$$J_V = (K_f \times [\Delta P - \sigma \Delta \Pi])$$

where J_V is the rate of fluid transfer between vascular and interstitial compartments, K_f is the water permeability, ΔP is the difference between capillary and interstitial hydrostatic pressure, $\Delta \Pi$ equals the difference between capillary and interstitial oncotic pressure, and σ is the reflection coefficient (albumin = 1).

Thus, an increase in the driving force for fluid movement into the interstitial compartment may result from a decrease in the colloid oncotic pressure of plasma, as may occur in hypoalbuminemia, or an increase in the capillary hydrostatic pressure, as occurs in congestive heart failure.

NORMAL VOLUME HOMEOSTASIS

The kidney plays a crucial role in regulating the constancy of extracellular fluid (ECF) volume. The response to a reduction in ECF volume consists of hemodynamic responses that adjust cardiac output and peripheral vascular resistance to maintain blood pressure, as well as primary renal responses that adjust external sodium and water balance. Together, this response has been termed the *integrated volume response* (Fig. 28-2). Hemodynamic alterations occur within minutes of a perceived volume reduction and are characterized by tachycardia, increased peripheral resistance from arterial vasoconstriction, and decreased venous capacitance from venoconstriction. Renal conservation of salt and water lags behind by 12 to 24 hours and involves the release of various hormones (see Fig. 28-2). Stimulation of the extrarenal baroreceptors also results in the release of antidiuretic hormone (ADH), which promotes water retention in the kidney. Vasoconstrictive factors, such as endothelins produced and released by vascular endothelial cells, also play a role in modulating systemic hemodynamics. Elevation of the efferent arteriolar resistance increases the filtration fraction, increases peritubular protein concentration, and increases sodium and water reabsorption in proximal tubules. Vasodilator prostaglandins, such as prostaglandin E_2, modulate these vasoconstrictive influences and maintain the glomerular filtration rate (GFR) by enhancing the renal blood flow in states associated with ECF volume depletion. This action is the reason that nonsteroidal anti-inflammatory drugs are so deleterious during volume depletion.

In response to volume expansion, the renal excretion of salt and water is increased because of the suppression of the aforementioned pathways. The release of atrial natriuretic peptide is a major factor promoting natriuresis in volume-expanded states. Atrial natriuretic peptide is released from the atrial myocytes in response to atrial stretch associated with volume expansion. This peptide release promotes natriuresis by increasing GFR and inhibiting collecting duct sodium reabsorption.

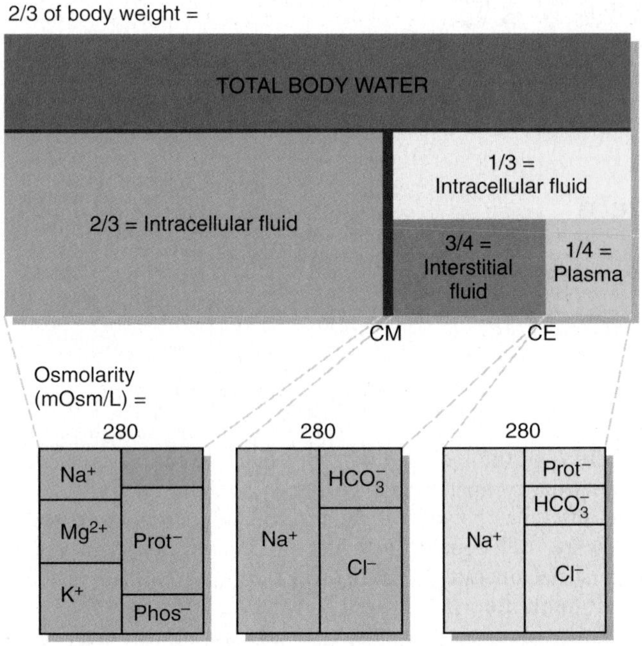

ABNORMAL VOLUME REGULATION

The integrated volume response depends on afferent mechanisms that sense changes in the *effective circulating volume* (ECV). ECV is difficult to define because it is not a measurable and distinct body fluid compartment. ECV relates to the *fullness* and tension within the arterial tree. Because only 15% of total blood volume is in the arterial compartment, arterial blood volume can be decreased in relation to the holding capacity of the arterial tree. In most circumstances, ECV correlates with the total ECF volume, except in certain disorders in which ECV is decreased in the presence of an increased total ECF volume (Table 28-1). In these disorders, the ECV is decreased as a result of either decreased cardiac output or arterial vasodilation, which decreases fullness and tension in the arterial circulation.

Because the afferent sensors respond to ECV rather than to the total ECF volume, in disease states such as congestive heart failure and hepatic cirrhosis, during which ECV is low, continued activation of the *integrated volume response* occurs and thus promotes further salt and water retention.

VOLUME DEPLETION

Disorders of extracellular volume result from alterations in sodium balance. The causes of true volume depletion (e.g.,

Figure 28-1 Composition of body fluid compartments. The compartments are anatomically defined by the cell membrane (CM) and capillary endothelium (CE). The osmolar concentration among compartments is equivalent despite wide variation in cation and anion composition.

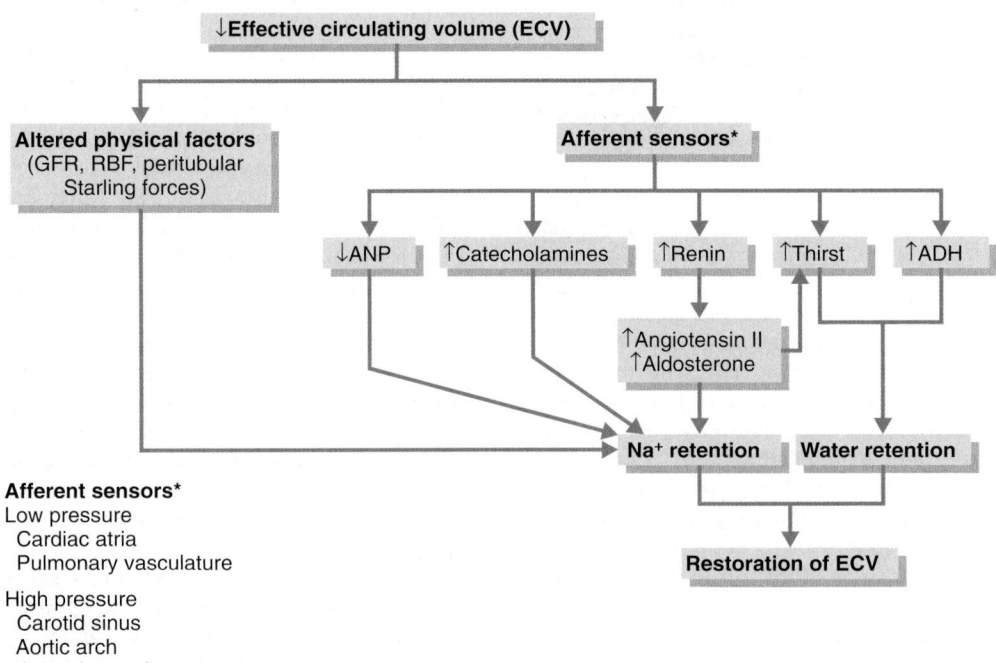

Figure 28-2 Volume repletion reaction. ADH, antidiuretic hormone; ANP, atriopeptin; GFR, glomerular filtration rate; RBF, renal blood flow.

Table 28-1 **Disorders Characterized by Decreased Effective Circulating Volume with Increased Total Extracellular Fluid Volume**
Congestive heart failure
Liver disease
Sepsis
Nephrotic syndrome (minority)
Pregnancy
Anaphylaxis

Table 28-2 **Causes of Volume Depletion**

Gastrointestinal Losses

Upper: bleeding, nasogastric suction, vomiting
Lower: bleeding, diarrhea, enteric or pancreatic fistula, tube drainage

Renal Losses

Salt and water: diuretics, osmotic diuresis, postobstructive diuresis, acute tubular necrosis (recovery phase), salt-losing nephropathy, adrenal insufficiency, renal tubular acidosis
Water: diabetes insipidus

Skin and Respiratory Losses

Sweat, burns, insensible losses

Sequestration Without External Fluid Loss

Intestinal obstruction, peritonitis, pancreatitis, rhabdomyolysis

Table 28-3 **Causes of Volume Excess**

Primary Renal Sodium Retention (Increased Effective Circulating Volume)

Oliguric acute renal failure
Acute glomerulonephritis
Severe chronic renal failure
Nephritic, nephrotic syndrome
Primary hyperaldosteronism
Cushing syndrome
Early stages of severe liver disease
Conn syndrome
Gordon syndrome
Liddle syndrome

Secondary Renal Sodium Retention (Decreased Effective Circulating Volume)

Heart failure
Later stages of severe liver disease
Nephrotic syndrome (minimal change disease)
Pregnancy

decreased ECV and total ECF volume) are listed in Table 28-2. Extrarenal losses are the most common clinical causes of volume depletion, and when they occur with normal renal function, the urine is highly concentrated, salt poor, and acidic. When volume depletion occurs from renal losses, the urine is inappropriately dilute and sometimes rich in salt. The syndrome of nephrogenic diabetes insipidus is one such cause, and in congenital forms of the syndrome, loss-of-function mutations occur in the V2 vasopressin receptor (X-linked), as well as autosomal dominant and recessive forms caused by inactivating mutations of the collecting duct water channel aquaporin-2. The clinical findings in states of true volume depletion are secondary to an underfilling of the arterial tree and to the renal and hemodynamic responses to this underfilling. Mild volume depletion may be associated with orthostatic dizziness and tachycardia. As the intracellular compartment becomes further depleted, recumbent tachycardia becomes evident, and urine output diminishes. Patients with severe volume depletion may exhibit vasoconstriction, hypotension, mental obtundation, cool extremities, and negligible urine output. Many of these clinical features can be explained based on effects of vasoconstrictor hormones, such as catecholamine and angiotensin II, that are released in response to hypovolemia.

Significant volume depletion can occur in the absence of classic clinical findings. States of volume depletion in patients receiving cardiovascular drugs and excess renal sodium loss from intrinsic renal disease or diuretics are examples of clinical circumstances in which an assessment of the state of hydration may be difficult. An appropriate clinical history is always mandatory, particularly prior knowledge of the patient's body weight. If doubt exists about the state of hydration, particularly in critically ill patients, measurement of the central venous pressure by means of catheterization permits assessment of the intravascular volume status.

The absolute quantity and the rate of fluid replacement depend on the severity of volume depletion, which is estimated by the clinical presentation. If fluid repletion is to involve parenteral infusions, the distribution of the infused fluid should be considered. Nearly all the volume of solutions containing 0.9% sodium chloride and colloid is retained in the extracellular space, and these are the preferred parenteral solutions for the treatment of hypovolemia. By contrast, only one third of infused 5% glucose in water (D_5W) remains in the extracellular compartment.

VOLUME EXCESS

Volume expansion occurs when salt and water intake exceeds renal and extrarenal losses. The causes are listed in Table 28-3. The underlying disturbance common to these disorders is sodium and water retention by the kidney. The sodium and water retention may be primary, resulting in increased ECV, or secondary, in response to a decreased ECV. The net result of renal sodium and water retention is an alteration of Starling forces that leads to increased capillary hydrostatic pressure and favors fluid shifts from the intravascular to interstitial space. Most patients with nephrotic syndrome have an increased ECV resulting from primary renal sodium retention. In advanced liver disease, the ECV is decreased because of arterial underfilling from vasodilation that results in secondary renal sodium retention. However, in early liver disease, the volume excess may result from primary renal sodium retention. Severe hypoalbuminemia associated with liver disease, nephrotic syndrome, or severe malnutrition may overwhelm the local capillary homeostatic mechanisms and may lead to edema formation.

The mainstay in treating volume excess is dietary sodium restriction in combination with diuretics (Table 28-4). Diuretics enhance natriuresis by inhibiting the reabsorption of sodium at various sites along the nephron. The cardinal example of a proximal tubular diuretic is acetazolamide, a *carbonic anhydrase inhibitor*, which blocks proximal

Table 28-4 **Characteristics of Commonly Used Diuretics**			
Agent	**Site**	**Primary Effect**	**Secondary Effect**
Carbonic anhydrase inhibitors (acetazolamide)	Proximal tubule	Blocking of ↓ Na^+-H^+ exchange	K^+, HCO_3^- loss
Loop diuretics (furosemide, bumetanide, ethacrynic acid)	Thick ascending limb of loop of Henle	↓ $Na^+/K^+/2\ Cl^-$ transport	K^+ loss ↑ H^+ secretion ↑ Ca^{2+} excretion
Thiazide Diuretics			
Thiazides	Distal convoluted tubule	↓ NaCl co-transport	↓ K^+ loss ↓ H^+ secretion ↓ Ca^{2+} excretion
Metolazone	Distal tubule, proximal tubule	↓ NaCl reabsorption	—
Aldosterone antagonists (spironolactone)	Cortical collecting duct	↓ Na^+ reabsorption	↓ K^+ loss ↓ H^+ secretion
Primary sodium channel blockers (triamterene, amiloride)	Cortical collecting duct	↓ Na^+ reabsorption	↓ K^+ loss ↓ H^+ secretion

Ca^{2+}, calcium; Cl^-, chloride; H^+, hydrogen; HCO_3^-, bicarbonate; K^+, potassium; Na^+, sodium; NaCl, sodium chloride.

reabsorption of sodium bicarbonate. Consequently, prolonged use of acetazolamide may lead to hyperchloremic acidosis. Metolazone, a member of the thiazide class of diuretics, in addition to blocking sodium reabsorption in the distal tubule, exerts its natriuretic effect in the proximal tubule. Because the proximal tubule is the major site for phosphate reabsorption, profound phosphaturia may accompany the use of metolazone. *Loop diuretics* such as furosemide and bumetanide inhibit the sodium, chloride, and potassium co-transporter of the thick ascending limb of the loop of Henle. *Thiazide diuretics* inhibit the sodium and chloride co-transporter of the distal tubule. The loop diuretics promote calcium excretion, and the thiazide diuretics decrease calcium excretion. Thus, the former are useful in managing hypercalcemia, whereas the latter are useful in preventing calcium stone formation. Spironolactone, an *aldosterone antagonist,* decreases sodium reabsorption in the cortical collecting duct. Primary *sodium channel blockers* such as amiloride also block sodium reabsorption in the cortical collecting duct by an aldosterone-independent mechanism. The last two groups of diuretics do not cause hypokalemia, which is a common complication associated with the use of other diuretics. In states of severe sodium retention and edema formation, such as severe congestive heart failure and nephrotic syndrome, a combination of diuretics working at different sites in the nephron may be more effective than the use of a single class of diuretics. Moreover, using potassium-sparing diuretics in combination with a potassium-wasting diuretic can minimize potassium and magnesium deficits. In patients with cirrhosis and ascites, abdominal paracentesis with concomitant intravenous infusion of some colloid has been used as a good therapeutic alternative to diuretics.

Osmolality Disorders

Body fluid osmolality, the ratio of solute to water in all fluid compartments, is maintained within an extremely narrow range. Because water moves freely across most cell membranes, changes in the ECF osmolality cause reciprocal changes in the intracellular volume. The ECF osmolality can be approximated by calculating the serum osmolality based on the major solutes in that compartment:

$$\text{Calculated osmolality} = (2 \times \text{sodium}) + (\text{glucose} \div 18) + (\text{BUN} \div 2.8)$$

where the glucose and blood urea nitrogen (BUN) concentrations are expressed as milligrams per deciliter and the serum sodium concentration is expressed as milliequivalents per liter.

Measured osmolality usually equals the calculated osmolality. However, in the presence of osmotically active substances, such as ethanol, methanol, or ethylene glycol, the measured osmolality is higher than the calculated osmolality. Under these circumstances, the *osmolar gap* (measured minus calculated osmolality) provides a clue to the presence of toxins and gives an estimated concentration of these solutes. Alterations in the plasma sodium concentration almost always reflect changes in water balance. Because sodium is the major cation in the ECF, disorders of osmolality are generally reflected by an abnormal sodium concentration in the ECF.

Regulation of osmolality involves changes in renal water excretion, and the sodium excretion is not affected by osmoregulatory factors unless concomitant ECV depletion exists. ECF osmolality is regulated by dual pathways in the *water repletion reaction* (Fig. 28-3). Osmoreceptor cells in the central nervous system that are located in the wall of the third ventricle sense minor changes in the osmolality of blood in the internal carotid circulation. Neuronal signals from osmoreceptors stimulate the release of ADH from the posterior pituitary gland and simultaneously stimulate the sensation of thirst. ADH causes renal water conservation by increasing water permeability and water reabsorption in the collecting ducts. Thirst leads to an increase in water intake. When the ECF volume is reduced by about 10%, water

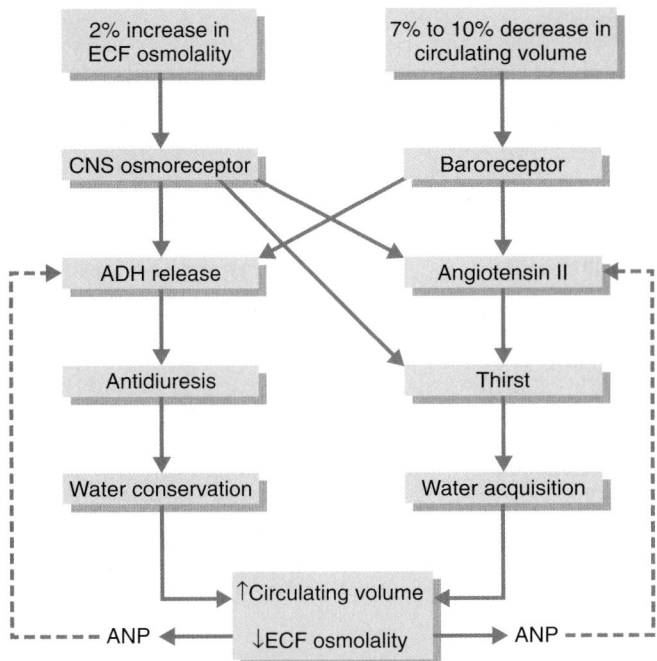

Figure 28-3 Water regulatory mechanisms. Alterations in extracellular fluid (ECF) osmolality or volume stimulate *(solid lines)* thirst and release of antidiuretic hormone (ADH). The net result is a positive water balance. Counter-regulation is provided by the inhibitory effects *(dashed lines)* of atriopeptin (ANP). CNS, central nervous system.

retention is activated as a means of replenishing ECF volume irrespective of osmolality. In this case, baroreceptors in the venous and arterial circulation stimulate ADH release through neuronal pathways. This *nonosmotic* stimulation of ADH release occurs independently of osmoreceptor function. Water repletion activates mechanisms that counter-regulate water conservation. Suppression of thirst and inhibition of ADH release lead to decreased water intake and increased renal water excretion.

Hyponatremia

PATHOPHYSIOLOGIC FACTORS

A diagnostic approach to hyponatremia, the most common electrolyte disorder in hospitalized patients, is outlined in Figure 28-4. The causes of hyponatremia show an association with normal, high, or low total-body sodium content. In some hyponatremic disorders, the serum osmolality is elevated; thus, the intracellular water content is not increased, and no risk for brain edema exists. Hyperglycemia and the use of hypertonic mannitol may result in hyponatremia because of water shift from the intracellular to extracellular space. Hyponatremia associated with normal serum osmolality may be seen in patients with extreme hyperlipidemia and hyperproteinemia, resulting from methodologic errors in techniques to measure serum electrolyte concentration. The increasing use of ion-selective electrodes for these measurements is making these causes of *pseudohyponatremia* uncommon. Hyponatremia may also be seen in patients who undergo transurethral resection of the prostate or hysteroscopic examination because of the absorption of large

amounts of hypo-osmolar glycine or sorbitol irrigating solutions.

Most hyponatremic disorders are associated with hypo-osmolality. In principle, hypo-osmolality can result from an increase in water intake or a decrease in renal water excretion, or both. Under normal circumstances, the kidneys can excrete 16 to 20 L of water free of solutes, or *free water,* per day. Water excretion may be impaired secondary to a reduced GFR, reduced ECV, impaired sodium-chloride reabsorption in the renal diluting segments of the distal nephron, which can be caused by severely reduced solute intake, and failure to suppress ADH secretion in response to hypotonicity (syndrome of inappropriate secretion of ADH [SIADH]). Finally, there is a rare congenital syndrome, the nephrogenic syndrome of inappropriate antidiuresis (NSIAD), which is caused by a gain in function mutation of the V2 vasopressin receptor, such that the latter is activated even in the absence of vasopressin. Marathon runners develop hyponatremia, which can be fatal, as a result of the inability to excrete ingested water during the race.

Because of the large capacity of normal kidneys to excrete free water, even in patients with *primary polydipsia,* the hyponatremia is caused by both large water intake and impaired water excretion. Hyponatremia may also occur with modestly increased water intake in the presence of impaired GFR or decreased solute intake. In patients with decreased GFR, renal water excretion is impaired because of decreased delivery of filtrate to the distal nephron. Patients with chronic starvation or beer potomania have deficient oral intake of solutes. Because renal water excretion depends on osmolar intake, these patients may develop hyponatremia at a modestly increased level of water intake.

More commonly, hyponatremia occurs as a result of the inability to dilute urine maximally because of reduction in the rate of salt absorption by the diluting segment, sustained nonosmotic release of ADH, or a combination of these two factors. In the disorders associated with decreased ECV, nonosmotic ADH release occurs and promotes water retention by the kidney. In addition, these patients have enhanced proximal sodium-chloride reabsorption with diminished distal delivery. These disorders may be associated with signs of either volume expansion or volume depletion.

SIADH is the prototype of the primary release of ADH or ADH-like substances. It occurs most often in association with pathologic processes of the central nervous system or pulmonary system. Many medications can enhance the release of ADH or can potentiate its effect (Table 28-5). The circulating ADH allows excessive water absorption in the collecting duct with a modest expansion of the ECF volume. With the increase in volume, renal perfusion is increased, and the kidney subsequently decreases sodium reabsorption in an attempt to reestablish euvolemia. Two infants have recently been described with apparent SIADH in which the serum vasopressin levels are suppressed. Evaluation revealed gain of function mutations of the V2 vasopressin receptor in these patients.

DIAGNOSIS AND TREATMENT

The signs and symptoms of hyponatremia are related to brain cell swelling caused by an increase in the brain water content resulting from water shift from a hypo-osmolar

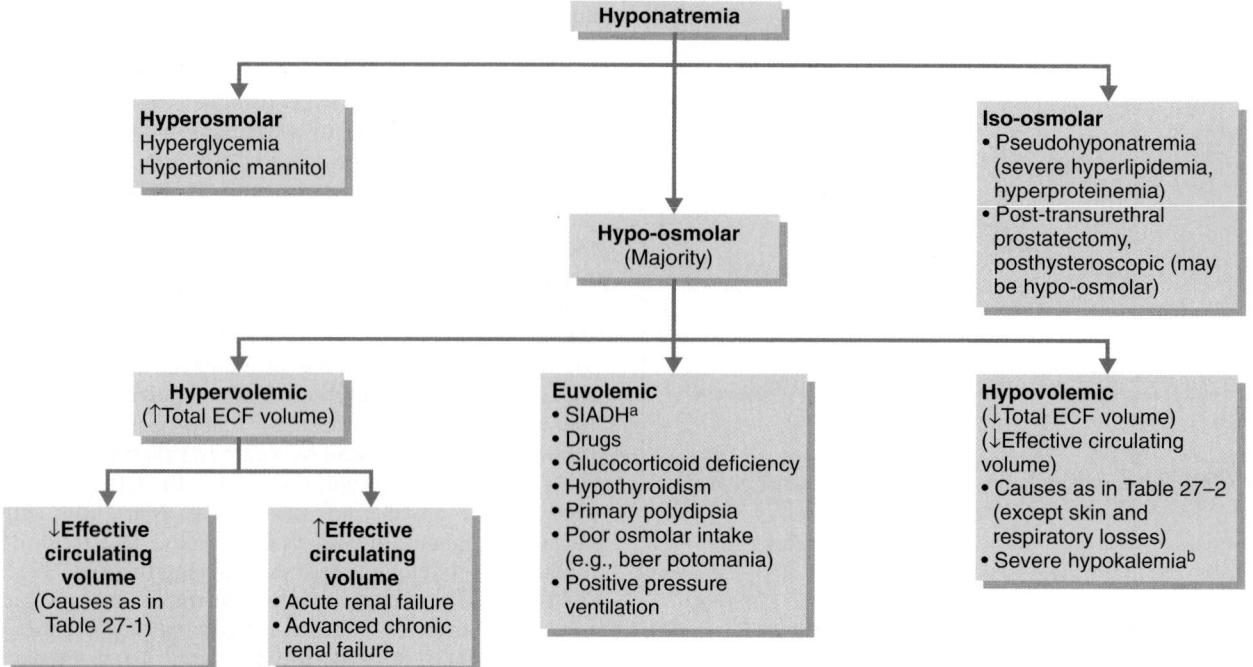

aSIADH patients may have modest volume expansion.
bSeen in patients with hypokalemia due to diuretic use and may be due to Na+ entry into the cells to replace K+ loss.

Figure 28-4 Diagnostic approach to hyponatremia. ECF, extracellular fluid; SIADH, syndrome of inappropriate secretion of antidiuretic hormone.

Table 28-5 **Causes of Syndrome of Inappropriate Secretion of Antidiuretic Hormone**

Central Nervous System Disorders

Trauma
Infection
Tumors
Porphyria

Pulmonary Disorders

Tuberculosis
Pneumonia
Positive pressure ventilation

Neoplasia

Carcinoma: bronchogenic, pancreatic, ureteral, prostatic, bladder
Lymphoma and leukemia
Thymoma and mesothelioma

Drugs

Increased antidiuretic hormone release
Chlorpropamide
Clofibrate
Carbamazepine
Vincristine
Potentiated antidiuretic hormone action
Chlorpropamide
Cyclophosphamide
Nonsteroidal anti-inflammatory agents

Modified from Andreoli TE: Disorders of fluid volume, electrolyte, and acid-base balance. In Wyngaarden JB, Smith LH Jr, Bennett JC (eds): Cecil Textbook of Medicine, 19th ed. Philadelphia: WB Saunders, 1992, p 509.

extracellular environment. Hence, hyponatremic disorders should be considered in any patient who has acute mental status changes. An assessment of the volume status by physical examination is the most important initial step in the diagnostic approach to patients with hyponatremia. The most difficult differential diagnosis among hyponatremic disorders involves the distinction between patients who have reduced ECV and those who have SIADH. In both instances, the urine osmolality may be inappropriately concentrated relative to the serum osmolality. In reduced ECV, the urine sodium concentration is negligible, whereas it is usually higher than 30 mEq/L in patients with SIADH. High BUN and serum uric acid levels also suggest reduced ECV. When hyponatremia is associated with a low BUN and uric acid level, SIADH is the most likely diagnosis.

Baseline data should include body weight, serum electrolytes, serum osmolality, urine electrolytes, and urine osmolality; frequent measurement of serum and urine electrolytes, intake, and urine output should be performed during the treatment of hyponatremia. As a general rule, the administration of sodium solutions with a tonicity greater than that of urine raises serum sodium concentrations. The treatment should depend on the underlying clinical disease and volume status of the patient. Sodium and water intake should be restricted in the volume-expanded patient. In patients with decreased ECV and true hypovolemia, secondary to extrarenal losses, treatment should include isotonic sodium chloride.

In patients with SIADH, restriction of water intake is the mainstay of therapy. However, this is difficult to achieve

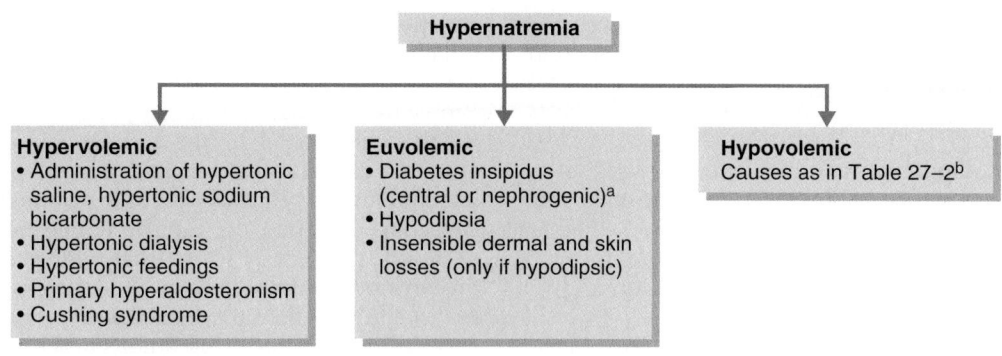

^aMay be hypovolemic.
^bUnder "sequestration," only rhabdomyolysis may cause hypernatremia owing to shift of water from extracellular to intracellular space.

Figure 28-5 Diagnostic approach to hypernatremia.

because patients are invariably thirsty, particularly in the southern regions of the United States. Demethylchlortetracycline and lithium, while proposed, are not generally acceptable. Hypertonic saline, particularly in patients with SIADH, will produce a profound natriuresis, and hyponatremia will develop rapidly. The most rational approach to therapy is the use of furosemide in combination with normal saline. Furosemide forces the excretion of a urine which is half-normal saline, whereas the administration of normal saline helps correct the hyponatremia. The vasopressin receptor antagonist conivaptan has been shown to be effective in treating hyponatremia as well.

When hyponatremia occurs acutely (<48 hours), cerebral edema can ensue. The typical signs and symptoms include headache, nausea, vomiting, weakness, incoordination with falls, delirium, and seizures. Patients in whom hyponatremia develops over days to weeks may exhibit more subtle neurologic signs and symptoms.

The rate of correction of serum sodium depends on the symptoms and duration of hyponatremia. The correction of serum sodium with acute hyponatremia may be achieved rapidly (up to 2.5 mEq/L per hour) until central nervous system symptoms and seizures subside. Even under these circumstances, an absolute change of serum sodium of more than 20 mEq/L/day should be avoided. In patients with chronic hyponatremia (>48 hours), the serum sodium concentration should be corrected at a rate of 0.5 mEq/L per hour until it reaches 120 mEq/L. Patients with asymptomatic hyponatremia (acute or chronic) do not need aggressive therapy. This caution is necessary because of the occurrence of central pontine myelinolysis with too rapid correction.

Hypervolemic hypotonic hyponatremia secondary to cirrhosis, congestive heart failure, or renal failure should be treated not only by measures directed at the underlying disease but also with loop diuretics to help promote the excretion of hypotonic urine. Water restriction should be maintained at less than 1 L per 24-hour period. For patients with chronic SIADH that is not responsive to treatment of the underlying cause, free-water restriction alone is often sufficient. In resistant cases and in patients with neurologic symptoms, a combination of furosemide and normal or high dietary sodium intake is necessary. V2-receptor antagonists are increasingly used in these cases as well.

Hypernatremia

PATHOPHYSIOLOGIC FACTORS

In most instances, hypernatremia is caused by excess water loss, rather than by sodium gain. Hypertonicity of the plasma is a powerful stimulus for thirst. Patients who are unable to sense thirst owing to diseases of the brain and patients who are physically unable to obtain water may develop hypernatremia. Most patients with hypernatremia, however, exhibit a primary defect in urinary concentrating ability along with insufficient administration of free water (Fig. 28-5).

Water can be lost in the urine, in excess of electrolytes, and in conditions characterized by the presence of large quantities of osmotically active solutes in the filtrate. This type of *osmotic diuresis* can occur in patients with hyperglycemia, after the infusion of mannitol, or in patients who are excreting excessive amounts of amino acids or urea. The last situation occurs in patients receiving high-protein tube feedings or total parenteral nutrition.

Diabetes insipidus is a disorder in which the collecting tubule is impermeable to water. Patients may have a central defect in the release of ADH or a defect in renal responsiveness to the hormone (nephrogenic).

In hypernatremia caused by osmotic diuresis, urine osmolality may be higher than serum osmolality because of the presence of solutes such as glucose, mannitol, or urea in the urine.

TREATMENT

Hypernatremia that is associated with hypovolemia implies a sodium deficit in addition to the water deficit and requires isotonic saline infusion. In other patients, hypotonic intravenous solutions (D₅W, half-normal saline, or quarter-normal saline) should be administered to correct hypernatremia. The water content of these fluids varies according to the electrolyte concentration. For example, 1 L of D₅W essentially equals 1 L of free water because glucose is eventually metabolized. However, 1 L of half-normal saline or quarter-normal saline contains 500 or 750 mL, respectively, of free water. In addition, if other solutes, such as potassium or magnesium, are added to the intravenous fluids, their contribution to the tonicity of the administered fluid should be taken into account. Administration of solutions that are hypotonic relative to the urine corrects hypernatremia.

The serum sodium concentration can be used as a guide to the replacement of free water by the following formula:

$$\text{Water deficit} = 0.6 \times \text{body weight (kg)} \times (1 - [140 / Na^+])$$

where Na^+ = plasma sodium, and body weight (kg) = estimated body weight when hydrated.

The treatment of patients with central diabetes insipidus is discussed in Chapter 65.

As is the case in patients with hyponatremia, the rate of correction of hypernatremia is important. In chronic hypernatremia (>36 to 48 hours), the brain generates compounds that raise the intracellular osmolality and thereby minimize cell shrinkage. This process is metabolically driven and is slow to return to normal. Thus, rapid correction of plasma osmolality may lead to a shift of water to the relatively hypertonic intracellular compartment and may result in brain edema. As a general rule, hypernatremia should be corrected over 48 hours at a rate not exceeding 0.5 mEq/L per hour, or 12 mEq/L per day.

Disturbances in Potassium Balance

The human body contains about 3500 mEq of potassium. With a normal concentration of 3.5 to 5 mEq/L, the ECF contains about 70 mEq of potassium, or only 2% of total-body stores. In response to a dietary potassium load, rapid removal of potassium from the extracellular space is necessary to prevent life-threatening hyperkalemia. For example, in the absence of a homeostatic mechanism, if a person ingests 50 mEq of dietary potassium in a single meal (the average daily American diet contains 100 to 120 mEq of potassium per day), the serum potassium might rise to 7 mEq/L (assuming an extracellular volume of 14 L with a baseline serum potassium of 4 mEq/L). Thus, the initial adaptation to a potassium load is the rapid redistribution of potassium from the extracellular space to the intracellular space. Various hormones, including insulin, aldosterone, and catecholamines, cause movement of potassium into cells. The acid-base status of the patient is another determinant of the serum potassium concentration because potassium moves across cell membranes driven by pH gradients between the cell and the ECF compartments. The greatest effect on the serum potassium concentration is associated with metabolic acidosis involving mineral acids. The cellular permeability to the anions of the mineral acids is low; consequently, the basolateral membrane is hyperpolarized, provoking potassium movement into the blood. By contrast, metabolic acidosis caused by organic acids, such as lactic acid and keto acids, does not cause hyperkalemia. The anions of these acids are relatively permeable and accompany hydrogen into the cell. This situation diminishes the electrochemical gradient favoring potassium efflux.

Although these mechanisms affect the distribution of potassium between the fluid compartments, other mechanisms are necessary to maintain overall potassium balance. People ingest about 100 mEq of potassium daily, the bulk of which is eliminated by the kidneys. Increased potassium excretion results from enhanced distal nephron potassium secretion by the principal cells of the connecting tubule and collecting duct into the tubular lumen down an electrochemical gradient. Factors that enhance this gradient promote potassium secretion. These factors include the rate of distal tubular flow, the distal delivery of sodium, the presence of poorly reabsorbable anions in the tubular fluid, and stimulation by aldosterone.

The ratio of extracellular to intracellular potassium establishes the resting membrane potential of the cell. Hence hyperkalemia or hypokalemia is associated with alteration of the resting membrane potential, which accounts for most of the symptoms and findings in these disorders.

DIAGNOSTIC APPROACH

A careful history with emphasis on the patient's diet and use of medications and laxatives should be obtained. Spurious hyperkalemia and hypokalemia must be excluded. In addition to serum electrolytes and magnesium, urine electrolytes and urine osmolality should be obtained. The next step should be to determine whether abnormal renal potassium handling is involved in the genesis of the disorder. This state may be determined by measuring the 24-hour urine potassium excretion. In extrarenal hyperkalemia, renal potassium excretion should be more than 200 mEq/day, and if hypokalemia is caused by extrarenal losses, the renal potassium excretion should be less than 20 mEq/day.

HYPERKALEMIA

The ratio of intracellular to extracellular potassium concentration is the major determinant of the resting potential of the cell membrane. As the extracellular potassium concentration increases, the cell membrane is partially depolarized, the sodium permeability is diminished, and the ability to generate action potentials is decreased. In muscle tissue, this change accounts for muscle weakness and paralysis. In the heart, hyperkalemia exhibits as changes in the electrocardiogram. These changes include peaked T waves, decreased amplitude or the absence of P waves, wide QRS complexes, sinus bradycardia, and conduction defects.

A pathophysiologic approach to the causes of hyperkalemia is outlined in Figure 28-6. Vigorous phlebotomy techniques can result in lysis of red blood cells, a process that releases intracellular potassium into the serum sample. Thrombocytosis ($>1 \times 10^6/\mu L$) and leukocytosis ($>60,000/\mu L$) may also be associated with *spurious hyperkalemia*. These disorders can be diagnosed rapidly by determining the plasma and serum concentrations of potassium. True hyperkalemia is present if these values differ by less than or equal to 0.2 mEq/L.

Chronic renal insufficiency does not cause hyperkalemia unless it is advanced, with a GFR ranging from less than 10 to 15 mL per minute. Thus, hyperkalemia in chronic renal insufficiency is usually caused by a distal nephron defect in potassium secretion rather than by the impaired GFR, as

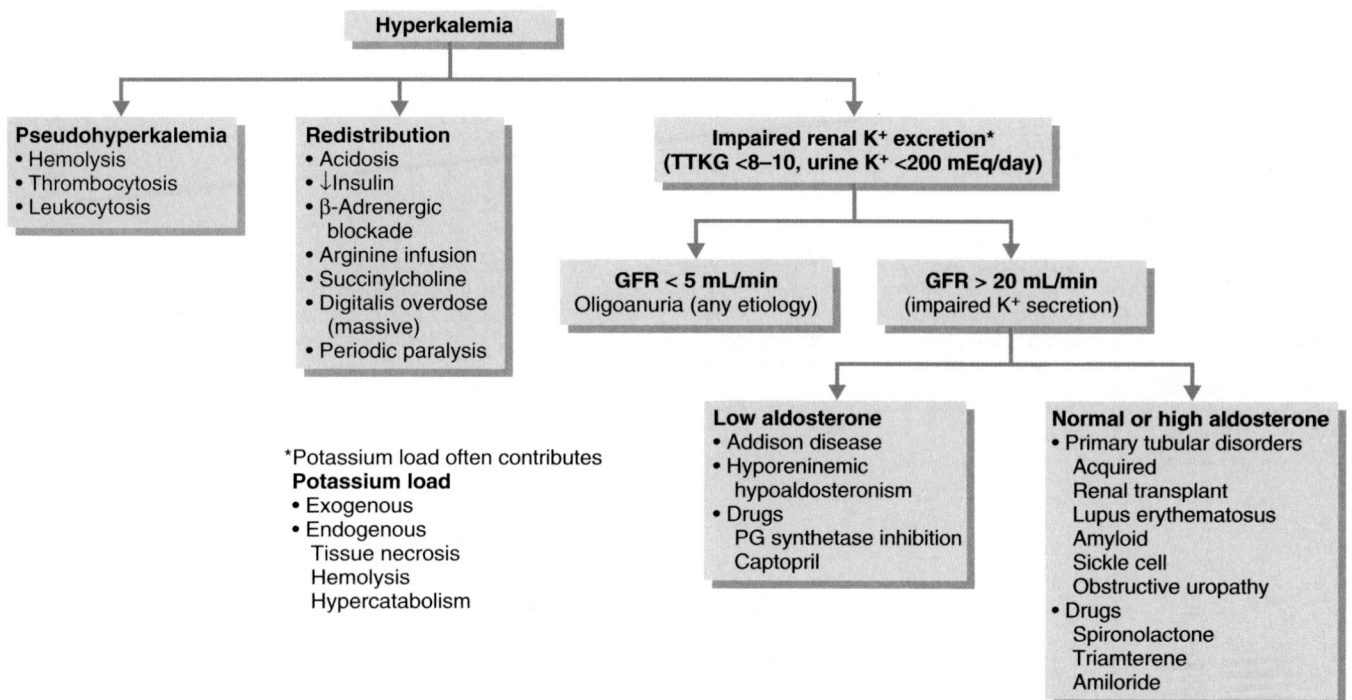

Figure 28-6 Diagnostic approach to hyperkalemia. GFR, glomerular filtration rate; PG, prostaglandin; TTKG, transtubular potassium gradient.

shown in Figure 28-6. Failure to increase plasma aldosterone by the administration of corticotropin or furosemide confirms the diagnosis of *hyporeninemic hypoaldosteronism.* Prostaglandin deficiency may play a role in the pathogenesis of this disorder. Determination of the urine potassium in response to a single dose of an oral mineralocorticoid (such as 9α-fludrocortisone) may help differentiate hypoaldosteronism from aldosterone resistance. In aldosterone resistance, no increase in urine potassium excretion occurs in response to the mineralocorticoid.

Treatment of hyperkalemia depends on the urgency of clinical findings. When electrocardiogram changes consistent with hyperkalemia are present, the most rapid method of reversing the effects of hyperkalemia is to reestablish the normal membrane potential. Calcium antagonizes the membrane effects of hyperkalemia and can provide rapid protection of the cardiac conduction system. This protection, however, is short lived and must be accompanied by other therapies to decrease the extracellular potassium concentration. The distribution of potassium into the intracellular compartment by administration of sodium bicarbonate, β_2-adrenergic agonists, or insulin rapidly decreases the serum concentration of potassium. The ultimate goal of the treatment is the net removal of potassium from the body. Exchange resins, such as sodium polystyrene sulfonate, can enhance potassium excretion from the gastrointestinal tract. Attempts can be made to enhance renal excretion by improving the distal delivery of sodium with sodium bicarbonate and administration of loop diuretics. Finally, dialysis can be used to remove excess extracellular potassium. For long-term management of patients with an aldosterone deficiency, an oral preparation of a mineralocorticoid can be used. Discontinuing any offending drug that may contribute to the patient's hyperkalemia is mandatory.

HYPOKALEMIA

Because potassium is the most abundant intracellular cation, its deficiency results in a wide variety of defects. For example, rhabdomyolysis and adynamic ileus have been associated with hypokalemia. Chronic hypokalemia stimulates thirst and may cause nephrogenic diabetes insipidus. However, the most prominent abnormalities relate to the cardiovascular system. Typically, hypokalemia is associated with flattening of the T waves and development of U waves. The most urgent abnormality is an association with arrhythmias, particularly in patients receiving digitalis. Hypokalemia, through stimulation of renal ammonia synthesis, may worsen hepatic encephalopathy in patients with hepatic cirrhosis.

A diagnostic approach to hypokalemia is outlined in Figure 28-7. As in hyperkalemia, spurious hypokalemia can also occur with leukocytosis (>60,000 cells/µL), resulting from active uptake of potassium by white blood cells from the serum. True hypokalemia is caused by redistribution, extrarenal potassium loss, poor intake, or renal potassium losses. Because only 2% of total-body potassium is distributed in the extracellular compartment, serum potassium measurements may not accurately reflect the total-body stores. In fact, hypokalemia can occur in the presence of normal total-body potassium stores. This state occurs when potassium shifts from the extracellular space to the intracellular space. Excess circulating catecholamines, insulin administration, and alkalosis are the major causes of redistribution of potassium from the extracellular space to the intracellular space. Redistribution hypokalemia is particularly important in the clinical setting of myocardial infarction and exacerbation of chronic obstructive pulmonary disease. These patients are especially prone to arrhythmias because excess catecholamines (in response to stress or

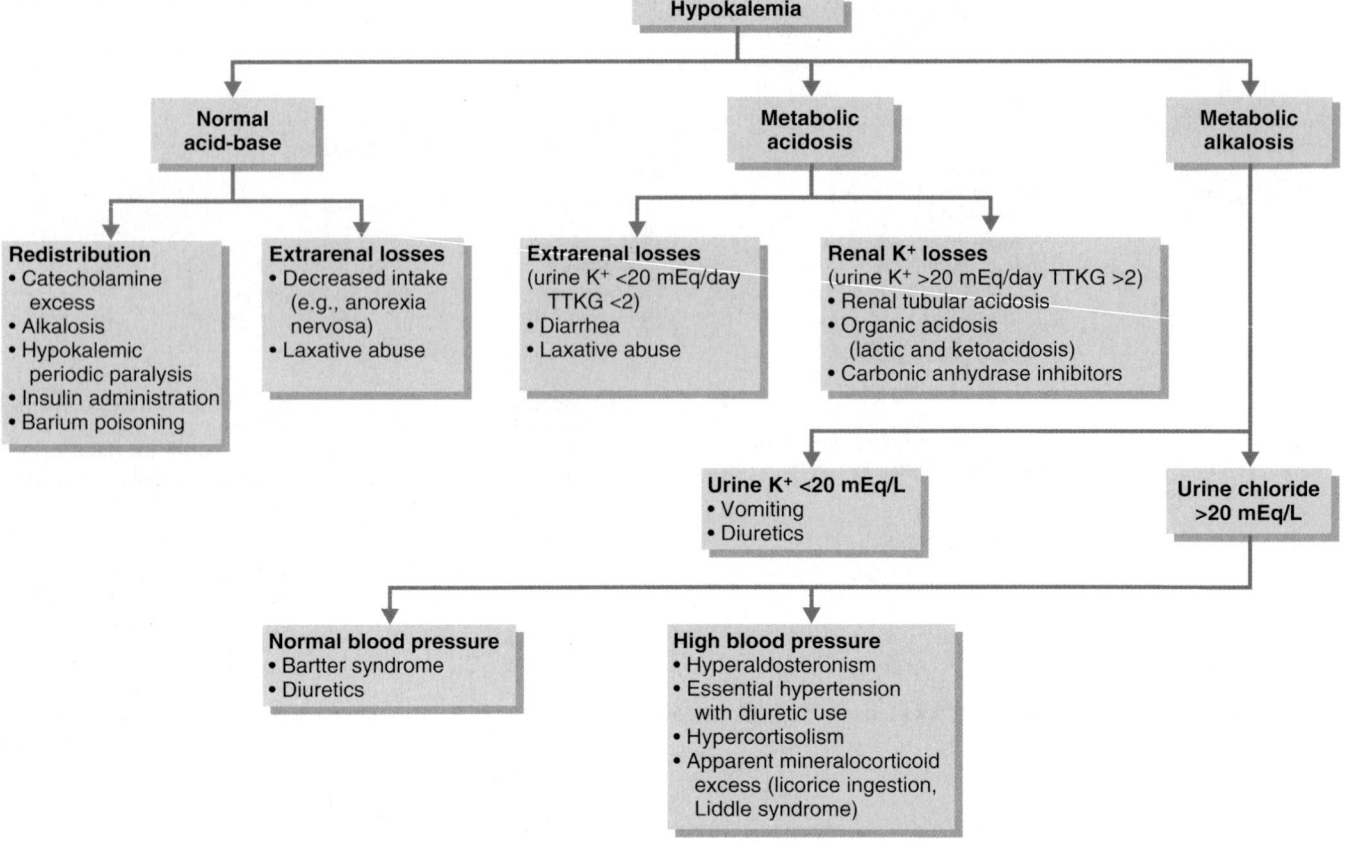

Figure 28-7 Diagnostic approach to hypokalemia. TTKG, transtubular potassium gradient.

inhaled β₂ agonists) cause potassium shifts in the setting of total-body potassium depletion from frequent diuretic usage.

In patients with hypokalemia, the acid-base status, the presence or absence of hypertension, and measurement of urinary chloride and potassium are helpful in narrowing the diagnostic possibilities. In patients with diuretic abuse (usually patients with eating disorders), the urine sodium and chloride concentrations are high in the presence of metabolic alkalosis, a profile similar to that of *Bartter syndrome,* which is a rare genetic defect usually seen in adolescents with other neurologic abnormalities and caused by reduced activity of the sodium, potassium, and chloride (NKCC2) co-transporters in the thick ascending limb (see later). In this setting, a urine screen for diuretics may be necessary to make the diagnosis. In comparison, patients with surreptitious vomiting have a low urinary chloride concentration. Patients who abuse laxatives have low urine sodium and chloride concentrations, with metabolic acidosis or normal acid-base status. Glycyrrhizic acid, the active ingredient in licorice, blocks 11β-dehydrogenase, an enzyme that inactivates glucocorticoids, and its inhibition results in unregulated activation of the mineralocorticoid receptors in the distal nephron.

Determination of serum magnesium should always be performed in a patient with hypokalemia. Hypokalemia that is associated with hypomagnesemia is resistant to therapy unless concomitant magnesium deficiency is corrected.

Given the factors that determine transmembrane potassium shifts, the net potassium deficit may be difficult to calculate. An estimate for a 70-kg man based on the serum concentration is a 100- to 200-mEq deficit in total-body potassium when the serum concentration decreases from 4 to 3 mEq/L. At less than 3 mEq/L, every 1-mEq/L decrease in the serum concentration of potassium reflects an additional 200- to 400-mEq deficit in total-body potassium. Hypokalemia should be treated with oral potassium supplementation. Intravenous potassium administration should only be used in urgent situations, such as in patients with arrhythmias or digitalis toxicity, and intolerance to oral formulations in patients with adynamic ileus. The rate of intravenous potassium administration generally should not exceed 10 mEq per hour; only under electrocardiographic monitoring, the potassium administration rate can be increased up to 20 mEq per hour. Hypokalemia associated with long-term diuretic therapy may be treated with the addition of a potassium-sparing diuretic.

Bartter and Gitelman Syndromes

A major advance in the study of inherited disorders of salt-wasting syndromes has been the demonstration that Bartter and Gitelman syndromes result from mutation of specific ion transport proteins expressed by cells of the distal nephron. The dysfunction of the thiazide-sensitive sodium-chloride co-transporter (NCCT) in Gitelman syndrome, and the bumetanide-sensitive sodium-potassium-chloride

Table 28-6 **Various Bartter Syndromes**

	Type 1	Type 2	Type 3	Type 4	Type 5
Gene name	*SLC12A1*	*KCNJ1*	*CLCNKB*	*BSND*	*CASR*
Protein name	NKCC2	ROMK	CLCNKB	Barttin	CaR
Major symptoms	Polyuria, hypocalcemia	As for type 1	Variable	As for type 1	—
Seizures	Dehydration	—	Mild to severe	+ Deafness	—
Urine Ca^{2+}	↑	↑	↑	↑	↑
Urine Mg^{2+}	↓	↓	↓	↓	↓
Nephrocalcinosis	+++	+++	±	−	+++

Ca^{2+}, calcium; Mg^{2+}, magnesium.

Table 28-7 **Known Pathophysiology of Gitelman Syndrome**

Loss of functional mutation: NCCT
NaCl wasting
Secondary hyperaldosteronism: K wasting
Cellular hyperpolarization secondary decreased Cl⁻ entry
↑ Apical ECaC entry
↑ Basolateral Na/Ca exchange
Net effect: hypocalciuria
Mg wasting: uncertain mechanism

(NKCC2) co-transporter in Bartter syndrome cause salt wasting, extracellular volume depletion, secondary hyperaldosteronism, and hypokalemia.

The various characteristics of the five different Bartter syndromes and the Gitelman syndromes are shown in Tables 28-6 and 28-7. Stated briefly, Bartter syndrome is a genetically heterogeneous disease. Based on molecular genetic studies, five different subtypes of Bartter syndromes can be distinguished. Type I, or neonatal Bartter syndrome, is caused by loss of function mutations in the sodium-potassium-chloride co-transporter NKCC2. NKCC2 is encoded by the *SCL12A1* gene on chromosome 15. This sodium-potassium-chloride co-transporter is expressed in the apical cell membranes of the thick ascending limb of the loop of Henle (TAL), and normally accounts for about 30% of total reabsorption of sodium filtered by the glomerulus. Patients with this syndrome present early in life with a severe systemic disorder characterized by marked sodium and potassium wasting, polyhydramnios, and significant hypercalciuria and nephrocalcinosis. Prostaglandin synthesis and excretion are significantly increased and may account for much of the systemic symptoms.

Bartter syndrome type II is due to loss of function mutation of the *KCNJ1* gene on chromosome 11, encoding the inward rectifier voltage-dependent potassium channel ROMK. The potassium channel ROMK is localized in the apical membrane of TAL but is also expressed in the cortical collecting duct. In the TAL, the potassium flow through this channel into the renal tubule is necessary for NKCC2 activity, which needs adequate luminal potassium supply. In the cortical collecting duct, this channel is also involved in the excretion of dietary potassium. In this syndrome, an aberrant ROMK channel leads to malfunction of the NKCC2 co-transporter and results in salt wasting, high tubular flow, and distal potassium wasting. Bartter syndrome type III is

caused by loss of function mutations of the *CLCNKB* gene on chromosome 1 encoding a chloride channel protein CLC-Kb. This protein is expressed in the basolateral cell membranes of the TAL and is responsible for the reabsorption of sodium chloride in the TAL.

The renal salt wasting in Bartter type III syndrome is less severe than types I and II. Recently, Bartter syndrome type IV was found to be caused by loss of function mutation of the *BSND* gene (Bartter syndrome and sensorineural deafness) on chromosome 1p31. The *BSND* gene encodes barttin, a protein expressed in the basolateral membrane of the TAL. Barttin is the β subunit of the ClC-Kb chloride channel; it is necessary for ClCKb delivery to the plasma membrane; and in the cochlea, it co-localizes with chloride channels ClCKa and ClCKb. These patients present also with sodium, potassium wasting, and impaired cochlear function and deafness. Recently, the presence of hypokalemic alkalosis due to Bartter syndrome type V was found in patients with autosomal dominant hypocalcemia. In this disease, hypocalcemia was related to gain of function mutation of the calcium-sensing receptor (CaSR). The CaSR is heavily expressed at the basolateral membrane of the TAL, where it is thought to play an important inhibitory role in regulating the transcellular transport of sodium, chloride, and calcium. Activation of the basolateral CaSR in the TAL reduces apical K^+ channel activity, which induces a Bartter-like syndrome. Genetic activation of the CaSR by these mutations is also expected to increase urinary calcium excretion by inhibiting the generation of the lumen positive potential difference that drives paracellular calcium transport in the TAL.

To date, Gitelman syndrome appears to be molecularly homogeneous. Although a loss of function mutation of the *SLC12A3* gene in chromosome 16q13 has been identified as one of the causes, recent genetic characterization of Gordon syndrome, a disease with clinical features opposite to Gitelman syndrome, suggests the possibility that similar mirror-image mutations and possibly more than one, might account for Gitelman syndrome. The *SLC12A3* gene encodes the renal thiazide-sensitive sodium-chloride co-transporter NCCT. NCCT is responsible for the sodium reabsorption in the distal tubule, which accounts for about 7% of the total filtered sodium. Although Gitelman syndrome is a milder disorder than Bartter syndrome, patients do report significant morbidity related to muscular symptoms, fatigue, and increased risk for cardiac arrhythmias in patients having a prolonged QT interval. Although plasma renin activity is increased, renal prostaglandin excretion is not elevated, another feature that distinguishes Gitelman syndrome from Bartter syndrome.

A major phenotypic difference between Bartter and Gitelman syndromes involves urinary calcium excretion. The hypercalciuria of Bartter syndrome is believed to result largely from dysfunction of thick ascending limb cells. Calcium absorption, which is passive and paracellular, is driven by lumen-positive transepithelial voltage that is generated by NKCC2 co-transport and luminal K^+ recycling. When NKCC2 co-transport is reduced or blocked by loop diuretics or genetic abnormality, the lumen positivity declines, and calcium reabsorption declines. What is not entirely clear is why the loss of luminal positivity does not lead to increased magnesium excretion. In addition to this mechanism, increased distal delivery of NaCl, as a result of dysfunction of the TAL raises intracellular chloride concentration, which in turns inhibits apical calcium channel of distal convoluted tubule (DCT) cells, further contributing to calcium retention and nephrolithiasis. In contrast to patients with Bartter syndrome, patients with Gitelman syndrome invariably demonstrate hypocalciuria.

The hypocalciuria of Gitelman syndrome resembles the clinical beneficial effects of DCT diuretics (thiazides and others) to reduce urinary calcium excretion. The mechanisms of hypocalciuria in Gitelman syndrome are well established. First, mild contraction of the ECF volume increases calcium reabsorption along the proximal tubule. Second, reduction in NaCl entry to DCT cells stimulates transepithelial calcium transport. When apical Na and Cl entry into DCT cells is inhibited, because of either diuretic treatment or genetic disease, the intracellular chloride concentration declines. Lower intracellular Cl activity hyperpolarizes the cell and activates calcium entry through the distinctive apical calcium channels ECaC and CaT2, expressed in the DCT cells. Because calcium movement from lumen to cell must be balanced, the increased calcium entry to DCT cells stimulates calcium efflux through the basolateral Na^+/Ca^+ exchanger and the Ca-ATPase. Therefore, the resultant effect is the development of hypocalciuria.

Although the pathogenesis of calcium disorders in Bartter and Gitelman syndromes is relatively clear, only recently has the pathogenesis of magnesium disorders associated with these syndromes been clarified. Gitelman syndrome is associated with severe hypomagnesemia, whereas Bartter syndrome is not. Recent observations in genetic disorders of hypomagnesemia, as well as clinical observations in patients undergoing chemotherapy with anti–epidermal growth factor (EGF) antibodies have helped to clarify the molecular mechanisms involved in magnesium transport. Magnesium is absorbed along the entire nephron, but the predominant site for reabsorption is along the distal tubule. In the medullary and cortical TAL, magnesium, along with calcium, is reabsorbed through a charge-selective paracellular path. Mutations in claudin-16 (also called paracellin) and claudin-19 cause severe hypomagnesemia and nephrocalcinosis. In the DCT, a specific channel, the transient receptor potential melastatin, subfamily 6 channel, TRPM6, mediates magnesium reabsorption. Mutations in the *EGF* gene, which is expressed in the distal tubule, cause hypomagnesemia, and anti-EGF antibodies induce hypomagnesemia. The latter observations suggest a regulatory role of EGF in the reabsorption of magnesium. Knockout of the thiazide-sensitive sodium chloride co-transporter and inhibition of this transporter with thiazides cause hypomagnesemia and reduce

TRPM6 expression. Thus, reduced expression of the TRPM6 channel is the most likely explanation of the hypomagnesemia seen in Gitelman syndrome.

Disturbances in Acid-Base Balance

Most metabolic processes occurring in the body result in the production of acid. The largest source of endogenous acid production is from the complete catabolism and oxidation of glucose and fatty acids ultimately to carbon dioxide and water. Pulmonary ventilation excretes the volatile acid produced by such cellular respiration, about 22,000 mEq of hydrogen daily, as carbon dioxide. Cellular metabolism of sulfur-containing amino acids, the oxidation of phosphoproteins and phospholipids, nucleoprotein degradation, and the incomplete combustion of carbohydrates and fatty acids result in the formation of nonvolatile acids. These processes produce about 1 mEq/kg body weight of hydrogen daily. Nonvolatile acid excretion is effected through the kidney. The primary factors regulating alteration in the rate of minute ventilation are changes in cerebrospinal fluid and arterial blood pH.

The normal concentration of hydrogen in arterial blood is 40 mEq/L, equal to a pH of 7.40. This concentration is maintained relatively constant despite variations in the endogenous and exogenous acid inputs. Circulating and intracellular buffers acutely neutralize an acid load. The capacity of these buffering systems is limited, however, and would be quickly depleted by normal endogenous acid production. Mechanisms for excreting acid must therefore be effective to regenerate these buffers to maintain acid-base homeostasis.

RENAL HYDROGEN ION EXCRETION

The kidney contributes to acid-base homeostasis by the reclamation of 4500mEq of bicarbonate filtered at the glomerulus daily and by the generation of new bicarbonate. This renal bicarbonate generation is given by the equation for net acid excretion (NAE):

$$E_{NAE} = ENH_4^+ + E_{TA} - EHCO_3^-$$

where $ENH_4^+ + E_{TA}$ is the rate of ammonium and titratable acid excretion, respectively, and $EHCO_3^{-1}$ is the rate of bicarbonate excretion. Although not difficult, measurement of NAE is not routinely done, and thus analysis of acid-base disorders has relied on indirect but more readily available measurements.

The principal process of renal bicarbonate generation is accomplished by urinary acidification and ammonia generation. Ammonia is generated from glutamine and secreted into the tubule fluid by the proximal tubule epithelium. Acidification is accomplished by proton secretion by distinct transporters uniquely distributed along the nephron. These transporters were highlighted in Chapter 26, and this chapter discusses how they modify the tubular fluid pH. The acidification profile of tubular fluid is shown in Figure 28-8. Tubule fluid pH falls slightly along the proximal tubule by

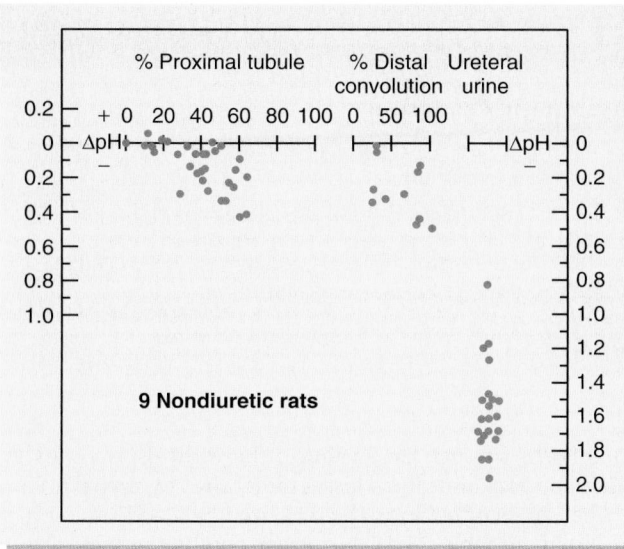

Figure 28-8 pH changes along the rat nephron.

Table 28-8 Systemic Approach to the Analysis of Acid-Base Disorders

Assess the accuracy of the acid-base parameters using the Henderson equation ($H^+ = 24 \times [Paco_2/HCO_3^-]$) or the Henderson-Hasselbalch equation ($pH = 6.1 + log[HCO_3^-/0.03] \times Paco_2$).

Obtain a good history and perform a complete physical examination, looking for clues to a particular acid-base disturbance.

Calculate the serum anion gap: $Na^+ - (HCO_3^- + Cl^-)$.

Identify the primary acid-base disturbance and assess whether a simple or mixed acid-base disturbance is present.

Examine serum electrolytes and ancillary laboratory data.

Measure urine pH and urine electrolytes, urine urea nitrogen, and glucose to calculate the urine anion gap ($Na^+ + K^+ - Cl^-$) or urine osmolal gap (measured osmolality − [2($Na^+ + K^+$) + [urea nitrogen/2.8] + [glucose/18]).*

*Measurement of urine Na^+ and Cl^- and urine pH should be obtained when metabolic alkalosis is present. Measurement of urine electrolytes, urine glucose, and urine pH should be obtained when an element of normal anion gap metabolic acidosis is present.

the operation of the sodium-hydrogen exchanger type 3 (NHE3) located at the luminal membrane. This proton secretion is linked to bicarbonate reabsorption, and nearly 90% of the filtered load of bicarbonate is reabsorbed from the tubule fluid during its course along the proximal tubule. The proximal tubule is a high-capacity bicarbonate reabsorption system whose rate results from the presence of carbonic anhydrase in the luminal membrane. Carbonic anhydrase in the luminal membrane rapidly catalyzes the dehydration of carbonic acid to carbon dioxide and water and thus restricts the fall in tubule fluid pH along the proximal tubule and prevents the development of too steep a pH gradient into which sodium-hydrogen exchange takes place. The distal tubule, on the other hand, lacks a luminal carbonic anhydrase and has a limited capacity to reabsorb bicarbonate. However, given that the bicarbonate concentration reaching these sites is low and the principal buffers in the tubule fluid along these sites are ammonia and phosphate ions, the continued operation of the distal proton pumps lowers the prevailing urinary pH to sometimes 1000-fold below the pH of the initial filtrate. Along these sites, however, the full operation of the kidney in acid-base homeostasis is observed as the urinary buffers are titrated by secreted protons from pumps distributed along the distal nephron and excreted into the urine.

The rate of bicarbonate generation is not fixed and responds to changes in volume and electrolyte status, hormones, and acid-base parameters. Proximal bicarbonate reabsorption is increased during volume depletion, by elevation in the partial pressure of carbon dioxide (Pco_2), as seen in chronic respiratory acidosis, and by hypokalemia. Conversely, volume expansion or the reduction of the Pco_2 lowers the proximal tubular reabsorptive rate for bicarbonate. Aldosterone and ambient Pco_2 affect the rate of distal nephron hydrogen ion secretion.

ASSESSMENT OF ACID-BASE STATUS

A systematic approach to assessing acid-base status consists of several steps, as summarized in Table 28-8. The initial step

is to obtain arterial and venous blood samples to measure blood pH and Pco_2, as well as serum electrolytes to determine the nature of the acid-base disturbance. Validation of the internal consistency of the calculated and measured bicarbonate should be carried out. Based on the pH, Pco_2, and serum bicarbonate, a minimum diagnosis should be established. Next, a measurement of the compensatory response and the anion gap should be performed. If the compensation of a primary acid-base defect is inappropriate, then a mixed acid-base disorder is considered (Table 28-9). The anion gap is useful in the diagnostic approach to metabolic acidosis. When an organic acid, such as lactic acid, is added to the ECF compartment, the bicarbonate concentration falls as the acid is buffered. The anion gap increases as the organic base is accumulated. Quantitatively, the increase in anion gap should be equivalent to the decrease in bicarbonate concentration. Thus, by adding the difference between the calculated and normal anion gap to the prevailing bicarbonate concentration, an estimate of the *starting* bicarbonate concentration can be made. An abnormally elevated initial bicarbonate concentration indicates concomitant metabolic alkalosis. After establishing the nature of the acid-base disorder and whether it is complex or simple, examination of the urine pH and urine anion or osmolal gap can also provide useful information.

METABOLIC ACIDOSIS

Metabolic acidosis is characterized by a decrease in the serum bicarbonate concentration. This decrease occurs either by excretion of bicarbonate-containing fluids or by utilization of bicarbonate as a buffer of acids. In the latter instance, the nature of the base may affect the electrolyte composition. Thus, considering metabolic acidosis by means of the anion gap is convenient (Table 28-10).

Metabolic acidoses with a normal anion gap is most commonly caused by extrarenal losses of bicarbonate, as occurs in diarrheal diseases, but may also be caused by abnormally high renal excretion of bicarbonate and by the addition of

Table 28-9 Nature of Adaptive Response to Primary Acid-Base Disorders

Primary Acid-Base Disturbance	Initiating Mechanism	Secondary Physiologic Response
Metabolic acidosis	$\downarrow$ plasma HCO_3^-	$\downarrow$ $Paco_2$ of 1.0-1.3 mm Hg for each 1 mEq/L fall in plasma HCO_3^- $Paco_2 = (1.5 \times HCO_3^-) + 8 + 2$
Metabolic alkalosis	$\uparrow$ Plasma HCO_3^-	$\uparrow$ $Paco_2$ of 0.4 to 0.7 mm Hg for each 1 mEq/L rise in plasma HCO_3^-
Respiratory acidosis	$\uparrow$ $Paco_2$	*Acute:* $\uparrow$ plasma HCO_3^- of 1 mEq/L for every 10-mm Hg rise in $Paco_2$ *Chronic:* $\uparrow$ plasma HCO_3^- of 3.5 mEq/L for every 100-mm Hg fall in $Paco_2$
Respiratory alkalosis	$\downarrow$ $Paco_2$	*Acute:* $\downarrow$ plasma HCO_3^- of 2 mEq/L for every 10-mm Hg fall in $Paco_2$ *Chronic:* $\downarrow$ plasma HCO_3^- of 4-5 mEq/L for every 10-mm Hg fall in $Paco_2$

Note: Rare cases with $Paco_2$ values greater than 55 mm Hg have been reported.

Table 28-10 Causes of Metabolic Acidosis

Normal Anion Gap

Bicarbonate losses
Extrarenal
Small bowel drainage
Diarrhea
Renal
Proximal renal tubular acidosis
Carbonic anhydrase inhibitors
Primary hyperparathyroidism
Failure of bicarbonate regeneration
Distal renal tubular acidosis
Aldosterone deficiency
Addison disease
Hyporeninemic hypoaldosteronism
Aldosterone insensitivity
Interstitial renal disease
Aldosterone antagonists
Ureteroileostomy (ileal bladder)
Acidifying salts
Ammonium chloride
Lysine or arginine hydrochloride
Diabetes mellitus (recovery phase)

Wide Anion Gap

Reduced excretion of acids
Renal failure
Overproduction of acids
Ketoacidosis
Diabetic
Alcoholic
Starvation
Lactic acidosis
Toxin ingestion
Methanol
Ethylene glycol
Salicylates

Modified from Andreoli TE: Disorders of fluid volume, electrolyte, and acid-base balance. In Wyngaarden JB, Smith LH Jr, Bennett JC (eds): Cecil Textbook of Medicine, 19th ed. Philadelphia: WB Saunders, 1992, p 523.

substances yielding hydrochloric acid, as when arginine hydrochloride is administered.

The urinary anion gap is defined as follows:

$$\text{Urinary anion gap} = (\text{sodium} + \text{potassium}) - \text{chloride}$$

The equation provides an approximate index of urinary ammonium excretion, as measured by a negative urinary anion gap. Thus, a normal renal response would be a negative urinary anion gap, generally in the range of 30 to 50 mEq/L. In such an instance, the acidosis is probably caused by gastrointestinal losses rather than by a renal lesion.

The causes of acidosis characterized by a wide anion gap are listed in Table 28-10. In severe *renal failure,* inorganic compounds such as phosphates and sulfates are the major contributors to the increased anion gap. Organic compounds also accumulate in patients with severe renal failure. *Ketoacidosis* results from accelerated lipolysis and ketogenesis caused by relative or absolute insulin deficiency. Alcoholic ketoacidosis and starvation ketoacidosis result from the suppression of endogenous insulin secretion caused by inadequate carbohydrate ingestion. In addition, in alcoholic ketoacidosis, insulin resistance contributes to ketone formation. The syndrome of *lactic acidosis* results from impaired cellular respiration. Lactate is produced from the reduction of pyruvate in muscle, red blood cells, and other tissues as a consequence of anaerobic glycolysis. In situations of diminished oxidative metabolism, excess lactic acid is produced. This anaerobic state also favors a shift of keto acids to the reduced form, β-hydroxybutyrate. The nitroprusside reaction, which is catalyzed by the keto acids acetoacetate and acetone, is thus nonreactive in the setting of lactic acidosis. Lactic acidosis occurs most commonly in disorders characterized by inadequate oxygen delivery to tissues, such as shock, septicemia, and profound hypoxemia. Certain toxins may also sufficiently alter mitochondrial function and establish an effective anaerobic state. Some of these toxins may undergo metabolism into organic acids that can contribute to the generation of acidosis characterized by a large anion gap. Methanol is metabolized by alcohol dehydrogenase to formic acid. Ethylene glycol is metabolized to glycolic and oxalic acids. Salicylates are themselves acidic compounds and can cause acidosis characterized by a wide anion gap.

The treatment of metabolic acidosis depends on the underlying cause and the severity of the manifestations. The rapid administration of parenteral sodium bicarbonate is generally indicated when the pH is less than 7.1 and hemodynamic instability is evident. Oral bicarbonate supplementation may be sufficient if the acidosis is caused by gastrointestinal bicarbonate loss or renal tubular acidosis (RTA). Treatment of organic acidosis should be directed at the underlying disorder. If the generation of the organic acid can be interrupted, the organic base pair may be metabolized, effectively regenerating bicarbonate. The acidemia of diabetic ketoacidosis, for example, can be effectively treated by administration of insulin, thereby inhibiting further ketogenesis. In lactic acidosis, therapy should be directed toward improving tissue perfusion. In alcoholic and starvation ketoacidosis, administration of dextrose-containing intravenous fluids corrects the acidosis.

RENAL TUBULAR ACIDOSIS SYNDROMES

Currently, three major RTA syndromes have been identified. These syndromes are discussed later, and their principal characteristics are described in Table 28-11.

Proximal Renal Tubular Acidosis Syndromes

Proximal RTA occurs either alone or as the full Fanconi syndrome, with glycosuria, aminoaciduria, and phosphaturia. In proximal RTA, the threshold is reduced from 25 mmol/L to about 18 to 20 mmol/L (Fig. 28-9). Thus, a single-pulse loss of bicarbonate of about 850 to 900 mEq takes place.

Proximal RTA occurs in a significant number of systemic diseases, most notably Wilson disease, cystinosis, and the gammopathies, especially light-chain disease; it is also seen in renal transplantation. Several molecular defects have been identified that also cause proximal RTA:

- Mutations in the carbonic anhydrase II gene, which reduce its expression. It is transmitted as an autosomal-recessive syndrome characterized by osteopetrosis, cerebral calcification, and mental retardation.
- Mutations in the *SCLC4A4b* gene that codes for the basolateral membrane sodium-bicarbonate transporter. This lesion is also an autosomal-recessive disease characterized by glaucoma, cataracts, band keratopathy, and psychomotor retardation.
- Mutations in the *SLC9A3* gene, which encodes the luminal NHE3 transport protein.
  Generalized Fanconi syndrome, which appears to be the consequence of a deficit in adenosine triphosphate (ATP) production in the proximal tubule, which reduces the activity of the basolateral sodium-potassium adenosine triphosphatase (Na^+,K^+-ATPase). This reduction is seen in severe phosphate depletion as well as in hereditary fructose intolerance.

The focus of treatment is to enhance proximal bicarbonate reabsorption by reducing ECF volume. This reduction is achieved most commonly by salt restriction. An attempt to raise serum bicarbonate by oral bicarbonate therapy is counterproductive because it raises extracellular volume, enhances bicarbonaturia, provokes kaliuresis and phosphaturia, and produces hypokalemia and hypophosphatemia. Supplemental potassium to correct the hypokalemia is often necessary.

Type	Locus	Defect
Proximal	S_1-S_3	↓HCO_3^- threshold
Hyperkalemic	CCD principal cell	↓V_M (−) leading to ↓H^+ secretion
Gradient limited	OMCD intercalated cells	Three specific defects in H^+ secretion

Table 28-11 Renal Tubular Acidosis Syndromes

CCD, cortical collecting duct; OMCD, outer medullary collecting duct; S, segment; V_M (−), negative transepithelial voltage in the OMCD.

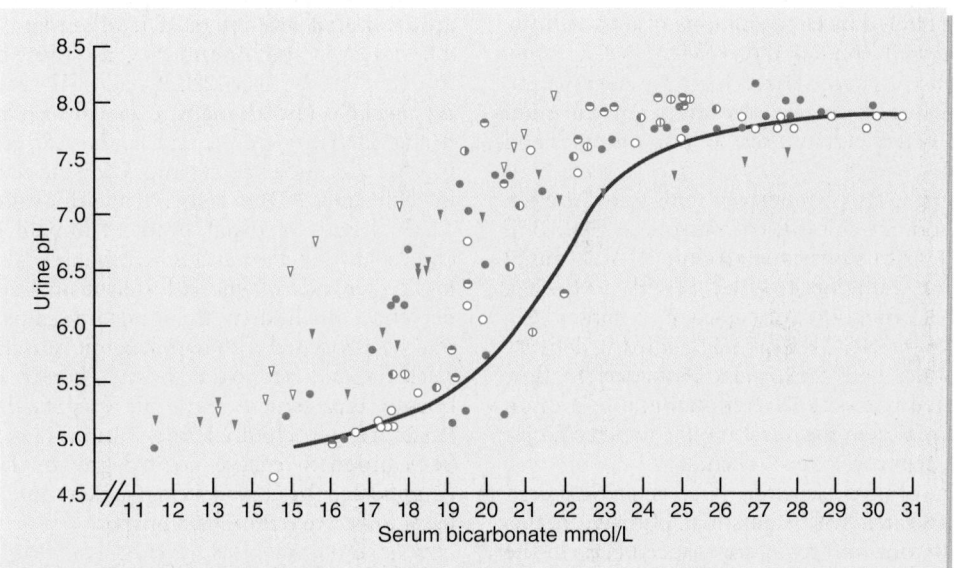

Figure 28-9 Bicarbonate titration curve in proximal renal tubular acidosis (RTA). Normal bicarbonate titration is shown by the *solid line*. Note that in patients with proximal RTA, bicarbonate excretion begins to appear in the urine when serum bicarbonate concentration exceeds 16 to 18 mmol/L, whereas in normal individuals, bicarbonate does not appear until serum bicarbonate is above 22 to 24 mmol/L. Below the threshold, patients with proximal RTA can reabsorb filtered bicarbonate nearly completely.

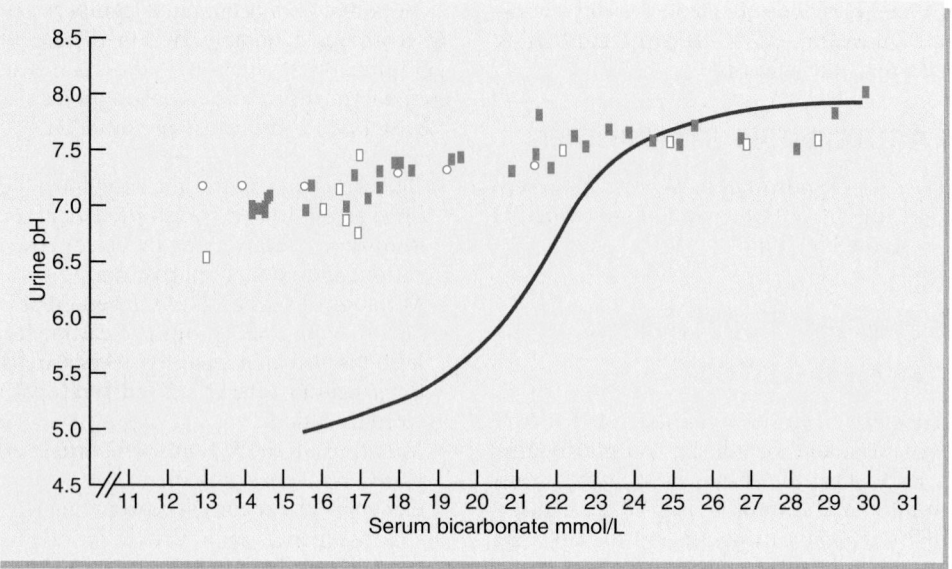

Figure 28-10 Bicarbonate titration curve in gradient-limit renal tubular acidosis. Note the fixed bicarbonate excretion at any level serum bicarbonate (compare with Fig. 28-9).

Hyperkalemic Renal Tubular Acidosis Syndromes

This second major group of RTA is theoretically caused by defects in principal cell function and takes three clinical forms. Pseudohypoaldosteronism I is inherited as an autosomal-recessive disease characterized by hyperkalemia, sodium wasting, and failure to thrive. Serum aldosterone is elevated, and the defect is unresponsive to administration of mineralocorticoids. A truncated form of epithelial sodium channel (ENaC) is found with low activity and massive sodium loss and is treated by large amounts of oral sodium. A second form, termed *familial hyperkalemic hypertension*, or *Gordon syndrome*, is characterized by hyperkalemia and sodium avidity, often accompanied by low renin and mild hypertension. The defect is responsive to loop diuretics and sodium restriction.

Gordon syndrome is also responsive to thiazide diuretics, which inhibit the sodium-chloride co-transporter (NCC) in the distal tubule. This form of hyperkalemic RTA is caused by a loss of function mutation in *WNK-4* (with no lysine), which inhibits NCC function (discussed in Chapter 26). Thus, the activity of the NCC is increased, reducing delivery to the collecting duct and consequent reduction in flow and voltage mediated potassium excretion. Because sodium reabsorption is increased in the distal tubule, hypercalciuria is prominent, and nephrocalcinosis occurs.

The third form of hyperkalemic RTA is an acquired disease usually associated with interstitial fibrosis. In this form, serum aldosterone and renin are reduced even in the presence of hyperkalemia. The reason for this defect in aldosterone secretion and responsiveness to administered mineralocorticoids is unknown but suggests defects in principal cell function. The disease responds partially to furo-

semide and cautious liberalization of salt intake without provoking hypertension.

The third major category of RTA is the so-called gradient-limited form and appears to be caused by a defect in outer medullary collecting duct function. Both principal and intercalated cell transports are defective. This disease is characterized by a fixed defect in bicarbonate excretion without apparent threshold (Fig. 28-10) and a fixed excretion of alkaline urine. Most commonly, the disease is the consequence of an inherited defect in the activity of the hydrogen-ATPase or potassium-hydrogen-ATPase. Acquired damage to the latter can also occur in autoimmune diseases, most notably Sjögren syndrome. This damage also occurs in sickle cell disease and primary hyperparathyroidism when these are associated with interstitial kidney damage. Drugs such as amphotericin and lithium may also cause damage. Impaired function of the basolateral band III chloride-bicarbonate exchanger is also thought to explain isolated cases because mutations have been found in the *AEI* gene that codes for it. Multiple mutations in the *AEI* gene may also occur, and in such cases, RTA is associated with ovalocytosis.

In all cases of distal, gradient-limited RTA, hyperchloremic acidosis occurs and is accompanied, because of sodium loss, by secondary hyperaldosteronism, leading to potassium depletion. In children, the syndrome impairs growth, and it may be associated with hypokalemic muscle paralysis, hypercalciuria, and nephrocalcinosis. Therapy consists of bicarbonate replacement as well as potassium replacement. Particularly in children, large amounts of bicarbonate may be required to ensure normal growth. Distal RTA is also complicated by a low urinary excretion of citrate, which leads to severe nephrocalcinosis.

METABOLIC ALKALOSIS

A gain in base or loss of acid increases the bicarbonate concentration of the ECF. Normally, an elevation of the serum bicarbonate concentration is corrected by excretion of the excess bicarbonate. The maintenance of *metabolic alkalosis,* therefore, implies a defect in the renal mechanism regulating bicarbonate excretion. This failure to excrete excess bicarbonate occurs by both physiologic responses to volume depletion, especially if hypercapnia and hypokalemia accompany the alkalosis, or by pathophysiologic responses, as occur in autonomous mineralocorticoid excess.

The most common cause of metabolic alkalosis is gastric loss of hydrochloric acid by vomiting or mechanical drainage. Diuretic (thiazide and loop) use is commonly associated with metabolic alkalosis. Volume depletion associated with vomiting and diuretic use enhances proximal bicarbonate reabsorption. Enhanced activity of sodium-hydrogen exchange at this site, and consequent enhanced volume reabsorption, results in enhanced bicarbonate reabsorption (see Chapter 26). Volume depletion also leads to aldosterone secretion, which stimulates distal nephron hydrogen secretion and augments potassium secretion. Repair of the alkalosis under these circumstances requires administration of sodium chloride and potassium. Endogenous or exogenous mineralocorticoid excess (see Fig. 28-7) is unresponsive to volume administration as extracellular volume is expanded. The stimulation of distal hydrogen secretion by aldosterone is sufficient to limit bicarbonate excretion and stimulate potassium secretion. Repair of this disorder requires removal of the excess mineralocorticoid. In all these disorders, concomitant hypokalemia promotes the maintenance of metabolic alkalosis.

Excessive alkali ingestion (e.g., milk-alkali syndrome) is an uncommon cause of metabolic alkalosis and results from impaired renal bicarbonate excretion caused by renal failure in the setting of excess alkali intake. In this instance, both hypercalcemia and vitamin D excess are thought to play roles in damaging the kidney. Removal of alkali often corrects the alkalosis, but renal function remains reduced if nephrocalcinosis is prominent.

The determination of urinary chloride concentrations is helpful in formulating a rational approach to the diagnosis and treatment of metabolic alkalosis. In patients with hypertension since childhood, alkalosis, hypokalemia, and low urinary chloride, consideration should be given to Liddle syndrome. These features resemble mineralocorticoid excess, but renin and aldosterone levels are suppressed (pseudohypoaldosteronism). The disorder is inherited as an autosomal recessive disorder with mutations in the *ENaC* gene that result in deletion of the C-terminal region of the protein. This condition results in reduced degradation and increased density of sodium channels in the luminal membrane of the principal cells of the collecting duct (see Chapter 26). The clinical features are a consequence of the enhanced salt reabsorption, resultant volume expansion, and increased distal nephron potassium and proton secretion.

Patients with high urinary chloride and alkalosis and who are hypertensive require work-up for hypercorticism, which may be autonomous, as in primary aldosteronism and Cushing disease or secondary to renal artery stenosis. Rarer still are the 11-β-hydroxylase deficiencies, or *apparent* m*in*eralocorticoid *excess* (AME), in which reduced conversion of glucocorticoids reaching the collecting duct leads to overstimulation of ENaC. Another such syndrome of congenital hypertension and alkalosis is glucocorticoid-remediable aldosteronism (GRA), which is caused by a gene duplication in which the promoter for the 11-β-hydroxylase gene drives the aldosterone synthase gene and leads to adrenocorticotropic hormone–responsive aldosterone synthesis. In each of these instances, hyperactivity of ENaC leads to all clinical features of the syndrome.

Normotensive or hypotensive conditions with alkalosis, hypokalemia, and high urinary chloride consist of two distinct forms: Bartter syndrome and Gitelman syndrome. Each syndrome involves distinct abnormalities in segment-specific sodium chloride reabsorption, as well as differences in calcium and magnesium excretion. In Bartter syndrome (see Table 28-6), several disabling mutations in genes affecting the reabsorption of sodium chloride across the TAL have been characterized, including loss-of-function mutations in the NKCC2 co-transporter, the ROMK channel protein, and the basolateral chloride channel, and a gain in function mutation of the calcium-sensing receptor. Each of these mutations causes salt wasting, including enhanced calcium excretion, volume depletion, and, in many instances, reduced blood pressure. The reduction in ECF volume causes a secondary hyperaldosteronism, which, when coupled with enhanced sodium delivery to the collecting duct, causes potassium wasting and enhanced proton excretion. In Gitelman syndrome, disabling mutations in the DCT thiazide-sensitive sodium-chloride co-transporter have been described. The phenotypic characteristics of Gitelman syndrome in contradistinction to Bartter syndrome are the reduced calcium excretion and hypercalcemia observed, as might be expected from inhibition of the sodium-chloride co-transporter (see Chapter 26). The cause of hypermagnesuria in Gitelman syndrome is reduced expression of TRPM6 channel in the DCT.

RESPIRATORY ACIDOSIS

Respiratory acidosis occurs with any impairment in the rate of alveolar ventilation. Acute respiratory acidosis occurs with a sudden depression of the medullary respiratory center (narcotic overdose), with paralysis of the respiratory muscles, and with airway obstruction. Chronic respiratory acidosis generally occurs in patients with chronic airway disease (emphysema), with extreme kyphoscoliosis, and with extreme obesity (pickwickian syndrome).

The serum bicarbonate concentration is increased, the magnitude of which depends on the acuity and the severity of the respiratory disorder. The compensatory increase in serum bicarbonate in prolonged hypercapnia (>1 week) is primarily a function of bone buffering as the kidney plays a relatively minor role in the increase. Acute increases in the P_{CO_2} result in somnolence, confusion, and, ultimately, carbon dioxide narcosis. Asterixis may be present. Because carbon dioxide is a cerebral vasodilator, the blood vessels in the optic fundi are often dilated, engorged, and tortuous. Frank papilledema may be present in patients with severe hypercapnic states.

The only practical therapy of acute respiratory acidosis involves treatment of the underlying disorder and ventilatory support. In patients with chronic hypercapnia who develop an acute increase in the P_{CO_2}, attention should be directed toward identifying the factors that may have aggravated the chronic disorder. Diuretics often exacerbate the increase in serum bicarbonate and result in a mixed disorder of metabolic alkalosis and respiratory acidosis. Under these circumstances, acidification of the serum may be necessary to improve ventilation.

RESPIRATORY ALKALOSIS

Respiratory alkalosis occurs when hyperventilation reduces the arterial P_{CO_2} and consequently increases the arterial pH. Acute respiratory alkalosis is most commonly a result of pregnancy; it may also occur in damage to the respiratory centers, in acute salicylism, in fever and septic states, in advanced liver disease, and when respiratory rate is increased in pneumonia, pulmonary embolism, and congestive heart failure. The disorder may be produced iatrogenically by injudicious mechanical ventilatory support. Chronic hyperventilation occurs in the acclimatization response to high altitudes cause by reduced ambient partial pressure of oxygen.

Acute hyperventilation is characterized by lightheadedness, paresthesias, circumoral numbness, and tingling of the extremities. Tetany occurs in severe cases. When anxiety provokes hyperventilation, air rebreathing with a paper bag generally terminates the acute attack.

Prospectus for the Future

- Identification of additional gene mutations informative about the renal regulation of water and solute transport

- Design of small molecules to inhibit salt and water transport in specific nephron segments for the treatment of hypertension and edema

References

Andreoli TE: Water: Normal balance, hyponatremia and hypernatremia. Ren Fail 22:711-735, 2000.

Cao G, Hoenderop JGJ, Bibdels RJM: Insight into the molecular regulation of the epithelial magnesium channel TRPM6. Curr Opin Nephrol Hypertens 17:373-378, 2008.

Gamba G: Role of WNK kinases in regulating tubular salt and potassium transport and in the development of hypertension. Am J Physiol Renal Physiol 288:F245-F252, 2005.

Ellison DH, Berl T: Clinical practice: The syndrome of inappropriate antidiuresis. N Engl J Med 356:2064-2072, 2007.

Kokko JP: Fluid and electrolytes. In Goldman L, Bennett JC (eds): Cecil Textbook of Medicine, 21st ed. Philadelphia, WB Saunders, 2000, pp 540-567.

Tannen RL: Dyskalemias. In Massry SG, Glasscock FJ (eds): Textbook of Nephrology, 4th ed. Philadelphia, Lippincott Williams & Wilkins, 2001, pp 295-307.

Glomerular Diseases

Jamie P. Dwyer and Julia B. Lewis

Each human kidney contains nearly 1 million glomerular capillary tufts, which derive from an afferent arteriole and are held together by the mesangial matrix. The glomerular capillary tufts drain into an efferent arteriole forming an arteriolar portal system. Fenestrated endothelial cells, the glomerular basement membrane (GBM), and delicate foot processes extending from epithelial podocytes, which are interconnected to each other by slit diaphragms (**Web Fig 29-1**), form a selective filtration barrier between the capillary blood and urinary space (**Web Fig 29-2A**). Each glomerular tuft has an associated renal tubule that drains into the urologic system. Nearly one fourth of the blood of each heartbeat is filtered by the kidney (about 120 to 180 L per 24 hours). Remarkably, despite the 12,000 to 18,000 g of protein filtered by the capillaries each day, less than 150 mg appears in urine. This is accomplished in part by the negatively charged GBM and the 4-nm slit-pore membranes restricting the movement of large or negatively charged proteins. Therefore, the glomerulus serves as a size- and charge-selective barrier to the movement of proteins and cells from the capillary blood into the urinary space.

The glomerulus can be injured by a variety of means, including genetic mutations producing familial diseases, immune-mediated inflammation, vascular injury, deposition of abnormal proteins, and infection. These injuries result in diverse glomerular diseases manifesting clinically as proteinuria, hematuria, pyuria, and vascular changes.

Clinical Syndromes

Glomerular diseases can have diverse clinical manifestations, including hematuria (**Web Fig. 29-3**), proteinuria, pyuria (**Web Fig. 29-4**), hypertension, fluid retention, edema, and a reduction in glomerular filtration rate (GFR). Glomerular diseases can be acute, developing over days; subacute, developing over weeks; or chronic, developing over months or years. Distinct clinical syndromes have been described; however, these syndromes are not always mutually exclusive (Table 29-1) The acute nephritic syndrome is characterized by hypertension, hematuria, edema, red blood cell (RBC) casts (Fig. 29-1) or dysmorphic RBCs (**Web Fig. 29-5**), modest proteinuria (1 to 2 g per 24 hours), and decreased

GFR. If the loss of GFR (seen as a rise in serum creatinine) occurs over days, acute nephritis is called rapidly progressive glomerulonephritis (RPGN) and is associated with crescentic glomerulonephritis on renal biopsy. Patients with the clinical syndrome of RPGN in whom the disease extends to the lungs are classified as having a pulmonary-renal syndrome (Table 29-2). In nephrotic syndrome, the patient excretes more than 3.5 g of protein in a 24-hour urine collection and has edema, hypoalbuminemia, and hypercholesterolemia. In long-standing nephrotic syndrome, decreased GFR and hypertension often develop (e.g., in diabetic nephropathy). Many glomerular diseases present with microscopic or gross hematuria and either no or mild proteinuria. Hematuria may be the only manifestation of some glomerular diseases throughout their course, as in thin basement membrane disease, or may be an early manifestation that progresses over time to involve other clinical signs such as decreased GFR, as in antineutrophil cytoplasmic antibody (ANCA)-associated vasculitis. When abnormal proteins, such as paraproteins, are deposited in or accumulate in the glomerulus in glomerular deposition diseases, the clinical manifestations can range from asymptomatic mild proteinuria to severe nephrotic syndrome. Glomerular vascular syndromes occur in patients in whom the injury is primarily

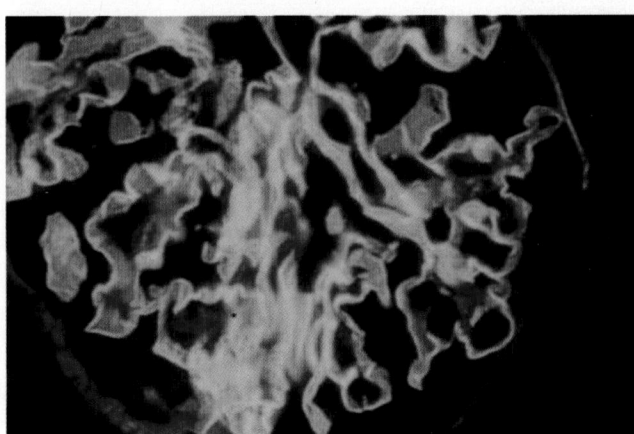

Figure 29-1 Immunofluorescence demonstrating a linear pattern of immunoglobulin G.

Table 29-1 Clinical Syndromes

Acute Nephritic Syndromes

Poststreptococcal glomerulonephritis
Subacute bacterial endocarditis
Lupus nephritis* (WHO class III or IV)
Anti-GBM disease, Goodpasture syndrome
ANCA-associated vasculitis (Wegener granulomatosis,
    microscopic polyangiitis, Churg-Strauss syndrome)*
Cryoglobulinemia*
IgA nephropathy
Henoch-Schönlein purpura
Membranoproliferative glomerulonephritis

Nephrotic Syndromes

Minimal change disease
FSGS
MGN
Diabetic nephropathy
Lupus nephritis (WHO class V)
ANCA-associated vasculitis
Deposition diseases
Nail-patella syndrome
Fabry disease
Syphilis (MGN)
Schistosomiasis (MPGN, FSGS, amyloid)

Primarily Hematuria Manifested Glomerular Diseases

IgA nephropathy
Thin basement membrane disease
Alport syndrome
MGPN
Lupus nephritis (WHO class II or III)
ANCA-associated vasculitis (early)*
Sickle cell disease

Glomerular Deposition Diseases

Light-chain deposition disease
Amyloidosis
Fibrillary glomerulonephritis, immunotactoid
    glomerulonephritis
Fabry disease

Glomerular Vascular Syndromes

Hypertensive nephrosclerosis
Cholesterol emboli
Sickle cell disease
Thrombotic thrombocytopenia purpura, hemolytic uremic
    syndrome
Antiphospholipid antibody syndrome
ANCA-associated vasculitis
Henoch-Schönlein purpura
Cryoglobulinemia*
Amyloidosis
Ischemic nephropathy

Infection-Associated Syndromes

Poststreptococcal glomerulonephritis
Subacute bacterial endocarditis
HIV (FSGS)
Hepatitis B and C (MGN and MPGN, respectively)
Syphilis
Leprosy
Malaria
Schistosomiasis

*May present as a pulmonary-renal syndrome.
  ANCA, antineutrophil cytoplasmic antibody; FSGS, focal segmental glomerulosclerosis; GBM, glomerular basement membrane; IgA, immunoglobulin A; MGN, membranous glomerulonephritis; MPGN, membranoproliferative glomerulonephritis; WHO, World Health Organization.

Table 29-2 Differential Diagnosis of Rapidly Progressive Glomerulonephritis

Linear Immune Staining

Anti-GBM disease
Goodpasture syndrome
Rarely membranous glomerulonephritis

Granular Immune Staining

Subacute bacterial endocarditis (past infectious)
Lupus nephritis
Cryoglobulinemia
Membranoproliferative glomerulonephritis (type II more
    than type I)
Immunoglobulin A nephropathy, Henoch-Schönlein purpura
Idiopathic

No Immune Staining (Pauci-immune)

Antineutrophil cytoplasmic antibody–associated vasculitis
    (Wegener granulomatosis, microscopic polyangiitis,
    Churg-Strauss syndrome)
Idiopathic

localized to the renal vasculature and is usually associated with hematuria and mild proteinuria. Lastly, a wide variety of infections can produce inflammatory reactions in the glomerulus, ranging from nephritic syndrome with RPGN to mild proteinuria or nephrotic syndrome.

The classification of glomerular diseases is hampered by the fact that an individual glomerular disease can present with more than one constellation of clinical signs or symptoms. For example, lupus nephritis can present as nephrotic syndrome, rapidly progressive glomerulonephritis, or asymptomatic hematuria. Hence, all classifications of glomerular diseases are complex and somewhat arbitrary. Each of the major glomerular diseases is discussed next, and potential alternate manifestations are noted (see Table 29-1).

Evaluation of Glomerular Diseases

A detailed history and physical examination can help clarify the differential diagnosis of glomerular lesions. Onset and timing may be important (e.g., nephrotic syndrome in a child suggests minimal change nephropathy). Associated physical examination findings may add to the diagnosis (e.g., Raynaud phenomenon in lupus nephritis, livedo reticularis in cholesterol emboli). Assessment for anemia, thrombocytopenia, eosinophilia, microangiopathic hemolysis, serologies for antinuclear antibody (ANA), ANCAs, anti-GBM antibody, antibodies to hepatitis B and C, HIV, rheumatoid factor, anti-DNAse B, antistreptolysin O (ASO) titer, cryoglobulin, and monoclonal proteins may help in narrowing the diagnostic possibilities. Urine microscopy is a critical element in the evaluation of a patient with glomerular diseases and may reveal hematuria, RBC casts, oval fat bodies or fatty casts (**Web Fig. 29-6**), or proteinuria. Measurement of 24-hour creatinine clearance and proteinuria helps distinguish the presence or absence of nephrotic syndrome and assesses GFR. Ultimately, a specific diagnosis may rely on a renal biopsy. Indications for renal biopsy vary from patient to patient and between countries. Renal biopsy allows one

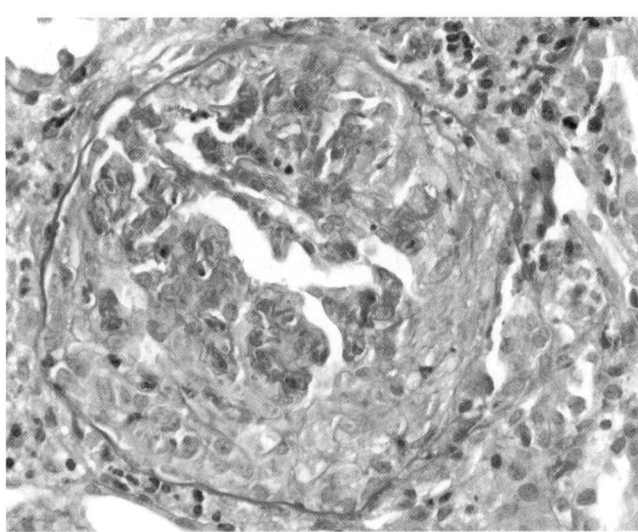

Figure 29-2 Glomerulus demonstrating crescent formation.

to make a diagnosis and can be determined by light micro-scopy if the disease is focal (involving <50% of glomeruli) or diffuse (involving >50% of glomeruli), segmental (involving a portion of a glomerulus) or global (involving the entire glomerulus). It can also demonstrate so-called crescent formation (Fig. 29-2), which is the pathologic hallmark of rapidly progressive glomerulonephritis. Immunofluorescence microscopy can identify types of immunoglobulin deposition and location (e.g., linear immunoglobulin G [IgG] staining in Goodpasture syndrome (Fig. 29-1). There may be minimal or no immune deposition (pauci-immune glomerulonephritis). Electron microscopy can show the location of electron-dense deposits (e.g., subepithelial deposits in poststreptococcal glomerulonephritis (**Web Fig. 29-7**) or subendothelial deposits in proliferative lupus nephritis (**Web Fig. 29-8**).

General Treatment Guidelines for Glomerular Disease

Specific therapies for the different glomerular disease are noted next. In all forms of glomerular disease, treatment of hypertension, if present, is indicated with a target blood pressure of 130/80 mm Hg. For many glomerular diseases, including all those associated with proteinuria, treatment with drugs that inhibit the renin-angiotensin system is recommended. It has also been suggested that accelerating therapy to maximally reduce proteinuria should be a goal. Volume overload, manifested by edema, should be treated by reduction in salt and water intake and judicious use of diuretics. Hypercholesterolemia should be controlled with dietary modification and pharmacologic therapy. If a hyper-coagulable state exists, anticoagulation may be necessary. Every effort should be made to avoid exposure to nephro-toxins because patients with glomerular disease may be at increased risk for acute kidney injury. Lastly, close monitoring of renal function by a specialist is indicated in most cases.

Table 29-3 **Glomerular Diseases Associated with Hypocomplementemia**
Poststreptococcal glomerulonephritis
Lupus nephritis (acute)
Cholesterol emboli
Membranoproliferative glomerulonephritis, hepatitis C
Subacute bacterial endocarditis
Cryoglobulinemia
Shunt nephritis

Acute Nephritic Syndromes

POSTSTREPTOCOCCAL GLOMERULONEPHRITIS

Poststreptococcal glomerulonephritis (PSGN) can occur as a postinfectious complication of skin and throat infections with particular M types (nephritogenic strains) of strepto-cocci. PSGN due to streptococcal pharyngitis occurs in fewer than 5% of people infected, typically 1 to 3 weeks after the pharyngitis. Streptococcal impetigo is a less common cause of PSGN than pharyngitis but leads to PSGN in as many as 50% of infected people 2 to 6 weeks after the impetigo. In undeveloped countries, PSGN can occur in a epidemic form, but in Western countries, it typically occurs sporadically in the summer and autumn. PSGN can occur in adults but usually occurs in children between the ages of 2 and 14 years.

Patients present classically with acute nephritis, characterized by hematuria, pyuria, RBC casts, edema, hypertension, systemic symptoms of headache and malaise, flank pain due to renal capsular swelling, and oliguric renal failure. Because the hematuria occurs after the pharyngitis, it is called *met-apharyngitic* or *postpharyngitic* hematuria. Five percent of children and 20% of adults have nephrotic range proteinuria. A subclinical disease has also been reported, characterized by asymptomatic microscopic hematuria. Early in the course, 90% of patients will have decreased levels of C_3 and CH_{50} with normal levels of C_4. Patients with PSGN must be distinguished from other glomerular diseases associated with hypocomplementemia (Table 29-3). Rheumatoid factor, cryoglobulins, and ANCA may all be positive. Increased titers of ASO antibodies (30%), anti-DNAase (70%) or antihyaluronidase antibodies (40%) can help confirm the diagnosis. Histologically, the kidney demonstrates a diffuse proliferative glomerulonephritis with hyper-cellularity of mesangial and endothelial cells (**Web Figs. 29-9 and 29-10**), glomerular infiltrates of polymorphonuclear leukocytes, and granular, "lumpy-bumpy" subendothelial and subepithelial deposits of IgG, IgM, and complement. Treatment is supportive and may require renal replacement therapy. Antibiotic therapy does not alter the course of PSGN. Immunosuppressive therapy is also ineffective. Complete recovery occurs in 90% to 95% of patients; in children, recovery is usually seen within 3 to 6 weeks of the onset of nephritis, whereas in adults, proteinuria and hematuria may continue for 1 to 2 years. End-stage renal disease (ESRD) is uncommon, occurring in 1% to 3% of adults and rarely in children.

SUBACUTE BACTERIAL ENDOCARDITIS

Endocarditis-associated glomerulonephritis is a complication of subacute bacterial endocarditis. Patients present with hematuria, pyuria, and mild proteinuria, or less commonly with RPGN. Laboratory examination reveals an elevated erythrocyte sedimentation rate, hypocomplementemia, a positive rheumatoid factor, cryoglobulinemia (type III), and anemia. Renal biopsy reveals a focal proliferative glomerulonephritis with abundant mesangial, subendothelial, and subepithelial deposits of IgG, IgM, and complement. Patients who present with RPGN have crescents on renal biopsy. Embolic infarcts or abscesses may also be present. Treatment is antibiotics for 4 to 6 weeks, and the prognosis is good.

Glomerulonephritis can also occur in patients with infected ventriculoatrial and ventriculoperitoneal shunts (shunt nephritis); pulmonary, intra-abdominal, pelvic, or cutaneous infections; and infected vascular prostheses. Treatment is eradication of the infection.

LUPUS NEPHRITIS

Sixty percent of adults and 80% of children with systemic lupus erythematosus (SLE) develop renal abnormalities. The clinical manifestations and treatment of lupus nephritis are closely linked to the renal pathology (Table 29-4). Clinical signs and laboratory data can include hematuria, proteinuria, RBC casts, hypertension, hypocomplementemia, and anti–double-stranded DNA (anti-dsDNA) antibodies. Renal biopsy is critical to distinguish the variants of lupus nephritis (**Web Fig. 29-11**), and patients with lupus often undergo multiple biopsies as their lupus-related renal lesions may vary over time. The World Health Organization (WHO) has outlined distinct patterns of lupus-related glomerular injury (see Table 29-4). WHO class I lesions have minimal clinical manifestations and either normal histology or minimal mesangial deposits. Prognosis is excellent, and no treatment is required. WHO class II nephritis demonstrates mesangial immune complex deposition with mesangial proliferation, but few clinical renal manifestations, normal renal function, and a good prognosis. Specific treatment is generally not necessary. WHO class III lesions demonstrate focal lesions with proliferation and scarring (focal proliferative lupus nephritis), and patients with class III lesions have diverse clinical courses. Patients can present with hypertension, hematuria, proteinuria, nephrotic syndrome (25% to 33%), or elevated serum creatinine (25%). Some patients with only mild focal proliferation involving a small percentage of glomeruli respond to steroid therapy alone with an excellent prognosis. Others with more severe proliferation involving a greater percentage of glomeruli have a worse prognosis, and therapy with steroids and other immunosuppressive drugs (cyclophosphamide, mycophenolate) is required. WHO class IV nephritis demonstrates global, diffuse proliferative lesions involving most of the glomeruli (diffuse proliferative lupus nephritis). Clinically, patients present with the most severe manifestations, including RPGN, hematuria, RBC casts, hypertension, proteinuria (50% nephrotic range), and declining renal function. Without treatment, WHO class IV lesions have the worst prognosis, and therapy with steroids and immunosuppressive drugs is recommended. If remission is achieved (defined as a return to near-normal renal function and proteinuria <330 mg per 24 hours), long-term renal outcomes are good. The WHO class V lesion has a membranous pattern with subepithelial immune deposits. Class V lesions may also have associated proliferative lesions and are subcategorized. Patients typically present with nephrotic syndrome (60%) and may also have hypertension, renal dysfunction, and renal vein thrombosis as manifestations. Unlike WHO class IV lesions, data on treatment of class V lesions are conflicting. This may reflect heterogeneity of the lesions in the WHO class V category. In patients with severe nephrotic syndrome or elevated serum creatinine, a course of steroids in combination with immunosuppressive agents will improve the disease course. The WHO class VI lesions have 90% scarred or sclerotic glomeruli, which implies ESRD. Importantly, if this lesion is found in biopsy, no further immunosuppressive therapy is indicated. Overall, about 20% of patients with lupus nephritis reach ESRD. Renal transplantation is an option but is usually performed only after 6 months of inactive lupus. Systemic lupus typically becomes quiescent with complete kidney failure, perhaps as a result of the immunosuppression associated with uremia.

Table 29-4 **Lupus Nephritis**			
World Health Organization Class	**Histology**	**Clinical Manifestations**	**Treatment**
1	Normal	Hematuria	None
2	Mesangial immune complexes with proliferation	Hematuria, mild proteinuria	With or without prednisone only
3	Focal endocapillary with or without extracapillary proliferation with subendothelial deposits	Hypertension, hematuria, proteinuria, variable decline in renal function	Mild: prednisone only Severe: prednisone plus cytotoxics or mycophenolate
4	Diffuse endocapillary and extracapillary proliferation with diffuse subendothelial deposits	Hematuria, red blood cell casts, proteinuria, declining renal function, possibly RPGN	Prednisone plus cytotoxics or mycophenolate
5	Membranous with diffuse subepithelial deposits	Nephrotic syndrome	Prednisone plus cytotoxics or mycophenolate
6	Global sclerosis	Near end-stage renal disease	Dialysis, transplantation

ANTIGLOMERULAR BASEMENT MEMBRANE DISEASE

Patients with anti-GBM disease have autoantibodies directed against epitopes in the quaternary structure of the α_3 NC1 domain of type IV collagen found in the GBM. This can present as an isolated glomerulonephritis (anti-GBM disease) or involve collagen IV in the lung, presenting as a pulmonary-renal syndrome called Goodpasture syndrome. It occurs in two age peaks, in young men in their 20s and in men and women in their 60s and 70s, and can be triggered by exposure to infection, smoking, or solvents. Patients can present with hemoptysis, anemia, fever, dyspnea, hematuria, and RPGN (see Table 29-2). About 10% of patients with RPGN have anti-GBM disease. Alternately, usually in older patients, it can present more indolently with isolated hematuria, anemia, and a more gradual loss of renal function. Urgent renal biopsy is diagnostic and reveals a characteristic linear pattern of staining of the capillary loops with IgG (Fig. 29-1) and C_3. Serum can also be tested for anti-GBM antibodies. Treatment consists of high-dose steroids, cyclophosphamide, and plasmapheresis.

ANTINUCLEAR CYTOPLASMIC ANTIBODY–ASSOCIATED SMALL VESSEL VASCULITIS

ANCAs are found in the serum of 80% to 85% of patients with pauci-immune glomerulonephritis. ANCA antibodies are of two types: anti-proteinase 3 (anti-PR3) or anti-myeloperoxidase (anti-MPO). ANCAs are implicated in the small vessel endothelial cell injury seen in Wegener granulomatosis, microscopic polyangiitis, and Churg-Strauss syndrome. Anti-PR3 ANCA is generally seen in a cytoplasmic pattern (c-ANCA) (**Web Fig. 29-12**) and is more common in Wegener granulomatosis. Anti-MPO ANCA is generally seen in a perinuclear pattern (p-ANCA) (**Web Fig. 29-12**) and is more common in microscopic polyangiitis or Churg-Strauss syndrome. Patients with Wegener granulomatosis may present with fever, rhinorrhea, nasal ulcers, sinus symptoms, pulmonary symptoms (hemoptysis), arthritis, microscopic hematuria, and mild proteinuria. It can present as limited disease with pulmonary and no renal involvement, pulmonary-renal syndrome, asymptomatic microscopic hematuria, or RPGN. Microscopic polyangiitis may present with many of the same symptoms as Wegener granulomatosis, but upper airway or pulmonary symptoms are rare. In Churg-Strauss syndrome, patients may have eosinophilia, purpura, mononeuritis multiplex, and respiratory involvement manifested as asthma or allergic rhinitis. The presentation may also be a pulmonary-renal syndrome with pulmonary infiltrates and RPGN. In most cases, renal biopsies associated with any of the above conditions reveal pauci-immune glomerulonephritis with only a few immune complexes in the small vessels and either a crescentic glomerulonephritis or a focal necrotizing glomerulonephritis. The biopsy is typically consistent with, but not diagnostic of, ANCA-associated vasculitis. Treatment is aggressive with plasmapheresis, high-dose steroids, and cyclophosphamide for induction therapy. Maintenance therapy appears important in these diseases to prevent relapse and usually involves lower doses of steroids and cytotoxic drugs.

CRYOGLOBULINEMIA

Cryoglobulinemia presents in middle age, more commonly in women than men, with manifestations of purpura, fever, Raynaud phenomena, arthralgias, fatigue, and renal involvement (40% to 50% of patients). Renal manifestations may range from mild (with isolated hematuria or proteinuria) to severe (with acute nephritic syndrome and RPGN). Serologic testing may reveal a positive rheumatoid factor, low levels of C_4, and evidence of hepatitis C infection. Up to 50% of patients with cryoglobulinemia have hepatitis C virus. Renal biopsy most commonly reveals a membranoproliferative pattern of injury with intraluminal hyaline thrombi. Treatment is not well established, but plasmapheresis and the use of cytotoxic agents have been reported to induce remissions; however, relapses are common. Often, treating the hepatitis C infection (if present) ameliorates the cryoglobulinemia.

IgA nephropathy, Henoch-Schönlein purpura, and membranoproliferative glomerulonephritis also may present as an acute nephritic syndrome or RPGN but are discussed later because acute nephritic syndrome is not their most common presentation.

Nephrotic Syndromes

MINIMAL CHANGE DISEASE

Minimal change disease (MCD) is the most common cause of nephrotic syndrome in children. Seventy to 90% of nephrotic syndrome cases in children and 10% to 15% in adults are due to MCD. MCD is typically idiopathic but can rarely be associated with Hodgkin disease or nonsteroidal anti-inflammatory drugs. MCD presents clinically with the abrupt onset of proteinuria in the nephrotic range, acellular urine, and edema. In children, the proteinuria is primarily albumin and is called *selective proteinuria*. Diagnosis in children is usually presumptive, and a renal biopsy is only done in nonresponders to steroid therapy. Renal biopsy is the only definitive diagnostic test and reveals normal light microscopy (**Web Fig. 29-13**), negative immunofluorescent microscopy, and effacement of the foot processes (**Web Fig. 29-2B**) supporting the epithelial podocytes on election microscopy. Although it has been reported that up to 30% of children will have a spontaneous remission, most children today are treated with steroids. Ninety to 95% of children develop a complete remission (<0.2 mg per 24 hours of proteinuria) after 8 weeks of steroid therapy. Eighty to 85% of adults achieve remission, but only after 20 to 24 weeks of therapy. Steroid-dependent patients relapse as their steroid dose is tapered. Other less common clinical features include hypertension (30% in children, 50% in adults), atopy (40% in children, 30% in adults), microscopic hematuria (20% in children, 30% in adults), and renal failure (<5% in children, 30% in adults). Relapses are common in children after the first remission. Frequent relapsers are defined as having two or more relapses in 6 months. The frequency of relapses decreases after puberty. In adults, relapses are less common but more resistant to therapy. Steroid-resistant patients fail to respond to steroid therapy. Cytotoxic drugs such as cyclophosphamide, chlorambucil, and mycophenolate mofetil are given to frequent relapsers and to steroid-dependent or

Table 29-5 **Etiology of Focal Segmental Glomerulosclerosis (FSGS)**
Primary idiopathic FSGS
Secondary FSGS
HIV (usually collapsing variant)
Reflux nephropathy
Heroin abuse
Sickle cell disease
Oligomeganephronia
Renal dysgenesis or agenesis (low nephron mass)
Radiation nephritis
Familial podocytopathies
NPHS1 (nephrin) mutation
NPHS2 (podocin) mutation
TRPC6 (cation channel) mutation
ACTN4 (α-actinin 4 mutation)

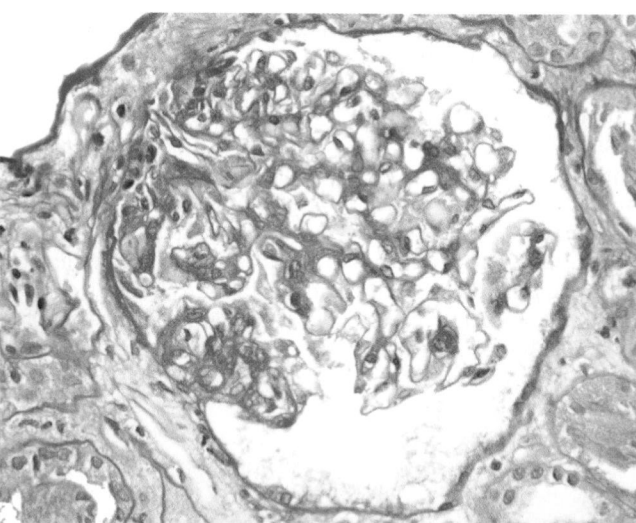

Figure 29-3 Glomerulus demonstrating a focus of sclerosis and hyalinosis.

steroid-resistant patients. Cyclosporine has been reported to induce remissions, but relapse is frequent when it is withdrawn. Overall, the prognosis is better in children than adults.

FOCAL SEGMENTAL GLOMERULOSCLEROSIS

Focal segmental glomerulosclerosis (FSGS) accounts for 10% to 15% of nephrotic syndrome in children, and in adults it represents one third of non–diabetes-associated nephrotic syndrome. It is even more common in African American adults, in whom it is the etiology of more than 50% of cases of nephrotic syndrome. FSGS can either be primary and idiopathic or secondary to either a familial or systemic process (Table 29-5). Patients present with proteinuria, frequently microscopic hematuria, hypertension, edema, and impaired kidney function. Although there is much overlap in clinical presentations, adults with FSGS are more likely to present with hematuria, hypertension, and impaired renal function than adults with MCD. Children with nephrotic syndrome who fail empiric steroid therapy often have FSGS on renal biopsy. Renal biopsy changes (Fig. 29-3) are most prominent in glomeruli located at the corticomedullary junction and include focal and segmental scarring. A cellular lesion with endocapillary hypercellularity and heavy proteinuria has also been described. A collapsing glomerulopathy with segmental or global glomerular collapse (**Web Fig. 29-14**), massive proteinuria, and rapidly advancing renal failure has been described in heroin users, patients with HIV, and African Americans. FSGS rarely remits spontaneously, and patients treated with steroids achieve remission far less often than patients with MCD. Treatment of primary FSGS should include inhibitors of the renin-angiotensin system and, in patients with a high risk for progressive loss of renal function, 6 to 9 months of steroid therapy. Patients at high risk include those with nephrotic range proteinuria, African Americans, males, and patients with renal insufficiency. It is estimated that 50% of these patients will reach ESRD in 6 to 8 years without treatment. With steroid therapy, proteinuria remits in 20% to 45% of patients. In secondary FSGS, the underlying cause should be treated, and steroid therapy is not indicated.

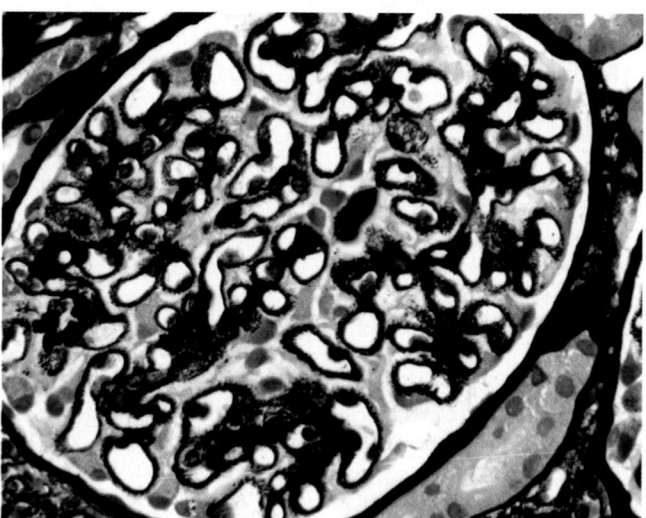

Figure 29-4 Membranous glomerulopathy showing "spikes" on capillary loops.

MEMBRANOUS GLOMERULONEPHRITIS

Membranous glomerulonephritis (MGN) accounts for 25% to 30% of nephrotic syndrome in adults and is the most common cause of nephrotic syndrome in elderly people. Most cases of MGN are idiopathic, but 20% to 30% of cases are associated with malignancies (solid tumors of the breast, lung, colon), infection (hepatitis B, schistosomiasis, malaria), or rheumatologic diseases (systemic lupus, rheumatoid arthritis). Eighty percent of patients present with nephrotic syndrome with nonselective proteinuria, and 50% of patients present with microscopic hematuria. Because of the thrombogenic conditions associated with nephrotic syndrome, thrombotic events can be a feature of many glomerular diseases. However, MGN has the highest reported incidence of renal vein thrombosis, pulmonary embolism, and deep vein thrombosis. The diagnosis of MGN relies on the renal biopsy. Light microscopy reveals uniform thickening of and "spike" formation in the basement membranes (Fig. 29-4) along the capillary loops, whereas immunofluorescence demonstrates granular glomerular deposits of IgG (**Web Fig. 29-15**) and C_3. Electron microscopy reveals electron-dense subepithelial deposits that distinguish MGN stages I to V. One third of patients with MGN have spontaneous remissions even 1 to 2 years after diagnosis. One third of patients have proteinuria without loss of renal function, and one third have nephrotic syndrome with a progressive decline in renal function. All patients should have treatment of edema, dyslipidemia, and hypertension and should receive drugs that inhibit the renin-angiotensin system. Patients with primary MGN who do not have a spontaneous remission should be treated with steroids and a cytotoxic agent or cyclosporine.

DIABETIC NEPHROPATHY

Diabetic nephropathy is the single most common cause of chronic kidney disease in the United States, representing 45% of all patients enrolled in the Medicare ESRD program. About 40% of patients with either type 1 or type 2 diabetes mellitus (DM) develop diabetic nephropathy. African American, Native American, Polynesian, and Maori patients with type 2 diabetes are far more likely to develop diabetic nephropathy than Caucasian patients with type 2 DM. The natural history of diabetic nephropathy is similar in patients with type 1 or type 2 DM. However, the time of onset of DM is often difficult to determine in patients with type 2 DM, and in newly diagnosed patients, even advanced diabetic nephropathy may be present. In patients with newly diagnosed diabetes, renal hypertrophy and glomerular hyperfiltration are present. Within 1.5 to 3 years, morphologic changes develop (Fig. 29-4), including glomerular basement thickening, mesangial expansion, hyaline arteriosclerosis, and in some patients, nodular glomerulosclerosis or Kimmelstiel-Wilson nodules. In the about 40% of patients with DM who develop clinically significant diabetic nephropathy, the earliest manifestation is an increase in urinary albumin excretion. Albuminuria in the range of 30 to 300 mg per 24 hours is arbitrarily referred to as *microalbuminuria*. Albuminuria greater than 300 mg per 24 hours is termed *overt nephropathy* or *proteinuria*. Current recommendations are to test patients with type 1 DM for microalbuminuria after 5 years of diabetes and yearly thereafter. Patients with type 2 DM should be tested at the time of diagnosis of DM and yearly thereafter.

Patients with microalbuminuria, if untreated, increase their urinary albumin losses and develop frank proteinuria. Proteinuria can be as little as 500 mg per 24 hours or greater than 20 g per 24 hours. Once proteinuria is present, renal function declines, with up to 50% of patients reaching ESRD in 5 to 10 years. However, many patients with microalbuminuria or proteinuria and type 2 DM die from adverse cardiovascular events before they reach ESRD. Ninety to 95% of patients with type 1 DM and diabetic nephropathy have diabetic retinopathy, whereas only 60% to 65% of patients with type 2 DM and nephropathy have retinopathy. In contrast to other glomerular diseases, patients with diabetic nephropathy often have normal-sized to enlarged kidneys despite even advanced renal disease. In the absence of other clinical or serologic data suggesting an alternate cause of glomerular disease, the diagnosis of dia-

betic nephropathy is usually a clinical one, not requiring a renal biopsy.

In type 1 DM, intensive blood sugar control has been unequivocally demonstrated to prevent both development and early progression of diabetic nephropathy. The data supporting intensive blood sugar control in type 2 DM are less compelling. Guidelines recommend controlling systemic blood pressure to about 130/80 mm Hg. Most patients with overt diabetic nephropathy require three or more antihypertensive drugs to achieve this goal. Multiple large clinical trials have demonstrated that drugs that inhibit the renin-angiotensin system slow the progression of early or overt nephropathy independent of their effect on systemic blood pressure.

Other glomerular diseases that can present as nephrotic syndrome, such as lupus nephritis (WHO class V), ANCA-associated vasculitis, deposition diseases, nail-patella syndrome, Fabry disease, and infection-associated glomerular disease are discussed in other sections.

Primarily Hematuria Manifested Glomerular Diseases

IMMUNOGLOBULIN A NEPHROPATHY AND HENOCH-SCHÖNLEIN PURPURA

IgA nephropathy is one of the most common causes of glomerulonephritis worldwide. There are well-described geographic and racial differences in the prevalence of IgA nephropathy. IgA nephropathy is more common in Asia and Southern Europe than in North America. In addition, IgA nephropathy is rarely familial (<10% of cases of IgA nephropathy), and clusters of cases have been associated with a founder effect. It has a peak incidence in the second and third decades of life and a male preponderance.

IgA nephropathy classically presents as recurrent episodes of gross hematuria during or immediately after an upper respiratory infection (synpharyngitic hematuria). Alternatively, it can present as persistent microscopic hematuria. Proteinuria, which can be in the nephrotic range, if it occurs at all, typically occurs late in the disease course. Rarely, IgA nephropathy can present as RPGN. In most patients, IgA nephropathy is a benign disease, with only 25% to 30% of patients progressing to ESRD over 20 years. Risk factors for progression include hypertension, the absence of macroscopic hematuria, proteinuria, and male gender. Specific diagnosis requires a renal biopsy that demonstrates characteristic dominant IgA mesangial staining on immunofluorescent microscopy (**Web Fig. 29-16**).

Inhibition of the renin-angiotensin system has been demonstrated to slow the progression of multiple glomerular diseases associated with proteinuria, including IgA nephropathy. There is no consensus on multiple other therapies that have been tried in small studies, including fish oil, tonsillectomy, steroid therapy, or cytotoxic therapy. The recommended treatment of IgA nephropathy when it presents as RPGN is plasmapheresis, steroids, and cytotoxic agents.

Henoch-Schönlein purpura is a closely related glomerular disease with indistinguishable biopsy findings. Clinically, it is distinguished from IgA nephropathy by prominent systemic symptoms (including arthralgias), a younger age of onset (usually in childhood), and abdominal complaints.

MEMBRANOPROLIFERATIVE GLOMERULONEPHRITIS

Membranoproliferative glomerulonephritis (MPGN) is a grouping of morphologically related but pathogenically distinct glomerular diseases. MPGN can be idiopathic or secondary to a systemic process. MPGN is rare in African Americans, and the idiopathic disease usually presents in childhood and adolescence. MPGN is subdivided into type I, type II (dense deposit disease), and type III disease. Type I MPGN is associated with hepatitis B, hepatitis C, cryoglobulinemia, systemic lupus, sickle cell anemia, antiphospholipid antibody syndrome, and less commonly, neoplastic diseases. Patients with MPGN type II or dense deposit disease commonly have C_3 nephritic factors, which are antibodies that stabilize the C_3 convertase and allow it to activate serum C_3. Type II is also associated with partial lipodystrophy and factor H deficiency. Type III disease has been reported with complement receptor deficiencies and may also have associated "nephritic factors." Patients with MPGN present with hematuria, proteinuria (nephrotic syndrome most common in type I), pyuria (30%), low C_3 levels (50% to 70%) (see Table 29-3), and in type I, frequent systemic symptoms of fatigue and malaise. Fifteen to 20% of patients with MPGN present with acute nephritis and RPGN (more common in type II). Renal biopsy findings include capillary loop thickening with basement membrane duplication and mesangial hypercellularity, often with lobular segmentation (**Web Fig. 29-17**). In type I, mesangial interposition between the capillary basement membrane and endothelial cells produces a double contour, "tram-tracking" appearance. Fifty percent of patients with MPGN develop ESRD within 10 years after diagnosis, and 90% have renal insufficiency after 20 years. In the presence of proteinuria, treatment with inhibitors of the renin-angiotensin system is indicated. In patients with RPGN, treatment with plasmapheresis, steroids, and cytotoxic agents is often empirically done. Patients with infection-associated MPGN have been reported to respond to treatment of the primary infection. Evidence for specific treatments for idiopathic MPGN is not well established.

THIN BASEMENT MEMBRANE DISEASE

Thin basement membrane disease (TBMD), also known as *benign familial hematuria*, is estimated to affect 1% of the general population. About 50% of patients with TBMD have an autosomal dominant pattern of transmission, and 40% to 50% of patients have mutations in either the COL4A3 or COL4A4 gene. These mutations cause subtle decreases in the $\alpha_3\alpha_4\alpha_5$ collagen IV networks in the GBM. This is in distinction to Alport syndrome, in which the collagen IV networks are lost or severely distorted, but has led some authors to view TBMN as a mild form of collagen IV glomerulopathy and Alport syndrome as a severe form. Patients present with isolated microscopic hematuria. Proteinuria is absent. The diagnosis is confirmed by a renal biopsy revealing attenuated GBM lamina densa, usually less than 250 nm in adults. Distinguishing classic TBMD from Alport syndrome is impor-

tant because in contrast to Alport syndrome, TBMD has a completely benign prognosis.

ALPORT SYNDROME

Alport syndrome, also known as *hereditary nephritis*, encompasses a spectrum of patients with mutations in collagen IV who present with hematuria. About 85% of patients have an X-linked mutation of COL4A5, causing a reduction or distortion in $\alpha_3\alpha_4\alpha_5$ (IV) and in $\alpha_5\alpha_5\alpha_6$ (IV) collagen. Female carriers have variable penetrance depending on the type of mutation or degree of mosaicism. Autosomal recessive disease with mutations in COL4A3 or COL4A4 causing loss of the $\alpha_3\alpha_4\alpha_5$ (IV) networks and autosomal dominant disease with mutations in COL4A3 or COL4A4 causing aberrations of the $\alpha_3\alpha_4\alpha_5$ (IV) network have been reported as well. Patients present with microscopic hematuria, mild proteinuria, and varying degrees of sensorineural deafness; some patients develop lenticonus of the anterior lens capsule. Rarely, mental retardation or leiomyomatosis is associated with Alport syndrome. Male patients are more affected than female patients and far more commonly progress to chronic glomerulosclerosis and ESRD. In the juvenile X-linked form of Alport syndrome, male patients reach ESRD before 30 years of age, and in the adult form, ESRD occurs after 30 years of age. Early severe deafness or lenticonus suggests a poorer prognosis. On skin biopsy, 80% of males with X-linked Alport syndrome have negative staining for α_5 (IV) in the epidermal basement membrane, and mosaic immunostaining is found in 50% of X-linked females with Alport syndrome. When skin biopsies are nondiagnostic in X-linked Alport syndrome (20% to 50%) and in patients with autosomal recessive or dominant Alport syndrome, renal biopsy is performed. Alport syndrome patients early in the disease have thin GBMs, which thicken over time into multilamellations surrounding lucent areas, the so-called split basement membrane. Primary treatment is control of systemic blood pressure using inhibitors of the renin-angiotensin system.

Sickle cell anemia–associated glomerulopathy, ANCA-associated vasculitis, and lupus nephritis can also present with hematuria but are discussed in other sections.

Glomerular Deposition Diseases

SYSTEMIC AMYLOID AND NONAMYLOID MONOCLONAL IMMUNOGLOBULIN DEPOSITION DISEASES

Of patients affected by systemic amyloidosis, about 63% have AL amyloid with deposits of immunoglobulin light chains, 29% have AA amyloid with deposits of serum amyloid A protein fragments, 2% have heredofamilial amyloid, and 5% are undetermined. In primary AL amyloidosis, light chains produced in excess by clonal plasma cell dyscrasias are most commonly of the lambda class (75%). About 10% of these patients have multiple myeloma. In AA amyloidosis, also known as *secondary amyloidosis*, serum amyloid A, an acute-phase reactant, forms deposits in patients with a chronic inflammatory process. Rheumatoid arthritis is the most common inflammatory process and is seen in 40% of patients with AA amyloidosis. Amyloid fibrils can infiltrate the liver, heart, peripheral nerves, carpal tunnel, and kidney. Patients with renal involvement present with proteinuria, often of nephrotic range, and associated renal vein thrombosis can occur. Biopsy of the kidney is diagnostic with positive Congo red staining, positive staining for monoclonal light or heavy chains (30% false-negative results), and 10- to 12-nm nonbranching fibrils seen on electron microscopy (**Web Fig. 29-18**). Hereditary amyloidosis is negative for both monoclonal heavy and lights chains and is diagnosed with stains specific for the abnormal protein deposited (e.g., fibrinogen, transthyretin, apolipoprotein, or lysozyme). Proper identification of hereditary amyloidosis is important because specific therapy such as liver transplantation may be indicated. Treatment of AA and AL amyloidosis is undergoing much change. In patients with AA amyloid, primary treatment of the systemic inflammatory process is critical (colchicine or anticytokine therapies), coupled with new therapeutic strategies such as eprodisate (an amyloid formation–inhibiting compound). AL amyloid treatment is directed at treating the underlying plasma cell dyscrasia, and although high-dose melphalan and steroid treatment with autologous stem cell transplantation have been used, they have been associated with significant toxicity in older patients and in patients with significant renal dysfunction. If multiple myeloma is present, therapy is directed towards this.

The nonamyloid monoclonal immunoglobulin deposition diseases (MIDDs) constitute a varied group of disorders that form Congo red negative deposits. Light-chain (light-chain nephropathy), light-heavy chain, and heavy-chain diseases represent disorders in which granular (not fibrillary) deposits that stain positive for monoclonal light or heavy chains are found on kidney biopsy. Light-chain nephropathy is most commonly seen and is associated with nephrotic syndrome, with 70% of patients progressing to ESRD. Light-chain nephropathy, in contrast to amyloidosis, is associated with predominant κ light chains. Treatment is directed at the plasma cell dyscrasia, and high-dose melphalan and prednisone with autologous stem cell transplantation have been used successfully. Thalidomide and its congeners have also been used as primary therapy. In immunotactoid and fibrillary glomerulonephritis, deposits of oligoclonal or oligotypic immunoglobulins form organized fibrils or tubules. Both disorders appear in adults in the fourth decade, with moderate to heavy proteinuria, hematuria, and a wide variety of associated renal histologic lesions. Treatment is control of systemic blood pressure and proteinuria with agents that block the renin-angiotensin system.

FABRY DISEASE

Fabry disease is an X-linked inborn error of globotriaosylceramide metabolism secondary to deficient lysosomal α-galactosidase A activity. Affected organs include the vascular endothelium, nerves, heart, brain, and kidneys. Renal manifestations of Fabry disease may include mild to moderate proteinuria and sometimes microscopic hematuria or nephrotic syndrome. Renal biopsy is diagnostic with enlarged glomerular visceral epithelial cells packed with vacuoles containing globotriaosylceramide, and focal and segmental scle-

rosis. Treatment with recombinant α-galactosidase A has been demonstrated to clear the microvascular endothelial deposits in the kidneys, heart, and skin.

Glomerular Vascular Syndromes

HYPERTENSIVE NEPHROSCLEROSIS

Although only about 6% of patients with systemic hypertension develop kidney disease, up to one third of patients with ESRD have hypertensive nephrosclerosis as a primary cause. The risk for ESRD from hypertension is far higher in African Americans than Caucasians. Patients present with hypertension, less than 1 to 2 g of proteinuria, and less commonly microscopic hematuria. Episodes of malignant hypertension can be associated with acute kidney injury, nephrotic range proteinuria, or a thrombotic microangiopathic picture that can accelerate the path to ESRD. The diagnosis of hypertensive nephrosclerosis is usually inferred without a renal biopsy. Treatment is blood pressure control. In African Americans with hypertensive nephrosclerosis, antihypertensive therapy initiated with an angiotensin-converting enzyme (ACE) inhibitor has been demonstrated to slow the rate of decline of renal function.

CHOLESTEROL EMBOLI

Patients with underlying atherosclerosis may shower cholesterol crystals into the circulation, most commonly in the presence of a precipitating factor such as angiography or systemic anticoagulation, or less commonly spontaneously. Clinical manifestations include hematuria, mild proteinuria, loss of renal function (often in a stepwise fashion), livedo reticularis, fever, eosinophilia, eosinophiluria, and hypocomplementemia. Biopsy reveals characteristic biconvex clefts in vessels (**Web Fig. 29-19**). Although no specific therapy is of demonstrated benefit, blood pressure control, lipid-lowering agents, and cessation of smoking are reasonable recommendations.

THROMBOTIC THROMBOCYTOPENIC PURPURA AND HEMOLYTIC UREMIC SYNDROME

Thrombotic thrombocytopenic purpura (TTP) and hemolytic uremic syndrome (HUS) share the clinical features of thrombocytopenic purpura and microangiopathic hemolytic anemia (the combination of which is called *thrombotic microangiopathy*) (Table 29-6), fever, acute renal failure, and neurologic disturbances. The differentiation between TTP and HUS is difficult and is sometimes based on prominent renal symptoms or an association with diarrheal illness (Shiga toxin–induced diarrhea) in HUS, in contrast to prominent neurologic symptoms in TTP. In renal biopsy specimens, there is evidence of glomerular capillary endotheliosis with platelet thrombi and the formation of fibrin in and around the glomeruli. The cornerstone of therapy is plasma exchange, which is hypothesized either to remove antibodies to ADAMTS13, a metalloprotease that cleaves large multimers of von Willebrand factor, or to replace a

Table 29-6 **Thrombotic Microangiopathic Glomerulopathies**
Thrombotic thrombocytopenic purpura
Hemolytic uremic syndrome
Malignant hypertension
Scleroderma renal crisis
Preeclampsia, eclampsia
HELLP syndrome (hemolysis, elevated liver enzymes, low platelets)
Antiphospholipid antibody syndrome
Drugs: oral contraceptives, quinine, cyclosporine, tacrolimus, ticlopidine, clopidogrel

deficiency of ADAMTS13. Decreased activity of ADAMTS13 has been implicated in the pathogenesis of TTP and HUS.

ANTIPHOSPHOLIPID ANTIBODY SYNDROME

Antiphospholipid antibody syndrome is a systemic disease etiologically related to the presence of antibodies to anionic phospholipids. It can be idiopathic or associated with systemic lupus, pregnancy, or another primary renal disease. Thrombocytopenia, spontaneous venous or arterial occlusions, and renal manifestations may occur. Kidney injury occurring in about 25% of patients with this syndrome can present as acute renal failure, acute flank pain with renal vein thrombosis, or subacute proteinuria (1 to 2 g per 24 hours) and hematuria. Renal biopsy characteristically reveals occluded vessels, ischemic mesangiolysis, and glomerulosclerosis. The mainstay of treatment is anticoagulation with warfarin.

SICKLE CELL DISEASE

Patients with homozygous SS sickle cell anemia develop chronic vaso-occlusive disease that manifests commonly in the kidney as hyposthenuria early in the disease. Over time, microscopic hematuria, gross hematuria, hypertension, FSGS, interstitial nephritis, renal infarction or MPGN may appear. Treatment involves reducing the frequency of sickle crises and administering inhibitors of the renin-angiotensin system.

Infection-Associated Syndromes

Viral infections can be associated with many different kidney diseases, including glomerulonephritis and the nephrotic syndrome, hematuria, and acute and chronic renal failure. Viruses involved in kidney disease include HIV, hepatitis C, hepatitis B, parvovirus, polyomaviruses, cytomegalovirus, hantavirus, and coronavirus.

HIV-associated nephropathy presents after at least 2 to 3 years of HIV infection and is more common in patients with low CD4 counts and in African Americans. Distinguishing features include the absence of hypertension and well-preserved kidney size despite advanced renal failure, nephrotic syndrome, and a relatively rapid decline in renal function. Renal biopsy most commonly reveals FSGS, typically the collapsing form, but MPGN, IgA nephropathy, MCD, and MGN have all been reported. Because HIV replicates in the kidney, aggressive management to reduce the HIV burden with antiretroviral therapy is indicated. Use of ACE inhibitors has also been reported to slow the rate of decline of renal function.

Chronic hepatitis C infection is strongly associated with MPGN type I with or without mixed IgG and IgM cryoglobulins. Chronic hepatitis B infection can be associated with polyarteritis nodosa, MGN, or less commonly MPGN. Treatment of both these conditions aims at reducing the level of infection.

A variety of other infections can be associated with one or more glomerular lesions. Syphilis can be associated with nephrotic syndrome from MGN; leprosy with focal glomerulonephritis or renal amyloidosis; malaria with mild proteinuria and a mesangioproliferative glomerulonephritis; and schistosomiasis with MPGN.

Prospectus for the Future

The most common cause of glomerular disease and progressive kidney disease is diabetic nephropathy. A strong effort is underway to detect patients at risk for diabetic nephropathy using genetic and other urinary biomarkers through proteomics. By early identification of individuals at risk for kidney failure, novel treatment strategies may be developed that can prevent the progressive loss of kidney function and ESRD.

Additionally, better understanding of the mechanisms of glomerular injury in the various forms of glomerulonephritis has paved the way for development of disease-specific therapy, rather than systemic immunosuppression, to limit the extensive side effects and result in higher remission and cure rates for the disease.

Major Nonglomerular Disorders

James L. Pirkle, Amanda W. Basford, and Roy Zent

The tubulointerstitial compartment comprises the majority of the tissue mass of the kidney and can be affected by a diverse group of disorders, including acute and chronic tubulointerstitial nephritis, stone and cyst formation, and tumors. These disorders can present as acute or chronic renal failure, severe pain, or as incidental radiographic findings. Primary vascular disorders and some forms of acute tubular injury will be discussed in separate chapters.

Acute Interstitial Nephritis

Acute interstitial nephritis (AIN) is a clinicopathologic entity defined as a sudden decrease in renal function caused by acute infiltration of inflammatory cells into the interstitial compartment of the kidney (**Web Figs. 30-1 and 30-2**). AIN accounts for up to 10% to 20% of all cases of acute kidney injury (AKI).

CLINICAL PRESENTATION

The typical presentation of AIN is a sudden decrease in renal function in an otherwise asymptomatic patient recently begun on a new medication. The classic clinical triad of fever, rash, and eosinophilia are manifestations of a systemic hypersensitivity reaction, and any or all of these may be seen in AIN. Another fairly common symptom is lumbar or flank pain, possibly due to distention of the renal capsule. It is important to note that most patients do not have any of these features, and their absence does not preclude the diagnosis of AIN. Importantly, hypertension and edema, features of acute glomerulonephritis, are uncommon in AIN.

Characteristic laboratory tests include elevation of serum creatinine, consistent with acute kidney injury, sterile pyuria, and white blood cell casts. Hansel stain of the urine may demonstrate eosinophils. Although eosinophiluria is strongly suggestive of AIN, it is often not observed. Patients com-monly have non-nephrotic range proteinuria (<1 g per day) and microscopic hematuria. Red blood cell casts are rarely seen. Eosinophilia may be seen on the peripheral blood smear.

ETIOLOGY

Drug reactions are the most common cause of AIN. Antibiotics are the most common offenders, most notably penicillins, cephalosporins, trimethoprim-sulfamethoxazole, and ciprofloxacin. Nonsteroidal anti-inflammatory drugs (NSAIDs) are a well-described cause of AIN, as are proton pump inhibitors such as omeprazole. The second most common cause of AIN is systemic infection. AIN may also be associated with acute pyelonephritis and autoimmune disease. A list of frequent causes of AIN is shown in Table 30-1.

TREATMENT AND PROGNOSIS

Treatment of AIN consists of removal of any suspected offending drug or treatment of the underlying infection or disorder. In cases in which antibiotics are being used to treat infection, another appropriate drug should be substituted. A short treatment with high-dose corticosteroids (prednisone, 1 mg/kg per day for a minimum of 2 weeks) may accelerate recovery if used early in the clinical course.

Most cases of AIN resolve completely after the offending factor has been removed. However, the longer the patient remains in renal failure, the less likely it is that complete recovery of renal function will occur.

Chronic Interstitial Nephritis

Chronic interstitial nephritis (CIN) is a clinicopathologic entity defined as slowly progressive renal insufficiency due to tubular cell atrophy and progressive interstitial fibrosis

Table 30-1 Causes of Acute Interstitial Nephritis

Drugs

Antibiotics

Penicillins
Cephalosporins
Sulfa drugs
Ciprofloxacin
Acyclovir

Nonsteroidal Anti-inflammatory Drugs

Diuretics

Thiazides
Furosemide
Triamterene

Other

Cimetidine
Omeprazole
Phenytoin
Allopurinol

Systemic Infections

Legionnaires disease
Leptospirosis
Streptococcal infection
Cytomegalovirus infection

Primary Kidney Infections

Acute bacterial pyelonephritis

Autoimmune Disorders

Sarcoidosis
Sjögren syndrome

Idiopathic

Table 30-2 Clinical Findings that Suggest Chronic Interstitial Nephritis

Hyperchloremic metabolic acidosis (out of proportion to the degree of renal insufficiency)

Hyperkalemia (out of proportion to the degree of renal insufficiency)

Reduced maximal urinary concentrating ability (polyuria, nocturia)

Partial or complete Fanconi syndrome (phosphaturia, bicarbonaturia, aminoaciduria, uricosuria, glycosuria)

Modest proteinuria (<2 g/day)

caused by a chronic interstitial mononuclear cell infiltrate (**Web Fig. 30-3**). CIN is responsible for 15% to 30% of all cases of end-stage renal disease (ESRD).

CLINICAL PRESENTATION

Patients with CIN are usually asymptomatic until they develop advanced chronic kidney disease (CKD), which is characterized by symptoms of uremia: fatigue, malaise, nausea, nocturia, and sleep disturbance. Patients, might, however present earlier with features of the primary disease that has caused the CIN (see "Etiology" below). CIN is sometimes found incidentally on routine laboratory work (Table 30-2).

Laboratory studies reveal a glomerular filtration rate (GFR) that falls over time, characterized by a slowly rising serum creatinine. Urinalysis commonly reveals non-nephrotic range proteinuria (<1 g per day) and may show microscopic hematuria and pyuria. Because CIN is primarily a disease of the tubules, specific findings of tubular dysfunction might be out of proportion to the degree of renal insufficiency. Examples include lead toxicity and multiple myeloma, which primarily affect the proximal tubule and may present as a proximal renal tubular acidosis (RTA), glycosuria, aminoaciduria, and uricosuria. Chronic urinary obstruction usually causes distal tubular damage and may result in distal RTA, salt wasting, and hyperkalemia. Diseases such as analgesic nephropathy, sickle cell disease, and polycystic kidney disease affect the medullary collecting tubules and may cause polyuria due to urinary concentrating defects.

ETIOLOGY

Many conditions are associated with CIN (Table 30-3). This section highlights the more common causes and describes the appropriate treatment and prognosis for each.

Metabolic Disturbances

Disorders of calcium metabolism that create hypercalcemia can lead to nephrocalcinosis, a deposition of calcium around the tubules and collecting ducts. Nephrocalcinosis may also occur in settings of acute hyperphosphatemia, as has been reported after the use of sodium phosphate solutions for bowel cleansing. CIN associated with nephrocalcinosis may be only slowly and incompletely reversible after the hypercalcemia is resolved.

Prolonged hyperuricemia is associated with chronic renal insufficiency, but it is unclear whether elevated serum urate levels per se result in CIN because chronic hyperuricemia is often associated with stones, hypertension, or renal ischemic disease, all of which may also cause CIN. Primary hyperoxaluria, an inborn error of metabolism, and enteric hyperoxaluria, a syndrome resulting from jejunoileal bypass or other cause of gastrointestinal malabsorption, may lead to progressive CIN and ESRD.

Analgesic Nephropathy

Analgesic nephropathy is a common condition that is caused by medications containing aspirin in combination with acetaminophen, phenacetin, caffeine, or codeine. Acetaminophen (a metabolite of phenacetin) is concentrated in the papillary tips and metabolized to reactive metabolites that can injure cells in the renal papilla, leading to papillary necrosis. The effect is worsened by NSAIDs, which decrease the supply of glutathione and thus decrease reducing potential. CIN usually accompanies the papillary necrosis in this entity. Analgesic nephropathy usually occurs in young women who have co-morbidities of emotional stress, neuropsychiatric disturbances, and gastrointestinal disturbances. Plain computed tomography (CT) of the kidneys may show papillary calcification and an abnormal contour of the renal cortex.

Treatment involves cessation of analgesic use. Progression of renal function loss is usually slowed or even arrested with discontinuation of the offending agents. These offending combination drugs are no longer available in North America or in many other parts of the world.

Table 30-3 Conditions Associated with Chronic Interstitial Nephritis

Hereditary Diseases

Autosomal dominant polycystic kidney disease

Metabolic Disturbances

Hypercalcemia, nephrocalcinosis
Hyperuricemia
Hyperoxaluria
Hypokalemia
Cystinosis

Drugs and Toxins

Analgesics, nonsteroidal anti-inflammatory drugs
Lead
Nitrosoureas
Cisplatin
Cyclosporine
Tacrolimus
Lithium
Chinese herbs

Immune Mediated

Wegener granulomatosis
Sjögren syndrome
Systemic lupus erythematosus
Vasculitis
Sarcoidosis

Hematologic Disease or Malignancy

Multiple myeloma
Sickle cell disease
Lymphoma

Infection

Chronic pyelonephritis, xanthogranulomatous
   pyelonephritis

Obstruction

Tumors
Stones
Bladder outlet obstruction
Vesicoureteral reflux

Miscellaneous

Radiation nephritis
Hypertensive arterionephrosclerosis
Renal ischemic disease

Lead Nephropathy

Occupational lead exposure has declined in the United States owing to strict governmental regulations. Lead can be ingested as a result of contaminated drinking water (from old lead pipes or crystal) or from drinking alcohol made in stills constructed with lead-soldered radiators. Lead is taken up by the proximal tubule cells, where it causes aminoaciduria, glycosuria, and CIN. The classic triad of hypertension, gout, and chronic renal insufficiency may suggest lead nephropathy as the cause. Diagnosis is made by the finding of elevated 24-hour urinary excretion of lead after administration of two 1-g doses of ethylenediaminetetraacetic acid (EDTA).

Treatment of this condition is accomplished using chelation therapy with EDTA, which may arrest or even reverse the CKD.

Chinese Herb Nephropathy

Chinese herb nephropathy (CHN) was first reported in 1992 in a cohort of women from Belgium who had ingested diet pills containing root extracts. Cases have since been reported around the world. CHN usually presents silently, with evidence of renal insufficiency found on routine laboratory studies. Some patients may present with Fanconi syndrome or fatigue from anemia, which tends to be marked in CHN. Aristolochic acid, found in the herb genus *Aristolochia*, was identified as the nephrotoxic component and has reproduced the findings of CHN when administered to rat models. The clinical course is that of a rapidly progressive CIN with accelerated interstitial fibrosis, often leading to ESRD. Treatment consists of discontinuing ingestion of the herbs. Patients should be monitored for urothelial malignancy, which has also been associated with aristolochic acid.

Sarcoidosis

The most common cause of renal dysfunction in patients with sarcoidosis is hypercalcemia. However, sarcoidosis can also cause a noncaseating granulomatous interstitial nephritis that may lead to renal insufficiency in a subset of patients. These patients may develop glycosuria, concentrating defects, and RTA.

Patients with CIN related to sarcoidosis often respond well to corticosteroid therapy. Repeat kidney biopsies after treatment have shown loss of granulomas and lymphocytic infiltrate.

Multiple Myeloma

Multiple myeloma may cause acute and chronic renal dysfunction in a variety of ways. This disease predominantly causes tubulointerstitial pathology, and the most common renal complication is light-chain cast nephropathy (myeloma kidney). Other tubulointerstitial complications include hypercalcemia with nephrocalcinosis, hyperuricemia, and amyloid deposition. In light-chain cast nephropathy, excess light chains produced by the myelomatous plasma cells become trapped in the tubules and associate with Bence Jones proteins to create casts. The tubular cells are damaged as they try to reabsorb the heavy load of filtered light chains. Casts clogging the tubules initiate a multinucleated giant cell inflammatory reaction.

Treatment of light-chain cast nephropathy requires chemotherapy to reduce excess light-chain production, volume repletion, and alkalinization of the urine.

Urinary Tract Obstruction

Urinary tract obstruction is discussed in more detail elsewhere in this chapter. Both acute urinary obstruction and chronic urinary obstruction are associated with a mononuclear cell interstitial infiltrate. Urinary obstruction causes CIN accompanied by impaired excretion of hydrogen ions and potassium and a vasopressin-resistant concentrating defect.

Treatment is relief of the obstruction, which results in halting the progression of loss of renal function.

Radiation Nephritis

Radiation nephritis develops in most patients whose kidneys are exposed to more than 2300 cGy. It may present as an acute severe form of injury within 1 year of the radiation and is associated with the development of hypertension, anemia, and edema. A more insidious chronic form presents with mild renal insufficiency, hypertension, and mild proteinuria.

The pathogenesis of this condition is primarily that of injury to the vascular endothelium, followed by vascular occlusion, tubular atrophy, and eventually interstitial fibrosis.

Hypertensive Arterionephrosclerosis

One of the most common causes of chronic kidney disease in the United States, hypertensive arterionephrosclerosis, begins with arteriolopathy in the afferent arterioles leading to interstitial and glomerular changes likely related to ischemia. Tubular atrophy and interstitial fibrosis are prominent causes of the loss of renal function in these patients. This topic is discussed in detail in Chapter 31.

Urinary Tract Obstruction

Obstruction to urine flow may occur at any point from the renal pelvis to the urethral meatus. Unilateral ureteral obstruction usually causes no detectable change in urine flow or serum creatinine levels, and renal failure occurs only if the drainage of both kidneys is significantly compromised. Total urinary tract obstruction is an important cause of ESRD.

CLINICAL PRESENTATION

A change in urinary habits is often the presenting symptom of urinary tract obstruction. The most common cause of true anuria is complete urinary obstruction and is usually observed in elderly males who present with anuria or symptoms of metabolic disturbance. These patients usually have AKI with markedly elevated creatinine levels accompanied by metabolic acidosis and significant hyperkalemia. Complete urinary obstruction should be considered in any patient who is anuric. Patients with partial bladder outlet obstruction present with urinary hesitancy, decreased urine flow rate, polyuria, and nocturia. This condition is typically found in an elderly male who complains of nocturia and may have a fluctuating serum creatinine. Tubular defects may or may not be evident. Physical examination often reveals an enlarged prostate.

In patients with complete urinary obstruction, renal ultrasound may demonstrate hydronephrosis or hydroureter. However, dilation of the urinary tract may not be evident within the first 24 hours of obstruction or in patients who are volume depleted. The bladder may not even appear distended in patients who have complete urinary obstruction at the bladder outlet. In patients with partial urinary obstruction, renal ultrasound may demonstrate chronically dilated urinary tract, but a normal study does not exclude the diagnosis. A postvoid residual of more than 200 mL is considered abnormal and may suggest bladder outlet obstruction.

ETIOLOGY

Table 30-4 lists the common causes of urinary tract obstruction. The most common cause in adults is prostatic hypertrophy in a male patient.

TREATMENT AND PROGNOSIS

Management of the acute urinary tract obstruction is directed toward identifying the site and cause of obstruction

Table 30-4 **Causes of Urinary Obstruction**
Congenital Urinary Tract Malformation
Meatal stenosis
Ureterocele
Posterior urethral valves
Intraluminal Obstruction
Calculi
Blood clots
Sloughed papillary tissue
Extrinsic Compression
Pelvic tumors
Prostatic hypertrophy
Retroperitoneal fibrosis
Acquired Anomalies
Urethral strictures
Neurogenic bladder
Intratubular precipitates

and alleviating it. In the case of bladder outlet obstruction, this usually involves placement of a urinary catheter. If a ureter is found to be obstructed, surgical intervention, either through a ureteral stent or percutaneous nephrostomy tube, is required. Infection behind an obstruction is considered a urologic emergency and must be relieved. After relief of a complete obstruction, a postobstructive diuresis may be observed and must be monitored closely and treated with volume repletion when necessary. This diuresis is caused partly by the sodium and urea retained during the obstruction and partly by the tubular concentrating defect. There is usually complete recovery of renal function after relief of the acute, complete obstruction.

Management of the chronic partial obstruction depends on the location of the obstruction. If the history and physical examination suggest prostatic hypertrophy, an α_1 antagonist such as tamsulosin or an α-reductase inhibitor such as dutasteride may be used to improve urine flow. This condition often requires surgery to relieve obstruction within the prostate.

Cystic Diseases of the Kidney

Renal cysts are epithelium-lined cavities filled with fluid or semisolid debris. Cysts result from genetic and nongenetic processes and occur in a variety of diseases in both adults and children. Cysts can be simple or complex, and a clear diagnosis of cyst type is required to plan intervention.

SIMPLE CYSTS

Simple cysts are benign, asymptomatic lesions commonly found in normal kidneys. Simple cysts are the most common renal mass, accounting for 65% to 70% of all renal masses, and there is an increasing incidence with age. Cysts may be solitary, multiple, and bilateral and range in size from less than 1 cm to greater than 10 cm.

On ultrasound, simple cysts appear anechoic, have a thin or almost invisible wall, and demonstrate through-transmis-

Table 30-5 Bosniak Renal Cyst Classification Scheme

Category	Description
I—Simple cyst	A benign simple cyst with a thin wall and no septa, calcifications, or solid components.
II—Minimally complicated	A benign cystic lesion with a few thin septa. The wall or septa may contain fine calcifications or short segment of a slightly thickened calcification. (This category also includes uniformly high-attenuating lesions that are less than 3 cm in diameter, well marginated, and nonenhancing.)
IIF—Complicated	Well-marginated cysts, but more complicated than category II. They have multiple thin septa or minimal smooth thickening of the septa or wall and may contain calcifications that may be thick and nodular. (This category also includes totally intrarenal, nonenhancing high-attenuating lesions that are more than 3 cm in diameter.)
III—Indeterminate	Indeterminate cystic masses that have thickened irregular or smooth walls or septa. These lesions are enhancing on computed tomography. Forty to 60% of these lesions are malignant (cystic renal cell carcinoma and multiloculated cystic renal cell carcinoma). The rest of these cysts are hemorrhagic, chronic infected cysts or multiloculated cystic nephroma and are benign.
IV—Malignancy	Eighty-five to 100% of these lesions are malignant. On computed tomography, they have characteristics of category III cysts and contain enhancing soft tissue components that are adjacent to and independent of the wall or septum on the cyst. These lesions should undergo surgical evaluation.

sion because of the rapid progression of the sound waves through fluid when compared with soft tissue.

EVALUATION OF THE COMPLEX CYST

Complex cysts contain calcifications, septations, and mural nodules. These cysts have internal echoes representing hemorrhage, pus, or protein. Complex cysts may be benign or malignant. Malignancy is more likely if the cyst has increased wall nodularity, septations, or vascularity.

With the increased use of various imaging procedures, more and more renal cysts are being identified. To help diagnose and manage these lesions, the Bosniak renal cyst classification system was created. Based on morphologic and enhancement characteristics on CT scanning, cystic renal masses are placed into one of five different categories (Table 30-5).

Category I and II cysts generally do not require further evaluation. In some instances, an ultrasound may be repeated in 6 to 12 months to ensure stability. There is no defined approach to renal cystic lesions with indeterminate findings on ultrasound and CT scanning. Category IIF cysts should be reimaged and followed. The absence of change would point toward a more benign process, whereas progression of the cyst would suggest a neoplastic process and should undergo surgical evaluation. Some authorities suggest all Bosniak category III lesions undergo surgical evaluation owing to the high incidence of malignancy.

Magnetic resonance imaging (MRI) is used to evaluate patients with indeterminate lesions. MRI is useful for characterizing the internal contents of the cysts, differentiating hemorrhage or mucin, and is more sensitive than ultrasound and CT in showing enhancement of the internal septations.

Renal masses are being increasingly identified with the wide use of CT and MRI, and as a result, the role of renal mass biopsy will likely increase. In patients with indeterminate imaging, percutaneous image-guided biopsy appears safe and can provide a diagnosis in up to 80% of cases. A biopsy is required before percutaneous cryoablation of all renal masses.

Autosomal Dominant Polycystic Kidney Disease

Autosomal dominant polycystic kidney disease (ADPKD) is the most common hereditary disorder that causes ESRD and accounts for 8% to 10% of all cases of ESRD. The disease is characterized by cyst formation in the ductal organs, especially the kidney and liver. Patients also have noncystic, extrarenal manifestations such as mitral valve prolapse, intracranial aneurysms, and hernias. Patients usually present in adulthood but may have disease manifestations in infancy.

Polycystic kidneys are diffusely cystic and enlarged. Diagnostic criteria for individuals with a 50% risk by positive family history include two cysts, either bilateral or unilateral, in patients younger than 30 years. The criteria expand to two cysts in both kidneys in patients 30 to 59 years old and at least four cysts in each kidney in patients older than 60 years.

CLINICAL PRESENTATION

ADPKD is a multisystem disorder. Patients can have a reduction in urinary concentrating ability and glomerular hyperfiltration early in the disease. The kidneys will increase in size with age, and the structural abnormalities can lead to pain, hematuria, hypertension, and renal insufficiency. Hematuria occurs in up to 40% of patients at some time during the disease process and can be due to cyst hemorrhage, stone, infection, or tumor. Occasionally, a hemorrhagic cyst will rupture, leading to a significant retroperitoneal bleed that necessitates transfusion. Urinary tract infections are a common occurrence in ADPKD, being more common in women than men. Cyst infections and abscess formation are usually due to retrograde flow of bacteria; therefore, cystitis and asymptomatic bacteriuria should be promptly treated. Nephrolithiasis due to uric acid and calcium oxalate stones occurs in 20% of patients with ADPKD. Urinary stasis in the cysts, along with decreased ammonia excretion, low urinary pH, and low urinary citrate concentration, precipitate stone formation.

Hypertension is a major complication of ADPKD and is present in at least 75% of patients. Undiagnosed hypertension can lead to end-organ damage and has been shown to significantly affect the life expectancy of patients with ADPKD. Hypertension also accelerates the loss of GFR.

Polycystic liver disease is the most common extrarenal manifestation of ADPKD and occurs in both *PKD-1* and non–*PKD-1* genotypes (see "Etiology" below). Liver cysts arise from abnormal development and differentiation of the bile ducts. There is usually preserved liver function, but patients may have biliary hamartomas, biliary fibroadenomas, cystic dilation of peribiliary glands, and dilation of intrahepatic and extrahepatic bile ducts. Estrogen likely contributes to cyst growth, but the use of oral contraceptive pills and hormone replacement therapy is contraindicated only in those patients with significant liver enlargement. Symptoms of polycystic liver disease are usually due to massive liver enlargement or mass effect from a single large or multiple dominant cysts.

Intracranial aneurysms occur in 8% of the ADPKD population and appear to cluster within families. Patients with ADPKD should be screened for intracranial aneurysms if there is a family history of intracranial aneurysm or subarachnoid hemorrhage, previous aneurysm rupture, preparation for elective surgery that may involve hemodynamic instability, or high-risk occupations. Other vascular abnormalities appear to exist, such as thoracic aortic and cervicocephalic arterial dissections and coronary artery aneurysms. Mitral valve prolapse is the most common valvular abnormality and has been found in up to 25% of patients with ADPKD.

ETIOLOGY

The disease is expressed in an autosomal dominant pattern with variable penetrance. Two genes have been identified; *PKD-1* and *PKD-2*, and a third gene may exist. The *PKD-1* and *PKD-2* genes encode the proteins polycystin 1 and polycystin 2, and both proteins are thought to play an important role in the regulation of intracellular calcium homeostasis (**Web Fig. 30-4**). Polycystin 1 is a membrane receptor protein capable of binding and interacting with many proteins, carbohydrates, and lipids and eliciting intracellular responses through phosphorylation pathways. Polycystin 2 is thought to act as a calcium-permeable channel.

Both ADPKD type I and II have similar pathologic and physiologic features, but type II usually has a later onset of symptoms and a slower disease progression. Patients with mutations in both the *PKD-1* and *PKD-2* genes (transheterozygotes) have a more severe clinical course than patients with a mutation in only one of the genes.

TREATMENT AND PROGNOSIS

Treatment is directed at preventing complications of the disease and preserving renal function. Patients with flank pain should be evaluated for infection of cysts, stones, or tumor. If multiple cysts are contributing to pain, surgical decompression is effective in 80% to 90% of patients at 1 year, and 62% to 77% have sustained relief for greater than 2 years. Laparoscopic and retroperitoneoscopic nephrec-

tomy and arterial embolization can be used to treat symptomatic polycystic kidneys.

Blood pressure control is essential to prevent end-organ damage and delay progression of CKD. ACE inhibitors or angiotensin receptor blockers may have renoprotective properties in addition to blood pressure lowering properties.

ESRD occurs in 50% of patients by the age of 57 to 73 years. Risk factors for progressive renal failure include *PKD-1* genotype, male gender, diagnosis before the age of 30 years, first episode of hematuria before 30 years old, and onset of hypertension before 35 years old.

Patients who progress to ESRD tend to have a better prognosis on dialysis than those patients with ESRD from other causes. Females also tend to have a better prognosis. Patients also have higher endogenous erythropoietin and have better maintenance of hemoglobin. Peritoneal dialysis can be performed despite renal size, but patients are at increased risk for inguinal and umbilical hernias.

Autosomal Recessive Polycystic Kidney Disease

Autosomal recessive polycystic kidney disease (ARPKD) is much rarer than the autosomal dominant form; the incidence is about 1 in 20,000 live births and often leads to fetal or neonatal death due to significant bilateral renal enlargement resulting in impaired lung function and pulmonary hypoplasia.

CLINICAL PRESENTATION

The diagnosis of ARPKD can be suggested on fetal ultrasound. The fetus may have enlarged echogenic kidneys and oligohydramnios, and decreased bladder urine may be seen as early as 16 weeks.

ETIOLOGY

ARPKD is due to mutations in the *PKHD-1* gene. The disease typically starts in utero, and cystic development is superimposed on a normal developmental sequence. The tubules develop a fusiform dilation of the collecting ducts. Patients present with biliary abnormalities due to defective remodeling of the ductal plate in utero, and primitive bile duct configuration will persist, leading to progressive portal fibrosis and congenital hepatic fibrosis.

TREATMENT AND PROGNOSIS

The estimated perinatal mortality rate is 30% to 50%. For infants who survive past 1 year of life, the mean 5-year patient survival rate is 80% to 95%. Progression to ESRD is highly variable. Hypertension usually develops in the first months of life and affects 70% to 80% of patients. Children who present later in childhood or adolescence frequently have portal hypertension as the predominant feature. These patients can develop hepatosplenomegaly and bleeding esophageal or gastric varices, thrombocytopenia due to hypersplenism, anemia, and leukopenia. In patients with

ESRD and severe portal hypertension, combined liver-kidney transplantation may be indicated.

Juvenile Nephronophthisis–Medullary Cystic Disease Complex

CLINICAL PRESENTATION

Juvenile nephronophthisis (NPHP) and medullary cystic disease complex share the same histopathologic features. These two disorders differ only in their mode of transmission and onset. Both are characterized by small, shrunken kidneys with cysts restricted to the medulla. Decreased urinary concentrating capacity, polyuria, and polydipsia are common symptoms in both.

Juvenile nephronophthisis is an autosomal recessive disorder that presents in childhood, and medullary cystic kidney disease is an autosomal dominant disorder that occurs in adults. Juvenile nephronophthisis is much more common than medullary cystic kidney disease.

ETIOLOGY

Six genes (*NPHP-1* to *NPHP-6*) have been identified in juvenile NPHP. The disease accounts for 6% to 15% of ESRD in children and adolescents. Three different forms have been described based on the age of onset of ESRD (infantile, juvenile, and adolescent). The juvenile and adolescent forms are nearly indistinguishable with regard to clinical, pathologic, and genetic analyses and therefore are referred to as *juvenile NPHP*.

TREATMENT AND PROGNOSIS

In juvenile NPHP, the most common form, ESRD occurs at a mean age of 13 years; the onset of ESRD in the infantile form usually occurs before 5 years old. Decreased urinary concentrating capacity usually precedes the decline in renal function; onset occurs in the school-aged child. Salt wasting develops in most patients with renal insufficiency, and sodium supplementation is often required until ESRD occurs.

Ten to 15% of children with juvenile NPHP have extrarenal abnormalities. Retinal abnormalities are the most common finding. Short stature, oculomotor apraxia (Cogan syndrome), mental retardation, and bone abnormalities have also been described. Congenital hepatic fibrosis occasionally occurs.

Acquired Cystic Kidney Disease

CLINICAL PRESENTATION

Acquired cystic kidney disease (ACKD) is a complication of CKD and is defined as more than three to five macroscopic cysts in each kidney of a patient who does not have a heredity cystic kidney disease. There is a high association with renal neoplasms, and it has been suggested that ACKD should be considered preneoplastic.

The prevalence of ACKD in dialysis patients ranges from 5% to 20%, and it is seen in about 80% to 100% of patients on dialysis for 10 years or longer. There is equal occurrence in patients on hemodialysis or peritoneal dialysis. The course of ACKD is variable after transplantation. If the renal allograft has good long-term function, cyst growth may slow or regress. However, if the graft function is impaired or failing, there may be further progression in the native kidneys and possible development of de novo ACKD in the graft.

ETIOLOGY

Various factors are thought be involved in the development of ACKD, but the slow, progressive parenchymal loss appears to be the most important process. The loss of nephrons with CKD stimulates compensatory growth of remaining, intact nephrons, which is characterized by initial hypertrophy followed by hyperplasia. A cyst will develop from these hyperplastic tubules if transepithelial fluid secretion continues with impairment of distal outflow.

TREATMENT AND PROGNOSIS

There is nearly a 40-fold increased risk for renal cell carcinoma (RCC) in patients with ACKD compared with the general population. There is an increased risk for malignant transformation in males, African Americans, long duration of dialysis, and severe ACKD with significant organ enlargement. Compared with sporadic RCC, ACKD-associated RCC is characterized by younger patient age, male predominance, more frequent multiple and bilateral manifestations, and less aggressive behavior.

Up to 25% of kidneys with acquired cystic disease harbor tumors, about one third of which are carcinomas. Because of the high risk for malignant transformation, screening for ACKD is advocated, but there is no consensus screening strategy. Screening during transplantation evaluation is recommended with ultrasonography followed by CT of suspicious lesions based on the prevalence of renal cancer in up to 4% of the patients and concerns about the role of immunosuppression in accelerating tumor growth.

Renal Tumors

RENAL CELL CARCINOMA

The most common primary renal neoplasm is RCC, and it accounts for 85% of all primary renal malignancies. RCC accounts for 2% to 3% of all cancers and 2% of cancer deaths worldwide.

The clinical presentation of RCC may vary widely, from an incidental finding on imaging obtained for other clinical indications to the classic clinical triad of flank pain, hematuria, and palpable abdominal renal mass. Fever occurs in up to 20% of patients with RCC and is one of the most common presenting symptoms. Other common presenting symptoms include anorexia, weight loss, and fatigue. Many RCCs are clinically occult for much of their courses and end up presenting with signs and symptoms of metastatic disease. Anemia is one of the most common laboratory findings, occurring in 20% to 40%. Paraneoplastic syndromes may occur with RCC, including hepatic dysfunction thought due to cytokine overproduction (Stauffer syndrome), hypercalcemia due to parathyroid-like hormone production, and erythrocytosis due to erythropoietin overproduction.

RCCs are classified according to cell type, of which there are five: clear cell, chromophilic, chromophobic, oncocytic, and collecting duct. The clear cell type is the most common, making up 75% to 85% of all RCCs. Clear cell carcinomas are characterized by a deletion in one or both copies of chromosome 3p. As mentioned later, patients with a mutated *VHL* tumor suppressor gene are at increased risk for clear cell RCC.

Treatment and prognosis are based on staging. Prognosis is excellent for disease that is confined to the kidney. The mainstay of treatment is nephrectomy, which has been shown to be beneficial even in locally invasive disease. Traditional chemotherapy has been largely ineffective in treating RCC. Immunotherapy using interleukin-2 (IL-2) gives somewhat better results, with response rates between 20% to 40%. IL-2 therapy is often limited by toxicity, with a major side effect being renal failure. Molecular targeted therapy directed against the vascular endothelial growth factor (VEGF) pathway and mammalian target of rapamycin (mTOR) have shown some promise in treating RCC. In general, if RCC can be completely surgically resected, the prognosis is good; however, if metastatic disease is present, prognosis is poor, with a 5-year survival rate of 10%.

TUBEROUS SCLEROSIS COMPLEX

Tuberous sclerosis complex is an autosomal dominant, tumor suppressor gene syndrome with tumor-like malformations, hamartomas, which can be found in the brain, kidneys, heart, lungs, and skin. TSC is due to an inactivating mutation in one of two genes, *TSC-1* on chromosome 9 and *TSC-2* on chromosome 16, adjacent to the *PKD-1* gene. Mutations lead to disruption of cell migration and differentiation of neural crest derivatives.

TSC affects 1 in 6000 people with variable disease penetrance. Two thirds of TSC cases appear to result from new mutations, and new mutations are more common in the *TSC-2* gene. The clinical manifestations of *TSC-2*–linked disease tend to be more severe. Patients may have seizures, mental retardation or autism, and skin lesions, and tumors in the brain, retina, kidney, and heart are common. Kidney involvement frequently occurs in TSC with angiomyolipomas, cysts, and renal malignancies. Angiomyolipomas are hamartomatous structures composed of abnormal, thick-walled vessels, varying amounts of smooth muscle cells, and adipose tissue. Angiomyolipomas are seen in about 80% of patients with TSC by the age of 10 years and increase in frequency and size with age. These tumors are benign and often require no treatment. However, they can grow and become locally invasive and may cause bleeding, pain, and hypertension. Annual evaluation with either ultrasound or CT is recommended. Female sex hormones may accelerate the growth of these lesions, and patients should be cautioned about the use of estrogen treatment and pregnancy.

Renal cysts occur less frequently than angiomyolipomas, but similarly increase in size and number with age. The occurrence of both cysts and angiomyolipomas is strongly suggestive of TSC. Strict blood pressure control is the mainstay of treatment for cystic disease.

Benign and malignant tumors of the kidney can occur in patients with TSC. The lifetime risk of a malignancy in the kidney in a patient with TSC is about 2% to 3%. TSC-associated renal carcinomas include clear cell, papillary, and chromophobe carcinomas. These carcinomas are often bilateral and occur with a higher frequency and earlier age of onset than in the general population.

CKD can occur but is rare. Decline in renal function is usually due to angiomyolipoma-parenchyma destruction, progressive renal cystic disease, interstitial fibrosis, and focal segmental glomerulosclerosis.

VON HIPPEL-LINDAU DISEASE

Von Hippel-Lindau disease (VHL) is an autosomal dominant disease that predisposes patients to tumors of the eyes, cerebellum, spinal cord, adrenal glands, pancreas, and epididymis, as well as renal and pancreatic cysts. RCC is one of the most common tumors in VHL, and reports indicate RCC occurs in up to 75% of patients by age 60 years. A germline mutation in the *VHL* tumor suppressor gene on chromosome 3 has been found; VHL is familial in 80% of cases and due to a new mutation in the remaining 20%. The incidence is 1 in 36,000 newborns.

The disease is subclassified by the risk for pheochromocytoma. Type I has a low risk for developing pheochromocytomas, whereas type II carries a high risk for developing pheochromocytomas. Type II is further divided according to the risk for developing RCC. There is a low risk for RCC in type 2A and a high risk in type 2B. In type 2C, patients will have familial pheochromocytoma without other VHL-associated malignancies.

In an individual at risk for VHL, the diagnosis is made if a single retinal or cerebellar hemangioblastoma, RCC, or pheochromocytoma is present. In presumed sporadic cases, diagnosis requires two or more retinal or central nervous system hemangioblastomas or a single hemangioblastoma and a characteristic visceral tumor.

The RCCs are usually the clear cell type, multiple and bilateral. They are often detected as an incidental finding on imaging or routine screening in patients with a family history of VHL. RCCs usually present by 35 to 40 years of age. VHL-associated RCC metastasizes to the lymph nodes, liver, lungs, and bones and accounts for about 50% of all VHL deaths.

Nephrolithiasis

Nephrolithiasis is a common disease, and the prevalence is rising in the United States and other developed countries. Up to 10% of all Americans will develop a stone in their lifetime. Lifestyle factors, medical conditions, and medications all contribute to stone formation. Population-based

Table 30-6 **Medications Associated with Stone Formation**	
Medication	**Mechanism**
Acetazolamide	Hypocitraturia
Vitamin C	Hypocitraturia
Calcium supplements	
Vitamin D	Hypercalciuria
Antacids	Hypercalciuria
Theophylline	Hypercalciuria
Nifedipine	Hypercalciuria
Probenecid, ASA	Hyperuricosuria
Topamax	Hypocitraturia
Indinavir	Precipitation within the tubule
Acyclovir	Precipitation within the tubule

Table 30-7 **Urinalysis and Radiographic Findings of Renal Calculi**		
Stone Type	**Urine Microscopic**	**Radiologic**
Calcium oxalate monohydrate Calcium oxalate dehydrate	Dumbbell shaped; under polarized light appear coarse, needle shaped Envelope shaped	Opaque, round, multiple calculi
Struvite, magnesium ammonium phosphate	Coffin lid	Opaque, may be staghorn
Uric acid	Pleomorphic, often rhombic plates or rosettes	Radiolucent
Cystine	Hexagonal	Opaque

studies suggest that diabetes mellitus, obesity, and hypertension are associated with nephrolithiasis. Kidney stone disease occurs more frequently in men than women and is more common in white than African American populations.

CLINICAL PRESENTATION

The risk for recurrence after the initial episode is about 50% within 5 years, and nearly two thirds of patients have recurrence by 10 years. Patients present with severe flank pain with or without hematuria, and a possible history of passing "gravel" in their urine. Nephrolithiasis may sometimes be associated with polyuria, dysuria, and vomiting.

When eliciting the patient's history, one should inquire about prior hematuria or kidney stones, urinary tract infection, past medical history, medications (Table 30-6), family history, and a lifestyle and dietary analysis. Laboratory examinations should include serum electrolytes, creatinine, calcium, phosphorous, and uric acid levels. Urinalysis is needed for determination of pH, hematuria, evaluation of possible infection, and identification of the type of crystal. Urinalysis findings seen in stone disease are indicated in Table 30-7. It is recommended to capture and analyze passed kidney stones.

The diagnosis is initially suspected by clinical presentation. A noncontrast helical CT scan with 3- to 5-mm sections is currently the preferred diagnostic test in patients with suspected nephrolithiasis and will also show urinary tract obstruction. Renal ultrasonography is an alternative in pregnant women, but routine ultrasound cannot localize ureteral stones, which can be detected by transvaginal ultrasonography.

There is disagreement on the extent of evaluation after the first episode of kidney stones; however, because of the high rate of recurrence, a full metabolic evaluation after the first episode should be completed in any patient willing to make lifestyle changes and should always be undertaken in those with recurrent stone disease. Routine chemistries, calcium, and parathyroid hormone level should be obtained. About 2 months after the initial stone episode, at least two separate 24-hour urine collections should be obtained while the patient maintains his or her usual diet and physical activities. The urine volume, pH, and excretion of calcium, uric acid, citrate, oxalate, sodium, and creatinine (to assess completeness of collection) should be measured. Monitoring kidney stones should be performed initially at 1 year, and if negative, every 2 to 4 years unless the patient develops new symptoms consistent with recurrent stones. If multiple stones are present, the radiologist should document the number of stones to monitor progression.

ETIOLOGY

Kidney stones are more likely to occur when one or more factors that lead to supersaturation of the urine, precipitation of crystals, and subsequent aggregation into a clinically detectable stone are present. The main nonsystemic causes of stones include idiopathic hypercalciuria, hypocitraturia, hyperoxaluria, hyperuricosuria, and low urine volume and low pH. The specific types of stones are outlined in more detail later.

TREATMENT AND PROGNOSIS

Stone size is the major determinant of the likelihood of spontaneous stone passage; however, location of stone is also important. Stones less than 4 mm in diameter pass spontaneously. As stone size increases above 4 mm, there is a progressive decrease in the spontaneous passage rate. Stones greater than 10 mm in diameter are unlikely to pass. Proximal ureter stones are also less likely to pass spontaneously.

All patients with stones should be instructed to drink enough fluid to make at least 2 L per day of urine. This will increase urine flow rate and lower the urine solute concentration, both of which protect against stone formation. Both calcium channel blockers (nifedipine) and α blockers (tamsulosin) have been shown to increase the likelihood of stone passage when compared with conservative treatment. Studies comparing the two medications have reported similar or slightly higher rates of stone passage with tamsulosin. Specific treatment modalities may be implemented when the metabolic risk factors for stone formation are identified (Table 30-8). Urgent urologic consultation is indicated in patients with urosepsis, acute renal failure, anuria, unyielding pain, nausea, or vomiting.

Table 30-8 Treatment Modalities for Different Nephrolithiasis Risk Factors

Urinary Abnormality	Dietary Change	Medication
High calcium	Adequate dietary calcium intake Reduce animal protein intake Reduce sodium intake to <3 g/day	Thiazide
High oxalate	Avoid high oxalate foods Adequate dietary calcium intake	Consider vitamin B_6
High uric acid	Reduce purine intake	Allopurinol
Low citrate	Increase fruit and vegetable intake Reduce animal protein intake	Alkali (K citrate)
Low volume	Increase total fluid intake; goal to produce at least 2 L/day of urine	N/A

Table 30-9 Principle Risk Factors for Calcium Stone Formation

Higher urine calcium

Higher urine oxalate

Lower urine citrate

Lower urine volume

Dietary factors, including a low intake of fluid, calcium, potassium, and phytate, and a high intake of sodium, sucrose, and protein

Medical conditions, including primary hyperparathyroidism, obesity, gout, diabetes, and medullary sponge kidney

Calcium Stones

About 80% of patients with kidney stone disease form calcium stones. These stones are predominantly made of calcium oxalate, but a majority also contain calcium phosphate, mainly as apatite. Calcium phosphate and calcium oxalate stones are associated with the same risk factors. These are shown in Table 30-9.

Hypercalciuria can occur in the presence or absence of hypercalcemia. Hypercalcemia can be due to primary hyperparathyroidism, sarcoidosis, immobilization, neoplasms, excess vitamin A, excess vitamin D, or calcium supplementation. However, about 50% of patients have hypercalciuria in the absence of any identifiable cause of hypercalcemia and exhibit normal serum calcium and parathyroid hormone levels. Hypercalciuria tends to be familial and can be due to increased intestinal absorption ("absorptive hypercalciuria"), increased bone resorption ("resorptive hypercalciuria"), and increased renal losses ("renal hypercalciuria"), in which there is a defect in renal tubular calcium reabsorption. Most individuals with hypercalciuria exhibit more than one abnormality. The underlying mechanisms for idiopathic hypercalciuria are unknown, but 1,25-dihydoxyvitamin D and the vitamin D receptor may play an important role.

The urine pH contributes to the likelihood of formation of certain stones. Acidic urine favors uric acid precipitation, and calcium stones can form around a uric acid stone nidus. Increased animal protein intake leads to an increased acid load and results in increased urinary calcium excretion. The high protein intake also increases urinary calcium excretion by increasing the GFR.

Low urinary citrate excretion is a risk factor for calcium stone formation. Urinary citrate binds to urinary calcium forming a soluble complex and decreasing free ionic calcium for calcium oxalate stone formation. Urinary citrate also acts as an inhibitor of calcium oxalate crystal aggrega-

tion and growth. Citrate is normally reabsorbed in the proximal tubule, and reabsorption is increased in the presence of acidosis. Hypocitraturia is defined as citrate excretion below 320 mg per day. Several causes of hypocitraturia have been identified, including RTA, chronic diarrhea and malabsorption, metabolic acidosis, and hypokalemia. Potassium depletion causes decreased intracellular potassium and decreased intracellular pH and increases hydrogen secretion into the tubular lumen, causing hypocitraturia. A diet high in animal protein can cause hypocitraturia due to increased acid generation and excretion. If a patient has hypocitraturia, supplementing citrate intake with potassium citrate will increase urinary citrate excretion. A higher potassium intake may increase urinary citrate excretion (potassium-rich foods tend to have a high alkali content), thereby increasing the inhibitory properties of urine.

Hyperoxaluria may be present in up to 40% of male and 15% of female stone formers and is usually only mildly elevated. Oxalate is a product of the normal metabolism of glycine and ascorbic acid. There is a significantly increased risk for stone formation with urinary oxalate excretion above 25 mg per day. Dietary calcium can decrease oxalate absorption in the gut by formation of insoluble calcium oxalate salts in the intestinal lumen. Dietary magnesium may also reduce the risk for stone formation by the same mechanism, but the effect may be minor.

Marked hyperoxaluria is usually associated with inflammatory bowel disease, jejunoileal bypass, or intestinal resection and malabsorption because these patients have malabsorption of fatty acids and bile salts. There is an increase in oxalate reabsorption and excretion due to binding of free calcium to fatty acids in the intestinal lumen and to increased colonic permeability to small molecules such as oxalate.

Patients with diarrhea and malabsorption may have additional risk factors for stone formation in addition to increased oxalate absorption. Diarrheal fluid losses can result in decreased urine volume and a metabolic acidosis, which leads to a low urine pH and a decrease in citrate excretion; low urine pH can also promote uric acid stone formation. Patients with partial ileal bypass for obesity may have an incidence of kidney stones as high as 4% per year. It is postulated that low urine volumes, high oxalate, and a high rate of other stone risk factors such as low citrate all contribute to the increased recurrence.

Primary hyperoxaluria is a rare disorder in which enzyme deficiencies lead to an overproduction of oxalate from glyoxylate.

Ingestion of high doses of vitamin C can cause increased oxalate generation due to metabolism of ascorbic acid. Metabolic studies have shown that ingestion of 2000 mg per day of vitamin C significantly increases oxalate excretion in a large proportion of calcium oxalate stone formers.

If hyperoxaluria is present, patients should be instructed to follow a low oxalate diet and limit vitamin C ingestion. A deficiency of oxalate degradation by *Oxalobacter formigenes* in the intestine may contribute to increased absorption and urinary excretion of oxalate.

If urine calcium is elevated, attempts to lower the urine calcium concentration should be instituted by using a thiazide diuretic. Thiazide diuretics, the drug of choice for treatment of hypercalciuria, work at the distal convoluted tubule to inhibit Na and Cl transport and increase renal calcium reabsorption. During chronic treatment with thiazide diuretics, patients develop extracellular fluid volume contraction, and patients will increase NaCl reabsorption, with an associated passive reabsorption of calcium in the proximal tubule. A high sodium intake will also enhance the excretion of calcium because passive reabsorption of calcium in the proximal tubule follows gradients established by NaCl and water reabsorption.

URIC ACID STONES

Uric acid stones are caused by the precipitation of uric acid in the urine. Risk factors include dehydration, persistently acidic urine, hyperuricosuria due to overproduction of uric acid, or increased secretion associated with RTA. Uric acid stones are radiolucent stones.

A high intake of animal protein may increase the risk for uric acid stone formation owing to its high purine content. Furthermore, metabolism of animal protein leads to increased acid production due to the higher sulfur-containing amino acid content of animal protein and subsequently lowers urinary pH.

Diabetes mellitus may be a risk factor for the development of uric acid stones. This hypothesis is based on the observation that patients with recurrent uric acid stones tend to have metabolic and clinical findings characteristic of metabolic syndrome, including obesity. In addition, insulin appears to stimulate ammoniagenesis and sodium-hydrogen exchange in the proximal tubule. Therefore, insulin resistance impairs renal ammoniagenesis, resulting in a net lower urinary pH and increased risk for uric acid stone formation.

Alkali therapy is the most effective treatment of existing uric acid stones. Pure uric acid stones dissolve if urine pH is maintained at or above 6.5. Low doses of alkali on a daily basis can prevent new uric acid stone formation. Allopurinol is an additional agent that can be used if a patient has marked hyperuricosuria.

STRUVITE STONES

Struvite stones are composed of magnesium ammonium phosphate with variable amounts of calcium carbonate-apatite. Struvite stones occur in the presence of chronic urinary tract infection with urease-producing bacteria (Table 30-10). Bacterial urease acts on urine urea to yield ammonia and carbon dioxide; these are further hydrolyzed into ammonium and carbonate, resulting in a urine pH greater

Table 30-10 **Urease Producing Bacteria**
Most species of *Proteus* and *Providencia*
Klebsiella
Pseudomonas
Serratia
Haemophilus
Staphylococcus
Corynebacterium

than 7.2. The alkaline urine is ideal for struvite stone formation.

Struvite stones account for less than 10% of all stones and most often occur in patients with increased frequency of urinary tract infection, such as patients with spinal cord injuries, neurogenic bladder, urinary diversion, or chronic indwelling Foley catheters.

Clinically, patients present with urinary tract infection, hematuria, flank pain, or obstructive uropathy. In rare instances, patients with chronic renal obstruction and infection can develop xanthogranulomatous pyelonephritis, which is a rare inflammatory condition in which the renal parenchyma becomes atrophic and is replaced by fat, pus, and cellular debris.

All struvite stones are infected because they occur in the region surrounding bacterial colonies. When struvite stones are calcified, they present radiographically with a characteristic multilobular shape and laminated appearance and may extend to involve all calyces, forming staghorn calculi. The only curative treatment is eradication of the infection with antimicrobials and removal of all stone material. Percutaneous nephrostolithotomy and extracorporeal shock-wave lithotripsy are the first-line treatment. Chronic antibiotic therapy may limit stone growth and may lead to partial dissolution in nonsurgical patients.

CYSTINE STONES

Cystinuria is an autosomal recessive trait in which patients have excess excretion of cystine into the urine and form cystine stones. The incidence of cystinuria varies from 1 in 20,000 to 1 in 15,000 live births and is highest in Scandinavia. The solubility of cystine in the urine is about 300 mg/L, and when overexcretion leads to higher concentrations than the solubility limit, cystine stones tend to form.

Clinically, patients present during the second or third decade of life with nephrolithiasis. Urinary tract obstruction, recurrent infection, and hypertension can occur, and on occasion the patient may have progressive kidney failure and require dialysis or transplantation. If transplantation is required, the disease does not appear to recur in the transplanted kidney.

Treatment is aimed at reducing the excretion and increasing the solubility of cystine. Lowering urinary cystine concentrations by increasing urinary volume reduces the likelihood of precipitation of cystine stones. An intake of more than 4 L per day may be required to reduce the solubility of cystine. The use of sulfhydryl agents to produce soluble mixed disulfides instead of cystine has been the mainstay of medical treatment. In the past, D-penicillamine was used for treatment because the drug forms a mixed disulfide with cystine and reduces cystine excretion. However, long-term use is limited by the undesirable side effects of D-penicillamine, including nephrotic syndrome, membranous nephropathy, serum sickness, fever, rash, and pancytopenia.

A newer drug, mercaptopropionylglycine (Thiola), is also capable of reducing the free cystine concentration of the urine; side effects are less common, making it the preferable choice for the treatment of cystinuria.

Captopril, a sulfhydryl-containing angiotensin-converting enzyme II inhibitor, has been studied in the treatment of cystine stones. Study results are mixed; some studies show a reduction in cystine excretion, whereas others do not. Cystine stones are refractory to extracorporeal shock-wave lithotripsy.

Cystinuria should not be confused with cystinosis. Cystinosis is also a genetic disorder, but patients have intracellular accumulation of cystine leading to widespread tissue damage, including renal failure. Patients with cystinuria only have increased excretion and accumulation of the amino acid in the tubular lumen.

Prospectus for the Future

- Vasopressin receptor antagonists may be a new treatment option in the future for polycystic kidney disease. Phase III, multicenter, randomized controlled trials are underway to evaluate the long-term safety and efficacy of oral tolvaptan in adults with PKD.
- Obstruction is a reversible cause of acute renal failure that can lead to CKD and should be evaluated as a possible cause in patients who present with renal insufficiency.

- Antibiotics and cytotoxic or immunosuppressive agents are useful therapeutic agents but can cause AIN. Patients should be monitored closely when these agents are used. Combination analgesics should be avoided. Efforts should be made to increase the public's awareness of the risk for AIN caused by over-the-counter and imported herbal remedies.

References

Debelle FD, Vanherweghem JL, Nortier JL: Aristolochic acid nephropathy: A worldwide problem. Kidney Int 74:158-169, 2008.

Floege J, Eitner, F: Acquired cystic kidney disease and malignancies in chronic kidney disease. In Johnson RJ, Feehally J (eds): Comprehensive Clinical Nephrology, 3rd ed. Philadelphia, Elsevier, 2007, pp 911-916.

Gabow PA: Autosomal dominant polycystic kidney disease [review]. N Engl J Med 329:332-342, 1993.

Guay-Woodford L: Other cystic kidney diseases. In Johnson RJ, Feehally J (eds): Comprehensive Clinical Nephrology, 3rd ed. Philadelphia, Elsevier, 2007, pp 519-534.

Hruska KA, Beck AM: Nephrolithiasis. In Schrier R (ed): Diseases of the Kidney and Urinary Tract, 8th ed. Philadelphia, Lippincott Williams & Wilkins, 2007, pp 575-576, 736-737.

Jonasch E, George DJ, Atkins MB: Renal neoplasia. In Brenner BM (ed): Brenner and Rector's The Kidney, 7th ed. Philadelphia, WB Saunders, 2004, pp 1895-1927.

Kelly CJ, Neilson EG: Tubulointerstitial diseases. In Brenner BM (ed): Brenner and Rector's The Kidney, 7th ed. Philadelphia, WB Saunders, 2004, pp 1483-1513.

Lieske JC, de la Vega LS, Gettman MT, et al: Diabetes mellitus and the risk of urinary tract stones: A population-based case-control study. Am J Kidney Dis 48:897-904, 2006.

Monk RD, Bushinsky DA: Nephrolithiasis and nephrocalcinosis. In Johnson RJ, Feehally J (eds): Comprehensive Clinical Nephrology, 3rd ed. Philadelphia, Elsevier, 2007, pp 641-656.

O'Sullivan DA, Torres VE: Autosomal dominant polycystic kidney disease. In Johnson RJ, Feehally J (eds): Comprehensive Clinical Nephrology, 3rd ed. Philadelphia, Elsevier, 2007, pp 505-518.

Odvina CV: Comparative value of orange juice versus lemonade in reducing stone-forming risk. Clin J Am Soc Nephrol 1:1269-1274, 2006.

Parks JH, Coward M, Coe FL: Correspondence between stone composition and urine supersaturation in nephrolithiasis. Kidney Int 51:894-900, 1997.

Rose BD, Post TW: Proximal tubule. In Rose BD, Post TW (eds): Clinical Physiology of Acid-Base and Electrolyte Disorders, 5th ed. New York, McGraw Hill, 2001, pp 92-94.

Seiner R, Ebert D, Nicolay C, Hesse A: Dietary risk factors for hyperoxaluria in calcium oxalate stone formers. Kidney Int 63:1037-1043, 2003.

Taylor EN, Curhan GC: Diet and fluid prescription in stone disease. Kidney Int 70:825-839, 2006.

Taylor EN, Curhan GC: Body size and 24-hour urine composition. Am J Kidney Dis 48:905-915, 2006.

Wilson PD: Mechanisms of disease: Polycystic kidney disease. N Engl J Med 350:151-164, 2004.

Zeidel ML, Pirtskhalaishvili G: Urinary tract obstruction. In Brenner BM (ed): Brenner and Rector's The Kidney, 7th ed. Philadelphia, WB Saunders, 2004, pp 1867-1895.

Vascular Disorders of the Kidney

James M. Luther and Gerald Schulman

Vascular disorders are the most common causes of chronic kidney disease (CKD) in the industrialized world, largely because of the increasing burden of diabetes and hypertension. Atherosclerotic renovascular disease is a common cause of CKD and hypertension, responsible for a syndrome of ischemic renal disease. Added to this are diseases of the vasculature that are mediated by inflammatory and immunologic processes.

Normal function of the microvasculature (arterioles, glomeruli, and capillaries) and vascular endothelium is essential for maintenance of all aspects of renal function but may be altered by a number of clinically important diseases. Preeclampsia, thrombotic thrombocytopenic purpura (TTP), hemolytic uremic syndrome (HUS), and cholesterol emboli are the principal diseases altering microvascular function, each with its own distinct pathogenesis and clinical characteristics. Advances in molecular biology have led to a more detailed understanding of these processes, and now laboratory tests are available to aid in the diagnosis of TTP that were not possible even a decade ago. Similar insights into the pathogenesis of preeclampsia and HUS have also deepened our understanding of renal and endothelial function.

Renal Vascular Anatomy

The renal arteries arise directly from the aorta and enter the renal hilum. The right renal artery must pass anterior to the inferior vena cava (IVC) and is longer than the left renal artery. In a significant minority of the population, an accessory renal artery may also arise from the aorta to provide blood supply to a portion of the kidney, which may become important when evaluating patients for renovascular hypertension. The renal arteries give rise to segmental, interlobar, and then arcuate arteries (Fig. 31-1). Arcuate arteries course along the corticomedullary junction and give rise to interlobular arterioles, which extend outward into the cortex and provide the afferent arterioles. The glomeruli arise from these afferent arterioles, and then efferent arterioles continue and dive toward the medulla as the vasa rectae. The vasa rectae provide the sole blood supply for the renal medulla, making this portion of the kidney particularly susceptible to ischemic insults. Venules form from the ascending vasa rectae and eventually empty into the renal veins. The left renal vein returns to the IVC anterior to the aorta and inferior to the inferior mesenteric artery, which may rarely cause compression of this vein. The left gonadal vein also empties into the left renal vein, and thus a left varicocele may be evident if the renal vein is occluded by thrombosis or tumor involvement. The right renal vein is much shorter and directly empties into the IVC, whereas the right gonadal vein empties directly into the IVC and is not typically affected by right renal vein obstruction.

Renovascular Disease

Renovascular disease is the most common form of secondary hypertension, affecting up to 5% of patients with hypertension. Any process that narrows the renal arterial lumen beyond a critical point will elicit a humoral response from the ipsilateral kidney to increase intravascular pressure in an attempt to normalize blood flow to the kidney. Although many clinicians define renal artery stenosis (RAS) as a stenosis of at least 50%, some have attempted to define criteria for a "hemodynamically significant" stenosis using direct flow measurements, although the clinical utility of these measurements is uncertain. The hormonal response to a critical stenosis is initially characterized by renin and aldosterone secretion (secondary hyperaldosteronism), renal sodium and fluid reabsorption, and resultant hypertension. The end result is to raise perfusion pressure in the affected kidney and maintain glomerular filtration rate (GFR). The contralateral kidney, which is initially unaffected, cannot prevent this humoral response from the ischemic kidney but may allow a pressure natriuresis. Hypertension is maintained by increased vasoconstriction due to angiotensin II, and a pressure natriuresis is induced in the normal contralateral kidney. If the renal arteries to both kidneys are

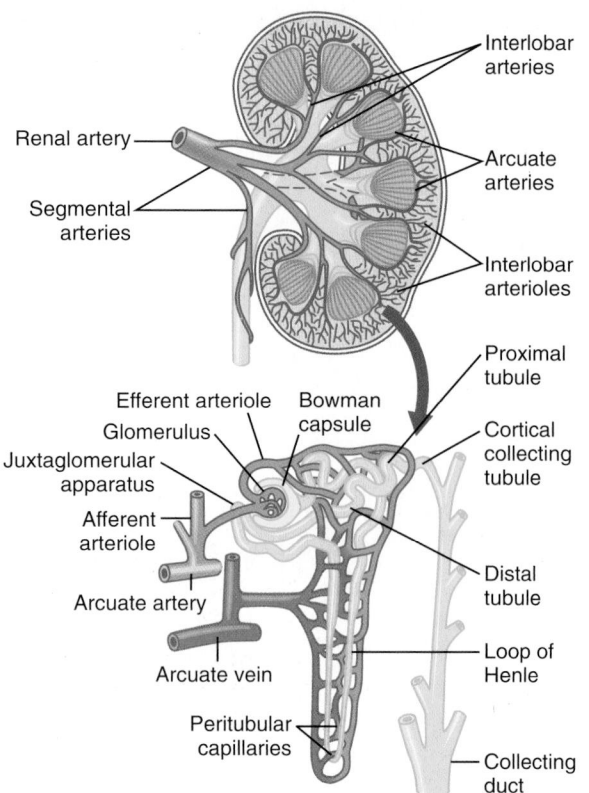

Figure 31-1 Section of the human kidney showing the renal arteries and a schematic of the microcirculation of each nephron. (From Guyton AC, Hall JE: Textbook of Medical Physiology, 11th ed. Philadelphia, Elsevier, Saunders, 2006, p 309.)

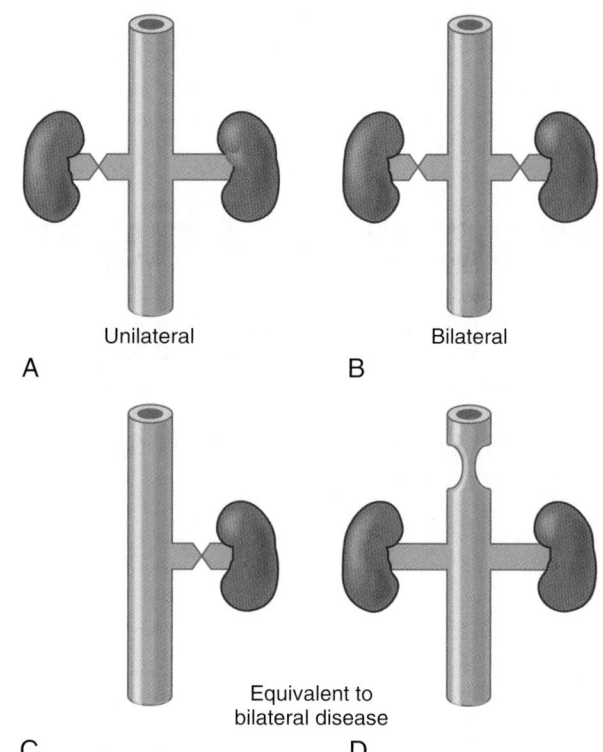

Figure 31-2 Anatomy of renal artery stenosis. Renal artery stenosis may be unilateral (**A**), bilateral (**B**), or unilateral with a solitary kidney (**C**). Aortic disease may also serve functionally as bilateral renal artery stenosis (**D**).

narrowed, there will be a period of sodium retention due to vasoconstriction and angiotensin II–stimulated aldosterone production. Hypertension will be mediated by volume expansion rather than by increased total peripheral resistance. The same situation is seen when the initially normal contralateral kidney suffers microvascular damage after long-term exposure to the hypertensive state.

Thus, ischemic renal disease may be seen with unilateral or bilateral stenosis of the renal arteries or with unilateral RAS and a contralateral kidney damaged by hypertension (Fig. 31-2). Stenosis of a single kidney leads to hypertension that is sensitive to blockade of angiotensin II. Stenosis of both renal arteries or microvascular damage to the contralateral kidney leads to hypertension that is sensitive to volume reduction and blockade of angiotensin II.

In addition, successful hypertension treatment may produce renal ischemia and reduce the glomerular filtration of the affected kidney, but this may not be detectable by measurement of the serum creatinine if the contralateral kidney is functioning normally. However, a decline in GFR may be evident if there is underlying renal dysfunction, as is often the case with long-standing hypertension, diabetes, or vascular disease. In the case in which either a solitary kidney or both kidneys (bilateral RAS) are affected, acute renal failure may result. Renal function may improve after stopping angiotensin I–converting enzyme (ACE) inhibitor or angiotensin II, type I receptor (ARB) treatment or revascularization if detected promptly.

Atherosclerosis is the primary cause of RAS, although any process that narrows one or both renal arteries may also cause renal ischemia. The cause of RAS is not necessarily distinguishable based on clinical or laboratory findings alone, but the history may provide important clues. Atherosclerotic disease is rarely present in patients younger than 40 years, and is more common in males (2:1) and Caucasians.

CLINICAL EVALUATION FOR RENAL ARTERY STENOSIS

RAS should be suspected in patients with refractory hypertension or new-onset hypertension in patients older than 50 years (Table 31-1). Evaluation should always begin with a thorough history and physical examination, including particular attention to blood pressure and pulse amplitude in each extremity. A significant discrepancy between extremities may indicate peripheral vascular disease and increase clinical suspicion for RAS. An abdominal bruit is present in about 50% of subjects but is not specific for RAS. Edema is not typically present unless significant renal insufficiency exists. Laboratory evaluation may reveal hypokalemia ($K^+ < 3.5$ mEq/L) or metabolic alkalosis ($HCO_3^- > 28$ mEq/L). Renal insufficiency may be present, but its absence does not rule out RAS. Plasma renin activity and aldosterone are typically elevated. Urinalysis is usually normal, but low-grade proteinuria (usually <1 g/day) may result from long-standing hypertension.

Table 31-1 **Clinical Findings Suggestive of Renovascular Disease**
Onset of hypertension at <30 years of age (FMD) or severe hypertension at >55 years of age (atherosclerotic RAS)
Accelerated, resistant, or malignant hypertension
Unexplained atrophic kidney or size discrepancy >1.5 cm between kidneys
Sudden, unexplained pulmonary edema
Unexplained renal dysfunction, including individuals starting renal replacement therapy
Development of new azotemia or worsening renal function after administration of an ACE inhibitor or ARB agent
Multivessel coronary artery disease or peripheral arterial disease
Unexplained congestive heart failure or refractory angina

ACE, angiotensin-converting enzyme; ARB, angiotensin II, type I receptor blocker; FMD, fibromuscular dysplasia; RAS, renal artery stenosis.
Adapted from Hirsch AT, Haskal ZJ, Hertzer NR, et al: ACC/AHA 2005 Practice Guidelines for the management of patients with peripheral arterial disease (lower extremity, renal, mesenteric, and abdominal aortic). Circulation 113:e463-e654, 2006.

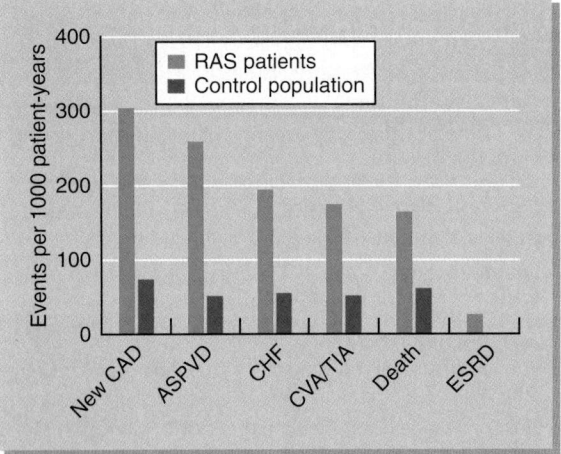

Figure 31-3 Incidence of cardiovascular outcomes in patients older than 65 years with atherosclerotic renal artery stenosis (RAS), compared with an age-matched population. ASPVD, atherosclerotic peripheral vascular disease; CAD, coronary artery disease; CHF, congestive heart failure; CVA/TIA, cerebrovascular event or transient ischemic attack; ESRD, end-stage renal artery disease requiring dialysis. (Data from Kalra PA, Guo H, Kausz AT, et al: Atherosclerotic renovascular disease in United States patients aged 67 years or older: Risk factors, revascularization, and prognosis. Kidney Int 68:293-301, 2005).

Radiologic evaluation of RAS is guided by the local expertise at the testing facility. Renal ultrasound provides only a limited window into the presence of RAS because this modality will likely only reveal a discrepancy in kidney size, which develops only after prolonged ischemia and irreversible renal injury. However, a change in kidney size on serial imaging in the setting of known RAS may be a harbinger of worsening renal function and should prompt the clinician to consider revascularization. Renal ultrasound provides an assessment of renal size, and when used with Doppler pulse wave analysis, may give information regarding flow velocity in the renal arteries. However, renal duplex ultrasound (US) is technically demanding and is best performed by an experienced ultrasonographer at a high-volume center. Despite a reported high sensitivity of renal duplex US in the literature, it is doubtful that most centers can reproduce these results.

Computed tomography (CT) with intravenous iodinated contrast permits evaluation of the arterial vasculature (CT angiography, CTA) and is more easily reproducible across centers, providing the highest resolution of the renal vasculature. However, the risk associated with intravenous contrast may preclude CTA in subjects with renal insufficiency. Magnetic resonance angiography (MRA) with intravenous contrast is also highly reproducible, but application is limited by implanted metallic medical devices. Gadolinium administration to patients with advanced renal insufficiency (GFR < 30 mL per minute) is also contraindicated owing to the potential risk for nephrogenic fibrosing dermopathy. Analyses of renal duplex, CTA, and MRA data suggest that CTA and MRA have similarly high sensitivity and specificity.

Nuclear imaging using technetium-DTPA or MAG3 can assess the uptake and excretion in each kidney, before and after the administration of a short-acting ACE inhibitor, captopril (captopril renogram). When unilateral RAS is present but is compensated by increased systemic pressure, captopril administration produces greater afferent arteriolar dilation and reduces renal perfusion to the ischemic kidney. However, this test has limited specificity and is insensitive in the case of bilateral RAS. The most sensitive and specific test, but also the most invasive, is renal arteriography. One added advantage of arteriography is that angioplasty or stenting can be performed during arteriography. Because of the frequent occurrence of accessory renal arteries, an aortogram must be performed rather than selective renal angiography to ensure that all vessels are visualized.

TREATMENT OF ATHEROSCLEROTIC RENAL ARTERY DISEASE

Patients with atherosclerotic RAS almost always have coexistent cerebrovascular, coronary, or other peripheral vascular disease. Clinicians should recognize and treat this high cardiovascular risk associated with atherosclerotic renal disease. The absolute risk for developing end-stage renal disease (ESRD) is increased in these patients compared with those without RAS, but remains much less than the risk for developing coronary disease, symptomatic peripheral vascular disease, heart failure, or stroke (Fig. 31-3). As with other manifestations of peripheral arterial disease, atherosclerotic RAS is recognized as an ischemic heart disease equivalent because of this increased risk, and clinical guidelines recommend intensive lipid lowering and aspirin use for this subgroup. Therefore, attempts to modify other cardiovascular risk factors (smoking cessation, hypertension and diabetes control, and antiplatelet therapy) are an essential component of therapy.

Intervention for atherosclerotic RAS is controversial and is the subject of several ongoing randomized clinical trials to investigate medical management versus intervention with renal artery stenting. Generally accepted guidelines for intervention have been reported, but decisions should still be made on a case-by-case basis (Table 31-2). Smaller clinical

Table 31-2 Indications for Renal Revascularization
Resistant Hypertension
Failure of medical therapy despite full doses of ≥3 drugs, including diuretic
Compelling need for ACE inhibitor or ARB therapy with angiotensin-dependent GFR
Progressive Renal Insufficiency
Salvageable kidneys
Recent rise in serum creatinine
Loss of GFR during antihypertensive therapy (especially ACE inhibitor or ARB)
Evidence of preserved diastolic blood flow (low resistive index)
Circulatory Congestion, Recurrent "Flash" Pulmonary Edema
Refractory Congestive Heart Failure with Bilateral Renal Arterial Stenosis

ACE, angiotensin-converting enzyme; ARB, angiotensin II, type I receptor blocker; GFR, glomerular filtration rate.
From Garovic VD, Textor SC: Renovascular hypertension and ischemic nephropathy. Circulation 112:1362-1374, 2005.

Table 31-3 Histologic Classification of Fibromuscular Dysplasia

Subtype	Proportion of Cases (%)	Radiologic Appearance
Medial fibroplasia	60-70	"String of beads" with aneurysms
Perimedial fibroplasia	15	"String of beads" without large aneurysms
Medial hyperplasia	5-15	Smooth tubular stenosis
Intimal fibroplasia	1-2	Focal or smooth stenosis
Adventitial fibroplasia	<1	Focal or smooth tubular stenosis

studies have suggested that percutaneous transluminal renal angioplasty with stenting may improve blood pressure control in atherosclerotic RAS, but carries a risk for worsening renal function in a significant percentage of patients. This may be due to atheroembolic disease, contrast nephropathy, or stent thrombosis and may lead to irreversible renal failure. Moreover, recent studies have failed to prevent the decline in renal function using distal protection devices or platelet inhibition to protect against atheroemboli.

FIBROMUSCULAR DYSPLASIA

Fibromuscular dysplasia (FMD) is a nonatherosclerotic, noninflammatory disease causing RAS in young female patients. The etiology of FMD is unclear, but it is believed to be a developmental abnormality. Depending on the population, FMD is responsible for 10% to 25% of renovascular hypertension cases. FMD affects the renal arteries most commonly (bilateral in about 35%), but carotid and vertebral arteries can also be affected and produce neurologic symptoms. The disease frequently afflicts younger patients, with a female preponderance, but may also come to clinical attention in patients older than 50 years.

Classification of FMD is based on the histologic layer of the artery involved (intima, media, or adventitia) (Table 31-3). Medial fibroplasia with mural aneurysm is the most common cause of FMD in adults (70% of cases), consisting of alternating fibromuscular ridges and aneurysmal segments in the distal two thirds of the renal artery and a classic "string-of-beads" appearance on angiography (Fig. 31-4). Perimedial fibroplasia of the outer half of the media produces severe multifocal stenosis and causes about 15% of FMD cases in adults. Medial subtypes of FMD generally have a benign course and are responsive to angioplasty. The intimal subtype may have a higher likelihood of ischemic events and multiorgan system involvement. Symptoms are usually precipitated by stenoses, but rarely FMD may cause dissection or macroaneurysms that require intervention.

Treatment for FMD depends on the severity of complications. Pharmacologic treatment alone may be adequate to control hypertension in simple cases. Intervention should be considered in patients with severe or difficult-to-control hypertension, or decreasing renal mass. Success may differ for various subtypes, but further research is needed. Balloon angioplasty without stenting is successful in most patients, but recurrence is not uncommon. For this reason, serial monitoring with renal duplex ultrasonography is needed to assess for restenosis. In selected cases in which percutaneous intervention is impossible, surgical intervention may be an appropriate option. Prompt intervention is important because improvement of hypertension is most achievable in those with shorter duration of hypertension, those with normal renal cortical thickness, and those younger than 50 years.

AORTIC DISSECTION

Aortic dissection occurs after injury to the intimal layer and propagation of blood flow "dissects" within the wall of the aorta, producing a false lumen and compressing the true vessel lumen. Aortic dissection is classified by either the site of origin (DeBakey classification) or the segment of the aorta involved (Stanford classification) (Fig. 31-5). DeBakey type I and II dissections originate in the ascending aorta, and type III dissections originate in the descending aorta. Stanford type A refers to dissections involving the ascending aorta, and type B to all others not involving the ascending aorta.

Major branch vessels of the aorta, including the renal arteries, may become obstructed as a result of extension or obstruction of the vessel by the false lumen. Aortic dissection frequently compromises the renal arteries when it extends into the abdominal aorta and causes renal failure in 21% of patients with type B dissections. The left renal artery is more commonly involved than the right because of anatomic circumstances. When disease is extensive enough to cause acute renal failure, vascular compromise to the intestinal or cerebral vasculature, or severe aortic regurgitation usually coexists and contributes to a high mortality rate. A similar clinical picture occurs with an isolated aortic intramural hematoma (IMH), which is thought to originate from a ruptured vasa vasorum. IMH is estimated to cause 5% to 10% of acute aortic syndromes and generally carries the same risks for organ ischemia, with a higher incidence of aortic rupture.

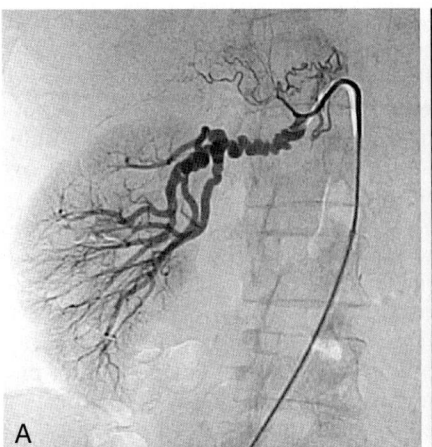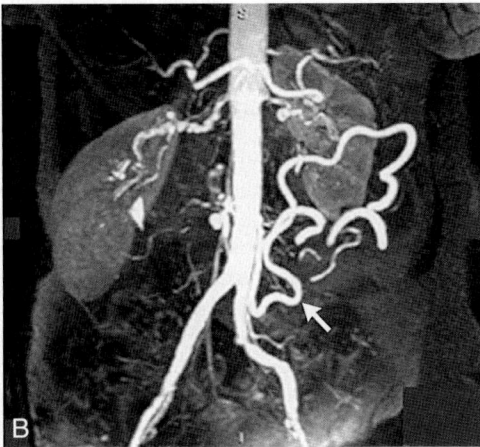

Figure 31-4 **A,** Typical medial fibroplasia ("string-of-beads" appearance) on angiogram of a right renal artery. **B,** Gadolinium-enhanced magnetic resonance angiography in the same patient, revealing bilateral medial fibroplasia of the renal arteries and a large marginal artery of Drummond (*arrow*), indicating that there is disease of the superior mesenteric artery. (From Slovut DP, Olin JW: Fibromuscular dysplasia. N Engl J Med 350:1862-1871, 2004.)

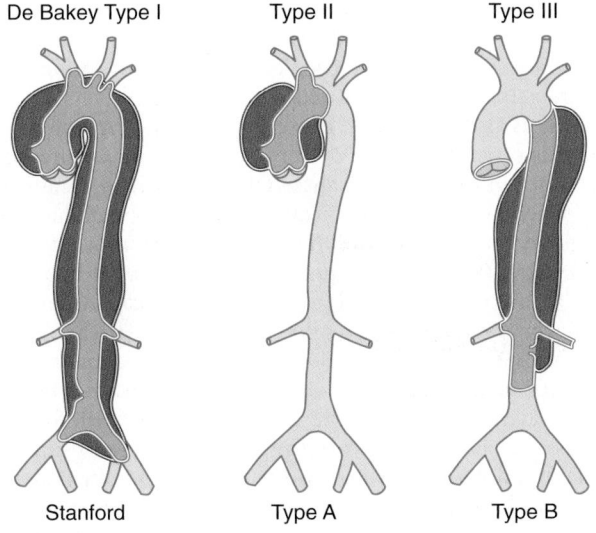

De Bakey

Type I — Originates in the ascending aorta, propagates at least to the aortic arch and often beyond it distally

Type II — Originates in and is confined to the ascending aorta

Type III — Originates in the descending aorta and extends distally down the aorta or, rarely, retrograde into the aortic arch and ascending aorta

Stanford

Type A — All dissections involving the ascending aorta, regardless of the site of origin

Type B — All dissections not involving the ascending aorta

Figure 31-5 Classification of aortic dissection according to involvement of the thoracic, abdominal, or both portions of the aorta by the Stanford and DeBakey systems. (From Nienaber CA, Eagle KA: Aortic dissection: New frontiers in diagnosis and management: Part I: From etiology to diagnostic strategies. Circulation 108:628-635, 2003.)

Aortic dissection most frequently affects older patients (50 to 70 years of age) with coexistent vascular risk factors such as male sex, hypertension, smoking, and atherosclerosis. Occasionally a genetic connective tissue defect such as Marfan syndrome or Ehlers-Danlos syndrome type IV (about 5% of cases) may cause aortic dissection, and these should be considered in younger patients (<40 years of age). Trauma or procedures (e.g., aortic catheterization) can also cause dissection of the aorta or renal artery. Rarely, isolated renal artery dissection may occur spontaneously, most commonly in the setting of polyarteritis nodosa or FMD. Renal failure occurs in about 20% of patients diagnosed with acute type B aortic dissection and is an independent predictor of in-hospital mortality.

The initial diagnosis of aortic dissection is frequently missed, partly because of the widely varying clinical presentations, and may be discovered incidentally on unrelated imaging studies. The most frequent symptom during aortic dissection is chest pain, which may be described as a "ripping" sensation. Isolated loss of pulse in one or more extremities may be a clinical clue, and number of arteries involved correlates with severity of dissection. Aortic dissection should also be considered in patients during evaluation of acute renal failure. A common clue to the diagnosis on routine chest radiograph is a widened mediastinum, with or without a pleural effusion (most frequently on the left). Once the diagnosis of aortic dissection is established, evaluation of renal artery involvement is best undertaken noninvasively, in order to minimize further vascular injury. Contrast-enhanced CT or magnetic resonance imaging (MRI) or MRA usually provides images capable of confirming or excluding renal involvement, although each modality carries the same limitations as outlined for evaluation of RAS. Transesophageal echocardiography is useful for establishing the diagnosis of aortic dissection but does not provide information below the diaphragm. Similarly, renal duplex ultrasonography may be useful for evaluating renal perfusion in the setting of aortic dissection but is not recommended for initial investigation of aortic dissection. Aortography alone is not a sensitive test for aortic dissection but could provide information regarding renal perfusion.

Aortic dissection is a hypertensive emergency and requires aggressive reduction of blood pressure into the normal range. Medical management of aortic dissection should focus on minimizing arterial blood pressure with antihypertensive agents. Medications that reduce the rate of increase in blood pressure during the cardiac cycle (dP/dT), such as β blockers, have theoretical benefit in aortic dissection to reduce the rate of progression. Surgical treatment options for renal involvement due to aortic dissection are dependent on individual circumstances, and careful evaluation by an experienced vascular surgeon is recommended. Thoracic aortic dissection requires surgical repair due to the high mortality rate if left untreated, but isolated abdominal aortic disease may be medically managed.

EMBOLIC DISEASE

Systemic arterial emboli, typically originating from the left atrium or left ventricle, may cause acute obstruction of the renal artery. Emboli usually originate in the heart, most commonly because of atrial fibrillation, bacterial endocarditis, valvular disease, or atrial myxoma. Rarely, a paradoxical embolus may occur from the venous system through an atrial septal defect. Symptoms of acute renal ischemia may include flank pain, hematuria, and fever. Laboratory findings are nonspecific but include elevated lactate dehydrogenase (LDH), microscopic hematuria, and leukocytosis. Diagnosis can be definitively made by presence of a focal nonenhancing region on contrast-enhanced CT. The area of affected kidney is usually not large enough to necessitate dialysis, although some worsening of renal function is commonly observed. The diagnosis of renal infarction is rarely made early enough to initiate treatment with intra-arterial thrombolysis, and it is questionable whether the risks and marginal benefit of this procedure warrant aggressive treatment. Therapy should instead address the underlying source of renal emboli.

LARGE VESSEL VASCULITIS

Systemic vasculitides such as Takayasu arteritis and polyarteritis nodosa (PAN) commonly affect large vessels such as the renal arteries but rarely cause glomerulonephritis.

Takayasu arteritis is commonly referred to as "pulseless disease" because of obstructing lesions of the large vessels of the aorta, most commonly the subclavian arteries, and frequently involves the main renal arteries (65% to 75% of cases), producing RAS, renal ischemia, or renal infarction. Takayasu arteritis is giant cell arteritis affecting mainly women of reproductive age. Common clinical features are constitutional symptoms, decreased pulses, claudication, bruits, and hypertension. Blood pressures are often unreliable in these patients because of the focal arterial lesions, and the arm with the highest obtainable blood pressure should be used. Diagnosis is made on clinical grounds, and treatment with corticosteroids may be beneficial.

PAN is a medium-large vessel vasculitis with no gender predilection, affecting predominantly older patients (40 to 60 years of age). It commonly causes both large vessel disease and necrotizing vasculitis of the renal parenchymal vessels, such as renal artery microaneurysms, which are evident on renal angiogram or CT angiography in 40% to 90% of cases. By definition, PAN does not involve the arterioles or glomeruli. Most patients present with fever, malaise, and weight loss in addition to specific organ complaints related to skin, joint, nerve, and gut involvement. Symptoms specific to renal involvement may include loin pain and hematuria. Rarely, a renal artery aneurysm may produce renal ischemia, renal artery dissection, or spontaneous rupture. Diagnosis is made on clinical grounds and by angiography; there are no confirmatory serologic tests. Progressive renal disease is not typical, and most patients have complications related to other organs, most notably the gastrointestinal tract. Treatment with corticosteroids and immunosuppressive drugs is effective in reducing disease severity and mortality.

HYPERTENSIVE NEPHROSCLEROSIS

Hypertension is highly prevalent in the U.S. population, increasing with age and affecting 50% of adults aged 60 to 69 years. Uncontrolled hypertension is responsible for about 60% of cerebrovascular disease and about 50% of ischemic heart disease in the United States and is the leading attributable risk for death worldwide. Renal failure due to hypertension is relatively rare in the general population, but owing to the high prevalence of disease, a large proportion of renal failure is thought to be due to hypertension.

CKD is also a common cause of secondary hypertension, and it is often difficult to determine which disease preceded the other. Hypertension causes CKD in African Americans at a much higher rate than Caucasians, even at similar levels of blood pressure control. This fact has been accepted by nephrologists and could cause an overestimate of hypertension as the cause of ESRD or CKD in African Americans. However, the renal biopsy pilot study of the African American Study of Kidney Disease (AASK) trial documented the accuracy of this diagnosis based on history alone. Pharmacologic treatment of hypertension reduces the risk for progression to ESRD and worsening of creatinine in multiple patient populations, providing further evidence for the causative role of hypertension. The markedly increased risk for hypertensive nephrosclerosis in African Americans is being intensely investigated for possible genetic factors.

Diagnosis is typically made on clinical grounds, with a history of long-standing or severe hypertension preceding the development of renal insufficiency. The urinary sediment is typically bland with only low-grade proteinuria (<1 g per day). Symmetrical loss of renal cortical thickness on renal imaging with a generally smooth surface is typically found. Renal biopsy findings include afferent arteriolar medial thickening and hyalinization, and intimal fibrosis. Glomeruli are focally or globally sclerotic, with wrinkled glomerular basement membrane due to glomerular ischemia. Hypertensive nephrosclerosis is often found on renal biopsy in patients with other vascular disorders (e.g. diabetes, atheroembolic disease, or RAS).

An accelerated or "malignant" phase of hypertension with progressively increasing blood pressure and development of end-organ damage may occur if hypertension is not treated. Renal biopsy in this situation reveals arteriolar fibrinoid necrosis and "onion-skinning" of the interlobular arteries. These pathologic findings can overlap somewhat with scleroderma renal crisis and thrombotic microangiopathy, although malignant hypertension tends to affect smaller arteries such as the afferent arterioles. The clinical history is necessary to differentiate these diseases.

Treatment is aimed at lowering blood pressure to levels recommended for other high-risk populations such as diabetics (<130/80 mm Hg) when CKD is present. Blood pressure reduction prevents future development of congestive heart failure, stroke, and ESRD. Many studies suggest that ACE inhibitors or ARBs are more effective in preventing morbidity, but other drug classes are almost always needed. Thiazide-type diuretics (e.g., hydrochlorothiazide) are recommended in most patients, and loop diuretics (e.g., furosemide) are needed when renal function worsens (GFR < 30 mL per minute).

ATHEROEMBOLIC DISEASE

Even the most astute clinician may fail to make the diagnosis of cholesterol emboli, and they are sometimes revealed only after renal biopsy or at autopsy. Cholesterol emboli originate from aortic atherosclerotic plaque, typically dislodged during an invasive arterial procedure (e.g., cardiac catheterization or vascular or cardiac surgery, particularly abdominal aortic aneurysm resection). In patients with severe atherosclerosis, cholesterol emboli may occur spontaneously or may even be precipitated by heparin anticoagulation. Because patients must have underlying atherosclerosis, the incidence increases with age and rarely occurs before age 40 years.

Cholesterol crystals are disrupted and lodge in small arterial vessels, including the arcuate or interlobular arteries of the kidney. In many cases, emboli also occur in the extremities, causing skin changes (livedo reticularis, digital ischemia), or the gastrointestinal tract, causing intestinal ischemia. Symptoms are typically related to organ ischemia but may also include fever by an unknown mechanism. Massive cholesterol embolization may cause acute renal ischemia leading to renin release and severe hypertension. If the embolic burden is lower, a decline in renal function typically occurs after 7 to 14 days as a result of the vascular inflammation and remodeling response to the cholesterol crystals. Typical laboratory findings include peripheral blood or urinary eosinophilia, elevated erythrocyte sedimentation rate, hypocomplementemia, and elevated amylase or liver enzymes. On renal biopsy, the fixation process washes out cholesterol crystals, leaving a typical needle-shaped disruption in the arterial lumen surrounded by reactive endovascular cells. These lesions may be seen on only a few sections, and even then may be overlooked by experienced pathologists. Cholesterol crystals may be visible on frozen sections if they are available because they do not undergo the same fixation process. Diagnosis is usually made clinically in the appropriate setting, but confounding features may necessitate renal biopsy.

The degree of renal insufficiency is determined by the magnitude of the embolic burden and the acuity of the process, owing to the degree of inflammation induced by the material from the plaque. Many patients may have stabilization after the insult, whereas others will progress to advanced renal failure or ESRD. There is no specific treatment for cholesterol emboli. Because an inflammatory reaction may be associated with the emboli, some researchers advocate corticosteroids, but their use is unproved for preventing progression of renal failure. Statin therapy is appropriate for most patients for treatment of underlying atherosclerotic disease. Treatment with ACE inhibitors is effective for hypertension control in the acute setting, but worsening renal function may limit their use. Supportive care for renal failure may necessitate acute or long-term dialysis.

PREECLAMPSIA

Preeclampsia affects 3% to 5% of pregnancies and causes about 50,000 worldwide maternal deaths each year. It is the principal renal complication of pregnancy, characterized by the onset of hypertension (blood pressure > 140/90 mm Hg) and proteinuria (>300 mg per day) typically in the third trimester. Earlier development (<20 weeks' gestation) of preeclampsia is associated with reduced placental blood flow, reduced fetal growth, and more severe maternal disease. Although hypertension and proteinuria are the principal signs of preeclampsia, it is a systemic vascular disease with potential central nervous system, gastrointestinal, hepatic, and hematologic involvement. In severe cases, the disorder may cause seizure (eclampsia, in about 2% of cases), cerebral hemorrhage, pulmonary edema, placental abruption, or renal failure. The HELLP syndrome, characterized by *h*emolysis, *e*levated *l*iver enzymes, and *l*ow *p*latelets, is thought to be a manifestation of severe preeclampsia and is also associated with increased maternal and fetal mortality. Clinicians should be aware that although most cases of eclampsia occur before delivery, one third of cases may occur during the immediate postpartum period.

Multiple risk factors have been identified for preeclampsia (Table 31-4), and recent progress has been made in the pathogenesis. Placenta-derived circulating antiangiogenic factors have been described that precede the onset of preeclampsia, such as soluble fms-like tyrosine kinase-1 (sFlt1), or soluble endoglin (sEng), which inhibit circulating angiogenic hormones. These factors may be causative of widespread endothelial injury, and their role in preeclampsia is being further investigated. Endothelial dysfunction in turn causes increased sensitivity to vasopressor agents, systemic vasoconstriction, and reduced fibrinolytic function. Renal biopsy reveals endothelial cell swelling (endotheliosis) and,

Table 31-4 **Risk Factors for Preeclampsia**
Primigravida
Multiple gestation
Hypertension
Renal disease
Diabetes
Hydatidiform disease
Preeclampsia in a previous pregnancy
Preeclampsia history in first-degree relative
Black race
Collagen vascular disease
Thrombophilia
Extremes of age
Note: Smoking has a protective effect.

Table 31-5 Antihypertensive Medications in Pregnancy

Medication	Serious Adverse Effects
Commonly Used	
Methyldopa	None definite
Clonidine	Fetal bradycardia
Hydralazine	None definitely reported
Labetalol, β blockers	Fetal bradycardia
Thiazide diuretics	Volume contraction
Calcium channel blockers	None definite
Contraindicated	
Angiotensin-converting enzyme inhibitors	Teratogenicity and fetal death
Angiotensin II receptor antagonists	Teratogenicity and fetal death

Note: There is a direct relationship between magnitude of blood pressure change and risk for small-for-gestational-age infants, regardless of drug choice. All drugs are category C for treatment of hypertension in pregnancy.

in severe cases, fibrin microthrombi with ischemia and necrosis.

Despite several clinical trials for the prevention of pre-eclampsia, no therapy is very effective. The only effective treatment for preeclampsia remains placental delivery. Proper obstetrical care is essential to balance the risk to the mother against the risk for prematurity of the fetus. Treatment of severe hypertension with antihypertensive agents can reduce cerebrovascular events due to elevated blood pressure, but will not treat the underlying disorder or reverse the disease. Methyldopa has long been the drug of choice for hypertension in pregnancy, whereas β blockers such as labetalol are common second-line drugs (Table 31-5). As with many medications in pregnancy, the risk profile of these medications is poorly defined. Treatment with magnesium sulfate in severe cases of preeclampsia effectively reduces the risk for progression to eclampsia, but does not reduce maternal or fetal mortality. The benefits of magnesium sulfate in mild or moderate cases of preeclampsia are less certain. Most cases gradually resolve after delivery of the placenta. However, even after delivery, preeclampsia is a risk factor for future hypertension, renal disease, and cardiovascular events.

SCLERODERMA RENAL CRISIS

Systemic sclerosis (scleroderma) is an idiopathic connective tissue disorder that produces inflammation and fibrosis of the skin and internal organs (skin, heart, lungs, and gastrointestinal tract). Proliferative endovascular lesions may lead to obliteration of the vascular internal lumina and renal ischemia, with severe hypertension, increased renin activity, angiotensin II, and aldosterone. In severe cases, microangiopathic hemolytic anemia may also occur. Acute oliguric renal failure or rapidly worsening hypertension in the setting of underlying scleroderma is clinically referred to as *scleroderma renal crisis*.

The annual incidence of renal crisis in patients with scleroderma is about 7% to 10%, primarily in patients with diffuse disease, rather than the more limited local cutaneous systemic sclerosis. The incidence of renal crisis also increases

with the severity of skin involvement and joint contractures and frequently occurs early in the course of disease (within first 1 to 2 years of diagnosis). Because this may occur early during the course of disease, or even before the clinical diagnosis of scleroderma is made, clinicians must be alert to this possibility.

The renin-angiotensin system appears to play an important role in the progression of the disease, although no clear trigger has been found. Clinical predictors of impending renal crisis include new-onset anemia, rapidly worsening skin findings, and cardiac involvement. There are presently no clinically recommended serologic tests that reliably predict or confirm the diagnosis of renal crisis. Renal biopsy may reveal interlobular artery involvement with intimal thickening, endothelial cell proliferation, and edema. In the afferent arterioles, fibrinoid necrosis may occur with intravascular fibrin accumulation extending into the glomeruli, often with ischemic collapse. The classic onion-skinning appearance of the larger arteries occurs in chronic disease.

Before the advent of ACE inhibitors and hemodialysis, renal crisis was almost universally fatal, even with multidrug antihypertensive regimens, and was a major cause of mortality in patients with scleroderma. If the diagnosis of scleroderma renal crisis is made before advanced renal failure is established, ACE inhibition may halt or even reverse the decline in renal function. Some experts recommend continuing ACE inhibitors even if renal function declines and temporary dialysis is necessary, citing increased chance of renal recovery even after temporary dialysis during continuation of treatment. With the advent of ACE inhibitor therapy, the mortality rate of scleroderma renal crisis has improved from near 90% to close to 10%.

Thrombotic Microangiopathy

Thrombotic microangiopathy encompasses the clinical syndromes of TTP, secondary TTP, diarrhea-related hemolytic uremic syndrome (D+HUS), and diarrhea-negative HUS (D−HUS, or atypical HUS). The common feature among these disorders is microvascular thrombosis that produces microangiopathic hemolytic anemia and organ dysfunction, although each syndrome has distinct clinical, pathophysiologic, and epidemiologic features (Table 31-6).

Although many processes cause microvascular endothelial injury (Table 31-7), these affect the vasculature at different levels. Thrombosis due to HUS and TTP primarily affects the glomeruli. Scleroderma often extends to the interlobular arteries, as opposed to malignant hypertension, which more often affects the afferent arterioles. However, there is significant overlap and similar histologic features among these diseases, making careful clinical evaluation essential for accurate determination of the etiology.

THROMBOTIC THROMBOCYTOPENIC PURPURA

TTP is characterized by microangiopathic hemolytic anemia and thrombocytopenia without an identifiable cause.

Table 31-6 Characteristics that Differentiate Shiga Toxin–Related HUS from TTP

Feature	Shiga Toxin–Related HUS	TTP
Epidemiology	Endemic areas (commonly, not exclusively)	Endemic regions not reported
Similar cases in family	If yes, synchronous	If yes, separated in time and space
Recurrences	Rare	Common
Gastrointestinal prodrome	Painful diarrhea, frequently bloody	Nondiarrheal abdominal symptoms predominate, but not as prodrome
von Willebrand factor profile	Increased degradation to smaller multimers	Ultralarge forms (assay not universally available); depletion of large and ultralarge forms in advanced stage
ADAMTS 13	Normal or slightly decreased	Deficient (<0.1 U/mL)
Characteristics of intravascular thrombi	Fibrin predominates	von Willebrand factor predominates
Endothelial cell appearance	Swollen	Not swollen
Response to plasma therapy	Not demonstrated	Yes
Diagnosis	Isolation of STEC; antibody response to *Escherichia coli* O157:H7 LPS antigen	ADAMTS 13 activity; inhibitors of ADAMTS 13 activity; genetic analysis for mutations of ADAMTS 13 gene

ADAMTS 13, a disintegrin and metalloproteinase, with thrombospondin-1-like domains; HUS, hemolytic uremic syndrome; LPS, lipopolysaccharide; STEC, Shiga-toxigenic *E. coli*; TTP, thrombotic thrombocytopenic purpura.
Data from Tarr PI, Gordon CA, Chandler WL: Shiga-toxin-producing Escherichia coli and haemolytic uraemic syndrome. Lancet 365:1073-1086, 2005.

Table 31-7 Disorders Associated with Thrombocytopenia and Microangiopathic Hemolysis

Condition	Example
Pregnancy	Preeclampsia, HELLP syndrome
Medications	Cyclosporine, tacrolimus, chemotherapeutic agents (e.g., mitomycin C), quinine, cocaine, ticlopidine, heparin, statins
Transplantation	Allogeneic bone marrow, solid organ
Neoplastic diseases	Metastatic cancers
Disseminated intravascular coagulation	Consumption of fibrinogen and other clotting factors
Prothrombotic disorders	Paroxysmal nocturnal hemoglobinuria, antiphospholipid antibody syndrome
Cardiovascular procedures	Cardiac catheterization, angioplasty, vascular bypass operations, artificial aortic valve with perivalvular leak
Infectious diseases	Rocky Mountain spotted fever, anthrax
Intravascular devices	Prosthetic heart valves, prosthetic aortic valve with perivalvular leak
Malignant hypertension	Blood pressure >200/120 mm Hg

Data from Tsai HM: Advances in the pathogenesis, diagnosis, and treatment of thrombotic thrombocytopenic purpura. J Am Soc Nephrol 14:1072-1081, 2003.

Patients may also have fever, renal dysfunction, and neurologic impairment, although these occur late in the disease and may be prevented by early diagnosis and treatment. Purpura is only rarely observed and is not necessary to make the diagnosis. Idiopathic TTP is thought to have an autoimmune mechanism in many cases. Other causes of hemolytic anemia with thrombocytopenia, such as autoimmune hemolysis, disseminated intravascular coagulation (DIC), cancer, eclampsia, drug toxicity (e.g., ticlopidine, cyclosporine, tacrolimus), stem cell transplantation, or malignant hypertension, may also have evidence of microangiopathic hemolysis and are classified as secondary TTP. The annual incidence of TTP is 4 cases per 1,000,000, with a 3:2 female ratio with a peak incidence in the third and fourth decades of life.

Idiopathic TTP is thought to be caused by a deficiency of ADAMTS 13 (a disintegrin-like and metalloproteinase with thrombospondin repeats), a plasma protease that normally cleaves von Willebrand Factor (vWF) and limits the extent of intravascular thrombosis (Fig. 31-6). Microthrombi composed primarily of platelets and vWF accumulate within the vascular bed of multiple organs, leading to microangiopathic hemolytic anemia. Deficiency in ADAMTS 13 may be either acquired (e.g., immunoglobulin G [IgG] autoantibodies) or genetic. Other laboratory abnormalities are reflective of microangiopathic hemolytic anemia, such as thrombocytopenia, elevated LDH, indirect bilirubin, reticulocyte count, and low haptoglobin. Coagulation laboratory tests (prothrombin time [PT], activated partial thromboplastin time [aPTT], fibrinogen) are typically normal, although fibrin split products may be elevated. Renal dysfunction may not occur, but microscopic hematuria and proteinuria are frequently present.

Without treatment, TTP has a mortality rate of about 90%, with most deaths occurring within 3 months of onset of symptoms. Treatment with plasma infusion normalizes ADAMTS 13, reducing intravascular hemolysis, and reduces mortality. Plasmapheresis and replacement with fresh-frozen plasma carries the advantage of removing inhibitory autoantibodies in addition to normalizing ADAMTS 13 levels because of the large volume of plasma that can be

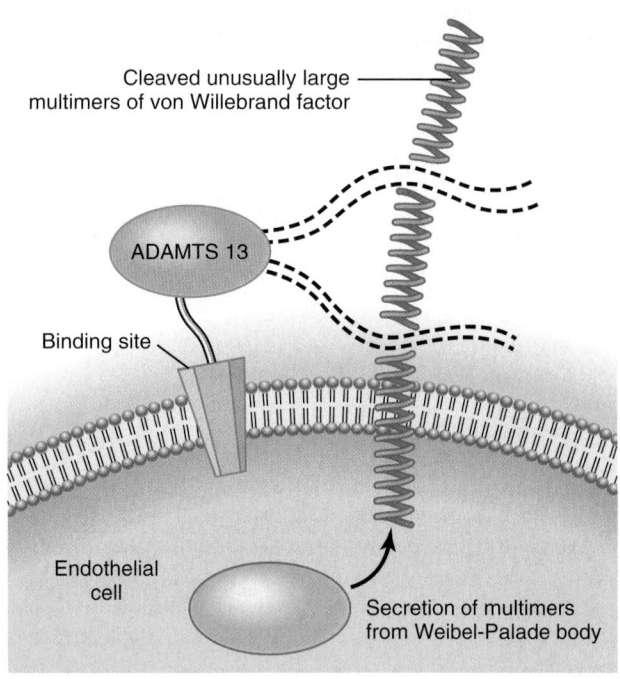

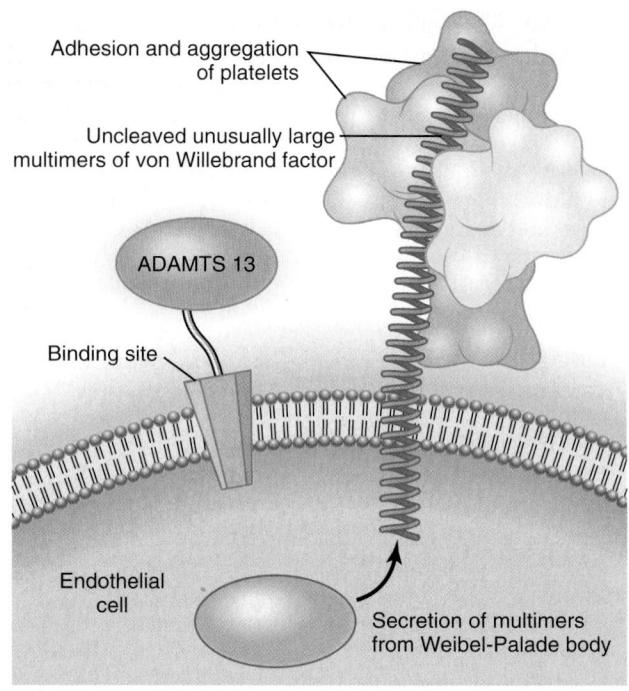

A   B

Figure 31-6 Relation between ADAMTS 13 activity, excessive adhesion and activation of platelets, and thrombotic thrombocytopenic purpura. **A,** In normal subjects, ADAMTS 13 (von Willebrand factor–cleaving metalloprotease) molecules attach to binding sites on endothelial cell surfaces and cleave unusually large multimers of von Willebrand factor as they are secreted by stimulated endothelial cells. The smaller von Willebrand factor forms that circulate after cleavage do not induce the adhesion and aggregation of platelets during normal blood flow. **B,** Absent or severely reduced activity of ADAMTS 13 in patients with thrombotic thrombocytopenic purpura prevents timely cleavage of unusually large multimers of von Willebrand factor as they are secreted by endothelial cells. The uncleaved multimers induce the adhesion and aggregation of platelets in flowing blood. (From Moake JL: Thrombotic microangiopathies. N Engl J Med 347:589-600, 2002.)

infused. Assay for ADAMTS 13 activity must be sent before therapy is initiated to obtain accurate results, but treatment should not be delayed for these results to return. Severity of ADAMTS 13 deficiency (<5%) is predictive of future relapse, although those with severe deficiency are just as likely to respond initially to plasmapheresis as those with mild deficiency. In patients with relapsing TTP, treatment with vincristine may reduce the need for plasmapheresis. Secondary TTP is not associated with ADAMTS 13 deficiency and will not respond to plasmapheresis or plasma infusion. Likewise, patients with HUS typically do not have severe ADAMTS 13 deficiency.

HEMOLYTIC UREMIC SYNDROME

Infection with the Shiga-toxigenic *Escherichia coli* strain O157:H7 may be complicated in about 15% of cases by thrombotic microangiopathy limited to the renal vasculature, termed the HUS. HUS is defined as anemia with schistocytes, thrombocytopenia, and renal dysfunction in the absence of other causes of coagulopathy. *Shigella dysenteriae* serotype 1 or other Shiga toxin–producing strains of *E. coli* may also cause HUS. HUS most commonly affects infants and children, although adults may also be affected. Cases of HUS often cluster owing to outbreaks of *E. coli* O157:H7, with peaks in summer and autumn. *E. coli* is endemic within the gastrointestinal tract of cattle, and cases are often tracked to undercooked meat, exposure to bovine

fecal matter, animal exposure, or other contaminated food products.

Shiga-toxigenic bacterial strains commonly produce a prodrome of painful, bloody diarrhea, which precedes the development of HUS by 2 to 12 days (median of 3 days). Shiga toxin is directly thrombogenic within the renal vasculature (Fig. 31-7). Although intravascular coagulation HUS is often limited to the kidney, the heart, gastrointestinal tract, and central nervous system (seizures, stroke, and coma) are also affected in a significant minority of cases and carry a worse prognosis.

Laboratory abnormalities in HUS commonly include elevated creatinine, anemia, schistocytes on peripheral smear, elevated reticulocyte count, and thrombocytopenia. In contrast to DIC, fibrinogen levels are normal or high, and the prothrombin time is normal or only slightly prolonged. Fresh stool should be sent for culture of *E. coli* O157:H7, which can potentially aid in tracing the source of an outbreak. Stool studies should also be performed in patients without diarrhea because *E. coli* O157:H7 may rarely cause HUS in the absence of intestinal symptoms. If *E. coli* O157:H7 is not detected on culture, then repeat culture for other Shiga-toxigenic organisms should be pursued. The pathologic renal lesions of HUS include vessel wall thickening with endothelial cell swelling and intraglomerular thrombosis with platelet- and fibrin-rich thrombi. Fragmentation of red blood cells may be seen within the renal vasculature and within the vessel wall.

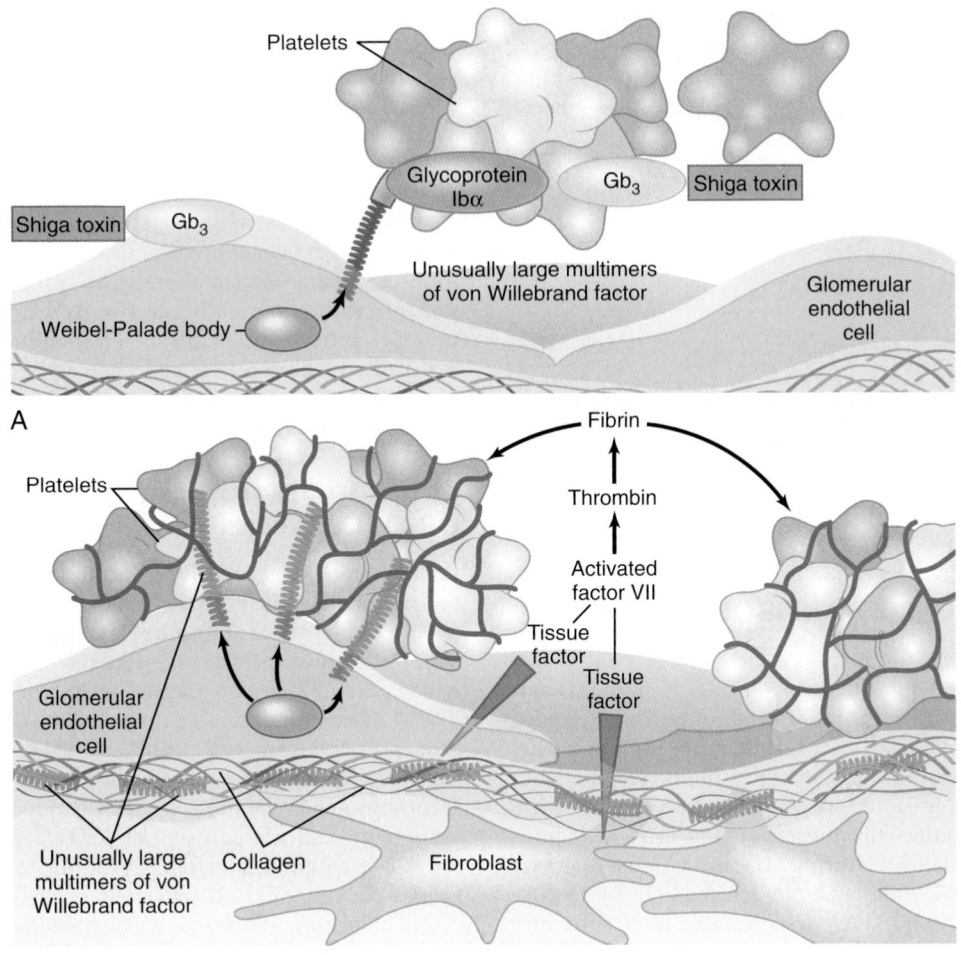

Figure 31-7 Mechanism of platelet-fibrin formation in hemolytic uremic syndrome. **A,** Platelets activated by Shiga toxin may adhere by means of the glycoprotein Ibα components of glycoprotein Ib/IX/V complexes to unusually large multimers of von Willebrand factor that are secreted from toxin-stimulated renal endothelial cells. The adherence of platelets to endothelial cells is especially likely if the cleavage of multimers extruding from endothelial cells by von Willebrand factor–cleaving metalloprotease, ADAMTS 13, is impaired by the interactions of Shiga toxin with globotriaosylceramide (Gb₃) receptors on endothelial cell surfaces. The activation of platelets that is mediated by Shiga toxin may contribute to the aggregation of additional platelets. **B,** Endocytosis and activation of the A subunits of Shiga toxin may cause the death and desquamation of endothelial cells, exposing unusually large multimers of von Willebrand factor entwined with collagen in the subendothelium. Platelets from flowing blood in the renal microcirculation may then adhere and aggregate on the exposed multimers and collagen. Local exposure of tissue factor and binding and activation of factor VII may occur on fibroblasts, invading phagocytic cells, and injured renal endothelial and epithelial cells. These actions may, in turn, induce the activation of factors IX and X, cleavage of prothrombin to thrombin by the complex of activated factor X and activated factor V, and the thrombin-induced formation of fibrin polymers, thus potentiating renal microvascular thrombosis. (From Moake JL: Thrombotic microangiopathies. N Engl J Med 347:589-600, 2002.)

Treatment of D+HUS is supportive, including adequate volume repletion with isotonic intravenous fluids, transfusion for severe anemia, and avoidance of other nephrotoxic agents (e.g., nonsteroidal anti-inflammatory drugs, aminoglycoside antibiotics, iodinated contrast). Platelet transfusion is generally not recommended because it may worsen the ongoing microvascular thrombosis. Antibiotic treatment of patients with bloody diarrhea is not recommended because it is not effective in reducing the incidence of HUS, and may actually increase the risk. Corticosteroids, anticoagulation (aspirin, heparin), thrombolytic agents, and plasma administration have also proved ineffective for the treatment of HUS. With supportive care alone, most patients with D+HUS will recover with normalization of renal func-

tion or only mild renal insufficiency, although about 25% may develop advanced renal failure or ESRD over the next 1 to 2 decades of life. Risk for chronic renal failure is increased with cortical necrosis and involvement of more than 50% of glomeruli on renal biopsy. The risk for complications and death increases with age, with mortality increasing from about 5% to 10% in children to about 30% in adults.

D–HUS (atypical HUS) accounts for a small percentage (about 5%) of cases and has a higher likelihood of recurrence, ESRD, or death. Many cases are due to genetic defects in the complement pathway (complement H, factor I, or CD46). With modern testing for ADAMTS 13 levels, laboratory testing may help distinguish cases of atypical HUS from TTP.

Table 31-8 Antiphospholipid Antibody Tests

Lupus Anticoagulants*

Activated partial thromboplastin time
Dilute Russell viper venom time
Kaolin clotting time
Dilute prothrombin time
Textarin time
Taipan time

Anticardiolipin Antibodies

Isotype specific enzyme-linked immunosorbent assay (IgG, IgM, or IgA)

Anti-β$_2$-Glycoprotein I Antibodies

*Nonspecific inhibitors that prolong in vitro clotting assays and fail to correct after addition of 1:1 mixture of normal plasma using the tests listed.
Data from Lim W, Crowther MA, Eikelboom JW: Management of antiphospholipid antibody syndrome: A systematic review. JAMA **295**: 1050-1057, 2006.

ANTIPHOSPHOLIPID ANTIBODY SYNDROME

Anti-phospholipid antibodies (APAs) refer to autoantibodies that interfere with phospholipid-binding proteins, such as lupus anticoagulants (LA) or anticardiolipin antibodies (aCL), that interfere with in vitro phospholipid-dependent clotting assays (Table 31-8). The diagnosis of APS is a clinical diagnosis that requires the presence of arterial or venous clotting events or fetal loss during pregnancy (after 10 weeks' gestation) because LA and aCL are detectable in up to 10% of healthy populations. APAs are detectable in 30% to 50% of patients with systemic lupus erythematosus (SLE), and renal involvement is often observed in this setting. In the absence of an underlying autoimmune disease, the syndrome is referred to as primary antiphospholipid antibody syndrome (APS), and secondary APS when associated with other diseases such as SLE.

The procoagulant effect of APAs may be due to interference with the anticoagulant β$_2$-glycoprotein 1, inhibition of fibrinolysis, direct endothelial injury, accelerated atherosclerosis, and activation of platelet, monocyte, and endothelial cells. APS has been associated with thrombotic events at any level within the renal vasculature (arteries, arterioles, glomeruli, or veins). The most commonly associated events are renal vein thrombosis, renal artery thrombosis, focal cortical atrophy, and thrombotic microangiopathy (including during pregnancy). APS nephropathy associated with SLE is often the only associated renal biopsy finding and appears to correlate more with the presence of LA than aCL.

Clinical signs of APS include livedo reticularis, thrombocytopenia, hemolytic anemia, and valvular heart disease. Laboratory screening for APAs is recommended in patients with unexplained venous or arterial thrombosis or multiple spontaneous abortions. One clinical clue to the presence of LA is a prolonged aPTT in the absence of heparin therapy or other anticoagulant therapy. Pathologic changes on renal biopsy of patients with primary APS are small vessel vaso-occlusive disease with fibrous intimal hyperplasia of interlobular arteries, recanalizing thrombi in arteries and arterioles, focal cortical atrophy, and thrombotic microangiopathy.

Long-term warfarin anticoagulation with a target international normalized ratio (INR) of 2 to 3 is indicated for patients with primary or secondary APS and prior DVT, arterial thrombosis, or recurrent spontaneous abortion. Warfarin is contraindicated during pregnancy, so heparin therapy with or without low-dose aspirin (81 mg) is necessary until the end of pregnancy in those cases. Treatment of APA-positive patients in the absence of prior clinical events is more controversial because of the high false-positive rate for these tests. Aspirin therapy for primary prevention in patients with persistently positive APA has been advocated, but not proved. In addition, plasmapheresis, prednisone, and hydroxychloroquine have been advocated for treatment of thrombotic microangiopathy due to APS and should be considered in severe cases.

RENAL VEIN THROMBOSIS OR OCCLUSION

Renal vein thrombosis (RVT) occurs rarely but is a potentially treatable cause of renal dysfunction. Although clinicians consider the diagnosis of RVT in the setting of nephrotic syndrome, most cases are associated with malignancy (66%), whereas a minority are caused by the nephrotic syndrome (20%) or an unidentifiable cause (12%). Other precipitating causes include surgery, trauma, and genetic or acquired hypercoagulable states (e.g., protein C or S deficiency, antithrombin gene mutation, factor V Leiden mutation). Most malignancy-associated cases of RVT (78%) are caused by renal cell carcinoma, often spreading to the contralateral kidney causing bilateral renal vein occlusion.

The nephrotic syndrome is associated with risk for venous thrombosis including RVT, which positively correlates with increasing severity of disease assessed by 24-hour urinary protein excretion and serum albumin (<2 g/dL). Some studies have documented about a 25% to 30% incidence of RVT in patients with nephrotic syndrome. Hypercoagulability is thought to be due to loss of antithrombotic proteins in the urine, increased procoagulant factors, or platelet activation. Glomerular diseases most commonly associated with RVT are membranous nephropathy, focal segmental glomerular sclerosis, membranoproliferative glomerulonephritis, and minimal change disease.

Patients may present with symptoms attributable to renal cell carcinoma, such as flank pain, gross hematuria, nausea, anorexia, or lower extremity swelling. In males, a left renal vein occlusion may cause a left varicocele, a result of the venous drainage of the left gonadal vein. In patients without a malignancy, symptoms of RVT depend on the acuity of the thrombosis. Acute, complete thrombosis is more likely to present with signs and symptoms, including hematuria, flank pain, abdominal distention, and acute renal failure. RVT in adults usually occurs gradually and allows time to develop collateral venous return. In gradual occlusion, most patients do not develop symptoms or acute renal failure, although a mild elevation of proteinuria and creatinine is often noted. Because patients often do not have symptoms, RVT is likely more common than reported in the literature, and some have suggested screening high-risk patients by CT scan.

The gold standard method for diagnosis is renal venography, but it has a risk for clot dislodgment, bleeding, and

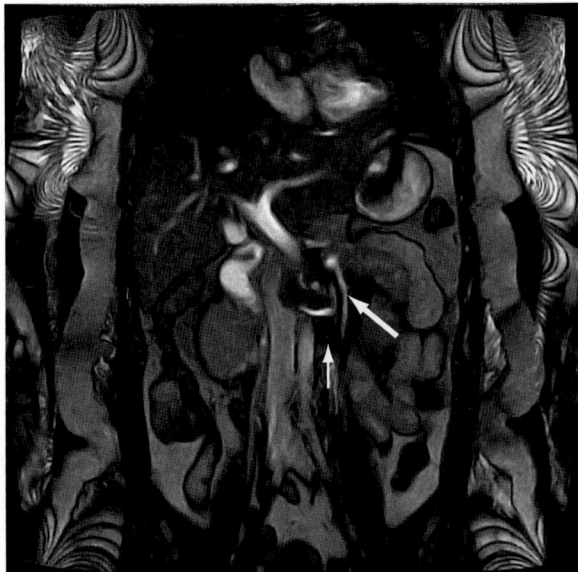

Figure 31-8 Magnetic resonance venography demonstrating left renal vein thrombosis in a patient with membranous glomerulonephritis and nephrotic syndrome (urine protein excretion 7 g per 24 hours). The thrombosis can be seen as a dark void within the left renal vein (*large arrow*) extending into the inferior vena cava (*small arrow*).

iodinated contrast, so less invasive methods are now commonly used. Contrast-enhanced CT appears to have a relatively high sensitivity and specificity, although it carries some risk for contrast nephropathy. MRI using either gadolinium-based contrast (Fig. 31-8) or "time-of-flight" sequencing is promising but needs further characterization. Intravenous pyelography may detect RVT but has a low sensitivity and specificity. Renal Doppler ultrasound is useful but is user dependent and has a lower sensitivity than CT venography.

Treatment with systemic anticoagulation (warfarin) is recommended in the absence of contraindications and may be associated with improved long-term survival. RVT does not appear to increase mortality in the absence of underlying malignancy. Most clinicians maintain anticoagulation for 6 to 9 months, similar to the approach with nonrenal deep vein thrombosis and pulmonary embolism. The long-term recurrence risk is low if the underlying predisposition is successfully treated, and patients are unlikely to require indefinite anticoagulation. Direct intravenous thrombolysis or operative thrombectomy may be considered in severe cases. Prophylactic anticoagulation in high-risk patients has been proposed and may be considered in appropriate candidates.

Prospectus for the Future

The burden of obesity, hypertension, and diabetes continues to increase at an alarming rate in the industrialized world, contributing significantly to the incidence of CKD. Atherosclerotic RAS remains a common cause of secondary hypertension and carries with it a markedly increased risk for future cardiovascular events. Revascularization should be used in limited situations until results from ongoing clinical trials are available. Other vascular disorders of the kidney are less commonly encountered but should be considered in the appropriate clinical setting in order to initiate early treatment.

References

Altman D, Carroli G, Duley L et al: Do women with pre-eclampsia, and their babies, benefit from magnesium sulphate? The Magpie Trial: A randomised placebo-controlled trial. Lancet 359:1877-1890, 2002.

Besbas N, Karpman D, Landau D, et al: A classification of hemolytic uremic syndrome and thrombotic thrombocytopenic purpura and related disorders. Kidney Int 70:423-431, 2006.

Chobanian AV, Bakris GL, Black HR, et al: Seventh Report of the Joint National Committee on Prevention, Detection, Evaluation, and Treatment of High Blood Pressure: The JNC 7 report. JAMA 289:2560-2572, 2003.

Chobanian AV, Bakris GL, Black HR, et al: Seventh Report of the Joint National Committee on Prevention, Detection, Evaluation, and Treatment of High Blood Pressure. Hypertension 42:1206-1252, 2003.

Cooper CJ, Haller ST, Colyer W, et al: Embolic protection and platelet inhibition during renal artery stenting. Circulation 117:2752-2760, 2008.

Estrera AL, Miller CC, III, Safi HJ, et al: Outcomes of medical management of acute type B aortic dissection. Circulation 114(1 Suppl):I384-I389, 2006.

Fogo A, Breyer JA, Smith MC: Accuracy in the diagnosis of hypertensive nephrosclerosis in African Americans: A report from the African American Study of Kidney Disease (AASK) trial. Kidney Int 51:244-252, 1997.

Gagnadoux MF, Habib R, Gubler MC, et al: Long-term (15-25 years) outcome of childhood hemolytic-uremic syndrome. Clin Nephrol 46:39-41, 1996.

Garovic VD, Textor SC: Renovascular hypertension and ischemic nephropathy. Circulation 112:1362-1374, 2005.

Glassock RJ: Prophylactic anticoagulation in nephrotic syndrome: A clinical conundrum. J Am Soc Nephrol 18:2221-2225, 2007.

Hirsch AT, Haskal ZJ, Hertzer NR, et al: ACC/AHA 2005 Practice Guidelines for the management of patients with peripheral arterial disease (lower extremity, renal, mesenteric, and abdominal aortic). Circulation 113:e463-e654, 2006.

Kalra PA, Guo H, Kausz AT, et al: Atherosclerotic renovascular disease in United States patients aged 67 years or older: Risk factors, revascularization, and prognosis. Kidney Int 68:293-301, 2005.

Kansal S, Feldman M, Cooksey S, Patel S: Renal artery embolism: A case report and review. J Gen Intern Med 23:644-647, 2008.

Levine RJ, Lam C, Qian C, et al: Soluble endoglin and other circulating antiangiogenic factors in preeclampsia. N Engl J Med 355:992-1005, 2006.

Levine RJ, Maynard SE, Qian C, et al: Circulating angiogenic factors and the risk of preeclampsia. N Engl J Med 350:672-683, 2004.

Levine RJ, Thadhani R, Qian C, et al: Urinary placental growth factor and risk of preeclampsia. JAMA 293:77-85, 2005.

Lim W, Crowther MA, Eikelboom JW: Management of antiphospholipid antibody syndrome: A systematic review. JAMA 295:1050-1057, 2006.

Maynard S, Epstein FH, Karumanchi SA: Preeclampsia and angiogenic imbalance. Annu Rev Med 59:61-78, 2008.

Moake JL: Thrombotic microangiopathies. N Engl J Med 347:589-600, 2002.

Nienaber CA, Eagle KA: Aortic dissection: New frontiers in diagnosis and management: Part I: From etiology to diagnostic strategies. Circulation 108:628-635, 2003.

Nochy D, Daugas E, Droz D, et al: The intrarenal vascular lesions associated with primary antiphospholipid syndrome. J Am Soc Nephrol 10:507-518, 1999.

Nzerue CM, Hewan-Lowe K, Pierangeli S, Harris EN: "Black swan in the kidney": Renal involvement in the antiphospholipid antibody syndrome. Kidney Int 62:733-744, 2002.

Pascual A, Bush HS, Copley JB: Renal fibromuscular dysplasia in elderly persons. Am J Kidney Dis 45:e63-e66, 2005.

Sadler JE: Von Willebrand factor, ADAMTS13, and thrombotic thrombocytopenic purpura. Blood 112:11-18, 2008.

Samarkos M, Loizou S, Vaiopoulos G, Davies KA: The clinical spectrum of primary renal vasculitis. Semin Arthritis Rheum 35:95-111, 2005.

Sibai B, Dekker G, Kupferminc M: Pre-eclampsia. Lancet 365:785-799, 2005.

Slovut DP, Olin JW: Fibromuscular dysplasia. N Engl J Med 350:1862-1871, 2004.

Steen VD, Costantino JP, Shapiro AP, Medsger TA Jr: Outcome of renal crisis in systemic sclerosis: Relation to availability of angiotensin converting enzyme (ACE) inhibitors. Ann Intern Med 113:352-357, 1990.

Steen VD, Medsger TA Jr: Long-term outcomes of scleroderma renal crisis. Ann Intern Med 133:600-603, 2000.

Tarr PI, Gordon CA, Chandler WL: Shiga-toxin-producing Escherichia coli and haemolytic uraemic syndrome. Lancet 365:1073-1086, 2005.

Tsai HM: The molecular biology of thrombotic microangiopathy. Kidney Int 70:16-23, 2006.

Tsai HM: Advances in the pathogenesis, diagnosis, and treatment of thrombotic thrombocytopenic purpura. J Am Soc Nephrol 14:1072-1081, 2003.

Tsai TT, Fattori R, Trimarchi S, et al: Long-term survival in patients presenting with type B acute aortic dissection: Insights from the International Registry of Acute Aortic Dissection. Circulation 114:2226-2231, 2006.

Vasbinder GB, Nelemans PJ, Kessels AG, et al: Diagnostic tests for renal artery stenosis in patients suspected of having renovascular hypertension: a meta-analysis. Ann Intern Med 135:401-411, 2001.

Witz M, Kantarovsky A, Morag B, Shifrin EG: Renal vein occlusion: A review. J Urol 155:1173-1179, 1996.

Wong CS, Jelacic S, Habeeb RL, et al: The risk of the hemolytic-uremic syndrome after antibiotic treatment of Escherichia coli O157:H7 infections. N Engl J Med 342:1930-1936, 2000.

Wysokinski WE, Gosk-Bierska I, Greene EL, et al: Clinical characteristics and long-term follow-up of patients with renal vein thrombosis. Am J Kidney Dis 51:224-232, 2008.

Acute Kidney Injury

Didier Portilla and Sudhir V. Shah

Definition and Etiology

Acute renal failure (ARF) is a syndrome that can be broadly defined as an abrupt decrease in glomerular filtration rate (GFR) sufficient to result in retention of nitrogenous waste products (blood urea nitrogen [BUN] and creatinine) and perturbation of extracellular fluid volume and electrolyte and acid-base homeostasis. In the absence of a universally accepted definition of acute renal failure, and in recognition that ARF as previously defined includes a spectrum of clinical conditions, the term *acute kidney injury* (AKI) has been proposed to reflect the entire spectrum of the syndrome. In addition, a consensus conference involving key societies in nephrology and critical care worldwide has recommended the diagnostic criteria for AKI as outlined in Box 32-1.

Despite technical advances in renal replacement therapy and supportive care during the past few years, the mortality rate of patients with AKI remains high. Several recent studies highlight the clinical importance of AKI (Table 32-1).

Acute kidney injury can result from (1) diseases that cause a decrease of renal blood flow *(prerenal azotemia)*, (2) diseases that directly involve renal parenchyma *(renal azotemia)*, or (3) diseases associated with urinary tract obstruction *(postrenal azotemia)* (Fig. 32-1).

The most common intrinsic renal disease that leads to AKI is an entity referred to as *acute tubular necrosis* (ATN), which is a clinical syndrome characterized by an abrupt and sustained decline in GFR occurring within minutes to days in response to an acute ischemic or nephrotoxic insult. The clinical recognition of ATN is largely predicated on exclusion of prerenal and postrenal causes of sudden azotemia, followed by exclusion of other causes of intrinsic AKI (glomerulonephritis, acute interstitial nephritis, and vasculitis). The other defined renal syndromes must be excluded before concluding that ATN is present. Although the name *acute tubular necrosis* is not an entirely valid histologic description of this syndrome, the term is ingrained in clinical medicine and is therefore used in this chapter.

> ### Box 32-1 Diagnostic Criteria for Acute Kidney Injury
>
> An abrupt (within 48 hours) reduction in kidney function, currently defined as an absolute increase in serum creatinine of more than or equal to 0.3 mg/dL ($\geq$26.4 μmol/L), a percentage increase in serum creatinine of more than or equal to 50% (1.5-fold from baseline), or a reduction in urine output (documented oliguria <0.5 mL/kg per hour for more than 6 hours). The above criteria include both an absolute and a percentage change in creatinine to accommodate variations related to age, gender, and body mass index and to reduce the need for a baseline creatinine, but do require at least two creatinine values within 48 hours. The urine output criterion was included based on the predictive importance of this measure but with the awareness that urine outputs may not be measured routinely in non–intensive care unit settings. It is assumed that the diagnosis based on the urine output criterion alone will require exclusion of urinary tract obstructions that reduce urine output or of other easily reversible causes of reduced urine output. The above criteria should be used in the context of the clinical presentation and following adequate fluid resuscitation when applicable. Note: Many acute kidney diseases exist, and some (but not all) may result in AKI. Because diagnostic criteria are not documented, some cases of AKI may not be diagnosed. Furthermore, AKI may be superimposed on or lead to chronic kidney disease.

From Mehta RL, Kellum JA, Shah SV, et al: Acute kidney injury network: Report of an initiative to improve outcomes in acute kidney injury. Crit Care 11:R31, 2007. Copyright © 2007 Mehta et al.; licensee BioMed Central Ltd.

Differential Diagnosis and Diagnostic Evaluation of the Patient

ACUTE AZOTEMIA DURING HOSPITALIZATION

AKI complicates about 5% of hospital admissions and up to 30% of admissions to intensive care units. Despite the exhaustive list of conditions that can cause acute azotemia in hospitalized patients, a thorough history and physical examination and simple laboratory tests often suffice for diagnosis. In hospitalized adults, prerenal azotemia is the single most common cause of acute azotemia, and ATN is the most common intrinsic renal disease that leads to AKI. Thus, the most important differential diagnosis is between prerenal azotemia (e.g., volume depletion) and ATN (secondary to ischemia or nephrotoxins). In the elderly male patient, bladder outlet obstruction must also be excluded. In addition, depending on the clinical setting, other diagnoses to be considered are acute interstitial nephritis (secondary to antibiotics), atheromatous emboli (from prior aortic surgery or aortogram), ureteral obstruction (pelvic or colon surgery), or intrarenal obstruction (acute uric acid nephropathy).

APPROACH TO DIAGNOSIS: CHART REVIEW, HISTORY, AND PHYSICAL EXAMINATION

Determination of the cause of AKI depends on a systematic approach, as depicted in Table 32-2. The difficulty in arriving at a correct diagnosis in a hospitalized patient is not the failure to identify a possible cause of the AKI; the problem is often just the opposite in that several causes of AKI may be possible. The correct diagnosis depends on a thorough analysis of available data concerning the patient with AKI

Table 32-1 Clinical Importance of Acute Kidney Injury

Increasing incidence of acute kidney injury

Even minor (0.3 mg/dL) increases in serum creatinine levels are associated with increased in-hospital mortality

Acute kidney injury indicates a poor prognosis associated with a poor, long-term morbidity and mortality

A relatively unrecognized effect of acute kidney injury is the subsequent development of chronic kidney disease and progression to dialysis dependency in about 15% of the patients

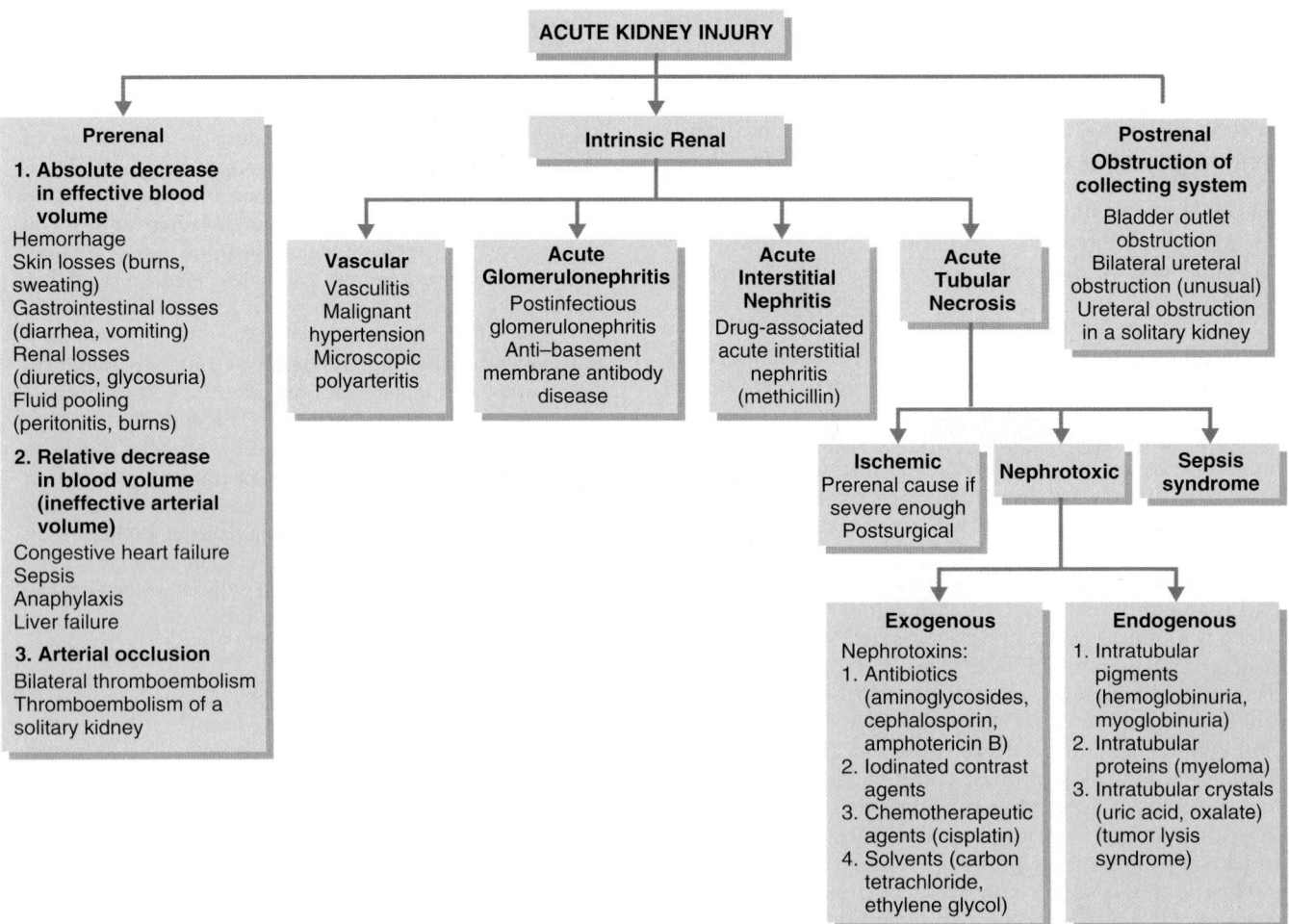

Figure 32-1 Causes of acute kidney injury.

and on examination of the sequence of deterioration in renal function in relation to chronology of the potential causes of AKI. The correct diagnosis also requires knowledge of the natural history of the different causes of AKI. Some of the important data that should be sought from the patient's chart review are presented in Table 32-3.

Reduced body weight, postural changes in blood pressure and pulse, and decreased jugular venous pulse all suggest a reduction in extracellular fluid volume. Prerenal azotemia may also develop in states in which extracellular fluids are expanded (cardiac failure, cirrhosis, and nephrotic syndrome), but the *effective* blood volume is decreased. Thorough abdominal examination may show a distended, tender bladder that indicates lower urinary tract obstruction. When lower urinary tract obstruction is suspected as a cause of acute azotemia, examination of the prostate and a sterile *in-and-out* diagnostic postvoid bladder catheterization

should be performed as a part of the physical examination. The urine volume should be recorded and a specimen saved for studies described later.

Additional findings that may be helpful are the occurrence of fever and rash in some patients with acute interstitial nephritis. A history of recent aortic catheterization and the finding of livedo reticularis are diagnostic clues for cholesterol or atheromatous emboli.

Differentiating prerenal azotemia from ATN may be difficult, partly because evaluation of volume status in a critically ill patient is not easy, and any cause of prerenal azotemia, if severe enough, may lead to ATN. Evaluation of the urine volume and urine sediment and of certain urinary indices is particularly helpful in making the correct diagnosis.

URINE VOLUME

The urine volume is often less than 400 mL per day in oliguric ATN. Normal urine output does not exclude the diagnosis of ATN because many patients with ATN have urine outputs as high as 1.5 to 2 L per day. This nonoliguric ATN is frequently associated with nephrotoxic antibiotic-induced AKI. In contrast, anuria (no urine output) should suggest a diagnosis other than ATN, the most important being obstruction. Widely varying daily urine outputs also suggest obstruction.

URINE SEDIMENT

In prerenal failure, a moderate number of hyaline and finely granular casts may be seen, but coarsely granular and cellular casts are infrequent. In ATN, the sediment is usually quite characteristic: *dirty* brown granular casts and renal tubular epithelial cells, free and in casts, are the most striking elements and are present in 70% to 80% of patients with ATN

Table 32-2 Diagnostic Approach to Acute Kidney Injury

1. Record review (see Table 32-3); special attention to evidence of recent reduction in glomerular filtration rate and sequence of events leading to deterioration of renal function to determine possible causative factors
2. Physical examination, including evaluation of hemodynamic status
3. Urinalysis, including thorough sediment examination
4. Determination of urinary indices
5. Bladder catheterization
6. Fluid diuretic challenge
7. Radiologic studies, particular procedure dictated by clinical setting (e.g., ultrasonography to look for obstruction)
8. Renal biopsy

Table 32-3 Record Review in a Hospitalized Patient Who Develops Acute Kidney Injury

Record Finding	Comments
Prior renal function	Determination of whether the azotemia is acute; patients with prior renal insufficiency particularly susceptible to AKI, secondary to contrast dyes
Presence of infection	Sepsis a possible cause of AKI, even in the absence of hypotension
Nephrotoxic agents	Aminoglycosides (e.g., gentamicin) important cause of ATN in hospitalized patients, typically nonoliguric ATN during first 2 wk of therapy; antibiotics possible cause of acute interstitial nephritis; cytotoxic drugs (e.g., cisplatin) possible cause of AKI
Contrast studies including oral cholecystography, intravenous pyelography, angiography	Important cause of ATN in hospitalized patients; typically causes oliguric ATN within 24 to 48 hr after study
Episodes of hypotension	Suggestion of prerenal azotemia or ischemic ATN
History of blood transfusions	Incompatible blood transfusion an unusual cause of ATN
Review of chart for history of loss or sequestration of extracellular fluid volume, intake-output, and serial weights	Important clues to the possibility of prerenal azotemia
Type of surgery	Patients who have had cardiac or vascular surgery or with obstructive jaundice particularly susceptible to ATN
Type of anesthesia	Methoxyflurane and the related less toxic enflurane causes of nonoliguric ATN
Amount of blood loss during surgery and whether associated with hypotension	Suggestion of prerenal azotemia or ischemic ATN

AKI, acute kidney injury; ATN, acute tubular necrosis.

(**Web Fig. 32-1A and B**). A benign sediment containing few formed elements should alert the physician to the possibility that obstruction is present. In AKI associated with intratubular oxalate (e.g., methoxyflurane anesthesia) or uric acid deposition (associated with acute hyperuricemia after chemotherapy of neoplastic disease), the sediment contains abundant oxalate or uric acid crystals.

URINARY INDICES

An important series of diagnostic tests relates to an assessment of renal tubular function. The most widely used and convenient tests are measurements of sodium and creatinine simultaneously obtained from plasma and urine serum samples to calculate the fractional excretion of sodium (Fe_{Na}). The rationale for the use of these indices is as follows: The ratio of urine to plasma creatinine (U/P_{Cr}) provides an index of the fraction of filtered water excreted. If the assumption is made that all of the creatinine filtered at the glomerulus is excreted into the urine and that relatively little is added by secretion (an oversimplification but an acceptable one), then any increment in the concentration of creatinine in urine over that in plasma must result from the removal of water.

In prerenal azotemia, owing to the reduction in the amount of glomerular filtrate entering each nephron and to an added stimulus to salt and water retention, U/P_{Cr} typically is considerably greater than it is in ATN, and urinary sodium concentrations characteristically are low (Table 32-4). In contrast, in the ATN variety of AKI, the nephrons excrete a large fraction of their filtered sodium and water, and the results are a lower U/P_{Cr} and a higher Fe_{Na}. An exception to the rule that low Fe_{Na} indicates prerenal and high Fe_{Na} indicates ATN is the use of a diuretic or the presence of glucosuria that decreases tubular sodium reabsorption and increases Fe_{Na}. Recent studies show that, in the presence of diuretics, the rate of fractional excretion of urea (Fe_{urea}) of less than 35 indicates intact tubular function, thus favoring prerenal rather than established ARF as a cause of the azotemia. Because of the adaptive responses, in a patient with advanced chronic kidney disease (CKD), prerenal azotemia may not be associated with a Fe_{Na} of less than 1%. Interpretations of these tests, therefore, must

be made in conjunction with other assessments of the patient because clinically important exceptions to these generalizations exist. For example, certain types of ATN, such as in the case of severe burns, sepsis, and radiographic dye-induced kidney injury, or conditions associated with vascular inflammation, such as acute glomerulonephritis, acute vasculitis, or kidney transplant rejection, may exhibit all of the clinical characteristics of ATN but with an Fe_{Na} of less than 1%.

INDICATIONS FOR OTHER DIAGNOSTIC TESTS AND RENAL BIOPSY

If the diagnosis of prerenal azotemia or ATN is reasonably certain, and if the clinical setting does not require the exclusion of other causes of acute azotemia, then no further diagnostic evaluation is necessary. Further assessment is indicated in the following situations: (1) when the diagnosis is uncertain, especially if the clinical setting, suggests other possibilities (obstruction or vascular accident); (2) when clinical findings make the diagnosis of prerenal azotemia or ATN unlikely (anuria); or (3) when oliguria persists beyond 4 weeks.

Ultrasonography of the urinary tract is a noninvasive way to determine the presence of dilation of the collecting system that would suggest postrenal AKI. Radionuclide methods are available to assess the presence or absence of renal blood flow, differences in flow to the two kidneys, and excretory (secretory) function. However, these studies have reduced accuracy in quantitating absolute rates of flow. Renal biopsy is useful in cases in which clinical and laboratory assessment suggest diagnoses other than ischemic or nephrotoxic injury that may respond to disease-specific therapy. These conditions include glomerulonephritis, vasculitis, hemolytic uremic syndrome (HUS), thrombotic thrombocytopenic purpura, and allergic interstitial nephritis.

Approach to the Patient with Renal Failure

Azotemia first discovered outside the hospital may be either chronic or acute in origin. Useful points in deciding whether renal failure is acute or chronic are summarized in Table 32-5. Most patients who have advanced azotemia have chronic renal failure. Before a detailed evaluation is carried out, priority should be given to identifying complications of renal failure that may be lethal without prompt treatment. Some of these complications, such as marked fluid overload and pericardial tamponade, may be detected on clinical examination. However, life-threatening complications such as severe hyperkalemia or extreme metabolic acidosis require laboratory evaluation.

Even before the nature of the underlying disease causing azotemia is known, a decision to initiate dialysis has to be made. Dialysis should be instituted promptly in patients with severe hyperkalemia, acidosis, marked fluid overload, or uremic manifestations. Many uremic manifestations are nonspecific. However, a pericardial rub and neurologic manifestations such as asterixis are indications for prompt dialysis.

Table 32-4 Urinary Diagnostic Indices

Index	Prerenal Azotemia	Acute Tubular Necrosis
Urine sodium (U_{Na}) (mEq/L)	<20	>40
Urine creatinine (U_{Cr}) (mg/dL)/P_{Cr} (mg/dL)	>40	<20
Urine osmolarity (U_{OSM}) (mOsm/kg H_2O)	>500	<350
Renal failure index (RFI) = $U_{Na}U_{Cr}/P_{Cr}$	<1	>1
Fractional excretion of filtered sodium (Fe_{Na}) $Fe_{Na} = U_{Na}P_{Cr}/P_{Na}U_{Cr}$ (100)	<1	>1

P_{Cr}, plasma creatinine; P_{Na}, plasma sodium; U_{Cr}, urine creatinine; U_{Na}, urine sodium.

Table 32-5 Useful Features that Suggest Acute or Chronic Kidney Disease

Feature	Acute Kidney Injury	Chronic Kidney Disease
Previous history	Normal renal function	History of elevated blood urea nitrogen or creatinine
Kidney size	Normal	Small, with exception of multiple myeloma, diabetes, amyloid, polycystic kidney disease
Bone film	No evidence of renal osteodystrophy	Possible evidence of renal osteodystrophy
Hemoglobin, hematocrit	Anemia possible, but normal hemoglobin level in a patient with advanced azotemia is presumptive evidence of acute renal failure	Anemia common

LABORATORY EVALUATION

In hospitalized adults in whom the diagnoses of prerenal and postrenal azotemia have been excluded, AKI is usually caused by ATN. By contrast, in an outpatient setting in which prerenal and postrenal causes have been excluded, other renal parenchymal diseases cause AKI more often. Examination of the urine for blood and protein and of the urine sediment can give valuable information that often helps narrow considerably the diagnostic possibilities and suggest further appropriate laboratory evaluation.

The presence of 3+ to 4+ protein, 2+ to 3+ blood, and an active sediment with red blood cells (RBCs) and RBC casts is characteristic of proliferative glomerulonephritis. A history of an underlying systemic disease and various laboratory tests such as complement levels, antinuclear factor, and protein electrophoresis may suggest the presence of glomerulonephritis, but a kidney biopsy is required for a definitive diagnosis (reviewed in Chapter 29).

The presence of only a few RBCs in the urine sediment with strongly heme-positive urine or a heme-positive supernatant (with the RBCs removed by centrifugation) most commonly results from myoglobinuria or hemoglobinuria. Patients with rhabdomyolysis have a marked increase in the muscle enzymes such as creatine phosphokinase (CPK). The urine sediment in patients with myoglobinuria may show RBCs, pigmented casts, granular casts, and numerous uric acid crystals.

IMAGING STUDIES

Kidney size gives important clues about whether the kidney failure is acute or chronic and whether obstruction is present. Renal ultrasonography is the initial procedure of choice because it is noninvasive and reliable. The finding of normal-sized kidneys in a patient with advanced azotemia generally suggests that the patient has acute rather than chronic kidney disease; however, several important causes of CKD, including diabetes mellitus, HIV nephropathy, multiple myeloma, and amyloidosis, may be associated with normal-sized kidneys. The renal ultrasound examination is also helpful in (1) making a diagnosis of polycystic kidney disease, (2) determining whether one or two kidneys are present, and (3) localizing the kidney for renal biopsy.

Normal kidney size in a patient with kidney failure is often an indication for renal biopsy. Before a renal biopsy is carried out, the patient's blood pressure must be controlled, bleeding and coagulation parameters must be checked, and the presence of two kidneys must be confirmed.

CYSTATIN C: A NEW MARKER FOR KIDNEY FUNCTION?

Cystatin C is a nonglycosylated 13-kD basic cysteine protease that all nucleated cells produce, and inflammatory conditions or muscle mass do not alter the production rate; only thyroid dysfunction has been shown to alter serum levels independent of glomerular filtration rate (GFR). Serum cystatin C levels increase before serum creatinine levels in patients with progressive CKD. Recent data also suggests that cystatin C levels increase 1 to 2 days before serum creatinine in patients developing AKI in the setting of radiocontrast nephropathy, kidney transplantation, and AKI in the intensive care unit. Cystatin C is excreted by glomerular filtration and then undergoes essentially complete tubular reabsorption and catabolism, without secretion, so that it is not normally found in urine in significant amounts. Based on these preliminary studies, cystatin C holds a promise as a potential novel diagnostic test to indicate the early development of acute tubular injury.

Clinical Presentation, Complications, and Management of Acute Tubular Necrosis

AKI produces signs and symptoms that reflect loss of the regulatory, excretory, and endocrine functions of the kidney. The loss of excretory ability of the kidney is expressed by a rise in the plasma concentration of specific substances that the kidney normally excretes. The most widely monitored indices are the concentrations of BUN and creatinine in the serum. In patients without other complications, the BUN rises by about 10 to 20 mg/dL per day, and the bicarbonate level falls to a steady-state level of 17 to 18 mEq/L. The serum potassium level need not rise appreciably, except in the presence of a hypercatabolic state, gastrointestinal bleeding, or extensive tissue trauma.

Because ATN is inherently a catabolic disorder, patients with ATN generally lose about 0.5 lb per day. Providing adequate calories (1800 to 2500 kcal or 35 kcal/kg body weight per day) and about 1 to 1.4 g/kg body weight of protein per day may minimize further weight loss. The use of hyperalimentation with 50% dextrose and essential amino acids has had little effect on minimizing mortality and morbidity in patients with ATN, except in patients who also have significant burns.

Hyperkalemia is a life-threatening complication of AKI and often necessitates urgent intervention. The electromechanical effects of hyperkalemia on the heart are potentiated by hypocalcemia, acidosis, and hyponatremia. Thus, the electrocardiogram, which measures the summation of these effects, is a better guide to therapy compared with a single potassium determination. The cardiac effects of hyperkalemia are primarily referable to blunting of the magnitude of the action potential in response to a depolarizing stimulus. The sequential electrocardiographic changes observed in hyperkalemia are peaked T waves, prolongation of the PR interval, widening of the QRS complex, and a sine wave pattern, and these changes are mandatory indications for prompt treatment. The most common biochemical abnormality responsible for death in patients with ATN is hyperkalemia.

Moderate acidosis is generally well tolerated and does not need treatment unless used as an adjunct to controlling hyperkalemia or when plasma bicarbonate levels fall to less than 15 mEq/L. Hyperkalemia and acidosis not easily controlled by medical therapy are indications for initiating dialysis.

In most patients, hypocalcemia is asymptomatic and does not require treatment. Phosphate-binding gels may be used in patients with significant hyperphosphatemia. Anemia regularly develops in patients with ATN and does not require treatment unless it is symptomatic or contributes to heart failure.

In a well-managed patient (with use of early dialysis), many of the uremic manifestations outlined in Table 32-6 either do not develop or are minimal. However, infection remains the main cause of death despite vigorous dialysis. Thus, meticulous aseptic care of intravenous catheters and wounds and avoidance of the use of indwelling urinary catheters are important in the management of such patients.

The indications for initiating dialysis are severe hyperkalemia and acidosis not easily controlled by medical treatment or fluid overload. In the absence of any of the foregoing conditions, most nephrologists advocate dialysis when the BUN reaches about 80 to 100 mg/dL because the goal of modern therapy is to avoid the occurrence of uremic symptoms. Therefore, the patient is dialyzed as frequently as is necessary to keep the BUN at less than 80 mg/dL. When this approach is used, most patients do not develop uremic symptoms, the diet and fluid intake can be liberalized, and the overall management of the patient is easier. Finally, the clinician must review thoroughly the indications for and the doses of all drugs administered to patients with ATN. Monitoring of blood concentrations of drugs is an important adjunct to effective treatment.

Outcome and Prognosis

The oliguric phase of ATN typically lasts for 1 to 2 weeks and is followed by the diuretic phase. About one fourth to

Table 32-6 **Major Complications of Acute Kidney Injury**	
Impairment of Fluid and Electrolyte Excretion	
Water	Hyponatremia
Sodium chloride	Volume expansion
	Congestive heart failure
Potassium	Hyperkalemia
	Arrhythmias
Hydrogen	Acidosis
Phosphate	Hyperphosphatemia
	Hypocalcemia
	Metastatic calcifications
Magnesium	Hypermagnesemia
Uric acid	Hyperuricemia
Retention of urea and other solutes	Uremia
	Cardiac: pericarditis
	Neurologic: asterixis, confusion, somnolence, coma, seizures
	Hematologic: anemia, coagulopathy, bleeding diathesis
	Infection
	Gastrointestinal: nausea, vomiting, gastritis, bleeding
	Skin: pruritus
	Glucose intolerance
Synthetic Impairment	
1,25-Dihydroxyvitamin D_3	Hypocalcemia
Erythropoietin	Anemia
Impaired drug metabolism and excretion	Drug toxicity, decreased diuretic effectiveness

one third of the deaths occur in the diuretic phase. This finding is not surprising because, with the availability of dialysis, the most important determinant of the outcome is not the uremia itself but rather the underlying disease that causes the ATN.

As noted previously, infection continues to be the most important cause of death in patients with ATN. In modern acute care hospitals, the outcome of patients who develop ATN is highly variable, and, depending on the nature of the underlying disease, mortality rates may be in excess of 50%. In patients who survive the acute episode, renal function returns essentially to normal, with the only residual findings being a modest reduction in GFR and an inability to concentrate and acidify urine maximally.

Prevention

The first principle of good management is prophylaxis. This approach requires recognition of the clinical settings in which ATN normally occurs (e.g., in patients undergoing cardiac or aortic surgery) and recognition of patients particularly susceptible to ATN. Useful measures include correcting fluid deficiencies before surgical procedures and keeping patients who are particularly at risk adequately hydrated before radiocontrast studies. Nephrotoxic drugs should be used only when essential and then only with careful monitoring of the patient. Finally, pretreatment with allopurinol before chemotherapy of massive tumors diminishes uric acid excretion.

Pathogenesis of Acute Tubular Necrosis

Although an initial decrease in renal blood flow appears to be a requisite for the development of ischemic ATN, blood flow returns to near normal within 24 to 48 hours after the initial insult. Despite adequate renal blood flow, tubular dysfunction persists, and the GFR remains depressed. Despite the common use of the term *acute tubular necrosis,* necrosis of the tubules is seen infrequently in either ischemic or nephrotoxic AKI. In addition, although two kinds of cell death, *apoptosis* and *necrosis,* are recognized, one of the major advances in the medical community's understanding of cell death has been the recognition that the pathways traditionally associated with apoptosis may be critical in the form of cell injury associated with necrosis. Thus, evidence indicates that apoptotic mechanisms, including increased mitochondrial membrane permeability resulting in the release and activation of apoptogenic factors such as endonuclease, are important in renal tubular injury and that certain mediators (increased fatty acids, oxidants, caspases, and ceramide) regulate this process. The pathway that the cell follows depends on both the nature and the severity of insults. Integral to the path that is followed is thought to be the expression of many genes involved in cell cycle regulation, as well as a group of genes that are proinflammatory and chemotactic. The cascades that lead to the apoptotic or necrotic mode of cell death probably are activated almost simultaneously and may share some common pathways (see Table 32-4).

Various biochemical changes have been implicated in proximal tubule cell injury in ARF. These changes include mitochondrial dysfunction, adenosine triphosphate (ATP) depletion, phospholipid degradation, elevation in cytosolic free calcium, decrease in sodium Na^+, K^+-ATPase activity, alterations in substrate metabolism, lysosomal changes, and the production of oxygen-free radicals. Which changes are causative and which may simply be byproducts of advanced cell injury is not yet clear.

Recent studies provide support for the role of microvascular endothelium and inflammatory cells in the pathophysiology of ischemic AKI. An early elevation on circulating levels of von Willebrand factor (a marker for endothelial cell injury) is seen, as well as increases in F-actin aggregates in the basolateral aspects of renal microvascular endothelial cells, accompanied by increased leukocyte and perhaps T-cell endothelial–adhesive interactions. Leakage of glomerular ultrafiltrate from the tubular lumen into the renal interstitium across the damaged renal tubular cells, obstruction to flow resulting from debris or crystals in the lumen of the tubules, and a decrease in the glomerular capillary ultrafiltration coefficient have all been proposed to play a pathophysiologic role in sustaining the clinical picture of ATN.

Specific Causes of Acute Renal Failure

EXOGENOUS NEPHROTOXINS
Radiographic Contrast Agents

Contrast media–associated AKI has been associated with increased mortality, permanent loss of kidney function, kidney failure requiring dialysis, prolonged hospitalization, and increased cost of medical care. Contrast media–associated AKI is rare in patients who are not at high risk for contrast nephropathy. Risk factors associated with contrast media nephropathy are listed in Table 32-7. Patients with a combination of advanced CKD and diabetes are considered at extremely high risk for developing acute kidney disease.

The exact mechanism by which contrast medium causes acute kidney disease is not well understood. Suggested mechanisms include severe vasoconstriction of renal medullary vessels and direct renal tubular toxicity likely related to release of oxidants.

Although acute kidney disease in this setting is usually defined as an increase in serum creatinine of 0.5 mg/dL or 25% or more from the baseline, an increase in serum creatinine of as little as 0.3 mg/dL is associated with unfavorable outcomes. Most patients develop acute kidney failure within 24 to 96 hours after parenteral administration of contrast media and, in most of these patients, kidney function recovers within 7 to 10 days. In a small proportion of patients, kidney function may not recover completely, or the patients may require dialysis. A diagnosis of contrast media–associated AKI is made on the temporal association of exposure to contrast media and kidney injury without any other obvious cause for AKI. Most patients have an Fe_{Na} of less than 1%. To date, no treatment for contrast media–associated renal failure is available, and therefore prevention is the key (Table 32-8). Hydration with saline has proved beneficial. In high-risk groups, intravenous administration of saline 4 to 12 hours before and 8 to 12 hours after

Table 32-7 **Major Risk Factors Associated with Contrast Media-Associated Nephropathy**
Chronic kidney disease
Diabetes mellitus
Age > 65 yr
Volume depletion
Study requiring large volume of contrast
High osmolar contrast media
Presence of more than one risk factor

Table 32-8 **Prevention of Contrast Media-Associated Nephropathy**
Identify high-risk patients
Avoid volume depletion
Use adequate saline hydration before and after the procedure
Limit contrast volume
Use iso-osmolar contrast media

administering contrast media is recommended. Hydration with a solution containing bicarbonate has been shown to decrease the incidence of contrast nephropathy, but until more data are available, normal saline is recommended. Iso-osmolar contrast media has also been shown to have lower incidence of contrast nephropathy. Prophylactic use of *N*-acetylcysteine has not shown to be of consistent benefit.

Aminoglycosides

One of the most important manifestations of aminoglycoside (e.g., tobramycin, gentamicin, amikacin) nephrotoxicity is AKI, which occurs in about 10% of patients receiving these drugs. Maintaining blood levels in the therapeutic range reduces but does not eliminate the risk for nephrotoxicity. AKI is usually mild and nonoliguric and produces a rise in the serum creatinine level after about 1 week of therapy with one of the aminoglycosides. The prognosis for recovery of kidney function after several days is excellent, although some patients may need dialysis support before recovery.

Nonsteroidal Anti-Inflammatory Drugs

Nonsteroidal anti-inflammatory drugs (NSAIDs) have several acute renal effects. NSAIDs are potent inhibitors of prostaglandin synthesis, a property that contributes to their nephrotoxic potential in certain high-risk patients in whom renal vasodilation depends on prostaglandins. The most frequent pattern of injury related to NSAIDs is prerenal azotemia, particularly in patients who either are volume contracted or have a reduced effective circulating volume. Susceptible persons include those with congestive heart failure, cirrhosis, CKD, and volume depletion. Hyperchloremic metabolic acidosis, often associated with hyperkalemia, has also been recognized as an effect of the NSAIDs, particularly in persons with preexisting chronic interstitial kidney disease. Hyporeninemic hypoaldosteronism occurs in these persons in states of renal prostaglandin inhibition. Finally, NSAIDs have been associated with the development of acute interstitial nephritis, often associated with renal insufficiency and nephrotic-range proteinuria. This complication appears to be an idiosyncratic reaction to propionic acid derivatives such as ibuprofen, naproxen, and fenoprofen. In contrast to acute interstitial nephritis associated with other drugs, the incidence of hypersensitivity symptoms and eosinophilia is low. Discontinuation of the offending agent usually results in resolution of this disorder.

Cyclo-oxygenase-2 Inhibitors

Cyclo-oxygenase-2 (COX-2) inhibitors have recently become a frequently used component of drug therapy in the adult population to treat acute inflammatory states, including arthritis and pain. Results from recent clinical trials have indicated that prostaglandins formed by COX-2 have important roles in renal physiology under certain conditions and that the effects of COX-2 inhibitors on kidney function are similar to those of traditional NSAIDs. Patients who are considered at elevated risk for adverse kidney events, including those with advanced age, kidney or hepatic disease, congestive heart failure, and diuretic or angiotensin-converting enzyme inhibitor therapy, should be monitored with the same caution when receiving therapy with COX-2 inhibitors

as they would be when receiving NSAIDs. A total of 15 cases of AKI associated with the use of these drugs have been reported to date: 9 with celecoxib and 6 with rofecoxib. All cases occurred in patients with the risk factors listed previously, and all patients returned to baseline renal function within 3 days to 3 weeks after discontinuation of COX-2 inhibitor therapy.

Cisplatin

Kidney injury is a well-recognized and dose-dependent complication of cisplatin, an antineoplastic agent used in the treatment of several carcinomas. Hypomagnesemia resulting from renal losses of magnesium may be severe and can occur in as many as 50% of patients. Patients should be well hydrated before they receive cisplatin, and simultaneous treatment with other known nephrotoxins should be avoided whenever possible. The usual lesion is that of ATN, but with severe damage or recurrent administration of the drug, chronic interstitial disease may ensue.

ETHYLENE GLYCOL TOXICITY

Ethylene glycol is a colorless, odorless, sweet liquid found in solvents and antifreeze. Ingestion of ethylene glycol, usually in the form of antifreeze, produces a characteristic syndrome of severe high anion gap $(Na^+) - [(Cl^-) + (HCO_3^-)]$ metabolic acidosis with a large osmolar gap $[(2)(Na^+) + (BUN)/2.8 + (glucose)/18 + (ethanol)/4.7]$. Ethylene glycol is metabolized by alcohol dehydrogenase to glycolic acid, which is believed to be the major contributor to acidosis. The key clinical findings in patients who have ingested ethylene glycol are disorientation and agitation initially, progressing to central nervous system depression, renal failure, metabolic acidosis, respiratory failure, and circulatory insufficiency. Hypocalcemia is a prominent feature attributed to the deposition of calcium oxalate in multiple tissues but may be aggravated by a decreased parathyroid hormone response. The typical urine sediment is calcium oxalate crystals. AKI generally follows after 48 to 72 hours.

Aggressive intervention with intravenous sodium bicarbonate to enhance renal clearance of glycolate through ion trapping, intravenous ethanol or fomepizole (Antizol) to block the metabolism of ethylene glycol, and hemodialysis for removing ethylene glycol and glycolate should be initiated at the time of diagnosis. Regular monitoring of the osmolar gap (corrected for ethanol level if intravenous ethanol is being used during treatment) and anion gap will help guide therapy during hemodialysis.

ANGIOTENSIN-CONVERTING ENZYME INHIBITORS

AKI associated with angiotensin-converting enzyme inhibitors is thought to be hemodynamic in origin, resulting from loss of autoregulation of renal blood flow and GFR, and has been typically reported when these drugs are given to patients with bilateral renal artery stenosis or with moderately advanced azotemia. Allergic acute interstitial nephritis similar to that observed with antibiotic administration has also been reported.

ENDOGENOUS NEPHROTOXINS

Rhabdomyolysis

Since the first description of the causative association between rhabdomyolysis and AKI in persons with crush injuries during World War II, the spectrum of causes of rhabdomyolysis, myoglobinuria, and renal failure has broadened. Rhabdomyolysis is most frequently the result of trauma or other injury, leading to muscle compression, ischemia, excess muscle activity associated with exercise or seizures, metabolic derangements (hypokalemia and hypophosphatemia), drugs, and infections. Cocaine use, neuroleptic malignant syndrome, and the use of hydroxymethylglutaryl coenzyme A reductase inhibitors (statin drugs) in the treatment of hypercholesterolemia also contribute to or cause rhabdomyolysis. Muscle pain and dark-brown orthotoluidine-positive urine without RBCs are important diagnostic clues, but the diagnosis must be confirmed by elevations of CPK and myoglobin. About one third of patients with rhabdomyolysis develop ARF, frequently associated with hyperkalemia, hyperuricemia, hyperphosphatemia, early hypocalcemia, and a reduced ratio of BUN to creatinine because of excessive creatinine release from muscle. Late hypercalcemia is also a typical feature of the disease.

The most important aspect of management will be rapid volume repletion. When patients are encountered in the field, intravenous fluids of normal saline at 200 to 300 mL per hour should be initiated. If urine output increases in 4 to 6 hours, the solution should be continued to match the urine output until the rhabdomyolysis resolves. However, if the patient continues to be oliguric (urine output < 400 mL per day), the infusion should be discontinued and the patient treated conservatively for AKI. Experience from recent disasters documents that early aggressive hydration and alkalinization (3 ampules of sodium bicarbonate to 1 L of 5% dextrose in water at 250 mL per hour) are capable of preventing myoglobinuric AKI by protecting the kidney from the nephrotoxicity of myoglobin and urate. The metabolic alkalosis induced will help protect the patient from hyperkalemia, which can be a lethal complication of rhabdomyolysis.

Hyperuricemic Acute Kidney Injury

AKI may occur in patients with *high-turnover* malignant diseases (acute lymphoblastic leukemia and poorly differentiated lymphomas) who either spontaneously or, more frequently, after cytotoxic therapy release massive amounts of purine uric acid precursors. This process leads to uric acid precipitation in the renal tubules. During massive cell lysis, phosphate and potassium are also released in large amounts, with resulting hyperphosphatemia and hyperkalemia. The peak uric acid level is often greater than 20 mg/dL, and a ratio of urinary uric acid to creatinine concentrations greater than 1:1 suggests the diagnosis of acute uric acid nephropathy. Prevention of AKI includes establishing a urinary output of 3 L or more per 24 hours, and treatment with allopurinol before cytotoxic therapy is instituted. More recent studies suggest that crucial to the management of tumor lysis syndrome (TLS) is the prompt initiation of a hypouricemic agent such as rasburicase. An established dose of 0.2 mg/kg of rasburicase is effective at decreasing uric acid levels significantly in 4 hours of administration and to undetectable levels in 48 hours of initiation. Rasburicase has excellent tolerability and is potentially cost-effective in patients at high risk for TLS. Rasburicase is a safe and effective hypouricemic agent for both adults and children at high risk for TLS and for this reason should be considered the uricolytic agent of choice in these patients.

Hepatorenal Syndrome

The hepatorenal syndrome (HRS) is defined as kidney failure in patients with severely compromised liver function in the absence of clinical, laboratory, or anatomic evidence of other known causes of kidney failure. It closely resembles prerenal failure, except it does not respond to conventional volume replacement. Type I HRS is characterized by rapid decline in renal function within weeks and is most often seen in patients suffering from acute liver failure, acute alcoholic hepatitis, or acute decompensation of chronic liver disease. These patients tend to have severe hyperbilirubinemia, prolongation of prothrombin time, hyponatremia, and clinical evidence of portal hypertension and hepatic encephalopathy. Arterial blood pressure is usually low. Acute decompensation in type 1 HRS may be precipitated by bacterial infections, that is, spontaneous bacterial peritonitis, abdominal paracentesis, use of nephrotoxic antibiotics or NSAIDs, overzealous use of diuretics, diarrhea, and gastrointestinal bleeding. If left untreated, it runs a rapid downhill course resulting in death of the patient within weeks. Type 2 HRS is characterized by insidious onset and slowly progressive deterioration of renal function. This is most often seen in patients with decompensated cirrhosis and portal hypertension. This group of patients has low to normal blood pressure, less jaundice, and also refractory ascites. It tends to run a slowly progressive downhill course over months. The hallmark of hepatorenal syndrome is oliguria with urine osmolality two to three times the concentration of plasma, as well as urine that is virtually sodium free, similar to that of patients with prerenal azotemia.

In patients with hepatorenal syndrome, there is marked splanchnic and systemic vasodilation that results in arterial hypotension, arteriolar baroreceptor unloading, and overstimulation of sympathetic nervous and renin-angiotensin systems. This reflex neurohumoral hyperactivity, through endogenous vasoconstrictors and vasopressors such as angiotensin II and noradrenaline, induces arterial vasoconstriction in different extrasplanchnic vascular beds, including preglomerular arteries in the kidney. Recent randomized clinical trials have shown that treatment with a combination of the vasopressin analogue terlipressin plus intravenous albumin improved renal function in patients with type 1 HRS.

Acute Kidney Injury Related to Pregnancy

AKI of pregnancy is presently a rare occurrence in industrialized nations, occurring in about 1 in 20,000 deliveries. This decreased incidence is directly related to legalization of abortion in many countries.

AKI associated with infection following an abortion may be precipitated by hypotension, hemorrhage, sepsis, and disseminated intravascular coagulopathy. Although many organisms can be involved, the most serious and common infection associated with AKI is that caused by *Clostridium* species. The clinical picture may be associated with hemolysis as a result of the production of a toxin. Aggressive management with broad-spectrum antibiotics and dialysis support are the mainstays of therapy for this group of patients.

Pyelonephritis, or urinary tract infection, is one of the most common medical complications of pregnancy. About 25% of patients can develop a transient decline in GFR during pyelonephritis. These patients should be treated initially with intravenous antibiotics followed by oral antibiotics for up to 2 weeks of therapy.

In the third trimester, AKI is associated with and is secondary to complications of pregnancy, including preeclampsia, postpartum hemorrhage, amniotic fluid embolism, placental abruption, and retained fetal and placental parts. A renal failure pattern resembling ATN is seen in patients suffering from preeclampsia and peripartum hemorrhage. Bilateral cortical necrosis may occur in association with any type of ischemic injury and appears to have a disproportionate incidence in pregnancy compared with the nonpregnant adult. Abruptio placentae can also cause ATN but is most commonly associated with renal cortical necrosis. The syndrome involving hemolysis, elevated liver enzymes, and low platelets (HELLP syndrome) in association with preeclampsia has been associated with ARF in up to 7.7% of patients.

Postpartum AKI, also known as *postpartum hemolytic uremic syndrome,* is characterized by hypertension and microangiopathic hemolytic anemia and occurs 1 day to several months after delivery, the most common time frame being from 2 to 5 weeks postpartum. The mainstay of treatment is plasma exchange, with a maternal survival rate of 70% to 80%, compared with the 90% mortality rate that existed before the use of plasma exchange. Elevation of lactate dehydrogenase in HUS versus elevated transaminases in HELLP syndrome may provide help in distinguishing these two syndromes.

Prospectus for the Future

Members representing key societies in nephrology and critical care worldwide have organized a group called the *Acute Kidney Injury Network* to address many of the critical issues facing this field. Consensus conferences and research initiatives, as well as establishment of a clinical trials network emerging from such initiatives, are likely to provide significant advances in the field in the next decade. It is generally accepted that many of the clinical trials in AKI have failed because of late intervention. There is urgent need to identify biomarkers that indicate early kidney injury and predict development of renal failure before the changes in serum creatinine. There are several groups in the United States and elsewhere critically evaluating biomarkers for this purpose and other biomarkers that may have prognostic and therapeutic implications. Patients at risk for AKI are likely to be identified by specific genetic differences that predispose patients to the development of AKI. For example, patients who develop repeated episodes of rhabdomyolysis-induced AKI have been found to have genetic polymorphisms of carnitine palmitoyltransferase enzymes, a series of mitochondrial enzymes involved in the metabolism of fatty acids. Similarly, it may be possible to detect why, for example, only about 15% of patients develop aminoglycoside nephrotoxicity. Thus, in the future, it may be possible to target specific therapies that minimize potential side effects.

References

Chertow GM, Burdick E, Honour M, et al: Acute kidney injury, mortality, length of stay, and costs in hospitalized patients. J Am Soc Nephrol 16:3365-3370, 2005.

Dangas G, Iakovou I, Nikolsky E, et al: Contrast-induced nephropathy after percutaneous coronary interventions in relation to chronic kidney disease and hemodynamic variables. Am J Cardiol 95:13-19, 2005.

Herget-Rosenthal S, Marggraf G, Hüsing J, et al: Early detection of acute renal failure by serum cystatin C. Kidney Int 66:1115-1122, 2004.

Lassnigg A, Schmidlin D, Mouhieddine M, et al: Minimal changes of serum creatinine predict prognosis in patients after cardiothoracic surgery: A prospective cohort study. J Am Soc Nephrol 15:1597-1605, 2004.

Moreau R, Lebrec D: Acute kidney injury: New concepts. Nephron Physiol 109:73-79, 2008.

Nash K, Hafeez A, Hou S: Hospital-acquired renal insufficiency. Am J Kidney Dis 39:930-936, 2002.

Portilla D, Kaushal GP, Basnakian AG, Shah SV: Recent progress in the pathophysiology of acute renal failure. In Runge MS, Patterson C (eds): Principles of Molecular Medicine, 2nd ed. Totawa, NJ, Humana Press, 2006, pp 643-649.

Schrier RW, Wang W, Poole B, Mitra A: Acute renal failure: Definitions, diagnosis, pathogenesis and therapy. J Clin Invest 114:5-14, 2004.

Uchino S, Kellum J, Bellomo R, et al: Acute renal failure in critically ill patients. JAMA 294:813-818, 2005.

Chronic Renal Failure

Kerri Cavanaugh and T. Alp Ikizler

Chronic kidney disease (CKD) is defined as progressive and irreversible loss of renal function. The spectrum of CKD ranges from proteinuria to elevated serum creatinine, representing a decrease in the glomerular filtration rate (GFR), and finally complete loss of kidney function, that is, end-stage renal disease (ESRD). According to the National Kidney Foundation Kidney Disease Outcomes Quality Initiative (K/DOQI), CKD is classified into stages 1 to 5, based on GFR and irrespective of the underlying etiology (Table 33-1). In stages 1 and 2, in which GFR is more than 60 mL/1.73 m^2 per minute, evidence of kidney damage, such as proteinuria, hematuria, or other abnormalities in blood, urine, or imaging tests, must be present to meet the diagnostic criteria of CKD. Additionally, evidence of kidney damage must be present and persistent for at least 3 months to differentiate CKD from acute kidney injury.

CKD is a worldwide public health problem. First, in the United States, the prevalence of CKD estimated by population-based studies is about 20 million people. Many people with CKD will progress to kidney failure and require dialysis or a kidney transplantation. ESRD is the term used in the United States to describe people with kidney failure who are eligible to receive either dialysis or a kidney transplantation. Trends in the incidence and prevalence of ESRD suggest a continuing increase in the numbers of patients requiring care at least for the next few decades (**Web Fig. 33-1**). Care of the ESRD patient is costly, accounting for $23 billion (6.4%) of the U.S. Medicare budget in 2006. Second, elevated serum creatinine has been increasingly recognized as an independent risk factor for cardiovascular disease and death. Thus, classification of CKD will identify the patient at risk not only for renal loss but also for decreased survival.

The most common causes of ESRD are listed in Table 33-2. During the evaluation of CKD, every attempt should be made to arrive at the specific cause of kidney disease. Laboratory measurements of the serum creatinine concentration over a period of time (at least 3 months) will help differentiate between acute kidney injury and CKD. Renal biopsy is the most specific tool to reach a definitive diagnosis and guides treatment of the underlying cause, assessment of the prognosis, and determination of suitability for kidney transplantation. However, the procedure itself has potential complications, and clinical information, including present, past, and family histories, serology, examination of the urine sediment, and renal imaging may be sufficient to provide a conclusive diagnosis.

Pathophysiology of Chronic Kidney Disease

To ensure adequate solute, water, and acid-base balance, the surviving nephrons must adjust by increasing their filtration and excretion rates. Patients with CKD, especially at stages 3 to 5, are vulnerable to edema formation and severe volume overload, hyperkalemia, hyponatremia, and azotemia. During progressive kidney disease, sodium balance is maintained by increasing fractional excretion of sodium by the nephrons. Acid excretion is maintained until the late stages of CKD, when the GFR falls to less than 15 mL per minute. Initially, increased tubular ammonia synthesis provides an adequate buffer for hydrogen in the distal nephron. Later, a significant decrease in distal bicarbonate regeneration results in hyperchloremic metabolic acidosis. Further loss of nephron mass leads to the retention of organic ions such as sulfates, which results in an anion gap metabolic acidosis.

It has been appreciated for several decades that once GFR has decreased to below a critical level, CKD tends to progress relentlessly toward ESRD, regardless of the initial insult. This observation suggests that loss of a critical number of nephrons provokes a vicious cycle of further nephron loss. Figure 33-1 shows how risk factors may interact with pathophysiologic mechanisms to accelerate CKD progression. Detailed studies have elucidated a number of interrelated mechanisms that together contribute to CKD progression, including glomerular hemodynamic responses to nephron loss, proteinuria, and proinflammatory responses. Tubular hypertrophy is associated with increased energy expenditure, a metabolic event related to generation of reactive oxygen metabolites. Reactive oxygen metabolites have been proposed as a mechanism of tubulointerstitial damage in animal models. In addition, hyperlipidemia is believed to play a role in progressive kidney disease through mesangial

Table 33-1 Classification of Chronic Kidney Disease and U.S. Prevalence Rates

Stage	Description	GFR, (mL/1.73 m²/min)	U.S. Prevalence* (millions) (%)	U.S. Prevalence
1	**Kidney damage†** with normal or increased GFR	≥90	3.6	1.8
2	**Kidney damage†** with mildly decreased GFR	60-89	6.5	3.2
3	Moderately decreased GFR	30-59	15.5	7.7
4	Severely decreased GFR	15-29	0.7	0.4
5	Kidney failure	<15 or dialysis	0.3	0.1

*Data from Coresh J, Selvin E, Stevens LA, et al: Prevalence of chronic kidney disease in the United States. JAMA 298:2038-2047, 2007.
  †As defined by the National Kidney Foundation, 2002. Kidney damage is defined as pathologic abnormalities or markers of damage, including abnormalities in blood or imaging studies.
  GFR, glomerular filtration rate.

Table 33-2 Incidence of End-Stage Renal Disease by Primary Diagnosis, 2002-2006

Primary Cause	Incidence (%)
Diabetes	44.8
Hypertension, large vessel disease	27.4
Glomerulonephritis	7.7
Interstitial nephritis; pyelonephritis	3.4
Cystic, hereditary, congenital disease	3.1
Neoplasms, tumors	2.4
Secondary glomerulonephritis, vasculitis	2.2
Miscellaneous conditions*	4.9
Cause unknown	7.5

*Including sickle cell disease, AIDS nephropathy, postpartum renal failure, traumatic loss, hepatorenal syndrome, and tubular necrosis.

proliferation and sclerosis. Activation of the renin-angiotensin-aldosterone system (RAAS) pathway and increased transforming growth factor-β (TGF-β) also play critical roles in leading to renal fibrosis. The observation that interventions that reduce intraglomerular pressure, such as protein restriction and the use of angiotensin-converting enzyme (ACE) inhibitors or angiotensin-receptor blockers (ARBs), help attenuate progression of renal disease further support the importance of glomerular hemodynamics and RAAS in progressive kidney disease.

Care of the Patient with Chronic Kidney Disease

Comprehensive care of kidney disease includes screening, diagnosing, and treating CKD and complications of CKD to prevent CKD development and progression (**Web Fig 33-2**). Screening for CKD is recommended in patients with high-risk co-morbid disease, including diabetes mellitus and hypertension, and also those with a family history of kidney disease. Once a diagnosis of CKD is established, management goals include (1) prevention of progression of CKD, (2) identifying and treating symptoms and complications of CKD, and (3) preparing patients for renal replacement therapy (RRT).

PREVENTION OF PROGRESSION

In addition to treatment of the specific underlying cause of kidney disease, methods used to slow progression of CKD include optimal control of hypertension, diabetes, and other cardiovascular disease risk factors (i.e. tobacco cessation), use of medications that block the RAAS pathway, diet modifications, avoidance of nephrotoxins, and addressing potentially reversible causes of acute kidney injury in the setting of CKD.

MANAGEMENT OF HYPERTENSION AND DIABETES

Several controlled trials have conclusively confirmed that aggressive management of hypertension attenuates the rate of progression of kidney disease, with significant benefits being shown in patients with diabetic kidney disease and other etiologies of CKD. The present recommendation is to target blood pressure to lower than 130/80 mm Hg in patients with diabetes or kidney disease. In addition, studies demonstrate that medications that block the production or effect of angiotensin II prevent the progression of CKD above and beyond control of hypertension in patients with diabetic and nondiabetic kidney disease and proteinuria. Dihydropyridine calcium channel blockers have not been shown to be as beneficial as ACE inhibitors or ARBs in slowing the progression of kidney disease. To reach optimal blood pressure control, an average of 2.7 antihypertensive medications will be needed per patient. When using a patient-centered multidisciplinary approach, it is important to evaluate the impact of therapy on a person's lifestyle to minimize side effects and maximize adherence to recommended therapies.

Diabetes mellitus is the leading cause of CKD in developed countries and is increasing in prevalence worldwide because of the epidemics of type 2 diabetes mellitus and obesity. For patients with diabetes mellitus, it is essential to screen annually for evidence of proteinuria as an indicator of CKD because an estimated GFR alone may not adequately reflect kidney damage due to diabetes. Adequate glycemic control in patients with diabetes mellitus and CKD is shown to prevent progression of CKD. Recommended goal glycosylated hemoglobin (A1C) measures are less than 7% irrespective of a concurrent diagnosis of CKD. For patients with diabetes mellitus and hypertension, ACE inhibitors and ARBs are the preferred medications for therapy because they

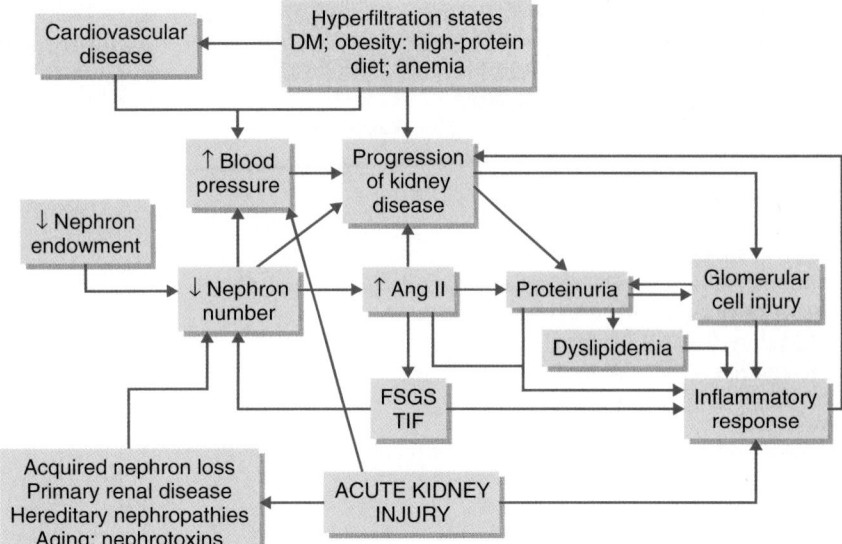

Figure 33-1 A simplified depiction of risk factors interacting with pathophysiologic mechanisms to accelerate chronic kidney disease progression. DM, diabetes mellitus; FSGS, focal segmental glomerulosclerosis; TIF, tubulointerstitial fibrosis. (Adapted from Taal MW, Brenner BM: Predicting initiation and progression of chronic kidney disease: Developing renal risk scores. Kidney Int 70:1694-1705, 2006.)

slow the progression of CKD. ACE inhibitors and ARBs may also be considered in patients with diabetes and proteinuria, but without hypertension, to slow CKD progression.

Diet

Dietary protein restriction is advocated to reduce uremic symptoms and slow progression of CKD. Several meta-analyses indicate that reduced protein diets may be modestly beneficial to slow CKD progression, but the largest clinical trial, the Modification of Diet in Renal Disease (MDRD) study, did not show a significant benefit. The recommended dietary protein intake in advanced CKD (stage 4 or 5) is 0.60 g/kg per day and, if this is not accepted or tolerated, can be increased to 0.75 g/kg per day, with at least 50% of the protein being of high biologic value (Table 33-3). The primary concern of applying a low-protein diet in patients with advanced CKD is the risk for predisposition to poor nutritional state, which is a strong predictor of increased mortality if present at the initiation of dialysis. The present consensus is that aggressive dietary management in patients with CKD, with proper restriction of sodium, potassium, phosphorus, and protein intake, may reduce progression of CKD, albeit to a small extent. Such dietary interventions should be instituted only under closely supervised patients in whom dietary behaviors such as protein and caloric intake can be monitored and maintained in conjunction with a specialized dietician.

Avoiding Toxic Drug Effects

Many drugs that are excreted by the kidney should be avoided, or their doses should be reduced, in patients with renal insufficiency, as shown in Table 33-4. Drugs may injure the kidney in many ways, including direct toxicity leading to acute tubular necrosis, induction of interstitial nephritis, or development of urinary crystals that may obstruct the kidney. Common classes of medications that injure the kidney include antibiotics, specifically aminoglycosides; nonsteroidal anti-inflammatory drugs, including cyclo-oxygenase-2 (COX-2) inhibitors; and antiretroviral

Table 33-3 Recommended Intake of Protein and Energy in Kidney Failure

Chronic Kidney Disease	Protein	Energy
Stage 1-3 (GFR > 30 mL/min)	No restriction	No restriction
Stage 4-5 (GFR < 30 mL/min)	0.60-0.75 g/kg/day*	35 kcal/kg/day†
Dialysis		
Hemodialysis	>1.2 g/kg/day	35 kcal/kg/day†
Peritoneal dialysis	>1.3 g/kg/day	35 kcal/kg/day†

*With close supervision and frequent dietary counseling.
†30 kcal/kg/day for individuals 60 years or older.
GFR, glomerular filtration rate.

medications. Over-the-counter herbal medications, including aristolochic acids, have been suggested to cause CKD and kidney failure. Herbal supplements, such as St. John's Wort, may interact with kidney transplant medications and should be avoided. Additionally, iodinated radiocontrast agents can cause acute or acute-on-chronic kidney injury. Iso-osmolar contrast agents are less toxic than high-osmolar agents. Risk factors for contrast-induced acute kidney injury include volume depletion and underlying CKD. Patients at high risk for contrast-induced kidney injury should receive intravenous fluid hydration with normal saline, and the volume of the contrast should be minimized. Some studies appear to indicate that 0.45% saline with 50 mEq of sodium bicarbonate per liter 8 to 10 hours before and after the procedure is beneficial, but large-scale controlled studies are still needed because a meta-analysis showed controversial results. Recent studies have also suggested a protective role of N-acetylcysteine, 600 mg orally given twice a day, the day before and the day of the contrast exposure, suggesting a role of reactive oxygen species in the injury. More recently, an association between the contrast agent gadolinium, used in magnetic resonance imaging (MRI), has been associated

Table 33-4 Drug Dosages in Chronic Kidney Disease

Major Dosage Reduction	Minor or No Reduction	Avoid Usage
Antibiotics		
Aminoglycosides	Erythromycin	
Penicillin	Nafcillin	Nitrofurantoin
Cephalosporins	Clindamycin	Nalidixic acid
Sulfonamides	Chloramphenicol	Tetracycline
Vancomycin	Isoniazid, rifampin	
Quinolones	Amphotericin B	
Fluconazole	Aztreonam, tazobactam	
Acyclovir, ganciclovir	Doxycycline	
Foscarnet		
Imipenem		
Others		
Digoxin	Antihypertensives	Aspirin
Procainamide	Benzodiazepines	Sulfonylureas
H_2 antagonists	Quinidine	Lithium carbonate
Meperidine	Lidocaine	Acetazolamide
Codeine	Spironolactone	NSAIDs
Propoxyphene	Triamterene	Phosphate-containing bowel-preps

NSAIDs, nonsteroidal anti-inflammatory drugs.

Table 33-5 Reversible Causes of Acute Kidney Injury in Chronic Kidney Disease

Decreased renal perfusion
    Intravascular volume depletion
    Heart failure
Obstruction
Infection
Nephrotoxins
    Endogenous: myoglobulin, hemoglobin, uric acid, calcium, phosphorus
    Exogenous: contrast media, drugs
Poorly controlled hypertension: malignant or accelerated hypertension

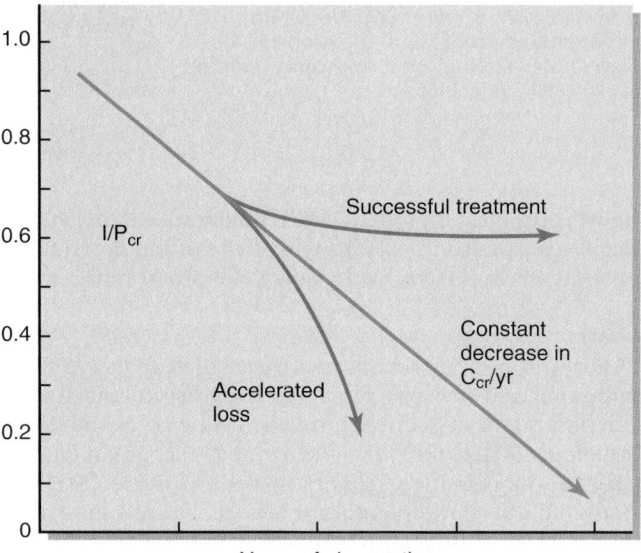

Figure 33-2 Use of the reciprocal of plasma creatinine concentration (1/P_{cr}) to follow the progress of glomerular disease in a patient. (Data from Sullivan LP, Grantham JJ: Physiology of the Kidney, 2nd ed. Philadelphia, Lea & Febiger, 1982).

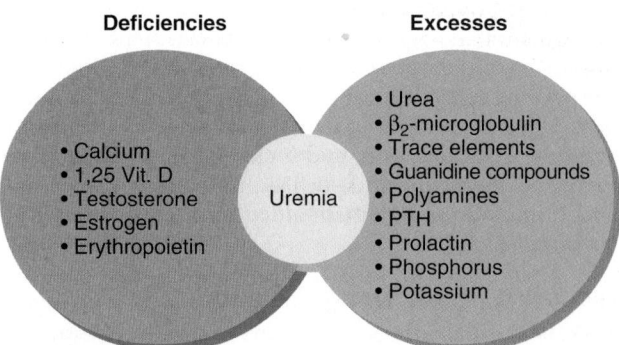

Figure 33-3 Etiologic factors of uremia. PTH, parathyroid hormone.

with the severe fibrotic skin condition of nephrogenic systemic fibrosis in patients with CKD, but with the majority with ESRD receiving dialysis therapy. Caution must be exercised when considering MRI evaluations requiring contrast in patients with advanced CKD.

Reversible Causes of Acute Deterioration in Kidney Function

The rate of decline in GFR for individual patients is log linear. Accordingly, plotting 1/serum creatinine against time usually predicts the rate at which a specific patient will reach ESRD, as shown in Figure 33-2. When such a patient suddenly shows acceleration of kidney failure, the differential diagnosis for such acceleration should be considered and investigated, as presented in Table 33-5. Recent evidence indicates that diagnosis of in-hospital acute kidney injury is associated with a higher rate of progression of kidney disease and increased incidence of ESRD, emphasizing the importance of detection and prevention of acute kidney injury.

CLINICAL MANIFESTATIONS

General Features of Uremic Syndrome

Patients with CKD usually do not become symptomatic until the GFR is less than 15 mL per minute. *Uremia* is a syndrome that affects every organ system. Uremic syndrome is likely the consequence of a combination of factors, including retained molecules, deficiencies of important hormones, and metabolic factors, rather than the effect of a single uremic

toxin (Fig. 33-3). Among these toxins, urea can cause symptoms of fatigue, nausea, vomiting, and headaches. Its breakdown product (cyanate) can result in carbamylation of lipoproteins and peptides and adverse effects, leading to multiple organ dysfunctions.

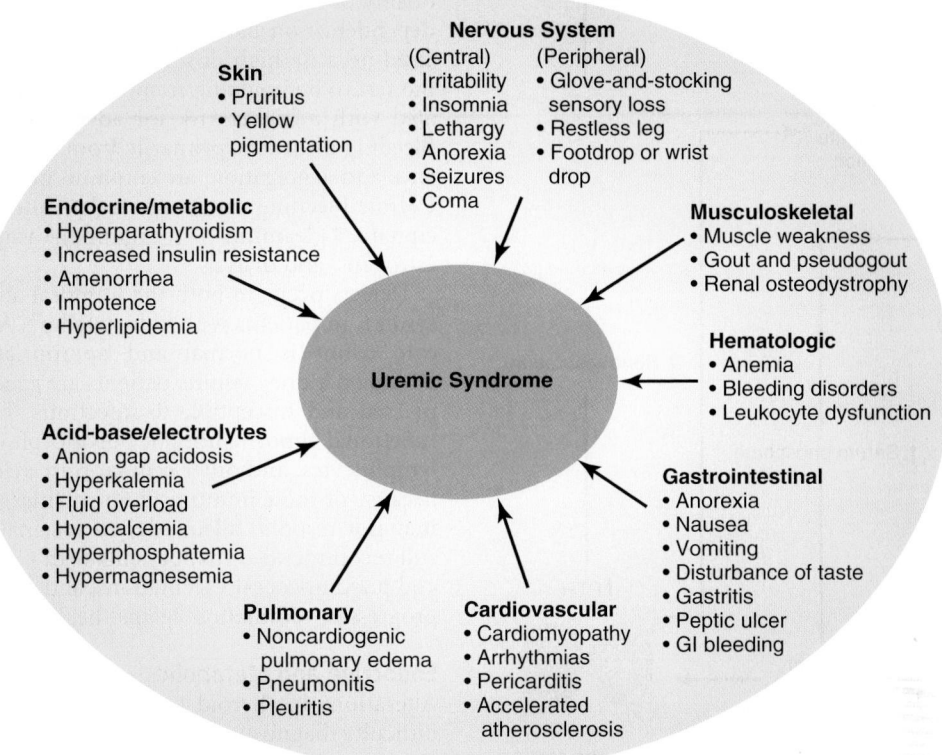

Skin
- Pruritus
- Yellow pigmentation

Nervous System
(Central)
- Irritability
- Insomnia
- Lethargy
- Anorexia
- Seizures
- Coma

(Peripheral)
- Glove-and-stocking sensory loss
- Restless leg
- Footdrop or wrist drop

Endocrine/metabolic
- Hyperparathyroidism
- Increased insulin resistance
- Amenorrhea
- Impotence
- Hyperlipidemia

Musculoskeletal
- Muscle weakness
- Gout and pseudogout
- Renal osteodystrophy

Uremic Syndrome

Hematologic
- Anemia
- Bleeding disorders
- Leukocyte dysfunction

Acid-base/electrolytes
- Anion gap acidosis
- Hyperkalemia
- Fluid overload
- Hypocalcemia
- Hyperphosphatemia
- Hypermagnesemia

Gastrointestinal
- Anorexia
- Nausea
- Vomiting
- Disturbance of taste
- Gastritis
- Peptic ulcer
- GI bleeding

Pulmonary
- Noncardiogenic pulmonary edema
- Pneumonitis
- Pleuritis

Cardiovascular
- Cardiomyopathy
- Arrhythmias
- Pericarditis
- Accelerated atherosclerosis

Figure 33-4 Diagrammatic summary of the major manifestations of the uremic syndrome. GI, gastrointestinal.

Guanidines, byproducts of exogenous or endogenous protein metabolism, are increased in renal failure. These byproducts can inhibit α_1-hydroxylase activity within the kidney and can lead to deficient calcitriol production and secondary hyperparathyroidism. High parathyroid hormone levels have been implicated in various manifestations of uremia, especially in cardiomyopathy and metastatic calcifications. β_2-microglobulin accumulation in patients with ESRD has been associated with neuropathy, carpal tunnel syndrome, and amyloid infiltration of the joints.

Signs and Symptoms of Uremia

Major manifestations of uremia are shown in Figure 33-4.

Cardiovascular

In addition to hypertension, cardiovascular disorders are common in patients with CKD. Mortality from cardiovascular disease in CKD patients, especially those with stage 3 to 5 disease, is 3.5 times that of an age-matched population (**Web Fig. 33-3**). Heart disease accounts for more than 50% of the deaths in ESRD patients. More than 60% of patients who start dialysis have echocardiographic manifestations of left ventricular hypertrophy, dilation, and systolic or diastolic dysfunction. Anemia and hypertension contribute to left ventricular hypertrophy and congestive heart failure. Secondary hyperparathyroidism can lead to metastatic calcification in the myocardium, cardiac valves, and arteries. Accelerated atherogenesis is responsible for the high prevalence of coronary artery disease in this population and the high rate of recurrent coronary artery stenosis after angioplasty. Arrhythmias, including those resulting in sudden death, may result from electrolyte abnormalities or are related to ischemic cardiovascular disease. Pericarditis can occur in patients with uremia before they start dialysis, as well as in patients who are already undergoing dialysis, usually related to inadequate dialysis. Initiation of dialysis or intensifying dialysis therapy usually successfully treats pericarditis.

Gastrointestinal

Gastrointestinal disturbances are among the earliest and most common signs of the uremic syndrome. Patients with kidney failure usually describe a metallic taste and loss of appetite. Later, they experience anorexia, nausea, vomiting, and weight loss, and those with severe uremia may also experience stomatitis and enteritis. Several pathologic processes due to uremia can lead to a higher risk for gastrointestinal bleeding. This may be caused by gastritis, peptic ulceration, and arterial venous malformations in addition to platelet dysfunction.

Neurologic

Central nervous system (CNS) manifestations are frequent and occur rather late, often with development of fatigue and anorexia. They are mostly characterized by changes in cognitive function and memory and by disturbances in sleep. Lethargy, irritability, asterixis, seizures, and frank encephalopathy with coma are late manifestations of uremia and are usually avoided by early initiation of dialysis. Peripheral neurologic manifestations appear as a progressive symmetrical sensory neuropathy in a glove-and-stocking distribution. Patients have decreased distal tendon reflexes and loss of vibratory perception. Peripheral motor impairment can result in restless legs, footdrop, or wristdrop. Optimal

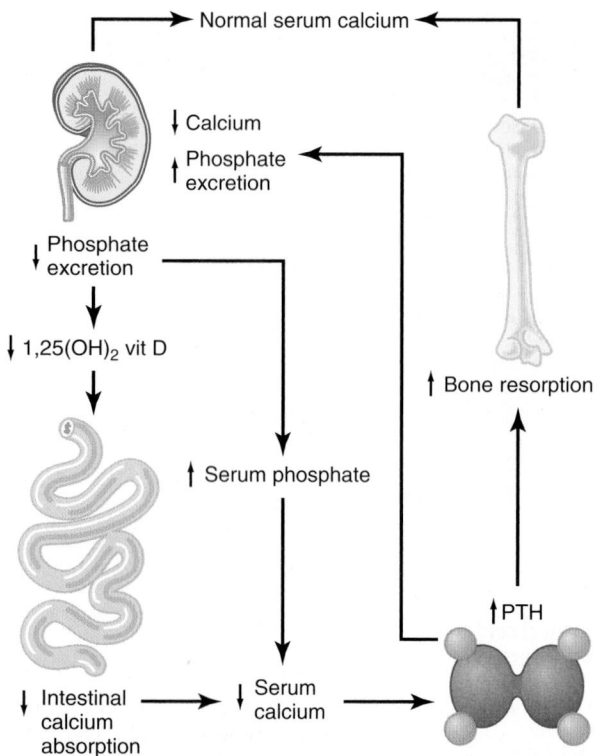

Normal serum calcium

↓ Calcium

↓ Phosphate excretion

↓ Phosphate excretion

↓ 1,25(OH)₂ vit D

↑ Serum phosphate

↑ Bone resorption

↓ Intestinal calcium absorption → ↓ Serum calcium

↑PTH

Figure 33-5 Calcium and phosphate homeostasis in the setting of renal failure. The decreased excretion of phosphate initiates the cycle directed at normalization of the serum calcium concentration. PTH, parathyroid hormone.

dialysis or transplantation has been shown to reverse most of the CNS peripheral neurologic manifestations.

Musculoskeletal

Alterations in calcium and phosphate homeostasis and renal osteodystrophy, with hyperparathyroidism and disturbance of vitamin D metabolism, are common manifestations of CKD and kidney failure. Hypocalcemia and secondary hyperparathyroidism are the results of phosphate retention and the lack of α_1-hydroxylase activity in the failing kidney, with consequent deficiency of the most active form of vitamin D. Over time, the adaptive parathyroid hypertrophy becomes maladaptive and leads to bone disease and tissue calcification. Calcium and phosphate homeostasis in the setting of kidney failure is demonstrated in Figure 33-5. Control of hyperparathyroidism is achieved with dietary phosphate restriction, oral phosphate-binding medications, calcium and vitamin D supplementation, and dialysis therapy. Calcimimetics are a novel class of drug that targets calcium-sensing receptors on the parathyroid gland and sensitizes them to the inhibitory effect of serum calcium. This action inhibits parathyroid hyperplasia and treats secondary hyperparathyroidism related to kidney disease.

Hematologic and Immunologic

Erythropoietin (EPO), a hormone produced by the kidney that regulates erythrocyte production, becomes progressively deficient as kidney failure progresses and renal mass declines. EPO and iron deficiency are common causes of anemia in CKD. Administration of synthetic EPO every 1 to 2 weeks to patients results in correction of anemia, improved

quality of life and anemia-related symptoms, and decreased dependence on blood transfusions. Caution must be exercised because high doses of EPO resulting in elevations of the serum hemoglobin to more than 13 g/dL may be associated with a higher risk for adverse cardiovascular events. Bleeding disorders, primarily from defects in platelet adherence and aggregation, are common in patients with uremia. Uremic bleeding can be generally controlled with cryoprecipitate, 1-deamino-(8-D-arginine)-vasopressin, conjugated estrogens, and dialysis.

Defects occur in both the humoral and cellular immune systems in patients with kidney failure. Although the leukocyte count is normal and appropriately responsive in advanced kidney failure, patients are generally immunosuppressed and susceptible to infections. This may be due to functional abnormalities of polymorphonuclear leukocytes, lymphocytes, and other cellular host defenses. Additionally, because of these immune abnormalities, patients with CKD may not respond adequately to vaccination. However, it is still recommended that patients with CKD receive influenza and pneumococcal vaccinations, and as their kidney disease progresses, vaccination against hepatitis B virus.

Endocrine and Metabolic

Alterations in thyroid function testing may contribute to difficulty diagnosing thyroid disease in patients with uremia. Common laboratory findings may include an increased triiodothyronine resin uptake, a low triiodothyronine level resulting from the impaired conversion of thyroxine to triiodothyronine peripherally, and normal thyroxine levels. Thyroid-stimulating hormone levels are usually normal. On occasion, the use of a thyrotropin-releasing hormone stimulation test may be needed for a diagnosis of thyroid disorders in uremia. Interestingly, goiter is present in up to one third of patients with chronic renal failure.

A deranged pituitary-gonadal axis can result in sexual dysfunction exhibited by impotence, decreased libido, amenorrhea, sterility, and uterine bleeding. Hyperprolactinemia may be responsible for some of the abnormalities of the pituitary-gonadal axis. Patients have decreased plasma levels of testosterone, estrogen, and progesterone, with normal or increased levels of follicle-stimulating hormone and luteinizing hormones. Pregnancy is uncommon in female patients who have a GFR of less than 30 mL per minute.

As renal function diminishes, many patients with diabetes have a decreased insulin requirement. This change is partly a result of the increased half-life of exogenously administered insulin secondary to decreased renal insulin clearance, which may lead to development of frequent episodes of hypoglycemia in a person with diabetes who was well controlled on a stable insulin regimen. However, increased peripheral insulin resistance in patients with uremia has also been described. Insulin resistance occurs secondary to tissue insensitivity to insulin due to a postreceptor defect, as well as metabolic acidosis and hyperparathyroidism, which impair insulin release and secretion.

Lipid abnormalities are common findings in the early course of kidney disease. They are most consistent with type IV hyperlipoproteinemia, with a marked increase in plasma triglycerides and less of an increase in total cholesterol. The activity of lipoprotein lipase is decreased in uremia, with a reduction in the conversion of very-low-density lipoprotein to low-density lipoprotein and thus hypertriglyceridemia. These abnormalities of lipid metabolism are considered contributors to accelerated atherosclerosis and contribute to mesangial proliferation and progressive kidney disease. The treatment of choice is the hydroxymethylglutaryl–coenzyme A reductase (HMG-CoA) inhibitor class of drugs because of their pluripotent effects on inflammation and atherosclerosis.

Acidosis and Electrolytes

As CKD progresses to a moderate impairment of kidney function, the kidney is unable to generate and excrete adequate acid, and a chronic metabolic acidosis may develop. This is typically an anion gap acidosis due to retained anions. Once the serum bicarbonate falls below 20 mEq/L, treatment with sodium bicarbonate or sodium citrate should be considered to prevent the exacerbation of bone disease or nutritional metabolic derangements.

Hyperkalemia occurs in patients with CKD as a result of progression of CKD resulting in oliguria and decreased renal clearance of potassium, intracellular to extracellular shifts of potassium in the setting of metabolic acidosis related to kidney failure, and also the concomitant use of medications such as ACE inhibitors, ARBs, or other medications that alter potassium clearance. The primary method of treatment is dietary reduction of potassium but may also include use of loop diuretics or potassium-binding medications. Hypokalemia is much less common in CKD but may occur in the setting of very poor nutritional intake or use of high-dose potassium-wasting diuretic medications.

Hyperphosphatemia is also very common as CKD progresses because of a reduction in renal clearance of phosphate. As described previously, this contributes to the development of secondary hyperparathyroidism in the kidney patient. Dietary reduction of phosphorus and use of phosphate-binding medications taken at each meal can successfully control serum phosphorus levels.

Skin

Uremic hue, a yellowish skin color, is likely the result of retained liposoluble pigments, such as lipochromes and carotenoids. Uremic hue usually responds to dialysis, control of hyperparathyroidism, improved calcium and phosphate balance, and, occasionally, ultraviolet rays. Calciphylaxis, or calcific uremic arteriolopathy, results in painful skin calcification and is often seen in patients with a serum calcium x phosphate product that exceeds 70 mg/dL in the presence of severe hyperparathyroidism. Nail findings include the half-and-half nail, characterized by red, pink, or brownish discoloration of the distal nail bed, pale nails, and splinter hemorrhages. Other common signs and symptoms include pruritus, pallor related to anemia, and ecchymoses due to disorders of bleeding.

Care of the Patient with End-Stage Renal Disease

As CKD progresses to kidney failure, it is important to prepare for the initiation of renal replacement therapies. Patients with moderately advanced kidney disease (CKD stage 4) should be referred to a nephrologist for co-management. This may include evaluation of risk for CKD progression, estimation of timing until kidney failure, and introduction of and preparation for the modalities of renal replacement therapy. Late referral (<3 months before ESRD) to a nephrologist is associated with a higher risk for death after initiation of renal replacement therapy.

RENAL REPLACEMENT THERAPIES

A plan for a modality of RRT should be discussed with the patient early in the course of kidney failure and before the appearance of uremic symptoms. The two primary treatments for ESRD are dialysis and transplantation. There are two types of dialysis, hemodialysis and peritoneal dialysis. Kidney transplants may be from either deceased or living donors. In the United States in 2006, 101,306 patients began hemodialysis, whereas only 6,758 (6%) elected peritoneal dialysis. First kidney transplantations were performed in 15,918 people, although most of these patients (83%) received dialysis for some period of time before receiving a kidney transplant. This distribution of patients on various modalities differs in other countries. Chronic dialysis is usually initiated when the GFR is 15 mL per minute or less and there are no apparent reversible causes of kidney failure. However, chronic dialysis may be started at any time when complications of ESRD, such as fluid balance and potassium levels, cannot be controlled medically. The choice of dialysis modality largely depends on the patient's physical characteristics, social support exposure to pre-ESRD patient education, and lifestyle choices. In medically eligible patients, kidney transplantation is encouraged because it allows a better quality of life, increased survival rate, and greater chance for rehabilitation.

Hemodialysis

As illustrated in Figure 33-6, blood is pumped from a temporary or permanent vascular access into tubing that leads to a large number of capillaries bundled together in a dialyzer (**Web Fig. 33-4**). The capillaries are made up of semisynthetic materials that are biocompatible. This membrane is semipermeable and is capable of allowing exchange of small molecules across the concentration gradient by diffusion. Moving in the opposite direction to blood is a dialysate solution that is passing through outside the capillaries, thus allowing countercurrent exchange. This solution contains sodium chloride, bicarbonate, and varying concentrations of potassium. Diffusion through the membrane allows low-molecular-weight substances such as urea, potassium, and organic acids to move across according to the concentration gradient. Fluid is removed by *ultrafiltration*, which is achieved by applying transmembrane hydrostatic pressure across the dialyzer.

In the setting of ESRD, an average patient undergoing *intermittent* chronic hemodialysis requires 4 hours of dialysis 3 times a week to adequately remove toxins. The treatment requires a blood flow of about 400 mL per minute from the access to the dialysis machine. Common complications associated with hemodialysis treatments include hypotension and muscle cramping. Avoiding excessive weight gain (more than 2 to 3 kg) between treatments can minimize these complications.

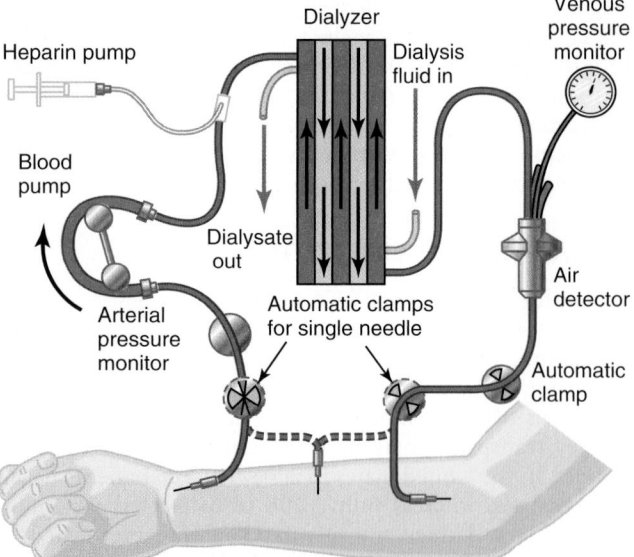

Figure 33-6 Essential components of a dialysis delivery system that, together with the dialyzer, make up an *artificial kidney.* In isolated ultrafiltration, no dialysis fluid is used (bypass mode). Also shown is the apparatus for using a single needle for inflow and outflow of blood from the patient (From Keshaviah PR: Hemodialysis monitors and monitoring. In Maher JF [ed]: Replacement of Renal Function by Dialysis, 3rd ed. Boston, Kluwer Academic Publishers, 1989. Reprinted by permission of Kluwer Academic Publishers.)

Access for Hemodialysis

The recommended access for hemodialysis is a permanent access such as an arteriovenous fistula (AVF) or arteriovenous graft (AVG) (**Web Fig. 33-5, Web Table 33-1**). In certain instances, a temporary or permanent indwelling catheter can be used for hemodialysis. Although the goal is for at least 66% of prevalent dialysis patients to use an AVF for dialysis access (http://www.fistulafirst.org), many patients continue to use AVGs or catheters. Temporary catheters are placed into internal jugular, subclavian, or femoral veins the way central venous lines are placed and can be used for a short time. Permanent catheters have a cuff around the outer wall of the tubing and tunnel under the chest wall skin for some distance before entering the internal jugular vein. The cuff causes local fibrosis in the subcutaneous tissue, thus sealing the access of skin flora into the catheter and reducing the infection rates. However, catheters have much higher rates of infection, lower blood flow rates, and a higher risk for mortality compared with AVF and AVG.

Peritoneal Dialysis

Peritoneal dialysis is a type of RRT in which the peritoneal capillaries act as a semipermeable membrane similar to a hemodialysis filter. This technique has several advantages over hemodialysis because it allows independence from the long time spent in dialysis units, it does not require as stringent dietary restrictions as in hemodialysis, and rehabilitation rates are better than those observed in hemodialysis, with more patients returning to full-time employment. Residual renal function is maintained for a longer period (e.g., 1 to 2 years) while the patient receives peritoneal dialysis, thus improving morbidity and mortality. In continuous ambulatory peritoneal dialysis, dialysate of 2- to 3-L volumes

is instilled through a peritoneal catheter (**Web Fig. 33-6**) into the peritoneal cavity for varying amounts of time and exchanged 4 to 6 times daily. In continuous cyclic peritoneal dialysis, the patient is connected to a machine referred to as a *cycler* that allows inflow of smaller volumes of dialysate with shorter dwell time overnight while the patient sleeps. This process allows patients to be actively working during the day. Several modifications in this regimen can be made to fit specific patients to achieve adequate clearance of toxins and fluid. The rate of removal of various solutes depends on the concentration gradient, surface area, and permeability of the peritoneal membrane to the solute. Smaller molecules move across the peritoneal membrane with ease and are influenced by ultrafiltration rates. Ultrafiltration is achieved through increasing dextrose concentration in the dialysate. The two major drawbacks of peritoneal dialysis are peritonitis and difficulty in achieving adequate clearances in patients with excess body mass. Peritonitis in patients undergoing peritoneal dialysis can be treated with intraperitoneal antibiotics, most often as outpatients. Catheter removal is indicated in some cases of peritonitis, for instance, bacterial peritonitis that is not responding to antibiotics and fungal peritonitis. Additionally, a slow deterioration occurs in the permeability of the membrane, especially after one or more peritonitis episodes, leading to inadequate dialysis and, ultimately, to the need to change the modality of RRT to hemodialysis.

Management of Complications in Dialysis

As with CKD, patients receiving dialysis therapy experience similar abnormalities in many related organ systems. The risk for cardiovascular disease, and cardiovascular events, remains very high in this complex patient population. Efforts to minimize cardiovascular risk, such as treatment of hypertension and screening for evidence of cardiac ischemia, are recommended. Tobacco cessation remains an important component of reducing cardiovascular risk. Recent studies in prevalent dialysis patients have not demonstrated that lowering lipid levels with statins reduces cardiovascular risk and mortality, although it may be that the greatest impact of lipid lowering can be made in the CKD patient before reaching ESRD. Anemia, hyperphosphatemia, and hyperparathyroidism are also common in patients receiving dialysis therapy, and treatment strategy is similar to that recommended for patients with CKD, albeit with minor differences in dosing and target levels.

Kidney Transplantation

Kidney transplantation is the preferred modality of RRT, although hemodialysis or peritoneal dialysis often is required before, during, or after transplantation. When cyclosporine became available in 1983, the success rate of kidney transplantation from deceased donors improved significantly, with an 85% to 90% 1-year graft survival rate, compared with 65% with azathioprine and steroids. A decrease in the incidence of acute rejection and some improvement in long-term allograft survival have been seen secondary to the introduction of newer immunosuppressive agents that include rapamycin, mycophenolate mofetil, tacrolimus, and anti–interleukin-2 receptor antibodies (daclizumab and basiliximab).

Table 33-6 **Comparison of Donor Sources for Kidney Transplantation**	
Advantages	**Disadvantages**
Living Donor	
Better tissue match with less likelihood of rejection	Small potential risk of operation to donor
Smaller doses of drugs for immunosuppression	Requirement of willing, medically suitable family member or other person
Waiting time for transplant reduced	
Sequelae of long-term dialysis avoided	
Elective surgical procedure	
Better early graft function with shorter hospitalization	
Better short-term and long-term success	
Deceased Donor	
Availability to any recipient	Tissue match not as similar
Availability of other organs for combined transplants (i.e., kidney-pancreas transplant)	Waiting time variable
	Operation performed urgently
Availability of vascular conduits for complex vascular reconstruction	Early graft function possibly compromised
	Short-term and long-term success not as good as from living donor

Types of Kidney Transplants

Kidney transplant donors may be deceased or living and, among those living, may be related or unrelated.

Advantages and disadvantages of deceased versus living donors are listed in Table 33-6. Because the deceased donor organ supply is inadequate, the pressure for living kidney donation has increased. Unrelated donors with a stable and close emotional relationship with the recipient or who have agreed to an equitable kidney exchange as part of a kidney transplant program may be appropriate for donation. Survival of grafts from living unrelated donors is better than survival of grafts from deceased donors, despite less histocompatibility matching of human leukocyte antigen (HLA). The main advantages of a living related donor transplant are less ischemic injury and histocompatibility matching. Figure 33-7 is a representation of the inheritance pattern of HLA within a family. HLA-identical matches consistently demonstrate superior graft survival and reduced chance for rejection than less well-matched living or deceased donor renal transplants. However, with procedures to reduce antibodies, including plasmapheresis and pre-transplantation immunosuppressive therapy, it is possible to successfully perform kidney transplantations in ABO blood group–incompatible pairs.

Immunosuppressant Drug Therapy

Prophylaxis against and treatment of graft rejection are at the heart of the success of kidney transplantation. All protocols for immunosuppression aim at disruption of the lymphocyte cell cycle, and many include some period of exposure to corticosteroids. Since the introduction of cyclosporine in the early 1980s, the number of drugs capable of suppressing the immune system has increased steadily. These agents, by virtue of their specific mode of action, have succeeded in preventing most patients from having early and irreversible graft rejections without severe toxic effects. The mechanism of action of some of the most commonly used immunosuppressants is illustrated in Figure 33-8.

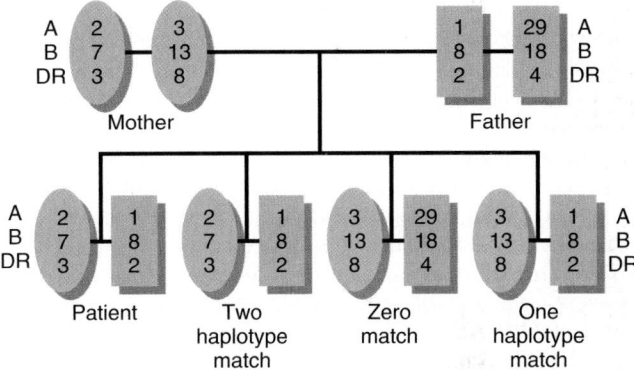

Figure 33-7 Diagrammatic representation of inheritance of human leukocyte antigen tissue types in a family with four siblings.

The hepatic cytochrome P-450 system is essential for cyclosporine, tacrolimus, and rapamycin metabolism. Significant changes in the levels of these drugs may occur when patients start or discontinue taking any of several drugs that can induce or inhibit this system. Therefore, evaluation for drug-drug interactions is critical to prevent toxic or even subtherapeutic effects of either the immunosuppressant drug or the other prescribed therapy.

Cyclosporine exerts its specific immunosuppressive activity by inhibiting immunocompetent lymphocytes in the G_0 and G_1 phases of the cell cycle. Some of the most important side effects of cyclosporine include hematologic suppression, hyperkalemia, seizures, exacerbation of gout, dyslipidemia, and gingival hypertrophy. Most effects respond to an appropriate dose reduction. The most significant of these effects is nephrotoxicity, and this is often related to decreased glomerular blood flow.

Tacrolimus has a mechanism of action and side-effect profile similar to those of cyclosporine but with the additional problems of hyperglycemia and an increased tendency

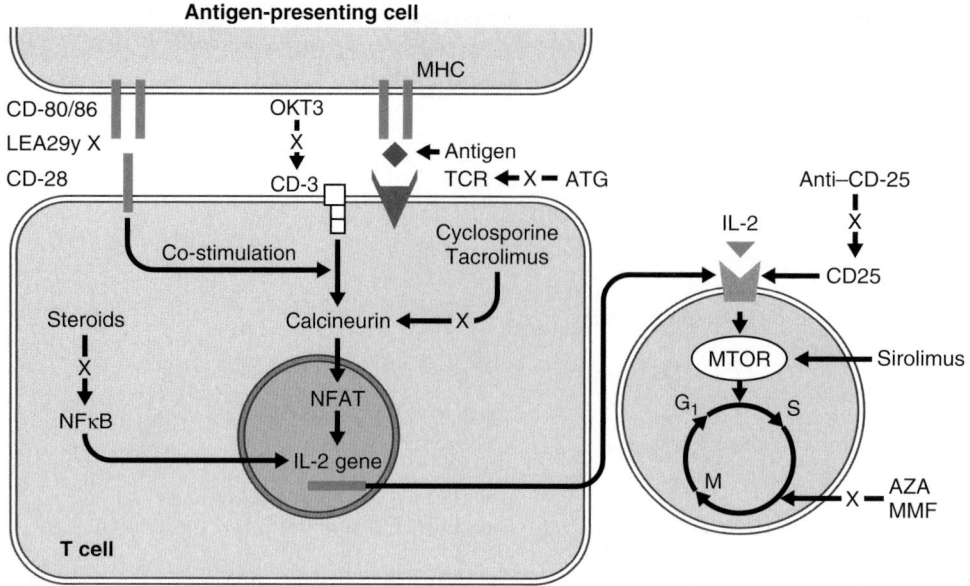

Figure 33-8 Pathways of T-cell activation and site of action of immunosuppressive agents. ATG, antithymocyte globulin; AZA, azathioprine; IL, interleukin; MHC, major histocompatibility complex; MMF, mycoplasma membrane fraction; MTOR, mammalian target of rapamycin; NFAT, nuclear factor of activated T-cells; TCR, T-cell receptor.

toward neurotoxicity. Both cyclosporine and tacrolimus can cause calcineurin inhibitor nephrotoxicity, which may contribute to chronic allograft nephropathy and ultimately graft loss.

Mycophenolate mofetil or *mycophenolic acid* specifically inhibits T-lymphocyte and B-lymphocyte proliferation by interfering with purine synthesis and thus DNA synthesis. Mycophenolate mofetil has been associated with a 60% to 70% reduction in acute transplant rejection compared with conventional therapies and thus promotes long-term graft survival. Side effects include anemia and leucopenia as well as gastrointestinal symptoms.

Rapamycin is a macrolide antibiotic produced by the fungus *Streptomyces hygroscopicus*. Rapamycin binds to the mTOR (mammalian target of rapamycin) receptor, thus blocking the phosphorylation of *p70(s6)* kinase and the eukaryotic initiation factor 4E–binding protein, PHAS-I. This action leads to the dampening of cytokine and growth factor activity on T, B, and nonimmune cells. The major side effects are thrombocytopenia and dyslipidemia (primarily hypertriglyceridemia).

Acute Rejection

T lymphocytes survey the human body and are capable of recognizing foreign antigens when these antigens are presented in association with HLA antigens, especially class II histocompatibility antigens. When the recipient's helper cells identify foreign HLA class II antigens presented by dendritic or other antigen-presenting cells in the transplanted kidney, lymphocyte activation occurs. Activated cytotoxic lymphocytes invade the tubular interstitial region of the transplanted kidney, with resulting tubulitis. Clinically, acute rejection is detected by graft tenderness, rise in serum creatinine levels, oliguria, and, in some instances, fever. Frequent monitoring of kidney function has allowed early detection of acute rejection based on rising serum creatinine before any clinical signs or symptoms become apparent.

Acute rejection episodes have a negative impact on long-term graft survival. Acute humoral rejection involves the intrarenal arteries and leads to vasculitis, carrying a poor prognosis. This type of rejection is usually resistant to steroids, thus necessitating antilymphocyte and possibly plasmapheresis therapy.

Post-transplantation Infection

Infection is second only to cardiovascular disease as the leading cause of mortality in kidney transplant recipients. Prophylaxis therapies are often used immediately after kidney transplantation to prevent infectious diseases that are of particularly high risk, including *Pneumocystis jirovecii* pneumonia, urinary tract infections, and cytomegalovirus infection. In addition to common community-acquired bacterial and viral infections, kidney transplant recipients are also susceptible to numerous viral, fungal, and other opportunistic infections that normally do not cause severe illness in the immunocompetent host. Fortunately, the timetable of these infections is predictable, and an educated guess based on the time of infection after transplantation, together with the specific set of syndromes associated with each infection, can help early recognition and prompt empirical treatment pending confirmatory tests. Figure 33-9 shows the temporal relationship of infections in renal transplantation.

Post-transplantation Malignant Disease

Immunosuppression increases the risk for developing malignant disease. Skin cancer (mostly squamous cell) has the highest incidence in transplant recipients compared with all other types of malignancy. Sun exposure is the most significant risk factor, and skin protection provides excellent primary prevention. With continuous surveillance and aggressive management, metastasis from skin cancers is rare.

Transplant recipients are also at high risk for developing non-Hodgkin lymphoma and Kaposi sarcoma, a rare

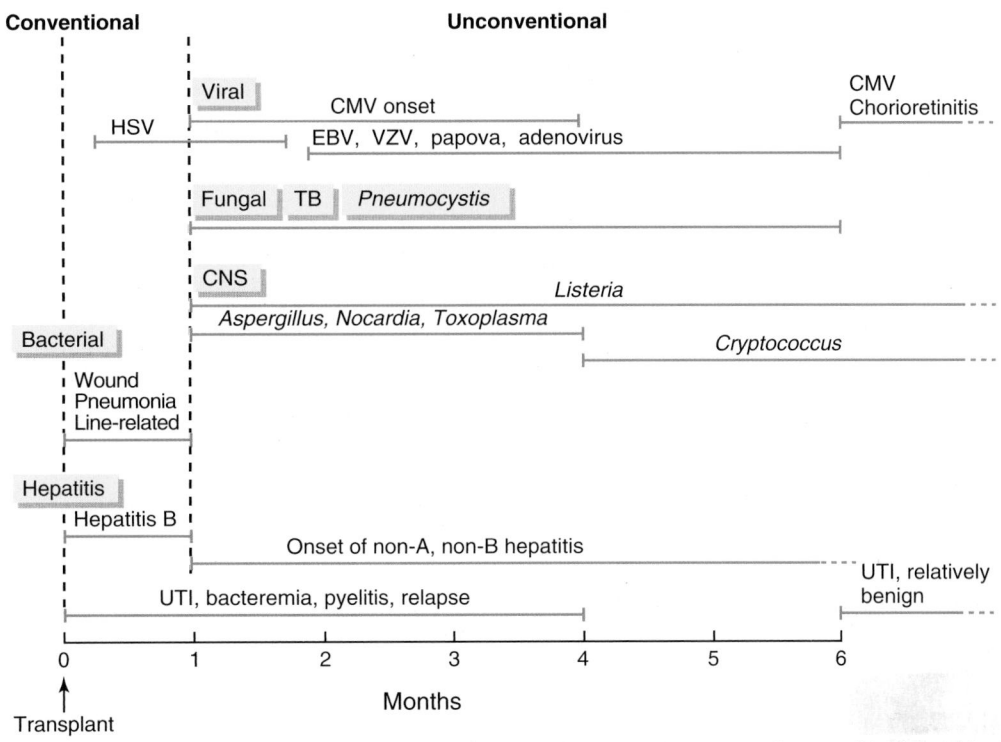

Figure 33-9 Timetable for the occurrence of infection in the renal transplant recipient. Exceptions to this timetable should initiate a search for an unusual hazard. CMV, cytomegalovirus; CNS, central nervous system; EBV, Epstein-Barr virus; HSV, herpes simplex virus; TB, tuberculosis; UTI, urinary tract infection; VZV, varicella-zoster virus. (From Rubin RH, Wolfson JS, Cosimi AB, et al: Infection in the renal transplant recipient. Am J Med 70:405-411, 1981. Copyright 1981 by Excerpta Medica, Inc.)

occurrence in the immunocompetent host. In addition to age-appropriate screening, cancer surveillance should be an essential part of post-transplantation follow-up. Transplant recipients should be educated to recognize and report early changes in bowel habits, respiratory symptoms, hematuria, musculoskeletal symptoms, skin changes, or weight changes.

Prospectus for the Future

In the CKD population, the major challenges will be to slow the progression of kidney disease by identifying novel targets and development of new immunosuppressive regimens or therapies to achieve tolerance after transplantation. Other efforts include the following:
- Biomarkers of chronic kidney disease
- More sensitive markers of kidney function such as serum cystatin-C
- Development of an artificial kidney
- Development of laboratory tests to measure the overall immune reactivity of solid organ transplant recipients in order to customize treatment protocols without the risk for rejection or opportunistic infections
- Genetic manipulation of animals to succeed in xenotransplantation

References

Abbate M, Remuzzi G: Progression of renal insufficiency: Mechanisms. In Massry SG, Glassock RJ (eds): Massry and Glassock's Textbook of Nephrology, 4th ed. Philadelphia, Lippincott, Williams & Wilkins, 2001, pp 1210-1217.

Coresh J, Selvin E, Stevens LA, et al: Prevalence of chronic kidney disease in the United States. JAMA 298:2038-2047, 2007.

Halloran PF: Drug therapy: Immunosuppressive drugs for kidney transplantation. N Engl J Med 351:2715-2729, 2004.

Luke RG: Chronic renal failure. In Goldman L, Bennett JC (eds): Cecil Textbook of Medicine, 21st ed. Philadelphia: WB Saunders, 2000, pp 571-577.

National Kidney Foundation: KDOQI clinical practice guidelines for chronic kidney disease: Evaluation, classification and stratification. Am J Kidney Dis 39(2 Suppl 1):S1-S266, 2002.

National Kidney Foundation: KDOQI clinical practice guidelines and clinical practice recommendations for diabetes and chronic kidney disease. Am J Kidney Dis 49(2 Suppl 2):S12-S154, 2007.

Rubin RH, Marty FM: Principles of antimicrobial therapy in the transplant patient [editorial]. Transpl Infect Dis 6:97-100, 2004.

Sarnak MJ, Levey AS, Schoolwerth AC, et al: Kidney disease as a risk factor for development of cardiovascular disease: A statement from the American Heart Association Councils on Kidney in Cardiovascular Disease, High Blood Pressure Research, Clinical Cardiology, and Epidemiology and Prevention. Circulation 108:2154-2169, 2003.

U.S. Renal Data System: USRDS 2008 Annual Data Report: Atlas of Chronic Kidney Disease and End-Stage Renal Disease in the United States. Bethesda, MD. National Institutes of Health, National Institute of Diabetes and Digestive and Kidney Diseases, 2008.

Wanner C, Krane V, Marz W, et al: Atorvastatin in patients with type 2 diabetes mellitus undergoing hemodialysis. N Engl J Med 353:238-248, 2005.

Section VII

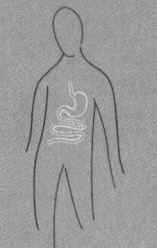

Gastrointestinal Disease

Chapter 34

Common Clinical Manifestations of Gastrointestinal Disease

A. Abdominal Pain

Charles M. Bliss, Jr. and M. Michael Wolfe

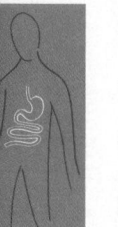

Abdominal pain is a frequent manifestation of intra-abdominal disease. Abdominal pain is difficult to localize or grade because the sensation of pain is colored by emotional and physical factors. Abdominal pain may be classified as acute or chronic. Acute pain occurs suddenly and suggests serious physiologic alterations. Conversely, chronic pain may be present for several months; although it does not mandate immediate attention, chronic pain may lead to prolonged evaluation. Appropriate evaluation of abdominal pain requires knowledge of pain mechanisms, close attention to history and physical examination findings, and recognition of important accompanying symptoms as well as awareness of the strengths and weaknesses of the tests that might be used.

Physiology

Abdominal pain results from stimulation of receptors specific for thermal, mechanical, or chemical stimuli. Once these receptors are excited, pain impulses travel through sympathetic fibers. Abdominal pain can be characterized as somatic or visceral. Somatic pain originates from the abdominal wall and parietal peritoneum, whereas visceral pain originates in internal organs and from the visceral peritoneum. Two types of neurons carry pain: A fibers, which have rapid conduction, and C fibers, which have slow conduction. Most visceral neurons are of the C type, and the pain resulting from their stimulation tends to be variable with regard to sensation and localization. In contrast, fibers originating from the parietal peritoneum and abdominal wall are of

both the A and the C types, and the pain tends to be sharp and distinctly localized.

Because of this pattern of innervation, abdominal viscera are not sensitive to cutting, tearing, burning, or crushing. However, visceral pain results from stretching of the walls of hollow organs, or of the capsule of solid organs, as well as from inflammation or ischemia.

Causes of Abdominal Pain

Multiple intra-abdominal and extra-abdominal disorders can produce abdominal pain. Distinguishing acute from chronic abdominal pain is helpful. The approach varies with each specific cause, but acute abdominal pain generally demands prompt intervention.

Clinical Features

HISTORY

The differential diagnosis of abdominal pain, whether acute or chronic, requires thorough history taking with regard to pain characteristics, location and radiation, timing, and the presence of any other accompanying symptoms.

Pain location often indicates the organ responsible for the problem. For instance, epigastric pain is usually typical of peptic ulcer or dyspepsia, whereas right upper quadrant pain

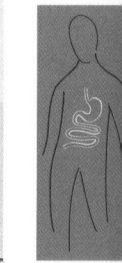

Table 34-1 **Key Abdominal Pain Syndromes**			
Condition	**Type**	**Location**	**Radiation**
Acute Abdominal Pain			
Appendicitis	Crampy, steady	Periumbilical, RLQ	Back
Cholecystitis	Intermittent, steady	Epigastric, RUQ	Right scapula
Pancreatitis	Steady	Epigastric, periumbilical	Back
Perforation	Sudden, severe	Epigastric	Entire abdomen
Obstruction	Crampy	Periumbilical	Back
Infarction	Severe, diffuse	Periumbilical	Entire abdomen
Chronic Abdominal Pain			
Esophagitis	Burning	Retrosternal	Left arm, back
Peptic ulcer	Gnawing	Epigastric	Back
Dyspepsia	Bloating, dull	Epigastric	None
IBS	Crampy	LLQ, RLQ	None

IBS, irritable bowel syndrome; LLQ, left lower quadrant; RLQ, right lower quadrant; RUQ, right upper quadrant.

is more suggestive of cholecystitis and other biliary disorders. Early in the course of illness, pain may be perceived in one location and subsequently felt in another; this pattern of progression may be suggestive of specific pain syndromes. In acute cases, abdominal pain tends to be sharp and severe. The pain of a perforated viscus is intense, and the pain from a dissecting aneurysm may be described as tearing or crushing. Chronic pain may be less severe; pain from irritable bowel or dyspepsia is constant and dull, and the pain of chronic peptic ulcer is described as gnawing or hunger pain. The pattern of pain relief is helpful for diagnosing some conditions. The physician should also inquire about whether pain is steady or intermittent and whether it occurs at night. For nocturnal pain, a distinction should be made between pain that awakens the patient and pain that is felt when the patient wakes up for other reasons.

Table 34-1 outlines characteristics, location, and radiation of pain for a few common acute and chronic abdominal conditions.

PHYSICAL EXAMINATION

Examination of the abdomen may provide invaluable clues to the diagnosis, but the examination should start with the general appearance of the patient. A patient writhing in bed and unable to find a comfortable position may be suffering from obstruction. In contrast, a patient lying with the lower extremities flexed and avoiding any motion may be suffering from peritonitis. Abdominal distention indicates obstruction or ascites. Visual inspection for peristalsis is helpful for the diagnosis of small bowel obstruction, but this sign is present only in the early stages. Focal areas of distention may indicate hernias; note should also be made of any scars from previous surgery.

Auscultation should be performed in several areas to evaluate the timber and pattern of bowel sounds as well as to search for bruits or hums. Absence of bowel sounds suggests ileus, whereas the presence of hyperactive, high-pitched sounds may indicate obstruction. Multiple bruits alert the examiner to the possibility of significant vascular disease, suggesting ischemia.

The abdomen should be palpated gently, starting in an area away from the area of pain. The physician searches for areas of localized tenderness and rebound as well as for masses and enlarged organs. Percussion is performed to identify size of organs or to determine the presence of ascites. Pain on percussion of the abdomen indicates peritoneal reaction, as does severe rebound tenderness.

A rectal examination is important for identifying a rectal tumor in the case of colon obstruction or tenderness high in the rectum in acute appendicitis. Pelvic examination should be performed in women to rule out pelvic inflammatory disease.

Acute Abdomen

The acute abdomen is a challenging condition in medical practice. The first question to be answered is whether immediate surgery is needed. Therefore, a quick evaluation is necessary to avoid undue delay in intervention for patients who require surgery. Early surgical consultation should be obtained, even in doubtful cases, rather than awaiting confirmation of the diagnosis via laboratory or radiologic studies.

The acute abdomen is caused by sudden inflammation, perforation, obstruction, or infarction of various intra-abdominal organs. However, many extra-abdominal conditions such as pneumonia, myocardial infarction, nephrolithiasis, and metabolic disorders may cause acute abdominal pain.

In some instances, the acute abdomen, in its early stages, may show few findings. The examiner should be aware that patients with benign chronic conditions might come to the emergency department with severe pain that is out of proportion to any physical findings. With the acute abdomen, inquiring about medical history, particularly previous abdominal surgery, is important. Indeed, a patient with sudden crampy pain and abdominal distention may have intestinal obstruction caused by adhesions or an incarcerated hernia. Performing an entire examination of the patient, looking for jaundice, skin lesions, or evidence of chronic liver disease, is also important.

A complete blood cell count with differential, a urinalysis, and measurements of serum amylase, lipase, bilirubin, and electrolytes are necessary components of the laboratory examination. Additional studies may be done but usually do not aid in the rapid decision making required in the evaluation of the acute abdomen. An elevated white blood cell count may indicate inflammatory disease, and extremely high values are quite typical of acute intestinal ischemia. An elevated serum amylase concentration usually indicates acute pancreatitis, although a perforated ulcer or mesenteric thrombosis may also cause hyperamylasemia.

Radiographic examination is an important part of the evaluation of the patient with an acute abdomen. An abdominal film is important in revealing the intra-abdominal gas pattern, and an upright film that includes the diaphragm or left lateral decubitus film may identify intra-abdominal air. Ultrasonography can be helpful in the diagnosis of acute cholecystitis or appendicitis. Computed tomography (CT) scans have become more helpful with technologic improvements in scanners; early CT scans allow prompt diagnosis of sometimes unsuspected abdominal diseases. Examination with a radiopaque medium should be used judiciously, especially if surgery is anticipated. **Web Figures 34-1 through 34-4** are CT images of appendicitis, diverticulitis, pancreatitis, and ulcerative colitis.

Chronic Abdominal Pain

Chronic abdominal pain poses a challenge for the physician to distinguish organic pain resulting from a specific pathologic process from functional pain. The location and characteristics of pain, as already discussed, serve as important guides, as do other accompanying symptoms. The presence of postprandial nausea and vomiting suggests chronic peptic ulcer, disorders of gastric emptying, or outlet obstruction. The documentation of weight loss mandates the search for an organic cause, such as inflammatory bowel disease or celiac disease. If anorexia accompanies weight loss, particularly in elderly patients, cancer must be excluded. If no cancer can be found and all objective tests are normal, the possibility of chronic depression must be entertained.

The most frequent causes of chronic abdominal pain are *functional*. Dyspepsia is characterized by chronic intermittent epigastric discomfort, sometimes accompanied by nausea or bloating. These symptoms are not always relieved by acid suppression and may be the result of an underlying motor disorder. Furthermore, the eradication of *Helicobacter pylori,* when found in a patient with dyspeptic symptoms, may not necessarily lead to the resolution of symptoms. Controversy thus presently exists regarding the most effective strategy for the treatment of dyspepsia when *H. pylori* organisms are found in the absence of peptic ulcer disease.

Irritable bowel syndrome (IBS) is a common disorder. Estimates are that 15% of Americans suffer from IBS on a regular basis and that 40% to 50% of referrals to gastroenterologists are related to IBS. The syndrome consists of abdominal distention, flatulence, and disordered bowel function. The abdominal pain of IBS tends to be in the left lower quadrant, but it can be located elsewhere or be more generalized. Any patient with weight loss, anemia, nocturnal symptoms, steatorrhea, or onset of symptoms after age 50 years should be carefully evaluated for organic disease. The Rome criteria, developed for research studies, may be helpful in the diagnosis of IBS. These criteria include pain associated with change in bowel habits, relieved with defecation or accompanied by distention or bloating. Patients are reassured, counseled, and treated with anticholinergic agents and stool softeners. Alosetron, a serotonin 5-HT$_3$ antagonist, has been shown to help relieve symptoms in patients with diarrhea-predominant IBS. Tegaserod, a serotonin 5-HT$_4$

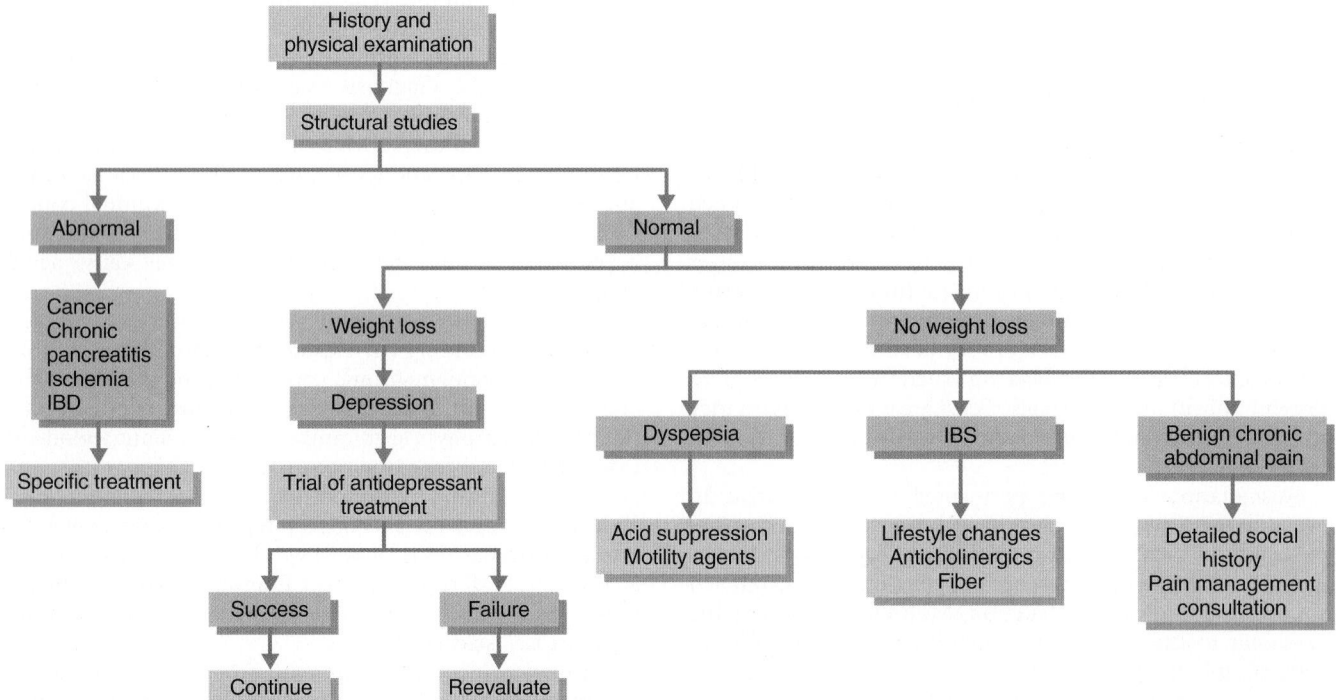

Figure 34-1 Approach to the patient with chronic abdominal pain. IBD, inflammatory bowel disease; IBS, irritable bowel syndrome.

agonist, has been found to be effective in relieving pain and constipation in constipation-predominant IBS and has recently been approved for use in both men and women.

The more challenging clinical problem is the one of functional abdominal pain syndrome. This term describes a condition in which the pain has been present for months or years. The complaints of pain are often not related to eating, defecation, or menses, unlike other causes of chronic pain. The patient is likely to be a woman who has undergone numerous examinations and diagnostic studies with negative findings and, in many cases, surgical operations without any relief. Lengthy or repeated diagnostic work-ups are counterproductive and only convince the patient that one more test is what is needed to determine the source of the pain. The physician must establish that organic disease is not present and must also realize that the pain is real. The patients are not malingerers despite the fact that the pain does not fit any familiar pattern. Depression may be the result rather than the cause of the pain.

Chronic abdominal pain is a clinical situation requiring as much tact, diplomacy, and compassion as it does scientific knowledge. An effort should be made to inquire about social factors, including history of physical and sexual abuse, particularly in women. Psychiatric evaluation may be necessary, but the suggestion for such a consultation may be interpreted by the patient as a belief from the physician that the "pain is in my head." A referral to a competent pain management specialist is helpful in a certain number of cases. This approach offers the possibility of providing relief with nerve blocks when the pain is localized or other pain-relieving devices. If this approach fails, referral to a psychologist or psychiatrist may be acceptable to the patient.

For a practical approach to chronic abdominal pain, see the algorithm in Figure 34-1.

References

Chang L, Ameen VZ, Dukes GE, et al: A dose-ranging, phase II study of the efficacy and safety of alosetron in men with diarrhea-predominant IBS. Am J Gastroenterol 100:115-123, 2005.

Drossman DA: Functional abdominal pain syndrome. Clin Gastroenterol Hepatol 2:353-365, 2004.

Johanson JF, Wald A, Tougas G, et al: Effect of tegaserod in chronic constipation: A randomized, double-blind, controlled trial. Clin Gastroenterol Hepatol 2:796-805, 2004.

Lembo A, Ameen VZ, Drossman DA: Irritable bowel syndrome: Toward an understanding of severity. Clin Gastroenterol Hepatol 3:717-725, 2005.

Ng CS, Watson CJE, Palmer CR, et al: Evaluation of early abdominopelvic computed tomography in patients with acute abdominal pain of unknown cause: Prospective randomized study. BMJ 325:1387-1390, 2002.

B. Gastrointestinal Hemorrhage

T. Carlton Moore, Chi-Chuan Tseng,* and M. Michael Wolfe

Acute Gastrointestinal Hemorrhage

Acute gastrointestinal (GI) bleeding remains a common and major medical problem, despite recent advances in diagnosis and treatment. Bleeding occurs as the result of a variety of diseases, and adequate treatment depends on assessing hemodynamic stability, determining blood loss, and identifying sources of bleeding. Although advancements in medical and surgical intensive care, pharmacologic therapy, and the prompt deployment of endoscopic therapies have significantly decreased the rate of rebleeding, the overall mortality rate from acute bleeding episode has remained essentially unchanged during the past half century, at about 5% to 10%, owing to an aging population and an increased prevalence of serious concomitant illnesses.

PRESENTATION OF GASTROINTESTINAL BLEEDING

When massive GI bleeding occurs, patients generally present with any combination of weakness, dizziness, lightheaded-ness, shortness of breath, postural changes in blood pressure or pulse, cramping abdominal pain, and diarrhea. The characteristics of bleeding may help to localize the source of bleeding to the upper or lower GI tract. Patients with acute bleeding commonly present with one of the following symptoms:

Hematemesis. The patient usually presents with vomiting of bright red blood or of material that resembles coffee grounds. After excluding swallowed blood from the nasopharynx or secondary to hemoptysis, the source of bleeding is likely proximal to the ligament of Treitz.

Melena. As little as 50 to 100 mL of blood in the stomach can produce melena. Black, tarry, usually foul-smelling stools are most often a manifestation of upper GI bleeding; however, a small bowel or proximal colonic source of bleeding may on occasion lead to melenic stools.

Hematochezia. The passage of bright-red blood or maroon stools per rectum frequently indicates a lower GI source of bleeding. However, about 10% to 15% of patients presenting with acute severe hematochezia have an upper GI source of bleeding. This group of patients commonly displays signs of hemodynamic instability.

*Deceased.

ETIOLOGY OF GASTROINTESTINAL BLEEDING

A major goal during early management of bleeding is to distinguish between upper and lower GI bleeding. In addition to the symptoms and signs stated previously, certain aspects of the history, physical examination, laboratory studies, and age of the patient may assist in localizing the site of bleeding. However, the site of bleeding frequently remains undetermined after initial evaluation. Common sources of acute GI hemorrhage are listed in Table 34-2.

APPROACH TO THE PATIENT WITH ACUTE GASTROINTESTINAL BLEEDING

Assessment of Vital Signs and Resuscitation

The first step in the evaluation and therapy for the patient with acute GI hemorrhage is to determine the severity of blood loss (Fig. 34-2). Vital signs with postural changes should be recorded immediately. If the systolic blood pressure drops more than 10 mm Hg or the pulse increases more than 10 beats per minute as the patient changes positions from supine to standing, it is likely the patient has lost at least 800 mL (15%) of circulating blood volume. Hypotension, tachycardia, tachypnea, and mental status changes in the setting of acute GI hemorrhage suggest at least a 1500-mL (30%) loss of circulating blood volume.

The goals of resuscitation are to restore the normal circulatory volume and to prevent complications from red blood cell loss, such as cardiac, pulmonary, renal, or neurologic consequences. Initially, at least two large-bore intravenous catheters are used to administer isotonic solutions (e.g., lactated Ringer solution, 0.9% NaCl), and blood products if indicated. If the patient is in shock, central venous access should be established. The amount of blood products to be transfused must be individualized, and in view of a potential risk for blood transfusion, it is not appropriate to simply transfuse until an arbitrary hematocrit is achieved. If coagulation studies are abnormal, as commonly observed in cir-

Table 34-2 Common Sources of Acute Gastrointestinal Hemorrhage

Source	Associated Clinical Features	Treatments
Upper Gastrointestinal Tract		
Esophagitis	Heartburn, dysphagia, odynophagia	Medication* Antireflux surgery or procedures
Esophageal cancer	Progressive dysphagia, weight loss	Chemoradiotherapy, surgery Palliative endoscopy procedures
Gastritis, gastric ulcer	Aspirin, NSAID use	Withdraw NSAIDs
Duodenitis, duodenal ulcer	Abdominal pain, dyspepsia *Helicobacter pylori* infection	Medication† Endoscopic therapy for acute bleeding
Gastric cancer	Early satiety, weight loss, abdominal pain	Surgery, chemotherapy
Esophagogastric varices	History of CLD Stigmata of CLD on examination	Variceal banding, sclerotherapy Vasopressin, octreotide TIPS or decompressive surgery
Mallory-Weiss tear	History of retching before hematemesis	Supportive (usually self-limited) Endoscopic therapy
Lower Gastrointestinal Tract		
Infection	History of exposure, diarrhea, fever	Supportive, antibiotics
Inflammatory bowel diseases	History of colitis, diarrhea, abdominal pain, fever	Steroids, 5-ASA, immunotherapy Surgery if unresponsive to medication
Diverticula	Painless hematochezia	Supportive Surgery for recurrent disease
Angiodysplasia	Painless hematochezia Often in ascending colon Commonly involves stomach and small bowel as well	Endoscopic therapy Supportive Surgery for localized disease
Colon cancer	Change in bowel habit, anemia, weight loss	Surgery
Colon polyp	Usually asymptomatic	Endoscopic or surgical removal
Ischemic colitis	Typically elderly patients History of vascular disease May produce abdominal pain	Supportive (self-limited)
Meckel diverticulum	Painless hematochezia in young patient Located at distal ileum	Surgery
Hemorrhoids	Rectal bleeding associated with bowel movement	Supportive Surgery, banding

*Proton pump inhibitors or histamine-2 receptor antagonists.
†Proton pump inhibitors or histamine-2 receptor antagonists in the absence of *H. pylori* infection; various combinations of antibiotics, proton pump inhibitors, and bismuth products in the presence of *H. pylori* infection.
CLD, chronic liver disease; NSAIDs, nonsteroidal anti-inflammatory drugs; TIPS, transjugular intrahepatic shunt; 5-ASA, 5-aminosalicylic acid compounds.

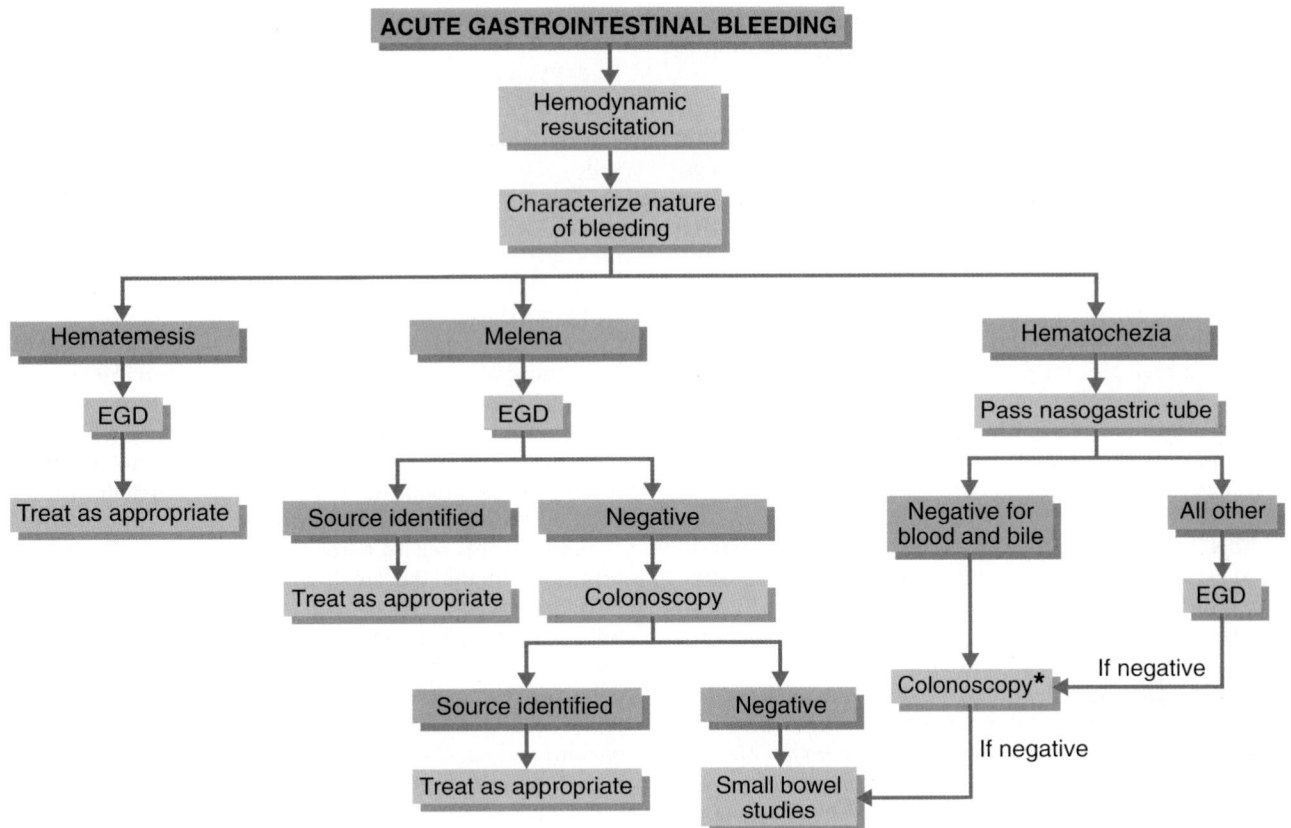

*If severe bleeding prevents endoscopic visualization, arteriography may be performed.

Figure 34-2 Approach to the patient with acute gastrointestinal bleeding. EGD, esophagogastroduodenoscopy.

rhotic patients, fresh-frozen plasma, platelets, or both may be required to control ongoing hemorrhage.

Initial Evaluation

As the patient is being fluid resuscitated, the following information should be obtained by history and physical examination in order to determine the source of bleeding:

1. The nature of bleeding: melena, hematemesis, hematochezia, or occult blood. A digital rectal examination is essential for the determination of stool color and the identification of anal fissures or rectal neoplasms.
2. The duration of GI bleeding, which helps dictate the appropriate pace of the evaluation to determine the bleeding source
3. The presence or absence of abdominal pain; for example, hematochezia caused by diverticula or angiodysplasia is typically painless, but when due to ischemia, it may be accompanied by abdominal pain.
4. Other associated symptoms, including fever, urgency or tenesmus, recent change in bowel habits, and weight loss
5. Current or recent medication use, particularly nonsteroidal anti-inflammatory drugs (NSAIDs) or aspirin (which may predispose to ulceration or gastritis; see Chapter 37), anticoagulants, and alcohol. Many over-the-counter products may contain aspirin or NSAIDs.
6. Relevant past medical and surgical history, including a history of GI bleeding, abdominal surgery (prior abdomi-

nal aorta repair should raise suspicion for an aortoenteric fistula), history of radiation therapy (radiation proctitis), history of major organ disease (including cardiopulmonary, hepatic, or renal disease), history of inflammatory bowel diseases, and recent polypectomy (postpolypectomy bleeding).

The physical examination must include an assessment of vital signs, cardiac and pulmonary examination, and abdominal and digital rectal examination. The initial laboratory examination should include complete blood cell count, blood typing and cross-matching, and measurements of serum electrolytes, blood urea nitrogen, creatinine, and coagulation factors. The first hematocrit measurement may not reflect the degree of blood loss, but it will decrease gradually to a stable level over 24 to 48 hours.

The initial disposition of the patient must also be considered. Patients older than 60 years, those with severe blood loss or with continued bleeding (as reflected by a significant decrease in hematocrit or postural changes in blood pressure or pulse rate), and those with significant comorbid illness are at the greatest risk for complications of GI hemorrhage and are best managed in an intensive care setting until stabilized.

Identification of the Bleeding Source

In about 80% to 90% of cases, acute GI hemorrhage resolves spontaneously without recurrence. Nevertheless, it is prudent to localize the bleeding source. Proper identification allows

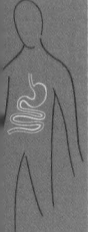

for direct treatment in cases in which bleeding does not spontaneously resolve and allows for the identification of the patient at risk for further bleeding. For example, in a patient with a bleeding gastric or duodenal ulcer, acid suppression with an intravenous proton pump inhibitor may maximize clot stability and enhance platelet aggregation. Proton pump inhibitors, in combination with appropriate endoscopic management, decrease the risk for ulcer rebleeding, the need for urgent surgery, and death. Direct visualization of the bleeding site by endoscopy can alter patient management because various stigmata of hemorrhage may be identified within the ulcer crater. Stigmata that carry a high risk for rebleeding are active bleeding and the presence of a pigmented protuberance (artery visible within the ulcer crater). The patient with a "clean base" ulcer exhibiting no such stigmata has an excellent prognosis for cessation of bleeding. The patient found to have high-risk stigmata is likely (>50%) to have continued or recurrent bleeding. In such a patient, the site of bleeding may be treated by injection therapy with vasoconstrictors or saline, thermal therapy by electrocautery, or mechanical therapy by placement of endoscopic clips. These endoscopic therapies decrease rates of rebleeding, mortality, need for transfusion, need for surgery, and length of hospital stay. Thermal or mechanical therapy applied alone, or in combination with injection therapy, is more effective than injection therapy alone.

An approach to the patient with acute GI bleeding is outlined in Figure 34-2. Historical points and objective findings often enable localization of the bleeding site to the upper GI tract (proximal to the ligament of Treitz) or to the lower GI tract (distal to that point). For the patient with melena or hematemesis, the upper GI tract should be examined first. Patients with hematochezia more commonly have lower GI bleeding, but when the pace of bleeding is brisk, an upper GI tract lesion may manifest with hematochezia. Placement of a nasogastric tube with aspiration of contents is a reasonable first step. The absence of blood does not by itself rule out the presence of an upper GI source because blood from a duodenal bulb ulcer may not flow back into the stomach and allow for sampling by the nasogastric tube. In general, in patients who present with acute GI hemorrhage and have significant blood loss, an upper endoscopy should be the initial step in the evaluation. Once the lower GI tract has been identified as the source of bleeding, sigmoidoscopy or colonoscopy is the test of choice. In cases of lower GI bleeding in which the pace of bleeding is so brisk as to preclude endoscopic visualization of the colon and rectum, scintigraphic ^{99m}Tc-sulfur colloid– or ^{99m}Tc-pertechnetate–labeled erythrocyte scans can localize the bleeding site if the rate of blood loss exceeds 0.5 mL per minute. Although the bleeding site identified by scintigraphic examination may not be accurate, it will direct visceral arteriographic search while minimizing the dye used. There is *no* role for barium studies in the evaluation of acute GI hemorrhage.

Chronic Gastrointestinal Hemorrhage

This condition may manifest as self-limited, recurrent episodes of melena or hematochezia, usually not with the degree of hemodynamic compromise discussed earlier. Patients may also have no overt evidence of blood loss, but rather may have persistent anemia and consistent occult blood loss.

The evaluation of this condition differs from that of acute GI hemorrhage. Obviously, the pace of the evaluation is less urgent. Furthermore, the likely causes for this bleeding differ from those of acute GI bleeding. Patients with this condition usually have undergone upper and lower endoscopy at least once, with no bleeding source identified. Therefore, the bleeding must have either an upper GI tract or colonic source that is difficult to identify or that emanates from the small intestine. The small intestine is a difficult area to examine in this regard because of its length and configuration. In general, the small intestine is initially evaluated radiographically. The patient may ingest barium, which is followed through the length of the small intestine. To distend the small bowel and give greater mucosal detail, an enteroclysis tube may be placed with its distal tip near the ligament of Treitz, allowing more forceful administration of barium and air. Computed tomographic and magnetic resonance enterography are rapidly replacing fluoroscopic imaging. However, all these imaging techniques have limited diagnostic utility. Flat mucosal lesions such as vascular ectasias, a common cause of obscure bleeding, may easily be missed. When radiographic studies are unrevealing, endoscopic evaluation of the small bowel may be attempted by push or double-balloon enteroscopy, or by "capsule endoscopy" (see Chapter 35). For the patient with persistent blood loss, no source of bleeding in the upper GI tract or colon as determined by endoscopy, and negative findings on radiologic studies, the entire small intestine may be examined at laparotomy with endoscopy in the operative suite. In addition, angiographic evaluation of the whole GI tract may reveal the source of chronic blood loss.

References

Barkun A, Bardou M, Marshall JK: Consensus recommendations for managing patients with nonvariceal upper gastrointestinal bleeding. Ann Intern Med 139:843-857, 2003.

Bounds BC, Friedman LS: Lower gastrointestinal bleeding. Gastroenterol Clin North Am 32:1107-1125, 2003.

Gralnek IM, Barkun AN, Bardou M: Management of acute bleeding from a peptic ulcer. N Engl J Med 359:928-937, 2008.

Huang CS, Lichtenstein DR: Nonvariceal upper gastrointestinal bleeding. Gastroenterol Clin North Am 32:1053-1078, 2003.

Manning-Dimmitt LL, Dimmitt SG, Wilson GR: Diagnosis of gastrointestinal bleeding in adults. Am Family Physician 71:1339-1346, 2005.

Marek TA: Gastrointestinal bleeding. Endoscopy 35:891-901, 2003.

Mitchell SH, Schaefer DC, Dubagunta S: A new view of occult and obscure gastrointestinal bleeding. Am Family Physician 69:875-881, 2004.

Rupp T, Singh S, Waggenspack W: Gastrointestinal hemorrhage: The prehospital recognition, assessment, and management of patients with GI bleed. J Emerg Med Serv 29:80-95, 2004.

C. Malabsorption†

Marcos C. Pedrosa and Elihu M. Schimmel

The main purpose of the GI tract is the digestion and absorption of major nutrients (fat, carbohydrate, and protein), essential micronutrients (vitamins and trace minerals), water, and electrolytes. Digestion involves both mechanical and enzymatic breakdown of food. Mechanical processes include chewing, gastric churning, and the to-and-fro mixing in the small intestine. Enzymatic hydrolysis is initiated by intraluminal processes requiring gastric, pancreatic, and biliary secretions and is completed at the intestinal brush border. The final products of digestion are absorbed through the intestinal epithelial cells. The regulation of gastric emptying, normal intestinal progression, and adequate intestinal surface area are additional important factors.

Most food components can be absorbed throughout the length of the small intestine, but some can be absorbed only at specific areas (e.g., vitamin B_{12} and cholesterol are absorbed only in the terminal ileum). Several molecules undergo an enterohepatic circulation with release into and reabsorption from the intestine, notably the bile acids needed for fat absorption. The primary absorptive function of the colon is the absorption of water and electrolytes; in addition, there is colonic salvage of much of the carbohydrate from indigestible fiber through bacterial enzymatic activity. This section discusses normal assimilation of the major nutrients and the approach to patients with maldigestion or malabsorption.

Digestion and Absorption of Fat

Dietary fat is composed predominantly of triglycerides (about 95%) with long-chain fatty acids (16- and 18-carbon molecules). In animal fat, the constituent fatty acids are mostly saturated (e.g., palmitic and stearic), whereas those of vegetable origin are rich in unsaturated fatty acids (i.e., having one or more double bond in the carbon chain; e.g., oleic and linoleic acids). Fats are insoluble (hydrophobic), and digestion begins with emulsification (i.e., fat droplets are dispersed in the aqueous medium of the lumen). Bile salts and pancreatic enzymes are bound to the surface of these globules by colipase, resulting in the release of fatty acids and a monoglyceride. These are taken up as mixed micelles with bile salts, allowing these hydrophobic particles to cross the unstirred water layer that overlies the epithelial brush border. Within the cell, the fatty acids are resynthesized into triglycerides and, together with cholesterol and phospholipids, are

†All material in this chapter is in the public domain, with the exception of borrowed figures or tables.

packaged into chylomicrons and very-low-density lipoproteins (VLDLs) to be exported through lymphatic channels. Bile salts remain in the lumen, are recycled into new micelles, and are finally reabsorbed in the terminal ileum with 95% efficiency. Most dietary lipids are absorbed in the jejunum, together with the fat-soluble vitamins (A, D, E, and K). Whereas fat constitutes up to 40% to 45% of diet calories in developed countries, a goal of 35% or less is set as a dietary recommendation for reduction of risk from cardiac disease and some cancers.

Digestion and Absorption of Carbohydrates

The bulk of dietary carbohydrates consist of starch, a glucose polymer, and the disaccharides sucrose and lactose, but only monosaccharides are absorbed. Salivary and pancreatic amylases release oligosaccharides from starch, and the final hydrolysis to glucose monomers occurs at the brush border, including disaccharide hydrolysis by sucrase and lactase. Glucose and galactose are actively transported in conjunction with sodium, whereas fructose absorption occurs by facilitated diffusion. About half of dietary energy is ordinarily derived from carbohydrate, with a nutritional goal of 55% and an increased component of insoluble fiber (i.e., that which is indigestible by mammalian enzymes, but variably broken down by colonic bacteria).

Digestion and Absorption of Proteins

Dietary proteins are the major source for amino acids and the only source for the essential amino acids. Digestion starts in the stomach with pepsins secreted by the gastric mucosa, but most of the hydrolysis is accomplished by pancreatic enzymes in the proximal small bowel. The pancreas secretes the proteases trypsin, elastase, chymotrypsin, and carboxypeptidase as inactive proenzymes. Enterokinase (more properly, enteropeptidase) is secreted by the intestinal brush border and splits trypsinogen to its active form, trypsin, which, in turn, converts the other proenzymes to their active forms. The products of luminal brush border peptidase digestion consist of amino acids and oligopeptides, which are transported across the epithelial cell. The transfer of most amino acids is sodium dependent and takes place in the proximal small bowel. Dietary need for amino acid nitrogen is met with about 15% of calories from protein.

Table 34-3 **Pathophysiologic Mechanisms in Malabsorption**		
Luminal Phase	**Mucosal Phase**	**Transport Phase**
Reduced nutrient availability	Extensive mucosal loss (resection or infarction)	Vascular conditions (vasculitis; atheroma)
Cofactor deficiency (pernicious anemia; gastric surgery)	Diffuse mucosal disease (celiac sprue)	Lymphatic conditions (lymphangiectasia; irradiation; nodal tumor, cavitation, or infiltrations)
Nutrient consumption (bacterial overgrowth)	Crohn disease; irradiation; infection; infiltrations; drugs: alcohol, colchicine, neomycin, iron salts	
Impaired fat solubilization	Brush border hydrolase deficiency (lactase deficiency)	
Reduced bile salt synthesis (hepatocellular disease)	Transport defects (Hartnup cystinuria; vitamin B_{12} and folate uptake)	
Impaired bile salt secretion (chronic cholestasis)	Epithelial processing (abetalipoproteinemia)	
Bile salt inactivation (bacterial overgrowth)		
Impaired cholecystokinin release (mucosal disease)		
Increased bile salt losses (terminal ileal disease or resection)		
Defective nutrient hydrolysis		
Lipase inactivation (Zollinger-Ellison syndrome)		
Enzyme deficiency (pancreatic insufficiency or cancer)		
Improper mixing or rapid transit (resection; bypass; hyperthyroidism)		

Adapted from Riley SA, Marsh MN: Maldigestion and malabsorption. In Feldman M, Scharschmidt BF, Sleisenger MH (eds): Sleisenger and Fordtran's Gastrointestinal and Liver Disease: Pathophysiology/Diagnosis/Management, 6th ed. Philadelphia, WB Saunders, 1998, pp 1501-1522.

Mechanisms of Malabsorption

The term *maldigestion* refers to defective hydrolysis of nutrients, whereas *malabsorption* refers to impaired mucosal absorption. In clinical practice, however, *malabsorption* refers to all aspects of impaired nutrient assimilation. Malabsorption can involve multiple nutrients or be more selective, and the clinical manifestations of malabsorption are thus highly variable. The complete process of absorption consists of a *luminal phase*, in which various nutrients are hydrolyzed and solubilized; a *mucosal phase*, in which further processing takes place at the brush border of the epithelial cell with subsequent transfer into the cell; and a *transport phase*, in which nutrients are moved from the epithelium to the portal venous or lymphatic circulation. Impairment in any of these phases can result in malabsorption (Table 34-3).

LUMINAL PHASE

Digestion is accomplished for the most part by pancreatic enzymes, particularly lipase, colipase, and trypsin; the gastric digestive enzymes do not play a major role. As a consequence, chronic pancreatitis can result in malabsorption, particularly for fat and protein. Deficiency in bile salts also contributes to fat malabsorption and may be the result of cholestatic liver disorders (impaired secretion of bile), bacterial overgrowth (resulting in luminal bile salt deconjuga-

tion), or ileal disease or resection (with loss of effective enterohepatic circulation of the bile acids). The major part of digestion occurs in the duodenum and most proximal jejunum.

MUCOSAL PHASE

Mucosal disease is a more common cause of malabsorption. It can occur because of diffuse small intestinal disease, such as in celiac sprue or Crohn disease, or from a decrease of surface area (e.g., after surgical resection for small bowel infarction). Selective defects in an otherwise normal intestine may result in specific entities such as lactase deficiency or abetalipoproteinemia.

TRANSPORT PHASE

After absorption, nutrients leave the cells through venous or lymphatic channels. Consequently, malabsorption may occur after mesenteric venous obstruction, lymphangiectasia, or lymphatic obstruction from malignancy or infiltrative processes (such as Whipple disease).

Multiple Mechanisms

Occasional disorders can impair the absorptive process at many stages. For example, patients with subtotal gastrectomy often have malabsorption. There are resultant defects at all phases: impaired gastric churning; premature emptying; and impaired mixing (in the jejunum) of food with bile and pancreatic enzymes. The latter is a consequence of anatomic changes (gastrojejunostomy bypassing the duodenum) and reduced production of pancreatic enzymes (because cholecystokinin and secretin release are blunted when gastric contents bypass the duodenum). Finally, stasis may lead to bacterial overgrowth in the afferent loop, with changes in the bile acids needed for fat absorption. Another example of manifold mechanisms is diabetes mellitus, with delayed gastric emptying, abnormal intestinal motility, bacterial overgrowth, and pancreatic exocrine insufficiency.

Clinical Manifestations of Malabsorption

The clinical manifestations of malabsorption are usually nonspecific. A change in bowel movements—usually diarrhea—and weight loss may occur early. Later, symptoms and signs of nutrient deficiency develop. Muscle wasting and edema result from protein malabsorption. Nutritional anemia, due to iron and vitamin deficiency (folate and B_{12}), contributes to fatigue. Bleeding tendency, such as ecchymosis, may be attributed to prolonged prothrombin time (high international normalized ratio) from vitamin K deficiency. Bulky, oily stools are the hallmark of steatorrhea resulting from fat malabsorption, whereas bloating (abdominal distention) and soft diarrheal movements occur as a result of carbohydrate malabsorption. Signs associated with malabsorption are presented in Table 34-4.

Clinical Tests for Malabsorption

Blood assays of albumin, carotene, cholesterol, calcium, and folic acid and of the prothrombin time are useful screening studies for malabsorption. These tests are helpful in assessing the severity of malabsorption, but are not specific for the differential diagnosis. Many tests are available in the work-up of malabsorption; those that have been most useful clinically are discussed next.

FECAL FAT ANALYSIS

The simplest qualitative method for detecting stool fat is the microscopic examination of a Sudan stain of a drop of stool. Sensitivity is limited, but it is quick and easy and correlates well with the quantitative measurement of fecal fat when moderate to severe steatorrhea is present. To quantify fat, stool is collected for 3 consecutive days while the patient is on a diet containing 100 g of fat per day, and the specimen is analyzed for fat content. Normal fat excretion should not exceed 6 g/day. Although the test is cumbersome and nonspecific, it offers an accurate quantification of fecal fat excretion provided fat consumption is appropriate.

TESTS OF PANCREATIC EXOCRINE FUNCTION

Intubation study of the duodenum with a fluoroscopically placed double-lumen tube may be the best index of pancreatic exocrine function. After stimulation of the pancreas, duodenal contents are aspirated and analyzed for bicarbonate and enzyme output. The test is invasive and time consuming; much experience is needed for its accurate interpretation; and it remains more of a research tool than a useful clinical test. The measurement of pancreatic enzymes in the blood (trypsinogen) or in the stool (chymotrypsin or elastase) is simple and provides helpful laboratory evidence for the diagnosis of moderate to severe pancreatitis. Pancreatic calcifications seen on abdominal films or computed tomography (CT) scan indicate the presence of chronic pancreatitis. Magnetic resonance cholangiopancreatography is a sensitive, noninvasive imaging procedure that may supplement CT scan for diagnostic purposes. Abnormal ductal anatomy can be best demonstrated by an endoscopic retrograde cholangiopancreatography (ERCP), but this test is invasive and has significant adverse side effects.

SMALL INTESTINAL BIOPSY

Peroral small intestinal mucosal biopsy is a key diagnostic test for diseases that affect the cellular phase of absorption. In some diseases, the histologic features are diagnostic; in others, the findings may be highly suggestive (Table 34-5). Endoscopic duodenal biopsies have largely replaced the more cumbersome jejunal sampling obtained by aspiration biopsy tubes. Several tissue samples should be taken from the distal duodenum to enhance the diagnostic accuracy.

D-XYLOSE TEST

D-xylose is a 5-carbon monosaccharide that is transported across the intestinal mucosa largely by passive diffusion. In this test, a patient ingests 25 g of D-xylose, and urine is collected for the next 5 hours. Healthy subjects excrete more than 4.5 g of D-xylose in 5 hours (or ≥20% of the ingested load). The test reflects intestinal transport function and surface area; it serves as an indicator of mucosal absorption. Abnormally low (false-positive) results may occur in the presence of impaired renal excretory function, massive peripheral edema, or ascites. Abnormal results can also be seen in the presence of bacterial overgrowth, but this "pseudomalabsorption" may be corrected after treatment with antibiotics serving as a therapeutic trial.

RADIOGRAPHIC STUDIES

Barium studies of the small bowel in malabsorption are usually nonspecific. Occasionally, however, distinct anatomic changes are seen in jejunal diverticulosis, lymphoma, Crohn disease, strictures, or enteric fistulas; also, there may be a distinctive barium pattern of thin-walled, dilated loops, suggestive of celiac sprue.

SCHILLING TEST

Absorption of vitamin B_{12} requires several steps. First, the ingested vitamin binds to salivary R-factor protein; gastric parietal cells secrete intrinsic factor that mixes with the ingested meal. In the duodenum, pancreatic trypsin hydro-

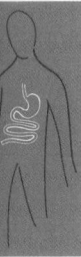

Table 34-4 Signs Associated with Malabsorption Syndromes

Signs	Associated Syndromes
Gastrointestinal	
Mass	Crohn disease, lymphoma, tuberculosis, glands
Distention	Intestinal obstruction, gas, ascites, pseudocyst (pancreatic), motility disorder
Steatorrheic stool	Mucosal disease, bacterial overgrowth, pancreatic insufficiency, infective or inflammatory, drug induced
Extraintestinal	
Skin	
Nonspecific	Pigmentation, thinning, inelasticity, reduced subcutaneous fat
Specific	Blisters (dermatitis herpetiformis), erythema nodosum (Crohn disease), petechiae (vitamin K deficiency), edema (hypoproteinemia)
Hair	
Alopecia	Gluten sensitivity
Loss or thinning	Generalized inanition, hypothyroidism, gluten sensitivity
Eyes	
Conjunctivitis, episcleritis	Crohn disease, Behçet syndrome
Paleness	Severe anemia
Mouth	
Aphthous ulcers	Crohn disease, gluten sensitivity, Behçet syndrome
Glossitis	Deficiencies of vitamin B_{12}, iron, folate, niacin
Angular cheilosis	Deficiencies of vitamin B_{12}, iron, folate, B complex
Dental hypoplasia (pitting, dystrophy)	Gluten sensitivity
Hands	
Raynaud phenomenon	Scleroderma
Finger clubbing	Crohn disease, lymphoma
Koilonychia	Iron deficiency
Leukonychia	Inanition
Musculoskeletal	
Monoarthropathy and polyarthropathy	Crohn disease, gluten sensitivity, Whipple disease, Behçet syndrome
Back pain (osteomalacia, osteoporosis, sacroiliitis)	Crohn disease, malnutrition, gluten sensitivity
Muscle weakness (low potassium, magnesium, vitamin D, generalized inanition)	Diffuse mucosal disease, bacterial overgrowth, lymphoma
Nervous System	
Peripheral neuropathy (weakness, paresthesias, numbness)	Vitamin B_{12} deficiency
Cerebral (seizures, dementia, intracerebral calcification, meningitis, pseudotumor, cranial nerve palsies)	Whipple disease, gluten sensitivity, diffuse lymphoma

From Riley SA, Marsh MN: Maldigestion and malabsorption. In Feldman M, Scharschmidt BF, Sleisenger MH (eds): Sleisenger and Fordtran's Gastrointestinal and Liver Disease: Pathophysiology/Diagnosis/Management, 6th ed. Philadelphia: WB Saunders, 1998, pp 1501-1522.

lyzes the R protein, freeing the vitamin to bind with intrinsic factor. The vitamin B_{12}–intrinsic factor complex is then absorbed by specific receptors found on enterocytes in the distal ileum. Consequently, malabsorption of vitamin B_{12} can occur because of lack of intrinsic factor (e.g., pernicious anemia or gastric resection), pancreatic insufficiency, bacterial overgrowth, or ileal resection or mucosal disease (i.e., Crohn disease). The Schilling test quantifies vitamin B_{12} absorption using radiolabeled vitamin B_{12} as a marker. The test may be expanded to several stages to amplify its diagnostic spectrum. In stage 1, after the injection of 1000 mcg of unlabeled vitamin B_{12} to saturate hepatic storage, the patient ingests 0.5 mcg of radiolabeled vitamin. Urine is then collected for the measurement of radioactivity; reduced radioactivity suggests B_{12} malabsorption. The test is repeated

(stage 2) with the addition of oral intrinsic factor to the ingested vitamin B_{12}; if urinary excretion of the radiolabel is corrected, pernicious anemia is diagnosed. If malabsorption is still present, the patient is given a short course of oral antibiotics (stage 3), and the test is repeated; correction of radiolabeled B_{12} excretion establishes bacterial overgrowth. If the test result remains abnormal, oral pancreatic enzymes are given (stage 4), and the test is repeated; correction of the abnormality implies pancreatic deficiency. Finally, if all these interventions fail, ileal disease or the absence of transcobalamin protein is determined by other diagnostic tests. This long outline serves more as an example of an algorithm of clinical analysis; the usual routine in clinical settings is to administer parenteral vitamin B_{12} while the etiology is delineated by other modalities.

BREATH TESTS

Breath tests rely on bacterial degradation of luminal compounds, which releases metabolic byproduct gases (such as hydrogen, methane, and CO_2) that can be measured in the exhaled breath. In the case of disaccharidase deficiency, a specific disaccharide (such as lactose) that is orally ingested but not properly absorbed in the small intestine is delivered to the colon, where bacterial fermentation liberates metabolites; hydrogen gas is the marker assayed in the breath. In the presence of bacterial overgrowth of the small intestine, orally ingested glucose ferments in the proximal small bowel (instead of being absorbed), resulting in increased breath hydrogen; here, the timing of exhaled hydrogen aids in the diagnosis. The measurement of radioactive CO_2 (tested with a nutrient labeled with ^{14}C) in the breath has been used to estimate the malabsorption of fat or bile acids and for measurement of bacterial overgrowth (^{14}C-xylose). The radioactive tests are cumbersome, and their usefulness in clinical practice is limited.

Approach to the Patient with Suspected Malabsorption

A large number of diagnostic tests are available for the work-up of malabsorption, necessitating the use of a rational algorithm (Fig. 34-3). The most accurate test for fat malabsorption remains the 72-hour fecal fat analysis; however, the test is difficult to carry out in clinical practice. Surrogate screening for steatorrhea is done with the qualitative stool fat examination (Sudan stain) and serum carotene. If the stool fat content is normal, the patient may still have selective impairment of the absorption of a specific carbohydrate. This latter condition should be suspected if the primary symptoms are cramps, flatulence, and diarrhea. The most common example of carbohydrate malabsorption is lactose intolerance; specific tests include the oral lactose tolerance test, but measurement of breath hydrogen is more sensitive

---

Table 34-5 Utility of Small Bowel Biopsy Specimens in Malabsorption

Often Diagnostic

Whipple disease
Amyloidosis
Eosinophilic enteritis
Lymphangiectasia
Primary intestinal lymphoma
Giardiasis
Abetalipoproteinemia
Agammaglobulinemia
Mastocytosis

Abnormal but Not Diagnostic

Celiac sprue
Systemic sclerosis
Radiation enteritis
Bacterial overgrowth syndrome
Tropical sprue
Crohn disease

Data from Trier JS: Diagnostic value of peroral biopsy of the proximal small intestine. N Engl J Med 285:1470, 1971.

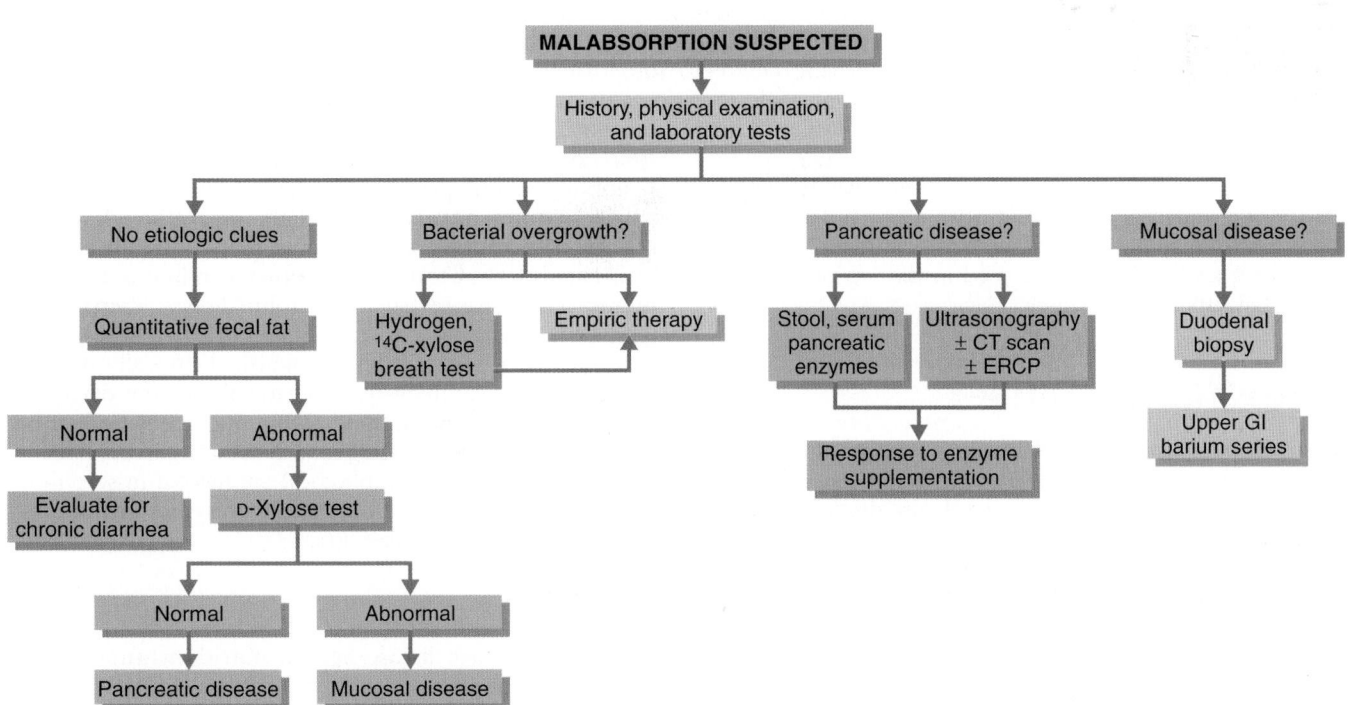

Figure 34-3 Approach to the patient with suspected malabsorption. CT, computed tomography; ERCP, endoscopic retrograde cholangiopancreatography; GI, gastrointestinal. (Adapted from Riley SA, Marsh MN: Maldigestion and malabsorption. In Feldman M, Scharschmidt BF, Sleisenger MH [eds]: Sleisenger and Fordtran's Gastrointestinal and Liver Disease: Pathophysiology/Diagnosis/Management, 6th ed. Philadelphia, WB Saunders, 1998, pp 1501-1522.)

and specific. More generally, an osmotic gap in fecal water suggests a dietary (rather than secretory) cause of the diarrhea related to luminal short-chain fatty acids or carbohydrates. The osmotic gap is calculated by the following formula: plasma osmolality − [2 × (fecal Na$^+$ + fecal K$^+$)]. The osmotic gap is not calculated by directly measuring stool osmolality because it increases with time in the specimen container. In addition, luminal osmolality is equal to serum osmolality because the colon cannot establish a gradient against the serum concentration of solutes.

When fat malabsorption is demonstrated (>6 g per 24 hours, or increased qualitative stool fat and decreased serum carotene), a D-xylose absorption-excretion test should be performed next. A normal D-xylose test makes diffuse mucosal disease unlikely and suggests maldigestion, principally pancreatic enzyme or bile salt deficiency. Clues to chronic pancreatitis include a history of alcohol abuse or previous episodes of pancreatitis; unusual causes of pancreatic malabsorption, such as cystic fibrosis, microlithiasis, or drug toxicity, require specific testing and a detailed history. In the search for maldigestion, serum enzyme tests and abdominal imaging (plain film or, with much greater sensitivity, abdominal CT scan) can be obtained next to identify pancreatic disease. If the urinary D-xylose excretion is abnormal, the breath hydrogen test may be used to diagnose bacterial overgrowth using glucose for the carbohydrate load. When no bacterial overgrowth is present, a mucosal biopsy should be performed (see Table 34-5). Radiologic studies of the small bowel with barium may be helpful on occasion.

When the etiology of malabsorption remains unclear, other considerations should include parasitic infection, such as *Giardia lamblia* or ascariasis involvement of the pancreatic duct (more common in undeveloped countries). These diagnoses require a careful stool examination for ova and parasites or fecal antigen studies. Occasionally, therapeutic trials for treatable conditions should be instituted, such as a gluten-free diet for celiac disease, pancreatic enzyme replacement for pancreatic exocrine function, metronidazole for *G. lamblia* infection, or broad-spectrum antibiotics for suspected bacterial overgrowth.

The specific treatment of malabsorption depends on identifying the underlying condition. Parenteral nutrition may have a role in maintaining an adequate nutritional status. Treatment modalities are discussed in the sections devoted to the corresponding diseases.

Specific Disorders

Malabsorption can be caused by a large number of disorders, some of them listed in Table 34-3. Two of these disorders, celiac sprue and bacterial overgrowth, are discussed in this section as illustrative of the pathophysiology. Cystic fibrosis of the pancreas may be the most common cause of malabsorption in the very young and is discussed in other sections.

CELIAC SPRUE (ALSO NONTROPICAL SPRUE, OR GLUTEN-SENSITIVE ENTEROPATHY)

Celiac disease is characterized by intestinal mucosal injury resulting from immunologic damage from gluten in persons genetically predisposed to this condition. The prevalence of the disease among relatives of patients with celiac sprue is about 10%. There is a strong association of celiac sprue with human leukocyte antigen (HLA) class II molecules, particularly HLA-DQ2 and HLA-DQ8. The disease is induced by exposure to storage proteins found in grain plants such as wheat (which contains gliadin), barley, and rye and their products. Oats are implicated not because of gliadin but because of contamination with wheat during packaging and transportation. The exposure initiates a cellular immune response that results in mucosal damage, particularly in the proximal intestine. Results of investigations suggest that an enzyme, tissue transglutaminase, may be the autoantigen of celiac sprue.

Clinical Presentation

Celiac disease can manifest with the classic constellation of symptoms and signs of a malabsorption syndrome. Not uncommonly, the manifestation may be atypical, with nonspecific GI symptoms such as bloating, chronic diarrhea (with or without steatorrhea), flatulence, lactose intolerance, or deficiencies of a single micronutrient, as in iron deficiency anemia. Extraintestinal complaints such as depression, weakness, fatigue, arthralgias, osteoporosis, or osteomalacia may predominate. A number of diseases, including dermatitis herpetiformis, type 1 diabetes mellitus, autoimmune thyroid disease, and selective immunoglobulin A (IgA) deficiency, are found in significant association with celiac disease.

Diagnosis

Although celiac disease is a leading consideration in every patient with the malabsorption syndrome, it should also be included in the differential diagnosis of patients with atypical manifestations. Fiberoptic or capsule endoscopy may show the typical features of broad and flattened villi; with the former instrument, tissue can be sampled for histology. Intestinal biopsy is the most valuable test in establishing the diagnosis, and the spectrum of pathologic changes ranges from normal villous architecture with an increase in mucosal lymphocytes and plasma cells (the infiltrative lesion) to partial blunting or total villous flattening. Although abnormal biopsy findings are not specific, they are highly suggestive, particularly because most other conditions that can mimic celiac disease (such as Crohn disease, gastrinoma, lymphoma, tropical sprue, graft-versus-host disease, or immune deficiency) may be distinguished clinically. A clinical response to a gluten-free diet establishes the diagnosis and precludes the need, in adults, to document healing by repeated biopsies. Serologic blood tests (antigliadin, antiendomysial, and reticulin antibodies) are helpful in screening of patients with atypical symptoms or asymptomatic relatives of patients with celiac sprue.

Treatment

Strict, lifelong adherence to a gluten-free diet is the only treatment for celiac disease. Specific nutritional supplementation should be provided to correct deficiencies, particularly those of iron, vitamins, and calcium. A clinical response may be seen within a few weeks. Patients should be monitored to ensure adequate response and proper adherence to the diet. The long-term prognosis is excellent in patients who adhere to the diet, although there may be a slight increase in the incidence of malignancies, particularly lymphoma.

BACTERIAL OVERGROWTH SYNDROME

The proximal small bowel normally contains fewer than 10^4 bacteria per milliliter of fluid, with no anaerobic *Bacteroides* organisms and few coliforms. Overgrowth of luminal bacteria can result in diarrhea and malabsorption by a number of mechanisms: (1) deconjugation of bile salts, which leads to impaired micelle formation and impaired uptake of fat; (2) patchy injury to the enterocytes (small intestinal epithelial cells); (3) direct competition for the use of nutrients (e.g., uptake of vitamin B_{12} by gram-negative bacteria or the fish tapeworm *Diphyllobothrium latum*); and (4) stimulated secretion of water and electrolytes by products of bacterial metabolism, such as hydroxylated bile acids and short-chain (volatile) organic acids.

Conditions Associated with Bacterial Overgrowth

The most important factors maintaining the relative sterility of the upper gut include (1) gastric acidity, (2) peristalsis, and (3) intestinal immunoglobulins (IgA). Thus, conditions that impair these functions can result in bacterial overgrowth. Impaired peristalsis can be caused by motility disorders (e.g., scleroderma, amyloidosis, or diabetes mellitus) or anatomic changes (e.g., surgically created blind loops, obstruction, jejunal diverticulosis). Achlorhydria (resulting from atrophic gastritis or the inhibition of gastric acid secretion), pancreatic insufficiency, and hypogammaglobulinemia are also associated with bacterial overgrowth, but uncommonly result in clinical steatorrhea.

Diagnosis

Direct culture of jejunal aspirate is the most definitive diagnostic test, but it is invasive, uncomfortable, and a costly laboratory undertaking. The ^{14}C-xylose breath test is an accurate and sensitive laboratory test, whereas breath hydrogen after an oral challenge with glucose is simpler, although not as sensitive or specific. Empirical therapeutic trial with antibiotics is an acceptable alternative to diagnostic testing.

Treatment

When appropriate, specific therapy, such as surgery for intestinal obstruction, should be provided. More commonly, patients are treated with antibiotics, the most appropriate being those effective against aerobic and anaerobic enteric organisms. Tetracycline, trimethoprim-sulfamethoxazole, or metronidazole, in combination with a cephalosporin or quinolone, is a suitable agent. A single course of therapy for 7 to 10 days may be therapeutic for months. In other patients, intermittent therapy (1 week of every 4 weeks) or even an extended period of continuous therapy may be the most effective management.

Malabsorptive Therapy

Cardiovascular disease and other consequences of obesity have reached epidemic proportions in the United States, and as a result, one approach to the problem has included the deliberate induction of malabsorption (primarily of fats) to reduce lipid levels and the body mass index (BMI). Medications used for this purpose include bile-acid binding resins, such as cholestyramine and colestipol, and more recently, the lipase inhibitors, orlistat (Xenical) and ezetimibe (Zetia). Surgical treatment usually consists of gastric partition combined with some degree of small intestinal bypass, which induces significant weight loss by several proposed mechanisms, including malabsorption, improved nutrient deposition, and enhanced satiety.

References

Alaedidni A, Green PH: Celiac disease: Understanding a complex disease [narrative review]. Ann Intern Med 142:289-298, 2005.

DiBaise JK, Young RJ, Vanderhoof JA: Intestinal rehabilitation and the short bowel syndrome. Am J Gastroenterol 99:1386-1395, 2004.

Goulet O, Ruemmele F: Causes and management of intestinal failure in children. Gastroenterology 130(Suppl 1):S16-28, 2006.

Green PH, Jabri B: Celiac disease. Annu Rev Med 57:207-221, 2006.

Gupta V, Toskes PP: Diagnosis and management of chronic pancreatitis. Postgrad Med J 81:491-497, 2005.

MacDonald TT, Montelone G: Immunity, inflammation, and allergy in the gut. Science 307:1920-1925, 2005.

Marth T, Raoult D: Whipple's disease. Lancet 361:239-246, 2003.

Owens SR, Greenson JK: The pathology of malabsorption: current concepts. Histopathology 50:64-82, 2007.

Pietzak MM, Thomas DW: Childhood malabsorption. Pediatr Rev 24(6):195-206, 2003.

Romanuglo J, Schiller D, Bailey RJ: Using breath tests wisely in a gastroenterology practice: An evidence-based review of indications and pitfalls in interpretation. Am J Gastroenterol 97:1113-1126, 2002.

Swallow DM: Genetics of lactase persistence and lactose intolerance. Annu Rev Genet 37:197-219, 2003.

D. Diarrhea

Satish K. Singh

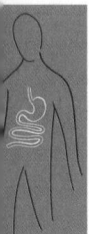

Definition

Diarrhea is both a symptom and a sign. As a symptom, diarrhea is most often reported as a decrease in stool consistency and an increase in stool volume; often, patients will use the term to describe frequency, urgency, and fecal incontinence as well. As a sign, diarrhea is defined as a stool weight (i.e., water content) that exceeds 200 g in 24 hours. This section discusses the physiologic aspects of intestinal solute and water transport and the pathophysiologic factors and management of diarrheal diseases.

Normal Physiology

About 8 to 9 L of fluid enter the small intestines daily: 1 to 2 L is derived from dietary intake, whereas the balance comes from normal salivary, gastric, pancreatic, biliary, and intestinal secretions. The small intestine absorbs most of this fluid so that only 1 to 1.5 L pass into the colon. In the colon, further water salvage results in a final stool output of only 100 to 200 mL per day.

Different types of specialized epithelial cells line the small and large intestines. However, all epithelial cells possess (1) polarity, in that they have distinct apical (facing the lumen) and basolateral (facing the blood) domains, (2) intercellular *tight* junctions that join their apical poles, and (3) a basolateral Na^+ pump (Na^+,K^+-ATPase) that maintains an electrochemical gradient. Among different small and large intestinal segments, epithelial cells mediate a range of different transport processes but share the fact that ions are moved across the epithelium by transport processes, while water follows along passive osmotic gradients. Movement of ions across the epithelium can be either passive, along electrochemical and concentration gradients, or active, against such gradients, requiring energy expenditure. Active ion transport is always transcellular, that is, it occurs *through* cells. Because of their charge, ions do not readily penetrate lipid bilayers and are moved through the plasma membrane in a regulated fashion through specialized proteins known as *pumps, carriers,* and *channels.*

Pumps are energy (adenosine triphosphate [ATP])-requiring transporters capable of moving ions and solutes against an electrochemical gradient. The most important pump in the intestinal epithelium is Na^+,K^+-ATPase, which removes Na^+ from the inside of the cell across the basolateral membrane against electrochemical gradients. With each cycle of the pump, three Na^+ ions are exported, and two K^+ ions are imported, creating an electronegative, Na^+-poor cell interior that ultimately drives transepithelial Na^+ and water absorption (Fig. 34-4).

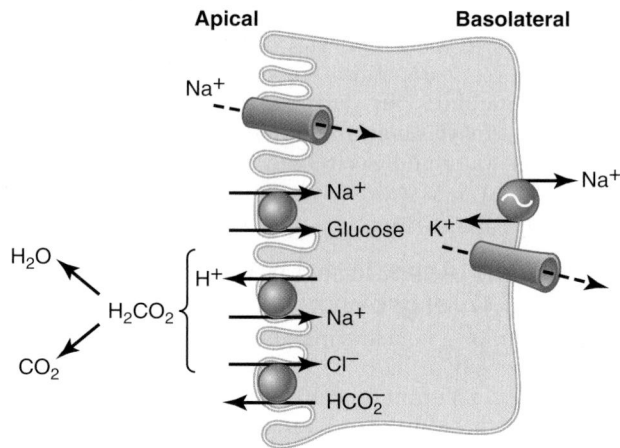

Figure 34-4 Apical sodium transporters. Sodium moves down its electrochemical gradient across the apical membrane of the epithelial cell. Pathways for apical sodium uptake include (1) channel proteins specific for sodium that can be blocked by amiloride, (2) carriers that couple the movement of sodium to the movement of nutrients such as glucose, and (3) antiport carriers that mediate electroneutral entry of sodium in exchange for intracellular hydrogen ion (i.e., acid). The common exit pathway across the basolateral membrane is the sodium pump. (From Sellin JH: Intestinal electrolyte absorption and secretion. In Feldman M, Scharschmidt BF, Sleisenger MH [eds]: Sleisenger and Fordtran's Gastrointestinal and Liver Disease: Pathophysiology/Diagnosis/Management, 6th ed. Philadelphia: WB Saunders, 1998, pp 1451-1471.)

Fluid secretion throughout the gut depends on electrogenic chloride (Cl^-) secretion. Active Cl^- secretion is predominantly mediated by cells within the crypts that possess tandem pathways for basolateral uptake and apical exit of Cl^-. Typically, basolateral Cl^--uptake mechanisms are coupled to the Na^+ gradient, thus maintaining intracellular Cl^- concentration above electrochemical equilibrium. As a result, increased apical Cl^- permeability following activation of an apical Cl^--channel protein causes Cl^- to exit the cell into the lumen, resulting in Cl^- and water secretion. One Cl^- channel, in particular, has been identified as a defective gene product in cystic fibrosis. Known as the *cystic fibrosis transmembrane regulator* (CFTR), it is activated by elevations in intracellular cyclic adenosine monophosphate (cAMP) as well as by several other mediators implicated in secretory diarrhea. The process of active chloride secretion is shown in Figure 34-5. Of note, secretory diarrheas produce a fluid rich in Cl^- *and* HCO_3^- anions. Basolateral HCO_3^- uptake (through Na-HCO_3^- cotransport [NBC] or Cl:HCO_3 exchange) in tandem with an apical exit pathway (through Cl:HCO_3 exchange or an HCO_3^- conductive pathway) have been implicated in the process of active bicarbonate secretion in animal models.

Although the small bowel and the colon share many basic mechanisms with regard to ion transport, differences exist. As a result, the small intestinal fluid that enters the colon has a plasma-like electrolyte composition, whereas fecal fluid contains twice as much K^+ as it does Na^+. At no time does either the small or the large intestine maintain standing osmotic gradients.

Pathophysiologic Factors

A significant number of mechanisms can cause diarrhea, and these mechanisms are listed in Table 34-6. However, most diarrheal states are caused by either inadequate absorption of ions, solutes, and water or by increased secretion of electrolytes that result in water accumulation in the lumen.

SECRETORY DIARRHEA

Secretory diarrhea is caused by abnormal ion transport across the intestinal epithelium, which results in decreased absorption, increased secretion, or both. Secretory diarrheas are typically caused by neurohumoral mediators or bacterial toxins that affect intracellular levels of cAMP, cyclic guanosine monophosphate (cGMP), and calcium. Elevated levels of these intracellular second messengers, in turn, typically inhibit electroneutral NaCl absorption and induce Cl^- secretion, the net result being increased water accumulation in the gut lumen. A classic example of a secretory diarrhea is cholera. A toxin produced by the bacterium binds to membrane receptors on enterocytes, irreversibly activating a guanine nucleotide-binding protein (G protein) that leads to enhanced cAMP production. The increased intracellular cAMP (1) inhibits apical electroneutral NaCl absorption (mediated by coupled Na^+-hydrogen ion [H^+] and Cl^--bicarbonate ion [HCO_3^-] exchange) and (2) simultaneously induces Cl^- secretion by activating apical Cl^- channels. These events result in massive diarrhea, intravascular volume loss, and, absent fluid resuscitation, eventual circulatory collapse. The hallmark of toxigenic and hormone-mediated secretory diarrheas is that there is no associated histopathologic

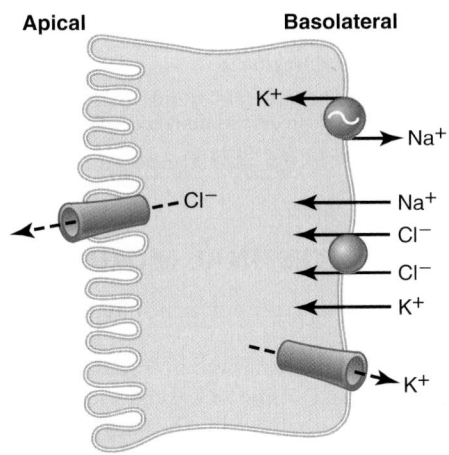

Figure 34-5 Chloride secretion. Discrete basolateral entry steps and apical exit steps are integral to chloride secretion. A carrier couples the movement of sodium, potassium, and chloride in a 1:1:2 stoichiometry and permits chloride to accumulate in the cell above its electrochemical equilibrium. Chloride exits the cell across the apical membrane by means of a chloride channel. The sodium and potassium that entered with the chloride are recycled by, respectively, the sodium pump and a basolateral potassium channel. (From Sellin JH: Intestinal electrolyte absorption and secretion. In Feldman M, Scharschmidt BF, Sleisenger MH [eds]: Sleisenger and Fordtran's Gastrointestinal and Liver Disease: Pathophysiology/Diagnosis/Management, 6th ed. Philadelphia, WB Saunders, 1998, pp 1451-1471.)

Table 34-6 **Classification of Diarrhea**

Type	Mechanism	Examples	Characteristics
Secretory	Increased secretion or decreased absorption of Na^+ and Cl^-	Cholera Vasoactive intestinal peptide–secreting tumor Bile salt enteropathy Fatty acid–induced diarrhea	Large-volume, watery diarrhea No gas or pus No solute gap Little or no response to fasting
Osmotic	Nonabsorbable molecules in gut lumen	Lactose intolerance (lactase deficiency) Generalized malabsorption (particularly carbohydrates) Mg^{2+}-containing laxatives	Watery stool; no blood or pus Improves with fasting Stool may contain fat globules or meat fibers and may have an increased solute gap
Inflammatory	Destruction of mucosa Impaired absorption Outpouring of blood, mucus	Ulcerative colitis Shigellosis Amebiasis	Small frequent stools with blood and pus Fever Variable
Decreased absorptive surface	Impaired reabsorption of electrolytes or nutrients	Bowel resection Enteric fistula	
Motility disorder	Increased motility with decreased time for absorption of electrolytes or nutrients	Hyperthyroidism	Variable
	Decreased motility with bacterial overgrowth	Irritable bowel syndrome Scleroderma Diabetic diarrhea	Malabsorption

Na^+, sodium; Cl^-, chloride; Mg^{2+}, magnesium.

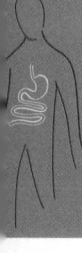

Table 34-7 **Some Causes of Secretory Diarrhea**
Infections
Bacterial toxins (enterotoxigenic *Escherichia coli*)
Stimulant Laxatives
Ricinoleic acid (castor oil), senna (Senokot), bisacodyl (Dulcolax)
Bile Acid and Fatty Acid Malabsorption
Intestinal Resection
Neuroendocrine Tumors
Zollinger-Ellison syndrome (gastrin)
Carcinoid syndrome (serotonin, substance P, prostaglandins)
Medullary carcinoma of the thyroid (calcitonin, prostaglandins)
Pancreatic cholera syndrome (vasoactive intestinal peptide)

Table 34-8 **Some Causes of Osmotic Diarrhea**
Laxatives Containing Poorly Absorbed Anion
Sodium phosphate (Phospho-Soda)
Laxatives Containing Poorly Absorbed Cation
Magnesium hydroxide (Phillip's Milk of Magnesia), magnesium citrate (Citrate of Magnesia)
Disaccharidase Deficiency
Lactose intolerance
Poorly Absorbed Carbohydrate
Lactulose, sorbitol ("sugar-free" gum), mannitol, congenital glucose-galactose or fructose malabsorption
General Malabsorption Syndromes

epithelial injury, leaving intact apical Na^+-coupled nutrient transporters (Na^+-glucose, Na^+–amino acid) that are not inhibited by intracellular second messengers. The persistence of these intact, alternative Na^+-absorption pathways can be exploited effectively by glucose and starch-based oral rehydration therapies.

Clinically, secretory diarrheas (1) are high output (often >1 L per day), (2) persist during fasting, and (3) display a minimal (<50 mOsm) stool osmotic gap (i.e., the amount by which stool osmolality exceeds what is accounted for by measured electrolytes, estimated from $2[Na^+] + 2[K^+]$) because salt secretion alone is causing the diarrhea. Some causes of secretory diarrhea are listed in Table 34-7. Although these features are classic for cases of pure secretory diarrhea, a more complex picture can result when mixed mechanisms coexist, for example, in malabsorptive syndromes such as celiac disease. Osmotic forces from malabsorbed fatty acids interfere with normal fluid absorption from both the small intestine and the colon, whereas bile acids interfere with absorption of water and electrolytes in addition to inducing Cl^- secretion in the colon. Thus, the component of water loss from fat malabsorption may fall substantially during fasting (see "Osmotic Diarrhea" next), an osmotic gap might be present as a result of carbohydrate malabsorption, fermentation and organic anion production, and a secretory component may exist as well if, for example, bile acids are substantially malabsorbed causing colonic Cl^- secretion.

OSMOTIC DIARRHEA

Water and solute movement is coupled throughout the GI tract, and no standing osmotic gradients are maintained across the mucosa. As a result, osmotic diarrhea is simply caused by excessive levels of poorly absorbed, osmotically active solutes in the lumen. Some causes of osmotic diarrhea are presented in Table 34-8. Osmotic diarrhea has two important clinical features. First, diarrhea stops when patients fast because they are no longer taking in poorly absorbed osmoles or the nutrients that they are malabsorbing. Second, stool analysis reveals an elevated osmotic gap because of the presence in stool of osmotically active or nonabsorbed agents.

ABNORMAL INTESTINAL MOTILITY

Altered GI motility can cause diarrhea by two mechanisms:

1. Enhanced motility, resulting in rapid gut transit and decreased contact time between luminal contents and absorptive epithelial cells. Decreased transit time and enhanced propulsive contractions contribute to postvagotomy, postgastrectomy, carcinoid, hyperthyroid, and diabetic diarrheas as well to diarrhea-predominant IBS.
2. Decreased motility, caused by diseases such as scleroderma or diabetes. These diseases promote small intestinal stasis that can result in overgrowth of largely anaerobic bacteria that inappropriately deconjugate bile acids, causing steatorrhea and diarrhea.

EXUDATIVE DIARRHEA

Inflammatory or infectious conditions that result in damage to the intestinal mucosa with disruption of the epithelial layer and intercellular junctions can cause diarrhea by numerous mechanisms. Blood, mucus, and serum proteins can be lost, the extent of which depends largely on the degree of injury. However, mucosal damage and attendant inflammation can interfere with absorption, induce secretion, and affect motility, all of which contribute to diarrhea.

Evaluation of Diarrhea
HISTORY AND PHYSICAL EXAMINATION

A thoroughly obtained history will yield valuable clues that guide appropriate and cost-effective investigation of diarrheal diseases. The *duration* of diarrhea is particularly useful because most acute diarrheas are caused by microbial pathogens and typically resolve independent of intervention. Chronic diarrhea, defined as lasting more than 4 weeks, is unlikely to be infectious. The presence of blood is also a useful clue because it suggests inflammation, neoplasm, ischemia, or infection by invasive organisms. Large-volume diarrhea suggests small bowel or proximal colonic disease; in contrast, frequent small stools with associated urgency suggest left-sided colonic or rectal disease. All current and recent medications (specifically new medications, antibiotics, and antacids) and alcohol intake should be reviewed. Intake of nutritional supplements should also be reviewed, including sugar substitutes that contain poorly absorbed carbohydrates, fat substitutes, milk products, shellfish, and heavy intake of fruits, fruit juices, and caffeine. The social history should include travel, source of drinking water (treated city water or well water), consumption of raw milk in rural populations, exposure to farm animals that may spread *Salmonella* or *Brucella,* and sexual practices. Familial occurrence of celiac disease, inflammatory bowel disease, or multiple endocrine neoplasia syndromes should be considered as well. Physical examination in acute diarrhea is helpful in determining severity of disease and hydration status. Physical findings are less helpful in chronic diarrhea, although certain findings have been associated with specific diseases: oral ulcers and pyoderma gangrenosum with inflammatory bowel disease, dermatitis herpetiformis with celiac disease, and lymphadenopathy with lymphoma.

Further evaluation with appropriate laboratory tests depends largely on the duration and severity of diarrhea and the presence of blood, overt or occult, in the stool.

ACUTE DIARRHEA

Acute diarrhea is defined as lasting less than 4 weeks and is most commonly caused by infectious organisms or toxins. It is usually self-limited and, in the absence of blood in the stool, usually remains undiagnosed. If a patient is seen early in the course of illness and has mild diarrhea without systemic symptoms or blood in the stool, expectant management with observation and follow-up is the most appropriate course of action. Otherwise, and certainly in the presence of blood, stool should be evaluated for infectious organisms, and antimicrobials should be initiated when appropriate. If organisms are not identified, sigmoidoscopy or colonoscopy should be performed and biopsies obtained. Further investigations should be guided by findings on sigmoidoscopy (e.g., if inflammatory bowel disease is suspected), severity of diarrhea, immunocompetence of the patient, and the presence of systemic toxicity. A general algorithm for the evaluation of acute diarrhea is shown in Figure 34-6.

CHRONIC DIARRHEA

Clinicians have numerous tests at their disposal for investigating a patient with chronic diarrhea, and a rational approach should be exercised in making the most appropriate choices. Duration of diarrhea, evidence of systemic involvement, nutritional deficiencies, and prior work-up should guide the evaluation of the patient. In contrast to acute diarrhea, infectious origin is uncommon with chronic diarrhea. However, certain persistent parasitic infections, such as giardiasis and postviral syndromes that result in persistently disturbed brush border enzyme, motility, and transport activities, can produce a chronic malabsorptive diarrheal picture.

Weight loss and evidence of nutritional deficiencies suggest malabsorption caused by a pathologic process in the small intestine or pancreas, the latter associated with a history of excessive alcohol intake or chronic pancreatitis. Chronic bloody diarrhea suggests inflammatory bowel disease, particularly ulcerative colitis. Chronic diarrhea with no evidence of nutritional or metabolic derangements suggests lactose intolerance (common); IBS, particularly when associated with abdominal pain (common); microscopic colitis (particularly in elderly women); eosinophilic enteritis (in young men); fecal incontinence; or surreptitious laxative abuse. Colon cancer should always be considered in older patients, especially those who have not had age-appropriate screening. Large-volume diarrhea in the absence of nutritional deficiencies, with features of a secretory process, usually prompts a search for hormone-producing tumors, although more often than not, they remain occult. Whenever possible, therapy is directed specifically toward the underlying cause. When no specific treatment is available (as in microscopic colitis) or no cause is determined, empiric therapies (e.g., antibiotics for possible bacterial overgrowth, *G. lamblia* infection, cholestyramine for bile acid malabsorption) with or without agents that decrease motility and secretion in general (e.g., loperamide, diphenoxylate and, in more severe cases, codeine, paregoric, long-acting somatostatin analogue), can be tried. A general algorithm for the approach to chronic diarrhea is presented in Figure 34-7.

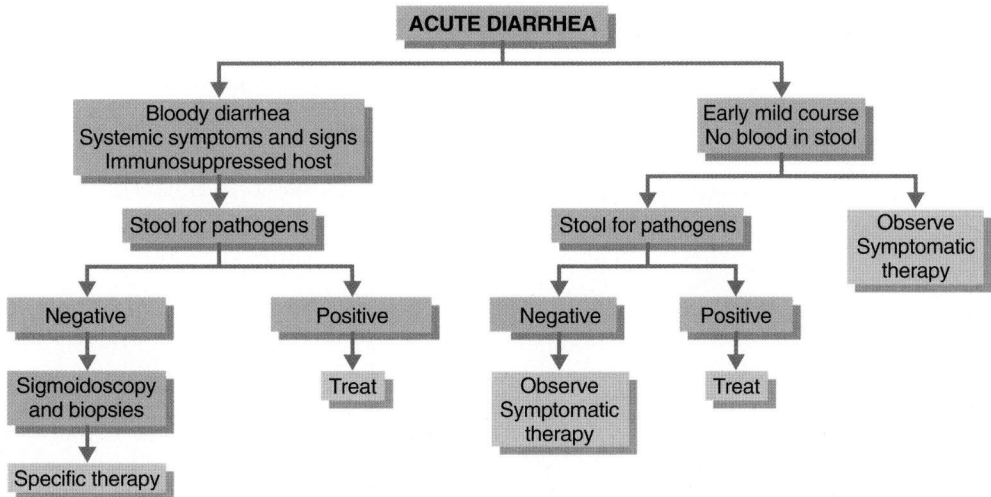

Figure 34-6 Algorithm for the evaluation of the patient with acute diarrhea.

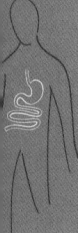

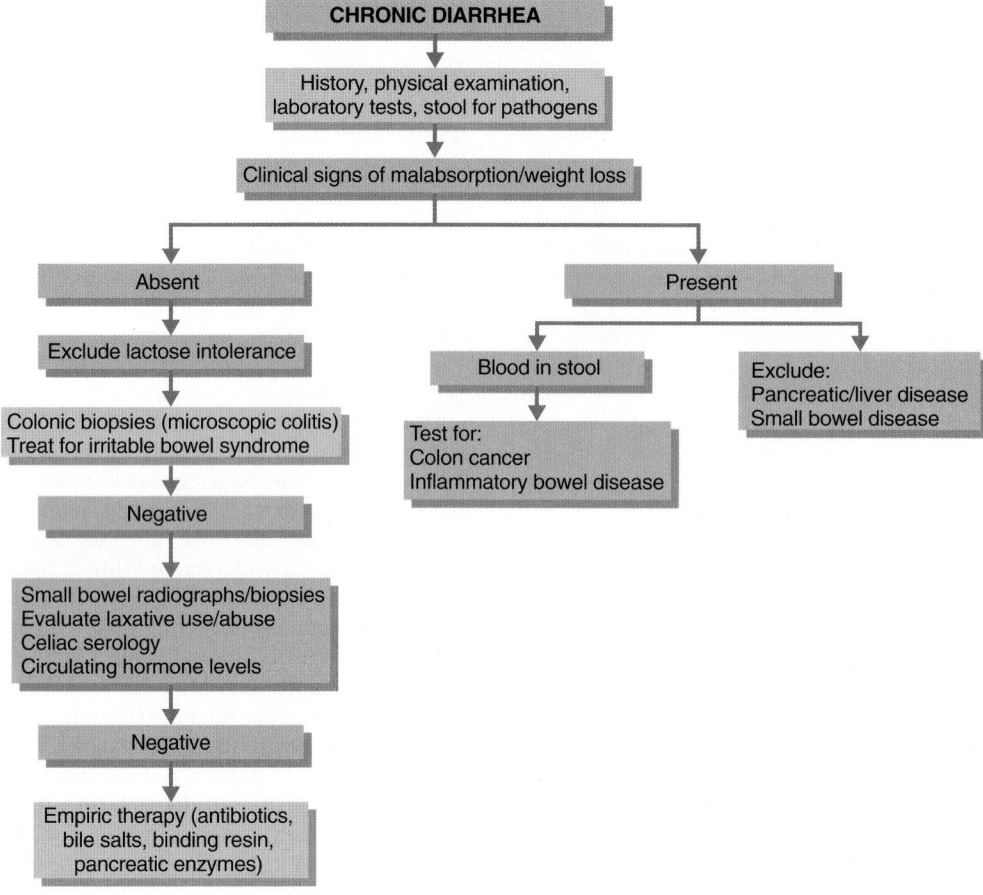

Figure 34-7   Algorithm for the evaluation of the patient with chronic diarrhea.

Prospectus for the Future

When viewed in a long-term perspective, the addition of diagnostic studies such as CT scanning, endoscopy, and most recently capsule endoscopy has clearly heightened diagnostic accuracy. The hope is that, in the future, even more sophisticated diagnostic instruments, including biochemical measurements, will enhance our understanding of the complex manifestations of abdominal pain.

References

Afzalpurkar RG, Schiller LR, Little KH, et al: The self-limited nature of chronic idiopathic diarrhea. N Engl J Med 327:1849, 1992.

Camilleri M. Chronic diarrhea: A review on pathophysiology and management for the clinical gastroenterologist. Clin Gastroenterol Hepatol 2:198-206, 2004.

Eherer AJ, Fordtran JS: Fecal osmotic gap and pH in experimental diarrhea of various causes. Gastroenterology 103:545, 1992.

Field M: Intestinal ion transport and the pathophysiology of diarrhea. J Clin Invest 111:931-943, 2003.

Fine KD, Schiller LR: AGA technical review on the evaluation and management of chronic diarrhea. Gastroenterology 116:1464-1486, 1999.

Harrell LE, Chang EB: Intestinal water and electrolyte Transport. In Feldman M, Friedman LS, Brandt LJ, Sleisenger MH (eds): Sleisenger & Fordtran's Gastrointestinal and Liver Disease, 8th ed. Oxford, UK, Elsevier, 2005.

Headstrom PD, Surawicz CM: Chronic diarrhea. Clin Gastroenterol Hepatol 3:734-737, 2005.

Mertz HR: Irritable bowel syndrome. N Engl J Med 349:2136-2146, 2003.

Schiller LR: Diarrhea. Med Clin North Am 84:1259-1274, 2000.

Schiller LR: Chronic diarrhea. Gastroenterology 127:287-293, 2004.

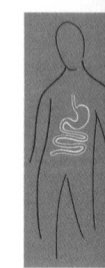

Endoscopic and Imaging Procedures

Brian C. Jacobson and Daniel S. Mishkin

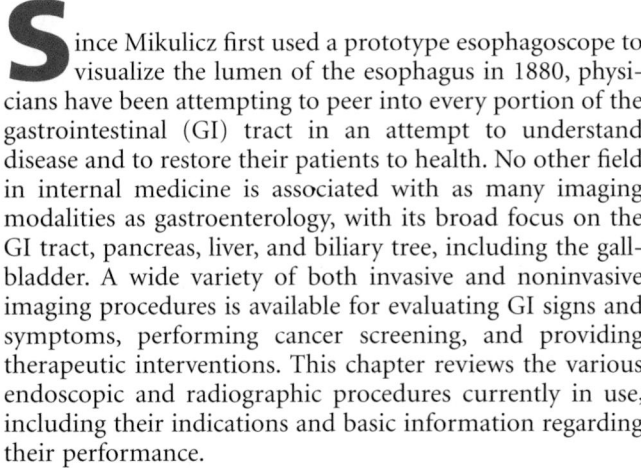

Since Mikulicz first used a prototype esophagoscope to visualize the lumen of the esophagus in 1880, physicians have been attempting to peer into every portion of the gastrointestinal (GI) tract in an attempt to understand disease and to restore their patients to health. No other field in internal medicine is associated with as many imaging modalities as gastroenterology, with its broad focus on the GI tract, pancreas, liver, and biliary tree, including the gallbladder. A wide variety of both invasive and noninvasive imaging procedures is available for evaluating GI signs and symptoms, performing cancer screening, and providing therapeutic interventions. This chapter reviews the various endoscopic and radiographic procedures currently in use, including their indications and basic information regarding their performance.

Gastrointestinal Endoscopy

The once-rigid endoscope has been supplanted by today's flexible instruments. These instruments are composed of long shafts 6 to 12 mm in diameter (Fig. 35-1) that house wires for deflecting the endoscope's tip in multiple directions, digital imaging equipment, and an accessory channel for the passage of biopsy forceps or other tools. The distal end contains lenses for both lighting and visualization, and the proximal end includes a series of knobs and buttons used to deflect or *steer* the endoscope's tip, insufflate air into the GI lumen, wash the lens, and suction air or liquid from the GI lumen.

GI endoscopy can be performed in dedicated endoscopy suites or at a patient's bedside in emergency situations. After positioning the patient appropriately and providing sedation, if necessary, the lubricated endoscope is passed through the intended orifice and advanced manually by the endoscopist. Bends and turns in the GI lumen are navigated by deflecting the endoscope tip and by applying torque

to the instrument shaft (i.e. rotating the shaft along the long axis of the instrument). Endoscopy is generally safe, with complications that include bleeding (0.3% to 1% after colonoscopic polypectomy), perforation (0.05% in general, but 0.1% to 0.5% after polypectomy), and sedation-associated hypotension and hypoxia (1% to 5%). Death related to endoscopic procedures is exceedingly rare (0% to 0.01%).

Technologic advances continue to affect endoscopic imaging, such as the recent introduction of high-definition instruments, magnification endoscopy, and narrow band imaging (NBI). NBI incorporates specific filters into the endoscope's light source to limit the instrument's lighting to narrow wavelengths in the blue and green range of the visible spectrum. By eliminating red light, endoscopic images demonstrate greater mucosal detail that may highlight subtle neoplastic changes.

ESOPHAGOGASTRODUODENOSCOPY

Esophagogastroduodenoscopy (EGD), often referred to as *upper endoscopy,* is performed with a *gastroscope* and allows the endoscopist to visualize the esophagus, stomach, and duodenum to its third and sometimes fourth portions (Fig. 35-2). Diagnostic indications for EGD include dysphagia and odynophagia, screening for and surveillance of Barrett esophagus, screening for esophagogastric varices, upper GI symptoms suggestive of ulcer disease or malignancy, suspected upper GI bleeding, and occasionally investigation of less common entities, such as celiac sprue or protein-losing enteropathy. The therapeutic interventions performed during EGD include the treatment of esophageal varices; dilation of esophageal strictures; rupture of esophageal rings and webs; dilation of the gastroesophageal junction in the setting of achalasia; removal or ablation of neoplastic lesions such as polyps, foci of high-grade dysplasia, or small malignancies; therapy for upper GI bleeding; and the placement of palliative stents for malignant obstruction of the esophagus, pylorus, or duodenum.

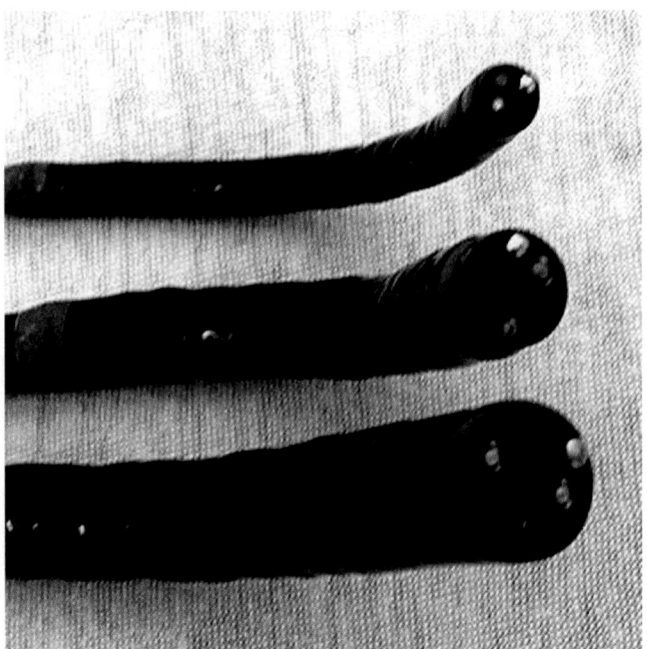

Figure 35-1 Endoscopes used for upper GI endoscopy. Endoscopes of varying sizes are available for use in different situations. The uppermost endoscope (6-mm diameter) can be used for unsedated endoscopy. The middle endoscope (9-mm diameter) is used for standard diagnostic endoscopy. The lowermost endoscope (12-mm diameter) is used for therapeutic endoscopy, such as the placement of enteral stents. (Courtesy of Brian C. Jacobson.)

ENTEROSCOPY

Examination of the small intestine beyond the ligament of Treitz is not feasible with a standard gastroscope. More recently, greater strides have been made to gain direct visualization of the 6 meters or 22 feet of the small intestine. *Push enteroscopy* using a long (>200 cm) endoscope allows the endoscopist to both image and biopsy or cauterize lesions in the small intestine. Advancing this instrument beyond the first 50 cm of jejunum can be difficult. Balloon-assisted enteroscopy is an exciting new technique that provides endoscopic access to most of the small bowel. This method employs balloons, incorporated into overtubes or the endoscope itself, to permit pleating of the small bowel onto the endoscope. By inflating and deflating the balloons in sequence, the enteroscope can be advanced through extremely long stretches of small intestine. Combining an anterograde (through the mouth) and retrograde (through the anus) approach, the entire small intestine can be visualized. Intraoperative enteroscopy is yet another means for obtaining visualization of the deeper portions of jejunum or ileum. In this procedure, a surgeon will make an incision in the patient's abdomen and then pleat the small bowel onto the enteroscope while the endoscopist visualizes the luminal surface. Once a lesion is identified, the surgeon may elect to proceed directly to a resection of the affected intestine.

VIDEO CAPSULE ENDOSCOPY

The desire to obtain visualization of the GI lumen in the least invasive way has resulted in the development of video capsule endoscopy, the use of pill-size wireless cameras that

the patient swallows (**Web Fig. 35-1; Web Video 35-1**). Currently, capsule endoscopes are available for the evaluation of the esophagus and small intestine. Capsules are 11 × 26 mm and can transmit images wirelessly to a data recorder as they travel through a patient's GI tract, without the need for sedation. At the end of the study, the data recorder allows for stored images to be uploaded into a computer for viewing while the capsule is ultimately passed in the patient's stool. The esophageal capsule is helpful in patients being screened for esophageal varices or individuals with suspected complications of acid reflux, such as reflux esophagitis or Barrett esophagus. The small bowel capsule has become the gold standard for visualizing the small intestine, most commonly for the purpose of investigating obscure GI bleeding (**Web Figs. 35-2 and 35-3; Web Videos 35-2 and 35-3**) and suspected inflammatory bowel disease (**Web Figs. 35-4 and 35-5**).

SIGMOIDOSCOPY AND COLONOSCOPY

Flexible sigmoidoscopy allows visualization of the rectum, sigmoid colon, and descending colon to the level of the splenic flexure. Enemas are given before the procedure to clear stool from the distal colon. Because sigmoidoscopy is quick (<10 minutes) and not particularly painful, sedation is typically not provided, making it a convenient tool for colorectal cancer screening. Additional indications for sigmoidoscopy include acute and chronic diarrhea and rectal bleeding and for evaluating responses to therapies for colitis.

Colonoscopy allows direct visualization of the entire large bowel and even several centimeters of terminal ileum. Bowel cleansing for colonoscopy requires the ingestion of osmotically active solutions, such as sodium phosphate or polyethylene glycol, coupled with a liquid diet for 24 hours before the procedure. Colonoscopy is more uncomfortable for the patient than sigmoidoscopy, which requires sedation. Indications for colonoscopy include those for sigmoidoscopy, as well as iron deficiency anemia, frank and occult GI blood loss, and assessing inflammatory bowel disease, including surveillance for dysplasia. Therapeutic interventions possible during colonoscopy include polypectomy, thermal ablation of vascular ectasias, decompression of colonic dilation associated with pseudo-obstruction, and occasionally the endoscopic control of lower GI bleeding.

ENDOSCOPIC RETROGRADE CHOLANGIOPANCREATOGRAPHY

Endoscopic retrograde cholangiopancreatography (ERCP) is a combined endoscopic and radiographic procedure for imaging the biliary and pancreatic ducts. A *duodenoscope* is a specially designed instrument for use during ERCP that includes an imaging lens oriented on the side of the endoscope's tip, allowing a direct view of the ampulla of Vater on the medial wall of the second portion of the duodenum. A tiny finger-like projection called an *elevator* helps the endoscopist guide a catheter into the duct of interest. Contrast is then injected through the catheter, filling the duct, and fluoroscopic images are obtained (Fig. 35-3). ERCP is indicated for evaluating obstructive jaundice with or without suppurative cholangitis, biliary colic with suspected bile duct stones, chronic or recurrent acute pancreatitis, and suspected

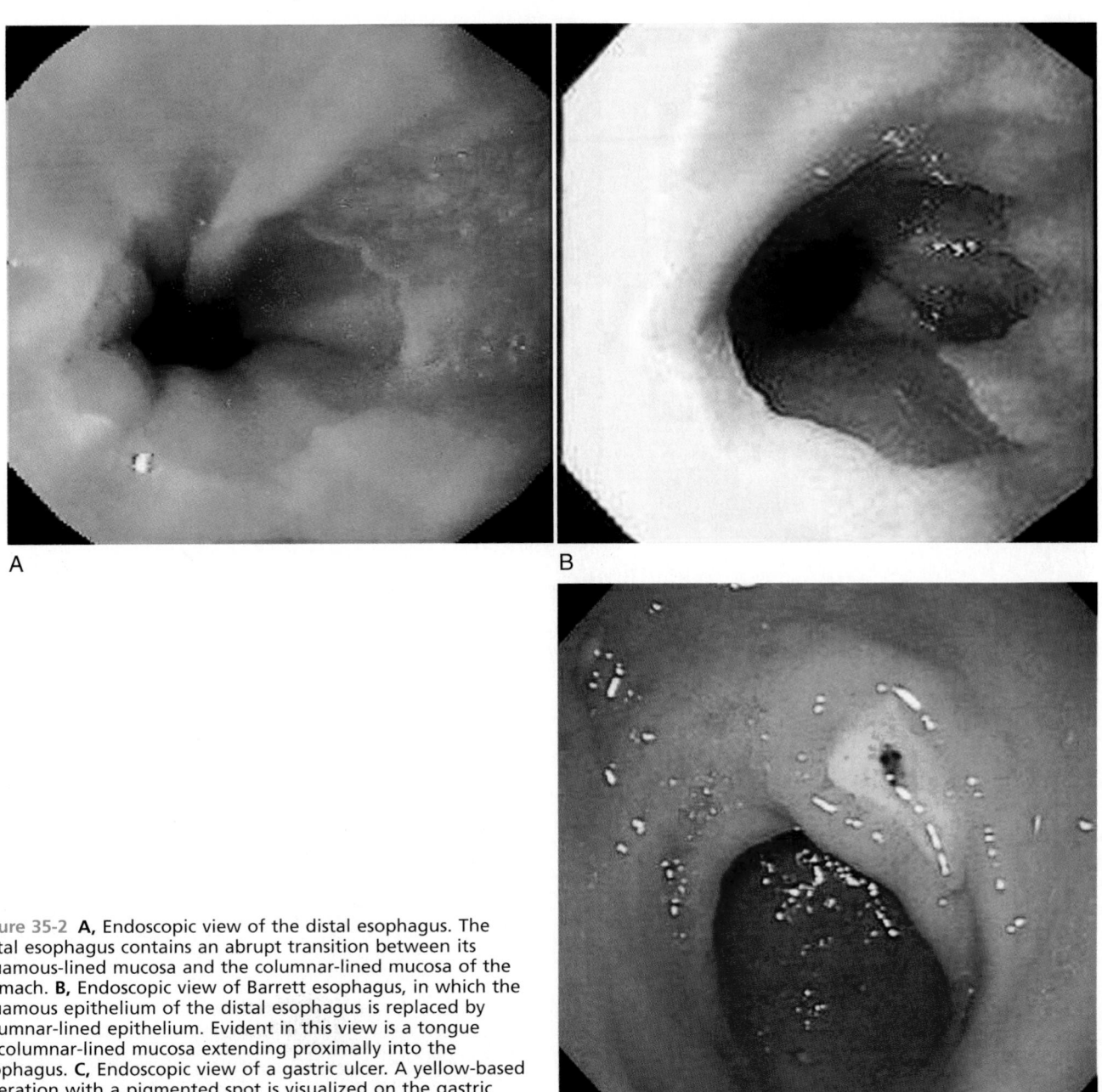

Figure 35-2 **A,** Endoscopic view of the distal esophagus. The distal esophagus contains an abrupt transition between its squamous-lined mucosa and the columnar-lined mucosa of the stomach. **B,** Endoscopic view of Barrett esophagus, in which the squamous epithelium of the distal esophagus is replaced by columnar-lined epithelium. Evident in this view is a tongue of columnar-lined mucosa extending proximally into the esophagus. **C,** Endoscopic view of a gastric ulcer. A yellow-based ulceration with a pigmented spot is visualized on the gastric wall at the transition between the corpus and the antrum. (Courtesy of M. Michael Wolfe.)

primary sclerosing cholangitis. Bile duct brushings and even biopsies may be obtained to determine whether a biliary stricture is neoplastic. With the use of a special manometry catheter, sphincter of Oddi pressures can also be measured in cases of suspected sphincter of Oddi dysfunction. Therapeutic interventions possible during ERCP include sphincterotomy (an incision through the sphincter of Oddi using a catheter with an electrocautery cutting wire), removal of bile duct stones, and placement of biliary or pancreatic duct stents to alleviate signs and symptoms of obstruction. ERCP carries a significant (5%) risk for complications, including pancreatitis, postsphincterotomy bleeding, and perforation.

Choledochoscopy and *pancreatoscopy* are techniques in which an endoscope 3 mm or less in diameter is passed through the accessory channel of a duodenoscope and into the bile or pancreatic ducts. The use of this small endoscope permits direct visualization of ductal abnormalities, guides electrohydraulic lithotripsy of large stones, and allows for direct sampling of ductal lesions.

ENDOSCOPIC ULTRASOUND

Endoscopic ultrasound (EUS) or endosonography is performed with an endoscope containing an ultrasound transducer in its tip. Because this transducer can be placed within

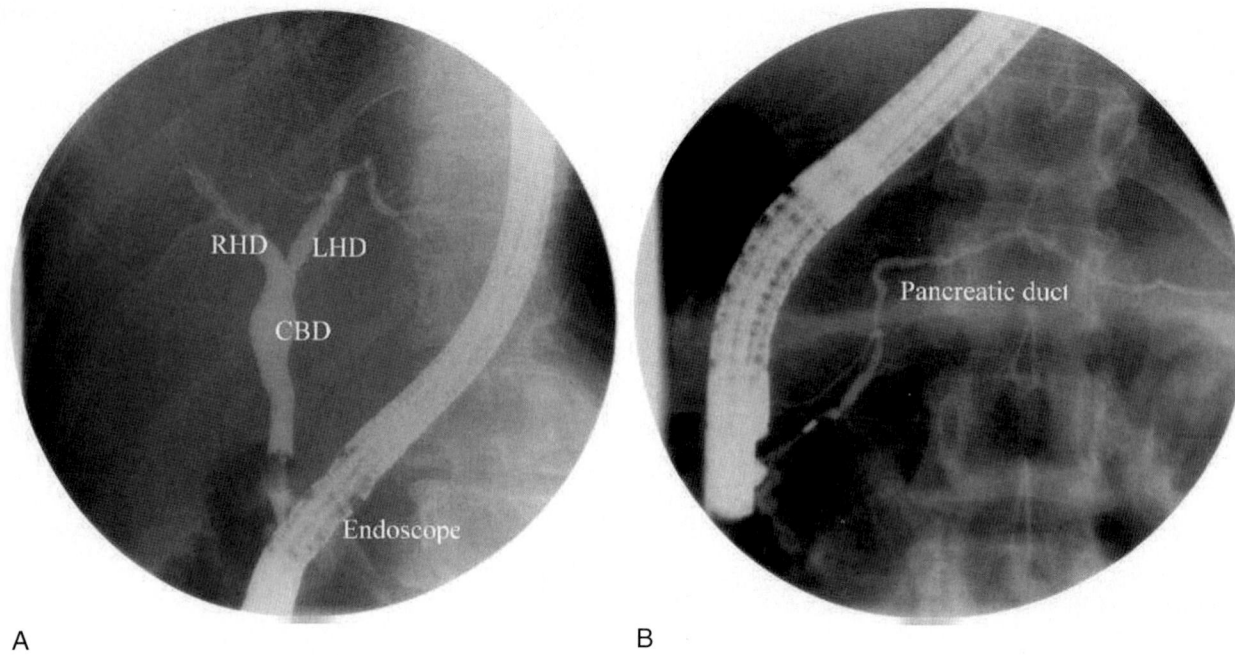

A   B

Figure 35-3 Endoscopic retrograde cholangiopancreatography (ERCP). **A,** Normal cholangiogram. Contrast injected into the biliary tree during ERCP demonstrates the intraductal anatomy of the common bile duct (CBD), right hepatic duct (RHD), left hepatic duct (LHD), and smaller intrahepatic biliary radicals. **B,** Normal pancreatogram. Contrast injected into the pancreatic duct during ERCP defines the intraductal anatomy throughout the length of the pancreas. (Courtesy of Brian C. Jacobson.)

the GI lumen, high-resolution images of the bowel wall can be obtained, revealing distinct layers that correspond to the mucosa, submucosa, muscularis propria, and serosa (Fig. 35-4). This technique allows the endoscopist to stage tumor depths and determine the layer of origin of subepithelial masses. In addition, EUS can penetrate the luminal wall, providing sonographic images of the mediastinum, pancreas, liver, gallbladder, and mesenteric vessels. Thin EUS probes can be passed through the accessory channel of a duodenoscope and into the biliary and pancreatic ducts to provide sonographic images of small tumors and stones. Fine-needle aspiration (FNA) can be performed under EUS guidance, enhancing the diagnostic capability of EUS. Tissue samples obtained by EUS-guided FNA are analyzed by cytopathologists and can distinguish benign from malignant lesions and metastatic spread of cancer to lymph nodes or the liver. FNA can also be performed to drain cystic lesions, such as pancreatic cystic neoplasms and pseudocysts.

Nonendoscopic Imaging Procedures

PLAIN ABDOMINAL RADIOGRAPHS

Plain abdominal radiographs include upright, supine, and lateral decubitus films obtained with standard x-ray equipment and without the use of contrast agents. Plain abdominal radiographs can reveal evidence of a pneumoperitoneum, dilated bowel loops and air-fluid levels, excessive amounts of stool, or displacement of bowel loops. These findings are indicative of a perforation, obstruction or ileus, constipation or fecal impaction, and volvulus or organ enlargement,

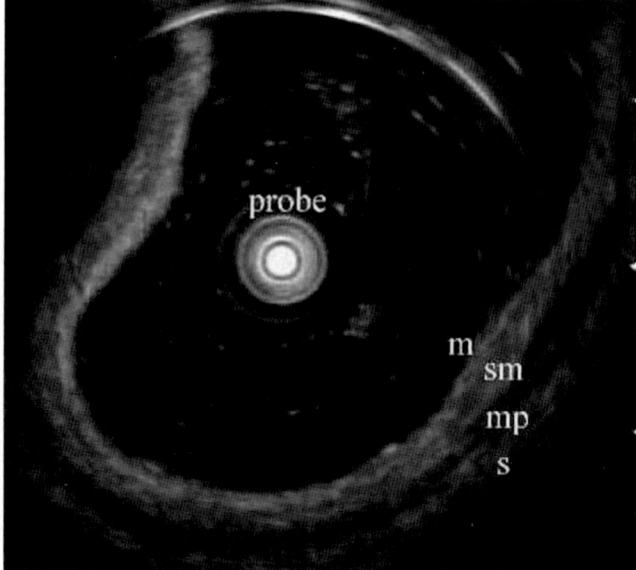

Figure 35-4 Endoscopic ultrasound of the gastrointestinal wall. A 12-MHz ultrasound probe, passed through the accessory channel of an endoscope, demonstrates the normal layers of the rectal wall. The mucosa (m) appears as a superficial, hyperechoic (white) band and a deeper hypoechoic (black) band. The submucosa (sm) appears as the next hyperechoic layer. The muscularis propria (mp) appears hypoechoic, and the serosa (s) appears as the outermost, hyperechoic layer. (Courtesy of Brian C. Jacobson.)

respectively (Fig. 35-5). Calcifications, such as those seen in chronic pancreatitis and gallstone disease, may also be visible on these radiographs. Plain films are most useful in the initial evaluation of abdominal pain or nausea and vomiting.

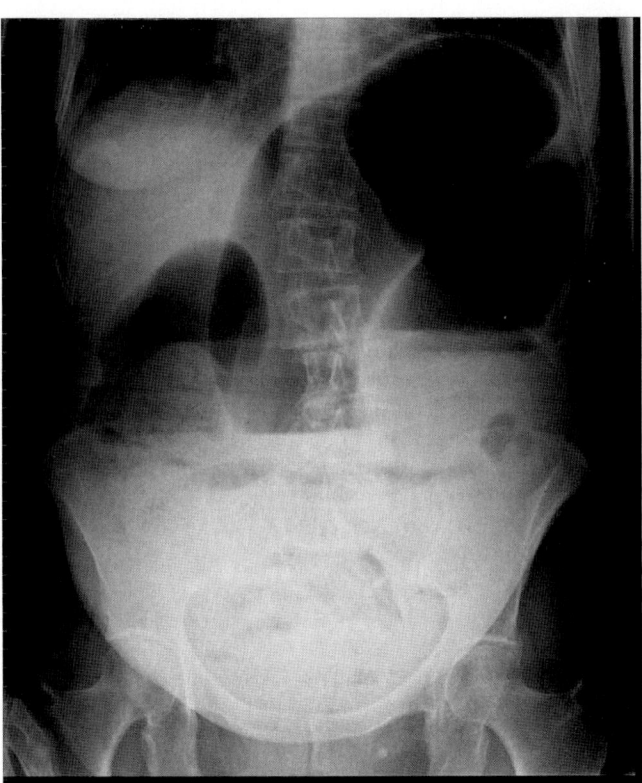

Figure 35-5 Upright plain radiograph of the abdomen. Air in dilated loops of colon and air-fluid levels can be seen in this patient with a sigmoid volvulus. (Courtesy of Brian C. Jacobson.)

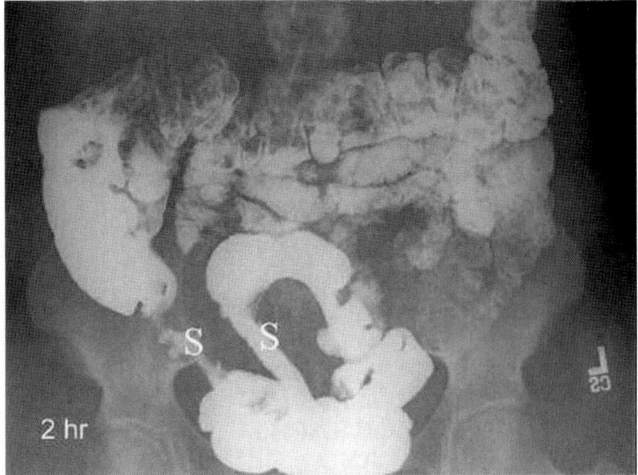

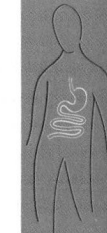

Figure 35-6 Small bowel follow-through. Ingested barium defines the contours of the small and large bowel lumen. A long stricture (S) of the terminal ileum can be seen in this patient with Crohn disease. (Courtesy of Brian C. Jacobson.)

CONTRAST STUDIES

Contrast agents such as barium or the water-soluble diatrizoate (e.g., Gastrografin) can be administered by mouth or rectum to detect mucosal abnormalities (ulcerations and masses), strictures, herniations, diverticula, and abnormal peristalsis. Contrast agents can be used alone *(single contrast)* or with the instillation of air or ingestion of gas-forming agents *(double contrast)*. The former method is more useful for detecting obstructing lesions and motility disturbances, whereas the latter method aids in detecting more subtle findings such as small ulcerations or polyps.

An *video esophagogram* entails the filming of a patient's oral cavity and pharynx during the ingestion of contrast materials of various thicknesses and textures. This imaging modality permits careful assessment of a patient's ability to manipulate a food bolus, swallow effectively, and avoid aspiration events. A video esophagogram is indicated for evaluating patients with oropharyngeal dysphagia and recurrent aspiration pneumonia. A more generalized *barium esophagogram* focuses attention on the esophagus during the ingestion of a bolus of contrast. This study can detect esophageal rings, webs, strictures, and motility problems that endoscopy might miss. A barium esophagogram may be useful for evaluating nonoropharyngeal dysphagia as well as odynophagia.

An *upper GI series* includes serial radiographic images as an ingested contrast agent travels through the esophagus, stomach, and duodenum. This study can define gastric abnormalities, such as ulcerations and mucosal thickening. It is indicated in evaluating abdominal pain and suspected gastric outlet obstruction. If radiographic imaging continues as the contrast agent traverses the jejunum and ileum, the study is called a *small bowel follow-through* (Fig. 35-6). During this more involved procedure, a radiologist will obtain multiple films, including *spot films,* or close-up views of regions that appear abnormal. Fluoroscopy can be used to follow a contrast agent during the journey through the small bowel. Attention is paid not only to structural findings but also to the length of time required for contrast to reach and enter the colon. For more detailed small bowel images, *enteroclysis* can be performed. This method requires the infusion of concentrated contrast directly into the small bowel through a nasojejunal tube placed under fluoroscopic guidance. Because of its invasive nature, enteroclysis is becoming less common in this era of wireless capsule endoscopy. Indications for a small bowel follow-through include suspected small bowel obstruction or partial obstruction from any cause, suspected small bowel mucosal diseases such as Crohn disease, and obscure GI blood loss.

Single- and double-contrast barium enemas can detect colonic strictures, diverticula, polyps, and colonic ulcerations, and they can reduce an intussusception. A barium enema may be used in conjunction with flexible sigmoidoscopy to provide screening for colorectal cancer, or it may be used to visualize the proximal colon when colonoscopy cannot be completed for various reasons. In general, the upper GI series and barium enema have been superseded by upper endoscopy and colonoscopy because the endoscopic procedures offer increased sensitivity for detecting mucosal abnormalities, the ability to obtain mucosal biopsies, and the potential for resection of identified lesions.

TRANSABDOMINAL ULTRASOUND

Ultrasonography is often the first imaging study obtained in the evaluation of suspected biliary colic, jaundice, and abnormal liver tests. Its use of sound waves to create an image avoids radiation exposure, and the addition of Doppler techniques permits the assessment of vascular patency. Ultrasound can detect parenchymal abnormalities, such as fatty liver or cirrhosis, focal masses or cysts, ascites, biliary ductal dilation, gallstones, and large vessel thromboses. It may detect thickening of the gut wall and areas of intussusception. Ultrasound is also used to guide needle placement for biopsies or fluid aspiration. Ultrasound cannot penetrate bone or air, preventing its use as a more general diagnostic tool for the GI tract.

COMPUTED TOMOGRAPHY, COMPUTED TOMOGRAPHY ENTEROGRAPHY, AND COMPUTED TOMOGRAPHY COLOGRAPHY

Computed tomography (CT) uses computer-aided reconstruction of multiple radiographic images obtained in a circular or helical course around a patient's vertical axis. Internal organs are visualized based on their inherent tissue densities compared with their surroundings. The GI lumen is usually opacified by having the patient drink an oral contrast agent. In addition, intravenous contrast agents can be administered to highlight regions with increased blood flow, thereby improving detection of pathologic lesions, such as tumors. CT can detect parenchymal lesions, such as tumors, cysts, and abscesses, as well as define the size, shape, and parenchymal characteristics of organs, such as the liver and spleen. Vascular abnormalities, such as perigastric varices or large vessel thromboses, and intra-abdominal fluid, such as ascites, can also be seen with CT. The caliber and contour of the GI tract wall are demonstrated by CT, aiding in the diagnosis of inflammatory lesions, such as colitis, diverticulitis, and appendicitis. CT can also be used to guide needle biopsies of abdominal masses and to place electrodes into tumors for ablative therapies such as radiofrequency ablation. The use of CT to guide placement of drainage catheters has made possible the percutaneous treatment of intra-abdominal abscesses, pseudocysts, and pancreatic necrosis.

CT enteroclysis and *CT enterography* are two emerging techniques developed to provide better images of the small intestine. CT enteroclysis uses a nasojejunal tube to deliver contrast into the small intestine, whereas CT enterography uses an orally ingested intraluminal contrast to highlight the small intestinal mucosa. With the advancement of this technology and its ability to reconstruct images in multiple planes, both luminal and extraluminal information can be obtained.

CT can also be used to obtain high-resolution images of the colon. CT colography, or *virtual colonoscopy,* makes use of special image reconstruction software to create accurate visualization of the colonic lumen, provided that the patient has completed a bowel-cleansing regimen identical to that used for colonoscopy. These CT images are 70% to 90% sensitive for detecting polyps or masses within the colon, helping to determine which patients need therapeutic colonoscopy. Virtual colonoscopy is presently being used in some centers to complete colonic visualization in the setting of an incomplete endoscopic colonoscopy.

MAGNETIC RESONANCE IMAGING AND MAGNETIC RESONANCE CHOLANGIOPANCREATOGRAPHY

Similar to CT, magnetic resonance imaging (MRI) provides multiple cross-sectional images of the abdomen and pelvis. These images are created using powerful field magnets to orient small numbers of nuclei within the body in such a way as to produce a measurable magnetic moment. MRI therefore avoids radiation exposure but requires the patient to lie nearly motionless, and often within a small enclosed tube, for prolonged periods. MRI can visualize parenchymal lesions such as masses and cysts and may better characterize abnormalities seen on CT, such as hemangiomas, hepatic focal nodular hyperplasia, and fatty liver. MRI is also helpful in better characterizing perirectal abscesses and fistulas in Crohn disease. Special rectal MRI probes or coils can provide detailed images of rectal cancer used for tumor staging.

MRI of the biliary and pancreatic ducts (*magnetic resonance cholangiopancreatography,* MRCP) is a noninvasive method that can detect ductal dilation, strictures, stones, pancreatic parenchymal changes in chronic pancreatitis, and congenital ductal abnormalities, such as pancreas divisum. Although MRCP techniques continue to improve, this technique fails to visualize small bile duct stones (<4 mm) and strictures, and it may be inaccurate for diagnosing primary sclerosing cholangitis. *Magnetic resonance angiography* is a magnetic resonance method for visualizing blood vessels and serves as an important noninvasive tool for evaluating patients with suspected mesenteric ischemia.

VISCERAL ANGIOGRAPHY

Angiography is an invasive technique whereby a catheter is introduced into a blood vessel, and intravascular contrast is injected during fluoroscopic imaging to visualize the vessel's lumen. Visceral angiography is used for evaluating mesenteric vessels in the setting of GI bleeding and suspected mesenteric ischemia. For GI bleeding, angiography is sensitive enough to detect 1 to 1.5 mL per minute of blood loss. Once the site of bleeding has been localized, the radiologist can infuse vasopressin (a vasoconstrictor) or embolize the vessel using tiny coals or gelatin sponges to ensure hemostasis. In the setting of mesenteric ischemia, angiography permits localization of a vascular stenosis or obstruction, followed by possible therapeutic interventions (e.g., balloon angioplasty, stent placement, infusion of vasodilators and thrombolytics). Other indications for angiography include the placement of transjugular intrahepatic portosystemic shunts (TIPS) in cirrhotic patients with intractable variceal bleeding or refractory ascites and for chemoembolization of liver tumors.

RADIONUCLIDE IMAGING

Technetium-99m (^{99m}Tc) is currently the major radionuclide used in GI imaging. Its 6-hour half-life and ready availability make it ideal for clinical use. ^{99m}Tc is used to label various substances for use in several imaging techniques. ^{99m}Tc-sulfur colloid scanning and ^{99m}Tc-labeled red blood cell scanning are two distinct methods that can be used to detect active GI bleeding. The latter uses the patient's own blood cells to carry the radionuclide throughout the body.

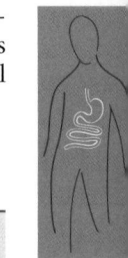

These methods can detect as little as 0.05 to 0.4 mL per minute of blood loss. However, localization of the site of bleeding is less accurate with these methods compared with angiography. ^{99m}Tc scans are often performed before angiography to document ongoing bleeding before subjecting a patient to the more invasive, less sensitive study. A ^{99m}Tc-labeled red blood cell scan can also be used to diagnose a hepatic hemangioma with an almost 100% positive predictive value.

Cholescintigraphy using ^{99m}Tc-iminodiacetic acid (IDA) analogs is the most commonly performed liver study in nuclear medicine. The radionuclide is taken up by the liver, is excreted into bile, and passes through the biliary tree into the gallbladder and duodenum. Failure to visualize the gallbladder during a hepatobiliary IDA scan may indicate cholecystitis secondary to cystic duct obstruction by a gallstone. Meckel diverticulum can be a source of abdominal pain and bleeding, but it can be difficult to visualize with standard endoscopic and radiographic imaging. The agent ^{99m}Tc-pertechnetate has a high affinity for gastric mucosa and is therefore used to demonstrate the presence of this congenital anomaly.

Prospectus for the Future

Through continued technologic advances, improvements in both endoscopic and radiologic image quality and resolution will also continue. In addition, the gastrointestinal lumen will no longer be regarded as a boundary to therapeutic endoscopy. Examples of expected innovations include:

- *The implementation of transgastric endoscopically guided surgical procedures.* With the use of recently introduced instruments, an endoscopist will be able to incise the gastric wall, advance an endoscope into the peritoneal cavity, and then perform surgical procedures such as elective cholecystectomy. A new field of *endosurgery* will develop to accompany these advances and will require training in both surgical principles and gastroenterology.
- *Commercial availability of new endoscopic imaging methods, such as confocal microscopy and fluorescence endoscopy.* Confocal microscopy allows an endoscopist to obtain magnified endoscopic images similar to those seen with a low-power microscope. Fluorescence endoscopy entails the use of special wavelengths of light to excite naturally occurring fluorophores in benign and neoplastic tissue. These fluorophores, such as collagen and nicotinamide adenine dinucleotide plus hydrogen (NADH), then fluoresce in a predictable manner, thereby providing a means of identifying, by endoscopy, otherwise microscopic changes, such as dysplasia without the need for a biopsy.
- *Video capsule endoscopes with advanced diagnostic and possibly therapeutic capabilities.* Through further advances in nanotechnology, video capsule endoscopes will be able to sample gastrointestinal secretions, measure intraluminal pressures, take biopsy samples, and perhaps even provide focal ablation of lesions using thermal energy or radiofrequency ablation.

References

Byrne MF, Jowell PS: Gastrointestinal imaging: Endoscopic ultrasound. Gastroenterology 122:1631-1648, 2002.

DiSario JA, Petersen BT, Tierney WM, et al: Enteroscopes. Gastrointest Endosc 66:872-880, 2007.

Fletcher JG, Huprich J, Loftus EV, et al: Computerized tomography enterography and its role in small-bowel imaging. Clin Gastroenterol Hepatol 6:283-289, 2008.

Gore RM, Levine MS: Textbook of Gastrointestinal Radiology, 2nd ed. Philadelphia, WB Saunders, 2000.

Mishkin DS, Chuttani R, Croffie J, et al: ASGE Technology Status Evaluation Report: Wireless capsule endoscopy. Gastrointest Endosc 63:539-545, 2006.

Thrall JH, Ziessman HA: Nuclear Medicine: The Requisites, 2nd ed. St. Louis: Mosby, 2000.

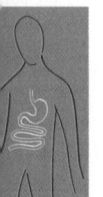

Esophageal Disorders

Robert C. Lowe and M. Michael Wolfe

The esophagus appears to be a simple organ with a single function, the transmission of ingested food and fluids to the stomach. This task is achieved, however, by a tightly coordinated pattern of motility, coupled with a protective barrier that prevents gastric secretions from entering the esophagus and pharynx. Derangement of these activities can cause a significant number of distressing symptoms that are among the most common reasons for patients to seek medical care.

Normal Function of the Esophagus

The esophagus is a hollow muscular tube designed to transport ingested materials from the mouth to the stomach in a coordinated fashion. It is composed of both striated muscle (the proximal one third) and smooth (the distal two thirds) muscle, bounded by two sphincters that are tonically contracted between swallows. The upper esophageal sphincter (UES) opens to admit a bolus into the esophagus and then closes rapidly to prevent aspiration of material into the trachea. The lower esophageal sphincter (LES) opens at the initiation of a swallow and remains open until the bolus passes into the stomach. It then closes to prevent reflux of ingested material into the esophageal body.

The act of swallowing begins with propulsion of the chewed bolus into the posterior oropharynx by the tongue. During the next phase of swallowing, several actions occur:

- The soft palate elevates to close off the nasopharynx.
- The epiglottis closes over the larynx, sealing off the trachea.
- The larynx is pulled upward to facilitate esophageal opening.
- The UES relaxes.
- The pharyngeal constrictors contract to propel the bolus into the esophagus.

Once the bolus has entered the esophagus, it is propelled downward by a series of coordinated contractions (primary peristalsis). The motility of the esophagus is mediated by local neurotransmitter release from enteric neurons. Con-traction of esophageal segments above a bolus is induced by acetylcholine, whereas relaxation of segments below the bolus is mediated by both nitric oxide (NO) and vasoactive intestinal peptide (VIP).

Symptoms of Esophageal Disease

Heartburn (pyrosis) is the most common symptom of esophageal disease, occurring in 44% of Americans at least once a month. About 10% of persons in the United States experience heartburn every day. It is most often described as a burning sensation in the epigastrium that rises into the chest. Patients often move their hand up and down between the xiphoid and sternal angle when describing this symptom. Given that heartburn is a cardinal sign of gastroesophageal reflux, it tends to occur after meals, when a patient is lying supine, or after an increase in intra-abdominal pressure (bending or lifting). Specific types of food, including fatty or spicy foods and chocolate, may also induce heartburn. Symptoms are often relieved temporarily by antacid preparations. Heartburn may be accompanied by regurgitation of bitter or sour fluid into the back of the throat or by excessive saliva production (the so-called water brash, which is caused by a vagal reflex induced by the presence of acid in the esophagus).

Dysphagia refers to a sensation of difficulty swallowing; patients report that a food bolus "gets stuck" or "goes down slowly." Although patients may point to their neck or chest when describing where the bolus gets held up, the location to which they point is poorly correlated with the actual level of obstruction. Dysphagia may result from a mechanical obstruction of the esophagus, inflammation of the esophageal mucosa, or an abnormality of motility of the esophagus.

Odynophagia, or pain on swallowing, needs to be differentiated from dysphagia in the patient history because it can be an important clue to the cause of the swallowing disorder. Painful swallowing is most often associated with infectious esophagitis or pill-induced esophageal ulcers but is only rarely present in acid-mediated esophageal disease.

Chest pain may also be a sign of esophageal disease, most often caused by gastroesophageal reflux or esophageal dysmotility. Unfortunately for the clinician, the symptoms of cardiac and esophageal chest pain overlap because of the shared neural pathways mediating pain sensation to these organs. Typical features of angina may occur in reflux-induced chest pain, including radiation to the neck and jaw, relief with nitrates, which modulate esophageal motility, and onset of symptoms with exertion. Chest pain that wakes a patient from sleep, however, is uncommon in true cardiac disease and may suggest an esophageal disorder, as does pain that is relieved with antacids or pain that lasts for several hours without associated symptoms. Esophageal chest pain is often thought to occur in response to esophageal spasm, but most data suggest that gastroesophageal reflux is responsible for most cases.

Gastroesophageal Reflux Disease

Gastroesophageal reflux disease (GERD) is the most common disorder of the esophagus, causing occasional heartburn in nearly one half of the population and daily symptoms in nearly 15% of Americans. GERD is responsible for about $10 billion to $12 billion in direct medication costs per year, and acid antisecretory therapies used in the treatment of GERD are among the most commonly prescribed drugs in the United States.

PATHOGENESIS

GERD occurs when the esophageal mucosa is bathed in acid-containing gastric secretions. Under normal conditions, several defensive mechanisms exist to minimize esophageal acid exposure. The most important of these mechanisms is the LES, which remains closed between swallows, separating the gastric and esophageal compartments. In a minority of patients with GERD, the LES is tonically weak, whereas the most common abnormality seen in these patients is an increase in transient LES relaxations (TLESRs). These brief relaxations occur in all persons, but those with GERD have a large number of episodes, allowing excessive acid exposure to the esophagus. The presence of a hiatal hernia contributes to deficient LES function by removing the added constriction of the diaphragmatic crura; thus, hiatal hernia is often noted in patients with GERD. However, reflux and hiatal hernia may occur independently of one another. Other factors contributing to esophageal protection include the following:

- Esophageal bicarbonate secretion
- Esophageal motility. Acid in the esophagus induces contractions (so-called secondary peristalsis) to clear the refluxate. Patients with motility disorders cannot empty refluxed acid into the stomach, leading to increased esophageal exposure to acid and symptoms of GERD.
- Saliva. Salivary bicarbonate helps neutralize refluxed acid. Patients with sicca syndrome, therefore, have an increased incidence of GERD symptoms.

These factors are summarized in Figure 36-1.

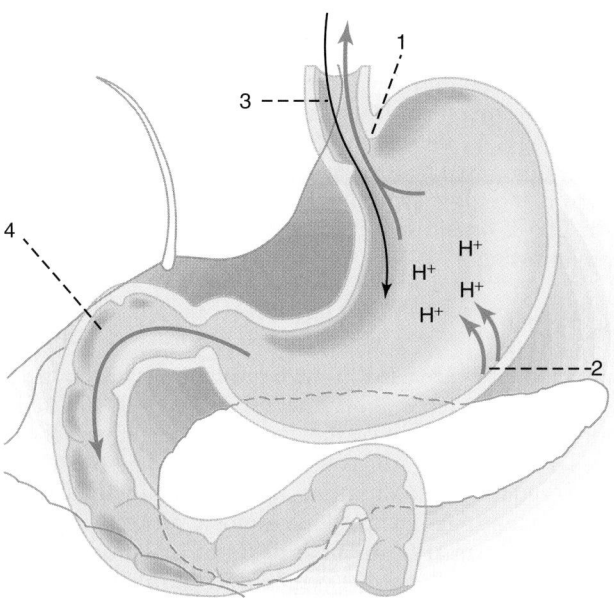
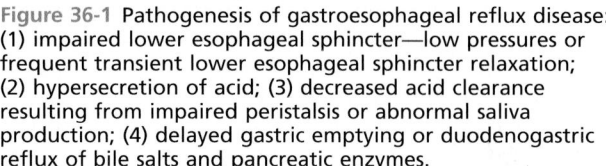

Figure 36-1 Pathogenesis of gastroesophageal reflux disease: (1) impaired lower esophageal sphincter—low pressures or frequent transient lower esophageal sphincter relaxation; (2) hypersecretion of acid; (3) decreased acid clearance resulting from impaired peristalsis or abnormal saliva production; (4) delayed gastric emptying or duodenogastric reflux of bile salts and pancreatic enzymes.

CLINICAL FEATURES

Heartburn is the cardinal clinical feature of GERD, and, when present, the diagnosis of GERD is made easily. Complaints of bitter regurgitation or water brash add to the diagnostic accuracy, but these features are not always present. In some cases, atypical symptoms dominate in patients with no history of heartburn. Most cases of noncardiac chest pain, which can mimic angina, are believed to be caused by GERD. In addition, a significant number of additional symptoms, including chronic cough, asthma, hoarseness, chronic sore throat, and globus sensation, may be the result of occult gastroesophageal reflux (**Web Table 36-1**).

DIAGNOSIS

The diagnosis of GERD is most often made on clinical grounds in patients with typical symptoms. Endoscopy is not a sensitive means of diagnosing GERD, given that only 15% of patients with GERD will have endoscopic evidence of esophagitis; endoscopy is useful, however, in identifying complications of GERD, including esophageal ulcers, strictures, and Barrett esophagus. A barium upper gastrointestinal series may demonstrate reflux of contrast material, but this, too, is insensitive as a diagnostic test for GERD. If a diagnosis of GERD is in question owing to the presence of atypical symptoms or comorbid illnesses, the appropriate diagnostic test is a 24-hour ambulatory pH study. In the past, this study was performed with a nasogastric probe that is placed into the stomach for 24 hours; transducers continuously monitor the pH of the esophagus while the patient participates in his or her usual daily routine. Symptomatic episodes are recorded in a diary and compared with the recorded pH values. More recently, an endoscopically placed esophageal probe has been developed that can measure pH for 48 hours; this probe is clipped to the esophageal mucosa, and the patient can perform his or her activities without the nuisance of a nasogastric tube. Although pH monitoring is the most accurate means of diagnosing GERD, it is not often used because an empiric trial of antisecretory therapy that leads to symptom resolution is considered diagnostic and is often used in place of expensive and invasive pH monitoring.

THERAPY

Many modalities are used in the treatment of GERD; these are outlined in Table 36-1. Therapy begins with lifestyle modifications that reduce the incidence of reflux. These maneuvers are often not completely successful, and most patients require the addition of medical therapy to achieve relief of symptoms. The pathophysiologic process underlying GERD is primarily an abnormality of LES motility, but current therapies directed at augmenting motility are rarely successful. Promotility agents such as metoclopramide have been used in GERD but with limited efficacy and a preponderance of side effects. Consequently, the mainstays of therapy for GERD are acid-neutralizing and antisecretory therapy, which neutralize or inhibit gastric acid secretion and render the refluxate less irritating to the esophageal mucosa. Magnesium and aluminum-based antacids (Mylanta, Maalox, Rolaids) offer temporary relief of symptoms, but lasting relief is better achieved with histamine-2 (H_2) receptor antagonists and proton pump inhibitors (PPIs). Provided their optimal administration, PPIs are the most effective preparations, controlling GERD symptoms in greater than 85% of patients with daily (before breakfast) or twice-daily (before breakfast and dinner) dosing.

SEQUELAE OF GASTROESOPHAGEAL REFLUX DISEASE

Common complications of GERD include esophagitis, ulceration, and esophageal stricture. Strictures typically produce progressive dysphagia to solids and often require endoscopic dilation to relieve the obstruction followed by intensive antisecretory therapy to prevent recurrence.

BARRETT ESOPHAGUS

Barrett esophagus is a condition in which the squamous mucosa of the esophagus undergoes metaplasia, becoming a columnar-lined epithelium with features of intestinal mucosa (goblet cells, Paneth cells). This specialized intestinal epithelium appears to occur as a result of years of acid exposure and is present in 5% to 15% of patients who undergo endoscopy for chronic GERD symptoms (**Web Fig. 36-1**). Barrett esophagus changes may be localized to the area of the gastroesophageal junction or may extend several centimeters proximally. The clinical significance of Barrett metaplasia lies in its propensity to undergo neoplastic change and develop into adenocarcinoma (**Web Fig. 36-2**). The risk for cancer in Barrett esophagus is estimated to be 40 to 100 times that of the general population, with a 0.5% risk for developing cancer per patient-year. Neither acid suppression therapy nor fundoplication leads to regression of Barrett metaplasia. At present, endoscopic surveillance is recommended for all patients with Barrett esophagus. Endoscopy is performed every 2 years, and biopsies are taken from the area of abnormal mucosa. If the biopsies reveal low-grade dysplasia, the frequency of endoscopies is increased. If high-grade dysplastic changes are seen and confirmed by a second pathologist, the risk for subsequent adenocarcinoma is greater than 25%, and surgical resection or ablative therapies should be considered.

Dysphagia

Evaluation of a patient complaining of difficulty swallowing begins with the discrimination between oropharyngeal and true esophageal disease. Oropharyngeal dysphagia is a disorder of initiation of swallowing caused by neurologic or muscular disease, including Parkinson disease, stroke, multiple sclerosis, myasthenia gravis, and amyotrophic lateral sclerosis (ALS). Patients with oropharyngeal dysphagia may complain of an inability to move the bolus to the back of the mouth and may note pooling of food in the cheeks after a swallow. Coughing or sputtering while eating may indicate aspiration of food, and nasal regurgitation is a classic sign of oropharyngeal dysphagia caused by a lack of coordination of the soft palate, which fails to close off the nasopharynx during swallowing. Treatment of oropharyngeal dysphagia consists of treating the underlying disorder, if possible, along with intensive speech and swallowing therapy that teaches patients techniques for improving their swallowing function.

Table 36-1 **Treatment of Gastroesophageal Reflux Disease**

Simple (Lifestyle) Measures

Elevation of the head of the bed
Avoidance of food or liquids 2 to 3 hr before bedtime
Avoidance of fatty or spicy foods
Avoidance of cigarettes, alcohol
Weight loss
Liquid antacid (aluminum hydroxide, magnesium hydroxide), 30 mL, 30 minutes after meals and at bedtime, *or* over-the-counter H_2 receptor blockers

Persistent Symptoms

Without Esophagitis

Alginic acid antacids (Gaviscon), 10 mL, 30 minutes after meals and at bedtime
Promotility drugs
Cisapride, 10 mg 4 times daily (qid)
Metoclopramide, 10 mg qid
H_2 receptor blockers
Cimetidine, 400 mg twice daily (bid)
Ranitidine, 150 mg bid
Famotidine, 20 mg bid
Nizatidine, 150 mg bid

With Esophagitis

H_2 receptor blockers—regular or double dose depending on severity
H_2 receptor blocker and promotility agent
Proton pump inhibitor
Omeprazole, 20 mg every morning
Lansoprazole, 30 mg every morning
Antireflux surgery

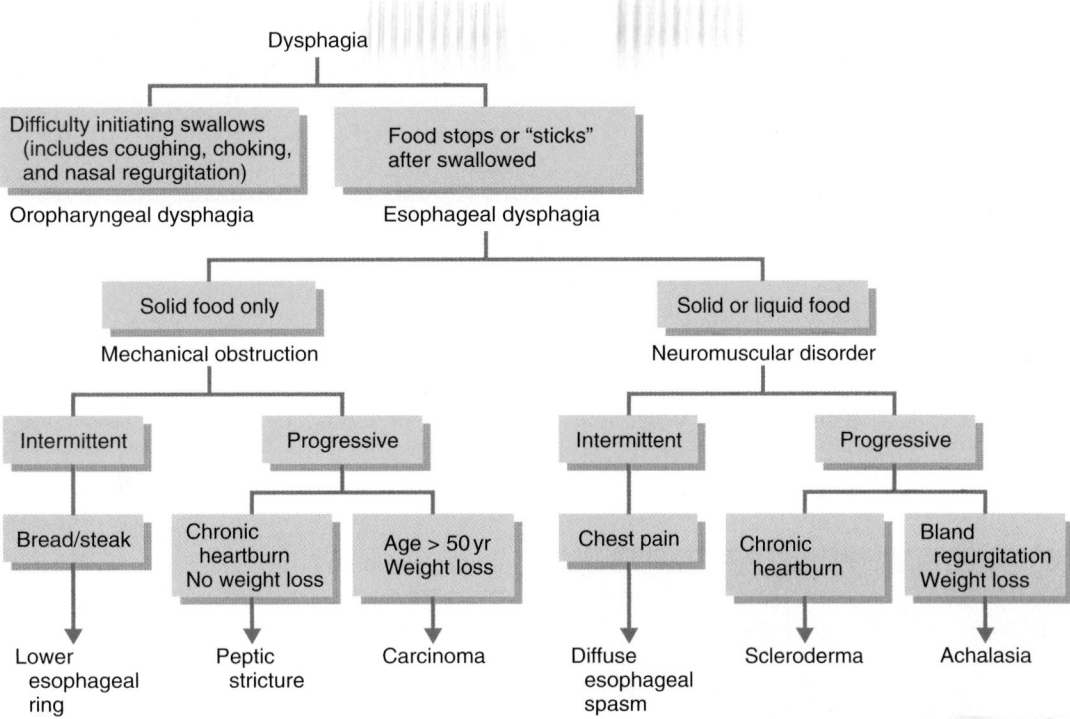

Figure 36-2 Algorithm for the differential diagnosis of dysphagia.

If a patient is found to truly have esophageal dysphagia, the next step in evaluation is to distinguish between mechanical obstruction of the esophagus and an abnormality of esophageal motility. Patients with motility disorders often describe dysphagia to both solids and liquids, whereas patients with obstruction generally have progressive obstruction only to solids until very late in their disease, when the obstruction becomes so narrow as to interfere with the passage of liquids. An important diagnostic feature in patients with dysphagia to solids is whether the dysphagia is intermittent or progressive. Intermittent dysphagia indicates the presence of an esophageal ring or web, whereas progressive symptoms are more likely to be caused by a stricture or mass lesion. A barium swallow is useful in outlining obstructive lesions of the esophagus, although endoscopy will then be necessary for purposes of biopsy and possible dilation; many gastroenterologists choose to evaluate dysphagia with an initial upper endoscopy to avoid numerous diagnostic tests.

If radiologic testing or endoscopic examination fails to demonstrate an obstructing lesion, the motility of the esophagus should be evaluated using esophageal manometry, a procedure in which a nasogastric tube with pressure transducers is placed in the esophagus, and pressures are measured during a specific number of swallows. This procedure permits diagnosis of motility disorders such as achalasia, diffuse esophageal spasm, or other nonspecific motility disorders. An algorithm for the management of patients with dysphagia is presented in Figure 36-2.

Esophageal Motility Disorders

Many patients with esophageal dysmotility have a nonspecific disorder that cannot be definitively characterized;

however, three of the more common disorders of esophageal motility are achalasia, diffuse esophageal spasm, and scleroderma. The features of these three diseases are outlined in Table 36-2.

ACHALASIA

Achalasia is a rare disorder of esophageal motility characterized by a tonically contracted LES that fails to relax appropriately during swallows, along with a dilated, aperistaltic esophagus. The disorder is caused by a degeneration of neurons in the myenteric plexus of the esophagus and in the vagal nuclei supplying the esophagus. Patients with achalasia typically have progressive dysphagia and weight loss and commonly experience chest pain and regurgitation of undigested food. Diagnosis is made using esophageal manometry, which reveals a tightly contracted LES that fails to relax with swallowing, along with poor or absent peristalsis in the esophageal body. Endoscopy is indicated to rule out an obstructing lesion of the lower esophagus or gastric cardia, which can mimic achalasia. Barium study in achalasia demonstrates a characteristic pattern shown in Figure 36-3. The widely dilated esophagus that tapers to a narrow "bird's beak" is highly suggestive of achalasia but does not obviate the need for endoscopy and manometric evaluation. Treatment is directed at opening the contracted LES, either by balloon dilation or by surgical myotomy. Botulinum toxin injections are also used to relax the LES, but relief is usually transient, and retreatment is almost always necessary.

DIFFUSE ESOPHAGEAL SPASM

Diffuse esophageal spasm is a motility disorder of the esophagus that usually produces episodes of chest pain and intermittent dysphagia to both solids and liquids. Manometric examination of the esophagus reveals uncoordinated,

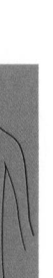

Table 36-2 Esophageal Motor Disorders

	Achalasia	Scleroderma	Diffuse Esophageal Spasm
Symptoms	Dysphagia Regurgitation of nonacidic material	Gastroesophageal reflux disease Dysphagia	Substernal chest pain (angina-like) Dysphagia with pain
Radiographic appearance	Dilated, fluid-filled esophagus Distal *bird-beak* stricture	Aperistaltic esophagus Free reflux Peptic stricture	Simultaneous noncoordinated contractions
Manometric findings			
Lower esophageal sphincter	High resting pressure Incomplete or abnormal relaxation with swallow	Low resting pressure	Normal pressure
Body	Low-amplitude, simultaneous contractions after swallowing	Low-amplitude peristaltic contractions or no peristalsis	Some peristalsis Diffuse and simultaneous nonperistaltic contractions, occasionally high amplitude

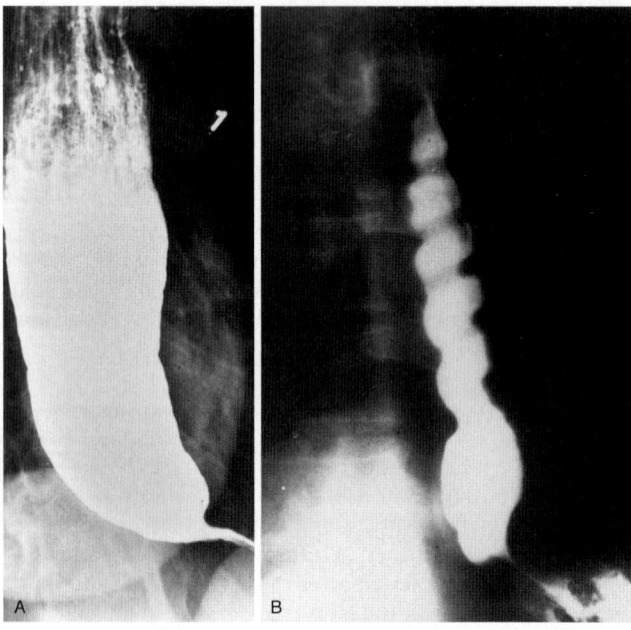

Figure 36-3 Radiologic appearance of achalasia (**A**) and diffuse esophageal spasm (**B**). In achalasia, the esophageal body is dilated and terminates in a narrowed segment or bird beak. The appearance of numerous simultaneous contractions is typical of diffuse esophageal spasm.

nonperistaltic contractions of normal or increased amplitude. This disorder is difficult to treat, given that pharmacologic therapy with nitrates and calcium channel blockers often proves minimally effective. Balloon dilation of the esophagus has been associated with relief in a minority of patients, as has surgical myotomy.

SCLERODERMA (PROGRESSIVE SYSTEMIC SCLEROSIS)

Esophageal dysmotility is a cardinal feature of scleroderma, occurring in up to 80% of patients. Scleroderma affects the distal two thirds of the esophagus (i.e., the smooth muscle portion), leading to fibrosis, atrophy, aperistalsis of the distal esophagus, and decreased LES tone. The manometric features of scleroderma include poor peristalsis in the distal esophageal body and a weak LES. As a result of this dysmotility, gastroesophageal reflux is typically present and is often severe; erosive esophagitis and peptic strictures are not uncommon, and patients may exhibit dysphagia caused by the primary dysmotility or to mechanical obstruction associated with stricture. The use of PPIs has significantly decreased the incidence of erosive GERD and its sequelae in patients with scleroderma.

Other Esophageal Disorders

ESOPHAGEAL RINGS AND WEBS

Esophageal rings (also called *Schatzki* or *B rings*) are rings of fibrous tissue that occur in the lower esophagus and cause intermittent dysphagia to solids. Classically, patients experience dysphagia when eating a large piece of meat or soft bread (leading to the name *steakhouse syndrome*). Between episodes of dysphagia, patients report normal swallowing and no associated symptoms. On endoscopic examination, rings are visible in the distal esophagus and may be partial or completely circumferential (**Web Fig. 36-3**). Treatment with balloon or bougie dilation is effective in relieving symptoms, although some patients require repeated dilations to remain symptom free. Esophageal webs are similar to rings but tend to occur in the proximal esophagus. An association between esophageal webs and iron deficiency anemia (sideropenic dysphagia) has been described (also known as *Plummer-Vinson* or *Patterson-Kelly syndrome*).

EOSINOPHILIC ESOPHAGITIS

Eosinophilic esophagitis (EE) is an inflammatory disorder of the esophagus characterized by a dense eosinophilic infiltration of the mucosa that leads to structural abnormalities in many patients. EE was originally described in the pediatric population but in recent years has been increasingly recognized in adults. The eosinophilia is believed to be the result of a delayed hypersensitivity reaction to food antigens or other allergens outside of the gastrointestinal tract. Dysphagia is the most commonly reported symptom, but patients may complain about heartburn, chest pain, or nausea; a food impaction may be the first presentation of EE. Endoscopic findings may include a narrowed esophageal lumen, longitudinal furrows or circular ridges in the mucosa, and discrete luminal strictures. The esophagus in EE is friable and prone to tearing with simple passage of the endoscope, during biopsy or after dilation. Diagnosis is established if biopsies from the proximal esophagus demonstrate 15 to 25 eosinophils per high-power field. Current treatment consists of swallowed topical steroids; fluticasone inhalers are used, but the contents are sprayed into the mouth and swallowed to coat the esophagus with the steroid preparation. This has proved effective in reducing symptoms and improving histology in pediatric clinical trials, and it is currently used in adults as well; oral steroids may be necessary in refractory cases.

ESOPHAGEAL INFECTIONS

Infections of the esophagus occur but are uncommon in patients who are immunocompetent. They are, however, a major source of morbidity in patients with compromised immunity, including organ transplant recipients, patients infected with HIV and patients on chronic steroids. Infectious esophagitis tends to produce both dysphagia and odynophagia, with the latter being the predominant symptom. Candida esophagitis is often associated with oral thrush and tends to produce dysphagia and only mild pain on swallowing. Candida has a characteristic appearance on endoscopic examination, and esophageal brushings and biopsies dem-

onstrate fungal hyphae (**Web Fig. 36-4**). Treatment with oral fluconazole is generally effective. Herpes simplex virus (HSV) causes multiple esophageal ulcers and exhibits clinically severe odynophagia. Acyclovir is the treatment of choice for herpes esophagitis. Cytomegalovirus (CMV) also causes esophageal ulceration and odynophagia. Endoscopic examination usually demonstrates a single large ulcer in the distal esophagus, and biopsies often detect viral inclusions that confirm the diagnosis. Both ganciclovir and foscarnet are effective treatments for CMV esophagitis. HIV infection is associated with esophageal ulceration and odynophagia, although much less commonly in the era of effective antiretroviral therapy.

PILL ESOPHAGITIS

Several medications can cause esophageal ulceration following prolonged contact with the esophageal mucosa. The most common medications associated with this condition include tetracyclines, potassium preparations, nonsteroidal anti-inflammatory drugs, iron sulfate, and the bisphosphonate alendronate. Patients report epigastric pain, sometimes radiating to the back, and both dysphagia and odynophagia. Treatment is symptomatic, and topical preparations such as viscous lidocaine may be helpful in relieving discomfort. Prevention of pill esophagitis is accomplished by ensuring that patients drink sufficient fluid (>120 mL) when taking oral medications. Patients should also be counseled to avoid lying down immediately after swallowing pills.

Prospectus for the Future

Our understanding of a significant number of issues regarding GERD, including extraesophageal manifestations and disease sequelae, will continue to evolve in the future, leading to progress in the treatment options for this common disorder. These issues include the following:

- The development of effective and safe prokinetic agents aimed at treating the pathophysiologic motor abnormalities underlying GERD and the development of new medication aimed at providing prompt and sustained improvement in symptoms associated with GERD, such as episodic heartburn
- Improvements in the understanding of the precise role and contribution of gastric contents to the development of noncardiac chest pain and tracheopulmonary symptoms attributed to GERD
- Improvement in the early detection of Barrett metaplasia, dysplasia, and early esophageal adenocarcinoma (including

chemoprevention) in patients with GERD. These improvements will include a better understanding of the cellular and molecular pathways that underlie metaplastic and neoplastic transformation and tumor progression, which will serve to provide additional targets for selective pharmacologic or immunologic forms of therapy.

- Technologic advances in the performance of both instrument and capsule endoscopic methods, including endoscopic spectrophotometry, for the diagnosis and treatment of Barrett esophagus–associated dysplasia and esophageal adenocarcinoma
- A better definition of the roles of surgical and endoscopic methods to treat GERD and its complications and the precise role of photodynamic therapy and other novel methods for the ablation of dysplastic and neoplastic mucosa

---

References

Baehr PH, McDonald GB: Esophageal infections: Risk factors, presentation, diagnosis, and treatment. Gastroenterology 106:509-532, 1994.

Barrison AF, Jarboe LA, Weinberg BM, et al: Patterns of proton pump inhibitor use in clinical practice. Am J Med 111:469-473, 2001.

Mittal RK, Balaban DH: The esophagogastric junction. N Engl J Med 336:924-932, 1997.

Shaheen N, Ransohoff DF: Gastroesophageal reflux, Barrett esophagus, and esophageal cancer: Scientific review. JAMA 287:1972-1981, 2002.

Shaker R, Castell DO, Schoenfeld PS, Spechler SJ: Nighttime heartburn is an under-appreciated clinical problem that impacts sleep and daytime function: The results of a Gallup survey conducted on behalf of the American Gastroenterological Association. Am J Gastroenterol 98:1487-1493, 2003.

Spechler SJ: Clinical practice: Barrett's esophagus. N Engl J Med 346:836-842, 2002.

Spechler SJ, Castell DO: Classification of oesophageal motility abnormalities. Gut 49:145-151, 2001.

Vakil N: Review article: New pharmacological agents for the treatment of gastro-oesophageal reflux disease. Aliment Pharmacol Ther 19:1041-1049, 2004.

Chapter 37

Diseases of the Stomach and Duodenum

Wanda P. Blanton, Jaime A. Oviedo, and M. Michael Wolfe

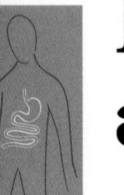

The stomach, a J-shaped dilation of the alimentary tract, acts as a reservoir for recently ingested food and initiates the process of digestion. By storing large quantities of food (1.5 to 2 L in the adult), the stomach allows intermittent feeding. Once solid particles have been reduced in size to accommodate the much smaller capacity of the duodenum, the gastric contents are released through the pylorus in a controlled fashion. This chapter focuses on the anatomy and physiology of the stomach and duodenum as well as on the most common disease processes that may involve these two organs.

Gastroduodenal Anatomy

The stomach is in continuity with the esophagus proximally and the duodenum distally. A circular smooth muscle structure, the *lower esophageal sphincter,* located at the distal end of the esophagus, creates a high-pressure zone that, under normal conditions, prevents gastric contents from refluxing into the esophagus. Similarly, the pyloric sphincter, the most distal portion of the stomach, plays an important role in the trituration of solid food particles and ensures the downstream propulsion of the food bolus, preventing duodenogastric reflux. The stomach is divided into four regions (Fig. 37-1; **Web Video 37-1**). The cardia is a poorly defined transition from the esophagogastric junction to the fundus. The dome-shaped fundus projects upward above the cardia and is the most superior part of the stomach in contact with the left hemidiaphragm and the spleen. The body, or corpus, located immediately below and continuous with the fundus, is the largest part of the stomach and is characterized by the presence of longitudinal folds known as rugae. The antrum extends from the incisura angularis, a fixed sharp indentation that marks the end of the gastric body, to the *pylorus,* or *pyloric channel,* a tubular structure that joins the stomach to the duodenum.

The mucosa, or inner lining of the stomach, is formed by a layer of columnar epithelium. The submucosa, immediately deep to the mucosa, provides a skeleton of dense connective tissue in which lymphocytes, plasma cells, arterioles, venules, lymphatics, and the myenteric plexus are contained. The third tissue layer, the muscularis propria, is a combination of an inner oblique, a middle circular, and an outer longitudinal smooth muscle layer. The serosa, a thin, transparent continuation of the visceral peritoneum, is the final layer of the stomach wall. The autonomic innervation of the stomach stems from both the sympathetic and parasympathetic nervous systems. The anterior and posterior trunks of the vagus nerve provide parasympathetic innervation, whereas the celiac plexus, coursing along the vascular supply of the stomach, provides sympathetic innervation.

The gastric mucosal surface is composed of a single layer of mucus-containing columnar epithelial cells. The surface lining is invaginated by gastric pits, which provide access to the gastric lumen for gastric glands. The gastric glands of different regions of the stomach are lined with different types of specialized cells. The oxyntic or acid-producing region of the stomach is found in the fundus and body, where gastric glands contain characteristic parietal cells, which secrete both acid and intrinsic factor. These glands also contain zymogen-rich chief cells, which synthesize pepsinogen, and enterochromaffin-like endocrine cells, which secrete histamine. Antral glands have different endocrine cells, including gastrin-secreting G cells and somatostatin-secreting D cells.

The duodenum, the most proximal portion of the small intestine, forms a C-shaped loop around the head of the pancreas and is in continuity with the pylorus proximally and the jejunum distally (see Fig. 37-1 and **Web Video 37-1**). Angular changes in course divide the duodenum into four portions. The first part of the duodenum is the duodenal bulb or cap and is characterized by a smooth, featureless luminal surface. The remainder of the duodenum has characteristic circular folds known as the *plica circularis* or *valvulae conniventes,* which increase the surface area available for digestion. Similar to the stomach, the duodenal wall is formed by mucosa, submucosa, muscularis, and serosa layers. The duodenal mucosa is lined with columnar cells forming villi surrounded by crypts of Lieberkühn. The

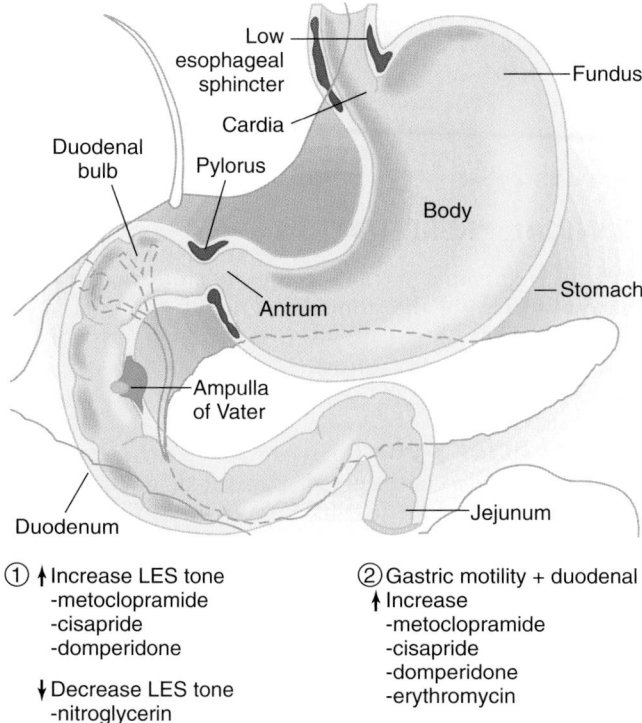

① ↑Increase LES tone
-metoclopramide
-cisapride
-domperidone

↓Decrease LES tone
-nitroglycerin
-calcium channel blockers
-progesterone
-theophylline
-benzodiazepines
-opioids
-chocolate
-coffee
-peppermint

② Gastric motility + duodenal
↑ Increase
-metoclopramide
-cisapride
-domperidone
-erythromycin

↓Decrease
-opioids
-anticholinergics
-hyperglycemia
-tricyclic antidepressants

Figure 37-1 Anatomic regions of the stomach and duodenum. Agents that affect lower esophageal sphincter (LES) tone and gastroduodenal motility.

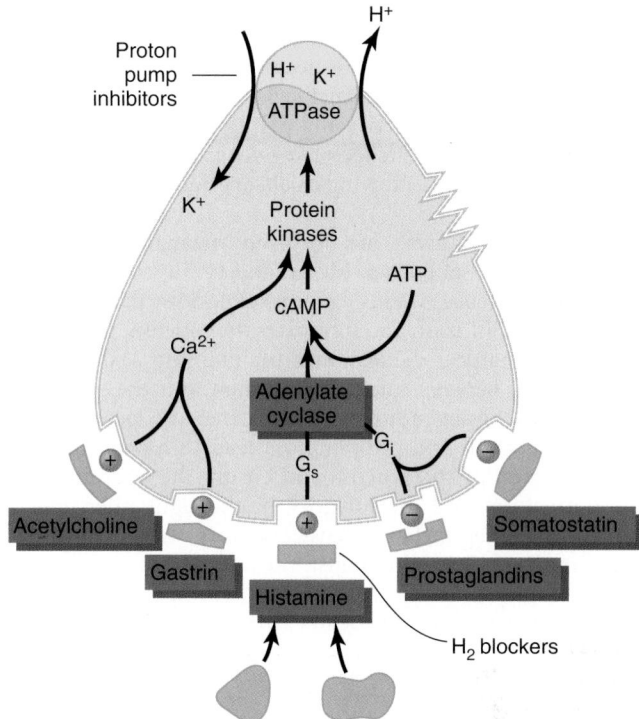

Figure 37-2 Schematic representation of acid secretion by the parietal cell. Each transmitter has a specific receptor located on the basolateral surface of the parietal cell. Stimulation of these receptors leads to activation of intracellular second messenger systems. Gastrin and acetylcholine promote the accumulation of intracellular calcium, whereas histamine causes a stimulatory G protein (G_s) to activate adenylate cyclase, which, in turn, generates cyclic adenosine monophosphate (cAMP). These intracellular messengers then activate protein kinases, which activate the proton pump (the H^+, K^+-ATPase enzyme), located at the apical surface of the parietal cell, to secrete H^+ ion in exchange for K^+ ions. Prostaglandins and somatostatin inhibit parietal cell function by binding to receptors that act through inhibitory G proteins (G_i) to inhibit adenylate cyclase. *Long arrows* indicate sites of action of various drugs that inhibit acid secretion. ECL, enterochromaffin-like endocrine cells.

submucosa includes characteristic Brunner glands that produce bicarbonate-rich secretions involved in acid neutralization. The innervation of the duodenum is also similar to that of the stomach.

Gastroduodenal Mucosal Secretions and Protective Factors

Although hydrochloric acid (HCl) is the primary gastric secretion, the stomach also secretes water, electrolytes (hydrogen [H^+], sodium [Na^+], potassium [K^+], chloride [Cl^-], and bicarbonate [HCO_3]), enzymes (pepsin and gastric lipase), and glycoproteins (intrinsic factors and mucin) to assist in a wide variety of physiologic functions. The digestion of proteins and triglycerides, as well as the complex process of vitamin B_{12} absorption, begins in the gastric lumen. Gastric acid also prevents the development of enteric colonization and systemic infections. The normal human stomach contains about 1 billion parietal cells that secrete H^+ ions into the gastric lumen in response to various physiologic stimuli. Parietal cells located in the oxyntic glands of the fundus and body of the stomach are stimulated

to secrete H^+ ions by three different pathways: neurocrine, paracrine, and endocrine (Fig. 37-2). The neurocrine pathway involves the vagal release of acetylcholine, which stimulates H^+ ion generation through a parietal cell muscarinic M_3 receptor. The paracrine pathway is mediated by the release of histamine from mast cells and enterochromaffin-like (ECL) cells in the stomach. Histamine binds to histamine-2 receptors on parietal cells, activating adenylate cyclase, which, in turn, leads to an increase in adenosine $3',5'$-cyclic monophosphate (cAMP) levels and subsequent generation of H^+ ions. The secretion of gastrin from antral G cells constitutes the endocrine pathway and stimulates H^+ ion generation both directly on the parietal cell and indirectly by stimulating histamine secretion from ECL cells. The hydrogen-potassium adenosine triphosphatase (H^+, K^+-ATPase) enzyme, or proton pump, located at the apical surface of the parietal cell, is the final step of acid secretion. A negative feedback loop governs both gastrin release and acid secretion, preventing postprandial acid hypersecretion. Somatostatin, produced by D cells in the gastric corpus and fundus, inhibits release of gastrin from G cells and may also reduce acid secretion from parietal cells and histamine release from ECL cells. Acid is necessary to convert pepsinogen, secreted from gastric chief cells, into pepsin, a proteolytic enzyme that is inactive at a pH greater than 4. Parietal cells also secrete intrinsic factor, a glycoprotein that binds to ingested vitamin B_{12}, allowing its absorption in the terminal ileum.

Several mechanisms are involved in maintaining the protective mucosal barrier. Mucus and HCO_3 constitute the first line of defense. Mucus forms a stable layer that prevents H^+ ion back-diffusion and lubricates the mucosa, protecting against mechanical damage and maintaining a significant pH gradient between the gastric lumen and the epithelial cell surface. Endogenous epithelial defensive factors, such as cell migration and proliferation, lead to a constant and rapid renewal of the mucosa and ensure the continuity of the epithelium and the integrity of the tight intercellular junctions. Subepithelial defensive factors such as an adequate mucosal blood flow constitute a second line of protection and play a crucial role in maintaining a normal pH environment and thereby the integrity of the gastroduodenal mucosa.

Gastroduodenal Motor Physiology

Based on electrophysiologic and functional characteristics, the stomach can be divided into two functional compartments. The proximal stomach (fundus and proximal third of the body) acts as a reservoir for recently ingested food, whereas the distal stomach grinds, mixes, and sieves food particles. The smooth muscle of the proximal stomach has a characteristic tonic contraction that allows for gastric accommodation, a process by which the fundus relaxes in response to incoming food and fluid, with little increase in intragastric pressure. In contrast, the distal stomach produces high-amplitude contractions originating from the pacemaker region in the midportion of the greater curvature.

Gastroduodenal motor events vary in response to fasting and food intake. During fasting, gastric motility is characterized by a pattern of phasic contractions known as the migrating motor complex (MMC). The MMC clears the stomach and small intestine of undigested food particles, mucus, and sloughed epithelial cells. The MMC begins in the stomach and migrates down the length of the small bowel with a combined duration of 84 to 112 minutes. Following a meal, irregular contractile activity propels the ingested material distally.

Gastric emptying of a mixed solid and liquid meal involves the coordinated actions of the distinct regions of the stomach with feedback from the small intestine. Although liquids empty from the stomach at a relatively linear rate, solids are propelled forward by gastric contractions toward the antrum, where particles are triturated by high-amplitude contractions. Once solids have been reduced in size to particles of 1 to 2 mm, they are emptied into the pylorus.

A variety of medications and foods that exert significant effects on gastroduodenal motility are described in Figure 37-1 (see Web Video 37-1). Agents that modify the lower esophageal sphincter and esophageal motility are explained in Chapter 36.

Gastritis

CLINICAL PRESENTATION

Gastritis represents a nonspecific inflammation of the mucosal surface of the stomach. Clinically, the three most common causes of gastritis are *Helicobacter pylori*, nonsteroidal anti-inflammatory drugs (NSAIDs), and stress-related mucosal changes.

Helicobacter pylori

Helicobacter pylori are curved, flagellated, gram-negative rods found only in gastric epithelium or in gastric metaplastic epithelium. It is the most common worldwide microbial infection, with an estimated 50% of the world's population being infected. *H. pylori* organisms clearly cause histologic gastritis and are found in 50% to 95% of patients with gastroduodenal ulcers. However, only a minority of patients with *H. pylori* gastritis develop peptic ulcer disease (PUD) or gastric cancer. In the Western world, a clear age-related prevalence of *H. pylori* infection exists in healthy individuals, increasing from 10% in those younger than 30 years to 60% in those older than 60 years, and the mode of transmission appears to be by the fecal-oral route. Improvements in sanitation and standards of living have been associated with a decline in the rate of infection. *H. pylori* colonization is more common in individuals in lower socioeconomic strata compared with other groups. In the developing world, infection is far more common, with more than 80% of the population being infected by age 20 years. *H. pylori* infection is typically lifelong, unless antimicrobial treatment is instituted.

H. pylori organisms reside in the mucus layer overlying gastric epithelium and are characterized as noninvasive organisms. Factors important in the organism's ability to colonize the stomach include its motility, production of urease, and bacterial adherence. Ammonia generated from urea by *H. pylori* urease neutralizes acid, creating a more hospitable microclimate in which the bacteria can survive. *H. pylori* also have the ability to bind specifically to gastric-type epithelium, which prevents the organisms from being shed during cell turnover and mucus secretion or gastric motility. Tissue injury is mediated by the production of lipopolysaccharide, leukocyte-activating factors, and CagA and VacA proteins, which have been associated with cytotoxic effects, inflammation, and cytokine activation. Colonization causes acute and chronic inflammation consisting of neutrophils, plasma cells, T cells, and macrophages accompanied by varying degrees of epithelial cell injury, all of which resolve after treatment.

Although predicting the ultimate outcome of *H. pylori* infection is impossible, the clinical manifestations can be correlated with various distributions of gastric histopathologic states. Antral-predominant *H. pylori* gastritis is associated with duodenal ulcers, whereas corporal and fundic colonizations are more likely to cause atrophic gastritis. Other important factors that may influence the outcomes of the infection include the host response, environmental factors, and age at the time of infection. Virtually all patients with *H. pylori* infection have a chronic superficial gastritis; however, duodenal and gastric ulcers develop in only 20% of infected patients. Patients with *H. pylori* infection and severe atrophic gastritis, corpus-predominant gastritis, or both, along with intestinal metaplasia, are at increased risk for intestinal-type gastric cancer. Finally, the mucosal lymphocytic response to *H. pylori* infection may lead to a monoclonal B-cell proliferation in mucosa-associated lymphoid tissue (MALT). MALT lymphomas, also known as *maltomas*, are rare, with about 1 in 1 million infected patients developing the disease. Complete histologic regression has been demonstrated in 50% to 80% of maltomas following eradication of *H. pylori*. Flat, localized, nonbulky lesions of the distal stomach are associated with greater rates of cure after antibiotic therapy.

Nonsteroidal Anti-inflammatory Drugs

NSAIDs are one of the most widely used classes of drugs. Although generally well tolerated, NSAIDs are associated with a small but significant percentage of adverse gastrointestinal (GI) events. Concepts about NSAID-induced gastroduodenal mucosal injury have evolved from a simple notion of topical injury to theories involving multiple mechanisms with both local and systemic effects. According to the dual-injury hypothesis, NSAIDs have direct toxic effects on the gastroduodenal mucosa and indirect effects through active hepatic metabolites and decreased synthesis of mucosal prostaglandins. Hepatic metabolites are excreted into the bile and subsequently into the duodenum, where they may cause mucosal damage to the stomach by duodenogastric reflux and to the small intestine by antegrade passage through the GI tract. Prostaglandin inhibition, in turn, leads to reduction in epithelial mucus, decreased secretion of HCO_3, impaired mucosal blood flow, reduced epithelial proliferation, and decreased mucosal resistance to injury. The impairment in mucosal resistance facilitates mucosal injury by endogenous factors, including acid, pepsin, and bile salts.

Prostaglandins are derived from arachidonic acid, which originates from cell membrane phospholipids through the action of phospholipase A_2. The metabolism of arachidonic acid to prostaglandins and leukotrienes is catalyzed by the cyclo-oxygenase (COX) pathway and the 5-lipoxygenase (LOX) pathway, respectively (Fig. 37-3). Two related but unique isoforms of COX, designated COX-1 and COX-2, have been demonstrated in mammalian cells. Despite their structural similarities, each is encoded by distinct genes that differ with regard to their distribution and expression in tissues; the COX-1 gene is primarily expressed constitutively, whereas the COX-2 gene is inducible. COX-1 appears to function as a housekeeping enzyme in most tissues, including the gastric mucosa, whereas the expression of COX-2 can be induced by inflammatory stimuli and mitogens in many different types of tissue. Theories have therefore suggested that the anti-inflammatory properties of NSAIDs are mediated through the inhibition of COX-2, whereas adverse effects, such as gastroduodenal ulceration, occur as a result of the effects on COX-1. The discovery of the two COX isoforms led to the development of COX-2–

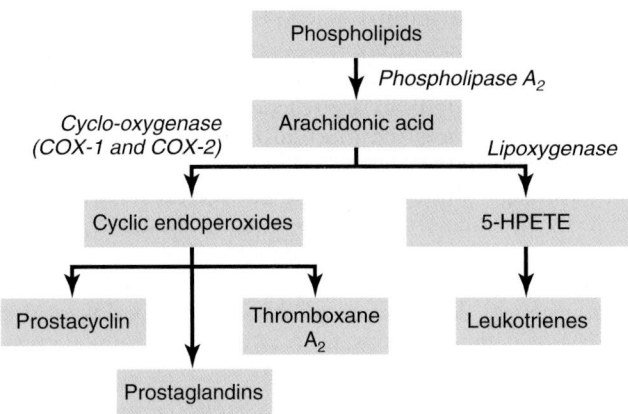

Figure 37-3 Biosynthesis of prostaglandins and leukotrienes through the cyclo-oxygenase and lipoxygenase pathways.

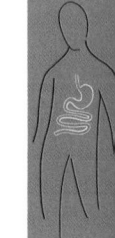

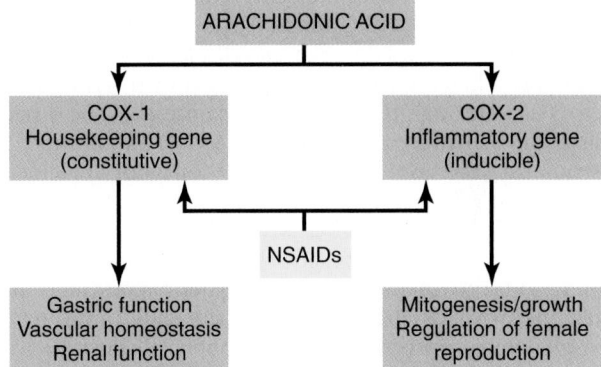

Figure 37-4 Depiction of the two cyclo-oxygenase (COX) isoenzymes that catalyze the synthesis of tissue prostaglandins from arachidonic acid.

specific inhibitors (e.g., celecoxib, rofecoxib, valdecoxib), drugs that maintain their anti-inflammatory properties while preserving the biosynthesis of protective prostaglandins (Fig 37-4).

The spectrum of NSAID-related mucosal injury includes a combination of subepithelial hemorrhages, erosions, and ulcerations that is often referred to as *NSAID gastropathy*. Erosions are likely to be small and superficial, whereas ulcers tend to be larger (more than 5 mm in diameter) and deeper. Although no area of the stomach is resistant to NSAID-induced mucosal injury, the most frequently and severely affected site is the antrum. Microscopically, a *reactive* pattern of injury can be found that is characterized by mucin depletion and little or no increase in inflammatory cells. Endoscopic studies have shown a prevalence of gastroduodenal ulcers of 10% to 25% in patients with chronic arthritis treated with NSAIDs, which is 5 to 15 times the expected prevalence in an age-matched healthy population.

Stress-Related Gastric Mucosal Damage

During critical illness, events such as shock, hypotension, and catecholamine release are associated with reduced blood flow and mucosal ischemia. When blood flow to the mucosa is inadequate, the normal mucosal protective mechanisms, including epithelial turnover and mucus and HCO_3 secretion, are altered. In addition, mediators such as cytokines and oxygen-free radicals are released. The combination of these events reduces the mucosal resistance to acid back-diffusion, causing erosions that may progress to ulceration and bleeding. Although mucosal damage develops in most critically ill patients, stress ulcers usually remain superficial and do not erode through the stomach wall to cause perforation. The major problem is blood loss, which is occult in most instances. Although occult stress ulcer bleeding occurs in 20% of patients in long-term intensive care units, gross hemorrhage occurs in only 5%.

TREATMENT

Aggressive volume resuscitation, control of sepsis, and adequate oxygenation in critically ill patients are important measures that may reduce the occurrence of low-flow states and subsequent mucosal damage. A wide variety of prophylactic strategies are used to prevent GI bleeding in critically ill patients. Pharmacologic agents used in this setting exert their effects through three main mechanisms: (1) acid neutralization, (2) mucosal protection, and (3) inhibition of gastric acid secretion. Acid neutralization with antacids is effective but requires administration every 1 to 2 hours through a nasogastric tube, which is inconvenient and increases nursing time. The side effects of magnesium-containing antacids include diarrhea, hypermagnesemia, and alkalemia, whereas aluminum-based antacids cause hypophosphatemia, constipation, and metabolic alkalosis, as well as potentially toxic plasma aluminum levels in patients with renal insufficiency. Mucosal protective agents such as sucralfate, an aluminum salt of sucrose sulfate, may improve mucosal blood flow through a prostaglandin-mediated mechanism. Sucralfate is well tolerated at doses of 1 g every 4 to 6 hours. Constipation occurs in 2% to 4% of patients, and aluminum toxicity has occurred in patients with chronic renal failure. Prostaglandin analogues (e.g., misoprostol) exert a protective effect on the gastric mucosa but have not been carefully studied for stress ulcer prophylaxis, and their use in this setting cannot be recommended. Antisecretory agents inhibit gastric acid secretion and are frequently used in the prevention of stress-induced mucosal damage in critically ill patients. Histamine-2 (H_2) receptor antagonists (e.g., cimetidine, ranitidine, famotidine, nizatidine), given either as a continuous infusion or by bolus injection, have been shown to reduce the incidence of clinically significant stress bleeding. An increase in intragastric pH to greater than 4 has been demonstrated with these agents; however, tolerance occurs rapidly and may limit their clinical efficacy. Although H_2 receptor antagonists are considered safe, they do possess both class-specific and individual side-effect potentials. The most prominent class-specific effect is central nervous system toxicity, which occurs more frequently in elderly patients compared with other age groups. Proton pump inhibitors (PPIs) irreversibly block parietal cell H^+,K^+-ATPase. These agents (e.g., omeprazole, lansoprazole, rabeprazole, pantoprazole, esomeprazole) are prokinetic agents that are normally activated following systemic absorption and localization to the highly acid milieu of the secretory canaliculus of *activated* parietal cells. Activation occurs after

Table 37-1 **Indications for Stress Bleeding Prophylaxis**
Coagulopathy
Respiratory failure
Central nervous system trauma
Burns
Organ transplantation
History of peptic ulcer disease with or without bleeding
Multiorgan failure
Trauma or major surgery

a meal, and because critically ill patients are generally fasting, PPIs administered orally or by nasogastric tube are significantly less active in this setting and are thus not recommended. However, in patients receiving enteral feeding, PPIs administered by the enteral route suppressed acid more effectively than intravenous PPIs. Pantoprazole, the first intravenous PPI available in the United States, has shown promising results in several small studies and may prove beneficial in stress bleeding prophylaxis. Intravenous preparations of lansoprazole and esomeprazole have recently become available.

Prophylaxis is recommended in patients with coagulopathy and in patients with respiratory failure requiring mechanical ventilation for more than 48 hours. Other patients in whom stress bleeding prophylaxis is indicated include those with central nervous system trauma, burns, organ transplantation, a history of PUD with or without bleeding, multiorgan failure, trauma, and major surgery (Table 37-1).

OTHER CAUSES OF GASTRITIS

Autoimmune atrophic gastritis exhibits an autosomal-dominant inheritance pattern and is associated with autoantibody formation. Histologically, autoimmune atrophic gastritis is characterized by chronic inflammation, gradual atrophy of glands, and loss of parietal cells. The process is usually confined to the corpus and fundus, where the gastric glands tend to undergo intestinal metaplasia. Loss of parietal cells results in achlorhydria, vitamin B_{12} deficiency, and megaloblastic anemia (pernicious anemia). These patients have an increased risk for carcinoma, especially in Scandinavian countries. No overall increased cancer risk has been documented in American patients, and routine surveillance has not been advocated in the United States.

Lymphocytic gastritis is characterized by a mononuclear infiltration of T cells, usually antral predominant, and is often associated with celiac disease, collagenous-lymphocytic colitis, and Ménétrier disease. Eosinophilic gastritis is characterized by an eosinophilic infiltration of the stomach, especially the antrum. All layers of the gastric wall may be affected, but selective predominance of eosinophilic infiltrates may be found in the submucosa, muscle layers, or subserosa, making biopsy diagnosis difficult. Clinical manifestations include delayed gastric emptying or manifestations of anemia from chronic blood loss caused by associated mucosal ulceration. Corticosteroids are used to control symptoms.

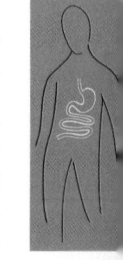

Ménétrier disease is a rare disease characterized by giant gastric folds in the fundus and the body of the stomach. Histologically, increased mucosal thickness, glandular atrophy, and an increase in the size of the gastric pits are characteristic findings. Hypochlorhydria and hypoalbuminemia are commonly seen. In children, Ménétrier disease is thought to be caused by cytomegalovirus (CMV), whereas overexpression of a tissue growth factor has been implicated in the adult form of the disease.

In addition to *H. pylori,* a variety of infectious pathogens may involve the stomach. Gastric infections are typically seen in patients who are immunocompromised in the settings of HIV infection, chemotherapy, and organ transplantation. Bacterial infections such as tuberculosis and syphilis rarely involve the stomach. CMV and herpesvirus infection, as well as fungal (e.g., *Candida,* histoplasmosis, mucormycosis, cryptococcosis, aspergillosis), and parasitic infections (e.g., *Cryptosporidium, Strongyloides*) are also possible. Other diseases such as sarcoidosis and Crohn disease may involve the stomach. The presence of granulomas on histologic specimens, along with systemic manifestations of the disease, confirms the diagnosis.

The stomach is occasionally involved by acute *graft-versus-host* disease. Gastric erosions or ulcers may be encountered in the investigation of bone marrow transplantation patients with abdominal pain or GI bleeding. Biopsy specimens should be obtained to rule out opportunistic infections (e.g., CMV).

Alcohol, drugs (e.g., cocaine, iron, potassium chloride), and physical agents (nasogastric tubes) are also associated with nonspecific forms of gastritis. Similarly, ischemia as a result of vascular injuries, embolization, vasculitis, and amyloidosis has been described as a cause of gastritis.

Peptic Ulcer Disease

Peptic ulcers are a common clinical problem characterized by mucosal defects of the GI mucosa of the stomach or the duodenum. The proteolytic enzyme pepsin and gastric acid were initially identified as the key factors involved in the pathogenesis of ulcers. Thus, the concept of *no acid, no ulcer* has been widely used and accepted for many years. However, in the past two decades, the roles of factors other than acid and pepsin in the development of ulcers have been recognized. Men and women are at equal risk for developing PUD, and the overall lifetime risk for both genders is 10%. Peptic ulcers are uncommon in children, but the risk increases with age. More than 70% of all ulcer cases occur in individuals between the ages of 25 and 64 years. However, whereas the incidence of PUD is decreasing in the young age groups, more persons 65 years and older are developing ulcers. These trends are likely related to the overall decrease in the prevalence of *H. pylori* infection and the increasing use of NSAIDs by the older population. The most important risk factors for the development of peptic ulcers are infection with *H. pylori* and use of NSAIDs. If neither of these factors is present, an alternative cause must be sought, such as hypersecretory states (e.g., Zollinger-Ellison syndrome [ZES]) or one of the other less common causes of ulcer disease, including Crohn disease, vascular insufficiency, viral infection, radiation therapy, and cancer chemotherapy.

Although a significant number of environmental factors, including stress, personality, occupation, alcohol consumption, and diet, have been linked to the development of ulcers, no convincing evidence suggesting that any of these factors by itself can cause PUD has been found.

PATHOPHYSIOLOGIC FACTORS

By killing ingested bacteria and other micro-organisms, gastric acid prevents the development of enteric colonization and ensures both efficient absorption of nutrients and prevention of systemic infections. Gastric acid is also an important factor in protein hydrolysis and digestion and, under various conditions, may play an etiologic role in inciting gastroduodenal mucosal injury. Postprandial gastric acid secretion is regulated primarily by increases in gastrin expression, which is controlled by a negative feedback loop wherein postprandial gastrin-mediated acid secretion stimulates the release of somatostatin from antral D cells. Somatostatin appears to act by a paracrine mechanism to inhibit further release of gastrin from G cells. Somatostatin produced by D cells in the gastric corpus and fundus may also directly inhibit acid secretion from parietal cells and may suppress histamine release from ECL cells. Although the presence of acid is necessary for ulcers to form, acid secretion is normal in nearly all patients with gastric ulcers and is increased in only one third of patients with duodenal ulcers. Therefore, acid is clearly not the only factor involved in the pathogenesis of peptic ulcers, and the balance between aggressive factors that act to injure the gastroduodenal mucosa and defensive factors that normally protect against corrosive agents is also important. When this delicate balance is disrupted for any reason, an ulcer may ensue.

In addition to the regulation of intragastric acidity, mechanisms involved in maintaining the protective mucosal barrier include mucus and HCO_3^- secretion, mucosal blood flow, cell restitution and repair, and changes in local immune factors. The mucosal defensive properties appear to be mediated to a large extent by endogenous prostaglandins, nitric oxide, and trefoil proteins. When the synthesis of any or all is diminished, the ability of the gastroduodenal mucosa to resist injury is reduced, and even normal rates of acid secretion may be sufficient to injure the mucosa. As stated previously, the pathogenesis of peptic ulcer is complex and involves an imbalance between defensive and aggressive factors. Individuals infected with *H. pylori* have been shown to have a diminished number of somatostatin-secreting D cells, which decreases the magnitude of the response to luminal acidification. Thus, in patients with *H. pylori* infection limited to the antrum, the negative inhibition of gastrin release is disrupted, resulting in higher postprandial gastrin levels and hypersecretion of acid. In addition, *H. pylori* organisms penetrate the mucous layer and adhere to surface epithelial cells by attaching to phospholipids and glycoproteins. Once attached, the bacteria synthesize and release phospholipases and proteases that are harmful to the mucous layers and the underlying cells. Interleukin-8 and other cytokines that contribute to mucosal injury are subsequently released from the gastric epithelium. About 65% of *H. pylori* isolates produce a vacuolating toxin. Toxin-producing strains may be more pathogenic than those that do not produce toxins, and their presence correlates with a more

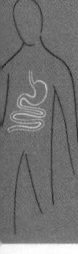

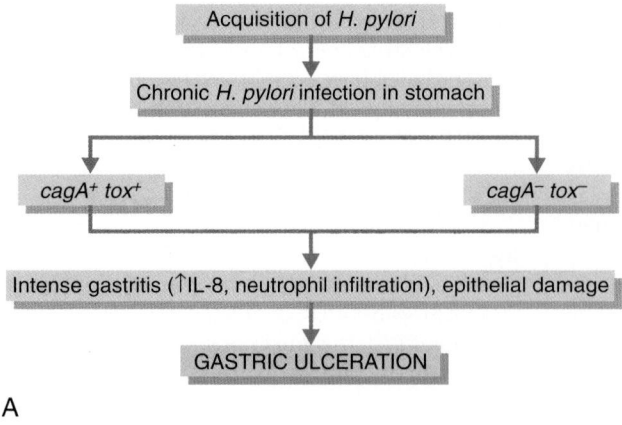

A

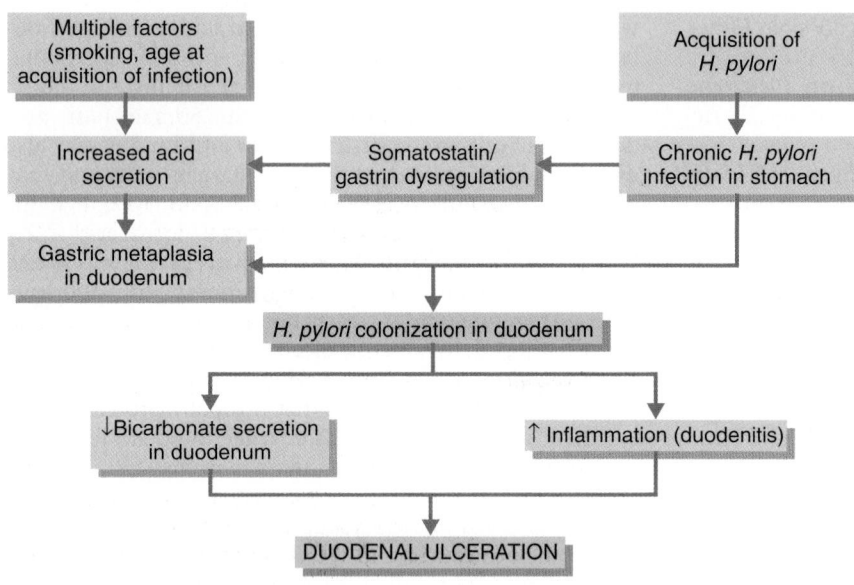

B

Figure 37-5 Mechanisms by which *Helicobacter pylori* may cause gastric ulcers (**A**) and duodenal ulcers (**B**). IL-8, interleukin-8. (From Peek RM, Blaser MJ: Pathophysiology of *Helicobacter pylori*-induced gastritis and peptic ulcer disease. Am J Med 102:200-207, 1997.)

intense polymorphonuclear cell infiltration. A cytotoxin-associated gene *(cagA)* has been found to be a marker for strains that make the vacuolating toxin. Patients infected with *cagA*-positive strains are more likely to develop ulcers (Fig. 37-5).

Although a large number of gastroduodenal ulcers are associated with *H. pylori* infection, at least 60% of individuals with complicated ulcers (e.g., hemorrhage, perforation) report the use of NSAIDs, including aspirin. Topical injury caused by NSAIDs certainly contributes significantly to the development of gastroduodenal mucosal injury. However, the systemic effects of these agents appear to play the predominant role, largely through the decreased synthesis of mucosal prostaglandins. NSAID-induced ulceration occurs with all traditional NSAIDs, regardless of enteric coating or delivery as a prodrug formulation. The risk for NSAID-induced ulceration and complications is dose related and increases with age older than 60 years, concurrent corticosteroid use, increasing duration and dose of therapy, anticoagulant therapy, and a history of prior ulcer disease.

ZES, produced by gastrin-secreting tumors, accounts for 0.1% of patients who have PUD and should be considered in patients with ulcers in unusual sites (e.g., distal duodenum, jejunum); multiple, recurrent, or complicated duodenal ulcers; or ulcers associated with chronic diarrhea.

CLINICAL PRESENTATION

Peptic ulcers can exhibit in a variety of forms ranging from asymptomatic iron deficiency anemia to abdominal pain, obstruction, perforation, and hemorrhage. Symptoms may mimic those of other diseases, including cholecystitis, pancreatitis, gastric cancer, and gastroesophageal reflux. Myocardial ischemia or infarction, especially of the inferior wall, can cause abdominal pain that resembles peptic ulcer. Abdominal pain is generally epigastric and is usually described as a dull ache but may be sharp or burning. Less than 20% of patients report the hunger-like pain traditionally associated with both gastric and duodenal ulcers. Similarly, the character of the symptoms and their relation with meals, specifically pain relief after food intake for duodenal ulcer and pain worsening for gastric ulcer, do not always correlate with endoscopic diagnosis and are less useful in predicting ulcer location. Nocturnal pain and pain relief with milk or antacids are common with duodenal ulcers but can also occur with gastric ulcers. NSAID-associated ulcers typically produce painless bleeding. Nausea and vomiting are commonly associated with peptic ulcers, being slightly more common with gastric ulcers. Gastric outlet obstruction may be caused by antropyloric or duodenal ulcers but should be differentiated from malignant obstruction resulting from gastric or pancreatic cancer. Weight loss, although suggestive of malignancy, is frequently reported by patients with peptic ulcers.

DIAGNOSIS

Because the clinical features of gastroduodenal ulcers may overlap with other disorders, and the physical examination is often not helpful in the diagnosis, imaging studies of the GI tract are required to confirm the presence of peptic ulcers. Although contrast radiology (barium upper GI series) can be used, endoscopy is usually preferred because, in addition to characterizing the ulcer, it allows tissue sampling to exclude malignancy, assessment of *H. pylori* infection, and, in cases of acute ulcer hemorrhage, delivery of endoscopic therapy for the control of hemorrhage.

DIAGNOSTIC TESTS FOR *HELICOBACTER PYLORI*

The fact that the eradication of *H. pylori* infection is associated with a significant reduction in ulcer recurrence is now recognized. *H. pylori* testing is thus essential in all patients with PUD. Diagnostic tests for detecting *H. pylori* infection and the indications for their use are summarized in Figure 37-6. Immunoglobulin G serologic testing is the noninvasive test of choice for diagnosing *H. pylori* infection in the untreated patient. However, because the antibodies may persist for several years, serologic analysis is not useful as a means to document cure of the infection. Positive results of antibody testing may thus indicate past exposure but not necessarily current infection with *H. pylori*. Another noninvasive mean of detecting *H. pylori* is the ^{13}C- or ^{14}C-labeled urea breath test. When present, *H. pylori* urease splits the urea, which may be detected as labeled carbon dioxide in the breath of a patient. The urea breath test is more accurate than serologic tests, and although more expensive and less widely available, it is the noninvasive test of choice to document successful *H. pylori* eradication after antibiotic therapy. Patients should not receive PPIs for at least 14 days before administration of breath tests to avoid false-negative results. Stool antigen testing is also available and useful in the initial diagnosis of *H. pylori* infection. If endoscopic examination is performed, the diagnosis is made by the rapid urease test or histologic testing. In the rapid urease test, mucosal biopsies are placed in a urea-containing medium with a pH-sensitive indicator that changes color when ammonia is produced from urea by the urease of the organism. The rapid urease test has high sensitivity and specificity equivalent to histologic analysis and is inexpensive. Recent treatment with antibiotics or PPIs may decrease the yield of the test. Histo-

logic analysis is frequently the standard for detecting *H. pylori* infection and can establish the degree, type, and location of inflammation. Gastric biopsy specimens should be taken from both the antrum and the corpus because the bacteria are not uniformly distributed throughout the stomach. The presence of chronic active gastritis is strongly suggestive of *H. pylori* infection, even if bacteria are difficult to identify.

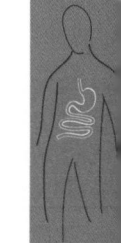

Complications of Peptic Ulcer Disease

BLEEDING

PUD is the leading cause of upper GI bleeding, accounting for about 50% of instances and more than 150,000 hospital admissions annually in the United States. Although bleeding ceases spontaneously in 80% of patients, the mortality rate associated with bleeding ulcers is 5% to 10%. Patients with bleeding ulcers exhibit hematemesis, melena, or hematochezia, often without abdominal pain. The major risk factor for bleeding ulcers is NSAID use. Predictors for an adverse outcome include hemodynamic instability at presentation, bright red blood from the rectum or through the nasogastric tube, age older than 60 years, ongoing transfusion requirements, and an increasing number of underlying medical illnesses. All patients with upper GI bleeding should undergo early upper endoscopic examination, which allows for both therapeutic intervention and the determination of other predictors for rebleeding. Rebleeding rates are about 5% for clean-based ulcers, 10% for ulcers with flat spots, 22% for adherent clots, 43% for nonbleeding visible vessels, and 55% for active oozing or spurting from an ulcer (Fig. 37-7). Patients with large ulcers, greater than 1 to 2 cm in diameter, also have increased rebleeding and mortality rates. Endoscopic therapy with techniques such as multipolar or thermal coagulation or injection with epinephrine clearly improves the outcome in patients with bleeding ulcers by decreasing mortality, length of hospital stay, number of blood transfusions, and need for emergency surgery.

Because most ulcer bleeding recurs within 3 days of initial presentation, patients with active bleeding or stigmata of hemorrhage, such as raised pigmented spots in an ulcer crater or clot, can be discharged within 2 to 3 days if they are stable. Given the excellent prognosis for patients with clean-based ulcers, discharge within 24 hours of presentation or immediately after endoscopic examination appears to be safe. About 20% of patients rebleed after endoscopic therapy, and 50% of these can be successfully retreated. The remainder may be treated angiographically with either intra-arterial vasopressin or embolization techniques. Surgery is generally reserved for instances in which all other measures have failed. Although endoscopic therapy is the first treatment modality in the management of actively bleeding gastroduodenal ulcers, some evidence also suggests that adjuvant use of acid suppression therapy can reduce recurrent bleeding after initial endoscopic control. A continuous infusion of intravenous omeprazole has been shown to reduce the incidence of recurrent ulcer hemorrhage following endoscopic therapy. Thus, patients with significant

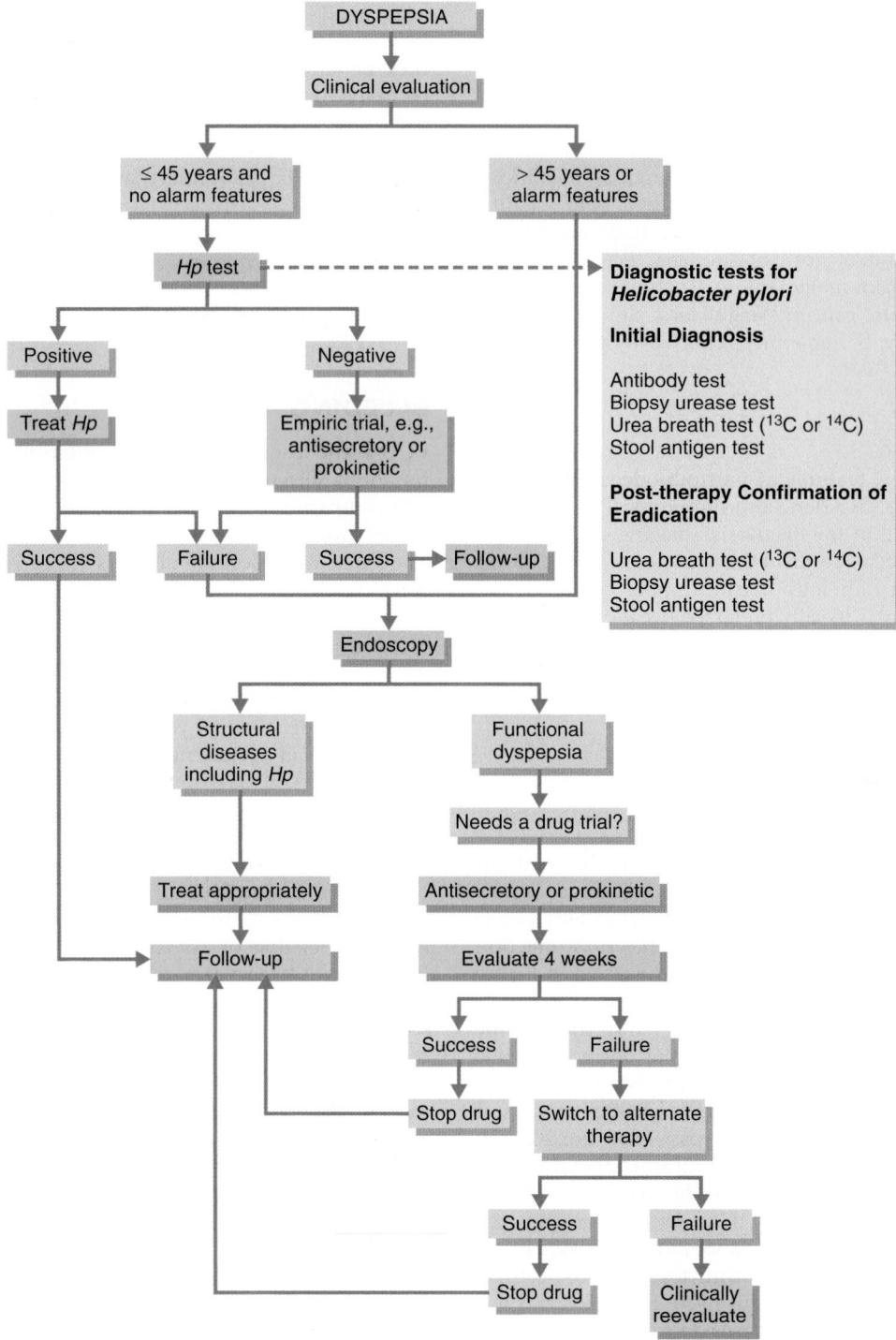

Figure 37-6 Diagnostic approach to patients presenting with uninvestigated dyspepsia. Alarm features include weight loss, vomiting, dysphagia, evidence of anemia, gastrointestinal bleeding, or an abdominal mass or lymphadenopathy. *Hp, Helicobacter pylori.* (Modified from American Gastroenterological Association medical position statement: Evaluation of dyspepsia. [No authors listed]. Gastroenterology 114:579-581, 1998.)

upper GI bleeding in whom a peptic ulcer is suggested should be treated with an intravenous PPI using a loading dose (80 mg of pantoprazole) followed by a continuous infusion (8 mg per hour of pantoprazole). If at the time of endoscopic examination, no evidence of recent or active bleeding can be found, and after feeding has been initiated, oral administration can be substituted for the parenteral route.

PERFORATION

Perforation, which occurs when a peptic ulcer erodes through the full thickness of the stomach or duodenum, is a far less common complication than bleeding. Ulcer perforation usually leads to peritonitis, which, if untreated, may result in sepsis and death. Patients exhibit sudden onset of

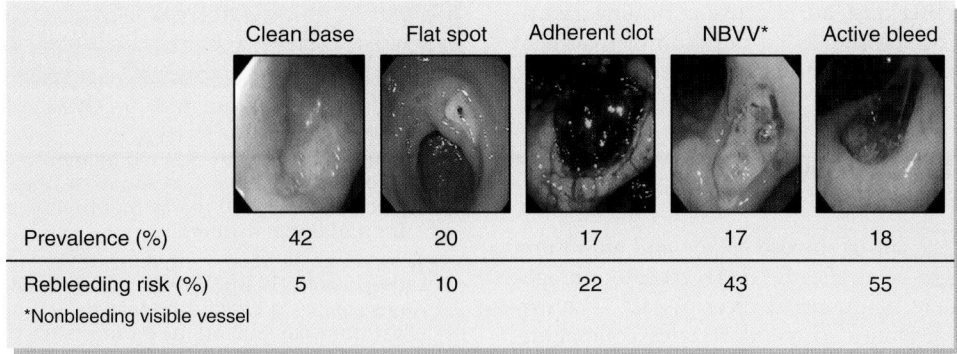

	Clean base	Flat spot	Adherent clot	NBVV*	Active bleed
Prevalence (%)	42	20	17	17	18
Rebleeding risk (%)	5	10	22	43	55

*Nonbleeding visible vessel

Figure 37-7 Endoscopic classification of peptic ulcers with prevalence and risk of rebleeding. (From Laine L, Peterson WL: Medical progress: Bleeding peptic ulcer. N Engl J Med 331:717-727, 1994.)

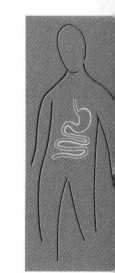

severe abdominal pain that typically begins in the epigastrium and radiates throughout the entire abdomen. When peritonitis has occurred, physical examination is remarkable for abdominal pain, guarding, rebound tenderness, and boardlike rigidity. The clinical suggestion of perforation may be confirmed in most cases by the presence of free intra-abdominal air (pneumoperitoneum) with either an upright chest radiograph or upright and supine abdominal radiographs. In less obvious instances, computed tomography (CT) or an upper GI water-soluble contrast study may be helpful. Perforation mandates surgical intervention. A perforated duodenal ulcer is typically repaired with an omental patch, whereas a perforated gastric ulcer necessitates either an omental patch or a resection.

GASTRIC OUTLET OBSTRUCTION

In the era before acid suppression and *H. pylori*, PUD accounted for 60% of the cases of gastric outlet obstruction. More recently, the incidence of both ulcers and obstruction requiring surgery has declined, and estimates indicate that fewer than 5% of patients with duodenal ulcer and less than 1% to 2% with gastric ulcer develop significant gastric outlet obstruction. Gastric outlet obstruction is typically caused by either pyloric channel or duodenal ulcers and may be seen in the setting of acute ulceration, in which edema, spasm, and inflammation lead to obstruction, or as a consequence of chronic ulceration with scarring and fibrosis. Patients usually exhibit symptoms of early satiety, bloating, nausea, vomiting, and weight loss. Endoscopy is the diagnostic test of choice but is frequently obscured by the presence of retained food residue. Patients in whom gastric outlet obstruction is suggested should undergo gastric decompression and lavage to remove retained gastric contents before endoscopic examination. Malignancy may now account for 50% of instances of gastric outlet obstruction and should be excluded with adequate biopsy and cytology samples. Occasionally, imaging techniques such as barium upper GI series and radionuclide gastric-emptying scans can also be used to determine the length of the obstructed area and to evaluate gastric emptying. In addition to the correction of fluid, electrolyte, and pH imbalances resulting from persistent vomiting, patients with gastric outlet obstruction should undergo nasogastric decompression for 3 to 5 days. During that time, acid suppression with an intravenous H₂ receptor antagonist or PPI should also be instituted. Adequacy of response may

be assessed empirically with a trial of refeeding. For patients failing to respond to medical therapy, treatment options include endoscopic balloon dilation and surgery.

Treatment of Peptic Ulcer Disease

HEALING ULCERS BY SUPPRESSING ACID SECRETION

Regardless of the cause, the inhibition of gastric acid secretion continues to be the cornerstone of therapy for PUD. Antacids are effective agents for healing ulcers and may provide some symptom relief. However, because of the need to take these drugs at least 4 times, and up to 7 times, every day, and the frequency of associated adverse effects, antacids are now rarely used in the healing of gastroduodenal ulcers.

H₂ receptor antagonists reduce acid secretion by competitively and selectively inhibiting the histamine receptor on the parietal cell. H₂ receptor antagonists increase intragastric pH and inhibit pepsin activity. In general, H₂ receptor antagonists are safe and well tolerated, although the occurrence of adverse effects is slightly increased with cimetidine because of binding to cytochrome P-450 and hence increased risk for drug interactions. H₂ receptor antagonists heal 90% to 95% of duodenal ulcers and 88% of gastric ulcers after 8 weeks. Given as a single full dose at bedtime, cimetidine (800 mg), ranitidine and nizatidine (300 mg), and famotidine (40 mg) have comparable efficacies for ulcer healing. The recommended duration of treatment is 4 weeks for duodenal ulcers and 8 weeks for gastric ulcers.

PPIs, the most potent inhibitors of gastric acid secretion available, heal gastroduodenal ulcers more rapidly than H₂ receptor antagonists. However, because they are most effective when the parietal cell is stimulated to secrete acid in response to a meal, PPIs should only be taken before a meal and should not be used in conjunction with H₂ receptor antagonists or other antisecretory agents. Moreover, because acid secretion must be stimulated for maximal efficacy, PPIs are administered before the first meal of the day. These agents are safe and well tolerated; adverse effects are unusual and include headache, diarrhea, and nausea. Single daily doses of omeprazole (20 mg), pantoprazole (40 mg), rabeprazole (20 mg), lansoprazole (30 mg), or esomeprazole

(40 mg), all before breakfast, are effective in healing gastroduodenal ulcers. The recommended duration of treatment is again 4 weeks for duodenal ulcers and 8 weeks for gastric ulcers.

HEALING BY ENHANCING MUCOSAL DEFENSE

Sucralfate, a complex salt of sucrose sulfate and aluminum hydroxide, appears to be as effective as H_2 receptor antagonists in the treatment of duodenal ulcer disease. The evidence for efficacy in healing of gastric ulcers is less compelling. Sucralfate has little or no effect on acid secretion and acts through several different mucosal protective mechanisms. In the gastroduodenal lumen, sucralfate becomes a gel-like substance that binds to both defective and normal mucosa, acting as a physical barrier to the diffusion of acid, pepsin, and bile acids. The recommended dose is 1 g 4 times daily, which makes it less convenient than other agents for treating PUD.

Although bismuth compounds and prostaglandin analogues have been shown to provide protective effects on the gastroduodenal mucosa and may have some effect on ulcer healing, these agents are not routinely used in the initial treatment of peptic ulcers.

TREATMENT OF *HELICOBACTER PYLORI* INFECTION

Eradication of *H. pylori* should be attempted in all patients with documented current or past PUD and evidence of infection. The various niches of *H. pylori* within the gastric mucosa provide a challenge for antimicrobial therapy. Successful therapy requires a combination of drugs that prevents the emergence of resistance and effectively reaches the bacteria. Therapy must be of sufficient duration to ensure that a small population of bacteria does not remain viable. Combinations of two antibiotics, plus either a PPI or ranitidine bismuth citrate, are used to maximize the chance of eradication. Current treatment regimens for *H. pylori* are shown in Table 37-2. Factors such as antibiotic resistance and noncompliance with therapy have been identified as predictors of treatment failure. Metronidazole resistance is most common, and both metronidazole and clarithromycin resistance are increasing in frequency, with rates of 37% and 10%, respectively. Because compliance is essential for treatment success, the current regimens offer simpler dosing than earlier options. A failed initial course of antibiotic therapy suggests antibiotic resistance, and it may be assumed that, if the patient received metronidazole or clarithromycin in the original regimen, resistance to that antibiotic is present. When possible, repeat use of the same antibiotic should be avoided. The recommended duration for repeat treatment courses is 14 days. An alternative initial approach involves a shorter, 10-day treatment course with PPI and sequential dosing of amoxicillin and clarithromycin, but further validation studies are needed before recommendation.

MAINTENANCE THERAPY

Before embarking on long-term maintenance therapy for PUD, careful attention must be paid to eliminating the most

---

Table 37-2 **Treatment Regimens for *Helicobacter pylori* Infection**

Triple therapy (cure rate, 85% to >90%)
BMT triple therapy for 14 days
  Bismuth subsalicylate, 524 mg by mouth 4 times daily
  Metronidazole, 250 mg by mouth 4 times daily
  Tetracycline HCl, 500 mg by mouth 4 times daily + H_2-RA
    for additional 4 weeks
LAC for 10 or 14 days
  Lansoprazole, 30 mg by mouth twice daily
  Amoxicillin, 1 g by mouth twice daily
  Clarithromycin, 500 mg by mouth twice daily
OAC for 10 or 14 days
  Omeprazole, 20 mg by mouth twice daily
  Amoxicillin, 1 g by mouth two times daily
  Clarithromycin, 500 mg by mouth twice daily
RBC-AC (cure rate, >90%)
  Ranitidine bismuth citrate + amoxicillin + clarithromycin
MOC (cure rate, >90% in the absence of metronidazole
  resistance)
  Metronidazole + omeprazole + clarithromycin

H_2-RA, histamine-2 receptor antagonist; HCl, hydrochloric acid.

---

important risk factors for ulcer recurrence: *H. pylori* infection and NSAID use. Moreover, hypersecretory states, including gastrinoma, should be excluded before considering maintenance therapy in individuals with recurrent ulcers without *H. pylori* infection. Patients with a history of ulcer complications, frequent ulcer recurrence, continued NSAID use, or *H. pylori*–negative ulcers, and those who fail to clear *H. pylori* infection despite appropriate therapy, should be considered candidates for maintenance antisecretory therapy. However, even patients who have had a complicated ulcer may not require maintenance therapy, provided *H. pylori* infection is cured. Maintenance regimens include an H_2 receptor antagonist at bedtime at one half the dose required for initial healing or a PPI taken before breakfast.

TREATMENT AND PROPHYLAXIS OF NSAID-INDUCED ULCERATION

The optimal treatment in patients with NSAID-induced gastroduodenal ulcers is the discontinuation of the offending agent. If NSAIDs must be continued, therapy with an antisecretory agent should be instituted. Based on their superior safety profile and their ability to heal gastroduodenal ulcers at an accelerated rate whether or not NSAID use is continued, PPIs are preferred over both H_2 receptor antagonists and misoprostol in the treatment of NSAID-associated gastroduodenal ulcers.

Because of the significant rate of serious complications associated with NSAIDs and the poor correlation of dyspeptic symptoms (e.g., abdominal pain, distention, nausea, heartburn) with the presence of gastroduodenal mucosal injury, prevention of ulceration has become the principal goal in the management of NSAID-related GI toxicity. Risk factors for NSAID-related injury have been identified and include advanced age (>60 years), prior history of PUD or ulcer hemorrhage, concomitant use of anticoagulants or corticosteroids, significant comorbid conditions, and use of high NSAID doses (Table 37-3). Two strategies have been used to prevent ulcers: (1) the concomitant use of

Table 37-3 **Risk Factors for Development of NSAID-Related Ulcers**
Definite
Advanced age
History of ulcer
Concomitant corticosteroid therapy
Concomitant anticoagulation therapy
High doses of NSAIDs
Serious systemic disorders
Possible
Concomitant infection with *Helicobacter pylori*
Cigarette smoking
Consumption of alcohol
NSAIDs, nonsteroidal anti-inflammatory drugs.

medications such as misoprostol or PPIs, and (2) the development of safer anti-inflammatory agents, such as COX-2–specific inhibitors. Misoprostol, a prostaglandin E_1 analogue, significantly reduces the development of both gastric and duodenal ulcers in patients using NSAIDs. By augmenting prostaglandin-dependent pathways, misoprostol reduces gastric acid secretion and enhances mucosal defenses. However, misoprostol is associated with significant adverse effects and a high frequency of therapy discontinuation as a result of these effects, especially when administered 4 times a day. The most frequent symptom is diarrhea, although symptoms such as abdominal pain, nausea, and bloating may also occur. A lower dose of misoprostol (200 mcg 3 times daily) is nearly as effective as 4 times daily dosing for preventing duodenal and gastric ulcers, with a slight reduction in the occurrence of adverse effects.

The second strategy to prevent NSAID-induced ulcers involves the co-administration of an antisecretory agent, usually a PPI, or the substitution of the traditional NSAID with one of the newer COX-2–specific inhibitors.

According to available evidence from clinical trials, PPIs are superior to H_2 receptor antagonists in preventing gastroduodenal ulceration as well as in improving dyspeptic symptoms during continued NSAID use. Similarly, PPIs provide protection against endoscopic NSAID ulcers at a rate at least comparable with that of misoprostol, with fewer associated GI symptoms. However, misoprostol, but not PPIs, has been shown in a prospective analysis to decrease the prevalence of ulcer complications.

COX-2–specific inhibitors (e.g., celecoxib, rofecoxib, valdecoxib) have shown an improved GI safety profile with reduced incidence of ulcers and ulcer complications and at least similar effectiveness when compared with traditional NSAIDs.

However, recent evidence suggesting an increased risk for cardiovascular events, specifically myocardial infarctions and strokes, associated with the use of selective COX-2 inhibitors, has led to significant public concern with subsequent market withdrawal of some of these agents and restricted use of others. These adverse effects are thought to be related, at least in part, to the inhibition of prostacyclin with the resultant unopposed *thrombogenic* effects of thromboxane A_2. Recommendations for use of nonselective NSAID versus COX-2 inhibitor and use of either PPI or misoprostol involve risk stratification of the patient's cardiovascular risk and GI risk by the clinician.

More recent meta-analysis demonstrated that concomitant *H. pylori* infection and NSAID use double the risk for ulcer complications. Therefore, in patients who require chronic NSAID use, the current recommendation is to test for and eradicate *H. pylori*, given that it is a treatable risk factor.

SURGERY

Because of the remarkable progress in pharmacologic acid suppression therapy and the recognition that ulcer disease can be cured by eliminating *H. pylori* infection and NSAIDs, surgery now plays a marginal role in treating uncomplicated PUD. Surgical intervention is now mostly reserved for managing the complications of peptic ulcers, especially gastric outlet obstruction and perforation. Some of the different surgical approaches are shown in Figure 37-8.

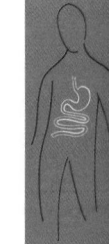

NONULCER DYSPEPSIA

Dyspepsia, a classic symptom of PUD, is a common clinical problem and may be seen in 25% to 40% of adults. However, only 15% to 25% of patients with dyspepsia are found to have a gastric or duodenal ulcer. The remainder of patients have nonulcer or functional dyspepsia, a condition most likely related to an abnormal perception of events in the stomach caused by afferent visceral hypersensitivity. Recent evidence suggests that about 40% of patients with nonulcer dyspepsia (NUD) have impairment in the fundic accommodation response of the stomach. Dyspeptic symptoms may be chronic, recurrent, or of new onset. The diagnostic work-up should focus on excluding other causes of dyspepsia such as gastroparesis and gastric cancer.

MANAGEMENT

Three possible strategies for managing patients with NUD have been formulated (see Fig. 37-6). Immediate endoscopic evaluation is indicated for individuals older than 45 years and persons exhibiting alarm features (*red flags*) such as weight loss, recurrent vomiting, dysphagia, GI bleeding, anemia, a strong family history of GI cancer, or an abdominal mass. Urgent endoscopic examination is indicated to exclude a serious underlying disease process, particularly gastric and esophageal carcinoma. If a gastric ulcer is found during endoscopic examination, multiple biopsies and cytologic analysis should be obtained to exclude malignancy. Ulcer treatment is subsequently employed, and ulcer healing should be confirmed with a follow-up endoscopic examination because nonhealing ulcers can occasionally be a manifestation of gastric carcinoma. Barium radiography offers poor sensitivity and specificity and is thus no longer recommended in the evaluation of dyspepsia.

The second option when treating patients younger than 45 years with NUD but without alarm features is an empirical trial of antisecretory therapy for 1 to 2 months. Endoscopy is indicated in patients who fail to respond to this regimen. Avoiding the introduction of long-term drug use in this situation is important, particularly because of the considerable benefit of placebo in such individuals.

The third strategy for managing NUD involves initial noninvasive testing for *H. pylori* followed by antimicrobial

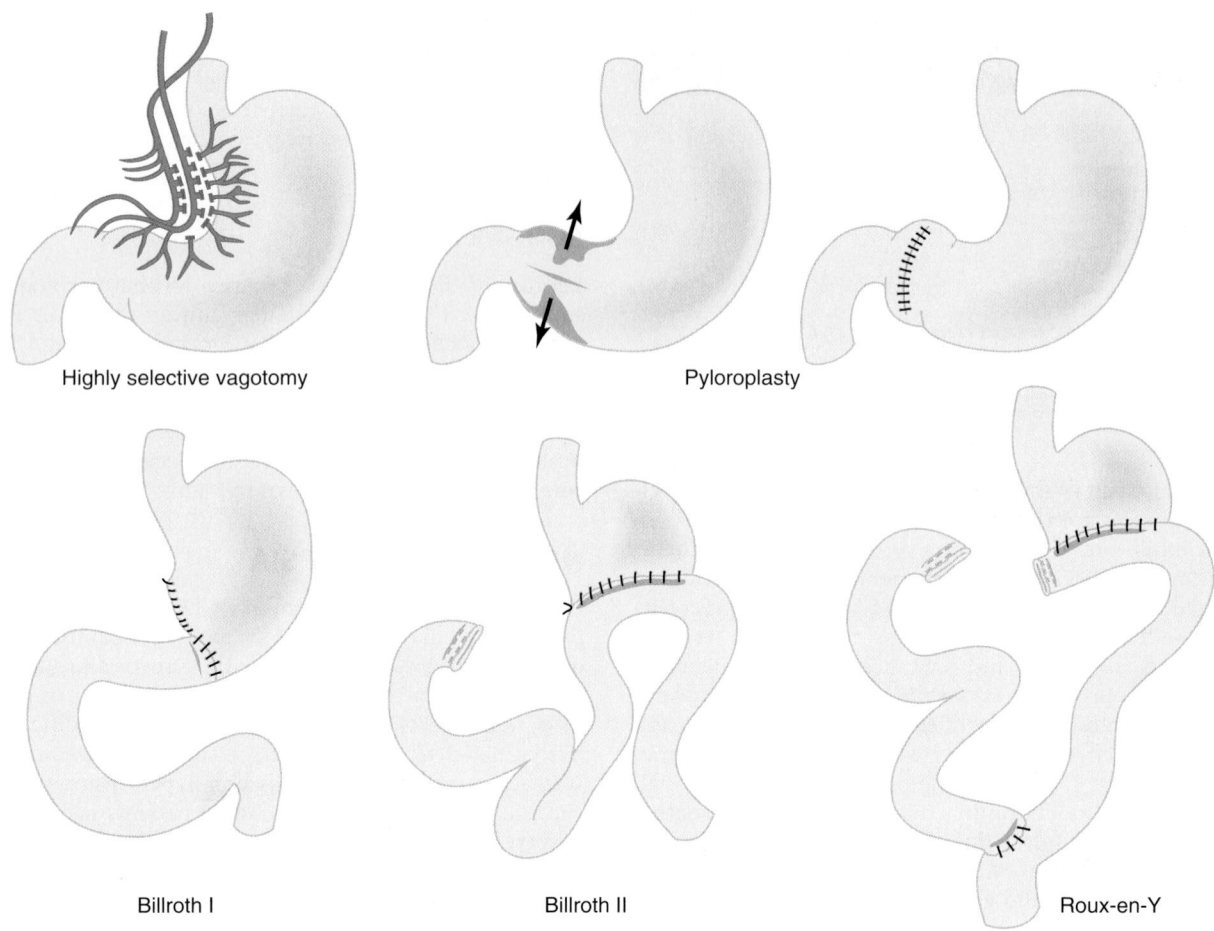

Highly selective vagotomy   Pyloroplasty

Billroth I   Billroth II   Roux-en-Y

Figure 37-8 Operations for peptic ulcer disease.

therapy in patients with positive tests. This strategy is presumed to heal ulcers if present, eliminate the ulcer diathesis, and save on resources, particularly in patients younger than 45 years without alarm symptoms. The frequency of *H. pylori* infection in the community should also be taken into account because noninvasive tests show decreased accuracy when the prevalence of *H. pylori* is less than 10%. This approach, although advocated by some physicians, has not been proved effective in relieving NUD. Moreover, indiscriminate use of antimicrobial therapy may be associated with altering normal intestinal flora, increasing resistance of *H. pylori* and other bacteria that are not a target of therapy, and producing a series of adverse events such as antibiotic-associated and *Clostridium difficile* colitis.

Zollinger-Ellison Syndrome

ZES is characterized by elevated levels of serum gastrin produced by gastrin-secreting tumors that are most often located in the pancreas and duodenum. Hypergastrinemia stimulates hypersecretion of gastric acid and pepsin, which may produce peptic ulcers, duodenojejunitis, esophagitis, and diarrhea. ZES is an uncommon cause of PUD, accounting for less than 1% of the instances. The gastrin-secreting

tumor in ZES, referred to as a *gastrinoma*, is frequently located in the *gastrinoma triangle*, an area encompassed by the second and third portions of the duodenum, the junction of the head and neck of the pancreas, and the cystic duct. Seventy-five percent of all gastrinomas are sporadic; the remaining 25% are part of the type I multiple endocrine neoplasia (MEN-I) syndrome, an autosomal-dominant condition with a locus on chromosome 11, typically associated with hyperparathyroidism and pituitary tumors. All patients with sporadic gastrinomas without evidence of liver metastases should be surgically explored with the intent of removing local and regional disease. Unfortunately, despite careful diagnostic testing, no tumor is found in at least 10% of diagnosed instances of ZES.

ZES should be anticipated in patients with recurrent PUD in the absence of *H. pylori* infection or NSAID use, as well as in patients with multiple duodenal ulcers, ulcers in unusual locations (distal duodenum or jejunum), or severe or refractory diarrhea or gastroesophageal reflux disease. Although peptic ulcer occurs in more than 90% of patients with ZES, as many as 35% of individuals exhibit only diarrhea. The diagnosis of ZES is made when a fasting gastrin concentration of more than 1000 pg/mL exists in the setting of gastric acid hypersecretion. In equivocal cases (e.g., gastrin < 1000 pg/mL), a positive secretin provocative test will confirm the diagnosis. The secretin test is positive ($\geq$200 pg/mL increase over the preinjection fasting gastrin level) in about 90% of patients with ZES and moderately elevated gastrin levels. Basal acid output is elevated (>15 mmol per hour without previous gastric acid–reducing surgery and >5 mmol per hour with prior surgery) in more than 90% of patients with ZES. Because gastrinomas constitute a relatively uncommon cause of hypergastrinemia, other causes should be considered. The most common causes of hypergastrinemia are antrum-dominant *H. pylori* infection or achlorhydria related to either decreased intraluminal acid in the setting of atrophic gastritis or antisecretory therapy with PPIs. Hypergastrinemia may be related to other causes, including retained gastric antrum (after ulcer surgery), massive small bowel resection, chronic gastric outlet obstruction, and chronic renal failure. Therefore, acid hypersecretion, as documented by gastric acid analysis, is necessary for the diagnosis of ZES.

Once hypergastrinemia has been established and obvious causes have been excluded, efforts should focus on localizing and resecting the gastrin-secreting tumor. The single best imaging test for gastrinoma is somatostatin-receptor scintigraphy (SRS), which is more sensitive than any conventional imaging study, including CT, magnetic resonance imaging (MRI), and ultrasonography, although endoscopic ultrasonography (EUS) is equally sensitive for localizing primary tumors of the pancreas. If liver metastasis is present, a CT- or ultrasound-guided liver biopsy should be performed. In patients without liver metastasis, SRS will localize a possible primary tumor in 60% of cases. If the patient is a surgical candidate and SRS is positive for a primary tumor, no additional localization studies are required. If the SRS is negative for a possible primary tumor, the use of MRI, angiography, or EUS will detect a possible primary tumor in an additional 15% of patients. Multiple pancreatic or duodenal tumors are generally detected in patients with MEN-I syndrome, and although the precise role of surgery in these patients is less certain, some physicians recommend surgery if a lesion larger than 3 cm is identified with preoperative imaging techniques to decrease the possibility of hepatic metastasis. However, successful and long-lasting remission of MEN-I syndrome occurs rarely, if at all.

All patients with ZES, whether sporadic or familial, require antisecretory therapy after the diagnosis is established and during initial evaluation as attempts are made to localize the gastrinoma. Patients with ZES should be treated initially with a PPI using twice the dose normally employed to treat common gastroduodenal ulcers. Intravenous PPIs such as pantoprazole in daily doses ranging from 80 to 240 mg can be used in patients who are unable to take medications by mouth, including those undergoing surgery. The goal of therapy is a basal acid output of less than 10 mmol per hour in the hour preceding the next dose of the drug. Chronic therapy with PPIs uniformly results in continued inhibition of acid secretion, good symptom control, complete healing of any mucosal lesions, and few adverse effects.

Gastroparesis

Gastroparesis is a syndrome characterized by delayed gastric emptying, resulting in impaired transit of food from the stomach to the duodenum in the absence of mechanical obstruction. Symptoms of gastric stasis include early or easy satiety, bloating, nausea, and vomiting. Because eating exacerbates symptoms, patients frequently exhibit anorexia, weight loss, and nutritional deficiencies. A wide range of clinical disorders is associated with impaired gastric emptying (Table 37-4). Diabetes mellitus is the most common cause of gastroparesis, and up to 60% of patients with diabetes complain of symptoms consistent with gastric stasis. Although gastroparesis is typically seen in individuals with long-standing (>10 years) type 1 diabetes who have other complications, such as peripheral and autonomic neuropathy, nephropathy, and retinopathy, GI complaints are also common within the first decade of diagnosis. Diabetic gastroparesis appears to occur as a result of permanent neuropathy of autonomic and enteric nerves, transitory variations in glycemic control, or a combination of both. Idiopathic gastroparesis is also common and comprises those instances with no clearly identifiable cause. Up to one third of these patients have virus-induced gastroparesis, with viral infiltration of the myenteric plexus in the stomach. Patients who have undergone gastric surgery, especially those having had preoperative gastric outlet obstruction as a complication of PUD, are also commonly affected by

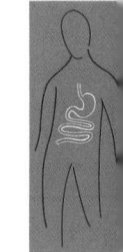

Table 37-4 **Causes of Delayed Gastric Emptying**
Mechanical Causes
Peptic ulcer disease, scarred pylorus
Malignancy: gastric cancer, gastric lymphoma, pancreatic cancer
Gastric surgery: vagotomy, gastric resection, roux-en-Y anastomosis
Crohn disease
Endocrine and Metabolic Causes
Diabetes mellitus
Hypothyroidism
Hypoadrenal states
Electrolyte abnormalities
Chronic renal failure
Medications
Anticholinergics
Opiates
Dopamine agonists
Tricyclic antidepressants
Abnormalities of Gastric Smooth Muscle
Scleroderma
Polymyositis, dermatomyositis
Amyloidosis
Pseudo-obstruction
Myotonic dystrophy
Neuropathy
Scleroderma
Amyloidosis
Autonomic neuropathy
Central Nervous System or Psychiatric Disorders
Brainstem tumors
Spinal cord injury
Anorexia nervosa
Stress
Miscellaneous
Idiopathic gastroparesis
Gastroesophageal reflux disease
Nonulcer (functional) dyspepsia
Cancer cachexia or anorexia

gastroparesis. Finally, Parkinson disease, rheumatologic disorders, hypothyroidism or hyperthyroidism, chronic intestinal pseudo-obstruction, and a variety of paraneoplastic syndromes can also produce gastroparesis.

The diagnostic evaluation of delayed gastric emptying should focus on excluding structural and metabolic abnormalities. Endoscopy is the preferred initial test to rule out mechanical gastric outlet obstruction, and a small bowel follow-through radiograph may be useful to exclude small bowel lesions. Serum electrolytes, blood cell counts, and thyroid studies should also be performed. When these studies are negative, radionuclide scintigraphy (gastric-emptying scan) using a mixed solid-liquid meal can quantitate delayed gastric emptying. Assessment of solid emptying is more clinically relevant than liquid emptying. In especially difficult cases, GI manometry and electrogastrography may help in the diagnosis.

Managing gastroparesis begins with identifying and treating potentially correctable causes. Medications that reduce gastric emptying, such as narcotics, anticholinergics, and tricyclic antidepressants, should be avoided. Because liquids empty easier than solids, and because liquid emptying is often preserved in patients with gastroparesis, simple dietary modifications may be helpful in treatment. The diet should be modified to include blenderized foods and liquid supplements. High-fat and fiber-rich foods should be avoided because they inhibit gastric emptying under normal conditions and are less likely to empty. Medical options are limited and involve the use of prokinetic drugs, which are agents that improve transit in the GI tract.

Metoclopramide is a dopamine-2 receptor antagonist that also facilitates the release of acetylcholine from cholinergic nerve terminals in the gut, thereby accelerating gastric emptying. The efficacy of metoclopramide is inconsistent, and adverse effects and the development of tolerance complicate long-term therapy. Adverse effects occur in up to 20% of patients and include drowsiness, anxiety, fatigue, insomnia, restlessness, agitation, extrapyramidal effects, galactorrhea, and menstrual irregularities. The typical dosage is 10 mg, 20 to 30 minutes before meals and at bedtime, although doses as high as 80 mg or as low as 20 mg may be used daily. Doses should be reduced for patients with renal failure. Domperidone, another dopamine receptor antagonist with prokinetic properties, has similar efficacy to metoclopramide in the treatment of delayed gastric emptying but is currently not available in the United States.

Cisapride, an agent that increases gastric motor activity by facilitating the release of acetylcholine at the myenteric plexus, is no longer routinely available in the United States and other countries because of serious adverse effects, including ventricular tachycardia, ventricular fibrillation, torsades de pointes, and prolongation of the QT interval, which have been reported when cisapride is administered with other drugs that inhibit cytochrome P-450.

Erythromycin is a macrolide antibiotic that stimulates smooth muscle motilin receptors located at all levels of the GI tract. The prokinetic effects of erythromycin are related to its ability to mimic the effect of the GI peptide motilin to stimulate smooth muscle contraction, which accounts for the acceleration of solid and liquid gastric emptying. Erythromycin may dramatically improve gastric emptying in patients with severe diabetic gastroparesis when given acutely at an intravenous dose of 1 to 3 mg/kg every 8 hours. Long-term use of the drug at a dose of 250 to 500 mg orally every 8 hours in patients with gastric stasis is of limited efficacy because of tachyphylaxis and side effects.

Endoscopic botulinum toxin A injection into the pyloric sphincter has also been reported in the treatment of delayed gastric emptying in small studies, but long-term benefit has not been proved.

In patients who are refractory to these measures, surgical placement of a jejunal tube, with or without a venting gastrostomy, may be necessary. Total parenteral nutrition is rarely indicated. Surgical gastrectomy should only be considered in patients with refractory postsurgical gastric stasis. Gastric pacemakers and other prokinetics, specifically new serotonin-receptor agonists, are under investigation and may be options in the future.

Rapid Gastric Emptying

Rapid gastric emptying is a far less common clinical problem than delayed gastric emptying. *Dumping syndrome* describes the alimentary and systemic manifestations of early delivery of large amounts of osmotically active food to the small intestine. Dumping syndrome is usually seen when the normal reservoir, grinding, and sieving properties of the stomach are disrupted, most commonly following surgery for obesity (Roux-en-Y gastric bypass) or PUD. The accelerated emptying of hypertonic boluses of nutrient material into the small intestine results in splanchnic vasodilation and release of vasoactive peptides. Early dumping symptoms, occurring about 30 minutes after a meal, include epigastric fullness and pain, nausea, vomiting, early satiety, and vasomotor features such as flushing, palpitations, and diaphoresis. Later symptoms, such as diaphoresis, tremulousness, and weakness, occur about 2 hours after a meal and may be caused by hypoglycemia from rebound hyperinsulinemia. Treatment of dumping syndrome involves dietary manipulation to decrease the volume and osmotic load emptied into the intestine. Frequent small feedings of meals low in carbohydrates, separation of liquid and solid intake, and avoidance of hypertonic fluids and lactose are usually helpful. When these measures fail, administration of octreotide at a dose of 25 to 50 mcg subcutaneously 30 minutes before meals may be helpful. Octreotide acts by slowing gastric emptying and intestinal transit as well as by inhibiting the release of insulin. Surgical procedures to slow gastric emptying have limited success.

Gastric Volvulus

Gastric volvulus occurs when the stomach twists on itself. This event may be transient, producing few if any symptoms, or may lead to obstruction or even ischemia and necrosis. *Primary gastric volvulus,* seen in one third of the patients, occurs below the diaphragm when the stabilizing ligaments are too lax as a result of congenital or acquired causes. *Secondary gastric volvulus* occurs above the diaphragm in association with paraesophageal hernias or other diaphragmatic defects. Acute gastric volvulus produces sudden, severe pain of the upper abdomen or chest, persistent retching producing scant vomitus, and the inability to pass a naso-gastric tube. This combination of symptoms, also known as Borchardt triad, should lead to a strong clinical suggestion of acute gastric volvulus. Chronic gastric volvulus may be associated with mild and nonspecific symptoms, such as epigastric discomfort, heartburn, abdominal fullness or bloating, and borborygmi, especially after meals. The diag-nosis of gastric volvulus is made by upper GI series demon-strating an abrupt obstruction at the site of the volvulus. Acute gastric volvulus requires emergency surgical evalua-tion because of the substantial risk for mortality related to gastric ischemia or perforation. Treatment consists of surgi-cal gastropexy and repair of any associated paraesophageal hernia.

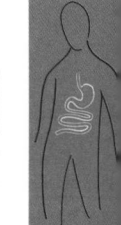

Prospectus for the Future

Our understanding of a significant number of issues involving gastroduodenal pathologic mechanisms and therapeutics will continue to evolve in the next few years. Select goals include the following:

- Development of variations in the structure and delivery of antisecretory therapy, leading to formulations designed to provide increased rapid onset of action and to improve effectiveness in individuals who are unable to take medications by mouth or those with dysmotility or malabsorption
- Further clarification of the optimal *H. pylori* treatment regimen given increased antibiotic resistance profiles

and the goal of improving patient compliance to treatment
- Procurement of evidence-based data to aid in managing stress-related mucosal ulcerations in critically ill patients
- Elucidation of the exact nature and strength of the association between COX-2–selective inhibitors and cardiovascular disease and future development of safer NSAIDs
- Further insight into the mechanism governing GI motility and the development of new agents for the treatment of motility disorders

References

Chan FK, Graham DY: NSAIDs, risks, and gastroprotective strategies: Current status and future. Gastroenterology 134:1240-1257, 2008.

Fuccio L, Minardi ME, Rocco MZ, et al: Meta-analysis: Duration of first-line proton-pump inhibitor-based triple therapy for *Helicobacter pylori* eradication. Ann Intern Med 147:553-562, 2007.

Olsen KM, Devlin JW: Comparison of the enteral and intravenous lansoprazole pharmacodynamic responses in critically ill patients. Aliment Pharmacol Ther 28:326-333, 2008.

Papatherodoridis GV, Sougioultzia S, Archimandritis AJ: Effects of Helicobacter pylori and nonsteroidal anti-inflammatory drugs on peptic ulcer disease: A systematic review. Clin Gastroenterol Hepatol 4:130-142, 2006.

Park MI, Camilleri M: Gastroparesis: clinical update. Am J Gastroeterol 101:1129-1139, 2006.

Vergara M, Catalan M, Gisbert JP, et al: Meta-analysis: Role of Helicobacter pylori eradication in the prevention of peptic ulcer in NSAID users. Aliment Pharmacol Ther 21:1411-1418, 2005.

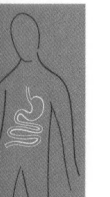

Inflammatory Bowel Disease

Christopher S. Huang and Francis A. Farraye

Although a significant number of infectious organisms and noninfectious processes (e.g., medications, radiation, ischemia) can result in intestinal inflammation, the term *inflammatory bowel disease* (IBD) generally refers primarily to two idiopathic diseases: ulcerative colitis and Crohn disease. The diagnosis of IBD is made by incorporating clinical, endoscopic, radiologic, and histologic information. Ulcerative colitis is characterized by inflammatory changes that involve the colonic mucosa in a continuous superficial fashion, generally starting in the rectum and extending proximally. Depending on the extent of the disease, ulcerative colitis can be divided into proctitis (rectum only), proctosigmoiditis, left-sided colitis (extending to the splenic flexure), or pancolitis. This classification is important for both prognostic and therapeutic reasons. Unlike ulcerative colitis, Crohn disease can involve any segment of the gastrointestinal system, often in a discontinuous fashion. It is characterized by transmural inflammation, which results in significant complications such as abscesses, fistulas, and strictures. Despite the chronic nature of these two diseases, new and emerging targeted anti-inflammatory treatments hold great promise in helping to reduce morbidity and improve the quality of life of individuals with IBD.

Epidemiology

In the United States, about 1.4 million individuals have IBD, and the overall incidence of new cases of IBD is about 3 to 10 new cases per 100,000 people. During the past several decades, the incidence of ulcerative colitis has remained stable, whereas the incidence of Crohn disease has gradually increased. The prevalence of IBD is essentially 10-fold higher, between 30 and 100 per 100,000 people. A bimodal age of presentation exists, with an initial peak between the second and fourth decades of life followed by another peak at about the sixth decade of life. Both sexes are equally affected.

The incidence and prevalence of IBD reflect the genetic and environmental factors that contribute to these disorders.

For example, both diseases are common in northern climates, among whites, particularly in populations with Northern European ancestry, including North Americans, South Africans, and Australians. Individuals of Ashkenazi Jewish descent have also been found to have a twofold to eightfold increased risk for these disorders compared with non-Jews. Although the prevalence and incidence rates of IBD are lowest in Hispanics and Asians, IBD can occur in any ethnic or racial group from anywhere in the world.

Causes

Although the causes of IBD remain unknown, recent advances in the understanding of the genetic, immunologic, and environmental factors are beginning to decipher the etiologic factors of these complex disorders. Currently, it is believed that IBD results from an inappropriate, overactive mucosal immune response to commensal intestinal bacteria in genetically susceptible individuals.

GENETIC FACTORS

About 5% to 20% of patients with IBD have a first-degree relative with the disease, and first-degree relatives of IBD patients have about a 10- to 15-fold increased risk for developing IBD, predominantly with the same disease as the proband. A positive family history is generally more frequently observed in patients with Crohn disease than in patients with ulcerative colitis, suggesting that genetic factors contribute more significantly in the etiology of Crohn disease. Through advances in genome-wide association studies, several susceptibility loci on multiple chromosomes have been linked to IBD, supporting a polygenic cause to these disorders. Polymorphisms in the *NOD-2* gene (also known as *CARD-15*, located on chromosome 16) were the first definitive genetic risk factors identified for Crohn disease. Homozygous mutations of the *NOD-2* gene are associated with a greater than 20-fold increase in susceptibility for Crohn disease. Defects in the NOD-2 protein appear

430

to result in abnormal intestinal immune responses to bacterial cell wall components. These gene mutations are estimated to account for about 15% to 25% of the cases of Crohn disease and are linked predominantly to fibrostenotic terminal ileal disease. Another gene of interest is the *IL-23R* gene on chromosome 1, which has also been shown to be strongly associated with IBD, particularly Crohn disease. Disease-associated *IL-23R* polymorphisms have also been reported in patients with ulcerative colitis, psoriasis, and ankylosing spondylitis. Many other genes have been uncovered by genome-wide association studies, such as *OCTN*, *DLG-5*, *ICAM-1*, and *TLR-4*, and are currently under investigation for their potential involvement in the pathogenesis of IBD.

IMMUNOLOGIC FACTORS

Profound alterations in mucosal immunology have been demonstrated in patients with IBD. In the normal immunologic state of the intestine, recently activated lymphoid tissue is abundant within the mucosal compartment. This state has been described as controlled, or *physiologic,* inflammation, which has likely developed in response to constant encounters with antigenic substances (derived from host microbial flora, or dietary and environmental sources) that have crossed the epithelial barrier from the luminal environment. Indeed, one of the main functions of the intestinal immune system is to discriminate noxious or harmful substances and organisms from nonharmful ones. As a result, a large and well-maintained network of many different mucosal immune cells exists, including cells involved in reducing immune responses (regulatory cells) and those involved in activating immune responses. In IBD, this homeostatic balance, or immune tolerance, is dysregulated, resulting in overactivation of the immune system. Crohn disease, for example, reflects an excessive and persistent CD4 helper T-cell subtype 1 (T_H1) immune response to components of commensal bacterial flora. The T_H1 cytokine profile, including interferon-γ, interleukin-2 (IL-2), IL-12, and tumor necrosis factor-α (TNF-α), is elevated in patients with Crohn disease. The cytokine profile of ulcerative colitis is atypical, with greater expression of IL-5 and IL-13 present, cytokines characteristically associated with a T_H2 response. More recently, non-T_H1/T_H2 pathways have been identified as being potentially important in the pathogenesis of IBD. IL-23, for example, has been recognized as an inducer of a subset of proinflammatory T cells (T_H17) that secrete high levels of IL-17 and play an important role in mediating inflammation in murine models of colitis. IL-17 expression has been shown to be upregulated in active IBD, both Crohn disease and ulcerative colitis.

ENVIRONMENTAL FACTORS

Although believed to be important, the role of environmental factors in IBD pathogenesis remains poorly understood. Many infectious agents, including *Mycobacteria paratuberculosis* and measles virus, have been implicated in IBD, but none fulfills the criteria of true pathogens. Environmental factors are suspected because the disease is more common in industrialized countries, and the frequency has been increasing in countries that are becoming more industrialized. It has been postulated that poor sanitation, food contamination, and crowded living conditions are associated with helminthic infection, which leads to regulatory T-cell conditioning and stimulation of IL-10 and transforming growth factor-β production by mononuclear cells, thereby preventing intestinal inflammation. However, to date, the only environmental factor clearly associated with IBD is tobacco smoking. Smoking seems to be protective against ulcerative colitis, whereas smokers with Crohn disease have more aggressive disease than do nonsmokers. No dietary triggers have been found to cause IBD, but elemental diets and diversion of the fecal stream can reduce recurrence of inflammation in Crohn disease.

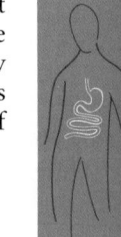

Clinical Features of Ulcerative Colitis

Ulcerative colitis is characterized by chronic inflammation of the mucosal surface that involves the rectum (proctitis) and extends proximally through the colon in a continuous manner. The extent and severity of the colonic inflammation determine prognosis and presentation (insidious versus acute onset).

Most patients initially exhibit diarrhea, abdominal pain, urgency to defecate, rectal bleeding, and the passage of mucus per rectum. Patients occasionally have extraintestinal manifestations (see later discussion) before they develop intestinal symptoms. About 40% to 50% of patients have proctitis or proctosigmoiditis, 30% to 40% have left-sided colitis (disease extending to the splenic flexure), and the remaining 20% to 25% have pancolitis. Of the patients who initially show proctitis or proctosigmoiditis, about 15% develop more extensive disease over time.

The typical clinical course is of chronic intermittent exacerbations, followed by periods of remission. Signs of a worsening clinical course include the development of abdominal pain, dehydration, fever, and tachycardia. Clinical features, including bowel frequency, fever, increased heart rate, and blood in stools, as well as the presence of anemia and an elevated erythrocyte sedimentation rate (ESR) or C-reactive protein, have been used to assess severity of ulcerative colitis.

MAJOR COMPLICATIONS

Toxic Megacolon and Perforation

Toxic megacolon is characterized by gross dilation of the large bowel associated with fever, abdominal pain, dehydration, tachycardia, and bloody diarrhea, which may require urgent surgical intervention. Perforation can occur in the setting of toxic megacolon or in patients with active colitis, especially those taking corticosteroids.

Gastrointestinal Hemorrhage and Anemia

Although massive hemorrhage is uncommon, this complication is an indication for surgical intervention. Anemia commonly occurs and is caused by chronic blood loss from the involved colonic mucosa as well as bone marrow suppression from the inflammatory condition.

Colonic Adenocarcinoma

The risk for colon cancer is increased in patients with ulcerative colitis, the magnitude of which is related to the extent and duration of disease. Colon cancer risk is increased 10- to 20-fold (if disease extends proximal to the sigmoid colon) after 8 years of disease compared with that in unaffected individuals. Colonoscopy with surveillance biopsies are recommended every 2 years after 8 to 10 years of disease in patients with pancolitis and after 12 to 15 years in patients with left-sided colitis, followed by yearly examinations after 20 years of disease. Proctitis is not associated with an increased cancer risk. Patients with IBD and primary sclerosing cholangitis (PSC) appear to be at particularly increased risk, and yearly surveillance is recommended after the initial diagnosis of PSC. A minimum of 33 "random" mucosal biopsy samples are recommended during the colonoscopic examination, in addition to targeted samples of circumscript lesions. The use of chromoendoscopy and other enhanced imaging techniques increases the detection of dysplastic lesions in patients with ulcerative colitis. Colectomy is indicated in patients with flat high-grade dysplasia, multifocal flat low-grade dysplasia, possibly unifocal flat low-grade dysplasia, or evidence of colorectal cancer. Polypoid dysplasia entirely removed by polypectomy without flat dysplasia elsewhere in the colon can be managed with continued surveillance colonoscopy.

Clinical Features of Crohn Disease

Crohn disease may involve any portion of the gastrointestinal tract, and it is the site of involvement, as well as the type of inflammation, that defines the clinical presentation. Unlike ulcerative colitis, the inflammation in Crohn disease is transmural, and the bowel wall can become thickened, fibrotic, and strictured. The mucosal surface may develop *cobblestoning* related to edema with linear ulcerations. Deep fissures can develop and result in microperforations and the formation of fistulous tracts. The disease may be continuous but often has *skip* lesions with intervening segments of normal intestine. The mesentery can become infiltrated with fat, known as *creeping fat*. The disease is often present for months or years before diagnosis, and, in children, growth retardation may be the sole presenting sign.

Distribution of Crohn disease is divided into three major patterns. The most common is ileocecal, which involves the distal portion of the small intestine (terminal ileum) and the proximal large bowel, and is observed in about 40% of patients. Ileocecal Crohn disease may mimic many other diseases, including acute appendicitis. Common symptoms include right lower quadrant abdominal pain, fever, weight loss, and sometimes a palpable inflammatory mass. Chronic inflammation, which leads to fibrosis and stricture formation, may result in partial or complete intestinal obstruction, as demonstrated by abdominal pain, distention, nausea, and vomiting. Because vitamin B_{12} and bile salts are absorbed in the terminal ileum, ileal Crohn disease or surgical resection of the terminal ileum may lead to B_{12} deficiency as well as deficiencies of the fat-soluble vitamins (A, D, E, and K) as a result of bile salt malabsorption.

The second major site of Crohn disease involves the small intestine, especially the terminal ileum, and is seen in about 30% of individuals at the time of presentation. Similar complications develop, including fistulas, which may form between different segments of bowel (e.g., enteroenteric, enterocolonic), bowel and skin (enterocutaneous), bowel and bladder (enterovesicular), and bowel and vagina (rectovaginal).

The third site of disease is confined to the colon and is observed in 25% of individuals at the time of presentation. Although the disease often spares the rectum, 30% to 40% of patients may develop disabling perianal involvement with fissures, fistulas, and abscesses. Diarrhea is the major consequence but usually with less bleeding than that seen in ulcerative colitis. Distinguishing Crohn colitis from ulcerative colitis can be difficult.

The remaining sites of Crohn disease are rare (5%) and include the esophagus, stomach, and duodenum.

MAJOR COMPLICATIONS

Stenosis (Stricture) of the Small Intestine or Colon

Stenosis may lead to bowel obstruction or stasis with subsequent small intestinal bacterial overgrowth.

Malabsorption

Extensive ileal mucosal disease may lead to malabsorption of vitamin B_{12} (resulting in a megaloblastic anemia and neurologic side effects if not corrected) and malabsorption of bile salts (resulting in diarrhea induced by unabsorbed bile salts and potential fat-soluble vitamin deficiency). Depletion of the bile salt pool can lead to the formation of gallstones. Weight loss may result from generalized malabsorption caused by loss of absorptive surfaces.

Fistulas

Transmural inflammation may lead to spontaneous drainage into adjacent bowel loops (enteroenteric fistula), bladder (enterovesical fistula), skin (enterocutaneous fistula), and vagina (rectovaginal), or it may lead to abscess formation around bowel or in other surrounding tissues.

Nephrolithiasis

Chronic fat malabsorption leads to luminal binding of free fatty acids to calcium, allowing oxalate, which normally is poorly absorbed because it complexes to calcium in the gut lumen, to be absorbed. This increase in oxalate absorption increases the risk for urinary calcium oxalate stone formation. Patients with an ileostomy or chronic volume loss from diarrhea are also at increased risk for uric acid stones.

Malignancy

For colonic Crohn disease, the risk for colorectal cancer is equivalent to ulcerative colitis of similar extent and duration. Therefore, screening and surveillance recommendations are similar to those for ulcerative colitis (see previous discussion). Patients with only small intestinal Crohn disease without colonic involvement are not thought to be at increased risk for colorectal cancer. The rates of small bowel carcinoma and lymphoma are increased in patients with Crohn disease.

Diagnosis

The diagnosis of IBD is based on a constellation of clinical features, laboratory tests, and endoscopic, radiographic, and histologic findings. Laboratory tests are not specific and usually reflect inflammation (leukocytosis) or anemia. Perinuclear antineutrophil cytoplasmic antibody (p-ANCA) is positive in up to 70% of patients with ulcerative colitis but rarely positive in patients with Crohn disease, whereas anti–*Saccharomyces cerevisiae* antibodies (ASCA) are common in Crohn disease and are rarely found in ulcerative colitis. Additional markers including anti–CBir-1 and anti–Omp-C may improve the sensitivity and specificity of serologic testing. Stool examination for ova and parasite identification and testing for *Clostridium difficile* toxin and enteric bacterial pathogens should be performed to exclude infections that can mimic IBD.

Colonoscopy in patients with ulcerative colitis reveals a granular mucosa, decreased vascular markings, decreased mucosal reflection, and superficial ulcerations (Fig. 38-1). In more severe cases, the mucosa is friable, with deeper ulcerations and exudate. Patients with long-standing disease have *pseudopolyps,* which represent islands of normal tissue in regions of previous ulceration. On endoscopic examination in Crohn disease (Fig. 38-2), the involved mucosa may show aphthoid ulcerations, deep linear or stellate ulcers, edema, erythema, exudate, and friability with intervening areas of normal mucosa (skip lesions).

In Crohn disease, small bowel radiography (i.e., small bowel follow-through) has traditionally been the best study with which to investigate the jejunum and ileum, although video capsule endoscopy has recently become increasingly used in this setting. Using this technology, small ulcerations and strictures that are undetectable on small bowel radiography can be visualized (**Web Fig. 38-1**), although patients with known or suspected strictures or fistulas should not undergo capsule endoscopy given the risk for capsule retention. On small bowel radiography, involved areas have edema and thickening of the bowel wall that lead to bowel loop separation and can also show ulcerations of the mucosa, fistulas, or strictures. A tight, long stricture in the small bowel is commonly called the *string sign* (Fig. 38-3). Linear ulcers with segments of edematous or uninvolved mucosa lead to the characteristic pattern referred to as *cobblestoning.* Computed tomographic (CT) scanning can often identify bowel wall thickening with surrounding inflammation as well as intra-abdominal abscesses and fistulas. The recent development of CT enterography and magnetic resonance enterography represent advances in small bowel imaging technology and will likely become primary imaging studies in patients with known or suspected Crohn disease.

Mucosal biopsies in ulcerative colitis reveal crypt architectural distortion, with crypt abscesses and infiltration by plasma cells, neutrophils, lymphocytes, and eosinophils (Fig. 38-4). In Crohn disease, the inflammation is transmural and more commonly focal. Granulomas are found in 25% to 30% of histologic specimens in Crohn disease, but not in ulcerative colitis, and can assist in the diagnosis of Crohn disease in the right clinical setting (Fig. 38-5).

Differential Diagnosis

The differential diagnosis of IBD includes infectious colitis, ischemic colitis, radiation enteritis, enterocolitis induced by nonsteroidal anti-inflammatory drugs, diverticulitis, appendicitis, gastrointestinal malignancies, and irritable bowel syndrome. In patients with acute onset of bloody diarrhea, infectious causes that must be excluded include *Salmonella enteritidis, Shigella* species, *Campylobacter jejuni, Escherichia*

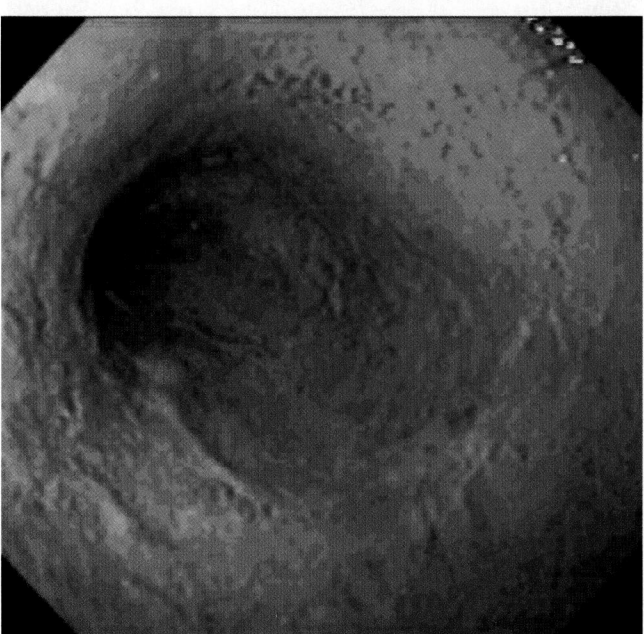

Figure 38-1 Endoscopic image in ulcerative colitis demonstrating diffuse inflammation characterized by erythema, edema, friability, and hemorrhage.

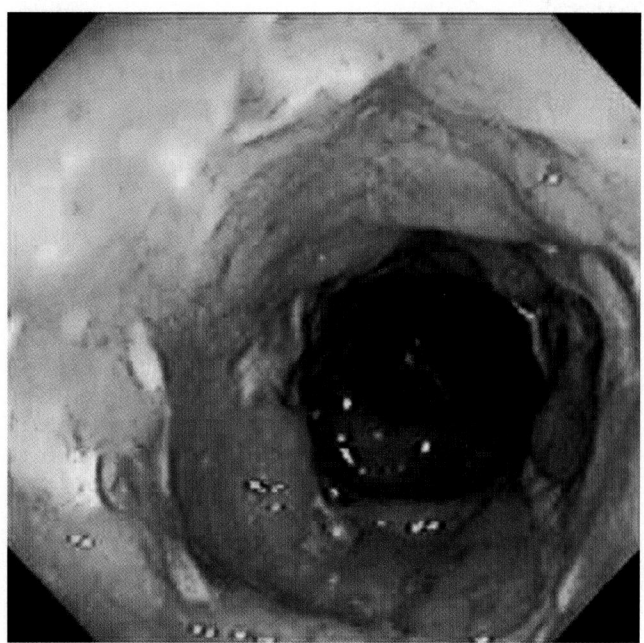

Figure 38-2 Endoscopic image in Crohn disease demonstrating linear ulcers in areas of otherwise normal mucosa.

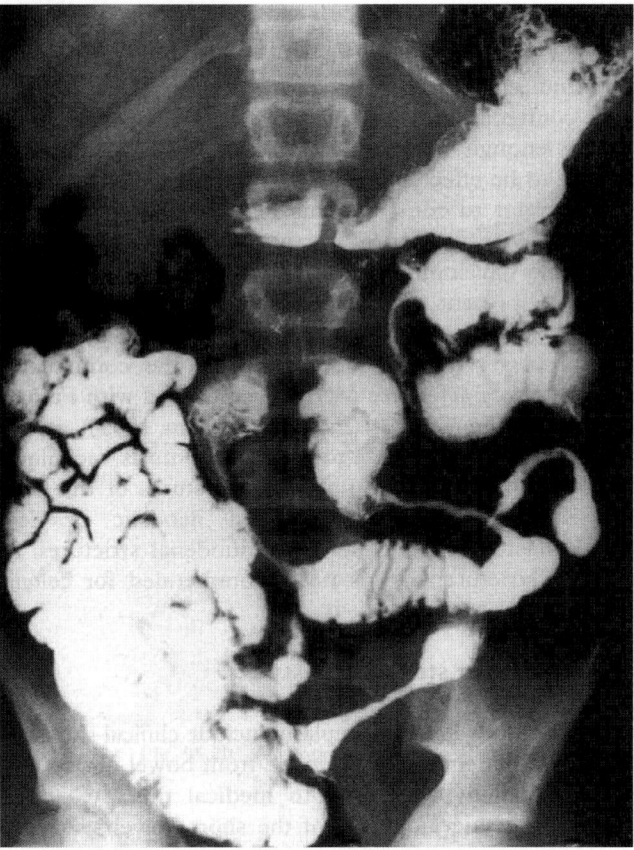

Figure 38-3 Radiograph demonstrating small bowel Crohn disease with skip areas and a string sign.

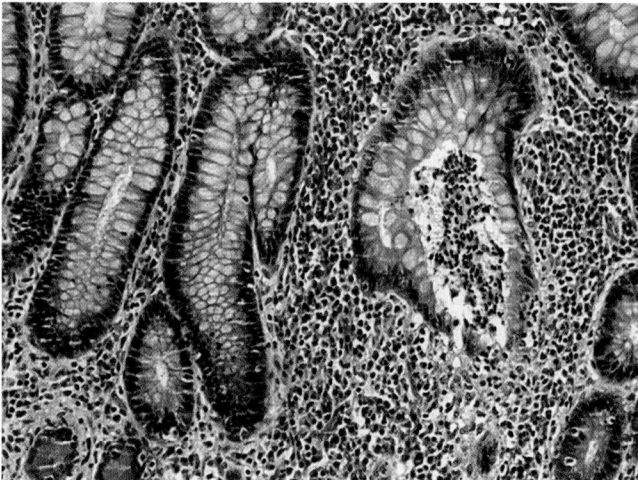

Figure 38-4 Mucosal biopsy demonstrating crypt branching and a crypt abscess characteristic of ulcerative colitis (hematoxylin and eosin stain). (Courtesy of Niall Swan, MD.)

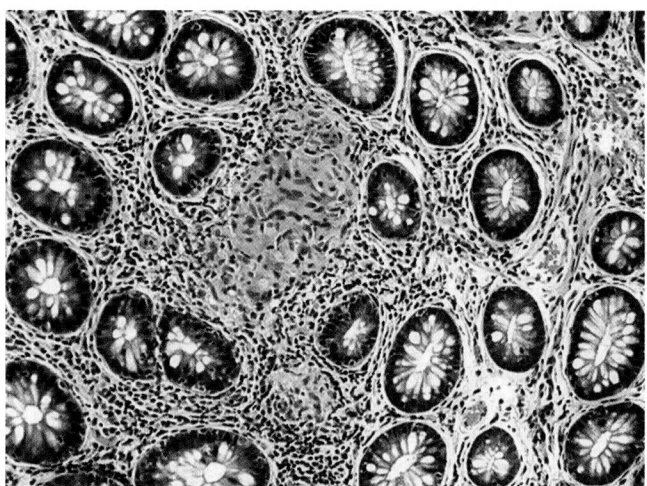

Figure 38-5 Colonic biopsy demonstrating chronic inflammatory infiltrate with a granuloma (hematoxylin and eosin stain; magnification 10×). (Courtesy of Niall Swan, MD.)

coli O157, and *C. difficile.* Among the infectious causes, *Yersinia enterocolitica* can mimic Crohn disease because the pathogen causes ileitis, mesenteric adenitis, fever, diarrhea, and right lower quadrant abdominal pain. *Mycobacterium tuberculosis,* strongyloidiasis, and amebiasis must be excluded in high-risk populations because these infections can mimic IBD, and treatment with corticosteroids can lead to disseminated infection and death.

Extraintestinal Manifestations

Although both ulcerative colitis and Crohn disease primarily involve the bowel, they are associated with inflammatory manifestations in other organ systems, reflecting the systemic nature of these disorders (Table 38-1). Most of these manifestations occur frequently when the bowel is involved, and, in some cases, they may become more difficult to treat than the bowel disease itself.

The most common extraintestinal manifestation is arthritis, of which two major types have been identified. The first is a peripheral, large joint, asymmetrical, seronegative, oligoarticular, nondeforming arthritis (about 20% of patients) that may involve the knees, hips, wrists, elbows, and ankles. This *peripheral arthropathy* usually parallels the course of the large bowel disease *(colitic arthritis)* and usually lasts for only

a few weeks. A second arthritis is axial in location, and its activity does not mirror that of the bowel disease. It consists of sacroiliitis or ankylosing spondylitis. Ankylosing spondylitis (about 5% to 10% of IBD patients) presents with low back pain and stiffness, usually worse during the night, in the morning, or after inactivity. Sacroiliitis alone (without ankylosing spondylitis) is common in IBD (up to about 80% of patients), but many of these patients are asymptomatic.

Liver complications of IBD include both intrahepatic and biliary tract diseases. Intrahepatic diseases include fatty liver, pericholangitis, chronic active hepatitis, and cirrhosis. Pericholangitis, also known as small-duct sclerosing cholangitis, is the most common of these diseases and usually is asymptomatic, identified only by abnormalities in alkaline phosphatase and γ-glutamyl transpeptidase on laboratory tests and histologically by portal tract inflammation and bile ductule degeneration. Small-duct sclerosing cholangitis may progress to cirrhosis.

Table 38-1 Extraintestinal Manifestations of Inflammatory Bowel Disease

Skin

Pyoderma gangrenosum
Erythema nodosum
Sweet syndrome

Hepatobiliary

Primary sclerosing cholangitis
Cholelithiasis
Autoimmune hepatitis

Musculoskeletal

Seronegative arthritis
Ankylosing spondylitis
Sacroiliitis

Ocular

Uveitis
Episcleritis

Miscellaneous

Hypercoagulable state
Autoimmune hemolytic anemia
Amyloidosis

Table 38-2 Differentiating Features

	Ulcerative Colitis	Crohn Disease
Site of involvement	Only involves colon Rectum almost always involved	Any area of the gastrointestinal tract Rectum usually spared
Pattern of involvement	Continuous	Skip lesions
Diarrhea	Bloody	Usually nonbloody
Severe abdominal pain	Rare	Frequent
Perianal disease	No	In 30% of patients
Fistula	No	Yes
Endoscopic findings	Erythematous and friable Superficial ulceration	Aphthoid and deep ulcers Cobblestoning
Radiologic findings	Tubular appearance resulting from loss of haustral folds	String sign of terminal ileum RLQ mass, fistulas, abscesses
Histologic features	Mucosa only Crypt abscesses	Transmural Crypt abscesses, granulomas (about 30%)
Smoking	Protective	Worsens course
Serology	p-ANCA more common	ASCA more common

ASCA, anti–*Saccharomyces cerevisiae* antibodies; p-ANCA, perinuclear antineutrophil cytoplasmic antibody; RLQ, right lower quadrant.

Biliary tract disease includes an increased incidence of gallstones and primary sclerosing cholangitis (PSC). PSC is a chronic cholestatic liver disease marked by fibrosis of the intrahepatic and extrahepatic bile ducts, occurring in 1% to 4% of patients with ulcerative colitis and less often in Crohn disease. Overall, about 70% of patients with PSC have ulcerative colitis. Fibrosis leads to strictures of the bile ducts, which, in turn, may lead to recurrent cholangitis (fever, right upper quadrant pain, and jaundice) and progression to cirrhosis. In addition, about 10% of patients develop cholangiocarcinoma. Medical or surgical therapy for the IBD does not modify the course of PSC, and most patients will progress to cirrhosis and liver failure over 5 to 10 years unless a liver transplantation is performed.

The two classic dermatologic manifestations of IBD are pyoderma gangrenosum and erythema nodosum. Pyoderma gangrenosum (about 5% of patients) exhibits as a discrete ulcer with a necrotic base, usually on the legs. The ulcer may spread and become large and deep, destroying soft tissues. Pyoderma parallels the activity of the IBD in 50% of cases. Treatment is usually with systemic or intralesional steroids, or both. Other treatment options include dapsone, cyclosporine, and infliximab. Erythema nodosum (10% of patients, usually with peripheral arthropathy) exhibits raised, tender nodules, usually over the anterior surface of the tibia. It heals without scarring and responds to treatment for the underlying bowel disease. A less common dermatologic manifestation of IBD is Sweet syndrome, or acute febrile neutrophilic dermatosis. This is a condition characterized by the sudden onset of fever, leukocytosis, and tender, erythematous, well-demarcated papules and plaques that show dense neutrophilic infiltrates on histologic examination.

Ocular manifestations of IBD include uveitis and episcleritis (5%). Uveitis (or iritis) is an inflammatory lesion of the anterior chamber and produces blurred vision, photophobia, headache, and conjunctival injection. Local therapy includes steroids and atropine. Episcleritis is less serious than uveitis, producing burning eyes and scleral injection, and is treated with topical steroids.

Other complications of IBD include chronic anemia (common), digital clubbing and hypertrophic osteoarthropathy (uncommon in adults), an increased incidence of thromboembolic disease (uncommon), and amyloidosis (rare).

Differentiation between Ulcerative Colitis and Crohn Disease

Generally, the diagnoses of ulcerative colitis and Crohn disease can be made based on the findings as described in their respective sections presented earlier and those outlined in Table 38-2. As noted, most Crohn patients have small bowel involvement, skip lesions, and pain, whereas most ulcerative colitis patients have bloody diarrhea with involvement of the rectum and a continuous, superficial spread of the disease. The endoscopic, radiologic, and histologic criteria aid in the phenotypic differentiation of these disease entities. However, occasionally, a diagnosis of *indeterminate colitis* is made as a result of an overlap of findings. For example, colonic Crohn disease may produce superficial continuous rectal involvement similar to ulcerative proctitis. Similarly, chronic ulcerative colitis can infrequently result in inflammation of the terminal ileum, called *backwash ileitis*. In many indeterminate cases, repeated examination is necessary, or complications develop that help identify the form of the disease.

Treatment (Induction and Maintenance of Remission)

As part of the initial management of patients with IBD, the clinician must determine the extent and assess the severity of the disease. Patients with mild or moderate disease can be managed as outpatients with close monitoring in association with a gastroenterologist. Patients with severe or fulminant disease, as indicated by abdominal pain, fever, tachycardia, anemia, and leukocytosis, require hospital admission and multidisciplinary team management. Because IBD is a chronic recurrent illness, treatment is centered on controlling the acute attack with induction of remission followed by maintenance of remission. Treatment options for ulcerative colitis and Crohn disease are reviewed in Table 38-3.

5-AMINOSALICYLIC ACID

The aminosalicylates are given either orally or topically (suppository and enema) and are safe and effective in the treatment of mild to moderate disease as well as in maintenance of remission of ulcerative colitis. The efficacy of most of these agents in the induction or maintenance of remission of Crohn disease is questionable. This category includes sulfasalazine (Azulfidine) at a dose of 4 to 6 g/day in divided doses, which consists of 5-aminosalicylic acid (5-ASA) linked to a sulfapyridine moiety and which is activated following the release of the 5-ASA after bacterial lysis in the colon. Side effects, including headache, nausea, and skin

reactions, may require discontinuation of sulfasalazine in about 30% of patients. Reversible oligospermia may occur with sulfasalazine, and rare serious side effects include pleuropericarditis, pancreatitis, agranulocytosis, interstitial nephritis, and hemolytic anemia. Patients who take sulfasalazine need folic acid supplementation. Newer derivatives of oral 5-ASA compounds, such as mesalamine (Pentasa, 4 g per day in divided doses; Asacol, 2.4 g per day in divided doses; Lialda, 2.4 to 4.8 g once daily), olsalazine (Dipentum, 1 to 2 g per day in divided doses), and balsalazide (Colazal, 6.75 g per day in divided doses), as well as topical forms of mesalamine (Canasa suppositories, 1000 mg once daily; or Rowasa enemas, 4 g once nightly), are being commonly used because of a favorable side-effect profile. In addition to their use in the primary treatment of IBD, several studies suggest that long-term use of 5-ASA medications may reduce the risk for colorectal cancer in patients with ulcerative colitis.

CORTICOSTEROIDS

Corticosteroids may be used topically, orally, or intravenously and are effective for controlling active disease but are not useful for maintaining remission. They are indicated for moderate or severe disease and in patients in whom treatment with 5-ASA fails. The most commonly used agent is prednisone, started in doses between 40 and 60 mg per day. Patients typically improve rapidly, and the medication is usually tapered down slowly, that is, 5 to 10 mg per week until discontinuation. Patients who do not improve after 1 week of oral treatment and those with more severe disease are best treated in the hospital with intravenous corticosteroids, such as intravenous hydrocortisone, 300 mg per day, or methylprednisolone, which can be given either by continuous infusion or in three divided doses. Corticosteroids have numerous side effects with long-term use. Budesonide (Entocort, 9 mg given once daily), a corticosteroid that undergoes extensive first-pass hepatic metabolism, is now available for inducing and maintaining remission of ileocolonic Crohn disease and may offer long-term benefits with decreased corticosteroid side effects. Controlled trials have shown that budesonide is more effective than placebo and oral 5-ASA, and has similar efficacy to prednisolone for the induction of remission in Crohn disease.

ANTIBIOTICS

Antibiotics are primarily used in patients with Crohn disease who have colonic, perianal, or fistulizing disease. Intravenous antibiotics are also part of the initial treatment in patients with severe, toxic, or fulminant colitis. The two commonly used antibiotics are metronidazole (Flagyl) and ciprofloxacin (Cipro). Ciprofloxacin is prescribed at a dosage of 500 mg twice a day. Metronidazole is prescribed at a dosage of 20 mg/kg per day in three divided doses. Patients should be warned of potential side effects, such as a disulfiram (Antabuse) effect and peripheral neuropathy.

IMMUNOMODULATORS

Included in this category are azathioprine (Imuran, 2 to 2.5 mg/kg per day) and its active metabolite 6-

Table 38-3	**Treatment Options**	
Disease Severity	**Ulcerative Colitis**	**Crohn Disease**
Mild	Oral and topical 5-ASA compounds	5-ASA compounds Antibiotics Elemental diet
Moderate	Oral and topical 5-ASA compounds Oral steroids Azathioprine, 6-MP Infliximab	5-ASA compounds Antibiotics Budesonide or oral steroids Azathioprine, 6-MP Methotrexate Infliximab, adalimumab, certolizumab, natalizumab
Severe	Intravenous steroids Cyclosporine Infliximab Surgery	Intravenous steroids Azathioprine, 6-MP Methotrexate Infliximab, adalimumab, certolizumab, natalizumab Surgery

5-ASA, 5-aminosalicylic acid; 6-MP, 6-mercaptopurine.

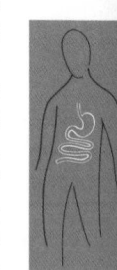

mercaptopurine (6-MP) (Purinethol, 1 to 1.5 mg/kg per day) as well as methotrexate and cyclosporine. Azathioprine and 6-MP are effective therapies for maintaining remission in both Crohn disease and ulcerative colitis and are used primarily as steroid-sparing agents. They have a slow onset of action (months) but are generally safe and well tolerated. Other regimens include subcutaneous or intramuscular methotrexate for induction (25 mg weekly) and maintenance of remission (15 to 25 mg weekly) in active Crohn disease and intravenous cyclosporine (2 to 4 mg/kg per day given over 24 hours) as *bridge* treatment for severe steroid-refractory ulcerative colitis. Given the potential for both short-term and long-term side effects, as well as the need for close follow-up, patients needing these medications are best managed by gastroenterologists.

BIOLOGIC THERAPY

Advances in our knowledge of the immunopathogenesis of IBD have led to a new class of therapies that target specific aspects of the immune system, collectively known as the *biologic agents*. The first such agent to be used in IBD was infliximab, a chimeric monoclonal antibody to TNF-α, which has been shown to be effective in the treatment of moderate to severe Crohn disease, including fistulizing disease. More recently, infliximab has also been shown to be beneficial in the treatment of ulcerative colitis that is refractory to conventional medical therapy. Because infliximab is a chimeric antibody, its toxicities include infusion reactions, delayed-type hypersensitivity reactions, and formation of autoantibodies (which can reduce its efficacy). Two newer anti-TNF agents, adalimumab (a fully human monoclonal antibody), and certolizumab pegol (a humanized anti-TNF antibody Fab fragment), have also proved efficacious in patients with moderate to severe Crohn disease who have not responded well to conventional treatments. These two agents are administered subcutaneously, and may have a lower toxicity profile. Natalizumab, a humanized anti-α_4-integrin antibody, blocks inflammatory cell migration and adhesion and has recently been approved for the treatment of moderate to severe Crohn disease in patients who have had an inadequate response to, or are unable to tolerate, conventional Crohn disease therapies including inhibitors of TNF-α.

Because of the potent effects these biologic agents have on the immune system, careful patient selection and monitoring for complications are necessary. Reactivation of latent tuberculosis and other serious infections have been reported with the anti-TNF agents, and there may be an increased risk for non-Hodgkin lymphoma and possibly solid tumors as well. Natalizumab has been linked to rare cases of progressive multifocal leukoencephalopathy caused by the human polyoma JC virus.

PROBIOTICS

Probiotics are viable nonpathogenic organisms that, after ingestion, may prevent or treat intestinal diseases. Probiotics are being explored in treatment of IBD and may help prevent recurrence after surgery for Crohn disease and to treat pouchitis after ileal pouch-anal anastomosis.

NUTRITIONAL SUPPORT

Nutritional support is an important adjunctive aspect in the management of patients with IBD. However, the role of nutrition as a primary treatment has been limited to patients with small bowel Crohn disease. These patients may achieve and maintain remission with total parenteral nutrition or elemental diets after prolonged periods (at least 4 weeks). Many patients with Crohn disease and ulcerative colitis experience weight loss during exacerbations of their illness and need caloric supplements. Vitamins and minerals can be given orally as a multivitamin with folic acid. Vitamin B_{12} should be supplemented parenterally in patients who have extensive ileal disease or an ileal resection. Patients taking corticosteroids require supplemental calcium and vitamin D, and individuals with extensive small bowel involvement can also develop malabsorption of fat-soluble vitamins (A, D, E, and K), iron deficiency, and rarely trace minerals. Lactose-free diets, as well as low-fiber diets, may be necessary in patients with active disease or strictures.

ANTIDIARRHEALS AND BILE SALT RESIN BINDERS

Antidiarrheal agents and bile salt resin binders are adjuncts used to manage diarrhea in patients with IBD. Antidiarrheal agents should be used cautiously during exacerbations of colitis because they can precipitate toxic megacolon. The main role of these medications involves controlling diarrhea in patients who have undergone previous resections. Generally, when less than 100 cm of terminal ileum has been resected, patients can develop a bile salt malabsorptive state during which bile salts enter the colon and result in a secretory diarrhea. Bile salt resin binders such as cholestyramine are an effective treatment in these cases. When patients have undergone one or more extensive resections, the bile salt pool is depleted, and fat malabsorption develops. These patients may require a low-fat diet supplemented with medium-chain triglycerides and antidiarrheal agents, but bile salt resin binders should not be used.

SURGICAL MANAGEMENT

Surgical intervention is indicated for patients with severe complications such as obstruction, perforation, massive gastrointestinal hemorrhage, and toxic megacolon not responsive to medical treatment. The other main indication for surgical treatment is the presence of dysplasia or cancer. For patients with ulcerative colitis, regardless of the extent of disease, the entire colon must be removed, and the operation is essentially curative. About 20% to 25% of patients have pancolitis, and one third to one half will require colectomy within 2 to 5 years of diagnosis, depending on the severity of their colitis. In contrast, less than 10% of individuals with mild disease or proctitis will undergo colectomy by 10 years after diagnosis. Historically, the initial operation for ulcerative colitis was a total proctocolectomy and Brooke ileostomy. More recently, the ileal pouch-anal anastomosis has become the operation of choice in most patients. In this operation, the colon is removed, and the small bowel is constructed into a reservoir (ileal pouch) that is anastomosed to the anus, allowing defecation through the anus. Complications of this operation include the development of pouchitis, fecal incontinence, reduced fertility, and need for reoperation.

Surgery is not curative in Crohn disease and is generally avoided, if possible. Nonetheless, 10 years after a diagnosis of Crohn disease, more than 60% of patients will require surgery. Many surgical procedures in patients with Crohn disease are performed to manage complications of the disease, including segmental resection, stricturoplasty, fistulectomy, and abscess drainage. Unfortunately, the recurrence rate is high, with 70% of patients having an endoscopic recurrence within 1 year of surgery and 50% having a symptomatic recurrence within 4 years.

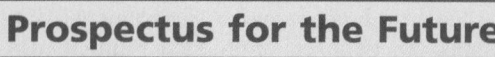

Prospectus for the Future

As our understanding of the etiologic and pathophysiologic aspects of inflammatory bowel disease increases, major advancements in diagnosis and treatment are anticipated. These advancements include the following:

- The use of molecular, genetic, and serologic tests to differentiate between subtypes of disease as well as identify individuals at high risk for developing complications of inflammatory bowel disease

- The increased, and earlier, use of biologic agents to specifically target aspects of the immune system and inflammatory pathways known to be involved in IBD pathophysiology
- Improvements in the detection of dysplasia and prevention of colorectal cancer (including chemoprevention) in patients with chronic colitis

References

Baumgart DC, Sandborn WJ: Inflammatory bowel disease: Clinical aspects and established and evolving therapies. Lancet 369:1641, 2007.

Brown SJ, Mayer L: The immune response in inflammatory bowel disease. Am J Gastroenterol 102:2058, 2007.

Cho JH: The genetics and immunopathogenesis of inflammatory bowel disease. Nat Rev Immunol 8:458, 2008.

Cima RR, Pemberton JH: Medical and surgical management of chronic ulcerative colitis. Arch Surg 140:300, 2005.

D'Haens G, Baert F, van Assche G, et al: Early combined immunosuppression or conventional management in patients with newly diagnosed Crohn's disease: An open randomised trial. Lancet 371:660-667, 2008.

Itzkowitz SH, Present DH: Crohn's and Colitis Foundation of America, Colon Cancer in IBD Study Group: Consensus Conference. Colorectal cancer screening and surveillance in inflammatory bowel disease. Inflamm Bowel Dis 11:314, 2005.

Katz S: Update in medical therapy of ulcerative colitis: Newer concepts and therapies. J Clin Gastroenterol 39:557, 2005.

Kornbluth A, Sachar DB: Ulcerative colitis practice guidelines in adults (update): American College of Gastroenterology, Practice Parameters Committee. Am J Gastroenterol 99:1371, 2004.

Peyrin-Biroulet L, Desreumaux P, Sandborn WJ, Colombel JF: Crohn's disease: Beyond antagonists of tumour necrosis factor. Lancet 372:67-81, 2008.

Sandborn WJ, Feagan BG, Lichtenstein GR: Medical management of mild to moderate Crohn's disease: Evidence-based treatment algorithms for induction and maintenance of remission. Aliment Pharmacol Ther 26:987-1003, 2007.

Siegel CA, Sands BE: Review article: Practical management of inflammatory bowel disease patients taking immunomodulators. Aliment Pharmacol Ther 22:1, 2005.

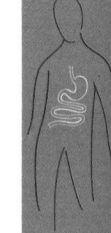

Neoplasms of the Gastrointestinal Tract

Paul C. Schroy III

Esophageal Carcinoma

Carcinoma of the esophagus is one of the most lethal of all cancers. The lack of early symptoms and serosal barrier, as well as the rich, bidirectional esophageal lymphatic flow, often results in advanced disease by the time of diagnosis. The American Cancer Society estimates that about 16,500 new cases of esophageal cancer and 14,530 esophageal cancer deaths will occur in the United States in 2009. Historically, squamous cell carcinoma (SCC) constituted 95% of all esophageal carcinomas. Since 1980, however, the incidence of adenocarcinoma of the esophagus has rapidly increased and now accounts for about 50% of newly diagnosed cases of esophageal carcinoma. The epidemiology of SCC differs from that of adenocarcinoma of the esophagus, but the symptoms, treatments, and prognoses are similar.

INCIDENCE AND EPIDEMIOLOGY

The incidence of SCC varies dramatically throughout the world. The highest rates are found in developing countries such as northern China, Iran, India, and parts of southern Africa. SCC is relatively uncommon in the United States, with an annual incidence of less than 5 cases per 100,000 population. Esophageal cancer is rare among individuals younger than 40 years, but thereafter increases in incidence with each subsequent decade. Men are affected more often than women, and African Americans have a fivefold increase in incidence compared with other racial and ethnic groups. The cause of SCC is unknown, but environmental, dietary, and local esophageal factors have been implicated. Heavy alcohol consumption and smoking are the predominant risk factors for SCC in the United States. In developing countries, nutritional deficiencies (e.g., selenium), betel nut chewing, human papillomavirus infection, and consumption of extremely hot drinks (e.g., tea), nitrates, and pickled vegetables, are also important risk factors. Predisposing conditions include lye strictures, radiation injury, Plummer-Vinson syndrome, achalasia, tylosis, and celiac disease.

Adenocarcinoma of the esophagus is primarily a disease of white men. The primary risk factor for adenocarcinoma is Barrett esophagus, a condition in which specialized intestinal-type columnar mucosa replaces the normal squamous mucosa in response to chronic gastroesophageal reflux disease. It is presumed that intestinal metaplasia progresses to low-grade dysplasia and then high-grade dysplasia and finally adenocarcinoma. The risk for developing adenocarcinoma in the setting of Barrett esophagus is about 0.5% per year. Long-standing gastroesophageal disease, obesity, and cigarette smoking have also been implicated as potential causative factors. Endoscopic surveillance with biopsy is recommended for Barrett esophagus but not chronic gastroesophageal reflux disease.

Clinical Presentation

Early and curable esophageal carcinoma is frequently asymptomatic and detected serendipitously. The presence of symptoms heralds an advanced and most often incurable stage of disease. Under careful questioning, most patients will have had symptoms for a few months before seeking medical attention. Dysphagia is the most common symptom of esophageal carcinoma. It occurs when the esophageal lumen has been compromised by about 75% of its normal diameter. Difficulty swallowing solid foods precedes dysphagia to liquids. With complete obstruction, regurgitation, aspiration, and cough or pneumonia may occur. Pulmonary symptoms may also occur if a tracheoesophageal fistula is present. Patients uniformly have weight loss and anorexia. Chest pain, hiccups, or hoarseness indicates involvement of adjacent structures such as the mediastinum, diaphragm, and recurrent laryngeal nerve, respectively. If gastrointestinal bleeding occurs, it is often occult or associated with iron deficiency anemia. Life-threatening gastrointestinal hemorrhage can occur if the tumor has invaded major vessels. Clubbing of the nails and paraneoplastic syndromes, such as hypercalcemia and Cushing syndrome, are rarely seen.

DIAGNOSIS

Patients with dysphagia or other suggestive symptoms should be evaluated by upper endoscopy or an esophageal barium study. The advantage of endoscopy includes the opportunity to obtain tissue of the cancer, either by biopsy or brush cytologic study. Esophageal carcinoma may appear as a plaque, an ulcer, a stricture, or a mass. Nearly 90% of adenocarcinomas develop in the distal esophagus, whereas 50% of SCCs occur in the middle third of the esophagus, and the other 50% are evenly distributed in the proximal and distal esophagus. Computed tomography (CT) scanning of the chest and abdomen is performed to detect invasion of local structures and metastases to the lung and liver. Endoscopic ultrasonography (EUS), with its ability to image the esophageal wall as a five-layer structure that correlates with histologic layers, is more accurate than CT for staging tumor depth, local invasion, and regional node involvement. EUS also permits targeted fine-needle aspiration of suspicious findings.

THERAPY

Stage is the most important prognostic factor for the survival of patients with esophageal cancer and influences the treatment options. Staging is based on the tumor-node-metastasis (TNM) classification system. Only localized tumors confined to the wall of the esophagus are potentially curable by surgery. Overall 5-year survival rates for patients undergoing curative resection, however, are just 5% to 20%. Preoperative chemotherapy with multidrug regimens combined with radiation therapy may reduce local recurrence rates and improve survival. Chemotherapy plus radiation therapy is also recommended for patients with locally unresectable disease, medical conditions that preclude surgery, and those who refuse surgery. Patients with metastatic disease should be considered for palliative treatment of dysphagia. Local treatment with endoscopic methods (such as malignant stricture dilation), placement of an endoprosthesis (stent), and tumor ablation by laser or photodynamic therapy are often the methods of choice for rapid palliation. More sustained palliation can be achieved using combined chemotherapy and radiation therapy.

Gastric Carcinoma

Gastric carcinoma is one of the leading causes of cancer-related deaths worldwide. For unknown reasons, the incidence of gastric cancer has declined dramatically in the United States since the 1930s. Despite its declining incidence, the American Cancer Society estimates that about 21,100 new cases and 10,620 gastric cancer deaths will occur in 2009. Unfortunately, gastric cancer is often advanced at the time of diagnosis; the 5-year survival rate is about 24%.

INCIDENCE AND EPIDEMIOLOGY

More than 90% of gastric cancers are adenocarcinomas. The incidence of gastric cancer varies widely throughout the world. The disease is more common in developing countries than industrialized nations and shows a predilection for

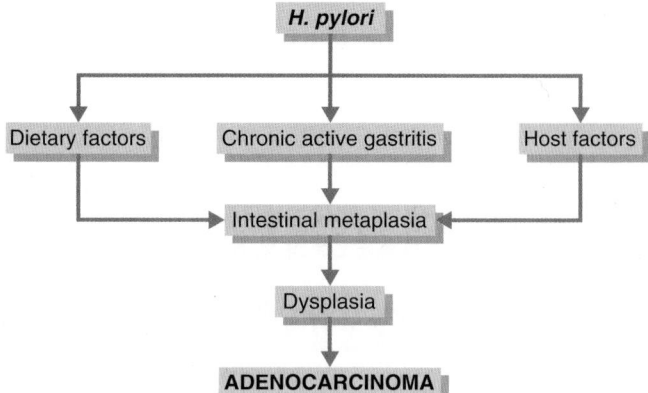

Figure 39-1 Model for the development of gastric adenocarcinoma.

urban and lower socioeconomic groups. Japan, China, the Andean regions of South America, and Eastern Europe exhibit the highest rates. The United States has among the lowest incidence rates at less than 10 cases per 100,000 population. Gastric cancer rarely occurs before age 40 years; thereafter, the incidence rises steadily, peaking in the seventh decade. Men are afflicted at a rate nearly twice that of women. African Americans, Hispanic Americans, and Native Americans are 1.5 to 2.5 times more likely to develop gastric cancer than whites. Migrants typically acquire the risk of their host countries, suggesting an important role for environmental factors. Low socioeconomic status, improper food storage, and other dietary and local gastric factors are associated with the disease. Dietary factors include deficiencies in fats, protein, and vitamins A and C and excesses in salted meat and fish, smoked foods, pickled vegetables, and nitrates. Predisposing conditions including atrophic gastritis, postgastrectomy states, achlorhydria, pernicious anemia, adenomatous polyps, and Ménétrier disease are also associated with an increased incidence. The World Health Organization has classified *Helicobacter pylori* as a carcinogen and epidemiologically linked to gastric adenocarcinoma (Fig. 39-1). However, only a small proportion of patients infected with *H. pylori* develop gastric adenocarcinoma.

Gastric lymphomas account for fewer than 5% of primary gastric malignancies. The stomach is the most common site of extranodal non-Hodgkin lymphoma, but Hodgkin lymphoma of the stomach is rare. Gastric mucosa-associated lymphoid tissue (MALT) lymphomas are associated with *H. pylori* infection in 90% of cases and are reported to regress in 60% to 70% of cases after eradication of *H. pylori*. MALT lymphomas can also occur in association with various autoimmune and immunodeficiency syndromes. Most develop in individuals older than 50 years, and there is a slight male predominance.

CLINICAL PRESENTATION

The location, size, and growth pattern of gastric malignancies may influence the presenting symptoms. Abdominal discomfort is the most frequent symptom; however, early satiety, nausea, and vomiting may occur, especially with gastric outlet obstruction. Gastrointestinal bleeding may manifest as iron deficiency anemia, occult bleeding, or

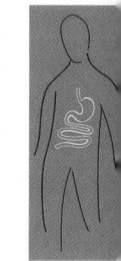

frank upper gastrointestinal hemorrhage. Anorexia and weight loss often accompany other symptoms. The signs of metastatic disease, which may be found on physical examination and signify incurability, include a Virchow (left supraclavicular) node, a Blumer shelf (mass in the perirectal pouch, found on digital rectal examination), and a Krukenberg tumor (metastasis to the ovaries). A variety of paraneoplastic syndromes have been associated with gastric adenocarcinoma and warrant an investigation for a gastrointestinal malignancy. They include Trousseau syndrome (thrombosis), acanthosis nigricans (pigmented dermal lesions), membranous nephropathy, microangiopathic hemolytic anemia, Leser-Trélat sign (seborrheic keratoses), and dermatomyositis.

DIAGNOSIS

The diagnostic tests for gastric malignancies include double contrast (barium) upper gastrointestinal radiography or endoscopy. Lesions detected on barium study require endoscopic biopsy and cytologic study for histologic evaluation. Gastric carcinomas may appear as ulcers, masses, enlarged gastric folds, or an infiltrative process with a nondistensible stomach wall (linitis plastica). The accuracy of endoscopic ultrasonography is in the range of 77% to 93% for determining the depth of invasion and 65% to 90% for predicting regional node involvement. CT scanning of the chest and abdomen may detect metastases in the lung and liver but is otherwise poor for staging. Laparoscopy is increasingly being used for staging and determination of resectability with high accuracy.

THERAPY

The standard treatment of gastric cancer is complete surgical resection with removal of all gross and microscopic disease. The postoperative local-regional recurrence rate remains 80%. A postoperative combination of chemotherapy plus radiation therapy reduces local recurrence rates and improves survival in patients undergoing curative resection. In the United States, nearly two thirds of patients present with advanced disease (stages III to IV), with a survival rate of less than 20%. Chemotherapy is the mainstay of treatment for such patients, but long-term survival is rare. Palliative resection may be performed to prevent obstruction or treat bleeding; radiation therapy and endoscopy may also be of palliative benefit in select patients. Treatment options for gastric lymphomas include some combination of chemotherapy, radiation therapy, and surgery, depending on stage of disease.

Colorectal Polyps and Carcinoma

Carcinoma of the colon and rectum is the third most common cancer and the second most common cause of cancer deaths in American men and women. More than 146,970 new cases and 49,920 colorectal cancer-related deaths will occur in 2009. Screening has been shown to be an effective strategy for reducing both colorectal cancer mortality, through early detection, and incidence, through the identification and removal of premalignant adenomas.

INCIDENCE AND EPIDEMIOLOGY

Worldwide incidence and mortality of colorectal cancer varies considerably. With the notable exception of Japan, industrialized countries are at greatest risk. In the United States, incidence rates have declined slightly during the past decade but remain in excess of 40 cases per 100,000 persons. About 6% of Americans will develop colorectal cancer during their lifetime. Age is an important determinant of risk. Although extremely uncommon in individuals younger than 35 years (except those with rare predisposing genetic syndromes), the incidence of colorectal cancer increases steadily with age, beginning at about 40 years of age, with an approximate doubling with each successive decade thereafter to about 80 years of age. Cancer of the colon affects men and women at similar rates, whereas cancer of the rectum is more common in men. Colorectal cancer does not appear to have a racial predilection; however, African Americans are more likely to present with advanced-stage disease. Epidemiologic studies have identified a number of modifiable risk factors related to colorectal cancer. Factors associated with an increased risk for the disease include obesity, red meat, alcohol, and tobacco; conversely, factors associated with a decreased risk include physical activity, nonsteroidal anti-inflammatory agents, and multivitamins.

Most colorectal cancers are believed to arise from benign adenomatous polyps (adenomas). The epidemiology of colorectal adenomas is similar to that of colorectal cancer. In general, the prevalence of colorectal adenomas in a given country parallels the prevalence of colorectal cancer. Age is an important determinant of prevalence in high-risk countries. In the United States, autopsy studies suggest an overall prevalence of 50%, ranging from about 30% at age 50 years to 55% at age 80 years. Fortunately, only a minority of adenomas progress to colorectal cancer. It is unknown how long an adenoma takes to develop into an invasive cancer, but data from multiple observational studies suggest at least 10 years. Insight into the molecular mechanisms responsible for the adenoma-carcinoma sequence suggests that colorectal carcinogenesis is a multistage process (Fig. 39-2) resulting from the accumulation of genetic alterations involving various oncogenes (e.g., K-*ras*), tumor suppressor genes (e.g., *APC* or *β-catenin*, *DCC*, *SMAD-4*, *SMAD-2*, and *p53*), or DNA mismatch repair genes (e.g., *hMLH-1*).

High-risk groups have been identified and include those with a personal or family history of colorectal cancer or adenomas, various genetic polyposis and nonpolyposis syndromes, and inflammatory bowel disease (Table 39-1). Hereditary nonpolyposis colorectal cancer (HNPCC) and familial adenomatous polyposis (FAP) are well-defined genetic syndromes associated with the highest risk for colorectal cancer. HNPCC (Lynch syndromes) is characterized by inherited mutations in one of the DNA mismatch repair genes (e.g., *hMLH-1* or *hMSH-2*), early-onset colorectal cancer (average age, 44 years) in the absence of polyposis, a predominance (60% to 70%) of tumors proximal to the splenic flexure, an excess of both colorectal and extracolonic (e.g., endometrial) cancers, and an estimated lifetime risk for colorectal cancer of 80% to 90%. In contrast, FAP is characterized by inherited mutations in the *APC* gene, the appearance of hundreds of colorectal adenomas during the second or third decade of life, and a risk for colorectal cancer

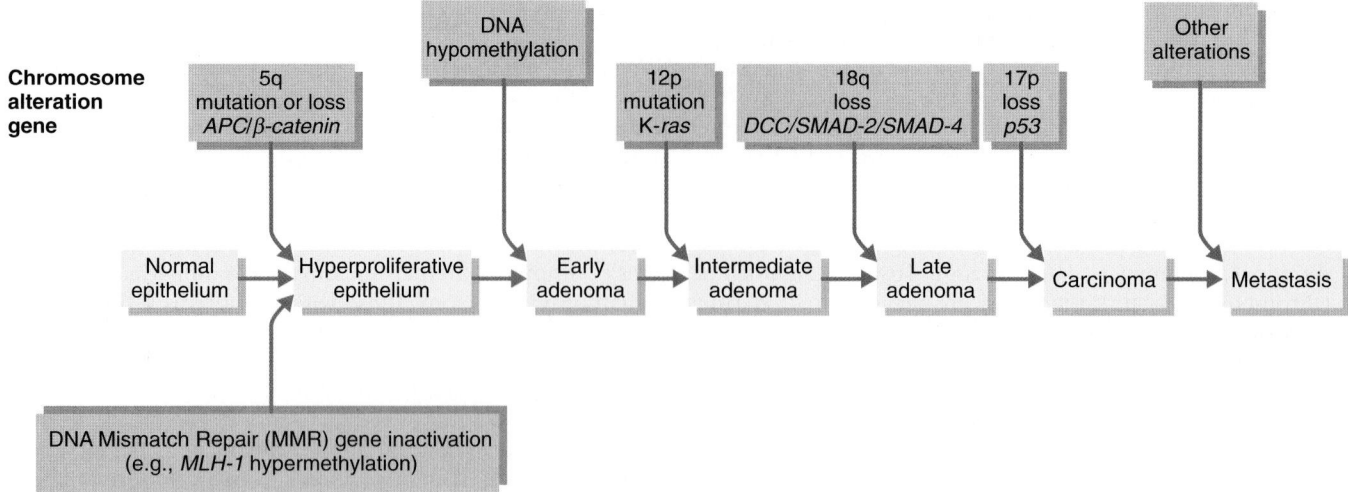

Figure 39-2 A genetic model for colorectal tumorigenesis.

Table 39-1 Risk Factors for Colorectal Cancer

Age ≥ 50 yr

Personal history of adenomatous polyps or colorectal cancer

Familial adenomatous polyposis or Gardner syndrome

MYH-associated adenomatous polyposis

Hereditary nonpolyposis colon cancer

Ulcerative colitis or Crohn colitis

First-degree relative with colon cancer or adenomatous polyps diagnosed before age 60 yr

Hamartomatous polyposis syndrome (Peutz-Jeghers syndrome, juvenile polyposis)

that approaches 100% by the fifth decade if left untreated. FAP is also associated with benign fundic gland polyps in the stomach and duodenal adenomas and adenocarcinomas that have a predilection for the periampullary region. Gardner syndrome is a variant of FAP in which affected probands also exhibit a variety of extraintestinal manifestations such as osteomas, desmoids, and other soft tissue tumors. Congenital hypertrophy of the retinal pigment epithelium is an early benign manifestation of both FAP and Gardner syndrome. *MYH*-associated adenomatous polyposis syndrome is indistinguishable from FAP clinically but caused by mutations of the base excision repair gene, mutY homologue (*MYH*) rather than *APC*.

Peutz-Jeghers syndrome is an autosomal dominant condition characterized by hamartomatous polyposis of both the small and large bowel and mucocutaneous pigmentation. Affected individuals are at increased risk for both gastrointestinal (stomach, small bowel, and colon) and extraintestinal (e.g., genital tract, pancreas, and breast) malignancies occurring at a young age. Generalized juvenile polyposis is another inherited hamartomatous polyposis syndrome associated with a small, albeit increased, risk for colorectal cancer.

CLINICAL PRESENTATION

Most colorectal neoplasms are asymptomatic until advanced. Gastrointestinal blood loss is the most common symptom

and may present as occult bleeding, hematochezia, or unexplained iron deficiency anemia. Other symptoms include abdominal pain from obstruction or invasion, change in bowel habits, or unexplained anorexia or weight loss. A palpable mass may be present in patients with advanced cancers of the cecum.

DIAGNOSIS

All patients with symptoms suggestive of colorectal neoplasia should undergo an evaluation of the colon by colonoscopy, flexible sigmoidoscopy, or double contrast barium enema. About 50% of colorectal adenomas and cancers are located between the rectum and splenic flexure; however, the prevalence of cancers proximal to the splenic flexure increases with increasing age, especially among women. Colorectal cancers may arise in sessile (flat) or pedunculated (on a stalk) polyps, or they may appear as a stricture, a fungating mass, or an ulcerated mass. Colonoscopy has greater accuracy than a barium enema study in the detection of small polyps and early cancers as well as the ability to remove neoplasms or biopsy lesions at the time of the examination. Lesions detected on barium enema study necessitate colonoscopic evaluation. CT scanning and of the abdomen and pelvis is used preoperatively to assess the extent of metastatic disease. Magnetic resonance scanning and positron emission tomography may also be useful in detecting metastatic disease in select patients. EUS is used for the preoperative staging of rectal cancer. Carcinoembryonic antigen level is measured preoperatively for a baseline value and, if elevated, monitored to detect tumor recurrence postoperatively.

Periodic screening by colonoscopy, CT colonography (virtual colonoscopy), flexible sigmoidoscopy, or double-contrast enema is recommended for asymptomatic, average-risk patients beginning at age 50 years. Stool blood testing and stool DNA testing are alternative screening methods for patients who refuse one of the preferred methods (Table 39-2). Screening recommendations for high-risk patients vary depending on the risk factor (see Table 39-2) but in general rely on colonoscopy performed at a younger age and at more frequent intervals than for those at average risk.

Table 39-2 Colorectal Cancer (CRC) Screening and Surveillance Recommendations*

Indication	Recommendations

Average risk	Beginning at age 50 yr:
	   Colonoscopy every 10 yr
	   Computed tomographic colonography every 5 yr
	   Flexible sigmoidoscopy every 5 yr
	   Double-contrast barium enema every 5 yr
	   (Stool blood testing annually or stool DNA testing acceptable but not preferred)

One or two first-degree relatives with CRC at any age or adenoma at age < 60 yr	Colonoscopy every 5 yr beginning at age 40 yr, or 10 yr younger than earliest diagnosis, whichever comes first
Hereditary nonpolyposis colorectal cancer	Genetic counseling and screening[†] Colonoscopy every 1 to 2 years beginning at age 25 yr and then yearly after age 40 yr[‡]
Familial adenomatous polyposis and variants	Genetic counseling and testing[†] Flexible sigmoidoscopy yearly beginning at puberty[‡]
Personal history of CRC	Colonoscopy within 1 yr of curative resection; repeat at 3 yr and then every 5 yr if normal
Personal history of colorectal adenoma	Colonoscopy every 3 to 5 yr after removal of all index polyps
Inflammatory bowel disease	Colonoscopy every 1 to 2 yr beginning after 8 yr of pancolitis or after 15 yr if only left-sided disease

*Recommendations proposed by the American Cancer Society and U.S. Multi-Society Task Force on Colorectal Cancer; recommendations for average-risk patients also endorsed by the American College of Radiology.
[†]Whenever possible, affected relatives should be tested first because of potential false-negative results.
[‡]Screening recommendation for individuals with positive or indeterminate tests as well as for those who refuse genetic testing.

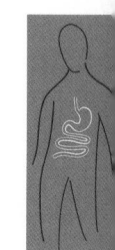

Colonoscopic surveillance is recommended for patients with a history of colorectal cancer or adenomas and inflammatory bowel disease.

THERAPY

The rate of survival of patients with colorectal carcinoma is based on the stage of disease (Table 39-3). Unfortunately, 45% of patients first come to medical attention with stage III or IV disease. Surgery alone is curative for early-stage colorectal cancers. Surgery and adjuvant chemotherapy with 5-fluorouracil and leucovorin ± oxiliplatin or capecitabine alone are recommended for stage III colon cancer. For patients with stage II and III rectal cancer, the combination of postoperative radiation and 5-fluorouracil (± leucovorin) has been found to significantly reduce the recurrence rate, cancer-related deaths, and overall mortality. Independent of nodal status, preoperative chemoradiotherapy followed adjuvant chemotherapy is recommended for patients with locally advanced rectal cancers. For patients with stage IV disease, palliative surgery, chemotherapy, and radiation therapy are the mainstays of therapy.

Carcinoid Tumors

The overall incidence of gastrointestinal carcinoid tumors in the United States is estimated at 1 to 2 cases per 100,000 people. The most common sites, in descending order of frequency, are the small intestine (ileum), rectum, appendix, colon, and stomach.

Carcinoid tumors arise from neuroendocrine cells and contain a variety of secretory granules containing various hormones and biogenic amines. Serotonin is synthesized

Table 39-3 Survival and Comparison of Dukes and TNM Staging in Colorectal Carcinoma

Dukes	TNM Stage	5-Year Survival Rate (%)
A	I	93
B	II	72-85
C	III	44-83
D	IV	8

from 5-hydroxytryptophan and metabolized in the liver to 5-hydroxyindoleacetic acid, which is biologically inert and secreted in the urine. The release of serotonin (hindgut tumors) and other vasoactive substances into the systemic circulation is thought to cause the carcinoid syndrome. Therefore, carcinoid metastases in the liver or other sites that drain into systemic veins may be associated with the carcinoid syndrome, as may primary carcinoids in the ovary or bronchus. The symptoms include episodic flushing, wheezing, diarrhea, right-sided valvular heart disease, and, potentially, vasomotor collapse. Localized tumors may present with gross or occult bleeding, obstructive symptoms, or abdominal pain depending on their location.

Most carcinoids are indolent; however, the malignant potential is variable and appears to be related to the site and, often, the size of the primary tumor. Carcinoids arising in the ileum and those 2 cm or larger have the greatest malignant potential. Surgical resection is the only curative treatment for carcinoid tumors. Somatostatin analogues are highly effective in the management of the symptoms of carcinoid syndrome.

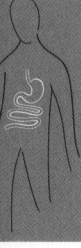

Prospectus for the Future

Further elucidation of the clinical and molecular epidemiologic mechanisms of gastrointestinal neoplasms will improve risk stratification and enable clinicians to tailor their use of screening and surveillance strategies, chemopreventive agents, and therapeutic options.

Progress in our understanding of the cellular and molecular pathways that underlie neoplastic transformation and tumor progression will provide additional targets for selective pharmacologic or immunologic therapies.

Technologic advances will facilitate the endoscopic diagnosis and treatment of premalignant and malignant diseases of the gastrointestinal tract.

References

Dicken BJ, Bigam DL, Cass C, et al: Gastric adenocarcinoma: Review and considerations for future directions. Ann Surg 241:27-39, 2005.

Houghton J, Wang TC: *Helicobacter pylori* infection and gastric cancer: A new paradigm for inflammation-associated epithelial cancers. Gastroenterology 1281567-1281578, 2005.

Levin B, Lieberman DA, McFarland B, et al: Screening and surveillance for the early detection of colorectal cancer and adenomatous Polyps, 2008: A joint guideline from the American Cancer Society, the US Multi-Society Task Force on Colorectal Cancer, and the American College of Radiology. CA Cancer J Clin 58:130-160, 2008.

Shaheen N: Advances in Barrett esophagus and esophageal adenocarcinoma. Gastroenterology 128:1554-1566, 2005.

Winawer SJ, Zauber AG, Fletcher RH, et al: Guidelines for colonoscopy surveillance after polypectomy: A consensus update by the US Multi-Society Task Force on Colorectal Cancer and the American Cancer Society. Gastroenterology 130:1872, 2006.

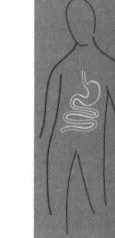

Diseases of the Pancreas

David R. Lichtenstein

Anatomy and Physiology

The pancreas is an organ located in the retroperitoneum (Fig. 40-1) that weighs between 70 and 120 g and is about 12 to 20 cm in length. The head of the pancreas is nestled in the C loop of the duodenum, and the tail extends obliquely posterior to the stomach toward the hilum of the spleen. The pancreas consists of the pancreatic acinus and islet cells. The acinar cells compose more than 95%, and the islets about 1% to 2%, of the pancreatic mass. Hormones that the islets produce include insulin, glucagon, somatostatin, and pancreatic polypeptide. The functional exocrine unit of the pancreas is the pancreatic acinus, which is composed of both acinar and ductal epithelial cells. Acinar cells synthesize proteolytic digestive enzymes, which are packaged separately in the Golgi region into condensing vacuoles and transported in an inactive form referred to as *zymogens* to the apical portions of the cell, where they are discharged into the central ductule of the acinus by exocytosis. The ductules coalesce to form larger ducts, which empty into the duodenum at the ampulla of Vater. Inactive enzymes secreted into the duodenum are converted to an active form by enterokinase secreted from small bowel enterocytes. Trypsinogen, converted to active trypsin in the duodenum by enterokinase, is the trigger enzyme that subsequently converts the other zymogens to active enzymes (Fig. 40-2). Enzymes secreted in an active form include lipase, amylase, and ribonuclease. The ductal cells secrete primarily water and electrolytes, which decrease the viscosity of the protein-rich acinar secretions and alkalinize gastric contents emptied into the duodenum to levels at which the pancreatic enzymes become catalytically active (pH ranges from >3.5 to 4).

Normal Pancreas Development

At about 4 weeks of gestation, the dorsal pancreas forms as an evagination from the duodenum, and shortly thereafter, the ventral pancreas forms from the hepatic diverticulum. Rotation of the duodenum places the two pancreatic buds in close proximity at 7 to 8 weeks of gestation, at which time

their main ducts begin to fuse. If fusion is incomplete, the duct of Wirsung drains only the ventral pancreas through the major ampulla, and the duct of Santorini drains the bulk of the pancreas (dorsal pancreas) through the relatively small accessory ampulla. This common anomaly, termed *pancreas divisum,* is present in 5% to 10% of the general population and may be associated with acute and chronic pancreatitis. Theories suggest that pancreatitis may result from relative outflow obstruction of the main dorsal duct through the small accessory ampulla. Endoscopic papillotomy or surgical sphincteroplasty are two therapeutic maneuvers that may reduce the incidence of recurrent pancreatitis by increasing drainage through the accessory papilla.

Acute Pancreatitis

Acute pancreatitis is best defined as an acute inflammatory process of the pancreas that may also involve peripancreatic tissues and remote organ systems. The overall incidence is 1 in 4000 for the general population. Most patients with acute pancreatitis have a mild course and recover with restoration of normal pancreatic function and gland architecture. However, in 10% to 20%, the various pathways that contribute to increased intrapancreatic and extrapancreatic inflammation result in what is generally termed *systemic inflammatory response syndrome* (SIRS). In some instances, SIRS predisposes to multiple organ dysfunction or pancreatic necrosis. Early steps in the management of patients with acute pancreatitis can decrease severity, morbidity, and mortality. Prevention of the septic and nonseptic complications in patients with severe acute pancreatitis depends largely on monitoring, vigorous hydration, and early recognition of pancreatic necrosis and choledocholithiasis.

CAUSES AND PATHOGENESIS

The pathogenesis of acute pancreatitis remains incompletely understood. Based on experimental models, the initiating event in acute pancreatitis is intra-acinar activation of trypsin from trypsinogen, resulting in acute intracellular injury, pancreatic autodigestion, and the potential for

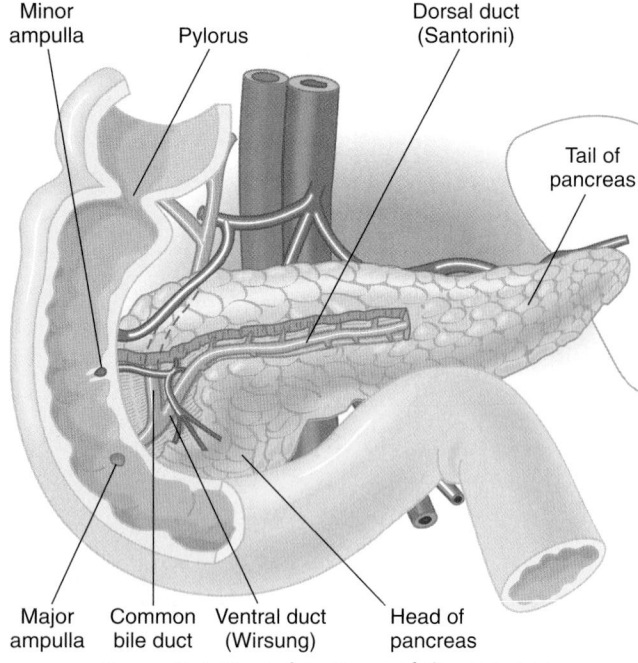

Figure 40-1 Normal anatomy of the pancreas.

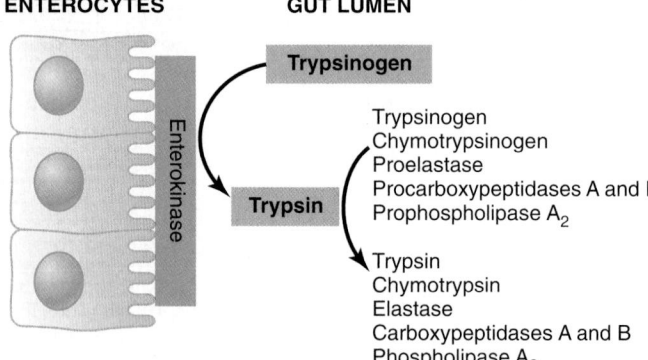

Figure 40-2 Mechanism of proenzyme activation in the intestinal lumen. (Adapted from Solomon TE: Exocrine pancreas: Pancreatitis. In The Undergraduate Teaching Project in Gastroenterology and Liver Disease, Unit 24. Bethesda, Md, American Gastroenterological Association, 1984.)

profound systemic complications once activated enzymes are leaked into the bloodstream. Initiating events may include obstruction of the pancreatic duct (e.g., gallstones, pancreatic tumor), overdistention of the pancreatic duct (e.g., from endoscopic retrograde cholangiopancreatography [ERCP]), reflux of biliary or duodenal juices into the pancreatic duct, changes in permeability of the pancreatic duct, ischemia of the organ, and toxin-induced cholinergic hyperstimulation.

During the initial hospitalization for acute pancreatitis, reasonable attempts to determine etiology is appropriate, particularly those causes that may affect acute management. The cause of acute pancreatitis is readily identified in 70% to 90% of patients after an initial evaluation consisting of history, physical examination, focused laboratory testing, and routine radiologic evaluation. Gallstones account for 45%, alcohol 35%, miscellaneous causes 10%, and idiopathic causes 10% to 20% of acute pancreatitis cases (Table 40-1).

Table 40-1 Causes of Acute Pancreatitis

Obstructive Causes

Gallstones
Tumors: ampullary or pancreatic tumors
Parasites: *Ascaris* or *Clonorchis* species
Developmental anomalies: pancreas divisum, choledochocele, annular pancreas
Periampullary duodenal diverticula
Hypertensive sphincter of Oddi
Afferent duodenal loop obstruction

Toxins

Ethyl alcohol
Methyl alcohol
Scorpion venom: excessive cholinergic stimulation causes salivation, sweating, dyspnea, and cardiac arrhythmias; seen mostly in the West Indies
Organophosphorus insecticides

Drugs

Definite association (documented with rechallenges): azathioprine/6-mercaptopurine, valproic acid, estrogens, tetracycline, metronidazole, nitrofurantoin, pentamidine, furosemide, sulfonamides, methyldopa, cytarabine, cimetidine, ranitidine, sulindac, dideoxycytidine
Probable association: thiazides, ethacrynic acid, phenformin, procainamide, chlorthalidone, L-asparaginase

Metabolic Causes

Hypertriglyceridemia, hypercalcemia, end-stage renal disease

Trauma

Accidental: blunt trauma to the abdomen (car accident, bicycle)
Iatrogenic: postoperative, endoscopic retrograde cholangiopancreatography, endoscopic sphincterotomy, sphincter of Oddi manometry

Infectious

Parasitic: ascariasis, clonorchiasis
Viral: mumps, rubella, hepatitis A, hepatitis B, non-A and non-B hepatitis, coxsackievirus B, echovirus, adenovirus, cytomegalovirus, varicella virus, Epstein-Barr virus, human immunodeficiency virus
Bacterial: mycoplasma, *Campylobacter jejuni*, tuberculosis, *Legionella* species, leptospirosis

Vascular

Ischemia: hypoperfusion (such as postcardiac surgery) or atherosclerotic emboli
Vasculitis: systemic lupus erythematosus, polyarteritis nodosa, malignant hypertension

Idiopathic

Ten to 30% of patients with pancreatitis; up to 60% of these patients have occult gallstone disease (biliary microlithiasis or gallbladder sludge). Other less common causes include sphincter of Oddi dysfunction and mutations in the cystic fibrosis transmembrane regulator.

Miscellaneous

Penetrating peptic ulcer
Crohn disease of the duodenum
Pregnancy associated
Pediatric association: Reye syndrome, cystic fibrosis

CLINICAL MANIFESTATIONS

Abdominal pain is virtually always present and may be severe and refractory to analgesics. Pain often radiates to the back and is usually worse when supine. The onset may be swift with pain reaching maximal intensity within 30 minutes, is frequently unbearable, and characteristically persists for more than 24 hours without relief. Physical examination usually reveals severe upper abdominal tenderness at times associated with guarding. Ileus occurs when the inflammatory process extends into the small intestinal and colonic mesentery or when a chemical peritonitis occurs. Other manifestations include nausea, vomiting, and fever caused by the significant inflammatory process and release of cytokines (Fig. 40-3).

In acute pancreatitis, a wide variety of toxic materials, including pancreatic enzymes, vasoactive materials (e.g., kinins), and other toxic substances (e.g., elastase, phospholipase A_2), are liberated by the pancreas and extravasate along fascial planes in the retroperitoneal space, lesser sac, and the peritoneal cavity. These materials cause chemical irritation and contribute to third-space losses of protein-rich fluid, hypovolemia, and hypotension. These toxic materials may also reach the systemic circulation by lymphatic and venous pathways and contribute to subcutaneous fat necrosis and end-organ damage, including shock, renal failure, and respiratory insufficiency (atelectasis, effusions, and acute respiratory distress syndrome [ARDS]). Grey Turner sign (ecchymosis of the flank) or Cullen sign (ecchymosis in the periumbilical region) may be seen in association with hemorrhagic pancreatitis.

Metabolic problems are common in severe disease and include hypocalcemia, hyperglycemia, and acidosis. Hypocalcemia is most commonly caused by concomitant hypoalbuminemia. Other mechanisms may include complexing of calcium to released free fatty acids, protease-induced degradation of circulating parathyroid hormone (PTH), and failure of PTH to release calcium from bone. Local spread of inflammation leads to effects on contiguous organs that include gastritis and duodenitis, splenic vein thrombosis, colonic necrosis, and external compression of the common bile duct, leading to biliary obstruction. Trypsin can activate

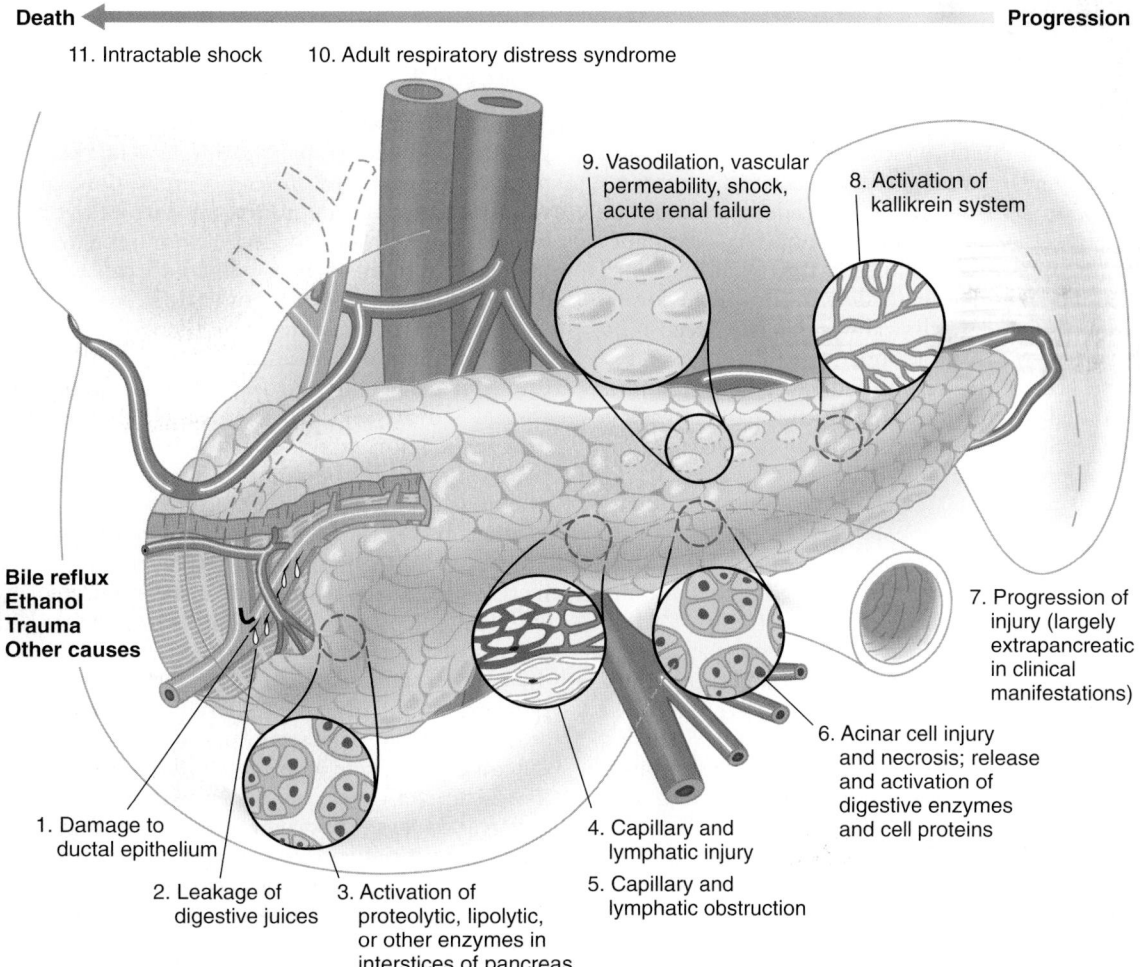

Figure 40-3 The pathophysiology of acute pancreatitis is not fully understood, but, as this schematic illustration implies, a cascade of events seems likely, beginning with the release of toxic substances into the parenchyma and ending with shock and death. Damage to the ductal epithelium or acinar cell injury may result from bile reflux, increased intraductal pressure, alcohol, or trauma. (Adapted from Grendell JH: The pancreas. In Smith LH Jr, Thier SO [eds]: Pathophysiology: The Biological Principles of Disease, 2nd ed. Philadelphia, WB Saunders, 1985, p 1228.)

plasminogen to plasmin and induce clot lysis. On the other hand, trypsin can activate prothrombin and thrombin and produce thrombosis, leading to disseminated intravascular coagulation. Extrapancreatic fluid collections occur when fluid extravasates from the pancreas or surrounding leaky tissues. They are located in or near the pancreas and lack a wall of granulation or fibrous tissue. Acute fluid collections occur more commonly with severe pancreatitis. Most of these lesions regress spontaneously, and almost all remain sterile. The older term *phlegmon* was used in the past to describe inflammatory collections, but it is too ambiguous and imprecise for current use, given that it does not differentiate acute fluid collections from areas of pancreatic necrosis nor infected from noninfected collections.

Pancreatic pseudocysts are defined as encapsulated nonepithelial lined collections of pancreatic juice, either pure or containing debris, single or multiple, small or large, and they can be located in or adjacent to the pancreas. Fluid collections must be present for a minimum of 4 weeks from the onset of pancreatitis to be termed a pseudocyst. Although most pseudocysts remain asymptomatic, presenting symptoms may include abdominal pain, early satiety, nausea, and vomiting due to compression of the stomach or gastric outlet. Rapidly enlarging pseudocysts may rupture, hemorrhage, obstruct the extrahepatic biliary tree, erode into surrounding structures, extend into the mediastinum, and become infected. Most pseudocysts less than 6 cm in diameter will resolve over time, and one third of lesions less than 10 cm in diameter remain asymptomatic or resolve. Indications for pseudocyst drainage include suspicion of infection or progressive enlargement with associated symptoms described previously. Asymptomatic pseudocysts should be followed. Pseudocysts can be drained surgically, percutaneously or endoscopically. The choice of treatment for symptomatic pseudocysts is frequently determined by the locally available expertise and by clinician preference because no method has been shown to be superior to the others. Pancreatic fistula occurs as a result of duct disruption and is treated with total parenteral nutrition, endoscopic stenting, and octreotide. Surgical intervention may be needed if the conservative approach is unsuccessful.

DIAGNOSIS

The diagnosis of acute pancreatitis is based on a combination of clinical, biochemical, and radiologic factors. There is general acceptance that a diagnosis of acute pancreatitis requires two of the following three features: (1) abdominal pain characteristic of acute pancreatitis, (2) serum amylase or lipase more than 3 times the upper limit of normal, and (3) characteristic findings of acute pancreatitis on computed tomography (CT) scan. Elevated serum pancreatic enzymes may occur in a wide variety of other conditions, including bowel perforation, intestinal obstruction, mesenteric ischemia, tubo-ovarian disease, and renal failure. Serum lipase is slightly more specific and remains normal in some conditions associated with an elevation of serum amylase, including macroamylasemia, parotitis, and tubo-ovarian disease. The serum amylase level usually rises rapidly, as does the serum lipase level, and may remain elevated for 3 to 5 days. Serum lipase remains elevated longer than amylase and thus may be helpful if patients seek medical attention several days after symptom onset. Repeated measurements of pancreatic enzymes have little value in assessing clinical progress, and the magnitude of serum amylase or lipase elevation does not correlate with the severity of pancreatitis. Macroamylase and macrolipase can occasionally cause isolated nonpathologic elevations of these enzymes, a situation in which the measurement of urinary clearance is useful.

Pancreatic imaging with CT scanning can be used to confirm a diagnosis of pancreatitis (pancreatic enlargement, peripancreatic inflammatory changes, and extrapancreatic fluid collections). Selective CT scanning may also be useful in evaluating complications and assessing severity of disease (see later discussion), although a normal CT scan is present in 15% to 30% of mild cases. Acute gallstone pancreatitis should be suspected in patients with gallstones on ultrasonography or elevated liver tests, in particular an aspartate aminotransferase level elevated greater than threefold. Magnetic resonance imaging (MRI) is similar to CT with respect to imaging the inflamed pancreas and may be preferred in individuals at risk for contrast-induced injury (e.g., contrast allergy or renal insufficiency). However, recent studies also indicate the potential for gadolinium-induced nephrotoxicity with MRI examinations. MRI is also sensitive for the detection of necrosis, small neoplasms of the pancreas, and stones in the pancreaticobiliary tree.

SEVERITY OF DISEASE

Supportive therapy alone is effective in treating 75% of all patients with acute pancreatitis. Twenty-five percent of patients, however, will suffer a complication, with one third succumbing to complications, yielding an overall mortality rate of 5% to 10%. Early deaths within the first 2 weeks are the result of multisystem organ failure caused by the release of inflammatory mediators and cytokines. Late deaths result from local or systemic infection. The risks for infection and death correlate with disease severity and the presence and extent of pancreatic necrosis. Therefore, a combination of clinical scoring and CT grade provides the most precise prognostic information.

Patients should be stratified into mild or severe levels of illness based on well-established clinical criteria such as Ranson criteria (Table 40-2) or Acute Physiologic and Chronic Health Evaluation (APACHE II) scores. With increasing scores, the likelihood of a complicated, prolonged, and fatal outcome increases. The mortality rate is about 1% when fewer than three Ranson signs exist, 10% to 20% when three to five signs exist, and more than 50% when six Ranson signs exist. Similarly, an APACHE II score greater than 8 has been shown to predict severe pancreatitis. Conversely, a fatal outcome is unlikely with an APACHE II score less than 8. The distinction between interstitial and necrotizing acute pancreatitis has important prognostic implications (Fig. 40-4). Interstitial pancreatitis is characterized by an intact microcirculation and uniform enhancement of the gland on contrast-enhanced CT scanning. About 20% to 30% of patients with acute pancreatitis have necrotizing pancreatitis. Necrotizing pancreatitis is characterized by disruption of the pancreatic microcirculation so that large areas do not enhance on CT (Fig. 40-5). The presence of pancreatic necrosis predicts a worse severity of pancreatitis, particularly infection in the necrotic pancreatic tissue, also termed

Table 40-2 **Signs Used to Assess Severity of Acute Pancreatitis**
At Time of Admission or Diagnosis
Age > 55 yr
White blood cell count > 16,000/mm³
Blood glucose > 200 mg/dL
LDH > 2 × normal
ALT > 6 × normal
During Initial 48 Hours
Decrease in hematocrit > 10%
Serum calcium < 8 mg/dL
Increase in blood urea nitrogen > 5 mg/dL
Arterial Po₂ < 60 mm Hg
Base deficit > 4 mEq/L
Estimated fluid sequestration > 600 mL

ALT, alanine aminotransferase; LDH, lactate dehydrogenase; Po₂, partial pressure of oxygen.

Data from Ranson JH, Rifkind KM, Turner JW: Prognostic signs and nonoperative peritoneal lavage in acute pancreatitis. Surg Gynecol Obstet 43:209-219, 1976. By permission of *Surgery, Gynecology and Obstetrics.*

infected necrosis. Infected necrosis develops in 30% to 50% of patients with acute necrotizing pancreatitis but rarely in those with interstitial disease (<1%). The mortality rate for infected necrosis approaches 30%, accounting for more than 80% of deaths from acute pancreatitis. In those individuals with necrotizing pancreatitis and suspected infection (fever, leukocytosis, organ failure), antibiotics should be administered while appropriate cultures (including culture of CT-guided percutaneous aspiration of the pancreas) are obtained. Antibiotics can be discontinued if no source of infection is found because the success of prophylactic antibiotics in patients with severe pancreatitis in reducing infectious complications (central line sepsis, pulmonary infection, urinary tract infection, and infected pancreatic necrosis) has not been demonstrated. Moreover, broad-spectrum antibiotic use in these individuals may lead to the emergence of resistant organisms and fungal infections in the necrotic pancreas. Because clinical and laboratory findings are often similar in patients with either sterile or infected necrosis, the diagnosis of infected necrosis is made by percutaneous

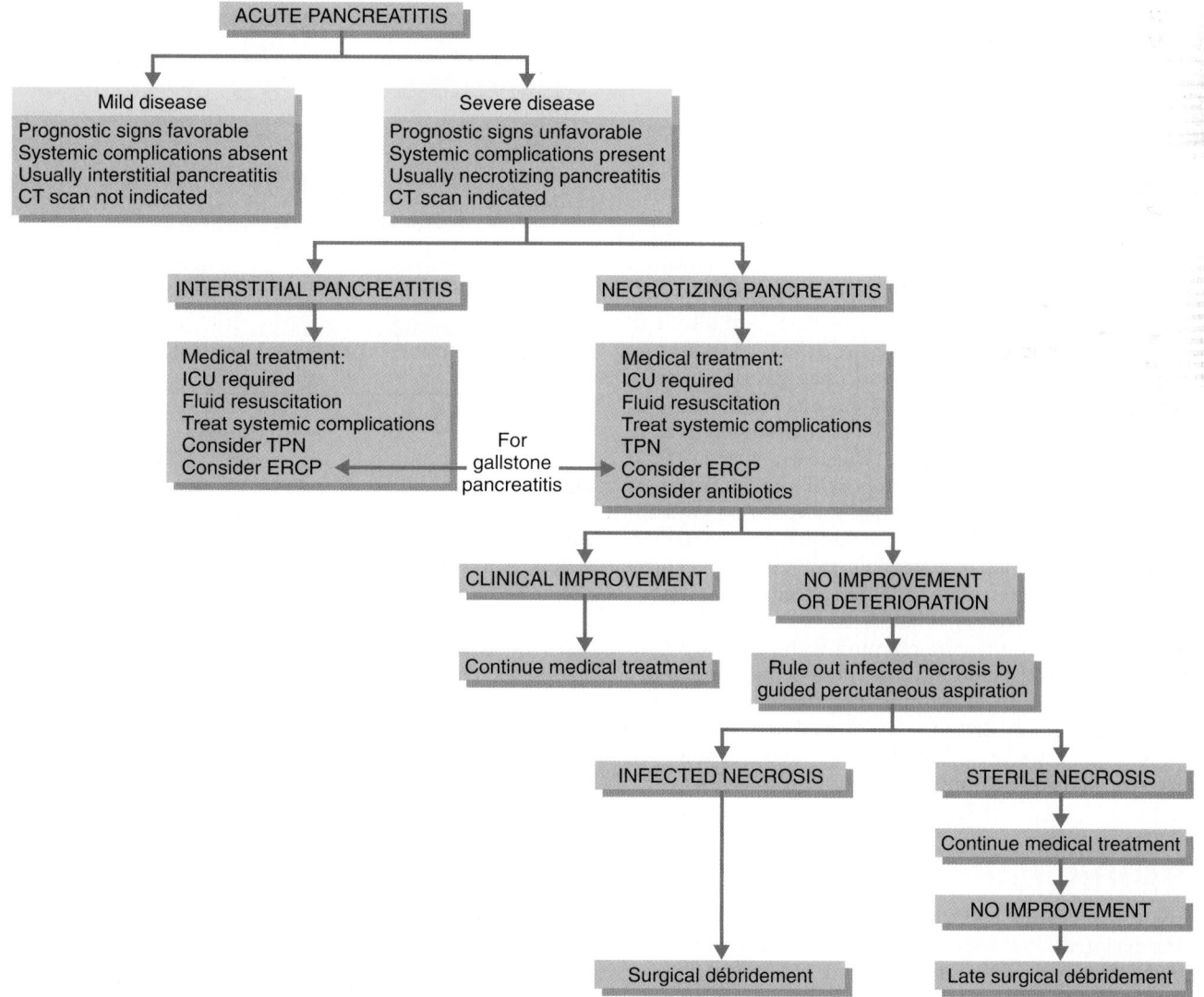

Figure 40-4 Therapeutic algorithm for evaluating acute pancreatitis. CT, computed tomography; ERCP, endoscopic retrograde cholangiopancreatography; ICU, intensive care unit; TPN, total parenteral nutrition. (From Banks PA: Acute and chronic pancreatitis. In Feldman M, Scharschmidt BF, Sleisenger MH [eds]: Sleisenger and Fordtran's Gastrointestinal and Liver Disease: Pathophysiology/Diagnosis/Management, 6th ed. Philadelphia, WB Saunders, 1998, p 833.)

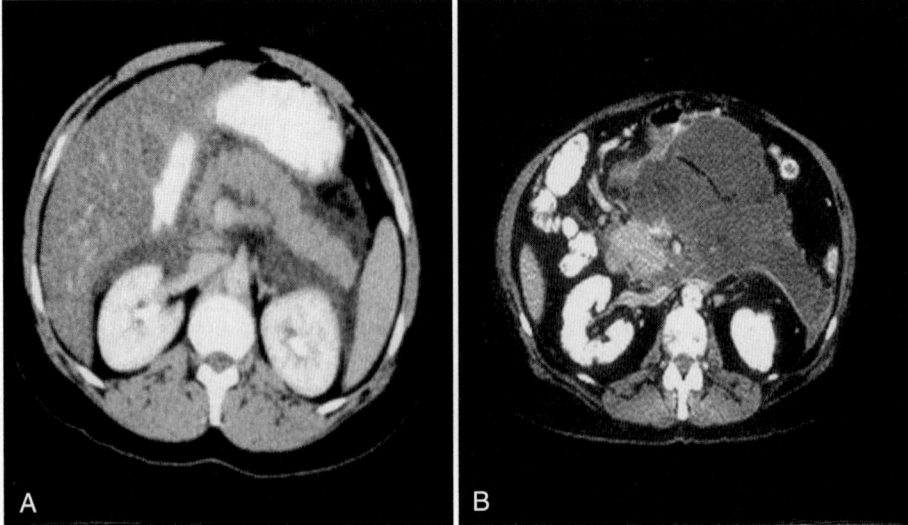

Figure 40-5 Contrast computed tomography scans demonstrating interstitial pancreatitis (**A**) and necrotizing pancreatitis (**B**).

CT-guided needle aspiration (Gram stain and culture), which is safe and accurate. Patients with infected necrosis require surgical débridement, whereas patients with sterile necrosis can be followed with supportive therapy, reserving surgical débridement for persistent end-organ failure.

TREATMENT

In addition to supportive care, the goals of medical therapy include limiting systemic complications and preventing pancreatic infection once necrosis takes place. No specific treatments have proved effective in lowering morbidity and mortality, including agents that put the pancreas to rest (e.g., somatostatin, calcitonin, glucagon, nasogastric suction, histamine-2 receptor blockers) and enzyme inhibitors (e.g., aprotinin, gabexate mesilate). All patients should receive close supportive care, including effective analgesia, fluid resuscitation, and nutritional support if oral nutrition is anticipated to be withheld for more than 7 to 10 days. To meet metabolic demands and rest the pancreas, nutrition can be provided by total parenteral nutrition through central venous access or preferably as enteral feeding through a jejunal nasoenteric feeding tube. Systemic complications are best managed in an intensive care unit with aggressive fluid administration and hemodynamic monitoring. Emergency ERCP (**Web Video 40-1**) for removing impacted gallstones or establishing biliary drainage is indicated for patients with evidence of biliary sepsis. This procedure should be followed by elective cholecystectomy.

Chronic Pancreatitis

Chronic pancreatitis is defined as an inflammatory disease of the pancreas characterized by irreversible morphologic changes that typically cause pain and permanent loss of function. Chronic pancreatitis can be classified into nonobstructive and obstructive types (Table 40-3). The most common nonobstructive cause is chronic alcoholism (70%). Alcohol can cause episodes of acute pancreatitis, but at the

Table 40-3 **Causes of Chronic Pancreatitis**
Nonobstructive
Alcohol
Idiopathic: 10%-20% of total cases
Tropical, nutritional
Inherited: cystic fibrosis, hereditary
Traumatic
Metabolic: hypertriglyceridemia, hypercalcemia
Obstructive
Benign obstruction: sphincter of Oddi dysfunction or papillary stenosis, pancreas divisum with obstruction of accessory ampulla
Neoplastic obstruction: tumors of the ampulla or ductal system

time of the initial attack, structural and functional abnormalities often exist indicative of underlying chronic pancreatitis. Because most alcoholics do not develop pancreatitis, the presumption is that other unidentified genetic, dietary, or environmental influences exist. If alcoholism is excluded, most patients with chronic pancreatitis in the United States have no demonstrable cause, termed idiopathic (20%). Gallstone pancreatitis, the major cause of acute pancreatitis, almost never leads to chronic pancreatitis. Calcific pancreatitis of the tropics is a major cause of chronic pancreatitis worldwide. Other miscellaneous causes (10%) include trauma, pancreas divisum, cystic fibrosis, hereditary pancreatitis, and metabolic disturbances such as hypercalcemia and hypertriglyceridemia.

PATHOGENESIS

Alcoholic pancreatitis is the result of abnormal secretion and necrosis fibrosis of the gland. The *abnormal secretion theory* notes that chronic alcohol ingestion induces hypersecretion of protein from the acinar cell, increased secretion of ionized calcium, concomitant defects in ductal bicarbonate (HCO_3^-) secretion decreasing the solubility of secretory proteins

(GP2), and reduced secretion of lithostathine (formerly called *pancreatic stone protein*), a low-molecular-weight, nonenzymatic protein that inhibits lattice formation by binding to growth sites of calcium carbonate crystals. These secretory defects favor the formation of calcium-protein complexes and ultimately lead to intraductal protein precipitates that obstruct ductules. Progressive blockage of both small ducts and the main pancreatic duct leads to further structural deterioration of ducts, acinar tissue, and eventually islets of Langerhans. The *necrosis fibrosis theory* suggests that alcohol may also have specific cytotoxic effects on acinar cells that act independently to cause tissue damage, possibly even acute pancreatitis. The acute attacks of pancreatitis lead to necrosis of the parenchyma and disruption of the ductal system. After the necrosis subsides and healing occurs, fibrosis of the main duct occurs, which obstructs the gland and leads to large duct disease.

Hereditary pancreatitis results from a mutation of a gene on chromosome 7q that encodes for an abnormal cationic trypsinogen, which cannot be inactivated by intracellular protective proteins. Normally active trypsin is degraded by cleavage of Arg at position 117. In hereditary pancreatitis, Arg is mutated to His, preventing cleavage and resulting in accumulation of active trypsin.

CLINICAL MANIFESTATIONS

Although several different clinical patterns can be seen, most patients with chronic pancreatitis experience pain that can be episodic or continuous. Pain may be accompanied by steatorrhea with symptoms of diarrhea and weight loss. On occasion, patients exhibit exocrine or endocrine insufficiency in the absence of pain. Other patients are asymptomatic and found to have chronic pancreatitis incidentally on imaging.

The pain of chronic pancreatitis is poorly understood. Possible causes include inflammation of the pancreas, increased intrapancreatic pressure, neural inflammation, or extrapancreatic causes, such as stenosis of the common bile duct and duodenum. Evidence in favor of pressure as a cause of pancreatic pain includes reports of pain relief following endoscopic or surgical decompression of a dilated main pancreatic duct. Steatorrhea does not occur until the output of lipase is decreased to less than 10% of normal. Diabetes mellitus is a late complication of chronic pancreatitis, becoming apparent only after 80% to 90% of the gland is severely damaged. The complications of chronic pancreatitis include the development of pseudocysts, pancreatic fistulas, biliary obstruction, pancreatic cancer, small bowel bacterial overgrowth, and gastric varices secondary to splenic vein thrombosis.

DIAGNOSIS

Because direct biopsy of the pancreas is considered too risky, the diagnosis of chronic pancreatitis is typically based on tests of pancreatic structure and function. Marked structural changes usually, but not always, correlate with severe functional impairment, as determined by pancreatic function tests. In early chronic pancreatitis, however, mild abnormalities of pancreatic function can precede any morphologic changes seen on imaging. Moreover, tests of pancreatic

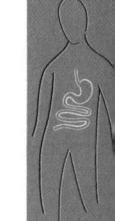

structure may remain normal even with advanced deterioration of pancreatic function and with severe structural deterioration. Laboratory evaluation, such as amylase and lipase, are frequently normal in the setting of well-established chronic pancreatitis, and serum pancreatic enzymes thus neither confirm nor exclude the diagnosis.

TESTS OF FUNCTION

The secretin stimulation test is considered the gold standard functional test for diagnosing chronic pancreatitis. The observation that HCO_3^- production is impaired early in chronic pancreatitis has led to the rationale for use of this test to diagnose chronic pancreatitis in the early stages of disease (sensitivity of 95%). This test involves the oral placement of a catheter into the duodenum for aspiration of pancreatic juice before and after stimulation with intravenous secretin. This quantitative measure of pancreatic secretion and enzyme activity is primarily performed in patients with chronic abdominal pain in whom the diagnosis of chronic pancreatitis is suspected and in whom results of imaging studies are negative or equivocal. The secretin test is not widely given because the study is labor intensive and is uncomfortable for patients.

Several less invasive tests have been developed, but they are all less accurate than the secretin test, especially in the diagnosis of early chronic pancreatitis. The 72-hour fecal fat determination is often regarded as the gold standard to document steatorrhea (fecal fat > 7 g per 24 hours); however, the test is not specific for pancreatic exocrine insufficiency. The test also lacks sensitivity because steatorrhea will not occur in chronic pancreatitis until pancreatic lipase output falls to less than 5% to 10% of normal. The serum trypsinogen level correlates with functioning acinar parenchyma. A low level (<10 ng/mL) is highly specific for exocrine pancreatic insufficiency. The sensitivity is 80% to 90% in patients with advanced chronic pancreatitis with steatorrhea but only 10% to 20% in those without steatorrhea. Fecal chymotrypsin or elastase levels may be used as a simple stool test of pancreatic function, but neither is commonly employed in the United States.

TESTS OF STRUCTURE

Findings that suggest chronic pancreatitis include ductal abnormalities (dilation, stones, duct irregularity), parenchymal abnormalities (calcification, inhomogeneity, atrophy), gland contour changes, and pseudocysts. Imaging studies may be normal in the early stages of disease. Plain film radiography of the abdomen for detecting pancreatic calcifications can be seen in 20% to 50% of individuals with alcohol-induced chronic pancreatitis. The test should be the first diagnostic test performed when pancreatitis is suspected because it is both simple and inexpensive. Calcifications not detected on plain films can be detected more readily by CT scanning (Fig. 40-6).

ERCP (**Web Video 40-2**) and endoscopic ultrasonography (EUS) are the most sensitive imaging studies to evaluate for structural abnormalities of the pancreatic parenchyma and ductular system. The major limitation of ERCP is the development of procedure-related acute pancreatitis in up to 5% of patients. As a result, ERCP should be reserved for

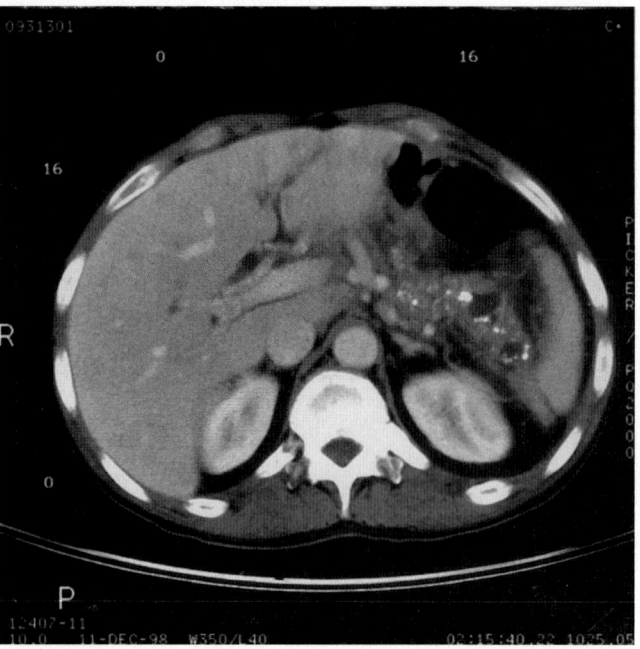

Figure 40-6 Computed tomography scan of a patient with calcifications and small pseudocysts in the pancreas consistent with chronic pancreatitis.

patients in whom the diagnosis cannot be established or for evaluating symptomatic complications (stones, strictures) associated with chronic pancreatitis. EUS appears to be promising, with early findings that may be more sensitive compared with other tests of structure or function. Magnetic resonance cholangiopancreatography (MRCP) is a noninvasive diagnostic imaging modality that provides visualization of the pancreatic and biliary systems with images similar to those seen by ERCP but without the risk for precipitating acute pancreatitis.

TREATMENT

Pancreatic enzyme preparations are effective at treating malabsorption and are clinically indicated if patients suffering from chronic pancreatitis lose more than 10% of their body weight, excrete more than 15 g per day of fat with their stool, or suffer from dyspepsia. Four types of pancreatic enzyme preparations are available. Most commercial preparations consist of pancreatin, which is the shock-frozen powdered extract of porcine pancreas containing lipase, amylase, trypsin, and chymotrypsin. Enzyme supplements are not absorbed from the gastrointestinal tract but rather are inactivated by enteral bacterial flora or digestive secretions and fecally eliminated. Administration of acid-stable, encapsulated microspheres or microtablets filled with pancreatic enzymes has greatly increased the efficacy of enzyme supplementation in chronic pancreatitis. Patients with documented exocrine insufficiency should eat three main meals a day and three snacks in between. In general, 25,000 to 50,000 IU of lipase should be ingested simultaneously along with a main meal and 25,000 IU of lipase with snacks; it should not be taken either before or after the meals. When gastric hyperacidity is present, proton pump inhibitors or histamine-2 receptor antagonists should be used to delay enzyme inacti-

vation. In cases of progressive maldigestion and steatorrhea, supplementing lipid-soluble vitamins parenterally may be necessary. In cases of severe exocrine insufficiency, one third of the daily caloric intake can be met by administering medium-chain triglycerides (MCTs), which do not require lipolysis by lipase for absorption. Although clinically effective, patients usually do not like MCT fat because of poor palatability. Symptom improvement, not laboratory tests, demonstrates the efficacy of enzyme supplementation. If these methods do not provide improvement, the next step is to decrease dietary fat intake to less than 50 g per day and to substitute MCTs, which do not require hydrolysis before absorption, for some dietary fat. Other factors may accentuate steatorrhea, including concomitant small bowel bacterial overgrowth, which can occur in up to 25% of patients with chronic pancreatitis. Bacterial overgrowth may be caused by hypomotility of the gut secondary to inflammatory diseases of the head of the pancreas or to chronic use of narcotic analgesics.

The greatest challenge in treating chronic pancreatitis is controlling abdominal pain. Pain is said to improve over time but may take years and is not uniform. Methods of pain relief initially include abstinence from alcohol, analgesics, and pancreatic enzyme supplements. Supplemental pancreatic enzymes are given to decrease cholecystokinin-mediated pancreatic secretion, an approach that alleviates pain in some patients with chronic pancreatitis. Therapy is initiated with large doses of pancrelipases (non–enteric-coated) pancreatic enzyme preparations because, in theory, the enteric-coated preparations release their enzymes further down the intestine away from the stimulatory cholecystokinin (CCK) enterocytes. Nerve blocks (celiac plexus block and splanchnicectomy) yield equivocal results. Endoscopic decompression of pancreatic duct obstruction secondary to strictures or stones may result in pain relief. Surgical ductal drainage, usually with lateral pancreaticojejunostomy (Puestow procedure), may effectively decrease pain in about 80% of patients. This procedure is safe and has an operative mortality rate of less than 5%; however, only 50% of patients are free of pain at 5-year follow-up. Patients with nonobstructed, nondilated ductal systems may require pancreatic resection.

Carcinoma of the Pancreas

Carcinoma of the pancreas is the fourth leading cause of cancer in adults, with about 28,000 new cases and 25,000 deaths annually. The prognosis is grim; less than 20% of all patients are alive beyond the first year of disease, and only 1% to 3% are alive beyond the fifth year. Carcinoma of the pancreas accounts for about 5% of cancer deaths in the United States. More than 90% of these tumors are adenocarcinomas and arise from the ductal cells.

CAUSES AND PATHOGENESIS

Contributing factors include age, gender (male risk ratio 1.4:1), carcinogens, cigarette smoking, hereditary pancreatitis, chronic pancreatitis, and possibly a high-fat diet. Occu-

Diagnosis and Staging of Pancreatic Cancer

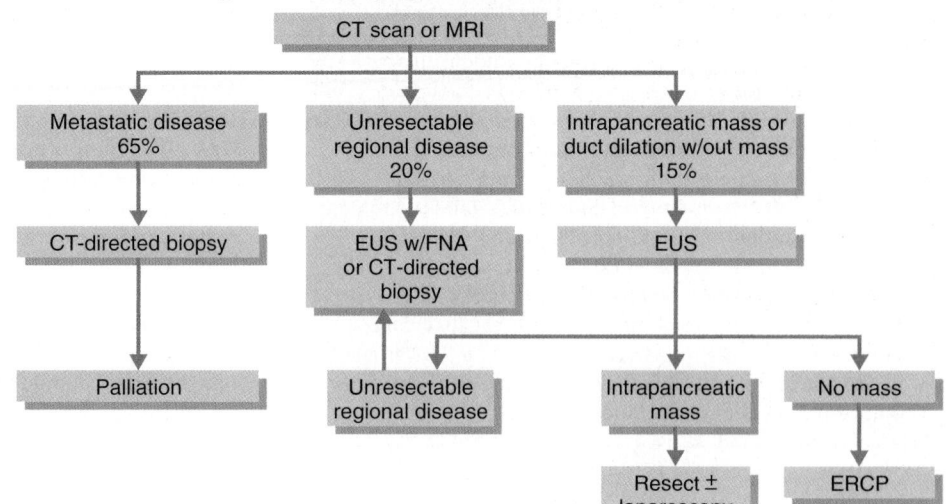

Figure 40-7 Diagnostic algorithm for evaluating a patient with suspected pancreatic carcinoma. CT, computed tomography; ERCP, endoscopic retrograde cholangiopancreatography. (From Cello JP: Pancreatic cancer. In Feldman M, Scharschmidt BF, Sleisenger MH [eds]: Sleisenger and Fordtran's Gastrointestinal and Liver Disease: Pathophysiology/Diagnosis/ Management, 6th ed. Philadelphia, WB Saunders, 1998, p 865.)

pational exposure to β-naphthylamine and benzidine are clear risk factors; however, these substances are not thought to be causative agents in most patients. Patients with long-standing diabetes may also be at a slightly increased risk. Neither alcohol nor coffee consumption appears to be a risk factor.

CLINICAL MANIFESTATIONS

The clinical manifestations of pancreatic carcinoma may be nonspecific and are often insidious. The tumor has usually reached an advanced stage by the time of diagnosis. Common presenting signs and symptoms of pancreatic cancer include jaundice, weight loss, and abdominal pain. The pain is usually constant, with radiation to the back. Because most cancers begin in the pancreatic head, patients may exhibit obstructive jaundice or a large, palpable gallbladder (Courvoisier sign). Painless jaundice is the most common presentation in patients with a potentially resectable and curable lesion. Anorexia, nausea, and vomiting may also occur, along with emotional disturbances, such as depression. Other, less common presenting symptoms include signs of migratory thrombophlebitis (Trousseau sign), acute pancreatitis, diabetes, paraneoplastic syndromes (Cushing syndrome), hypercalcemia, gastrointestinal bleeding, splenic vein thrombosis, and a palpable abdominal mass.

DIAGNOSIS AND STAGING

Diagnosis of pancreatic cancer is frequently suggested by the presence of a pancreatic mass on imaging studies. Evidence of a dilated pancreatic duct, hepatic metastases, invasion of vessels, or a dilated common bile duct in the setting of biliary obstruction may also be found. The appearance on imaging may be impossible to distinguish from benign causes of pancreatic masses such as focal pancreatitis. CT and MRI are the best initial studies to define a mass and assess for liver metastasis or vascular invasion. ERCP should be considered if

pancreatic cancer is suspected but a mass is not found on other imaging studies. ERCP will show a main pancreatic duct stricture in at least 97% of such cases (Fig. 40-7).

The use of tumor markers to diagnose carcinoma of the pancreas has yielded disappointing results. The tumor marker CA 19-9 has a sensitivity of 80% to 90% and a specificity of 85% to 95% in diagnosing pancreatic cancer in patients exhibiting signs and symptoms suggestive of pancreatic cancer. EUS, when compared with other imaging studies (spiral CT, MRI, and angiography), is the most accurate diagnostic and staging technique, providing information of tumor location, vascular invasion, and lymph node involvement. The major determinant of both operative resectability and long-term survival is the presence of vascular invasion (superior mesenteric artery or vein, portal vein) or metastatic disease. Unfortunately, only 10% to 20% of carcinomas in the head of the pancreas and essentially no cancers of the body and tail are resectable for cure. If evaluation is conclusive that a pancreatic tumor is not resectable, the first objective is to confirm the cell type, which can be done accurately by CT- or EUS-guided biopsy. When nonoperative staging suggests a resectable tumor, some centers prefer a staging laparoscopy before attempted curative resection.

TREATMENT

Surgery for resectable carcinoma of the head of the pancreas usually involves a Whipple operation. If resection cannot be done at the time of laparotomy, biliary diversion should be done to relieve jaundice, and gastrojejunostomy is performed if duodenal invasion is present to relieve duodenal obstruction. Surgery offers the only chance for cure. The rate of operative mortality is less than 5%. Attempts at radiation and chemotherapy have met with little success and only modest improvements in patient survival. For patients with inoperable lesions, palliative interventions to alleviate jaundice, pain, and intestinal obstruction often become the focus of therapy.

Prospectus for the Future

Our understanding of the pathophysiologic mechanisms responsible for pancreatitis and pancreatic malignancy will continue to evolve. This improved understanding will lead to early diagnosis and improved treatment options.

- Improvements in our understanding of the genetic predisposition for developing pancreatitis will lead to the identification of at-risk individuals and ultimately treatment options to prevent pancreatic injury.
- Elucidation of inciting factors and subsequent inflammatory mediators responsible for the local and systemic injuries seen in acute pancreatitis will offer early treatment options to reduce tissue injury and thereby reduce the severity of the disease process.

- Technologic advances in the endoscopic and minimally invasive surgical treatment of pancreatic necrosis will facilitate care and reduce morbidity and mortality.
- New modalities to evaluate tissue characteristics in early chronic pancreatitis will provide a gold standard for diagnosis and thereby allow for early detection and more appropriate treatment when pain is the presenting symptom.
- Further characterization of the early biologic changes that precede the development of symptomatic pancreatic malignancy will result in prevention, early detection, and new nonsurgical modalities for treatment.

References

American Gastroenterological Association: Medical position statement: Epidemiology, diagnosis, and treatment of pancreatic ductal adenocarcinoma. Gastroenterology 117:1463-1484, 1999.

Avgerinos C, Delis S, Rizos S, Dervenis C: Nutritional support in acute pancreatitis. Dig Dis Sci 21:214-219, 2003.

Banks PA, Freeman ML, and the Practice Parameters Committee of the American College of Gastroenterology: Practice guidelines in acute pancreatitis. Am J Gastroenterol 101:2379-2400, 2006.

Chowdhury RS, Forsmark CE: Pancreatic function testing [review]. Aliment Pharmacol Ther 17:733-750, 2003.

Draganov P, Forsmark CE: "Idiopathic" pancreatitis. Gastroenterology 128:756-763, 2005.

Ellis I, Lerch MM, Whitcomb DC: Consensus Committees of the European Registry of Hereditary Pancreatic Diseases, Midwest Multi-Center Pancreatic Study Group, International Association of Pancreatology. Genetic testing for hereditary pancreatitis: Guidelines for indications, counseling, consent and privacy issues. Pancreatology 1:405-415, 2001.

Etemad B, Whitcomb DC: Chronic pancreatitis: Diagnosis, classification, and new genetic developments. Gastroenterology 120:682-707, 2001.

Forsmark CE, Baillie J: AGA Institute technical review on acute pancreatitis. Gastroenterology 132:2022-2044, 2007.

Lockhart AC, Rothenberg ML, Berlin JD: Treatment for pancreatic cancer: Current therapy and continued progress. Gastroenterology 128:1642-1654, 2005.

Pandol SJ, Saluja AK, Imrie CW, Banks PA: Reviews in basic and clinical gastroenterology. Acute pancreatitis: Bench to bedside. Gastroenterology 132:1127-1151, 2007.

Rosch T, Daniel S, Scholz M, et al: Endoscopic treatment of chronic pancreatitis: A multicenter study of 1000 patients with long-term follow-up. Endoscopy 34:765-771, 2002.

Schneider G, Siveke JT, Eckel F, Schmid RM: Pancreatic cancer: Basic and clinical aspects. Gastroenterology 128:1606-1625, 2005.

Tenner S: Initial management of acute pancreatitis: Critical issues during the first 72 hours. Am J Gastroenterol 99:2489-2494, 2004.

Vege SS, Baron TH: Management of pancreatic necrosis in severe acute pancreatitis. Clin Gastroenterol Hepatol 3:192-196, 2005.

Warshaw AL, Banks, PA, Fernandez-Del Castillo C: AGA technical review: Treatment of pain in chronic pancreatitis. Gastroenterology 115:765-776, 1998.

Wray CJ, Ahmad SA, Matthews JB, Lowy AM: Surgery for pancreatic cancer: Recent controversies and current practice. Gastroenterology 128:1626-1641, 2005.

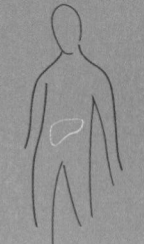

Section VIII

Diseases of the Liver and Biliary System

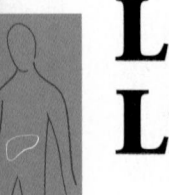

Laboratory Tests in Liver Disease

Rajan Kochar and Michael B. Fallon

The liver, the largest internal organ in the body, plays a central role in many essential physiologic processes, including glucose homeostasis, plasma protein synthesis, lipid and lipoprotein synthesis, bile acid synthesis and secretion, and vitamin storage (B_{12}, A, D, E, and K). In addition, the liver is vital in biotransformation, detoxification, and excretion of a vast array of endogenous and exogenous compounds. The clinical manifestations of liver disease are varied and can be quite subtle. Clues to the existence, severity, and origin of liver disease may be obtained from a thorough history and physical examination as well as by routine laboratory screening tests.

Laboratory Tests of Liver Function and Disease

Understanding the utility of different types of laboratory tests of the liver is extremely important in characterizing the underlying liver disease. Unlike tests used to assess function of other organ systems (e.g., arterial blood gas, creatinine clearance), many so-called liver function tests do not directly measure hepatic function and may not accurately reflect the cause or severity of the liver disease process. Specific diagnostic tests such as serologic tests for viral, autoimmune, and inherited liver disease are covered in other chapters.

Tests of Hepatic Function

The great variety of functions that the liver performs has made it difficult to devise a simple, inexpensive, reproducible, and noninvasive test that accurately reflects hepatic capacity for all functions. Instead, currently available tests of liver function are indirect, static measurements of serum levels of compounds that are synthesized, metabolized, or excreted by the liver. The liver has a large reserve capacity, and therefore results of *function* tests may remain relatively normal until liver dysfunction is severe.

The most widely available and useful liver function tests are outlined in Table 41-1. The serum albumin level and prothrombin time both reflect the hepatic capacity for protein synthesis. The prothrombin time is dependent on coagulation factors II, V, VII and X and responds rapidly to altered hepatic function because of the short serum half-lives of factors II and VII (about 6 hours). This makes the prothrombin time a useful marker of hepatic synthetic function that can be followed as frequently as daily. However, because serum levels of factors II, VII, IX, and X are dependent on vitamin K, coexistent vitamin K deficiency must be excluded or treated before using the prothrombin time as a measure of hepatic function. In contrast, the serum half-life of albumin is 14 to 20 days, and serum levels fall with prolonged liver dysfunction or in acute liver impairment. Malnutrition and renal or gastrointestinal losses merit consideration in the setting of significant hypoalbuminemia, especially if the prothrombin time is relatively well preserved. Serum globulins may be increased in some patients with chronic liver disease such as hepatitis C and cirrhosis. Elevations of individual gamma-globulins can be indicative of specific disease processes such as autoimmune hepatitis (total immunoglobulin G [IgG]), primary biliary cirrhosis (IgM), and alcoholic liver disease (IgA).

Serum ammonia may be elevated in liver disease. Although it is a poor marker of hepatic function, it is used frequently in the diagnosis of portosystemic encephalopathy.

Quantitative tests of liver function, including indocyanine green clearance, galactose elimination capacity, aminopyrine breath test, antipyrine clearance, monoethylglycinexylidide, and caffeine clearance may be superior to conventional biochemical tests in predicting prognosis. However, the clinical utility of these tests has not been established, and they are limited primarily to research centers.

Screening Tests of Hepatobiliary Disease

Screening tests of hepatobiliary disease (see Table 41-1) may be divided into two categories: (1) tests of biliary obstruction

Table 41-1 **Laboratory Tests of Hepatic Function**

	Property Examined	**Causes of Abnormal Results**
Tests of Hepatic Function (Normal Values)		
Serum albumin (3.5-5.5 mg/dL)	Protein synthetic capacity (over days to weeks)	Decreased synthetic capacity Protein malnutrition Increased protein loss (nephrotic syndrome, protein-losing enteropathy) Increased extracellular fluid volume
Prothrombin time (10.5-13 sec)	Protein synthetic capacity (hours to days)	Decreased synthetic capacity (especially factors II and VII) Vitamin-K deficiency Consumptive coagulopathy
Screening Tests of Hepatobiliary Disease		
Tests of Biliary Obstruction or Impaired Bile Flow		
Serum bilirubin (0.2-1 mg/dL) (3.4-17.1 mmol/L)	Extraction of bilirubin from blood; conjugation and excretion into bile	Hemolysis Diffuse liver disease Cholestasis Extrahepatic bile duct obstruction Congenital disorders of bilirubin metabolism
Serum alkaline phosphatase (also 5'-nucleotidase and γ-glutamyl transpeptidase) (56-176 U/L)	Increased enzyme synthesis and release	Bile duct obstruction Cholestasis Infiltrative liver disease (neoplasms, granulomas) Bone destruction, remodeling Pregnancy
Tests of Hepatocellular Damage		
Aspartate aminotransferase (AST) (10-30 U/L)	Release of intracellular enzyme	Hepatocellular necrosis Cardiac or skeletal muscle necrosis
Alanine aminotransferase (ALT) (5-30 U/L)	Release of intracellular enzyme	Same as AST; however, more specific for liver cell damage

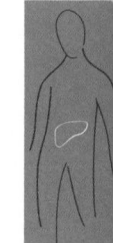

and cholestasis, and (2) tests of hepatocellular damage, based on the mechanisms responsible for the abnormal test. However, none of the tests is specific for either category, and the overall pattern and the relative magnitude of abnormalities in these two categories of tests often provide diagnostic clues to the type of liver disease present.

Bilirubin is present in the serum in two forms: unconjugated (indirect) and conjugated (direct). Normal serum bilirubin level is less than 1 mg/dL, with the conjugated fraction representing up to 30% of the total. The *serum bilirubin* level reflects a balance between bilirubin production and its conjugation and excretion into bile by the liver. The differential diagnosis for hyperbilirubinemia (see Chapter 42) requires consideration of an extensive list of disorders in which bilirubin production (hematologic disorders with predominantly unconjugated hyperbilirubinemia), hepatic metabolism (congenital abnormalities of bilirubin conjugation, liver disease), or excretion (congenital abnormalities of bilirubin excretion or biliary obstruction with predominantly conjugated hyperbilirubinemia) is altered. Hence, an elevated serum bilirubin determination is not specific for any cause of liver disease. However, such an abnormality, especially in association with predominant elevations in other tests of biliary obstruction, should prompt an evaluation for potentially treatable biliary abnormalities. Recognizing that serum bilirubin levels may not return promptly to normal after relief of biliary obstruction or improvement in liver disease is important because some bilirubin binds covalently to albumin and is removed from the circulation only as albumin is catabolized.

Serum alkaline phosphatase activity reflects a group of isoenzymes derived from liver, bone, intestine, and placenta.

Serum levels are elevated in association with a variety of conditions, including cholestasis, partial or complete bile duct obstruction, bone regeneration, pregnancy, and neoplastic, infiltrative, and granulomatous liver diseases. An isolated elevated alkaline phosphatase level may be the only clue to partial obstruction of the common bile duct, to obstruction of ducts in a single lobe or segment of liver, or to neoplastic or granulomatous hepatic disease. In cholestasis, serum alkaline phosphatase levels rise as a result of retention of bile acids in the liver, which solubilize alkaline phosphatase off the hepatocyte plasma membrane, as well as stimulate its synthesis. 5'-Nucleotidase and γ-glutamyl transpeptidase, other hepatocyte plasma membrane enzymes, are similarly released into the circulation during bile duct obstruction or cholestasis and are used to confirm that an elevated alkaline phosphatase level is caused by hepatobiliary disease. An isolated elevated serum alkaline phosphatase with normal 5'-nucleotidase and γ-glutamyl transpeptidase enzymes suggests a nonhepatic cause, and electrophoretic fractionation of alkaline phosphatase isoenzymes may be useful to confirm alternate sources.

Aspartate (aspartate aminotransferase [AST] or serum glutamic-oxaloacetic transaminase [SGOT]) and *alanine* (alanine aminotransferase [ALT] or serum glutamic-pyruvic transaminase [SGPT]) *aminotransferases* are intracellular amino-transferring enzymes present in large quantities in hepatocytes. After injury or death of liver cells, these enzymes are released into the circulation. In general, the serum aminotransferases are sensitive (albeit nonspecific) tests of liver damage, and the height of the serum aminotransferase activity level reflects the severity of hepatic necrosis, with important exceptions. For instance, both enzymes require pyridoxal

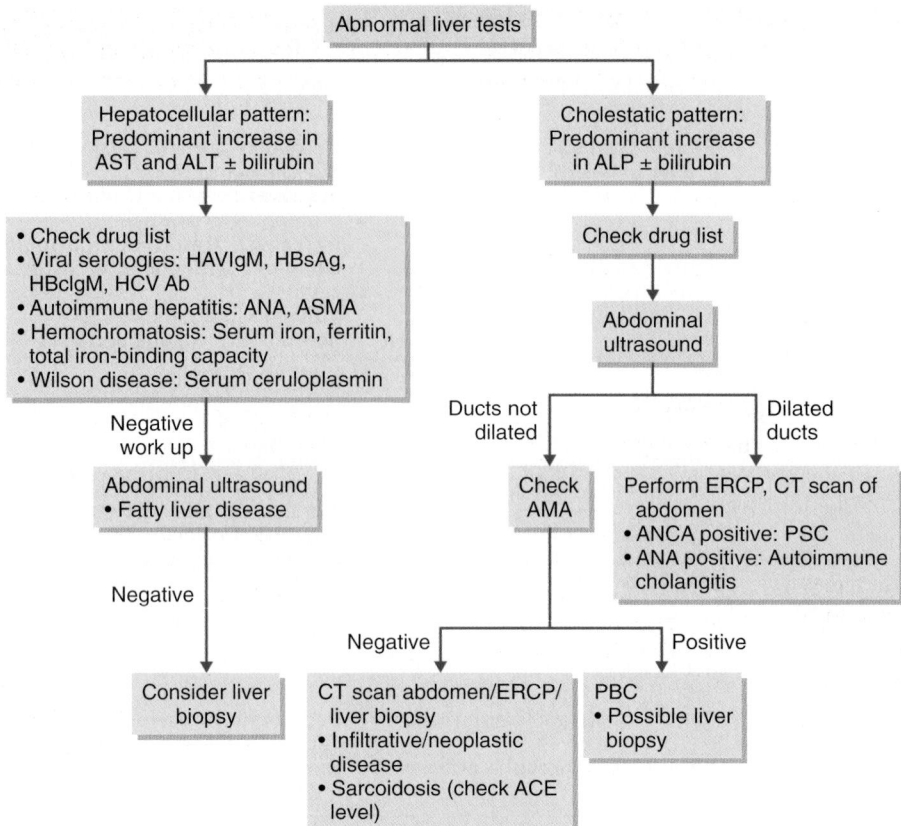

Figure 41-1 Abnormal liver function test patterns and diagnostic approach. ACE, angiotensin-converting enzyme, ALT, alanine aminotransferase; AST, aspartate aminotransferase; ALP, alkaline phosphatase; ANCA, antineutrophil cytoplasmic antibody; ANA, antinuclear antibody; AMA, antimitochondrial antibody, ASMA, anti–smooth muscle antibody; ERCP, endoscopic retrograde cholangiopancreatography; CT, computed tomography; HAVIgM, hepatitis A immunoglobulin M; HBsAg, hepatitis B surface antigen; HBcIgM, hepatitis B core immunoglobulin M; HCVAb, hepatitis C virus antibody; PBC: primary biliary cirrhosis; PSC, primary sclerosing cholangitis.

5′-phosphate as a cofactor, and the relatively low serum aminotransferase values seen in patients with severe alcoholic hepatitis (usually 300 U/L) may reflect deficiency of this cofactor. ALT is found primarily in hepatocytes and an elevation in ALT is more specific than AST for liver disease. In most hepatocellular disorders, ALT is higher than or equal to the AST, with the exception of alcoholic liver disease, in which the ratio is reversed, and an AST/ALT ratio of more than 3 is highly suggestive of alcohol as the underlying cause. Lower ALT levels are due to a deficiency of pyridoxal 5′-phosphate. Although aminotransferase levels are increased in a wide array of liver diseases, extremely high levels (15 times the upper limit of normal) generally indicate acute hepatocellular necrosis from viral or toxic causes (such as acetaminophen toxicity) or, less frequently, indicate acute bile duct obstruction or hepatic ischemia (*shock liver*). Patients who have isolated asymptomatic elevations of AST and ALT may have nonalcoholic fatty liver disease (caused by obesity, insulin resistance and diabetes, or hyperlipidemia), alcohol-induced liver disease, or hepatocellular disease, such as hemochromatosis or chronic viral hepatitis. These patients should be screened for treatable diseases. Some patients may require liver biopsy.

Individual liver function tests frequently do not indicate the nature of the underlying liver disease. However, the overall *pattern* of liver test abnormalities and the relative magnitude of abnormalities in individual tests often provide significant insight into whether the nature of the liver disease is primarily hepatocellular or cholestatic. Figure 41-1 outlines common patterns of liver test abnormalities and a diagnostic evaluation. Isolated elevation in indirect bilirubin and, rarely, total bilirubin levels greater than 5 mg/dL will occur in hemolysis or Gilbert syndrome. Bile duct obstruction rarely increases AST and ALT above 500 U/L or alkaline phosphatase above 4 to 5 times higher than the upper limits of normal. Ischemic hepatitis often produces ALT and AST levels above 1000 mg/dL, with rapid resolution after fluid resuscitation, excluding other causes of acute hepatocellular necrosis.

Common liver function test patterns in patients with cirrhosis include mildly elevated enzymes (AST and ALT) and elevated bilirubin (primarily conjugated) and alkaline phosphatase associated with thrombocytopenia and prolonged prothrombin time. Specific causes of cirrhosis influence the liver function abnormalities observed (see Chapter 45).

Liver Biopsy

Biopsy and histologic examination of liver tissue are frequently valuable in the differential diagnosis, staging, and consideration of treatment of diffuse or localized parenchy-

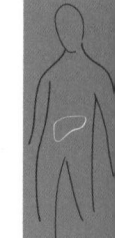

mal diseases (e.g., cirrhosis, hepatitis, hemochromatosis, tumors) or hepatomegaly. Liver biopsies can be performed either by a percutaneous or by a transjugular approach. Tissue from a biopsy represents 1/50,000 of total liver tissue, and sampling variability has been noted. Although generally safe, serious complications such as bleeding (1 per 1000) and death (1 per 10,000) may occur. Absolute contraindications include uncooperative patient, prothrombin time greater than 3 to 5 seconds, platelets under 50,000/mm^3, nonsteroidal anti-inflammatory drug use in previous 7 to 10 days, and suspected echinococcal cysts in the liver. Recently, noninvasive serum markers and ultrasound and magnetic resonance elastography have been increasingly studied as alternatives to liver biopsy to assess hepatic fibrosis.

Prospectus for the Future

In a significant number of liver disorders that exhibit abnormal liver tests (e.g., hepatitis C, nonalcoholic fatty liver disease), an important diagnostic consideration is the degree of hepatic fibrosis. In general, liver biopsy has been the gold standard for staging disease based on the amount of fibrosis found. Recently, transient elastography and a large number of panels of serum markers have been used to predict the degree of hepatic fibrosis noninvasively, particularly in hepatitis C infection. *Transient elastography* is a sonographic technique based on the theory that a "shear wave" moves faster in a less elastic liver (more fibrosis and scarring) than a normal or less fibrotic liver. A low-frequency shear wave is emitted from a probe, and the amount of time it takes to progress through a set "window" of tissue is measured and used as an index of tissue elasticity and fibrosis. This technique has shown accurate results in advanced fibrosis (stages 3 and 4). Several serum markers of fibrosis have also been evaluated and found to be good for ruling out advanced fibrosis but not for confirming mild or intermediate fibrosis. Using transient elastography and serum markers together has shown increased accuracy in assessing hepatic fibrosis. The use of such tests to predict hepatic fibrosis is likely to increase both in viral and in nonviral liver disease in the near future and may eventually replace liver biopsy as the primary means of assessing degree of hepatic fibrosis.

Another area of active investigation in liver disease is the use of genetic testing to predict susceptibility to drug-induced hepatotoxicity and to predict therapeutic response to specific therapies for liver disease. These pharmacogenomic techniques have the potential to detect genetic markers that may guide the use of drug therapies for liver disease and prevent drug-induced liver disease.

References

Green RM, Flamm S: AGA technical review on the evaluation of liver chemistries. Gastroenterology 123:1367-1384, 2002.

Berk PD: Approach to the patient with jaundice or abnormal liver tests. In Goldman L, Ausiello D (eds): Cecil Textbook of Medicine, 22nd ed. Philadelphia: WB Saunders, 2004, pp 897-906.

Kotlyar DS, Blonski W, Rustgi V: Noninvasive monitoring of hepatitis C fibrosis progression. Clin Liver Dis 12:557-571, viii, 2008.

Chapter **42**

Jaundice

Klaus Mönkemüller, Helmut Neumann, and Michael B. Fallon

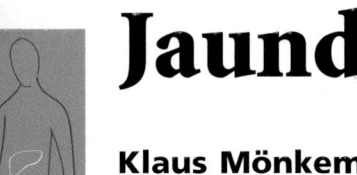

Jaundice, also known as *icterus* (Greek for yellow), connotes the yellow pigmentation of skin, sclerae, and mucous membranes that is caused by elevated serum bilirubin levels (hyperbilirubinemia). The word jaundice derives from the French *jaune*, meaning yellow. Jaundice per se is not a pathologic condition but rather a sign of various illnesses such as liver diseases and various hematologic disorders. There is one exception for which bilirubin can be pathologic: in newborns, hyperbilirubinemia can cause severe cerebral damage in neonates due to deposition of unconjugated bilirubin in the cerebral basal ganglia or nuclei. This completely preventable and treatable disease is known as kernicterus (from the German *Kern*, meaning nucleus). Normal serum bilirubin levels range from 0.5 to 1 mg/dL, and jaundice becomes clinically evident at levels higher than 2.5 to 3 mg/dL. Typically, plasma bilirubin concentration must exceed 1.5 mg/dL for the discoloration to be easily visible.

Bilirubin Metabolism

Hyperbilirubinemia can be classified based on the three phases of hepatic bilirubin metabolism: (1) uptake, (2) conjugation, and (3) excretion into the bile, the last step being rate limiting. However, a more practical way to categorize jaundice is into prehepatic, hepatic, and posthepatic causes (Table 42-1). This latter classification is useful for the practicing clinician.

Most of the bilirubin (80%) is derived from the breakdown of senescent red blood cells, whereas the remainder derives from ineffective erythropoiesis and catabolism of myoglobin and hepatic hemoproteins such as cytochrome P-450. The normal rate of bilirubin production is about 4 mg/kg body weight daily (Fig. 42-1). After erythrocytes have completed their normal life span of 120 days, or sooner in cases of hematologic disorders, they are destroyed within the reticuloendothelial system and release their contents into the bloodstream, where it is ingested by macrophages, which in turn split the hemoglobin into heme and globin. The heme ring is cleaved by the enzyme microsomal heme oxygenase to form biliverdin (from the Latin *viridis*, meaning green, i.e., green color pigment), which is then converted to

the tetrapyrrole pigment bilirubin by the cytosolic enzyme biliverdin reductase. This unconjugated (or "indirect," see later discussion of the *van der Bergh reaction*) bilirubin is released into the plasma, where it is tightly bound to albumin and then transported to the liver. Because unconjugated bilirubin is insoluble in water, it cannot be excreted in urine or bile. However, it will dissolve in lipid-rich environments and thus traverses the blood-brain barrier and placenta.

After dissociating from albumin in the space of Disse, unconjugated bilirubin is transported across the liver cell plasma membrane and attaches to intracellular binding proteins (ligandin). It is then conjugated with glucuronic acid by the enzyme uridine diphosphate (UDP) glucuronyl transferase to form bilirubin monoglucuronide and diglucuronide, which are water soluble. Conjugated bilirubin is excreted into bile by active transport across the canalicular membrane by a multispecific canalicular transporter. When biliary excretion of conjugated bilirubin is impaired, the pigment regurgitates from hepatocytes into plasma, causing an increase in the plasma level. Because conjugated bilirubin is water soluble and less tightly bound to albumin than is unconjugated bilirubin, it is readily filtered by the glomerulus and appears in the urine, giving it a dark color (choluria). Once in bile, bilirubin enters the intestine, where bacteria convert it to colorless tetrapyrroles (urobilinogens) that are excreted in feces. Up to 20% of urobilinogen is reabsorbed and undergoes enterohepatic circulation or excretion in urine.

Laboratory Measurement of Bilirubin

The *van den Bergh reaction*, which is the most commonly used test for detecting bilirubin in biologic fluids, combines bilirubin with diazotized sulfanilic acid to form a colored compound. The direct-reacting fraction is roughly equivalent to conjugated bilirubin and the indirect-reacting fraction (total minus direct fraction) to unconjugated bilirubin. This characteristic provides a means for classifying jaundice into two categories: unconjugated hyperbilirubinemia and conjugated hyperbilirubinemia.

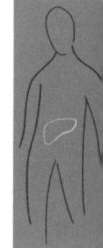

Table 42-1 **Classification of Jaundice**

Prehepatic (Predominantly Unconjugated Hyperbilirubinemia)

Overproduction

Hemolysis (e.g., spherocytosis, sickle cell disease, hemolysis of the newborn, autoimmune disorders)
Ineffective erythropoiesis (e.g., megaloblastic anemias)
Hematomas
Pulmonary emboli

Hepatic (Unconjugated Hyperbilirubinemia)

Decreased Hepatic Uptake

Gilbert syndrome
Drugs (e.g., rifampin, radiographic contrast agents)
Neonatal jaundice
Posthepatitis
Decreased cystolic binding proteins (e.g., newborn or premature infants)
Portocaval shunt
Prolonged fasting

Decreased Conjugation Due to Limited Glucuronyl Transferase Activity

Gilbert syndrome
Crigler-Najjar syndrome types I and II
Neonatal jaundice
Breast-milk jaundice
Chronic persistent hepatitis
Wilson disease
Noncirrhotic portal fibrosis
Drug inhibition (e.g., chloramphenicol)

Predominantly Conjugated Hyperbilirubinemia

Impaired Hepatic Excretion

Familial disorders (Dubin-Johnson syndrome, Rotor syndrome, benign recurrent cholestasis, cholestasis of pregnancy)
Hepatocellular infiltrative disorders
Liver metastasis
Liver cirrhosis
Hepatitis (viral, bacterial, parasitic, autoimmune, ethanol and drug induced)
Drug-induced cholestasis (especially chlorpromazine, erythromycin estolate, isoniazid, halothane)
Primary biliary cirrhosis
Primary sclerosing cholangitis
Pericholangitis
Congestive heart failure
Shock
Toxemia of pregnancy
Sarcoidosis
Hepatic trauma
Amyloidosis
Autoimmune cholangiopathy
Vanishing bile duct syndrome
Sepsis
Postoperative complications

Extrahepatic

Extrahepatic Biliary Obstruction

Gallstones, choledocholithiasis
Cholecystitis
Tumors of the head of the pancreas (adenocarcinoma, mucinous duct ectasia, neuroendocrine tumors, metastasis)
Tumors of bile ducts (cholangiocarcinoma, Klatskin tumor: cholangiocarcinoma at the bifurcation)
Gallbladder cancer
Tumors of the ampulla of Vater (adenoma, adenocarcinoma)
Tumors of the duodenum (adenocarcinoma, lymphoma)
Hemobilia (blood in the biliary tree)
Biliary strictures (postcholecystectomy, post–liver transplantation, primary sclerosing cholangitis)
Congenital disorders (biliary atresia, idiopathic dilation of common bile duct, cystic fibrosis)
Metastasis to the hepatic hilum
Primary bile duct lymphoma
Cholangiopathy of acquired immunodeficiency syndrome
Choledochal cysts
Infectious cholangiopathy *(Clonorchis sinensis, Ascaris lumbricoides, Fasciola hepatica)*
Chronic pancreatitis (fibrosis of the head of the pancreas)

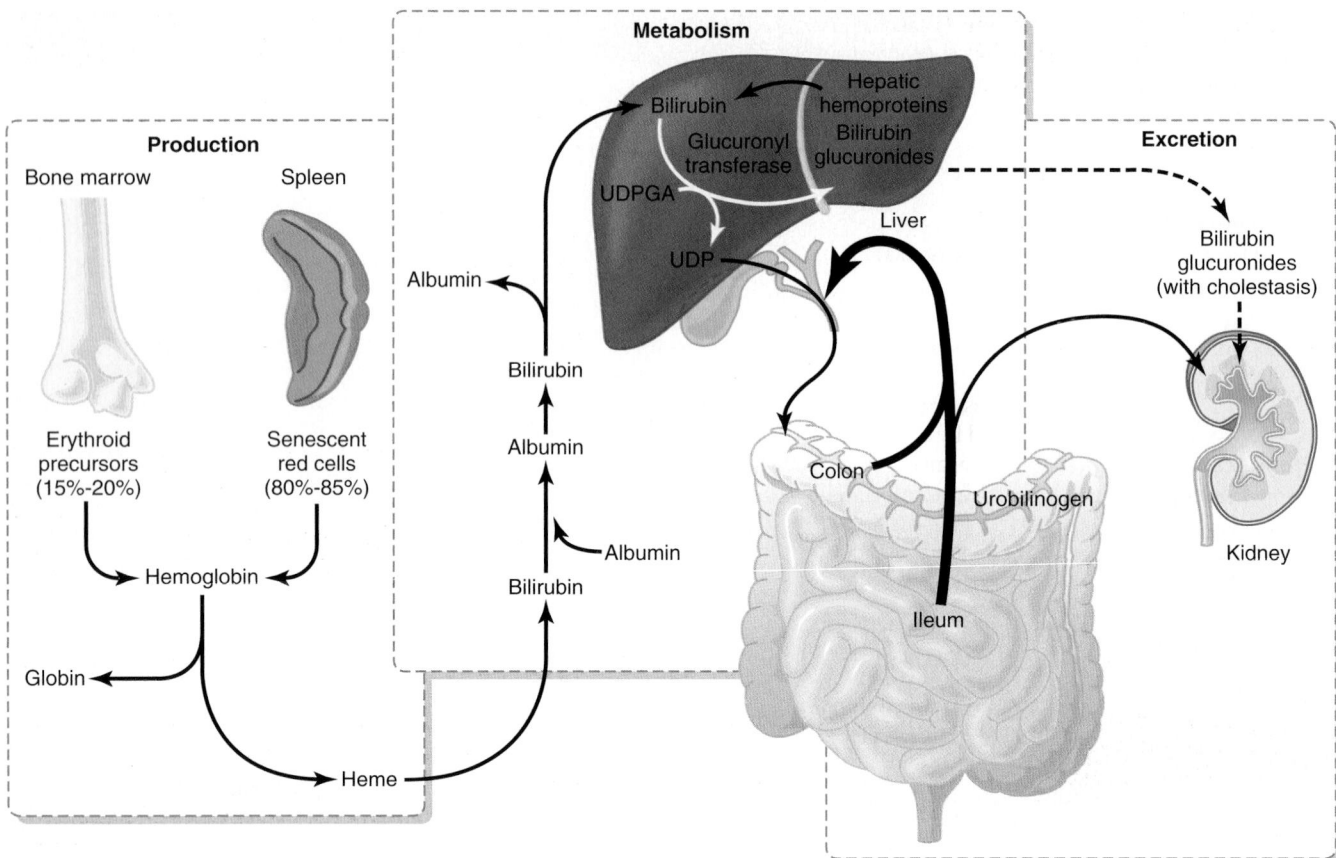

Figure 42-1 Bilirubin production, metabolism, and excretion (see text for detailed description). UDP, uridine diphosphate; UDPGA, uridine diphosphate glucuronic acid.

Unconjugated Hyperbilirubinemia

Mechanisms that cause unconjugated hyperbilirubinemia are (1) overproduction, (2) impaired hepatic uptake, and (3) decreased conjugation of bilirubin. These disorders are not usually associated with significant hepatic disease.

ETIOLOGY OF HYPERBILIRUBINEMIA

Prehepatic

Prehepatic jaundice can be caused by any condition resulting in excessive bilirubin production or hepatic uptake. These conditions include an increased production of bilirubin that may result from hemolysis (intravascular or extravascular), hematomas, or pulmonary emboli. Furthermore, certain genetic diseases can lead to an increased red cell lysis and therefore hemolytic jaundice. Examples are glucose 6-phosphate dehydrogenase deficiency, sickle cell anemia, and spherocytosis. Infectious diseases like malaria can also cause jaundice by breakdown of red blood cells. Jaundice resulting from hemolysis is characteristically mild, and serum bilirubin levels rarely exceed 5 mg/dL in the absence of coexisting hepatic diseases. Ineffective erythropoiesis, which may be significantly increased in megaloblastic anemias, also leads to mild jaundice. Hemolysis can be investigated by examining the peripheral blood smear (and in some cases the bone marrow smear) and measuring the reticulocyte count, haptoglobin, lactate dehydrogenase (LDH), erythrocyte fragility, and Coombs test.

Hepatic

Every condition resulting in hepatic injury can cause hepatic jaundice. These conditions include any causes of hepatitis, such as infectious diseases (viral, bacterial), toxic metabolites (alcohol, carbon tetrachloride, amanita), drugs (rifampin, flavaspidic acid, iodinated contrast agents), autoimmune disorders (autoimmune hepatitis, primary biliary cirrhosis, primary sclerosing cholangitis), and liver tumors (mostly metastasis). Other, less common causes included Gilbert syndrome, Crigler-Najjar syndrome, and Niemann-Pick disease type C (a metabolic disorder in which cholesterol and glycolipids are stored in the body rather than sphingomyelin, resulting in progressive neurologic damage).

IMPAIRED HEPATIC UPTAKE

Impaired hepatic uptake causes jaundice that occurs after administering certain drugs, such as rifampin (competition for bilirubin uptake) and those involved in treating Gilbert syndrome. Gilbert syndrome is a benign disorder that affects up to 7% of the population, with male predominance. It commonly exhibits during the second or third decade of life as mild unconjugated hyperbilirubinemia that is exacerbated by fasting or is noted on routine laboratory testing. Most patients have a bilirubin level that is less than 3 mg/dL. The genetic defect is usually a homozygous abnormality in the TATAA element of the promoter region of the UDP glucuronyl transferase gene. The diagnosis is strongly suggested by unconjugated hyperbilirubinemia in which normal hepatic enzymes exist and overt hemolysis is absent. Liver biopsy is generally not indicated. Therapy is not usually given, but the bilirubin level does decrease significantly with phenobarbital administration.

IMPAIRED CONJUGATION

Crigler-Najjar syndrome occurs as a result of impaired conjugation of bilirubin that is caused by genetically determined decrease or absence of UDP glucuronyl transferase activity. Conjugation may also be impaired by mild, acquired defects of UDP glucuronyl transferase induced by drugs such as chloramphenicol.

Neonatal Jaundice

In neonates, jaundice develops for two main reasons. First, the relative immature hepatic metabolic pathways are unable to conjugate bilirubin as efficiently and quickly as in adults. Second, bilirubin production is increased. Of those two mechanisms, the major defect is in bilirubin conjugation, which may cause mild to moderate unconjugated hyperbilirubinemia between the 2nd and 5th days of life, lasting until the 8th day in normal births or to about the 14th day in premature births. This neonatal jaundice is usually harmless and does not require any kind of therapy. Severe pathologic unconjugated hyperbilirubinemia in the neonate is usually caused by a combination of hemolysis secondary to blood group incompatibility and defective conjugation. This neonatal jaundice is a serious condition that requires immediate attention because severe hyperbilirubinemia is associated with a risk for permanent neurologic damage *(kernicterus)*. Phototherapy is the treatment of choice. If jaundice does not improve using phototherapy, other etiologies of neonatal jaundice should be sought (Table 42-2).

Conjugated Hyperbilirubinemia

Conjugated hyperbilirubinemia is generally associated with impaired formation or excretion of *all* components of bile, a situation termed *cholestasis*. The two major mechanisms of conjugated hyperbilirubinemia are (1) a defect in the excretion of bilirubin from hepatocytes into bile (intrahepatic cholestasis) or (2) a mechanical obstruction to the flow of bile through the bile ducts.

IMPAIRED HEPATIC EXCRETION (INTRAHEPATIC CHOLESTASIS)

Intrahepatic cholestasis can result from a wide range of conditions, including those that impair canalicular transport (e.g., drugs) and those that cause destruction of the small

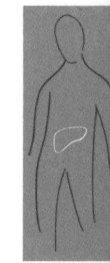

Table 42-2 **Neonatal Jaundice**

Prehepatic

Hereditary spherocytosis
Nonspherocytic hemolytic anemia (glucose 6-phosphate dehydrogenase deficiency, α-thalassemia, vitamin K_3–induced hemolysis, pyruvate kinase deficiency)

Hepatic

Crigler-Najjar syndrome types I and II
$α_1$-antitrypsin deficiency
Sepsis
Drug-induced
Hypothyroidism
Breast-milk jaundice
Fetomaternal blood group incompatibility (Rhesus, Landsteiner groups ABO)

Posthepatic

Extrahepatic biliary obstruction
Biliary atresia
Bile duct paucity
Alagille syndrome

intrahepatic bile ducts (e.g., primary biliary cirrhosis, tumors).

Primary biliary cirrhosis is a chronic, progressive liver disease that occurs primarily in women and is characterized by the destruction and subsequent disappearance of small lobular bile ducts. The gradual decrease in the number of bile ducts leads to progressive cholestasis, portal inflammation, fibrosis, and eventually cirrhosis.

Drug-induced cholestasis may be caused by a wide array of drugs. Culprits include but are not limited to nitrofurantoin, oral contraceptives, anabolic steroids, erythromycin, cimetidine, gold salts, chlorpromazine, prochlorperazine, imipramine, sulindac, tolbutamide, ampicillin, and other penicillin-based antibiotics.

Postoperative jaundice typically occurs 1 to 10 days after surgery and has an incidence of 15% after heart surgery and 1% after elective abdominal surgery. It is multifactorial in origin. In hepatocellular disease, all three steps of hepatic bilirubin metabolism are impaired. Excretion, the rate-limiting step, is usually the most affected, leading to predominantly conjugated hyperbilirubinemia. Jaundice may be profound in acute hepatitis (see Chapter 43) without adverse prognostic implications. In contrast, in chronic liver disease, persistent jaundice usually implies irreversible decrease in hepatic function and a poor prognosis.

POSTHEPATIC

Posthepatic jaundice is also called *obstructive jaundice* and results from a complete or partial obstruction of the intrahepatic or extrahepatic bile ducts. The most common causes are gallstones in the common bile duct or pancreatic head tumors. Not infrequently, the first sign of pancreatic cancer is jaundice. Other causes include strictures of the common bile duct, biliary atresia, ductal carcinoma, pancreatitis, pancreatic pseudocysts, or parasites named *liver flukes* (e.g., *Clonorchis sinensis, Dicrocoelium dendriticum,* or *Opisthorchis viverrini*). *Mirizzi syndrome* is a rare cause of posthepatic jaundice affecting up to 0.7% to 1.4% of all cholecystectomies in which the common bile duct obstruction is caused by an extrinsic compression from an impacted stone in the cystic duct (see Table 42-1).

Clinical Approach to Jaundice

Because the differential diagnosis of jaundice is broad, a thorough history and physical examination and a judicious use of laboratory and imaging studies are needed to define its cause. Jaundice appears as yellowing of the skin and sclera. Other conditions may cause yellowing or darkening of the skin (e.g., carotinemia, Addison disease, quinacrine ingestion), but scleral and mucosal discolorations are absent in these conditions. The most important initial step is to define whether the jaundice is predominantly caused by an elevation of unconjugated or of conjugated bilirubin. If jaundice is primarily the result of unconjugated bilirubin, evaluation for hemolysis is appropriate. In patients with elevated conjugated bilirubin, the clinical challenge lies in distinguishing whether biliary obstruction or impaired hepatic excretion is the cause (see Chapter 41).

In cholestatic jaundice caused by biliary obstruction or impaired hepatic excretion, the alkaline phosphatase level is typically increased more than 3 times normal, whereas serum transaminases are usually elevated less than 5-fold to 10-fold (see Chapter 40). Patients with cholestasis also may develop pruritus and malabsorption of fat and fat-soluble vitamins (A, D, E, and K). Recurrent abdominal pain and nausea (gallstones) and epigastric pain radiating to the back with weight loss and gallbladder distention (carcinoma of the pancreatic head) suggest the presence of specific causes of biliary obstruction. In complete biliary obstruction, conjugated hyperbilirubinemia is prominent and usually peaks at about 30 mg/dL in the absence of renal failure. Eosinophilia may accompany drug-induced jaundice. Inquiry about the use of drugs known to cause cholestasis, serologic testing for antimitochondrial antibody for primary biliary cirrhosis, and endoscopic retrograde cholangiopancreatography (ERCP) or magnetic resonance cholangiopancreatography to evaluate primary sclerosing cholangitis may be helpful.

In jaundice produced by hepatocellular disease resulting from a variety of causes (see Chapters 43 and 45), serum transaminases are characteristically elevated more than 10-fold, and alkaline phosphatase levels are less than 3 times normal. Evidence of hepatocellular damage and disease is also frequently present and includes a prolonged pro-

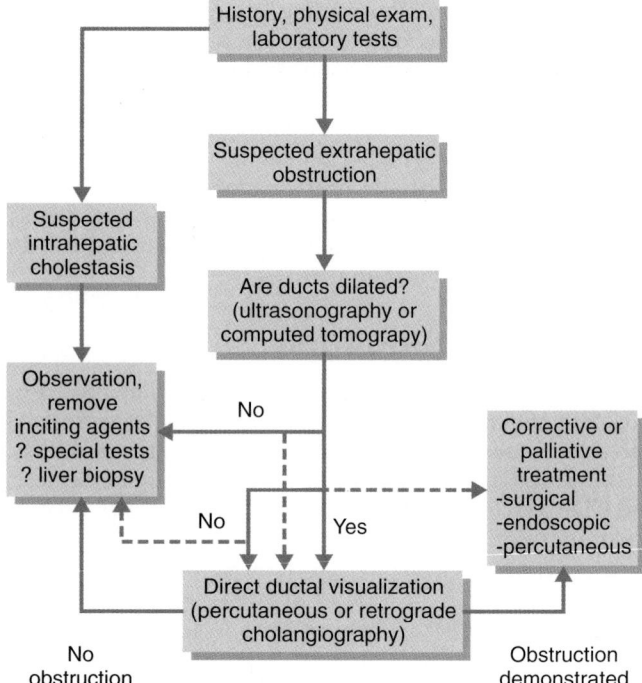

Figure 42-2 Approach to the patient with cholestatic jaundice. The algorithm demonstrates the systematic consideration of the available diagnostic options.

thrombin time, hypoalbuminemia, and clinical features of hepatic dysfunction (i.e., palmar erythema, spider angiomas, gynecomastia, and ascites). An inquiry about the use of drugs known to cause hepatocellular injury, alcohol, risk factors for viral hepatitis, and preexisting liver disease, along with serologic testing for hepatitis (see Chapter 43), may be useful.

A diagnostic approach to jaundice is outlined in Figure 42-2. If extrahepatic obstruction is suspected, noninvasive studies such as ultrasound or computed tomography should be used to determine whether bile ducts are dilated. If dilated ducts are found on noninvasive imaging, direct cholangiography (either endoscopic or radiologic) will provide the most reliable approach to management and potential treatment of cholestatic jaundice. If intrahepatic cholestasis is suggested clinically and extrahepatic obstruction is excluded by noninvasive means or by direct cholangiography, liver biopsy will sometimes be useful in determining the cause of cholestasis.

Prospectus for the Future

Important issues regarding both the diagnosis of and therapy for jaundice remain. A fundamental diagnostic issue is distinguishing obstructive jaundice from intrahepatic diseases. During the past 5 to 10 years, both magnetic resonance cholangiopancreatography and endoscopic ultrasound (EUS) technology have greatly improved. Increasing experience with these modalities and continuing technical advances have reduced dramatically ERCP as a common diagnostic modality. Furthermore, the use of EUS-based techniques to enhance capabilities in therapeutic ERCP is likely to expand.

Another rapidly advancing area involves understanding the molecular mechanisms and regulation of bile secretion both under normal conditions and in the setting of specific causes of jaundice. These insights, as well as new information regarding the genetic predisposition to drug-induced cholestasis, will likely lead to novel therapeutic options to diminish the adverse effects of jaundice as well as provide a means to decrease the incidence of drug-induced cholestatic liver disease.

References

Akobeng A: Neonatal jaundice. Clin Evid 12:501-507, 2004.

Berk PD: Approach to the patient with jaundice or abnormal liver tests. In Goldman L, Ausiello D (eds): Cecil Textbook of Medicine, 22nd ed. Philadelphia, WB Saunders, 2004, pp 897-905.

Bloomer JR, Risheg H: Bilirubin and porphyrin metabolism. In Maddrey WC, Feldman M (eds): Atlas of the Liver, 3rd ed. Philadelphia, Current Medicine 1-17, 2003.

Trauner M, Wagner M, Fickert P, Zollner G: Molecular regulation of hepatobiliary transport systems: Clinical implications for understanding and treating cholestasis. J Clin Gastroenterol 39(4 Suppl 2):S111-S124, 2005.

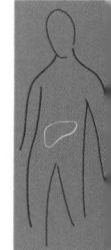

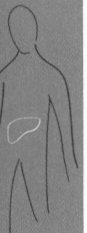

Acute and Chronic Hepatitis

Rajan Kochar, Aasim M. Sheikh, and Michael B. Fallon

The term *hepatitis* denotes inflammation of the liver. It is applied to a broad category of clinicopathologic conditions that result from the damage produced by viral, toxic, metabolic, pharmacologic, or immune-mediated attack on the liver. The common pathologic features of hepatitis are hepatocellular necrosis, which may be focal or extensive, and inflammatory cell infiltration of the liver, which may predominate in the portal areas or may extend into the parenchyma.

Acute hepatitis implies a condition lasting less than 6 months, culminating either in complete resolution of the liver damage with return to normal liver function and structure or a rapid progression of the acute injury toward extensive necrosis and a fatal outcome. Physical examination is usually unremarkable but may show enlarged, tender liver and icteric mucous membranes. Laboratory evidence of hepatocellular damage in the form of elevated aminotransferase (aspartate aminotransferase [AST] and alanine aminotransferase [ALT]) levels are the hallmark and may show elevations 20- to 100-fold normal values. Independent of the cause of hepatitis and the level of biochemical abnormality, the clinical course may range from subclinical to severe hepatocellular dysfunction, with evidence of impairment of coagulation, marked jaundice, and disturbance of neurologic function (see Chapter 44).

Chronic hepatitis is defined as a sustained inflammatory process in the liver reflected by liver function test abnormalities lasting longer than 6 months and is often difficult to differentiate from acute hepatitis on clinical or histologic criteria alone. Patients are typically asymptomatic and generally have lower aminotransferase abnormalities compared with those with acute hepatitis. Histologically, a diagnosis of chronic hepatitis requires the presence of inflammatory cells in the biopsy but also typically has evidence of significant fibrous deposition, disruption of hepatic lobular architecture, and possibly progression toward cirrhosis.

Acute Hepatitis

The causes of acute hepatitis include viral hepatitis (hepatitis A through E), drugs (prescription, nonprescription, and illicit), alcohol, toxins, autoimmune hepatitis, and Wilson disease. The mechanisms whereby these agents produce hepatic damage include direct toxin-induced necrosis (e.g., acetaminophen, *Amanita phalloides* toxin) and host immune-mediated damage (e.g., viral hepatitis). Massive hepatic necrosis is the dominant process in cases of *Amanita* poisoning, and the clinical course is more aptly described as fulminant hepatic failure (see Chapter 44) than as acute hepatitis. Such a course is less common but well recognized with all other causative agents. **Web Figure 43-1** is an algorithm detailing diagnostic approach to acute hepatitis.

Acute Viral Hepatitis
ETIOLOGY

Five hepatotropic viruses cause acute viral hepatitis (Table 43-1). Hepatitis viruses A (HAV), B (HBV), C (HCV), D (HDV), and E (HEV) have all been characterized at the molecular level. All are RNA viruses except HBV, which is an enveloped DNA virus. HAV is the most common cause of acute viral hepatitis in the United States, followed by HBV. HBV has been extensively characterized. The complete HBV virion (Dane particle) consists of several components that elicit distinct antibody responses from the host (Fig. 43-1). Clinically relevant is the surface envelope (hepatitis B surface antigen [HBsAg]), a core of partially double-stranded circular DNA (HBV DNA) to which is attached a DNA polymerase, and a nucleocapsid (hepatitis B core antigen [HBcAg] and hepatitis B early antigen [HBeAg]) that encloses the DNA and the polymerase. HCV is the most

Table 43-1 Characteristics of Common Causative Agents of Acute Viral Hepatitis

	Hepatitis A	Hepatitis B	Hepatitis C	Hepatitis D	Hepatitis E
Causative agent	28-nm RNA virus	42-nm DNA virus; core and surface components	30-nm enveloped/ RNA virus	36-nm hybrid particle with HBsAg coat	30- to 32-nm nonenveloped RNA virus
Transmission	Fecal-oral; water-borne or food-borne; sexual transmission	Parenteral inoculation, sexual and vertical; direct contact	Similar to HBV but vertical transmission; poor sexual transmission	Similar to HBV	Similar to HAV
Incubation period	2-6 wk	4 wk-6 mo	5-10 wk	Similar to HBV	2-9 wk
Period of infectivity	2-3 wk in late incubation and early clinical phase	During HBsAg positivity (occasionally only with anti-HBc positivity)	During HCV RNA positivity	During HDV RNA or anti-HDV positivity	Similar to HAV
Onset	Acute	Acute, insidious	Insidious	Acute, insidious	Acute
Massive hepatic necrosis	Rare	Uncommon	Rare	Yes	Yes
Carrier state	No	Yes	No	Yes	No
Chronic hepatitis	No	1% to 10% (90% in neonates)	Common (85%)	Common	No
Cancer	No	Yes	Yes	Yes/No	No
Treatment	Supportive	Supportive Lamivudine in select cases	Interferon-α $\pm$ ribavirin	Treat hepatitis B	Supportive
Prophylaxis	Hygiene, immune serum globulin, vaccine	Hygiene, hepatitis B immune globulin, vaccine	Hygiene	Hygiene, HBV vaccine	Hygiene, sanitation, vaccine

HAV, hepatitis A virus; HBc, hepatitis B core; HBsAg, hepatitis B surface antigen; HBV, hepatitis B virus; HCV, hepatitis C virus; HDV, hepatitis D virus.

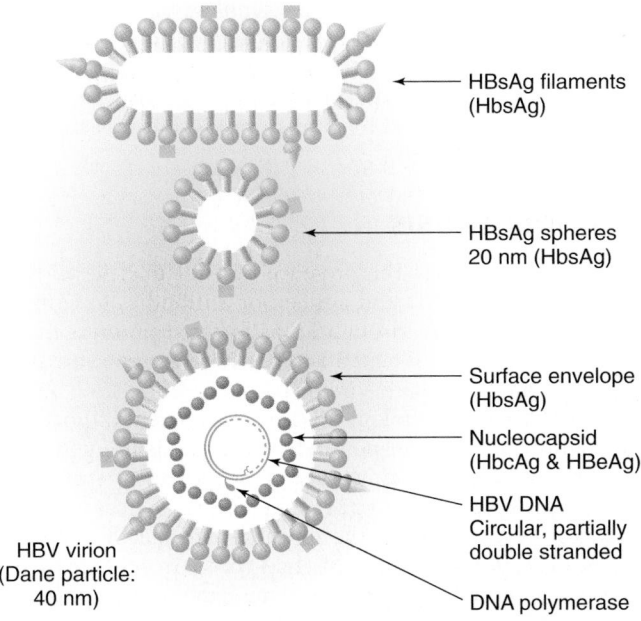

HBsAg filaments (HbsAg)

HBsAg spheres 20 nm (HbsAg)

Surface envelope (HbsAg)

Nucleocapsid (HbcAg & HBeAg)

HBV DNA Circular, partially double stranded

DNA polymerase

HBV virion (Dane particle: 40 nm)

Figure 43-1 Schematic diagram of hepatitis B virus (HBV)-related particles in serum and the associated antigens *(in parentheses)*. The spheres and filaments consist of only hepatitis B surface glycoproteins (HBsAg). They are 20 nm in diameter and are 10,000-fold greater in concentration than the complete virion (Dane particle: 40 nm diameter).

prevalent hepatitis virus worldwide but is an infrequent cause of symptomatic acute hepatitis. It accounts for most cases of acute hepatitis previously designated non-A, non-B. Cytomegalovirus and Epstein-Barr virus only occasionally cause acute hepatitis. HDV is an incomplete RNA virus that requires HBsAg for transmission from cell to cell; thus it causes hepatitis only in patients with hepatitis B, both acute (HDV co-infection) and chronic (HDV superinfection). Seven to 10% of presumed acute viral hepatitis cases have as yet unidentified cause or causes.

TRANSMISSION

The modes of transmission of the hepatitis viruses are noted in Table 43-1.

HAV and HEV are both excreted in the feces before onset of symptoms and are transmitted by the fecal-oral route (Fig. 43-2). They are thus implicated in most instances of water-borne and food-transmitted infection and in epidemics of viral hepatitis. HEV is linked to outbreaks in East Asia, Central Africa, the Middle East, and Mexico. It has a high rate of attack in young adults in these endemic areas and can lead to fulminant hepatitis, particularly in pregnant women.

HBV and HCV are both transmitted parenterally. HBV is present in virtually all body fluids and excreta of carriers. Transmission occurs most commonly through blood and blood products, contaminated needles, and sexual contact. High-risk transmission groups include the following: sexual partners of acutely and chronically infected persons, with male homosexuals being at particularly high

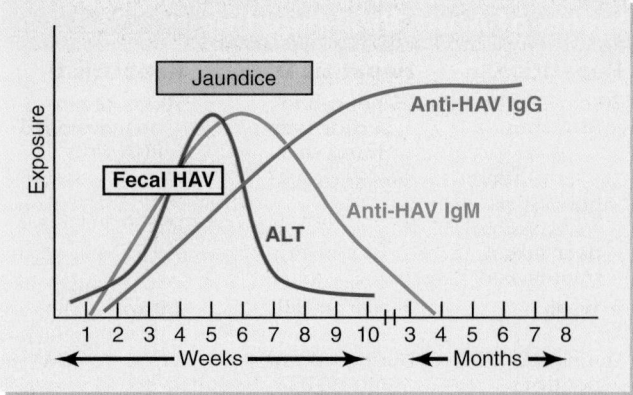

A

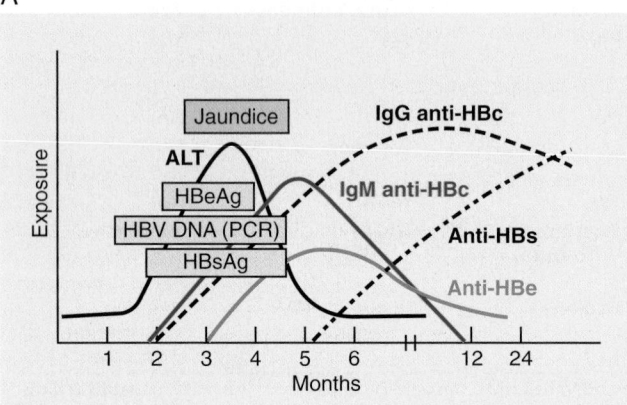

B

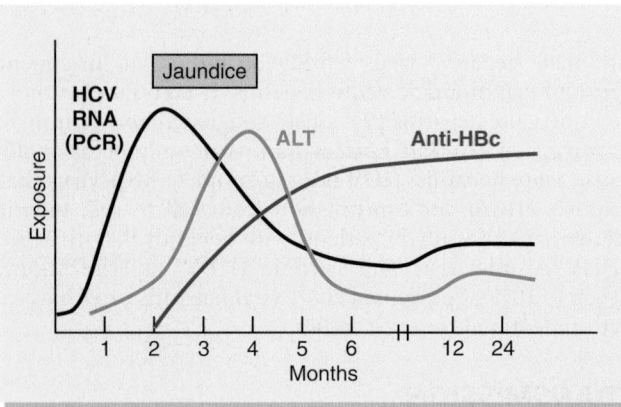

C

Figure 43-2 Sequence of clinical and laboratory findings in (A) a patient with acute hepatitis A virus (HAV) infection, (B) a patient with hepatitis B virus (HBV) infection, and (C) a patient with hepatitis C virus (HCV) infection. ALT, alanine transaminase; HBc, hepatitis B core; HBe, hepatitis B early; HBeAg, hepatitis B early antigen; HBs, hepatitis B surface; HBsAg, hepatitis B surface antigen; IgG, immunoglobulin G; PCR, polymerase chain reaction.

risk, intravenous drug abusers, infants of infected mothers *(vertical transmission),* and health professionals. Patients with increased exposure to blood or blood products or with impaired immunity (e.g., patients undergoing dialysis and patients with leukemia, hemophilia, or trisomy 21 syndrome) are also highly susceptible to HBV.

HCV was the main cause of post-transfusion hepatitis before 1992. It is presently the most common cause of hepatitis in intravenous drug users, and it accounts for a substan-

tial number of cases of sporadic, community-acquired hepatitis. The risk for vertical and sexual transmission of hepatitis C is much lower than with hepatitis B.

CLINICAL AND LABORATORY MANIFESTATIONS

Acute viral hepatitis typically begins with a prodromal phase lasting several days and characterized by constitutional and gastrointestinal symptoms including malaise, fatigue, anorexia, nausea, vomiting, myalgia, and headache. A mild fever may be present. Symptoms suggestive of influenza may be prominent. Arthritis and urticaria resembling serum sickness, attributed to immune complex deposition, may be present in 5% to 10% of cases of acute hepatitis B and C. Taste and smell alteration may occur. Jaundice soon appears with bilirubinuria and acholic (pale) stools, often accompanied by an improvement in the patient's sense of well-being. The liver is usually tender and enlarged; splenomegaly is found in about one fifth of patients. Notably, large proportions of all patients with acute viral hepatitis are asymptomatic or have symptoms without jaundice *(anicteric hepatitis).* In such instances, medical attention is often not sought.

Aminotransferases (ALT and AST) are released from the acutely damaged hepatocytes, and serum levels rise often to greater than 20-fold normal and as high as 100-fold normal. An elevated serum bilirubin (>2.5 to 3 mg/dL) results in jaundice and defines *icteric hepatitis.* Values higher than 20 mg/dL are uncommon and approximately correlate with the severity of disease. Elevations in serum alkaline phosphatase are usually limited to 3 times normal levels, except in cases of cholestatic hepatitis. A complete blood cell count most commonly shows mild leukopenia with atypical lymphocytes. Anemia and thrombocytopenia may also be present. The icteric phase of acute viral hepatitis may last days to weeks, followed by gradual resolution of symptoms and laboratory values.

SERODIAGNOSIS

The ability to detect the presence of viral nucleic acids in hepatitis B, C, and D and antigen or antibodies to components of hepatitis A through E has fostered progress in the epidemiology of viral hepatitis. These viral markers are used in the diagnosis of acute viral hepatitis (see Fig. 43-2; Tables 43-2 and 43-3). An etiologic diagnosis is of great importance in planning preventive and public health measures pertinent to the close contacts of infected patients and in evaluating prognosis. Epstein-Barr virus and cytomegalovirus hepatitis may also be diagnosed by the appearance of specific antibodies of the immunoglobulin M (IgM) class. In acute hepatitis B, HBsAg and HBeAg are present in serum. Both are usually cleared within 3 months, but HBsAg may persist in some patients with uncomplicated cases for 6 months to 1 year. Clearance of HBsAg is followed after a variable "window" period by emergence of anti-HBs, which confers long-term immunity. Anti-HBc and anti-HBe appear in the acute phase of the illness, but neither provides immunity. Uncommonly, during the serologic window period, anti-HBc IgM, a marker of active viral replication suggesting recent infection, may be the only evidence of HBV infection. HDV infec-

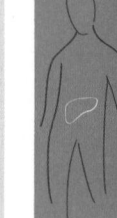

Table 43-2 **Serologic Markers of Viral Hepatitis**

Agent	Marker	Definition	Significance
Hepatitis A virus (HAV)	Anti-HAV	Antibody to HAV	—
	IgM type	—	Current or recent infection or convalescence
	IgG type	—	Current or previous infection; conferring immunity
Hepatitis B virus (HBV)	HBsAg	HBV surface antigen	Positive in most cases of acute or chronic infection
	HBeAg	HBe antigen; a component of the HBV core	Transiently positive in acute hepatitis B
			May persist in chronic infection
			Reflection of presence of viral replication, whole Dane particles in serum, high infectivity
	HBV DNA	Infectious viral genomic material	Serum level reflects degree of viral replication; predicts response to therapy
	Anti-HBe	Antibody to HBe antigen	Transiently positive in convalescence
			Persistently present in some chronic cases
			Usually a reflection of low infectivity
	Anti-HBc (IgM or IgG)	Antibody to HBV core antigen	Positive in all acute and chronic cases
			Reliable marker of infection, past or current IgM anti-HBc a reflection of active viral replication and acute infection
			Not protective
Anti-HBs	Positive in late convalescence in most acute cases	Antibody to HBV surface antigen and after vaccination	Confers immunity
Hepatitis C virus (HCV)	Anti-HCV	Antibodies to a group of recombinant HCV peptides	Positive on average 12 wk after exposure; not protective
			Persistent in acute, chronic, or past infection
	HCV RNA	Infectious viral genomic material	Reflects ongoing infection, level inversely linked to treatment response
Hepatitis D virus (HDV)	Anti-HDV (IgM or IgG)	Antibody to HDV antigen	Acute or chronic infection seen with positive HBsAg; not protective
	HDV antigen	Viral peptide	IgM and IgG clear in resolving infection
	HDV RNA	Infectious viral genomic material	IgG persists in chronic infection
			Persists in chronic infection
			Most reliable test for acute or chronic infection
Hepatitis E virus (HEV)	Anti-HEV (IgM or IgG)	Antibody to HEV antigen	Acute or chronic infection
			IgM may persist up to 6 months

IgG, immunoglobulin G; IgM, immunoglobulin M.

tion superimposed on HBV infection is most reliably detected by polymerase chain reaction (PCR) testing for HDV RNA. Other possible tests include HDV antigen and anti-HDV (IgM and IgG antibodies). Acute hepatitis C can be detected using a sensitive PCR assay for HCV RNA within 2 weeks of exposure. Serum antibodies to HCV develop within 12 weeks of exposure or within 4 to 5 weeks after biochemical abnormalities are discovered. At onset of symptoms, 30% of patients will be missed if checked by serum enzyme immunoassay (EIA) for HCV antibody alone. Commercial EIAs for hepatitis E to detect both IgM and IgG class antibodies are also available but may lack general sensitivity and specificity. The HEV IgM antibody is present for up to 6 months after exposure.

COMPLICATIONS

Cholestatic Hepatitis

In some patients, most commonly during HAV infection, a self-limited period of cholestatic jaundice may supervene that is characterized by marked conjugated hyperbilirubinemia, elevation of alkaline phosphatase, and pruritus. Investigation may be required to differentiate this condition from mechanical obstruction of the biliary tree (see Chapter 45).

Fulminant Hepatitis

Massive hepatic necrosis occurs in less than 1% of patients with acute viral hepatitis and leads to a devastating and often

Table 43-3 Interpretation of Serologic Markers and Serum DNA in Hepatitis B

	HBsAg	HBeAg	Anti-HBc IgM	Anti HBc IgG	Anti-HBs	Anti-HBe	HBV DNA*
Acute hepatitis	+	+/−	+				+
Acute hepatitis, window period			+				
Recovery from acute hepatitis			+	+	+	+/−	
Chronic hepatitis	+	+					+
Chronic hepatitis (precore mutant)	+					+	+
Inactive carrier	+					+/−	
Vaccinated					+		

HBsAg, hepatitis B surface antigen; HBeAg, hepatitis Be antigen; anti-HBc IgM, hepatitis B core antibody (IgM type); anti-HBc IgG, hepatitis B core antibody (IgG type); anti-HBs, hepatitis B surface antibody; anti-HBe, hepatitis Be antibody; HBV DNA, hepatitis B viral DNA.
*HBV DNA > 10^5 copies/mL.

fatal condition called *fulminant hepatic failure*. This condition is discussed in detail in Chapter 44.

Chronic Hepatitis

Hepatitis A does not progress to chronic liver disease, although occasionally it has a relapsing course. Persistence of aminotransferase elevation and viral antigens or nucleic acids beyond 6 months in patients with hepatitis B and C suggests evolution to chronic hepatitis, although slowly resolving acute hepatitis may occasionally lead to such test abnormalities for up to 12 months, with eventual complete resolution. Chronic hepatitis is considered in detail later in this chapter.

Rare Complications

Acute viral hepatitis may be followed by *aplastic anemia*, which affects mostly male patients and results in a mortality rate of greater than 80%. Pancreatitis, myocarditis, pericarditis, pleural effusion, and neurologic complications, including Guillain-Barré syndrome, aseptic meningitis, and encephalitis, have also been reported. Cryoglobulinemia and glomerulonephritis are associated with hepatitis B and C, and polyarteritis nodosa with hepatitis B.

MANAGEMENT

All cases of acute hepatitis A, B, and E, unless complicated by fulminant hepatitis, are self-limited (see Table 43-2). Treatment of acute hepatitis C is important, and recent data support that early treatment within 12 weeks of diagnosis with pegylated interferon-α induces high sustained virologic response rates. Studies of antiviral therapy in acute hepatitis B have not shown clear benefit, although many experts advocate use of nucleoside or nucleotide analogues, specifically in the setting of acute liver failure due to hepatitis B. The treatment in all other cases is largely supportive and includes rest, maintenance of hydration, and adequate dietary intake. Most patients show a preference for a low-fat, high-carbohydrate diet. Alcohol should be avoided. Vitamin supplementation is of no proven value, although vitamin K may be indicated if prolonged cholestasis occurs. Nausea can be treated with small doses of metoclopramide and hydroxyzine. Hospitalization is indicated for patients with severe nausea and vomiting and for those with evidence of deteriorating liver function, such as hepatic encephalopathy or pro-

longation of the prothrombin time. In general, hepatitis A and E may be regarded as noninfectious after 3 weeks, whereas hepatitis B is potentially infectious to sexual contacts throughout its course, although the risk is low once HBsAg has cleared.

PREVENTION

Both feces and blood from patients with hepatitis A and E contain virus during the prodromal and early icteric phases of the disease (see Fig. 43-2). Raw shellfish concentrate the HAV from sewage pollution and may serve as vector of the disease. General hygienic measures should include hand washing by contacts and careful handling, disposal, and sterilization of excreta and contaminated clothing and utensils. Close contacts of patients with hepatitis A should receive anti-HAV serum immunoglobulin as soon as possible after exposure. HAV vaccination is appropriate for children and travelers to endemic areas, individuals with immunodeficiency or chronic liver disease, and those with high-risk behaviors or occupations. Recently, a recombinant vaccine for HEV has been shown to be safe and effective in a high-risk population (healthy adults in an endemic area) in a randomized controlled trial, but formal guidelines for its use have not been established. Hepatitis B is rarely transmitted by body fluids other than blood. However, it is highly infectious, and strict adherence to universal precautions is mandatory. Efforts at preventing hepatitis B have involved the use of immunoglobulin-enriched anti-HBs (HBIG) and recombinant HBV vaccines. Postexposure prophylaxis with HBIG after blood or mucosal exposure (e.g., needlestick, eye splash, sexual contacts of patients with acute hepatitis B, neonates born to mothers with acute or chronic infection) should be given within 7 days along with HBV vaccine. Preventive vaccination is currently recommended for high-risk groups and individuals (health care professionals, patients undergoing dialysis, patients with advanced liver disease or hemophilia, residents and staff of custodial care institutions, sexually active homosexual men) and is advocated universally for children.

No accepted prevention strategies are available for HCV. Serum immunoglobulin is not useful for postexposure prophylaxis. The advent of widespread blood product screening for anti-HCV has made post-transfusion hepatitis a rarity.

Alcoholic Fatty Liver and Hepatitis

Alcohol abuse is a major cause of liver disease in the Western world. Three major pathologic lesions resulting from alcohol abuse are (1) fatty liver, (2) alcoholic hepatitis, and (3) cirrhosis. These lesions are not mutually exclusive, and there may be features of all three lesions in the same patient. The first two lesions are potentially reversible and may sometimes be confused clinically with viral hepatitis or gallbladder or biliary tract disease. Alcoholic cirrhosis is discussed in Chapter 45.

MECHANISM OF INJURY

Mechanisms of liver injury caused by alcohol are complex. Ethanol and its metabolites, acetaldehyde and nicotinamide adenine dinucleotide phosphate (NADP), are directly hepatotoxic and cause a large number of metabolic derangements. Induction of cytochrome P-450 (CYP2E1) and cytokine pathways, particularly tumor necrosis factor-α (TNF-α), is also critical in initiating and perpetuating hepatic injury and producing the lesions of alcoholic hepatitis.

Hepatotoxic effects from alcohol vary considerably among individuals. Nevertheless, consumption by men of 40 to 80 g of ethanol per day (one beer or one mixed drink = 10 g of ethanol) for 10 to 15 years carries a substantial risk for the development of alcoholic liver disease, whereas women appear to have a lower threshold of injury. Malnutrition and presence of other forms of chronic liver disease may potentiate the toxic effects of alcohol on the liver, and genetic factors may contribute to individual susceptibility.

CLINICAL AND PATHOLOGIC FEATURES

Alcoholic fatty liver may exhibit as incidentally discovered tender hepatomegaly. Some patients consult a physician because of pain in their right upper quadrant. Jaundice is rare. Aminotransferases are mildly elevated (<5 times normal). Liver biopsy shows diffuse or centrilobular fat occupying most of the hepatocyte.

Alcoholic hepatitis, a severe and prognostically ominous lesion, is characterized by the following histologic triad: (1) Mallory bodies (intracellular eosinophilic aggregates of cytokeratins), usually seen near or around the cell nuclei of hepatocytes; (2) infiltration by polymorphonuclear leukocytes; and (3) a network of interlobular connective tissue surrounding hepatocytes and central veins (*pericellular, perivenular,* and *perisinusoidal fibrosis*). Patients with this histologic lesion may be asymptomatic or extremely ill with hepatic failure. Anorexia, nausea, vomiting, weight loss, and abdominal pain are common symptoms. Hepatomegaly is present in 80% of patients with alcoholic hepatitis, and splenomegaly is often present. Fever is common, but bacterial infection should always be excluded because patients with alcoholic liver disease are prone to develop pneumonia, as well as infection of the urinary tract and the peritoneal cavity, when ascites is present. Jaundice is commonly present and may be pronounced, with cholestatic features that require differentiation from biliary tract disease

(see Chapter 42). Cutaneous signs of chronic liver disease may be found, including spider angiomas, palmar erythema, and gynecomastia. Parotid enlargement, testicular atrophy, and loss of body hair may be prominent (see Chapter 45). Ascites and encephalopathy may be present and indicate severe disease. The white blood cell count may be strikingly elevated, whereas aminotransferase levels are only modestly increased (range, 200 to 400 U/L), which is an important differentiating feature from other forms of acute hepatitis in which aminotransferases are significantly increased (invariably in the thousands). The ratio of AST to ALT nearly always exceeds 2:1, in contrast to viral hepatitis, in which the aminotransferase levels are usually increased in parallel. Prolonged prothrombin time, hypoalbuminemia, and hyperglobulinemia may be found.

DIAGNOSIS

A history of excessive prolonged alcohol intake is often difficult to obtain from patients with alcoholic liver disease. However, historical, clinical, and biochemical features of alcoholic hepatitis are often sufficient to establish the diagnosis. Many patients suspected or found to imbibe alcohol excessively may have causes other than alcohol for their liver disease (e.g., chronic viral hepatitis). Thus, when other causes of liver disease are suggested and the patient's alcohol intake is uncertain, appropriate serologic testing and a liver biopsy may be needed to establish a diagnosis.

COMPLICATIONS AND PROGNOSIS

Alcoholic fatty liver disease completely resolves with cessation of alcohol intake. Alcoholic hepatitis can also resolve, but more commonly it progresses either to cirrhosis, which may already be present at the time of initial presentation, or to hepatic failure and death. The development of encephalopathy, ascites, deteriorating renal function (*hepatorenal syndrome*), and gastrointestinal bleeding from varices often complicates alcoholic hepatitis (see Chapter 45). Patients with a hepatic discriminant function (DF) higher than 32 (DF = 4.6 × [prothrombin time (in seconds) − control (in seconds)] + total bilirubin [mg/dL]) have high risk for mortality.

TREATMENT

Fatty liver and early stages of alcoholic hepatitis (without extensive fibrosis) are reversible conditions, and therefore complete abstinence from alcohol is the most important step. The cornerstone of treatment of acute alcoholic hepatitis is meticulous supportive care. A high-calorie diet with vitamin (particularly thiamine) and protein supplementation is instituted and may require administration by nasogastric tube in patients with severe anorexia. In the absence of infection, gastrointestinal bleeding, or renal failure, specific patients with alcoholic hepatitis with DF greater than 32 and hepatic encephalopathy may benefit from corticosteroids. Because TNF-α plays a role in the pathogenesis of alcohol induced liver injury, several strategies for TNF-α inhibition have been evaluated as treatment options. Pentoxifylline (an oral TNF-α antagonist) has in a single randomized trial shown benefit in severe alcoholic

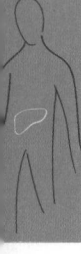

hepatitis by diminishing the risk for renal failure. Recent studies using infliximab (monoclonal antibody) and etanercept (TNF-α receptor blocker) in alcoholic hepatitis have shown an increased frequency of severe infections and higher mortality, and these agents are not recommended for therapy.

Drug-Induced and Toxin-Induced Hepatitis

A broad spectrum of hepatic disease may result from a variety of therapeutic drugs or toxins (Table 43-4). The pathophysiologic mechanisms whereby these hepatic lesions are produced are complex. At one end of the spectrum is a predictable, dose-dependent, direct toxic effect on hepatocytes that leads to frank centrilobular hepatocellular necrosis, typical of acetaminophen and carbon tetrachloride toxicity. Other reactions are generally not predictable and usually occur for unknown reasons in susceptible persons (*idiosyncratic drug reaction*). In some instances, genetically determined differences in pathways of hepatic drug metabolism may result in metabolites with greater toxic potential. Classic examples include viral hepatitis–like reactions (halothane and isoniazid), cholestatic hepatitis (chlorpromazine),

Table 43-4 Classification of Drug-Induced Liver Disease

Category	Examples
Predictable hepatotoxins with zonal necrosis	Acetaminophen
	Carbon tetrachloride
Nonspecific hepatitis	Aspirin
	Oxacillin
	Herbs (chaparral, germander)
Viral hepatitis-like reactions	Halothane
	Isoniazid
	Phenytoin
Cholestasis	Estrogens
	Erythromycin
	Amoxicillin, clavulanic acid
Noninflammatory	17α-substituted steroids
Inflammatory	Chlorpromazine
	Antithyroid agents
Fatty liver: large droplet	Ethanol
	Corticosteroids
Fatty liver: small droplet	Amiodarone
	Allopurinol
Chronic hepatitis	Methyldopa
	Nitrofurantoin
Tumors	Estrogens
	Vinyl chloride
Vascular lesions	6-Thioguanine
	Anabolic steroids
	Herbs (senna, comfrey)
Fibrosis	Methotrexate
Granulomas	Allopurinol
	Sulfonamides

granulomatous hepatitis (allopurinol), chronic hepatitis (methyldopa), and pure cholestasis without inflammation or hepatocellular necrosis (estrogens and androgens). Immune-mediated hepatic damage may contribute in some cases, possibly when the drugs or their metabolites act as a hapten on the surface of hepatocytes. A few important classes of drugs that cause hepatitis are discussed here.

ANALGESICS

Acetaminophen overdose is the leading cause of acute liver failure in the United States, accounting for 40% to 50% of all cases, and carries a mortality rate close to 30%. Acetaminophen is metabolized by the hepatic cytochrome P-450 system to a potentially toxic metabolite that is subsequently rendered harmless through conjugation with glutathione. When massive doses are taken (>10 to 15 g), the formation of excess toxic metabolites depletes the available glutathione and produces necrosis. Acetaminophen overdose, commonly taken in a suicide attempt, leads to nausea and vomiting within a few hours. These symptoms subside and are followed in 24 to 48 hours by clinical and laboratory evidence of hepatocellular necrosis (raised aminotransferase levels) and hepatic dysfunction (prolonged prothrombin time and hepatic encephalopathy). Similar findings may occur with therapeutic doses of acetaminophen in patients with chronic alcoholism or malnutrition. Extensive liver necrosis may lead to fulminant hepatic failure and death. In a patient with nonstaggered overdose, a serum acetaminophen level should be drawn 4 to 24 hours after ingestion. If plotted on a treatment nomogram of plasma drug concentration against time, it can predict the severity of outcome and need for therapy. Treatment with *N*-acetylcysteine given orally (140-mg/kg bolus followed by 70 mg/kg × 17 doses) or intravenously, thought to promote hepatic glutathione synthesis, may be life saving.

Nonsteroidal anti-inflammatory drugs (NSAIDs) as a class are an important cause of drug-induced liver disease. *Salicylates* cause dose-dependent hepatocellular injury that is usually clinically mild and easily reversible. *Diclofenac*, one of the most commonly prescribed NSAIDs worldwide, has been linked to asymptomatic elevation of aminotransferases, acute hepatitis, and fulminant hepatic failure. *Sulindac* is considered the most likely NSAID to produce hepatic injury and causes a damage spectrum ranging from hepatocellular to mixed to pure cholestatic injury. Whether the newer cyclo-oxygenase-2–selective NSAIDs have a lower risk for hepatotoxicity is uncertain.

ANTIBIOTICS AND ANTIVIRALS

Antimicrobials as a class are the most frequently incriminated agents causing drug-induced liver injury. Amoxicillin–clavulanic acid is the leading cause of antibiotic-related liver injury and results in a cholestatic hepatitis. Men appear to be more susceptible than women. Other common agents include nitrofurantoin, isoniazid, trimethoprim-sulfamethoxazole, and fluoroquinolones. Isoniazid, as a single-drug prophylaxis against tuberculosis, commonly produces raised serum aminotransferase levels in 20% of patients. This effect appears to be transient and self-limited in most patients. However, a 1% incidence exists of clinical hepatitis, which progresses to fatal hepatic necrosis in 10% of affected patients. Individual and age-related differences in hepatic acetylation of potentially toxic isoniazid metabolites may be important in this injury. Thus, the incidence of severe hepatic damage increases with age such that significant elevation of aminotransferase levels in persons who are older than 35 years is an indication for discontinuing the drug. Erythromycin is an established agent causing cholestatic injury. Trimethoprim-sulfamethoxazole characteristically causes cholestatic or mixed injury. A large number of agents used to treat HIV infection have been linked with hepatic injury of various forms. Important among these agents are nevirapine, ritonavir, and indinavir.

CENTRAL NERVOUS SYSTEM AGENTS

Central nervous system agents are second only to antimicrobials as a frequent cause of drug-induced liver injury. Important categories are anticonvulsants and anesthetics. Other common agents include duloxetine, bupropion, and fluoxetine. Among anticonvulsants, sodium valproate, phenytoin, carbamazepine, and lamotrigine are the most common drugs causing liver injury. Phenytoin and carbamazepine have been implicated in an *antiepileptic hypersensitivity syndrome,* characterized by a triad of rash, fever, and hepatocellular injury that may lead to fulminant hepatic failure. Lymphadenopathy and a mononucleosis-like picture with atypical lymphocytes may be present. Renal and pulmonary involvement may also occur. Historically, the anesthetic agent halothane caused an uncommon acute viral hepatitis–like reaction several days after exposure in susceptible persons. Hepatic injury was caused in part by an allergic response to hepatic neoantigens produced by halothane metabolism, and the severity of this reaction increased with repeated exposure. Newer, commonly used halogenated anesthetic agents (e.g., isoflurane, enflurane) are hepatotoxic in a much smaller number of patients, though cross-sensitivity does exist.

HERBS

Herbal supplements are taken throughout the world, and about $5 billion per year is spent in the United States alone on herbal agents. Incorrectly considered to be safe because they are *natural,* many herbs are hepatotoxic. *Senecio, Heliotropium, Crotalaria,* and comfrey contain pyrrolizidine alkaloids that cause hepatic veno-occlusive disease. Hepatotoxicity ranging from mild hepatitis to massive necrosis and fulminant hepatic failure has been associated with the use of chaparral, germander, pennyroyal oil, mistletoe, valerian root, comfrey, and Ma huang. Milk thistle, often taken by patients with chronic hepatitis and cirrhosis, has not been associated with hepatotoxicity, but its benefit is undefined because of a lack of controlled studies.

Chronic Hepatitis

Chronic hepatitis is defined as a hepatic inflammatory process that fails to resolve after 6 months and, in those with acute viral hepatitis, by persistence of serum viral antigens and nucleic acids beyond a similar period.

ETIOLOGY

Acute viral hepatitis can ultimately lead to chronic hepatitis, with the notable exceptions of HAV and HEV. Nonalcoholic steatohepatitis (NASH) is now considered the most frequent cause of chronic hepatitis in the United States and Western Europe. Several drugs may produce chronic hepatitis, the best recognized being methyldopa. In contrast to acute hepatitis, an etiologic agent is sometimes difficult to identify in cases of chronic hepatitis. The pathogenesis of these idiopathic forms may represent quiescent autoimmune disease, undetected past drug-induced injury or NASH, antibody-negative viral infections, or misdiagnosed cholestatic liver injury (e.g., primary biliary cirrhosis, primary sclerosing cholangitis).

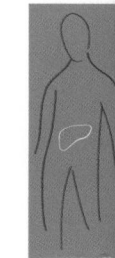

CLASSIFICATION

Current classification of chronic hepatitis is based on the *etiologic agent* responsible for disease, the *grade* of injury (determined by the numbers and location of inflammatory cells), and the *stage* of disease on liver biopsy (determined by the degree, location, and distortion of normal architecture by fibrosis). This classification allows integration of knowledge of the natural history of specific causes with histologic features of hepatic damage to assess the severity and prognosis of the process. Thus, in general, biochemical and serologic studies along with liver biopsy are used in the diagnosis and management of chronic hepatitis.

Chronic Viral Hepatitis

Chronic hepatitis B follows acute hepatitis B in 5% to 10% of adults in the United States. HBV infection without evidence of any liver damage may persist, resulting in asymptomatic or *healthy* hepatitis B carriers. In Asia and Africa, many such carriers appear to have acquired the virus from infected mothers during infancy (vertical transmission). Patients who are HBsAg and HBeAg positive and have high serum HBV DNA (>20,000 IU/mL or >100,000 copies/mL), coupled with increased serum aminotransferases (ALT, 2 times normal) are in a high replicative phase (see Table 43-3). In contrast, patients in a low replicative phase are HBsAg and anti-HBe positive, have low serum HBV DNA (<20,000 IU/mL or <100,000 copies/mL), and near-normal or normal aminotransferases. Such patients can go into high replicative phase and exhibit acute or chronic hepatitis B. A subgroup of patients with chronic hepatitis B may be HBeAg negative but still be in a high replicative phase, as evidenced by high HBV DNA levels in serum. These patients have a precore or core mutant form of hepatitis B. Patients infected with HBV in high replicative phase are at highest risk for developing cirrhosis and hepatocellular carcinoma. Such patients and those who have already progressed to early cirrhosis are the primary targets of anti-HBV therapy. Currently, seven drugs are approved as single agents for treating hepatitis B in the United States, including injectable interferon-α (pegylated and nonpegylated) and oral nucleoside or nucleotide analogues (e.g., lamivudine, telbivudine, adefovir, tenofovir, entecavir). All these drugs lead to suppression of serum viral DNA to a variable amount as well as seroconversion from HBeAg to anti-HBe in 10% to 30% of patients. Resistance to the oral agents with prolonged use is a major concern and is highest for lamivudine among the current agents. Interferon, on the other hand, has numerous side effects and may not be well tolerated. In general, patients without cirrhosis with active replication may be treated with interferon-α or more commonly with nucleoside and nucleotide analogues. In patients with cirrhosis, interferon-α is not an appropriate therapy, and long-term nucleoside or nucleotide analogue therapy is recommended in patients even with lower levels of viral replication.

Chronic hepatitis C develops in up to 75% of individuals acutely exposed to HCV and is estimated to affect 1.8% of the U.S. population. More than 20% of these patients may develop cirrhosis in about 30 years. Hepatitis C has six major genotypes, of which, in the United States, genotype 1 is the most common, followed by genotypes 2 and 3. Genotype has no impact on course of illness but is the most important determinant of successful outcome of treatment. Chronic hepatitis C is currently treated with a combination of pegylated interferon-α injections and oral ribavirin. Durable suppression of viral activity (sustained virologic response [SVR], defined as undetectable HCV RNA 6 months after therapy) occurs in as many as 80% of all patients infected with genotype 2 or 3 when treated for 24 weeks and in 50% of those infected with genotype 1 when treated for 48 weeks. Recent studies indicate that patients with a rapid virologic response (RVR, defined as undetectable HCV RNA at 4 weeks, particularly genotypes 2 or 3, may be treated with a shorter duration of therapy. Both interferon and ribavirin have numerous side effects, which contraindicates their use in 50% or more of patients currently infected with HCV. Of the remaining 50%, therapy is usually advised for patients with favorable genotypes or those who demonstrate moderate to high fibrosis on liver biopsies. Newer agents in development for hepatitis C include protease inhibitors as part of a new class of agents called *specifically targeted antiviral therapy for hepatitis C* (STAT-C). Successful treatment of chronic hepatitis B and C may lead to a decrease in hepatic inflammation and fibrosis and to a reduced risk for progression to cirrhosis and the development of hepatocellular carcinoma.

Autoimmune Hepatitis

Autoimmune liver disease has several forms; however, the typical disease occurs in young women and is characterized by significant hepatic inflammation with a preponderance of plasma cells and fibrosis. The presence of hypergammaglobulinemia, as well as antinuclear antibody (ANA) or anti–smooth muscle antibody (anti-SMA), represents the most common classic or type 1 variant. Type 2 autoimmune hepatitis is characterized by the presence of anti–liver-kidney microsomal antibodies (anti-LKM) and the absence of ANA and anti-SMA. Type 2 autoimmune hepatitis occurs most commonly in girls and young women. A third type of autoimmune hepatitis with antibodies to soluble liver antigen or liver-pancreas antigen (anti-SLA/LP) is no longer considered a unique entity because these antibodies can be found in type 1 and type 2 autoimmune hepatitis as well. There are

no pathognomonic features of autoimmune hepatitis, and the diagnosis is made by a combination of factors. Recently, a simplified diagnostic algorithm that includes the presence of autoantibodies, hypergammaglobulinemia, typical liver histology, and absence of viral hepatitis has proved useful in identifying patients with autoimmune hepatitis. Extrahepatic manifestations that include amenorrhea, rashes, acne, vasculitis, thyroiditis, and Sjögren syndrome are common. Evidence of hepatic failure and the presence of chronic disease on biopsy at the time of diagnosis are frequent. Indications for treatment include abnormal liver function tests and significant hepatic inflammation on biopsy. Corticosteroids are the mainstay of treatment, typically in combination with azathioprine to minimize long-term use of high-dose steroids. This regimen is efficacious in most patients (>80%) and, in many instances, prolongs survival.

Nonalcoholic Fatty Liver Disease

Nonalcoholic fatty liver disease (NAFLD), a term that encompasses steatosis (fatty liver), nonalcoholic steatohepatitis (NASH), and cirrhosis secondary to NASH, has become increasingly recognized as the most common reason for abnormal liver function tests among adults in the United States and Western Europe. Although NAFLD most commonly occurs in persons who are overweight, have diabetes, and have hyperlipidemia, it can also occur in persons of normal weight. Estimates indicate that about 30 million Americans have NAFLD, and of these, 8.6 million have NASH, with nearly 20% having signs of advanced disease (i.e., bridging fibrosis, cirrhosis) on histologic examination. Noninvasive modalities for diagnosis of NAFLD include radiologic imaging and serum markers of hepatic fibrosis. However, liver biopsy with histologic examination is the most accurate test for determining presence of NASH and defining the degree of fibrosis. Histologic criteria for NASH include macrovesicular fatty infiltration (mainly triglyceride); inflammation, including polymorphonuclear leukocytes; and hepatocyte injury (ballooning degeneration or necrotic hepatocytes), with or without fibrosis. The pathogenesis is still under investigation, but insulin resistance plays an essential role leading to lipolysis and hyperinsulinemia, upregulation of cytochrome P-450 pathways, and impaired mitochondrial and peroxisomal fatty acid oxidation. This state leads to excessive oxidative stress, cytokine induction, and inflammation. Weight reduction and exercise are established to improve liver histology in NASH. Clinical trials assessing lipid-lowering agents and drugs that improve insulin resistance (e.g., thiazolidinediones and metformin) are ongoing, but efficacy and safety are not yet established.

Genetic and Metabolic Hepatitis

Wilson disease and α$_1$-antitrypsin deficiency generally occur before the age of 35 years, and a family history of liver disease

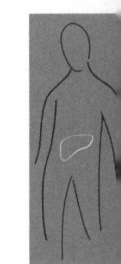

may be present. Wilson disease is caused by mutation in the *WD* gene and is autosomal recessive. A resultant accumulation of copper in various tissues occurs, including liver, brain, and the corneas, with neuropsychiatric signs and symptoms and liver disease ranging from steatosis to chronic hepatitis to fulminant liver failure. Diagnostic evaluation for Wilson disease includes low serum ceruloplasmin and high urinary and hepatic copper levels. Therapy is indefinite and includes copper chelation, typically with trientine, followed by diminishing copper absorption with zinc supplementation. α_1-antitrypsin deficiency is also inherited as an autosomal recessive disorder. The normal gene product is designated as PiM, and the deficiency variants are PiS (50% to 60% α_1-antitrypsin expression) and PiZ (10% to 20% α_1-antitrypsin expression). The most common carrier phenotypes are PiMS and PiMZ, and the disease phenotypes are PiZZ, PiSS, and PiSZ. A low serum α_1-antitrypsin level and diastase-positive staining of hepatocellular inclusions on liver biopsy suggest α_1-antitrypsin deficiency. Phenotypic testing has been considered the gold standard for the diagnosis. However, genotypic testing is now available. Intravenous pooled human plasma α_1-antitrypsin and recombinant gene therapy are options for patients with emphysema but are not useful for patients with liver disease.

Prospectus for the Future

A better understanding of the molecular genetics and replication cycles of hepatitis B and C, as well as the role of cell-mediated and humoral immunity (or lack thereof) in various forms of chronic viral and nonviral hepatitis, has led to an expansion of therapeutic options for patients with these diseases. Therapeutic vaccines designed to boost humoral immunity against specific HCV and HBV epitopes are currently in clinical trials. Several STAT-C agents that target specific enzymes involved in hepatitis C replication, including protease inhibitors such as telaprevir and boceprevir and other non-nucleoside inhibitors, are in various stages of development, including ongoing clinical trials. At least five new drugs targeting hepatitis B replication are on the horizon. The next step is to assess, in combination, the numerous anti-HBV drugs, both old and new, to enhance their efficacy while diminishing the risk for viral resistance. Increasing experience with the use of newer immunosuppressive agents with novel mechanisms of action such as mycophenolate mofetil, tacrolimus, and cyclosporine opens avenues for studying these agents in patients with autoimmune hepatitis. Finally, recognition of the central role of TNF-α in the pathogenesis of alcoholic hepatitis has led to investigation of a significant number of TNF-α antagonists, currently in use for rheumatologic and autoimmune diseases, in this disorder.

References

Chalasani N, Fontana RJ, Bonkovsky HL, for the Drug Induced Liver Injury Network (DILIN): Causes, clinical features, and outcomes from a prospective study of drug-induced liver injury in the United States. Gastroenterology 135:1924-1934, 2008.

Hennes EM, Zentya M, Czaja AJ, et al: Simplified criteria for the diagnosis of autoimmune hepatitis. Hepatology 48:169-176, 2008.

Lee WM, Squires RH, Jr., Nyberg SL, et al: Acute liver failure: Summary of a workshop. Hepatology 47:1401-1415, 2008.

Levitsky J, Mailliard ME: Diagnosis and therapy of alcoholic liver disease. Semin Liver Dis 24:233, 2004.

Lindsay KL, Hoofnagle JH: Acute viral hepatitis. In Goldman L, Ausiello D (eds): Cecil Textbook of Medicine. Philadelphia, WB Saunders, 2004, pp 911-917.

Lok ASF, McMahon BJ: Chronic hepatitis B. Hepatology 45:507-539, 2007.

Fulminant Hepatic Failure

Brendan M. McGuire and Michael B. Fallon

Fulminant hepatic failure (FHF) is defined as the onset of encephalopathy occurring within 8 weeks of the onset of jaundice in a patient with hepatic injury and no prior history of liver disease. *Late-onset hepatic failure* is recognized as the development of encephalopathy in patients between 8 and 24 weeks after the onset of jaundice. The pathogenesis of FHF involves severe widespread hepatic necrosis, commonly resulting from acute viral infection with hepatitis A, B, C, D, or E viruses (see Chapter 43). It may also result from exposure to hepatotoxins such as acetaminophen, isoniazid, halothane, valproic acid, or mushroom toxins (e.g., those of *Amanita phalloides*). Reye syndrome (a disease predominantly of children) and acute fatty liver of pregnancy, both of which are characterized by microvesicular fatty infiltration and little hepatocellular necrosis, often resemble FHF. Other rare causes of FHF include Wilson disease, hepatic ischemia, autoimmune hepatitis, and malignancy. In a significant number of patients with FHF, no cause is found, although a viral infection is usually presumed to be responsible (**Web Figs. 44-1 and 44-2**).

Diagnosis

The diagnosis of FHF is based on the combination of hepatic encephalopathy and liver failure. It is characterized biochemically by significantly elevated serum bilirubin and transaminase levels and marked prolongation of the prothrombin time.

Treatment

Treatment of FHF remains supportive because the underlying cause of liver failure is rarely treatable. However, most processes that result in widespread liver cell necrosis and FHF are transient events, and liver cell regeneration with recovery of liver function often occurs if patients do not die from the complications of liver failure in the interim. Meticulous supportive treatment in an intensive care unit setting has been shown to improve survival. Patients with FHF should be treated in centers with experience with this disease and with a liver transplantation program. Numerous complications result from FHF, and thorough identification and treatment of each are essential (Table 44-1).

Hepatic encephalopathy is often the first and most dramatic sign of liver failure. The pathogenesis of hepatic encephalopathy remains unclear. Hepatic encephalopathy that accompanies FHF differs from that associated with chronic liver disease in two important aspects: (1) it often responds to therapy only when liver function improves, and (2) it is frequently associated with two other potentially treatable causes of coma: hypoglycemia and cerebral edema. Therapy for hepatic encephalopathy in FHF differs slightly from the principles outlined in Chapter 45. Lactulose may be given orally, per nasogastric tube, or rectally, but the oral route should not be used if the patient is at risk for aspiration. Lactulose should be discontinued if no improvement is noted after several doses are administered. Intubation is often necessary to protect the airway from aspiration and to allow ventilation in patients with advanced encephalopathy.

Cerebral edema, the pathogenesis of which is unknown, is a common complication and the leading cause of death in FHF. Clinically, differentiating FHF from hepatic encephalopathy is difficult, and computed tomography of the head is often unreliable. Therefore, measuring intracranial pressure is important. The goal is to maintain an intracranial pressure of less than 20 mm Hg. Management includes control of agitation, head elevation of 20 to 30 degrees, hyperventilation, administration of mannitol, barbiturate-induced coma, and urgent liver transplantation.

Hypoglycemia is a common complication of liver failure resulting from impaired hepatic gluconeogenesis and insulin degradation. All patients should receive 10% glucose intravenous infusions with frequent monitoring of blood glucose levels. Other metabolic abnormalities commonly occur, including hyponatremia, hypokalemia, respiratory alkalosis, and metabolic acidosis. Thus, frequent monitoring of blood electrolytes and pH is indicated.

Bleeding occurs frequently and is commonly caused by gastric erosions and impaired synthesis of clotting factors. All patients should receive vitamin K and prophylactic gastric acid suppression. Fresh-frozen plasma should be used if clinically significant bleeding occurs or if major pro-

Table 44-1 Management of Selected Problems in Fulminant Hepatic Failure

Complications	Pathogenesis	Management
Hepatic encephalopathy	Liver failure	Search for treatable causes (e.g., hypoglycemia, drugs used for sedation, sepsis, gastrointestinal bleeding, electrolyte imbalance, decreased P_{O_2}, increased P_{CO_2}); lactulose
Cerebral edema	Unknown	Elevate head of bed 20-30 degrees; hyperventilate (P_{CO_2}, 25-30 mm Hg); mannitol, 0.5-1 g/kg intravenous bolus over 5 min; pentobarbital infusion; urgent liver transplantation
Coagulopathy and gastrointestinal hemorrhage	Decreased synthesis of clotting factors Gastric erosions	Vitamin K; fresh-frozen plasma if actively bleeding and for prevention of bleeding; gastric acid suppression
Hypoglycemia	Decreased gluconeogenesis Decreased insulin degradation	Intravenous 10% dextrose, monitor every 2 hr; 30%-50% dextrose may be needed
Agitation	May be caused by: Encephalopathy Intracranial pressure Hypoxemia	Search for treatable causes (e.g., P_{O_2}, skin ulcers, lacerations, abscesses); soft restraints; if severely agitated and a concern for injury, consider sedation along with mechanical ventilation to protect airway
Infection	Liver failure and invasive monitoring	Surveillance cultures and low threshold for empiric antibiotics

P_{CO_2}, partial pressure of carbon dioxide; P_{O_2}, partial pressure of oxygen.

cedures, including intracranial pressure monitoring and central line placement, are performed.

Infection is one of the leading causes of death in FHF. As many as 80% of patients with FHF develop infection (80% bacterial, 20% fungal). Patients are at higher risk for infection as a result of impaired immunity resulting from liver failure and of the need for invasive monitoring. Severe infection may occur without fever or leukocytosis. Therefore, frequent cultures and a low threshold for beginning antibiotics are required.

Hepatic Transplantation

Hepatic transplantation (see Chapter 45) has been performed with success in patients with FHF and is the treatment of choice for patients who appear unlikely to recover spontaneously. Because of the urgent need for transplantation, potential candidates should be transferred to trans-plantation centers before significant complications develop (e.g., coma, cerebral edema, hemorrhage, infection). Transplantation is usually indicated in patients with severe encephalopathy or coagulopathy.

Prognosis

The cause of FHF and the degree of hepatic encephalopathy are important in determining prognosis. Patients with FHF from acetaminophen overdose or viral hepatitis A or B have a better survival rate than do patients with Wilson disease or without a known cause. The short-term survival rate for patients with FHF in coma is 20% without liver transplantation. The 1-year survival rate of patients with FHF after liver transplantation is 80% to 90%. Patients who survive without a transplant also have an excellent prognosis because liver tissue usually regenerates normally, regardless of the cause of FHF.

Prospectus for the Future

The development of effective therapy for FHF has been an ongoing focus of clinical and basic investigators for many years. Recently, a significant number of advances suggest the potential for improved treatments. Specifically, basic insights into the mechanisms of hepatocyte cell death and regeneration have defined specific pathways that may be manipulated to decrease hepatocyte loss and improve hepatocyte regeneration in response to acute injury. Such therapies are effective in animal models and are likely to be explored in humans. In addition, ongoing clinical trials with the use of hypothermia in FHF suggest that cooling may decrease cerebral injury and improve overall survival. Multicenter trials will be needed to confirm the efficacy of such an approach.

References

Stravitz R, Kramer AH, Davern T, et al, for the Acute Liver Failure Study Group: Intensive care of patients with acute liver failure: Recommendations of the U.S. Acute Liver Failure Study Group. Crit Care Med 35: 2498-2508, 2007.

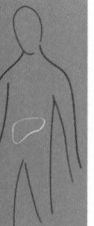

Cirrhosis of the Liver and Its Complications

Rajan Kochar, Miguel R. Arguedas, and Michael B. Fallon

Definition and Etiopathogenesis

Cirrhosis is the irreversible end result of a variety of inflammatory, toxic, metabolic, and congestive insults to the liver. These insults lead to the formation of interconnecting bands of fibrous tissue that surround *nodules* consisting of foci of regenerating hepatocytes. These regenerative nodules may be small (<3 mm; *micronodular cirrhosis*), a typical feature of alcoholic cirrhosis, or large (>3 mm; *macronodular cirrhosis*), more commonly seen as a sequela to chronic active hepatitis. The disruption of the normal hepatic lobular architecture distorts the vascular bed and contributes to portal hypertension and intrahepatic shunting. Normal hepatocyte function is disturbed by the resulting inadequacy of blood flow and ongoing inflammatory, toxic, or metabolic damage to hepatocytes. In addition, disturbances in cellular regulation and differentiation during hepatocyte regeneration may lead to the development of hepatocellular carcinoma. Therefore, the clinical features of cirrhosis and its complications arise from portal hypertension, hepatocellular dysfunction, and altered cellular differentiation (Table 45-1). These disturbances are associated with significant morbidity and mortality, with more than 25,000 deaths occurring annually in the United States as a result of chronic liver disease. Alcohol consumption, hepatitis C virus infection, and nonalcoholic fatty liver disease are the most common causes of cirrhosis in Western industrialized nations, whereas hepatitis B is a major cause in Asia and in developing countries. Other important causes include biliary cirrhosis (primary and secondary), autoimmune hepatitis, cardiac cirrhosis, inherited diseases, and metabolic disorders. Cryptogenic cirrhosis remains a diagnosis of exclusion. Chronic active hepatitis, nonalcoholic fatty liver disease, and α_1-antitrypsin deficiency are discussed in Chapter 43. Hemochromatosis and Wilson disease are covered in Chapter 63. Common and uncommon conditions that may lead to cirrhosis are listed in Table 45-2.

Diagnosis

Patients with cirrhosis are often asymptomatic, and the diagnosis is incidentally established at the time of physical examination, laboratory testing, or radiologic testing for unrelated purposes. Alternatively, patients may present with specific complications of cirrhosis such as variceal bleeding, ascites, spontaneous bacterial peritonitis, and hepatic encephalopathy.

Liver biopsy is considered the gold standard for the diagnosis of cirrhosis. In most cases, however, the diagnosis can be made reliably by a combination of clinical, laboratory, and radiologic findings, and liver biopsy is done more often to assess the stage and severity of disease, prognosis, and response to treatment.

CLINICAL FEATURES

Symptoms are often nonspecific and include fatigue, malaise, weakness, weight gain or weight loss, anorexia, nausea, increased abdominal girth, and abdominal discomfort. Physical findings include jaundice, abnormal liver span or consistency, splenomegaly, ascites, lower extremity edema, spider angiomas, palmar erythema, nail changes (Terry nails—proximal nail plate discoloration; and Muehrcke lines—white horizontal lines), gynecomastia, caput medusae, asterixis, and testicular atrophy. Table 45-1 highlights the pathogenetic mechanisms underlying these signs and symptoms.

LABORATORY FINDINGS

Hepatocellular dysfunction leads to impaired protein synthesis (hypoalbuminemia and prolongation of prothrombin

Table 45-1 Clinical Features and Pathogenesis of Cirrhosis

Signs and Symptoms	Pathogenesis
Constitutional	
Fatigue, anorexia, malaise, weakness, weight loss	Liver dysfunction
Cutaneous	
Spider angiomas, palmar erythema	Altered estrogen and androgen metabolism
Jaundice	Decreased bilirubin excretion
Caput medusae	Portosystemic shunting due to PH
Endocrine	
Gynecomastia, testicular atrophy, decreased body hair in men; decreased libido virilization and menstrual irregularities in women	Altered estrogen and androgen metabolism
Gastrointestinal	
Abdominal pain	Hepatomegaly, hepatocellular carcinoma
Abdominal swelling	Ascites due to PH
Gastrointestinal bleeding	Variceal hemorrhage due to PH
Hematologic	
Anemia, leukopenia, thrombocytopenia	Hypersplenism secondary to PH
Ecchymosis	Decreased synthesis of coagulation factors
Neurologic	
Altered sleep pattern, somnolence, confusion, asterixis	Hepatocellular dysfunction and portosystemic shunting

PH, portal hypertension.

Table 45-2 Causes of Cirrhosis

Alcohol
Nonalcoholic steatohepatitis
Viral hepatitis
   Hepatitis B, C, and D
   Cytomegalovirus
   Epstein-Barr virus
Cardiac cirrhosis
   Chronic right heart failure
   Constrictive pericarditis
Drugs and toxins
Autoimmune hepatitis
Primary biliary cirrhosis
Secondary biliary cirrhosis
   Bile duct strictures
   Tumors of the bile ducts
   Biliary atresia
   Cystic fibrosis
   Primary sclerosing cholangitis
   Choledochal cyst
Chronic hepatic congestion
Budd-Chiari syndrome
Inherited and metabolic disorders
   Hemochromatosis
   Wilson disease
   α_1-antitrypsin deficiency
   Galactosemia
   Glycogen storage disorders

time), hyperbilirubinemia, low blood urea nitrogen levels, and elevated serum ammonia levels. *Portal hypertension* is responsible for thrombocytopenia and leukopenia resulting from splenic sequestration (hypersplenism). Anemia may result from hypersplenism or gastrointestinal blood loss. Patients with ascites may have dilutional hyponatremia. The levels of liver enzymes may vary with the etiology and stage of cirrhosis.

RADIOLOGIC FEATURES

Current radiologic modalities include ultrasound (with and without Doppler of the portal and hepatic venous vasculature), computed tomography, and magnetic resonance imaging. Imaging findings supportive of the diagnosis of cirrhosis include relative enlargement of the left hepatic and caudate lobes as a result of right lobe atrophy, surface nodularity, and features of portal hypertension such as ascites, intra-abdominal varices, and splenomegaly. These findings in the presence of clinical and laboratory features of cirrhosis preclude the need for a diagnostic liver biopsy, and it is considered only when the cause of liver disease is in doubt.

Major Complications of Cirrhosis

The major sequelae of cirrhosis are as follows:

1. As a consequence, predominantly of *hepatocellular dysfunction*:
   a. Jaundice
   b. Coagulopathy
   c. Hypoalbuminemia
2. As a consequence, predominantly of *portal hypertension*:
   a. Variceal hemorrhage
   b. Ascites
   c. Spontaneous bacterial peritonitis
   d. Hepatorenal syndrome
   e. Hepatic encephalopathy
   f. Hepatopulmonary syndrome
3. Hepatocellular carcinoma

The pathophysiologic interrelationships among these complications are shown diagrammatically in Figure 45-1.

HEPATOCELLULAR DYSFUNCTION

Cirrhosis results in impaired synthesis of proteins by hepatocytes, which leads to disturbances in the conjugation and excretion of bilirubin, hypoalbuminemia, deficient production of coagulation factors, and diminished capacity for hepatic detoxification (see Chapters 41 and 44).

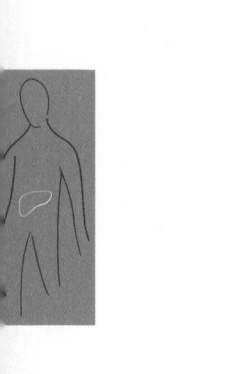

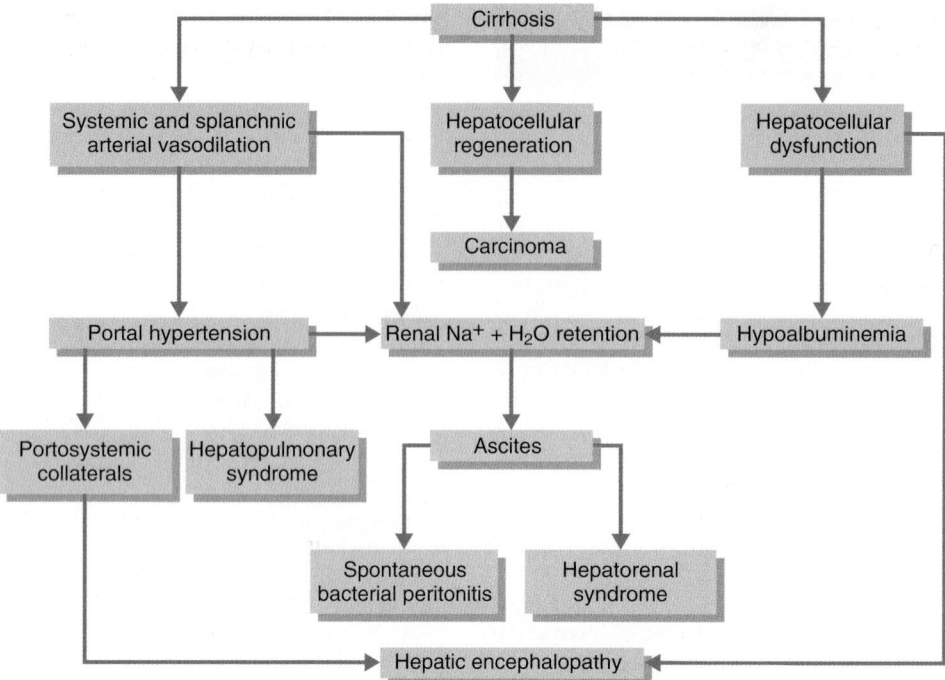

Figure 45-1 Inter-relationships among the complications of cirrhosis.

PORTAL HYPERTENSION

The normal portal venous pressure is low (5 to 10 mm Hg), and the hepatic venous pressure gradient (HVPG), which reflects sinusoidal pressure, is less than 5 mm Hg. In cirrhosis, the distortion of hepatic architecture by fibrous tissue and regenerative nodules, as well as a dynamic component caused by an increase in intrahepatic vascular tone, leads to increased resistance to portal venous flow, resulting in increased portal venous pressure (>10 mm Hg). The HVPG is measured using a transvenous approach by subtracting free hepatic venous pressure from the wedged hepatic venous pressure.

Although cirrhosis is the most important cause of portal hypertension, any process leading to increased resistance to portal blood flow into (presinusoidal) or through (sinusoidal) the liver or to hepatic venous outflow from the liver (postsinusoidal) may result in portal hypertension (Table 45-3). In addition, cirrhosis is associated with increased cardiac output, which leads to greater splanchnic blood flow, further aggravating portal hypertension. It is important to recognize that the HVPG is reliably increased only in sinusoidal portal hypertension.

In an attempt to decompress the portal system, venous collaterals form between the portal and systemic circulations. Major sites of collateral vessel formation include the gastroesophageal junction, retroperitoneum, rectum, and falciform ligament of the liver (abdominal and periumbilical collaterals). Clinically, the most important collaterals are those connecting the portal vein to the azygos vein through dilated, tortuous veins (varices) in the submucosa of the gastric fundus and esophagus.

Table 45-3 **Causes of Portal Hypertension**
Increased Resistance to Flow
Presinusoidal
Extrahepatic
• Portal or splenic vein occlusion (thrombosis, sclerosis, tumor)
Intrahepatic
• Schistosomiasis
• Congenital hepatic fibrosis
• Sarcoidosis
Sinusoidal
Cirrhosis (many causes)
Alcoholic hepatitis
Postsinusoidal
Intrahepatic
• Veno-occlusive disease
Extrahepatic
• Budd-Chiari syndrome
• Cardiac causes: constrictive pericarditis
Increased Portal Blood Flow
Splenomegaly not caused by liver disease
Arterioportal fistula

Variceal Hemorrhage

Gastroesophageal varices may develop when the portal pressure gradient exceeds 10 mm Hg, and the risk for variceal rupture leading to hemorrhage occurs when the gradient is greater than 12 mm Hg. Hemorrhage develops in 10% to 30% of patients every year, and each episode of variceal hemorrhage is associated with a mortality rate as high as

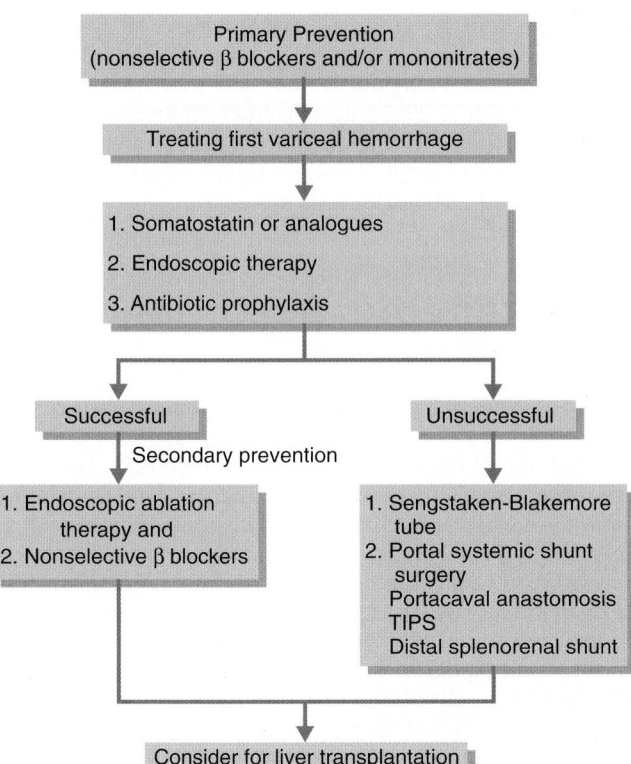

Figure 45-2 Prevention and treatment of variceal bleeding. TIPS, transjugular intrahepatic portosystemic shunt.

15% to 30%. Bleeding occurs most commonly from large varices in the esophagus when high tension in the walls of these vessels leads to rupture. Among gastric varices, fundal varices have the highest rate of bleeding and may bleed with portal pressure gradients of less than 12 mm Hg. Variceal bleeding usually causes painless hematemesis, melena, or hematochezia, which typically leads to hemodynamic compromise (see Chapter 34), further aggravated by impaired hepatic synthesis of coagulation factors (from hepatocellular dysfunction) and thrombocytopenia (from hypersplenism).

The management of gastroesophageal varices includes the treatment of acute variceal hemorrhage, the prevention of rebleeding (secondary prophylaxis), and the prevention of the initial episode of bleeding (primary prophylaxis) (Fig. 45-2). In the setting of acute variceal hemorrhage, the initial intervention consists of hemodynamic resuscitation with colloids such as blood or fresh-frozen plasma and airway protection and ventilatory support, if necessary. Combined pharmacologic and endoscopic therapy is superior to either therapy alone, especially if pharmacologic therapy is instituted immediately. In addition, prophylactic intravenous antibiotics should be administered early because they reduce the risk for infection, rebleeding, and death. Current pharmacologic therapy consists of somatostatin or its synthetic analogues (i.e., octreotide, vapreotide). These agents are best instituted before endoscopic examination. Endoscopic therapy includes band ligation and/or sclerotherapy (**Web Video 45-1**). Prospective studies have demonstrated that band ligation is the preferred modality given the lower inci-

dence of adverse effects and complications. In patients with gastric variceal hemorrhage, endoscopic variceal ablation with cyanoacrylate glue is superior to band ligation, although this therapy is not approved in the United States. Balloon tamponade (Sengstaken-Blakemore tube, Linton tube, or Minnesota tube) is a temporary measure reserved for patients in whom endoscopic therapy fails in the setting of massive hemorrhage. These patients may need to undergo portal decompression through a surgical shunt or transjugular intrahepatic portosystemic shunt (TIPS) placement. After an initial episode of variceal bleeding, recommendations for secondary prophylaxis include a combination of nonselective β blockers (propranolol and nadolol) and variceal obliteration through repeated courses of endoscopic band ligation. However, individual patient characteristics may dictate whether nonselective β blockers can be used. There are no formal recommendations on frequency and duration of follow-up endoscopy, although it is generally done at 1- to 6-month intervals after obliteration of varices. Endoscopic screening has been recommended to identify patients at high risk for variceal bleeding (i.e., those with large varices) so that primary prophylaxis can be instituted. Several studies suggest that certain clinical features (e.g., thrombocytopenia, ascites, telangiectasias) may help predict patients who are likely to have large varices, but given the poor predictive values of these features, endoscopic screening should be performed in all patients newly diagnosed with cirrhosis. Capsule endoscopy has been evaluated as a less invasive screening alternative to upper endoscopy but is currently less sensitive in diagnosing varices. Primary prophylaxis should be instituted for all patients with large varices and in those with advanced liver disease (Child class B and C) with small varices. Nonselective β blockers are the agents of choice for primary prophylaxis because they reduce portal blood flow and vascular resistance and hence portal pressure. In patients with contraindications or intolerance to β blockers, variceal obliteration through endoscopic band ligation is the best alternative.

Ascites

Ascites is the accumulation of excess fluid in the peritoneal cavity. Although cirrhosis is the most common cause of ascites, this condition may have numerous other causes (Table 45-4). The serum ascites-albumin gradient has replaced the exudative-transudative classification of ascites. An elevated serum ascites-albumin gradient (>1.1 g/dL, serum albumin concentration–ascites albumin concentration) signifies the presence of portal hypertension. Ascites becomes clinically detectable with fluid accumulation greater than 500 mL. Shifting dullness to percussion is the most sensitive clinical sign of ascites, but ultrasonography can readily detect smaller fluid volumes (250 mL).

The precise sequence of events leading to the development of cirrhotic ascites remains debated. However, both excess renal sodium and water retention resulting from portal hypertension and splanchnic vasodilation resulting in overflow of fluid into the peritoneum (*overflow theory*) and decreased effective circulating blood volume resulting from systemic arterial vasodilation leading to activation of neurohumoral systems and sodium and water retention (*underflow theory*) play a role.

Management of cirrhotic ascites consists initially of sodium restriction, preferably to less than 2 g per day. Restricted fluid intake may be necessary if hyponatremia (<125 mEq/L) is present. The administration of spironolactone, an aldosterone antagonist, supplemented with a loop diuretic (e.g., furosemide), is effective in about 90% of patients. Diuresis should be monitored closely because aggressive diuretic therapy may result in electrolyte disturbances (i.e., hyponatremia, hypokalemia) and hypovolemia, leading to impaired renal function and potentially precipitating hepatic encephalopathy. *Refractory ascites* occurs in about 10% of patients with cirrhosis and is defined as persistent tense ascites despite maximal diuretic therapy (spironolactone, 400 mg per day, and furosemide, 160 mg per day) or the development of azotemia or electrolyte disturbances at submaximal doses of diuretics. Treatment in these patients includes repeated large-volume paracentesis and colloid volume expansion with albumin, TIPS placement, and liver transplantation (Fig. 45-3). In recent years, vaso-pressin receptor antagonists called *aquaretics* (they promote electrolyte-free water excretion) are increasingly being studied for use in hyponatremia and may have a role in refractory ascites. These agents downregulate *aquaporin-2* channels in the collecting ducts and reduce water reabsorption. *Conivaptan* is an aquaretic recently approved by the U.S. Food and Drug Administration.

Spontaneous Bacterial Peritonitis

Cirrhotic patients may develop infection of ascitic fluid leading to acute spontaneous bacterial peritonitis (SBP) without an obvious source of contamination. The most common organisms include *Escherichia coli* and other Enterobacteriaceae such as *Klebsiella* species. Gram-positive organisms such as *Streptococcus, Enterococcus,* and *Pneumococcus* species may also be found. The microbiology of SBP is distinct from secondary peritonitis. Anaerobes are rarely found, and typically a single organism is isolated. Clinical features include fever, abdominal pain, and signs of peritoneal irritation. Often, the infection may be clinically silent or may be demonstrated by the development of hepatic encephalopathy or renal insufficiency. Therefore, diagnostic paracentesis should be considered in any patient with cirrhotic ascites who deteriorates clinically. The diagnosis is strongly suggested if the ascitic fluid polymorphonuclear leukocyte count is greater than 250 cells/mL and is confirmed by culture, preferably inoculated into blood culture bottles at the time of paracentesis. The use of rapid bedside diagnostic methods such as leukocyte esterase reagent strips is not routinely recommended in view of low sensitivity. Treatment is directed at the offending organism, and empiric therapy can be initiated with a third-generation cephalosporin to cover gram-negative bacilli and gram-positive cocci, and should be narrowed to the specific pathogen. Response to treatment is usually seen within 72 hours, and duration

Table 45-4 **Causes of Ascites**	
Serum Ascites-Albumin Gradient	
High: >1.1 g/dL	**Low: <1.1 g/dL**
Cirrhosis	Peritoneal carcinomatosis
Chronic hepatic congestion	Peritoneal tuberculosis
Right ventricular heart failure	Pancreatic and biliary disease
Budd-Chiari syndrome	Nephrotic syndrome
Constrictive pericarditis	
Massive liver metastases	
Myxedema	
Mixed ascites	

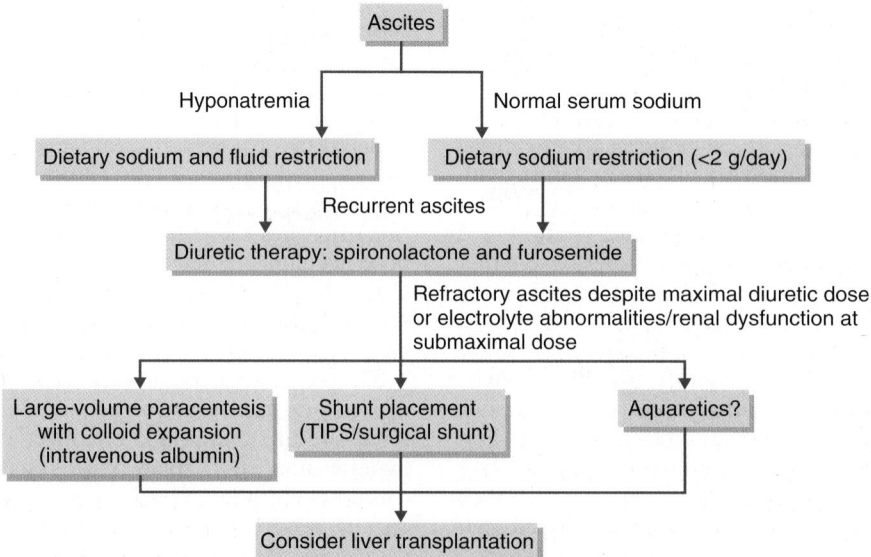

Figure 45-3 Management of ascites in cirrhosis. TIPS, transjugular intrahepatic portosystemic shunt.

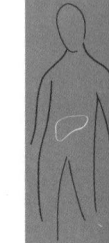

of therapy can be limited to 5 days unless bacteremia is present, in which case a 2-week course is recommended. The administration of intravenous albumin has been shown to decrease the incidence of renal dysfunction and to improve short-term survival. Given the high rates of recurrence (up to 70% within 1 year), long-term antibiotic prophylaxis is indicated in patients with a prior episode of spontaneous bacterial peritonitis (recurrence rate reduction to <20%) and also in patients without a previous episode but with advanced liver failure and low ascitic protein levels (<1 g/dL), whereas short-term prophylaxis should be considered in patients with cirrhosis and ascites who are hospitalized with upper gastrointestinal bleeding. Common prophylactic regimens for SBP include fluoroquinolones (ciprofloxacin, 750 mg per week; norfloxacin, 400 mg per day) and trimethoprim-sulfamethoxazole (1 double-strength tablet daily). Long-term antibiotic prophylaxis can increase susceptibility to severe gram-positive bacterial infections.

Hepatorenal Syndrome

Serious liver disease from any cause may be complicated by a form of functional renal failure, termed the *hepatorenal syndrome,* which almost invariably occurs in the presence of significant hepatic synthetic dysfunction and ascites. This syndrome occurs in about 4% of patients with decompensated cirrhosis, and some prospective series have determined that the probability of developing this syndrome in patients admitted to the hospital for the treatment of ascites may be as high as 30% to 40% at 2 years. Typically, the kidneys are histologically normal, with the capacity of regaining normal function in the event of recovery of liver function such as after liver transplantation. Severe cortical vasoconstriction has been demonstrated angiographically, and it reverses when these kidneys have been transplanted into patients who do not have cirrhosis. The renal dysfunction is characterized by a declining glomerular filtration rate, oliguria, low urine sodium (<10 mEq/L), normal urinary sediment, and azotemia, often with a disproportionately high ratio of blood urea nitrogen to creatinine. Two types of hepatorenal syndrome have been described. Type I is characterized by rapidly progressive renal failure that occurs within 2 weeks and is associated with a dismal prognosis. In type II, renal dysfunction occurs more slowly and is associated with a better prognosis. The decline in renal function often follows one of three events in a patient with cirrhosis and ascites: infection, overdiuresis, or large-volume paracentesis.

Hepatorenal syndrome should be diagnosed only after plasma volume depletion (a common cause of reversible, prerenal azotemia in patients with cirrhosis, particularly in patients receiving diuretics) and other forms of acute renal injury have been excluded. Mortality is high in hepatorenal syndrome; therefore, in all patients with cirrhosis, precipitating factors should be avoided (overdiuresis, dehydration from lactulose, nephrotoxic agents such as nonsteroidal anti-inflammatory drugs [NSAIDs]) and treated (diagnosis and treatment of spontaneous bacterial peritonitis and alcoholic hepatitis) as rapidly as possible.

Recently, several medical therapies have been studied and may have some benefit, including octreotide in combination with midodrine (α-adrenergic agonist), vasopressin analogues (terlipressin), and intravenous albumin. TIPS has also been reported to stabilize or even improve renal function, but liver transplantation has become the accepted treatment for hepatorenal syndrome.

Hepatic Encephalopathy

Hepatic encephalopathy is a complex neuropsychiatric syndrome that may complicate severe or advanced liver disease or extensive portosystemic collateral formation *(shunting).* Two major forms of hepatic encephalopathy are recognized: acute and chronic.

Acute hepatic encephalopathy usually occurs in the setting of fulminant hepatic failure. Cerebral edema plays an important role in this setting, progression to coma is common, and mortality is extremely high (see Chapter 44). *Chronic hepatic encephalopathy* usually occurs in the setting of cirrhosis and is often reversible. It commonly produces disturbances in the sleep-wake cycle, subtle neurologic dysfunction, and behavioral changes.

The pathogenesis of hepatic encephalopathy in the setting of cirrhosis is thought to involve the inadequate hepatic removal of predominantly nitrogenous compounds or other toxins ingested or formed in the gastrointestinal tract. Ammonia, derived from both amino acid deamination and bacterial hydrolysis of nitrogenous compounds in the gut, has been implicated in the pathogenesis of hepatic encephalopathy, but venous ammonia blood levels correlate poorly with the presence or degree of encephalopathy. Other potential contributors to hepatic encephalopathy have been investigated, including γ-aminobutyric acid, mercaptans, short-chain fatty acids, benzodiazepine-like compounds, imbalance between plasma branched-chain and aromatic amino acids, altered cerebral metabolism (disturbed sodium-potassium adenosine triphosphatase [Na^+,K^+-ATPase] activity), zinc deficiency, and deposition of manganese in the basal ganglia.

The clinical features of hepatic encephalopathy include disturbances of higher neurologic function (e.g., intellectual and personality disorders, dementia, inability to copy simple diagrams *[constructional apraxia],* disturbance of consciousness), disturbances of neuromuscular function (e.g., asterixis, hyperreflexia, myoclonus), and rarely a Parkinson-like syndrome and progressive paraplegia. One of the earliest manifestations is the alteration of the normal sleep-wake cycle. Hepatic encephalopathy is usually divided into stages according to its severity (Table 45-5). Hypoglycemia, subdural hematoma, meningitis, and drug overdose should be considered in the differential diagnosis of hepatic encephalopathy.

Treatment of hepatic encephalopathy is based on identifying and addressing precipitating factors (Table 45-6), short-term restricting of dietary protein, reducing and eliminating substrates for the generation of nitrogenous compounds, and preventing ammonia absorption from the bowel. Gastrointestinal bleeding and increased protein intake may provide increased substrate for the bacterial or metabolic formation of nitrogenous compounds that induce encephalopathy. Patients prone to develop hepatic encephalopathy have increased sensitivity to drugs that depress the central nervous system, and the use of these drugs should be avoided

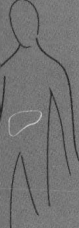

Table 45-5 **Stages of Hepatic Encephalopathy**	
Stage*	**Clinical Manifestations**
I	Apathy
	Restlessness
	Reversal of sleep rhythm
	Slowed intellect
	Impaired computational ability
	Impaired handwriting
II	Lethargy
	Drowsiness
	Disorientation
	Asterixis
III	Stupor (arousable)
	Hyperactive reflexes, extensor plantar responses
IV	Coma (response to painful stimuli only)

*Stage 0 encephalopathy is used to describe subclinical impairment of intellectual function.

Table 45-6 **Hepatic Encephalopathy: Precipitating Factors**
Gastrointestinal bleeding
Increased dietary protein
Constipation
Infection
Central nervous system depressant drugs (benzodiazepines, opiates, tricyclic antidepressants)
Deterioration in hepatic function
Hypokalemia: most often induced by diuretics
Azotemia: most often induced by diuretics
Alkalosis: most often induced by diuretics
Hypovolemia: most often induced by diuretics

in these patients. Protein restriction may be considered in patients with severe encephalopathy, but long-term restriction is associated with worsening malnutrition. Treatment with formulas rich in branched-chain amino acids has shown no benefit in improving encephalopathy or mortality. Reduction and elimination of nitrogenous compound substrates can be achieved by administering enemas and using antibiotics that reduce colonic bacteria (i.e., neomycin, metronidazole, rifaximin). Nonabsorbable disaccharides (i.e., lactulose) are fermented to organic acids by colonic bacteria, lowering stool pH and trapping ammonia in the colon, and thereby preventing absorption. In addition, the cathartic effect of lactulose eliminates ammonia and other nitrogenous compounds, and patients are usually directed to achieve two to three soft stools per day as the goal of lactulose therapy.

Hepatopulmonary Syndrome

Hepatopulmonary syndrome occurs in 10% to 30% of patients with cirrhosis and is characterized by gas exchange abnormalities (increased alveolar-arterial gradient and hypoxemia) as a result of intrapulmonary vascular dilation. The vascular dilation leads to impaired oxygen transfer from alveoli to the central stream of red blood cells within capillaries, resulting in a *functional* intrapulmonary right-to-left shunt that improves with 100% oxygen. Intrapulmonary shunting can be demonstrated through contrast echocardiography. In this modality, agitated saline, which creates microbubbles, is injected into a peripheral vein while performing two-dimensional echocardiography. Delayed visualization (after the third heartbeat following injection) of microbubbles in the left cardiac chambers indicates intrapulmonary vasodilation, whereas early visualization occurs with intracardiac shunting. Clinical features range from subclinical abnormalities in gas exchange to profound

hypoxemia causing significant dyspnea. The presence of hepatopulmonary syndrome significantly increases mortality and worsens functional status and quality of life. No proven medical therapy exists, but supplemental oxygen improves arterial oxygen levels. The treatment of choice is liver transplantation, which often leads to complete reversal of the syndrome.

HEPATOCELLULAR CARCINOMA

Hepatocellular carcinoma (HCC) accounts for less than 2.5% of all malignancies in the United States. Recent epidemiologic studies, though, have demonstrated a 71% relative increase in the age-adjusted incidence rate of this malignancy over the past 20 years. In other areas of the world, including sub-Saharan Africa, China, Japan, and Southeast Asia, HCC is one of the most frequent malignancies and is an important cause of mortality, particularly in middle-aged men. HCC often arises in a cirrhotic liver and is closely associated with chronic viral hepatitis. Hepatitis B virus DNA has been shown to integrate in the host cell genome, where it may disrupt tumor suppressor genes and activate oncogenes. In areas of high prevalence, vaccination to prevent infection with hepatitis B virus has reduced the incidence of this disease. The exact pathophysiologic mechanisms leading to tumorigenesis in patients with other causes of cirrhosis (e.g., hemochromatosis, alcohol, hepatitis C viral infection) remain poorly understood. Risk factors for development of HCC, as well as its clinical manifestations, are listed in Table 45-7. Currently used imaging techniques for detecting HCC and the most common appearance of the tumor are listed in Table 45-8. A tissue specimen may be necessary to confirm the diagnosis of HCC in some cases but may not be needed if characteristic clinical and radiologic features are present, especially when accompanied by a rise in serum α-fetoprotein levels. Diagnosis of small, treatable tumors is possible with intensive screening programs that employ imaging studies and serum α-fetoprotein levels, although the long-term outcomes and cost-effectiveness of these strategies remain unclear. Patients with well-compensated cirrhosis may undergo surgical resection or liver transplantation, whereas, in patients with advanced cirrhosis, liver transplantation should be considered. Nonsurgical options include percutaneous ethanol injection, arterial

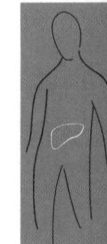

Table 45-7 **Hepatocellular Carcinoma**
Incidence
From 1 to 7 per 100,000 to >100 per 100,000 in high-risk areas
Sex
4:1 to 8:1 male preponderance
Associations
Chronic hepatitis B infection
Chronic hepatitis C infection
Hemochromatosis (with cirrhosis)
Cirrhosis (alcoholic, cryptogenic)
Aflatoxin ingestion
Thorotrast
α_1-Antitrypsin deficiency
Androgen administration
Common Clinical Presentations
Abdominal pain
Abdominal mass
Weight loss
Deterioration of liver function
Unusual Manifestations
Bloody ascites
Tumor emboli (lung)
Jaundice
Hepatic or portal vein obstruction
Metabolic effects
Erythrocytosis
Hypercalcemia
Hypercholesterolemia
Hypoglycemia
Gynecomastia
Feminization
Acquired porphyria
Clinical and Laboratory Findings
Hepatic bruit or friction rub
Serum α-fetoprotein > 400 ng/mL

Table 45-8 **Ultrasonographic, Radiographic, and Magnetic Resonance Imaging Characteristics of Hepatocellular Carcinoma**
Ultrasonography
Mass lesion with varying echogenicities but usually hypoechoic
Dynamic Computed Tomography
Arterial phase: tumor enhances quickly
Venous phase: quick de-enhancement of the tumor relative to the parenchyma
Magnetic Resonance Imaging
T1-weighted images: hypointense
T2-weighted images: hyperintense
After gadolinium administration, the tumor increases in intensity

chemoembolization, and radiofrequency ablation. In patients with widespread, multifocal disease and in those with vascular invasion, the prognosis is poor, with median survival from the time of diagnosis of less than 6 months. However, recently, sorafenib (angiogenesis inhibitor) has been approved for use in unresectable HCC and has been shown to prolong survival in such patients.

HEPATIC TRANSPLANTATION

Liver transplantation is a highly successful procedure in patients with progressive, advanced, and otherwise untreatable liver disease. Advances in surgical techniques and supportive care, the use of cyclosporine and tacrolimus for immunosuppression, and careful selection of patients have all contributed to the excellent results of liver transplantation. From 70% to 80% of patients undergoing liver transplantation survive at least 3 years, usually with good quality of life. The most common indication for liver transplantation in the United States is chronic liver disease resulting from hepatitis C virus infection. Other liver diseases for which transplantation is commonly performed include cirrhosis from alcoholic liver disease, nonalcoholic fatty liver disease, autoimmune hepatitis, primary biliary cirrhosis, and primary sclerosing cholangitis. Patients with hepatitis B are candidates for liver transplantation if they can be given hepatitis B immunoglobulin or nucleoside analogues (i.e., lamivudine) to help prevent recurrence. Excellent results have also been obtained in selected patients with fulminant hepatic failure (see Chapter 44). Liver transplantation for malignant hepatobiliary disease has been less successful because of recurrent disease in the transplanted liver.

The timing of liver transplantation presents a particular challenge given the insufficient availability of donor organs. Liver-assist devices for temporary support until an organ becomes available are being evaluated. Recently, the United Network for Organ Sharing has accepted the Model for End-Stage Liver Disease (MELD) system for determining organ allocation. The MELD system consists of a prognostic model that predicts mortality according to selected clinical and laboratory variables, therefore prioritizing organ availability to patients with more advanced disease in whom predicted mortality is high.

VASCULAR DISEASE OF THE LIVER

Disorders of the hepatic vasculature are uncommon and include portal vein thrombosis, hepatic vein thrombosis (Budd-Chiari syndrome), and veno-occlusive disease. Affected patients usually have portal hypertension with or without associated liver dysfunction, which may mimic the presentation of cirrhosis.

Portal Vein Thrombosis

Thrombosis of the portal vein may develop after abdominal trauma, umbilical vein infection and neonatal sepsis, intra-abdominal inflammatory diseases (e.g., pancreatitis), hypercoagulable states, or in association with cirrhosis. In most cases, however, particularly in children, the cause is unknown. The disease produces the manifestations of portal hypertension; however, liver histology is usually normal. The diagnosis is established by angiography, but noninvasive imaging modalities such as Doppler ultrasonography, computed tomography, and magnetic resonance imaging may reveal thrombus, collateral circulation near the porta hepatis, and splenomegaly. In long-standing portal vein thrombosis, tortuous venous channels develop within the organized clot, leading to *cavernous transformation.*

In acute portal vein thrombosis, thrombolysis may be attempted, but anticoagulation with warfarin remains the mainstay of therapy. In most patients, recanalization of the thrombus occurs within 6 months of initiating anticoagulation. Recommendations for duration of anticoagulation following an acute event vary and are usually 3 to 6 months. Long-term anticoagulation may be used in chronic thrombosis, especially when associated with hypercoagulable states. Concern exists that anticoagulation may precipitate hemorrhage from varices that arise as a consequence of portal hypertension, although studies have not shown an increased risk for variceal bleeding in anticoagulated patients with chronic portal vein thrombosis. If variceal hemorrhage occurs, it is best managed with endoscopic obliteration. Prophylaxis with β blockers to prevent variceal bleeding may decrease portal pressure and potentially propagate thrombus and is generally not recommended. If endoscopic treatment fails, surgical management with portosystemic shunting may be attempted, but this approach is often difficult because of the absence of suitable patent vessels.

Budd-Chiari Syndrome

The occlusion of the major hepatic veins or the inferior vena cava, especially in the intrahepatic and suprahepatic segments, causes Budd-Chiari syndrome. Most cases are caused by hematologic disease (e.g., polycythemia vera, paroxysmal nocturnal hemoglobinuria, essential thrombocytosis, and other myeloproliferative disorders), pregnancy, oral contraceptive use, tumors (especially hepatocellular carcinoma), hypercoagulable states (e.g., factor V Leiden mutation, protein C and S deficiency), abdominal trauma, and congenital webs of the vena cava. About 20% of cases are idiopathic, but many of these patients may have early, subclinical myeloproliferative disease or genetic mutations associated with a hypercoagulable state.

The presentation of Budd-Chiari syndrome can be acute, which may be associated with fulminant liver failure, or it may exhibit as a subacute or chronic illness. Acute disease produces right upper quadrant abdominal pain, hepatomegaly, ascites, and jaundice, whereas the subacute or chronic form produces primarily portal hypertension. Elevation of serum bilirubin and transaminase levels may be mild, but liver function is often poor, with profound hypoalbuminemia and coagulopathy. The diagnosis can be established noninvasively with Doppler ultrasonography, which may show decreased or absent hepatic vein blood flow, and computed tomography, which shows delayed or absent contrast filling of the hepatic veins and hypertrophy of the caudate lobe. Magnetic resonance angiography may also demonstrate the previously mentioned findings. Hepatic venography is especially useful in cases in which the results of the noninvasive modalities are inconclusive. Venography often shows an inability to catheterize and visualize the hepatic veins; the characteristic *spider web pattern*

of collateral vessels may also be demonstrated, and the inferior vena cava may appear compressed, owing to hepatomegaly or an enlarged caudate lobe. On liver biopsy, centrilobular congestion, hemorrhage, and necrosis (*nutmeg liver*) are seen, with cirrhosis developing in patients with chronic obstruction.

Treatment should be individualized and is dependent on the mode and severity of presentation and the potential cause of the disease. Supportive therapy to relieve ascites and edema (e.g., dietary sodium restriction, diuretics) and chronic anticoagulation may be considered in patients with chronic Budd-Chiari syndrome in whom methods to decompress congestion are not feasible. Thrombolysis followed by anticoagulation is most useful in patients with acute forms. In selected patients (e.g., those with venous webs or strictures or single-vessel thrombosis), angioplasty with or without stent placement may be used. Decompressive modalities are most useful before the development of cirrhosis and include transjugular intrahepatic portacaval and side-to-side portacaval shunts. In patients with cirrhosis, liver transplantation followed by continued anticoagulation is often considered the best option.

Veno-occlusive Disease

Veno-occlusive disease, also called *sinusoidal obstruction syndrome*, is characterized by jaundice, painful hepatomegaly, and fluid retention that most often occurs after cytoreductive therapy and before bone marrow transplantation but may also follow exposure to other drugs and herbal preparations (e.g., azathioprine, pyrrolizidine alkaloids). Endothelial cell injury leads to obstruction at the level of the hepatic venules and the sinusoids.

The diagnosis is clinically suspected when weight gain, epigastric–right upper quadrant abdominal pain, and jaundice develop within the first 3 to 4 weeks after bone marrow transplantation. Laboratory abnormalities include hyperbilirubinemia, elevated transaminases, and in severe cases, profound synthetic dysfunction. Clinical manifestations may be rapidly progressive and may lead to multiorgan dysfunction and death in 20% to 25% of patients. Doppler abdominal ultrasonography may reveal ascites, reversal of portal vein flow, and an elevated hepatic artery resistance index. Liver biopsy is diagnostic and is usually obtained using the transjugular approach. The advantages of this approach compared with the percutaneous route include measurement of the hepatic venous pressure gradient (typically elevated in veno-occlusive disease) and a lower incidence of bleeding.

Mild forms of the disease may favorably respond only to supportive therapy. In moderate to severe disease, treatment has been attempted with tissue plasminogen activator and heparin, antithrombin III, prostaglandin E_1, and glutamine plus vitamin E, although their efficacy has not been clearly established. Recently, defibrotide (a mixture of porcine-derived single-stranded phosphodiester oligonucleotides) has been evaluated as a potential treatment option for severe veno-occlusive disease. It is an attractive option because of lack of severe adverse effects, but convincing evidence for its efficacy has not been established.

Prospectus for the Future

For many years, cirrhosis has been viewed as an irreversible fibrotic reaction to chronic liver injury. However, as the mechanisms of hepatic fibrosis have been explored and treatments for chronic liver disease have been implemented, cirrhosis has been increasingly seen as an imbalance of multiple factors that regulate the generation and degradation of collagen. Among the consequences of the increased understanding of hepatic fibrogenesis is the potential for development of specific agents that influence collagen production and those that may prevent and even diminish hepatic fibrosis. A significant number of antifibrotic agents have been successfully used in animal models of liver injury, and these agents are likely to enter clinical use in the near future.

Another key issue in the therapy of complications of cirrhosis is defining the effectiveness of medical treatment of esophageal varices. Noncardioselective β-adrenergic blockers decrease the risk for variceal bleeding. This effect is established to occur in the subgroup of patients who have a significant reduction in portal pressure measured by hepatic venous pressure recordings. Currently, direct measurement of hepatic venous pressures is not routinely used to assess efficacy of noncardioselective

β-adrenergic blockers in lowering portal pressure. The development of noninvasive means to measure portal pressures or targeted measurement of hepatic venous pressure recordings in patients treated with noncardioselective β-adrenergic blockers are likely to help guide treatment of esophageal varices.

During the past few years, several artificial liver support systems have been proposed and studied in acute liver failure (ALF) and acute on chronic liver failure (ACLF). The system currently being evaluated extensively in the United States and Europe is the molecular adsorbents recirculating system (MARS), which is based on the principles of extracorporeal albumin dialysis (ECAD). Because a large number of toxins that accumulate in liver failure are bound to albumin, using an albumin-rich dialysate across an albumin-enriched polymer membrane has shown significant biochemical and clinical improvement in patients with ALF or ACLF. Patients receiving ECAD have reduced serum bilirubin levels, bile acid levels, and improvement in encephalopathy and synthetic function (increased serum albumin). These findings are promising, but a survival benefit has not been assessed, and these systems are not standard of care yet.

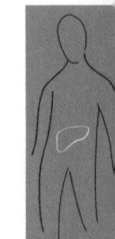

References

Arguedas MR: The critically ill liver patient: The variceal bleeder. Semin Gastrointest Dis 14:34-38, 2003.

Carbonell N, Pauwels A, Serfaty L, et al: Improved survival after variceal bleeding in patients with cirrhosis over the past two decades. Hepatology 40:652-659, 2004.

Cardenas A, Gines P: Management of complications of cirrhosis in patients awaiting liver transplantation. J Hepatol 42:S124-S133, 2005.

Chaparro M, Gonzalez Moreno L, Trapero-Marugán M, et al: Pharmacological therapy of hepatocellular carcinoma with sorafenib and other oral agents [review article]. Aliment Pharmacol Ther 28:1269-1277, 2008.

De Franchis R, Dell'Era A, Iannuzzi F: Diagnosis and treatment of portal hypertension. Dig Liver Dis 36:787-798, 2004.

Fallon MB, Krowka MJ, Brown RS, et al: Impact of hepatopulmonary syndrome on quality of life and survival in liver transplant candidates. Gastroenterology 134:1764-1776, 2008.

Fernandez J, Navasa M, Planas M, et al: Primary prophylaxis of spontaneous bacterial peritonitis delays hepatorenal syndrome and improves survival in cirrhosis. Gastroenterology 133:818-824, 2007.

Garcia-Tsao G, Bosch J, Groszmann RJ: Portal hypertension and variceal bleeding: Unresolved issues. Summary of an American Association for the Study of Liver Diseases and European Association for the Study of the Liver single-topic conference. Hepatology 47:1764-1772, 2008.

Marrero JA: Screening tests for hepatocellular carcinoma. Clin Liver Dis 9:235-251, 2005.

Menon KV, Shah V, Kamath PS: The Budd-Chiari syndrome. N Engl J Med 350:578-585, 2004.

Sanyal AJ, Boyer T, Garcia-Tsao G, et al: A randomized, prospective, double-blind, placebo-controlled trial of terlipressin for type 1 hepatorenal syndrome. Gastroenterology 134:1360-1368, 2008.

Valla DC: Thrombosis and anticoagulation in liver disease. Hepatology 47:1384-1393, 2008.

Valla DC: Budd-Chiari syndrome and veno-occlusive disease/sinusoidal obstruction syndrome. Gut 57:1469-1478, 2008.

Wadleigh M, Ho V, Momtaz P, Richardson P: Hepatic veno-occlusive disease: Pathogenesis, diagnosis, and treatment. Curr Opin Hematol 10:451-462, 2003.

Webster GJ, Burroughs AK, Riordan SM: Portal vein thrombosis: New insights into aetiology and management. Aliment Pharmacol Ther 21:1-9, 2005.

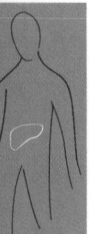

Chapter **46**

Disorders of the Gallbladder and Biliary Tract

Shyam Varadarajulu, Rudolf Garcia-Gallont, and Michael B. Fallon

The main role of the biliary tract and gallbladder is to transport bile into the intestines, which, in turn, is essential for digesting fat. Diseases of the gallbladder and the biliary tract are among the most common afflictions of humankind. This chapter examines the most common gallbladder and biliary tract disorders, focusing on cholelithiasis. The reader is referred to Chapter 42 for a detailed discussion of bilirubin metabolism and the diagnostic approach to jaundice and to Chapter 35 for a review of the various imaging techniques used to study the biliary tract.

Normal Biliary Anatomy and Physiology

Figure 46-1 outlines the normal anatomy of the liver and biliary tract. The liver produces 500 to 1500 mL of bile per day. Bile passes through the canaliculi to the hepatic bile ducts and then into the common hepatic duct. Tonic contraction of the sphincter of Oddi, located in the region of the ampulla of Vater, during fasting diverts about one half of the bile through the cystic duct into the gallbladder, where it is stored and concentrated. Cholecystokinin, released after food is ingested, causes the sphincter of Oddi to contract and then to relax, allowing delivery of a timed bolus of bile, rich in bile acids, into the intestine. Bile acids, detergent molecules possessing both fat-soluble and water-soluble moieties, convey phospholipids and cholesterol from the liver to the intestine where cholesterol undergoes fecal excretion (see Chapter 42, Fig. 42-1). In the intestinal lumen, bile acids solubilize dietary fat and promote its digestion and absorption. Bile acids are, for the most part, efficiently reabsorbed by the small intestinal mucosa, particularly in the terminal ileum, and are recycled to the liver for re-excretion, a process termed *enterohepatic circulation*.

Gallstones (Cholelithiasis)

In studies performed in the United States, Europe, and South America, about 10% to 15% of adults have gallstones. In the United States, gallstone disease leads to more than 500,000 cholecystectomies annually, with estimated costs of $4.5 billion per year. Gallstones are of two types: (1) cholesterol (75%) and (2) pigmented (black or brown) (25%), the latter being composed of calcium bilirubinate and other calcium salts. The risk factors for cholelithiasis are shown in Table 46-1.

PATHOGENESIS OF CHOLELITHIASIS

The three main factors that lead to cholesterol gallstone formation are (1) cholesterol supersaturation of bile, (2) nucleation, and (3) gallbladder hypomotility. The liver is the most important organ in regulating total-body cholesterol stores. Once secreted, cholesterol, which is insoluble in water, is solubilized in bile by forming mixed micelles with bile acids and phospholipids. In most individuals, many of whom do not develop stones, more cholesterol is in bile than can be maintained in stable solution (supersaturated bile). As bile becomes more supersaturated, aggregation of microscopic cholesterol molecules into coalescent vesicles that crystallize (nucleation) takes place. Gradual deposition of additional layers of cholesterol leads to the appearance of macroscopic stones. Factors that influence nucleation include bile transit time, gallbladder contraction, bile composition (concentration of cholesterol, phospholipids, and bile salts), and presence of bacteria, mucin, and glycoproteins, which act as a nidus to initiate cholesterol crystal formation. The interplay between *pronucleating* and *antinucleating* factors in the gallbladder may determine whether cholesterol gallstones will form from supersaturated bile.

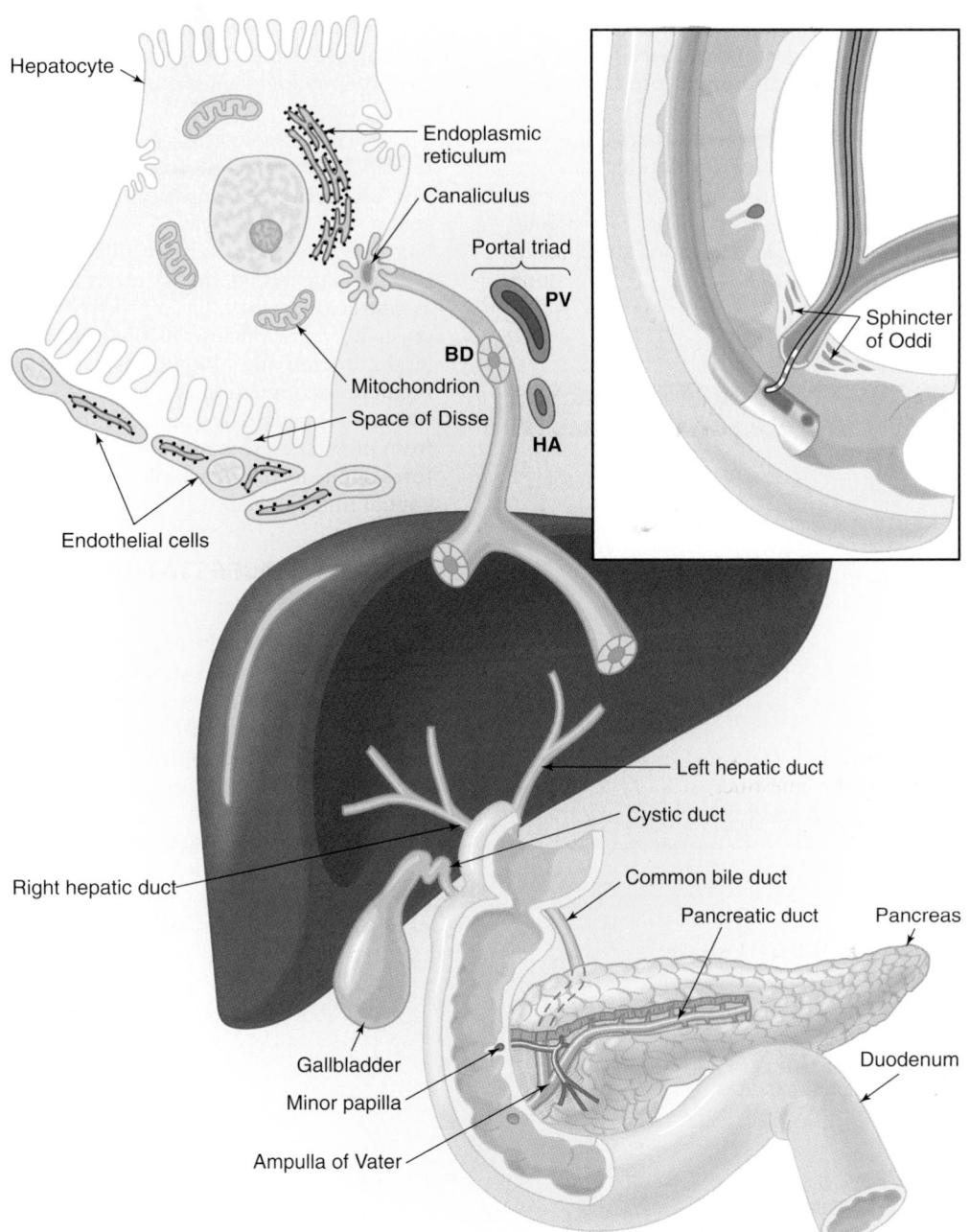

Figure 46-1 Normal anatomy and histology of the liver and biliary tract. Materials destined for metabolism or excretion by the liver (such as unconjugated bilirubin) enter the sinusoidal bed and cross the endothelial barrier and the space of Disse. Unconjugated bilirubin is taken up by the hepatocyte, conjugated with glucuronide to become water soluble, and excreted into bile across the canalicular membrane of the hepatocyte. The canaliculi empty into bile ductules (BD), which, in turn, lead to the interlobular (small), septal (medium), and large intrahepatic bile ducts and finally to the main branches of the common bile duct. The portal areas, or portal triads, are composed mainly of portal vein (PV), hepatic artery (HA), and BD branches *(left side, magnification)*. Tonic contraction of the sphincter of Oddi, located in the region of the ampulla of Vater, during fasting diverts about one half of the bile through the cystic duct into the gallbladder, where it is stored and concentrated to be released later during meal times. Diseases at any level of the biliary tree can lead to cholestasis and obstructive jaundice; for example, primary sclerosing cholangitis is caused by inflammatory obstruction of the interlobular bile ducts, whereas stones, cancer of the ampulla of Vater, or pancreatitis can cause distal obstruction of the common bile duct. Investigation of the bile duct is best accomplished using a side-viewing endoscope to insert a catheter into the ampulla of Vater, with injection of contrast to obtain an endoscopic retrograde cholangiogram *(right side, inset)*. If pathology is detected (e.g., cholangitis, stricture, stone), therapeutic maneuvers such as stone removal, stenting, or sphincterotomy to enlarge the distal opening of the common bile duct can be performed.

Gallbladder sludge is a superconcentrated mixture of bile acids, bilirubin, cholesterol, mucus, and proteins that exhibits various degrees of fluidity and is prone to precipitate into semisolid or solid form.

The pathophysiologic factors of pigment stones is less well understood compared with gallstone formation; however, increased production of bilirubin conjugates (hemolytic states), increased biliary calcium (Ca^{2+}) and bicarbonate (HCO_3^-), cirrhosis, and bacterial deconjugation of bilirubin to a less soluble form are all associated with pigment stone formation.

Many of the recognized predisposing factors for cholelithiasis and gallbladder sludge can be understood in terms of the pathophysiologic scheme outlined previously:

1. Biliary cholesterol saturation is increased by estrogens, multiparity, oral contraceptives, obesity, rapid weight loss, and terminal ileal disease, which decreases the bile acid pool.
2. Nucleation is enhanced by biliary parasites, recurrent bacterial infection of the biliary tract, and antibiotics such as ceftriaxone, which has a proclivity to concentrate and crystallize with calcium in the biliary tree. Total parenteral nutrition and blood transfusions also promote bile pigment accumulation and *gelfaction* of sludge.
3. Bile stasis is caused by gallbladder hypomotility (resulting from pregnancy, somatostatin, or fasting), bile duct strictures, choledochal cysts, biliary parasites, and total parenteral nutrition.

Table 46-1 Risk Factors for Cholelithiasis

Primary

Age
Obesity
Female sex
Rapid weight loss
Race (e.g., Native American)

Secondary

Use of oral contraceptives
Pregnancy
Diabetes mellitus
Use of insulin
Low socioeconomic status
Sedentary lifestyle
Total parenteral nutrition
Hemolysis
Biliary parasites (e.g., *Clonorchis sinensis*)

CLINICAL MANIFESTATIONS OF GALLSTONES

Most individuals with gallstones remain asymptomatic (50% to 60%), about one third develop biliary colic or chronic cholecystitis, and 15% develop acute complications. The natural history of gallstone disease is outlined in Figure 46-2. Obstruction of the biliary tract at any level by stones or sludge is the underlying cause of all manifestations of gallstone disease. Obstruction by gallstones can occur at the level of the cystic duct, common hepatic duct, common bile

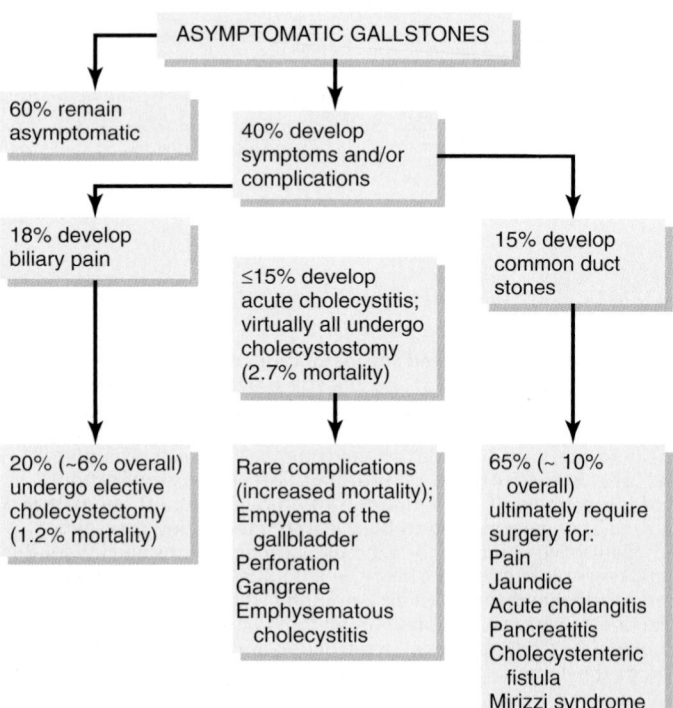

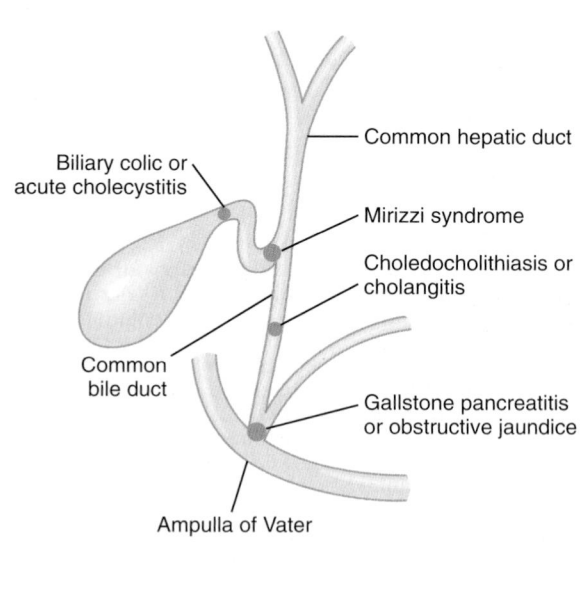

Figure 46-2 Natural history of asymptomatic gallstones. **A,** The clinical syndromes associated with gallstones are shown here, and the numbers represent the approximate percentage of adults who develop one or more of these symptoms or complications over a 15- to 20-year period. Over this period, about 30% of individuals with gallstones undergo surgery. (The risk for developing complications of gallstones varies considerably among series. The figures shown here represent those derived from more recent studies). **B,** Clinical manifestations of symptomatic gallstones.

Table 46-2 **Differential Diagnosis of Cholelithiasis**
Peptic ulcer disease
Gastroesophageal reflux disease
Nonulcer dyspepsia
Irritable bowel syndrome
Sphincter of Oddi dysfunction
Hepatitis and perihepatitis (Fitz-Hugh-Curtis syndrome)
Hepatic abscess
Nephrolithiasis
Pyelonephritis
Perinephric abscess
Pneumonia
Pulmonary infarction
Pulmonary embolism
Angina pectoris
Pancreatitis
Ruptured ectopic pregnancy
Appendicitis

duct, and ampulla of Vater (see Fig. 46-1). Symptoms arise from contraction of the gallbladder during transient obstruction of the cystic duct by gallstones, whereas persistent obstruction of the cystic duct leads to superimposed inflammation or infection of the gallbladder (i.e., acute cholecystitis). Obstruction of the distal common bile duct may result in abdominal pain, cholangitis (infection of the biliary tract), or pancreatitis (resulting from pancreatic duct obstruction). The presence of a large stone in the cystic duct can cause common bile duct obstruction and is referred to as *Mirizzi syndrome*. Common conditions to consider in the differential diagnosis of gallstone disease are listed in Table 46-2.

Asymptomatic Gallstones

Asymptomatic patients should be followed expectantly. Prophylactic cholecystectomy is considered in groups at increased risk for developing complications: (1) patients with diabetes who have a greater morbidity and mortality from acute cholecystitis; (2) persons with a calcified (porcelain) gallbladder or large gallbladder polyps, which are associated with an increased risk for carcinoma of the gallbladder; (3) persons with sickle cell anemia, in whom hepatic crises may be difficult to differentiate from acute cholecystitis; (4) children with gallstones because they frequently develop symptomatic disease; and (5) Native Americans, who are predisposed to developing gallbladder cancer in the setting of gallstones.

Biliary Colic

The term *chronic cholecystitis* has been used to denote recurrent and *nonacute* symptoms caused by the presence of gallstones over a period of days to several years. A better term for this condition is *biliary colic* because the presence of symptoms correlates poorly with pathologic findings in the gallbladder wall. Biliary colic is typically a steady ache in the epigastrium or right upper quadrant, of sudden onset, reaching a plateau of intensity over a few minutes, which subsides gradually over 30 minutes to several hours. Referred

pain may be felt at the tip of the scapula or right shoulder. Nausea and vomiting may occur, whereas fever and a palpable mass (signs of acute cholecystitis) are not evident. Other symptoms such as dyspepsia, fatty food intolerance, bloating and flatulence, heartburn, and belching may occur in patients with gallstones; however, these symptoms are nonspecific and frequently occur in individuals with normal gallbladders.

Gallstones can be best demonstrated by transabdominal ultrasonography (sensitivity and specificity, >95%), which has become the initial test to evaluate cholelithiasis. Ultrasound accuracy drops to 20% for visualization of stones within the common bile duct. This limitation of transabdominal ultrasound has been overcome by endoscopic ultrasound (**Web Video 46-1** shows gallstones on endoscopic ultrasonography) and magnetic resonance cholangiopancreatography (MRCP), both of which have an accuracy of 90% to 95% for detecting cholelithiasis and common bile duct stones. Oral cholecystography is no longer used for the routine evaluation of gallstones.

Laparoscopic cholecystectomy has replaced open cholecystectomy as the treatment of choice for recurrent biliary pain. Open cholecystectomy is generally reserved for selected high-risk patients (e.g., those with prior abdominal surgery with adhesions, obesity, or cirrhosis). Laparoscopic cholecystectomy may be accompanied by intraoperative endoscopic retrograde cholangiopancreatography (ERCP) (see Chapter 35 and Fig. 46-1) or transoperative radiologic examination of the common bile duct if concomitant choledocholithiasis is suspected. Factors that may predict the presence of choledocholithiasis include jaundice, pancreatitis, abnormal liver tests, and bile duct dilation.

Cholecystectomy relieves symptoms of biliary pain in virtually all patients with gallstone disease and prevents development of future complications. Dissolution of cholesterol gallstones by orally administered chenodeoxycholic acid or ursodeoxycholic acid is successful in highly selected patients but is slow and costly and requires lifelong administration. Alternative methods to eliminate gallstones, including contact dissolution and fragmentation of stones, are used rarely.

Acute Cholecystitis

Acute cholecystitis refers to distention, edema, ischemia, inflammation, and secondary infection of the gallbladder, generally resulting from obstruction of the cystic duct by gallstones or less commonly by cancer or sludge. The clinical hallmark of acute cholecystitis is the acute onset of upper abdominal pain that lasts for several hours. The pain gradually increases in severity and typically localizes to the epigastrium or right hypochondrium with radiation to the right lumbar, scapular, and shoulder area. Nausea and vomiting, anorexia, and low-grade fever are common. Unlike biliary pain, the pain of acute cholecystitis does not subside spontaneously. The findings on physical examination in patients with acute cholecystitis may include inspiratory arrest on palpation of the right upper quadrant (Murphy sign), fever, and less commonly mild jaundice or a palpable gallbladder.

Complications of acute cholecystitis include emphysematous cholecystitis (in people with diabetes, older adults, and individuals who are immunosuppressed), empyema, gangrene, and perforation of the gallbladder. Gallbladder perforation may be *free* into the peritoneum or through a cholecystenteric fistula with gallstone migration and bowel obstruction (gallstone ileus). Mirizzi syndrome is the occurrence of profound jaundice resulting from extrinsic compression of the common hepatic duct by an impacted stone in the cystic duct at the gallbladder neck.

The diagnostic modalities employed for acute cholecystitis are similar to those for biliary pain. An ultrasound examination that shows the presence of gallstones, along with pericholecystic fluid, gallbladder wall thickening, and localized tenderness over the gallbladder (ultrasonographic Murphy sign), provides strong supportive evidence for acute cholecystitis. Radionuclide scanning after intravenous administration of technetium-99m (^{99m}Tc)-diisopropyl iminodiacetic acid or hepatobiliary iminodiacetic acid (HIDA) scan is the most accurate test to confirm the clinical impression of acute cholecystitis. If the gallbladder fills with the isotope, acute cholecystitis is highly unlikely, whereas if contrast enters the bile duct and duodenum, but the gallbladder is not visualized, the clinical diagnosis of acute cholecystitis is strongly supported.

Because of the high risk for recurrent acute cholecystitis, most patients need to undergo cholecystectomy, often performed within the first 24 to 48 hours after presentation or, less often, 4 to 8 weeks after an acute episode (Fig. 46-3). Cholecystostomy may be performed on patients with a high operative risk. Antibiotics are generally used when fever or leukocytosis are present. Expectant management is reserved for patients with uncomplicated disease who are not good operative candidates or those in whom the diagnosis is not clear.

Acalculous Cholecystitis

Acalculous cholecystitis accounts for 5% of cases of acute cholecystitis and carries higher morbidity and mortality rates than acute calculous cholecystitis. It is classically associated with the triad of prolonged fasting, immobility, and hemodynamic instability such as occurs in critically ill patients, especially if they have required total parenteral nutrition or blood transfusions. Gallbladder ischemia and sludge may be important in the pathogenesis. Acalculous cholecystitis is also seen in patients with AIDS, in whom it is usually caused by infectious agents such as cytomegalovirus or *Cryptosporidia*. Ultrasonographic features include absence of gallstones, thickened gallbladder wall, and a positive Murphy sign. As in acute cholecystitis, the gallbladder is not visualized on HIDA scan. Management includes antibiotics and cholecystectomy. If the patient is seriously ill, the gallbladder can be drained percutaneously to relieve the obstruction (cholecystostomy).

Choledocholithiasis and Acute Cholangitis

In the United States, most stones in the common bile duct (choledocholithiasis) originate from the gallbladder, occurring in up to 15% of persons with cholelithiasis (see Fig 46-4). Less commonly, stones may form de novo in the biliary tree. Common bile duct stones may be asymptomatic (30% to 40%), or they may produce biliary colic, jaundice, cholangitis, or pancreatitis.

Acute (suppurative) cholangitis is defined as life-threatening infection and inflammation of the biliary tract as the result of choledocholithiasis. The classic clinical manifestations of acute cholangitis are abdominal pain, jaundice, and fever (Charcot triad). Clinical findings may be absent in elderly or immunosuppressed patients. Cholangitis is a medical-surgical emergency that can lead rapidly to sepsis,

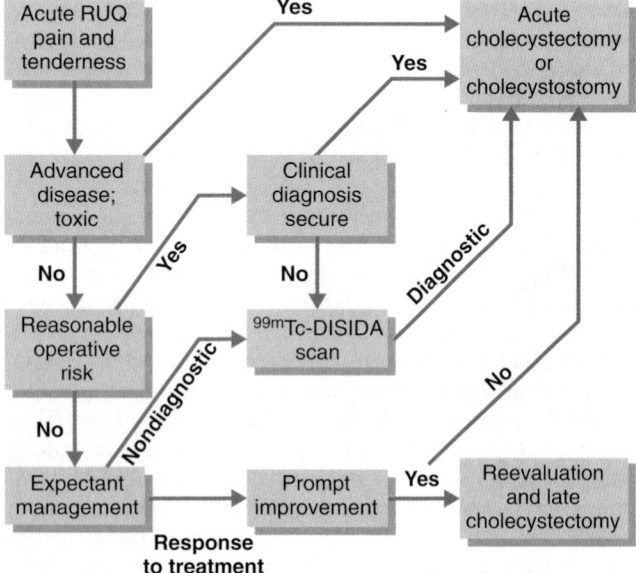

Figure 46-3 Scheme for managing patients with right upper quadrant (RUQ) pain and tenderness who are thought to have acute cholecystitis. This scheme is based on a policy of early operation (conventional or laparoscopic) for appropriate patients and use of cholecystostomy (operative or percutaneous) for patients who are poor operative risks.

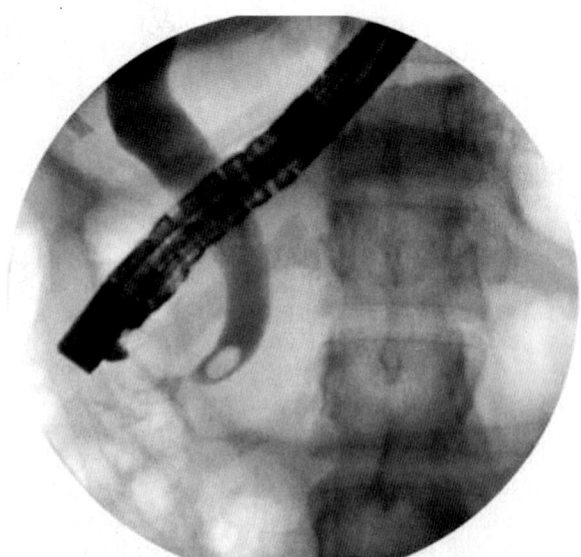

Figure 46-4 Cholangiogram at ERCP demonstrating a common bile duct stone.

shock, and death. Diagnosis is based on a compatible clinical and laboratory picture (abnormal liver function tests and leukocytosis) and radiologic or endoscopic evidence of common bile duct stones.

Treatment of acute cholangitis includes administration of broad-spectrum antibiotics and prompt removal of stones, typically with ERCP (see Fig. 46-1) and endoscopic sphincterotomy (**Web Video 46-2**). Cholecystectomy is subsequently performed when the patient has stabilized.

Gallstone Pancreatitis

Considering that gallstone pancreatitis recurs in 25% of patients, a cholecystectomy should be performed once the patient has recovered clinically from an attack of pancreatitis. If the patient remains jaundiced during an attack of presumed gallstone pancreatitis, suggestive of a stone in the bile duct, an ERCP is performed so that stones can be extracted by sphincterotomy.

Primary Sclerosing Cholangitis

Primary sclerosing cholangitis is an idiopathic condition of nonmalignant, nonbacterial, chronic inflammatory fibrosis and obliteration of the intrahepatic and extrahepatic bile ducts. It most commonly occurs in young men (two thirds are younger than 45 years), often in association with ulcerative colitis (70% of patients with primary sclerosing cholangitis have ulcerative colitis). The clinical spectrum of primary sclerosing cholangitis is broad, ranging from asymptomatic patients with abnormal liver enzymes (typically an elevated alkaline phosphatase) to recurring episodes of fever, chills, abdominal pain, and jaundice. The diagnosis of primary sclerosing cholangitis is made by ERCP or MRCP, which shows characteristic changes (beading) of the intra-

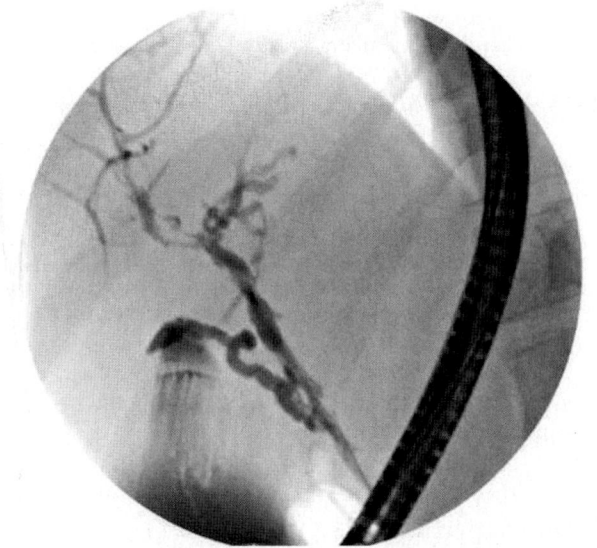

Figure 46-5 Cholangiogram at ERCP demonstrating the characteristic beading of the intra- and extra-hepatic bile ducts in a patient with PSC.

hepatic or extrahepatic bile duct, or both (see Fig 46-5). No proven therapy exists for primary sclerosing cholangitis, although ursodeoxycholic acid and methotrexate are being used in some centers. Other forms of therapy include prophylactic antibiotics for prevention of recurrent bacterial cholangitis, treatment of pruritus, and repletion of fat-soluble vitamins. Endoscopic dilation of a *dominant* biliary stricture during ERCP is an effective treatment of cholestasis in selected patients. Most patients with advanced primary sclerosing cholangitis eventually progress to end-stage liver disease, and evaluation for liver transplantation is appropriate in advanced disease. One third of patients with primary sclerosing cholangitis will develop cholangiocarcinoma; therefore, thorough clinical, laboratory (liver function tests and cancer markers such as CA 19-9), and radiologic follow-up are warranted.

Other Disorders of the Biliary Tree

BILIARY STRICTURES

Benign biliary strictures usually result from surgical injury or chronic pancreatitis. Biliary strictures resulting from surgical injury may cause symptoms days to years later. Early diagnosis is important because strictures that partially obstruct are clinically asymptomatic and may cause secondary biliary cirrhosis. Biliary stricture should be suspected in any patient with a history of surgery of the right upper quadrant or chronic pancreatitis (typically caused by alcohol) with a persistently elevated serum alkaline phosphatase and γ-glutamyl transpeptidase. Endoscopic balloon catheter dilation with or without stenting or surgical repair is useful in selected patients.

OTHER NONMALIGNANT CAUSES OF BILIARY OBSTRUCTION

Structural abnormalities such as choledochal cysts, Caroli disease (congenital saccular intrahepatic bile duct dilation), and duodenal diverticula may also cause bile duct obstruction, often with secondary choledocholithiasis resulting from bile stasis. Hemobilia, with intermittent bile duct obstruction by blood clots, may be caused by hepatic injury, neoplasms, or hepatic artery aneurysms. Biliary parasites should always be considered as a cause of biliary strictures in the appropriate epidemiologic setting. *Ascaris lumbricoides* is a common cause of cholangitis and jaundice in South America, Africa, and the Indian subcontinent. *Clonorchis sinensis* is the etiologic agent of oriental cholangiohepatitis in Korea and Southeast Asia and in immigrants to the United States. The liver fluke *Fasciola hepatica* is a leading cause of biliary strictures and cholangitis worldwide, most commonly in the Bolivian Andes.

BILIARY NEOPLASMS

Biliary neoplasms such as gallbladder cancer, cancer of the ampulla of Vater, and cholangiocarcinoma are uncommon in the United States, but gallbladder cancer is common in other parts of the world, such as Chile and Southeast Asia.

Risk factors for developing these cancers include primary sclerosing cholangitis, chronic ulcerative colitis, choledochal cysts, gallstones, *C. sinensis* infection, hepatolithiasis, and α_1-antitrypsin deficiency. Cholangiocarcinoma and cancer of the ampulla of Vater usually exhibit as unremitting painless jaundice, although necrosis and sloughing of the tumor may cause intermittent biliary obstruction and the appearance of occult fecal blood. If cholangiocarcinoma is present at the bifurcation of the extrahepatic bile duct (50% of cases), the condition is known as *Klatskin tumor* (see Fig 46-6). Carcinoma of the gallbladder often produces advanced disseminated disease with weight loss, jaundice, pruritus, and a large right upper quadrant mass. Symptoms of gallbladder cancer also may resemble those of acute or chronic cholecystitis, particularly when the tumor is small. Although early-stage tumors can be treated surgically, most cases are diagnosed at an advanced stage and are hence incurable.

GALLBLADDER POLYPS

Gallbladder polyps are outgrowths of the gallbladder mucosal wall. Most of these lesions are not neoplastic but are hyperplastic or represent lipid deposits (cholesterolosis). Patients who have gallbladder polyps and concomitant gallstones should undergo cholecystectomy regardless of the polyp size or the presence of symptoms because gallstones are a risk factor for gallbladder cancer in patients with gallbladder polyps. Cholecystectomy should also be recommended for patients who have biliary colic or pancreatitis. Patients with gallbladder polyps larger than 1 cm should undergo cholecystectomy because of their malignant potential. Polyps smaller than 1 cm should be monitored with periodic imaging.

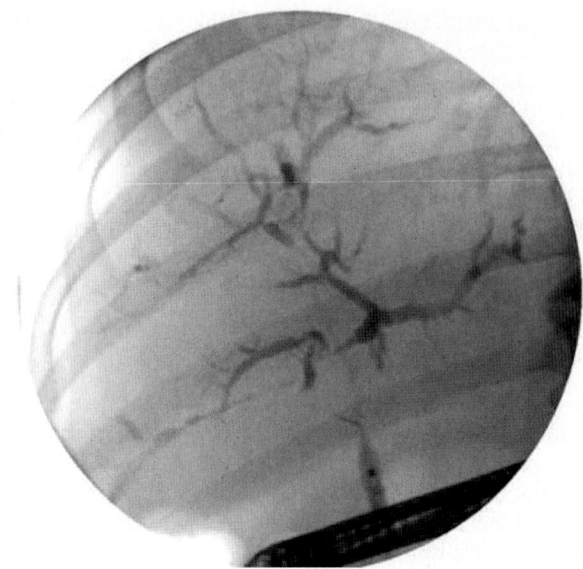

Figure 46-6 Cholangiogram at ERCP demonstrating Klatskin tumor at the bile duct bifurcation.

SPHINCTER OF ODDI DYSFUNCTION

Sphincter of Oddi dysfunction is a benign motility disorder leading to noncalculous obstruction to the flow of bile or pancreatic juice at the level of the pancreatobiliary junction. Patients typically have unexplained abdominal pain (biliary-type pain), with or without elevations of the liver tests. In a selected group of patients, endoscopic or surgical sphincterotomy is of value.

Prospectus for the Future

Imaging of the biliary tract is a critical component of the diagnosis and treatment of biliary disorders. MRCP and endoscopic ultrasound are increasingly used to define which patients require more invasive evaluation and treatment by ERCP. These modalities may also provide important additional information not obtainable by ERCP. As technology improves, these alternate techniques are likely to become the mainstay of diagnosis for biliary disorders, allowing ERCP to be targeted to patients who require specific diagnostic and therapeutic interventions.

A second area of focus in biliary tract disorders is the accurate diagnosis of cholangiocarcinoma, particularly in the setting of primary sclerosing cholangitis. A significant number of novel genetic and immunologic approaches for analysis of bile and biliary epithelium have recently been exploited. These markers may provide a means for significantly enhancing the sensitivity and specificity of detecting cholangiocarcinoma.

References

Browning JD, Horton JD: Gallstone disease and its complications. Semin Gastrointest Dis 14:165-177, 2003.

Chattopadhyay D, Lochan R, Balupuri S, et al: Outcome of gallbladder polypoidal lesions detected by transabdominal ultrasound scanning: A nine-year experience. World J Gastroenterol 11:2171-2173, 2005.

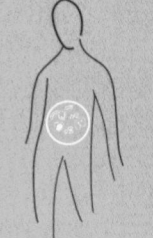

Section IX

Hematologic Disease

Chapter 47

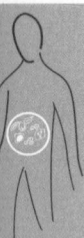

Hematopoiesis and Hematopoietic Failure

Eunice S. Wang and Nancy Berliner

Hematopoiesis

Hematopoiesis is the process that determines the formation and development of the wide variety of cellular elements of the blood. The constituents of peripheral blood arise by a complex and carefully regulated process of ontogeny. The pluripotent hematopoietic stem cell both maintains itself by self-renewal and undergoes multilineage differentiation to generate the appropriate numbers and types of cells within the circulating blood compartment (Table 47-1). The hematopoietic system is unique in that it is constantly undergoing this full cycle of maturation by which a primitive cell develops into a variety of highly specialized end-stage cells, all of which have different life spans and are present in different quantities. The bone marrow must have the capacity to produce cells to compensate for the normal rapid turnover of hematopoietic cells resulting from senescence, utilization, and migration into tissue spaces. Furthermore, it must have a reserve capacity to produce additional cells in response to unusual demands that arise from bleeding, infection, or other stresses. Understanding the repeated cycle of cellular ontogeny and self-renewal that meets these challenges provides important insights into normal and pathologic mechanisms in hematology.

HEMATOPOIETIC TISSUES

Hematopoiesis commences in the embryonic yolk sac, in which early erythroblasts in blood islands form the first hemoglobinized cells. After 6 weeks of gestation, the fetal liver begins producing primitive lymphocytoid cells, megakaryocytes, and erythroblasts, and the spleen becomes a secondary site of erythropoiesis. Hematopoiesis then shifts to its definitive long-term site in the bone marrow, the principal site for lifelong hematopoiesis in the normal host. Early in life, all fetal bones contain this regenerative bone marrow, but the marrow becomes progressively replaced by fat with age. In adults, active marrow resides only in the axial skeleton (sternum, vertebrae, pelvis, and ribs) and in the proximal ends of the femur and humerus. Consequently, bone marrow samples, needed for many hematologic diagnoses, are usually obtained from the iliac crest or sternum. Under pathologic conditions that stress the capacity of the marrow space, as seen in diseases associated with marrow fibrosis (myeloproliferative diseases) or in severe inherited hemolytic anemia (thalassemia major), extramedullary hematopoiesis may be reestablished in sites of fetal hematopoiesis, especially the spleen.

STEM CELL THEORY OF HEMATOPOIESIS

All mature hematopoietic cells are hypothesized to originate from a small population of pluripotent stem cells. Comprising less than 1% of all cells in the bone marrow, these cells bear no distinctive morphologic markings and are best defined by their unique functional properties. Stem cells have two distinctive characteristics. First, they are highly resilient and productive, capable of continuously replenishing huge numbers of granulocytes, lymphocytes, and erythrocytes throughout life. The demand for a continuous fluctuating supply of blood cells requires a hematopoietic system capable of producing large numbers of selected cells in a short time. For example, overwhelming infection by invading microorganisms triggers the release of neutrophils, whereas hypoxia or acute blood loss leads to increased red blood cell production. Second, hematopoietic stem cells (HSCs) represent a self-renewing cell population that is able to maintain its numbers while also providing a continued supply of progenitor cells of multiple different lineages.

Despite their vast proliferative potential, under normal conditions, most HSCs are quiescent, and few cells undergo expansion or differentiation at any one time. However, their ability to proliferate is striking. Studies with lethally irradiated mice have demonstrated the ability of a few transplanted cells (termed *colony-forming unit-spleen cells* [CFU-S]) to regenerate multilineage hematopoiesis.

The signals regulating the differentiation of pluripotent stem cells into committed progenitors are unknown. Data suggest that the first step toward lineage commitment is a *stochastic* (chance) event; subsequent stages of maturation

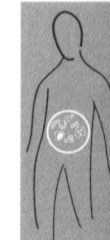

are hypothesized to occur under the influence of growth factors, or cytokines (Table 47-2). Cytokines act on different cells through specific cytokine receptors. Activation of these receptors induces signal-transduction pathways that lead to changes in gene transcription and eventual cell proliferation and differentiation. These growth factors have also been shown to act as survival factors for the developing hematopoietic cells by preventing *apoptosis* (programmed cell death). This process occurs in the cellular milieu of the bone marrow, and the well-recognized fact is that hematopoiesis also depends in part on the nonhematopoietic cells (fibroblasts, endothelial cells, osteoblasts, and fat cells) that make up the bone marrow microenvironment. Recent research in HSC biology has focused on how these cells are regulated by growth factors in the marrow local microenvironment and by unique cell surface ligand interactions between stem cells and the surrounding stromal cells in well-defined sites termed *stem cell niches*.

HEMATOPOIETIC DIFFERENTIATION PATHWAY

Traditionally, hematopoiesis has been hypothesized to proceed along a tightly regulated hierarchy (Fig. 47-1) governed by effects of intrinsic transcription factors and cytokines in the bone marrow microenvironment. As more primitive cells mature under the influence of specific regulatory cytokines, they undergo several cell divisions and become *progenitor cells* committed to one lineage. They also lose their self-renewal capacity. Morphologically, these cells are transformed from nonspecific blastlike cells into cells that can be identified by their color, shape, and granular and nuclear content. Functionally, they acquire distinguishing cell surface receptors and responses to specific signals. Maturing *granulocytes* and *erythroid cells* undergo several more cell divisions in the bone marrow, whereas *lymphocytes* travel to the thymus and lymph nodes for further development. *Megakaryocytes* cease cellular division but continue with nuclear replication. Eventually, these cells are released from the marrow as fully functional *erythrocytes, mast cells, granulocytes, monocytes, eosinophils, macrophages,* and *platelets*.

Table 47-1 Normal Values for Peripheral Blood Cells

Cell Type and Size	Mean	Range
Hemoglobin	Women: 14 g/dL Men: 15.5 g/dL	Women: 12-16 g/dL Men: 13.5-17.5 g/dL
Hematocrit	Women: 41% Men: 47%	Women: 36%-46% Men: 41%-53%
Reticulocyte	1%	0.5%-1.5%
Count	60,000/mcL	35,000-85,000/mcL
Mean corpuscular volume	80-100	
Platelet count	250,000/mcL	150,000-400,000/mcL
Total white count	7400/mcL	4500-11,000/mcL
Neutrophils	4400/mcL (40%-60%)	1800-7700/mcL
Lymphocytes	2500/mcL (20%-40%)	1000-4800/mcL
Monocytes	300/mcL (<5%)	

Table 47-2 Cytokines and Their Activities

Abbreviation	Name	Effects on Hematopoiesis
EPO	Erythropoietin	Stimulation of proliferation and maturation of erythroid progenitors; produced by the kidney in response to anemia and hypoxia; important clinically for treatment of anemia associated with low EPO levels (renal failure, anemia of chronic disease)
G-CSF	Granulocyte colony-stimulating factor	Stimulation of proliferation and maturation of granulocytes; more broad-based effect because also increases release of *stem cells* in peripheral blood; clinically important for treatment of neutropenia and mobilization of stem cells for transplantation
GM-CSF	Granulocyte-monocyte colony-stimulating factor	Proliferation of granulocyte and monocyte precursors; role unclear in steady-state hematopoiesis because knockout has no hematopoietic phenotype
TPO	Thrombopoietin	Proliferation of megakaryocytes; results disappointing in clinical studies
M-CSF	Monocyte colony-stimulating factor	Proliferation of monocytes
IL-2	Interleukin-2	Proliferation of T cells
IL-3	Interleukin-3 (multi-CSF)	Proliferation of granulocytes, monocytes; broad-based effects, appearing to increase the proliferation of *stem cells;* not in use clinically
IL-4	Interleukin-4	Proliferation of B cells
IL-5	Interleukin-5	Proliferation of T cells, B cells; proliferation and differentiation of eosinophils
IL-11	Interleukin-11	Proliferation of megakaryocytes; undergoing clinical testing
LIF	Leukemia inhibitory factor	Proliferation of stem cells and megakaryocytes
SCF	Stem cell factor (kit ligand)	Proliferation of progenitor cells; broad-based effects on multiple lineages

CSF, colony-stimulating factor.

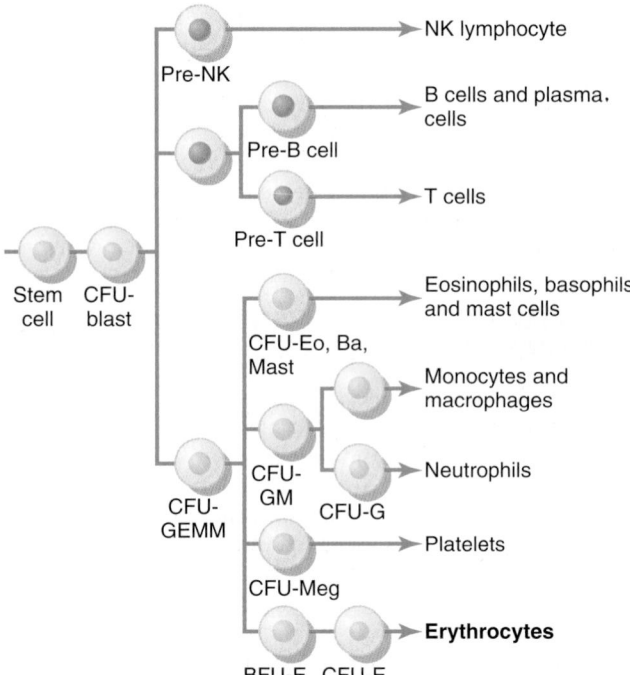

Figure 47-1 Schema of the development of the cells of the bone marrow. Ba, basophil; BFU, blast-forming unit; CFU, colony-forming unit; E, erythroid; Eo, eosinophil; G, granulocyte; GEMM, granulocyte-erythrocyte-macrophage-megakaryocyte; GM, granulocyte-macrophage; Meg, megakaryocyte; NK, natural killer.

Pluripotent Stem Cells

The pluripotent HSC is morphologically indistinguishable and is best identified by its expression of the cell differentiation antigen, CD34, and by its ability to form pluripotent colonies in vitro. Under the influence of interleukin-1 (IL-1), IL-3, IL-6, fms-like tyrosine kinase 3 (flt-3), and a specific stem cell factor (c-kit ligand, or steel factor), this cell matures into either a myeloid-lineage stem cell (CFU–granulocyte-erythrocyte-macrophage-megakaryocyte [CFU-GEMM]) or a lymphoid-lineage stem cell. In the presence of granulocyte-macrophage colony-stimulating factor (GM-CSF) and IL-3, the myeloid stem cell will further differentiate into daughter cells of its named lineages (see Fig. 47-1). The lymphopoietic stem cell, in contrast, will become either a pre-B cell or a prothymocyte (pre-T cell) and will leave the marrow for further maturation.

Erythroid Lineage

Primitive erythroid precursors arising from the myeloid stem cell are called burst-forming unit–erythroid cells. These cells then differentiate into CFU-erythroid (CFU-E) cells, which are the committed progenitor cells of erythrocytes. CFU-E cells express receptors for erythropoietin (EPO), an 18-kD molecule produced by renal interstitial cells in response to low oxygenation states or anemia. EPO upregulates proliferation of CFU-E cells and promotes their maturation into proerythroblasts and reticulocytes, which begin to synthesize hemoglobin (see Table 47-2).

Granulocyte and Monocyte Lineages

Human GM-CSF acts early in the hematopoietic pathway to regulate maturation of the CFU-GEMM stem cell. Differen-tiation of this myeloid precursor into specific committed progenitors occurs under the direction of granulocyte-CSF (G-CSF) and monocyte-CSF (see Table 47-2). CFU-granulocyte cells undergo sequential transformation into easily recognizable myeloblasts, myelocytes, and eventually early polymorphonuclear neutrophils with their characteristic polysegmented nuclei. CFU-monocyte cells, in contrast, retain a single nucleus as they mature from monoblasts to promonocytes to monocytes and sometimes macrophages.

Other Lineages

Eosinophils and basophils develop from CFU-GEMM cells under the influence of IL-5 and IL-3–IL-4, respectively. The acquisition of their specific granular contents helps in distinguishing their precursors from those of early monocytes. The development of platelets is morphologically distinct from the other lineages. CFU-GEMM cells differentiate into CFU-megakaryocyte cells, so named because these cells cease cell division early but not nuclear replication. Megakaryocytes are the only cells in the body with the capacity to double their DNA content (termed *endomitosis*). Over the course of several cell cycles, the maturing megakaryocyte eventually acquires several times the nuclear content of other cells in preparation for its eventual dissolution into platelets with a fraction of the cytoplasm of other hematopoietic cells. Two growth factors, thrombopoietin (TPO) and IL-11, have been shown to increase platelet counts by promoting megakaryocyte development (see Table 47-2).

Stem Cell Plasticity

Provocative recent data have challenged the conventional paradigm of hierarchical hematopoietic stem differentiation. Experts have proposed that hematopoietic stem cells can not only differentiate back into more immature progenitors, but can also cross lineages and transdifferentiate into nonlymphohematopoietic cells such as myocytes, hepatocytes, gastrointestinal epithelial cells, and neurons. Whether this *plasticity* of hematopoietic stem cells is truly an intrinsic property of adult stem cells or is caused by contaminating cells of other populations, fusion of hematopoietic cells with other tissue cells, or artifacts introduced by ex vivo stem cell isolation techniques remains controversial. Nevertheless, the suggestion that adult hematopoietic stem cells may be a dynamic renewable resource for tissue repair and regeneration holds great future promise.

Primary Hematopoietic Failure Syndromes

Diseases of the hematopoietic stem cell that disrupt the normal regulated pattern of stem cell development can result in underproduction of mature progeny *(aplastic anemia)*, overproduction of mature progeny *(myeloproliferative disease)*, or failed differentiation with the production of excess immature forms *(myelodysplasia* and *acute leukemia)*. *Hematopoietic failure*, defined as the inability of hematopoietic stem cells to produce normal numbers of mature blood cells, manifests clinically as peripheral pancytopenia (decreased production of all blood cell lineages). Although marrow dysfunction causing pancytopenia can arise from a

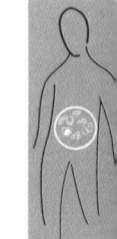

Table 47-3 **Differential Diagnosis of Pancytopenia**
I. Primary Bone Marrow Disorders
Aplastic anemia (AA)
Congenital aplastic anemia syndromes
Fanconi anemia
Shwachman-Diamond syndrome
Dyskeratosis, congenital
Acquired aplastic anemia
Hypocellular myelodysplastic (MDS) syndrome
Myelofibrosis (MF)
Paroxysmal nocturnal hemoglobinuria
Acute leukemias (acute lymphocytic leukemia [ALL], acute myeloid leukemia [AML])
Hairy cell leukemia
II. Systemic Diseases with Secondary Bone Marrow Effects
Metastatic solid tumor to marrow
Autoimmune disorders (systemic lupus, Sjögren syndrome)
Nutritional deficiencies (vitamin B_{12}, folate, alcoholism)
Infections (overwhelming sepsis from any cause, viruses, brucellosis, ehrlichiosis [mycobacteria])
Storage diseases (Gaucher disease, Niemann-Pick disease)
Anatomic (hypersplenism)

number of causes, both hematologic and nonhematologic (Table 47-3), primary bone marrow failure disorders are characterized by a profound impairment of the ability of the HSC to replenish the stem cell pool. Rarely, marrow failure syndromes are found to be due to intrinsic HSC defects. In most cases, these disorders are the result of extrinsic damage to inherently normal HSC. The most common treatment modalities for primary hematopoietic failure disorders consist of exogenous growth factor administration and stem cell transplantation.

GROWTH FACTORS IN CLINICAL USE

The discovery of the factors that influence normal hematopoiesis has led to important applications to the treatment of patients with defects in hematopoietic cell production. The discovery that committed hematopoietic cells of each lineage can be stimulated to proliferate and differentiate in the presence of specific cytokines (see Table 47-2) has been of great clinical utility. Advances in DNA technology have led to the synthesis and purification of recombinant human (rh) proteins with similar biologic activity in vivo. The administration of these products to patients has allowed the successful manipulation of the numbers of mature cells in the peripheral blood. For example, exogenous erythropoietin is now considered a mainstay in the management of anemia caused by renal failure, chemotherapy, and marrow failure syndromes. The use of G-CSF or GM-CSF in patients with febrile neutropenia and documented infection or sepsis after chemotherapy or radiation therapy has been demonstrated to reduce hospital stays and to shorten the period of high infection risk. Administration of GM-CSF has also been hypothesized to improve host immune responses to fungal infections. High-dose G-CSF also is routinely used to mobilize CD34$^+$ marrow stem cells into the peripheral blood for collection before and after stem cell transplantation in patients with delayed stem cell engraftment (see later). Early trials of TPO growth factors to stimulate platelet production

were halted owing to development of antihuman platelet antibodies in some patients. Second-generation thrombopoietic agents bearing no structural resemblance to TPO but designed to bind and activate the TPO receptor are in clinical trials. Treatment with romiplostim, a recombinant protein defined as a peptibody and given as a weekly subcutaneous injection, was recently approved for patients with chronic immune-mediated thrombocytopenia based on studies showing a doubling of platelet counts and decreased platelet transfusion requirements in treated patients. Eltrombopag, an orally available small organic TPO agonist, was given daily to similar patients and also induced platelet elevations with little reported toxicity. The potential application of TPO agonists for management of thrombocytopenia in marrow failure syndromes awaits the results of ongoing phase III clinical trials.

HEMATOPOIETIC STEM CELL TRANSPLANTATION

Types of Transplantations

Our understanding of HSC biology has fostered the development of techniques to manipulate these cells for therapeutic purposes. The fact that the antitumor effects of most chemotherapeutic drugs and radiation therapy are dose dependent and that both cause a major dose-limiting toxicity of myelosuppression has long been known. Hematopoietic stem cell transplantation permits the administration of intense myeloablative doses of chemotherapy and total-body radiation intended to eradicate malignant cells followed by the infusion of stem cells (either from a donor or from the same patient) to replete the ablated marrow. Although historically used in the treatment of primary stem cell disorders such as leukemia, the therapeutic potential of transplantation is now being employed for patients with nonmalignant hematologic malignancies (e.g., aplastic anemia, sickle cell anemia, congenital immunodeficiencies), solid tumors (e.g., renal cell carcinoma, melanoma), and nonmalignant autoimmune diseases (e.g., amyloidosis, systemic lupus). In general, younger patients (<50 years of age) are considered the best candidates for this intensive therapy, although this too is changing in the setting of newer supportive modalities. Several modes of stem cell transplantation have been developed. In *autologous transplantation,* the patient's bone marrow or peripheral blood stem cells are collected during remission following high-dose chemotherapy or rhG-CSF administration. These cells are cryopreserved, thawed, and reinfused. Such an approach incurs a higher risk for relapse as a result of reinfusion of a stem cell product that may remain contaminated with tumor. *Allogeneic stem cell transplantation* is a procedure whereby abnormally functioning hematopoietic bone marrow is eradicated and is replaced with normal bone marrow or stem cells from a compatible source, either a related or an unrelated donor. High-dose chemotherapy with or without total-body radiation is administered to destroy the patient's bone marrow, followed by the infusion of new stem cells that engraft and restore normal hematopoiesis. Treatment-related morbidity is significant, with a procedure-related mortality of 10% to 30%; however, improvements in supportive care and immunomodulatory therapy designed to suppress *graft-versus-host*

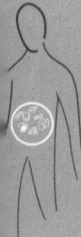

disease (GVHD), an autoimmune phenomenon in which intact lymphocytes in the transplanted marrow attack the host tissues, are continuing to improve outcome. Donor and patient are tested for compatibility of human leukocyte antigen (HLA) and major histocompatibility complex (MHC) proteins expressed on all cells. Three major HLA class I antigens (A, B, and C) and three MHC class II antigens (DP, DQ, and DR) have been developed. The six HLA gene loci are tightly linked on chromosome 6 and are almost always inherited on a single cluster of genes, or *haplotype.* Therefore, all children are a *half-match (haploidentical)* to each of their parents, and full siblings have a 25% probability of being HLA identical to one another. HLA-matched non-related transplants have higher rates of GVHD than transplants from HLA-matched related donors as a result of other minor HLA incompatibilities. Patients who receive *HLA-mismatched* stem cell transplantation risk acute GVHD, marrow rejection, and fatal marrow aplasia. Morbidity and mortality associated with non–HLA-compatible transplants can be prohibitive.

Increasing evidence indicates that the excellent response of some patients to HSC transplantation is partly related to the active suppression of the patient's original or residual or relapsing disease by cells from the newly transplanted donor graft, referred to as the *graft-versus-leukemia* (GVL) *effect.* Studies have documented the compelling observation that infusion of donor lymphocytes can restore remission in patients with evidence of relapse after allogeneic transplantation for chronic myelogenous leukemia (CML). Conversely, procedures that minimize the reactivity between donor and host increase disease relapse. For example, the rate of relapse in patients who receive *syngeneic* (identical twin) *stem cell transplantation* and in patients who receive T-cell–depleted marrow in an attempt to reduce GVHD is increased.

The observation of the effectiveness of donor lymphocyte infusions in controlling CML has led to the conclusion that the immunologic effects of transplanted allogeneic cells may be as important as (or more important than) cytoreduction for the cure of some hematologic malignancies. To further exploit these effects, *nonmyeloablative stem cell transplantations* are now performed, whereby patients receive conditioning and immunosuppressive regimens in doses sufficient to permit donor stem cell engraftment without aggressive cytoreduction. These *mini-transplants* result in chimeric marrows (part patient, part donor) without significant periods of cytopenias or hematopoietic compromise, although most responding patients convert to a fully donor-derived marrow over time. Although still experimental, these procedures are increasingly being used in patients who are otherwise ineligible for traditional myeloablative transplantation regimens (age >50 to 55 years or other comorbidities) or in individuals with nonmalignant autoimmune or congenital disorders.

Hematopoietic Stem Cell Sources for Transplantation

Historically, stem cell transplantations have employed allogeneic *bone marrow* (BM) *stem cells* aspirated from the posterior iliac crest of the donor and intravenously infused into the patient following myeloablation and immunosuppressive therapy. The process of engraftment or reconstitution of normal hematopoietic function takes several weeks. Patients often require almost daily platelet and red blood cell transfusions and are hospitalized during this period of prolonged neutropenia to minimize life-threatening bacterial, viral, and fungal infections. Other complications include severe mucositis, hemorrhagic cystitis, GVHD, relapsed disease, and graft failure. The discovery that high-dose rhG-CSF treatment results in the mobilization of large numbers of CD34+ hematopoietic progenitor and stem cells from bone marrow sites into circulating blood (up to 10- to 15-fold increase over baseline levels) has led to the use of *peripheral blood stem cells* (PBSC) collected by apheresis procedures in place of bone marrow stem cells for allogeneic transplantation. When compared with marrow-derived stem cells, PBSC engraft more rapidly after myeloablation. Patients receiving allogeneic PBSC transplants have decreased neutrophil recovery time, lower transfusion requirements, and fewer inpatient hospital days with similar rates of acute GVHD and long-term survival outcomes as traditional marrow transplanted patients. Because PBSC collections often contain threefold to fourfold more CD34+ stem cells and 10-fold more lymphoid cells than do harvested marrow grafts, higher rates of chronic GVHD may occur. *Umbilical cord blood* (UCB) *stem cells* have also been found to be a rich source of immature CD34+ HSCs. The less stringent HLA compatibility requirements of UCB-HSC matches have led to the increasing use of these transplants as a therapy for patients lacking full compatible HLA-matched PBSC or BM donors. Although still considered experimental, some transplantation centers have reported similar long-term outcomes following UCB transplants as conventional marrow or peripheral blood stem cell transplants for primary hematologic diseases. However, the relatively fewer (and limited) numbers of CD34+ stem cells found in harvested umbilical cord units accounts for a much slower hematopoietic recovery following UCB and a statistically higher risk for nonengraftment compared with other stem cell sources. For this reason, UCB transplantation procedures have been limited to pediatric patients and smaller adults or to adult patients for whom there is more than one HLA-compatible UCB unit.

APLASTIC ANEMIA
Etiology and Pathogenesis

Aplastic anemia (AA) is a rare disorder characterized by pancytopenia with a markedly hypocellular bone marrow. This disease was first described by Paul Ehrlich in 1888, who noted that autopsy bone marrow specimens from a young woman who died of severe anemia and neutropenia were extremely hypoplastic. More recent studies demonstrate that patients with severe AA possess only a fraction of normal pluripotent stem cell numbers despite normal functional marrow stromal cells and normal or even elevated levels of stimulatory cytokines. AA is an uncommon disease. The incidence ranges from 1 to 5 cases per million in the general population, found predominantly in young adults (20 to 25 years of age) and older adults (60 to 65 years of age). Interestingly, the incidence is threefold higher in developing countries (Thailand and China) compared with industrialized Western nations (Europe and Israel), a fact that is not

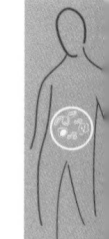

Table 47-4 **Causes of Acquired Aplastic Anemia**
Drugs (dose related): chemotherapeutic agents, antibiotics (chloramphenicol, trimethoprim-sulfamethoxazole)
Idiosyncratic (many unproven): chloramphenicol, quinacrine, nonsteroidal anti-inflammatory drugs, anticonvulsants, gold, sulfonamides, cimetidine, penicillamine
Toxins: benzene and other hydrocarbons, insecticides
Viral infection: hepatitis, Epstein-Barr virus, human immunodeficiency virus
Immune disease: graft-versus-host disease in immunodeficiency, hypogammaglobulinemia
Paroxysmal nocturnal hemoglobinuria (PNH)
Radiation
Pregnancy

explained by differences in drug or radiation exposure. A small proportion of AA cases occur in the context of a congenital bone marrow failure disorder, such as Fanconi anemia, Shwachman-Diamond syndrome, and dyskeratosis congenita. The most common congenital AA, Fanconi anemia, is an autosomal recessive disorder arising from mutations in genes encoding DNA repair proteins.

The known causes of acquired AA are numerous (Table 47-4) and range from myeloablative radiation exposure to common viruses and medications. Prior bone marrow toxicity from drugs, chemicals (benzene, cyclic hydrocarbons found in petroleum products, rubber glue, insecticides, chemical dyes), or radiation predisposes to AA because these agents directly injure proliferating and differentiating HSC by inducing DNA damage. In contrast, therapies such as cytotoxic chemotherapy (especially with alkylating agents) and radiation target all rapidly cycling cells and often induce reversible bone marrow aplasia. Despite these many causes of acquired AA, most AA cases are idiopathic.

Acquired and congenital AA appear to be linked etiologically through abnormal telomere maintenance. Telomeres are repeated nucleotide sequences, which cap and protect chromosome ends from degradation. Cell division leads to normal telomere erosion; when telomeres reach a critically short length, cells cease to proliferate, senesce, and undergo apoptosis, often with accompanying DNA damage and genomic instability. The presence of the telomerase enzyme in normal HSC preserves long telomeres and promotes quiescence and prolonged cellular life span. Patients with autosomal dominant dyskeratosis congenita have mutations in genes for telomerase complexes, predisposing to premature aging and enhanced marrow failure in the setting of accelerated telomere shortening. One third of patients with acquired AA also have short telomeres likely due to a combination of genetic, environmental, and epigenetic factors.

Autoreactive host lymphocytes also function as culprits in destroying normal hematopoiesis in AA. Bone marrow stromal cells and cytokine levels in patients with AA are normal. The fact that AA also occurs in diseases of immune dysregulation and after viral infections further suggests an immune-mediated mechanism for the disease. One hypothesis is that antigens presented to the immune system by viruses or drugs trigger cytotoxic T-cell responses that then persist to destroy normal stem cells. In rare instances, 1 in 100,000 patients will develop a severe AA as an idiosyncratic

drug reaction. Whether these individuals unknowingly possess a certain genetic predisposition to sensitivity to exposures (such as nonsteroidal anti-inflammatory drugs, sulfonamides, or the Epstein-Barr virus) commonly found in the general population is unknown.

Clinical Features

The clinical onset of AA can be insidious or abrupt. Patients often complain of symptoms related to their cytopenias: weakness, fatigue, dyspnea, or palpitations resulting from anemia; gingival bleeding, epistaxis, petechiae, or purpura caused by low platelet counts; or recurrent bacterial infections caused by low or nonfunctioning neutrophils. Physical examination is often normal except in patients with congenital AA who may have various abnormalities.

Laboratory Studies

Diagnostic confirmation of AA requires bone marrow biopsy to confirm hypocellularity and to rule out other marrow processes. Normal bone marrow cellularity ranges from 30% to 50% up to age 70 years and is under 20% after age 70 years (**Web Fig. 47-1A**). In contrast, bone marrow cellularity in patients with AA usually ranges from 5% to 15% cellularity with increased fat accumulation and few, if any, hematopoietic cells (primarily plasma cells and lymphocytes) (**Web Fig. 47-1B**). In AA, hematopoietic progenitor and precursor cells are morphologically normal but number less than 1% of normal levels and have been shown to be markedly dysfunctional with a decreased ability to form differentiated progenitor cell colonies in vitro. Evidence of increased blasts, dysplastic hematopoietic cells (such as pseudo-Pelger-Huët abnormalities or micromegakaryocytes) (**Web Fig. 47-2**), or clonal cytogenetically abnormal cells in the peripheral blood or marrow are diagnostic of acute leukemia or myelodysplasia and not AA, even in the setting of a hypocellular marrow. In young patients, a diagnosis of Fanconi anemia is made by demonstrating enhanced sensitivity of cultured cells to mitomycin or diepoxybutane-induced chromosomal damage. Although patients with AA typically have a low reticulocyte count from low red blood cell production with a paucity of blood cells (**Web Fig. 47-3A**) and macrocytic red cells (**Web Fig. 47-3B**) on the peripheral smear, patients with other primary marrow disorders may also exhibit similar findings.

Treatment

Treatment of AA is based on the severity of disease. Patients with mild cytopenias can be monitored expectantly. However, patients with severe AA based on peripheral blood cells counts (defined as a neutrophil count <500/μL, platelet count <20,000/μL, anemia with corrected reticulocyte count <1%, and marrow cellularity 5% to 10%) have a poor median survival rate of 2 to 6 months without treatment. Because most of these patients die from overwhelming infections, supportive care with broad-spectrum antibiotics, antifungal agents, and antiviral agents is warranted in patients with advanced neutropenia. Red blood cell and platelet transfusions are helpful in patients who are profoundly symptomatic (with care given to patients eligible for transplantation).

Current therapeutic approaches to AA are focused on either replacing the defective HSC by stem cell transplanta-

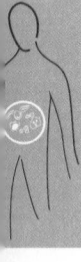

tion or controlling an overactive immune response. All young patients with severe AA and an HLA-compatible bone marrow donor should be considered for allogeneic bone marrow transplantation, which offers the best chance for definitive cure. Although long-term survival is excellent in patients younger than 30 years transplanted from a sibling donor (75% to 90%), morbidity from the transplant itself and the management of long-term transplant-related complications are continuing problems. Outcome in patients older than 40 years or in patients without an HLA-matched related donor are poor.

The presumed immune mechanisms for drug-induced aplasia have provided the impetus for immunosuppressive approaches to the treatment of AA in older patients, in patients who are unable to find a compatible stem cell donor, and in those who are otherwise ineligible for stem cell transplantation. Treatment with a combination of antithymocyte globulin (ATG) and cyclosporine (a specific T-cell inhibitor) allows for restoration of marrow function (i.e., independence from red blood cell or platelet transfusions) in 70% to 80% of patients, with a 5-year survival rate in responders of 90%. Side effects of ATG include anaphylaxis and serum sickness as a result of foreign antigens in the antisera, which are generally self-limited. Patients often relapse and recur with this disease and may warrant retreatment with repeat ATG, newer immunosuppressive agents (such as mycophenolate mofetil), androgens, and experimental agents. Treatment with traditional chemotherapies such as cyclophosphamide has usually proved too toxic. Because endogenous cytokine production is usually high in patients with AA, the routine use of growth factors such as rhG-CSF, EPO, or stem cell factor is generally ineffective; however, in patients with refractory disease, long-term administration of combination cytokines appears to have some effects in sustaining blood cell counts. Patients who survive the initial treatment of aplasia, however, remain at increased risk for the emergence of other primary hematologic disorders, such as myelodysplasia, leukemia, and paroxysmal nocturnal hemoglobinuria (PNH). The relationship of such clonal disorders to the pathogenesis of the original aplastic anemia is controversial.

PAROXYSMAL NOCTURNAL HEMOGLOBINURIA

Etiology and Pathogenesis

PNH is an uncommon disease characterized by intravascular hemolysis and venous thrombosis in association with bone marrow failure. The disease arises from expansion of pluripotent hematopoietic stem cells containing a somatic mutation in the phosphatidylinositol glycan complementation class A (*PIG-A*) gene. Loss of *PIG-A*, which codes for a membrane lipid moiety (glycosyl phosphatidylinositol [GPI]), leads to abnormal hematopoietic cells deficient in dozens of proteins that are normally attached to the cell surface by the GPI anchor. Disease manifestations of PNH result from lack of the GPI-linked proteins (CD55 and CD59) that usually protect red blood cells and platelets from complement-mediated attack. Loss of CD55 or CD59 leads to increased immune destruction of blood cells. Blood cells arising from abnormal PNH clones can have complete (type

III cells) or partial (type II cells) GPI deficiency. The degree of GPI deficiency is associated with the severity of the clinical symptoms. Of note, GPI-deficient cells almost always coexist in the marrow with varying populations of normal GPI-expressing cells (type I cells). The presence of small numbers of abnormal PNH clones in patients with AA or myelodysplastic syndrome (MDS, discussed later) suggest significant overlap in the etiologies of all three of these diseases. This has led to the reclassification of PNH into "classic PNH disease" and "PNH in the setting of another specified bone marrow disorder." Mechanistically, it is postulated that suppression of normal hematopoiesis by the host immune system, directly or indirectly by a preceding or coexistent disorder, provides a marrow environment favoring selective expansion of PNH stem cell clones and their deficient blood cell progeny over normal hematopoiesis.

Clinical Features and Laboratory Studies

Patients are typically younger individuals who present with chronic complaints of abdominal pain, dysphagia, erectile dysfunction, and intense lethargy due to smooth muscle dystonia resulting from depletion of circulating nitric oxide levels by free hemoglobin. Acute exacerbations often occur on an intermittent to frequent basis and are difficult to manage. The diagnosis of PNH is made by identification of complete or partial GPI protein deficiency on red cells and granulocytes, usually identified by loss of CD59, CD55, CD16, or CD24 expression in a clonal population. Laboratory tests reveal ongoing low-grade intravascular hemolysis with increased LDH levels correlating with severity of hemolysis and symptoms. Cytopenias, particularly anemia, often render patients transfusion dependent with ongoing hemoglobinuria due to the release of free plasma hemoglobin from intracellular compartments. Median survival from diagnosis is usually 10 to 15 years. Venous thrombosis involving the cerebral and intra-abdominal veins occurs in about half of patients and is the cause of death in up to one third, although the etiology of the increased thrombotic risk is not entirely understood. Other causes of morbidity and mortality are side effects of progressive aplastic anemia (see AA, discussed earlier) and a 5% long-term risk for leukemic transformation. About 15% of PNH patients have spontaneous resolution of disease without long-term sequelae, suggesting that *PIG-A* mutations may appear transiently and disappear spontaneously in normal hematopoietic cell populations for unknown reasons.

Treatment

Treatment of PNH ranges from supportive care with transfusions and iron and folic acid supplementation to allogeneic stem cell transplantation in select patients for curative intent. Documented venous thrombosis is treated with lifelong full anticoagulation. *Eculizumab* is a humanized antibody that binds with high affinity to the complement protein C5, preventing terminal complement-mediated intravascular hemolysis in patients with PNH. Results from multiple clinical trials have shown that eculizumab therapy decreases hemolysis and hemoglobinuria, reduces requirements for red blood cell transfusions, and is associated with significant improvement in quality of life for PNH patients. Therapy is generally well tolerated with a theoretical increased risk for meningococcal infections due to complement-mediated blockade. Eculizumab therapy may also result in decreased risk for life-threatening thrombosis, which would ultimately improve long-term survival in this disease.

MYELODYSPLASTIC SYNDROME

Etiology and Pathogenesis

Myelodysplastic syndrome (MDS) is a heterogeneous group of blood disorders characterized by ineffective and disordered hematopoiesis in one or more of the major myeloid cell lines: erythroid cells, neutrophils and their precursors, and megakaryocytes. Patients have one or more cytopenias despite the presence of normal or increased numbers of hematopoietic cells in the bone marrow. Disordered maturation is accompanied by increased intramedullary *apoptosis* (programmed cell death), which contributes to the decreased release of mature cells into the periphery.

Primary MDS is predominantly a disease of elderly persons and occurs in about 1 in 500 patients between the ages of 60 and 75 years. Most cases are idiopathic. Although often considered "preleukemic" disease, the overall risk for MDS transformation to acute myeloid leukemia (AML) is only 25% to 30%. However, the identification of characteristic gene deletions (5q–) and translocations diagnostic of both MDS and AML subtypes (see Chapter 48) underline the likelihood of similar mechanisms of clonal myeloid stem cell injury in both disorders.

Persons with prior exposure to radiation, chemotherapy, and organic chemicals (benzene) are at increased risk for developing secondary MDS. This disorder may occur at any age and comprises 10% to 15% of all diagnosed MDS cases. MDS arising months to years after prior chemotherapy (involving any cytotoxic agent but particularly after alkylating agents and anthracyclines), ionizing radiation, radiolabeled antibody therapy, or stem cell transplantation for cancer is termed therapy-related MDS (t-MDS). Because t-MDS typically swiftly evolves to more aggressive disease, these cases have recently been reclassified with therapy-related acute myeloid leukemia (t-AML) and treated accordingly (see Chapter 48).

Clinical Features

Most patients with MDS are referred for evaluation of an incidental finding of peripheral cytopenias. Symptomatic patients usually exhibit findings related to the secondary effects of cytopenias: bleeding and bruising caused by thrombocytopenia, infection caused by leukopenia, or fatigue and dyspnea related to anemia. Physical examination is usually unremarkable, although 25% or more of patients may have splenomegaly. In some patients with MDS, development of skin lesions with fever (acute febrile neutrophilic dermatosis, or Sweet syndrome) may herald the transformation of MDS into acute leukemia. The disease course of MDS varies widely. Some patients may live normal life spans, but most die prematurely of cytopenia-related complications, marrow failure, or evolution to AML. Median survival is usually less than 2 years.

Laboratory Studies

Dysplasia of myeloid hematopoietic cells is evident in the blood and marrow of MDS patients. Review of the periph-

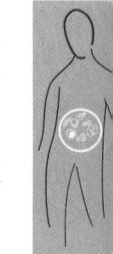

eral blood smear may show characteristic morphologic abnormalities in addition to cytopenias. Erythroid cells are usually macrocytic, often with basophilic stippling. Neutrophils are often hypogranular and hypolobulated, with a characteristic bilobed nuclear morphology termed *pseudo–Pelger-Huët abnormality.* Pelger-Huët anomaly should be anticipated when automated differential cell counts report unusually large numbers of bands. The bone marrow in MDS is usually normocellular or hypercellular, although 10% of patients may have a hypocellular marrow. Dysplastic changes usually occur in all three cell lines. Erythroid cells appear megaloblastic, with multinucleated cells or asynchronous nuclear-cytoplasmic development. Extremely small *micromegakaryocytes* and agranular megakaryocytes may also be present. The myeloid series shows poor maturation with a *left shift* to earlier hypogranulated myeloid forms. Although elevated numbers of myeloid blasts are common, increasing blasts are indicative of progression toward acute leukemia. Electron microscopy of the marrow shows cellular changes (prominent nuclear chromatin, cytoplasmic vacuoles, and blebs) characteristic of increased apoptosis (**Web Fig. 47-3**).

The natural history (and treatment of) some MDS subtypes is correlated with specific cytogenetic abnormalities, and hence careful molecular studies of the marrow should be performed at initial evaluation. For example, MDS associated with deletion of the short arm of chromosome 7 (7p–) or complex cytogenetic abnormalities such as monosomy 7 or trisomy 8 often have poor clinical outcomes. Presence of an isolated deletion in the long arm of chromosome 5 may have a well-characterized clinical course (termed the *5q– syndrome*). Patients are predominantly older women with a refractory macrocytic anemia, normal or elevated platelet counts, and an overall better clinical prognosis. These patients often live for several years with intermittent red blood cell transfusions and have a low risk for eventual leukemic transformation. The presence of multiple or complex cytogenetic aberrations carries a worse prognosis.

Although one third to one half of patients presenting with cytopenia and myeloid dysplasia will have diagnostic clonal cytogenetic abnormalities in marrow cells, in many cases, the marrow karyotype is normal. For these patients, the diagnosis of MDS should be one of exclusion with other potential causes of marrow failure and pancytopenia evaluated (see Table 47-3). MDS should never be diagnosed in acute disease states, during chronic hospitalization, or within 6 months of known myelotoxic therapy (radiation, chemotherapy). Causes such as vitamin B_{12} or folate deficiency, alcohol use, and HIV infection should be considered. A patient with possible MDS and a hypocellular bone marrow must be evaluated for aplastic anemia. In general, the presence of (1) consistent cytopenia in one of more myeloid lineages, (2) no other obvious etiologies, and (3) dysplasia of at least 10% myeloid marrow cells or 5% to 19% blast cells should be considered MDS.

In the past, MDS was classified based on dysplastic marrow morphology and percentage of blasts into five subtypes: refractory anemia, refractory anemia with ringed sideroblasts, refractory anemia with excess blasts, refractory anemia with excess blasts in transformation, and chronic myelomonocytic leukemia (CMML). More recently, these five subtypes were expanded to eight subtypes, with recognition of

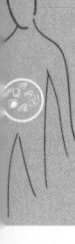

Table 47-5 **World Health Organization Classification of Myelodysplastic Syndromes**
Refractory Anemia (RA)
Blood: anemia, no or rare blasts
BM: erythroid dysplasia only, <5% blasts, and <15% ringed sideroblasts
Refractory Anemia with Ringed Sideroblasts (RARS)
Blood: anemia, no blasts
BM: ≥15% ringed sideroblasts, erythroid dysplasia only, <5% blasts
Refractory Cytopenia with Multilineage Dysplasia (RCMD)
Blood: cytopenias (bicytopenia or pancytopenia), no or rare blasts, <1 × 10⁹/L monocytes
BM: dysplasia in ≥10% of the cells of two or more myeloid cell lines, <5% blasts, no Auer rods, <15% ringed sideroblasts
Refractory Cytopenia with Multilineage Dysplasia and Ringed Sideroblasts (RCMD-RS)
Blood: cytopenias (two or more), no or rare blasts, no Auer rods, and <1 × 10⁹/L monocytes
BM: dysplasia in ≥10% of the cells of two or more myeloid cell lines, <5% blasts, ≥15% ringed sideroblasts, no Auer rods
Refractory Anemia with Excess Blasts—1 (RAEB-1)
Blood: cytopenias, <5% blasts, no Auer rods, and <1 × 10⁹/L monocytes
BM: unilineage or multilineage dysplasia, 5%-9% blasts, and no Auer rods
Refractory Anemia with Excess Blasts—2 (RAEB-2)
Blood: cytopenias, 5%-19% blasts, Auer rods ±<1 × 10⁹/L monocytes
BM: unilineage or multilineage dysplasia, 10%-19% blasts, ± Auer rods
Myelodysplastic Syndrome—Unclassified (MDS-U)
Blood: cytopenias, no or rare blasts, no Auer rods
BM: unilineage dysplasia in one myeloid line, <5% blasts, and no Auer rods
MDS Associated with Isolated del(5q)
Blood: anemia, usually normal or increased platelet count, and <5% blasts
BM: normal to increased megakaryocytes with hypolobulated nuclei, <5% blasts, isolated cytogenetic abnormality of deletion 5q, and no Auer rods

BM, bone marrow.

multilineage dysplasia as an important feature (i.e., refractory cytopenia with multilineage dysplasia, refractory cytopenia with multilineage dysplasia and ringed sideroblasts) and the reclassification of CMML as myeloproliferative-myelodysplastic syndrome (Table 47-5). The presence of an isolated 5q– cytogenetic abnormality in MDS was established as a distinct clinical syndrome. Evidence of marrow dysplasia following prior chemotherapy, radiation, or other myeloablative therapy is now considered therapy-related AML (t-AML). Although in general, MDS patients with refractory anemia and excess blasts or refractory cytopenias with multilineage dysplasia fare poorly, morphologic classification of MDS correlates only approximately with overall survival.

Classification of MDS into clinical prognostic categories remains a work in evolution. In 1998, the International Prognostic Scoring System (IPSS) was developed by an inter-national working group to better predict clinical outcomes in MDS. The IPSS divides patients with MDS into three prognostic categories based on cytogenetic abnormalities, cytopenias, advanced age, and percentage of bone marrow blasts and provides median survival and time to leukemia transformation for each IPSS stage (Table 47-6). Based on criticism that the IPSS relies only on characteristics of patients at disease onset and includes cases now considered to be AML by the World Health Organization (WHO) criteria, a new WHO classification–based prognostic scoring system (WPSS) was devised emphasizing WHO morphology, karyotype, and transfusion dependence at any time during MDS disease course. Division of MDS patients into five new risk categories was validated to predict for overall survival and leukemic evolution for MDS at any follow up time (Table 47-7).

Treatment

New insights into the pathophysiology of ineffective hematopoiesis characterizing MDS has led to a number of therapeutic options for this disease, allowing for individualized therapy based on patient preference, performance status, disease biology, and prognostic risk category.

Supportive Therapy

Most patients with MDS are elderly individuals who may not tolerate or desire aggressive intervention without hope of cure. Many who are considered low risk for disease transformation are either transfusion independent or are managed supportively with chronic red blood cell and platelet transfusions to maintain quality of life. One complication of chronic transfusion therapy is iron overload caused by the delivery of between 200 and 250 mg of iron with each unit of transfused red blood cells. Excess iron is stored in macrophages and eventually accumulates in the hepatic parenchyma, myocardium, skin, and the pancreas, leading to secondary hemochromatosis or transfusional iron overload. Clinical symptoms include liver dysfunction, heart failure, hyperpigmentation, or diabetes mellitus. To prevent these, patients who develop marked elevations in transferrin saturation or serum ferritin levels should undergo iron chelation therapy with deferoxamine or an oral agent (deferiprone). Chronic administration of recombinant EPO has also been shown to reduce transfusion needs in some MDS patients, particularly those with low endogenous serum EPO levels and few transfusion requirements. Individuals with recurrent or refractory neutropenic infections also often receive G-CSF and GM-CSF treatment alone or in addition to EPO and antibiotic regimens. All these treatments are supportive in nature and do not affect overall survival.

Intensive Therapy

Patients with high-risk MDS (defined as MDS with cytogenetic abnormalities predisposing to leukemia transformation or high levels of circulating blasts with IPSS scores of Int-2 or higher, see Table 47-7) are candidates for aggressive AML-based chemotherapy (see Chapter 48). These standard regimens are designed to eradicate rapidly proliferating blast cells, not dysfunctional MDS cells, and therefore unsurprisingly are associated with a high relapse rate (within 12 to 18 months) and no significant prolongation of overall survival, even in patients who achieve remission. As in other

Table 47-6 International Prognostic Scoring System (IPSS) for Myelodysplastic Disorders

Score	Blasts	Karyotype	Cytopenias*	Overall Score	Median Survival (yr)
0	<5%	Normal, Y–, 5q–, 20q–	0-1 cytopenias	0	5.7
0.5	5%-10%	All other abnormalities	2-3 cytopenias	0.5-1.0	3.5
1.0		Abnormal 7, >3 abnormalities		1.5-2.0	1.2
1.5	11%-20%			2.5 or higher	0.4
2.0	21%-30%				

*Cytopenias are defined as hemoglobin < 10q/dL; neutrophils < 1500/µL; platelets < 100,000/µL.

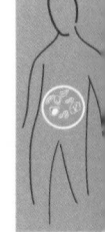

Table 47-7 World Health Organization (WHO) Classification-Based Prognostic Scoring System (WPSS) for Myelodysplastic Disorders

Variable	0	1	2	3
WHO category	RA, RARS, 5q–	RCMD, RCMD-RS	RAEB-1	RAEB-2
Karyotype*	Good	Intermediate	Poor	—
Transfusion requirement†	No	Regular	—	—

Note: Risk groups were as follows: very low (score = 0), low (score = 1), intermediate (score = 2), high (score = 3 to 4), and very high (score = 5 to 6).

MDS, myelodysplastic syndrome; RA, refractory anemia; RARS, refractory anemia with ringed sideroblasts; RCMD, refractory cytopenia with multilineage dysplasia; RCMD-RS, refractory cytopenia with multilineage dysplasia and ringed sideroblasts; RAEB-1, refractory anemia with excess of blasts—1; RAEB-2, refractory anemia with excess of blasts—2; 5q–, myelodysplastic syndrome with isolated del(5q) and marrow blasts less than 5%.

*Karyotype was as follows: good: normal, –Y, del (5q), del (20q); poor: complex (≥3 abnormalities), chromosome 7 anomalies; and intermediate: other abnormalities.

†Red blood cell (RBC) transfusion dependency was defined as having at least one RBC transfusion every 8 weeks over a period of 4 months.

hematologic stem cell disorders, the only curative therapy is allogeneic stem cell transplantation, ideally performed at complete remission. AML-based chemotherapy may be offered to such patients before transplantation. All patients younger than 40 years with MDS and a HLA-matched sibling donor should be offered transplantation at diagnosis. Long-term disease-free survival rates for such patients with low-risk disease are more than 50%. The high transplant-related mortality, morbidity, and relapse rates associated with mismatched or unrelated donor transplants or with transplantation in older MDS patients have led these types of transplantation to be held in reserve until development of high-risk disease.

Targeted Therapeutic Agents

Although not curative, a panoply of novel therapeutic agents targeting the unique biologic features of MDS have been shown to improve outcomes for many MDS patients ineligible for or unwilling to pursue stem cell transplantation or supportive care. These agents, administered largely in the outpatient setting, have induced disease remissions, retarded leukemia evolution, and for the first time, prolonged overall survival of MDS patients.

The recognition that epigenetic modifications of the abnormal HSC clones in MDS affect cell growth and apoptosis and are central to disease pathogenesis led to the clinical application of two DNA methyltransferase inhibitors (5-azacytidine and decitabine) to the treatment of the disease. These agents are hypothesized to reverse the abnormal hypermethylation and gene silencing in abnormal HSC. 5-Azacytidine has been shown to delay time to leukemia transformation in two thirds of patients with transfusion-dependent MDS, decrease transfusion requirements, and improve quality of life compared with transfusion support

alone. A phase III clinical trial comparing 5-azacytidine with conventional care regimens for higher-risk MDS patients showed a superior overall survival advantage favoring 5-azacytidine treatment. These results are the first to demonstrate that any therapy can alter the natural history of this disease and renders 5-azacytidine the new standard of care for transfusion-dependent MDS patients. Decitabine is a related compound to 5-azacytidine and represents an alternative treatment option for patients with high-risk MDS. Decitabine therapy has been shown to induce remission and reduce transfusion needs in MDS patients compared with supportive care and historical controls; however, the survival benefit of decitabine use in MDS has yet to be demonstrated. One unique feature of DNA methyltransferase inhibitor therapy with either hypomethylating agent is the observation that most therapeutic responses occur 4 to 6 months after treatment initiation. Moreover, MDS patients treated with 5-azacytidine who did not achieve a defined complete remission in the marrow nevertheless still survived significantly longer than patients treated with supportive care alone. These data suggest that, in contrast to AML, the best treatment for MDS is not cytotoxic-mediated eradication of abnormal HSC clones but chronic (epigenetic) modification of cells resulting in restoration of normal hematopoiesis. It remains to be seen whether achievement of remission after hypomethylation modulation in MDS equates with long-term disease control.

Certain MDS disease subgroups appear to have hematopoietic failure mediated at least in part by autoimmune cells selectively targeting the destruction of normal HSC. These disease subsets exhibit significant overlap with AA and PNH (described earlier in this chapter). For instance, a proportion of young patients with low-risk MDS disease and a HLA-DR15 haplotype have demonstrated a 30% to 50%

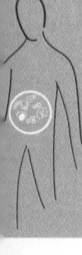

improvement in counts after T-cell immunosuppressive therapy with ATG or cyclosporine. MDS patients with isolated trisomy 8 or the demonstrated presence of PNH clones, or both, have also been reported to respond to treatment with immunosuppressive agents.

Some patients with MDS characterized by deletions in the long arm of chromosome 5 (5q– aberration) have a disease that is extraordinarily sensitive to therapy with lenalidomide, an immunomodulatory agent shown to exert antigrowth effects on MDS cells and the MDS marrow microenvironment. Complete and durable responses occur in up to 66% of 5q– syndrome MDS patients after lenalidomide therapy and are accompanied by disappearance of the abnormal cytogenetic clone in the marrow in some patients.

Defects in ribosomal protein function, specifically the ribosomal subunit protein RPS-14, have been identified as the etiology of 5q– syndrome MDS, paralleling findings implicating a different ribosomal subunit (RPS-19) in the congenital bone marrow syndrome Diamond-Blackfan anemia. This suggests a common link between these diseases. How lenalidomide works to correct hematologic abnormalities in 5q– MDS patients remains an area of active investigation. Lenalidomide also induces responses in up to one third of non-5q– MDS patients demonstrating a specific defect in erythroid differentiation on gene expression profiling. Whether unique gene signatures or other biologic markers in MDS patients can be used to further tailor therapy for MDS patients remains to be seen.

Prospectus for the Future

The field of stem cell biology is rapidly changing. The study of hematopoietic stem cell function in marrow failure syndromes provides hints of specific molecular pathways disturbed in many diseases of hematopoietic and nonhematopoietic stem cells. These observations are also furthering our understanding of the complex interplay among AA, PNH, and MDS. Understanding of stem cell plasticity and the stem cell niche in regulating disease may open promising new avenues for therapies of a wide array of disease. Umbilical cord blood stem cells represent a potential source of donor cells for allogeneic stem cell transplantation in patients with primary hematologic diseases lacking other HLA-matched marrow donors. Nonmyeloablative stem cell transplantations (mini-transplants) employing low-dose conditioning and immunosuppressive regimens represent another emerging treatment option for older patients with primary marrow failure syndromes. Thrombopoietin agonists that effectively stimulate platelet production in chronic immune thrombocytopenic states are likely to play an increasing role in the treatment of primary marrow failure syndromes. Novel agents targeting the unique biologic features of ineffective hematopoiesis in marrow failure syndromes have improved outcomes for many patients over the past few years: eculizumab in PNH; 5-azacytidine in transfusion-dependent MDS; immunosuppressive drugs in AA and MDS subsets; lenalidomide in 5q– MDS. The finding that therapeutic responses to lenalidomide in patients with MDS lacking 5q– can be predicted by the presence of a specific erythroid differentiation gene signature strongly suggests that future research may result in delineation of additional unique biologic pathways to further tailor therapeutic options for this disease.

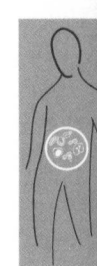

Clonal Disorders of the Hematopoietic Stem Cell

Eunice S. Wang and Nancy Berliner

Malignant transformation involves combined defects in cellular maturation and differentiation. The multistep theory of oncogenesis suggests that these defects are often separable and may contribute to a stepwise progression from a normal to a fully transformed cell. The continuous cycling of hematopoietic cells provides a milieu for the development of clonal genetic abnormalities that support this model. Clonal defects of the hematopoietic stem cell give rise to an array of preleukemic and leukemic disorders. Primary defects of maturation give rise to the *myelodysplastic disorders* (discussed in Chapter 47), whereas loss of normal control of proliferation results in *myeloproliferative disease*. All of these disorders are preleukemic, with a variable but definite rate of transformation to acute leukemia.

Myeloproliferative Neoplasms

ETIOLOGY AND PATHOGENESIS

Myeloproliferative neoplasms (MPNs), also known as chronic myeloproliferative diseases (MPDs), are clonal stem cell disorders characterized by leukocytosis, thrombocytosis, erythrocytosis, splenomegaly, and bone marrow hypercellularity. The hallmark of MPN is the failure of a transformed multipotent stem cell to respond to normal feedback mechanisms regulating hematopoietic cell mass. Stem cells from patients with MPN demonstrate clonal colony growth in vitro when these cells are grown in the presence of serum without the addition of exogenous cytokines, and this technique has been used as a diagnostic test for MPN. MPNs have traditionally been divided into four classic disorders based on the predominant hyperproliferative cell type: polycythemia vera (PV), essential thrombocytosis (ET), primary myelofibrosis (PMF; also known as idiopathic myelofibrosis or agnogenic myeloid metaplasia), and chronic myelogenous leukemia (CML). Hypereosinophilic syndrome (HES),

mast cell disease, and other less common diseases are also included (Table 48-1).

Complications of MPN arise from the overproduction of one or more lineages in the blood. All can be associated with clonal evolution and blastic transformation to acute leukemia (**Web Fig. 48-1**), although, with the exception of CML, this is an infrequent and late complication. In most patients with MPN, the pathogenesis of disease is now attributed to dysfunctional kinases. In CML, a reciprocal translocation between chromosomes 9 and 22 (termed the *Philadelphia chromosome*) results in a breakpoint cluster region—the Abelson leukemia *(bcr-abl)* fusion protein with constitutive kinase activity. In PV, PMF, and ET, a mutation involving the substitution of a valine for phenylalanine at position 617 (V617F) in the Janus kinase 2 (JAK2) has been identified in most patients and may account for the abnormal growth properties that characterize these stem cell disorders. Identification of somatic JAK2 mutations in all MPNs has led to the clinical development and testing of orally bioavailable small molecule inhibitors that selectively target JAK2 for treatment of MPN. Results from these trials are eagerly awaited.

Polycythemia Vera

ETIOLOGY AND PATHOGENESIS

PV, literally meaning *increased red blood cells in the blood*, is a syndrome of increased red blood cell mass in the peripheral blood resulting from a clonal multipotent hematopoietic stem cell defect. When patients are first diagnosed with an elevated hemoglobin per unit volume *(erythrocytosis)*, initial evaluation should focus on whether this increase reflects an enhanced red cell mass (i.e., *absolute erythrocytosis or polycythemia*) or a normal red cell mass in the presence of a decreased plasma volume (i.e., *relative erythrocytosis* caused by dehydration or other causes). The latter condition is not true polycythemia (Table 48-2). Polycythemia or absolute erythrocytosis is defined as *an absolute increase in red cell*

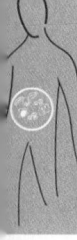

Table 48-1 World Health Organization 2008 Classification Scheme for Myeloid Neoplasms

1. Acute myeloid leukemia
2. Myelodysplastic syndrome (MDS)
3. Myeloproliferative neoplasms (MPNs)
   a. Chronic myelogenous leukemia
   b. Polycythemia vera
   c. Essential thrombocythemia
   d. Primary myelofibrosis
   e. Chronic neutrophilic leukemia
   f. Chronic eosinophilic leukemia, not otherwise categorized
   g. Hypereosinophilic syndrome
   h. Mast cell disease
   i. MPNs, unclassifiable
4. MDS, MPD
5. Myeloid neoplasms associated with eosinophilia and abnormalities of PDGF-RA, PDGF-RB, or FGF-R1

FGF-R1, fibroblast growth factor receptor-1; PDGF-RA, platelet-derived growth factor receptor alpha polypeptide; PDGF-RB, platelet-derived growth factor receptor beta polypeptide.

Table 48-2 Causes of Erythrocytosis

I. Relative or spurious erythrocytosis (normal red cell mass)
   A. Hemoconcentration secondary to dehydration (diarrhea, diaphoresis, diuretics, water deprivation, emesis, ethanol, hypertension, preeclampsia, pheochromocytoma, carbon monoxide intoxication)
II. True or absolute erythrocytosis
   A. Polycythemia vera
   B. Primary congenital polycythemia
   C. Secondary erythrocytosis caused by:
      1. Congenital causes (e.g., activating mutation of erythropoietin receptor)
      2. Hypoxia caused by carbon monoxide poisoning, high oxygen affinity hemoglobin, high-altitude residence, chronic pulmonary disease, hypoventilation syndromes such as sleep apnea, right to left cardiac shunt, neurologic defects involving the respiratory center
      3. Nonhypoxic causes with pathologic erythropoietin production
         a. Renal disease (cysts, hydronephrosis, renal artery stenosis, focal glomerulonephritis, renal transplantation)
         b. Tumors (renal cell cancer, hepatocellular carcinoma, cerebellar hemangioblastoma, uterine fibromyoma, adrenal tumors, meningioma, pheochromocytoma)
      4. Drug-associated causes
         a. Androgen therapy
         b. Exogenous erythropoietin growth factor therapy

Adapted from Hoffman R, Benz EJ, Shattil SJ, et al (eds): Hematology: Basic Principles and Practice, 2nd ed. New York, Churchill Livingstone, 1995.

mass caused by increased red blood cell production. Under normal conditions, the body's ability to increase red blood cell production in states of hypoxemia, anemia, hemolysis, and acute blood loss ensures continuous oxygen delivery to tissues. In response to physiologic stimuli, pluripotent stem cell precursors are activated by erythropoietin (EPO) to differentiate into erythroid progenitor cells and eventually hemoglobin-carrying erythrocytes. When numbers of mature red blood cells are adequate, a negative feedback mechanism suppresses further EPO production, and the serum hemoglobin level remains normal.

PV is a primary clonal stem cell disorder of unknown origin that is characterized by predominant erythrocytosis associated with other hematopoietic abnormalities. Although one half of all patients have concurrent leukocytosis or thrombocytosis, erythrocytosis is the hallmark and the cause of the most serious clinical complications of this disease. Diagnosis of PV was formerly one of *exclusion* based on an elevated red cell mass, splenomegaly, thrombocytosis, leukocytosis, lack of hypoxemia and other secondary causes of polycythemia, and elevated levels of leukocyte alkaline phosphatase and serum vitamin B_{12}-binding protein levels. More recent information on the disease pathophysiology has led to new diagnostic criteria (Table 48-3) based on the discovery of JAK2 mutations in virtually all patients with PV. Identification of low serum EPO levels and EPO-independent erythroid colony growth are now regarded as the only secondary criteria helpful in establishing a primary PV diagnosis.

Table 48-3 World Health Organization 2008 Diagnostic Criteria for Polycythemia Vera

Major Criteria

1. Hemoglobin (Hgb) >18.5 g/dL (men), >16.5 (women); *or* Hgb or hematocrit (Hct) >99% reference range for age, sex, or altitude of residence; *or* Hgb >17 g/dL (men), >15 g/dL (women) if associated with a sustained increase of ≥ 2g/dL from baseline that cannot be attributed to correction of iron deficiency; *or* elevated red cell mass (>25% above mean normal predicted value)
2. Presence of JAK2 V617F or similar mutation

Minor Criteria

1. Bone marrow trilineage myeloproliferation
2. Subnormal serum erythropoietin level
3. Endogenous erythroid colony formation in vitro

Either both major criteria and one minor criterion *or* the first major criterion and two minor criteria must be met for diagnosis of polycythemia vera.

CLINICAL FEATURES AND LABORATORY STUDIES

PV occurs in 1 to 3 of 100,000 people, with a median age at onset of 65 years. Early recognition and treatment of PV are important because untreated patients with PV suffer significant morbidity and mortality from thromboembolic disease in the cerebral, coronary, and mesenteric circulations.

Twenty percent of patients show symptoms of arterial and venous thrombosis, and thrombosis remains the most common cause of death. Typically, patients complain of headache, visual problems, mental clouding, and pruritus after bathing. Occlusive vascular events such as stroke, transient ischemic attacks, myocardial ischemia, and digital pain, paresthesias, or gangrene are common. In addition, pulmonary, deep vein, hepatic, and portal vein thromboses may occur. Paradoxically, patients are also predisposed to hemorrhagic events, which are presumably caused by abnormal platelet function, and such patients may exhibit gastrointestinal bleeding. Physical examination often shows retinal vein occlusion, ruddy cyanosis, and splenomegaly.

Peripheral blood often appears microcytic, with or without iron deficiency. Bone marrow examination shows a hypercellular marrow with pronounced hyperplasia of erythroid lineage cells (see **Web Fig. 48-2E**). Cytogenetic features at the time of diagnosis are usually normal; the development of clonal cytogenetic abnormalities heralds transformation in the later stages of disease. The incidence of the JAK2 V617F mutation in patients with PV ranges up to 97% in various studies.

TREATMENT

Without treatment, one half of all patients with PV die of thrombotic complications within 18 months of diagnosis. With therapy, PV is a chronic, progressive disease. The risk for transformation to myelofibrosis and myeloid leukemia is 5% to 20% over 20 years. Patients with advanced age, prior history of thrombosis, and high hematocrit values are at high risk for subsequent vascular events. Therefore, intermittent phlebotomy is the mainstay of treatment and usually results in iron deficiency anemia, which further reduces the rate of red blood cell production. Cytoreductive therapy is indicated for patients with intolerant or failing phlebotomy, with a prior history of or risk factors for thrombosis, or with symptomatic splenomegaly. Low-dose chemotherapeutic agents (such as chlorambucil, busulfan) and radioactive phosphorus (^{32}P) used in the past to treat leukocytosis and thrombocytosis have been associated with increased toxicity and risk for secondary AML. Current therapies include hydroxyurea (a low-dose cytotoxic agent that does not appear to increase leukemic risk), interferon-α (used in young patients and women during pregnancy), and anagrelide (a megakaryotoxic agent used for treating refractory thrombocytosis). Goals of therapy are hematocrit values less than 45% in men and less than 42% in women. As with all myeloproliferative disorders, initiation of cytoreductive therapy may precipitate hyperuricemia (resulting in secondary gout and uric acid stones), warranting treatment with allopurinol. Low-dose aspirin and treatment of asymptomatic thrombocytosis has been demonstrated to decrease thromboembolic events in patients with PV and is especially important in older patients with significant cardiac risk factors. In younger patients, nonsteroidal anti-inflammatory drugs and antiplatelet agents should be used judiciously because of the risk for gastrointestinal hemorrhage. With effective therapy, the long-term survival of these patients is excellent.

Essential Thrombocythemia

ETIOLOGY, PATHOGENESIS, AND LABORATORY STUDIES

ET (also known as *primary thrombocythemia*) is a pluripotent stem cell disorder resulting in elevated levels of platelets

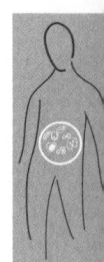

Table 48-4 **World Health Organization (2008) Diagnostic Criteria for Essential Thrombocythemia**
Major Criteria
1. Platelet count ≥ 450 × 10⁹/L
2. Megakaryocyte proliferation with large and mature morphology. No or little granulocytic or erythroid proliferation
3. Not meeting WHO criteria for CML, PV, PMF, MDS or other myeloid neoplasm
4. Demonstration of JAK2 V617F or other clonal marker or no evidence of reactive thrombocytosis
Diagnosis of essential thrombocytopenia requires meeting all four major criteria.
CML, chronic myelogenous leukemia; MDS, myelodysplastic syndrome; PMF, primary myelofibrosis; PV, polycythemia vera; WHO, World Health Organization.

and white blood cells. Platelet function and length of survival remain normal. Because elevated platelet counts (termed *thrombocytosis*) can occur secondary to other underlying causes (including bacterial infections, sepsis, iron deficiency, autoimmune diseases, and other malignant diseases), these other causes must be excluded before a diagnosis of ET is considered. In general, diagnosis requires a platelet count exceeding 450,000 × 10⁹/L with JAK2 mutation or no evidence of reactive thrombocytosis. In addition, bone marrow histology displays predominant proliferation involving the megakaryocytic lineage with increased mature megakaryocytes and little, if any, granulocytic or erythroid proliferation. Marrow immunohistochemical and cytogenetic studies to exclude diagnoses of myelodysplasia, myelofibrosis, or the Philadelphia chromosome diagnostic of CML are essential (Table 48-4). Although no genetic or biologic marker that is 100% specific for ET has been found, the presence of the JAK2 V617F mutation is found in more than one half of samples of patients with ET. Unlike other MPNs, bone marrow cells from patients with ET frequently do not show factor-independent colony growth, and the precise cause of this disease (and relationship with JAK2 mutational status) is under intense investigation.

CLINICAL FEATURES

ET is an uncommon disorder with an increasing number of cases found in patients who are asymptomatic on routine laboratory testing. Although the median age at onset is 60 to 65 years, 10% to 25% of patients are younger than 40 years of age. Up to two thirds of patients are symptomatic. Vasomotor symptoms include headache, dizziness, visual changes, and *erythromelalgia* (burning pain and erythema of feet and hands). Serious arterial thrombotic complications such as transient ischemic attacks, strokes, seizures, angina, and myocardial infarcts may occur. Patients may rarely have purpuric skin lesions or hematomas. The risk for gastrointestinal bleeding is less than 5%.

TREATMENT

In general, patients with this disorder have long-term survival rates similar to those of age-matched control patients.

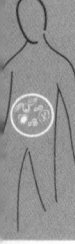

The risk for leukemic transformation is extremely low (3% to 4%) in comparison with other MPNs. However, morbidity from recurrent hemorrhagic and thrombotic complications is high and cannot be reliably predicted from the platelet count or platelet function abnormalities. Because treatment requires lifelong administration for disease control, assessment of risk factors and prior history of clinical signs and symptoms dictate therapeutic choices. All patients benefit from aggressive management of cardiovascular risk factors (such as smoking, hypertension, obesity, and hypercholesterolemia). Low-dose enteric aspirin may be used in all patients to relieve neurologic symptoms and carries a minimal risk for bleeding. Although young and pregnant patients are often not treated until they become symptomatic, older patients (>60 years) and those with a prior history of thrombosis or long disease duration may benefit from the addition of platelet-lowering agents. Hydroxyurea, a nonspecific myelosuppressive agent, is the most common first-line agent and is generally well tolerated with low long-term leukemogenic risks. Anagrelide (an oral antiplatelet agent that inhibits platelet aggregation and megakaryocyte maturation) is also used, primarily as a second-line agent after hydroxyurea failure resulting from associated acute side effects (fluid retention, palpitations), hemorrhage (with concomitant aspirin use), and risk for myelofibrosis transformation. Both of these agents are known teratogens and therefore cannot be used in the significant fraction of patients with ET who are young women of childbearing age. Because patients with ET have a high incidence of fetal wastage, interferon-α (a cytokine that alters the biologic mechanisms of the malignant clone but does not cross the placenta), in addition to heparin or aspirin, has been recommended to improve pregnancy outcomes in these patients.

Primary Myelofibrosis

ETIOLOGY, PATHOGENESIS, AND LABORATORY STUDIES

PMF (also known as *idiopathic myelofibrosis* or *agnogenic myeloid metaplasia*) is a clonal stem cell disorder characterized by abnormal excessive marrow fibrosis leading to marrow failure. An abnormal myeloid precursor is believed to give rise to dysplastic megakaryocytes that produce increased levels of fibroblast growth factors. These cytokines act on normal fibroblasts and other stromal cells, a process that stimulates excessive proliferation and collagen deposition. Over time, increasing fibrosis of the bone marrow leads to premature release of multipotent hematopoietic precursors into the periphery. These cells then migrate and reestablish themselves in other sites, thereby shifting hematopoiesis out of the bone marrow and into other tissues, especially the spleen and liver. This process is termed *extramedullary hematopoiesis*.

Early in the disease, patients may be asymptomatic with incidental findings of abnormal blood counts on routine laboratory tests. Although low blood counts may be present, overall platelet and red blood cell numbers at onset may be increased or normal depending on the degree of compensatory extramedullary hematopoiesis. Review of the peripheral

Table 48-5 Causes of Bone Marrow Fibrosis

I. Neoplastic causes
  a. Chronic myeloproliferative disorders: chronic idiopathic myelofibrosis, chronic myelogenous leukemia, polycythemia vera
  b. Acute megakaryoblastic leukemia (FAB-M₇)
  c. Myelodysplasia with myelofibrosis
  d. Hairy cell leukemia
  e. Acute lymphoblastic leukemia
  f. Multiple myeloma
  g. Metastatic carcinoma
  h. Systemic mastocytosis
II. Non-neoplastic causes
  a. Granulomatous diseases: mycobacterial infections, fungal infections, sarcoidosis
  b. Paget disease of bone
  c. Hypoparathyroidism or hyperparathyroidism
  d. Renal osteodystrophy
  e. Osteoporosis
  f. Vitamin D deficiency
  g. Autoimmune diseases: systemic lupus erythematosus, systemic sclerosis

FAB-M₇, French-American-British acute myeloid leukemia classification subtype 7.

Table 48-6 World Health Organization 2008 Diagnostic Criteria for Primary Myelofibrosis

Major Criteria

1. Megakaryocyte proliferation and atypia accompanied by reticulin and/or collagen fibrosis; *or* in the absence of reticulin fibrosis, the megakaryocytic changes must be accompanied by increased marrow cellularity, granulocytic proliferation, and often decreased erythropoiesis (i.e., prefibrotic primary myelofibrosis)
2. Not meeting World Health Organization criteria for chronic myelogenous leukemia, polycythemia vera, myelodysplastic syndrome, or other myeloid neoplasm
3. Demonstration of JAK2 V617F or other clonal marker or no evidence of reactive marrow fibrosis

Minor Criteria

1. Leukoerythroblastosis
2. Increased serum lactate dehydrogenase level
3. Anemia
4. Palpable splenomegaly

Diagnosis of primary myelofibrosis requires meeting all three major criteria and two minor criterion.

blood will commonly reveal leukoerythroblastic changes characterized by teardrop-shape erythrocytes, giant platelets, and nonleukemic immature myeloid, erythroid, and leukocyte cells. Diagnosis of PMF is made by demonstration of bone marrow fibrosis with markedly increased reticulin or collagen fibers (see **Web Fig. 48-1**) or increased marrow cellularity. Other underlying causes of bone marrow fibrosis, both neoplastic and non-neoplastic (Table 48-5), should be ruled out. Testing for JAK2 or other clonal markers should also be performed (Table 48-6).

CLINICAL FEATURES

PMF is a rare chronic disease, usually seen in elderly persons, with an annual incidence of 0.5 cases per 100,000. Although

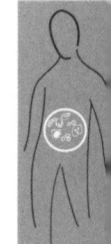

many patients are asymptomatic at diagnosis, most will complain over time of progressive fatigue and dyspnea related to anemia or early satiety and left upper quadrant pain associated with splenomegaly and splenic infarction. More than one half of these patients develop massive hepatosplenomegaly. In more advanced disease, patients may have constitutional symptoms such as fever, weight loss, and night sweats. As bone marrow failure evolves, complications of neutropenia and thrombocytopenia develop. Bleeding from occult disseminated intravascular coagulation is a risk. Extramedullary hematopoiesis in the peritoneal and pleural cavities, as well as in the central nervous system (CNS) and spinal cord, may also cause symptoms.

TREATMENT

Median survival in PMF is poor, ranging from 2 to 5 years. The most commonly accepted adverse prognostic factors at onset include hemoglobin less than 10g/dL, leukocyte count less than 4000/mcL or more than 30,000/mcL, a high percentage of circulating blasts, and the presence of constitutional symptoms. Other clinical factors of note are age greater than 60 years, thrombocytopenia, massive hepatosplenomegaly, and cytogenetic abnormalities. Over time, the disease may progress from a chronic phase to an accelerated phase, with acute leukemic transformation in 8% to 10% of patients. Treatment of PMF-related AML is usually ineffective. Other causes of nonleukemic death include heart failure, infection, intracranial hemorrhage, and pulmonary embolism.

At present, no medical therapy has been shown to prolong overall survival or retard disease progression significantly in PMF. Young patients with HLA-matched sibling donors may be considered for potentially curative experimental allogeneic stem cell transplantation (SCT) at academic medical centers. All patients with symptomatic anemia benefit from palliative transfusions and administration of recombinant erythropoietin, androgens (danazol), or low-dose thalidomide to maintain red blood cell levels. Symptoms caused by excess thrombocytosis and leukocytosis or progressive extramedullary hematopoiesis may be managed with hydroxyurea (as a first-line agent), interferon-α (in younger patients), or low-dose chemotherapeutic agents such as busulfan, interferon-α, or melphalan (with long-term leukemogenic potential). Splenectomy is offered to patients with symptomatic splenomegaly, refractory thrombocytopenia, hypermetabolic symptoms, and portal hypertension but may be associated with significant operative morbidity and mortality. Patients who are not surgical candidates may benefit from palliative splenic irradiation or from new biologic agents under development that target the abnormal marrow microenvironment.

Chronic Myelogenous Leukemia

ETIOLOGY AND PATHOGENESIS

CML is characterized by a predominant increase in the granulocytic cell line associated with concurrent erythroid and platelet hyperplasia. It is unique among the MPN in its characteristic natural history, including an inevitable transformation to acute leukemia. CML was the first hematologic malignant disease shown to be associated with a specific chromosomal abnormality. More than 95% of patients with CML have a clonal expansion of a stem cell that has acquired the Philadelphia chromosome, a balanced translocation between chromosomes 9 and 22 designated t(9;22)(q34;q11). This translocation fuses the *abl* virus gene on chromosome 9 to the *bcr* gene on chromosome 22 and generates a novel *bcr-abl* oncogene. The gene product, the *bcr-abl* protein, is a constitutively active cytoplasmic tyrosine kinase that has been found to induce leukemia in hematopoietic stem cells. The expression of the *bcr-abl* fusion protein activates multiple downstream signal transduction pathways to permit proliferation independent of cytokine and stromal regulation and render cells resistant to chemotherapy and normal programmed cell death *(apoptosis)*. A subset of patients with CML but lacking a detectable Philadelphia chromosome have subsequently been found to possess detectable *bcr-abl* fusion products by reverse transcriptase–polymerase chain reaction (RT-PCR), indicating a subchromosomal translocation resulting in the same pathologic gene product. The diagnosis of CML is made by detection of the Philadelphia chromosome using karyotype, PCR, or fluorescent in situ hybridization (FISH) analysis. Identification of the Philadelphia chromosome has allowed for easier diagnosis and monitoring of disease. Exquisitely sensitive and quantitative RT-PCR procedures not only allow for detection of up to a single *bcr-abl*-positive cell in 10^5 to 10^6 peripheral cells but also permit measurement of disease status in both peripheral blood and marrow samples. Responses to treatment regimes in CML are now defined as hematologic (restoration of normal peripheral blood cell counts), cytogenetic (loss of the Philadelphia chromosome by normal karyotypic or FISH analysis), and molecular (log reduction of detectable *bcr-abl* transcripts below a standard baseline by RT-PCR) remissions.

CLINICAL FEATURES

CML is the most common MPN, accounting for 15% to 20% of all leukemias and occurring in 1 of 100,000 people. The median age of onset is 53 years, but patients of any age may be affected. Up to 40% of patients are initially asymptomatic. Other patients exhibit fatigue, lethargy, shortness of breath, weight loss, easy bruising, and early satiety. Physical examination usually shows splenomegaly.

The natural history of CML is characterized by a *chronic phase* that evolves into an acute blast crisis. Patients are typically diagnosed during the chronic phase, an indolent stage lasting 3 to 5 years. Peripheral white blood cell counts are elevated with eosinophilia and basophilia (>20%) but few blasts (<5%). With control of peripheral blood cell counts, patients are essentially asymptomatic during this period. Eventually, the disease enters an *accelerated phase* characterized by fever, weight loss, worsening splenomegaly, and bone pain related to rapid marrow cell turnover. Despite therapy, the white blood cell count rises with increased numbers of circulating blasts (between 10% and 19%). The presence of increased peripheral blood basophils (>20%) results in histamine production, with symptoms of pruritus, diarrhea, and flushing. During accelerated phase, patients may also develop increasing splenomegaly, persistent thrombocytopenia, or thrombocytosis and leukocytosis, with new clonal cytogenetic abnormalities in marrow cells. The last phase of CML, termed *blast crisis,* marks an evolution to acute leukemia, in which marrow is replaced by 20% or more blasts, with accompanying loss of normal mature cellular elements in the marrow and periphery and extramedullary blast proliferation. Death occurs in a few weeks to months. Two thirds of patients develop AML, whereas the rest develop acute lymphoid leukemia, a finding confirming that the initial neoplastic cell is an early stem cell capable of multilineage differentiation.

LABORATORY STUDIES

Laboratory tests in CML patients typically demonstrate a markedly elevated white blood cell count (median, 170×10^9/L), with low leukocyte alkaline phosphatase levels, high uric acid and lactate dehydrogenase levels, and thrombocytosis. Review of the peripheral smear in chronic-phase CML demonstrates a full complement of myeloid cells in all stages of granulocytic development, including immature myeloblasts (usually numbering <5%), myelocytes, metamyelocytes, basophils, eosinophils, bands, and neutrophils. In contrast, the peripheral blood smear in reactive granulocytic hyperplastic states (termed *leukemoid reaction*) caused by acute infection or sepsis, consists predominantly of mature neutrophils and bands with few myelocytes, basophils, or eosinophils. The bone marrow in CML is densely hypercellular, with an overwhelming predominance of myeloid cells at all developmental stages and reticulin fibrosis (see **Web** 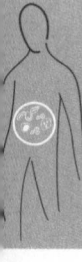 **Fig. 48-2**). Detection of the Philadelphia chromosome or abnormal *bcr-abl* transcripts by conventional or molecular testing will often confirm the diagnosis of CML.

TREATMENT

Historically, oral chemotherapeutic agents such as hydroxyurea and busulfan were used to reduce myeloid cell numbers in patients during the chronic phase of CML. Although these drugs decreased the rate of acute disease complications, they did not alter long-term prognosis or prevent progression to blast crises. Treatment with interferon results in hematologic remissions in 60% to 80% of patients with chronic-phase CML and was the first agent to induce cytogenetic responses in 20% to 30% of these patients. Achievement of cytogenetic remissions using interferon-α was associated with prolonged survival, with higher response rates obtained by combining chemotherapy with interferon. Although most patients treated with interferon still possessed cells with detectable *bcr-abl* translocation by PCR and remained at risk for disease relapse, many remained in hematologic and cytogenetic remission for several years. The mechanism by which the disease is controlled with interferon despite detectable *bcr-abl*–positive cells remains unknown. Unfortunately, patients with accelerated or blast crisis CML did poorly with interferon, and high-dose chemotherapy regimens in these patients induced only transient responses, with durations of less than 6 months.

The development of imatinib mesylate (Gleevec, formerly known as STI-571) for treatment of CML has been heralded as the first successful targeted therapy for cancer. Gleevec is a rationally designed competitive inhibitor of multiple tyrosine kinases, including *abl, bcr-abl,* platelet-derived growth factor receptor, and *c-kit.* Inhibition of phosphorylation of *bcr-abl* results in blockade of downstream signaling and growth pathways and induces apoptosis of *bcr-abl* positive cells. Preclinical studies demonstrated that Gleevec potently inhibited the growth of *bcr-abl*–expressing CML cell lines and progenitor cells in vitro and prolonged survival in animal tumor models. Initial early clinical trials of this orally active drug were begun in 1998 in CML patients who had failed interferon-α. Not only was the drug well tolerated with manageable side effects, but also 96% of patients receiving a dose greater than 300 mg per day for 4 weeks achieved hematologic remissions, with 33% obtaining cytogenetic remissions after 8 weeks. These striking results have been confirmed in multiple trials, and Gleevec was subsequently shown to be superior to interferon-α and cytarabine in untreated patients with newly diagnosed chronic-phase CML. At a median of 5 years' follow-up, initial therapy with Gleevec was shown to result in complete cytogenetic responses in 87% of chronic phase CML patients with an estimated overall survival of 89%. Only 7% of patients progressed to accelerated or blast-phase CML, and both response rates and adverse events from Gleevec treatment diminished over time of therapy. No patient achieving a complete cytogenetic response and molecular remission (defined as a three-log reduction in *bcr-abl* transcripts) after 12 to 18 months of Gleevec therapy was found to have disease progression after 5 years. Based on this study, Gleevec therapy is now the standard of care for treatment of chronic-phase CML.

Despite these results, this agent does not cure disease. Similar to those receiving interferon treatment, most of patients achieving CCR on Gleevec still demonstrate persistence of *bcr-abl*–positive leukemic CML stem cells by sensitive molecular testing. Therefore, lifelong Gleevec therapy is required to control disease, and even patients with excellent control of chronic-phase CML on Gleevec therapy remain at risk for eventual disease progression and therapy failure. Although Gleevec at high doses can induce transient hematologic and cytogenetic responses in patients with accelerated or blast-phase CML, these responses are short lived at best, and resistance to Gleevec in these advanced disease stages is well documented. In half of patients with clinical resistance to Gleevec, single nucleotide mutations in the *bcr-abl* gene result in conformational changes in the *bcr-abl* kinase, which alter the binding of drug and hence its inhibitory effects. Finally, a small percentage of patients with CML are unable to tolerate the side effects of Gleevec, primarily gastrointestinal in nature. To address these issues, newer *bcr-abl* kinase inhibitors have been developed, specifically dasatinib (Sprycel) and nilotinib (Tasigna) for treatment of Gleevec-resistant or intolerant CML patients. Both agents display increased potency against the *bcr-abl* kinase in vitro than Gleevec and have demonstrated activity in CML cells expressing the majority of known *bcr-abl* mutations. Early-phase clinical trials with single-agent dasatinib or nilotinib in previously treated imatinib-failure patients have consistently resulted in cytogenetic responses up to 40% of patients. However, the lack of clinical trials directly comparing both agents and the need to await long-term clinical outcome data

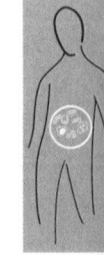

for either drug currently leave the choice of a second-line *bcr-abl* inhibitor to individual patients and practitioners. Toxicity profiles for both drugs are largely nonoverlapping with Gleevec.

Presently, the only treatment modality known to result in complete eradication of all detectable *bcr-abl*–expressing cells remains allogeneic SCT. Before the advent of targeted *bcr-abl* kinase inhibitor therapy, young patients with an HLA-matched donor were routinely offered potentially curative allogeneic bone marrow transplantation at the time of diagnosis of chronic-phase CML. Up to 50% to 75% of such patients achieved long-term survival following transplantation, with an improved outcome (for reasons that are not clear) in patients undergoing the procedure within 1 year of diagnosis. Evidence indicated that the excellent response of patients with CML to SCT is partly related to the active suppression of the disease by the newly transplanted graft, referred to as the *graft-versus-leukemia* (GVL) effect. However, the excellent control and low overall toxicity of long-term *bcr-abl* inhibitors for chronic-phase CML as compared with 20% to 30% mortality and morbidity rates following SCT has effectively rendered SCT a therapeutic option only for those chronic phase CML patients failing upfront Gleevec (e.g., blast crisis, intolerance). The only notable exception to this is individuals with CML disease expressing *bcr-abl* kinase mutations (such as T3151) known to be resistant to all *bcr-abl* inhibitor therapy. These patients should be identified early in the disease process for consideration for curative SCT versus treatment with upfront experimental options. Transplantation continues to remain the only curative therapeutic option for advanced-stage CML. Patients with accelerated-phase CML may be treated with high-dose Gleevec while awaiting allogeneic transplantation (if feasible) or experimental therapies, whereas those in blast-phase CML should undergo induction chemotherapy based on acute leukemia regimens followed by transplantation or clinical trials.

Overall, the transformation of CML, from a progressively fatal cancer to one in which almost 90% of patients are alive with stable disease on oral kinase therapy after 5 years, remains one of the crowning achievements in cancer therapy in the past decade. The median overall survival for CML patients has risen dramatically from a few months to a few years in the first half of the 20th century, to 6 years for interferon-treated patients, and has not yet been reached for *bcr-abl* inhibition therapy. Nevertheless, the search for a CML disease cure and for better treatment for those CML patients with disease refractory to Gleevec remains a therapeutic challenge for the years ahead.

Acute Leukemias

ETIOLOGY AND PATHOGENESIS

The *acute leukemias* are clonal hematopoietic malignant diseases that arise from the malignant transformation of an early hematopoietic stem cell. Leukemias occur in 8 to 10 of 100,000 people (in comparison with 42 of 100,000 for prostate cancer and 62 of 100,000 for breast cancer). Acute leukemias are classified by cell lineage into *acute myeloid/myelogenous leukemia* (AML) and *acute lymphoblastic/lymphocytic leukemia* (ALL) based on morphology, cytogenetics, cell surface and cytoplasmic markers, and molecular studies. Eighty to ninety percent of adult leukemia diagnoses are AML (with the rest being ALL), whereas most childhood leukemias are ALL (with 10% being AML).

The distinction between AML and ALL is crucial diagnostically, therapeutically, and prognostically. AML can be distinguished from ALL by cell morphology and by the presence of *Auer rods,* formed by the aggregation of myeloid granules (**Web Fig. 48-3**). Further immunophenotyping of blast cells using cell surface antigens, cytochemistry, and immunohistochemistry confirms cells as being of either myeloid or lymphoid origin (Table 48-7). Morphologic subgroups of both ALL and AML were originally defined by the French-American-British (FAB) group and, more recently, revised by the World Health Organization (WHO), incorporating newer biologic information (Table 48-8).

The pathogenesis of acute leukemia is under intense investigation. Many patients with acute leukemia have detectable characteristic clonal chromosomal abnormalities; however, the role of all but a few of these aberrations in malignant transformation is unknown. In general, unregulated proliferation of immature cells incapable of further differentiation (*blasts*) results in marrow replacement and hematopoietic failure. Known risk factors for leukemia are

Table 48-7 **Laboratory Aids to Distinguish between Acute Myeloblastic Leukemia and Acute Lymphoblastic Leukemia**		
	Acute Myeloblastic Leukemia (AML)	**Acute Lymphoblastic Leukemia (ALL)**
Morphology of blasts	Granules in cytoplasm Auer rods* Multiple nucleoli	Agranular basophilic cytoplasm Regular, folded nucleolus
FAB subclassification	L_1-L_3	M_1-M_7
Histochemistry	Myeloperoxidase positive	Myeloperoxidase negative, PAS positive
Cytoplasmic markers	—	Tdt positive
Surface markers (% of cases)	—	B-cell markers (5%) T-cell markers (15%-20%): CD2, CD3, or CD5 CALLA (50%-65%): CD10
Cytogenetic and oncogenetic	M_3: t(15;17) M_5: t(9;11)	L3: t(8;14) Abnormal ALL: Ph¹*bcr-abl*

*Auer rods are a linear coalescence of cytoplasmic granules that stain pink with Wright's stain.
CALLA, common acute lymphoblastic leukemia antigen; FAB, French-American-British classification system; PAS, periodic acid–Schiff stain.

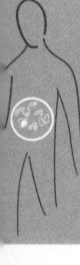

Table 48-8 French-American-British (FAB) and World Health Organization (WHO) Classifications of Acute Leukemia

FAB Classification of Acute Myeloid Leukemia (AML)

M_0—Acute myelocytic leukemia with minimal differentiation
M_1—Acute myelocytic leukemia without maturation
M_2—Acute myelocytic leukemia with maturation (predominantly myeloblasts and promyelocytes)
M_3—Acute promyelocytic leukemia
M_4—Acute myelomonocytic leukemia
M_5—Acute monocytic leukemia
M_6—Erythroleukemia
M_7—Megakaryocytic leukemia

FAB Classification of Acute Lymphoblastic Leukemia (ALL)

L_1—Predominantly *small* cells (twice the size of normal lymphocyte), homogeneous population; childhood variant
L_2—Larger than L_1, more heterogenous population; adult variant
L_3—*Burkitt-like* large cells, vacuolated abundant cytoplasm

WHO 2001 Classification of Acute Leukemia

I. Acute myeloid leukemia (AML)
   a. AML with recurrent genetic abnormalities
      AML with t(8;21)(q22;q22); (AML [CBF-α/ETO])
      AML with abnormal bone marrow eosinophils inv(16) (p13;q22) or t(16;16) (p13;q22); (CBF-α/*MYH-11*)
      Acute promyelocytic leukemia [AML with t(15;17) (q22;q12) (PML/RAR-α)] and variants
      AML with 11q23 (MLL) abnormalities
   b. AML with multilineage dysplasia
   c. AML and MDS, therapy related
      Alkylating agent related
      Topoisomerase II inhibitor related
   d. AML not otherwise defined
      AML minimally differentiated
      AML without maturation
      AML with maturation
      Acute myelomonocytic leukemia
      Acute monoblastic and monocytic leukemia
      Acute erythroid leukemia
      Acute megakaryoblastic leukemia
      Acute basophilic leukemia
      Acute panmyelosis with myelofibrosis
      Myeloid sarcoma
   e. Acute leukemia of ambiguous lineage
      Undifferentiated acute leukemia
      Bilineal acute leukemia
      Biphenotypic acute leukemia
II. Acute lymphocytic leukemia
   a. Precursor B-lymphoblastic leukemia/lymphoblastic lymphoma
   b. Precursor T-lymphoblastic leukemia/lymphoblastic lymphoma

CBF, core binding factor; ETO, "eight twenty-one"; MDS, primary myelodysplastic syndrome; MLL, mixed lineage leukemia; *MYH-11*, myosin heavy chain gene; PML, promyelocytic leukemia; RAR-α, retinoic acid α receptor.

high-dose radiation exposure and occupational exposure to benzene. Patients with secondary AML after exposure to prior chemotherapy have usually received alkylating agents (such as chlorambucil, melphalan, and nitrogen mustard) or topoisomerase II inhibitors (epipodophyllotoxins). An increased incidence of leukemia is also found in patients with chromosomal instability disorders such as Bloom syndrome, Fanconi anemia, Down syndrome, and ataxia telangiectasia.

CLINICAL FEATURES

Patients exhibit clinical evidence of bone marrow failure (similar to other hematopoietic disorders). Complications of disease include anemia, infection, and bleeding from peripheral cytopenias. In addition, proliferating blasts infiltrating the bone marrow may cause bone pain. Blasts also invade other organs and lead to peripheral, mediastinal, and abdominal lymphadenopathy, hepatosplenomegaly, skin infiltration, and meningeal involvement.

TREATMENT

Therapy of acute leukemias is divided into several stages. *Induction therapy* is directed at reducing the number of leukemic blasts to an undetectable level and restoring normal hematopoiesis (*complete remission*). At complete remission, however, significant subclinical disease persists, requiring further therapy. Subsequent *consolidation therapy* involves continuing chemotherapy with the same agents to induce elimination of further leukemic cells. With development of a wider range of effective agents, *intensification therapy* has been introduced, involving the use of high-dose therapy with different *non–cross-reactive* drugs, to eliminate cells with potential primary resistance to the induction regimen. *Maintenance therapy* employs low-dose intermittent chemotherapy given over a prolonged period to prevent subsequent disease relapse. The goal of therapy is to induce remission (defined as the presence of less than 5% blasts in the bone marrow and recovery of normal peripheral blood counts).

Adverse clinical prognostic factors for AML and ALL are similar despite widely different treatment approaches. In general, age exceeding 35 years, secondary or therapy-related disease, antecedent hematologic disorder, high initial leukocyte count, and prolonged time to achieve response to initial treatment are associated with poorer outcomes. Cytogenetic abnormalities represent the best independent predictor of overall survival in both acute leukemias (Tables 48-9 and 48-10).

Acute Myeloid Leukemia

CLINICAL FEATURES

AML represents a biologically heterogeneous group of neoplasms with widely divergent clinical outcomes. Long-term cure rates (defined as length of survival >5 years) range from 5% to 60% following chemotherapy alone, with an overall cure rate of 20% to 30%. AML occurs primarily in older adults, with a median age at diagnosis of 65 years. Patients most often present with complications related to progressively severe cytopenia, such as infection due to leukopenia, shortness of breath or fatigue due to anemia, or bleeding due to thrombocytopenia. AML patients may also exhibit unique acute clinical emergencies requiring immediate stabilization. *Leukostasis* (also called *hyperleukocytosis syndrome*) caused by high levels of circulating blasts (>80,000 to 100,000) leads to diffuse pulmonary infiltrates and acute respiratory distress. Blast cells may also injure surrounding vasculature, causing life-threatening CNS bleeding and thromboses. In addition, high blast cell numbers result in the release of cellular breakdown products (termed *tumor lysis syndrome*),

Table 48-9 Prognostic Factors in Acute Myeloid Leukemia

Clinical

Age >60 yr (median age for acute myeloid leukemia, 65 yr)
Therapy related or with antecedent hematologic disorder
(e.g., myelodysplastic syndrome, myeloproliferative
neoplasm, aplastic anemia)
Poor performance status
White blood cell count >20,000-30,000/mm³
Presence of extramedullary disease sites

Biologic

Karyotype: favorable, intermediate, poor (see below)
Immunophenotype: biphenotypic
Abnormal fms-like tyrosine kinase 3 caused by mutation or
internal tandem duplication
Multidrug resistance protein expression

Cytogenetic

Favorable
t(15;17)(q22;q12-21)
inv(16) or t(16;16) or del(16q)
t(8;21)(q22;q22)
Intermediate
Normal karyotype
Trisomy +8 only
t(9;11)(p22;q23)
Adverse
Complex (≥3 abnormalities)
Inv(3)(q21q26) or t(3;3)(q21;q26)
Deletion (5q– or 7q–), minus 5, minus 7
Translocations (6;9) or (9;22)
Abnormalities of 11q23 excluding t(9;11)

Table 48-10 Prognostic Factors in Acute Lymphoblastic Leukemia

Factor	Favorable	Unfavorable
Age	2-10 yr	<2 yr or >10 yr
White blood cell count at diagnosis	<30,000	>50,000
Phenotype	Precursor B	Precursor T
Chromosome number	Hyperdiploidy	Pseudo/hypodiploidy, near tetraploidy
Chromosome abnormality	t(12;21)	c-myc Alterations: t(8;14), t(2;8), t(8;22) mixed lineage leukemia alterations (11q23); Ph chromosome t(9;22)
Central nervous system disease at diagnosis	No	Yes
Sex	Women	Men
Ethnicity	Caucasian	African American, Hispanic
Time to remission	Short (7-14 days)	Prolonged time to remission or failure to achieve remission

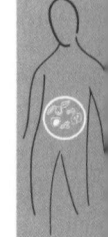

leading to hypokalemia, acidosis, and hyperuricemia with resultant renal failure. Treatment of leukostasis should be instituted as soon as possible in all patients with white blood cell counts in excess of 100 to 200 × 10⁹/L and consist of leukapheresis, hydroxyurea, and initiation of induction chemotherapy to inhibit further production of circulating tumor cells. Hydration, urine alkalinization to reduce urine crystallization, allopurinol, or rasburicase, or a combination, should be initiated as indicated. Red blood cell transfusions are often contraindicated in patients with high numbers of circulating blast cells because of the risk for further increases in blood viscosity. CNS complications such as intracranial bleeding, cranial nerve invasion, and leukemic meningitis are treated with emergency whole-brain irradiation or directed radiation to affected sites.

LABORATORY STUDIES

Laboratory evaluation of patients with AML typically shows white blood cell counts ranging from neutropenic levels (<1 × 10⁹/L) to extreme leukocytosis (>100,000 to 200,000 × 10⁹/L). Severe thrombocytopenia, normocytic anemia, and circulating peripheral blasts are common. Bone marrow aspirate and biopsy typically show a profusion of myeloblasts numbering 20% to 100% with depressed production of normal mature cells.

Diagnostic marrow aspirates are typically evaluated using morphology, flow cytometry, and routine cytogenetic-molecular analyses to (1) distinguish between AML and ALL, and (2) determine AML disease subsets. In the past, AML was divided based largely on morphologic criteria and immuno-

histochemical staining into FAB subtypes M₀ to M₇ defined by the stage of cellular differentiation of the abnormal cells (see Table 48-8 and **Web Fig. 48-3**). Some of these FAB subsets correlate with specific clinical syndromes that help determine treatment approaches as well as prognosis. The most common FAB subtype in adult AML is M₂. Patients with AML-M₃ (acute promyelocytic leukemia) often exhibit spontaneous bleeding from disseminated intravascular coagulation (see later). Patients with AML-M₄ or -M₅ disease (representing acute monocytic-myelomonocytic leukemias) have high levels of circulating white blood cells and may present with swollen gums resulting from tissue infiltration with leukemic blasts. Patients with megakaryoblastic leukemia (AML-M₇) have significant marrow fibrosis and usually exhibit organomegaly and pancytopenia similar to those seen in patients with myelofibrosis and myeloid metaplasia.

In 2001, AML was reclassified into new distinct subtypes defined by the presence of unique karyotypic abnormalities [specifically t(8;21), inv(16), and t(15;17)] in a dysplastic bone marrow, *independent of number of marrow blasts*. Because the presence of these specific cytogenetic abnormalities is crucial for diagnosis, therapy, and prognosis of AML patients, karyotypic analysis is now considered an essential part of any suspected AML diagnosis. In addition, any evidence of marrow dysplasia following prior chemotherapy, radiation, or other myeloablative therapy is now considered therapy-related AML (rather than MDS) independent of blast count (see Table 48-8).

TREATMENT

Chemotherapy for AML involves induction chemotherapy (administered in the inpatient setting) followed by multiple

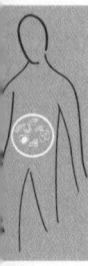

cycles (two to four) of consolidation chemotherapy administered over 4 to 6 months. Standard induction regimens employing cytosine arabinoside (cytarabine) with high-dose anthracycline (daunorubicin or idarubicin) lead to complete remission in 60% to 80% of younger adults with de novo AML. Lower remission rates are achieved in older adults (>65 years of age) and in those patients with antecedent hematologic diseases evolving into AML. After achieving complete remission after induction, patients may be offered additional consolidation chemotherapy versus allogeneic or autologous SCT (see Chapter 47). Patients whose AML fails to respond to initial induction therapy have a grim overall prognosis and may be retreated with experimental agents or non–cross-reactive chemotherapy drugs such as epipodophyllotoxins, or both, to obtain remission.

AML prognosis can be predicted to some degree based on patient age, disease presentation (specifically white blood cell count), or history of antecedent hematologic or therapy-related disease (see Table 48-9). However, diagnostic AML cytogenetics remains the most robust independent prognostic indicator of clinical outcome after standard AML therapy and often constitutes the most crucial determinant of an appropriate therapeutic strategy for individual patients. AML cytogenetics is divided into three categories: favorable, intermediate, and poor. AML characterized by t(8;21), inv(16) or del(16q), or t(8;21) aberrations are unusually responsive to induction chemotherapy followed by two to four cycles of high-dose cytosine arabinoside consolidation. Long-term 5-year survival rates of 55% to 60% can be obtained. AML subtypes associated with poor prognosis include those with known deletions in chromosome 5 or 7, 11q23 aberrations, inv(3q), t(3;3), t(6;9), t(9;22) (the Philadelphia chromosome), or the presence of three or more karyotypic abnormalities (termed *complex karyotype*). Remission rates in these AML disease subtypes are low; if remission is achieved, patients remain at high risk for AML relapse with chemotherapy-refractory disease. Overall survival rates for poor prognosis AML are 5% to 15%. The remaining AML patients have intermediate-risk cytogenetics [defined as normal karyotype, trisomy 8, t(9;11), or other cytogenetic abnormalities not included in the other groups]. These patients demonstrate a 30% to 45% long-term survival rate with standard chemotherapy. Cytogenetically normal AML constitutes 40% to 49% of all AML diagnoses. Recent data have revealed that up to one third of patients with normal karyotype AML have constitutive activation of the fms-like tyrosine kinase 3 (FLT-3) receptor as a result of point mutations or internal tandem duplications (not seen on routine karyotypic testing) in FLT-3 kinase. Presence of FLT-3 aberrations in AML predicts for poor remissions, high relapse rates, and shorter overall survival compared with FLT-3–negative AML patients. The development and clinical use of FLT-3 inhibitors for AML therapy has not resulted in the impressive results seen with Gleevec in CML; the presence of multiple signaling pathways in AML cells and rapid proliferation of AML clones leads to rapid development of drug resistance over a short period of time. Combination FLT-3 inhibition with chemotherapy for relapsed and newly diagnosed FLT-3–positive AML patients is under active investigation.

Given that the median age at presentation of AML is 65 years, a sizable proportion of AML patients are elderly individuals with major comorbidities or antecedent hematologic or malignant diseases rendering them poor candidates for induction chemotherapeutic regimens. Infectious complications remain the major cause of morbidity and mortality during intensive inpatient chemotherapy despite recent advances in prophylactic growth factor support, antibiotics, and antifungal agents. The low expected remission rates (30% to 50%) and high mortality and morbidity associated with induction are additional reasons for many patients to decline such therapy. For these patients, therapeutic options include supportive therapy with hydroxyurea, transfusion support alone, and hospice. Patients unfit for and those who choose not to receive intensive therapy have been treated with low-dose subcutaneous cytarabine with remission rates of up to 18%; alternatively, hypomethylating agents (5-azacytidine, decitabine) have been administered to AML and high-risk MDS patients with some responses.

Once remission is achieved after induction, AML patients are offered additional therapy in the form of consolidation chemotherapy, autologous, or allogeneic SCT. Decisions about the best time to perform bone marrow transplantation in patients are probably best guided by cytogenetic and clinical data (see Table 48-9). Clinical outcomes are improved when patients undergo bone marrow transplantation after initial induction chemotherapy (i.e., during the first complete remission) rather than after disease relapse for multiple reasons. However, chemotherapeutic regimens are also more effective in first remission than they are after transplantation, and the cure rate from transplantation performed during second remissions is still 25%. In general, patients with known poor prognostic AML are recommended to undergo early transplantation, whereas those with favorable disease features potentially responsive to high-dose cytarabine chemotherapy are encouraged to delay SCT until time of relapse. Allogeneic SCT represents the best chance for long-term cure for AML associated with complex or unfavorable cytogenetics, antecedent hematologic disease, or therapy-related or primary refractory disease. Cure rates following conventional chemotherapy in these patients range from 5% to 20%. In contrast, AML patients younger than 60 years undergoing allogeneic bone marrow transplantation from a matched donor are reported to have long-term overall survival rates up to 40% to 60%, with a procedure-related mortality rate of 10% to 25%. Intermediate to high-risk AML patients based on clinical or cytogenetic data who are ineligible for allogeneic transplantation because of advanced age or lack of compatible HLA donors may be offered autologous SCT instead. Whether autologous transplantation improves AML outcomes compared with chemotherapy alone is still under debate. However, the long-term survival rates after autologous transplantation range from 20% to 40% and are at least equivalent to consolidation chemotherapy regimens employing single-agent cytarabine therapy.

AML patients with relapsed or refractory disease after standard therapy should be considered for allogeneic SCT and therapy on experimental protocols. Older patients with relapsed CD33+ AML may be treated with gemtuzumab ozogamicin (Mylotarg) an anti-CD33 antibody chemically linked to a cytotoxic agent calicheamicin, which binds to CD33-expressing myeloid leukemia and normal hematopoietic cells and induces cell death. Unfortunately, complete remission rates after Mylotarg therapy are low (5% to 15%), and side effects include prolonged pancytopenia with risks for infectious complications and veno-occlusive liver disease due to CD33$^+$ liver parenchyma cells. Experimental therapies for AML, particularly nonmyeloablative (mini-transplants) SCT (see Chapter 47), have resulted in durable long-term remissions in a proportion of older AML patients and should be pursued based on patient preference, overall health status, and availability of an appropriate HLA-matched donor.

Acute Promyelocytic Leukemia

ETIOLOGY AND PATHOGENESIS

Acute promyelocytic leukemia (APL), formerly known as AML FAB-M3 (see Table 48-8), represents 10% to 15% of adult AML, with an increased incidence in younger patients (median age, 40 years). APL differs from other acute leukemias because of its unique disease biology. Morphologically, APL blasts are distinctive immature promyelocytic cells containing large granules and typically high numbers of Auer rods diagnostic for AML. APL cells possess a chromosomal translocation, t(15;17)(q22; q12), which results in a fusion protein composed of a nuclear transactivation protein (PML) on chromosome 15 with the retinoic acid α receptor on chromosome 17. Sequestration of the PML RAR-α fusion protein with other proteins results in a complex that represses transcription of genes essential for granulocytic differentiation, effectively resulting in differentiation arrest of leukemia cells at the promyelocytic stage.

CLINICAL FEATURES

Clinically, patients with APL often exhibit life-threatening bleeding caused by disseminated intravascular coagulation related to high procoagulant factor levels released from APL granules. Even today, bleeding complications in the CNS and other sites can be rapidly fatal if the disease is not recognized and treated as a medical emergency. All patients suspected of an APL diagnosis should be started empirically on ATRA (discussed later) therapy and treated aggressively with transfusions of fresh-frozen plasma, fibrinogen, and platelets until resolution of coagulopathy and disease confirmation.

TREATMENT

Treated appropriately, APL is the most curable acute leukemia in adults. The centerpiece of APL treatment is all-*trans*-retinoic acid (ATRA), a biologic agent shown to overcome growth arrest and permit differentiation of immature APL blast cells into neutrophils by altering the configuration of PML RAR-α to allow normal gene transcription. Although ATRA alone induces clinical remissions in up to 90% of patients, high relapse rates observed after monotherapy have led to the standard practice of combining ATRA with anthracycline chemotherapy in upfront induction regimens. Patients initiated on ATRA with or without chemotherapy must be closely observed for development of *retinoic acid* or

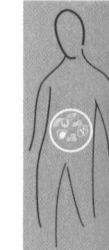

APL differentiation syndrome, life-threatening acute cardiopulmonary distress characterized by bilateral pulmonary effusions and infiltrates in the setting of high levels of circulating leukocytes with leukostasis. This serositis-like syndrome is attributed to adhesion of differentiating neoplastic cells to the pulmonary vasculature and carries a 5% to 10% mortality rate. Treatment consists of early initiation of corticosteroids and aggressive diuresis. In severe cases, ATRA should be temporarily held. Complete remission rates in APL are 90% to 95%, and more than two thirds of patients with APL treated with standard ATRA-containing induction, consolidation, and maintenance chemotherapy regimens achieve long-term remission. Relapsed APL patients can be treated with *arsenic trioxide*, a naturally occurring compound used as both a poison and a drug in many countries. Low-dose arsenic therapy promotes APL cell differentiation and apoptosis and induces remission rates in up to 90% of relapsed APL cases. Both APL differentiation syndrome and prolongation of the QT interval are common side effects of arsenic therapy. Arsenic has also been used for consolidation therapy in APL patients with improved clinical outcome. Patients achieving a second remission after arsenic therapy and those who have residual PML RAR-α–positive cells after standard induction and consolidation therapy should be considered for autologous or allogeneic SCT, or both. Mylotarg (anti-CD33 antibody-toxin) therapy has also been used for APL therapy with some success because most APL cells express CD33 antigens.

Acute Lymphoblastic Leukemia

ETIOLOGY AND PATHOGENESIS

ALL is a neoplasm of immature lymphoblasts expressing markers of B- or T-cell lineage. The prior FAB classification system divided ALL into three subtypes (L_1, L_2, and L_3) based on the morphology of malignant cells (see **Web Fig. 48-4**). More recently, the WHO system has reclassified the disease as either precursor B or T ALL, based on the lineage of specific cell surface antigens found on these cells during normal maturation (see Table 48-7). T ALL represents 15% to 25% of ALL diagnoses and is traditionally associated with superior clinical outcomes compared with B ALL. More than 50% of T ALL cases have activating mutations in Notch1, a key regulator of T-cell fate, and trials of inhibitors of the Notch pathway for treatment of relapsed disease are already underway.

CLINICAL FEATURES

ALL is predominantly a pediatric malignancy, with most cases occurring in children younger than 6 years of age. Progress in the understanding and treatment of this disease in the 1990s has led to cure rates of up to 80% in children with ALL but only 20% to 40% in adult patients with ALL. These poorer outcomes in adults are attributed to differences in the biologic mechanisms of disease in these different age groups as well as the inability of older patients to tolerate the intensive chemotherapy or transplantation procedures required to achieve long-term responses. Clinical and biologic features, particularly cytogenetics, at diagnosis have been identified as important prognostic factors (see Table 48-10). Of note, up to 50% of adult ALL (versus only 20% of pediatric ALL) cases are associated with presence of a Philadelphia chromosome abnormality, t(9; 22) (see earlier). Philadelphia chromosome expressing ALL is notoriously chemoresistant, with an increased risk for CNS involvement and overall 5-year survival rate of less than 10%.

TREATMENT

Treatment of ALL is lengthy and involves multiple chemotherapy agents given over a period of 2 to 3 years. Induction chemotherapy typically includes vincristine, corticosteroids, and L-asparaginase, with the addition of an anthracycline, cytarabine, or cyclophosphamide, or a combination, in adult patients. Given the propensity of ALL cells to reside in the CNS and testes (so-called sanctuaries for leukemia cells because standard systemic chemotherapy does not penetrate into these sites), most ALL patients undergo lumbar puncture at time of diagnosis, followed by routine administration of intrathecal methotrexate or whole-brain irradiation, or both, as a necessary adjunct to systemic induction and consolidation chemotherapy. Complete remission rates are 97% to 99% in children and 75% to 90% in adults. After normal hematopoiesis returns, patients then undergo consolidation and intensification therapy with multiple drugs to eradicate disease. For unknown reasons, ALL tends to relapse several months to years after initial remission. Studies have shown that the frequency of relapse is reduced by maintenance chemotherapy given for up to 2 to 3 years after initial remission achievement. Such prolonged treatment may eliminate slow-growing leukemic clones, prevent further transformation, or destroy occult disease in other (particularly CNS) sites. In addition to conventional chemotherapy, patients with Philadelphia chromosome–positive ALL also receive therapy with high-dose Gleevec, the oral *bcr-abl* tyrosine kinase inhibitor used in CML. High-risk patients with B ALL may benefit from anti-CD20 antibodies (rituximab) directed against B-cell antigens on abnormal lymphoblasts.

In ALL, as in AML, the worse the prognosis, the earlier transplantation should be offered. Studies have shown that high-risk ALL patients (defined as older patients, Philadelphia chromosome–positive disease, high presenting white blood cell count, or prolonged time to first remission) clearly benefit from SCT, preferably from an HLA-matched sibling, in first remission. Early transplantation in adults has achieved 5-year survival rates of 40% to 44%, in comparison with 20% with other therapies. Unfortunately, outcomes for high-risk ALL patients without an available HLA-matched donor are poor, and these individuals should pursue HLA-matched unrelated donor allogeneic SCT or experimental therapies. No significant benefit has been seen with autologous transplantation over standard chemotherapy for these patients. Whether Philadelphia chromosome–positive ALL patients lacking SCT donors benefit more from conventional chemotherapy plus Gleevec or other *bcr-abl* inhibitors compared with autologous SCT remains to be determined. Standard-risk ALL patients, particularly pediatric patients, with high long-term remission rates after conventional chemotherapy and maintenance need not undergo allogeneic SCT unless disease recurs.

Most ALL relapses arise within 2 years of initial diagnosis, with recurrence of leukemic cells in the bone marrow, CNS, or testes. Although relapsed disease may respond to further chemotherapy and local irradiation, the duration of second remissions is usually less than 6 months. All patients with relapsed ALL should be considered for allogeneic SCT (which represents the only known cure for disease) or experimental treatment. Autologous SCT for refractory or relapsed ALL is not routinely recommended because ALL blasts appear to be more chemoresistant, with higher failure rates after treatment.

Prospectus for the Future

Our molecular understanding of the pathogenesis of MPN and acute leukemia is progressing rapidly and is already having a critical impact on the development of novel therapeutic approaches that promise to transform our clinical approach to these diseases in the coming years.

Myeloproliferative Disease

The importance of the spectacular success of Gleevec as targeted therapy of CML cannot be overstated. As the first successful therapy based on an understanding of pathogenesis, Gleevec has become emblematic of the translation of our understanding of disease pathogenesis into tangible clinical care innovations. Second-generation tyrosine kinase inhibitors with activity against Gleevec-resistant CML are now available, and SCT is now only rarely offered to patients with CML. Similarly, the discovery of the JAK 2 mutations in non-CML myeloproliferative diseases opens new avenues for targeted intervention in these diseases for which previous therapy has been largely supportive. JAK 2 kinase inhibitors are already under development and will be a major focus of research in the coming years.

Acute Leukemia

Once again, molecular understanding of the pathogenesis of acute leukemia has led to important therapeutic advances in the treatment of disease. The discovery of the link between the retinoic acid receptor and the origins of APL has provided important insight into the unique sensitivity of this disease to ATRA. Gleevec and other oral *bcr-abl* kinase inhibitors has now been added to the armamentarium for treatment of Philadelphia chromosome–positive ALL. Identification of Notch-1 activating mutations in T ALL and FLT-3 kinase mutations in normal karyotype AML have led to ongoing clinical trials of targeted inhibitors for these pathways in both newly diagnosed and relapsed patients. Similar approaches may soon provide therapeutic entry points into the treatment of other acute leukemias associated with pathognomonic chromosomal translocations and genetic and molecular aberrations.

References

Aifantis I, Raetz E, Buonamici S: Molecular pathogenesis of T-cell leukemia and lymphoma. Nat Rev Immunol 8:380-390, 2008.

Baxter EJ, Scott LM, Campbell PJ, et al: Acquired mutation of the tyrosine kinase JAK2 in human myeloproliferative disorders. Lancet 365:1054-1061, 2005.

Byrd J, Mrozek K, Dodge R, et al: Pretreatment cytogenetic abnormalities are predictive of induction success, cumulative incidence of relapse, and overall survival in adult patients with de novo acute myeloid leukemia. Blood 100:4325-4336, 2002.

Druker BJ, Guilhot F, O'Brien SG, et al: Five-year follow-up of patients receiving imatinib for chronic myeloid leukemia. N Engl J Med 355:2408-2417, 2006.

Harrison CN, Campbell PJ, Buck G, et al: Hydroxyurea compared with anagrelide in high-risk essential thrombocythemia. N Engl J Med 353:33-45, 2005.

Jaffe ES, Harris NL, Stein H, Vardiman JW (eds): WHO Classification: Pathology and Genetics of Tumours of the Haematopoietic and Lymphoid Tissues. Lyon, France, IARC Press, 2001.

Landolfi R, Marchioli R, Kutti J, et al: Efficacy and safety of low-dose aspirin in polycythemia vera. N Eng J Med 350:114-124, 2004.

Maziarz RT: Who with chronic myelogenous leukemia to transplant in the era of tyrosine kinase inhibitors? Curr Opin Hematol 15:127-133, 2008.

Pardanani A: JAK2 inhibitor therapy in myeloproliferative disorders: Rationale, preclinical studies, and ongoing clinical trials. Leukemia 22:23-30, 2008.

Pullarkat V, Slovak ML, Kopecky KJ, et al: Impact of cytogenetics on the outcome of adult acute lymphocytic leukemia: Results of the Southwest Oncology Group 9400 study. Blood 111:2563-2572, 2008.

Ravandi F, Burnett AK, Agura ED, et al: Progress in the treatment of acute myeloid leukemia. Cancer 110:1900-1910, 2007.

Rowe JM, Goldstone AH: How I treat acute lymphocytic leukemia in adults. Blood 110:2268-2275, 2007.

Sanz MA, Tallman M, Lo-Coco F: Practice points, consensus, and controversial issues in the management of patients with newly diagnosed acute promyelocytic leukemia. Oncologist 10:806-814, 2005.

Schiffer CA: BCR-ABL tyrosine kinase inhibitors for chronic myelogenous leukemia. N Eng J Med 357:258-265, 2007.

Tefferi A, Vardiman JW: Classification and diagnosis of myeloproliferative neoplasms: The 2008 World Health Organization criteria and point-of-care diagnostic algorithms. Leukemia 22:14-22, 2008.

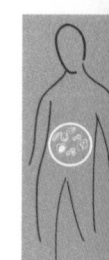

Chapter 49

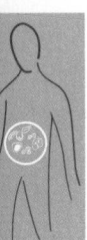

Disorders of Red Blood Cells

Michal G. Rose and Nancy Berliner

Normal Red Blood Cell Structure and Function

The red blood cells (RBCs, erythrocytes) deliver oxygen to all the tissues in the body and carry carbon dioxide back to the lungs for excretion. The erythrocyte is uniquely adapted to these functions. The RBC has a biconcave disk shape that maximizes the membrane surface area for gas exchange, and it has a cytoskeleton and membrane structure that allow it to deform sufficiently to pass through the microvasculature. Passage through capillaries that have a diameter that may be one fourth the resting diameter of the erythrocyte is made possible by interactions between proteins in the membrane (band 3 and glycophorin) and underlying cytoplasmic proteins that make up the erythrocyte cytoskeleton (spectrin, ankyrin, and protein 4.1).

The mature red cell contains no nucleus and is dependent throughout its life span on proteins synthesized before extrusion of the nucleus and release from the bone marrow into the peripheral circulation. About 98% of the cytoplasmic protein of the mature erythrocyte is hemoglobin. The remainder is mainly enzymatic proteins, such as those required for anaerobic metabolism and the hexose monophosphate shunt.

As discussed in the text that follows, defects in any of the intrinsic structural features of the erythrocyte can result in hemolytic anemia. Abnormalities of the membrane or cytoskeletal proteins are the causes of alterations in erythrocyte shape and flexibility. Inborn defects in the enzymatic pathways for glucose metabolism decrease the resistance to oxidant stress, and inherited abnormalities of hemoglobin structure and synthesis lead to polymerization of abnormal hemoglobin (sickle cell disease) or to the precipitation of unbalanced hemoglobin chains (thalassemia). All these changes result in decreased red cell survival.

Oxygen is transported by hemoglobin, a tetramer composed of two α chains and two β-like (β, γ, or δ) chains. In fetal life, the main hemoglobin is fetal hemoglobin (HbF [α_2, γ_2]); the switch from HbF to adult hemoglobin (HbA [$\alpha_2\beta_2$]) occurs in the perinatal period. By 4 to 6 months of age, the level of HbF falls to about 1% of total hemoglobin. HbA_2 ($\alpha_2\gamma_2$) is a minor adult hemoglobin, representing about 1% of adult hemoglobin (Table 49-1).

Clinical Approach to Anemia

Anemia, the reduction in red cell mass, is an important sign of disease. It may reflect decreased production of erythrocytes, because of nutritional deficiencies or primary hematologic disease or in response to systemic illness. Alternatively, anemia may reflect increased blood loss or cellular destruction from hemolysis. Hemolysis may occur as a result of intrinsic abnormalities of the red cell or immune-mediated red blood cell destruction, or as a part of a systemic vascular process. The investigation of anemia is a critical component of the evaluation of the patient and commonly provides valuable insight into systemic illness. Figure 49-1 provides an overview of the differential diagnosis of anemia.

CLINICAL PRESENTATION

The symptoms of anemia reflect both the severity and the rapidity with which the reduction in erythrocyte mass has occurred. Patients with acute hemorrhage or massive hemolysis may exhibit symptoms of hypovolemic shock. However, most patients develop anemia more slowly and may have few symptoms. Usual complaints are fatigue, decreased exercise tolerance, dyspnea, and palpitations. In patients with coronary artery disease, anemia may precipitate angina. On physical examination, the major sign of anemia is pallor. Patients may be tachycardic and often have audible flow murmurs. Patients with hemolysis often exhibit jaundice and splenomegaly.

LABORATORY EVALUATION

The key components of the laboratory evaluation of anemia are the reticulocyte count, peripheral blood smear, erythro-

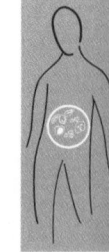

cyte indices, nutritional studies, and bone marrow aspirate and biopsy.

The *reticulocyte count* allows the critical distinction between anemia arising from a primary failure of red cell production and anemia resulting from increased red cell destruction or bleeding. Erythrocytes newly released from the marrow still contain small amounts of RNA; these are termed *reticulocytes* and can be detected by staining the peripheral blood smear with methylene blue or other supravital stains. In response to the stress of anemia, erythropoietin (EPO) production increases and promotes the production and release of increased numbers of reticulocytes. The number of reticulocytes in the peripheral blood therefore reflects the response of the bone marrow to anemia. The reticulocyte count can be expressed either as a percentage of the total red cell number or as an absolute number.

In patients without anemia, a normal reticulocyte count is 1%, with an absolute count of 50,000/mcL. When anemia is caused by decreased RBC survival, appropriate marrow response results in a reticulocyte count of more than 2%, with an absolute reticulocyte count of more than 100,000/mcL. When the reticulocyte count is not elevated, a search should begin for a cause of the failure of red cell production. Reticulocyte counts that are expressed as a percentage of total RBCs must be corrected for anemia because decreasing the number of circulating cells will increase the reticulocyte percentage without any increase in release from the marrow. The corrected reticulocyte count is calculated by multiplying the reticulocyte count by the ratio of the patient's hematocrit to a normal hematocrit. The advantage of the absolute reticulocyte count is that this correction is not necessary. The absolute reticulocyte count is becoming increasingly available and will probably supersede the standard reticulocyte count.

Evaluation of the *peripheral blood smear* (Fig. 49-2) may provide important clues to the causes of anemia. Red cell morphologic examination is especially critical in the evaluation of anemia associated with reticulocytosis, wherein an examination of the smear is essential to distinguish between immune hemolysis (which results in spherocytes) and microangiopathic hemolysis (which causes schistocytes or erythrocyte fragmentation). Changes associated with other causes of anemia include sickle and target cells that are characteristic of hemoglobinopathies, teardrop cells and nucleated red cells associated with myelofibrosis and marrow infiltration, intracorpuscular parasites in malaria and

Table 49-1 Structure and Distribution of Human Hemoglobins

Name of Hemoglobin (Hb)	Distribution	Structure
A	95%-98% of adult Hb	$\alpha_2\beta_2$
A$_2$	1.5%-3.5% of adult Hb	$\alpha_2\delta_2$
F	Fetal, 0.5%-1.0% of adult Hb	$\alpha_2\gamma_2$
Gower 1	Embryonic	$\zeta_2\epsilon_2$
Gower 2	Embryonic	$\alpha_2\epsilon_2$
Portland	Embryonic	$\zeta_2\gamma_2$

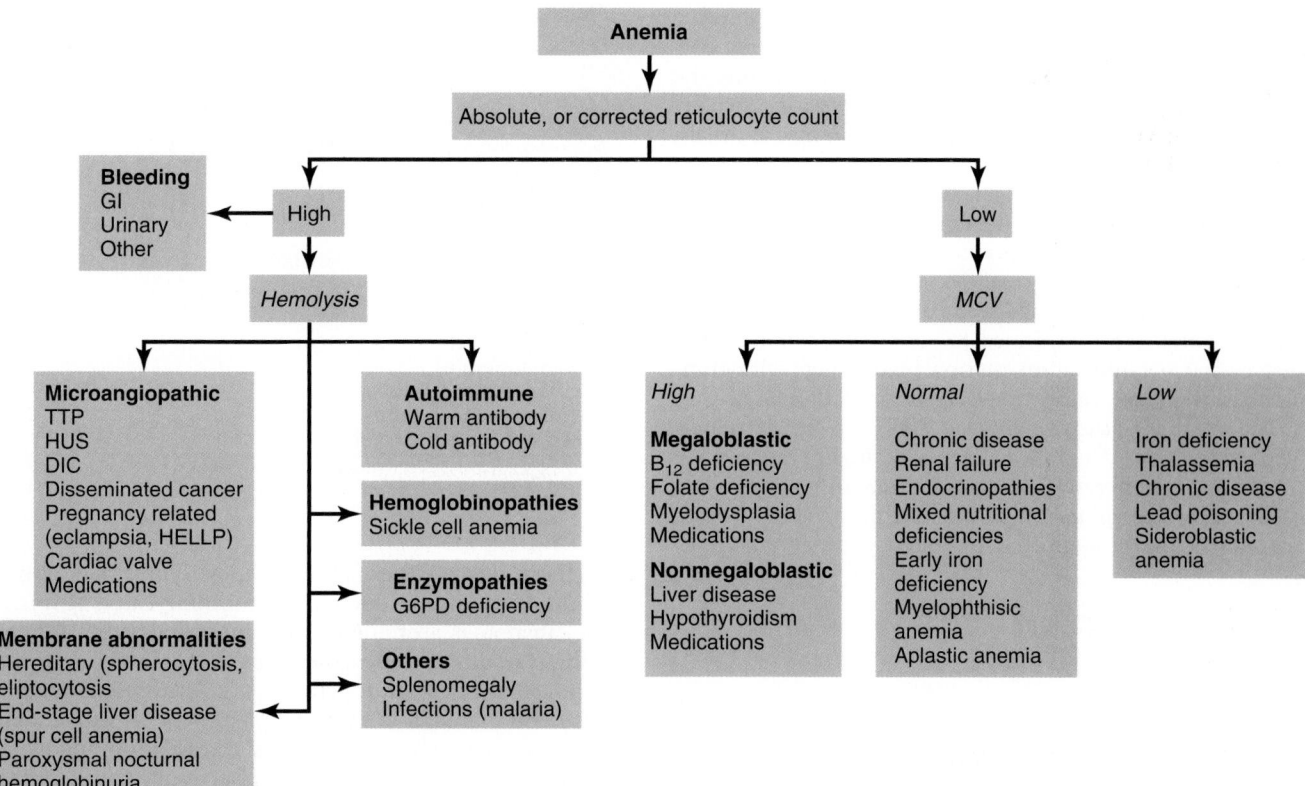

Figure 49-1 Overview of the differential diagnosis of anemia. DIC, disseminated intravascular coagulation; G6PD, glucose-6-phosphate dehydrogenase; GI, gastrointestinal; HELLP, hemolysis, elevated liver enzymes, and low platelet count; HUS, hemolytic uremic syndrome; MCV, mean corpuscular volume; TTP, thrombotic thrombocytopenic purpura.

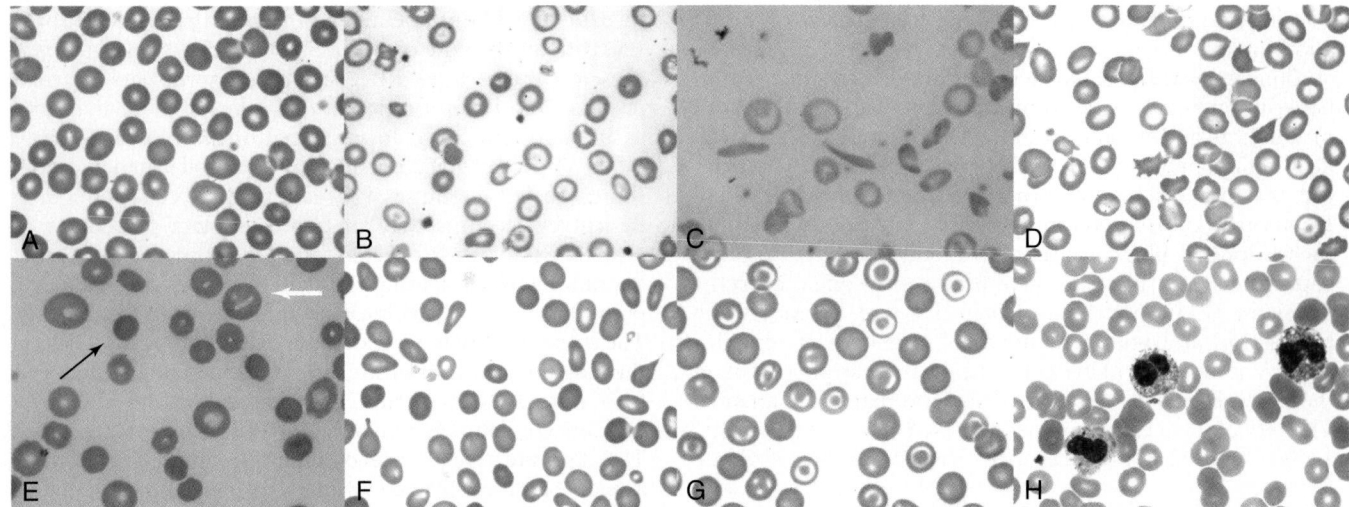

Figure 49-2 Peripheral blood smears in patients with anemia. **A,** Normal red blood cells. **B,** Iron deficiency anemia. **C,** Sickle cell anemia. **D,** Microangiopathic hemolytic anemia. **E,** Spherocytosis in autoimmune hemolytic anemia. **F,** Teardrops in myelofibrosis. **G,** Target cells. **H,** Pseudo–Pelger-Huet anomaly in myelodysplasia.

babesiosis, and pencil-shaped deformities associated with severe iron deficiency. In addition, examination of myeloid cells and platelets may also be helpful. Hypersegmented neutrophils and large platelets support the diagnosis of megaloblastic anemia, and the presence of immature blast forms may be diagnostic of leukemia. Figure 49-2 visualizes some common peripheral blood smear findings in patients with anemia.

In patients with anemia and an elevated reticulocyte count, the vigorous production of new erythroid cells suggests that marrow function is normal and is responding appropriately to the stress of the anemia. Bone marrow examination in this situation is rarely indicated because the marrow will simply show erythroid hyperplasia, usually without revealing any primary marrow pathologic anomaly. Evaluation should be focused on determining whether the cause of red cell consumption is either bleeding or hemolysis. In contrast, bone marrow examination is often required for the evaluation of hypoproliferative anemia. In patients in whom common abnormalities such as iron and other nutritional deficiencies have been ruled out, marrow aspiration and biopsy are indicated to search for abnormalities such as marrow infiltration, marrow involvement with granulomatous disease, marrow aplasia, or myelodysplasia.

The *mean corpuscular volume* (MCV) is an extremely helpful tool in the diagnosis of anemia with a low reticulocyte count (hypoproliferative anemia). The size of the red cells is used to characterize the anemia as microcytic (MCV < 80), normocytic (MCV 80 to 100), or macrocytic (MCV > 100).

Evaluation of Hypoproliferative Anemia

EVALUATION OF MICROCYTIC ANEMIA

The differential diagnosis of microcytic anemia is outlined in Table 49-2. Microcytosis and hypochromia are the hallmarks of anemias caused by defects in hemoglobin synthesis,

Table 49-2 **Differential Diagnosis of Anemia with Low Reticulocyte Count**
Microcytic Anemia (MCV < 80)
Iron deficiency
Thalassemia minor
Anemia of chronic disease
Sideroblastic anemia
Lead poisoning
Macrocytic Anemia (MCV > 100)
Megaloblastic Anemias
Folate deficiency
Vitamin B$_{12}$ deficiency
Drug-induced megaloblastic anemia
Myelodysplasia
Nonmegaloblastic Macrocytosis
Liver disease
Hypothyroidism
Reticulocytosis
Normocytic Anemia (MCV 80-100)
Early iron deficiency
Aplastic anemia
Myelophthisic disorders
Endocrinopathies
Anemia of chronic disease
Anemia of renal failure
Mixed nutritional deficiency
MCV, mean corpuscular volume.

which can reflect either failure of heme synthesis or abnormalities in globin production. The leading cause of microcytic anemia is iron deficiency, in which lack of heme synthesis results from the absence of iron to incorporate into the porphyrin ring (iron deficiency is discussed in detail in the section that follows). Up to 30% of patients with anemia of chronic disease have microcytosis. Lead poisoning blocks incorporation of iron into heme, also resulting in a microcytic anemia. Sideroblastic anemias arise from failure to synthesize the porphyrin ring, usually as a result of inhibition of the heme synthetic pathway enzymes. Congenital sidero-

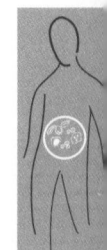

blastic anemia may respond to pyridoxine, a cofactor for several of the heme synthetic pathway enzymes. A more common cause of acquired sideroblastic anemia is alcohol abuse; ethanol inhibits most of the enzymes in the heme synthetic pathway. Failure of globin synthesis occurs in thalassemic syndromes, as described in detail in this chapter's section titled "Hemoglobinopathies." All these disorders lead to decreased mean corpuscular hemoglobin concentration, causing hypochromia and a decrease in red cell size (low MCV).

Iron Deficiency Anemia

Iron deficiency is the leading cause of anemia worldwide. Although the presentation of classic iron deficiency anemia is linked with a microcytic anemia, early iron deficiency is associated with a normocytic anemia. Consequently, iron deficiency should be considered in all patients with anemia, and iron indices should be a part of the evaluation of any patient with hypoproductive anemia, regardless of the MCV.

Iron is acquired in the diet from either heme (found in meat) or nonheme (derived from vegetables such as spinach) sources. Iron from heme is better absorbed than nonheme iron. Iron absorption is increased in iron deficiency and in patients with ineffective erythropoiesis. Iron is absorbed from the proximal small intestine bound to transferrin, which mediates its uptake into red cell precursors through the transferrin receptor. The iron is released and incorporated into heme. Iron outside of hemoglobin-producing cells is stored in ferritin. Men and women have total-body iron of 50 mg/kg and 40 mg/kg, respectively. Between 60% and 75% of the iron is found in hemoglobin. A small amount (2 mg/kg) is found in heme and nonheme enzymes, and 5 mg/kg is found in myoglobin. The remainder is stored in ferritin, which resides primarily in liver, bone marrow, spleen, and muscle. The capacity for excreting iron is limited, and iron overload occurs in patients with excessive absorption from the gastrointestinal tract (as a result of ineffective erythropoiesis or congenital hemochromatosis) or from chronic transfusions. Iron overload leads to increased iron deposition in these tissues and secondary deposition in endocrine organs, resulting in liver dysfunction, diabetes, and other endocrine abnormalities.

The most frequent cause of iron deficiency is occult blood loss. All men and postmenopausal women who are found to be iron deficient should have an evaluation for a source of gastrointestinal blood loss, regardless of the detection of occult blood. In premenopausal women, iron deficiency is most frequently secondary to loss of iron with menstruation (about 15 mg per month) and during pregnancy (about 900 mg per pregnancy). *Helicobacter pylori* infection has also recently been recognized as a cause of iron deficiency even in the absence of intestinal bleeding. Dietary deficiency of iron is most commonly seen in young children whose growth outstrips their intake of iron and in babies who drink mostly milk at the expense of an intake of iron-containing foods.

Laboratory Evaluation

As previously stated, early iron deficiency does not exhibit the hallmark microcytosis and hypochromia that characterize classic iron deficiency. Evaluation of the blood smear in advanced iron deficiency often demonstrates hypochromic RBCs, target cells, and pencil-shaped elongated cells.

Early iron deficiency is frequently associated with reactive thrombocytosis.

The mainstay of the diagnosis of iron deficiency is the peripheral blood iron indices. These include iron and total iron-binding capacity (TIBC) and ferritin. The transferrin saturation is the ratio of serum iron to transferrin concentration (TIBC), and is normally at least 20%. Iron deficiency results in a decrease in serum iron and an increase in iron-binding capacity, leading to a decrease in this ratio to less than 10%. Chronic inflammatory conditions (e.g., infection, inflammation, malignancy) often decrease both iron and TIBC, but the transferrin saturation usually remains above 20%.

The ferritin level is a reflection of total-body iron stores. The liver synthesizes ferritin in proportion to total-body iron, and a level of less than 12 ng/mL strongly supports a diagnosis of iron deficiency. Unfortunately, ferritin is an acute-phase reactant, and levels rise in the setting of fever, inflammatory disease, infection, or other stresses. However, ferritin levels in response to stress do not often rise above 50 to 100 ng/mL; therefore ferritin levels higher than 100 ng/mL usually rule out iron deficiency.

If the indirect measurement of iron indices does not definitively confirm or refute a diagnosis of iron deficiency, a bone marrow examination can be performed to provide a direct assessment of marrow iron stores. Presence of iron in the marrow excludes iron deficiency anemia because marrow iron stores will be depleted before any fall in red cell production resulting from iron deficiency; conversely, complete absence of marrow iron confirms the diagnosis of iron deficiency.

Treatment

Oral iron supplementation, with administration of ferrous sulfate or ferrous gluconate 2 to 3 times daily, is the treatment for iron deficiency. Side effects include diarrhea or constipation, and patients should be treated symptomatically. Reduction of the dose and gradual reinstitution of full doses may allow oral therapy to be continued. Iron should be administered for several months after resolution of anemia to allow for the reconstitution of iron stores.

In patients with malabsorption, a complete inability to tolerate oral iron, or iron demands that outstrip replacement with oral supplements, parenteral iron may be administered. The parenteral administration of iron, especially iron dextran, has been associated with anaphylaxis. However, newer preparations such as sodium ferric gluconate and iron sucrose are significantly safer. As previously stated, all male patients and postmenopausal women with iron deficiency require evaluation for a source of gastrointestinal bleeding.

EVALUATION OF MACROCYTIC ANEMIA

Two categories of hypoproductive macrocytic anemias exist: megaloblastic anemia and nonmegaloblastic macrocytic anemia. Megaloblastic anemia arises from a failure of DNA synthesis and results in lack of synchrony between the maturation of the nucleus and the cytoplasm of hematopoietic cells. Nonmegaloblastic macrocytic anemias usually reflect membrane abnormalities resulting from abnormalities in cholesterol metabolism and are most commonly found in patients with advanced liver disease or severe hypothyroidism. Reticulocytosis greater than 10% will also cause an elevated MCV on automated blood counts because reticulocytes are larger than mature RBCs.

Megaloblastic Anemia

Megaloblastic anemia results from a block to synthesis of critical nucleotide precursors of DNA, which leads to a cell cycle arrest in S phase. Cytoplasmic maturation occurs, but maturation of the nucleus is arrested. Cells take on a bizarre appearance, with large immature nuclei surrounded by more mature-appearing cytoplasm. Interference with DNA synthesis affects all rapidly dividing cells, and therefore patients with megaloblastic syndromes often have pancytopenia and gastrointestinal symptoms such as diarrhea and malabsorption. In women, megaloblastic changes of the cervical mucosa occur and may cause abnormal Papanicolaou smears. The most common causes of megaloblastic anemia are deficiencies of vitamin B_{12} or folate, medications that inhibit DNA synthesis or that block folate metabolism, and myelodysplasia.

Vitamin B_{12} (Cobalamin) Deficiency

Cobalamin (Cbl) is absorbed from animal protein in the diet. The process of Cbl absorption and metabolism is complex because Cbl is always bound to other proteins. In the stomach, protein-bound vitamins are released by digestion with pepsin and are bound to transcobalamin I. Transcobalamins I and III, termed *R binders* because of their rapid electrophoretic mobility, are found in all secretions, in plasma, and within the secondary granules of neutrophils. Although presumed to be involved with the storage of Cbl, their function is unknown, and isolated congenital deficiency of R binders is clinically silent. Within the proximal duodenum, pancreatic proteases digest Cbl away from the R binder proteins, and Cbl binds to intrinsic factor (IF). IF is secreted by the parietal cells of the stomach and mediates absorption of Cbl through IF-specific receptors in the distal ileum. Within the ileal mucosal cell, the IF-Cbl complex is again digested, and Cbl is released into the plasma bound to transcobalamin II (TCII), the carrier protein that mediates cellular uptake of Cbl by TCII-specific receptors.

Within the cell, Cbl is a cofactor for two intracellular enzymes, methylmalonyl–coenzyme A (CoA) mutase, and homocysteine-methionine methyltransferase (Fig. 49-3). Methylmalonyl-CoA mutase is a mitochondrial enzyme that functions in the citric acid cycle to convert methylmalonyl-CoA to succinyl-CoA. The cytoplasmic enzyme homocysteine–methionine methyltransferase is necessary for the transfer of methyl groups from *N*-methyltetrahydrofolate to homocysteine to form methionine. Demethylated tetrahydrofolate is necessary as a carbon donor in the conversion of deoxyuridine to deoxythymidine. Absence of Cbl results in a *trapping* of tetrahydrofolate in its methylated form and blocks the synthesis of thymidine 5′-triphosphate for incorporation into DNA. The megaloblastic changes induced by Cbl deficiency are mediated through this functional folate deficiency, which explains the similarity in the hematologic abnormalities induced by Cbl and folate deficiency.

Causes of Cobalamin Deficiency

The most common cause of Cbl deficiency is pernicious anemia, an autoimmune disease associated with gastric pari-

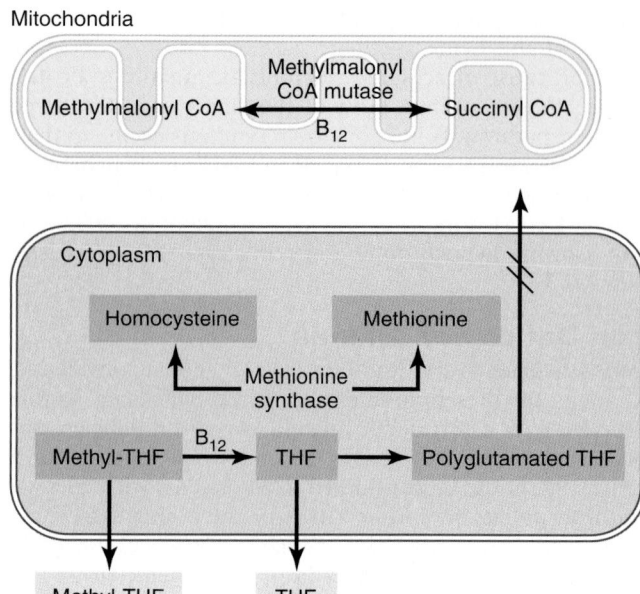

Figure 49-3 Metabolic pathways of folic acid and cobalamin. CoA, coenzyme A; THF, tetrahydrofolate.

Table 49-3 **Causes of Cobalamin Deficiency**
Malabsorption of Vitamin B_{12}
Pernicious anemia
Partial or total gastrectomy
Pancreatic insufficiency
Bacterial overgrowth
Diseases of the terminal ileum
Tapeworm infection
Nutritional (vegans)
Congenital Intrinsic Factor or Transcobalamin II Deficiency

etal cell atrophy, defective gastric acid secretion, and absence of IF. Antiparietal cell and anti-IF antibodies are frequently found in patients with pernicious anemia and other autoimmune conditions such as Graves disease, Addison disease, and hypoparathyroidism. Many other lesions in the gastrointestinal tract can interfere with the absorption of Cbl (Table 49-3). Gastrectomy causes loss of parietal cell function and IF secretion. Pancreatic insufficiency interferes with the digestion of the R binder–Cbl complex, hindering the binding of Cbl to IF and ileal absorption. Resection of the terminal ileum prevents vitamin B_{12} absorption, as do diseases that affect ileal mucosal function, such as Crohn disease, sprue, intestinal tuberculosis, and lymphoma. Because the body stores of Cbl are large and daily loss of Cbl is low, the stores of Cbl are adequate for 3 to 4 years if intake stops abruptly; signs of Cbl deficiency do not develop until defective absorption has occurred for several years. Nutritional Cbl deficiency is rare and is only seen in individuals who have been on strict vegan diets, excluding all animal products for many years. Infants born to vegan mothers who are breastfed are also at risk for developing Cbl deficiency.

Folate Deficiency

Folate is widely present in food such as leafy vegetables, fruits, and animal protein. However, because it is destroyed

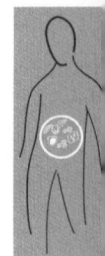

Table 49-4 **Causes of Folate Deficiency**
Dietary Insufficiency
Increased Folate Requirements
Pregnancy
Lactation
Hemolysis
Exfoliative dermatitis
Malignancy
Malabsorption
Sprue
Crohn disease
Short bowel syndrome
Antifolate Medications
Methotrexate
Sulfa drugs

by prolonged cooking, fresh fruits and vegetables are the most reliable source of folate. Consequently, nutritional folate deficiency is common in malnourished individuals who eat very little fresh fruits and vegetables. Folate deficiency can also be caused by increased demand, as occurs with pregnancy, hemolysis, and exfoliative dermatitis, and by increased losses, which occur with dialysis (Table 49-4). Folate is absorbed in the proximal small intestine, and malabsorption of folate can also lead to folate deficiency.

Other Causes of Megaloblastic Anemia

Drugs and toxins are common causes of megaloblastic anemia. Some drugs, such as methotrexate and sulfa drugs, act as direct folate antagonists and mimic folate deficiency. Purine and pyrimidine analogue chemotherapeutic agents (e.g., azathioprine, 5-fluorouracil) are direct DNA-synthesis inhibitors. Antiviral agents cause megaloblastic changes by unclear mechanisms. Alcohol interferes with folate metabolism, increasing the effect of frequent concomitant nutritional folate deficiency. Myelodysplasia commonly appears as a macrocytic anemia, with megaloblastic changes primarily in the erythroid series.

Clinical Manifestations of Megaloblastic Anemia

The development of megaloblastic anemia is usually gradual, allowing adequate time for concomitant plasma expansion to prevent hypovolemia. Consequently, patients are frequently severely anemic at presentation. They may have yellowish skin as a result of a combination of pallor and jaundice. Some patients have glossitis and cheilosis. With severe anemia, patients usually have an MCV above 110, although concomitant iron deficiency, caused by malabsorption secondary to megaloblastic changes in the intestinal tract, may decrease the macrocytosis. Patients frequently have pancytopenia.

A peripheral smear demonstrates large, oval cells (macro-ovalocytes), hypersegmented neutrophils, and large platelets. The bone marrow is hypercellular, with megaloblastic changes and abnormally large precursors. In addition, intramedullary destruction of erythrocytes (ineffective hematopoiesis) causes elevated bilirubin and lactate dehydrogenase.

Cbl deficiency is associated with neurologic abnormalities that are not seen with other causes of megaloblastic anemia.

The neurologic signs may range widely from a subtle loss of vibratory sensation and position sense caused by demyelination of the dorsal columns to frank dementia and neuropsychiatric disease. The neurologic changes may be present without anemia, especially if a patient with Cbl deficiency is treated with folate, which may correct the hematologic manifestations of megaloblastic anemia but does not treat the neurologic abnormalities. The neurologic manifestations of Cbl deficiency are thought to be secondary to loss of function of the mitochondrial enzyme methylmalonyl-CoA mutase. One proposed explanation is that the failure to metabolize odd-chain fatty acids, which results in their improper incorporation into myelin, causes the neurologic dysfunction. This explains why these findings are uniquely seen in patients with Cbl deficiency and are not seen in those with the megaloblastic anemias caused by abnormalities in the folate pathway.

Measuring levels of Cbl and folate in the peripheral blood confirms the diagnosis of megaloblastic anemia. Because megaloblastic changes in the gut mucosa can cause concomitant malabsorption of folate in the presence of Cbl deficiency, and vice versa, both levels should be measured in the patient with megaloblastic hematopoiesis. RBC folate levels better reflect the body folate stores and should be measured when a deficiency is clinically suggested but the *serum* folate levels are normal. Homocysteine levels are elevated in Cbl and folate deficiency, and methylmalonic acid levels are elevated in Cbl deficiency. These levels can be measured when Cbl deficiency is suggested, but serum Cbl levels are in the low-normal range.

In the setting of Cbl deficiency, a Schilling test may help establish the cause of the deficiency. Radioactive Cbl is given orally with a large parenteral dose of unlabeled Cbl. The absorption of orally administered Cbl is then measured by determining the excretion of radioactivity into the urine. Cbl bound to IF and labeled with a different isotope can be given simultaneously. Selective absorption of IF-bound Cbl supports a diagnosis of pernicious anemia. If neither isotope is absorbed, the test may be repeated after a course of antibiotics to treat potential bacterial overgrowth or after administering pancreatic enzymes to rule out pancreatic insufficiency. The use of the Schilling test has decreased with the availability of assays for antiparietal cell antibodies and anti-IF antibodies, particularly because the necessity of an adequate urine collection makes it frequently unreliable.

Treatment of Megaloblastic Anemia

Patients with Cbl deficiency should initially receive daily or weekly parenteral therapy with 1 mg subcutaneously or intramuscularly for four to eight doses. Maintenance therapy should then be instituted with 1 mg parenterally monthly. Oral therapy with high-dose crystalline vitamin B_{12} may overcome blocks to normal Cbl absorption, and oral therapy may be an option in patients who refuse parenteral supplementation. Therapy with Cbl should be accompanied by folate therapy because concomitant secondary folate deficiency may develop when RBC production increases with the availability of Cbl.

Patients with folate deficiency should receive replacement with 1 to 5 mg per day of oral folate. As previously noted, it is critical to be certain that patients are not Cbl deficient because replacement of folate may correct the hematologic parameters in patients with Cbl deficiency, but it will not improve the neurologic sequelae.

After treating megaloblastic anemia, a rapid response usually occurs. Reticulocytosis is seen as early as 2 days after therapy and peaks within 7 to 10 days. Despite rapid resolution of neutropenia, hypersegmentation of neutrophils may persist for several days. During this period, rapid cellular proliferation and turnover occur, which may precipitate hypokalemia, hyperuricemia, or hypophosphatemia. Patients should also be monitored for the development of iron deficiency in the face of increased demand with the rapid cellular proliferation in response to replacement. Anemia and other cytopenias should respond completely within 1 to 2 months, but the neurologic manifestations of Cbl deficiency improve slowly and may be irreversible.

EVALUATION OF NORMOCYTIC ANEMIA

The differential diagnosis of a normocytic hypoproductive anemia is extensive. Most nutritional anemias that cause microcytosis or macrocytosis begin as a normocytic anemia. Combined nutritional deficiencies may also cause normalization of the MCV. The measurement of EPO levels may be helpful in the diagnosis of normocytic anemia. In addition to helping in the diagnosis of anemia resulting from renal failure, many of the anemias associated with chronic inflammation and endocrinopathies exhibit a depressed EPO level. However, interpretation of EPO levels may be difficult in patients with mild anemia because the levels do not usually rise above the normal range until the hematocrit is depressed below 30%. Even below a hematocrit level of 30%, the EPO level will often be in the normal range, but such levels are inappropriately low in the setting of anemia. An elevated EPO level suggests inadequate marrow response to anemia and increases the likelihood of myelophthisis or primary bone marrow failure. In patients for whom the diagnosis is not clear upon routine nutritional and endocrine studies, a bone marrow examination is indicated to rule out primary marrow pathologic conditions.

Anemia of Chronic Disease

The anemia of chronic disease (now preferentially termed the *anemia of inflammation*) occurs in patients with chronic inflammatory, infectious, malignant, and autoimmune diseases. Patients have low-serum iron levels, but, in contrast to the iron indices in iron deficiency, the iron-binding capacity is also reduced, and the transferrin saturation is usually greater than 10%. Ferritin levels are often elevated, both as an acute-phase reactant and as a reflection of decreased iron incorporation. Recent studies have demonstrated that these patients have inappropriately high levels of hepcidin, a peptide produced by the liver, which is responsible for regulating intestinal iron absorption and iron mobilization from macrophages. Other abnormalities in patients with anemia of chronic disease include an absolute or relative EPO deficiency, poor iron incorporation into developing erythrocytes, and shortened erythrocyte survival.

Treatment of Normocytic Anemias

The mainstay of treatment of the anemia of chronic renal failure is EPO and iron replacement. The anemia of chronic disease will resolve if the underlying chronic condition is

treated. In the absence of primary treatment, anemia will often respond to therapy with EPO. EPO levels may be helpful in predicting which patients are likely to respond. Therapy with EPO may be successful in patients with levels below 150 U/L, although it is most successful if the level is below 50 U/L. Responses to EPO replacement are most dramatic in patients with multiple myeloma, rheumatoid arthritis, and in the anemia associated with HIV infection.

Treatment of other causes of normocytic anemia is dictated by the primary causes of the disorder. The evaluation and treatment of primary marrow failure syndromes and hematologic malignancies are discussed in Chapters 47 and 48, respectively.

Evaluation of Anemia with Reticulocytosis

An elevated reticulocyte count in the setting of anemia signals a compensatory response of a normal marrow to premature loss of erythrocytes. Hemolysis is the premature destruction of RBCs in the reticuloendothelial system (extrinsic hemolysis) or in blood vessels (intrinsic hemolysis). The only other condition that causes anemia with reticulocytosis is acute bleeding. The differential diagnosis of hemolytic anemia is outlined in Table 49-5.

Table 49-5 **Differential Diagnosis of Hemolytic Anemia**
Immune Hemolytic Anemia
Immunoglobulin G (warm antibody)–mediated hemolysis
Immunoglobulin M (cold antibody)–mediated hemolysis
Other Causes of Hemolysis from Causes Extrinsic to the Erythrocyte
Microangiopathic Hemolysis
Disseminated intravascular coagulation
Thrombotic thrombocytopenic purpura
Preeclampsia, eclampsia, HELLP
Drugs (mitomycin, cyclosporine)
Valvular hemolysis
Splenomegaly
Infection
Hemolytic Anemia Caused by Disorders of the Erythrocyte Membrane
Inherited Membrane Abnormalities
Hereditary spherocytosis
Hereditary elliptocytosis
Hereditary pyropoikilocytosis
Acquired Membrane Abnormalities
Paroxysmal nocturnal hemoglobinuria
Spur cell anemia
Hemolysis Caused by Erythrocyte Enzymopathies
Glucose-6-phosphate dehydrogenase deficiency
Other enzyme deficiencies
Hemoglobinopathies
Sickle cell disease
Other sickle syndromes
Thalassemia

HELLP, hemolysis, elevated liver enzymes, and low-platelet count in association with preeclampsia.

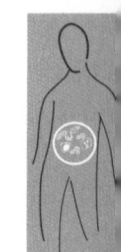

Table 49-6 Drug-Induced Autoimmune Hemolytic Anemia

Type	Mechanism	Common Drugs Implicated	Direct Coombs Test–Positive Hemolytic Anemia	Indirect Coombs Test–Positive Hemolytic Anemia
1	Hapten mediated	Penicillin Cephalothin	IgG positive Complement positive or negative	Positive only in the presence of drug
2	Immune complex mediated	Quinine Quinidine Phenacetin Rifampin Isoniazid Tetracycline Chlorpromazine	IgG negative Complement positive	Positive only in the presence of drug
3	True anti-RBC antibody	Methyldopa Levodopa Procainamide Ibuprofen Interferon-α	IgG positive Complement negative	Positive also in absence of drug

Although examination of the peripheral blood smear is frequently helpful in characterizing any anemia, it is absolutely critical in the evaluation of patients with hemolytic anemia. As previously noted, the morphologic examination of the erythrocytes is helpful in distinguishing immune hemolysis from microangiopathic hemolytic anemia. In addition, other red cell morphologic abnormalities are characteristic for specific diseases such as sickle cell disease (sickled cells), enzyme defects (*bite* cells), or erythrocyte membrane abnormalities (spherocytes and elliptocytes).

IMMUNE HEMOLYTIC ANEMIA

Immune-mediated hemolysis results from the coating of the erythrocyte membrane with antibodies or complement, or both. It may be mediated by immunoglobulin G (IgG) antibodies (*warm* antibody) or by IgM antibodies (*cold* antibody). The designations *warm* and *cold* denote the temperature at which maximal antibody binding takes place, and the clinical syndromes caused by the two types of antibodies are distinct.

The diagnosis of hemolytic anemia is based on the direct and indirect antiglobulin (Coombs) tests. To perform a direct Coombs test, patient erythrocytes are mixed with rabbit antisera directed against either human IgG or human complement. The cells are then monitored for agglutination, the presence of which confirms the presence of antibody or complement on the patient's red cells. The indirect Coombs test is performed by mixing patient serum with ABO-compatible erythrocytes and then combining this mixture with rabbit antisera against IgG; the Coombs test allows for the evaluation of antibody in the patient's serum.

IgG-Mediated (Warm) Immune Hemolysis

Classic autoimmune hemolytic anemia (AIHA) is caused by IgG antibody directed against erythrocyte antigens. Warm-type hemolysis may be primary (idiopathic) or associated with autoimmune disease, lymphoproliferative disorders, or drugs. Patients exhibit acute anemia, jaundice, and an elevated reticulocyte count. Some patients have splenomegaly. The peripheral blood smear demonstrates spherocytes (see

Fig. 49-2E). Laboratory analysis confirms the presence of IgG on the erythrocyte membrane, as demonstrated by a positive Coombs test; in some patients, the erythrocytes will also be coated with complement. The occasional patient will not have reticulocytosis; in such patients, the antibody destroys reticulocytes and mature erythrocytes.

The mainstay of therapy for AIHA is corticosteroids. Patients are usually treated with 1 to 2 mg/kg of prednisone, and in responding patients, doses are tapered slowly over several months. Patients who fail to respond to prednisone or cannot be tapered off the prednisone can be treated with other immunosuppressive agents, such as cyclophosphamide, azathioprine, or chlorambucil. The occasional patient will respond to intravenous immunoglobulin. Splenectomy may be effective in some patients who are steroid refractory or steroid resistant; however, patients who do not respond and who have ongoing hemolysis after splenectomy are at high risk for secondary thromboembolic events.

Warm antibodies mediate *drug-induced hemolysis*. Several mechanisms exist through which drugs may induce AIHA (Table 49-6). Penicillin produces hemolysis by binding to erythrocytes and acting as a hapten; the antibody is directed against the drug, and hemolysis occurs only in the presence of the drug. Type 2 hemolysis is caused by the formation of an antibody-drug complex that binds to the erythrocyte membrane and activates complement. Drugs associated with this type of hemolysis include quinidine, quinine, and rifampin. Still other drugs, including methyldopa and procainamide, cause hemolysis by inducing the production of *true* antierythrocyte antibodies directed against Rh and other RBC antigens. Antibody may persist in the absence of the drug, but not all patients with a positive Coombs test will have evidence of hemolysis.

IgM-Mediated (Cold) Hemolytic Anemia

Cold-type immune hemolysis is usually postinfectious. The most common associated illnesses are *Mycoplasma pneumoniae* and Epstein-Barr virus (EBV). IgM antibodies are produced that are directed against the RBC antigen I (*Mycoplasma*) or i (EBV). The antibodies bind at lower temperatures, present in fingers and toes, and bind complement. During the return to the central circulation, the IgM falls off the red cell, leaving complement bound. The Coombs test is negative for IgG or IgM but positive for complement. Hemolysis is self-limited, is rarely severe, and resolves with supportive therapy. In cases of severe hemolysis requiring transfusion, patients should be kept warm, and blood should be administered through a blood warmer to minimize further hemolysis.

Cold agglutinin disease is a chronic IgM antibody–mediated hemolysis usually seen in association with lymphoproliferative disease. Hemolysis is usually low grade; however, if severe, it responds poorly to steroids and splenectomy. Acute severe IgM-mediated hemolysis may respond to plasmapheresis. Supportive therapy includes avoidance of exposure to the cold. In the setting of lymphoproliferative disease, patients may respond to immunotherapy with rituximab (anti-CD20 antibody).

HEMOLYSIS FROM CAUSES EXTRINSIC TO THE ERYTHROCYTE

Microangiopathic Hemolysis

Microangiopathic hemolytic anemia (MAHA) is caused by traumatic destruction of RBCs as they pass through small vessels. The leading causes of MAHA include disseminated intravascular coagulation (DIC) and thrombotic thrombocytopenic purpura/hemolytic uremic syndrome (TTP/HUS) (see Table 49-5 and Fig. 49-1). Other causes include pregnancy-related syndromes such as preeclampsia, eclampsia, and the HELLP syndrome (hemolysis, elevated liver enzymes, and low platelets in association with preeclampsia); drugs; and metastatic cancers. A similar hemolytic picture can be seen in traumatic hemolysis on a damaged cardiac valve.

Finding schistocytes (fragmented erythrocytes) on the peripheral blood smear confirms the diagnosis of MAHA (see Fig. 49-2D). The presence of a normal prothrombin time and partial thromboplastin time supports a diagnosis of TTP/HUS over that of DIC. Diagnosis and management are described further in Chapter 53.

Infection

Hemolysis can be caused by direct infection of RBCs by parasites, as seen in malaria, babesiosis, and bartonellosis. Severe, overwhelming hemolysis can be seen in clostridial sepsis, in which bacterial toxins directly damage the membrane.

HEMOLYTIC ANEMIAS CAUSED BY DISORDERS OF THE ERYTHROCYTE MEMBRANE

Inherited Membrane Abnormalities

Hereditary spherocytosis (HS) is caused by heterogeneous congenital abnormalities in proteins of the erythrocyte cytoskeleton (Table 49-7). Most patients with HS have dominantly inherited mutations in spectrin or ankyrin. HS is characterized by hemolytic anemia, splenomegaly, and the presence of prominent spherocytes in the peripheral blood. Spherocytes are the result of *conditioning* of the erythrocytes in the spleen, whereby reticuloendothelial cells remove portions of the abnormal membrane that are the result of the

Table 49-7 Congenital Red Blood Cell Membrane Abnormalities

Name of Condition	Abnormal Membrane Proteins	Inheritance
Spherocytosis	Spectrin, ankyrin, band 3, protein 4.2	Autosomal dominant Recessive (rare)
Elliptocytosis	Spectrin, protein 4.1	Autosomal dominant Recessive (rare)
Pyropoikilocytosis	Spectrin	Recessive
Stomatocytosis	Sodium channel permeability defect	Autosomal dominant

disordered cytoskeleton. Spherocytes reflect membrane loss that decreases the membrane-to-cytoplasm ratio. Because a high membrane-to-cytoplasm ratio is responsible for the flexible, biconcave shape of the normal erythrocyte, the erythrocyte loses its biconcave morphologic characteristics and assumes a spherocytic shape with loss of membrane. Spherocytes are less flexible and may be destroyed in the microvasculature. The laboratory finding characteristic of HS is increased osmotic fragility, caused by the loss of distensibility associated with a decrease in surface membrane. HS is usually a mild disorder with well-compensated hemolysis. Patients typically have exacerbations during infections or when given marrow-suppressing medication. Patients with significant hemolysis should receive folate supplementation. Many patients require cholecystectomy for pigment stones. Severe, symptomatic anemia is treated with splenectomy.

Hereditary elliptocytosis (HE) is caused by dominantly inherited mutations affecting the interaction between membrane proteins and underlying cytoplasmic proteins (see Table 49-7). The most common abnormalities affect the interactions with spectrin and protein 4.1, which causes the RBCs to assume an elliptical shape. As in HS, patients usually have mild hemolysis and splenomegaly. *Hereditary pyropoikilocytosis* (HPP) is a rare recessive disorder that is frequently caused by the inheritance of two different membrane disorders (e.g., one allele for HS and one for HE). Patients have severe hemolysis with microspherocytes and elliptocytes on the smear. As with HS, treatment for symptomatic anemia in HE and HPP is splenectomy (see Table 49-7).

Acquired Membrane Abnormalities
Paroxysmal Nocturnal Hemoglobinuria

Paroxysmal nocturnal hemoglobinuria (PNH) is an acquired clonal disease that is associated with an abnormality of complement regulation. Normal erythrocytes are protected from complement-mediated cell lysis by the presence of membrane proteins, including delay-accelerating factor (DAF, CD55) and membrane inhibitor of reactive lysis (MIRL, CD59). Both these proteins are members of a family of proteins that are anchored to the membrane by a glycosylphosphatidylinositol (GPI) anchor. Patients with PNH have clonal mutations in phosphatidylinositolglycan A (PIG-A), the enzyme required for the synthesis of GPI. These mutations arise in the hematopoietic stem cell, and all hematopoietic cells lack GPI-anchored proteins. Absence of GPI-anchored proteins from erythrocytes renders these erythrocytes susceptible to complement-mediated lysis. Traditional tests for PNH are functional assays based on the increased susceptibility of erythrocytes to lysis by acidic serum (Ham test) or hypotonic medium (sucrose lysis test). Now that the underlying molecular abnormality in PNH has been defined, diagnosis can be made by flow cytometric documentation of the absence of CD55 or CD59 on the surface of RBCs or leukocytes.

PNH is a clonal stem cell disorder with several unique characteristics. Patients suffer from episodic acute intravascular hemolysis with a release of free hemoglobin that results in the hemoglobinuria for which the disease is named. Patients are also susceptible to venous thrombotic complications, including Budd-Chiari syndrome, portal vein thrombosis, cerebrovascular thrombosis, and peripheral veins. The disease is associated with a risk for developing myelodysplasia, myelofibrosis, acute leukemia, or aplastic anemia. Furthermore, patients with aplastic anemia who respond to immunosuppressive therapy frequently develop PNH-like clones. In the past, treatment has been largely supportive. However, treatment with eculizumab, a monoclonal antibody that binds to the C5 component of complement, has been shown to reduce hemolysis, transfusion requirements, and thromboembolic events in this disease and was recently approved by the U.S. Food and Drug Administration for this indication. Young patients, however, should be considered for allogeneic stem cell transplantation.

Spur Cell Anemia

Spur cells (acanthocytes) are cells with abnormal morphologic membrane found in patients with advanced liver disease, severe malnutrition, malabsorption, and asplenia. The membrane acquires protrusions as a result of abnormal lipids present in the membrane. The changes may be associated with mild hemolysis, although in patients with advanced liver disease, separating hemolysis from hypersplenism is difficult. Similar changes may be observed in patients with abetalipoproteinemia.

HEMOLYTIC ANEMIAS CAUSED BY DISORDERS OF ERYTHROCYTE ENZYMES

Glucose-6 Phosphate Dehydrogenase Deficiency

Glucose-6-phosphate dehydrogenase (G6PD) is a critical enzyme in the hexose monophosphate shunt pathway. By maintaining intracellular stores of reduced glutathione, it protects erythrocytes from membrane and hemoglobin oxidation (Fig. 49-4). The gene for G6PD resides on the X chromosome, and therefore nearly all patients with G6PD deficiency are male. Most G6PD mutations are found in African and Mediterranean populations, likely because they confer resistance to malaria. The African form of G6PD deficiency is relatively mild, whereas the Mediterranean form is severe.

Absence of G6PD renders erythrocytes sensitive to oxidative stress. In the setting of infection, acidosis, or oxidant drugs, hemoglobin may precipitate within the cells, causing

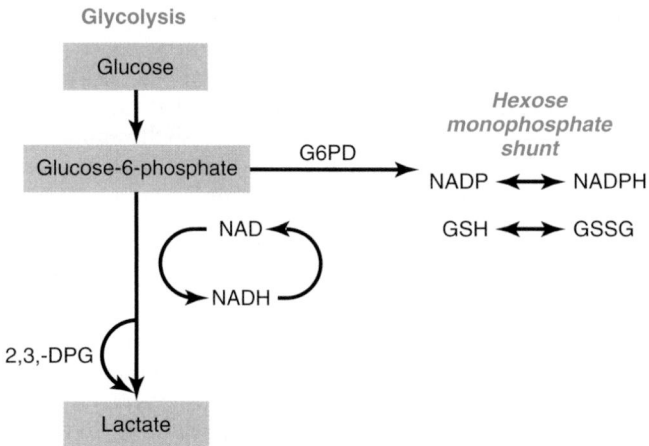

Figure 49-4 Metabolism of the red blood cell. 2,3-DPG, 2,3-diphosphoglycerate; G6PD, glucose-6-phosphate dehydrogenase; GSH, reduced glutathione; GSSG, reduced and oxidized glutathione; NAD, nicotinamide adenine dinucleotide; NADH, reduced form of NAD; NADP, nicotinamide adenine dinucleotide phosphate; NADPH, reduced form of NADP.

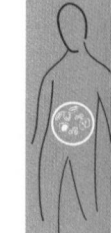

hemolysis. Many drugs are associated with hemolysis in the setting of G6PD deficiency, including sulfonamides, antimalarials, dapsone, aspirin, and phenacetin. Diagnosis should be considered in male patients of African American or Mediterranean extraction who have evidence of hemolysis in the setting of acute infection or recent exposure to oxidant drugs. Patients with the Mediterranean variant of G6PD deficiency may develop hemolysis on exposure to fava beans (favism). Cells with precipitated hemoglobin contain Heinz bodies that can be visualized with crystal violet staining of the peripheral blood smear. These inclusions are removed in the spleen, resulting in the additional finding of bite cells in the blood smear. Diagnosis can be confirmed with measurement of G6PD levels in the peripheral blood. However, reticulocytes and young RBCs in patients with G6PD deficiency have a higher enzyme level; consequently, if the diagnosis is probable, the patients with a normal G6PD level should be retested at a time removed from the acute episode, when the percentage of young RBCs is high. The mainstay of preventing hemolysis in these patients is the avoidance of oxidative stress, especially drugs implicated in causing hemolysis. Splenectomy is recommended only for patients with severe episodic or chronic hemolysis.

Other Enzyme Deficiencies

Enzyme deficiencies as rare causes of hemolytic anemia have been reported involving nearly all of the enzymes of the glycolytic pathway. The most common of these is pyruvate kinase deficiency. Autosomal genes encode these enzymes, and the pattern of inheritance is therefore autosomal recessive.

HEMOGLOBINOPATHIES

Hemoglobinopathies are mutations that result in the synthesis of quantitatively or qualitatively abnormal hemoglobins. The most common of these are the sickle syndromes and the thalassemias, which, like G6PD deficiency, arose in areas of the world in which malaria is endemic.

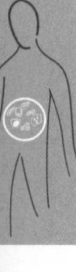

Sickle Cell Disease

Sickle cell disease is the most common of the sickle syndromes and arises from a point mutation that causes a glutamic acid-to-valine substitution in the sixth amino acid of the β-globin gene. It has arisen as an independent mutation in diverse populations in Africa, India, the Mediterranean, and the Middle East. The substitution of a hydrophobic for a hydrophilic residue renders the deoxygenated sickle hemoglobin (HbS) less soluble and therefore susceptible to polymerization and precipitation. The rate of precipitation of HbS is exquisitely sensitive to the intracorpuscular concentration of deoxygenated hemoglobin. Sickling is therefore increased in settings in which that concentration is increased either by changes in cellular hydration (dehydration) or by changes in the oxygen dissociation curve (e.g., hypoxia, acidosis, high altitude).

Acute Manifestations of Sickle Cell Disease

Most of the acute complications of sickle cell disease are related to vaso-occlusion (Table 49-8). Painful crises, secondary to occlusions of the microvasculature and ischemia of organs and tissues, can occur anywhere, with pain most common in the extremities, chest, abdomen, and back. Painful crises are commonly precipitated by infections, dehydration, rapid changes in temperature, and pregnancy. However, no obvious precipitating cause is often found for an acute painful crisis. Vaso-occlusion in the pulmonary circulation can be a particularly ominous complication of sickle cell disease, resulting in the *acute chest syndrome*, which is characterized by chest pain, hypoxemia, and pulmonary infiltrates. The roles of infection, infarction, and in situ thrombosis in the acute chest syndrome are indistinguishable, but all patients should receive antibiotics for presumed pneumonia. Because hypoxemia predisposes to further sickling and increasing respiratory compromise, the acute chest syndrome is life-threatening and is an indication for emergent exchange transfusion.

Neurologic events are a major cause of morbidity in patients with sickle cell disease. Acute large vessel occlusions occur in children, with a recurrence rate of 70% if untreated; such strokes are an indication for long-term exchange transfusion, which has been shown to decrease the rate of repeated occlusions. For reasons that are poorly understood, such large vessel occlusions rarely occur in adults. Adults may suffer hemorrhagic strokes as a result of aneurysmal dilation of proliferative vessels that form in response to repeated micro-occlusions in the cerebral vessels.

Any toxic or infectious insult that transiently suppresses bone marrow activity may cause an *aplastic crisis*. The shortened survival of the RBC in sickle cell disease renders the patients highly dependent on vigorous ongoing marrow activity, and short intervals of decreased reticulocyte formation can cause profound anemia. Most dramatic are infections associated with parvovirus B19, which directly infects erythroid precursors. Supportive care is usually all that is required. However, some patients may go on to develop bone marrow necrosis, with a leukoerythroblastic picture; this development may be further complicated by bone marrow embolization to the lungs.

Certain vascular beds are especially prone to complications of sickle cell disease. The renal medulla is highly susceptible to damage by vaso-occlusion because high tonicity and low oxygen tension both significantly increase the concentration of HbS. All patients with sickle cell disease develop defects in urinary concentration ability, and by adulthood, they are uniformly isosthenuric. Acute episodes of hematuria secondary to papillary necrosis are common.

The spleen is also a site in which recurrent sickling uniformly occurs. By adulthood, all patients have become functionally asplenic from repeated infarctions of the microvasculature. This contributing factor increases the susceptibility of patients with sickle cell disease to infections with encapsulated organisms. Acute infection remains a significant cause of death in patients with sickle cell disease. For unclear reasons, patients with sickle cell disease are particularly prone to osteomyelitis, with an unusually high incidence of *Salmonella* as the responsible organism.

Chronic Manifestations of Sickle Cell Disease

Sickle cell disease used to be a disease of childhood. As more patients with sickle cell disease survive to adulthood, it has become clear that repeated episodes of vaso-occlusion lead to damage to nearly every end organ (see Table 49-8). Renal failure and pulmonary failure are leading causes of death in adult patients with sickle cell disease. Other long-term complications include chronic skin ulcers, retinopathy, and liver dysfunction. In addition, most patients require cholecystectomy for pigment stones.

Treatment of Sickle Cell Disease

Treatment of sickle cell disease remains largely supportive. Painful crises are treated with fluid, oxygen supplementation, and analgesics. Patients with any indication of infection should receive antibiotics. Patients with symptomatic anemia should be transfused. Exchange transfusion is indicated for chest syndrome, stroke, bone marrow necrosis, and priapism. More controversial indications for exchange transfusion include intractable pain and slow response to other supportive measures. The goal of exchange transfusion is to

Table 49-8 **Clinical Manifestations of Sickle Cell Disease**
Acute Manifestations
Vaso-occlusive crisis
Painful crisis
Acute chest syndrome
Priapism
Cerebrovascular events
Thrombotic stroke
Hemorrhagic stroke
Aplastic crisis
Splenic sequestration
Osteomyelitis
Chronic Manifestations
Chronic renal disease
Isosthenuria
Chronic renal failure
Chronic pulmonary disease
Sickle hepatopathy
Proliferative retinopathy
Avascular necrosis
Skin ulcers

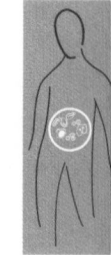

Table 49-9 **Thalassemic Syndromes**

Disorder	Genotypic Abnormality	Clinical Phenotype
β-thalassemia		
Thalassemia major (Cooley anemia)	Homozygous β^0-thalassemia	Severe hemolysis, ineffective erythropoiesis, transfusion dependency, iron overload
Thalassemia intermedia	Compound heterozygous β^0- and β^+-thalassemia	Moderate hemolysis, severe anemia, but not transfusion dependent; iron overload
Thalassemia minor	Heterozygous β^0- or β^+-thalassemia	Microcytosis, mild anemia
α-thalassemia		
Silent carrier	α-/αα	Normal complete blood count
α-thalassemia trait	αα/- - (α-thalassemia 1); *or* α-/α- (α-thalassemia 2)	Mild microcytic anemia
Hemoglobin H	α-/- -	Microcytic anemia and mild hemolysis; not transfusion dependent
Hydrops fetalis	- -/- -	Severe anemia, intrauterine anasarca from congestive heart failure; death in utero or at birth

achieve a level of 30% to 40% HbS. As previously noted, patients who have sustained a thrombotic large vessel stroke should undergo chronic exchange transfusion.

Treatment with hydroxyurea, an agent that increases the concentration of HbF in patients with sickle cell disease, reduces the incidence of vaso-occlusive crises. The efficacy of hydroxyurea in patients with recurrent crises has been demonstrated in a randomized study, and follow-up studies have revealed a survival advantage for patients treated with hydroxyurea. The effect is attributed to the formation of hemoglobin tetramers containing one B^s chain and one γ chain ($\alpha_2\beta^s\gamma$), which do not undergo polymerization. Studies have also suggested that response is related to decreases in leukocyte count and changes in endothelial adherence properties.

Other Sickle Syndromes
Hemoglobin C
Hemoglobin C (HbC) is caused by another substitution, glutamic acid to lysine, in the sixth position of the β-globin chain. Homozygous HbC causes very mild anemia symptoms and is usually clinically silent. Patients with hemoglobin S-C (HbSC) are compound heterozygotes for HbS and HbC. These patients are symptomatic, although the clinical manifestations are milder than in patients with homozygous HbS (HbSS). Patients have a higher hematocrit, and the higher viscosity increases the degree of retinopathy. They do not sustain splenic infarctions; unlike patients with HbSS, they usually have splenomegaly. Consequently, they occasionally have episodes of acute splenomegaly associated with profound decrease in hemoglobin and hematocrit (splenic sequestration crisis). Although such crises can also occur in children with HbSS, functional asplenia prevents this complication in adults with HbSS.

Sickle Cell β-Thalassemia
Patients who are double heterozygotes for HbS and β-thalassemia have a spectrum of disease dependent on the level of β globin that they produce. Sickle cell β^+-thalassemia is a milder disease than HbSS, probably because of the decreased intracorpuscular concentration of HbS. Patients with sickle cell β^0-thalassemia (see discussion that follows)

produce no normal β chains and have essentially the same phenotype as patients with HbSS.

Thalassemia
The thalassemic syndromes (Table 49-9) are a heterogeneous group of disorders associated with decreased or absent synthesis of either α- or β-globin chains. Severe thalassemic syndromes are associated with severe hemolytic anemia and are diagnosed in early childhood. However, mild forms of thalassemia minor frequently cause mild microcytic anemia with little or no evidence of hemolysis. These syndromes are often confused with iron deficiency because of the decreased MCV.

β-Thalassemia
Over 100 mutations have been described that lead to β-thalassemia, causing a decrease or absence of expression from the β-globin locus. The decreased expression of β globin can be caused by structural mutations in the coding region of the gene, resulting in nonsense mutations, truncated messenger RNA (mRNA), and no expression of intact globin from the affected allele (β^0-thalassemia). However, a large number of mutations that result in decreased transcription or translation or altered splicing of the β-globin mRNA may result in reduction but not elimination of globin-chain expression from the affected allele (β^+-thalassemia).

Defective globin-chain synthesis in β-thalassemia causes both decreased normal hemoglobin production and the production of a relative excess of α chains. The decrease in normal hemoglobin synthesis results in a hypochromic anemia, and the excess α chains form insoluble α-chain complexes and cause hemolysis. In mild thalassemic syndromes, the excess α chains are insufficient to cause significant hemolysis, and the primary finding is a microcytic anemia. In severe forms of thalassemia, hemolysis occurs both in the periphery and in the marrow, with intense secondary expansion of the marrow production of red cells. The expansion of the marrow space causes severe skeletal abnormalities, and the ineffective erythropoiesis also provides a powerful stimulus to absorb iron from the intestine.

The clinical spectrum of β-thalassemia reflects the heterogeneity of the molecular lesions causing the disease (see

Table 49-9). β-thalassemia major results from homozygous β⁰-thalassemia, leading to severe hemolytic anemia; such patients are diagnosed in infancy and are transfusion dependent from birth. β-thalassemia intermedia patients also have two β-thalassemia alleles, but at least one of them is a mild β⁺ mutation. These patients have severe chronic hemolytic anemia but do not require transfusions. Because of ineffective erythropoiesis, these patients chronically hyperabsorb iron and may develop iron overload in the absence of transfusions. β-thalassemia minor is usually due to heterozygous β-thalassemia, although it may reflect the inheritance of two mild thalassemic mutations. These are the patients in whom iron deficiency is often misdiagnosed. Iron studies will show normal to increased iron with normal iron saturation. Documenting a compensatory increase in HbA_2 and HbF will confirm the diagnosis.

α-Thalassemia

α-thalassemia is nearly always caused by mutations that delete one or more of the α-chain loci on chromosome 16. Four α-chain loci exist with two nearly identical copies of the α-globin gene on each chromosome. The spectrum of α-thalassemia therefore reflects whether the patient lacks one, two, three, or all four α-globin genes (see Table 49-9).

In general, the clinical manifestations of α-thalassemia are milder than those of β-thalassemia for two reasons. First, the presence of four α-chain genes allows for adequate α-chain synthesis unless three or four loci are deleted. Second, β-chain tetramers are more soluble than their α-chain counterparts and do not cause hemolysis. Patients with the loss of a single α-chain gene are silent carriers and have a normal hematocrit and MCV. Patients with the deletion of two α chains, either on the same chromosome (- -/αα; α-thal 1) or on different chromosomes (α-/α-; α-thal 2), are microcytic and mildly anemic. Patients who inherit one α-thal 1 allele and one α-thal 2 allele (- -/α-) have hemoglobin H disease. Hemoglobin H is the product of excess β-chain production, specifically $β_4$; it causes mild hemolytic anemia and minimal or no intramedullary erythrocyte destruction. Inheritance of the homozygous α-thal 2 allele results in no functional α-chain loci and is incompatible with life. The fetus is unable to make any functional hemoglobin beyond embryonic development because HbF also requires α chains. Free γ chains form tetramers, termed *hemoglobin Barts*. Hemoglobin Barts have an extremely high oxygen affinity, and failure to release oxygen in peripheral tissues results in severe congestive heart failure and anasarca, a clinical picture termed *hydrops fetalis*. Affected fetuses are stillborn or die soon after birth.

Prospectus for the Future

Anemia is increasingly recognized as a marker of increased morbidity and mortality in adults with a wide range of medical conditions, including renal failure, malignancy, cardiac disease, inflammatory conditions, and other chronic diseases. Studies are ongoing to evaluate the effect of treating anemia on patients' outcome and quality of life. Furthermore, advances in our pathophysiologic understanding of anemia of chronic disease are contributing to our knowledge of iron metabolism and the role cytokines play in hematopoiesis. These developments are paving the way for the development of new therapies for patients with anemia or iron overload. Ongoing progress in prenatal diagnosis and stem cell transplantation will contribute to our ability to prevent and treat the thalassemic syndromes and other hemoglobinopathies.

References

Andrews NC: Forging a field: The golden age of iron biology. Blood 112;219-230, 2008.

Bain BJ: Diagnosis from the blood smear. N Engl J Med 353:498-507, 2005.

Marks PW, Glader B: Approach to anemia in the adult and child. In Hoffman R, Benz EJ, Shatill SJ, et al (eds): Hematology: Basic Principles and Practice, 4th ed. New York, Churchill Livingstone, 2005, pp 455-464.

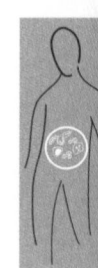

Clinical Disorders of Neutrophils

Michal G. Rose and Nancy Berliner

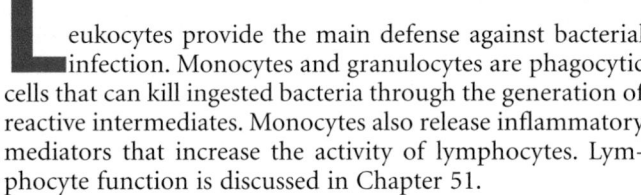

Leukocytes provide the main defense against bacterial infection. Monocytes and granulocytes are phagocytic cells that can kill ingested bacteria through the generation of reactive intermediates. Monocytes also release inflammatory mediators that increase the activity of lymphocytes. Lymphocyte function is discussed in Chapter 51.

Normal Granulocyte Development, Structure, and Function

NEUTROPHILS

Neutrophils (*polymorphonuclear leukocytes*) are the predominant white blood cell in the peripheral blood. They are morphologically recognizable by their characteristic segmented nucleus. They also contain various cytoplasmic granules that give them a characteristic appearance and are functionally important (Fig. 50-1).

Neutrophil killing of bacteria requires chemotaxis, phagocytosis, and intracellular killing (Fig. 50-2). *Chemotaxis* is the ordered movement of the cell toward an attracting stimulus, such as bacterial formyl peptides or complement fragments (C3b and C5a). Neutrophils adhere to endothelial cells by interaction of neutrophil surface glycoproteins (CD11b/CD18) with endothelial adhesion molecules (intracellular adhesion molecule-1 and endothelial leukocyte adhesion molecule-1), a process termed *margination*. In response to a chemotactic stimulus, these adherent neutrophils move toward the target along the endothelial surface. The syndrome of leukocyte-adhesion deficiency underscores the importance of neutrophil adhesion as the first step in bacterial killing. This rare congenital disease is caused by the absence of surface expression of the CD11b/CD18 complex on neutrophils. Neutrophils fail to adhere to endothelium, are unable to undergo chemotaxis, and do not phagocytose or kill bacteria. Patients have severe, life-threatening bacterial infections despite high levels of circulating neutrophils.

Phagocytosis requires recognition of target bacteria or debris by the neutrophil. Targets are *opsonized* by the surface binding of immunoglobulin or complement factor C3b. The neutrophil has surface receptors for C3b and the Fc portion of immunoglobulin G, which allows recognition and binding to the opsonized target. The target then becomes engulfed in a phagocytic vacuole, which fuses with neutrophil granules inside the cell.

Intracellular killing occurs by both oxygen-dependent and oxygen-independent mechanisms. Contents of the primary granules, including cathepsin G, defensins, and lysozyme, act to break down the bacterial cell wall and kill the target organism. The major mechanism of bacterial killing, however, is the *respiratory burst*. Stimulation of the neutrophil activates a membrane-bound oxidase complex, which generates superoxide through the transfer of an electron from reduced nicotinamide-adenine dinucleotide phosphate (NADPH). The interaction of superoxide with water generates hydroxyl ions. In addition, myeloperoxidase catalyzes the formation of hypochlorite ion from hydrogen peroxide and chloride. The NADPH oxidase is a multisubunit enzyme. Absence or decreased activity of any one subunit impairs bacterial killing and results in chronic granulomatous disease, another congenital illness in which patients are predisposed to life-threatening bacterial infections.

The granules that give neutrophils their characteristic appearance have important functions in the process of neutrophil-mediated activation and killing. *Primary granules* arise early in myeloid differentiation and are found in both neutrophils and monocytes. They contain a large number of proteins, including myeloperoxidase, acid hydrolases, and neutral proteases. These granules fuse with the phagocytic vacuole and aid in the digestion of ingested bacteria. *Secondary granules* arise later in the differentiation pathway and give the neutrophil its characteristic granular appearance. These granules contain lactoferrin, transcobalamin, and the matrix-modifying enzymes collagenase and gelatinase. On neutrophil stimulation, these granules are released into the extracellular space. Lactoferrin and transcobalamin act as antibacterial proteins by sequestering iron and vitamin B_{12}

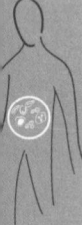

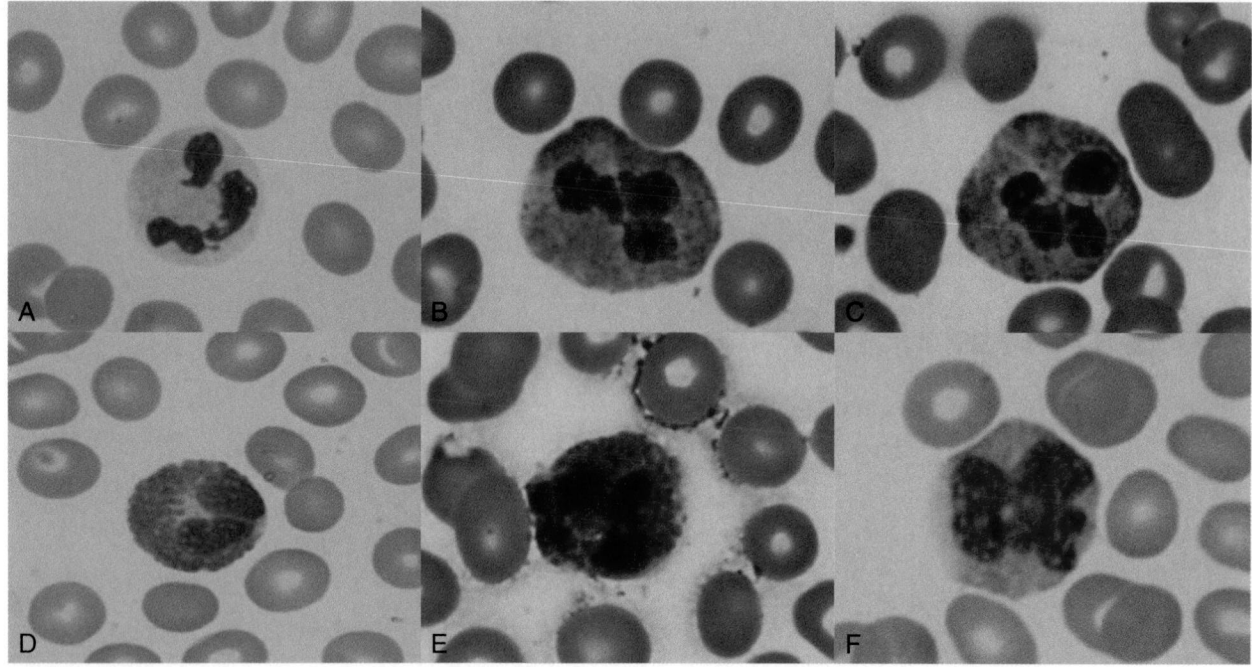

Figure 50-1 Normal granulocytes and monocytes in peripheral blood. **A to C,** Neutrophils (polymorphonuclear cells). **D,** Eosinophils. **E,** Basophils. **F,** Monocytes. (Courtesy of Robert J. Homer, MD, PhD.)

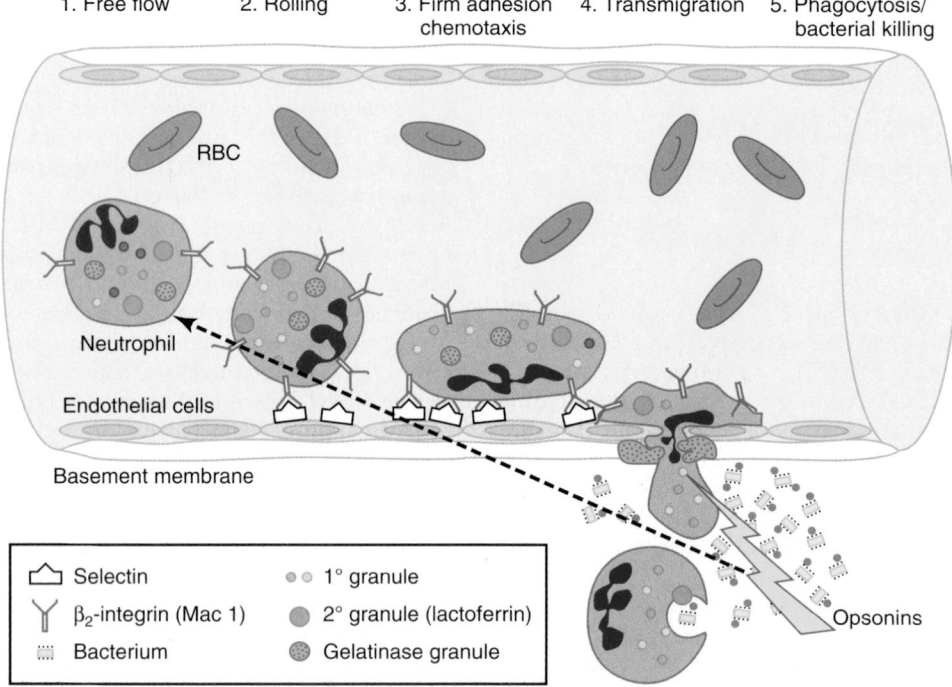

Figure 50-2 Sequence of neutrophil activation that shows the process of rolling, engagement with the vessel wall, attachment, diapedesis, and phagocytosis.

away from bacteria, and collagenase and gelatinase break down connective tissues at the site of inflammation. Abnormalities in neutrophil granules have been described in rare clinical syndromes. Absence of myeloperoxidase produces surprisingly mild symptoms and may be associated with defects in control of fungal infection. Secondary granule deficiency is extremely rare and is associated with a slight increase in the risk for bacterial infections.

EOSINOPHILS AND BASOPHILS

Eosinophils and basophils arise from myeloid precursors in the bone marrow. They transit rapidly from the marrow to the blood and into the peripheral tissues, where they play a role in allergic and inflammatory reactions. Like neutrophils, they have secondary granules that give them their characteristic appearance and are also functionally impor-

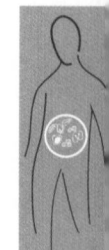

Table 50-1 **Differential Diagnosis of Eosinophilia**

Reactive

Infection

Especially parasites; more rarely mycobacteria

Allergic Diseases

Drugs, asthma, allergic rhinitis, atopy, urticaria

Pulmonary Diseases

Churg-Strauss disease, Loeffler pneumonia, pulmonary infiltrates with eosinophilia (PIE)

Drug Reactions

Usually disappears when drug discontinued

Malignancy

Paraneoplastic, angioimmunoblastic T-cell lymphoma, Hodgkin and non-Hodgkin lymphoma

Connective Tissue Diseases

Rheumatoid arthritis, eosinophilic fasciitis, vasculitis

Primary Hypereosinophilic Syndrome

More than 6 months with eosinophils >1500, with no other apparent cause

tant. Both cell types are present in small numbers under normal conditions.

Although eosinophils are capable of phagocytosis, most of the activity of these cells is mediated through the release of their granules. Their numbers are elevated in parasitic and helminthic infections, in which these cells are thought to play a role in the allergic response to those organisms. Numbers of these cells are also elevated in allergic reactions and in collagen vascular diseases, again linking their function to immunomodulation. *Hypereosinophilic syndromes*, in which extremely high levels of eosinophils can be seen, are rare, and they can be associated with damage to the lung, peripheral nervous system, and endocardial tissues. The differential diagnosis of eosinophilia is outlined in Table 50-1. Basophils appear to play a role in immediate hypersensitivity reactions and chronic inflammatory conditions. Their levels are increased in chronic myeloid leukemia.

MONOCYTES

Monocytes arise from a common myeloid precursor with granulocytes, under the influence of granulocyte-macrophage colony-stimulating factor (GM-CSF) and macrophage colony-stimulating factor (M-CSF). Most circulating monocytes are marginated along the walls of vessels. They migrate from the vessels into tissues, where they develop into macrophages. The monocyte-macrophage lineage has many diverse functions. These phagocytic cells perform chemotaxis, phagocytosis, and intracellular killing in much the same manner as neutrophils. They are especially important in the killing of mycobacteria, fungi, and protozoal species.

In addition to their role in killing of infectious organisms, monocytes have important interaction with other components of the immune system. They are antigen-presenting cells for T lymphocytes, they are capable of cellular cytotoxicity, and they secrete certain cytokines. The macrophages that process antigens and present them to T lymphocytes take on different forms in different tissues. They include the

Langerhans cells of the skin, the interdigitating cells of the thymus, and the dendritic cells in the lymph nodes. Antigen-presenting cells are nonphagocytic, and the process by which they internalize antigen is not fully understood. Protein antigens are partially digested and expressed on the cell surface in association with human leukocyte or Ia antigens. This feature permits interaction with and activation of helper T cells. Other macrophages, such as Kupffer cells of the liver and alveolar macrophages of the lung, play an important role in removing particulate and cellular debris and senescent erythrocytes from circulation.

Monocytes also have a role in tumor cell cytotoxicity. They are capable of both antibody-dependent and antibody-independent cytotoxicity against tumor cells. The cytotoxicity is increased by tumor necrosis factor, interleukin-1, and interferon, all of which are also secreted by monocytes. Monocytes secrete a large number of proteins. These include immunomodulatory proteins (tumor necrosis factor, interleukin-1, and interferon), cytokines (granulocyte colony-stimulating factor [G-CSF] and GM-CSF), coagulation proteins, cell adhesion proteins, and proteases.

Determinants of Peripheral Neutrophil Number

Most granulocyte precursors are in the bone marrow, where maturation occurs over 6 to 10 days. Marrow precursors represent 20% of the granulocyte mass, and the storage pool represents 75% of the granulocyte mass. Therefore, peripheral neutrophils represent only 5% of the total granulocyte mass. Furthermore, neutrophils circulate in transit between the marrow and peripheral tissues. Of the circulating neutrophils, more than one half are adherent to the vascular endothelium. Again, this process is termed *margination*. The half-life of a neutrophil in the circulation is short, usually only 6 to 12 hours; the neutrophil may then migrate into tissues, where it survives another 1 to 4 days. Therefore, the peripheral neutrophil count represents a sampling of less than 5% of the total granulocyte pool and is taken during a period of less than 5% of the total neutrophil life span. The peripheral white cell count is therefore a poor reflection of granulocyte kinetics. Abnormalities in neutrophil number can occur rapidly and may reflect either a change in marrow granulocyte production or a shift among various cellular compartments. An elevated peripheral white cell count may result from increased marrow production, or it may reflect mobilization of neutrophils from the marginated pool or release from the marrow storage pool. Similarly, a low granulocyte count may reflect decreased marrow production, increased margination or sequestration in the spleen, or increased destruction of peripheral cells.

The *total peripheral white cell count* represents the sum of lymphocytes and granulocytes. The significance of an elevated or depressed leukocyte count therefore depends on the nature of the cellular elements that are increased or decreased. *Leukocytosis* is a nonspecific term that may denote an increase in either lymphocytes (*lymphocytosis*) or neutrophils (*granulocytosis*). In rare cases, increases may reflect excessive numbers of monocytes or eosinophils.

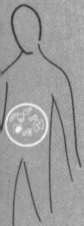

Leukocytosis related to an elevation in the neutrophil count is referred to as *neutrophil leukocytosis,* or *neutrophilia.* Extreme elevation of the white blood cell count to more than 50,000/mcL with the premature release of early myeloid precursors is termed a *leukemoid reaction;* this reaction may be associated with inflammatory reactions and infections, but it requires consideration of a diagnosis of myeloproliferative disease, especially chronic myelogenous leukemia. Evaluation of the peripheral blood smear may reveal characteristic changes that provide clues to the underlying disorder. A *leukoerythroblastic* smear shows the presence of immature granulocytes, teardrop-shaped erythrocytes, nucleated erythrocytes, and increased platelets. Such changes are reflective of marrow infiltration (*myelophthisis*) by fibrous tissue, granulomas, or neoplasm. As with leukocytosis, *leukopenia* may reflect either lymphopenia or *neutropenia.* Neutropenia is defined as an absolute neutrophil count of less than 1500/mcL.

Evaluation of Leukocytosis (Neutrophilia)

Leukocytosis is usually secondary to other processes, and it rarely indicates a primary hematologic disorder (Table 50-2). However, patients with persistent elevation of the neutrophil count, especially in association with elevation of the hematocrit or platelet count, should be evaluated to rule out a primary myeloproliferative disorder. A leukocyte alkaline phosphatase determination is helpful in ruling out chronic myelogenous leukemia because it tends to be low in this condition and normal or high in other myeloproliferative disorders and in leukemoid reactions.

Neutrophilia related to acute infection, stress, or acute steroid administration primarily reflects demargination and is usually transient. Persistent neutrophilia usually reflects chronic bone marrow stimulation. Nevertheless, bone

marrow aspirate and biopsy are rarely indicated in the workup of neutrophilia. The exception is in those patients who demonstrate leukoerythroblastic changes, in which a bone marrow examination and culture may be indicated to rule out tuberculosis or fungal infection, marrow infiltration with tumor, or marrow fibrosis. Cytogenetic and molecular studies should also be performed to help eliminate the diagnosis of chronic myelogenous leukemia and other myeloproliferative disorders.

Evaluation of Leukopenia (Neutropenia)

DIFFERENTIAL DIAGNOSIS OF NEUTROPENIA

Neutropenia can reflect decreased production, increased sequestration, or peripheral destruction of neutrophils (Table 50-3). Patients should first be evaluated for splenomegaly to rule out the possibility of sequestration. In patients who are completely asymptomatic and in whom previous studies are unavailable, the possibility of *constitutional* or *cyclic neutropenia* should be entertained and can be evaluated by serial peripheral blood counts. The normal neutrophil count varies among ethnic groups and is lower in African Americans (*constitutional neutropenia*) than it is in Caucasians. *Cyclic neutropenia* is a relatively benign disorder, in which cyclical changes occur in all hematopoietic cell lines but are most dramatic in the neutrophil lineage. At the nadir of the neutrophil counts, patients may have infections, but the disease is often clinically silent. In contrast, patients with congenital agranulocytosis or *severe congenital neutropenia* (SCN) exhibit profound neutropenia and infections in the perinatal period. *Kostmann syndrome* is a subset of SCN that was described 50 years ago as an autosomal recessive disorder; more recent studies have demonstrated that SCN may be autosomal dominant, autosomal recessive, and sporadic, and that the etiologies are also heterogeneous. About 50%

Table 50-2 **Differential Diagnosis of Neutrophilia**
Primary Hematologic Disease
Congenital
Myeloproliferative disorders
Secondary to Other Disease Processes
Infection
Acute
Chronic
Acute stress
Drugs
Steroids
Lithium
Cytokine stimulation (e.g., granulocyte colony-simulating factor)
Chronic inflammation
Malignancy
Myelophthisis
Marrow hyperstimulation
Chronic hemolysis, immune thrombocytopenia
Recovery from marrow suppression
Postsplenectomy
Smoking

Table 50-3 **Differential Diagnosis of Neutropenia**
Decreased Production of Neutrophils
Congenital and/or constitutional
Constitutional neutropenia
Benign chronic neutropenia
Kostmann syndrome
Benign cyclic neutropenia
Postinfectious
Nutritional deficiency (B_{12}, folate)
Drug induced
Primary marrow failure
Aplastic anemia
Myelodysplasia
Acute leukemia
Increased Peripheral Destruction
Overwhelming infection
Immune destruction
Drug related
Associated with collagen vascular disease
Isoimmune (in newborn)
Large granular lymphocyte leukemia
Hypersplenism and/or sequestration

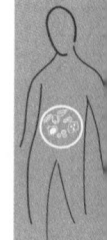

of autosomal dominant SCN, as well as virtually 100% of cyclic neutropenia, is associated with inherited mutations in the neutrophil elastase gene. These mutations are thought to result in the production of misfolded neutrophil elastase protein, which accumulates in the endoplasmic reticulum and activates the unfolded protein response. This complex cellular stress response coordinates the degradation of misfolded protein in the endoplasmic reticulum and can trigger cellular apoptosis if the stress is severe. Evidence suggests that different neutrophil elastase mutations activate the unfolded protein response to varying degrees, thus explaining how mutations in the same gene can cause both congenital agranulocytosis and the more benign cyclic neutropenia. More recent studies have established that autosomal recessive SCN (Kostmann syndrome) is caused by mutations in the *HAX-1* gene, a mitochondrial protein that is required for stabilization of the mitochondrial membrane. Absence of *HAX-1* results in loss of mitochondrial membrane potential and induction of apoptosis.

Until G-CSF became available, most patients with SCN died in early childhood, but the availability of cytokine therapy has prolonged survival. However, SCN is also associated with a significantly increased incidence of the development of acute leukemia, a complication that has become apparent as patients survive longer. Up to 20% of patients with SCN will develop acute myelogenous leukemia over 10 years. Acute myelogenous leukemia in these patients is often associated with truncation mutations in the G-CSF receptor. These are acquired somatic mutations that may contribute to the pathogenesis of leukemia but do not contribute to the congenital neutropenia. The role of these G-CSF receptor mutations in the pathogenesis of leukemic transformation is controversial.

Neutropenia may occur during or after viral, bacterial, or mycobacterial infections. *Postviral neutropenia* is especially common in children and probably reflects both increased neutrophil consumption and a viral suppression of marrow neutrophil production. Neutropenia may be seen as a complication of *overwhelming sepsis* and is associated with a poor prognosis.

Drug-induced neutropenia may reflect either dose-dependent marrow suppression or an idiosyncratic immune response. The former is one of the most common complications of chemotherapeutic drugs and is also common with antibiotics such as trimethoprim-sulfamethoxazole. Chloramphenicol causes dose-dependent marrow suppression, although its more ominous complication is the rare idiosyncratic reaction that gives rise to marrow aplasia. The drugs that are most commonly associated with neutropenia include clozapine, sulfasalazine, ticlopidine, and the thionamide antithyroid agents. Most drug-induced neutropenias respond rapidly to discontinuation of the offending agent. The administration of G-CSF speeds recovery.

Autoimmune neutropenia may be seen as a primary disease or as a secondary manifestation of systemic autoimmune disease or lymphoproliferative disease. Primary autoimmune neutropenia is a disorder of infants and young children that resolves spontaneously in more than 90% of patients within 2 years. Secondary autoimmune neutropenia is a common accompaniment to systemic lupus. Although not usually clinically severe, neutropenia is often a marker of disease activity. Neutropenia in rheumatoid arthritis is seen in association with splenomegaly (Felty syndrome) and also as part of the spectrum of large granular lymphocyte leukemia (LGL). LGL leukemia is a clonal expansion of suppressor T cells. Patients who develop LGL in association with rheumatoid arthritis share a common HLA-DR4 haplotype with patients with Felty syndrome, suggesting that these are in a common spectrum of disease. LGL is also a relatively common cause of acquired neutropenia in elderly patients in the absence of rheumatoid arthritis.

LABORATORY EVALUATION OF NEUTROPENIA

Unless the diagnosis of benign or cyclic neutropenia is likely, the evaluation of the patient with neutropenia should include stopping all potentially offending drugs and performing serologic studies to rule out collagen vascular disease. Unlike in patients with leukocytosis, bone marrow examination is indicated early in the evaluation and is frequently diagnostic. Neutropenia more often reflects primary hematologic disease, and bone marrow examination enables one to diagnose marrow failure syndromes, leukemia, and myelodysplasia. In the absence of bone marrow failure, other causes of neutropenia also may give a characteristic bone marrow picture. Drug-induced neutropenia produces a characteristic *maturation arrest* of the myeloid series. Rather than an actual inhibition of neutrophil maturation, this feature reflects the immune destruction of myeloid precursors that leaves only the earliest cells behind. All patients should have cytogenetic studies performed to aid in the diagnosis of myelodysplasia.

MANAGEMENT OF NEUTROPENIA

The therapeutic approach to patients with neutropenia depends on the degree of depression of the neutrophil count. Neutrophil counts between 1000 and 1500/mcL are not usually associated with any significant impairment in the host response to bacterial infection and require no intervention beyond what is demanded for diagnosis and indicated therapy of the underlying cause. Patients with neutrophil counts between 500 and 1000/mcL should be alerted to their slightly increased risk for infection, although serious problems are rarely encountered in patients with functional neutrophils and counts higher than 500/mcL. Patients with neutrophil counts lower than 500/mcL are at significant risk for infection. Such patients must be instructed to notify the physician at the first signs of infection or fever, and they must be managed aggressively with intravenous antibiotics regardless of the documentation of a source or infecting organism. Patients with a significantly depressed neutrophil count may exhibit few signs of infection because much of the inflammatory response at the site of infection is generated by the neutrophils themselves. In patients with severe immune-mediated neutropenia, steroids and intravenous immunoglobulin may be helpful in elevating the neutrophil count and in preventing infectious complications. G-CSF may increase the peripheral white cell count and may help resolve infections in neutropenia induced by drugs, including chemotherapy. It has also been efficacious in some patients with immune neutropenia as well as in patients with myelodysplasia.

Prospectus for the Future

Significant progress has been made in recent years regarding the elucidation of the molecular pathogenesis of severe congenital neutropenia and cyclic neutropenia. Compounds that modulate the unfolded protein response may play a role in the treatment of these disorders. Other studies aimed at elucidating the molecular basis for myeloid differentiation are establishing the importance of transcription factor function in neutrophil maturation and are providing insights into the pathogenesis of leukemia and myelodysplasia. Such insights may delineate pathways with entry points for therapeutic intervention in myeloid malignancy.

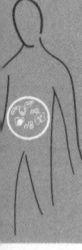

References

Baehner R: Normal phagocyte structure and function. In Hoffman R, Benz EJ, Shattil SJ (eds): Hematology: Basic Principles and Practice, 4th ed. New York, Churchill Livingstone, 2005, pp 737-762.

Berliner N, Horwitz M, Loughran TP Jr: Congenital and acquired neutropenia. Hematology (American Society of Hematology Education Program) 1:63-79, 2004.

Dinauer MC, Coates TD: Disorders of phagocyte function and number. In Hoffman R, Benz EJ, Shattil SJ (eds): Hematology: Basic Principles and Practice, 4th ed. New York, Churchill Livingstone, 2005, pp 787-830.

Rose MG, Berliner N: T-cell suppressor disorders. Oncologist 9:247-258, 2004.

Xia J, Link DC: Severe congenital neutropenia and the unfolded protein response. Curr Opin Hematol 15:1-7, 2008.

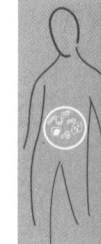

Disorders of Lymphocytes

Jill Lacy and Stuart Seropian

The central cell of the immune system is the lymphocyte. Lymphocytes mediate the adaptive immune response, providing specificity to the immune system by responding to specific pathogens and conferring long-lasting immunity to reinfection. Lymphocytes are derived from pluripotent hematopoietic stem cells that reside in the bone marrow and give rise to all of the cellular elements of the blood. Two major functional classes of lymphocytes have been developed: (1) B lymphocytes, or B cells, and (2) T lymphocytes, or T cells, which are distinguished by their site of development, antigenic receptors, and function. The major disorders of lymphocytes include (1) neoplastic transformation of specific subsets of lymphocytes resulting in an array of lymphomas or leukemias, (2) congenital and acquired defects in lymphocyte development or function with resultant immunodeficiency syndromes, and (3) physiologic responses to infection or antigenic stimulation that may lead to lymphadenopathy, lymphocytosis, or lymphocytopenia.

Cells of the Immune System: Lymphocyte Development, Function, and Localization

B CELLS

B cells are characterized by the presence of cell surface immunoglobulin (or antibody). Their major function is to mount a humoral immune response to antigens by producing antigen-specific antibody. B cells develop in the bone marrow in a series of highly coordinated steps that involve sequential rearrangement of the heavy- and light-chain immunoglobulin genes and expression of B-cell–specific cell surface proteins (Fig. 51-1). Rearrangement of the immunoglobulin genes results in the generation of a huge repertoire of B cells that are each characterized by an immunoglobulin molecule with unique antigenic specificity. Mature B cells migrate from the bone marrow to lymphoid tissue throughout the body and are readily identified by the presence of cell surface immunoglobulin and antigens that are B-cell specific, including CD19, CD20, and CD21. In response to antigen binding to cell surface immunoglobulin, mature B cells are activated to proliferate and undergo differentiation into end-stage plasma cells, which lose most of their B-cell surface markers and produce large quantities of soluble antibodies. Neoplastic disorders of B cells arise from B cells at different stages of development, and thus B-cell lymphomas can be highly varied in their morphologic mechanisms and cell surface expression of B-cell antigens, or immunophenotype.

T CELLS

T cells perform an array of functions in the immune response, including those that are classically regarded as cellular immune responses. T-cell precursors migrate from the bone marrow to the thymus, where they differentiate into mature T-cell subsets and undergo selection to eliminate autoreactive T cells that respond to self-peptides. In the thymus, T-cell precursors undergo a coordinated process of differentiation that involves rearrangement and expression of the T-cell receptor (TCR) genes and acquisition of cell surface proteins that are unique to T cells, including CD3, CD4, and CD8. As T cells mature in the thymus, they ultimately lose either the CD4 or CD8 protein, and thus mature T cells are composed of two major groups: CD4$^+$ and CD8$^+$ cells. After T-cell maturation and selection in the thymus, mature CD4 and CD8 T cells leave the thymus and migrate to lymph nodes, spleen, and other sites in the peripheral immune system. Mature T cells constitute about 80% of peripheral blood lymphocytes, 40% of lymph node cells, and 25% of splenic lymphoid cells.

Mature CD4 and CD8 T-cell subsets mediate distinct immune functions. CD8$^+$ cells kill virus-infected or foreign cells and suppress immune functions; thus, CD8 cells are designated cytotoxic T cells. CD4$^+$ cells activate other

CENTRAL HEMATOPOIETIC TISSUES   PERIPHERAL TISSUES

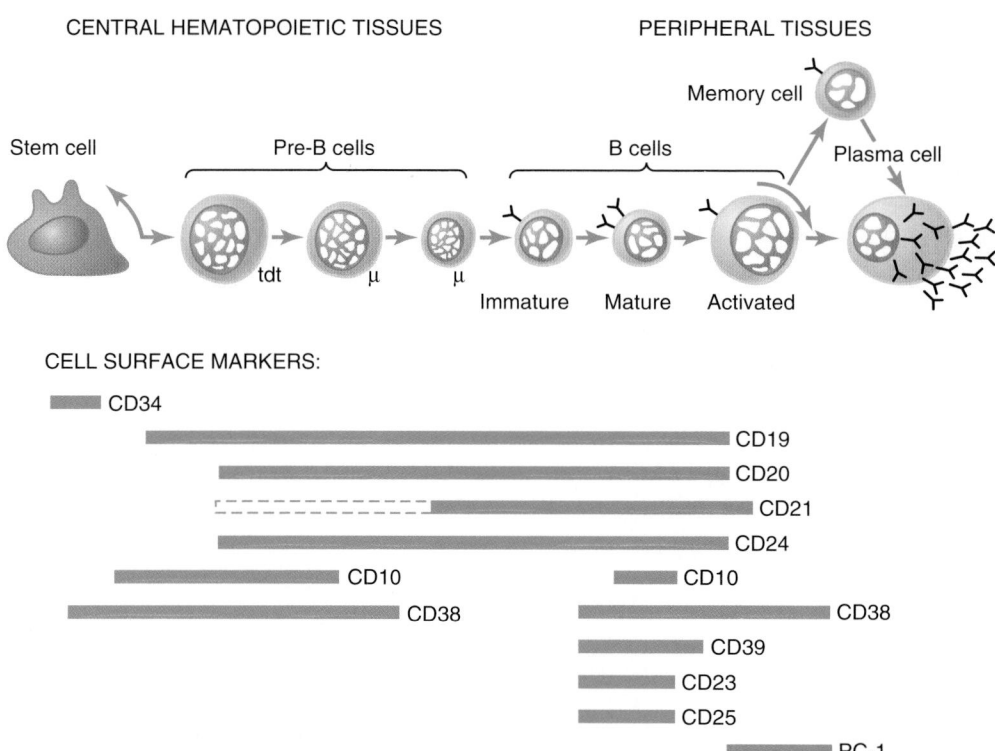

Figure 51-1 The maturation of B lymphocytes. *Top,* The changes in immunoglobulin production and maturation. *Bottom,* The appearance and disappearance of surface markers. (Adapted from Ferrarini M, Grossi CE, Cooper MD: Cellular and molecular biology of lymphoid cells. In Handin RI, Lux SE, Stossel TP [eds]: Blood Principles and Practice of Hematology. Philadelphia, JB Lippincott, 1995, p 643.)

immune response cells such as B cells and macrophages by producing cytokines and direct cell contact; thus, CD4 cells are considered helper T cells. Similar to B cells, T cells express unique TCR molecules that recognize specific peptide antigens. In contrast to B cells, T cells only respond to peptides that are processed intracellularly and bound to (or presented by) specialized cell surface antigen-presenting proteins, designated major histocompatibility complex (MHC) molecules. Furthermore, CD4 and CD8 T cells are MHC class restricted in their response to peptide-MHC complexes. CD4 cells recognize antigenic peptide fragments only when they are presented by MHC class II molecules, and CD8 cells recognize antigenic peptide fragments only when they are presented by MHC class I molecules. Antigenic peptides complexed with MHC class I and class II molecules originate from different sources. MHC class I molecules generally produce intracellular or endogenous antigens that are processed in the cytosol and traffic through the endoplasmic reticulum. MHC class II molecules generally produce antigens derived from extracellular sources taken up by endocytosis and processed in intracellular vesicles. Binding of the TCR by a specific peptide-MHC complex triggers activation signals that lead to the expression of gene products that mediate the wide diversity of helper functions in CD4$^+$ cells or cytotoxic effector functions in CD8$^+$ cells.

LYMPHOID SYSTEM

Lymphocytes localize to the peripheral lymphoid tissue, which is the site of antigen-lymphocyte interaction and lymphocyte activation. The peripheral lymphoid tissue is com-posed of lymph nodes, the spleen, and mucosal lymphoid tissue. Lymphocytes circulate continuously through these tissues through the vascular and lymphatic systems.

The lymph nodes are highly organized lymphoid tissues that are sites of convergence of the lymphatic drainage system that carries antigens from draining lymph to the nodes, where they are trapped. A lymph node consists of an outer cortex and an inner medulla (Fig. 51-2). The cortex is organized into lymphoid follicles composed predominantly of B cells; some of the follicles contain central areas or germinal centers, where activated B cells are undergoing proliferation after encountering a specific antigen, surrounded by a mantle zone. The T cells are distributed more diffusely in paracortical areas surrounding the follicles. The spleen traps antigens from blood rather than from the lymphatic system and is the site of disposal of senescent red cells. The lymphocytes in the spleen reside in the areas described as the white pulp, which surround the arterioles entering the organ. As in lymph nodes, the B and T cells are segregated into a periarteriolar lymphoid sheath that is composed of T cells and flanking follicles composed of B cells. The mucosa-associated lymphoid tissues (MALTs) collect antigen from epithelial surfaces and include the gut-associated lymphoid tissue (tonsils, adenoids, appendix, and Peyer patches of the small intestine) as well as more diffusely organized aggregates of lymphocytes at other mucosal sites.

Lymphocytes circulate in the peripheral blood and represent 20% to 40% of peripheral blood leukocytes in adults (the proportion is higher in newborns and children). Eighty to 90% of peripheral blood lymphocytes are T cells, and the remainder are largely B cells. Most peripheral blood

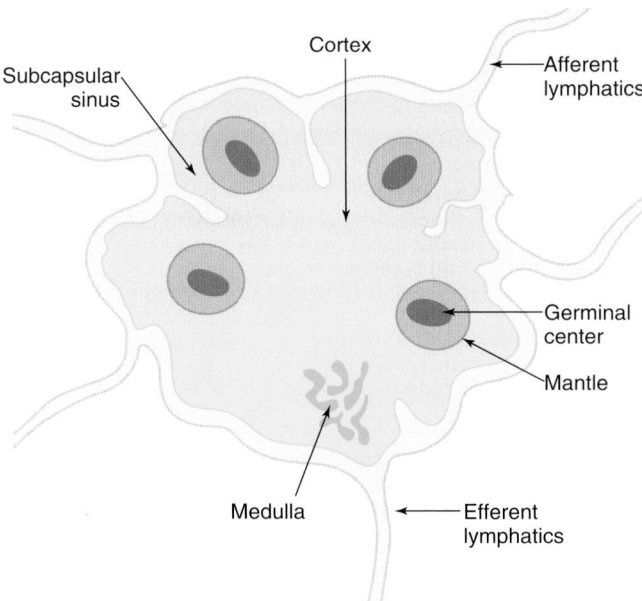

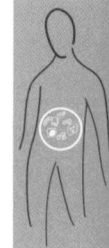

Figure 51-2 The structure of the normal lymph node. The cortical area contains the follicles, which consist of a germinal center and a mantle zone. The medulla contains a complex of channels that lead to the efferent lymphatics.

Table 51-1 **Causes of Lymphadenopathy**
Infectious Diseases
Viral: infectious mononucleosis syndromes (cytomegalovirus, Epstein-Barr virus), acquired immunodeficiency syndrome, rubella, herpes simplex, infectious hepatitis *Bacterial*: localized infection with regional adenopathy (streptococci, staphylococci), cat-scratch disease, brucellosis, tularemia, listeriosis, bubonic plague *(Yersinia pestis)*, chancroid *(Haemophilus ducreyi)* *Fungal*: coccidioidomycosis, histoplasmosis *Chlamydial*: lymphogranuloma venereum, trachoma *Mycobacterial*: scrofula, tuberculosis, leprosy *Protozoan*: toxoplasmosis, trypanosomiasis *Spirochetal*: Lyme disease, syphilis, leptospirosis
Immunologic Diseases
Rheumatoid arthritis Systemic lupus erythematosus Mixed connective tissue disease Sjögren syndrome Dermatomyositis Serum sickness Drug reactions: phenytoin, hydralazine, allopurinol
Malignant Diseases
Lymphomas Metastatic solid tumors to lymph nodes: melanoma, lung, breast, head and neck, gastrointestinal tract, Kaposi sarcoma, unknown primary tumor, renal, prostate
Atypical Lymphoid Proliferations
Giant follicular lymph node hyperplasia Transformation of germinal centers Castleman disease
Miscellaneous Diseases and Diseases of Unknown Cause
Dermatopathic lymphadenitis Sarcoidosis Amyloidosis Mucocutaneous lymph node syndrome Multifocal Langerhans cell (eosinophilic) granulomatosis Lipid storage diseases: Gaucher and Niemann-Pick diseases

lymphocytes are mature, resting lymphocytes that morphologically are small, with scant cytoplasm and inconspicuous nucleoli. A small percentage of peripheral blood lymphoid cells represent a third category of lymphoid cells that are referred to as natural killer (NK) cells. These cells do not bear the characteristic cell surface molecules of B or T cells, and their immunoglobulin or TCR genes have not undergone rearrangement. Morphologically, these cells are large, with abundant cytoplasm containing azurophilic granules, and thus they are often called *large granular lymphocytes*. Functionally, they are part of the innate immune system, responding nonspecifically to a wide range of pathogens without requiring prior antigenic exposure.

Neoplasia of Lymphoid Origin

Malignant transformation of lymphocytes can lead to a diverse array of neoplasms of lymphoid origin, including tumors that arise from T cells or B cells and tumors that represent different stages of lymphocyte development. Lymphoid malignancies usually involve lymphoid tissues, but they can arise in or spread to any site. The major clinical groupings of lymphoid malignancies include non-Hodgkin lymphomas (NHLs), Hodgkin disease (HD), lymphoid leukemias, and plasma cell dyscrasias.

The most common clinical presentation of a lymphoid malignancy in adults is painless enlargement of lymph nodes, or lymphadenopathy. Many causes of lymphadenopathy exist, in addition to lymphoid malignancies (Table 51-1). Thus, taking a thorough history and performing a careful physical examination is important before performing a lymph node biopsy. The investigation of lymphadenopathy can be organized according to the location of the enlarged nodes (localized or generalized) and the presence of clinical symptoms. Cervical lymphadenopathy is most often caused by infections of the upper respiratory tract, including infectious mononucleosis syndromes and other viral syndromes, as well as bacterial pharyngitis. Unilateral axillary, inguinal, or femoral adenopathy may be caused by skin infections involving the extremity, including cat-scratch fever. Generalized lymphadenopathy may be caused by systemic infections, such as HIV or cytomegalovirus infection, drug reactions, autoimmune diseases, one of the systemic lymphadenopathy syndromes, or lymphoma. If the cause of persistent lymphadenopathy is not apparent after a thorough evaluation, an excisional lymph node biopsy should be undertaken. An enlarged supraclavicular lymph node is highly suggestive of malignancy and should always be sampled.

The accurate diagnosis of lymphoma requires excisional biopsy of a lymph node or generous biopsy of involved lymph tissue. Fine-needle aspiration or needle biopsy is rarely sufficient for diagnosing malignant lymphoma. Analysis of the pathologic specimen should include routine histologic examination and immunophenotyping. Immunophenotyping involves the characterization of the immunologic cell surface antigens that are expressed on the malignant

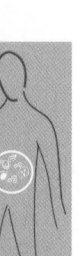

lymphocyte by means of a panel of monoclonal antibodies. Immunophenotyping permits a determination of cell of origin (B cell, T cell, NK cell, or nonlymphoid cell) and the pattern of cell surface antigens. In the case of B-cell NHLs, immunophenotyping can also reveal whether the process is monoclonal in origin (i.e., neoplastic) by determining whether the surface immunoglobulin is restricted to either κ or λ light chains. Immunophenotyping has become an essential aspect of the diagnosis and classification of lymphomas and can be accomplished by flow cytometric analysis or by immunohistochemical studies on tissue specimens. In some cases, cytogenetic analysis or molecular studies for immunoglobulin or TCR gene rearrangement may be required to determine the pathologic subtype of lymphoma or to establish a monoclonal (i.e., malignant) process. If a lymph node biopsy is nondiagnostic and unexplained lymph node enlargement persists, the biopsy should be repeated.

Non-Hodgkin Lymphomas

The NHLs comprise a heterogeneous group of lymphoid malignancies that differ with respect to their histologic appearance, cell of origin and immunophenotype, molecular biologic factors, clinical features, prognosis, and outcome with therapy. In view of the heterogeneity of NHLs, classification systems have been devised to identify specific pathologic subtypes that correlate with distinct clinical entities. These systems have evolved steadily over the past 50 years, as correlations between histopathologic and biologic behavior have emerged. Until recently, the most widely used classification system in North America was the Working Formulation (WF). The WF classified NHLs based on the architecture of the node (the presence of follicles versus diffuse infiltrate) and the morphologic features of the malignant lymphocyte (small cell versus large cell, with cleaved or noncleaved nucleus) and organized the pathologic subtypes into low, intermediate, or high grade based on their natural history and clinical behavior. In general, the low-grade histologies were associated with an indolent course and relatively long survival but were incurable, whereas the intermediate- and high-grade histologies were biologically aggressive (i.e., short natural history if left untreated) but were potentially curable with appropriate treatment. With the advent of immunophenotyping and molecular characterization of lymphomas, it became apparent that the WF did not adequately define specific pathologic and clinical entities. The Revised European-American Lymphoma (REAL) classification system, introduced in 1994, incorporated not only histologic features as described by the WF but also immunophenotype, cytogenetics, and epidemiologic and etiologic factors. Thus, the REAL classification identified several NHL subtypes that were not easily classified within the WF. These subtypes included the mantle cell lymphomas—the MALT lymphomas, and monocytoid B-cell lymphomas, which are both derived from cells in the marginal zone of lymph nodes; and the various T-cell lymphomas, including human T-cell leukemia virus type 1 (HTLV-1)–associated leukemia and lymphoma, cutaneous T-cell lymphoma (mycosis fungoides or Sézary syndrome), and the biologically aggressive peripheral T-cell lymphomas. The REAL classification was updated in 2001 by the World

Table 51-2 **Revised European-American Lymphoma/World Health Organization Classification of Lymphoid Neoplasms**
B-Cell Neoplasms
Precursor B-cell neoplasm
Precursor B-lymphoblastic leukemia/lymphoma (precursor B-cell acute lymphoblastic leukemia)
Mature (peripheral) B-cell neoplasms
B-cell chronic lymphocytic leukemia/small lymphocytic lymphoma
B-cell prolymphocytic leukemia
Lymphoplasmacytic lymphoma
Splenic marginal zone B-cell lymphoma (± villous lymphocytes)
Hairy cell leukemia
Plasma cell myeloma/plasmacytoma
Extranodal marginal zone B-cell lymphoma of MALT type
Nodal marginal zone B-cell lymphoma of MALT type
Follicular lymphoma
Mantle cell lymphoma
Diffuse large B-cell lymphoma
Mediastinal large B-cell lymphoma
Primary effusion lymphoma
Burkitt lymphoma/Burkitt cell leukemia
T- and NK-Cell Neoplasms
Precursor T-cell neoplasm
Precursor T-lymphoblastic lymphoma/leukemia (precursor T-cell acute lymphoblastic leukemia)
Mature (peripheral) T-cell neoplasms
T-cell prolymphocytic leukemia
T-cell granular lymphocytic leukemia
Aggressive NK-cell leukemia
Adult T-cell lymphoma/leukemia (HTLV-1)
Extranodal NK-/T-cell lymphoma, nasal type
Enteropathy-type T-cell lymphoma
Hepatosplenic gamma-delta T-cell lymphoma
Subcutaneous panniculitis-like T-cell lymphoma
Mycosis fungoides/Sézary syndrome
Anaplastic large cell lymphoma, T-/null cell, primary cutaneous type
Peripheral T-cell lymphoma, not otherwise characterized
Angioimmunoblastic T-cell lymphoma
Anaplastic large cell lymphoma, T-/null cell, primary systemic type

Only major categories are included. Common entities are shown in **bold type**.
B- and T-/NK-cell neoplasms are grouped according to major clinical presentations (predominantly disseminated/leukemic, primary extranodal, predominantly nodal).
HTLV-1, human T-cell leukemia virus; MALT, mucosa-associated lymphoid tissue; NK, natural killer.

Health Organization (WHO), and the REAL/WHO classification has replaced all previous classification systems (Table 51-2). The most common NHLs encountered in the United States are the follicular lymphomas, small lymphocytic lymphoma or leukemia (also known as *chronic lymphocytic leukemia* [CLL]), mantle cell lymphoma, and diffuse large B-cell lymphoma.

The cause of most NHLs is not known. In most patients with NHL, no apparent genetic predisposition or epidemiologic or environmental factor can be identified. Many of the NHL subtypes carry pathognomonic chromosomal translocations that often involve an immunoglobulin locus (or *TCR* locus in the case of T-cell–derived NHLs) and an oncogene or growth regulatory gene. The cause of these aberrant chromosomal rearrangements is unknown. Patients with congenital immunodeficiency syndromes or autoimmune disorders are at increased risk for developing NHL. Oncogenic human viruses play a causal role in some of the less common NHL variants. Epstein-Barr virus (EBV) is associated with several biologically aggressive NHLs, including AIDS-related diffuse aggressive lymphomas, the lymphoproliferative disorders that arise in patients who are immunosuppressed after organ transplantation, and the form of Burkitt lymphoma that is endemic in Africa. HTLV-1 is causally linked with an aggressive form of T-cell leukemia or lymphoma that is endemic in areas of Japan and the Caribbean basin. The herpesvirus of Kaposi sarcoma has been implicated in a variant of diffuse aggressive NHL that arises in serosal cavities and is encountered almost exclusively in patients infected with HIV. *Helicobacter pylori* infection is causally linked to gastric MALT lymphomas, and eradication of infection with antibiotics is often associated with regression of the lymphoma.

CLINICAL PRESENTATION, EVALUATION, AND STAGING

As described in the preceding section, most patients with NHL exhibit painless lymphadenopathy involving one or more of the peripheral nodal sites. Additionally, NHL can involve extranodal sites, and thus patients can exhibit a variety of symptoms reflective of the site of involvement. The most common sites of extranodal disease are the gastrointestinal tract, bone marrow, liver, and Waldeyer ring, although virtually any site potentially can be involved with NHL. In general, the aggressive subtypes of NHL (diffuse large cell, lymphoblastic, and Burkitt) are more likely than are the indolent lymphomas to involve extranodal sites. Central nervous system involvement, including leptomeningeal spread, rarely occurs in the indolent subtypes but does occur in the aggressive variants. The most aggressive NHLs (Burkitt and lymphoblastic) have a particular propensity to spread to the leptomeninges. Constitutional symptoms such as fever, weight loss, or night sweats occur in about 20% of patients with NHL at the time of onset, and these symptoms are more common in patients with aggressive subtypes of NHL.

The diagnosis of NHL requires an adequate biopsy of the involved nodal tissue or extranodal site. In patients with bone marrow and peripheral blood involvement, such as small lymphocytic lymphoma or CLL, making the diagnosis from immunophenotyping of peripheral blood lymphocytes by flow cytometry is often possible. Once the diagnosis of a lymphoma has been made, patients should undergo a complete staging evaluation (Table 51-3). Staging determines the extent of involvement, provides prognostic information, and may influence the choice of therapy. The modified Ann Arbor staging classification is used to stage patients with both NHL and Hodgkin disease (Table 51-4). Standard staging evaluation includes a thorough history to elicit symptoms referable to the lymphoma, including the presence of constitutional symptoms (fevers, night sweats, or weight loss, designated as *B* symptoms); a complete physical examination, with documentation of the size and distribution of enlarged lymph nodes; blood work, including lactate dehydrogenase (LDH) evaluation; computed tomography

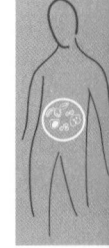

Table 51-3 Staging Evaluation for Lymphomas

Required Evaluation Procedures

Biopsy of lesion with review by an experienced hematopathologist

History with attention to the presence or absence of *B* symptoms

Physical examination with attention to node-bearing areas (including Waldeyer ring) and size of liver and spleen

Standard blood work, including:
  Complete blood cell count
  Lactate dehydrogenase and β_2-microglobulin
  Evaluation of renal function
  Liver function tests
  Calcium, uric acid

Bilateral bone marrow aspirates and biopsies

Radiologic studies, including:
  Chest radiograph (posteroanterior and lateral)
  Chest, abdomen, and pelvic CT scan
  PET scan (in Hodgkin and intermediate- and high-grade lymphomas)

Procedures Required under Certain Circumstances

Bone scan if bone symptoms

Plain bone radiographs of symptomatic sites or abnormal areas on bone scan

Brain or spinal CT or MRI if neurologic signs or symptoms

Serum and urine protein electrophoresis

Lumbar puncture with cerebrospinal fluid cytology (Burkitt and lymphoblastic lymphoma)

CT, computed tomography; MRI, magnetic resonance imaging; PET, positron emission tomography.

Table 51-4 Staging System for Lymphomas

Stage	Description
I	Involvement of a single lymph node region or structure (I) or a single extralymphatic site (IE)
II	Involvement of two or more lymph node regions on the same side of the diaphragm (II) or localized involvement of a contiguous extralymphatic site and lymph node region (IIE)
III	Involvement of lymph node regions on both sides of the diaphragm (III), which may be accompanied by localized involvement of one extralymphatic site (IIIE) or spleen (IIIS) or both (IIISE)
III₁	With or without involvement of splenic, hilar, celiac, or portal nodes
III₂	With involvement of para-aortic, iliac, and mesenteric nodes
IV	Diffuse or disseminated involvement of one or more extralymphatic organs with or without associated lymph node involvement

Identification of the presence or absence of symptoms should be noted with each stage designation: A, asymptomatic; B, fever, sweats, weight loss >10% of body weight.

(CT) scans of chest, abdomen, and pelvis; and bone marrow aspirate and biopsy. Positron emission tomographic (PET) scans or gallium scans can be helpful in assessing response to therapy in lymphomas that are metabolically active (usually the aggressive subtypes such as diffuse large cell lymphoma, lymphoblastic lymphoma, and Burkitt lymphoma) and are often included in the staging evaluation of

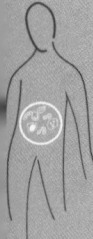

the aggressive NHLs. Lumbar puncture for cytologic analysis should be performed only in patients who are at risk for leptomeningeal disease, which includes all patients with Burkitt and lymphoblastic lymphoma and patients with diffuse large cell lymphoma with involvement of bone marrow, testes, or structures directly abutting the central nervous system (e.g., paranasal sinus, calvarium). A variety of ancillary tests may be performed in specific situations. For example, a test for HTLV-1 or HIV should be performed if adult T-cell leukemia or lymphoma or AIDS-related lymphoma is thought to exist, respectively. A gastrointestinal series or endoscopic evaluation may be warranted in all patients with gastrointestinal symptoms or in patients at risk for gastrointestinal tract involvement (lymphomas involving the Waldeyer ring). Serum protein electrophoresis and determination of β_2-microglobulin and quantitative immunoglobulins should be performed in patients who are thought to have plasma cell dyscrasias. A laparotomy for the sole purpose of staging patients with NHL is never performed because it rarely influences therapeutic decision making.

A variety of prognostic variables have been identified for NHL. In general, the predictors for poor survival in most subtypes of NHL include advanced stage at onset (stage III or IV), involvement of multiple extranodal sites of disease, elevated LDH levels, the presence of B symptoms, and poor performance status.

NATURAL HISTORY, PROGNOSIS, AND TREATMENT

Indolent Non-Hodgkin Lymphomas

The common low-grade or indolent histologic conditions include the follicular lymphomas (small cleaved cell and mixed cell types) and small lymphocytic lymphoma (the latter is identical to CLL and is discussed later), which account for about 30% and 5% of all NHLs, respectively. The low-grade follicular lymphomas are mature clonal B-cell neoplasms with an immunophenotype that is positive for surface immunoglobulin (κ- or λ-chain restricted) and the mature B-cell markers (CD19, CD20, CD21) and negative for CD5. Follicular lymphomas are characterized cytogenetically by the t(14;18) translocation that juxtaposes the immunoglobulin heavy chain with the antiapoptotic gene BCL-2; BCL-2 is uniformly expressed in follicular lymphomas. Although the follicular lymphomas are low grade, indolent neoplasms with a long natural history (median survival approaches 10 years), most patients (80% to 90%) exhibit an advanced stage (stage III or IV), often with bone marrow involvement and cannot be cured with standard treatment modalities. Factors associated with shortened survival include older age, advanced stage, anemia, multiple lymph node sites (more than four), and elevated LDH. Patients with three or more of these factors have a median survival of 5 years, roughly one half that of patients with zero or one risk factor. Most patients with follicular NHL eventually experience transformation of their disease to a more aggressive lymphoma, characterized pathologically by a diffuse large cell infiltrate and clinically by rapidly expanding nodes or other tumor masses, rising LDH levels, and the onset of disease-related symptoms.

The management of the follicular lymphomas is determined by the stage. For the few patients who are considered to have early-stage (I or nonbulky II) disease after clinical staging, the appropriate treatment is radiation therapy. With the use of subtotal or total lymphoid irradiation, more than one half of patients with early-stage disease will achieve a durable remission and appear to be cured. For patients with advanced-stage disease, the management is more controversial. Although advanced-stage indolent NHL is responsive to a variety of treatment modalities, the incurability and the long natural history has led to the practice of deferring treatment until the patient develops symptoms. This strategy is referred to as the *watch and wait* approach. Indications for treatment include cosmetic or mechanical problems caused by enlarging lymph nodes, constitutional symptoms, and evidence of marrow compromise. The appropriate treatment of advanced-stage disease, when necessary, is systemic chemotherapy. The follicular lymphomas are responsive to a variety of single and multidrug programs. Single alkylating agents (cyclophosphamide or chlorambucil), multidrug regimens containing an alkylating agent (e.g., cyclophosphamide, vincristine, and prednisone [CVP]), or fludarabine-based regimens (i.e., fludarabine and mitoxantrone, fludarabine, and cyclophosphamide) are all effective initial regimens for this disease. The addition of the chimeric (mouse-human) anti-CD20 monoclonal antibody rituximab to chemotherapy regimens has become commonplace and is associated with improvements in response rate and duration of remission. Most patients respond to treatment, and at least one third achieves a clinical complete remission that may last 1 to 3 years. Treatment should be discontinued when the maximum response has been achieved to minimize cumulative toxicity. Once a patient relapses, subsequent remissions may be achieved but are usually less durable compared with the first remission. Therapeutic options for patients who relapse include retreatment with chemotherapy, often with a different drug or combination than that used initially. Patients in relapse can also be treated with rituximab as a single agent. Rituximab is a highly effective nontoxic agent for use in patients with relapsed follicular lymphoma, inducing responses that are often durable in over one half of patients. Patients who respond to rituximab are often successfully retreated with rituximab at subsequent relapse, and, in contrast to the experience with second- or third-line chemotherapy, these patients may experience remissions that actually exceed the duration of their first remission from rituximab. Two radioactively labeled anti-CD20 antibodies, ibritumomab tiuxetan (yttrium-labeled) and iodine-131 tositumomab are now also in use for patients with relapsed or refractory follicular lymphoma and have been associated with a high response rate. For patients who have clinical or pathologic evidence of transformation to a higher grade of lymphoma, treatment that is appropriate for a diffuse aggressive histology should be offered (discussed later). The role of high-dose chemotherapy with autologous or allogeneic stem cell transplantation for follicular NHLs remains unclear and should be considered experimental. Long-term follow-up of patients undergoing allogeneic transplantation suggests that some patients are cured with this modality. However, the morbidity associated with allogeneic transplantation has limited its widespread use for refractory indolent lymphomas.

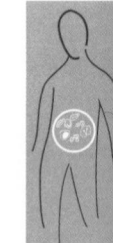

In addition to the follicular NHLs, the MALT lymphomas and closely related marginal zone lymphomas are also considered low-grade, indolent subtypes. Given the excellent prognosis, localized nature, and long natural history of the MALT lymphomas, they are generally managed conservatively with local treatment modalities (irradiation or surgery) and avoidance of systemic chemotherapy. Importantly, the gastric MALT lymphomas are highly associated with *H. pylori* infection, and remissions can often be achieved with eradication of this infection. Thus, antibiotic therapy is the first-line treatment for early gastric MALT lymphoma.

Diffuse Aggressive Non-Hodgkin Lymphomas

The aggressive NHLs are characterized by effacement of lymph node architecture with a diffuse infiltrate of large lymphocytes and include the diffuse large B-cell lymphoma (accounting for about one third of all NHLs), anaplastic large cell lymphoma, and peripheral T-cell lymphoma. Most of the diffuse aggressive large cell lymphomas are B cell in origin (diffuse large B-cell lymphoma); the T-cell diffuse aggressive lesions, or peripheral T-cell lymphomas, are managed similarly but have an overall worse prognosis compared with their B-cell counterparts. Burkitt lymphoma and lymphoblastic lymphoma are among the most aggressive lymphomas and are discussed separately later in this chapter (see "High-Grade Non-Hodgkin Lymphomas").

Diffuse aggressive NHLs exhibit clinically aggressive behavior, and, if left untreated, the median survival is less than 1 to 2 years. Compared with the follicular NHLs, a higher percentage of patients with diffuse aggressive histology will exhibit early-stage disease (30% to 50%) or involvement of an extranodal site (50%). The outcome and likelihood of cure of patients with diffuse aggressive histology is directly related to the total number of adverse prognostic features at onset: age older than 60 years, advanced stage (III or IV), elevated LDH levels, poor performance status, and the presence of two or more extranodal sites of disease. The likelihood of cure and long-term disease-free survival ranges from more than 75% in patients with one or fewer adverse factors to less than 30% in patients with four or more adverse factors.

In contrast to patients with low-grade follicular NHLs, all patients with diffuse aggressive histology should be offered immediate therapy because these lymphomas are potentially curable. The standard initial therapy for all patients with diffuse aggressive NHL is a multidrug chemotherapy regimen that includes an anthracycline in combination with the anti-CD20 monoclonal antibody rituximab. The most widely used chemotherapy regimen is a combination of cyclophosphamide, doxorubicin, vincristine, and prednisone (designated as CHOP). This regimen appears to be equivalent to more complex and intensive regimens such as m-BACOD, Pro-MACE, and MACOP-B, and thus CHOP plus rituximab remains standard initial therapy. Patients with early-stage disease (I or nonbulky stage II) may be treated with local radiation therapy after a minimum of three cycles of CHOP if exposure to chemotherapy is limited. Patients with advanced-stage disease require six cycles of CHOP plus rituximab; the role of local radiation to sites of bulky disease in the setting of advanced-stage disease is not established. Complete remissions can be achieved with CHOP plus ritux-imab or similar regimens, and more than 50% of patients are cured. Patients who experience relapse after achieving a remission often can be cured with high-dose chemotherapy with autologous peripheral blood stem cell support, or *transplantation*, particularly if their relapsed disease remains responsive to standard doses of chemotherapy. The morbidity and mortality of this procedure have diminished substantially since 1990 with the use of peripheral blood stem cells and colony-stimulating factor support, and transplantation can be safely performed in patients without serious comorbid conditions. High-dose chemotherapy with autologous stem cell transplantation is superior to standard doses of a salvage regimen and is considered standard therapy for patients with relapsed chemosensitive diffuse aggressive NHL.

Mantle Cell Lymphoma

Mantle cell lymphoma has been recognized with increasing frequency since immunophenotyping has become standard practice for classifying NHLs, and it is included in the REAL/WHO classification. Mantle cell NHL was not recognized in the WF and was often designated as a diffuse small cleaved cell or diffuse mixed cell lymphoma in the WF classification. It accounts for 5% to 8% of all NHLs. Mantle cell lymphomas are mature B-cell neoplasms that appear to arise in the mantle zone of the lymphoid follicle and display a highly characteristic immunophenotype. Mantle cells express the CD5 antigen, as well as the mature B-cell markers (CD19, CD20, and CD21), but typically are negative for CD23 expression. Because mantle cell lymphomas can be easily confused pathologically and clinically with CLL, which is the only other B-cell NHL that is CD5+, the absence of CD23 is important for distinguishing mantle cell lymphoma from CLL, which is typically CD23+. Mantle cell lymphomas are also characterized by a pathognomonic t(11;14) chromosomal translocation that juxtaposes the immunoglobulin heavy chain with the *BCL-1* or *PRAD-1* gene, which encodes the growth-promoting protein cyclin D1. Mantle cell lymphomas are in many ways similar to indolent lymphomas in that patients usually exhibit advanced-stage disease with frequent bone marrow involvement. These lymphomas are far more common in men than women and have a peculiar propensity to involve the Waldeyer ring and gastrointestinal tract. As with the low-grade follicular lymphomas, mantle cell lymphomas are treatable but not curable. However, in contrast to the indolent lymphomas, these neoplasms are biologically aggressive, with a median survival of only 2 to 3 years. These patients are generally treated with systemic chemotherapy with rituximab at diagnosis, because of the more aggressive nature of mantle cell lymphomas compared with follicular lymphomas, but durable remissions are difficult to achieve. The optimal therapy for this challenging subtype remains to be established, and these patients should be considered for experimental therapies, including immunotherapy or transplantation.

High-Grade Non-Hodgkin Lymphoma

The two high-grade subtypes, Burkitt or small noncleaved cell and lymphoblastic lymphoma, are quite rare in the adult population. Nonetheless, these subtypes are important because they are potentially curable with appropriate therapy and often require urgent, inpatient treatment at the time of

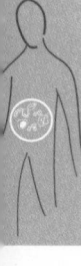

diagnosis because of their highly aggressive nature, rapid growth, and tendency to develop tumor lysis on initiation of therapy. Lymphoblastic lymphoma is an aggressive lymphoma that is closely related to T-cell acute lymphocytic leukemia and readily distinguished from most NHLs by its T-cell immunophenotype and the presence of terminal deoxynucleotide transferase. It usually afflicts young adult males and involves the mediastinum and bone marrow, with a propensity to relapse in the leptomeninges. Burkitt, or small noncleaved cell, lymphoma is a rare B-cell lymphoma in adults that is highly aggressive, with a propensity to involve the bone marrow and central nervous system. Burkitt lymphoma is characterized cytogenetically by the pathognomonic t(8;14) translocation that juxtaposes the *Ig* locus with the *myc* oncogene. In central Africa, where Burkitt lymphoma is endemic in children, it is usually associated with EBV. However, in the United States, it is uncommon for sporadic Burkitt lymphoma to be EBV positive. Burkitt lymphoma and lymphoblastic lymphomas both require treatment with intensive multiagent chemotherapy, including intrathecal chemotherapy to prevent leptomeningeal relapse. These lymphomas undergo rapid tumor lysis on initiation of chemotherapy, and all patients must receive prophylaxis against tumor lysis syndrome before and during their first course of chemotherapy. Prophylaxis includes hydration, alkalinization of the urine, and allopurinol.

Hodgkin Disease

HD is the most common lymphoma in young adults. It has a bimodal age distribution in the United States and industrialized countries, with the larger peak occurring between ages 15 and 35 years and a second smaller peak occurring in patients older than 50 years. The cause of HD remains enigmatic. Although EBV is frequently present in the malignant cell of HD, a direct causal link between EBV and HD has not been established. HD does not appear with increased frequency in patients with congenital immunodeficiency syndromes or in immunosuppressed organ transplant recipients, and the risk for HD does not appear to increase in patients infected with HIV.

The diagnosis of HD is made by identifying the Reed-Sternberg (RS) cell in involved lymphoid tissue. The classic RS cell is large and binucleate, with each nucleus containing a prominent nucleolus, suggesting the appearance of *owl eyes*. Although the cellular origin of the RS cell was debated for many decades, molecular studies have confirmed that RS cells are B cell in nature with clonal rearrangement of the germline *Ig* locus, despite the absence of cytoplasmic or cell surface immunoglobulin. In contrast to NHL and other malignancies, the bulk of the infiltrate in lymph nodes involved with HD is usually composed of benign reactive inflammatory cells, and often the diagnostic RS cells can be difficult to find. Immunophenotyping of classic RS cells reveals that they are CD30 (Ki-1) and CD15 positive and are negative for CD20, CD45, and cytoplasmic or surface immunoglobulin; EBV is identified in the RS cells in about one half of patients with HD.

Four pathologic variants of HD have been identified. Nodular sclerosing (NS) is by far the most common (80% of patients with HD) and is characterized by the presence of fibrous bands separating the node into nodules and the *lacunar* type of RS cells. It is the predominant type encountered in adolescents and young adults and typically involves the mediastinum and other supradiaphragmatic nodal sites. In the mixed cellularity (MC) type, which accounts for about 15% of patients with HD, band-forming sclerosis is absent, and RS cells are easily identified in a diffuse infiltrate that is more heterogeneous compared with that seen in the NS variant. The MC variant may be encountered in any age group, and advanced-stage disease with subdiaphragmatic involvement is more common with MC-variant HD than it is with NS-variant HD. The lymphocyte-depleted type is rare, accounting for less than 1% of the HD cases, and is characterized by sheets of RS cells with a paucity of inflammatory cells. This variant is most common in older adults, in patients infected with HIV, and in persons in nonindustrialized countries. The lymphocyte-predominant (LP) type has emerged as a distinct entity that may be more closely related to indolent NHL than it is to HD, although it is managed as true HD. The LP type is characterized by a nodular growth pattern with variants of RS cells that have polylobated nuclei and are referred to as *popcorn* cells; classic RS cells are usually absent. The immunophenotype of the atypical cells is distinct from classic RS cells, with expression of B-cell antigens (CD19 and CD20) and CD45 but absence of the classic RS markers CD15 and CD30. The presence of CD20 on the surface of LP-type Hodgkin cells has allowed therapeutic use of the monoclonal antibody rituximab, an agent not typically active in other subtypes of HD. The LP type of HD accounts for about 5% of cases, has a strong male preponderance, and tends to involve peripheral nodes with sparing of the mediastinum. The prognosis is excellent, although late relapses are more common than they are in the other types of HD.

HD arises in lymph nodes, most commonly in the mediastinum or neck, and spreads to adjacent contiguous or noncontiguous nodal sites, including retroperitoneal nodes and the spleen. As the disease progresses, it spreads hematogenously to involve extranodal sites, including bone marrow, liver, and lung. In contrast to NHL, HD rarely arises in extranodal sites, although HD can involve extranodal sites by contiguous spread from an adjacent lymph node (e.g., involvement of vertebrae from adjacent retroperitoneal lymph nodes, involvement of pulmonary parenchyma from adjacent hilar nodes).

HD usually produces painless enlargement of lymph nodes, most often in the neck. Mediastinal adenopathy may be found incidentally in a patient who is asymptomatic on routine chest radiography. Massive mediastinal or hilar adenopathy, with or without adjacent pulmonary involvement, may cause respiratory symptoms such as cough, shortness of breath, wheezing, or stridor. About one third of patients with HD have constitutional symptoms of fever, night sweats, or weight loss (*B* symptoms), which can be the presenting complaint. In addition to the *B* symptoms, generalized pruritus is also associated with HD and correlates with the NS type. Occasionally, patients give a history of troubling pruritus for months to years before the diagnosis of HD. Although HD is associated with functional T-lymphocyte defects, exhibited as cutaneous anergy to intradermal skin tests, patients rarely have opportunistic infections. If left untreated, the natural history of HD is one

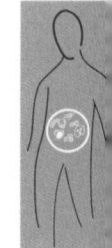

of inexorable, albeit often slow, progression to involve multiple nodal sites, followed by hematogenous spread to bone marrow, liver, and other viscera. As the disease advances, patients experience *B* symptoms, malaise, cachexia, and infectious complications, and patients with progressive HD ultimately die from complications of bone marrow failure or infection.

Accurate staging of patients with newly diagnosed HD is important for treatment planning, prognosis, and assessing response to therapy. A modification of the Ann Arbor classification is used (see Table 51-4), and the suffix *A* or *B* is appended to denote the absence or presence, respectively, of fever, night sweats, or weight loss. The staging work-up of a patient with newly diagnosed HD is similar to that of patients with NHL (see Table 51-3). Patients should undergo a thorough history and physical examination; complete blood work, including an erythrocyte sedimentation rate; chest radiography; CT scan of the chest, abdomen, and pelvis; bone marrow aspirate and biopsy; and PET scan (or gallium scan if PET scan is not available). Lymphangiograms have been used historically in assessing subdiaphragmatic adenopathy; however, the expertise to perform and interpret this test is no longer widely available and has been replaced by the combination of CT scanning and nuclear imaging techniques. Additional tests, such as bone films, bone scan, and spinal magnetic resonance imaging (MRI), should be obtained only if symptoms suggest involvement of these structures. The information derived from this noninvasive work-up defines the clinical stage of a patient with HD. The role of the staging laparotomy to determine involvement below the diaphragm waned substantially during the 1990s as therapy for early-stage disease evolved. This procedure entails a laparotomy with splenectomy, liver biopsy, and a sampling of retroperitoneal nodes. The information derived from this procedure defines the pathologic stage of the disease, and occult HD can be found below the diaphragm in as many as 30% of patients with clinical stage I or II disease, mandating treatment with chemotherapy. Staging laparotomy has largely been abandoned, given that treatment has evolved away from the use of primary radiotherapy (discussed later). However, if a patient with clinical stage I or II supradiaphragmatic disease will be treated with radiation therapy as the sole modality, a staging laparotomy is an option to rule out occult involvement of the spleen and retroperitoneal nodes. Patients who do undergo staging laparotomy with splenectomy are at risk for overwhelming bacterial infection with encapsulated organisms and should receive pneumococcal and *Haemophilus influenzae* vaccine before surgery.

A variety of prognostic factors that influence risk for relapse or survival have been identified in HD. The most important adverse prognostic factors are MC or lymphocyte-depleted histology, male sex, large number of involved nodal sites, advanced stage (age >40 years), presence of *B* symptoms, high erythrocyte sedimentation rate, and bulky disease (widening of the mediastinum by more than one third or the presence of a nodal mass measuring more than 10 cm in any dimension). The presence of any of these factors in patients with early-stage disease places the patients at increased risk for occult abdominal involvement or relapse after primary radiation therapy and thus influences the decision to include chemotherapy in the initial treatment.

The treatment of HD has evolved considerably since 1980. HD is highly curable; the cure rate exceeds 80% with the use of current treatment modalities. Because most patients with HD are young adults and will experience long-term disease-free survival, the emphasis has shifted toward using therapies that minimize treatment-related morbidity and mortality without sacrificing curative potential. Radiation therapy in moderate doses (>35 Gy) to involved sites of disease plus contiguous nodal regions is curative for most patients with low-risk, early-stage disease (nonbulky stage I and IIA without adverse risk factors) and remains a viable treatment option for these patients. However, the long-term follow-up of patients treated with standard doses of radiation therapy has revealed a substantially increased risk for developing a variety of solid tumors within or at the margin of the radiation field more than a decade later. Chest irradiation for HD is associated with a particularly high risk for breast cancer in women and for lung cancer in both men and women. Additional long-term sequelae of standard radiation therapy for HD include thyroid dysfunction (usually hypothyroidism) and accelerated coronary artery disease. Thus, enthusiasm for primary radiation therapy in standard doses for low-risk, early-stage HD is diminishing in patients who will require chest irradiation, which represents the overwhelming majority of patients in the early stage.

In response to the recognition of the long-term carcinogenic effects of standard-dose radiation, the approach to treating patients with low-risk, early-stage HD is evolving. Increasingly, the trend has been to combine chemotherapy (e.g., doxorubicin [Adriamycin], bleomycin, vinblastine, and dacarbazine, designated as the [ABVD] regimen) with a low dose of radiation therapy (<30 Gy), which has not been associated with an increased risk for secondary solid tumors. The optimal duration of chemotherapy in combination with low-dose irradiation for early-stage HD remains unsettled.

Patients with advanced-stage HD (III or IV) or with early-stage disease with adverse risk factors (e.g., bulky disease, *B* symptoms, MC type) are not candidates for radiation therapy as the sole treatment modality because of the high rate of relapse. These patients should be treated with chemotherapy. The multiagent chemotherapy program nitrogen mustard, vincristine (Oncovin), procarbazine, and prednisone (designated as MOPP) was demonstrated to be highly curative in patients with advanced-stage disease in the 1970s. MOPP remains a highly effective regimen, but it is rarely used in current practice because of the long-term toxic effects associated with MOPP. These effects include sterility in nearly all men and infertility in a significant percentage of women who receive MOPP and a high risk for developing acute myeloid leukemia. The ABVD regimen is now the most widely used program in the United States. ABVD is as effective as is MOPP but does not cause sterility, infertility, or treatment-induced leukemias. Roughly 60% of patients with stage III or IV disease are cured with ABVD. ABVD has been associated with pulmonary fibrosis in a small percentage of patients (<5%) because of the inclusion of bleomycin in this regimen; the risk for pulmonary fibrosis is highest in patients who have underlying lung disease or who receive chest irradiation as a part of the treatment program. Patients who have an underlying cardiomyopathy are not candidates for ABVD because of the potential risk for further cardiac injury from doxorubicin, and alternate regimens are required

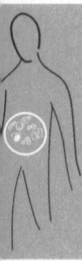

in these patients. More recently, the intensive regimen BEACOPP (Bleomycin, etoposide, Adriamycin, cyclophosphamide, vincristine, prednisolone, and procarbazine) has been associated with higher rates of complete response and freedom from treatment failure in patients with advanced disease and may be appropriate for selected patients. Infertility is a common side effect of treatment with BEACOPP, however, and further long-term follow-up is needed to study late sequelae of this effective regimen. Radiation therapy in combination with chemotherapy is not generally used to treat advanced-stage HD. However, in patients with bulky mediastinal disease, consolidative radiation to the mediastinum after completion of chemotherapy has been shown to decrease the rate of relapse. Thus, combined-modality therapy (chemotherapy plus radiation therapy) is considered standard for patients with bulky mediastinal disease.

Evaluating the patient's response to therapy in HD involves repetition of the staging evaluation (physical examination, CT, PET scan, and bone marrow biopsy if positive at diagnosis) during and at the completion of treatment. The presence of PET-avid disease, as measured after two cycles of ABVD therapy, has been shown to correlate with eventual resistance or relapse of disease. Conversely, patients may be cured despite the presence of a residual radiographic abnormality on chest radiography or CT (e.g., enlarged nodes, residual mediastinal mass) when the apparent residual disease is PET negative. Patients with residual radiographic abnormalities after an initial response to therapy should not be subjected to salvage therapy without additional corroborating evidence of persistent HD, such as biopsy confirmation or radiographic progression over time. A persistently positive PET scan after treatment in patients with residual radiographic abnormalities is also associated with a high rate of subsequent relapse, and these patients should be monitored closely or considered for immediate repeat biopsy or salvage therapy, or both. Most patients destined to relapse will do so within 2 years; relapses after 5 years are exceedingly rare.

Patients who relapse or fail to respond after initial therapy should be offered salvage therapy, given that many of these patients can now be cured if treated appropriately. About 20% of patients with early-stage HD who receive standard-dose radiation therapy (without chemotherapy) will relapse. These patients can be salvaged with standard chemotherapy (e.g., ABVD). Patients who relapse after standard chemotherapy should be treated with high-dose chemotherapy with autologous peripheral stem cell support. More than 50% of patients with recurrent, chemosensitive HD can be cured with this approach.

Lymphoid Leukemias

ACUTE LYMPHOCYTIC LEUKEMIAS

The acute lymphocytic leukemias that arise from precursor B or T cells are described in detail in Chapter 48.

CHRONIC LYMPHOCYTIC LEUKEMIA

B-cell CLL is a malignant disorder of lymphocytes characterized by expansion and accumulation of small lymphocytes

of B-cell origin. CLL is essentially identical to B-cell small lymphocytic lymphoma in the REAL and WF classifications but represents the leukemic form of the disease. CLL is the most common form of leukemia in the United States and affects twice as many men as it does women. Although it can occur at any stage of life, the incidence increases with age, and more than 90% of cases are diagnosed in adults older than 50 years of age. The cause of CLL is unknown. No apparent genetic basis for the disease has been found, and environmental factors, such as radiation and exposure to carcinogens, have not been implicated.

The common form of CLL is a clonal proliferation of mature B cells, expressing characteristic mature B-cell markers and low levels of surface immunoglobulin M (IgM) that is light-chain restricted, reflecting the clonal origin of this malignancy. In addition, CLL B cells express the CD5 molecule, which marks a minor subset of normal B cells, and CD23 (the Fc receptor for IgE). Thus, the diagnostic immunophenotype of CLL is that of a mature B-cell population that is clonal (by light-chain restriction or *Ig* gene rearrangement studies) expresses the characteristic mature B-cell markers (CD19, CD20, and CD21) and is positive for both CD5 and CD23. Although a pathognomonic chromosomal abnormality has not been identified in CLL, 30% to 50% of patients have cytogenetic abnormalities. The most frequent abnormalities involve chromosome 12 (often trisomy 12), 13, or 14. The presence of cytogenetic abnormalities of chromosomes 17 and 11 is associated with a very poor prognosis. Smears of the bone marrow or peripheral blood reveal a predominance of small lymphocytes with inconspicuous nucleoli, and involved lymph nodes reveal a diffuse infiltrate of these cells ablating normal architecture.

CLL cells accumulate in bone marrow, peripheral blood, lymph nodes, and spleen, resulting in lymphocytosis, decreased bone marrow function, lymphadenopathy, and splenomegaly. CLL is also frequently associated with immune dysregulation, exhibiting as hypogammaglobulinemia with an increased risk for bacterial infections and autoimmune phenomena such as Coombs-positive hemolytic anemia or immune thrombocytopenia. The diagnosis is often made incidentally on a routine blood cell count that shows a leukocytosis with a predominance of small lymphocytes; flow cytometric analysis of peripheral blood or a bone marrow aspirate will reveal the characteristic clonal B-cell population that is CD5 and CD23 positive. Some patients exhibit lymphadenopathy, symptoms related to cytopenias, or, occasionally, recurrent infections. As the disease progresses, patients develop generalized lymphadenopathy, hepatosplenomegaly, and bone marrow failure. Death often results from infectious complications or bone marrow failure in patients who have become refractory to treatment. In about 5% of instances, CLL transforms to a highly malignant diffuse large cell lymphoma, which is usually rapidly fatal; this transformation is commonly referred to as *Richter syndrome.*

CLL is a low-grade leukemia or lymphoma that is typically characterized by a long natural history with slow progression over years or even decades; median survival is in excess of 6 years. The extent of disease, or stage, at onset is the best predictor of survival. Table 51-5 shows the widely used Rai and Binet staging systems for CLL; most patients exhibit stage 0, I, or II disease. Given that standard therapy

Table 51-5 **Staging System for Chronic Lymphocytic Leukemia**					
Stage	Lymphocytosis	Lymphadenopathy	Hepatomegaly or Splenomegaly	Hemoglobin (g/dL)	Platelets (×10³/μL)
RAI System					
0	+	−	−	≥11	≥100
I	+	+	−	≥11	≥100
II	+	±	±	≥11	≥100
III	+	±	±	<11	≥100
IV	+	±	±	Any	<100
BINET System					
A	+	± (<3 lymphatic groups* positive)	±	≥10	≥100
B	+	± (≥3 lymphatic groups* positive)	±	≥10	≥100
C	+	±	±	<10	<100

*Cervical, axillary, inguinal nodes, liver, and spleen are each considered one group whether unilateral or bilateral.

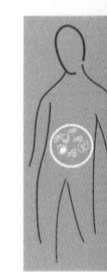

is not curative, and because CLL may have a long asymptomatic phase lasting years, specific treatment can be withheld until the patient develops symptoms (e.g., bulky lymphadenopathy, constitutional symptoms such as fevers, cytopenias caused by either bone marrow infiltration or autoimmune phenomenon). When treatment is required, initial therapy is begun either with the nucleoside analogue fludarabine or an alkylating agent such as chlorambucil or bendamustine. Most patients respond to either of these interventions with significant reductions in tumor burden. Fludarabine therapy is associated with a higher rate of complete remissions compared with therapy with chlorambucil, and combination regimens (e.g., fludarabine, cyclophosphamide, and rituximab) have shown particularly encouraging results. Patients with recurrent or refractory disease may respond to alemtuzumab, a humanized monoclonal antibody to the CD52 molecule, which is present on most lymphocytes. Rituximab is also an active agent for patients with recurrent CLL. Patients with poor-risk cytogenetic abnormalities are more likely to demonstrate resistance to standard therapies and have shortened survival. Such patients may be candidates for allogeneic transplantation, which appears to exert therapeutic effect through a strong immune or "graft-versus-leukemia" phenomenon. Patients who develop autoimmune phenomena require treatment with corticosteroids, and intravenous gamma-globulin may be used to reduce the frequency of infections in patients who have developed hypogammaglobulinemia. The development of a rapidly enlarging mediastinal mass, constitutional symptoms, and high serum LDH suggests transformation of disease to a diffuse large cell lymphoma, which is associated with a poor prognosis.

HAIRY CELL LEUKEMIA

Hairy cell leukemia is a rare biologically indolent neoplastic lymphoid disorder characterized by an accumulation of neoplastic B cells in the bone marrow, peripheral blood, and spleen that morphologically have a characteristic appearance described as *hairy*. Hairy cells are lymphoid cells with fine cytoplasmic projections that are readily identified by the presence of tartrate-resistant acid phosphatase, B-cell immu-

nophenotype, and rearranged heavy- and light-chain immunoglobulin genes. The diagnosis is made by identifying typical hairy cells in the peripheral blood or on bone marrow biopsy. The bone marrow is often inaspirable because of the extensive reticulin fibrosis typically present.

This disease may resemble CLL superficially, but it has unique clinical features and requires different therapy. Hairy cell leukemia may be diagnosed in a patient who is asymptomatic on routine blood cell count; patients who are symptomatic usually exhibit symptoms referable to splenomegaly, infection caused by impaired host defenses, or associated autoimmune syndromes such as vasculitis or arthritis. Osteolytic bone lesions can occur and may cause pain. *B* symptoms are rare. On examination, splenomegaly is present in more than 80% of patients; hepatomegaly is less common, and lymphadenopathy is distinctly unusual. Pancytopenia is typically present at diagnosis. The course of hairy cell leukemia is generally indolent, with slowly progressive pancytopenia and splenomegaly. However, a considerable variability can be found in severity and rate of disease progression. Before effective therapy, bacterial and fungal infections occurred frequently and were the major cause of death.

Asymptomatic patients without significant cytopenias or other complications of the disease require no immediate therapy and can be monitored closely for progression or infectious complications. Patients who exhibit moderate cytopenias, history of infections, rapidly progressive disease, symptomatic splenomegaly, bone involvement, or autoimmune syndromes should undergo therapy. First-line therapy is the purine nucleoside analogue 2-chlorodeoxyadenosine (2-CDA). In 90% of patients, one course of treatment given as a continuous infusion over 7 days results in a complete response that is often durable. Relapse may occur but may respond to retreatment with 2-CDA or an alternative purine analogue, pentostatin. Because the malignant cells express the cell surface antigen CD20, the anti-CD20 antibody rituximab may also be employed. Splenectomy or treatment with interferon-α is rarely required. The availability of several effective therapies and the indolent nature of hairy cell leukemia have resulted in survival that is similar to the age-matched population.

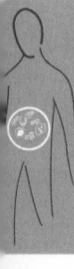

Plasma Cell Disorders

The plasma cell disorders, or *dyscrasias,* represent a group of B-cell neoplasms that are related to each other by virtue of their production and secretion of monoclonal immunoglobulin (or part of an immunoglobulin molecule), or M protein. The tumor cell of these disorders exhibits features of a differentiated plasma cell that is adapted to synthesize and secrete immunoglobulin at a high rate. The laboratory hallmark of plasma cell dyscrasias is the presence of a homogeneous immunoglobulin molecule (or part of an immunoglobulin molecule) that can be detected in the serum or urine by protein electrophoresis. Clinically, these disorders are often characterized by the systemic effects of the M protein as well as by the direct effects of bone and bone marrow infiltration. The classification of plasma cell dyscrasias is determined in part by the immunoglobulin class (IgG, IgA, IgD, IgE, or IgM) or component of immunoglobulin (heavy chain or light chain) that is produced (Table 51-6). The most common plasma cell neoplasms are multiple myeloma and the closely related plasmacytoma, which is a solitary myeloma of bone or extramedullary soft tissue; other less common plasma cell neoplasms include

Waldenström macroglobulinemia, heavy-chain disease, and primary amyloidosis.

M proteins can be found in benign and malignant conditions other than the plasma cell dyscrasias (see Table 51-6). About 10% of patients with CLL have detectable monoclonal IgG or IgM in their serum. M proteins can be detected in a variety of autoreactive or infectious disorders. In addition, an M protein can be found on serum protein electrophoresis in individuals with no apparent associated disease and in the absence of any other laboratory or clinical evidence of a plasma cell dyscrasia. This finding is designated *monoclonal gammopathy of unknown significance* (MGUS) and is defined by the presence of low levels of serum M protein (<3 g/dL), no urinary Bence Jones protein, less than 10% bone marrow plasma cells, and absence of anemia, hypercalcemia, renal failure, and lytic bone lesions. MGUS is more common than myeloma and increases in frequency with aging, occurring in 1% to 2% of the population older than 50 years. MGUS is often considered a premalignant condition, and these patients are at increased risk (sevenfold) for developing overt myeloma or related malignant plasma cell neoplasms compared with the general population. Nonetheless, progression of MGUS to a frank plasma cell neoplasm only

Disorder	M Protein	Antibody Activity of M Protein
Table 51-6 Classification of Disorders Associated with Monoclonal Immunoglobulin (M Protein) Secretion		
Plasma Cell Neoplasms		
Multiple myeloma	IgG > IgA > IgD; ±< free light chain or light chain alone (κ > λ)	
Solitary myeloma of bone	IgG > IgA > IgD; ± free light chain or light chain alone (κ > λ)	
Extramedullary plasmacytoma	IgA > IgG > IgD; ± free light chain or light chain alone (κ > λ)	
Waldenström macroglobulinemia	IgM ± free light chain (κ > λ)	
Heavy-chain disease	γ, α, or μ heavy chain or fragment	
Primary amyloidosis	Free light chain (λ > κ)	
Monoclonal gammopathy of unknown significance	IgG > IgM > IgA, usually without urinary light-chain secretion	
Other B-Cell Neoplasms		
Chronic lymphocytic leukemia	M protein occasionally secreted; IgM > IgG	
B-cell non-Hodgkin lymphomas; Hodgkin disease	M protein occasionally secreted; IgM > IgG	
Nonlymphoid Neoplasms		
Chronic myelogenous leukemia	No consistent patterns	
Carcinomas (e.g., colon, breast, prostate)	No consistent patterns	
Autoimmune or Autoreactive Disorders		
Cold agglutinin disease	IgM κ most common	Anti-I antigen
Mixed cryoglobulinemia	IgM or IgA	Anti-IgG
Sjögren syndrome	IgM	
Miscellaneous Inflammatory, Storage, or Infectious Disorders		
Lichen myxedematosus	IgG λ	
Gaucher disease	IgG	
Cirrhosis, sarcoid, parasitic diseases, renal acidosis	No consistent pattern	

IgA, immunoglobulin A; IgD, immunoglobulin D; IgG, immunoglobulin G; IgM, immunoglobulin M.
Modified from Salmon SE: Plasma cell disorders. In Wyngaarden JB, Smith LH Jr (eds): Cecil Textbook of Medicine, 18th ed. Philadelphia, WB Saunders, 1988, p 1026.

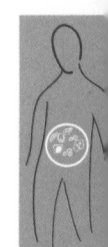

occurs in about 1% of patients per year. Distinguishing patients with stable, nonprogressive MGUS from patients in whom multiple myeloma will eventually develop is difficult. The risk for progression is greater in patients with IgA or IgM M proteins and in patients with initial concentrations of M protein in excess of 1.5 g/dL. Although no definitive evidence has been found that monitoring patients with the diagnosis of MGUS improves survival, patients should undergo annual evaluation, including serum electrophoresis, to detect progression to multiple myeloma before the onset of overt symptoms or complications.

MULTIPLE MYELOMA

Multiple myeloma is a malignant plasma cell disorder characterized by neoplastic infiltration of the bone marrow and bone and the presence of monoclonal immunoglobulin or light chains in the serum or urine. The diagnosis of multiple myeloma is made by identifying an increase in the number of plasma cells in the bone marrow (>30%) and a serum M protein other than IgM exceeding 3 g/dL for IgG or 2 g/dL for IgA or a urine M protein exceeding 1 g per 24 hours. Patients with lower levels of M protein or less than 30% bone marrow plasmacytosis may still be diagnosed with myeloma based on the presence of a combination of other features such as hypogammaglobulinemia, lytic bone lesions, or plasmacytoma. For patients lacking these features, the major differential diagnosis is usually between MGUS and myeloma; in some cases, the distinction can only be made by serial follow-up of the patient with evidence of rising M protein levels or the development of associated clinical manifestations of myeloma. About 20% of patients with multiple myeloma do not have detectable serum M protein by standard electrophoresis but have circulating free light chains that appear in the urine (Bence Jones protein) that can be detected in a 24-hour urine collection by urine protein electrophoresis *(light-chain disease)*. In rare cases, patients with *nonsecretory* myeloma have neither detectable serum nor urine M protein. However, in these patients, a monoclonal population of plasma cells can be detected by immunohistochemical identification of cytoplasmic light-chain–restricted immunoglobulin. Quantitative assays for detection of free light chains in the serum of patients with multiple myeloma have now become widely available and may be used to assess disease in a similar fashion to electrophoretic measurements. These assays are quite sensitive and may provide measurement of clonal protein in patients thought to have nonsecretory disease by other methods. Free light chains have a relatively short half-life in the circulation, 2 to 6 hours, in comparison with weeks for intact immunoglobulin molecules and may therefore be used to obtain a more rapid assessment of disease response for patients on therapy.

The clinical manifestations of multiple myeloma relate to the direct effects of bone marrow and bone infiltration by malignant plasma cells, the systemic effects of the M protein, or the effects of the concomitant deficiency in humoral immunity that occurs in this disease. The most common symptom in multiple myeloma is bone pain. Bone radiographs typically show pure osteolytic *punched-out* lesions, often in association with generalized osteopenia and pathologic fractures. Bony lesions can show as expansile masses

associated with spinal cord compression. Hypercalcemia caused by extensive bony involvement is common in myeloma and may dominate the clinical picture. Anemia occurs in most patients as a result of marrow infiltration and suppression of hematopoiesis and results in fatigue; granulocytopenia and thrombocytopenia are less common. Patients with myeloma are susceptible to bacterial infections because of impaired production and increased catabolism of normal immunoglobulins. Respiratory tract infections from *Streptococcus pneumoniae*, *Staphylococcus aureus*, *H. influenzae*, and *Klebsiella pneumoniae*, and gram-negative urinary tract infections are common. Renal insufficiency occurs in about 25% of patients with myeloma. The cause of renal failure in these patients is often multifactorial; hypercalcemia, hyperuricemia, infection, and amyloid deposition can contribute. However, direct tubular damage from light-chain excretion is invariably present. M proteins can also cause a host of diverse effects because of their physicochemical properties. These effects include cryoglobulinemia, hyperviscosity, amyloidosis, and clotting abnormalities resulting from interaction of the M protein with platelets or clotting factors.

Several staging or classification systems exist for myeloma. The three-tier staging system for myeloma is a functional system that correlates with survival (Table 51-7). In contrast to the anatomic staging systems used for lymphomas and solid tumors, myeloma staging is based on clinical tests (bone radiographs) and laboratory tests (hemoglobin, serum calcium, serum or urine M protein levels, and serum creatinine) that correlate with tumor burden. Adverse prognostic factors include advanced stage, impaired renal function, elevated LDH levels, abnormal bone marrow cytogenetics, depressed serum albumin levels, and elevated β_2-microglobulin levels. The last is the single most powerful predictor of survival. Recently, a simplified prognostic scheme, the International Staging System for Myeloma, identified three stages with distinct prognosis based on only two variables: β_2-microglobulin and albumin levels. A classification system proposed by the International Myeloma

Table 51-7 **Myeloma Staging System**	
Stage	**Criteria**

I	All of the following:
	1. Hemoglobin >10 g/dL
	2. Serum calcium <12 mg/dL
	3. Normal bone radiograph or solitary lesion
	4. Low M-component production
	   a. IgG level <5 g/dL
	   b. IgA level <3 g/dL
	   c. Urine light chain <4 g/24 hr

II	Fitting neither I nor III

III	One or more of the following:
	1. Hemoglobin <8.5 g/dL
	2. Serum calcium >12 mg/dL
	3. Advanced lytic bone lesions
	4. High M-component production
	   a. IgG level >7 g/dL
	   b. IgA level >5 g/dL
	   c. Urine light chains >12 g/24 hr

Subclassification:
  A Serum creatinine <2 mg/dL.
  B Serum creatinine <2 mg/dL.

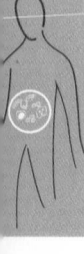

Working group divides patients with myeloma into two groups—asymptomatic and symptomatic myeloma—based on the presence or absence of four basic features termed myeloma-*related organ or tissue impairment* (ROTI). These factors include hypercalcemia, renal insufficiency, bone lesions, and anemia, and their presence provide sufficient evidence to initiate therapy.

Most patients with myeloma exhibit symptomatic, advanced-stage disease and require therapy. However, about 10% of patients have stage I disease or asymptomatic myeloma and an indolent course. These patients do not require immediate therapy, but they should be monitored for disease progression by serial quantification of the M protein. For patients with solitary bone or extramedullary plasmacytomas, particularly in the head and neck region, local radiation therapy can induce long-term remissions and is the treatment of choice. Patients with a solitary plasmacytoma of bone are often found on routine MRI of the spine to have asymptomatic bone disease and are at higher risk for subsequent development of myeloma.

Patients with symptomatic, advanced-stage (II or III) myeloma require systemic therapy as well as meticulous attention to supportive care. Although myeloma is not a curable malignancy, systemic therapy can prolong survival and dramatically improve quality of life. Options for treatment have expanded in the past decade to include three potent nonchemotherapeutic agents: thalidomide and lenalidomide (referred to as *immunomodulatory agents* or *Imids)* and bortezomib (a proteosome inhibitor), all of which are typically administered in combination with dexamethasone. These agents have largely supplanted traditional chemotherapeutic agents as initial and secondary therapies because they are efficacious and generally well tolerated.

The most commonly employed initial therapy is the combination of thalidomide and dexamethasone. Thalidomide was initially used as a sedative in the United Kingdom in the 1960s but was found to cause birth defects when used to combat nausea during pregnancy. The antiangiogenic properties of thalidomide subsequently led to its development as an anticancer agent. Although the mechanism of action of thalidomide in myeloma is unclear, one third of patients with recurrent or refractory disease following transplantation responded to thalidomide. In contrast to chemotherapy, thalidomide is infrequently myelosuppressive and has a unique side-effect profile, including peripheral neuropathy, constipation, somnolence, and rash. The combination of thalidomide and dexamethasone is highly active as initial therapy in treating myeloma and has the advantage of an all-oral treatment program. A troublesome unique side effect of the combination is the development of deep vein thrombosis in up to 25% of patients, and some form of preventative therapy is typically prescribed.

Lenalidomide, which is chemically related to thalidomide, is a more potent agent with a side-effect profile distinct from thalidomide. Myelosuppression is the main side effect of lenalidomide, and this drug is therefore not administered continuously. Lenalidomide therapy is also associated with an increased risk for deep vein thrombosis. Lenalidomide is indicated as second-line therapy for myeloma and is often employed as an alternate to thalidomide if troublesome side effects, such as neuropathy, dictate a change in therapy.

Bortezomib may be used as initial therapy for myeloma in combination with the alkylating agent melphalan plus prednisone. Because melphalan causes stem cell injury, this therapy may typically be avoided in patients who are eligible for stem cell transplantation. Bortezomib, in combination with dexamethasone, is an active drug for patients with recurrent or refractory disease and is associated with neuropathy, asthenia, and thrombocytopenia.

Most patients respond to initial therapy with a reduction in bone pain, hypercalcemia, and anemia in association with a decline in the M protein level. The use of high-dose chemotherapy with alkylating agents followed by autologous peripheral stem cell infusion has been shown to improve survival and quality of life compared with standard doses of chemotherapy. Although this approach is not curative, it does represent an important treatment option for some patients and has been shown to have an acceptable toxicity profile, even in older patients. Allogenic bone marrow transplantation may represent the only potentially curative treatment for myeloma, but the associated excessive morbidity and mortality in elderly patients and heavily pretreated patients have limited its use in this disease.

Patients who experience relapse after standard therapy or transplantation may be treated with alternate chemotherapy regimens or with novel combination therapies including both new agents (thalidomide, lenalidomide, bortezomib) and chemotherapy drugs.

Supportive care directed toward anticipated complications of myeloma is an important aspect of the management of this disease. Bone resorption can be reduced with regular injections of the diphosphonates zoledronic acid or pamidronate, reducing pain and pathologic fractures. Bony lesions, particularly those involving weight-bearing bones, may require palliative radiation for controlling pain and preventing pathologic fractures. Vertebral bony lesions may lead to spinal cord compression, with increasing back pain and neurologic symptoms. Any symptoms suggestive of cord compression require prompt evaluation with spinal MRI and, if necessary, local radiation to involved areas. Avoidance of nephrotoxins, including intravenous dyes, is important to prevent renal failure. Acute renal failure caused by light-chain deposition may improve with plasmapheresis to acutely reduce protein load. All patients should receive pneumococcal and *H. influenzae* vaccines, and intravenous gamma-globulin may be useful in preventing recurrent infections in patients with profound hypogammaglobulinemia. Use of erythropoietin may alleviate anemia and decrease the need for blood transfusions.

WALDENSTRÖM MACROGLOBULINEMIA

Waldenström macroglobulinemia is a malignancy of plasmacytoid lymphocytes that secrete large quantities of IgM. It is a chronic disorder affecting elderly patients (median age is 64 years) that shares features of the low-grade lymphomas and myeloma. In contrast to myeloma, Waldenström macroglobulinemia is associated with lymphadenopathy and hepatosplenomegaly, and, although bone marrow involvement is invariably present, lytic lesions and hypercalcemia are distinctly rare. The major clinical manifestation of Waldenström macroglobulinemia is usually the hyperviscosity syndrome caused by the physical properties of IgM. In contrast to IgG, IgM remains largely confined to the intravascular space, and, as IgM levels rise, plasma viscosity increases. Epistaxis, retinal hemorrhages, dizziness, confusion, and congestive heart failure are common symptoms of the hyperviscosity syndrome. About 10% of IgM proteins have properties of cryoglobulins, and these patients show symptoms of cryoglobulinemia or cold agglutinin syndrome demonstrated as acrocyanosis, Raynaud phenomenon and vascular symptoms, or hemolytic anemia precipitated by exposure to cold. Some patients with Waldenström macroglobulinemia may develop a peripheral neuropathy that may antedate the appearance of the neoplastic process.

The approach to and treatment of Waldenström macroglobulinemia are similar to those of other low-grade B-cell lymphomas. The use of nucleoside analogues (2-CDA and fludarabine) or an alkylating agent, alone or in combination with prednisone, is effective in decreasing adenopathy and splenomegaly and controlling the M spike but is not curative. Rituximab has been found to have activity in Waldenström macroglobulinemia as has the novel proteosome inhibitor bortezomib. Plasmapheresis is highly effective in acutely decreasing serum IgM levels and is often needed initially to treat hyperviscosity. Although complete remissions are rare, patients who respond to therapy have median survivals of 4 years, and some patients survive more than a decade.

RARE PLASMA CELL DISORDERS

Heavy-chain disease is a rare lymphoplasmacytoid neoplasm characterized by production of a defective heavy chain of the γ, α, or μ type. The clinical manifestations vary with the type of heavy chain secreted. γ heavy-chain disease is associated with lymphadenopathy, Waldeyer ring involvement with palatal edema, and constitutional symptoms. α heavy-chain disease, also known as *Mediterranean lymphoma*, is characterized by lymphoid infiltration of the small intestine with associated diarrhea and malabsorption. μ heavy-chain disease is associated with CLL. Primary amyloidosis is a systemic illness characterized by deposition of immunoglobulin light chain in organs and tissue, resulting in an array of symptoms caused by organ dysfunction. Congestive heart failure, bleeding diathesis, nephrotic syndrome, and peripheral neuropathy are common complications. Patients with primary amyloidosis respond poorly to the treatments used for myeloma. Encouraging results have been reported with high-dose chemotherapy and autologous stem cell support, particularly if patients are treated before the development of significant end-organ dysfunction such as cardiomyopathy.

CONGENITAL AND ACQUIRED DISORDERS OF LYMPHOCYTE FUNCTION

A significant number of congenital disorders affect lymphocyte maturation or function, resulting in immunodeficiency disorders. Acquired disorders of lymphocyte function are far more common compared with congenital disorders. HIV infection is the most important infectious cause of acquired immunodeficiency and is discussed in Chapter 109. Patients

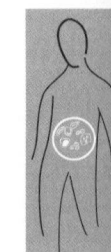

with HIV infection are at increased risk for developing NHL. NHLs that occur in the setting of HIV have the diffuse aggressive B-cell histology and include diffuse large B-cell lymphoma and Burkitt lymphoma; they are also frequently associated with EBV and are often advanced stage (III or IV) at initial diagnosis, with extranodal sites of involvement. Patients with HIV-associated NHL are potentially curable with the multidrug chemotherapy regimens used for treating these NHL subtypes in the general population. In addition, treatment of the underlying HIV infection with highly active antiretroviral therapy has improved the outcome and prognosis of patients with HIV-associated NHL.

Patients who have undergone an allogeneic organ transplantation require potent immunosuppressive drugs (e.g., cyclosporine, tacrolimus, mycophenolate, corticosteroids, methotrexate) to prevent graft-versus-host disease in the case of bone marrow transplantation or allograft rejection in the case of solid organ transplantation. These medications can cause profound defects in T-cell function with an associated acquired immunodeficiency state, and transplant recipients are susceptible to a host of viral and protozoal infections. In addition, patients who receive potent immunosuppressive drugs are at risk for developing a lymphoproliferative disorder (post-transplantation lymphoproliferative disorder [PTLD]) that can behave clinically as an aggressive lymphoma. PTLD is an EBV-associated lymphoproliferative disorder characterized by a polymorphous or monomorphous population of B cells that can be monoclonal or polyclonal. Patients who develop PTLD are treated by reducing the doses of immunosuppressive drugs whenever possible; this intervention alone will result in regression of PTLD in about one half of the patients, obviating the need for cytotoxic therapy. Patients who are not candidates for withdrawal of immunosuppression because of allograft rejection or who fail to respond to this strategy can be treated with rituximab alone or in combination with chemotherapy.

INFECTIOUS DISORDERS

Lymphocytes play an essential role in the adaptive response to infection. This response can be shown clinically with an increase in lymphocytes in the peripheral blood (reactive lymphocytosis) and lymph node enlargement. Reactive lymphocytosis is always polyclonal, usually predominantly T cell, and usually easily distinguishable from the common monoclonal B-cell neoplastic processes. Some infections are typically associated with a prominent lymphocytosis (e.g., EBV-associated infectious mononucleosis, cytomegalovirus, toxoplasmosis in immunocompetent hosts, viral hepatitis). Enlargement of lymph nodes, either local-regional or generalized lymphadenopathy, is a common manifestation of some infections (see Table 51-1). Lymph node enlargement may be striking and associated with tenderness. In most cases, the adenopathy is reactive, and the organism cannot be readily cultured from the node; in other cases (e.g., tuberculosis, fungal disease), culture or appropriate staining in lymph node tissue can identify the organism. Biopsy of the node generally will confirm the non-neoplastic nature of the process, showing a normal architecture and cellular pattern and absence of a monoclonal population of lymphoid cells.

Prospectus for the Future

Further advances in our understanding of lymphoproliferative diseases are likely to come from molecular studies such as DNA microarray analyses used to create profiles of gene expression in malignant cells. Such analyses will aid in further subclassifying lymphoproliferative diseases and will help define prognosis and response to therapy; such data are already available in limited form for diffuse large B-cell lymphoma and CLL. An understanding of gene expression profiles unique to specific disease will also provide additional targets for pharmacologic or immunologically based therapies.

The advent of humanized chimeric monoclonal antibodies targeted to CD20 has changed the therapy of some lymphomas, and antibodies to other cell surface antigens, including radiolabeled antibodies, are in development.

For multiple myeloma, combinations of both new agents (thalidomide, lenalidomide, bortezomib) and chemotherapeutic agents are likely to improve outcomes by achieving higher rates of complete remissions.

For allogeneic transplantation, reduced-intensity conditioning regimens are improving the therapeutic index of this procedure for curative treatment of multiple myeloma and lymphomas.

References

Armitage JO, Mauch PM, Harris NL, Bierman P: Non-Hodgkin's lymphomas. In DeVita VT Jr, Hellman S, Rosenberg SA (eds): Cancer-Principles and Practice of Oncology. Philadelphia, Lippincott, Williams & Wilkins, 2001, pp 2256-2315.

Canellos GP, Anderson JR, Propert KJ, et al: Chemotherapy of advanced Hodgkin's disease with MOPP, ABVD, or MOPP alternating with ABVD. N Engl J Med 327:1478-1484, 1992.

Diehl V, Mauch PM, Harris NL: Hodgkin's disease. In DeVita VT Jr, Hellman S, Rosenberg SA (eds): Cancer-Principles and Practice of Oncology. Philadelphia, Lippincott, Williams & Wilkins, 2001, pp 2339-2388.

Fisher RI, Gaynor ER, Dahlberg S, et al: Comparison of a standard regimen (CHOP) with three intensive chemotherapy regimens for advanced non-Hodgkin's lymphoma. N Engl J Med 328:1002-1006, 1993.

Gaidano G, Dalla-Favara R: Molecular biology of lymphomas. In DeVita VT Jr, Hellman S, Rosenberg SA (eds): Cancer-Principles and Practice of Oncology. Philadelphia, Lippincott, Williams & Wilkins, 2001, pp 2215-2235.

Harris N, Jaffe E, Diebold J, et al: World Health Organization classification of neoplastic diseases of the hematopoietic and lymphoid tissues: Report of the Clinical Advisory Committee Meeting, Airlie House, Virginia, November 1997. J Clin Oncol 17:3835-3849, 1999.

Kyle RA, Therneau TM, Rajkumar SV, et al: A long-term study of prognosis in monoclonal gammopathy of undetermined significance. N Engl J Med 346:564-569, 2002.

Maloney DG, Grillo-Lopez AJ, White CA, et al: IDEC-C2B8 (rituximab) anti-CD20 monoclonal antibody therapy in patients with relapsed low-grade non-Hodgkin's lymphoma. Blood 90:2188-2195, 1997.

McSweeney PA, Niederwieser D, Shizuru JA, et al: Hematopoietic cell transplantation in older patients with hematologic malignancies: Replacing high-dose cytotoxic therapy with graft-versus-tumor effects. Blood 97:3390-3400, 2001.

Munschi NC, Tricot G, Barlogie B: Plasma cell dyscrasias. In DeVita VT Jr, Hellman S, Rosenberg SA (eds): Cancer-Principles and Practice of Oncology. Philadelphia, Lippincott, Williams & Wilkins, 2001, pp 2465-2498.

Philip T, Guglielmi C, Hagenbeek A, et al: Autologous bone marrow transplantation as compared with salvage chemotherapy in relapses of chemotherapy-sensitive non-Hodgkin's lymphoma. N Engl J Med 33:1540-1545, 1995.

Singhal S, Mehta J, Desikan R, et al: Antitumor activity of thalidomide in refractory multiple myeloma. N Engl J Med 341:1565-1571, 1999.

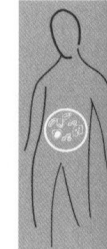

Normal Hemostasis

Christine S. Rinder and Henry M. Rinder

Hemostasis is the physiologic balance of procoagulant and anticoagulant forces that maintain both liquid blood flow and the structural integrity of the vasculature. Vascular damage results in initiation of clotting with the goal of producing a *localized* platelet-fibrin plug to prevent blood loss; this action is followed by processes that lead to clot containment, wound healing, clot dissolution, tissue regeneration, and remodeling. In healthy persons, all these reactions occur continuously and in a balanced fashion such that bleeding is contained, yet blood vessels simultaneously remain patent to deliver adequate organ blood flow. When any of these hemostatic processes is disrupted because of inherited defects or acquired abnormalities, disordered hemostasis may result in either bleeding or thromboembolic complications.

Blood flow in the arterial and venous systems is disparate and imposes different needs on the coagulation system. In the pressurized arteries, relatively minor vascular damage can rapidly result in massive blood loss; thus, the procoagulant response in arteries must rapidly arrest bleeding. Platelets are critical to this arterial response; they initially contain blood loss and then provide an active surface for soluble coagulation factors to both localize and accelerate fibrin and, ultimately, clot formation. By contrast, in the venous circulation, the slower flow rates produce slower bleeding, a feature that makes platelets less critical; instead, controlling the balance of venous hemostasis is most dependent on the rate of thrombin generation. These differences are further underscored clinically by the anticoagulant agents used in these distinct settings, that is, antiplatelet agents such as aspirin and clopidogrel to prevent coronary and cerebral artery thrombus, compared with interventions that inhibit thrombin, including the heparins and warfarin, for treatment and prophylaxis of venous thromboembolic disease.

This chapter briefly details the physiologic and interdependent mechanisms of vascular hemostasis, including the normal balance of procoagulant and anticoagulant functions of the blood vessel wall, platelet physiologic factors and receptor-ligand interactions critical for hemostasis, and the highly complex, interwoven pathways that represent the coagulation cascade.

Vascular Wall Physiology

Vascular endothelial cells (ECs) are capable of orchestrating both procoagulant and anticoagulant events depending on circumstances. When the vasculature is intact, healthy ECs exert tonic anticoagulant activity, helping to maintain blood fluidity. This is partially due to a passive barrier function separating the blood from subendothelial procoagulants such as collagen and tissue factor (TF). In addition, healthy ECs actively regulate the hemostatic balance of activity in their microenvironment through their secreted products (Table 52-1). These include prostacyclin and nitric oxide, both of which induce vascular smooth muscle relaxation and reduced shear when released in an abluminal direction. When secreted into the blood, they promote platelet cyclic adenosine monophosphate (cAMP) generation, thus inhibiting platelet activation and aggregation. ECs also secrete adenosine diphosphatase (ADPase), which degrades extracellular platelet-released adenosine diphosphate (ADP), thereby inhibiting platelet recruitment into the growing platelet clot. Soluble coagulation factors are also regulated by ECs in both tonic and inducible fashion. Tissue factor pathway inhibitor (TFPI) in its nascent circulating form blunts initiation of coagulation; TFPI is subsequently primed for increased activity by exposure to small amounts of factor Xa. Quiescent thrombomodulin and tissue plasminogen activator are localized at the EC extracellular matrix, ready to be activated by local formation of thrombin and fibrin, respectively, to carry out their anticoagulant and fibrinolytic functions.

When ECs are physically damaged or become activated, their balance of coagulant properties is shifted to favor a procoagulant state. This function is mediated both by the ECs themselves and by the underlying subendothelial matrix that is exposed by vascular injury. Activated (e.g., by toxins or secreted factors) ECs express adhesive ligands on their surface, including the selectins (both E-selectin and

P-selectin), β₁ and β₂ integrins, platelet endothelial cell adhesion molecule-1 (PECAM-1), and von Willebrand factor (vWF) multimers (see Table 52-1). On the EC surface, vWF multimers localize and promote platelet adhesion, whereas integrins mediate adhesion and subsequent transendothelial migration of leukocytes into the tissues. Exposed subendothelial matrix also binds vWF multimers (Fig. 52-1) and contains other procoagulant, adhesive proteins, including thrombospondin, fibronectin, and collagen. These moieties function both as ligands to capture platelets and as activators of adherent platelets; collagen, in particular, is both a platelet ligand and a strong platelet agonist; the latter capability causes platelets to undergo dense granule release and to express conformationally active ligands such as glycoprotein IIb/IIIa (GPIIb/IIIa; see later discussion). Another critical procoagulant mediator exposed by EC damage is TF, which is constitutively expressed by subendothelial smooth muscle cells and fibroblasts. As outlined later (see "Soluble Coagulation"), TF is the major initiator of the soluble coagulation system that, with activated platelets, results in the formation of a definitive platelet-fibrin clot (Fig. 52-2).

Platelet Physiology

The platelet functions as the cellular-based platform for hemostasis. Platelet surface receptors mediate primary

hemostasis and allow platelets to bind directly to endothelium and subendothelium at sites of damage. Platelet interaction with their ligands causes transmembrane signaling through surface receptors to induce platelet activation and promote procoagulant function through pathways, including translocation of additional receptors to the membrane surface, receptor conformational change to active forms, release of granule contents that recruit platelet adhesion, and exposure of procoagulant membrane phospholipids. The procoagulant surface of the platelet then serves as a platform for enhanced assembly of the coagulation cascade to generate thrombin, which (1) feeds back on platelets and the clotting cascade to amplify the procoagulant response, and (2) produces fibrin to provide secondary, long-lasting hemostasis. Finally, the platelet further assists thrombin in clot consolidation and protection from fibrinolysis by contributing factor XIII and platelet factor 4, respectively, to the clot milieu (Table 52-2).

PLATELET HEMOSTASIS

Platelets are anucleate cells between 2 and 4 μm in diameter with a volume between 6 and 11 fL. Platelets are derived from the megakaryocyte cytoplasm after a maturation time of about 4 days, with each megakaryocyte contributing about 1000 circulating platelets in its lifetime. When platelets are released into the circulation, they survive between 7 to 10 days; platelets leave the circulation through a combination of senescence and the normal maintenance of vascular structural integrity. For the latter, very few platelets are needed; approximately 7100 platelets/mcL are required for hemostasis per day when vascular structures are intact (e.g., no recent surgery or trauma) and when there is no increase in normal platelet consumption (e.g., sepsis). The normal platelet count range is between 150,000 and 450,000/mcL. With platelet counts in the normal range and normal platelet function, the bleeding time, an in vivo measure of platelet function, is generally less than 8 minutes. However, when normal functioning platelets are less than 100,000/mcL, the bleeding time is prolonged. Thus, in the presence of thrombocytopenia, the bleeding time cannot be used to determine whether bleeding is caused by abnormal platelet function or

Table 52-1 **Endothelial Cell Coagulant Properties**	
Procoagulant	**Anticoagulant**
Collagen	Vasodilation
Factor VIII	Adenosine diphosphatase
Fibronectin	Heparan sulfates
Integrins	Nitric oxide
Platelet-endothelial cell adhesion molecule-1	Prostacyclin Thrombomodulin
Selectins (E and P) Vasoconstriction	Tissue factor pathway inhibitor
von Willebrand factor	Tissue plasminogen activator

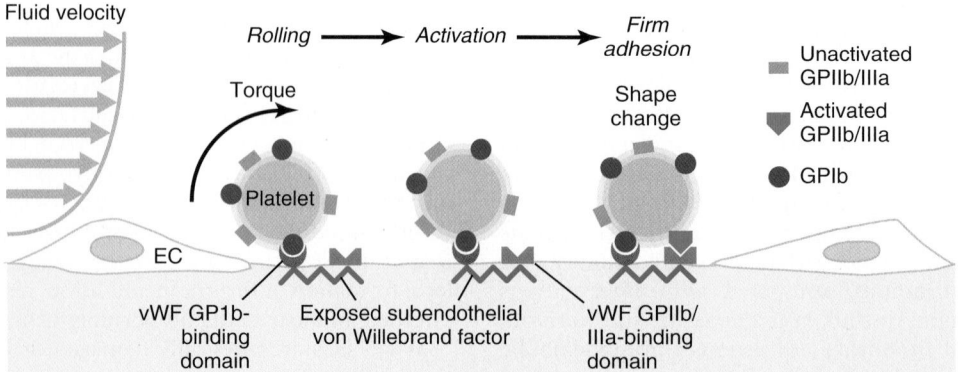

Figure 52-1 The adhesive interactions producing stable platelet attachment to subendothelial von Willebrand factor (vWF). The initial attachment between platelet glycoprotein Ib (GPIb) and its binding domain on vWF is rapid but has a short half-life, and the result is a rolling movement from torque generated by flowing blood. The vWF-GPIb interaction produces transmembrane signaling that activates the platelet to undergo shape change and simultaneously transforms GPIIb/IIIa into an activated conformation capable of binding to a distinct arginine-glycine-aspartate domain on vWF. This secondary adhesion causes the platelet to firmly adhere to the exposed subendothelial vWF. EC, endothelial cell.

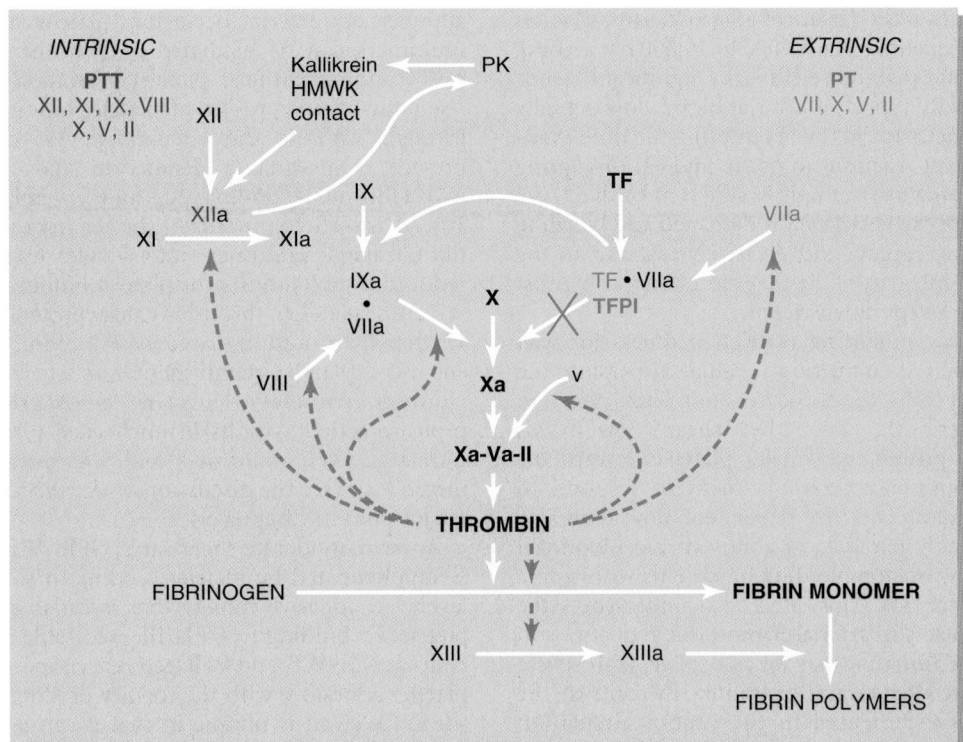

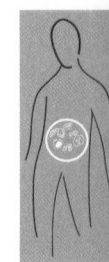

Figure 52-2 The coagulation cascade. The laboratory-defined *extrinsic* and *intrinsic* pathways allow monitoring of anticoagulation by the prothrombin time (PT) and partial thromboplastin time (PTT), respectively. The PT primarily monitors factor VII activity, whereas the PTT is the best measure of XI and the hemophilic factors IX and VIII; both assays will detect deficiency of the common pathway factors (X, V, and II). Initiation of clotting begins with TF exposure, which then combines with small amounts of circulating VIIa to form the extrinsic Xase complex and generate Xa. Xa forms the prothrombinase complex with Va and II, generating small amounts of thrombin, which begin to cleave fibrinogen into weak fibrin monomers in the initiation phase of coagulation. Thrombin's ability to activate factors, especially when carried out on the activated platelet surface, is responsible for propagation of the coagulant response. Thrombin generates XIa, which, in turn, activates IX; the TF-VIIa complex (before its shutdown by TFPI) also generates IXa. Thrombin-activated VIIIa then combines with IXa to form the intrinsic Xase complex, generating large amounts of Xa and prothrombinase complex on the platelet surface to further amplify thrombin generation. The large amounts of thrombin now generate enough fibrin monomers to form stable polymers and fibrin clot. HMWK, high-molecular-weight kininogen; PK, prekallikrein; TF, tissue factor; TFPI, tissue factor pathway inhibitor.

Table 52-2 Procoagulant Properties of Platelets

Receptor-Ligand Interactions Promoting Adhesion

GPIb/IX/V–vWF
GPIIb/IIIa–fibrinogen and GPIIb/IIIa–vWF
GPIa/IIa–collagen
P selectin–P selectin glycoprotein ligand-1

Receptor-Ligand Interactions Mediating Activation

GPV–thrombin
GPVI–collagen

Secreted α-Granule Proteins

Ligands (fibrinogen, fibronectin, thrombospondin, vitronectin, vWF)
Enzymes (α_2-antiplasmin, factors V, VIII, and XI)
Antiheparin (platelet factor 4)

Secreted Dense-Granule Agonists

ADP, serotonin

Secreted Cytosolic Factor XIII—Membrane Components

Thromboxane A$_2$ formation, phosphatidylserine expression

ADP, adenosine diphosphate; GP, glycoprotein; GPIa/IIa, complex of glycoprotein Ia and CD29; GPIb/IX/V complex, CD42; GPIIb/IIIa (α_2-β_3) complex, CD41; P selectin, CD62P; P selectin glycoprotein ligand-1, CD162; vWF, von Willebrand factor.

connective tissue disease. The bleeding time is an operator-dependent, highly variable in vivo assay that can leave scars; many laboratories have therefore switched to a so-called in vitro bleeding time test, for example, the Platelet Function Analyzer-100 (PFA-100), which uses anticoagulated whole blood to examine "closure time." However, the PFA-100 and other like-minded tests are similar to the bleeding time test in that they are unable to distinguish between thrombocytopenia and abnormal platelet function when platelet counts are below 100,000/mcL.

SHEAR-INDUCED ADHESION

Platelet–vessel wall interaction has been well characterized at the high flow velocities of the arterial circulation. The interaction between the vasculature and flowing blood, as shown on the left side of Figure 52-1, creates parallel planes of blood moving at different velocities; the blood closest to the vessel wall moves slower than blood closer to the center of the vessel. These different velocities create shear stress that is greatest at the vessel wall and is least at the center of the vessel. Shear rate therefore changes inversely with the vessel diameter, with levels estimated to vary between 500 per second in larger arteries and 5000 per second in the smallest arterioles. Shear rates at the surface of atherosclerotic plaques with modest (50%) stenosis reach 3000 to 10,000 per second, with even greater shear in more clinically significant stenoses. The high-velocity aspect of arterial blood flow actually opposes the tendencies to clot by (1) limiting the time available for procoagulant reactions to occur, and (2) disrupting cells and proteins that are not tightly adherent to the vessel wall. However, once the vessel wall is damaged and bleeding occurs, platelets can rapidly and decisively respond to the loss of endothelial integrity while they simultaneously resist the tendency to be swept downstream.

One of the forces enhancing platelet readiness for wall adhesion in the arterial circulation is radial dispersion, the tendency of larger cells (erythrocytes and leukocytes) to stream in the center of the vessel, where shear is lowest; this process effectively pushes the smaller platelets toward the vessel wall and optimally positions them to respond to hemostatic challenges. This size-dependent flow may also explain the seemingly paradoxical ability of red blood cell transfusions to slow or stop bleeding in patients with severe uremia (see Chapter 53). This effect also underscores the importance of platelets in arterial hemostasis; reductions in platelet number or function may be associated with severe arterial hemorrhage after surgery or trauma. By contrast, the lesser shear forces experienced in the venous circulation permit more random cell movement and greater time for coagulation reactions to occur; thus, the minimum requirements for platelet number and function in venous hemostasis are correspondingly less stringent.

In the setting of high-velocity blood flow at an arterial bleeding site, platelets must activate and adhere to the injured vessel nearly instantaneously. Two molecules present in the subendothelium are critical for this process: vWF and collagen. Control of bleeding in vessels under the highest shear stresses absolutely depends on the presence and function of vWF. vWF is a large molecule synthesized as multimeric *strings* in ECs and megakaryocytes, and multimeric vWF is both constitutively secreted into blood and stored in Weibel-Palade bodies of ECs. The *ultralarge* vWF multimers are the most active at binding platelets, particularly when *unfolded* by either shear stress or after tethering to the vessel surface. The multimeric forms of vWF, which are immobilized by adherence to exposed subendothelial collagen, bind to the GPIb/IX-V complex on the platelet surface when normally cryptic loci are exposed by high shear stress (see Fig. 52-1). This binding is extremely rapid but low affinity, thus slowing the platelets at this interface but leaving them only weakly adherent to subendothelial vWF. With platelets no longer streaming by, but instead tumbling or sliding over the subendothelium, the high shear stress in tandem with transmembrane signaling produced by the GPIb-V-IX-vWF interaction results in loss of the normal platelet discoid shape (shape change) and conformational change in another platelet receptor, GPIIb/IIIa.

LIGANDS

The activated GPIIb/IIIa receptor now binds either to fibrinogen or to the larger vWF multimers at a site distinct from the GPIb/IX-V-binding site. This secondary adhesion is a higher-affinity interaction than the latter, thereby securing platelets firmly to the subendothelium. At shear rates that approximate arterial occlusion, platelet adhesion to vWF multimers can be mediated entirely through GPIb-V-IX-vWF binding without platelet activation. One important regulator of this process of platelet binding and activation through vWF is the circulating vWF-cleaving protease present in plasma: a disintegrin and metalloproteinase with a thrombospondin type 1 motif, member 13 (ADAMTS-13). ADAMTS-13 modulates the activity of vWF by cleaving the ultralarge multimers into smaller fragments that have reduced overall affinity for platelet binding. Besides directly activating platelets, thrombin causes proteolysis of ADAMTS-13, thereby promoting large vWF multimer persistence and enhanced platelet recruitment into areas of vessel injury. However, pathologic loss of the ADAMTS-13 cleaving protease activity results in unchecked platelet adhesion to ultralarge vWF multimers and widespread microvascular thrombosis (see the discussion of *thrombotic thrombocytopenic purpura* in Chapter 54).

At more moderate shear rates, GPIb-V-IX-vWF adhesion is supplemented by platelet binding to subendothelial collagen, an adhesive moiety that is capable of arresting the platelet by binding to GPIa/IIa (see Table 52-2). Thus, subendothelial vWF and collagen act cooperatively to initiate platelet adhesion, with the former predominating at higher shear. Collagen is unique in that it can anchor platelets at one locus by binding to platelet GPIa/IIa and can activate platelets at a second locus by binding to platelet GPVI, and both platelet receptors are critical for physiologic platelet function. Indeed, the congenital absence of any of the critical platelet adhesion receptors—GPIIb/IIIa, GPIb/IX-V, GPVI, or GPIa/IIa—results in a significant hemostatic defect, correctable only by platelet transfusion. This finding is further reinforced by the α chain of GPIb normally serving as a cofactor for thrombin activation of platelets through both the GPV receptor and the protease activated receptor (PAR). Similarly to defects in platelet receptors, decreases in the vWF ligand, especially the larger multimeric forms, can lead to bleeding.

Once a layer of platelets is adherent to the site of injury, vWF bound to GPIb/IX-V on the luminal side of the adherent platelets serves to recruit additional platelets from the flowing blood into the growing platelet plug. Platelet recruitment is further enhanced by platelet activation and release of serotonin and ADP, which serve to activate and adhere platelets from the circulation to the growing platelet clot. Platelet activation is actually a series of interdependent processes with five major effects: (1) local release of ligands essential to stabilizing the platelet-platelet matrix, (2) continued recruitment of additional platelets, (3) vasoconstriction of smaller arteries to slow bleeding, (4) localization and acceleration of platelet-associated fibrin formation, and (5) protection of the clot from fibrinolysis.

The basis of the platelet plug is a platelet-ligand-platelet matrix with fibrinogen, fibronectin, and vWF serving as bridging ligands (Fig. 52-3). Both fibrinogen and vWF are endocytosed from plasma and stored in α granules inside the resting platelet. Both molecules are released with activation, and both can bind to a GPIIb/IIIa receptor on each of two platelets, thereby linking them. As mentioned earlier, platelet GPIIb/IIIa undergoes a calcium-dependent conformational change that allows it to bind to a locus containing the amino acid sequence arginine-glycine-aspartate (RGD)

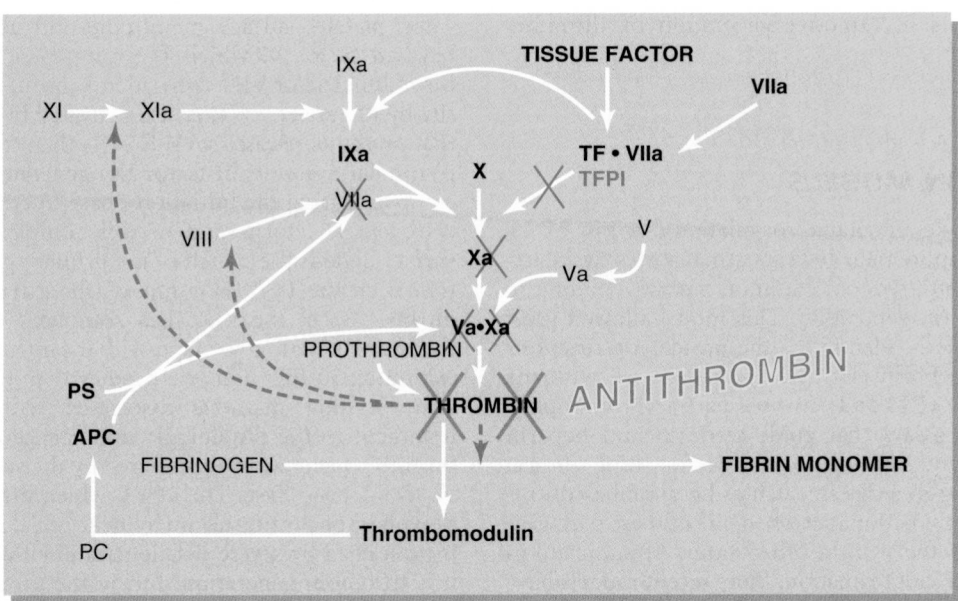
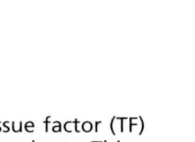

Figure 52-3 Endogenous anticoagulant pathways. In addition to tissue factor pathway inhibitor (TFPI) shutting off tissue factor (TF) stimulation and blocking the TF-VIIa-X complex, the clotting cascade is further downregulated by the natural anticoagulants. This inhibition is partly generated by thrombin, which activates thrombomodulin. Circulating antithrombin inhibits thrombin activity and Xa generation of thrombin. The complex of thrombin and thrombomodulin activates protein C (APC), which combines with protein S (PS) to cleave and inactivate VIIIa and Va, further blocking thrombin generation.

on fibrinogen, fibronectin, or vWF. Each fibrinogen molecule has two RGD sites on its polar ends, and the larger vWF multimers have several RGD sites, all capable of binding to conformationally altered GPIIb/IIIa and creating the platelet-ligand-platelet matrix. GPIIb/IIIa is the most abundant glycoprotein on the platelet surface, with about 50,000 copies on the *resting* platelet and additional GPIIb/IIIa receptors within the platelet cytosol that are mobilized to the surface after activation.

ACTIVATION

Platelets are also recruited into the platelet plug by local agonists (collagen, epinephrine, and thrombin) and by platelet release of agonists into the local microenvironment. Both collagen (as noted previously) and thrombin interact with their specific platelet receptors to activate platelets strongly; although epinephrine alone is not a powerful platelet agonist, stimulation of the α-adrenergic receptor on platelets primes them for synergistic activation by even relatively weak agonists such as ADP. Activating compounds released directly from the platelet include thromboxane A_2 (TXA_2), which is formed in the platelet cytosol after cyclooxygenase-1 (COX-1)–mediated cleavage of arachidonic acid and then released into the clot milieu. TXA_2 is both a platelet agonist and a vasoconstrictor, and it is rapidly degraded to its inert by-product, thromboxane B_2. Platelet COX-1 activity is *irreversibly* inhibited by aspirin, thereby blocking TXA_2 formation for the lifetime of that platelet. Aspirin irreversibly and covalently binds to a specific serine residue on COX-1 and causes steric hindrance of the active site, a tyrosine molecule across from the serine residue. Nonsteroidal anti-inflammatory drugs (NSAIDs) do not covalently bind through acetylation at serine. Instead, they reversibly and competitively bind at the active, catalytic tyrosine site. Thus, the antiplatelet

effects of NSAIDs are dependent on the continual presence of plasma levels of the NSAID, unlike aspirin. COX-2 is an induced isoform within leukocytes that mediates inflammation and pain. Because mature platelets do not appear to possess COX-2 activity, one rationale for development of the highly selective COX-2 inhibitors for inflammatory diseases was the avoidance of bleeding caused by platelet dysfunction by not affecting platelet COX-1 activity. However, it appears that vascular ECs use COX-2 activity to synthesize the antithrombogenic compound, prostacyclin (see Table 52-1 and Chapter 55). Downregulation of EC prostacyclin, coupled with preserved platelet prothrombotic function, may tip the hemostatic balance in favor of clot formation, and large-scale clinical trials have now shown that some highly selective COX-2 inhibitors increase the likelihood of hypertension and vascular arterial events, including myocardial infarction and stroke.

Other platelet agonists are liberated into the extracellular fluid by fusion of the dense and α granules with the platelet canalicular membrane, and the result is extrusion of granule contents. The dense granules contain serotonin that, similar to TXA_2, is both a platelet agonist and a vasoconstrictor. Another dense granule constituent, ADP, acts purely as a platelet agonist through the G-protein–linked $P2Y_{12}$ receptor and has no vasoactive properties (see Table 52-2). The importance of TXA_2- and serotonin-induced vasoconstriction is not entirely clear. However, vasoconstriction, by decreasing the vessel diameter, may increase shear stress and thereby facilitate recruitment of platelets to the injured site. The importance of dense granule release to the maintenance of hemostasis is underscored by the severe bleeding seen in congenital dense granule deficiencies (e.g., Hermansky-Pudlak syndrome). Platelet activation therefore serves to amplify platelet adhesion and, as detailed later, optimize the platelet surface for interaction with soluble coagulation

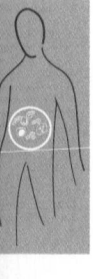

factors that results in explosive generation of thrombin and fibrin.

Soluble Coagulation

COAGULATION MODELS

The "cascade" model of soluble coagulation (see Fig. 52-2), as first described more than 40 years ago, features two starting points that converge to a common pathway leading to thrombin and fibrin generation. This model allowed great strides to be made in identifying the proteolytic reactions that culminate in fibrin clot and dovetailed well with the prothrombin time (PT) and activated partial thromboplastin time (aPTT) assays that guide warfarin and heparin dosing, respectively. Although workable for some clinical scenarios, bleeding in a disease such as hemophilia contradicts the model's prediction that when one of these pathways is dysfunctional, activity of the other should be sufficient to maintain adequate clot formation. More recent models have made significant strides in clarifying the dynamics of coagulation. Regulation of coagulation proteins is characterized by continuous low-grade factor activation and coordinated assembly of enzyme complexes, which are downregulated by circulating inhibitor proteins. These enzyme complexes consist of serine proteases, their cofactors, and zymogen substrates. In the absence of overt blood vessel disruption, enzyme complex formation and the resultant thrombin generation are both minimal and relatively slow; circulating anticoagulants are sufficient to inactivate these procoagulant complexes and prevent clot formation. However, once a procoagulant stimulus occurs that generates significant amounts of activated factors, formation of these enzyme complexes is rapidly amplified (partly by its assembly on a favorable membrane (phospholipid) surface), leading to intense thrombin, and subsequent fibrin, formation.

CLOT INITIATION

Coagulation in vivo follows exposure of the blood to a source of TF, typically on the surface of a fibroblast coming into contact with blood through a break in the vessel wall. The intrinsic or contact pathway of coagulation has no role in the earliest events in clotting. TF-initiated coagulation has two phases: an *initiation* phase and a second referred to as the *propagation* phase (see Fig. 52-2). The initiation phase begins as the exposed TF binds to factor VIIa, picomolar amounts of which are present in the circulation at all times. This VIIa-TF complex catalyzes the conversion of very small amounts of factor X to Xa, which in turn, generates nanomolar amounts of thrombin. The seemingly trivial amount of thrombin formed during the initiation phase sparks the inception of the propagation phase, successful completion of which culminates in explosive thrombin generation and, ultimately, fibrin deposition. More than 96% of the total thrombin that is generated during clotting occurs during the propagation phase.

CLOT PROPAGATION

Thrombin generated during the initiation phase is a potent platelet activator, supplying the developing clot with an acti-

vated platelet surface membrane and abundant platelet-released factor V, which is promptly activated to Va by thrombin. Factor VIII, conveniently brought to the bleeding site by its carrier, vWF, is also activated by thrombin, a step that causes its release by vWF. VIIIa then complexes with the picomolar amounts of factor IXa generated by the TF-VIIa complex during the initiation phase to create the VIIIa-IXa complex. The formation of this complex on the platelet surface heralds the switch of the primary path of Xa generation from the TF-VIIa complex (the extrinsic Xase) to the intrinsic Xase (the VIIIa-IXa complex). This switch is of significant kinetic advantage, with the intrinsic Xase complex exhibiting 50-fold higher efficiency than the extrinsic Xase. The bleeding diathesis associated with hemophilia is testament to the physiologic importance of the exuberant thrombin generation engendered by the switch from extrinsic to intrinsic Xase. The aPTT, which measures the initiation phase of clotting begun by an artificial in vitro stimulant, is prolonged by severe deficiencies in either VIII or IX, but it is thrombin generation during the propagation phase, a function not evaluated by the aPTT, that is most impaired in hemophilia.

The activated platelet expresses receptors for VIIIa, and IXa, and binding of these active proteases in complex with membrane phosphatidylserine enhances the binding of the enzyme's substrate, factor X, enhancing the kinetic efficiency of the intrinsic Xase complex. Assembly of the prothrombinase complex is similarly dependent on the activated platelet surface for optimal activity. Like the Xase complex, the membrane-bound prothrombinase complex activates prothrombin with a rate enhancement 300,000-fold higher than free Xa acting on prothrombin in solution. Platelet-bound Xa is the rate-limiting enzyme in prothrombin cleavage for both the initiation and propagation phases of clotting; its substrate, prothrombin, binds to GPIIb/IIIa on both activated and unactivated platelets. The net kinetic advantage conferred by platelet binding is such that assembly of the entire reaction on the platelet membrane is a 13 million–fold increase in catalytic efficiency over that of proteases free in solution.

What role do other intrinsic pathway factors play in coagulation? Evidence is growing that factor XI further amplifies the propagation phase of coagulation. Factor Xa is particularly rate limiting once the switch is made to the intrinsic Xase. Although small amounts of IXa are generated by the TF-VIIa complex, IXa generation in this manner is limited by TFPI. To generate Xa in amounts sufficient to fuel the propagation phase, a kinetically superior source of IXa is required. Factor XI is another zymogen activated by very small amounts of initiation phase–generated thrombin, but this activation is restricted to the activated platelet surface. Platelet-bound XIa activates IX on the platelet surface, thereby favoring assembly of the intrinsic Xase complex. Moreover, binding to the platelet surface protects XIa from its inhibitor, protease nexin 2. Thus, XIa generation on the activated platelet is instrumental for providing IXa in amounts sufficient to maintain peak Xa generation through the efficient intrinsic Xase complex.

LIMITING SOLUBLE COAGULATION

Endogenous anticoagulants can either inactivate formed thrombin or prevent thrombin generation. The most impor-

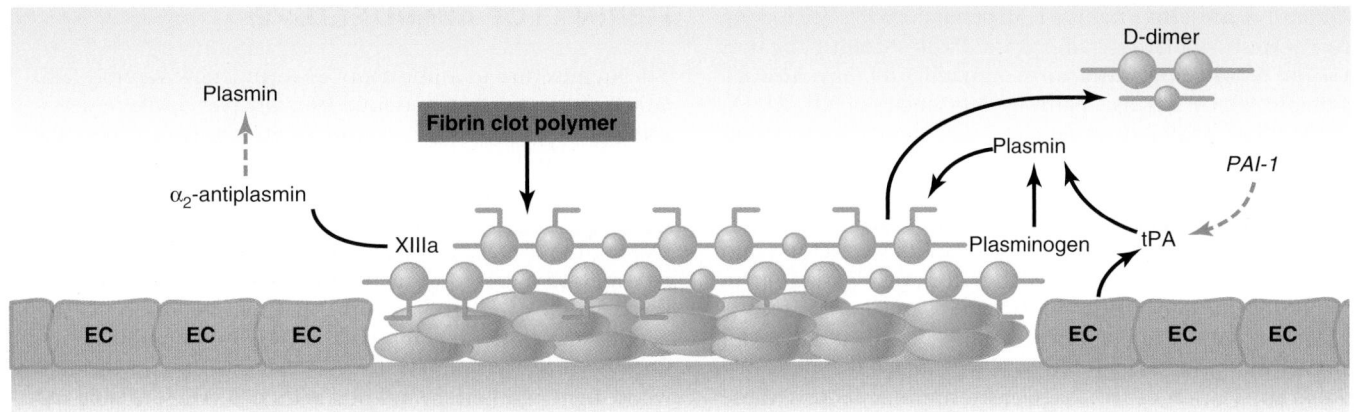
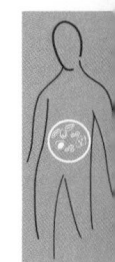

Figure 52-4 Balanced fibrinolysis limiting the platelet-fibrin clot. The platelet plug and fibrin matrices are strengthened by incorporating factor XIIIa into the fibrin clot. Factor XIIIa also binds α_2-antiplasmin to the clot to protect it from plasmin-mediated fibrinolysis. At the same time, nearby intact endothelial cells (ECs) secrete tissue-type plasminogen activator (t-PA). t-PA that evades plasminogen activator inhibitor-1 (PAI-1) converts clot-bound plasminogen to plasmin and leads to fibrin clot degradation and release of soluble fibrin peptides and D-dimer. Thus, detection of circulating D-dimer generally indicates active fibrinolysis.

tant of the former is antithrombin (AT). AT is physiologically present at over twice the concentration (3.2 $\mu mol/L^{-1}$) of the highest local thrombin concentration (1.4 $\mu mol/L^{-1}$) that can be reached during clotting, and AT activity against thrombin is potentiated 1000-fold by endogenous EC-associated heparan sulfate proteoglycans. Platelet surface membranes and platelet-released platelet factor 4 protect thrombin from inactivation at the clot. However, any thrombin that escapes into the circulation is immediately (<1 minute) inhibited by plasma AT, and in the microenvironment of healthy ECs that bind about 60,000 molecules of AT per cell, free thrombin is neutralized almost instantaneously. Thus, early thrombin generation is critically dependent on protection by the activated platelet membrane for sufficient time to transition from initiation to the propagation phase.

Among endogenous anticoagulants that target thrombin generation, the earliest in the coagulation process is TFPI, mentioned previously, which inactivates factor Xa and the TF-VIIa complex. TFPI is constitutively released by EC into the microvasculature. Under normal conditions, TFPI is largely localized to the endothelial surface by binding to EC-associated glycosaminoglycans but can be displaced by heparin. Nascent TFPI has direct activity only against Xa, but following exposure to Xa, TFPI acquires activity against the TF-VIIa complex. During the initiation phase, platelet-bound Xa is protected from inactivation by both TFPI and antithrombin. Preservation of the small amounts of Xa that are generated during this early stage of coagulation is critical to formation of the nanomolar amounts of thrombin needed to begin the propagation phase of clotting.

Activated protein C (APC) has anticoagulant, anti-inflammatory, and profibrinolytic properties that make it an important regulator of both thrombosis and inflammation. Like TFPI, protein C becomes activated only after coagulation is underway. Formed thrombin binds to thrombomodulin, a proteoglycan associated with endothelial and monocyte cell surfaces. Thrombomodulin-bound thrombin loses its ability to activate platelets and instead activates protein C. On the EC surface, nascent protein C binds to endothelial cell protein C receptor (EPCR), which posits it for activation by the adjacent thrombomodulin-bound

thrombin. In a reaction that is enhanced by EPCR and protein S, APC inactivates factors VIIIa and Va, components of the Xase and prothrombinase complexes, respectively, thereby limiting procoagulant self-amplification (Fig. 52-4). As with other coagulation factors, the activated platelet membrane protects VIIIa and Va from APC inactivation. In addition to its effects on thrombin generation, APC neutralizes plasminogen activator inhibitor-1 (PAI-1) to enhance clot remodeling. APC has anti-inflammatory properties as well; recombinant APC reduces tumor necrosis factor-α production after endotoxin challenge, and protein C–deficient mice (heterozygotes) exhibit higher levels of pro-inflammatory cytokines with systemic endotoxemia.

The liver is the major site of synthesis of all coagulation factors. In liver disease, however, factor VIII levels are not generally diminished because VIII is also produced by EC and the reticuloendothelial system. The subset of coagulation factors dependent on vitamin K for synthesis include prothrombin (II), VII, IX, and X, and the anticoagulants, proteins C and S. Post-translational modification (through a vitamin K–dependent carboxylase) of the amino-terminal domain of these proteins adds 10 to 12 γ-carboxyglutamate residues; these residues are critical for calcium binding and for determining the functional three-dimensional structure of the proteins and their proper binding orientation to membrane surfaces. Warfarin blocks vitamin K epoxide reductase and thereby decreases generation of vitamin K (from vitamin K epoxide) in the vitamin K cycle.

LABORATORY TESTING OF COAGULATION

For purposes of laboratory testing, the coagulation cascade is artificially divided into extrinsic (PT) and intrinsic (PTT) pathways, which converge to form a common pathway leading to thrombin and fibrin generation (see Fig. 52-2). In the laboratory, the *extrinsic* pathway (PT) is assessed by measuring the interaction of circulating VIIa with exogenously added TF (also known as *thromboplastin*). The PT is highly sensitive to deficiencies of factors VII, V, X, and II, all of which are associated with significant bleeding. Because II,

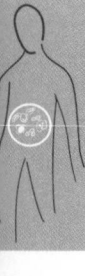

VII, and X are also vitamin K dependent, with VII having the shortest circulating half-life, the PT is currently the best test for monitoring warfarin (Coumadin) therapy. The PT is unaffected by intrinsic pathway deficiencies of XII, XI, IX, or VIII. The degree of prolongation of the PT by warfarin depends on the strength of the particular thromboplastin (based on its international sensitivity index [ISI]) and the specific coagulation instrument used for the assay. The international normalized ratio (INR) takes these factors into account to standardize among laboratories for variations in the prolongation of the PT induced by warfarin. The INR is calculated for each patient as follows: (patient PT/mean control PT^{ISI}). Therapeutic INRs with warfarin allow for global application of anticoagulant recommendations; these vary according to the specific disease indication and are covered in Chapter 53. In contrast to warfarin, the PT is relatively insensitive to therapeutic anticoagulation with unfractionated heparin.

The PTT measurement is based on *in vitro* contact activation (e.g., plasma stimulation with a negatively charged compound such as kaolin). The PTT is sensitive to deficiencies of contact factors (prekallikrein [PK], high-molecular-weight kininogen [HMWK], and factor XII), and coagulation factors of the intrinsic (XI, IX, and VIII) and common pathways (V, X, and prothrombin). Deficiencies of PK, HMWK, and XII prolong the PTT but do not result in clinical bleeding, implying that these factors are irrelevant to physiologic hemostasis. By contrast, severe deficiencies of XI, and especially IX and VIII, cause significant bleeding. The PTT is also highly sensitive to unfractionated heparin and is used to monitor therapeutic heparin anticoagulation. Unlike the INR for anticoagulation with warfarin (Coumadin), the range for therapeutic PTT levels with unfractionated heparin is much wider and not as easily standardized. Therapeutic unfractionated heparin levels can be measured by sensitive assays of anti-Xa activity; therapeutic levels of 0.3 to 0.7 anti-Xa U/mL generally correspond to a PTT of between 1.8 and 2.5 times either the patient's baseline PTT (before starting heparin) or the mean PTT of a control population.

It is worth noting that most of the commonly used laboratory tests of soluble coagulation measure the kinetics of the initiation phase only. The PT and PTT have as their endpoints the first appearance of fibrin gel, which occurs with less than 5% of the total reaction complete, and only minimal levels of prothrombin have been activated. The PT and PTT are very sensitive for detecting congenital abnormalities associated with severe factor deficits (e.g., hemophilia) and for guiding heparin and warfarin therapy. However, these tests fail to give information relevant to thrombin generation during the propagation phase, which determines whether a persistent clot forms or the endogenous anticoagulants and fibrinolytic regulators constrain it from excess growth.

Clot Viability and Maturation

Evidence is growing that initial formation of a thrombus does not ensure sustained hemostasis. Events initiated during thrombus generation that are critical to its stability operate after the clot is formed, whether fibrin rich in the venous or platelet rich in the arterial circulation.

FIBRIN CLOT ARCHITECTURE

The architecture of a fibrin clot is surprisingly variable, and although genetic factors unquestionably play a role in determining clot structure, two dominant factors are the local thrombin and fibrinogen concentrations, whose reaction yields the fibrin strands. A thrombin-rich microenvironment typically results in thinner, more tightly cross-linked fibers, making the overall fibrin clot virtually impermeable to lytic enzymes, as opposed to thrombin-poor locations where the fibrin strands are thicker and the structure more porous, making the clot vulnerable to thrombolysis. Similarly, high fibrinogen concentrations are associated with large thrombi whose tight, rigid meshwork makes them less deformable and more lysis resistant. Low fibrinogen concentrations, by contrast, produce a less compact clot that is highly lysis prone.

FIBRIN CROSS-LINKING BY FACTOR XIIIA

Factor XIII also plays a critical role in stabilizing the forming clot. XIII circulates in the plasma and is also stored within platelets; indeed, fully 50% of total fibrin-stabilizing activity in blood resides in the platelet and is released by activation. In plasma, XIII is a tetrameric molecule consisting of two α subunits, containing the active site of the enzyme, and two β subunits, which increase the zymogen's plasma half-life but must be dissociated for full enzyme activity. Platelet factor XIII, by contrast, is a dimer that contains only the two α subunits. Both forms of the zymogen require thrombin cleavage and fibrin as a cofactor, but plasma XIII activation proceeds at a considerably slower rate owing to the need for dissociation of the β subunits. Thrombin-activated XIIIa binds to fibrin and cross-links the fibrin units, thereby rendering them less permeable and more resistant to lysis. Furthermore, XIIIa cross-links the major plasmin inhibitor, α$_2$-antiplasmin, directly to fibrin, positing it for neutralization of any invading plasmin.

FIBRINOLYSIS

The fibrinolytic system operates to prevent fibrin from occluding healthy vessels. During clot formation, Xa and thrombin stimulate healthy ECs to release tissue plasminogen activator (t-PA) and urokinase-type plasminogen activator (u-PA), both capable of cleaving plasminogen into plasmin. The vast excess of plasminogen present in the plasma dictates that under normal circumstances, the concentration of these enzymes is rate limiting for plasmin formation. The kinetic efficiency of t-PA is improved by at least an order of magnitude by the presence of fibrin, thus helping keep t-PA most active in the microenvironment of the clot. By contrast, u-PA appears to require binding to activated platelets for its ability to liberate plasmin.

Acting to contain fibrinolysis are plasma mediators that either inactivate formed plasmin (e.g., α$_2$-antiplasmin and possibly α$_2$-macroglobulin) or block plasmin formation, foremost of which is PAI-1. PAI-1 is present in several-fold molar excess in the plasma and is also released by activated platelets, thereby protecting clots from premature lysis. PAI-1 plasma levels can be highly variable, in part because of its circadian pattern of secretion, but also because of polymorphisms of the PAI-1 gene. The 4G promoter region polymorphism of PAI-1 is associated with higher PAI-1 levels and a higher risk for thromboembolic disease (see Chapter 54). Another mediator that limits fibrinolysis in the vicinity of the clot is thrombin activator fibrinolysis inhibitor (TAFI). TAFI is synthesized in an inactive form by the liver and circulates in the plasma, possibly in a complex with plasminogen. TAFI cleaves specific fibrin lysine residues that would otherwise promote binding of fibrinolytic enzymes (e.g., plasmin). TAFI requires either plasmin or thrombin for activation; however, thrombin activation of TAFI requires extraordinarily large amounts of *free* thrombin. By contrast, EC-associated thrombomodulin potentiates thrombin-induced TAFI activation 1250-fold, making this an essential cofactor and one that is predominantly available only at the blood-vessel interface. In addition to the EC surface, macrophages are also critical to fibrinolysis. Macrophages degrade fibrin clot through lysosomal proteolysis by a plasmin-independent mechanism. The macrophage binds to fibrin and fibrinogen through its surface integrin receptor, CD11b/CD18; this binding is followed by internalization of the complex into the lysosome, where fibrin and fibrinogen are degraded.

Tissue repair and regeneration are the physiologic endpoints of clotting, eventually leading to dissolution of the fibrin-based clot. Besides t-PA and urokinase, the intrinsic pathway activators kallikrein, XIIa, and XIa also generate active plasmin from plasminogen. Plasminogen binding to cell surface receptors promotes its own activation to plasmin by placing it in proximity to t-PA and fibrin clot and protects plasmin from inactivation by circulating (not clot-bound) α_2-antiplasmin (see Fig. 52-4). Plasmin eventually dissolves the fibrin matrix to produce soluble fibrin peptides and D-dimer and also activates metalloproteinases that further degrade damaged tissue. Fibroblasts and leukocytes migrate into the wound, the latter mediated by selectin binding, and these inflammatory cells act in concert with growth factors secreted by leukocytes and activated platelets (e.g., transforming growth factor-β) to enhance vascular repair and tissue regeneration.

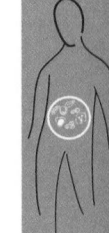

Prospectus for the Future

Interindividual Variability and the Extremes of "Normal"

The understanding of hemostasis physiology has been advanced by kinetic models using the interplay of cells and soluble coagulation factors. In such models, thrombin is clearly an important, if not central, coordinator of hemostatic function and thus is a target for measurement to assess hemostatic function and risk. However, as noted previously, the PT and PTT do not begin to measure the full physiology of the hemostatic response, and the platelet contribution to clotting is absent in such tests. It remains to be seen whether newer measurements such as endogenous thrombin potential or older methods such as thromboelastography can better quantitate global hemostatic function. Furthermore, the concept of the normal range for hemostasis factors may not be adequate for predicting outcomes. Indeed, measuring an individual's capacity to generate activated mediators and their kinetics has shown an extreme range of biologic variability. For example, total amounts and peak rate of thrombin formation and platelet amplification of thrombin generation demonstrate a remarkable breadth of "normal." The evolution of more sophisticated coagulation testing may demand more than a simple normal range, perhaps paralleling our clinical understanding of risk factors instead as a continuous predictor of a patient's response to hemostatic challenge. The goal would be to better identify patients whose coagulation response, although appropriate for most situations, may be insufficient to protect them, under stress, from either excessive bleeding or pathologic thrombosis.

References

Antman EM, DeMets D, Loscalzo J: Cyclooxygenase inhibition and cardiovascular risk. Circulation 112:759-770, 2005.

Brummel-Ziedins K, Vossen CY, Rosendaal FR, et al: The plasma hemostatic proteome: Thrombin generation in healthy individuals. J Thromb Haemost 3:1472-1481, 2005.

Jackson SP: The growing complexity of platelet aggregation. Blood 109:5087-5095, 2007.

Lane DA, Phillippou H, Huntington JA: Directing thrombin. Blood 106:2605-2612, 2005.

Lijnen HR: Pleiotropic functions of plasminogen activator inhibitor-1. J Thromb Haemost 3:35-45, 2005.

Oliver JJ, Webb DJ, Newby DE: Stimulated tissue plasminogen activator release as a marker of endothelial function in humans. Arterioscler Thromb Vasc Biol 25:2470-2479, 2005.

Scott EM, Ariens R, Grant PJ: Genetic and environmental determinants of fibrin structure and function: Relevance to clinical disease. Arterioscler Thromb Vasc Biol 24:1558-1566, 2004.

Chapter 53

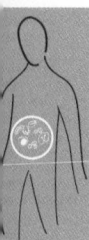

Disorders of Hemostasis: Bleeding

Christopher A. Tormey and Henry M. Rinder

Clinical Evaluation of Bleeding

The evaluation of bleeding requires a careful history, physical examination, and laboratory evaluation. The patient's history should include a description of bleeding (e.g., epistaxis, menorrhagia, hematoma formation), the circumstances under which bleeding occurs (e.g., association with trauma, surgery, dental procedures), and whether any blood products (and what kind) are required to staunch bleeding. The temporal addition of medications, such as aspirin, can be associated with bleeding, as can concomitant medical illnesses such as infection or liver disease. Finally, determining a family history of bleeding is critical; the physician may need to query several generations and second-degree relations, such as maternal uncles, when hemophilia is suggested in the proband.

The physical examination may yield some clues as to the origin of bleeding by distinguishing between small vessel bleeding, such as petechial (pinpoint) hemorrhage, from larger vessel bleeding, which usually produces hematomas and purpura (large bruises). Small vessel bleeding in the skin, in the mucous membranes, or in the gastrointestinal (GI) tract tends to occur more often in patients with thrombocytopenia, qualitative platelet defects, vascular abnormalities, and von Willebrand disease (vWD). In women, menorrhagia may be the only symptom of a bleeding disorder and should never be assumed to be solely attributed to a gynecologic etiology. Large vessel bleeding in organs, joints, or muscles is more commonly associated with factor deficiencies, such as hemophilia. Screening laboratory assays are useful in the initial assessment of the bleeding patient (Table 53-1) and should include (1) *blood cell counts* (especially the platelet count) and examination of the peripheral blood smear; (2) *prothrombin time* (PT), which is highly sensitive to defects in vitamin K–dependent coagulation factors; and (3) *partial thromboplastin time* (PTT), which detects deficiencies in factors VIII, IX, and XI. Abnormalities of factors X, V, and II (prothrombin) result in elevations of both the PT and the PTT. If the PT or PTT is prolonged, the patient's plasma should be combined with normal plasma (*mixing study*) and the clotting time study repeated. The mixing study distinguishes between factor deficiency (the PT or PTT corrects into the normal range) and a circulating inhibitor (the clotting time remains prolonged). Another readily available test for the patient with bleeding is the *thrombin time*, which assays the functional fibrinogen level.

Platelet function has been traditionally assessed by the in vivo *bleeding time*, an invasive measure of the time to halt bleeding in a skin incision. The bleeding time is prolonged by qualitative platelet defects and by rare connective tissue disorders. The bleeding time test is dependent on the expertise of the technician performing the test, and its poor reproducibility and the difficulty of performing the test in infants and neonates have limited its use. Several instruments use phlebotomized whole blood for in vitro assessment of platelet function. One such instrument that delivers an *in vitro bleeding time* is the Platelet Function Analyzer-100 (PFA-100); in this instrument, citrate-anticoagulated whole blood is passed through a small orifice in a cartridge impregnated with platelet activators such as collagen, adenosine diphosphate (ADP), and epinephrine. As the platelets activate and adhere, the orifice gradually becomes obstructed, and the time to complete occlusion by the platelet plug is measured as the closure time. The closure time is prolonged by qualitative platelet defects such as caused by aspirin and by vWD. Although thrombocytopenia (<100,000 platelets/mcL) obviates use of the closure time similar to the in vivo bleeding time, these in vitro tests are gradually supplanting the bleeding time.

Another laboratory study for evaluation of a prolonged PTT, especially in the inpatient setting, is performing the PTT with an added substance (polybrene, protamine, heparinase) to neutralize any contaminating heparin as a result of drawing the blood through an intravenous line. A prolonged PTT that does not correct with the mixing study may also be observed in patients with a lupus anticoagulant (often in the context of thrombosis). In this setting, the diagnosis of a lupus anticoagulant can be confirmed by documenting the correction of the PTT with the addition of

Table 53-1 **Screening Hemostasis Assays**

Laboratory Test	Aspect of Hemostasis Tested	Causes of Abnormalities
Blood counts and peripheral blood smear	Platelet count and morphologic features	Thrombocytopenia; thrombocytosis; gray platelet and giant platelet syndromes
Prothrombin time	Factor VII–dependent pathways	Vitamin K deficiency and warfarin; liver disease; DIC; factor deficiency (VII, V, X, II), factor inhibitor
Partial thromboplastin time	Factor XI–, IX–, and VIII–dependent pathways	Heparin; DIC; lupus anticoagulant*; vWD; factor deficiency (XI, IX, VIII, V, X, II), factor inhibitor
Thrombin time	Fibrinogen	Heparin; DIC; hypofibrinogenemia; dysfibrinogenemia
Platelet function analysis	Platelet and vWF function	Aspirin; vWD; storage pool disease
Mixing study	Presence of an inhibitor	Abnormal clotting time corrects with a deficiency; does not correct with an inhibitor

*Lupus anticoagulant is not associated with bleeding.
  DIC, disseminated intravascular coagulation; vWD, von Willebrand disease; vWF, von Willebrand factor.

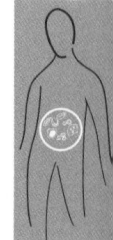

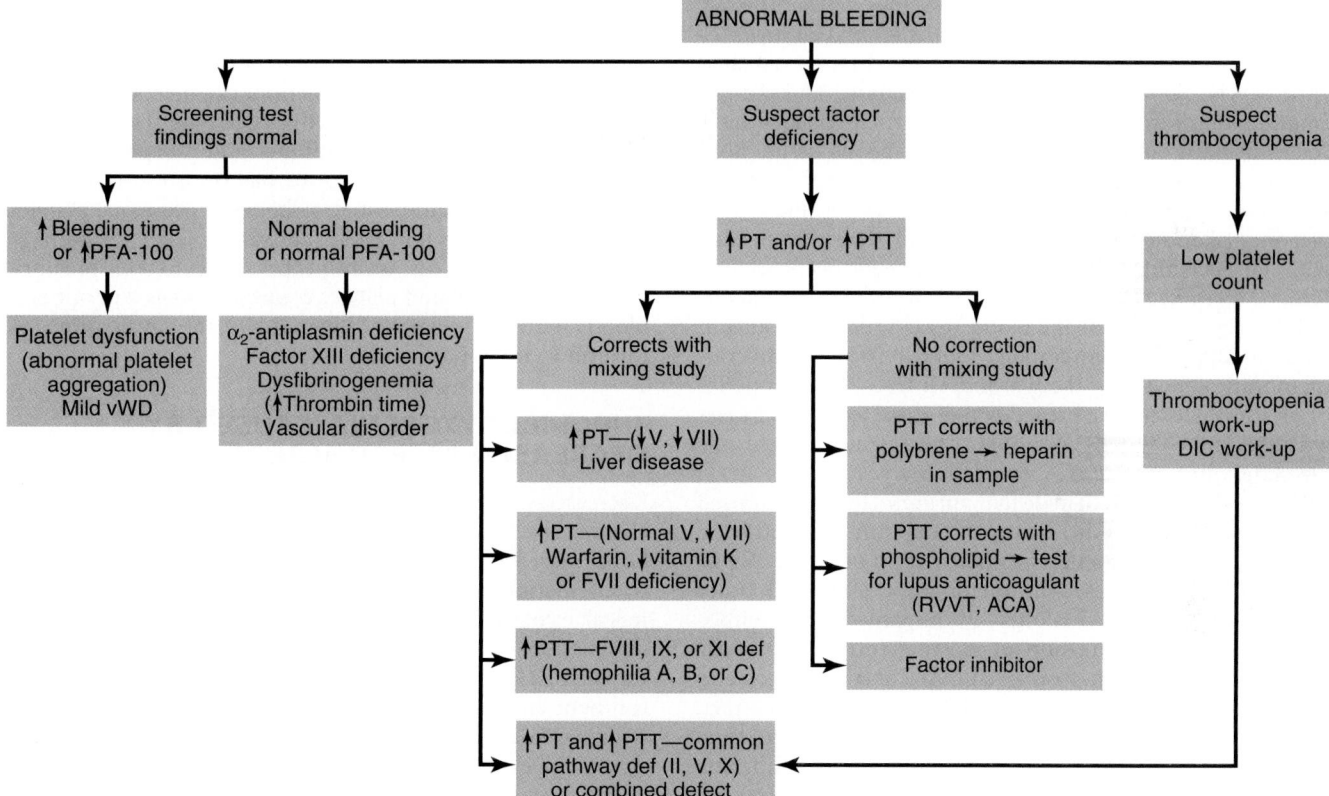

Figure 53-1 Algorithm for the evaluation of bleeding. Screening laboratory tests for platelet and factor deficiencies are used to narrow the work-up for bleeding, followed by specific factor and other coagulation studies (e.g., mixing studies, D-dimer) to confirm the diagnosis. ACA, anticardiolipin antibody; DIC, disseminated intravascular coagulation; FVIII, factor VIII; PFA-100, Platelet Function Analyzer-100; PT, prothrombin time; PTT, partial thromboplastin time; RVVT, Russell viper venom time; vWD, von Willebrand disease.

excess phospholipid as well as other specific tests for lupus anticoagulant (see "Antiphospholipid Antibody Syndrome" in Chapter 54).

A rapid approach to identifying possible causes of bleeding (Fig. 53-1) should consider the following major disease categories: (1) vWD, thrombocytopenia, or abnormal platelet function; (2) low levels of multiple coagulation factors resulting from vitamin K deficiency, liver disease, or disseminated intravascular coagulation (DIC); (3) single-factor deficiency, generally inherited; and more rarely, (4) an

acquired inhibitor to a coagulation factor such as factor VIII. The laboratory evaluation is most efficient when performed in this context.

Vascular Causes of Bleeding

Vascular purpura (bruising) is defined as bleeding caused by intrinsic structural abnormalities of blood vessels or

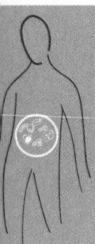

by inflammatory infiltration of blood vessels (*vasculitis*). Although vascular purpura usually causes bleeding in the setting of normal platelet counts and normal coagulation studies, vasculitis and vessel damage may be severe enough to cause secondary consumption of platelets and coagulation factors. Collagen breakdown and thinning of the subcutaneous tissue that overlies blood vessels is often observed in older patients and is termed *senile purpura*; similar atrophic skin changes are also common effects of steroid therapy. Another acquired cause of vascular purpura is scurvy, or vitamin C deficiency. *Scurvy* is characterized by bleeding around individual hair fibers (*perifollicular hemorrhage*) and corkscrew-shaped hairs. Bruising occurs in a classic *saddle* pattern, distributed over the upper thighs. The bleeding gums with scurvy are caused by gingivitis and not by the subcutaneous tissue defect. Thus, edentulous patients with scurvy do not have bleeding gums, and scurvy should not be excluded on this basis.

Congenital defects of the vessel wall may cause bruising. These rare syndromes include *pseudoxanthoma elasticum*, a defect of the elastic fibers of the vasculature that is associated with severe GI and genitourinary bleeding, and *Ehlers-Danlos syndrome*, characterized by abnormal collagen molecules in both blood vessels and subcutaneous tissue. Both syndromes exhibit bruising in the skin, but only patients with pseudoxanthoma elasticum develop significant GI bleeding. Another inherited vessel wall defect associated with GI bleeding is *hereditary hemorrhagic telangiectasia (Osler-Weber-Rendu syndrome)*. This disorder is characterized by degeneration of the blood vessel wall that results in angiomatous lesions resembling blood blisters on mucous membranes, including the lips and GI tract. The frequency of bleeding caused by a breakdown of these lesions increases with age, and GI lesions commonly cause significant, chronic bleeding, often resulting in iron deficiency.

The sudden onset of *palpable purpura* (localized, raised hemorrhages in the skin) in association with rash and fever may be caused by vasculitis, either aseptic or septic. *Septic vasculitis* may be caused by meningococcemia and other bacterial infections and is often accompanied by thrombocytopenia and prolongation of clotting times. One cause of aseptic vasculitis in young children and adolescents is *Henoch-Schönlein purpura*, a vasculitis of the skin, GI tract, and kidneys, which is usually accompanied by abdominal pain caused by bleeding into the bowel wall. This syndrome may occur after a viral prodrome and appears to be caused by an immunoglobulin A (IgA) hypersensitivity reaction, as evidenced by serum IgA immune complexes and renal histopathologic features resembling IgA nephropathy. *Drug hypersensitivity,* for example, to allopurinol can exhibit extensive cutaneous purpura as well.

The therapy of bleeding from vascular disorders is straightforward. Senile purpura and steroid-induced purpura do not usually require treatment. Scurvy is corrected by oral ascorbic acid. In the case of congenital disorders, including Ehlers-Danlos syndrome, hereditary hemorrhagic telangiectasia, and pseudoxanthoma elasticum, patients should avoid medications that may aggravate their bleeding tendencies (e.g., aspirin), and they should receive supportive therapy (e.g., iron supplementation, red blood cell transfusion). Systemic administration of estrogen in hereditary hemorrhagic telangiectasia may help decrease

epistaxis by inducing squamous metaplasia of the nasal mucosa and thereby protecting lesions from trauma. Treatment of septic vasculitis focuses on appropriate antibiotic therapy; in the case of aseptic vasculitis, steroids and immunosuppressive agents are most effective. When vasculitis is severe enough to cause consumption of platelets and coagulation factors (see discussion of DIC), transfusions of platelets, cryoprecipitate, or fresh-frozen plasma (FFP) may be indicated.

Bleeding Caused by Platelet Disorders: Thrombocytopenia

Thrombocytopenia (platelet count <150,000/mcL) is one of the most common problems in hospitalized patients. The initial diagnostic approach to thrombocytopenia involves classifying whether the low platelet count is caused by (1) decreased platelet production, (2) increased platelet sequestration, or (3) increased platelet destruction (Fig. 53-2). An evaluation of the number and morphologic features of marrow megakaryocytes has been the traditional diagnostic test for differentiating between decreased platelet production and peripheral sequestration (e.g., splenomegaly) or destruction (e.g., immune thrombocytopenic purpura [ITP]). The reticulated platelet count is used as a peripheral blood index of platelet kinetics in the evaluation of thrombocytopenia.

THROMBOCYTOPENIA CAUSED BY DECREASED MARROW PRODUCTION

Decreased production of platelets from the bone marrow is characterized by decreased or absent megakaryocytes on the bone marrow aspirate and biopsy and a low percentage of circulating reticulated platelets. Suppression of normal megakaryocytopoiesis occurs after (1) marrow damage and destruction of stem cells, such as with cytotoxic chemotherapy; (2) destruction of the normal marrow microenvironment and replacement of normal stem cells by invasive malignant disease, aplasia, infection (e.g., miliary tuberculosis), or myelofibrosis; (3) specific but rare intrinsic defects of the megakaryocytic stem cells; and (4) metabolic abnormalities affecting megakaryocyte maturation.

Thrombocytopenia may result from cytotoxic or immunosuppressive chemotherapy for malignant or autoimmune disease. Thrombocytopenia is usually reversible, and platelet production rebounds as megakaryocytic stem cells eventually recover and regenerate. However, repeated or intensive chemotherapy (e.g., stem cell transplantation) may permanently damage the megakaryocytic stem cells and supporting stromal environment and may cause chronic thrombocytopenia. This condition may be accompanied by leukopenia and anemia, similar to the presentation of de novo *myelodysplasia*. Commonly used drugs such as thiazide diuretics, alcohol, and estrogens may also damage bone marrow megakaryocytes. Nutritional disorders, especially alcoholism and abnormal folate or vitamin B_{12} metabolism, are also commonly associated with thrombocytopenia; platelet counts

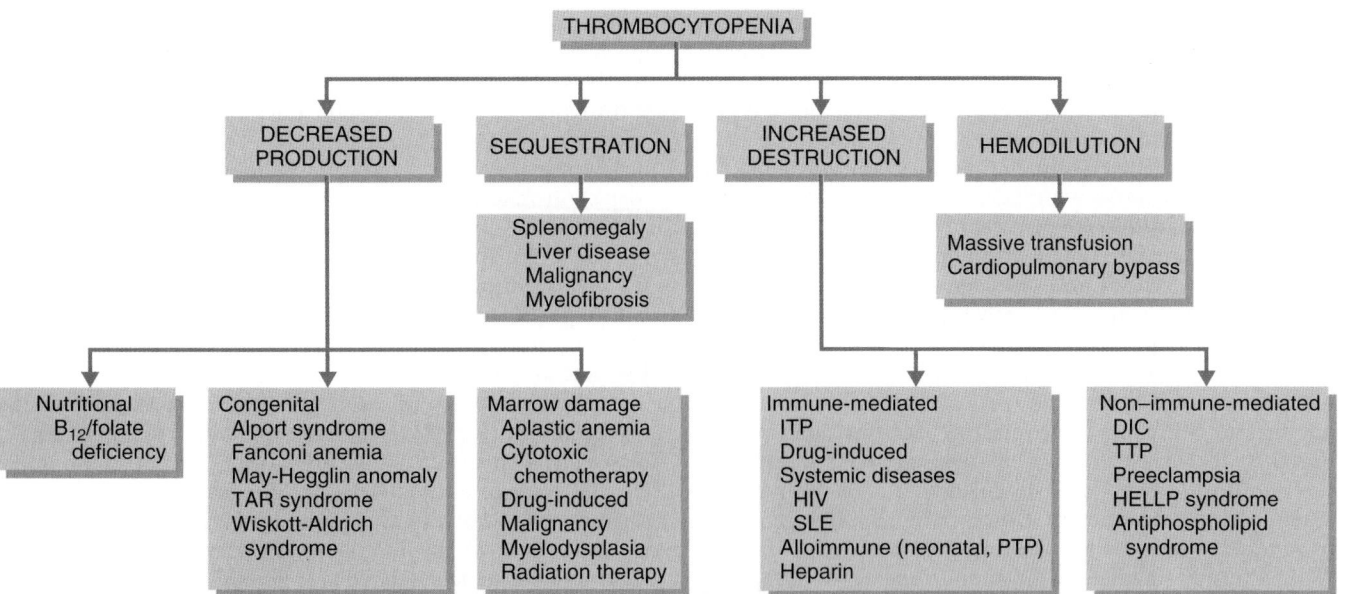

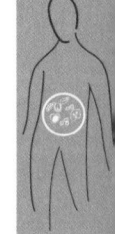

Figure 53-2 Differential diagnosis of thrombocytopenia. Disorders resulting in a decrease in circulating platelet number can be divided into four main pathophysiologic mechanisms: hypoproduction, sequestration, peripheral destruction, and hemodilution. The history, physical examination, and bone marrow evaluation usually narrow the range of possible causes. DIC, disseminated intravascular coagulation; HELLP, hemolysis, elevated liver enzymes, and low-platelet count in association with pregnancy; HIV, human immunodeficiency virus; ITP, immune thrombocytopenic purpura; PTP, post-transfusion purpura; SLE, systemic lupus erythematosus; TAR, thrombocytopenia-absent radius syndrome; TTP, thrombotic thrombocytopenic purpura.

respond to abstinence from alcohol and to appropriate multivitamin replacement therapy. Thrombocytopenia is also observed in patients with severe aplastic anemia, and the bone marrow shows decreased or absent megakaryocytes with other cell lineages similarly affected.

Platelet production is suppressed by intrinsic malignant diseases of the bone marrow such as leukemia and multiple myeloma and by malignant diseases that secondarily invade the bone marrow (non-Hodgkin lymphoma, small cell lung cancer, breast and prostate cancers, among others). The bone marrow aspirate under these circumstances shows decreased megakaryocytes and, occasionally, malignant cells; bone marrow biopsy has a much higher yield for diagnosing malignant involvement of the marrow. Flow cytometric evaluation for clonal B cells in the marrow aspirate is highly sensitive for detecting monoclonal B-cell lymphoproliferative disease (non-Hodgkin lymphoma).

Myelofibrosis, an increase in the reticulin fibers (and sometimes collagen) of the marrow, may lead to thrombocytopenia or pancytopenia. Myelofibrosis occurs most commonly in myeloproliferative disorders, in mastocytosis, and in mycobacterial and other infections involving the marrow. It may also occur occasionally in patients with myelodysplasia or acute megakaryocytic leukemia and rarely on a congenital basis (*osteogenesis imperfecta*).

Thrombocytopenia in children can result from congenital defects of megakaryocyte production as seen with *thrombocytopenia-absent radii syndrome, congenital amegakaryocytic thrombocytopenia* (secondary to a mutation in the thrombopoietin receptor), and *Fanconi anemia* (congenital aplastic anemia with renal hypoplasia and skin hyperpigmentation). Other disorders that are intrinsic to the bone marrow include the *May-Hegglin anomaly* and related myosin IIa/MYH9 gene diseases, characterized by giant platelets and Döhle

bodies (basophilic inclusions in leukocytes and platelets). Thrombocytopenia with small platelets is characteristic of *Wiskott-Aldrich syndrome*, an X-linked disorder with eczema and immunodeficiency that can be diagnosed by the lack of CD43 expression on T lymphocytes. When accompanied by nerve deafness and nephritis, congenital hypoproductive thrombocytopenia is termed *Alport syndrome*.

THROMBOCYTOPENIA CAUSED BY SEQUESTRATION

Up to 30% of circulating platelets are normally sequestered within the spleen at any given time. Conditions that lead to splenomegaly cause increased trapping of platelets and thrombocytopenia, often dropping the platelet count into the range of 50,000 to 100,000/mcL but rarely lower. Thrombocytopenia from sequestration is common in advanced liver disease, myeloproliferative disorders accompanied by splenomegaly (e.g., chronic myelogenous leukemia, chronic idiopathic myelofibrosis), and malignant disease involving the spleen. Splenectomy may be indicated in the latter but is rarely used to treat thrombocytopenia resulting from portal hypertension. The decision to perform splenectomy for thrombocytopenia in patients with myeloproliferative syndromes must be individualized and weighed against surgical complications, loss of the spleen's extramedullary hematopoietic ability, and even rebound thrombocytosis.

THROMBOCYTOPENIA CAUSED BY PLATELET DESTRUCTION

Increased platelet destruction can be caused by immune and nonimmune mechanisms. Autoimmune thrombocytopenia may be a primary disorder directed only at platelets or a

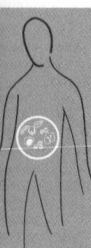

secondary complication of another autoimmune disease, such as systemic lupus erythematosus. Immune platelet destruction is caused by increased levels of polyclonal antiplatelet antibodies directed against platelet membrane glycoprotein receptors, most often cryptic neoepitopes of glycoprotein IIb/IIIa (GPIIb/IIIa) and less commonly GPIb. Coating of the platelet with these antibodies leads to opsonization of the platelets by Fc receptors on cells of the reticuloendothelial system (RES). Antibody-coated platelets are cleared by the spleen and, to a lesser extent, by the liver. These disorders generally involve a dramatic increase in marrow platelet production reflected by increased numbers of marrow megakaryocytes. The younger platelets produced have relatively high granule contents, providing increased hemostatic function. Bone marrow examination for the presence of increased or normal megakaryocyte numbers is the traditional means of distinguishing platelet destruction from decreased production. However, increased percentages of *reticulated platelets* are associated with destructive, especially immune-mediated, thrombocytopenia and may be sufficient for diagnosing platelet destruction. Thrombocytopenia resulting from immune clearance may be severe, and platelet survival is often reduced from the normal 7 to 10 days to less than 1 day. Despite severe thrombocytopenia, serious bleeding or hemorrhagic death is uncommon, partly because the function of young platelets is increased and partly because the number of circulating platelets required to maintain vascular integrity is relatively low, estimated at 7100/mcL per day.

IMMUNE THROMBOCYTOPENIC PURPURA

In children, acute ITP is often preceded by a viral infection, such as varicella. Patients with ITP exhibit petechial hemorrhage and mucosal bleeding; platelet counts are often lower than 20,000/mcL. The blood smear shows large platelets but no other abnormal cells such as blasts, which would accompany childhood leukemia. The bone marrow demonstrates increased or occasionally normal numbers of megakaryocytes. The diagnosis of ITP is partly made by exclusion. Fever, organomegaly, pancytopenia, lymphadenopathy, or abnormal peripheral blood cells should prompt an evaluation for malignant disease, such as leukemia, neuroblastoma, or Wilms tumor, or other bone marrow disorders. Laboratory tests may complement the clinical evaluation but are not required to make the diagnosis of ITP. These tests include the demonstration of an increased percentage of reticulated platelets in the peripheral blood or the detection of platelet autoantibodies in serum or on the platelet (*platelet-associated immunoglobulin*). However, assays of platelet-associated antibodies, though sensitive, are not specific for ITP because immunoglobulins that bind nonspecifically to platelets are often increased in patients with thrombocytopenia secondary to liver disease or HIV infection. In contrast, techniques that measure serum antibodies to specific platelet glycoproteins have greater specificity but are relatively insensitive. An increase in mean platelet volume is also a relatively insensitive indicator of destructive thrombocytopenia, in part because of the wide range of normal values. An increase in the reticulated platelet percentage is consistent with increased platelet destruction but cannot distinguish between ITP and other causes of platelet destruction such as heparin-induced thrombocytopenia (HIT) and thrombotic thrombocytopenic purpura (TTP) (both discussed in greater detail in Chapter 54). Thus the diagnosis of ITP remains largely clinical and does not require laboratory confirmation.

Acute ITP in children can resolve without therapy, but most clinicians prefer to treat children with steroids or intravenous immunoglobulin (IVIG). IVIG therapy for ITP is thought to work by multiple mechanisms: (1) high IgG concentrations block Fc receptors on phagocytes of the RES and on cellular effectors of antibody-dependent cytotoxicity; (2) infusion of IgG increases the fractional rate of IgG catabolism and thereby increases the destruction of antiplatelet IgG in direct proportion to its concentration; and (3) clearance of antiplatelet immunoglobulin may increase through anti-idiotypic effects (i.e., generating an immunologic response to the ITP antibodies). More than 80% of children with acute ITP have a rapid remission, and ITP does not recur. A subset of 10% to 20% of children eventually develops recurrent thrombocytopenia (i.e., chronic ITP); however, more than 70% of such children respond completely to splenectomy. For those with chronic courses after splenectomy, episodic IVIG, RhoGAM (see later discussion in this chapter), and in severe cases, immunotherapy with rituximab (Rituxan) are used. Hemorrhagic deaths are rare in acute childhood ITP (<2%), but some mortality (2% to 5%) is associated with chronic, refractory ITP.

As with children, the diagnosis of ITP in adults is made largely by exclusion, but unlike with children, acute ITP in adults rarely remits spontaneously and is more likely to become a chronic disorder, evolving to chronic ITP in more than 50% of patients. Petechial hemorrhage and mucosal bleeding are accompanied by platelet counts commonly lower than 20,000/mcL and often as low as 1000 to 2000/mcL. Hemorrhagic deaths occur in fewer than 10% of adults with ITP. In adults, ITP may be associated with other diseases, such as HIV or hepatitis C infection. ITP may be the presenting manifestation of HIV infection, whereas thrombocytopenia in more advanced stages of HIV infection is more often caused by bone marrow failure resulting from megakaryocyte infection with HIV, mycobacterial infection of the bone marrow, and nutritional deficiencies of end-stage HIV disease. ITP also occurs in patients with autoimmune disorders such as systemic lupus erythematosus, inflammatory bowel disease, and nonviral hepatitis. In some patients, ITP is accompanied by autoimmune hemolytic anemia, otherwise termed *Evans syndrome*; the direct Coombs test is usually positive indicating the presence of a warm-reactive autoantibody. Initial treatment may not be significantly different from that for ITP alone, but chronic Evans syndrome is thought to generally respond poorly to splenectomy, unlike ITP alone. In the setting of systemic lupus erythematosus, ITP may be secondary to factors associated with the autoimmune disease itself, including immune complex deposition on the platelet surface, as well as active vasculitis, both of which may lead to increased platelet clearance and low counts. Therapy of both ITP and the underlying autoimmune disorder is usually complementary. When the lupus anticoagulant or anticardiolipin antibody is present

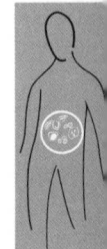

in association with systemic lupus erythematosus and thrombocytopenia, the diagnosis of secondary antiphospholipid antibody syndrome is made; this entity is most commonly associated with thromboembolic complications (see Chapter 54).

The first-line treatment of acute ITP in adults is steroids, usually prednisone, 1 to 2 mg/kg per day. Recent studies have suggested that high-dose dexamethasone given in pulses every 14 or 28 days for six to eight doses may result in superior control of disease. Platelet transfusions are not generally used in ITP because transfused-platelet survival is brief and bleeding complications are uncommon. However, in patients with significant bleeding or requiring surgery, platelet transfusions have been safely used and may transiently increase the platelet count, although usually for less than 24 hours. In patients with acute ITP with severe thrombocytopenia (<5000/mcL) or with life-threatening bleeding, high-dose methylprednisolone (1 g per day for 3 days) may be administered alone or in combination with IVIG (2 g/kg in divided doses over 2 to 5 days) and platelet transfusion. In recurrent ITP, chronic steroid treatment is often necessary but is usually accompanied by significant side effects. High-dose pulse dexamethasone given for 4 days every 2 weeks is associated with prolonged responses in about two thirds of chronic ITP patients. Children and adults with chronic ITP who initially respond to IVIG therapy generally respond well to splenectomy, whereas those who do not respond to IVIG are less likely to have disease remission after splenectomy. For all chronic ITP patients, more than 50% have some degree of disease remission after splenectomy. If ITP does recur after splenectomy, the presence of an accessory spleen must be ruled out, usually by liver and spleen scanning, because Howell-Jolly bodies may still be present. Recurrent disease may often be episodic, especially after viral infections, and these patients can be treated with IVIG. Alternatively, patients who are positive for the blood group Rh(D) antigen can be treated with Rh immunoglobulin (RhoGAM), a preparation of IgG class anti-Rh(D) antibodies. Anti-D induces red cell hemolysis (usually mild), thereby presumably causing Fc receptor blockade of the RES and decreased platelet uptake by the spleen and liver. Some patients with ITP, especially those with HIV infection, have experienced significant, even fatal, hemoglobinemia or hemoglobinuria after anti-D therapy, and this therapy should be carefully monitored. RhoGAM is generally ineffective in patients who have undergone splenectomy. In patients who fail to respond to splenectomy, steroid dose may be spared by the addition of a combination of IVIG, vincristine, and anti-D, with danazol and immunosuppressive therapy (e.g., azathioprine). Some patients with chronic ITP have responded to infusions of the anti-CD20 monoclonal antibody rituximab. Finally, chronic ITP with normal marrow cellularity can respond to stimulation of thrombopoiesis using thrombopoietin mimetics and agonist antibodies, which are showing promise in late-phase trials. However, because many patients with chronic ITP will never achieve normal platelet counts, the goal for therapy is often to keep platelet counts higher than 30,000/mcL to avoid significant bleeding. About 5% of adults with ITP die from chronic, refractory disease and the complications of its therapy.

DRUG-INDUCED IMMUNE THROMBOCYTOPENIA

Immune-mediated platelet destruction associated with specific drugs is an often overlooked cause of thrombocytopenia. One mechanism of drug-induced immune thrombocytopenia is the development of an antibody response against soluble drug molecules. When these soluble drugs bind to the platelet membrane, drug-induced antibodies subsequently act to destroy circulating platelets through the RES. Other mechanisms of drug-induced thrombocytopenia include formation of an immunogenic neoantigen through drug-platelet interactions (also known as the *hapten response*) with autoantibodies directed against drugs that cross-react with platelet antigens. Regardless of the mechanism of induction, development of thrombocytopenia is temporally related to exposure to the drug and is usually rapid. Discontinuation of the offending drug generally results in an equally rapid rise in the platelet count. Occasionally, for patients with prolonged thrombocytopenia after drug removal, immunosuppression with agents like IVIG (2 g/kg in two to three divided doses) or steroids may restore baseline platelet counts. Although confirmation of drug-induced thrombocytopenia can often be made by testing for the presence of antibodies with drug specificities, these tests are generally only routinely performed by specialty reference laboratories. Therefore, in cases in which drug-induced thrombocytopenia is suspected, clinicians should not await specific antibody testing before discontinuing potential offending agents.

Historically, quinidine or quinine-based formulations were among the first classes of drugs to be associated with platelet antibodies; such antibodies can be detected by tests using drug coupled to a carrier protein. As awareness of drug-induced thrombocytopenia has grown, scores of drugs including antibiotics, anticonvulsants, psychotropic drugs, and antiplatelet agents have been reported to mediate platelet destruction (Table 53-2). Heparin is also well known to induce thrombocytopenia; however, unlike other drugs, this reaction paradoxically leads to a prothrombotic state. The mechanism of heparin-induced thrombocytopenia and its prothrombotic effects are discussed in greater detail in Chapter 54. Overall, when eliciting the medical history from patients with acute-onset thrombocytopenia, a careful review of all medications, particularly those initiated just before the development of low platelet counts, may help to deduce more quickly the cause and reverse the platelet count decline.

ALLOIMMUNE THROMBOCYTOPENIA

Neonatal alloimmune thrombocytopenia occurs when the mother is homozygous for an uncommon platelet alloantigen, most often human platelet antigen 1b (HPA-1b) on the platelet GPIIIa receptor, and the child expresses the HPA-1a haplotype inherited from the father. The pathogenesis of alloimmune thrombocytopenia is analogous to the mechanism by which Rh(D) sensitization induces hemolytic disease of the newborn. The mother is exposed to the HPA-1a antigen during a first pregnancy, and during that or subsequent pregnancies, she produces high-titer IgG antibody against HPA-1a. These antibodies cross the placenta, react with HPA-1a–positive fetal platelets and cause peripheral-platelet destruction by the RES. Neonatal alloimmune thrombocytopenia may be severe, but the presence of antibody does not necessarily predict whether bleeding will occur in utero, at delivery, or in the first days of life. Transfusion of maternal platelets or random platelets lacking the HPA-1a antigen and IVIG are used to treat bleeding and to restore platelet count.

Alloimmune thrombocytopenia can also occur in adults after transfusion (*post-transfusion purpura*). As in neonates, this condition is based on exposure to a common platelet alloantigen such as HPA-1a that is not present on the patient's native platelets. This disorder can occur after transfusion of any blood product in a female who is homozygous for HPA-1b and who is alloimmunized to HPA-1s as a result of a previous pregnancy, or, more rarely, in any patient alloimmunized because of prior transfusions. More than

95% of blood donors express HPA-1a, and this antigen is shed by platelets. Consequently, any blood product can contain HPA-1a. The anamnestic response to the blood product causes destruction of residual donor platelets and, even more interestingly, destruction of native platelets *that do not express the HPA-1a alloantigen*. The pathophysiology of post-transfusion purpura is unclear, although evidence suggests that native platelets may be destroyed either nonspecifically by the RES or by adsorption of HPA-1a onto host platelets. As with neonates, these patients are treated with IVIG, and any further transfusions must be derived from homozygous HPA-1b donors. Although HPA-1a is the most common cause of alloimmune thrombocytopenia, other platelet alloantigens have been found to cause this clinical syndrome (Table 53-3).

Thrombocytopenia in neonates can also be caused by maternal ITP. Antiplatelet antibodies are commonly IgG class and may cross the placenta inducing thrombocytopenia in the fetus. However, significant neonatal thrombocytopenia is rare with maternal ITP and occurs in fewer than 10% of those at risk, although some evidence indicates that the incidence of neonatal thrombocytopenia is increased when the mother has ITP and maternal platelet counts are lower than 75,000/mcL. Sometimes, the mother needs to be treated for ITP with a secondary goal of decreasing placental transfer of the maternal autoantibody, although in most instances of maternal ITP, fetal thrombocytopenia is uncommon or mild, and safe vaginal delivery may be accomplished.

DISSEMINATED INTRAVASCULAR COAGULATION

One of the most common and potentially life-threatening causes of nonimmune platelet destruction is DIC, which is associated with sepsis, malignancy, advanced liver disease, and other disorders that trigger endotoxin release or cause severe tissue damage (Table 53-4). In DIC caused by bacterial sepsis, circulating endotoxin induces expression of tissue factor on circulating monocytes and endothelial cells, a process leading to overwhelming thrombin and fibrin generation. Deposition of fibrin occurs throughout the vasculature, with relatively inadequate concurrent fibrinolysis leading to a thrombotic or microangiopathic vasculopathy and subsequent organ damage. Thrombin activation of platelets and circulating factors eventually overwhelms the bone marrow and liver synthetic capability, respectively, resulting in thrombocytopenia and prolongation of the PT

Table 53-2 Commonly Used Drugs Associated with Immune Thrombocytopenia

Drug Class	Examples
Antibiotics	Penicillins
	Cephalosporins (cephalothin, ceftazidime)
	Vancomycin
	Sulfonamides (sulfisoxazole)
	Rifampin
	Linezolid
	Quinine
Antiepileptics, antipsychotics, and sedative-hypnotics	Benzodiazepines (diazepam)
	Haloperidol
	Carbamazepine
	Lithium
	Phenytoin
Antihypertensives	Diuretics (chlorothiazide)
	Angiotensin-converting enzyme inhibitors (ramipril)
	Methyldopa
Analgesics and anti-inflammatories	Acetaminophen
	Ibuprofen
	Naproxen
Antiplatelet agents	Abciximab
	Tirofiban
Anticoagulants	Heparin
	Low-molecular-weight heparin

Table 53-3 Molecular Basis for Alloimmune Thrombocytopenia

Glycoprotein	Alleles (Alloantigens)	Phenotype/Frequency	Amino Acid and Location
IIIa	HPA-1a/1b	0.98/0.25	Leucine/proline; 33
Ib	HPA-2a/2b	0.99/0.14	Threonine/methionine; 145
IIb	HPA-3a/3b	0.91/0.70	Isoleucine/serine; 843
IIIa	HPA-4a/4b	0.99/0.01	Arginine/glutamine; 143
Ia	HPA-5a/5b	0.99/0.21	Glutamic acid/lysine; 505
IIIa	HPA-6a/6b	NA	Proline/glutamic acid; 407
IIIa	HPA-7a/7b	NA	Proline/glutamic acid; 407
IIIa	HPA-8a/8b	NA	Arginine/cystine; 636

HPA, human platelet antigen; NA, data not available.

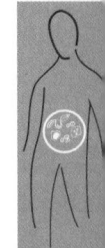

Table 53-4 **Causes of Disseminated Intravascular Coagulation**
Sepsis or Endotoxin
Gram-negative bacteremia
Tissue Damage
Trauma
Closed-head injury
Burns
Hypoperfusion or hypotension
Malignant Disease
Adenocarcinoma
Acute promyelocytic leukemia
Primary Vascular Disorders
Vasculitis
Giant hemangioma (Kasabach-Merritt syndrome)
Aortic aneurysm
Cardiac mural thrombus
Exogenous Causes
Snake venom
Activated-factor infusions (prothrombin-complex concentrate)

and PTT. Thus, although the primary lesion of DIC is thrombin and clot generation, the clinical endpoint is usually a *consumptive coagulopathy* with depletion of platelets and coagulation factors. Mucosal bleeding, especially in the GI tract, and oozing from intravenous puncture sites are early signs of DIC.

Fibrinogen levels are usually low but may be normal or even slightly high in DIC because the acute-phase reaction to sepsis or the underlying disorder may increase fibrinogen secretion. Therefore, DIC should not be ruled out because fibrinogen is in the normal range. Fibrinolysis in DIC is triggered by fibrin clot formation and the action of tissue-type plasminogen activator; laboratory testing shows increased levels of fibrin split products to more than 40 mcg/mL (cleavage of fibrin monomers) and D-dimer to more than 0.5 mg/mL (cleavage of fibrin-fibrin bonds). Although fibrin split products are usually elevated in patients with DIC, this finding is nonspecific; in contrast, an elevated D-dimer is more specific for DIC and is often used to confirm (and even replace) the elevated fibrin split product screening assay. The blood smear may also help in the diagnosis of DIC by showing significant numbers of schistocytes; however, this finding is not specific to DIC and is present in other micro-angiopathies such as TTP (see Chapter 54).

Chronic DIC may be triggered by consumption of platelets and factors in large clots associated with aneurysms, hemangiomas, and mural thrombi. Another unique cause of chronic DIC is malignant disease, often adenocarcinoma or acute promyelocytic leukemia; malignant cells in these disorders promote thrombin formation through (1) secretion of tissue factor; (2) elaboration of cysteine proteases that activate factor X; (3) induction of platelet-ligand binding; and (4) upregulation of endothelial cell plasminogen activator inhibitor-1 (PAI-1) or cyclo-oxygenase-2 (COX-2) (see later discussion of COX-2 prothrombotic effects). Chronic DIC associated with malignancy usually causes enough factor consumption that both the PT and the PTT are prolonged. Clinically, such patients exhibit *migratory thrombo-*

phlebitis (*Trousseau syndrome*) or *nonbacterial thrombotic* (*marantic*) *endocarditis*.

Therapy of DIC should be aimed at (1) treatment of the underlying disorder, such as antibiotics for sepsis or chemotherapy for malignant disease; (2) supportive hemostatic therapy, including platelets, cryoprecipitate (for fibrinogen), and FFP; and (3) disrupting activation of coagulation factors and platelets. For the last approach, anticoagulation is generally not indicated unless the balance of procoagulant versus anticoagulant activity actively favors clotting, such as arterial thromboemboli with mural thrombus or migratory thrombophlebitis with Trousseau syndrome. These specific thrombotic complications of chronic DIC are often resistant to warfarin therapy and generally require more intensive antithrombin and anti-Xa therapy with heparin (either unfractionated or low-molecular-weight heparin). In DIC precipitated by sepsis, pharmacologic activated protein C has been shown to significantly decrease mortality.

THROMBOCYTOPENIA WITH PREGNANCY-INDUCED HYPERTENSION

Mild thrombocytopenia in pregnant women is related to hemodilution, the normal physiology of pregnancy, that can bring platelet counts into the range of 100,000 to 150,000/mcL; these counts are not associated with maternal or fetal complications. In contrast, autoimmune causes of platelet destruction during pregnancy (as noted earlier) and pregnancy-induced hypertension can result in platelet counts lower than 100,000/mcL, and these conditions can be associated with complications. The spectrum of *pregnancy-induced hypertension* includes hypertension progressing to proteinuria and renal dysfunction (*preeclampsia*) and even to cerebral edema and seizures (*eclampsia*). Thrombocytopenia may appear as a late finding accompanying pregnancy-induced hypertension, often at the time of delivery or late in the third trimester. The related *HELLP syndrome* in pregnancy is characterized by hemolysis, elevated liver enzymes, and low platelet counts occasionally in association with hypertension. The thrombocytopenia associated with pregnancy-induced hypertension or HELLP may be related to abnormal vascular prostaglandin metabolism or placental dysfunction that leads to platelet consumption, vasculopathy, and microvascular occlusions. Both disorders are usually reversed by delivery of the fetus and placenta. Occasionally, IVIG or plasmapheresis has been required when the disorder does not resolve postpartum.

There are several other conditions, sometimes associated with pregnancy, which mediate nonimmune platelet destruction such as TTP, hemolytic uremic syndrome (HUS), and antiphospholipid syndrome. However, these platelet consumptive processes generally yield a thrombotic state rather than a tendency to bleed. More detailed discussion of these medical problems associated with thrombocytopenia can be found in Chapter 54.

DILUTIONAL THROMBOCYTOPENIA

In addition to sequestration, hypoproductive, and destructive causes of thrombocytopenia, low platelet counts can occasionally result from *hemodilution*. This circumstance usually follows resuscitative efforts after trauma and results

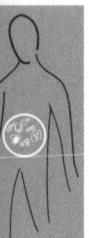

Table 53-5 Disorders Causing Abnormal Platelet Aggregation

	Response to Agonist				
	Epinephrine	**ADP**	**Collagen**	**Arachidonic Acid**	**Ristocetin**
Aspirin and NSAIDs	#	#	NL, ↓*	↓	NL
Glanzmann disease	Absent	Absent	Absent	Absent	#
Bernard-Soulier syndrome	NL	NL	NL	NL	Absent
Storage pool disease	↓	#	↓	NL, ↓	#
Hermansky-Pudlak syndrome	↓	#	↓	NL	#
Gray platelet syndrome	↓	↓	↓	NL	NL
von Willebrand disease	NL	NL	NL	NL	↓, NL†

*Aspirin results in decreased aggregation with low-dose collagen, but aggregation is normal with high-dose collagen.
†In von Willebrand disease type 2B, patients have increased aggregation with low-dose ristocetin, and decreased or normal aggregation with standard doses of ristocetin.
↓, Decreased; #, primary wave aggregation only; ADP, adenosine diphosphate; NL, normal; NSAIDs, nonsteroidal anti-inflammatory drugs.

from the infusion of massive volumes of intravenous solutions, red blood cells, and FFP. Hemodilution is also commonly seen during or immediately following cardiopulmonary bypass in which significant dilution occurs by the addition of the extracorporeal circuit volume to the normal circulatory system. Moreover, in addition to the hemodilution of bypass, platelets exposed to the cardiopulmonary bypass circuit can be cleared, whereas those that remain in the circulation become temporarily dysfunctional because of activation and loss of membrane receptors. This bypass defect may be mild and transient but occasionally is severe enough to lead to platelet-related bleeding, especially after long bypass procedures. After the conclusion of bypass or once the acute trauma is resolved, the platelet count rebounds within 48 to 72 hours; however, platelet transfusions may be needed to treat significant bleeding in such patients until the platelet count recovers. In trauma patients, recent data suggest that platelet transfusions may provide greatest benefit when given in higher ratios with red blood cell and plasma transfusions (see later discussion of FFP).

Table 53-6 Drugs Affecting Platelet Function

Strong Inhibitors

Abciximab (and other anti-GPIIb/IIIa or anti-RGD compounds)
Aspirin (often contained in over-the-counter medications)
Clopidogrel, ticlopidine (ADP-receptor blockers)
Nonsteroidal anti-inflammatory drugs

Moderate Inhibitors

Antibiotics (penicillins, cephalosporins, nitrofurantoin)
Dextran
Fibrinolytics
Heparin
Hetastarch

Weak Inhibitors

Alcohol
Nitroglycerin
Nitroprusside

ADP, adenosine diphosphate; GP, glycoprotein; RGD, arginine-glycine-aspartate.

Bleeding Caused by Qualitative Platelet Defects

ASPIRIN AND ACQUIRED CAUSES OF PLATELET DYSFUNCTION

The ability of platelets to adhere to damaged vasculature and to recruit additional platelets into the clot is critical for primary hemostasis, especially when patients are challenged by trauma or surgery. One critical question in the patient history or for preoperative screening is whether patients are taking medications that interfere with platelet function, such as aspirin. *Aspirin* irreversibly blocks normal arachidonic acid metabolism such that all exposed platelets are irreversibly affected and do not respond to arachidonic acid even after aspirin is discontinued. The characteristic aspirin-induced platelet aggregation pattern is shown in Table 53-5. In contrast, other *nonsteroidal anti-inflammatory drugs* (NSAIDs) (e.g., indomethacin) *reversibly* inhibit COX, and platelet function is restored within 24 to 48 hours after discontinuing the drug. Bleeding after most surgical procedures

that is associated with aspirin or NSAIDs is usually mild, and aspirin may not need to be discontinued before surgery, especially because aspirin-induced platelet dysfunction is desirable in patients at risk for stroke or myocardial infarction. However, when bleeding caused by aspirin requires treatment, infusion of desmopressin acetate (DDAVP) has been shown to be effective at decreasing the bleeding time; occasionally, transfusion of platelets is also appropriate. In most cases, a single-platelet transfusion of 4 to 6 random donor units contributes enough normal platelets (>10% of total circulating number) to restore primary hemostasis. Platelet dysfunction and bleeding caused by other drugs is similarly treated by discontinuing the drug and platelet transfusion when needed (Table 53-6).

Whereas the aspirin effect is restricted to COX-1, the different NSAIDs have variable relative affinity for COX-1 and COX-2. COX-2 is an inducible enzyme synthesized in endothelial cells in response to inflammatory cytokines. Suppression of COX-2 results in a reduction of endothelial cell prostaglandin I_2 (prostacyclin), a molecule that, among other functions, has antithrombotic effects through inhibition of platelet aggregation. The net effect of nonselective NSAIDs on the prothrombotic or antithrombotic balance favors bleeding because NSAID-induced COX-1 inhibition means that thromboxane A_2 (TXA_2) production in platelets is blocked. By contrast, the increase in cardiovascular risk seen with the more selective COX-2 inhibitors is probably attributable to the COX-2–induced lack of endothelial cell prostacyclin production, coupled with intact platelet function (no inhibition of TXA_2 by COX-2 blockade). Recent data also show that NSAIDs given before aspirin will compete for COX-1 binding sites and diminish aspirin's antiplatelet effect, another possible factor in the coagulant balance of concomitant NSAID and aspirin use.

Uremic platelet dysfunction is caused by toxic proteins that accumulate in renal failure, most importantly guanidinosuccinic acid (GSA), which induces high levels of nitric oxide formation by vascular endothelial cells; it is nitric oxide that inhibits platelet function. Control of renal failure with dialysis and maintenance of the hematocrit are usually adequate to preserve platelet function. However, uremic bleeding is a common inpatient problem, especially in the setting of acute renal failure. Short-term treatment of uremic platelet dysfunction includes DDAVP, which has been shown to shorten the bleeding time significantly, and cryoprecipitate. Conjugated estrogens are of some benefit for long-term treatment. Platelet transfusions may be useful in patients with life-threatening bleeding and acute renal failure, but the effect of this treatment is short lived because the transfused platelets rapidly acquire the uremic defect.

CONGENITAL PLATELET DYSFUNCTION

Inherited qualitative platelet defects include abnormalities of platelet receptors and granules. Two rare but well-characterized platelet receptor disorders are *Bernard-Soulier syndrome* and *Glanzmann thrombasthenia*. Bernard-Soulier syndrome is caused by decreased surface expression of platelet GPIb (the primary von Willebrand factor [vWF] receptor) and more rarely by diminished GPIb function. The syndrome is characterized by mild thrombocytopenia, increased bleeding time, large platelets, and mild-to-moderate bleeding symptoms. The diagnosis is usually made in children but may not show symptoms until adulthood. Laboratory testing for Bernard-Soulier syndrome shows an absent platelet aggregation response to ristocetin (see Table 53-5) despite adequate vWF levels and function, such as normal ristocetin cofactor (Rcof) activity. Glanzmann thrombasthenia is characterized by an increased bleeding time and abnormally low levels of expression of platelet GPIIb/IIIa (the receptor for both vWF and fibrinogen) or, more rarely, normal expression but absent GPIIb/IIIa function. Patients commonly exhibit bleeding in childhood. Platelet aggregation testing in Glanzmann thrombasthenia shows an absent or a diminished response to all agonists except ristocetin (see Table 53-5). Platelet transfusions correct the bleeding in both Bernard-Soulier syndrome and Glanzmann thrombasthenia. However, because of the high risk for alloimmunization with frequent platelet transfusions, this therapy should be used sparingly.

Inherited platelet granule disorders are defined by the type of granule that is absent or defective. *Storage pool disease* is characterized by a relative decrease or absence of dense granules and correspondingly moderate to severe mucosal bleeding. Release of dense granule constituents that recruit

and activate platelets is impaired. Thus, storage pool disease is characterized by a diminished or absent secondary wave of aggregation in response to most agonists (see Table 53-5). *Hermansky-Pudlak syndrome* is dense granule deficiency associated with oculocutaneous albinism and mild thrombocytopenia; patients have significant bleeding, which may occur spontaneously but more often occurs in association with surgical procedures. *Chédiak-Higashi syndrome* is a rare general granule disorder characterized by mild bleeding, partial albinism, and recurrent pyogenic infections; large, irregular, gray-blue inclusions are seen in neutrophils and monocytes. Gray platelet syndrome is characterized by colorless or gray platelets that lack normal staining on the peripheral smear; electron microscopy confirms the loss of α granules or their contents. Patients with gray platelet syndrome have a mild bleeding history, and aggregation testing exhibits diminished responses to epinephrine, ADP, and collagen. All the platelet granule disorders are successfully treated by avoiding aspirin and other antiplatelet drugs, by hormonal control of menses in women, and by platelet transfusions when bleeding occurs.

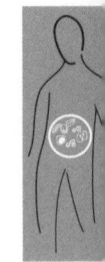

PLATELET TRANSFUSION THERAPY

Platelet transfusions, derived from the whole blood of healthy donors, can be used to stop or prevent bleeding. There are two broad categories of platelet transfusion support based on the conditions discussed in this chapter: (1) *prophylactic* platelet transfusions for thrombocytopenia in nonbleeding patients, and (2) platelet transfusion for the acutely bleeding patient. For the nonbleeding thrombocytopenic patient, there are several "triggers" that prompt platelet transfusion in the absence of frank hemorrhage. Patients receiving chemotherapy may be severely thrombocytopenic and should be transfused when their platelet counts are less than 10,000/mcL to prevent spontaneous bleeding. This is a safe and appropriate threshold for patients with relatively uncomplicated clinical pictures, without fever, sepsis, or GI bleeding. This threshold of 10,000/mcL significantly decreases the frequency of platelet transfusion and thereby reduces risks associated with multiple blood product exposures. If complicating circumstances are present, or if the patient is being managed on an outpatient basis, prophylactic transfusions should be given when platelet counts are lower than 20,000/mcL. For patients undergoing invasive procedures, such as a surgical intervention, it is reasonable to transfuse platelets when counts are lower than 50,000/mcL. Higher platelet counts are suggested for patients undergoing neurologic or ophthalmologic surgeries; platelet counts higher than 100,000/mcL are recommended, if possible, owing to the catastrophic nature of bleeding in these anatomic locations.

For the acutely bleeding patient, the decision to transfuse platelets should depend on several factors, but thrombocytopenia is the most straightforward. Platelet counts higher than 50,000/mcL are a reasonable goal for most cases of acute bleeding, whereas counts higher than 100,000/mcL might be necessary for neurologic bleeds. Congenital or acquired platelet dysfunction must also be considered for the acutely bleeding patient. Patients with significant bleeding who have taken an antiplatelet drug, such as aspirin, may benefit from platelet transfusion regardless of baseline counts. Another consideration for the acutely bleeding patient is the volume of blood products and fluids received. It is not uncommon for trauma patients to receive more than 10 units of red blood cells by transfusion in addition to plasma, volume expanders, and saline. As mentioned previously, the effects of large fluid volume resuscitation are reductions in the platelet count to less than 50% of baseline, resulting in a significant *dilutional coagulopathy*. In these scenarios, it is vitally important to obtain repeated platelet counts and to liberally transfuse platelets to maintain adequate hemostasis.

When the decision to transfuse platelets has been made, platelet units can be requested from the blood bank or transfusion service. In general, blood banks provide *pooled platelets,* which consist of 4 to 6 random donor platelet concentrates combined into one large dose. For the patient with uncomplicated thrombocytopenia, each unit of random donor-platelet concentrate ideally raises the platelet count by about 10,000/mcL. Thus, 6 pooled units of platelets transfused into a patient with a platelet count of 10,000/mcL would be expected to raise the count to nearly 50,000 to 60,000/mcL. Another commonly used platelet product is the *apheresis platelet* unit, which is a large single dose collected from one donor using apheresis technology. The dose from these *single-donor* or apheresis platelets is nearly equivalent to that of a 6-unit platelet pool and is estimated to increase platelet counts by up to 60,000/mcL in the uncomplicated patient. Usually, 1 platelet pool or 1 single-donor platelet unit should sufficiently raise platelet counts to correct thrombocytopenia. These doses should also be sufficient to stop or prevent bleeding associated with platelet dysfunction or invasive procedures. For the complicated patient, additional platelet doses may be necessary over time to achieve adequate hemostasis.

PLATELET TRANSFUSION FAILURE AND PLATELET REFRACTORINESS

Platelet transfusions in thrombocytopenic patients will not be successful in all cases. Uremia, as mentioned previously, will cause dysfunction of transfused platelets, limiting their function in vivo. Patients who are thrombocytopenic due to conditions like ITP will not generally show increases in platelet counts after transfusion because circulating autoantibodies cause rapid destruction of both endogenous and infused platelets. Many other underlying conditions can severely limit the effectiveness of platelet transfusion. This phenomenon, known as *platelet refractoriness,* can be caused by a wide variety of recipient problems, including fever, sepsis, splenomegaly, and DIC. These conditions generally decrease transfused platelet survival but not *immediate platelet recovery.* Thus, the patient with fever may have an initial increase in platelet count 1 hour after transfusion, but a subsequent decline in platelet counts at a steeper rate than expected owing to concomitant factors. For patients with this type of platelet refractoriness, addressing the underlying illness will often cause platelet transfusions to be more effective.

Platelet refractoriness can also be immune mediated. In a patient who is chronically transfused with platelets, alloantibodies against platelet antigens (e.g., human leukocyte antigen [HLA]), can be formed. Over time, and with multiple transfusion exposures, these antibodies can increase

sharply in titer and cause the rapid destruction of platelets after infusion. For the *alloimmunized patient,* platelet counts performed 1 hour after transfusion show virtually no change above baseline, pretransfusion levels. Generally, immunosuppression fails to decrease platelet alloantibodies, and efforts to improve platelet recovery are focused on finding compatible platelet units. The first step in transfusion management of the alloimmunized patient is to provide ABO antigen-matched platelets to minimize any clearance caused by naturally occurring ABO antibodies. If this step fails to yield increases in platelet counts, donor platelets that lack target antigens for the alloantibodies can be transfused. One such strategy is to use patient serum to *cross-match* for platelet donor units, with selection of those units most compatible for transfusion. If cross-match compatible platelets fail to induce an adequate platelet recovery, blood banks ultimately must provide platelets that are matched to the recipient's HLA system in the hope of evading HLA-based antibodies.

VON WILLEBRAND DISEASE

Disorders of the functional ligands for platelet adhesion to the vasculature cause bleeding that clinically resembles the bleeding associated with platelet or vascular disorders (e.g., epistaxis, GI bleeding). vWF is synthesized in endothelial cells and megakaryocytes and functions in plasma to mediate platelet adhesion to the damaged site (see Fig. 53-1). vWF is a large multimeric protein of varying size; the largest multimers contain the greatest number of adhesive sites and thus confer greater hemostatic ability than smaller vWF molecules. In patients with abnormal or low vWF levels, platelet adhesion to damaged vessels is delayed and results in mucosal bleeding and a prolonged bleeding time. vWF also serves as the carrier protein for factor VIII; deficiency of vWF or abnormal vWF-VIII binding leads to rapid clearance of factor VIII, decreased factor VIII levels, and a prolonged PTT. Many mutations in the vWF gene have been described; these have been phenotypically grouped into three major subtypes of vWD (Table 53-7).

Most patients have *type 1 vWD,* a mild-to-moderate *quantitative* decrease in all vWF multimers. This condition is commonly caused by a heterozygous mutation and shows a dominant pattern of inheritance. Type 1 vWD is characterized by equivalent decreases in factor VIII, vWF antigen, and Rcof activity; Rcof measures the ability of patient plasma (which contains vWF) to agglutinate normal platelets in the presence of ristocetin. Patients with type 1 vWD usually have mild to moderate bleeding, often only in relation to surgery or dental procedures. Patients with type 1 vWD are treated with DDAVP, which stimulates endothelial cells to release stored vWF and leads to an increase in plasma vWF antigen, Rcof, and factor VIII levels. DDAVP, at 0.3 mcg/kg given subcutaneously, usually yields excellent results. However, tachyphylaxis to DDAVP occurs because endothelial cells require time to synthesize new vWF after repeated DDAVP dosing. Thus, vWF concentrates must sometimes be used in patients with more severe type 1 vWD or in those who are undergoing a more prolonged hemostatic challenge (see later for details). Bleeding in type 1 vWD during pregnancy is exceedingly rare. Because vWF rises significantly in pregnancy, vWF antigen and Rcof levels

Table 53-7 **Classification of von Willebrand Disease (vWD)**

	Type 1	Type 2A	Type 2B	Type 2M	Type 2N	Type 3	Pseudo-vWD	BSS
Inheritance	AD	AD, AR	AD, AR	AD	AR	AR, AD	AD	AR
Platelet count	NL	NL	NL, ↓	NL	NL	NL	↓, NL	↓, NL
Bleeding time	NL, ↑–	↑	↑	↑	NL, ↑	↑↑	↑	↑
PTT	NL, ↑	↑, NL	↑, NL	↑	↑↑	↑↑	↑, NL	NL
VIII	NL, ↓	NL, ↓	↓, NL	NL, ↓	↓↓	↓↓	↓, NL	NL
vWF:Ag	NL, ↓	NL, ↓	↓, NL	NL	NL	Absent	↓, NL	NL
vWF:Rcof	NL, ↓	↓↓	↓, NL	↓↓	NL	Absent	↓, NL	NL
Multimers	NL, ↓	↓ H/I	↓↓ H	NL	NL	Absent	↓↓ H	NL
RIPA	NL, ↓	↓↓	↑*	↓	NL	↓↓	↑*	↓↓

↑, Increased; ↓, decreased; ↑*, increased agglutination in response to low-dose ristocetin; AD, autosomal dominant; AR, autosomal recessive; BSS, Bernard-Soulier syndrome; H, high-molecular-weight multimers; I, intermediate-molecular-weight multimers; NL, normal; PTT, partial thromboplastin time; RIPA, ristocetin-induced platelet agglutination; vWF:Ag, von Willebrand factor antigen level; vWF:Rcof = von Willebrand factor:ristocetin cofactor activity.

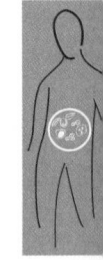

usually normalize during the second or third trimester and eliminate the bleeding risk for that time. Most pregnant women with type 1 vWD have no bleeding complications with delivery and do not require therapy during pregnancy or in the early postpartum period.

Type 2 vWD is characterized by heterozygous mutations of variable penetrance that produce a *qualitative* defect in the vWF molecule; the most common type 2 disorders are characterized by a relative lack of the larger vWF multimers (see Table 53-7). High-molecular-weight vWF multimers are absent in *type 2A disease*, and patients with type 2A vWD show disproportionately low Rcof activity compared with the vWF antigen level. The molecular defect is related to mutations in the A2 domain of vWF that render the molecule more susceptible to the vWF-cleaving protease (ADAMTS-13). Patients with type 2A vWD respond to vWF concentrate and less commonly to DDAVP. The abnormal vWF molecule in *type 2B vWD* has increased affinity for platelets, a situation that causes loss of high-molecular-weight multimers from the circulation and often produces thrombocytopenia. Platelet aggregometry in type 2B vWD (see Table 53-7) shows an abnormal increase in low-dose ristocetin-induced platelet agglutination; in the laboratory, the addition of patient vWF to normal platelets similarly increases ristocetin-induced platelet agglutination and confirms the abnormal vWF. DDAVP induces release of the abnormal vWF in patients with type 2B vWD, causing thrombocytopenia, and therefore is contraindicated; vWF concentrate should be used instead.

Type 2M vWD demonstrates laboratory findings similar to those in type 2A, but high-molecular-weight multimers are present. The defect in this rare type of vWF is most often a mutation in vWF *reducing* binding to its platelet ligand GPIbα. Some patients with type 2M vWD respond to DDAVP, but most require vWF concentrate. In *type 2N vWD*, the abnormal vWF molecule has decreased binding affinity for *factor VIII*, a characteristic that decreases factor VIII survival and produces a bleeding phenotype similar to hemophilia A. The low factor VIII levels do not respond to high-purity factor VIII infusions, unlike in true hemophilia A, but they improve with vWF concentrate. Rcof and vWF antigen levels are normal in type 2N vWD because the mutation in the factor VIII binding site does not affect vWF function or survival. Type 2N vWD should be

considered in females who present with hemophilia A; tests for vWF binding to factor VIII are available in reference laboratories.

The rare patient with *type 3 vWD* has a complete deficiency of vWF, often as a result of the inheritance of two abnormal vWF alleles (compound heterozygote). Patients with type 3 vWD have absent or extremely low levels of both Rcof and vWF antigen and factor VIII levels of 3% to 10% and usually have severe bleeding that may mimic hemophilia. Type 3 vWD does not respond to DDAVP and requires vWF concentrates for bleeding.

vWD can appear as an acquired defect, usually as a severe, type 2A–like defect with absent larger vWF multimers in a patient with no history of bleeding. *Acquired vWD* is caused by abnormal clearance of the larger vWF multimers and is associated with monoclonal gammopathies, lymphoproliferative disorders, myeloma, and other malignant and myeloproliferative diseases characterized by thrombocytosis. In these cases, acquired vWD has been successfully treated with IVIG and therapy of the underlying disease. One other cause of abnormal vWF multimer clearance resulting in acquired vWD is critical aortic stenosis, which is corrected with successful surgical repair.

FIBRINOGEN DISORDERS

Fibrinogen functions as a bridging ligand for the platelet receptor GPIIb/IIIa in the platelet-platelet matrix at sites of vascular damage. Fibrinogen also functions in the final steps of the coagulation cascade to form fibrin clot. Low fibrinogen levels are most commonly seen with consumptive disorders such as *DIC*, although rare congenital hypofibrinogenemias and afibrinogenemias are recognized. *Dysfibrinogenemia* is defined as an abnormal fibrinogen protein. Patients with dysfibrinogenemia usually bleed because of decreased adhesive function, but some patients have a hypercoagulable state. Dysfibrinogenemia is occasionally inherited, but it is more often acquired with liver disease. Both the PT and the PTT are prolonged by abnormalities of fibrinogen quantity or function (Table 53-8). A prolonged thrombin time is more specific for a low fibrinogen level or abnormal molecule, although inhibitors such as heparin and fibrin split products also prolong the thrombin time. The *reptilase time*, which is insensitive to heparin, can be used to

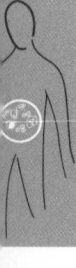

Table 53-8	**Screening Laboratory Results in Coagulation Factor Deficiencies**			
Deficient Factor	**Frequency**	**PT**	**PTT**	**TT**
I (Fibrinogen)	Rare	↑	↑	↑
II (Prothrombin)	Very rare	↑	↑	↑
V	1:1,000,000	↑	↑	NL
VII	1:500,000	↑	NL	NL
VIII	1:5000 (male patient)	NL	↑	NL
IX	1:30,000 (male patient)	NL	↑	NL
X	1:500,000	↑	↑	NL
XI	Rare*	NL	↑	NL
XII† or HMWK† or PK†	Rare	NL	↑	NL
XIII	Rare	NL	NL	NL

*Except in those of Ashkenazi Jewish descent (about 4% are heterozygous for factor XI deficiency).
†Not associated with clinical bleeding.
↑, Increased over normal range; HMWK, high-molecular-weight kininogen; NL, normal; PK, prekallikrein; PT, prothrombin time; PTT, partial thromboplastin time; TT, thrombin time.

eliminate the possibility of an increased thrombin time resulting from heparin contamination of the sample.

Bleeding Caused by Coagulation Factor Disorders

HEMOPHILIA AND OTHER INHERITED FACTOR DEFICIENCIES

Normal platelet hemostasis initiates plugging of vascular lesions and maintains mucosal integrity. However, if abnormalities of coagulation factors are present, the initial platelet plug is not solidified by secondary hemostasis, and the effects are clot breakdown and bleeding. This bleeding differs from platelet-type bleeding; coagulation factor deficiencies lead to bleeding in deep tissues and joints, and milder deficiencies result in bleeding in a delayed fashion after surgery. Most patients with significant factor deficiencies exhibit abnormal results of screening laboratory tests (see Table 53-8 and Fig. 53-1), although patients with mild deficiencies can still exhibit bleeding and normal coagulation screens.

The X-linked deficiencies of factor VIII (*hemophilia A*) and factor IX (*hemophilia B*) are the most common factor deficiencies after vWD. Hemophilia A is about 6 times more frequent than hemophilia B. About 50% or more of cases of severe hemophilia A arise as a result of an inversion of a major portion of the gene that results in complete loss of activity. Other mutations tend to result in milder disease. Most patients with hemophilia B have mutations that result in a functionally abnormal factor IX with absent activity. The combined results of antigenic and functional assays can resolve whether deficiency is due to loss of the protein or loss of its normal function. Both hemophilia A and hemophilia B are categorized by their factor levels: severe deficiency is characterized by absent (<1%) factor VIII or IX, whereas patients with moderate and mild hemophilia have factor levels of 1% to 5% and more than 5%, respectively.

Symptoms and signs of severe hemophilia A and hemophilia B develop in childhood with bleeding into muscles, joints, and soft tissue. Because they are X-linked disorders, they are observed primarily in male patients; the mother of an affected male patient is a carrier, and 50% of maternal uncles have the disease. About 25% to 30% of cases of hemophilia, however, result from new mutations and hence have no relevant family history. In exceedingly rare instances, a female carrier with extremely skewed X-inactivation may have a mild bleeding disorder with factor levels lower than 30%. Bleeding in severe hemophilia is often spontaneous and is also common after any type of surgery or even mild trauma. Bleeding in hemophilia frequently occurs in joints and in the retroperitoneum; hematuria and mucosal and intracranial bleeding also occur. Patients with moderate hemophilia have less spontaneous bleeding, but they are still at significant risk for hemorrhagic complications of surgery or trauma. Patients with mild hemophilia may be undetected into adulthood and diagnosed only with bleeding after major surgery. The complications of hemophilia stem from chronic bleeding into joints and muscles, which leads to severe deformities, arthritis, muscle atrophy, and contractures; these complications require intensive physical therapy and orthopedic care, often culminating in joint replacement. In addition, patients with hemophilia who received pooled-factor concentrates before the era of viral inactivation have complications related to transfusion-transmitted infections, including HIV and hepatitis B and C. Current therapy uses factor concentrates that are virally inactivated or recombinant.

INHERITED FACTOR DEFICIENCIES OTHER THAN HEMOPHILIA A OR B

Inherited bleeding disorders caused by deficiencies of coagulation factors V, VII, X, and XI (see Table 53-8) are much rarer than hemophilia A and B. Patients with *factor V deficiency* usually lack both plasma factor V and platelet factor V and have joint and muscle bleeding similar to patients with hemophilia. Some patients who are plasma V deficient are asymptomatic until they are challenged with the stress of surgery or trauma, and these patients are thought to have normal platelet factor V levels. Rarely, patients inherit factor deficiencies in tandem, such as combined factors V and VIII deficiencies.

Patients with *factor XI deficiency* generally have a milder bleeding disorder (even with factor XI levels <5%) than patients with hemophilia A or B, whereas *factor X deficiency* is usually more severe. *Factor XI deficiency* is an autosomal recessive disorder seen with increased frequency among Ashkenazi Jews, often manifesting late in adulthood and in clinical settings of increased fibrinolysis such as after prostate surgery. *Acquired factor X deficiency* can occur in association with amyloidosis, a condition in which the abnormal circulating light chains adsorb to and clear factor X and produce low levels and occasional bleeding.

ACQUIRED COAGULATION FACTOR DISORDERS

Factor Inhibitors

About 25% of patients with hemophilia A develop antibodies to transfused factor VIII. An inhibitor acts functionally

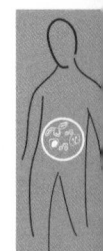

and can be measured in the laboratory as Bethesda units (BU); 1 BU is defined as the amount of inhibitor that neutralizes 50% of factor activity. High-level inhibitors (>10 BU) completely neutralize the activity of infused factor concentrates, negating their effectiveness in bleeding episodes. Bleeding therefore requires therapy using different regimens such as factor VIII inhibitor bypass activity (FEIBA) or recombinant factor VIIa (see later for details). For long-term treatment, suppression of an inhibitor is accomplished by a combination of IVIG, immunosuppressive therapy, plasmapheresis, and induction of *immune tolerance* using high-dose concentrate infusions. Patients with hemophilia B have a lower incidence of inhibitors (2% to 6%), but these inhibitors are treated in a similar fashion with high-dose FEIBA or recombinant VIIa and with similar strategies for long-term suppression of the antibody.

Acquired inhibitors to factor VIII (and more rarely to other coagulation factors) occasionally occur in patients (usually older) who do not have a history of bleeding. Acquired factor VIII inhibitor titers in this setting can be extremely high and are sometimes associated with pregnancy, autoimmune disorders, and malignant diseases, especially lymphoproliferative disorders. Patients with acquired inhibitors to factor VIII are similarly treated with factor VIIa or FEIBA. Intensive immunosuppressive therapy (Rituxan, an anti-CD20 agent) has become the mainstay of successful treatment and should be started as soon as possible to eradicate the inhibitor.

Vitamin K Deficiency

Inpatients and outpatients who are severely ill may have bleeding resulting from acquired coagulation factor deficiencies. Foremost among the causes of low factor levels is vitamin K deficiency. Vitamin K deficiency may be caused by (1) biliary tract disease interfering with enterohepatic circulation, leading to decreased absorption of vitamin K; (2) drugs, especially antibiotics, that sterilize the gut and reduce bacterial sources of vitamin K or other drugs (cholestyramine) that directly block vitamin K absorption—this category also includes cephalosporins, which interfere with intrahepatic metabolism of fat-soluble vitamin K; and (3) poor nutritional status induced by malabsorption, chronic disease, or poor oral intake in patients who are acutely ill. As noted previously, factors II, VII, IX, and X are vitamin K–dependent procoagulant factors, as are proteins C and S. Warfarin blocks vitamin K–dependent γ-carboxylation of these factors and causes an acute decrease in functional factor VII levels because factor VII has the shortest half-life (6 hours) of all vitamin K–dependent factors in vivo.

Dilutional Coagulopathy

As with platelets, coagulation factors can also be depleted through the dilutional effects of pure red blood cell transfusion, or with administration of massive amounts of volume expanders or saline solutions. It has been demonstrated that for every 10 units of red cells acutely transfused, there is a concomitant increase in INR to greater than 2. This is also occurring in conjunction with depletion and consumption of circulating coagulation factors secondary to the acute bleed. Therefore, in the setting of trauma, it is important to maintain adequate coagulation factor activity through plasma transfusion. In fact, there is recent evidence from the trauma literature to suggest that transfusion ratios of red cells to plasma should approach 1:1 to optimize hemostasis. The best means to monitor for the effects of dilutional coagulopathy is through repeated testing of PT and PTT with a liberal plasma transfusion strategy.

Bleeding in Patients with Liver Disease

Unlike patients with vitamin K deficiency or those receiving warfarin, patients with liver disease have low levels of nearly all factors, not just the vitamin K–dependent factors; the exception is factor VIII. Although liver transplantation increases factor VIII levels in patients with hemophilia, factor VIII levels are usually normal or increased with liver disease, a finding corresponding to RES and megakaryocytic sources of factor VIII production. If factor VIII levels are decreased in liver disease, consideration should be given to superimposed DIC. When a prolonged PT is evaluated for its cause, measurement of factor VII and a non–vitamin K–dependent factor, such as factor V, is most useful. In vitamin K deficiency, factor VII is low, and factor V is normal; both factors are low in patients with generalized liver disease. The PT is a sensitive measure of liver function and becomes elevated in patients with even mild liver disorders; this elevation precedes a significant decrease in the albumin or prealbumin levels and is usually coincident with transaminase changes. In patients with mild to moderate liver disease, the PT is prolonged, but the PTT usually remains within the normal range. When severe liver disease is present, the PT becomes even more prolonged, and the PTT becomes abnormal as well. Causes of bleeding in liver disease other than decreased factor synthesis include (1) decreased clearance of fibrin split products or associated DIC, (2) inhibition of platelet function, and (3) increased tissue plasminogen activator levels.

Bleeding in Patients with a Normal Laboratory Screen

Occasional patients with factor- or platelet-dependent bleeding disorders do not exhibit any abnormalities in screening laboratory assays (e.g., PT, PTT, platelet count). Besides vascular purpuras, other bleeding variants exhibit in this fashion (see Fig. 53-1). Patients with bleeding caused by mild vWD may have a normal PTT, but additional studies usually show mild decreases in factor VIII, vWF antigen, or vWF Rcof; multimeric analysis may also be abnormal in patients with mild type 2A vWD. Similarly, mild factor deficiencies (factor II, V, VII, VIII, IX, or XI) may not prolong the PT or PTT, but specific-factor assays demonstrate levels lower than the normal range. Mild bleeding, often with a delayed onset after surgery or trauma, may occur in patients with clot instability resulting from factor XIII deficiency or dysfibrinogenemia; in neonates, XIII deficiency presents with late umbilical stump bleeding. Factor XIII deficiency is diagnosed in the laboratory by screening for increased clot solubility in urea; if the clot dissolves

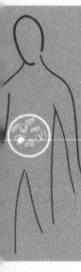

abnormally quickly in 8 mol/L urea, then an enzyme-linked immunosorbent assay for the actual XIII level should be performed. Factor XIII deficiency is currently treated with FFP, but recombinant factor XIII-A2 domain has promise for future therapy. Low fibrinogen levels or abnormal fibrinogen function will prolong both the thrombin time and the heparin-independent reptilase time. Low fibrinogen levels and dysfunction are treated with cryoprecipitate. Finally, bleeding in patients with normal platelet counts and clotting times should be evaluated by testing platelet qualitative function using platelet aggregometry or platelet function analysis. Inherited deficiencies of platelet receptors or granules and platelet abnormalities acquired with drugs or uremia can be diagnosed by demonstrating abnormal platelet aggregation or prolonged closure time results, respectively.

PLASMA AND COAGULATION FACTOR TRANSFUSION THERAPY

For patients with one or multiple defects in coagulation proteins, there are several options for replacement therapy. The most widely used product for replacement of coagulation factors is *FFP*. This product from healthy blood donors is frozen within a few hours of collection. As such, it contains normal (i.e., therapeutic) levels of all coagulation factors necessary to maintain hemostasis. FFP is the best choice for replacement of coagulation factors for a number of conditions, including liver failure or deficiencies of factors II, V, X, and XI. As such, FFP is commonly used for the reversal of warfarin therapy before invasive procedures or with the advent of bleeding. Appropriate dosing of FFP should be weight based and not dependent on the extent of prolongation of coagulation studies alone. Dosing of FFP at 10 to 15 mL/kg should be sufficient to replace deficient coagulation factors and correct abnormal coagulation studies. Thus, assuming a volume of about 200 mL per unit of FFP, a reasonable dose for a 70 kg individual would be 3 to 4 units of FFP. It is also important to recognize that dosing is time sensitive in that coagulation factors will degrade at standard half-lives upon infusion. Therefore, appropriate dosing of FFP also includes providing this product immediately before an intended procedure to ensure adequate hemostasis.

In some cases, patients may not be able to tolerate the infusion of large volumes of FFP required to reverse coagulopathic states. In these cases, other treatment modalities are available. One such product, *prothrombin complex concentrate* (PCC), quickly reverses prolonged PT studies without the need for large volumes of FFP. PCC is concentrated, lyophilized human-derived factors II, VII, IX and X that can

be reconstituted in small volumes and provided by intravenous bolus injection. A variant human-derived PCC, *FEIBA*, contains factors II, IX, and X and activated factor VII and is administered in doses of 75 U/kg every 8 to 12 hours, not to exceed 200 U in 24 hrs. Both products can be used effectively for vitamin K–dependent factor replacement when FFP is not a feasible option. Vitamin K should also be considered as an alternative to plasma infusion. Oral or parenteral replacement of vitamin K (1 to 10 mg per day for 3 days) restores coagulation factor synthesis in the presence of normal liver function and can be effectively used in the coagulopathic patient.

For patients with hemophilia A or B, several virally inactivated and recombinant factor VIII and IX concentrates are available. These products were developed because of the high rates of morbidity and mortality secondary to HIV and hepatitis viruses arising from pooled products used during the 1980s. For hemophilia, factor replacement is the key to effective therapy. Patients with severe hemophilia often infuse themselves with low doses of prophylactic factor on a regular basis (25 to 40 U/kg 3 times per week) and boost their dose or frequency of infusion when they sense internal bleeding, sustain trauma, or undergo dental procedures (Table 53-9). Patients with mild hemophilia A may not need factor infusions for minor surgery; indeed, such patients are often managed with ε-aminocaproic acid, 4 g every 4 to 6 hours, with or without infusions of DDAVP, 0.3 mcg/kg. However, most patients with hemophilia require factor infusions, if not prophylactically, then at times of surgery or trauma. Factor VIII products are infused every 8 to 12 hours, and 1 U/kg of factor VIII concentrate raises plasma factor VIII activity by 2%; thus, 50 U/kg of factor VIII theoretically will yield 100% factor VIII activity in a patient with severe hemophilia A. Factor IX has a longer half-life and is infused every 18 to 24 hours; factor IX requires 2 U/kg for a 2% increase in factor IX activity (i.e., 100 U/kg for 100% activity). Major surgery in patients with hemophilia requires intensive factor therapy to achieve normal factor levels (>80%) in both the intraoperative period and the early postoperative period to prevent wound hematoma formation. The dosing of factors (see Table 53-9) is adjusted downward from this intensity, depending on the severity of the insult, the patient's response to previous factor infusions, and whether inhibitors to factors have developed.

Unfortunately, as previously noted, patients with severe hemophilia A or B can develop inhibitors, antibodies directed against factor VIII or IX. In these cases, provision of standard doses of factor does not reverse coagulopathy, and bleeding persists. No specific factor product is clearly less immunogenic than others. Fortunately, several therapies have been developed to overcome, or bypass, the intrinsic

Table 53-9 **Factor Replacement Guidelines in Hemophilia A and B**				
Injury	**Initial Dosing**	**Maintenance**	**Factor VIII (U/kg) Initial Dosing**	**Factor IX (U/kg) Maintenance**
Dental prophylaxis	20	10-20 every 12 hr	10-20	20 every 12 hr
Hemarthrosis	10-20	10-20 every 12 hr	30-60	20 every 24 hr
Muscle hematoma	20-30	20 every 12 hr	30-50	30 every 24 hr
Trauma or surgery	50	20-30 every 8 hr	60-100	40-80

pathway of coagulation, thereby eliminating the need for active factor VIII or IX in the coagulation cascade. The previously discussed agent, FEIBA, has been employed for this purpose at doses of 50 to 100 U/kg. Another widely used bypass agent is activated factor VII (fVIIa), a recombinant factor protein. For a patient with hemophilia A and B and a strong factor inhibitor who presents with bleeding, fVIIa is generally dosed at 90 to 120 mcg/kg every 2 hours (and sometimes more frequently in pediatric patients) until the bleeding is controlled. This agent has been quite successful at controlling bleeding in hemophilia inhibitor populations as well as in patients with congenital factor VII deficiency and those with acquired coagulation factor inhibitors. Based on its success in treating bleeding associated with hemophilia, trials of fVIIa have been performed for non–hemophilia-associated bleeding with varied success. To date, the U.S. Food and Drug Administration has approved use of fVIIa only in the setting of factor VII deficiency (15 to 20 mcg/kg) or for treatment of bleeding associated with a factor inhibitor.

Several virally inactivated, *intermediate-purity* factor VIII concentrate products (not recombinant or monoclonal antibody purified) are also available for use. These factors generally contain large amounts of vWF (e.g., Humate-P) and are particularly useful for bleeding or prophylaxis in severe vWD, as effective replacement immediately before major invasive procedures, or in vWD patients who have failed DDAVP therapy.

CRYOPRECIPITATE TRANSFUSION THERAPY

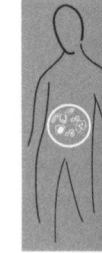

Cryoprecipitated antihemophiliac factor (better known as *cryoprecipitate*) is an underused but important blood product for the treatment of a variety of bleeding disorders. Cryoprecipitate is prepared by thawing frozen plasma at very cold temperatures and removing the precipitated portion. As such, it contains relatively high levels of fibrinogen, fibronectin, factor VIII, vWF, and factor XIII. A major advantage of cryoprecipitate is that the average single unit is only 10 to 15 mL. Based on its contents and small volume, cryoprecipitate is very useful for the replacement of fibrinogen in DIC or in patients demonstrating hypofibrinogenemia or dysfibrinogenemia. The product may be helpful for isolated factor XIII deficiency or factor XIII consumption in DIC. There is also mounting evidence to suggest that the vWF/factor VIII in cryoprecipitate can be used to overcome bleeding in uremia by enhancing the adhesive properties of circulating platelets.

Cryoprecipitate is most appropriately dosed by considering a patient's plasma volume and baseline fibrinogen levels. However, from a practical standpoint, for a 70-kg adult, a 10-unit pool (total volume, 150 mL) should be sufficient to provide adequate fibrinogen and enhance other hemostatic properties. For more advanced dosing protocols, consultation with the transfusion service is strongly recommended.

Prospectus for the Future

Novel modalities continue to be developed for the diagnosis of patients with bleeding disorders. For instance, application of assays measuring thrombin generation represents a distinct, and more specific, view of coagulation from a laboratory standpoint that may provide greater insight into the source of abnormal bleeding than current tests. Alternatives to transfusion are also being developed. For thrombocytopenic patients, this includes fibrin-coated albumin particles that could evade immune-mediated platelet destruction while yielding important therapeutic impact. Additionally, there has been renewed interest in chemical and cytokine-based stimulation of the bone marrow to produce endogenous platelets. These newer agents, known as *nonpeptide platelet growth factors*, appear to have none of the side effects associated with earlier generations of thrombopoietic drugs. Progress also continues to be made in the development and application of recombinant coagulation factors for the treatment of hemophilia with a focus on preparation of factors that are less immunogenic and therefore less prone to induce the development of significant inhibitors.

References

Aster RH, Bougie DW: Drug-induced thrombocytopenia. N Engl J Med 357:580-587, 2007.

Borgman MA, Spinella PC, Perkins JG, et al: The ratio of blood products transfused affects mortality in patients receiving massive transfusions at a combat support hospital. J Trauma 63:805-813, 2007.

Bussel JB, Cheng G, Saleh MN, et al: Eltrombopag for the treatment of chronic idiopathic thrombocytopenic purpura. N Engl J Med 357:2237-2247, 2007.

DiNisio M, Middeldorp S, Buller HR: Direct thrombin inhibitors. N Engl J Med 353:1028-1040, 2005.

Gomperts ED, Astermark J, Gringeri A, et al: From theory to practice: Applying current clinical knowledge and treatment strategies to the care of hemophilia A patients with inhibitors. Blood Rev 22:S1-S22, 2008.

Hedges SJ, Dehoney SB, Hooper JS, et al: Evidence-based treatment recommendations for uremic bleeding. Nat Clin Pract Nephrol 3:138-153, 2007.

Hod E, Schwartz J: Platelet transfusion refractoriness. Br J Haematol 142:348-360, 2008.

Levesque LE, Brophy JM, Zhang B: The risk for myocardial infarction with cyclooxygenase-2 inhibitors: A population study of elderly adults. Ann Intern Med 142:481-489, 2005.

Mazzucconi MG, Fazi P, Bernasconi S, et al: Therapy with high-dose dexamethasone (HD-DXM) in previously untreated patients affected by idiopathic thrombocytopenic purpura: A GIMEMA experience. Blood 109:1401-1407, 2007.

Pabinger I, Brenner B, Kalina U, et al: Prothrombin complex concentrate (Beriplex P/N) for emergency anticoagulation reversal: A prospective multi-national clinical trial. J Thromb Haemost 6:622-631, 2008.

Sadler JE: New concepts in von Willebrand disease. Annu Rev Med 173-191, 2005.

Salles II, Feys HB, Iserbyt BF, et al: Inherited traits affecting platelet function. Blood Rev 22:155-172, 2008.

Slichter SJ: Platelet transfusion therapy. Hematol Oncol Clin North Am 21:697-729, 2007.

Spence RK: Clinical use of plasma and plasma-fractions. Best Pract Red Clin Haematol 19:83-96, 2006.

Wolberg AS: Thrombin-generation assays: understanding how the method influences the results. Thromb Res 119:663-665, 2007.

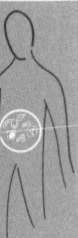

Disorders of Hemostasis: Thrombosis

Richard Torres and Henry M. Rinder

Clinical Evaluation of Thrombosis

The approach to patients with thromboembolism is defined by clinical history, laboratory studies, and occasionally physical findings. Events that trigger venous thromboembolic (VTE) disease include immobilization, orthopedic and other surgical procedures, use of oral contraceptives, and pregnancy. VTE that is recurrent (thrombophilia) may present at an early age or at unusual thrombotic sites (e.g., cerebral vessels) or be accompanied by a family history of VTE suggesting an inherited disorder. Acquired VTE risk may be associated with systemic disorders such as hemolysis (paroxysmal nocturnal hemoglobinuria and autoimmune hemolytic anemia), collagen vascular disorders (lupus), or various malignant diseases (adenocarcinoma). In contrast, arterial thromboembolic (TE) disease is more commonly superimposed on ruptured atherosclerotic plaque (e.g., coronary artery disease) and atheroembolic disorders (e.g., ischemic stroke, peripheral arterial disease). Arterial vascular disease is mainly associated with metabolic risk factors including hypertension, hypercholesterolemia, and diabetes, but arterial event risk may also be compounded by a congenital propensity to clot. The clinical approach to thrombotic disease is tailored to the location of the disease (arterial versus venous and the specific vascular bed) and whether there are abnormalities of the vascular endothelium, platelets, or soluble coagulation factors that predispose the patient to TE risk.

Vascular Causes of Thrombosis

The Virchow triad defines the pathologic mechanisms underlying thrombosis: diminished blood flow, damage to the vascular wall, and an imbalance favoring procoagulant over anticoagulant factors. The first two factors are clearly localized to specific vascular beds; although the last element of the triad may be systemic, data now show at least partial vascular bed–specific regulation of the hemostatic balance. For example, congenital deficiencies of antithrombin (AT), protein C, or protein S generally lead to VTE of the lower extremities. In contrast, the inherited hypercoagulable disorders associated with factor V Leiden (FVL) and the prothrombin G20210A mutation not only produce lower extremity VTE but also are associated with thrombosis of the cerebral veins and sinuses. This hemostatic regulation in vascular tissues is mediated by multiple factors that include (1) microenvironmental signals, such as shear stress, that affect endothelial cell (EC) expression of thrombomodulin, tissue factor, and nitric oxide synthase; (2) EC subtype-specific signaling (e.g., shear stress upregulates aortic, but not pulmonary artery, nitric oxide synthase); (3) differences in EC transcriptional regulation of proteins such as von Willebrand factor (vWF) and its cleaving protease, ADAMTS-13; and (4) the increasingly important link between inflammation and thrombosis that is mediated by selectin and integrin ligands functioning in both physiologies.

Atherothrombosis

This section briefly discusses hematologic factors that predispose to thrombosis in the setting of atherosclerotic plaque (atherothrombosis); the pathophysiologic mechanisms of atherogenesis are discussed in Chapter 9.

FIBRINOLYTIC SYSTEM

In addition to EC-intrinsic regulation of hemostasis, the interaction of EC with the fibrinolytic system is important in the development of atherothrombotic disease because it affects the balance point of clot propagation. The breakdown of stable fibrin polymers into fibrin split products (FSPs) is mediated by plasmin. Plasmin is converted from its inactive form, plasminogen, by tissue-type plasminogen activator (t-PA), the activity of which is regulated in turn by plasminogen activator inhibitor-1 (PAI-1). Abnormalities of

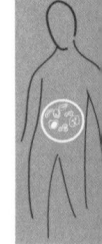

both t-PA and PAI-1 are associated with an increased risk for arterial thrombosis, but the degree to which absolute levels contribute to arterial thrombosis remains controversial. Curiously, it is high t-PA levels that are associated with higher rates of atherothrombosis, specifically acute myocardial infarction and stroke. This phenomenon may be a manifestation of upregulation of t-PA serving as a surrogate marker for high de novo PAI-1 levels, although a direct correlation of PAI-1 levels and overall arterial thrombosis rates remains weak. Still, there exists a strong association between abnormal hemostasis and high PAI-1 levels in patients with the metabolic syndrome or vascular disease in type II diabetes. Furthermore, the risk for acute myocardial infarction is elevated in the subset of angina pectoris patients with increased PAI-1 activity levels, and there is evidence for the direct contribution of PAI-1 to stent restenosis after angioplasty. From a genetic risk standpoint, the 4G isoform of PAI-1 (versus the 5G form) results in higher levels of PAI-1, but the association of the 4G isoform with increased relative risk for arterial thrombosis is small. Even in those instances in which there is a stronger link, the role of testing for fibrinolytic component levels in arterial thrombosis evaluation remains largely prognostic because directed therapies are not available. Aprotinin, which decreases blood loss during cardiopulmonary bypass through its antifibrinolytic effects, is also associated with increased risk for vein graft occlusion and myocardial infarction after bypass. For their part, t-PA polymorphisms and plasminogen levels do not correlate with atherothrombotic risk. Controversy remains as to any role in arterial thrombosis for thrombin activatable fibrinolysis inhibitor (TAFI), a fibrinolysis modulator (see "Prospectus for the Future" for the potential role of TAFI in VTE).

HYPERHOMOCYSTEINEMIA

Increased levels of plasma homocysteine (HCY) are linked to atherothrombosis. Extremely high plasma HCY levels, as are found in rare congenital syndromes characterized by homocysteinuria and hyperhomocysteinemia (e.g., cystathionine β-synthase deficiency), are associated with thromboembolism and severe premature atherosclerosis. Elevated HCY induces EC dysfunction and apoptosis, triggering normal coagulation pathways designed to respond to EC damage but without the corresponding upregulation of EC-dependent anticoagulant function such as activated protein C. However, epidemiologic studies support the assertion that even moderate elevations in HCY contribute to coronary, peripheral, and cerebral arterial disease. HCY in plasma can be measured after patients have fasted or after they have received a methionine load. Evidence indicates that both measures are important in that they are affected by different abnormalities of HCY metabolism, involving either the remethylation cycle or the trans-sulfuration pathway, respectively. In some cases, elevated HCY levels are partly due to a thermolabile form of the methylene tetrahydrofolate reductase (MTHFR) enzyme resulting from a polymorphism (C677T) in the coding region of the MTHFR binding site. This isoform occurs in up to 30% to 40% of the general population and introduces a higher set point for regulating HCY concentration (the substrate for MTHFR), particularly with relative folate deficiency. In fact, deficiency of any of the vitamin cofactors of HCY metabolism (folate, vitamin B_6, and vitamin B_{12}) may lead to mild hyperhomocysteinemia. Reduction in HCY levels by supplementation with vitamin B_6, vitamin B_{12}, and folate is probably the most effective therapy for reducing the HCY level, but multiple randomized studies have shown that supplementation does not decrease atherothrombotic risk, regardless of the cause of hyperhomocysteinemia and the presence of the MTHFR polymorphism.

ROLE OF PLATELETS

Although EC-associated abnormalities clearly influence hemostasis, platelet activation and adhesion are also critical to the development of atherothrombosis, especially in patients with acute coronary syndromes and ischemic stroke. In addition, antiplatelet therapies are primary modalities for maintaining short- and long-term patency after coronary revascularization. Antiplatelet therapy can be targeted against specific platelet functions, including cyclo-oxygenase–mediated thromboxane A_2 formation, interaction of adenosine diphosphate (ADP) with its platelet receptor, and glycoprotein IIb/IIIa (GPIIb/IIIa)-fibrinogen binding for aggregation (Table 54-1). Aspirin has long been a mainstay in treatment of myocardial infarction, angina, and stroke because of its irreversible inhibition of platelet cyclo-oxygenase, a process leading to blockade of thromboxane A_2 release. Aspirin effectively blocks platelet aggregation to weak physiologic agonists over the lifetime of a platelet of about 7 to 10 days (see Chapter 53, Table 53-5); however, aspirin is only partially inhibitory to platelet stimulation by thrombin and strong agonists such as collagen. Thus, blockade of platelet activation pathways other than through thromboxane A_2 has become an important modality for therapy of patients at risk for arterial thrombosis. Some drugs used to treat stroke and coronary disease specifically block the platelet P2Y12 ADP receptor from interaction with ADP in the clot milieu and thereby blunt platelet recruitment by preventing locally released ADP from activating additional platelets. Two thienopyrimidine derivatives, ticlopidine and clopidogrel, antagonize ADP-induced

Table 54-1 **Antiplatelet Therapies**
Inhibitors of Cyclo-oxygenase
Aspirin
Nonaspirin nonsteroidal anti-inflammatory drugs (not COX-2 selective)
ADP Receptor Antagonist
Clopidogrel
Phosphodiesterase Inhibitors
Dipyridamole
Prostacyclin
GPIIb/IIIa and RGD Blockers
Abciximab
Integrilin (or generic eptifibatide)
Lamifiban
Tirofiban
Xemilofiban

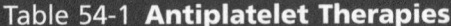

ADP, adenosine diphosphate; COX-2, cyclo-oxygenase 2; RGD, arginine-glycine-aspartate amino acid sequence.

platelet effects through their metabolites, which block ADP from binding to the platelet receptor. Both drugs are highly inhibitory to platelet function and produce bleeding times that are more prolonged than those produced with aspirin. Both are effective in combination with aspirin for preventing ischemic stroke and for blocking stent thrombosis after revascularization; however, the hematologic side effects of ticlopidine (TTP) have made clopidogrel the favored drug in this category. Some patients appear to have resistance to clopidogrel, defined as the lack of inhibition of platelet function; there is some evidence that this patient subset is heterozygous for a loss of function polymorphism in the *CYP2C19* gene.

A third avenue for blocking platelet activation targets GPIIb/IIIa, the primary platelet receptor for binding to fibrinogen and vWF. The modified monoclonal antibody abciximab prevents GPIIb/IIIa from binding to fibrinogen and blocks platelet aggregation after angioplasty, stent placement, and pharmacologic thrombolysis. Abciximab has been shown to reduce the incidence of recurrent acute ischemic events after percutaneous coronary revascularization in myocardial infarction and unstable angina patients mainly by decreasing the incidence of platelet-mediated thrombosis within the infarct related vessel during and after the procedure. Other GPIIb/IIIa blockers (e.g., eptifibatide [Integrilin] and tirofiban [Aggrastat]) that interfere with the GPIIb/IIIa arginine-glycine-aspartate (RGD) binding sites are also effective in treating acute coronary syndrome. Currently, GPIIb/IIIa inhibitors are indicated for acute parenteral use in patients with acute coronary syndromes and for maintaining coronary patency after revascularization. Thrombocytopenia is an uncommon (<2%) complication with all of the GPIIb/IIIa inhibitors, most likely related to exposure of neoepitopes on the receptor and immune-mediated platelet destruction. Clearance of the drug typically resolves the thrombocytopenia within 1 week. Platelet transfusion should be considered only if there is significant thrombocytopenic bleeding because of platelet transfusion's association with a high incidence of stent thrombosis after stent implantation.

Oral anti-GPIIb/IIIa formulations are not available because of two randomized trials in which mortality was increased in the GPIIb/IIIa inhibitor arms.

Not only is GPIIb/IIIa clearly critical for platelet-dependent atherothrombosis, it is apparent that a specific platelet GPIIb/IIIa allotype, human platelet antigen-1b (HPA-lb; see Chapter 53, Table 53-3), is a risk factor for coronary thrombosis. Studies have shown that the HPA-lb allotype of the GPIIIa molecule is associated with an increased incidence of coronary events, both myocardial infarction and unstable angina, as well as with coronary and cerebral injury after cardiac surgery. A large, long-term Danish study has shown that homozygosity for the HPA-lb allotype confers a threefold to fourfold increased risk for myocardial infarction in men. Evidence suggests that this and other platelet receptor allotypes associated with thrombosis promote increased platelet responsiveness to agonists and shear.

Inherited Risk Factors for Venous Thrombosis

The balance between thrombin formation and anticoagulant pathways has been extensively studied in patients with inherited deficiencies of naturally occurring anticoagulants (Table 54-2). These patients are predisposed to venous thromboembolism (VTE) and pulmonary embolism (PE).

FACTOR V LEIDEN

The most common inherited disorder leading to VTE is the FVL mutation. About 5% of individuals with European ancestry are heterozygous for FVL. The FVL mutation occurs at a site where activated protein C (APC) cleaves and inactivates normal factor Va (Arg506); abolition of this cleavage site results in APC resistance. Failure to inactivate the mutant factor Va allows the prothrombinase complex to be relatively uninhibited and leads to increased thrombin generation and

Table 54-2 Prevalence and Thrombotic Relative Risk (RR) Associations of Laboratory Findings		
Prevalence in General Population	**Venous RR**	**Arterial RR**
Hyperhomocysteinemia ± MTHFR homozygosity C677T (10%-15%)*	3	1.16
Activated protein C resistance (5%)*		
Heterozygous FVL	7	1
Homozygous FVL	20-80	1
Prothrombin G20210A (1%-2%)		
Heterozygous G20210A	2-5	1
Homozygous G20210A	>5	1
Platelet GPIIb/IIIa HPA-lb homozygosity (2%-3%)		4 (MI in men)
Protein C deficiency (0.2%-0.5%)	7	1
Protein S deficiency (0.1%)	8.5	1
Antithrombin III deficiency (0.02%-0.05%)	8	1
t-PA (very high level/low activity) (rare)	~1	2 (stroke)/10 (MI) Plasminogen activator inhibitor (PAI-1) excess (rare)
Dysfibrinogenemia (rare)	~1	1.5?

Note: Data on prevalence and relative risk vary widely, often with conflicting results. This information represents an interpretation of data collected from various sources, mainly meta-analyses.
*MTHFR frequency in European-American population.
FVL, factor V Leiden; HPA-1b, human platelet antigen-1b; MI, myocardial infarction; MTHFR, methylene tetrahydrofolate reductase; PAI-1, plasminogen activator inhibitor-1; t-PA, tissue-type plasminogen activator.

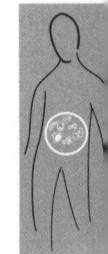

a thrombophilic phenotype. About one fourth of patients with an initial occurrence of VTE or PE will have heterozygous FVL, and this percentage increases to nearly 60% in those with recurrent VTE or a strong family history of VTE or PE. APC resistance can be demonstrated by specialized clotting tests showing that the addition of APC fails to prolong the partial thromboplastin time (PTT). Genotyping can then confirm whether FVL is present and whether heterozygous or homozygous.

Inheritance of heterozygous FVL conveys an about sevenfold increased risk for VTE or PE. However, at 50 years of age, only 25% of persons with heterozygous FVL have had VTE or PE compared with much higher percentages in persons with other inherited thrombophilias. It is with concomitant *acquired* risk factors such as immobilization, pregnancy, or oral contraceptive use that the risk for VTE or PE in persons with FVL becomes more significant. Parenthetically, MTHFR mutations do not demonstrate a synergistic effect with FVL, but the prothrombin mutation (see below) does. Homozygotes for FVL have an increased risk for VTE that is estimated to be between 20- and 80-fold. Only occasional reports exist of patients with homozygous FVL who are asymptomatic into old age. It is worth noting that APC resistance *without* the FVL mutation can occur rarely. Factor V Cambridge, although much less common than FVL, has a similar mutation at an APC cleavage site (Arg306) and is associated with APC resistance and thrombosis. *Acquired* APC resistance can also occur and may be caused by the presence of a lupus anticoagulant or cancer and can also be seen with pregnancy, hormone replacement therapy, and oral contraceptives.

PROTHROMBIN G20210A

Another mutation associated with inherited thrombophilia is the prothrombin G20210A mutation, which occurs in the 3′-untranslated region of the prothrombin gene; this mutation leads to higher than normal prothrombin levels and about a twofold increased risk for VTE or PE. The heterozygous mutation is present in about 3% of European-derived populations but is identified in about 15% of patients with VTE or PE. Homozygous prothrombin G20210A patients are rare, but their relative risk for VTE is thought to be about 10-fold. How the prothrombin mutation exactly affects thrombus development has not been fully defined, but it appears to be related to changes in polyadenylation of the prothrombin messenger RNA (mRNA) during transcription. The diagnosis of the G20210A genotype is made by examining DNA for this specific mutation; no screening or functional assays are available.

INHERITED DEFICIENCY OF NATURAL ANTICOAGULANT PROTEINS

Deficiencies in the naturally occurring anticoagulants (AT, protein C, and protein S) are less common than FVL or prothrombin G20210A, but they are more likely to produce symptomatic venous thrombosis at an earlier age. Only about one half the thromboses that occur with these deficiencies are associated with acquired risk factors such as pregnancy, surgery, or immobilization. Deficiencies of AT, protein C, or protein S are detected by functional or anti-

genic assays because some mutations cause a quantitative decrease in the factor, whereas others produce a dysfunctional protein. Many gene mutations have been associated with these deficiencies, but none is predominant. Deficiencies of AT, protein C, and protein S in the aggregate account for fewer than 5% to 10% of all patients with VTE or PE.

AT is a naturally occurring anticoagulant that complexes with endogenous heparan sulfates to inhibit both formed thrombin and factor Xa. Heterozygous AT deficiency leads to AT levels of less than 50% and is generally associated with VTE or PE. However, reports have noted a homozygous mutation in the heparin-binding site of AT that results in arterial thrombosis. Thrombosis occurs by the age of 25 years in 50% of patients who are heterozygous for AT deficiency. AT has a low molecular weight and is lost in the proteinuria of nephrotic syndrome, leading to symptomatic acquired AT deficiency. Acquired AT deficiency (as well as protein C deficiency) may also be associated with severe hepatic veno-occlusive disease after stem cell transplantation; AT and protein C may be excessively consumed in the damaged hepatic microvasculature. It is not surprising, then, that low levels of AT are associated with poor outcomes in such severely ill patients. AT replacement with or without heparin appears to be useful in resolving both platelet consumption and the fluid disorders of veno-occlusive disease after stem cell transplantation. Successful treatment of symptomatic patients with heterozygous AT deficiency has included short-term replacement of AT with fresh-frozen plasma or the recombinant AT protein, usually coupled with unfractionated heparin (UFH) anticoagulation; prophylaxis studies of recombinant AT in deficient patients are ongoing. Long-term therapy for congenitally deficient patients has consisted primarily of warfarin.

The complex of thrombin and thrombomodulin on the EC surface activates protein C; APC coupled with its cofactor, protein S, cleaves and inactivates factors Va and VIIIa. These actions downregulate the prothrombinase and tenase complexes, respectively, to slow the rate of thrombin generation. Similar to AT deficiency, heterozygous protein C and protein S deficiencies are observed with venous, and occasionally arterial, thrombosis at a young age (median occurrence, 20 to 40 years). Homozygous protein C deficiency does occur and presents in the neonate as *purpura fulminans* with widespread venous thrombosis and skin necrosis. A similar clinical presentation has been reported in heterozygous protein C–deficient adults after instituting warfarin therapy *without* simultaneous heparinization, called *warfarin-induced skin necrosis*. About one third of these patients are deficient in protein C on a hereditary basis, whereas the rest appear to have acquired protein C deficiency. Warfarin inhibits production of vitamin K–dependent protein C synthesis, and because of the factor's short half-life, protein C levels rapidly fall before a decline in the levels of the procoagulant factors II, IX, and X. This imbalance shortly after starting warfarin may favor a procoagulant state and occasionally results in widespread microvascular thrombosis. Although protein C deficiency, either inherited or acquired, is infrequent, guidelines recommend that patients with active VTE be fully anticoagulated with UFH or low-molecular-weight heparin (LMWH) before concurrent warfarin therapy is begun, and heparin should be continued until warfarin is therapeutic for at least

48 hours. Inherited deficiency of protein S has similarly been implicated in warfarin-induced skin necrosis. Protein S deficiency is commonly acquired in acute illness. Protein S circulates in a free form and is bound to C4b-binding protein; only free protein S is active as a cofactor for protein C. C4b-binding protein is an acute-phase reactant, and thus, increased C4b-binding protein levels with severe illness can decrease free protein S levels. A similar effect is seen in normal pregnancy. Short-term therapy for homozygous C deficiency or doubly heterozygous protein C or S deficiency, especially in the setting of neonatal *purpura fulminans,* has included plasma or protein C concentrate with full-dose UFH anticoagulation. Functional levels of AT, protein S, and protein C are readily measured in clinical laboratories. Antigenic levels of these proteins can also be assessed to define whether a functional deficiency is caused by a dysfunctional protein versus diminished synthesis. As with AT deficiency, long-term treatment with warfarin has been successful in heterozygous protein C or S deficiency. As expected, both protein C and S levels are decreased during warfarin therapy, rendering their evaluation invalid when warfarin has been instituted.

Acquired Risk Factors for Venous Thrombosis

SURGERY

Medical and surgical illnesses convey increased thrombotic risk; these *acquired* risk factors are acknowledged, even though the pathophysiologic features favoring thrombosis may be uncertain (Table 54-3). Stasis of blood flow is a clear risk factor for thrombus formation (e.g., in the left atrial appendage with nonvalvular atrial fibrillation) and for systemic thromboembolism (e.g., stroke in this case) in non-anticoagulated patients. Other high-risk situations, including surgery (especially orthopedic) and trauma, are associated with immobilization with resultant stasis of lower extremity blood flow. When evidence of thrombosis is actively sought,

Table 54-3 **Acquired Causes of Thrombosis**
Medical and Surgical Illnesses
Antiphospholipid antibody, lupus anticoagulant
Artificial heart valves
Atrial fibrillation (nonvalvular)
Hemolytic anemias (autoimmune hemolysis, sickle cell, thrombotic thrombocytopenic purpura, paroxysmal nocturnal hemoglobinuria)
Hyperlipidemia
Immobilization
Malignancy
Myeloproliferative disorders with thrombocytosis
Nephrotic syndrome
Orthopedic procedures
Pregnancy
Trauma, fat embolism
Medications
Heparin-induced thrombocytopenia
Oral contraceptives, hormone replacement therapy
Prothrombin complex concentrates

both surgery and trauma can be shown to be associated with extremely high (>50%) incidences of VTE. Besides immobilization, other pathophysiologic factors may contribute to the risk for VTE with surgery and trauma, including fat embolism and tissue damage, the latter especially after closed head injuries that result in massive tissue factor release. Prophylactic, permanent or temporary, inferior vena cava (IVC) filters are often placed in trauma patients to protect against PE, especially in high-risk patients in whom anticoagulation is contraindicated because of the increased risk for bleeding.

PREGNANCY AND FETAL LOSS

Pregnancy is a hypercoagulable state associated with venous stasis; increases in procoagulant proteins, such as fibrinogen, vWF, and factors VII, VIII, and X; decreased protein S; and increased fibrinolytic inhibitors, PAI-1, and TAFI. VTE can occur at any time during pregnancy or the puerperium. Inherited maternal thrombophilia can compound the procoagulant state of pregnancy and, in addition to the VTE risk in the mother, may predispose to fetal loss. The principal associated risk factors for fetal loss or stillbirth are FVL, the G20210A prothrombin mutation, AT deficiency, and protein C or S deficiency. Relative risks are markedly higher in mothers with a history of prior VTE, and the risk for fetal loss appears restricted to after 9 weeks of gestation. In fact, inherited thrombophilia appears to be protective against fetal loss in the first 9 weeks, possibly by means of limiting oxygen toxicity to the early embryo. As such, recommended indications for evaluating for inherited thrombophilia risk in women seeking to become pregnant are a history of VTE or recurrent fetal loss after 9 weeks of gestation when no specific cause can be identified. Both AT deficiency and hyperhomocysteinemia have also been associated with placental abruption. Aside from fetal loss due to thrombophilia, the risk for VTE and PE during pregnancy and in the postpartum period for women with identified thrombophilia is about fivefold higher than it is for nonpregnant women.

ORAL CONTRACEPTIVES AND HORMONE REPLACEMENT

Oral contraceptive use conveys an increased risk for VTE and PE, and a similar increased risk is seen early after instituting hormone replacement therapy (HRT). Concomitant heterozygosity for FVL further increases the risk for VTE and PE in women who take oral contraceptives or HRT. Cigarette use in women using oral contraceptives also significantly increases thrombosis risk, and this increase is thought to result from increased platelet reactivity, mediated in part by increased thromboxane synthesis. On the arterial side, epidemiologic evidence clearly points to smoking as the main cardiovascular risk factor but similarly implicates some risk attributable to long-term use of both the estrogen and progestin components of oral contraceptives and HRT; third-generation pharmaceuticals have not erased the thrombosis risk. As noted previously, acquired activated protein C resistance can be seen both in pregnancy and with oral contraceptive use, and both free and functional protein S levels decrease throughout pregnancy and with oral contraceptive use.

PROTHROMBOTIC DISEASE STATES

As noted earlier, thrombosis in nephrotic syndrome is associated with loss of AT through the kidneys. Hemolysis is a general prothrombotic state that appears to be mediated through blood cell destruction, perhaps by increasing exposure to procoagulant membrane phospholipids; hemolysis with TE complications has been noted with artificial heart valves, sickle cell disease, and other hemolytic anemias, including Coombs-positive autoimmune hemolytic anemia. In the case of paroxysmal nocturnal hemoglobinuria (PNH), complement activation may directly mediate platelet activation, and therapy with the complement inhibitor eculizumab has significantly decreased the rate of TE disease in PNH. Platelet activation and clearance appear to be the primary prothrombotic manifestations of heparin-induced thrombocytopenia and thrombotic thrombocytopenic purpura (TTP; see later). Although chronic disseminated intravascular coagulation is present in some malignancies (Trousseau syndrome), malignant diseases in general are associated with an increased risk for VTE and PE that is not related to disseminated intravascular coagulation. Such malignancies are not limited to mucinous adenocarcinomas or promyelocytic leukemia, and thrombosis occurs in a wide spectrum of malignancies, especially lung, breast, gastrointestinal, and any metastatic solid tumor. When idiopathic VTE or PE occurs in a cancer-free individual, an intensive work-up to find an occult malignancy is not warranted because this does not affect any subsequent cancer-related morbidity and mortality. However, once a cancer diagnosis is established in patients with prior VTE, they are at increased risk for subsequent VTE events, especially if the FVL or G20210A prothrombin mutation is present. UFH therapy in malignancy-associated VTE or PE appears to achieve outcomes superior to those provided by treatment with LMWH, direct thrombin inhibitors, or warfarin, possibly because of multiple beneficial anticoagulant effects mediated by the longer glycosaminoglycan sequences in UFH. In the special case of myeloproliferative disorders (e.g., essential thrombocythemia), abnormal platelet physiologic mechanisms causing hyperaggregability are often present and require platelet-specific inhibition (See "Hypercoagulability and Platelet Disorders" later).

ANTIPHOSPHOLIPID ANTIBODY SYNDROME

Another acquired prothrombotic disorder is the antiphospholipid (aPL) syndrome. The aPL syndrome may exhibit as a primary disorder, or it may be associated with other autoimmune diseases such as systemic lupus erythematosus (SLE). The etiologic character of this connection with lupus has not been fully defined, but replacement of the host immune system after hematopoietic stem cell transplantation for refractory SLE has the potential to eradicate the lupus anticoagulant and TE risk. All the manifestations of aPL syndrome are related to hypercoagulability, including recurrent venous or arterial thrombosis, thrombocytopenia caused by microcirculatory platelet clearance, and recurrent fetal loss resulting from placental vascular insufficiency. The serologic markers of aPL syndrome include *anticardiolipin antibodies, anti-β₂ glycoprotein I antibodies,* or the *lupus anti-*

coagulant. The Sydney Consensus Criteria for Antiphospholipid Syndrome is the current standard for diagnosis of aPL. It includes the clinical criteria of radiologically or pathologically confirmed thrombosis or fetal loss when thrombosis is the etiology, and the laboratory criteria of at least one of the three potential laboratory findings being positive on two or more occasions at least 12 weeks apart. The anticardiolipin antibodies are usually detected by enzyme-linked immunosorbent assay (ELISA), whereas lupus anticoagulants are defined by prolongation of a phospholipid-dependent clotting test (prothrombin time [PT], PTT, or Russell viper venom clotting time), which is then corrected by the addition of excess phospholipid. Thus, *lupus anticoagulant* is actually a misnomer because its presence predisposes the patient to clotting rather than to bleeding. Another misleading aspect of this nomenclature is that phospholipid-reactive antibodies are actually directed against phospholipid-binding proteins in plasma, β₂-GPI, annexin V, and prothrombin. The anti–β₂-GPI can be detected by immunoassay, and this marker is most correlated with TE risk. The risk for thrombosis correlates best with the presence of the lupus anticoagulant and is highest if all three serologic markers are present when the relative risk has been estimated to be greater than 50.

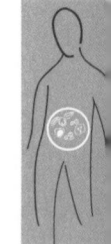

Hypercoagulability and Platelet Disorders

Essential thrombocythemia and polycythemia vera are clonal myeloproliferative disorders associated with the *Jak-2* mutation. They are wholly (essential thrombocythemia) or partially (polycythemia vera) characterized by thrombocytosis, and patients with these disorders are at increased risk for thrombosis. Platelet aggregometry in these disorders often shows abnormal responses, especially to epinephrine and ADP; however, the abnormal aggregation does not correspond to either bleeding or thrombosis risk. Patients with polycythemia vera in particular have a high incidence of thrombosis in the mesenteric, portal, and hepatic venous circulation. Thrombotic complications, both arterial and venous, occur in essential thrombocythemia, even in young patients. However, no clear clinical risk factors predict which myeloproliferative patients will develop thrombosis. Platelet counts greater than 1,000,000/mcL are thought to increase the risk for thrombosis, and increased platelet turnover in thrombocytosis is also associated with thromboembolic complications. The latter has been demonstrated by radioactive platelet survival studies and an increase in the percentage of reticulated platelets. Antiplatelet agents may cause bleeding in patients with myeloproliferative disorders; thus, aspirin is indicated only in patients with *symptomatic* thrombosis, including those with erythromelalgia. Successful treatment of symptomatic patients with aspirin increases platelet survival by decreasing platelet clearance. Concomitant therapy to prevent thrombotic complications of thrombocytosis includes lowering the platelet count with hydroxyurea. Evidence suggests that patients with essential thrombocythemia who are at high risk for arterial thrombosis are most effectively treated with the combination of hydroxyurea and low-dose aspirin and should not receive anagrelide, which

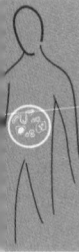

may actually increase the incidence of arterial thromboses. Patients with reactive (secondary) thrombocytosis resulting from iron deficiency anemia, chronic infection, rheumatoid arthritis, or the postsplenectomy state do not generally have increased thrombotic risk.

HEPARIN-INDUCED THROMBOCYTOPENIA

Although also immune in nature, heparin-induced thrombocytopenia (HIT) must be distinguished from other drug-induced forms of thrombocytopenia because of its potentially catastrophic *thrombotic* complications and its unique pathophysiologic features. Nearly 25% of patients who are exposed to UFH will develop antibodies (detected by ELISA) that recognize the complex of heparin and platelet factor 4 (PF4), the latter being released from activated platelets. When such patients receive heparin again, between 5% and 10% will develop HIT, most with platelet counts between 50,000 and 100,000/mcL. HIT rarely occurs in patients who have not been previously exposed to heparin (0.3% incidence). Surgery is a specific risk factor for HIT; the incidence of HIT in surgical patients is about 2.6%, compared with 1.7% in medical patients. HIT antibodies occur with high frequency in patients undergoing either cardiac surgery with cardiopulmonary bypass or orthopedic procedures like hip replacement. In contrast to UFH, the incidence of HIT in patients who have received only LMWH is far lower—only about one-tenth the rate seen with UFH. However, the mechanism of thrombocytopenia for both UFH and LMWH appears to be similar: platelet Fc-receptor binding of the heparin-PF4 antibody complex causes signal transduction and platelet activation with an enhanced ability for thrombin generation on the platelet surface. The diagnosis is predominantly clinical, but the rapid ELISA test will detect heparin-PF4 antibodies in serum. The main drawback of ELISA is that it does not indicate whether the antibody complex is a functional activator of platelets; thus, it is sensitive but not specific for HIT. The serotonin release assay is the functional test for HIT, detecting platelet activation after exposure to serum antibody in the presence of a therapeutic heparin level.

The thrombin-based procoagulant response in HIT incorporates platelets into microcirculatory clots, leading to thrombocytopenia; about 30% of HIT patients have overt TE complications, which may be severe or life-threatening. TE events can occur before, concurrent with, and after development of thrombocytopenia in HIT, with about equal frequency. Although thrombosis is more frequent in patients with both HIT and concomitant cardiovascular disease and in those receiving full-dose heparin, any heparin dose (even heparin flushes) can result in thrombosis in HIT. Arterial and venous TE can even occur weeks after heparin has been discontinued, an effect perhaps mediated by EC glycosaminoglycan binding to PF4 serving as a target for circulating HIT antibodies. Discontinuation of heparin, however, is critical; moreover, although the antibody may have been induced by treatment with UFH, more than 80% of these antibodies cross-react with LMWH. Thus, the preferred therapy for short-term anticoagulation in patients with HIT is a direct thrombin inhibitor (DTI), such as lepirudin

and argatroban, which are not targets for the heparin-PF4 antibodies. Indeed, because the event rate for subsequent thrombosis, limb amputation, and death is increased in HIT patients even if they do not present with thrombosis, the case can be made for always instituting DTI therapy after discontinuing heparin. Lepirudin is given intravenously at 0.10 mg/kg per hour and adjusted to prolong the PTT to 1.5 to 2.5 times the baseline value. Renal insufficiency slows lepirudin clearance, increasing the level for a given dose and corresponding to an increase in PTT and bleeding risk. The alternative to decreasing the lepirudin dose is to substitute argatroban, which is cleared by hepatic metabolism. In patients who develop HIT after warfarin has already been started, vitamin K should be administered to correct the levels of protein C and to ensure adequate dosing of DTIs.

The current recommendation for HIT management is to continue DTI therapy until the platelet count is higher than 150,000/mcL. Warfarin can then be added, and the two therapies should overlap for at least 5 days. The DTI should not be stopped until the INR is therapeutic for at least 48 hours. Because DTIs prolong the INR, therapeutic warfarin will result in a supertherapeutic INR (usually >4); once DTIs are stopped, it is essential to repeat the INR 4 to 6 hours later to confirm that the INR is in the therapeutic range. If there is no thrombosis with HIT, the total duration of anticoagulation should be 4 weeks. When thrombosis is present, anticoagulation should be continued for 3 to 6 months. Warfarin should never be used primarily to treat HIT and should not be instituted without simultaneous DTI coverage; warfarin may induce acquired protein C deficiency in HIT, similar to the skin necrosis syndrome, resulting in venous limb gangrene. One hallmark of protein C depletion in HIT after warfarin is a too rapid rise in the INR to more than 3.5; in that circumstance, warfarin should be discontinued and the patient repleted with vitamin K. Patients with a history of HIT who need surgery requiring cardiopulmonary bypass can be safely re-exposed to brief systemic UFH if ELISA testing is negative for the antibody at least 100 days from the previous UFH exposure. Another important consideration in retreating patients with a history of HIT is the development of antibodies against lepirudin in at least one third of exposed patients; because fatal anaphylaxis has been reported, lepirudin cannot be used twice. Argatroban does not, by contrast, provoke an antibody response.

THROMBOTIC THROMBOCYTOPENIC PURPURA

Another nonimmune cause of thrombocytopenia resulting from platelet activation and clearance is TTP. In patients with congenital or familial TTP, mutations in the vWF-cleaving protease, ADAMTS-13, abrogate its activity. Patients with acquired TTP without a family history usually have an antibody, often immunoglobulin G (IgG), that blocks the normal function of this vWF-cleaving protease to less than 10% of normal. Ultralarge vWF multimers released by EC normally anchor to EC through P-selectin and form long strings that adhere and aggregate platelets in the microcirculation. ADAMTS-13 downregulates the size of these multimers by docking to the A1/A3 vWF domains and cleaving within the A2 site. Deficient cleaving protease function in TTP leads to higher circulating levels of the larger, high-molecular-weight vWF multimers; these, in turn, cause increased platelet adhesion and clearance *without* activating the coagulation cascade. Therefore, both the PT and PTT are normal in TTP, unlike DIC. TTP after chemotherapy (mitomycin C) and in association with pregnancy, stem cell transplantation, lupus, or HIV infection appears to have a similar pathogenic mechanism of thrombosis. Thrombocytopenia (often severe) is accompanied by microangiopathy with schistocytes on the peripheral smear and increased serum lactate dehydrogenase. Microvascular occlusions in multiple organs cause many of the symptoms, especially in the kidney and brain. The classic pentad of signs (fever, thrombocytopenia, microangiopathic hemolysis, neurologic symptoms, and renal insufficiency) is present in fewer than 25% of patients with TTP. The diagnosis is generally made on the clinical assessment of thrombocytopenia and microangiopathic hemolytic anemia; assays for ADAMTS-13 activity and inhibitor are not yet widely available and do not have a rapid turn-around time.

Treatment of familial TTP is based on replenishment of cleaving protease activity with plasma transfusion; acquired TTP additionally requires removal of the antibody. The latter is accomplished by plasma exchange, whereby patient plasma is removed (plasmapheresis) and replaced with fresh-frozen plasma, often "cryo-poor" to reduce ultralarge vWF multimers in transfused plasma. Steroids and antiplatelet drugs (e.g., aspirin, dipyridamole) are often administered simultaneously, but the added benefit to plasma exchange remains unclear. Platelet transfusions are contraindicated in TTP because fatal thrombosis (e.g., myocardial infarction) has occurred in association with platelet transfusion. When plasma exchange fails to remit acquired TTP or when early relapse occurs, immunosuppressive therapy with anti-CD20 may be successful. The associated mortality of severe TTP (defined as undetectable ADAMTS-13 activity) is still significant, nearly 10% at 18 months after therapy with steroids and plasma exchange. Recombinant and purified forms of ADAMTS-13 are being investigated as potential therapeutic agents for treatment.

The *hemolytic uremic syndrome* (HUS) is part of the TTP spectrum of disease; however, the hemolytic anemia and renal failure of HUS are not usually accompanied by neurologic impairment, and HUS generally does not have the same degree of thrombocytopenia or schistocytosis as TTP. Moreover, less than 3% of HUS cases are associated with decreased vWF-cleaving protease activity. Unlike TTP, HUS is primarily diagnosed in children, and less commonly in adults, presenting with hemorrhagic colitis caused by Shiga-like, toxin-producing bacteria, especially the *Escherichia coli* 0157.H7 serotype. Atypical HUS (i.e., no diarrhea or Shiga-like toxin) is rarely associated with complement dysregulation due to mutations or polymorphisms in factors H, I, and B; these appear to increase platelet activation through complement (C3) deposition on the platelet surface. The similar pathophysiologic features of microvascular platelet thrombi place HUS within the TTP continuum, and indeed, some HUS patients, especially those with atypical disease, respond to plasmapheresis with plasma exchange as well as to maintenance hemodialysis until renal function recovers.

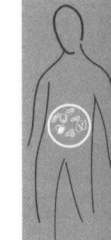

Table 54-4 **Laboratory Evaluation of Venous Thrombosis**
Activated protein C resistance, factor V Leiden
Lupus anticoagulant
Anticardiolipin, anti–β_2-GPI antibodies
Homocysteine level: fasting or following methionine load
Prothrombin 20210A mutation
Antithrombin III activity
Protein C activity
Protein S activity, if abnormal reflex antigenic levels (total/free)

Laboratory Evaluation of Thrombosis

Recurrent venous thromboembolism (VTE) is a strong indication for laboratory testing for causes of thrombophilia, especially in patients younger than 50 years of age, in patients with unexplained VTE, and in those with a family history of venous thrombosis. In these patients, any risk factors that may predispose the individual to recurrence must be defined, as well as any inherited disorders that may necessitate family counseling or avoidance of additional environmental risks. The current assays in the work-up of venous thrombophilia include the following: (1) APC resistance using a dilute factor V method, (2) genotyping for prothrombin G20210A, (3) lupus anticoagulant assay and anticardiolipin and anti–β_2-GPI antibodies, (4) functional AT level, and (5) functional protein C and protein S levels (Table 54-4). Genotyping for the FVL mutation should be done when APC resistance is present to define whether FVL is truly present and, if so, to determine whether the patient is heterozygous or homozygous. There has been little standardization of lupus anticoagulant testing. Hence, testing for antibodies specific to β_2-GPI can be helpful when the aPL syndrome is strongly suspected and no lupus anticoagulant is detected.

The utility of laboratory testing in the setting of atherothrombosis and arterial thromboembolism is unclear. Platelet-specific risk factors for both arterial and venous thrombosis have not been defined adequately for available laboratory tests to give meaningful or prognostic data. Therefore, platelet aggregation studies and examination of platelet receptor allotypes are not routinely indicated. In the setting of a myeloproliferative disorder, the platelet count and platelet aggregation, as well as platelet closure times, are the only available useful tests that might additionally justify hydroxyurea therapy. In patients with recurrent thromboses or a strong family history, other assays can be justified, including testing for t-PA and PAI-1 levels, and dysfibrinogenemia (prolonged thrombin or reptilase time), all of which should be done in consultation with specialists in hemostasis.

Therapy for Venous Thromboembolism

Prophylaxis for VTE should be administered in patients undergoing surgical procedures that carry an increased risk for producing venous thrombosis, especially orthopedic procedures or major operations requiring significant postoperative immobilization. Prophylactic therapies include lower extremity intermittent compression and pharmacologic treatment with UFH or LMWH. Once thromboembolism is diagnosed, immediate therapy is required. In most patients with venous thrombosis, anticoagulation is accomplished on a short-term basis with heparin compounds and on a long-term basis with warfarin. Thrombolytic therapy is indicated for patients with extensive proximal venous clots or PE. IVC filters are used in patients with contraindications to anticoagulation, complications of anticoagulation (usually active bleeding), or failure of anticoagulation (recurrent PE). IVC filters clearly decrease the incidence of early PE, but their use is also associated with thrombosis at the insertion site and late complications of IVC thrombosis and a 10% to 20% incidence of postphlebitic syndrome; whether simultaneous low-dose anticoagulation will prevent these complications is unknown. Temporary IVC filters are often used in trauma patients and appear to be most efficacious when they are placed for fewer than 7 to 10 days.

UFH is often the inpatient therapy of choice for acute anticoagulation because of its low cost, ease of monitoring, and short half-life. Heparin is begun as a bolus intravenous infusion of 80 U/kg, followed by a continuous infusion of 18 U/kg per hr; heparin doses in excess of 30,000 U per day have been shown to be most efficacious at preventing recurrent thrombosis. Heparin is monitored by the PTT. A therapeutic PTT for heparin is between 1.8 and 2.5 times the patient's initial PTT value. This PTT range should correspond to therapeutic anti-Xa levels of 0.3 to 0.7 U/mL. Adjustment of the heparin infusion should be based on the patient's weight and the PTT (Table 54-5); discontinuation of the heparin infusion, even for a brief period, may allow the PTT to normalize because of heparin's short half-life (about 4 hours). UFH should be continued for 4 days or more (longer in patients with extensive clots), and UFH can be discontinued when patients are fully anticoagulated with warfarin (INR ≥ 2 for 2 consecutive days). Some patients may receive large doses of heparin (usually >40,000 U per day), and yet the PTT does not become therapeutic. This *heparin resistance* is caused by a dissociation of the PTT and the true heparin activity; thus, monitoring of anti-Xa levels is generally indicated in heparin resistance. Heparin resis-

tance is only rarely caused by AT deficiency; more often, heparin resistance occurs in patients with coexistent inflammatory disease and is caused by increased plasma levels of factor VIII and other heparin-binding proteins.

LMWH is an excellent alternative to UFH in the management of thromboembolism and acute coronary events. The advantages of LMWH over UFH include the following: (1) reduced binding to macrophages and EC, a process that increases the plasma half-life of LMWH; (2) less nonspecific binding to plasma proteins that leads to a more predictable dose response and allows for intermittent fixed dosing; (3) reduced binding to platelets and PF4, with a resulting lower de novo incidence of HIT (10% to 20% of the rate for UFH); and (4) reduced bone loss. Although the incidence of HIT is lower with initial use of LMWH than with UFH, once HIT is established, antibody cross-reactivity with all the LMWH preparations precludes subsequent use of LMWH in HIT (see earlier). All the LMWH preparations (dalteparin, enoxaparin, nadroparin, and tinzaparin) have been shown to be as safe and effective as UFH in prophylaxis for VTE, treatment of uncomplicated VTE, and treatment of symptomatic PE when given in a subcutaneous, weight-adjusted dose. In particular, outpatient therapy with LMWH for uncomplicated VTE provides a significant cost saving (when compared with hospitalization for intravenous UFH) without compromising patient outcome. Because of its predictable dose-response curve, LMWH therapy does not require monitoring. LMWH therapy does not prolong the PTT and can only be monitored (e.g., in renal failure) by anti-Xa levels. Peak anti-Xa levels generally occur between 3 and 5 hours after subcutaneous LMWH injection. LMWH anti-Xa levels at that time point are 0.5 to 1 U/mL for twice-daily dosing and 1 to 2 U/mL for once-daily dosing; significant anti-Xa activity persists in plasma for 12 hours after subcutaneous injection. As with UFH, switching from LMWH to warfarin for long-term management can be accomplished after therapeutic INR values are present for 2 to 3 days.

Warfarin is still the current treatment of choice for long-term anticoagulation and for preventing early recurrence of thrombus. Warfarin should be begun in the first 24 hours after presentation with VTE, concurrent with heparin treatment. The PT is prolonged within hours by warfarin because of a rapid decrease in factor VII levels; however, therapeutic warfarin anticoagulation does not occur until other vitamin K–dependent factors (II, IX, and X) also decrease. Therapeutic warfarin anticoagulation usually requires at least 4 to 5 days of adequate warfarin dosing starting at 5 mg daily for 2 to 3 days; UFH or LMWH can be discontinued after at least 4 days of therapy and only when the INR is more than 2 for at least 2 consecutive days. One long-standing problem with warfarin anticoagulation is the interindividual variability in INR response to the same dosing among similar-sized individuals; at least 50% of this variability in sensitivity to warfarin may be explained by polymorphisms in the *CYP2C9* and *VKORC1* genes (see "Prospectus for the Future"). Accounting for genetic differences in these enzymes that metabolize and clear warfarin, as well as for age and body surface area, has yielded useful models for predicting safe and therapeutic warfarin dosing.

The intensity of warfarin dosing, evaluated by the INR, depends on the condition predisposing the patient to thromboembolism. Treatment of uncomplicated VTE in a patient

Table 54-5 **Unfractionated Heparin Dose Adjustment Based on Partial Thromboplastin Time (PTT) and Weight***	
PTT Value (Times Baseline)	**Heparin Adjustment**
1.2-1.5	40 U/kg bolus, ↑ infusion by 4 U/kg/hr
>1.5-2.4	No change
>2.4-3.0	↓ Infusion by 2 U/kg/hr
>3.0	Hold infusion for 1 hr, ↓ infusion by 3 U/kg/hr

*After initial therapy with 80 U/kg bolus and 18 U/kg/hr infusion.
↑, Increase; ↓, decrease.

Table 54-6	**Therapeutic International Normalized Ratio (INR) Ranges for Warfarin According to Patient Subgroup**
Subgroup	**INR Range**
Venous Thrombosis	
Treatment	2.0-3.0
Prophylaxis	1.5-2.5
Artificial Heart Valves	
Tissue	2.0-2.5
Mechanical	3.0-4.0
Atrial Fibrillation (Nonvalvular)	
Prophylaxis	1.5-2.5
Lupus Anticoagulant	
Treatment, prophylaxis	2.0-3.0
Refractory thromboembolism	3.0-4.0

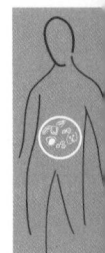

Table 54-7	**Guidelines for Duration of Anticoagulation in Venous Thromboembolism**
Condition	**Duration of Therapy**
Distal or superficial vein thrombus	3 mo
First Proximal VTE/PE	
No risk factors	Long-term*
Correctable risk factor (e.g., surgery, trauma)	3-6 mo
Malignancy	Long-term
Antiphospholipid syndrome	Long-term
Inherited risk factor[†]	>6 mo
Recurrent VTE/PE	Lifelong

*Long-term therapy must be adjusted individually according to other diseases, risks for bleeding, presence of transient risk factors, and ease of compliance.
[†]Inherited risk factors include factor V Leiden; prothrombin 20210A; deficiencies of antithrombin III, protein C, or protein S.
VTE/PE, venous thromboembolism/pulmonary embolism.

without known risk factors does not require an INR exceeding 3; in contrast, warfarin for recurrent thrombosis in treated patients with aPL syndrome may require INR values between 3 and 4 (Table 54-6).

The duration of warfarin treatment also varies depending on the circumstances of the VTE, the estimated clinical risk for bleeding, and the potential for recurrence. In general, the longer the period of anticoagulation with warfarin, the less the chance of recurrence; short-term warfarin (6 weeks) is not as effective at preventing recurrence compared with longer courses (6 months). Patients with definite, transient risk factors such as orthopedic surgery have low recurrence rates, even with short-term therapy; in contrast, patients with idiopathic thromboembolism have significant recurrence rates, even after 3 to 6 months of warfarin. Recent studies suggest that patients with idiopathic thromboembolism can be monitored for recurrence risk using the D-dimer measurement. For patients who have had their first unprovoked VTE episode, an elevated D-dimer 1 month after stopping anticoagulation conveys an increased risk for VTE recurrence compared with matched patients with a normal result. Resuming anticoagulation in that patient subset should decrease the D-dimer into the normal reference range. Evidence also indicates that inherited hypercoagulable disorders, such as FVL, probably confer a lifelong increased risk for VTE or PE. Some studies have shown that the bleeding risks incurred by long-term, but low-intensity, warfarin use are favorably balanced by the decreased incidence of recurrent thrombosis. Therefore, the presence of inherited thrombophilia may warrant continuing warfarin for a longer period, depending on the patient's other medical illnesses and whether transient circumstances may have predisposed the patient to VTE. Patients who develop recurrent VTE after discontinuation of warfarin should receive long-term anticoagulation, regardless of whether they have a defined cause of thrombophilia. Patients with aPL syndrome and a first episode of VTE are at very high risk for recurrent VTE (up to 50% per year) after anticoagulation is discontinued, clearly supporting the rationale for testing for aPL. Table 54-7 suggests broad guidelines for the duration of warfarin therapy in specific patient subgroups. Because

Table 54-8	**Drugs that Affect Warfarin Levels**
Drugs that Increase Warfarin Levels: Prolonged INR	
↓ Warfarin clearance	
Disulfiram	
Metronidazole	
Trimethoprim-sulfamethoxazole	
↓ Warfarin-protein binding	
Phenylbutazone	
↑ Vitamin K turnover	
Clofibrate	
Drugs that Decrease Warfarin Levels: Subtherapeutic INR	
↑ Hepatic metabolism of warfarin	
Barbiturates	
Rifampin	
↓ Warfarin absorption	
Cholestyramine	

↑, Increased; ↓, decreased; INR, international normalized ratio.

warfarin is a teratogen; effective contraception should be used concurrently in women of childbearing age.

Supratherapeutic INR levels commonly occur with warfarin therapy, with or without bleeding. In patients with moderately elevated INR values (>5) with little or no bleeding, temporary discontinuation of warfarin and reinstitution of the drug at a lower maintenance dose may be sufficient. Patients with higher INR values (5 to 9) without serious bleeding should have warfarin withheld and receive low doses (1 to 2.5 mg per day) of oral vitamin K to reach therapeutic INR levels; parenteral vitamin K can be given if gastrointestinal function is problematic. When serious active bleeding occurs with high INR values, especially if surgery is required to correct the bleeding, a combination of vitamin K and transfusion of plasma (see Chapter 53) will rapidly correct the INR. The INR can become elevated as a result of concurrent use of drugs that increase free warfarin levels (Table 54-8). Whenever bleeding occurs as a complication of anticoagulation, serious consideration must be given to

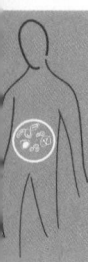

future bleeding risks and to whether the patient requires prophylactic IVC filter placement.

Antithrombotic Therapy during Pregnancy

Heparins, both UFH and LMWH, are the safest therapy for venous thrombosis during pregnancy; heparin does not cross the placenta, unlike warfarin, which causes a characteristic fetal embryopathy. Warfarin also causes fetal hemorrhage and placental abruption and should be avoided during pregnancy. VTE or PE during pregnancy should be treated with intravenous UFH for 5 to 10 days, followed by an adjusted-dose regimen of subcutaneous UFH, starting with 20,000 U every 12 hours and adjusted to achieve a PTT higher than 1.5 times baseline at 6 hours after injection. An attractive alternative to UFH during pregnancy is LMWH, which can be given subcutaneously once or twice daily and does not require monitoring. Suprarenal IVC filters have also been used successfully during pregnancy without significant morbidity. In women with aPL syndrome who become pregnant, therapy is critical to prevent fetal loss; aspirin (160 mg) is combined with prophylactic doses of either subcutaneous UFH (10,000 to 15,000 U per day in divided doses) or LMWH (to achieve an anti-Xa level of 0.1 to 0.3 U/mL). When such women have a history of TE disease, therapeutic doses of LMWH or UFH plus aspirin are employed.

Heparin should be discontinued at the time of labor and delivery, although the risk for hemorrhage is not high during delivery, especially if anti-Xa levels are less than 0.7 U/mL. One concern with residual anticoagulation at delivery is the risk for spinal hematoma with epidural anesthesia; this concern has been reported with both UFH and LMWH. The anti-Xa level that is safe for an epidural procedure is not known. Protamine sulfate can be used to neutralize UFH if the PTT is prolonged during labor and delivery; however, LMWH is only partially (10%) reversed by protamine.

Anticoagulation during the postpartum period can be carried out with heparin or warfarin; neither drug is contraindicated during breastfeeding. Women receiving long-term warfarin therapy (e.g., for valvular heart disease) who wish to become pregnant need to be switched to a fully anticoagulating dose of UFH or LMWH; warfarin treatment can be restarted postpartum.

Perioperative Anticoagulation

A common clinical problem is the management of anticoagulation in patients who require surgery. The principles of care in this situation reflect the need for adequate hemostasis during and immediately after surgical procedures and the critical importance of restarting anticoagulation as soon as possible postoperatively, especially because surgery itself represents a relative hypercoagulable state. In patients with VTE who are anticoagulated on a short-term basis (<1 month), elective surgical procedures should be postponed; if such patients must undergo surgery, discontinuation of anticoagulation and placement of a temporary IVC filter may be the best option. In most patients receiving long-term anticoagulation for VTE, preoperative heparin is not generally used; warfarin should be discontinued for at least 4 days preoperatively to allow the INR to decrease gradually to less than 1.5, a level that is safe for surgery. Postoperatively, intravenous heparin can be safely used for anticoagulation until therapeutic INR levels are reached after restarting warfarin. These guidelines obviously should be tailored to individual patient care. Patients with arterial thromboembolic disease may need heparin therapy right up until the time of the surgical procedure and shortly thereafter. In contrast, heparin therapy immediately after a major surgical procedure may be contraindicated because of the high risk for hemorrhage; anticoagulation may need to be delayed in this instance for 12 to 24 hours postoperatively.

Prospectus for the Future

Therapy for hypercoagulable states is increasingly being tailored to individual needs, that is, "personalized medicine":

- New labeling of warfarin includes information about how variations in the *CP2C9* and *VKORC1* genes account for differences in drug metabolism. Optimal maintenance dosing of warfarin will likely drive testing for these polymorphisms as part of future practice.
- Abnormalities in platelet aggregability and vWF multimer distribution have been noted in cancer, autoimmune disease, and pregnancy, with the potential for using these measures for overall thrombotic risk assessment.
- Similar stratification of thrombosis risk may involve TAFI, which inhibits fibrinolysis by protecting fibrin from the

cleaving effect of t-PA. High TAFI levels correlate with cardiovascular disease and stroke, and polymorphisms may be responsible.

With respect to therapy, an antithrombotic effect of C1q-TNF receptor protein (CTRP) has been demonstrated in animal models. CTRP blocks vWF binding sites on collagen, thereby preventing platelet interaction with collagen at arterial shear rates, and CTRP may also inhibit platelet aggregation directly. Because CTRP preserves overall hemostatic function as assessed by the activated clotting time, it has promise for treating arterial vascular disease.

References

Bates SM, Weitz J: New anticoagulants: Beyond heparin, low-molecular-weight heparin, and warfarin. Br J Pharmacol 144:1017-1028, 2005.

Harrison CN, Campbell PJ, Buck G, et al: Hydroxyurea compared with anagrelide in high-risk essential thrombocythemia. N Engl J Med 353:33-45, 2005.

Keijzer MBAJ, Borm GR, Blom HJ, et al: No interaction between factor V Leiden and hyperhomocysteinemia or MTHFR 677TT genotype in venous thrombosis. Thromb Haemost 97:33-37 2007.

Meltzer ME, Doggen CJM, de Groot PG, et al: Fibrinolysis and the risk of venous and arterial thrombosis. Curr Opin Hematol 14:242-248, 2007.

Miyakis S, Lockshin MD, Atsumi T, et al: International consensus statement on an update of the classification criteria for definite antiphospholipid syndrome (APS). J Thromb Haem 4:295-306, 2006.

Rieder MJ, Reiner AP, Gage BF, et al: Effect of VKORC1 haplotypes on transcriptional regulation and warfarin dose. N Engl J Med 352:2285-2293, 2005.

Stam J: Thrombosis of the cerebral veins and sinuses. N Engl J Med 352:1791-1798, 2005.

Tsantes AE, Nikolopoulos GK, Bagos PG, et al: The effect of the plasminogen activator inhibitor-1 4G/5G polymorphism on the thrombotic risk. Thromb Res 122:736-742, 2008.

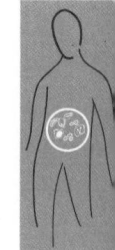

Section X

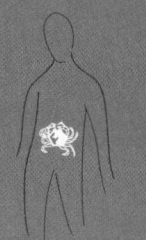

Oncologic Disease

Cancer Biology and Etiologic Factors

Alok A. Khorana and Barbara A. Burtness

Cancer is primarily a genetic disease. For most human cancers, a complex succession of multiple genetic mutations is necessary for the transformation of a normal cell into a tumor cell. Tremendous strides have been made in understanding the classes of genes responsible for the pathogenesis of cancers, epigenetics, the principles governing aberrant signal transduction in cancer cells, and cancer stem cells. This revolution in the understanding of cancer biology has led to a new wave of research into the design of drugs directed against specific targets and pathways in the cancer cell. This chapter reviews the cancer phenotype and principles of cancer biology.

Hallmarks of the Cancer Phenotype

More than 100 distinct types and subtypes of human cancer exist, involving nearly every organ and tissue of the body. Pathologically, these cancers may resemble the tissue from which they have arisen, for example, adenocarcinomas of the gastrointestinal tract show glandular formation similar to normal gastrointestinal mucosa. Despite this diversity, most cancers share essential traits that must be acquired for malignant growth. In this sense, tumor cells resemble other tumor cells much more than they resemble the normal cells of their tissue of origin. Hanahan and Weinberg have described the six essential acquired capabilities essential for tumor growth (Table 55-1). *Autonomy*, or self-sufficiency in growth signals, is most apparent when cells are grown in culture: normal cells require the addition of mitogenic growth factors, whereas tumor cells generate many of their own growth signals, and proliferate with little dependence on exogenous growth stimulation. In normal tissues, tight control of proliferation is achieved by the use of multiple growth inhibitors. Tumor cells, in contrast, display *insensitivity to antigrowth signals*. In addition, tumor cell populations maintain continued expansion by reducing the rate of cell attrition—primarily by acquiring *resistance to apoptosis*, or programmed

cell death. Normal cells stop growing after a certain number of doublings. Tumor cells, in contrast, are immortalized in culture because of the acquisition of *limitless replicative potential*. The induction of *angiogenesis*, or the establishment of a blood supply, is essential for tumors to grow beyond a size of 1 to 2 mm. This process is regulated by a balance between proangiogenic and antiangiogenic molecules. The proangiogenic vascular endothelial growth factor (VEGF-A) is a major mediator of tumor angiogenesis. Most human cancers express VEGF, as do various host cells. Bevacizumab, an anti-VEGF antibody, and sorafenib and sunitinib, oral small molecule VEGF receptor tyrosine kinase inhibitors, are all U.S. Food and Drug Administration–approved antiangiogenic agents used in a variety of cancers (see Chapter 59). Finally, the capacity for *invasion and metastasis* allows tumor cells to escape their primary sites and establish colonies at sites where nutrients and space are not limiting. Metastatic disease is the cause of death in more than 90% of cancer patients. Separate mutations are not required to acquire each of these characteristics (e.g., loss of the *p53* tumor suppressor gene can confer both uncontrolled growth and resistance to apoptosis). In the following section, the alterations in genes that are responsible for the acquisition of these common tumor characteristics are discussed.

Cancer Genetics: The Pathways to Cancer

The development of most human cancers is a multistep process, involving a complex succession of multiple genetic mutations (with some notable "one-hit" exceptions, e.g., *bcr-abl* translocation in chronic myelogenous leukemia). At each step, the cell undergoing transformation acquires a capability that provides a growth or survival advantage relative to the other, normal cells in the population, similar to darwinian evolution. Most invasive cancers develop only when several genes are mutated; this differentiates cancer from other genetic diseases such as cystic fibrosis in which mutations in one gene alone cause disease. Studies suggest that four to seven mutational events must occur for progression to the malignant phenotype. Mutations can occur upon exposure to environmental carcinogens, in the setting of dysregulated DNA repair, as a consequence of random replication errors, or, occasionally, in families with hereditary germline mutations in a cancer gene. Broadly, mutations in three classes of genes are responsible for cancer: oncogenes, tumor suppressor genes, and stability or caretaker genes. Table 55-2 shows the clinical consequences of selected mutations in these classes of genes.

ONCOGENES

Oncogenes are evolutionarily conserved genes that play an important role in normal cellular proliferation. Oncogene activation can result from chromosomal translocations, gene amplifications, or intragenic mutations. Activation of an oncogene leads to increased activity of the gene product. For example, chronic myelogenous leukemia (CML) occurs when the proto-oncogene *abl* from chromosome 9 translocates to the *bcr* gene on chromosome 22. The new protein formed by the union of the *bcr* and *abl* oncogenes, called *bcr-abl*, plays a role in coupling cell surface receptors to the signal transduction pathway, with resulting unchecked growth-promoting signals to the nucleus. An activating mutation in one allele of an oncogene is generally sufficient for enhancing tumorigenesis. Oncogene research has led to the use of oncogenes as targets of specifically designed drugs. Oncogenes are also used as biomarkers to predict prognosis and select therapy. The presence of t(8;21) or inv(16) translocations in patients with acute myelogenous leukemia

(AML) is usually predictive of a good response to standard antileukemic therapy. In patients with breast cancer, overexpression of *HER-2* is overall predictive of a poor prognosis but also of an excellent response to the anti–*HER-2* monoclonal antibody, trastuzumab.

Certain classes of signaling proteins are targeted much more frequently by oncogenic mutations. Recent research has focused particularly on *protein tyrosine kinases* (TKs), enzymes that catalyze the transfer of phosphate from adenosine triphosphate (ATP) to tyrosine residues in polypeptides. TKs normally regulate important cellular processes, including proliferation, survival, differentiation, function, and motility. Mutations in this small group of genes are responsible for a significant portion of human tumors. TKs can be perturbed in cancer by multiple mechanisms: overexpression of a normal receptor TK or its ligand, constitutive activation of receptor TK (in absence of ligand), or fusion of TK with a partner protein as a consequence of a chromosomal translocation or deletion (common in hematologic malignancies, such as the *bcr-abl* translocation in CML discussed previously). Inhibition of TK activity has emerged as a leading avenue for new cancer drug development. Imatinib, a small molecule directed against the kinase domain of the *bcr-abl* oncoprotein has been remarkably successful in inducing responses in patients with chronic-phase CML (see Chapter 59). Other anti-TK drugs include antibodies against receptor TKs or their ligands to interrupt TK signaling.

TUMOR SUPPRESSOR GENES

Tumor suppressor genes are recessive genes that keep cellular growth in check. When tumor suppressor genes undergo mutation or deletion, the rate of neoplastic transformation is much higher. Tumor suppressor genes are targeted in a different way than oncogenes: mutations in these genes result in a decreased activity of the gene product. Unlike oncogene activation, mutations in both alleles of a tumor suppressor gene are required to induce tumorigenesis. For instance, a germline (inherited) mutation in a single retinoblastoma gene (*RB-1*, a tumor suppressor gene) may not, by itself, cause retinoblastoma in a young child. However, if that child's genome suffers a "second hit" after birth (an *RB-1* somatic mutation), multiple tumors including bilateral retinoblastomas may occur. Single mutations in

Table 55-1 **Hallmarks of the Cancer Phenotype**
Self-sufficiency in growth signals
Insensitivity to antigrowth signals
Evasion of apoptosis
Limitless replicative potential
Induction of angiogenesis
Tissue invasion and metastasis

Table 55-2 **Cancers Associated with Selected Genetic Mutations**

Gene	Associated Hereditary Syndrome	Major Tumor Types
A. Oncogenes		
bcr-abl Translocation	—	Chronic myelogenous leukemia
BCL-2	—	Chronic lymphocytic leukemia
KIT, PDGF-RA	Familial gastrointestinal stromal tumors	Gastrointestinal stromal tumors
B. Tumor Suppressor Genes		
p53	Li-Fraumeni syndrome	Breast, sarcoma, adrenal, brain, multiple others
APC	Familial adenomatosis polyposis	Colon, stomach, intestine
VHL	von Hippel-Lindau syndrome	Kidney
C. Stability Genes		
BRCA-1, BRCA-2	Hereditary breast cancer	Breast, ovary
MSH-2, MLH-1	Lynch syndrome	Colon, uterus, stomach

the *RB-1* tumor suppressor gene may predispose to osteosarcoma, soft tissue sarcoma, melanoma, and brain tumors later in life. The tumor suppressor gene *p53* is the most commonly mutated gene in sporadic human cancers. This gene deletion can also be inherited, and progeny have a much higher rate of a variety of cancers, including breast and brain tumors, leukemia, and sarcoma, a pattern termed the *Li-Fraumeni syndrome*. If an environmental insult results in mutation or deletion and loss of function of the remaining normal copy of *p53* in any cell, a tumor may arise in that organ; this mechanism of carcinogenesis has been described for breast cancer, leukemia, and sarcoma, among other cancers. Suppressor gene mutations are also the most common cause of hereditary cancer.

STABILITY GENES

Accumulating evidence suggests that, in addition to oncogenes and tumor suppressor genes, mutations in a third class of genes called *stability or caretaker genes* can also promote tumorigenesis. Stability genes are responsible for the repair of errors in normal DNA replication and include mismatch repair genes, base-excision repair genes, and nucleotide-excision repair genes. Mutations in stability genes lead to increased errors in replication. Eventually, mutations in oncogenes and tumor suppressor genes occur, and this drives malignant transformation. The Lynch syndrome, or hereditary nonpolyposis colon cancer, is an example of an inherited syndrome of defects in DNA mismatch repair genes. Colon and endometrial cancers are two of the most commonly observed cancers in families afflicted by the Lynch syndrome. Somatic mutations in these genes are responsible for 10% to 15% of sporadic colon cancers as well. Similar to tumor suppressor genes, both alleles of stability genes must be inactivated for tumorigenesis to occur.

ADENOMA-TO-CARCINOMA SEQUENCE

The cascade of genetic events that leads to the transformation of normal colonic mucosa through development of preneoplastic polyps into colon cancer provides an excellent example of tumorigenesis in an epithelial organ (Fig. 55-1). The earliest change, or "gatekeeper" mutation, associated with adenomatous polyps is in the tumor suppressor *APC* gene. K-*ras* mutations occur relatively early and appear to correlate with early to late adenomas. Mutations in *p53* occur later in this sequence and may mark the transition from adenoma to carcinoma. As discussed previously, mutations in DNA mismatch repair genes create a mutator phenotype in which mutations in APC can occur, initiating neoplastic transformation and subsequent mutations. The genetic pathway responsible for tumorigenesis has clinical consequences: colon cancers that are initiated by defects in stability genes (the so-called microsatellite instability pathway) are characterized by a better prognosis but possible resistance to adjuvant 5-fluorouracil chemotherapy, in contrast to those primarily initiated by APC mutations (the so-called chromosomal instability pathway).

CANCER EPIGENETICS

The term *epigenetics* refers to changes in gene expression without alteration in the DNA sequence. Epigenetic changes in gene expression are hallmarks of malignancy. For instance, tumor suppressor genes can be silenced by DNA hypermethylation. Gene expression can also be altered by histone acetylases, which influence how tightly genomic DNA is spooled around histones, and alter the interaction of chromatin proteins with DNA. These epigenetic patterns are being studied as diagnostic, prognostic, and predictive markers and are also emerging as therapeutic targets. The demethylating agents 5-azacytidine and decitabine have activity in myelodysplastic syndromes and leukemia. Histone deacetylase inhibitors have modest activity in certain lymphomas.

Cancer Stem Cells

A newer view of cancer biology suggests that only a rare subpopulation of cancer cells has the capacity for self-renewal, differentiation, and unlimited proliferation. These rare cells have been termed *cancer stem cells*. In hematologic malignancies and some solid tumors, these cancer stem cells have the ability to re-form the tumor, whereas most other malignant cells do not. This has important consequences for understanding cancer biology, drug resistance, prognosis, and treatment. Cancer stem cell biology is an area of intense research.

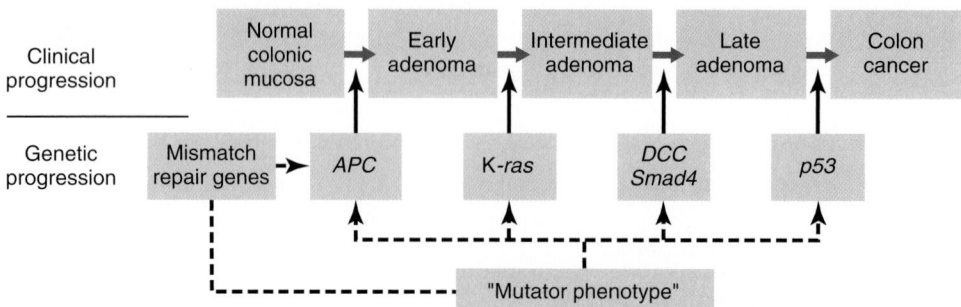

Figure 55-1 Adenoma to carcinoma sequence. Development of colon cancer from normal colonic epithelium is an example of multistep progression of neoplasia. In most patients, mutation of the tumor suppressor *APC* gene is the initial step, followed by mutations in K-*ras, DCC,* and *p53* genes. However, defects in DNA mismatch repair genes (hereditary or acquired), as shown on the left, can create a mutator phenotype, which can initiate and possibly accelerate this multistep progression.

Prospectus for the Future

The completion of the human genome project and continued advances in technologies for gene discovery will allow further rapid progress in cancer molecular genetics. Transforming these discoveries into meaningful advances in therapies for cancer patients, so-called translational research, remains, however, an extraordinary challenge for which no clear road map exists. Research endeavors that bridge gaps in knowledge between the bench and bedside will preoccupy oncologists for the next generation. In addition, discoveries in cancer genetics and epigenetics will be used even more effectively to develop sophisticated diagnostic tests (such as fecal DNA analysis or detection of circulating tumor cells) that can lead to discovery of cancers at much earlier, curative stages. In the meantime, cancer-related mortality continues to rise worldwide, and cancer is expected to becoming the leading cause of death in the United States in the next decade. Despite recent promising successes, we are only at the threshold of understanding and treating the complex and heterogenous group of diseases collectively known as cancer.

References

Esteller M: Epigenetics in cancer. N Engl J Med 358:1148-1159, 2008.

Jordan CT, Guzman ML, Noble M: Cancer stem cells. N Engl J Med 355:1253-1261, 2006.

Moscow JA, Cowan KH: Biology of cancer. In Goldman L, Ausiello DA (eds): Cecil Textbook of Medicine. Philadelphia, Elsevier, 2007.

Vogelstein B, Kinzler KW: Cancer genes and the pathways they control. Nat Med 10:789-799, 2004.

Weinberg RA, Hahn WC: Rules for making human tumor cells. N Engl J Med 347:1593-1603, 2002.

Chapter 56

Cancer Epidemiology and Cancer Prevention

Paula M. Lantz and Jennifer J. Griggs

Cancer Epidemiology

Each year, there are more than 11 million cancer cases diagnosed, 7 million cancer deaths, and 22 million cancer survivors worldwide, with significant increases projected because of population aging. Population-based estimates of cancer incidence are derived from tumor registry data. *Cancer incidence rates* are expressed as the number of new cases per 100,000 people. The risk for developing a particular type of cancer can be described as a *lifetime risk* or as an *age group–specific risk* (Table 56-1). Population-based estimates of cancer mortality are derived from cause of death information on death certificates. *Disease-specific mortality rates* are also expressed as rate per 100,000. Because age distributions change both within and across populations over time, cancer incidence and mortality rates are age adjusted.

Survival rates are usually expressed as relative survival rates, which consider mortality from other causes when describing cancer survival. For example, the 5-year *relative survival rate* is the percentage of people who did not die from their specific type of cancer within 5 years of diagnosis, taking into account expected age-specific mortality from other causes. Survival rates are reported by the stage of disease at diagnosis. People who have limited-stage disease (confined to the organ of origin) have higher 5-year survival rates than those with regional disease (involving regional lymph nodes), and people with regional disease have higher survival rates than do people with metastatic disease.

Cancer mortality rates in the United States and most other developed countries are consistently greater among people of lower socioeconomic position and among those from racial and ethnic minority groups, especially African Americans. Differences in mortality and survival rates across racial and ethnic groups are not fully accounted for by differences in the stage at diagnosis; even within the same stage, mortality differences persist. Socioeconomic factors, differences in treatment, and comorbidities are likely the greatest determinants of racial and ethnic disparities in cancer mortality and survival.

Cancer Prevention

The three levels of disease prevention are primary, secondary, and tertiary. *Primary* prevention keeps a disease from occurring by reducing exposure to risk factors. *Secondary* prevention detects a disease before it is symptomatic and when early intervention can change the natural history of the disease. *Tertiary* prevention reduces the complications of a disease once it becomes clinically evident. Tertiary prevention measures are addressed in Chapters 58 and 59.

It is estimated that more than 50% of cancer deaths in the United States could be prevented through behavioral risk factor modifications and increased use of proven cancer screening tests. Studying the effectiveness of cancer prevention measures requires large numbers of participants in both intervention and control groups, close monitoring for adherence in the intervention group and "contamination" of the control group, long-term follow-up, and appropriate ascertainment of disease and disease-free status. Such studies are challenging because of the effort and cost involved in the enrollment, retention, and treatment of study participants. Nonetheless, a significant number of effective cancer prevention and control strategies have been identified, many through controlled trials.

PRIMARY PREVENTION

Primary prevention of cancer is achieved either by avoiding a causative exposure or by using an agent that prevents the development of the malignant process. Primary prevention includes reductions in behavioral or lifestyle risks (e.g., avoidance of tobacco exposure; use of sunscreen; adherence to a low-fat, high-fiber diet), avoidance of occupational or environmental risks, and chemoprevention (Table 56-2).

The main *behavioral and lifestyle risk factors* targeted for the primary prevention of cancer include tobacco, alcohol, dietary factors, and physical activity (see Table 56-2). Tobacco is the single greatest contributor to cancer incidence and mortality worldwide, and this burden is prevent-

Table 56-1 Probability of Developing Cancer by Age Group and Sex, United States, 2003-2005

	Lifetime	Ages 40-59 Years	Ages 60-79 Years
All Sites			
Male	44%	8%	33%
Female	37%	9%	22%
Lung Cancer			
Male	8%	1%	6%
Female	6%	0.7%	4%
Colorectal Cancer			
Male	6%	1%	4%
Female	5%	0.7%	3%
Breast Cancer			
Female	14%	4%	7%
Prostate Cancer			
Male	16%	2%	13%

Table 56-2 Major Targets of Primary Prevention of Cancer

Behavioral Targets	Associated Cancers
Tobacco	Lung, bronchus, esophagus, head and neck, stomach, pancreas, kidney, bladder, cervical
High alcohol consumption	Liver, rectum, breast, oral cavity, pharynx, larynx, esophagus
Obesity, high dietary fat	Colon, breast, endometrium, kidney, pancreas, esophagus, prostate
Low dietary fiber	Colon
Sedentary lifestyle	Colon, breast
Other Agents and Exposures	
Human papillomavirus 16 and 18	Cervical
Hepatitis B and C viruses	Liver and hepatocellular cancers
Asbestos	Mesothelioma and other types of lung cancer
Radon	Lung
Ultraviolet radiation	Melanoma, basal and squamous cell carcinomas
Ionizing radiation	Leukemia, thyroid, lung, breast

able. More than 1 million people die from tobacco-induced cancers globally each year, and tobacco accounts for one third of all cancer diagnoses in the United States. Cigarette smokers have a 20-fold risk for developing cancer compared with nonsmokers, with smoking being the single largest cause of lung cancer. Smoking and chewing tobacco are major risk factors for head, neck, mouth, and esophageal cancers. Second-hand smoke exposure increases the risk for lung cancer in nonsmokers. Significant investments in tobacco prevention and control at the local, state, and national levels have led to a decline in smoking prevalence in the United States through both smoking cessation and

primary prevention among youth. Tobacco use, however, continues to be high (especially among men) and has been increasing in a number of countries.

High consumption of alcohol is a significant risk factor for liver, rectal, and breast cancers. Alcohol abuse, especially among smokers, is associated with squamous cell cancers of the oral cavity, pharynx, larynx, and esophagus. Epidemiologic studies suggest that the increased cancer risk is associated with all type of alcoholic beverages.

Diet and body weight appear to play a role in cancer etiology, although it is difficult in epidemiologic studies to isolate specific dietary components (e.g., fat, total calories, fiber content, nutrient deficiencies) and to sort out the role of diet versus weight, obesity, distribution of adipose tissue, or sedentary lifestyle. Dietary fat and obesity are associated with colon and breast cancers, but the exact nature of the relationship is still under investigation. Central or visceral adiposity in both men and women is associated with increased incidence and mortality from a number of cancers, including endometrium, breast in postmenopausal women, kidney, gallbladder, pancreas, esophagus, colon, and prostate. Sufficient dietary intake of fruits and vegetables reduces the risk for gastric and esophageal cancers. Low dietary fiber is strongly associated with colon cancer in epidemiologic studies; however, interventions to increase fiber intake have not shown a reduction in colon adenomas in clinical trials.

There is strong evidence from epidemiologic studies that 30 to 60 minutes per day of moderate to vigorous physical activity reduces the risk for colon and breast cancer. The evidence is suggestive but mixed for prostate, lung, and endometrial cancers. Potential mechanisms for a link between physical activity and cancer prevention are enhanced immune function, reduced body fat, and hormonal changes.

Reducing exposure to certain infectious agents and chronic inflammation can contribute to the primary prevention of cancer. Viral agents are a prominent cause of human cancers. Chronic hepatitis B and C viral infections have been linked with the development of liver cancer. Evidence suggests that hepatitis B vaccination can reduce the incidence of hepatocellular cancer. Human papillomaviruses 16 and 18 have been linked with cervical cancer, with vaccines against these virus strains and those causing genital warts both on the market and in development (see Chapter 57). Other viral agents implicated in cancer include the Epstein-Barr virus (nasopharyngeal cancer and Burkitt lymphoma) and human T-cell leukemia virus type I (HTLV-1). Chronic inflammation as the result of exposure to a specific chemical or microbial agent or ultraviolet or ionizing radiation may promote carcinogenesis susceptibility through a number of mechanisms. For example, chronic infection with the bacterium *Helicobacter pylori* can cause certain gastric lymphomas and gastric adenocarcinoma.

Various pharmacologic agents have been associated with an increased risk for specific cancers. Unopposed estrogen use in postmenopausal women increases the risk for endometrial cancer, although rates drop significantly when combined estrogen-progesterone therapy is substituted. Synthetic estrogens such as diethylstilbestrol (DES), which was given to mothers during pregnancy, may result in the development of vaginal cancer in their offspring.

In regard to occupation and environmental exposures, asbestos is the most common cause of occupational cancer

Table 56-3 Cancer Chemopreventive Agents

Cancer	Chemopreventive Agent
Breast cancer	Selective estrogen receptor modulators (e.g., tamoxifen, raloxifene) Statin drugs
Ovarian cancer	Oral contraceptives
Colon cancer	Folic acid Nonsteroidal anti-inflammatory agents Statin drugs
Melanoma	Topical sunscreens
Prostate cancer	Lycopene Statin drugs
Cervical cancer	Human papillomavirus vaccine
Liver cancer	Hepatitis B vaccine

Table 56-4 Cancer Screening Tests with Demonstrated Early Detection Benefit

Cancer	Screening Recommendations for People at Average Risk
Breast	Screening mammography every 1-2 yr starting at age 40 yr Annual clinical breast examination (in conjunction with mammography)
Cervical	Papanicolaou smear screens every 1-3 yr for women with a cervix Begin within 3 years of onset of sexual activity but no later than age 21 yr
Colon	Tests that detect polyps and cancer: Flexible sigmoidoscopy every 5 yr Colonoscopy every 10 yr Virtual colonoscopy (computed tomographic colonography) every 5 yr Double-contrast barium enema every 5 yr Tests that detect cancer: Fecal occult blood test every year Fecal immunochemical test every year

because of its link with the development of mesothelioma and other types of lung cancer. Radon exposure is the second leading cause of lung cancer, although there is a strong interaction between smoking and radon such that most radon-induced lung cancers are among smokers. Several other chemical compounds have been linked to human cancers including benzene (leukemia), benzidine (bladder), arsenic, soot and coal tars (lung and skin), and wood dusts (nasal). Carcinogens have been identified in air and water pollution as well. However, quantification of the association of these pollutants with development of cancer has proved difficult. Exposure to ionizing radiation, either accidental or therapeutic, is associated with an increased risk for leukemia as well as a variety of solid tumors. Exposure to ultraviolet radiation from the sun is a major cause of melanoma and basal and squamous cell carcinomas.

Chemopreventive agents are drugs, vaccines, or micronutrients (e.g., minerals, vitamins) used to prevent the development of cancer. Many agents have been shown through epidemiologic studies and randomized controlled trials to prevent some common types of cancer (Table 56-3). Chemopreventive agents usually have side effects and associated costs, and most are considered for people at high risk for developing the disease. The vaccine directed against specific strains of the human papillomavirus (HPV), offers the strong promise of preventing cervical cancer.

SECONDARY PREVENTION

Secondary prevention of cancer is achieved with screening tests to detect disease in asymptomatic patients at early stages of the disease progression. Proven cancer screening tests include mammography to detect breast cancer, Papanicolaou (Pap) smears to detect cervical dysplasia or cancer, and colonoscopy to detect polyps or colon cancer (Table 56-4). Screening tests do not prevent disease and are not diagnostic on their own. Instead, they identify patients who need additional diagnostic tests and may need treatment, with the intent of catching the disease at an earlier and thus more treatable stage. For most types of cancers, no effective screening tests exist.

For screening to be recommended for a disease, certain criteria must be met: (1) the disease must have a long asymptomatic (preclinical) phase, during which time intervention is likely to be beneficial, (2) an effective intervention must be available, (3) early treatment must reduce morbidity and mortality and be more effective than later treatment, and (4) the test should be highly sensitive and specific, and safe.

The *sensitivity* of a screening test is the likelihood of a positive test result in a person with the disease. A 100% sensitive test is never negative in a person who has the disease; that is, it has a 0% false-negative rate. The *specificity* of a test is the likelihood of a negative test result in a person who does not have the disease. A 100% specific test is never positive in a person without the disease and has a 0% false-positive rate. The *positive predictive value* of a test is the likelihood that a person with a positive test result has the disease, and the *negative predictive value* of a test is the likelihood that a person with a negative test result does not have the disease. Both values depend on the sensitivity and specificity of the test and the prevalence of the disease in the population screened.

Two main types of bias may occur in studies of screening effectiveness: (1) lead-time bias and (2) length-time bias. *Lead time* is the time between detection of disease by screening and the actual appearance of symptomatic disease. For rapidly progressive diseases with a short asymptomatic period, such as pancreatic cancer, treatment of disease detected by screening does not alter the outcome. Diagnosing the disease earlier with screening may make it appear that the patient lived longer, but the survival of the patient from the onset of disease is not altered. *Length-time bias* occurs when subsets of the cancer under study have different growth rates. Screening is more likely to detect cancers that grow slowly because of the greater prevalence of asymptomatic people with slow-growing tumors than with fast-growing tumors. Thus patients with cancer that is detected with screening appear to have longer survival as a result of screening, when in fact the longer course of their disease results from the behavior of the tumor itself. Randomized controlled trials are needed to address both lead time and length time bias. These trials, however, require large numbers of participants and years to complete, and are vulnerable to biases including "contamination" (i.e., screening among participants randomized to the nonscreening arm of the study).

Screening tests have risks and benefits. False-negative results miss the diagnosis, and the patient does not benefit from having had the screening test. False-positive results are expensive, inconvenient, may have health risks, and can cause the patient to be labeled with a disease that is not truly present. Screening tests also have monetary costs. For mass screening to be recommended, the screening test should be cost-effective across the entire age spectrum being recommended for routine screening.

Genetic Screening for Inherited Susceptibility to Cancer

DNA testing is available to test for inherited susceptibility to several types of cancer. In general, this testing is reserved for people with a strong family history of the disease (Table 56-5). If a mutation is found in an affected family member, other family members can be tested to assess their risk for developing the disease. Most genes associated with a predisposition to cancer are large, and mutations can occur anywhere within the gene.

Patients having genetic testing should receive counseling before and after the test to ensure that they know the test limitations, the prevention options available if the test result is positive, and the risks associated with having a positive test result. The potential side effects of prevention measures, psychosocial issues, and the impact of genetic testing on the family should all be fully discussed with patients before testing. Patients who receive a negative test result must understand that their risk for cancer is not zero but is similar to that of the general population, and the possibility of guilt over not being affected should also be explored.

Table 56-5 Hereditary Cancer Syndromes for which Genetic Testing Is Available

Cancer and Involved Genes	Prevention Measures
Breast: BRCA-1, BRCA-2 PTEN, STK-11, TP53	Prophylactic mastectomy
	Selective estrogen receptor modulators (tamoxifen, raloxifene)
	Lifestyle measures
	Increased intensity of screening, including breast MRI
Lobular breast cancer and gastric cancer	Prophylactic gastrectomy
	Prophylactic mastectomy
CDH-1 (E-cadherin)	Increased intensity of screening, including breast MRI
	Selective estrogen receptor modulators (tamoxifen, raloxifene)
Ovarian: BRCA-1, BRCA-2	Prophylactic oophorectomy
	Oral contraceptives
Colon:	
Familial adenomatous Polyposis (FAP)	Prophylactic colectomy
	Nonsteroidal anti-inflammatory drugs
APC	Lifestyle measures
Hereditary nonpolyposis	Lifestyle measures
Colon cancer (HNPCC)	Nonsteroidal anti-inflammatory drugs
MLH-1, MSH-2	Increased surveillance
MSH-6, PMS-2	Prophylactic total abdominal hysterectomy and oophorectomy
MYH-associated polyposis	Lifestyle measures
MYH	Nonsteroidal anti-inflammatory drugs
	Prophylactic colectomy
Uterine:	Prophylactic hysterectomy
PTEN, MLH-1, MSH-2, MSH-6, PMS-2	Increased surveillance

FAP, familial adenomatous polyposis; HNPCC, hereditary nonpolyposis colorectal cancer; MRI, magnetic resonance imaging; MYH, mutY homologue.

Prospectus for the Future

Advances in molecular epidemiology are poised to make significant contributions to both cancer epidemiology and prevention. Epigenetic modifications, or changes in gene expression that are stable between cell divisions but do not change the nucleotide sequence, are increasingly recognized as playing an important role in the tumorigenic process. Increased understanding of epigenetic processes (DNA methylation, histone modification, and chromatin remodeling) holds great promise for increasing understanding of gene-environment interactions, and for the future development and testing of new diagnostic and treatment technologies. In addition, the use of new technologies and biomarkers (e.g., epigenomics, proteomics, and metabonomics) will become very useful for longitudinal epidemiologic studies of cancer risk, susceptibility, etiology, and prevention and early detection. An example of a promising application is the recognition of genetic polymorphisms that identify smokers at a particularly high risk for lung cancer. Patients found to be at high risk

would be candidates for screening or chemoprevention-based clinical trials.

At the population level, developing cost-effective strategies through which to disseminate behavioral, screening, vaccine, and chemoprevention measures to those at highest risk is critical to realizing the full potential of such prevention measures. Answers regarding the efficacy of several cancer screening tests (including prostate-specific antigen screening for prostate cancer and computed tomography screening for lung cancer) are forthcoming from studies currently underway. For screening tests with proven benefits, public health interventions and policy remain challenged with optimal utilization. Mammography use has leveled off and even declined in some populations, and colon cancer screening remains underused. Although tobacco control efforts have had a great impact, cigarette smoking remains the number one preventable cause of morbidity and mortality worldwide.

References

Colditz GA, Sellers TA, Trapido E: Epidemiology-Identifying the causes and preventability of cancer. Nat Rev Cancer 6:75-83, 2006.

Giarelli E: Cancer vaccines: A new frontier in prevention and treatment. Oncology 21(11 Suppl Nurse Ed):11-17, 2007.

Kumar S, Mohan A, Guleria R: Biomarkers in cancer screening, research and detection: Present and future [review]. Biomarkers 11:385-405, 2006.

Schottenfeld D, Beebe-Dimmer JL: Advances in cancer epidemiology: Understanding causal mechanisms and the evidence for implementing interventions. Annu Rev Public Health 26:37-60, 2005.

Schottenfeld D, Beebe-Dimmer J: Alleviating the burden of cancer: A perspective on advances, challenges and future directions. Cancer Epidemiol Biomarkers Prev 15:2049-2055, 2006.

Vineis P, Perera F: Molecular epidemiology and biomarkers in etiologic cancer research: The new in light of the old. Cancer Epidemiol Biomarkers and Prev 16:1954-1965, 2007.

Solid Tumors

Robert F. Todd III and Jennifer J. Griggs

Lung Cancer

Lung cancer is a devastating malignant disease. Although the rate of increase of new lung cancers has leveled off, lung cancer remains the leading cause of cancer-related death in the world.

EPIDEMIOLOGY

Apart from nonmelanomatous skin cancer, lung cancer is now the most common malignant disease in the United States. More than 215,000 new cases of lung cancer are estimated to have occurred in 2008, and more than 161,840 deaths occur each year from lung cancer.

Tobacco smoke accounts for more than 90% of all lung cancers. One metabolite of cigarette smoke, benzopyrene diolepoxide, binds to areas near the *TP53* suppressor gene. This finding provides a link between the genetics of lung cancer and the epidemiologic association between smoking and cancer. Second-hand smoke is also associated with a higher risk for lung cancer than in the general population. A nonsmoking spouse of a smoker has a relative risk for lung cancer of 1.5 to 2 compared with nonexposed control individuals.

In addition to cigarette smoke, household exposure to radon seeping through the ground into enclosed spaces, as well as asbestos exposure, increase cancer risk. Cigarette smoking enhances the risk for cancer from both these toxic exposures. Although chest radiographs and computed tomographic (CT) screening of high-risk individuals may detect cancers at early stages of the disease, the value of systematic screening to reduce lung cancer mortality has not been proved.

PATHOLOGY

The two major types of lung cancer are *non–small cell lung cancer* (NSCLC) and *small cell lung cancer* (SCLC). NSCLC comprises several histologic subtypes, including squamous cell carcinomas, adenocarcinomas, and large cell tumors.

Squamous cell carcinoma usually exhibits a centrally located endobronchial lesion and is the subtype most commonly associated with paraneoplastic hypercalcemia. *Adenocarcinomas* are the most common lung cancers and are the type most often diagnosed in nonsmokers. Adenocarcinomas often exhibit a peripheral lung nodule. *Bronchioalveolar lung cancer* is a histologic variant of adenocarcinoma, characterized by multiple nodules and noninvasive growth along the peripheral airways of the lung. Sputum production with this subtype can be prolific. *Large cell tumors* are the least common; some have histologic features of neuroendocrine tumors. Although differences are noted in the clinical presentation of various subtypes, the natural history and response to conventional treatment are similar. However, with the advent of newer, molecularly targeted therapies, differences in response among the histologic subtypes are being observed.

SCLC is significantly linked to cigarette smoke exposure. The cell of origin is derived from the neuroendocrine family, which probably explains its proclivity to cause paraneoplastic syndromes such as the syndrome of inappropriate antidiuretic hormone production (SIADH) and Cushing syndrome. SCLC nearly always exhibits a large, central tumor with mediastinal involvement.

GENETICS

Many genetic abnormalities are associated with lung cancer. Representative examples include chromosomal deletions (loss of 3p alleles in most SCLCs and about half of NSCLCs), oncogene amplification (e.g., K-ras, c-erbB-1, and c-erbB-2 in NSCLC), tumor suppressor gene loss or mutation (e.g., p53 and Rb), and telomerase activation. Changes in the expression of lung cancer–associated molecular markers may have prognostic or therapeutic significance and may represent potential targets of novel therapy.

CLINICAL PRESENTATION

Signs and symptoms of all types of lung cancer commonly include cough, hemoptysis, chest pain, radiographic

Table 57-1 Staging Work-Up for Lung Cancer

Tumor	Staging Tests
Non–small cell lung cancer	Computed tomographic scans of chest through adrenal glands Bronchoscopy and mediastinoscopy if enlarged lymph nodes Positron-emission tomography if considering resection
Small cell lung cancer	Computed tomographic scans of chest, abdomen, and head Bone scan Positron-emission tomographic scan may also be useful for detecting cancer outside the chest

Table 57-2 Staging System for Lung Cancer

Stage	Criteria
Non–Small Cell Lung Cancer	
IA	Tumor size is ≤3 cm and located more than 2 cm from the carina. No lymph nodes are involved.
IB	Tumor size is >3 cm, ≤7 cm, and located more than 2 cm from the carina. No lymph nodes are involved.
IIA	Tumor size is ≤7 cm and located more than 2 cm from carina. Peribronchial and/or hilar nodes may be involved.
IIB	Tumor size is ≤7 cm located more than 2 cm from carina with peribronchial and/or hilar nodes involved; or tumor size >7 cm (or satellite tumors within the same lobe) with invasion of chest wall, diaphragm, mediastinal pleura, pericardium, or located less than 2 cm from the carina, without lymph node involvement.
IIIA	Any size tumor is present and may have invaded chest wall, carina, heart, great vessels, trachea, and esophagus. Tumor may involve ipsilateral peribronchial, hilar, mediastinal, and/or subcarinal nodes.
IIIB	Any size tumor is present and may have invaded any structure. Nodal involvement is always present and may extend to contralateral mediastinum or supraclavicular or scalene area.
IV	Metastases are present (including a malignant pleural effusion).
Small Cell Lung Cancer	
Limited	Tumor is confined to one lung. Nodes may involve contralateral lung, but all cancer must be encompassed in one radiation portal.
Extensive	Metastatic disease is present or disease is not limited to one radiation field.

evidence of a mass or pneumonia, and weight loss in the chronic smoker. About 60% to 70% of patients with SCLC exhibit metastatic disease. Common metastatic sites include the brain, liver, skeleton, adrenal glands, and bone marrow. SCLC may also cause the superior vena cava syndrome as well as paraneoplastic syndromes. NSCLC exhibits metastatic disease in 35% to 40% of patients at the time of diagnosis, most often in the liver, lung, bone, and adrenal glands. NSCLC is associated with paraneoplastic syndromes such as pulmonary hypertrophic osteoarthropathy and hypercalcemia.

STAGING

Table 57-1 describes the tests usually required for a thorough work-up of the patient with lung cancer. Because treatment substantially differs between NSCLC and SCLC, the testing strategies are discussed separately.

Non–Small Cell Lung Cancer

The goals of staging for NSCLC are to find patients who may be cured by resection. Therefore, attention to the mediastinum, a common site of lymph node spread, and a search for metastatic disease are both performed as soon as possible after diagnosis. Testing usually begins with a CT scan extending through the liver and adrenal glands, common sites of metastases. Bronchoscopy or fine-needle aspiration is frequently used to make the histologic diagnosis. Patients with NSCLC who have enlarged mediastinal lymph nodes should undergo mediastinoscopy or bronchoscopic transbronchial biopsy to determine resectability (mediastinal nodes are rarely resectable). If an adrenal gland is enlarged, biopsy of the adrenal gland should be performed. In patients with resectable disease, surgical treatment may offer a chance for cure. Positron-emission tomography (PET) is a useful test during the work-up of the patient with NSCLC, but positive findings require pathologic or more precise radiologic corroboration before deciding against lung cancer surgery.

Small Cell Lung Cancer

The goal of staging in SCLC is to determine which patients have limited-stage disease (about 30% to 40% of SCLC patients at the time of diagnosis) who can be potentially cured by the administration of combined chemoradiotherapy, compared with patients with extensive-stage metastatic

disease who cannot be cured but who can enjoy significant palliation with extension of survival as a result of chemotherapy. Limited-stage SCLC is defined as regional intrathoracic disease that can be encompassed within a single radiation field. Conversely, extensive disease represents locally advanced or widely metastatic disease that extends beyond a reasonable radiation field. Because common sites of metastatic disease include brain, liver, bone, and adrenal glands, diagnostic tests are performed to target these areas.

The staging system for each type of lung cancer is shown in Table 57-2. For the patient with NSCLC, tumor size, proximity to central structures, and location of lymph nodes are the most important features. Because surgery is rarely performed for the patient with SCLC, nodal detail is seldom obtained. The regional extent of the cancer and the ability to encompass the involved areas within a single radiation field determine treatment planning (Table 57-3).

TREATMENT

Non–Small Cell Lung Cancer

Because complete removal of the tumor provides the best chance for long-term survival, the focus of the primary treat-

Table 57-3 **Treatment and Outcomes for Lung Cancer**		
Tumor	**Standard Treatment by Stage**	**Outcome**
Non–small cell lung cancer	Early stages: surgery only (I); surgery followed by adjuvant chemotherapy (II, IIIA)	Early stages: patients with stage II lung cancer have a 40%-50% survival rate with surgery and adjuvant chemotherapy
	Later stage (unresectable): Combined chemotherapy and radiation or chemotherapy alone	Late stage: patients with stage IV lung cancer have 1-yr survival rate near 20% with chemotherapy
Small cell lung cancer	Limited: cisplatin-based chemotherapy with concurrent chest radiation Prophylactic cranial radiation is considered	Limited: 20%-30% 5-yr survival rate
	Extensive: chemotherapy palliates symptoms and prolongs survival but is not curative	Extensive: median survival rate is 10 mo with treatment

ment for the patient with NSCLC should begin with an assessment of resectability. Resectability depends on the anatomic location of the tumor as well as the patient's medical condition and pulmonary reserve. In general terms, the risk for pneumonectomy is small if the patient has a forced expiratory volume in 1 second greater than 2 L, carbon dioxide diffusing capacity of more than 60%, a maximal voluntary ventilation of more than 50% of predicted values, or the ability to walk up three flights of stairs. Lesser resections (e.g., lobectomy) may require less stringent criteria. Occasionally, patients with severe obstructive disease cannot undergo a curative procedure because they lack pulmonary reserve.

Patients with stage I and II tumors (localized lesions or involvement limited to hilar lymph nodes) should undergo surgical treatment. Peripheral tumors are removed by lobectomy; more central tumors, if resectable, may require pneumonectomy. Stage III tumors may be operable in some patients, particularly if they are treated with chemotherapy and radiation therapy (i.e., neoadjuvant therapy) before resection. In patients with significant mediastinal lymph node involvement detected during tumor resection or at the time of mediastinoscopy, the chance of long-term survival is less than 20% even with surgical treatment. Although postoperative radiation therapy is seldom useful, recent reports show a survival benefit when patients with stages II and IIIA undergo adjuvant chemotherapy. Chemotherapy using a variety of agents combined with cisplatin or carboplatin improves survival after surgery by about 5%.

Almost 80% of lung cancers are unresectable. If the tumor cannot be resected and has not spread to distant organs (stages IIIA and IIIB), chemotherapy is administered concurrently with radiation. This treatment leads to better median survival and 5-year disease-free survival rates than with radiation alone, but combined therapy for unresectable disease should be reserved for patients with good functional status. Aggressive treatment is much less effective (due to unacceptable toxicity) in patients who have lost more than 5% of their body weight or who are active less than 50% of the day. The median survival for patients with locally advanced, unresectable lung cancer who are candidates for combined modality therapy is now 15 to 18 months, and nearly 20% achieve a 5-year disease-free survival.

Patients with metastatic disease may benefit from chemotherapy. The most active agents are platinum derivatives such as cisplatin and carboplatin, taxanes such as paclitaxel and docetaxel, gemcitabine, vinorelbine, irinotecan, and pemetrexed. About 20% to 30% of patients achieve a greater than 50% reduction in their tumor volume after chemotherapy. For patients with advanced-stage lung cancer (stages IIIB with pleural effusion and IV), chemotherapy improves survival from an average of 8.5 to 11 months; quality-of-life studies show that chemotherapy delays symptoms and reduces their severity compared with no treatment. New agents that target neoplastic angiogenesis such as bevacizumab or the epidermal growth factor receptor antagonists such as erlotinib and cetuximab have shown therapeutic benefit either as single agents (e.g., erlotinib) or, more commonly, in combination with chemotherapy (bevacizumab) for these cancers.

Small Cell Lung Cancer

Patients with limited-stage SCLC are treated with curative intent with combined (concurrent) modality chemotherapy and radiotherapy. It is common practice to treat these patients with four to six cycles of chemotherapy (most commonly with cisplatin or carboplatin and etoposide) along with radiation therapy delivered to a radiation field encompassing the intrathoracic disease. About 50% to 60% of patients experience a complete response, and another 20% to 30% have a partial shrinkage of their cancer. Because 50% to 60% of patients with SCLC will ultimately develop brain metastases, prophylactic cranial radiation should be considered for those patients who have a complete response in the lung to primary chemoradiotherapy. About 20% to 30% of treated patients with limited-stage SCLC are alive and free of disease 3 years after diagnosis, and a proportion of these individuals are cured. Although patients with extensive-stage SCLC cannot be cured with existing therapy, chemotherapy can cause rapid tumor shrinkage with resolution of symptoms resulting in significant prolongation of life compared with supportive care alone.

Recurrent Lung Cancer

Both NSCLC and SCLC have high relapse rates. The use of second-line chemotherapy for these patients may palliate symptoms, but its use is not curative. Although these cancers may respond to subsequent agents such as docetaxel, pemetrexed, and erlotinib (NSCLC) or the camptothecins, the taxanes, and oral etoposide (SCLC), the use of these drugs should be limited to patients with good performance status, preferably on a clinical trial.

Head and Neck Cancers

EPIDEMIOLOGY AND NATURAL HISTORY

Most cancers of the head and neck, including cancers of the larynx, oral cavity, oropharynx, and sinuses, are squamous cell carcinomas. In 2008, an estimated 35,310 new cases were diagnosed, and 7590 deaths occurred. Tobacco use, alcohol consumption, and poor oral hygiene have all been linked to the development of cancers of the head and neck. Nasopharyngeal cancers are associated with Epstein-Barr viral infection. Infection with human papillomavirus (HPV), in particular HPV-16, is now an established risk factor for oropharyngeal cancer.

The major determinant of prognosis is the tumor burden, or the thickness of the tumor, and the presence or absence of regional lymph node involvement. The cure rate with small tumors is as high as 75% to 95% with radiation therapy or surgery. Continued use of tobacco after a diagnosis of a head and neck cancer is associated with a poor prognosis. People who have had cancer of the head and neck are at high risk for having a primary lung or esophageal cancer.

SYMPTOMS

Symptoms of cancers of the head and neck are related to the location of the tumor. For example, supraglottic laryngeal cancers cause pain with swallowing and a change in voice quality. Cancers of the oral cavity may exhibit a mass under the tongue or red or white patches in the mouth. Bleeding in the mouth or ill-fitting dentures may also be symptoms of cancer in the oral cavity. Symptoms of cancers of the sinus include sinusitis that does not resolve with appropriate treatment. Ear pain may be present with cancers of the oropharynx or hypopharynx.

DIAGNOSIS

Diagnosis of head and neck cancers require histologic confirmation with biopsy. Magnetic resonance imaging (MRI) or a CT scan of the head and neck is performed to determine a precise estimate of the extent of the tumor. Thorough examination of the entire aerodigestive tract with endoscopy will demonstrate a synchronous second primary tumor, for example, in the esophagus, in up to 15% of patients. Staging of the tumor is based on clinical and radiographic assessment.

TREATMENT

Small tumors that have not spread to regional lymph nodes are treated with radiation or surgery. Primary radiation therapy may allow preservation of organ function of, for example, the larynx, with surgical resection used in the case of recurrence. Locally advanced disease is treated with a combination of surgery and radiation therapy (with or without chemotherapy), or with a combination of radiation therapy and cisplatin-containing chemotherapy regimens. Most relapses occur within 2 to 3 years after therapy. Close surveillance is therefore warranted. Good-performance status patients with locally advanced, unresectable disease may also derive palliative benefit from combined modality chemotherapy (or cetuximab) and radiotherapy.

Gastrointestinal Cancers

Cancers of the gastrointestinal tract are among the most common tumors, with more than 271,000 new cases occurring in 2008. Advances in the treatment of colorectal cancer have improved survival and quality of life for patients with these diseases. Table 57-4 outlines the common signs and symptoms, treatments, and prognosis of gastrointestinal tumors.

ESOPHAGEAL CANCER

Epidemiology and Natural History

The two types of esophageal cancer are squamous cell and adenocarcinoma. *Squamous cell cancers* are most common in the cervical and thoracic esophagus, and *adenocarcinomas* commonly occur in the lower esophagus down to the gastroesophageal junction. Squamous cell cancers are more common in African Americans and are associated with predisposing factors that include smoking, caustic injury, achalasia, and alcohol intake. Squamous cell cancers are associated with other tobacco-related cancers in the upper airways and digestive tract. The rate of adenocarcinoma is increasing; this increase is related in part to Barrett esophagus, an adenomatous metaplasia of the distal esophagus often caused by gastroesophageal reflux disease, but other factors are likely. Almost 25% of patients with severe Barrett esophagus eventually develop esophageal adenocarcinoma. The most useful intervention for patients with Barrett esophagus is frequent endoscopic screening and biopsy; pharmacologic treatment of acid reflux disease does not prevent neoplastic transformation.

Symptoms

The most common symptom of esophageal cancer is dysphagia. As the lumen of the esophagus narrows, the patient loses normal swallowing capacity and has a sensation that solid food becomes "stuck." Eventually, the patient may be unable to swallow liquids. Patients commonly become afraid to eat because of frequent regurgitation at mealtime, resulting in significant weight loss.

Diagnosis

An upper gastrointestinal radiographic series or endoscopy will demonstrate an esophageal lesion, which should then undergo biopsy. The most effective staging tool is endoscopic ultrasonography, an accurate tool in assessing local depth of penetration and lymph node metastases. CT and positron-emission tomographic (PET) scanning are also required to ensure that the tumor has not already metastasized to the chest or liver, the two most common sites of spread.

Treatment

The most common treatment of esophageal cancer is surgery. Resection of the involved esophagus includes a wide margin

Table 57-4 **Gastrointestinal Cancers**

Tumor Site	Common Findings	Standard Treatments	Expected Outcome
Esophageal	Dysphagia, chest pain, weight loss	Early stage: neoadjuvant chemoradiotherapy and surgery Later stages: combination chemotherapy and radiation therapy and/or surgery	Stage II/III stage: about 30% 5-yr survival Average survival for metastatic disease is <9 mo
Gastric	Pain, supraclavicular adenopathy, vomiting, melena	Stage I: surgery alone Stage II and III: surgery if possible, followed by chemotherapy and/or radiation Metastatic disease: chemotherapy alone	Early stage: >90% 5-yr survival Positive nodal involvement: 20%-75% 5-yr survival for tumors <2 cm
Hepatocellular	Elevated α-fetoprotein; pain or change in liver function test	Resection for early lesions Unresectable: chemoembolization or tyrosine kinase inhibitor therapy for palliation	Always fatal in later stages of disease
Pancreas	Weight loss, boring midline pain through back, jaundice	Early stage: Whipple procedure and/or radiation therapy Late stage: chemotherapy with radiation or chemotherapy alone	Resectable: median survival 10-20 mo Radical surgery: 25% with negative nodal involvement and 10% with positive nodal involvement may be cured by surgery Unresectable: median survival 4-6 mo
Colon, rectal	Abdominal pain, occult or overt bleeding in stool, change in bowel habits	Early stage: resection alone If nodal involvement, add chemotherapy Chemotherapy and radiation therapy before and after surgery for patients with rectal cancers	Early stage: >70% at 5 yr Nodal involvement: 50%-70% at 5 yr Metastatic: median 14-24 mo
Anal	Constipation, bleeding, rectal pain and urgency	Early stage: chemotherapy with radiation therapy Later stage: abdominoperineal resection	Localized: 70% at 5 yr

on either side. The stomach is then pulled up to join the remainder of the esophagus. Alternatively, part of the intestine may be transposed to the chest to create another digestive pathway. About 10% to 30% of patients with stage II disease who are treated by surgical resection alone are alive and free of cancer 5 years after diagnosis. The results of recent studies indicate that administration of chemoradiotherapy before surgical resection ("neoadjuvant chemoradiotherapy") may offer survival benefit over surgery alone. If surgical treatment is not possible, either because the cancer is technically unresectable or the patient is medically unfit for surgery, the standard of care for these patients is to provide chemotherapy and radiation. This approach may cure 20% to 30% of patients. Whether the outcomes of combined chemotherapy and radiation are as favorable as surgical resection alone is not clear.

For patients with metastatic esophageal cancer, systemic chemotherapy using platinum-based combination regimens are effective in palliation and extending survival. For patients with severe dysphagia that does not resolve with radiation or surgery, endoscopic placement of a metal or plastic stent may permit adequate nutrition and resumption of a normal lifestyle.

GASTRIC CANCER
Epidemiology and Natural History
Gastric cancer rates are highest in developing countries that use smoked meats and meats high in nitrates. Other predis-

posing conditions include pernicious anemia, achlorhydria, gastric ulcers, and prior gastric surgery. Except for cancers of the gastroesophageal junction, gastric cancer rates have decreased in the United States (21,500 new cases occurring in 2008). A recognized risk factor for gastric cancer is infection with *Helicobacter pylori*. Whether early treatment of *H. pylori* infection changes the rate of cancer in infected populations is not clear.

Diagnosis
Patients with gastric cancer commonly experience abdominal pain, early satiety, anemia, hematemesis, weakness, and weight loss. Frequently, the cancer has already involved local lymph nodes by the time the diagnosis is made. Physical examination may show a gastric mass, an umbilical node (Sister Mary Joseph node), or a left supraclavicular node (Virchow node). Pathologic analysis shows an adenocarcinoma that can be localized or spread throughout the gastric lining *(linitis plastica)*. Required staging includes a CT scan to search for obvious nodal or metastatic involvement of the liver, upper gastrointestinal endoscopic examination, and endoscopic ultrasonography to determine depth of invasion and biopsy abnormal lymph nodes.

Treatment
Gastric cancer is most often treated surgically. When the tumor and all relevant lymph nodes have been removed, patients have a 20% to 60% chance of a 5-year survival, depending on the pathologic stage. If gastric cancer recurs,

the most common sites are local extension or hematogenous spread through the portal vein to the liver. Patients undergoing a complete resection for gastric cancer benefit from the addition of 5-fluorouracil (5-FU) and leucovorin chemotherapy and postoperative radiation therapy. This combination improves median survival by about 15 months compared with no adjuvant therapy. Patients with metastatic gastric cancer may elect chemotherapy to palliate symptoms. Active agents include platinum compounds, fluoropyrimidines, anthracyclines, taxanes, and irinotecan. Combination chemotherapy provides a 20% to 40% response rate and may extend survival.

COLORECTAL CANCER

Epidemiology and Natural History

About 1 in 20 people in the United States will be diagnosed with colon cancer (lifetime risk is 6%). An estimated 148,700 new cases were diagnosed in 2008, and in the same year, nearly 50,000 deaths occurred. Known predisposing factors are a history of ulcerative colitis and a strong family history of colon cancer. Several mutations, whether inherited or spontaneous, play a major role in the predisposition to colon cancer (see Chapter 55, Fig. 55-1 and Table 55-2). For example, familial polyposis is transmitted in an autosomal dominant manner. Individuals have mutations in the *APC* gene, which may be associated with periampullary and thyroid cancers or non-neoplastic growth such as osteomas, sebaceous cysts, and gastric polyps. Hereditary nonpolyposis colorectal cancer (HNPCC) is a more common autosomal disorder associated with microsatellite instability and mutations in h*MSH-2,* h*MLH-1, PMS-1, PMS-2,* and h*MSH-6.* Patients with HNPCC usually have colon or endometrial cancer when younger than 50 years and have first-degree relatives with colon cancer or other HNPCC-related cancers derived from the stomach, ovary, small bowel, biliary tract, ureter, or renal pelvis.

Whether the predisposing risk for colon cancer is genetically transmitted or sporadically acquired, a clear relationship exists between adenomatous polyps and the later development of colon cancer. Because the removal of polyps is probably the most important way to prevent the development of invasive colon cancer, the most reliable way to reduce colon and rectal cancer mortality is to perform regular screening. Colonoscopy is the most commonly used screening test. Studies using sigmoidoscopy and regular fecal occult blood testing also show reductions in the incidence and mortality of colorectal cancer. Patients with a proven mutation (Gardner syndrome, HNPCC) or a strong family history (familial adenomatous polyposis), and those who acquire other diseases associated with colorectal cancer, such as ulcerative colitis, should begin colonoscopy earlier than suggested for the general population. For patients with familial adenomatous polyposis, screening should start in the teenage years. For patients with HNPCC, screening for colon cancer should start 10 years before the age of diagnosis in the youngest family member with colorectal cancer. Research efforts are underway in the primary prevention of colorectal cancers using interventions such as diet, daily aspirin, cyclo-oxygenase-2 inhibitors, calcium and vitamin D supplementation, and other chemopreventive agents to reduce cancer incidence. Enthusiasm for promoting a high-fiber diet to reduce the risk for colon cancer has waned. Lifestyle changes are still considered important—fresh fruits and vegetables, regular exercise, fewer than two red meat servings per week—based on epidemiologic association.

Symptoms

Rectal bleeding commonly occurs with colon and rectal cancers. Patients with left-sided colon lesions often complain of a change in stool color or caliber or pelvic pain and transient bloating. Right-sided lesions may become friable and may result in occult bleeding. Occasionally, patients with colon and rectal cancers are asymptomatic until the tumor totally obstructs the bowel or perforates the peritoneal cavity. Colon and rectal cancers tend to spread hematogenously to the lungs and liver. Rectal cancer is more likely than colon cancer to recur locally because it is more difficult to get a wide margin of normal tissue and lymph nodes within the tight confines of the pelvis.

Diagnosis

The work-up for colon cancer requires measurement of serum carcinoembryonic antigen (CEA), an abdominal-pelvic CT scan, a chest radiograph, and endoscopic imaging of the colon to ensure that all polyps and cancers are removed near the time of the primary operation. Table 57-5 describes the staging system for colon and rectal cancers.

Treatment

In patients with stages I, II, and III colon cancer, surgical resection of the primary carcinoma along with any regional lymph node metastases is routinely performed; multiagent, adjuvant chemotherapy is recommended for all patients with stage III cancer (which reduces the rate of recurrence by about 40%) and for selected high-risk individuals with stage II cancer. For patients with rectal cancer, either primary resection (which may require colostomy) or neoadjuvant chemoradiotherapy is performed. Because of the higher likelihood of local recurrence in rectal cancer, any lesion that invades the muscle or lymph nodes is also treated with radiation therapy (if not given before surgery) and adjuvant chemotherapy. Surgical resection of the primary lesion in patients with advanced (stage IV) colorectal cancer

Table 57-5 **Staging for Colon and Rectal Cancer**			
Stage	**Tumor Size**	**Nodal Status**	**Metastases**
0	In situ	No	No
I	Invades mucosa only	No	No
II	May invade muscularis or through serosa	No	No
III	Any size tumor or any level of invasion	Yes	No
IV	Any size or depth	Positive nodal involvement present or absent	Yes

may be recommended to palliate or avoid symptoms of obstruction, bleeding, and pain.

Significant advances have been made in the use of chemotherapy for colorectal cancer. Regimens proved successful in prolonging survival for colon cancer include 5-FU with leucovorin or its oral analogue, capecitabine, alone. The addition of oxiliplatin to 5-FU–based adjuvant therapy has recently been shown to further improve survival after surgery. In the setting of metastatic cancer, infusions of chemotherapy with FOLFOX (5-FU, leucovorin, oxiliplatin), or FOLFIRI (5-FU, leucovorin, irinotecan) with the addition of antibodies targeting the vascular endothelial growth factor (VEGF; bevacizumab) or the epidermal growth factor receptor (cetuximab) prolong median survival beyond 20 months, almost twice the survival expected in the early 1990s. Despite improvements in survival, metastatic colon and rectal cancers are incurable unless the metastatic lesions can be surgically resected.

ANAL CARCINOMA

Anal cancers are increasing in frequency (currently about 5000 new cases per year). Persons infected with HPV and HIV are more likely to develop anal cancer. Patients with anal cancer usually experience rectal bleeding or complain of rectal fullness.

Combined chemotherapy with 5-FU and mitomycin and radiation therapy make up the standard approach to a patient with localized anal cancer. Results with combined therapy are superior to those with surgery, with the additional benefit of sparing the anal sphincter. Abdominoperineal resection is reserved for patients in whom chemoradiotherapy fails.

PANCREATIC CANCER
Epidemiology and Natural History

Pancreatic cancer, which is diagnosed in more than 37,000 people living in the U.S. each year, is strongly associated with cigarette smoking. A small proportion of pancreatic cancers are inherited from mutations in the *p16* and *BRCA-2* genes. Epithelial pancreatic cancer is an adenocarcinoma with an extremely high mortality rate because it is usually diagnosed when the tumor is beyond the capability of surgical resection. A less common type of pancreatic cancer, islet cell carcinoma, originates in the endocrine cells. Symptoms related to secretion of peptides such as gastrin, vasointestinal polypeptide, and insulin characterize these tumors.

Symptoms

The most common presentation of epithelial pancreatic cancer is abdominal pain accompanied by rapid weight loss. Characteristically, the pain is located in the periumbilical region and pierces or stabs through to the back. The pain is often explained by the frequent invasion of the celiac plexus deep in the retroperitoneum. Other symptoms of pancreatic cancer are the recent onset of diabetes, intestinal angina reflecting encasement of the superior mesenteric artery, a palpable gallbladder (Courvoisier sign), and jaundice from blockage of the distal common bile duct. Migrating thrombophlebitis (Trousseau sign) is a paraneoplastic complication of pancreatic adenocarcinoma. The tumor

marker CA-19-9 is elevated in up to 75% of patients with pancreatic cancer.

Treatment

The only curative treatment for pancreatic cancer is pancreaticoduodenectomy (Whipple procedure), an extensive operation requiring three anastomoses that carries a high mortality rate in centers with less experience with the procedure. The 5-year survival for surgically treated patients with localized pancreatic cancer is 25% for node-negative cancer but only 10% when lymph nodes are involved. Accordingly, it has become standard practice to offer adjuvant chemoradiotherapy or gemcitabine chemotherapy alone, which may provide a survival advantage. Patients with unresectable disease may benefit from local radiation therapy with concurrent 5-FU; more than 30% of patients treated with this combination have some improvement in their symptoms. Alternatively, gemcitabine-based chemotherapy alone may have palliative benefit. When patients have progressive or metastatic disease, the use of palliative chemotherapy with weekly gemcitabine has been shown to improve quality of life and survival to a small degree (5.7 months with gemcitabine, 4.4 months without gemcitabine, or 20% 1-year survival versus 5%). Recent meta-analyses suggest that certain gemcitabine-based chemotherapy combinations offer limited survival advantage over gemcitabine alone.

HEPATOCELLULAR CARCINOMA

Although uncommon in the United States (about 21,000 new cases per year), hepatocellular carcinoma (HCC) is one of the most common cancers throughout the world; more than 1 million cases are diagnosed each year. The common causes of HCC are chronic viral hepatitis (both B and C) and cirrhosis related to alcohol use or hemochromatosis. Although this approach is unproved, considerable interest exists in screening patients who are at extremely high risk with serial measurement for α-fetoprotein (AFP) levels. AFP levels are commonly elevated even in early-stage HCC.

Treatment of early-stage HCC is surgery. Cure rates are more than 75% for patients with tumors smaller than 2 cm. Patients with severe cirrhosis and who have small liver cancers may benefit from liver transplantation. Chemoembolization may provide palliative benefit for patients with unresectable tumors, but conventional cytotoxic chemotherapy is generally ineffective. However, recent findings suggest that molecularly targeted tyrosine kinase inhibitors such as sorafenib offer a survival advantage over supportive care.

Breast Cancer
EPIDEMIOLOGY

Breast cancer is the most common nonskin cancer in women and the second leading cause of cancer death (after lung cancer) among women in the United States. In 2008, an estimated 182,460 women were diagnosed with invasive breast cancer, and more than 40,000 died from breast cancer. Breast cancer in men is rare.

Risk factors for breast cancer include older age, a family history of breast cancer, early menarche, late menopause, first-term pregnancy after age 25 years, nulliparity, prolonged use of exogenous estrogen, and postmenopausal obesity. Exposure to ionizing radiation, as is used in the treatment of Hodgkin disease, also increases the risk for breast cancer. Only 5% to 10% of patients with breast cancer are associated with the breast cancer-susceptibility genes, *BRCA-1* and *BRCA-2*. Patients with multiple affected family members or those with a personal or family history of male breast cancer, bilateral breast cancer, or ovarian cancer should be offered genetic counseling and genetic testing for *BRCA-1* and *BRCA-2*. Mammographic screening in both average- and high-risk populations has been shown to reduce breast cancer mortality.

PATHOLOGY

Most breast cancers are infiltrating ductal adenocarcinomas. A smaller proportion of breast cancers are infiltrating lobular adenocarcinomas. Tubular and mucinous carcinomas, which are a subtype of infiltrating ductal cancers, are associated with a better prognosis. The estrogen and progesterone receptor status of the primary tumor should be assessed in all cases of invasive breast cancer. The oncoprotein-oncogene *HER-2/neu* (*human epidermal growth factor receptor*) is important in defining prognosis and treatment. Tumors that are negative for the estrogen and progesterone receptor and for overamplification of the *HER-2* oncogene (i.e., the so-called *triple-negative* tumors) are associated with a poorer prognosis. Such tumors are characteristic of those that develop in women who have the *BRCA-1* breast cancer susceptibility gene. Ductal carcinoma in situ (DCIS), also called *intraductal carcinoma*, is increasing in frequency, most likely because of increased mammographic screening.

CLINICAL PRESENTATION

Breast cancer is most often diagnosed through screening mammography or after a patient or her physician notices a palpable mass. Fewer than 10% of women have metastatic disease at diagnosis. Recurrent breast cancer most commonly exhibits metastases in the bone, liver, lung, and central nervous system, but breast cancer can recur in any organ of the body. Women with a history of breast cancer are also at increased risk for breast cancer in the contralateral breast. Inflammatory breast cancer is a clinical diagnosis in a woman with breast induration and erythema, often without a palpable mass. The skin findings are due to tumor emboli in the dermal lymphatics; skin biopsy is negative for cancer in 50% of patients.

STAGING

Breast cancer staging requires removal of the primary tumor and ipsilateral axillary lymph node assessment. Women with tumors larger than 5 cm and those with positive axillary lymph node involvement may have additional radiographic tests, including a chest radiograph, bone scan, and CT scan of the abdomen. Patients with smaller tumors and negative lymph node involvement do not need these tests unless they exhibit symptoms (e.g., skeletal pain) suggestive of metastatic involvement.

TREATMENT

For women with small breast tumors, breast-conserving therapy with lumpectomy followed by radiation therapy is standard therapy. Women with large tumors or with two or more tumors in separate quadrants of the breast should undergo mastectomy. Some women who are candidates for breast-conserving therapy choose to have a mastectomy, with or without breast reconstruction. Women who have had previous radiation to the breast, either for a previous breast cancer or other malignancies, are generally treated with mastectomy. Chemotherapy administered before surgical treatment (*primary* or *neoadjuvant chemotherapy*) may allow breast conservation in women with large tumors who would otherwise not be able to undergo a lumpectomy. Preoperative hormone therapy can be considered in frail patients with hormone receptor–positive tumors, but hormone therapy does not replace surgical treatment for most patients. Adjuvant therapy with chemotherapy and hormonal therapy improves relapse-free and overall survival rates in premenopausal and postmenopausal women who are at high risk for metastatic relapse. The monoclonal antibody trastuzumab, directed at the *HER-2* pathway, improves disease-free survival in patients with tumors that have overamplification (or high levels of overexpression) of the *HER-2* oncoprotein.

Treatment decisions in women with metastatic disease are based on the hormone receptor status, sites of disease, presence and severity of symptoms, time since initial diagnosis, and previous treatments. The monoclonal antibody trastuzumab may be used in combination with chemotherapy, hormonal therapy, or as a single agent. Life expectancy is longer in women with hormone-responsive disease and with lymph node or bone metastases, rather than liver, lung, or central nervous system metastases. Patients with metastatic breast cancer may live for many years, often responding to hormonal therapy for years before requiring chemotherapy for disease control. Many chemotherapeutic agents (singly or in combination), including the anthracyclines, taxanes, alkylating agents, fluoropyrimidines, vinca alkaloids, gemcitabine, and epithilones, demonstrate activity against breast cancer. Bisphosphonates, such as zoledronate and pamidronate, are given intravenously to decrease the pain associated with bone metastases and the risk for fracture in women with skeletal metastases.

DCIS is treated with either lumpectomy followed by radiation therapy or mastectomy. Women with multifocal or palpable DCIS should have assessment of lymph node status because a small but measurable proportion will have positive lymph node involvement that suggests the presence of invasive cancer. In these patients, systemic treatment is identical to that given to women with a clearly invasive breast primary tumor.

Prophylactic bilateral mastectomy is offered to women with the *BRCA-1* or *BRCA-2* breast cancer susceptibility genes. An alternative approach is close clinical surveillance, including monthly self-examination, frequent examination by a physician, and regular mammography or MRI. Oophorectomy or antiestrogen therapy can be used to decrease the risk for breast cancer in these women and in other women at high risk for the disease (see Chapter 56).

Table 57-6 Genitourinary Cancers

Tumor Site	Common Findings	Standard Treatments	Expected Outcomes
Testicle	Testicular swelling, pain, back pain Cough with metastatic presentation	Inguinal (not scrotal) orchiectomy Node-positive seminoma: radiation therapy Node-positive NSGCT: RPLND or chemotherapy	Early-stage seminoma: >90% 5-yr survival Stage III NSGCT: about 75% 5-yr survival Poor-risk tumors: <50%
Prostate	Elevated prostate-specific antigen, decreased urinary stream Bone pain with metastatic presentation	Early-stage: prostatectomy, radiation therapy, or watchful waiting Treatment recommendations depend on age, likelihood of spread, and tumor grade Later-stage tumors: hormone therapy, radiation therapy and/or chemotherapy	Early-stage: about 80%-90% 5-yr survival with surgery and radiation Stages C and D2: worse prognosis, time to relapse is variable
Bladder	Hematuria, cystitis	Superficial cancers: cystoscopic resection, biopsy, and intravesical chemotherapy Muscle invasion: neoadjuvant chemotherapy and cystectomy or bladder-sparing chemotherapy and radiation	Ten to 30% of superficial tumors progress to invasive cancer Muscle invasive disease: 50%-80% 5-yr survival; <40% of patients with positive nodal involvement live 5 yr
Renal cell	Hematuria, abdominal pain, and flank mass	Early-stage: radical nephrectomy Advanced or metastatic disease: high-dose IL-2, α-interferon, VEGF, or mTOR inhibitors	Confined to organ: 74%-100% 5-yr survival; Metastatic disease: 16%-32% 5-yr survival

IL-2, interleukin-2; mTOR, mammalian target of rapamycin; NSGCT, nonseminomatous germ cell tumor; RPLND, retroperitoneal lymph node dissection; VEGF, vascular endothelial growth factor.

Genitourinary Cancers

See Table 57-6 for a summary of genitourinary cancers.

PROSTATE CANCER AND TESTICULAR CANCER

These cancers are addressed in Chapter 72.

BLADDER CANCER

Epidemiology and Natural History

About 68,000 patients are diagnosed with bladder cancer each year in the United States. The disease is much less common in women than in men. About one fifth of affected patients will die of their disease. The most important risk factor is cigarette smoking, which accounts for at least two thirds of all cases. Other risk factors include exposure to polycyclic hydrocarbons in the dye, rubber, and paint industries, as well as long-term exposure to cyclophosphamide and phenacetin and chronic infection with *Schistosoma haematobium*.

Urothelial (transitional cell) carcinoma is the most common histologic type of bladder cancer. These tumors can occur anywhere urothelial lining exists, from the renal pelvis through the bladder and urethra. Squamous cell cancers, adenocarcinomas, and small cell carcinomas of the bladder and renal pelvis are less common and account for only 10% of all tumors in this region.

Symptoms

The most common presentation is gross or microscopic hematuria. About 30% of patients with bladder cancers experience symptoms of bladder irritation or spasms. When this cancer extends beyond the confines of the bladder, the symptoms relate to compression of local structures and may include leg swelling, pelvic pain, and compression of the nerves in the pelvic plexus.

Diagnosis

Bladder cancers are divided into superficial, invasive, and metastatic tumors. The evaluation of bladder cancer requires direct imaging and biopsy to determine the level of tumor invasion. Depth of invasion correlates with prognosis and determines the type of treatment required. Therefore, cystoscopy is the most important diagnostic tool. In patients at high occupational risk for developing the disease, urine cytologic examination may be helpful in the absence of symptoms that require cystoscopy. Furthermore, an intravenous pyelogram may be needed if cystoscopy does not localize a tumor in the bladder or ureters.

The most important determinant of prognosis and treatment is whether the tumor has invaded the muscular wall of the bladder. Because the relationship between the depth of invasion detected by cystoscopy and that detected by cystectomy is only 50%, other tools such as a CT scan, MRI, and a bone scan are important to help define the presence of invasion, nodal involvement, or metastasis. Histologic grade is important because low-grade tumors rarely invade muscle, whereas high-grade cancers do so frequently.

Treatment

Superficial low-grade tumors are treated by transurethral resection of the bladder (TURB). Cystoscopy is performed every 3 months to assess response and perform resections when required. For frequent relapses or when superficial cancer involves most of the surface of the bladder, intravesical therapy is recommended. For these patients, immunomodulators such as bacille Calmette-Guérin (BCG) vaccine or interferon or chemotherapeutic agents such as thiotepa or mitoxantrone are instilled in the bladder through a Foley catheter, allowed to dwell for a short time, and then voided. This process is repeated every week for 6 weeks and is followed by cystoscopy to assess response.

Tumors that invade the muscle require more aggressive surgical treatment. If the tumor has invaded muscle but is not through the bladder wall, the standard approach is neo-adjuvant chemotherapy followed by radical cystectomy. In this procedure, the bladder is removed along with the prostate, seminal vesicles, and proximal urethra in men; in women, a hysterectomy is performed along with a bilateral salpingo-oophorectomy and partial removal of the anterior vaginal wall. Because the bladder is removed, a pouch is created from the small bowel, often called an *ileal conduit,* to store and expel urine. In selected patients, an orthotopic neobladder connected to the native urethra can be constructed. Not all patients with tumors that invade the bladder wall require removal of the bladder. Bladder preservation and a combination of TURB followed or preceded by chemotherapy and radiation may be considered for patients with localized tumors away from the trigone or for those who are unable to tolerate aggressive surgery, although the outcomes of this approach may not be equivalent to radical cystectomy. Chemotherapy after surgery is recommended when bladder cancer is found in lymph nodes or when patients have metastatic disease. Patients with metastatic disease frequently respond to combination chemotherapy containing cisplatin or other agents such as gemcitabine and a taxane, but the tumor invariably relapses.

RENAL CELL CARCINOMA

Epidemiology and Natural History

Renal cell carcinoma, one of the least common tumors of the genitourinary system, accounts for about 3% of all cancers (an estimated 68,810 new cases in 2008). Some relationship exists between kidney cancer and exposure to cadmium, perhaps in cigarette smoke. Renal cell carcinoma occurs commonly in von Hippel-Lindau disease, in which synchronous, bilateral renal carcinomas occasionally occur. Abnormalities of the long arm of chromosome 3 are observed in more than 90% of patients. Most renal cell carcinomas are adenocarcinomas; a subtype called *clear cell carcinoma* represents more than 75% of all the tumors removed.

The natural history of kidney cancers is variable. Some tumors progress relentlessly and are refractory to all interventions whereas some patients can have spontaneous regression of metastases.

Symptoms

The classic presentation, consisting of hematuria, flank pain, and an abdominal mass, is observed in only 10% of patients. More often, hematuria alone or persistent back pain prompts the patient to seek attention. Many renal cell carcinomas are found during a CT scan performed for unrelated reasons. Occasionally, bilateral lower extremity edema occurs when the tumor has completely occluded the inferior vena cava. Renal cell carcinoma is also associated with unusual paraneoplastic syndromes, including fever, polycythemia from erythropoietin production, and hypercalcemia from ectopic production of parathyroid hormone (PTH).

Diagnosis

The most common tool to diagnose renal cell carcinoma is CT scanning of the abdomen. A large, dense, contrast-enhancing mass occupies a substantial amount of one kidney and is frequently accompanied by nodal or venous involvement. An MRI or direct injection of dye is recommended to assess inferior vena cava involvement. Because renal cell carcinoma commonly spreads to lungs and liver, a CT evaluation of the chest should be included in the staging procedures.

Treatment

Resection is the most common treatment for cancer limited to the kidney. Surgical treatment may be possible even if parts of the renal vein and vena cava are involved.

Renal cell carcinoma is notably resistant to chemotherapy and radiation. However, renal tumors may respond to biologic response modifiers such as interleukin-2 (IL-2) in about 10% to 15% of patients. Occasionally, IL-2 induces a complete response. Similar dramatic events have spontaneously occurred. Clinical trials have suggested that nonmyeloablative allogeneic bone marrow transplantation may be effective in some patients with renal cell cancer refractory to other conventional immunotherapy, but the usefulness of this approach is limited by its toxicity and by availability of a suitable donor. New agents that target the VEGF pathway (and other tyrosine kinase-dependent receptors), such as bevacizumab, sunitinib, and sorafenib, and the mTOR inhibitor temsirolimus have recently shown significant promise in extending the progression-free survival of patients who are not eligible for high-dose IL-2 therapy.

OVARIAN CANCER

Epidemiology

Ovarian cancer occurs in 1 in 60 women in the United States. More than 21,650 cases are expected to be diagnosed in the United States in 2008, with an estimated 15,520 deaths. As with most cancers, the incidence of ovarian cancer increases with age. Other risk factors include nulliparity, estrogen replacement (without progestin) therapy, obesity, and a family history of ovarian cancer. Ovarian cancer is more common in women who have one of the breast cancer susceptibility genes (see Chapter 56) and Lynch syndrome. Exposure to talc may increase the risk for ovarian cancer. Use of oral contraceptives decreases the risk for ovarian cancer, as do more than one pregnancy, breastfeeding, tubal ligation, and hysterectomy.

Pathology

Most malignant ovarian tumors arise from celomic epithelium. Tumors can arise in any part of the peritoneal cavity; thus, prophylactic oophorectomy reduces but does not eliminate the risk for ovarian cancer. Epithelial ovarian tumors are classified histologically as benign, malignant, or borderline. The most common histologic types of ovarian cancer are serous, mucinous, and endometrioid. Stromal tumors, most often granulosa cell tumors, and germ cell tumors account for fewer than 15% of ovarian tumors. Cancers from sites such as the breast and gastrointestinal tract can metastasize to the ovaries.

Clinical Presentation

Symptoms of early ovarian cancer include vague pelvic or abdominal pain, early satiety, and indigestion, but the symptoms are nonspecific; most patients with ovarian cancer are not diagnosed until the disease is advanced. No effective screening tests exist for ovarian cancer, although transvaginal ultrasound and the tumor marker CA-125 may be helpful in high-risk women with an affected first-degree relative and in women who carry a breast cancer susceptibility gene. Advanced ovarian cancer often causes abdominal swelling and pain, intestinal obstruction, and vaginal bleeding.

Staging and Treatment

Ovarian cancer is surgically staged with a total abdominal hysterectomy and bilateral salpingo-oophorectomy, omentectomy, lymph node sampling, and peritoneal biopsies. Stage I disease involves only the ovaries; stage II disease involves extension to the uterus, fallopian tubes, and pelvic structures; and peritoneal spread outside the pelvis, or retroperitoneal and inguinal lymph node involvement, is stage III disease. Many patients have clearly visible peritoneal tumor implants; however, in those who do not, representative biopsy specimens from all areas of the peritoneum, omentum, and retroperitoneal lymph nodes should be removed for microscopic examination. Disease outside the abdomen and in the liver parenchyma is stage IV disease. Patients with malignant pleural effusions also have stage IV disease.

The mainstay of treatment for ovarian cancer is surgery. Women whose total residual disease after surgery is less than 2 cm in diameter have an improved prognosis compared with women who have greater amounts of residual disease; thus, every effort should be made to debulk the patient to minimal residual disease.

Combination chemotherapy with paclitaxel and carboplatin is administered postoperatively to women with most stages of epithelial ovarian cancer, with the notable exception of those women with grade 1, stage IA or IB disease. If first-line therapy fails, additional chemotherapy is undertaken with a variety of agents whose response rate is affected by time since completion of first-line therapy. Platinum-resistant disease is almost universally fatal in a short time. Pleural effusions can be palliated with chemotherapy.

ENDOMETRIAL CANCER

Epidemiology

Endometrial cancer is the fourth most common malignant disease among women in the United States; more than 40,000 cases are diagnosed each year, leading to an estimated 7470 deaths in 2008. The tumor is usually found with early-stage disease and is usually curable, with 5-year survival rates higher than 80%. Those with localized disease at diagnosis have a 95% 5-year survival rate. Risk factors for endometrial cancer include increasing age, late menopause, nulliparity, obesity, and Lynch syndrome. Women who are treated with estrogen without concomitant progesterone or with tamoxifen and those who do not ovulate are also at increased risk for the disease. Most endometrial cancers are endometrioid adenocarcinomas.

Clinical Presentation

Most women with endometrial carcinoma have abnormal uterine bleeding. Even minimal postmenopausal bleeding should prompt an evaluation for endometrial cancer. Advanced disease can cause urinary symptoms or back or pelvic pain.

Staging and Treatment

Staging is achieved by surgical exploration. Most endometrial cancers are stage I, with invasion into less than half the uterine wall. More advanced tumors involve the cervix, vagina, pelvic or periaortic lymph nodes, bladder, and rectal mucosa. Metastases outside the pelvis (stage IV disease) are less commonly observed in patients with endometrioid pathology. However, more aggressive histologic subtypes, such as uterine papillary serous tumors and carcinosarcomas, are more likely to present with extrapelvic disease and to spread similarly to ovarian cancers.

Treatment of endometrial cancer consists of total hysterectomy, bilateral salpingo-oophorectomy, pelvic and para-aortic lymph node dissections, and peritoneal washings for histologic examination. Omentectomy is performed in patients with high-grade tumors. Radiation therapy is given to women with histologically high-grade tumors and those with deep myometrial involvement. Chemotherapy is added to the adjuvant treatment of women with stage III disease and to most stages of disease with more aggressive subtypes. Women with progressive or metastatic disease are treated with megestrol acetate, chemotherapy, or palliative radiation therapy.

CERVICAL CANCER

Because of widespread screening for cervical cancer with the Papanicolaou (Pap) smear, the incidence of invasive cervical cancer and mortality from cervical cancer have continued to decline in the United States. An estimated 11,000 cases of cervical cancer were diagnosed in 2008 with an estimated 3870 women dying of the disease. Cervical cancer and its precursor, cervical intraepithelial neoplasia, are more common in women with HIV infection and those infected with HPV subtypes 16, 18, 31, 33, and 35. Smoking, high parity, immunosuppression, and the long-term use of oral contraceptives may affect the persistence of HPV infection and the progression to cervical cancer. The cervical cancer vaccine directed against HPV offers promise of preventing cervical cancer worldwide when administered to women before the onset of sexual activity and before the acquisition of HPV infection (see Chapter 56). Most women with cervical intraepithelial neoplasia or cervical cancer are asymptomatic and are found to have the disease by Pap smear. Vaginal bleeding, postcoital bleeding, vaginal discharge, and pelvic pain may occur in women with invasive disease. Signs and symptoms of advanced disease are local pelvic involvement, including leg edema, or back and leg pain. Metastatic disease is rare.

Biopsy of the cervix confirms the diagnosis of cervical cancer in a woman with an abnormal Pap smear or a cervical lesion. Some women may need a cone biopsy if the colposcopy-directed biopsy is inconclusive, does not confirm invasive disease, or shows cervical dysplasia, or if the sample is inadequate. The use of other staging tests depends on the extent of local involvement, as determined by pelvic and rectal examination.

Treatment of cervical cancer depends on the stage of the disease. Cone biopsy may be sufficient in women with minimal microscopic invasion into the cervix who desire fertility. Women with more advanced disease that is still confined to the cervix can undergo radical hysterectomy with lymph node dissection, radiation with chemosensitization, or radical trachelectomy (in select cases of women still desiring fertility options). Combination chemotherapy with cisplatin and radiation therapy is recommended for women with locally advanced disease. Those with widely metastatic disease are treated with chemotherapy with or without palliative radiation therapy. A paclitaxel and cisplatin regimen is now the preferred treatment of recurrent, metastatic disease that is not amenable to radiation or pelvic exenteration.

Skin Cancer

BASAL CELL AND SQUAMOUS CELL CARCINOMA

Epidemiology and Natural History

Basal cell and squamous cell carcinomas are the most common cancers of the skin (in excess of one million unreported cases per year in the United States). Mortality from these cancers is exceedingly low, however, accounting for less than 0.1% of cancer deaths. Both types of cancer are more common on parts of the body exposed to sun and in people with light complexions. Although the most significant risk factor is exposure to ultraviolet radiation in sunlight, patients with immunosuppressive disorders (e.g., recipients of organ transplantation) or AIDS, as well as those with genetic disorders such as xeroderma pigmentosum, have a rate of skin cancer incidence that is many times higher than the rate of the general population. Unlike basal cell cancers, which rarely metastasize, squamous cell cancers can spread to regional lymph nodes. Thorough examination of regional lymph nodes is therefore necessary in patients with squamous cell cancer, particularly with squamous cell cancers of the lips, ears, and perianal and genital regions.

Treatment

Treatment options for basal cell and squamous cell cancers include surgical excision, radiation therapy, and cryosurgery. Topical fluorouracil may be used for treatment of superficial basal cell carcinomas or in situ squamous cell carcinomas. Dermatologists use Mohs micrographic surgery, which is a technique that examines serial frozen sections to achieve negative margins on each tumor border. This specialized approach offers the highest local control rates and is indicated for tumors with ill-defined borders and for those occurring in areas where maximal preservation of unaffected tissues is desirable, such as the eyes, nose, and genitalia.

MELANOMA

Epidemiology

The incidence of melanoma is increasing at a rate of 4% per year in the United States. Each year, more than 60,000 new cases are diagnosed, and more than 8000 deaths occur. Incidence rates increase with age and are 10-fold higher in white persons than in black individuals. Melanoma risk factors are similar to those of basal cell and squamous cell skin cancers (see previous discussion) but also include a genetic component, such as a personal history of dysplastic nevi and a family history of melanoma.

Pathology

Most melanomas are superficial-spreading melanomas. The antigenic markers S-100 and homatropine methylbromide (HMB-45) can be used to confirm the diagnosis of undifferentiated melanomas, although S-100 is nonspecific and HMB-45 is not 100% sensitive. Ulceration indicates a worse prognosis.

Clinical Presentation

Patients with melanoma most often report a change in a pigmented skin lesion on a sun-exposed surface. Characteristic changes include *a*symmetry, *b*order irregularities, *c*olor variation, *d*iameter more than 6 mm, and *e*nlargement (the ABCDE system). Although 90% of melanomas arise in the skin, melanomas can arise from any area where melanocytes reside, including the choroid of the eye. About 5% of melanomas arise from unknown primary sites. Melanoma can present with metastatic disease in lymph nodes, lung, bone, liver, or brain.

Staging

Melanoma is staged according to the thickness of the primary tumor, as measured both in millimeters of the tumor and in depth of invasion into the skin. The tumor thickness is the single most important prognostic factor. Even without nodal involvement, a melanoma more than 4 mm thick on the trunk has more than a 50% chance of distant metastasis. Sentinel lymph node analysis is indicated in patients with high-stage melanomas.

Treatment

Surgical excision with wide margins is required for cure of primary cutaneous lesions. The location and thickness of the lesion determine the optimal surgical margin. Locally recurrent lesions are surgically resected if possible; radiation therapy is given if surgical resection is not possible. In patients with regional lymph node involvement, adjuvant immunotherapy with 12 months of interferon-α may improve relapse-free survival rates. Many patients have severe side effects with interferon-α, such as myalgias and fever, and elect to discontinue treatment early.

When metastatic melanomas recur, the best treatment is high-dose IL-2. Although 5% to 10% of patients receiving this treatment may become long-term survivors, the toxicity of this approach precludes most patients from receiving it. In such patients, lower-dose interleukin treatments, oral temozolomide, intravenous dacarbazine, or multiagent chemotherapy (often administered with biologic agents like IL-2 and interferon) may be offered but are not curative. Radiation therapy is used to treat metastases to the brain, spinal cord, and bone, but melanoma is relatively resistant to radiation therapy.

Cancer of Unknown Primary

About 5% of people with cancer have metastatic disease in the absence of an identifiable primary tumor. Cancer of unknown primary most commonly exhibits disease in the bone, liver, lungs, or lymph nodes. Detailed pathologic examination, aided by immunohistochemical stains, electron microscopy, and chromosomal analysis, will usually distinguish between lymphomas and carcinomas. Such a distinction is important to make because lymphomas tend to be more responsive to therapy, and treatment of lymphomas differs from that of carcinomas. In patients with *adenocarcinoma of unknown primary origin*, limited radiographic examination, such as CT scans of the chest and abdomen, may help identify the site of the primary tumor. Other features of the metastatic disease may be revealing as well. For example, bone metastases are common in prostate and breast cancers, axillary lymphadenopathy is commonly seen in a woman with breast cancer, and liver metastases frequently occur in patients with lung, colon, and pancreatic cancers. Most tumor markers are nonspecific; therefore, reliance on a tumor marker alone in identifying a primary source of the cancer is not recommended. However, an elevated tumor marker level may provide supporting evidence for a primary cancer if risk factors for the tumor are present and the clinical pattern of spread is consistent.

Treatment of cancer of unknown primary is geared at palliation of symptoms with surgery, radiation therapy, combination chemotherapy with a broad spectrum of activity (active against a variety of cancers), or hormonal therapy (if the tumor is thought to be from an endocrine-responsive primary source such as prostate or breast cancer). Some people with cancer of unknown primary, such as people with only lymph node involvement, may live free of disease for many years and may be considered cured.

Metastases from Solid Tumors

Most patients who die from cancer generally die from metastatic spread of the primary tumor to distant sites. The process of invasion and metastasis requires each of the following steps: (1) development of the tumor's own vascular supply through angiogenesis, (2) tumor cell invasion through the host tissue basement membrane, (3) tumor embolization through either the lymphatic system or the bloodstream (hematogenous spread), (4) arrest and invasion into the basement membrane of the distant organ, (5) reestablishment of blood vessels to sustain growth of the metastatic cells, and (6) proliferation within the target organ. The processes of invasion and metastasis are highly selective, with only 0.01% of circulating cells forming a metastatic focus.

Advances in cancer therapeutics, such as the use of antibodies to the angiogenic molecule VEGF receptor, are targeted at disrupting neovascularization within malignant tumors or at interfering with tumor cell proliferation. The hope is that targeted therapies used alone or with cytotoxic chemotherapy will improve outcome while minimizing the toxicity to normal tissues (see Chapters 55 and 59).

Surgery for metastatic disease is generally reserved for palliation of symptoms because surgical resection is usually not curative and is associated with morbidity. In selected patients with metastatic colon cancer to the liver or lung, resection of the metastatic disease may offer a chance for cure.

Prospectus for the Future

Advances in our understanding of cancer causation and epidemiology, disease staging, tumor heterogeneity, and tumor and patient factors involved in response to treatment will all increase our ability to prevent and treat cancer. For example, polymorphisms in drug-metabolizing enzymes may explain differences in response to chemotherapy and survival among women with breast cancer. Similarly, microarray technology, which allows analysis of hundreds of genes involved in cell proliferation, can elucidate pathways of resistance to treatment and allow for more precise selection of cytotoxic therapy. The emerging concept of "cancer stem cells"—a small subpopulation of malignant cells capable of self-renewal that give rise to the bulk of more differentiated epithelial cancers—offers hope for the development of targeted therapies that attack this critical subset of tumor cells. Advances in imaging techniques may allow for detection of minimal residual disease, identifying patients who are likely to benefit from additional treatment. Finally, the increasing interest in measuring and improving quality of care will expand the reach of cancer therapies, improving cancer-specific outcomes at the population level.

References

D'Souza G, Kreimer AR, Viscidi R, et al: Case-control study of human papillomavirus and oropharyngeal cancer. N Engl J Med 356:1944-1956, 2007.

Lièvre A, Bachet JB, Boige V, et al: KRAS mutations as an independent prognostic factor in patients with advanced colorectal cancer treated with cetuximab. J Clin Oncol 26:374-379, 2008.

Liu S, Ginestier C, Charafe-Jauffret C, et al: BRCA1 regulates human mammary stem/progenitor cell fate. Proc Natl Acad Sci U S A 105:1680-1685, 2008.

Motzer RJ, Hutson TE, Tomczak P, et al: Sunitinib versus interferon alfa in metastatic renal-cell carcinoma. N Engl J Med 356:115-126, 2007.

Schatton T, Murphy GF, Frank NY, et al: Identification of cells initiating human melanomas. Nature 451:345-349, 2008.

Weir BA, Woo MS, Getz G, et al: Characterizing the cancer genome in lung adenocarcinoma. Nature 450:893-898, 2007.

Weir BA, Woo MS, Getz G, et al: Characterizing the cancer genome in lung adenocarcinoma. Nature 450:893-898, 2007.

Chapter 58

Complications of Cancer and Cancer Treatment

Alok A. Khorana and Jennifer J. Griggs

Cancer patients can experience a variety of medical problems related either to the cancer itself or to anticancer therapies. These can include the so-called paraneoplastic syndromes, which occur in cancer patients but cannot be directly attributed to invasion or metastases from the tumor. The management of these various cancer complications requires a multidisciplinary approach.

Cancer-Associated Thrombosis

SIGNIFICANCE

Cancer patients are at increased risk for both venous and arterial thrombotic events, the second leading cause of death. Venous events include deep vein thrombosis (DVT) and pulmonary embolism (PE), together called venous thromboembolism (VTE). Arterial events include stroke and myocardial infarction. VTE can occur in up to one fifth of cancer patients and is associated with decreased survival. The hypercoagulable state in patients with cancer is the result of the activation of the coagulation system by neoplastic cells. Certain cancers, such as pancreas, stomach, lung, and lymphoma, are particularly associated with VTE. Cancer chemotherapy further increases the risk for VTE, as does tamoxifen, which is commonly used in the treatment of breast cancer (see Chapter 57). Other risk factors associated with VTE include central venous catheters, obesity, prior history of VTE, and use of erythropoiesis-stimulating agents. Recent studies have suggested that elevated platelet and leukocyte counts, tissue factor levels, and P-selectin levels may be predictive of VTE. A risk model for VTE has recently been proposed.

CLINICAL PRESENTATION

The suspicion for VTE should be high in patients with cancer who present with dyspnea, cough, wheezing, chest pain, tachycardia, upper abdominal pain, or leg swelling. Even in patients who are ambulatory or on adequate anticoagulation, VTE should remain a consideration. The evaluation of patients with possible VTE is described in Chapter 54. Incidental PE may be identified on imaging studies conducted for staging of cancer, but these continue to be associated with adverse outcomes for cancer patients and should be treated appropriately.

TREATMENT

VTE can be effectively prevented with the use of prophylaxis in the hospitalized cancer patient. Unfractionated heparin, low-molecular-weight heparins (LMWHs), and fondaparinux have all been shown to be effective. Unfortunately, use of thromboprophylaxis continues to be low worldwide and requires a concerted systems-based approach. Cancer patients with established VTE should be treated with anticoagulation. In these patients, oral anticoagulation with warfarin is complicated by interactions with chemotherapeutic agents, variable nutrition status, and relative resistance. LMWHs given for up to 6 months are more effective than warfarin for preventing recurrent VTE in this setting and represent the preferred approach. Vena caval interruption using filters should be considered only in the presence of a clear contraindication to anticoagulation or after failure of LMWH anticoagulation. Chapter 54 addresses the use of anticoagulation therapy.

Febrile Neutropenia

SIGNIFICANCE

Febrile neutropenia (FN) is a common complication of chemotherapy and is defined as a blood neutrophil count lower than 0.5×10^9/L with body temperature higher than 101° F. The risk for infectious complications depends on the severity and duration of neutropenia. FN is associated with increased hospitalization rates, use of broad-spectrum antibiotics, interruption of chemotherapy, increased morbidity, worsened quality of life, and increased mortality.

TREATMENT

Most patients with FN are initially managed in the hospital setting with broad-spectrum antibiotics while awaiting culture data. Antibiotic therapy can subsequently be tailored based on identification of organisms. Myeloid growth factors may be used to hasten neutrophil recovery. Highly selected low-risk patients may be managed in the outpatient setting. The incidence of FN can be reduced with the use of prophylactic growth factors (with or without prophylactic antibiotics) or chemotherapy dose reductions or delay.

Spinal Cord Compression

SIGNIFICANCE

After brain metastases, spinal cord compression is the most common neurologic complication of cancer. About 20,000 patients develop spinal cord compression each year, and most of these patients already have a known diagnosis of a malignant disease. Lung and breast cancers cause about 20% of patients to develop spinal cord compression. Lymphoma, sarcoma, multiple myeloma, and prostate and renal cell cancers each account for 6% to 7% of the patients with spinal cord compression. In only 10% of patients is spinal cord compression the first manifestation of cancer. Although the risk for spinal cord compression in a patient with cancer is only 1%, the effects can be devastating. Early recognition of symptoms and intervention usually prevent a complete loss of motor function.

Most compressive tumors occur at the anterior aspect of the spinal cord. Tumor cells disseminate through the bloodstream to the bone marrow, where they multiply within the vertebral body and eventually extend posteriorly. Tumors cause necrosis and demyelination of predominantly the lateral and posterior white-matter columns. This observation suggests that the obstruction of venous outflow is the cause of the congestion, edema, and hemorrhage within the spinal cord.

CLINICAL PRESENTATION

About 70% of cases of spinal cord compression are thoracic, 20% are lumbosacral, and 10% occur in the cervical region. In 50% of patients, only one vertebral body is involved; in 25% of people, contiguous vertebral bodies are involved. In the remaining patients, multiple noncontiguous vertebral bodies are involved. Most patients complain of back pain that is constant, dull, aching, and progressive. Sneezing, coughing, or neck flexion often exacerbates the pain. In contrast to the pain associated with disk herniation, the pain is usually worse when the patient is in the supine position. Radicular pain may be constant or intermittent and usually localizes to the level of the compression. Bilateral bandlike pain is more common with thoracic disease, whereas unilateral radicular pain is more common with lumbosacral lesions.

Neurologic signs develop insidiously: (1) weakness, particularly exhibiting difficulty with proximal leg function, which causes difficulty in climbing stairs and occurs in about 80% of patients; (2) paresthesias; (3) ataxia, which is the result of proprioceptive impairment; and (4) autonomic dysfunction, including loss of bowel and bladder function. Weakness, sensory loss, ataxia, and autonomic dysfunction can all progress rapidly and may lead to paraplegia if treatment is not rapidly instituted.

DIAGNOSIS

Physical examination usually suggests the diagnosis and may help identify the level of spinal cord involvement. Radiologic tests should initially focus on the suspected area of involvement but should also include a thorough evaluation of the entire spine. The rapidity and severity of symptoms and signs determine how quickly diagnostic tests should be performed.

Plain radiographs are abnormal in 70% of patients with spinal cord compression. Among patients with pain, more than 80% will have abnormal radiographs. Typical radiographic findings include destruction of the pedicle and vertebral body collapse. Magnetic resonance imaging and computed tomography (CT) provide more information than do plain radiographs, and CT scans are superior in evaluating vertebral stability and bone destruction in patients undergoing surgical decompression.

TREATMENT

Loss of ambulation or sphincter function before treatment predicts a poor response to treatment. Goals of treatment are to prevent loss of neurologic function, palliate pain, prevent local recurrence, and preserve spinal stability.

Corticosteroids should be administered immediately. An intravenous bolus of dexamethasone 10 mg, with subsequent doses of 4 to 24 mg every 6 hours, is recommended for most patients. In highly selected patients with a single area of metastatic epidural spinal cord compression, immediate and direct decompressive surgical resection followed by radiation therapy is superior to radiation therapy alone. In patients with multiple sites of spinal cord compression and in those with highly radiosensitive cancers (e.g., lymphoma, multiple myeloma, germ cell tumors), radiation therapy is preferred. Surgical treatment is clearly needed in patients with spinal instability, in those without a histologic diagnosis, and in those who again develop epidural compression after or during radiation therapy.

Superior Vena Cava Syndrome

SIGNIFICANCE

The superior vena cava (SVC) syndrome is the result of obstruction of blood flow caused by compression or invasion of the SVC. The SVC is a thin-walled, low-pressure vessel surrounded by rigid structures that make it vulnerable to metastatic disease in adjacent lymph nodes. The SVC collateral vessels, including the azygos vein and the internal mammary, paraspinous, lateral thoracic, and esophageal veins, lessen the obstruction of flow. The azygos vein is the most important of these collateral vessels; SVC obstruction below the level of the azygos vein is not well tolerated.

Cancer is the cause of SVC syndrome in 65% of patients. Lung cancer is responsible for 80% of these cases, and lymphoma, breast cancer, and germ cell tumors account for most of the others. Nonmalignant causes include mediastinal fibrosis (e.g., histoplasmosis) and thrombosis of central venous catheters and pacemakers.

CLINICAL FINDINGS

Symptoms begin insidiously and are often worse on bending, stooping, or lying down. Symptoms include dyspnea, occurring in 60% to 70% of patients, and facial fullness, which occurs in 50% of patients. Cough, arm swelling, chest pain, and dysphagia may occur. Physical findings include venous distention of the neck and chest wall (60%), facial edema (50%), plethora and cyanosis (each in 20% of patients), and arm edema (10%).

DIAGNOSIS AND TREATMENT

Chest radiography shows mediastinal widening in two thirds of these patients and a pleural effusion in one fourth. A right hilar mass is observed in up to 15% of patients. CT scans can demonstrate the size, shape, and location of a mass; the extent of obstruction; and options for biopsy. Venography is not routinely obtained, but it may show patency of an SVC initially thought to be completely obstructed.

Treatment of the SVC syndrome requires a histologic diagnosis of the tumor before radiation or chemotherapy. Radiation to an occlusive mass can alter the tumor enough to preclude identification of the tumor type. Biopsy of a palpable supraclavicular or cervical node, thoracentesis, sputum cytologic analysis, mediastinoscopy, thoracoscopy, and percutaneous needle biopsy of the obstructing tumor are options for diagnosis.

The goals of treatment are to alleviate the obstruction and to attempt a cure. SVC occlusion does not change the prognosis of the underlying tumor. Small cell lung cancer, lymphoma, and germ cell tumors are best treated with chemotherapy alone or chemotherapy combined with radiation therapy.

Intravascular stents may successfully relieve a venous obstruction, even in patients with SVC thrombus. Percutaneous placement of stents should be considered in patients with severe symptoms requiring urgent relief because this can be done even before tissue diagnosis. Corticosteroids may improve symptoms in patients with cancers that respond to the cytolytic effects of steroids, such as breast cancer, lymphoma, and, occasionally, germ cell tumors. Corticosteroids are not effective in relieving symptoms in patients with lung cancer.

Hypercalcemia

SIGNIFICANCE

Hypercalcemia occurs with all types of cancer but most commonly in multiple myeloma and breast cancer. In patients with extensive osteolytic bone disease, the secretion of the parathyroid hormone–related polypeptide by the tumor, along with other cytokines such as transforming growth factor, interleukin-6, and tumor necrosis factor, causes hypercalcemia. The possibility of hypercalcemia should be considered in all patients with cancer who exhibit a change in mental status.

CLINICAL FINDINGS

The symptoms of hypercalcemia depend less on the absolute serum calcium level than on the time course over which the hypercalcemia develops. Common symptoms are constipation, polydipsia, polyuria, fatigue, nausea, vomiting, and bradycardia. Most patients with hypercalcemia have volume depletion. Patients are often confused and may be obtunded. Muscle stretch reflexes are often hyperactive.

TREATMENT

Treatment of hypercalcemia uses two strategies: increasing urinary calcium excretion and decreasing bone resorption (Table 58-1). Drugs such as thiazide diuretics, those that decrease renal blood flow (e.g., histamine blockers, nonsteroidal anti-inflammatory drugs), calcium-containing drugs, and vitamins A and D should be stopped immediately.

Fluid replacement at a rate of 300 to 400 mL per hour for 3 to 4 hours should be given with frequent monitoring of electrolytes. Such rapid fluid replacement should be seen as rehydration rather than as primary therapy. Drugs that decrease bone resorption should be administered as soon as the patient is rehydrated. Bisphosphonates are the most commonly used antiresorptive drugs; pamidronate, at a dose of 60 to 90 mg, is administered over 2 to 4 hours. The major side effects of pamidronate are fever and myalgias. Finally, furosemide, which inhibits calcium absorption in the thick ascending loop of Henle, is a useful calciuretic agent.

Gallium nitrate is a more potent inhibitor of bone resorption and induces normocalcemia in 70% to 90% of patients. Calcitonin, at a dose of 6 to 8 U/kg intramuscularly every 6 hours for 48 hours, is a weak hypocalcemic agent but has a rapid onset of action. Calcitonin can be used concurrently with pamidronate and gallium. Corticosteroids can be used to treat hypercalcemia caused by hematologic malignancies; patients with breast cancer occasionally respond to steroids.

Patients can be treated as outpatients if (1) the serum calcium concentration is less than 12 mg/dL, (2) they have

---

Table 58-1 **Management of Hypercalcemia**

Outpatient Management of Hypercalcemia

Preferably administer therapy for hypercalcemia with cytotoxic therapy (e.g., chemotherapy, radiation therapy)
Provide clear instructions about oral intake of fluids
Avoid thiazide diuretics; furosemide is acceptable
Administer pamidronate once a week
Administer gallium nitrate subcutaneously daily to minimize rebound hypercalcemia after acute normalization

Inpatient Management of Hypercalcemia

Administer intravenous fluids immediately
Administer antiresorptive therapy once good urine output is established
Administer pamidronate twice every 48-72 hr
Administer gallium nitrate (5-day infusion)
Cross over to another therapy if no response occurs
Administer calcitonin for the comatose patient or for the patient with cardiac irritability
Administer mithramycin for nonresponding patients only
Consider dialysis in patients with renal insufficiency

Table 58-2 **Paraneoplastic Syndromes**		
Syndrome	**Associated Tumors**	**Mechanism**
Ectopic ACTH production	Small cell lung cancer, pancreatic cancer, pheochromocytoma	Tumor secretion of ACTH precursor
SIADH	Lung cancer, head and neck tumors, brain tumors	Ectopic production of antidiuretic hormone
Cerebellar degeneration and peripheral neuropathy	Lung, ovarian, breast cancers, lymphoma (especially Hodgkin disease)	Autoantibodies, including antibodies to Purkinje cells (anti-YO antibodies and anti-Hu antibodies
Opsoclonus-myoclonus	Lung cancer / Neuroblastoma (in children)	No consistent findings; some patients have anti-HU antibodies
Lambert-Eaton myasthenic syndrome	Small cell lung cancer	Antibody production against calcium channels in presynaptic nerve terminal
Erythrocytosis	Renal cell carcinoma, hepatoma	Tumor production of erythropoietin
Thrombophlebitis	Pancreatic cancer, adenocarcinomas	Uncertain

ACTH, adrenocorticotropic hormone; SIADH, syndrome of inappropriate secretion of antidiuretic hormone.

no significant nausea and only mild constipation, (3) they are able to take fluids orally, (4) mentation is intact, (5) creatinine levels are normal, (6) they have a stable cardiac rhythm, and (7) a companion is available to observe them. Immediate inpatient management is indicated in all other situations.

Unless the underlying malignant disease is treated, hypercalcemia will persist or recur. Appropriate management of hypercalcemia therefore requires an attempt to control the cancer itself. Hypercalcemia that responds poorly to the previously discussed measures indicates a poor prognosis.

In patients with metastatic breast cancer undergoing effective treatment, hypercalcemia can develop as part of a treatment flare. Typically, such a response is characterized by bone pain and hypercalcemia, sometimes severe, occurring within 2 to 6 weeks of starting a new therapy. If symptoms are due to successful treatment, resolution typically occurs within 12 weeks. Technetium imaging with a bone scan may show greater activity than at baseline and may even demonstrate new bone lesions.

Paraneoplastic Syndromes

Tumors have disease manifestations through immunologic and metabolic factors that are not the direct result of invasion by neoplastic cells. These *paraneoplastic syndromes* may appear before the diagnosis of cancer is made. Because detection and treatment of the underlying malignant disease may improve the syndrome and occasionally may facilitate cure of the cancer, recognition of paraneoplastic syndromes is important.

Several of the paraneoplastic syndromes are the result of autoantibodies produced in response to the tumor, whereas others are the result of the hormonal production of ectopic peptide by the tumor. Tumor cells may also secrete hormones that are structurally distinct from the normal hormone; some of these are less active biologically than the normal hormone. The most common paraneoplastic syndrome is humoral hypercalcemia of malignancy, a condition usually caused by secretion by the tumor of the parathyroid hormone–related polypeptide. Table 58-2 lists the endocrinologic, neurologic, and hematologic paraneoplastic syndromes. Cutaneous syndromes, such as necrotizing

Table 58-3 **Examples of Long-Term Complications of Cancer Treatment**	
Treatment	**Examples of Long-Term Complications**
Surgery	Loss of vocal function after laryngectomy for laryngeal cancer
	Malabsorption after bowel resection
	Erectile dysfunction and incontinence after radical prostatectomy
	Premature menopause after oophorectomy
	Postmastectomy pain and upper extremity lymphedema
Radiation therapy	Pulmonary fibrosis after mediastinal or lung radiation
	Esophageal stricture after esophageal radiation
	Secondary malignancies (e.g., breast cancer after radiation therapy for Hodgkin disease)
	Chronic breast fibrosis after breast radiation
	Neurocognitive deficits after whole-brain radiation
	Loss of salivary gland function after radiation for cancers of the head and neck
	Premature atherosclerosis after mediastinal radiation
Chemotherapy	Cardiac dysfunction from prolonged exposure to anthracycline treatments
	Peripheral neuropathy from taxanes, cisplatin, and vinca alkaloids
	Ototoxicity from cisplatin
	Pulmonary toxicity from bleomycin
	Secondary leukemia from cyclophosphamide and etoposide
	Premature menopause
Hormonal therapy	Endometrial cancer from tamoxifen
	Thromboembolic events related to tamoxifen
	Loss of bone mineral density related to aromatase inhibitors and luteinizing hormone–releasing hormone agonists

migratory erythema and dermatomyositis, and gastrointestinal syndromes can also occur.

Long-Term Effects of Cancer and Cancer Treatment

People who have been successfully treated for cancer may experience long-term effects of the cancer and its treatment. Surgery, chemotherapy, radiation therapy, hormonal therapy, and biologic therapies can all have adverse effects that persist long after disease control, remission, or cure is achieved. Such long-term sequelae of cancer treatments are increasingly important as the number of cancer survivors increases and as the indications for chemotherapy and radiation broaden. Table 58-3 lists some of the long-term physical complications of cancer therapies.

In addition to the physical effects of cancer treatments, people who have survived cancer face a number of other issues, such as psychological consequences, persistent concerns about cancer recurrence, sexual dysfunction, and employment and insurance discrimination. Although most people can expect to return to their previous activities, most survivors report being affected in at least one of these areas. The impact of cancer on the family, including parents and siblings, partner, and children, persists long after cancer treatment is complete. Most people who have had cancer indicate that the disease and its treatment are life-changing events.

Prospectus for the Future

Advances in the management of cancer are likely to decrease the risk for catastrophic and permanent complications of cancer treatment. Selection of patients who are likely to reap the survival benefits of treatment will decrease the numbers of patients living with the long-term effects of treatment. Similarly, identifying patients at high risk for complications, such as venous thromboembolism, will lead to prevention strategies for those most likely to benefit from such strategies.

References

Khorana AA, Kuderer NM, Culakova E, et al: Development and validation of a predictive model for chemotherapy-associated thrombosis. Blood 111:4902-4907, 2008.

Rugo HS: Paraneoplastic syndromes and other non-neoplastic effects of cancer. In Goldman L, Ausiello DA (eds): Cecil Textbook of Medicine. Philadelphia, Elsevier, 2007.

Patchell RA, Tibbs PA, Regine WF, et al: Direct decompressive surgical resection in the treatment of spinal cord compression caused by metastatic cancer: A randomized trial. Lancet 366:643-648, 2005.

Wilson LD, Detterbeck FC, Yahalom J: Superior vena cava syndrome with malignant causes. N Engl J Med 356:1862-1869, 2007.

Principles of Cancer Therapy

Alok A. Khorana and Barbara A. Burtness

The treatment of cancer is in the midst of a quiet revolution. Chemotherapy continues to be the mainstay of systemic treatment, but the explosion of knowledge regarding cancer biology has allowed research efforts to focus on the development of more specific "targeted" agents. The annual number of new drugs approved for cancer treatment has increased several-fold since the 1990s. In addition, there are now nearly 400 anticancer agents in clinical trials, more than for any other class of medicine. Surgery and radiation therapy techniques continue to be refined, and these are safe and effective treatments for localized cancers. Despite these advances, cancer is still the second-leading cause of death in the United States, and considerable resources are devoted to the palliative care of cancer patients. The treatment of cancer involves multiple disciplines and requires that surgeons and medical and radiation oncologists work in an integrated fashion to deliver the best possible care to the patient. This chapter reviews the principles of surgical, radiation, and medical approaches to cancer at various points during its natural history. Prerequisites to starting treatment, such as diagnosis and staging, as well as supportive care interventions that can improve the safety of cancer treatments, are also discussed.

Diagnosis and Staging

Definitive treatment for cancer must not commence without a histologic diagnosis except under urgent circumstances. This typically involves an invasive biopsy that obtains sufficient material to evaluate morphology, invasiveness of the tumor, and expression of various molecular markers using immunohistochemistry. Noninvasive tests, such as radiologic imaging, are generally not accepted as substitutes for tissue diagnosis. There are occasional exceptions, such as elevated α-fetoprotein levels along with imaging evidence, which can be used to make a diagnosis of hepatocellular carcinoma.

Once the diagnosis of cancer has been made, the next step is to systematically determine the extent of tumor spread, a process called *staging*. Tumor staging can be clinical or pathologic. Staging for some of the solid tumors is described in Chapter 57. *Clinical staging* involves physical examination, and imaging studies including computed tomography scans, whole-body positron-emission tomography scans, radionuclide scans, or a combination thereof. The choice of studies for particular tumors is based on our knowledge of their propensity to spread to particular organs. *Pathologic staging* is more definitive and follows the tumor-node-metastasis (TNM) method developed by the American Joint Committee on Cancer and the International Union against Cancer. This system requires a careful evaluation of the primary resection specimen for three measurements: (1) the size and extent of invasion of the primary tumor (the T score), (2) the number and location of histologically involved regional lymph nodes (the N score), and (3) the presence or absence of distant metastases (the M score). The M score is based on information derived from both clinical and pathologic staging. TNM scores are then grouped into categories of stages from I through IV, reflecting an increasing burden of disease. The final TNM stage has both prognostic and therapeutic implications. For instance, a resected colon cancer that invades the muscularis propria, involves 2 of 16 lymph nodes, but has no evidence of distant metastases is staged as a T2 N1 M0 (stage III) colon cancer. The likelihood of tumor recurrence is 40% to 50%, and the patient is recommended to undergo 6 months of chemotherapy after surgery. On the other hand, if no lymph nodes are involved (T2 N0 M0, stage I), the likelihood of recurrence is less than 10%, and no chemotherapy is recommended.

Biomarkers provide additional prognostic information, such as the absence of hormone receptors or expression of *HER-2* in breast cancer, which are indicative of a poor prognosis. Such markers can also be predictive; for example, presence of *HER-2/neu* predicts for response to trastuzumab, and presence of hormone receptors predicts for response to tamoxifen. Prognostic and predictive biomarkers are available for different cancers, but these are not standardized, and most biomarkers have not been integrated into formal staging. Gene expression signatures that provide prognostic information beyond that already available from formal staging have been identified for certain cancers. A 21-gene signature is commonly used for clinical decision making regarding adjuvant therapy in patients with node-negative, estrogen receptor–positive breast cancer. For certain tumors, measurement of serum levels of tumor markers, such as carcinoembryonic antigen in colon cancer or α-fetoprotein in testicular and liver cancers, can also be of prognostic importance.

An evaluation of the patient's major organ function and other illnesses must also be conducted before treatment can commence. In addition, when the intent of treatment is palliative and not curative, the patient's functional ability, termed *performance status*, must be assessed. This can be done using various history-based methods, such as the Eastern Cooperative Oncology Group or Karnofsky scales. Patients with poor performance status or significant comorbid conditions may not derive a benefit from chemotherapy and are at greater risk for significant adverse events.

Principles of Cancer Surgery

The surgeon is involved in the cancer patient's care at various times: preventing cancer by removal of precancerous lesions or of organs at high risk for cancer (e.g., bilateral mastectomy in those with hereditary defects that can lead to breast cancer); making the diagnosis of cancer by biopsy; providing definitive treatment by removing the primary tumor; assisting in staging by sampling lymph nodes; reconstructing the limb or organ sacrificed; and, finally, providing palliative treatment of cancer (e.g., intestinal bypass for obstruction, cord decompression, or orthopedic procedures to prevent or treat pathologic fractures). Invasive biopsies and certain minor surgical procedures, such as inserting permanent intravenous access devices or temporary feeding tubes, are increasingly being performed by interventional radiologists rather than surgeons.

When cancer is localized, surgery is the most effective curative treatment available. The intent is to completely remove the tumor, regional lymph nodes, and adjacent involved tissue, with a safe margin of normal tissue. At surgery, the tumor is isolated and almost never opened during the procedure. Refinements in cancer surgery include an increasing use of laparoscopic procedures in selected cancers and the identification of a sentinel lymph node by injecting a dye during surgery and foregoing a full lymph node dissection if the sentinel node is uninvolved by cancer.

Principles of Radiation Therapy

More than half of all cancer patients receive radiation therapy at some point during the course of their disease. Radiation therapy can be used as definitive treatment, either alone or in combination with chemotherapy. Unlike surgery, locoregional treatment with radiation can preserve organ structure and function, thereby resulting in enhanced quality of life for patients. For example, use of radiation with chemother-

apy for treatment of localized laryngeal cancer has similar outcomes compared with surgery but allows preservation of the larynx. Radiation therapy is also effective in the palliative setting in relieving many symptoms of advanced cancer, particularly pain.

Ionizing radiation damages cellular DNA directly or indirectly through free radical intermediates. Cells are most susceptible to radiation during the M and G_2 phases of the cell cycle. The aim of radiation therapy is to deliver the highest dose possible to the tumor with minimal toxicity to adjacent normal tissues. Dividing the total planned radiation dose into small daily fractions takes advantage of the difference in repair capability between normal and malignant tissue and improves the tolerance of normal tissue. The biologic effects of radiation can be modified by numerous factors, including the amount of oxygen in the irradiated tissue and the use of chemotherapy for sensitizing tissue to radiation.

The goals of treatment planning for radiation therapy is to precisely define the dose and volume irradiated. The dose of radiation is measured in units of absorbed dose, Gray (Gy), which has replaced the older unit rad (1 Gy = 100 rad). Conventional radiation treatments deliver 1.8 to 2 Gy per day, 5 days per week, over 5 to 6 weeks. For palliative treatment, higher doses per fraction are used to deliver an effective dose over a shorter period of time.

Ionizing radiation can be administered as external-beam therapy using a linear accelerator to generate electrons or high energy x-rays. Electrons have a limited depth of penetration and are useful for superficial tumors. High energy x-rays deliver the radiation deep in the body while reducing the dose to the skin as they enter. Brachytherapy uses radioactive sources to deliver ionizing radiation (gamma rays) directly to the tumor. An example of this is implantation of iodine-125 seeds into the prostate as definitive therapy for early prostate cancer. Current approaches to improving radiation therapy include the use of advanced technology that allows delivery of a higher dose of radiation to specific areas of the tumor and sparing of normal tissue (conformal and intensity-modulated radiation therapy).

Normal tissue response to radiation therapy can be acute or late (Table 59-1). Acute effects occur within days to weeks of irradiation and are seen primarily in rapidly proliferating tissues such as skin and gastrointestinal mucosa. The severity depends on the total dose, but the damage can usually be repaired. Late effects, such as necrosis, fibrosis, or organ failure appear months or years after irradiation and are dependent on fraction size. Another late complication of radiation therapy is the development of secondary malignancies. This has been documented after radiation for breast cancer and Hodgkin disease.

Principles of Medical Therapy

The term *chemotherapy* refers to the use of cytotoxic agents, singly or in combination, for the systemic treatment of cancer. Most such agents are general antiproliferative agents that are more effective against rapidly growing tumors and have significant adverse effects on normal tissues that also

Table 59-1 Acute and Late Effects of Radiation Therapy

Organ	Acute	Late	Dose (Gy) Associated with Adverse Effects
Bone marrow	Aplasia	Leukemia, myelodysplasia	25
Spinal cord	None	Myelopathy	45
Heart	None	Pericarditis, cardiomyopathy, coronary artery disease	45
Rectum	Diarrhea, tenesmus	Stricture, obstruction	60
Eye	Conjunctivitis	Retinopathy	55
Lung	Pneumonitis	Chronic pneumonitis	25

Table 59-2 Commonly Used Chemotherapy Agents

Drug	Cancers Treated	Specific Class/ Mechanism of Action	Common Side Effects
A. Cell Cycle Specific			
5-Fluorouracil	Colorectal and other gastrointestinal, head and neck, breast	Antimetabolite, inhibits thymidylate synthase	Myelosuppression, mucositis, diarrhea
Gemcitabine	Pancreas, lung, breast, bladder	Antimetabolite, deoxycytidine analogue	Myelosuppression, N/V
Methotrexate	ALL, choriocarcinoma, breast, bladder, head and neck, lymphoma	Antimetabolite, folic acid antagonist	Myelosuppression, mucositis, acute renal failure
Doxorubicin	Breast, lung, NHL	Anthracycline, intercalates into DNA	Myelosuppression, N/V, mucositis, cardiomyopathy
Irinotecan	Colorectal, lung	Camptothecin, topoisomerase I inhibitor	Myelosuppression, diarrhea
Paclitaxel	Breast, lung, Kaposi sarcoma, ovarian	Plant alkaloid, inhibits microtubule formation	Myelosuppression, hypersensitivity reaction, sensory neuropathy
Vincristine	ALL, lymphomas, myeloma, sarcoma	Plant alkaloid, disrupts microtubule assembly	Peripheral neuropathy, constipation
B. Cell Cycle Nonspecific			
Cyclophosphamide	Breast, NHL, CLL, sarcoma	Alkylating agent, cross-links DNA	Myelosuppression, hemorrhagic cystitis, N/V, alopecia
Cisplatin	Lung, bladder, ovarian, testicular, cervical, head and neck	Alkylating agent, cross-links DNA	Nephrotoxicity, N/V, myelosuppression, sensory neuropathy

ALL, acute lymphoblastic leukemia, CLL, chronic lymphocytic leukemia; NHL, non-Hodgkin lymphoma; N/V, nausea and vomiting.

divide rapidly, such as bone marrow and digestive tract mucosa. Newer agents, including monoclonal antibodies and signal transduction inhibitors, are directed against targets that are relatively specific to tumor cells and therefore have less toxicity. These drugs are classified separately from chemotherapy as *targeted therapy* agents.

MECHANISMS OF CHEMOTHERAPY

Chemotherapeutic agents can be cell cycle specific or cell cycle nonspecific. Cell cycle nonspecific agents have a greater effect on cells traversing the cell cycle but also affect non-cycling cells whereas cell cycle–specific agents affect only cycling cells. Chemotherapy agents are further classified according to their mechanism of action into alkylating agents, antimetabolites, antitumor antibiotics, and mitotic spindle inhibitors. Commonly used chemotherapy agents and their mechanisms of action, major indications, and common side effects are described in Table 59-2. A prominent side effect of most chemotherapy agents is bone marrow suppression. This, in turn, can lead to infections from neu-

tropenia and life-threatening bleeding from thrombocyto-penia. For most drugs, treatment schedules have been developed whereby successive doses are given every 3 to 4 weeks. This interval between successive doses, called a *cycle* of chemotherapy, allows recovery of blood counts and other side effects before administration of the next dose. The concept of *dose intensity* is also important. Cellular killing with chemotherapy follows first-order kinetics: a given dose of drug kills only a fraction of tumor cells. The dose-response curve for chemotherapy drugs is steep. Thus, the greater the dose administered, the greater the kill: a 2-fold increase in dose can lead to a 10-fold increase in tumor cell kill. Unfortunately, this also means that dose reductions could impact on the eventual cure rate. Arbitrary reductions in doses of chemotherapy to spare patients toxicity should be avoided. Shortening the duration of cycles of chemotherapy using growth factor support, a "dose-dense" approach, has been shown to improve survival in selected patients when compared to traditional chemotherapy for breast cancer.

With rare exceptions, single chemotherapy agents cannot cure cancer. Combination chemotherapy regimens have therefore been developed for a variety of cancers. Combination therapy provides maximal cell kill, broader coverage of resistant cells, and may prevent or slow the development of resistant cells. Drugs used in a combination are chosen based on known efficacy as a single agent but with differing mechanisms of action and nonoverlapping toxicity profiles. These regimens are commonly referred to by acronyms, such as CHOP (cyclophosphamide, doxorubicin, vincristine, and prednisone) for lymphoma or FOLFOX (5-fluorouracil, leucovorin, and oxiliplatin) for colon cancer.

INDICATIONS FOR CHEMOTHERAPY

Chemotherapy is used in localized or advanced cancers for a variety of indications (Table 59-3). *Adjuvant* chemotherapy refers to its use after the primary tumor has been resected. Here, chemotherapy is directed against presumed systemic micrometastases in patients believed to be at high-risk for recurrence. In the example of stage III colon cancer cited previously, 6 months of adjuvant chemotherapy after colonic resection can reduce the patient's likelihood of developing recurrent cancer from 50% to 25%. Adjuvant chemotherapy has been shown to increase cure rates in breast and lung cancers as well. *Neoadjuvant* or *primary* chemotherapy refers to the use of chemotherapy before surgery, sometimes in combination with radiation therapy. If successful, neoadjuvant therapy can reduce the size of the tumor and consequently permit lesser surgery, for example, a lumpectomy instead of a mastectomy in breast cancer, or limb-sparing surgery instead of amputation in extremity sarcoma. In certain tumor sites, such as larynx or anal canal, neoadjuvant therapy can be so successful that it can lead to a complete obliteration of the tumor and avoid the need for surgery altogether. Chemotherapy is most often employed in the treatment of metastatic disease for which surgery or radiation therapy is ineffective. In this setting, chemotherapy can be occasionally curative, such as in certain lymphomas or testicular cancers. Even when it is not curative, however, chemotherapy can often extend survival and improve cancer-related symptoms and the patient's quality of life.

EVALUATION OF RESPONSE

The efficacy of chemotherapy is gauged by various methods and has been granted its own vocabulary. In patients with metastatic disease, all known sites of disease are followed by physical examination and serial radiologic imaging. Responses are judged according to the internationally accepted Response Evaluation Criteria in Solid Tumors (RECIST) rules. Disappearance of all known lesions is called a *complete response*, whereas a 30% or greater reduction in long diameter is called a *partial response*. Appearance of new lesions or an increase in the size of known lesions by 20% is termed *progression* and implies failure of treatment. A tumor that is neither responding nor progressing is termed *stable disease*. The percentage of patients who experience a response is called the *response rate* to the agent or agents being given. New drugs are often evaluated on the basis of response rates. It is important for both patient and physician to realize, however, that a response does not imply cure. A drug with even a 100% response rate is not curative if all patients relapse within, say, 6 months. Therefore, the gold standard for measuring the efficacy of a drug is considered to be an improvement in *survival*, or its surrogate, *disease-free survival*—the time interval when no disease is present. The use of effective second-line therapies may minimize the survival differences between two treatments prescribed as initial therapy, and in this context, disease-free survival can serve as an important endpoint in evaluating new regimens. Increasingly, quality-of-life endpoints such as use of pain medications or analysis of patient-filled questionnaires are being used to assess efficacy of drugs given with palliative intent. In patients receiving adjuvant therapy, response rates cannot be measured because there is no clinically evident disease: disease-free and overall survival rates are the only endpoints of efficacy in this setting. Serial measurement of tumor markers can also be useful in identifying recurrence of cancer and monitoring response to therapy in patients with some cancers.

LIMITATIONS OF CHEMOTHERAPY

Despite the wide use of chemotherapy, it is now understood that it can be curative only under certain circumstances. Several reasons exist for the inability of standard doses of chemotherapy to cure cancer. First, tumor cell kinetics naturally protect against chemotherapy. When chemotherapy was initially developed, it was believed that tumors contained a very high percentage of cells traversing the cell cycle. However, we now know that most human tumors display gompertzian growth kinetics, that is, the rate of tumor cell doubling *slows* progressively as tumor size increases. Thus, the growth fraction of tumors is greatest when a tumor is clinically undetectable. However, when the patient is symptomatic and has clinically evident disease, the growth fraction of tumors is less than 5%. This partly explains why chemotherapy can be successful in the adjuvant setting (when the burden of disease is minimal), but rarely results

---

Table 59-3 **Efficacy of Medical Therapy in Selected Cancers**
Cure Possible in Advanced Setting
Testicular cancer
Acute leukemias: lymphocytic, promyelocytic, selected myelocytic
Lymphomas: Hodgkin, selected non-Hodgkin
Childhood solid tumors: rhabdomyosarcoma, Ewing sarcoma, Wilms tumor
Choriocarcinoma
Small cell lung cancer
Cure Possible in Adjuvant Setting
Breast cancer
Colorectal cancer
Osteosarcoma
Non–small cell lung cancer
Increased Survival and Palliation in Advanced Disease
Colorectal cancer
Breast cancer
Ovarian cancer
Head and neck cancer
Bladder cancer
Small cell lung cancer
Hepatocellular cancer
Renal cancer
Multiple myeloma

in cures in the metastatic setting. Second, cancer cells can be resistant to chemotherapy. One of the most important forms of resistance is intrinsic and is mediated by an evolutionarily conserved cell membrane efflux pump called *P-glycoprotein*. Resistance can also be acquired after a period of exposure to chemotherapy agents by a variety of mechanisms; for example, tumor cells can decrease the uptake of methotrexate by decreasing the expression of the folate transporter, or amplify expression of the target enzyme thymidylate synthase when treated with 5-fluorouracil. Finally, mutations in the *p53* gene are quite common in various cancers. The P53 protein causes cell-cycle arrest and mediates apoptosis when DNA damage occurs. In the absence of a functioning P53, cancer cells are protected from chemotherapy-induced apoptosis.

STEM CELL TRANSPLANTATION

One way of overcoming the limitations of chemotherapy is to increase the dose given to patients. A major obstacle to delivering higher doses, however, is the possibility of life-threatening complications that can result from bone marrow suppression. Stem cell transplantation is a procedure whereby patients are given myeloablative doses of chemotherapy (sometimes with radiation therapy) and then "rescued" with infusions of peripheral blood or bone marrow stem cells that reconstitute the ablated bone marrow. The source of stem cells can be patients themselves (*autologous* transplantation) or a human leukocyte antigen–matched related or unrelated donor (*allogeneic* transplantation). Stem cell transplantation has been shown to improve survival in selected patients with chronic myelogenous leukemia, relapsed Hodgkin and non-Hodgkin lymphoma, refractory acute myelogenous leukemia, and multiple myeloma. Allogeneic transplantations are more successful in inducing cures than autologous transplantations, owing to the immunologic response mounted by the donor cells, termed *graft-versus-malignancy* effect. Newer approaches to stem cell transplantation take advantage of this phenomenon by using lower, nonmyeloablative doses of chemotherapy and relying on the graft-versus-malignancy effect to achieve tumor remissions. However, allogeneic transplantations can only be offered to a minority of patients because of the limited availability of matched donors (particularly in ethnic minorities) and the inability of older patients and those with comorbid illnesses to tolerate this procedure. To increase the availability of donors, umbilical cord blood is increasingly being studied as a source of stem cells. The complications of stem cell transplantation are primarily related to the toxicity of chemotherapy and radiation therapy to vital organs, including lungs and liver. Long-term morbidity and mortality after allogeneic transplantation can result from *graft-versus-host disease* and from complications of immunosuppressive agents used to treat it.

TARGETED THERAPY

The limitations of chemotherapy, coupled with a greater understanding of cancer cell biology, led to the development of a new class of drugs that are directed against targets that are relatively specific to cancer cells. These targets include growth factors and signaling molecules that are essential for proliferation of tumor cells, cell cycle proteins, regulators of apoptosis, and molecules that promote interactions between the tumor and host tissues, such as angiogenesis. Agents developed against these targets are also quite diverse and include monoclonal antibodies directed against cell surface antigens or growth factors, specific or multitargeted receptor tyrosine kinase inhibitors, specific pathway signal transduction inhibitors, antisense oligonucleotides, and gene therapies. Many of these agents are still in drug development. The usual side effects associated with chemotherapy such as myelosuppression, nausea and emesis, and alopecia are not observed with these drugs. However, other unique toxicities are seen. Commonly used targeted therapy agents, their mechanisms of action, major indications, and common side effects are described in Table 59-4.

The best-known targeted therapy agent is imatinib, which inhibits *bcr-abl*, the constitutively active fusion product arising from the Philadelphia chromosome of chronic myelogenous leukemia (CML) as well as *c-kit* (CD117), which is overexpressed in gastrointestinal stromal tumors (GIST) (Fig. 59-1). The daily oral administration of imatinib results in complete hematologic responses in more than 90% of patients in chronic-phase CML, and partial responses in more than 50% of patients with metastatic GIST. Although a major advance over traditional treatment for these malignancies, imatinib is not considered curative in most patients. Drug resistance to imatinib, in the form of a mutation in the kinase domain of *abl* that leads to poor binding of the drug, has been observed.

The success of imatinib as a single agent is unlikely to be replicated in many other malignancies, in which multiple redundant signaling pathways are dysregulated. Increasingly, tyrosine kinase inhibitors with multiple (as opposed to specific) targets are being studied. Sorafenib and sunitinib are two examples of such agents that inhibit various pathways, including vascular endothelial growth factor (VEGF), platelet-derived growth factor, and *c-KIT*. Initial studies have shown these drugs to be effective in renal and liver cancers. Furthermore, targeted therapy drugs can increase the efficacy of chemotherapy through various mechanisms. For instance, bevacizumab, an antiangiogenic agent directed against the proangiogenic VEGF increases both response rates and survival when combined with standard chemotherapy in advanced colon cancer. Similarly, the epidermal growth factor receptor (EGFR) antagonist cetuximab increases the efficacy of irinotecan-based chemotherapy in colon cancer and of definitive radiation therapy for oropharyngeal cancers. The availability of these agents has increased the number of drug combinations that can be used in particular cancers. Multiple combinations of chemotherapy and targeted therapy are now available for the treatment of advanced colon cancer. Correspondingly, median survival of patients with this disease has doubled. Another heartening aspect of targeted therapy agents has been (ironically) their broad applicability because many cancers utilize similar processes for growth and metastasis. For instance, bevacizumab may also be effective in lung and breast cancers.

Despite the excitement surrounding targeted therapy, much work is necessary to understand how and when these agents should be used. An example of how this might be done comes from recent research identifying specific molecular changes in EGFR, which are present in only 10% of lung

Table 59-4 Commonly Used Targeted Therapy Agents

Drug	Cancers Treated	Mechanism of Action	Common Side Effects
A. Monoclonal Antibodies			
Rituximab	NHL	Anti–CD-20	Infusional reaction, tumor lysis syndrome, skin reactions
Tositumomab	NHL	Anti–CD-20 radiolabeled with iodine-131	Infusional reaction, myelosuppression, infections
Bevacizumab	Colorectal, renal, lung, breast	Anti-VEGF	Hypertension, proteinuria, epistaxis, thromboembolism
Cetuximab, panitumumab	Colorectal	Anti-EGFR	Rash
Trastuzumab	Breast	Anti-*HER-2/neu*	Infusional reaction, congestive heart failure
B. Signal Transduction Inhibitors (Oral)			
Imatinib	CML, GIST	Inhibits *bcr-abl* and other receptor tyrosine kinases	N/V, diarrhea, fluid retention, myelosuppression
Erlotinib	Lung, pancreas	Anti-EGFR tyrosine kinase	Rash, diarrhea
Gefitinib	Lung	Anti-EGFR tyrosine kinase	Rash, hypertension, mild N/V
Sunitinib	Renal, GIST	VEGF, PDGF, *c-KIT*	Rash, diarrhea, fatigue
Sorafenib	Liver, renal	VEGF, PDGF, *c-KIT*	Hypertension, fatigue, diarrhea, hand-foot syndrome
Bortezomib	Lymphoma, myeloma	Proteasome inhibitor	Rash, N/V, neuropathy
C. Others			
Tretinoin (all-*trans*-retinoic-acid)	Acute promyelocytic leukemia	Differentiating agent	Vitamin A toxicity, retinoic acid syndrome, hyperlipidemia

CML, chronic myelogenous leukemia; EGFR, epidermal growth factor receptor; GIST, gastrointestinal stromal tumor; NHL, non-Hodgkin lymphoma; N/V, nausea and vomiting; VEGF, vascular endothelial growth factor.

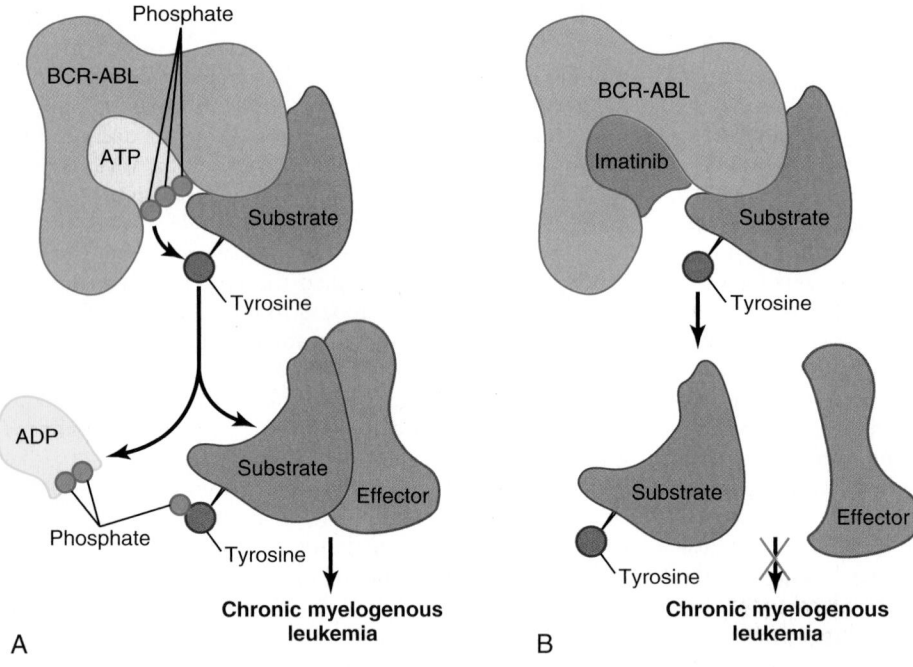

Figure 59-1 Mechanism of action of *bcr-abl* and of its inhibition by imatinib. **A,** The *bcr-abl* oncoprotein with a molecule of adenosine triphosphate (ATP) in the kinase pocket. The substrate is activated by the phosphorylation of one of its tyrosine residues. It can then activate other downstream effector molecules. **B,** When imatinib occupies the kinase pocket, the action of *bcr-abl* is inhibited, preventing phosphorylation of its substrate. ADP, adenosine diphosphate. (Reproduced from Savage DG, Antman KH: Imatinib mesylate: A new oral targeted therapy. N Engl J Med 346:683-693, 2002).

cancer patients. Although gefitinib is ineffective in most lung cancer patients, advanced lung cancer patients with these activating EGFR mutations have an extremely high likelihood of response. Similarly, the EGFR antagonists cetuximab and panitumumab appear to be ineffective in patients with colorectal cancer whose tumors carry mutations in the K-*ras* gene.

ENDOCRINE THERAPY

Cancers originating from tissues that are regulated by hormones, such as breast and prostate, continue to be susceptible to hormonal control mechanisms even when metastatic. Endocrine therapy includes the use of both hormones and antihormonal agents that work as antagonists or partial agonists. Many patients with metastatic breast cancer express hormone receptors (estrogen or progesterone) in tumor cells. More than 60% of these patients respond either to tamoxifen, an estrogen receptor modulator, or to aromatase inhibitors (letrozole, anastrozole, or exemestane), which inhibit adrenal steroid production. Similar responses are observed in men with metastatic prostate cancer treated with the luteinizing hormone–releasing hormone agonists leuprolide or goserelin, which decrease testosterone to castrate levels. In selected breast and prostate cancer patients, metastatic disease can be controlled for years with endocrine therapy only. Tamoxifen and the aromatase inhibitors are also highly effective in the adjuvant treatment of resected breast cancer. Furthermore, tamoxifen has been shown to reduce the incidence of breast cancer by 50% in healthy women at high-risk for developing breast cancer, making it a highly effective chemoprevention agent.

BIOLOGIC THERAPY

A diverse group of cytokines that use host immunomodulatory effects as their primary mechanism of action are classified as *biologic response modifiers* or *biologic agents*. Monoclonal antibodies are sometimes classified as biologic agents, although here they have been reviewed under targeted therapy. Interferons are used most commonly in chronic myelogenous leukemia, although they are not as successful as imatinib in inducing responses. Interferons are also used for the treatment of hairy cell leukemia, Kaposi sarcoma, and selected cases of melanoma and renal cell carcinoma. Interleukin-2 (IL-2) functions as a T-cell growth factor and induces lymphokine-activated and natural killer cell activity. IL-2 can induce responses in 10% to 20% of patients with metastatic melanoma or renal cell carcinoma. In a minority of these patients, responses are complete and last for years. However, IL-2 is associated with considerable toxicity, in particular, a capillary leak syndrome that leads to hypotension, edema, renal insufficiency, and even death.

Supportive Care

Supportive care interventions can improve the safety and tolerability of chemotherapeutic treatments. A diverse array of drugs is available for the treatment of chemotherapy-related side effects. Serotonin receptor antagonists and neurokinin-1 receptor antagonists, in combination with older antiemetic drugs, have made it possible to achieve complete control of chemotherapy-induced nausea and vomiting in nearly all settings. Erythropoietin and darbepoetin stimulate division and differentiation of erythroid precursors and are used for the treatment of chemotherapy-induced anemia. These agents are associated with increased thrombotic complications and, in some studies, with worse outcomes for cancer patients. Granulocyte-colony stimulating factor (filgrastim) and granulocyte-macrophage colony-stimulating factor (sargramostim) stimulate the proliferation and differentiation of myeloid progenitor cells and are used to shorten the duration of chemotherapy-induced neutropenia in patients with neutropenic fever. These agents are also used to mobilize and collect stem cells for transplantation. Filgrastim can also be used to shorten the duration of cycles of chemotherapy, permitting the dose-dense approach in adjuvant treatment of breast cancer discussed previously. Recombinant human keratinocyte growth factor (palifermin) helps protect against chemotherapy and radiation therapy–induced mucositis.

Palliative care is an integral part of the treatment of cancer, particularly in noncurative settings. Palliative aspects of treating cancer address not only physical symptoms, in particular pain syndromes, but also psychosocial and spiritual concerns. It is important to note that chemotherapy and radiation therapy are often employed with palliative intent and can improve quality of life. The oncologist usually provides palliative care along with active therapy for cancer, although end-of-life issues are more appropriately dealt with in a hospice setting.

Prospectus for the Future

Advances in cancer biology and the first wave of targeted therapy agents are just beginning to affect cancer mortality. Many changes in cancer drug development and use are necessary to achieve sustained improvement in cancer outcomes.

Drug Development

Currently, it can take up to $1 billion and 10 years to develop a single new drug. Given the plethora of new agents and limited resources to test them, preclinical validation of drug targets must be improved. The use of RNAi technology as well as development of more sophisticated preclinical models will allow vetting of new agents before they enter clinical trials. More rational selection of patients based on an understanding of the drug target should also accelerate drug development. Many targeted therapies affect processes important for early tumor development, such as angiogenesis. The paradigm of cancer drug development therefore requires change: instead of first testing drugs in patients with advanced and heavily pretreated disease, clinical trials should focus on early-stage cancers. Finally, optimizing clinical trial endpoints so that the efficacy of the drug can be discovered in real-time using biomarkers or functional imaging techniques (such as positron-emission tomography) will hasten the clinical trials process.

Rational Drug Therapy

The selection of agents to treat an individual patient is based primarily on histologic diagnosis and staging. Yet even within a given histologic classification and stage, there is enormous heterogeneity in tumor behavior. Molecular profiling of tumors using newly available genomic and proteomic technology will soon be incorporated into formal staging. This will permit rational, individualized therapy right at the bedside, rather than the one-size-fits-all approach currently being used.

References

Barker AD: Cancer Biomarkers. In Goldman L, Ausiello DA (eds): Cecil Textbook of Medicine. Philadelphia, Elsevier, 2007.

Ciardiello F, Tortora G: EGFR antagonists in cancer treatment. N Engl J Med 358:1160-1174, 2008.

Krause SD, Van Etten RA: Tyrosine kinases as targets for cancer therapy. N Engl J Med 353:172-187, 2005.

Meyerhardt JA, Mayer RJ: Drug therapy: Systemic therapy for colorectal cancer. N Engl J Med 352:476-487, 2005.

Paik S, Shak S, Tang G, et al. A multigene assay to predict recurrence of tamoxifen-treated, node-negative breast cancer. N Engl J Med 351:2817-2826, 2004.

Perry MC: Principles of Cancer Therapy. In Goldman L, Ausiello DA (eds): Cecil Textbook of Medicine. Philadelphia, Elsevier, 2007.

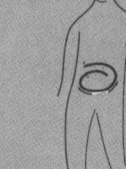

Section XI

Metabolic Disease

Chapter 60

Obesity

Osama Hamdy and Robert J. Smith

Definition and Assessment of Obesity

Obesity is usually defined as a body mass index (BMI) higher than 30 kg/m² (weight [kg]/(height [m])²). A person with a BMI of 25 to 29 is considered overweight. Severe obesity is defined as a BMI of more than 40. The old term *morbid obesity* refers to individuals weighing 45 kg more than desirable body weight (about 100 lb or about 60% above ideal body weight). There is increasing recognition of limitations to the interpretation of BMI, especially in individuals who are muscular or have a low BMI. Many clinicians prefer, at least conceptually, to define obesity not strictly by BMI but as an excess of body fat sufficient to confer risk. However, the BMI value is still useful for estimating overall health risks of obesity and comparing outcomes between clinical trials.

Population data in the United States indicate that adverse health consequences increase progressively with a BMI at or above 27 kg/m². In considering the cardiometabolic risk of obesity, individuals who accumulate visceral fat and have higher waist circumferences are at much higher risk for cardiovascular disease than those with the same BMI or a similar percentage of body fat but lower waist circumferences. The National Cholesterol Education Program Adult Treatment Panel III (ATP III) has included a waist circumference greater than 40 inches (102 cm) in American men and 35 inches (88 cm) in American women among five criteria that define the cardiometabolic syndrome. As an alternative mode of assessment, central and probably visceral obesity is likely with a waist-to-hip circumference ratio greater than 1 in men and 0.6 in women. Dual-energy x-ray absorptiometry and abdominal computed tomography or magnetic resonance imaging can be used to quantify visceral obesity, but these measurements typically are used in research studies and are not routine in clinical care.

Epidemiology of Obesity

During the past 20 years, the prevalence of overweight and obesity has increased sharply for both adults and children in the United States. Comparison of data from two National Health and Nutrition Examination Survey (NHANES) reports shows that among adults aged 20 to 74 years, the prevalence of obesity increased from 15% in the 1976-1980 survey to 32.9% in 2003-2004. According to the U.S. Centers for Disease Control and Prevention, after a quarter century of increases, obesity prevalence has stabilized, but levels are still high at 34% of U.S. adults older than 20 years in 2007. Because the adverse consequences of obesity develop over multiple years, it can be expected that the complications of obesity will continue to increase in prevalence. Overweight and obesity and their associated health problems have a significant economic impact on the U.S. health care system, accounting for about 9% of total medical expenditures. An epidemic of obesity and its complications similar to that in the United States is occurring throughout the world.

Pathogenesis of Obesity

Obesity exemplifies a genetic-environment interaction in which genetically prone individuals who lead a sedentary lifestyle and consume a larger amount of food are particularly at risk. Children of obese parents are 80% more likely to become obese through the combined effects of genetic and shared environmental factors.

In considering genetic factors, obesity may result from the effects of a single gene or the effects of multiple genes acting in concert. An example of a single gene defect is leptin deficiency. Leptin is a hormone produced in fat cells and is a potent inducer of satiety. Rare individuals with inactivating leptin mutations have been identified. They are characterized by increased food seeking and marked obesity, which can be substantially ameliorated by the administration of leptin. Mutations in a number of other genes that encode appetite regulatory proteins also have been identified as causes of obesity. However, these monogenic causes of obesity are rare, and the genes that contribute to common forms of human obesity have not yet been clearly identified. In addition to appetite regulation, there appears to be a heritable component associated with metabolic rate, spontaneous physical

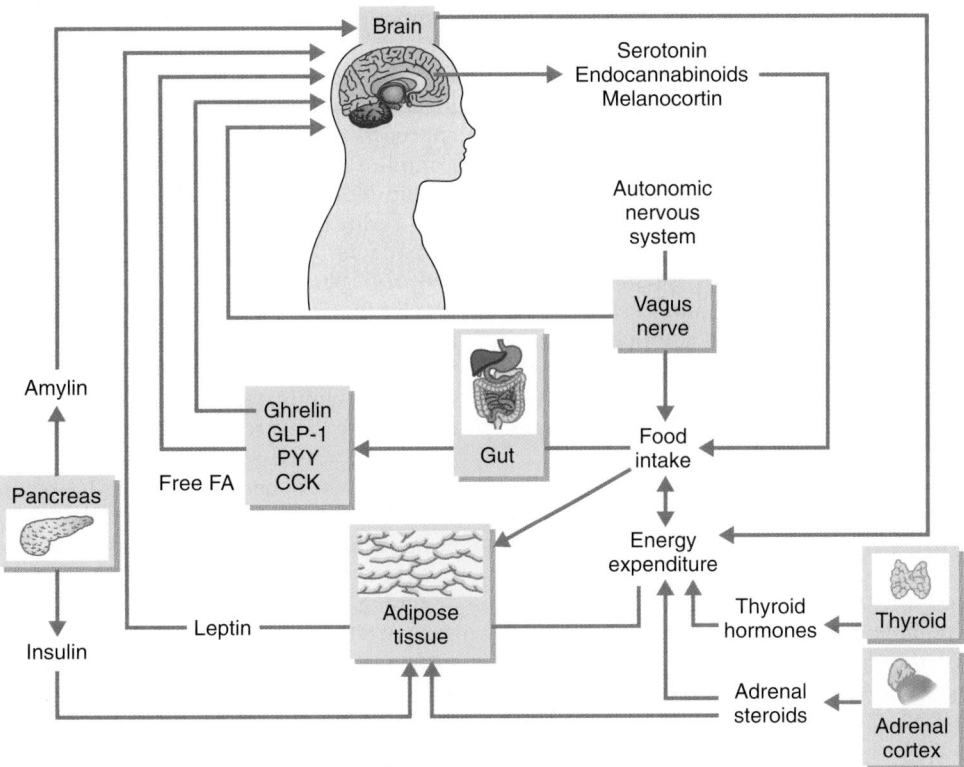
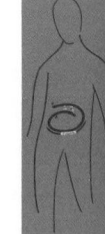

Figure 60-1 Hormonal and neurogenic control of appetite and food intake. CCK, cholecystokinin; FA, fatty acid; GLP-1, glucagon-like peptide-1; PYY, peptide YY.

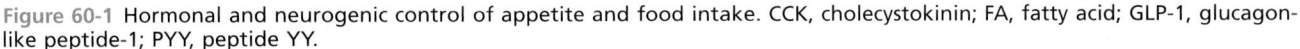

activity, and thermal responses to food. Polymorphisms in several candidate genes, including the melanocortin-4 receptor, the β₃-adrenergic receptor, and peroxisome proliferator–activated receptor-γ2 (PPAR-γ2), have been linked in population studies to obesity. Genome-wide association scans recently have identified additional genes linked to obesity, and it is thought that genetic risk in most individuals derives from the synergistic or additive effects of multiple genes. Although the specific genetic factors still are not well understood, the heritability of obesity clearly is evident in twin and adoptee studies, in which obese individuals generally follow the weight pattern of their identical twins and biologic parents even when raised apart.

Many hormones, neurotransmitters, and neurogenic signals affect appetite and food intake, as shown in Figure 60-1. Endocannabinoids increase appetite, enhance nutrient absorption, and stimulate lipogenesis. Melanocortin hormone, through its effect on several receptors, modifies appetite. Multiple gut hormones play significant roles in inducing satiety, including glucagon-like peptide-1 (GLP-1), peptide YY (PYY), and cholecystokinin. Leptin and pancreatic amylin are other potent satiety hormones. On the other hand, ghrelin, which is secreted from the stomach fundus, functions as an orexigenic or hunger-inducing hormone.

Although the genetic determinants of obesity clearly are significant, it is important to recognize the equal influence of environmental and socioeconomic factors. Lower socioeconomic status, lower education level, cessation of smoking, and consumption of high glycemic index carbohydrates all are associated with increased prevalence of obesity. The current worldwide epidemic of obesity undoubtedly is driven by changes in environmental and socioeconomic factors operating on a relatively stable background of genetic influences within a given population.

Pathogenesis of Obesity-Associated Risk

Recent evidence indicates that adipocytes in fat tissue function as an endocrine organ, producing secretory products with a major role in whole-body metabolism. The relationship of obesity to insulin resistance and endothelial dysfunction (the early stage of atherosclerosis) is mediated through the release of several hormones from adipose tissue. These hormones, designated adipocytokines or adipokines, include adiponectin, leptin, tumor necrosis factor-α (TNF-α), interleukin-6 (IL-6), resistin, plasminogen activator inhibitor-1 (PAI-1), angiotensinogen, and monocyte chemoattractant protein-1 (MCP-1). Many of these factors have actions that are proinflammatory or alter blood coagulation. Their production is influenced by both the overall amount of adipose tissue and its distribution between central and peripheral body regions. The differences in adipokine gene expression between visceral and subcutaneous fat likely have an important role in the high cardiometabolic risk of visceral obesity.

Risks Associated with Obesity

Overweight and obese individuals are at increased risk for multiple clinical disorders. A partial list of obesity-related conditions is provided in Table 60-1. Obese individuals often manifest more than one of these disorders, and such secondary consequences of obesity account for much of the morbidity and mortality of the obese state. The "metabolic syndrome" as defined by a National Cholesterol Education Program Expert Panel refers to a state of particularly high cardiometabolic risk that characterizes individuals with at least three of five individual risk factors: abdominal obesity (waist circumference >40 inches in men and >35 inches in women), glucose intolerance (fasting plasma glucose ≥100 mg/dL), hypertension (≥130/≥85 mm Hg), elevated plasma triglycerides (≥150 mg/dL), and low high-density lipoprotein (HDL) cholesterol (<40 mg/dL in men and <50 mg/dL in women). Even modest weight loss (7% to 10% of body weight) can result in substantial reduction in many if not all of these risks.

Treatment of Obesity

Current guidelines for treatment approaches to obesity are summarized in Table 60-2. The major options are lifestyle modification (diet and exercise), behavior modification, pharmacologic intervention, and bariatric surgery. In general, a combination of approaches is more effective than a single modality.

LIFESTYLE MODIFICATION

Managing overweight and obesity by lifestyle modification requires a multidisciplinary strategy and teamwork. Key components include a structured dietary intervention and a physical activity program. Evidence-based dietary guidelines should be used to design individualized patient plans in consultation with a registered dietitian. As a general approach, daily caloric intake initially should be reduced by a modest 250 to 500 calories. Calories from carbohydrate should be decreased to about 40 percent of total calories, with a daily intake of no less than 130 g carbohydrate. Except in patients with renal impairment (creatinine clearance <60 mL per minute) or significant microalbuminuria, protein may represent 20% to 30% of daily caloric intake to minimize lean mass loss during weight reduction. The remaining 30% of calories should come from fat. *Trans*-fats should be eliminated, and saturated fat should be reduced to 7% to 10% of total fat calories. Meal plans should also include increased soluble fiber (e.g., from fresh fruits and vegetables) and healthy carbohydrate consumption, especially foods with a low glycemic index. Caloric intake should be adjusted progressively as needed until weight loss is achieved. Underlying all these steps should be the goal of designing individualized plans that can be maintained over the long term. Many patients find it helpful to receive a structured dietary intervention that includes specific suggestions for daily meals. This may increase adherence and can be easier to follow than a list of general guidelines. Nutritionally complete meal replacement (e.g., in the form of shakes or bars) can be useful for some patients at the start of the weight reduction program.

Patients should meet with an exercise physiologist to construct an individualized plan that is responsive to their capabilities and lifestyle. A balanced exercise plan will incorporate a mix of cardiovascular, stretching, and strength exercises, and it should be graded to increase gradually in both duration and intensity. Patients can start with 10 to 20 minutes of daily stretching and aerobic exercise, with a gradual increase as tolerated. Any exercise should be preceded by a warm-up period to minimize injuries. Cardiovascular evaluation and oversight during implementation of exercise (e.g., through a cardiac rehabilitation program) should be considered based on individual risk. Current guidelines recommend an ultimate goal of 60 to 90 minutes of daily exercise, with a minimum of 150 to 175 minutes per week for weight loss benefits to be realized. Emphasis should be placed on moderate-intensity exercise, such as walking 20-minute miles, rather than strenuous exercise. Because patients who are not accustomed to exercising may find it difficult to incorporate physical activity into daily practice, it is also important to emphasize variety of exercises to avoid boredom.

Table 60-1 **Clinical Conditions Associated with Obesity**
Diabetes mellitus
Dyslipidemia
Hypertension
Ischemic heart disease
Stroke
Reproductive dysfunction
Cholelithiasis
Gastroesophageal reflux disease
Sleep apnea
Degenerative arthritis
Cancer (endometrial, breast, prostate)
Incontinence (women)

Table 60-2 Guide to Selecting Treatment Based on Body Mass Index

Treatment	Body Mass Index				
	25-26.9	27-29.9	30-34.9	35-39.9	≥40
Diet, physical activity, behavior therapy	Yes with comorbidities	Yes with comorbidities	Yes	Yes	Yes
Pharmacotherapy		Yes with comorbidities	Yes	Yes	Yes
Weight-loss surgery				Yes with comorbidities	Yes

"Yes" indicates that the treatment is indicated regardless of comorbidities.
Data from NIH/NHLBI/NAASO. October 2000, NIH Publication No. 00-4084.

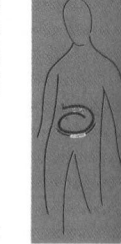

BEHAVIOR MODIFICATION AND PATIENT EDUCATION

Cognitive-behavioral intervention and patient education are important components of successful weight loss programs. Whenever possible, cognitive-behavioral intervention should be conducted by an experienced psychologist. The fundamental principals of intervention should include behavioral goal setting, stimulus control techniques, cognitive restructuring, assertive communication skills, stress management, and relapse prevention. Cognitive behavioral support conducted in a group setting with weekly meetings is frequently successful. Patients should learn how to set realistic goals for weight loss over a specific period of time. They also should receive guidance and support in dealing with specific challenges, such as social eating, coping with craving, and managing relapses.

PHARMACOLOGIC OPTIONS

Three antiobesity drugs—sibutramine, orlistat, and phentermine—are approved for use in the United States. Only sibutramine and orlistat are approved for long-term use. Rimonabant, an endocannabinoid receptor antagonist, is used in many countries but has not been approved in the United States because of concern about its common psychiatric side effect of depression. A recent meta-analysis of 30 placebo-controlled trials of 1 to 4 years' duration has provided evidence for significant weight loss with sibutramine (4.2 kg average weight loss, 10 studies, 2623 participants), orlistat (2.9 kg, 16 studies, 10,631 participants), and rimonabant (4.7 kg, 4 studies, 6365 participants).

Sibutramine

Sibutramine is an oral serotonin- and noradrenaline-reuptake inhibitor that controls appetite by inducing satiety. Sibutramine-assisted weight loss has been accompanied by improved serum concentrations of triglycerides, but adverse effects of lowered concentrations of HDL cholesterol and increased blood pressure and pulse rate. It therefore is recommended that blood pressure be monitored during sibutramine treatment. There typically is a gradual rebound of weight gain on discontinuation of sibutramine.

Orlistat

Orlistat limits caloric intake through inhibition of the lipase-mediated breakdown of fat in the gastrointestinal tract. This typically decreases fat absorption by about 30% and increases fecal fat content. In addition to its weight loss effect, there is evidence that orlistat can decrease the incidence of diabetes, improve concentrations of total and low-density lipoprotein (LDL) cholesterol, and improve blood pressure and glycemic control in patients with diabetes. Conversely, HDL cholesterol may be slightly lowered by orlistat, and there is an increased risk for cholelithiasis. Most patients develop some degree of side effects that range from diarrhea, flatulence, oily stools, and fecal urgency to fecal incontinence (rare). Gastrointestinal side effects are usually proportional to the amount of fat intake. Possible deficiency of fat-soluble vitamins A, D, E, and K mandates their routine supplementation in patients on orlistat. The usual dose of orlistat is 120 mg before each meal. A 60-mg dose is currently available over-the-counter. This dose is less effective but is associated with fewer adverse side effects.

Phentermine

Phentermine is approved for the short-term treatment of obesity. In addition to appetite suppression, it can cause elevated blood pressure, increased heart rate, and insomnia, owing to its sympathomimetic properties. Combining phentermine with tricyclic antidepressants or monoamine oxidase inhibitors may result in a marked increase in blood pressure and other serious side effects because of elevated serotonin levels.

BARIATRIC SURGERY

Bariatric surgery involves the use of one of several different techniques to modify the gastrointestinal tract in a manner that results in a decrease in calorie intake or absorption. The most common bariatric surgical procedures in the United States at present are Roux-en-Y gastric bypass (RYGB) and laparoscopic placement of an adjustable gastric band (LAGB) (Fig. 60-2). The number of bariatric procedures performed in the United States has increased about 15-fold over the past 10 years to nearly 200,000 in 2007. Bariatric surgery is indicated for individuals with a BMI of more than 40 kg/m² or with a BMI of more than 35 kg/m² plus high-risk comorbid conditions, such as severe sleep apnea, obesity-related cardiomyopathy, or uncontrolled type 2 diabetes. Bariatric surgery is not uniformly a low-risk procedure, and judicious patient selection and diligent perioperative care are mandatory. Contraindications include high operative risk (e.g., severe congestive heart failure or unstable angina), active substance abuse, and significant psychopathology.

LAGB is associated with substantially better maintenance of weight loss than lifestyle intervention alone and carries a very low operative mortality rate (0.1%). As a less invasive procedure than RYGB, it may be preferred in patients older than 55 years. LAGB is associated with significantly less loss of fat-free mass, but less excess weight loss than RYGB at 5 and 10 years. Complications associated with LAGB include band slippage, band erosion, balloon failure, port malposition, band and port infections, and esophageal dilation. Overall, complication and mortality rates are much lower for LAGB than those observed with RYGB.

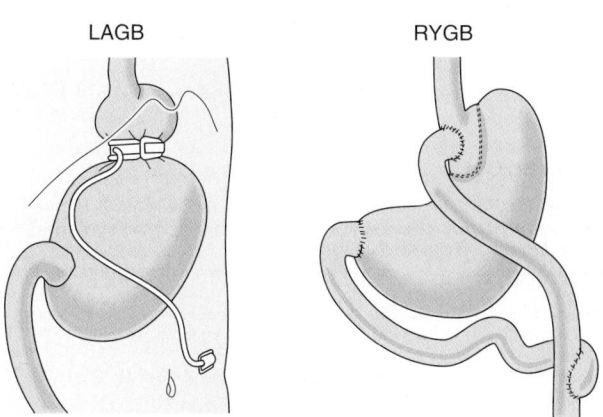

Figure 60-2 Common bariatric procedures. LAGB, laparoscopic adjustable gastric band; RYGB, Roux-en-Y gastric bypass.

RYGB is currently the most commonly performed bariatric procedure in the United States. In RYGB, the upper stomach is transected, creating a very small proximal gastric pouch with a capacity of 10 to 30 mL. The gastric pouch is anastomosed to a Roux-en-Y proximal jejunal segment, bypassing the remaining stomach, duodenum, and a small portion of jejunum. The operative mortality rate for RYGB is 0.5%. The resulting foregut bypass appears to have benefits beyond just calorie intake reduction and weight loss. These include improvement in the physiologic responses of gut hormones involved in glucose regulation and appetite control, such as ghrelin, GLP-1, and PYY. Mechanical improvements from decreased adiposity include less weight bearing by lower extremity joints and improved lung compliance and reduced fatty tissue around the neck, which relieves obstruction to breathing and sleep apnea.

A meta-analysis of 22,000 bariatric surgery patients demonstrated an average excess body weight loss of 61% accompanied by significant improvements in type 2 diabetes, hypertension, sleep apnea, and dyslipidemia. The beneficial effect of obesity surgery on type 2 diabetes is one of the most important outcomes, with resolution of diabetes in most patients (range, 40% to 100% of patients in various studies). Independent predictors of diabetes reversal following bariatric surgery include selection of RYGB as the bariatric procedure, a shorter duration of diabetes, and greater weight loss after surgery. Insulin-treated patients usually experience significant decreases in insulin requirements, and improvements in fasting blood glucose levels often occur before significant weight loss. Most type 2 diabetic patients are able to discontinue insulin therapy by 6 weeks after surgery, and euglycemia has been maintained up to 14 years after RYGB.

It is important to recognize that the altered gastrointestinal dynamics of gastric bypass surgery result in substantial risk for developing deficiencies of vitamins and minerals, including iron, calcium, vitamin B_{12}, vitamin D, and other fat-soluble vitamins. Supplements of multivitamins, iron, and calcium should be provided postoperatively, and there should be periodic screening for acquired deficiencies. Inadequate protein intake and absorption may occur after RYGB and lead to protein malnutrition. An infrequent but serious complication of RYGB that recently has been recognized is hyperinsulinemic hypoglycemia, which appears to result from induced changes in pancreatic β-cell mass and insulin secretion. This requires careful diagnostic evaluation to confirm hyperinsulinemia and rule out insulinoma. Affected patients may be responsive to diet modifications (frequent, low carbohydrate feedings), but when symptoms are severe, patients may require partial or total pancreatectomy.

Prognosis

Although a small percentage of obese individuals are able to achieve and maintain weight loss for a long period after nonsurgical intervention, most regain weight over the following months or years. Weight regain even after bariatric surgery is not uncommon, with regain occurring typically after reaching maximum weight loss about 2 years after surgery. Weight reduction of 10% to 20% in an obese individual from any intervention results in a decrease in total and resting energy expenditure, and this may prevent further weight loss at a given level of reduced calorie intake. In considering the underlying causes of obesity, there currently is substantial support for the concept of a biologic set point or control mechanism that may target a body weight in the overweight or obese range. Whether the set point is determined by genetic or environmental factors, this concept lends support to the theory that behavior is not the sole determinant of obesity. Further understanding of the genetic and hormonal regulation of obesity and their roles in establishing a functional set point may help in creating long-lasting and effective treatment strategies.

Prospectus for the Future

- The fundamental behavioral, environmental, and genetic determinants of appetite, satiety, and obesity will be better understood.
- New medications will be developed that more effectively modulate appetite and satiety control mechanisms, likely with a greater emphasis on the use of multiple medications in combination.

- The environmental factors promoting obesity, including influences on food choice and total calorie intake, will be better understood and will need to be addressed as population-level determinants of obesity.

References

Angrisani L, Lorenzo M, Borrelli V: Laparoscopic adjustable gastric banding versus Roux-en-Y gastric bypass: 5-year results of a prospective randomized trial. Surg Obes Relat Dis 3:127-134, 2007.

Bosello O, Zamboni M: Visceral obesity and metabolic syndrome. Obes Rev 1:47-56, 2000.

Centers for Disease Control and Prevention: State-specific prevalence of obesity among adults—United States, 2005. MMWR Morb Mortal Wkly Rep 55:985-988, 2006.

Farooqi IS, O'Rahilly S: Genetics of obesity in humans. Endocr Rev 27:710-718, 2006.

Hamdy O, Carver C: The Why WAIT program: Improving clinical outcomes through weight management in type 2 diabetes. Curr Diab Rep 8:413-420, 2008.

Hamdy O: The role of adipose tissue as an endocrine gland. Curr Diab Rep 5:317-319, 2005.

Kushner RF, Manzano H: Obesity pharmacology: Past, present, and future. Curr Opin Gastroenterol 18:213-220, 2002.

Maggard MA, Shugarman LR, Suttorp M, et al: Meta-analysis: Surgical treatment of obesity. Ann Intern Med 142:547-559, 2005.

Neovius M, Johansson K, Russner S: Head-to-head studies evaluating efficacy of pharmacotherapy for obesity: A systematic review and meta-analysis. Obes Rev 9:420-427, 2008.

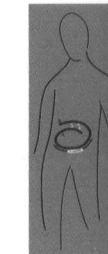

Anorexia Nervosa and Bulimia Nervosa

Michelle P. Warren

norexia nervosa is characterized by a classic triad of amenorrhea, weight loss, and psychiatric disturbance. The *Diagnostic and Statistical Manual of Mental Disorders* further defines criteria for anorexia as weighing less than 85% of ideal body weight and having missed at least 3 consecutive menstrual periods (Table 61-1). Anorexic patients are subdivided into those who just restrict food and those who purge. In addition, these patients may be hyperactive and exercise compulsively. There is a relatively high incidence of anorexia in athletes, particularly in groups in which there is an advantage to be thin, such as ballet dancers and gymnasts. Diabetic patients with anorexia nervosa may purposefully avoid good control in order to initiate weight loss. Bulimia nervosa is often related to previous anorectic behavior and is characterized by gorging followed by periods of severe food restriction. Unusual means are employed to lose weight, including vomiting and abuse of diuretics or laxatives. Weight may fluctuate, generally not to dangerously low levels, but many associated metabolic problems cause serious health issues. Bulimia is often associated with impulsive behavior, alcohol or drug use, promiscuity, and stealing or shoplifting.

Prevalence

The prevalence of these disorders has been increasing, with the lifetime prevalence of anorexia nervosa in women at 0.3% to 1%, and prevalence rates of 1% to 1.5% for bulimia in the United States. An even larger number of women (3% to 5%) have disordered eating that does not fulfill strict criteria for anorexia nervosa or bulimia nervosa, but instead meets criteria for an eating disorder "NOS" (not otherwise specified). All these conditions are much more common in women, with a ratio favoring females of 10:1 for anorexia. Although bulimia is more common in men than anorexia, most patients with this disorder are also women, with an incidence of 2% in female community-based samples and 4% to 13% in college-aged women. The physical consequences of extreme caloric restriction (<85% of ideal body

weight) or the metabolic insults resulting from overexercise or rarely bulimia include hypothalamic amenorrhea, low peak bone mass, bone loss, stress fractures, and infertility. The diagnostic criteria for anorexia nervosa and bulimia nervosa are summarized in Table 61-1.

Anorexia Nervosa

CLINICAL FEATURES

There is no blood test or specific physical finding that establishes the diagnosis of anorexia nervosa. Rather, the diagnosis is based on a symptom complex that includes severe weight loss and behavioral changes such as hyperactivity or preoccupation with food. There typically are perceptual changes with a distorted view of the body and generally an unreasonable concern about being too fat. Food intake may include large amounts of raw vegetables and diet soda, with avoidance of fat and meat. Most female patients present with amenorrhea, and this may be the first complaint to bring the patient to a physician. Constipation may be extreme, with bowel movements once a week and accompanying abdominal pain. Intolerance to cold is common, as are dry skin and hair loss. Lanugo-type hair may be present on the body. Hypercarotenemia may give a yellowish tinge to the skin. Petechiae, pedal edema, and acrocyanosis can occur. Bradycardia, hypotension, and hypothermia are common. Laboratory tests can be normal, but leukopenia accompanied by a relative lymphocytosis is common. Azotemia may develop secondary to dehydration; electrolyte abnormalities, including hyponatremia, hypokalemia, and hypophosphatemia, may occur; there may also be hypoglycemia. Typical endocrine abnormalities include hypothalamic amenorrhea characterized by low gonadotropins (especially luteinizing hormone) and also hypoestrogenism when amenorrhea is present. Low leptin and high ghrelin levels not infrequently are observed in anorexia nervosa. It is thought that these peptides, secreted by the adipose tissue and small bowel, respectively, serve as signals reflecting nutritional status and

Table 61-1 Diagnostic Features of Anorexia Nervosa and Bulimia Nervosa

Anorexia Nervosa

A. Refusal to maintain body weight at or above a minimally normal weight for age and height (e.g., weight loss leading to maintenance of body weight less than 85% of that expected; or failure to make expected weight gain during period of growth, leading to body weight less than 85% of that expected)
B. Intense fear of gaining weight or becoming fat, even though underweight
C. Disturbance in the way in which one's body weight or shape is experienced, undue influence of body weight or shape on self-evaluation, or denial of the seriousness of the current low body weight
D. In postmenarchal females, amenorrhea (i.e., the absence of at least three consecutive menstrual cycles; a woman is considered to have amenorrhea if her periods occur only after hormone, e.g., estrogen, administration)

Bulimia Nervosa

A. Recurrent episodes of binge eating. An episode of binge eating is characterized by both of the following:
  1. Eating, in a discrete period of time (e.g., within any 2-hour period), an amount of food that is definitely larger than most people would eat during a similar period of time and under similar circumstances
  2. A sense of lack of control over eating during the episode (e.g., a feeling that one cannot stop eating or control what or how much one is eating)
B. Recurrent inappropriate compensatory behavior in order to prevent weight gain, such as self-induced vomiting; misuse of laxatives, diuretics, enemas, or other medications; fasting; or excessive exercise
C. Binge eating and inappropriate compensatory behaviors that occur, on average, at least twice a week for 3 months
D. Self-evaluation unduly influenced by body shape and weight
E. Disturbance that does not occur exclusively during episodes of anorexia nervosa

From American Psychiatric Association: Diagnostic and Statistical Manual of Mental Disorders, 4th ed. Washington, DC, American Psychiatric Association, 1994, pp 549-550.

in turn appropriateness for reproductive function. Low T_4 and T_3 with normal thyroid-stimulating hormone can occur, and serum cortisol levels may be high as a consequence of decreased clearance and prolonged half-life. Diurnal variation of cortisol still occurs, but at a higher set point. Insulin-like growth factor type I levels usually are low, and this may contribute to growth compromise in young patients. Numerous associated medical problems may occur, including hypoglycemia with coma, cardiac arrest, liver dysfunction, pancreatitis, and kidney stones. By far the most ubiquitous and persistent problem is osteoporosis, which may be accompanied by fractures (especially stress fractures in patients who exercise heavily). The fractures until recently were believed to be secondary to hypoestrogenism, but recent work indicates that the problem is nutritional in origin and will not reverse with estrogen or oral contraceptives.

TREATMENT AND PROGNOSIS

Patients with a body mass index of less than 18 should be evaluated by both a medical physician and a psychiatrist or psychologist with experience in eating disorders. Patients who continue to lose weight, have complicating medical problems, or weigh less than 75% of ideal should be considered for inpatient treatment. Younger patients with intense family therapy can sometimes be managed as outpatients. Parenteral nutrition may be necessary in some patients to initiate weight gain and prevent severe medical problems. Because the mortality rate of anorexia nervosa is high (10%), the patient may need intensive monitoring in a specialized unit.

Most of the endocrine abnormalities resolve promptly with weight gain, but amenorrhea may take up to a year to resolve after recovery and may persist in up to 30% of patients. Osteoporosis and osteopenia will improve, and the occurrence of new fractures will decrease in proportion to BMI increases. Hormone replacement or oral contraceptives can be used if the amenorrhea persists. The return of menses is a hallmark of recovery, though this indicator will be lost in patients taking oral contraceptives. The recurrence rate of anorexia nervosa is high (up to 30%). In some patients, anorexia is chronic or, with partial improvement, takes the form of "eating disorder not otherwise specified." If infertility is an issue in weight-recovered patients, induction of ovulation often is successful with injectable gonadotropins or, in some cases with adequate estrogen secretion, oral clomiphene citrate. Ovulation has been induced by the administration of leptin in hypothalamic amenorrhea in an experimental protocol, and the administration of pulsatile gonadotropin-releasing hormone is effective but not currently available.

Bulimia Nervosa

CLINICAL FEATURES

The purge-gorge syndrome of bulimia may occur alone, but more commonly the bulimic behavior evolves from a restrictive anorexia nervosa–type syndrome. Thus, the medical problems induced by purging and gorging may be superimposed on the clinical abnormalities associated with anorexia. Bulimia patients often are secretive about their behavior and thus may be difficult to diagnose in the absence of weight loss or menstrual irregularity. Problems resulting from bulimia include severe tooth decay, parotid enlargement, stomach rupture, metabolic alkalosis, carpopedal spasm, hypercarotenemia, subcutaneous emphysema, pneumomediastinum, and pancreatitis. Evidence exists for hormonal defects in gonadotropin-releasing hormone and cholecystokinin regulation. The incidence of menstrual irregularity is highly variable, and patients with bulimia may have anovulation with normal estrogen secretion. Body weight also is variable and generally normal. Most associated medical problems are due to the vomiting, although hypokalemia has been seen with diuretic abuse, and myopathic weakness and electrocardiographic abnormalities are from ipecac abuse.

TREATMENT AND PROGNOSIS

Bulimia is often associated with depression, drug and alcohol abuse, and antisocial behavior such as stealing and promiscuity. All these problems need to be treated with appropriate psychiatric therapy as well as interventions to address drug dependency when it is present. Antidepressants have been used with variable success, and cognitive behav-ioral therapy may be effective. Bulimia has a high rate of chronicity and relapse (30%), although risk for relapse declines after 4 years. Long-term therapy is usually required, and fortunately, mortality is low.

Prospectus for the Future

- Identification of the molecular mechanism of bone loss in anorexia nervosa, which could lead to appropriate pharmacologic intervention when there is resistance to weight gain and the occurrence of fractures
- Development of tests that better assess bone quality and identify patients at risk for fracture

- Identification of genes that predispose to anorexia and bulimia nervosa
- Development of pharmacologic interventions that better control bulimic behavior and prevent chronicity

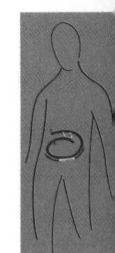

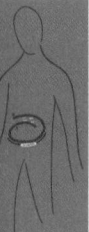

Chapter **62**

Malnutrition, Nutritional Assessment, and Nutritional Support in Adult Patients

Thomas R. Ziegler

Malnutrition

Protein-energy malnutrition and depletion of specific micronutrients are common in adult patients with chronic illnesses and in those requiring hospitalization, with a typical prevalence of 20% to 40%. Illness-associated anorexia, gastrointestinal symptoms, depression or anxiety, and other morbidities often lead to decreased food intake. These factors, in addition to disrupted meal scheduling, frequently result in inadequate nutrient intake in hospitalized patients that may cause or worsen malnutrition. Some patients have abnormal nutrient losses due to diarrhea, vomiting, polyuria, wound drainage, and dialysis. Drugs, including corticosteroids, chemotherapeutic agents, antirejection drugs, and diuretics are associated with skeletal muscle breakdown, gastrointestinal injury, and electrolyte or water-soluble vitamin losses. Bedrest itself induces skeletal muscle wasting and impaired muscle protein synthesis. Stressful illnesses are associated with increased blood concentrations of catabolic hormones (cortisol, catecholamines, and glucagon), release of pro-inflammatory cytokines (interleukins [e.g., IL-1, IL-6, and IL-8]) and tumor necrosis factor-α [TNF-α], and the development of tissue resistance to anabolic hormones (insulin and insulin-like growth factor-I [IGF-I]). The combination of decreased nutrient intake and increased tissue nutrient losses, coupled with increased energy, protein, and micronutrient needs due to inflammation, infection, and cytokinemia, leads to the wasting and micronutrient depletion common in medical patients with acute and chronic illness. Significant loss of lean body mass or deficiency of specific vitamins and minerals is associated with weakness and fatigue, increased rates of infection, impaired wound healing, and delayed convalescence.

Nutritional Status

Accurate nutritional assessment is essential for detecting preexisting depletion of body protein, energy reserves, and micronutrients, identifying risk factors for malnutrition, and defining steps needed to prevent or reverse nutrient deficiencies and depletion of lean body mass. Blood concentrations of specific micronutrients (e.g., copper, thiamine, 25-hydroxyvitamin D, vitamin B_6, folate, and vitamin B_{12}) and electrolytes (e.g., magnesium, potassium, and phosphorus) are important to guide needs and repletion responses. Unfortunately, there is not a practical, simple test that can be used as an index of general protein-energy nutritional status. Therefore, nutritional assessment involves the consideration of multiple measures and determinants, as outlined in Table 62-1. Integration of this information ultimately provides reliable insight into whether patients are likely to have mild, moderate, or severe protein-energy malnutrition and depletion or deficiency of specific vitamins, minerals, or electrolytes. Patients with an involuntary body weight loss of 5% to 10% or more of their usual body weight in the previous few weeks or months and those weighing less than 90% of their ideal body weight (e.g., a body mass index (BMI) <18.5 kg/m^2) should be carefully evaluated.

In hospitalized patients, especially those with severe illnesses, circulating concentrations of proteins (e.g., albumin, prealbumin, and transferrin) are generally quite low. These are not useful as protein nutritional status biomarkers, since they are markedly affected by non-nutritional factors, such as fluid status, capillary leak, iron status (transferrin), decreased hepatic synthesis, and increased clearance from the circulation. Because of its long circulating half-life (18 to 21 days), plasma albumin levels often remain low despite adequate feeding and are slow to respond to nutritional repletion. Prealbumin has a much shorter circulating half-life than albumin (several days), and serial plasma prealbumin levels therefore can provide a rough indication of protein status in clinically stable outpatients.

Nutritional Requirements

Energy requirements can be estimated using indirect calorimetry or the Harris-Benedict equation to calculate basal energy expenditure (BEE) in kilocalories (kcal) per 24 hours:

$$\text{Males: BEE} = 66.5 + (13.8 \times \text{kg body weight}) + (5.0 \times \text{height in cm}) - (6.8 \times \text{age in years})$$

$$\text{Females: BEE} = 655 + (9.6 \times \text{kg body weight}) + (1.8 \times \text{height in cm}) - (4.7 \times \text{age in years})$$

The maintenance energy requirement is about 1.3 times BEE in ambulatory subjects. Caloric need for patients receiving specialized nutrition support can be estimated as 25 to 30 kcal/kg per day (using ideal body weight from standard tables). Lower amounts of calories typically are given in intensive care unit (ICU) patients (15 to 20 kcal/kg per day) to avoid complications of overfeeding. In obese subjects, adjusted body weight should be used in the calculation of energy and protein needs as defined by the following equation:

$$\text{Adjusted body weight} = (\text{current weight} - \text{ideal body weight}) \times 0.25 + \text{ideal body weight}$$

Guidelines for protein requirements in adult patients are given in Table 62-2. For most catabolic or malnourished patients requiring specialized feeding, a generally recommended protein dose is 1.5 g/kg per day in individuals with normal renal function. This is about twice the recommended dietary allowance (RDA) for healthy adults of 0.8 g/kg per day. The administered protein dose should be adjusted downward as a function of the degree and tempo of azotemia (in the absence of dialysis therapy) and hyperbilirubinemia (see Table 62-2).

Nutritional Support

Nutritional support beyond usual oral feeding should be considered when patients have evidence of protein-energy malnutrition or a clinical condition likely to result in malnutrition. Major indications for specialized oral or enteral nutrition (EN) and parenteral nutrition (PN) support are summarized in Table 62-3. Consultation with a multidisciplinary nutrition support team, if available, has been shown to reduce complications and costs, and to increase the appropriate use of EN and PN in hospital settings.

ORAL NUTRITION SUPPORT

Oral nutrition supplementation includes provision of balanced oral diets of usual foods supplemented with complete liquid or solid nutrient products. These may include protein

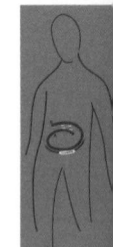

Table 62-1 Comprehensive Nutritional Assessment of Adult Medical Patients

- Review past medical and surgical history and current illness
- Obtain body weight loss history
- Estimate energy (calorie), protein, and micronutrient needs
- Determine dietary intake pattern in relation to nutrient needs
- Perform detailed physical examination (consider skeletal muscle wasting, skin lesions indicative of micronutrient deficiency)
- Evaluate gastrointestinal tract function
- Determine ambulatory and mental functional status
- Evaluate serial standard biochemical tests of organ function
- Consider consultation with multidisciplinary nutrition support team

---

Table 62-2 Estimated Protein Requirements in Adult Medical Patients

Clinical Condition	Protein Dose (g/kg/day)
Well-nourished with acute illness	1.2-1.5
Malnourished and/or severe catabolic stress	1.5-1.8
Postoperative	1.2-1.5
Hepatic failure	0.6-1.0 (based on estimated function)
Encephalopathy	0-0.6
Acute renal failure, not on renal replacement therapy	0.6-1.0 (based on estimated renal function/azotemia)
Renal failure, on renal replacement therapy	1.2-1.5

Table 62-3 Major Indications for Specialized Oral/Enteral or Parenteral Nutrition

- Evidence of moderate to severe protein or protein-energy malnutrition or deficiency of one or more essential micronutrients
- Involuntary loss of 5% to 10% or more of usual body weight
- Dietary food intake likely to be <50% of needs for more than 5 to 10 days
- Severe catabolic stress (e.g., intensive care unit care, serious infection, major operation), prolonged gastrointestinal dysfunction (>5-10 days), or intestinal failure (short bowel syndrome)
- Chronic obstructive lung disease, chronic infection, and other chronic inflammatory or catabolic disorders with documented poor nutrient intake and recent weight loss

---

supplements (e.g., hydrolyzed whey or casein powder that can be mixed with dietary beverages), high-potency multivitamin and mineral supplements, and specific micronutrients required to treat a diagnosed deficiency (e.g., zinc, copper, and vitamins B_6, B_{12}, and D). Several studies show that convalescence is enhanced with addition of 1 to 2 cans per day of complete liquid nutrient supplements to meals following stress such as total hip replacement. It is prudent to place patients with significant illnesses who can tolerate oral medications on a potent oral multivitamin and mineral preparation, at least for several months, although this is not specifically evidence supported.

TUBE FEEDING (ENTERAL NUTRITION)

Patients with intact gastrointestinal (GI) function may be unable to consume adequate diet orally due to medical or surgical conditions. Although PN is commonly administered in these settings, this practice is not evidence based. Current guidelines strongly favor oral nutritional supplements or EN if specialized nutrition support is indicated in patients with a functional GI tract. From extensive data primarily derived from animal studies, EN is associated with improved gut barrier function, decreased infectious complications, less hypermetabolism, and decreased morbidity and mortality in catabolic models compared with PN.

When delivered in appropriate amounts, commercially available tube feedings provide complete nutrition for most patients, although some severely stressed patients and those with malabsorption may have special needs. The feedings can be delivered by conventional nasogastric tubes into the stomach, small-bore nasogastric or nasojejunal tubes, percutaneous gastrostomy or jejunostomy tubes, or percutaneous gastrojejunostomy tubes. Gastric feedings can be by either continuous or bolus feeds, whereas small bowel feeds must be by continuous slow infusion using an infusion pump to avoid diarrhea. Tube feedings should be initiated at a slow rate (e.g., 10 to 20 mL per hour) for 8 to 24 hours and slowly advanced to the goal rate at 8- to 24-hour intervals. If subcutaneous insulin is being given, standing orders should be in place to ensure provision of dextrose-containing intravenous fluids whenever tube feedings are stopped for more than 1 to 2 hours. In managing an EN regimen, it should be recognized that numerous studies have shown that patients commonly receive only 50% to 70% of prescribed tube feedings due to gastrointestinal intolerance or discontinuation for medical tests and procedures.

Most outpatients and hospitalized patients tolerate standard enteral formulas delivered by gastric or intestinal routes that provide between 1 and 1.5 kcal/mL. A large variety of enteral tube feeding products are available for clinical use. The specific product chosen should be based both on clinical conditions and underlying organ function, with the assistance of a dietitian or other nutrition support professional.

Diarrhea is common in hospital patients receiving tube feedings but is typically due to factors independent of the feeding, including administration of antibiotics, sorbitol-containing or hypertonic medications (e.g., acetaminophen elixir), and infections. Diarrhea due to tube feeding can occur as a result of rapid formula administration, underlying gut mucosal disease, or severe hypoalbuminemia with associated bowel wall edema. Use of a fiber-containing enteral formula is sometimes a useful maneuver to decrease diarrhea. Other complications of tube feeding include aspiration, discomfort or sinusitis with nasally placed feeding tubes, pharyngeal or esophageal mucosal erosion due to local tube trauma, and entrance site leakage, skin breakdown, cellulitis, and pain with percutaneous feeding tubes. Metabolic complications of tube feeding include fluid imbalances, hyperglycemia, electrolyte abnormalities, azotemia, and occasionally refeeding syndrome. In general, if tube feedings are deemed to be required for more than 4 to 6 weeks, a percutaneous feeding tube should be placed.

Hospital patients receiving tube feedings should generally have blood glucose monitored at least daily, and blood electrolytes (including magnesium and phosphorus), renal function indices, and other blood chemistries at least weekly. There should be close monitoring of intake and output (including urine, stool, and drainage outputs), gastrointestinal tolerance, vital signs, physical findings, and changes in clinical course that may necessitate adjustments in the feeding regimen. When patients are able to consume oral food, tube feeding should be decreased incrementally and then discontinued when oral intake is clearly established (e.g., based on daily calorie counts by a dietitian).

PARENTERAL NUTRITION

PN support includes administration of complete nutrient mixtures, which contain dextrose, L-amino acids, lipid emulsion, electrolytes, vitamins, and minerals (plus certain medications as indicated, such as insulin or octreotide) by either peripheral or central vein. PN is lifesaving in patients with intestinal failure (e.g., short bowel syndrome). Unfortunately, in patient subgroups with lesser degrees of intestinal failure, only limited objective data from randomized, controlled studies are available on the efficacy of PN. Existing data indicate that PN benefits patients with preexisting moderate to severe malnutrition or with critical illness by decreasing overall morbidity and possibly mortality compared with patients receiving inadequate EN or hydration (intravenous dextrose) therapy alone.

The basic principle is to consider PN therapy in patients with a need for nutrition support who are unable to achieve adequate nutrient intake by the enteral route. Compared with PN, EN is less expensive, appears to better maintain intestinal mucosal structure and function, has fewer mechanical and metabolic complications, and is associated with reduced rates of nosocomial infections. Thus, the enteral route of feeding should be used and advanced whenever possible, and the amount of administered PN correspondingly reduced. Generally accepted indications for PN include (1) short bowel syndrome or other conditions causing intestinal failure that prohibit adequate intake or absorption of enteral nutrients (e.g., motility disorders, obstruction, severe ileus, severe inflammatory bowel disease), especially in patients with preexisting malnutrition; (2) inadequate enteral feeding (<50% of needs) that is likely to extend for 7 to 10 days due to an underlying illness; and (3) severe catabolic stress (e.g., requiring ICU care) with inadequate enteral nutrient intake likely to extend for 3 to 7 days or longer. In patients who meet these qualifications, PN is contraindicated if (1) the extra intravenous fluid required for PN cannot be tolerated; (2) there are severe electrolyte abnormalities or hyperglycemia on the planned day of PN initiation; (3) there is uncontrolled bloodstream infection or severe hemodynamic instability; or (4) placement of an intravenous line for PN poses undue risks.

PN can be delivered either as peripheral vein or central vein solutions. To diminish the risk for phlebitis, typical peripheral vein PN solutions provide low concentrations of dextrose (5%) and amino acids (<3.5%) with a large proportion of energy given as fat emulsion (50% to 60% of total calories). Because fluid restriction or organ dysfunction often precludes use of large fluid volumes, peripheral vein PN is generally not indicated in ICU patients. Intravenous lipid emulsions (typically added to PN as a 20% soybean oil–based solution) provide both essential linoleic and α-linolenic fatty acids and energy (10 kcal/g). The maximal recommended rate of fat emulsion infusion is about 1 g/kg per day. Most patients clear triglyceride from intravenous fat emulsion effectively from plasma, but it is important to monitor plasma triglyceride levels at baseline and then about weekly. Triglyceride levels should be maintained below 400 to 500 mg/dL to decrease risk for pancreatitis or compromised pulmonary diffusion capacity in patients with severe chronic obstructive lung disease.

Central venous administration of PN allows higher concentrations of dextrose and amino acids to be delivered as hypertonic solutions and thus decreases the amount of fat emulsion needed to reach caloric goals. Requirements for potassium, magnesium, and phosphorus are typically higher with central vein PN compared with peripheral vein PN owing to the increased dextrose provided (insulin-mediated intracellular electrolyte shift) and needs related to increased glucose metabolism and adenosine triphosphate (ATP) production. The higher concentrations of dextrose and amino acids allow most patients to achieve caloric and amino acid goals with only 1 to 1.5 L of PN per day. In central vein PN, initial orders typically provide 60% to 70% of non–amino acid calories as dextrose and 30% to 40% of non–amino acid calories as fat emulsion. These percentages are adjusted as indicated depending on blood glucose and triglyceride levels. Based on comprehensive data associating hyperglycemia with hospital morbidity and mortality, expert panels now recommend close blood glucose monitoring and control in ICU settings (goal of 80 mg/dL to 130 to 150 mg/dL). The dextrose amount in central vein PN should be reduced or regular insulin added to the PN bag, or both, to maintain blood glucose within the desired range. Separate intravenous insulin infusions should usually be used in acutely ill patients receiving central vein PN who develop hyperglycemia. Specific requirements for intravenous trace elements and vitamins have not been rigorously defined for patient subgroups, and therapy is directed at meeting published recommended doses that maintain blood levels in the normal range in most stable patients using standardized intravenous preparations.

The most common complication of peripheral vein PN is local phlebitis due to the catheter. Abnormalities in blood electrolytes can be corrected with adjustment of concentrations in the peripheral PN prescription. Hypertriglyceridemia typically responds well to lowering of the total PN lipid dose. Central vein PN is associated with a much higher rate of mechanical, metabolic, and infectious complications than peripheral vein PN. Mechanical complications include those related to insertion of the central venous catheter (e.g., pneumothorax, hemothorax, malposition of the catheter, and thrombosis). Infectious complications include catheter-related bloodstream infections and non–catheter-related

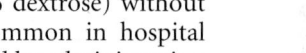

infections by bacteria and fungal species, which may in some cases be due to endogenous bacterial translocation from the gut lumen. The risk for these infections appears to be increased with use of non–subclavian vein central venous access (e.g., jugular, femoral veins) and multiple-use catheters with nondedicated PN infusion ports used for additional purposes such as blood drawing or medication administration. Poorly controlled blood glucose (>130 to 150 mg/dL) is not uncommon in patients requiring central vein PN, and this is associated with an increased risk for nosocomial infection. Risk factors for hyperglycemia include (1) poorly controlled blood glucose at PN initiation, (2) use of high dextrose concentrations (>10%) in the initial few days of PN administration or too rapid an increase in total dextrose load, (3) insufficient exogenous insulin administration, (4) inadequate monitoring of blood glucose responses to central vein PN administration, and (5) administration of corticosteroids and pressor agents such as norepinephrine (which stimulate gluconeogenesis and cause insulin resistance).

Overfeeding can induce severe metabolic complications, including carbon dioxide overproduction, azotemia, hyperglycemia, electrolyte alterations, and hepatic steatosis and injury (Table 62-4). Dextrose and lipid doses in PN should be advanced over several days after initiation, and blood glucose, electrolytes, triglycerides and organ function tests, intake and output measurements, and the clinical course must be closely monitored. Refeeding syndrome with central vein PN administration is relatively common in patients at risk, including those with preexisting malnutrition, electrolyte depletion, or alcoholism, or after prolonged periods of intravenous hydration therapy (e.g., 5% dextrose) without nutrition support, all of which are common in hospital patients. Refeeding syndrome is mediated by administration of excessive intravenous dextrose (>150 to 250 g, such as given in 1 L of PN with 15% to 25% dextrose). This markedly stimulates insulin release, which rapidly lowers blood potassium, magnesium, and especially phosphorus concen-

Table 62-4 **Common Metabolic Complications of Parenteral Nutrition**	
Parenteral Nutrition Prescription Problem	**Metabolic/Clinical Consequence**
Excess kcal, CHO, fat	Abnormal liver function tests
Excess kcal, CHO, fat	Hepatic steatosis
Excess CHO	Hypercapnia
Excess fluid, kcal, CHO, fat	Respiratory insufficiency
Excess amino acids	Azotemia
Excess sodium and fluid	Sodium and fluid retention
Excess CHO, inadequate insulin	Hyperglycemia-mediated immune cell dysfunction, infection
Inadequate or excessive electrolytes	Abnormal blood electrolyte levels
Excess fluid, kcal, sodium, CHO, inadequate electrolytes	Cardiac failure, arrhythmias
Excess CHO, inadequate electrolytes, thiamine	Refeeding syndrome

CHO, carbohydrate; kcal, calories.

trations due to intracellular shift and utilization in carbohydrate metabolic pathways. Administration of high doses of carbohydrate also consumes thiamine, which is required as a cofactor for carbohydrate metabolism and can precipitate thiamine deficiency. Hyperinsulinemia tends to cause sodium and fluid retention at the level of the kidney. Together, fluid and sodium retention, the drop in electrolytes (which can cause arrhythmias), and hypermetabolism due to excessive calorie provision can result in heart failure, especially in patients with preexisting heart disease. Prevention of refeeding syndrome requires vigilance to identify patients at risk, use of initially low PN dextrose concentrations, provision of higher doses of potassium, magnesium, and phosphorus based on current blood levels and renal

function, and supplemental thiamine (100 mg per day for 3 to 5 days).

For patients in whom home PN is indicated, physicians should consult with social service professionals to identify appropriate home care companies and nutrition support professionals to assess intravenous line access, metabolic status, and the home PN order and to ensure follow-up care and monitoring of PN. It is important not to arrange for rapid hospital discharge in patients newly started on PN. Securing reliable venous access and monitoring of fluid and electrolyte status over a 2- to 3-day period is an important aspect of care for most patients started on PN and imperative in those with severe malnutrition and at risk for refeeding syndrome.

Prospectus for the Future

- Optimal levels for vitamins (e.g., vitamin D) and micronutrients will be better defined, thus making clearer the circumstances under which they should be measured and provided.

- Better evidence will be generated on target blood glucose levels that achieve optimal benefit compared with adverse consequences in hospitalized, acutely ill patients with various disorders.

References

ASPEN Board of Directors and the Clinical Guidelines Task Force: Guidelines for the use of parenteral and enteral nutrition in adult and pediatric patients. JPEN J Parent Ent Nutr 26(1 Suppl):1SA-138SA, 2002.

Heyland DK, Dhaliwal R, Drover JW, et al, for the Canadian Critical Care Clinical Practice Guidelines Committee: Canadian clinical practice guidelines for nutrition support in mechanically ventilated, critically ill adult patients. JPEN J Parent Ent Nutr 27:355-373, 2003.

Kreymann KG, Berger MM, Deutz NE, et al: ESPEN guidelines on enteral nutrition: Intensive care. Clin Nutr 25:210-223, 2006.

Montejo JC: Enteral nutrition-related gastrointestinal complications in critically ill patients: A multicenter study. The Nutritional and Metabolic Working Group of the Spanish Society of Intensive Care Medicine and Coronary Units. Crit Care Med 27:1447-1453, 1999.

Singer P, Berger MM, Van den Berghe G, et al: ESPEN guidelines for parenteral nutrition: Intensive care. Clin Nutr 28(4):387-400, 2009.

Zaloga GP: Parenteral nutrition in adult inpatients with functioning gastrointestinal tracts: Assessment of outcomes. Lancet 367:1101-1111, 2006.

Ziegler TR, Evans ME, Fernández-Estívariz C, Jones DP: Trophic and cytoprotective nutrition for intestinal adaptation, mucosal repair, and barrier function. Annu Rev Nutr 23:229-261, 2003.

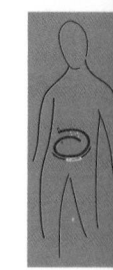

Disorders of Lipid Metabolism

Geetha Gopalakrishnan and Robert J. Smith

Lipids such as free fatty acids (FFAs), cholesterol, and triglycerides are hydrophobic molecules that bind protein for transport. Nonesterified FFAs travel as anions complexed to albumin. Esterified complex lipids are transported in lipoprotein particles. Lipoproteins have a hydrophobic core (cholesteryl esters and triglycerides) and an amphiphilic surface monolayer (phospholipids, unesterified cholesterol, and apolipoproteins). Ultracentrifugation separates lipoproteins into five classes based on their density (Table 63-1). Proteins on the surface of lipoproteins, apolipoproteins (apo), activate enzymes and receptors that guide lipid metabolism. Defects in the synthesis and catabolism of lipoproteins result in dyslipidemia. Two classes of lipids, triglyceride and cholesterol, play a significant role in the pathogenesis of atherosclerosis and therefore are the focus of this chapter.

Lipid Metabolism

In the intestinal lumen, dietary triglycerides and cholesterol esters are hydrolyzed by pancreatic lipase to produce glycerol, FFAs, and free cholesterol. Formation of micelles enables the absorption of glycerol and FFAs into the intestinal cell. The transport of free cholesterol is mediated by a cholesterol gradient that exists between the lumen and intestinal cell. Within the cell, glycerol combines with three fatty acid chains to form triglycerides, and cholesterol is esterified to form cholesterol esters. Triglycerides (85% of chylomicron mass) and cholesterol esters are assembled with surface lipoproteins to form chylomicrons. After entering the circulation, chylomicrons acquire more surface apolipoproteins such as apo C-II and apo E from high-density lipoprotein (HDL) particles (Fig. 63-1). Apo C-II activates lipoprotein lipase (LPL) located on the capillary endothelium. LPL hydrolyzes the core chylomicron triglycerides to release FFAs, which function as an energy source. Excess fatty acids are stored in adipose tissue or used in hepatic lipoprotein synthesis. The triglyceride-poor chylomicron remnant is then cleared from the circulation by hepatic LDL receptors.

These receptors are activated by apo E located on the surface of chylomicrons.

Very-low-density lipoproteins (VLDL) are synthesized by the liver (see Fig. 63-1). FFA and cholesterol obtained from the circulation or synthesized by the liver are incorporated into VLDL particles. Any condition that increases the flux of FFA to the liver, such as poorly controlled diabetes, will increase VLDL production. The liver assembles triglycerides (55% of VLDL mass), cholesterol (20%), and surface apolipoproteins to form VLDL particles. Apo C-II on the VLDL surface activates LPL, which hydrolyzes the triglyceride core of VLDL particles to generate VLDL remnant or intermediate-density lipoprotein (IDL). The IDL, deplete of triglycerides (25%), can be cleared from the circulation by apo E–mediated LDL receptors or can be hydrolyzed further to form low-density lipoproteins (LDLs). LDLs are triglyceride-poor (5%) particles composed of cholesterol esters (60%) and apolipoproteins. Apo B-100 on the surface of LDL binds LDL receptors and facilitates LDL clearance from the circulation. Internalized LDL cholesterol is used to synthesize hormones, produce cell membranes, and store energy.

In the liver, LDL cholesterol is used to synthesize bile acids (see Fig. 63-1), which are secreted into the intestinal lumen along with free cholesterol. Bile acids help transport fat. About 50% of the cholesterol and 97% of the bile acid entering the lumen is reabsorbed back into the circulation. The reabsorbed cholesterol regulates cholesterol and LDL receptor synthesis.

Many cells in the body, including liver parenchymal cells, synthesize cholesterol (Fig. 63-2). Acetate is converted to 3-hydroxy-3-methylglutaryl-coenzyme A (HMG-CoA). HMG-CoA reductase converts HMG-CoA to mevalonic acid, which is then converted to cholesterol through a series of steps. HMG-CoA reductase is the rate-limiting step in the cholesterol synthesis pathway. Drugs that inhibit this enzyme decrease cholesterol biosynthesis and cellular cholesterol pools. Internalization of LDL particles into cells is regulated by negative feedback (see Fig. 63-2). A negative cholesterol balance increases the expression of LDL receptors and

Table 63-1 **Properties of Lipoproteins**				
Lipoprotein Class	**Density (g/mL)**	**Origin**	**Apolipoproteins**	**Lipid**
Chylomicrons	<0.95	Intestine	C-II, E	TG (85%), cholesterol (10%)
VLDL	<1.006	Liver	B-100, C-II, E	TG (55%), cholesterol (20%)
IDL	1.006-1.019	VLDL catabolism	B-100, E	TG (25%), cholesterol (35%)
LDL	1.019-1.063	IDL catabolism	B-100	TG (5%), cholesterol (60%)
HDL	1.063-1.25	Liver, intestine	A-I, E	TG (5%), cholesterol (20%)

HDL, high-density lipoprotein; IDL, intermediate-density lipoprotein; LDL, low-density lipoprotein; TG, triglyceride; VLDL, very-low-density lipoprotein.

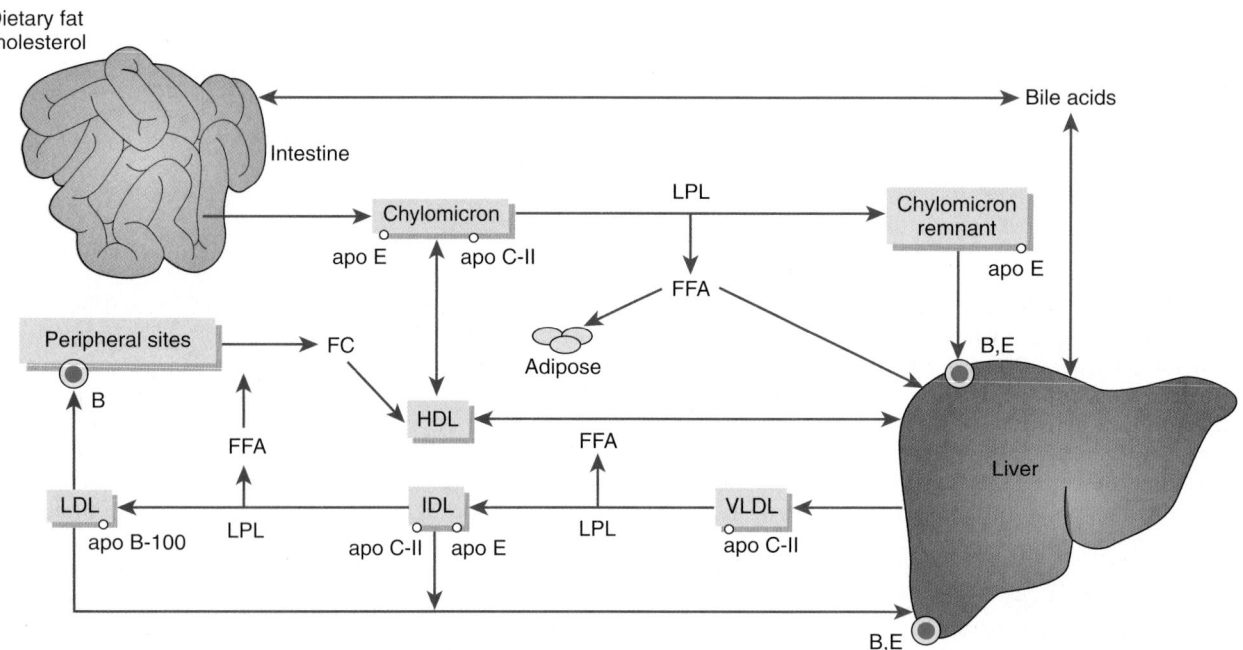

Figure 63-1 Normal metabolism of plasma lipoproteins (see text for details). B,E, membrane receptor for lipoproteins containing apo B and apo E (synonymous with the LDL receptor); apo, apolipoprotein; FFA, free (unesterified) fatty acids; FC, free (unesterified) cholesterol; HDL, high-density lipoprotein; IDL, intermediate-density lipoprotein; LDL, low-density lipoprotein; LPL, lipoprotein lipase; VLDL, very-low-density lipoprotein.

subsequent uptake of cholesterol from the circulation. A positive cell cholesterol balance suppresses LDL receptor expression and decreases uptake of LDL cholesterol into cells. Circulating LDL particles then enter macrophages and other tissues through scavenger receptors. Scavenger receptors are not regulated; therefore, these cells accumulate excess intracellular cholesterol resulting in the formation of foam cells and atheromatous plaques.

The antiatherogenic effect of HDL is attributed to the removal of excess cholesterol from tissue sites and other lipoproteins. HDL is synthesized in the liver and intestine (see Fig. 63-1). Excess phospholipids, cholesterol, and apolipoproteins on remnant chylomicrons, VLDL, IDL, and LDL are transferred to HDL particles and thus increase HDL mass. Apo A-I, a surface lipoprotein on HDL particles, mobilizes cholesterol from intracellular pools and accepts cholesterol released during lipolysis of triglyceride-rich lipoproteins. It also activates lecithin:cholesterol acyltransferase (LCAT), an enzyme that esterifies cholesterol. These cholesterol esters then move from the hydrophilic HDL surface to the hydrophobic HDL core. Cholesterol ester transfer protein (CETP) transfers core HDL cholesterol esters to

other lipoproteins such as VLDL. These lipoproteins deliver cholesterol to peripheral sites for hormone and cell membrane synthesis.

Diagnostic and Therapeutic Approach to Dyslipidemia

Disorders of lipid metabolism result from genetic and acquired defects in the production and removal of lipoproteins. A total cholesterol, triglyceride, or LDL level above the 90th percentile or an HDL level below the 10th percentile for the general population defines dyslipidemia. Total cholesterol, triglyceride, and lipoprotein assessments must be made in the fasting state. Chylomicrons, which are present in plasma for up to 10 hours after a meal, otherwise confound these measurements. It is advisable to confirm dyslipidemia with two separate determinations. Total cholesterol, triglyceride, and HDL levels can be measured directly. VLDL and LDL levels are calculated. If the triglyceride level is

LDL Cholesterol Uptake from Circulation

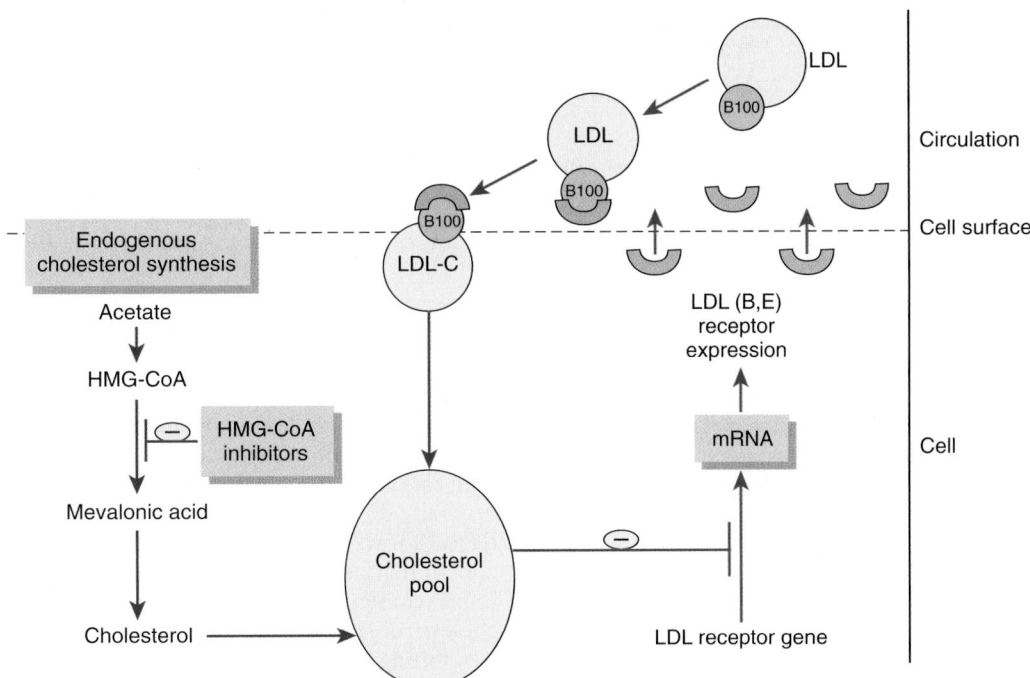
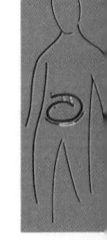

Figure 63-2 Regulation of low-density lipoprotein (LDL) receptor expression (see text for details). B,E, membrane receptor for lipoproteins containing apo B and apo E (synonymous with the LDL receptor); HMG-CoA, 3-hydroxy-3-methylglutaryl-coenzyme A; mRNA, messenger RNA.

less than 400 mg/dL, VLDL is calculated by dividing the triglyceride level by 5. LDL cholesterol is estimated by subtracting VLDL and HDL from the total cholesterol. VLDL and LDL cannot be determined if triglyceride levels are greater than 400 mg/dL. In this case, the lipoprotein abnormality can be identified by inspecting the serum. When the triglyceride level exceeds 350 mg/dL, the serum is cloudy. After refrigeration, a white surface layer depicts excess chylomicrons, whereas a dispersed opaque infranant reflects elevated VLDL.

The cost-effectiveness of screening and treating the general population for lipid disorders is continuously debated. Current guidelines do not recommend routine screening in children unless a lipoprotein abnormality or premature vascular disease is identified in a first-degree relative. A screening lipid panel is recommended for the general population at age 20 years, with fasting or nonfasting total cholesterol and HDL measurements as the initial screen (Table 63-2). If the total cholesterol value is greater than 200 mg/dL or the HDL value is less than 40 mg/dL, a repeat fasting lipid panel is required. If the total cholesterol value is less than 200 mg/dL and HDL is greater than 40 mg/dL, retesting is recommended every 5 years. Individuals with coronary heart disease (CHD), risk factors for CHD, or a CHD equivalent (symptomatic carotid artery disease, peripheral arterial disease, abdominal aortic aneurysm, or diabetes) should be screened more frequently based on risk assessment and LDL levels as shown in Table 63-2. CHD risk factors include age (men >45 years, women >55 years), family history of premature CHD (affected male first-degree relative <55 years or female first-degree relative <65 years), smoking, hypertension, and HDL less than 40 mg/dL. HDL greater than 60 mg/dL is cardioprotective. LDL treatment strategies are based on these risk indicators (Table 63-3).

Table 63-2 **Recommendations for Screening***
1. Initial fasting lipid profile is recommended at age 20 years

2. Rescreen every 5 years if:
  a. LDL <160 mg/dL in patients with 0-1 risk factor
  b. LDL <130 mg/dL in patients with ≥2 risk factors

3. Rescreen every 1-2 years if:
  a. LDL >160 mg/dL in patients with 0-1 risk factor
  b. LDL >130 mg/dL in patients with ≥2 risk factors
  c. LDL >100 mg/dL in patients with CHD or CHD equivalent

*Recommendations of the Adult Treatment Panel, National Cholesterol Education Program III, as modified in 2004. Coronary heart disease (CHD) risk factors include age (men >45 yr, women >55 yr), family history of premature CHD (male first-degree relative <55 yr, female first-degree relative <65 yr), smoking, hypertension, and high-density lipoprotein cholesterol (HDL) <40 mg/dL. Subtract a risk factor if HDL is >60 mg/dL. Coronary heart disease risk equivalents include symptomatic carotid artery disease, peripheral arterial disease, abdominal aortic aneurysm, and diabetes mellitus.
LDL, low-density lipoprotein cholesterol.

Treatment of elevated total and LDL cholesterol can slow the development and progression of CHD. Meta-analysis of primary and secondary prevention trials indicates that CHD mortality decreased by about 15% for every 10% reduction in serum cholesterol.

The impact of triglycerides on vascular disease is less clear. Metabolic factors such as diabetes and obesity are often associated with vascular disease and hypertriglyceridemia, and the atherogenic impact of these factors is difficult to separate from the effect of hypertriglyceridemia. However, in several population-based studies, abnormal triglyceride levels correlate with increased risk for CHD. Marked hypertriglyceridemia (>1000 mg/dL) is associated with the chylomicronemia

Table 63-3 Therapeutic Approach to Low-Density Lipoprotein Cholesterol Levels*

Risk Category	Treatment Goal: LDL (mg/dL)	Lifestyle Changes: LDL (mg/dL)	Drug Therapy: LDL (mg/dL)
≤One risk factor	<160	≥160	≥160-190
≥Two risk factors	<130	≥130	≥130-160
CAD or CAD risk equivalent	<100 (optional <70)	≥100	≥100-130

*Recommendations of the Adult Treatment Panel, National Cholesterol Education Program III, as modified in 2004. Coronary heart disease (CHD) risk factors include age (men >45 yr, women >55 yr), family history of premature CHD (male first-degree relative <55 yr, female first-degree relative <65 yr), smoking, hypertension, diabetes mellitus, and high-density lipoprotein cholesterol (HDL) <40 mg/dL. Subtract a risk factor if HDL is >60 mg/dL. Coronary heart disease (CHD) risk equivalents include symptomatic carotid artery disease, peripheral arterial disease, abdominal aortic aneurysm, and diabetes mellitus.
LDL, low-density lipoprotein cholesterol.

Table 63-4 Adult Treatment Panel III Nutrition Composition

Nutrient	Recommended Intake

Total fat
  Saturated (<7%)
  Polyunsaturated (<10%)
  Monounsaturated (<20%)
	25%-35% of total calories

Carbohydrates	50%-60% of total calories
Protein	15% of total calories
Cholesterol	<200 mg/day
Fiber	20-30 g/day

syndrome, characterized by pancreatitis and xanthomas. A fasting lipid panel is required to diagnose hypertriglyceridemia. Triglyceride levels above 200 mg/dL are classified as abnormal. Borderline triglyceride levels range from 150 to 200 mg/dL, and normal values are less than 150 mg/dL. A diet and exercise program is recommended for all individuals with abnormal triglyceride levels. Pharmacologic treatment can be considered if fasting triglycerides are greater than 200 mg/dL, especially if individuals are at risk for CHD or pancreatitis. Low HDL (<40 mg/dL) can also increase the risk for CHD. In the Framingham Heart Study, every 5 mg/dL decrease in HDL increased the risk for myocardial infarction. Lifestyle modifications (e.g., exercise) can be prescribed to improve HDL levels.

Management of Dyslipidemia

Treatment is initiated after two abnormal lipid findings. Dietary modifications can reduce LDL cholesterol and triglyceride levels (Table 63-4). If *target goals* are not achieved, pharmacologic therapy is considered (Table 63-5). Treatment effect can be assessed after 1 to 2 months and additional agents prescribed if goals are not achieved with maximal drug dosing.

LIFESTYLE MODIFICATION

Lifestyle modification should be the initial step in the management of hyperlipidemia (see Table 63-4). Restricting dietary intake of fat from 45% to 25% of total calories has been shown to lower total cholesterol by about 15% and LDL cholesterol by 25%. Low-fat diets that limit saturated fat content promote LDL receptor expression and increase the uptake of LDL cholesterol from the circulation. By contrast, saturated fat downregulates hepatic LDL receptors and increases circulating LDL. Unsaturated fats (poly and mono) generally do not have this effect and, therefore, are the preferred form of fat intake. However, polyunsaturated fats containing fatty acids with a *trans* rather than *cis* double bond configuration (*trans* fatty acids) increase plasma cholesterol levels similar to saturated fat.

Limiting the intake of saturated and *trans* unsaturated fatty acids requires appropriate calorie substitutions. Increasing carbohydrate content to achieve this goal can increase hepatic synthesis of triglyceride. Dietary substitution with soluble fibers (e.g., oat bran) has been recommended because these fibers have a limited effect on triglyceride levels. They also bind bile acids in the gut and thus decrease cholesterol levels. Other polyunsaturated fats such as omega-3 fatty acids are cardioprotective. They are abundant in fatty fish, flaxseed oil, canola oil, and nuts. They reduce VLDL production, inhibit platelet aggregation, and decrease CHD. Even two servings per week of fatty fish such as salmon can be beneficial.

Dietary fat increases the influx of triglyceride into plasma. LPL hydrolyzes the triglyceride core of chylomicrons and VLDL particles. This enzyme reaches kinetic saturation at triglyceride levels greater than 1000 mg/dL. At this point, any increase in triglyceride-rich lipoproteins results in an exaggerated increase in triglyceride levels. Therefore, dietary restriction of fat (<10%) is essential for the treatment of marked hypertriglyceridemia. Other factors such as carbohydrate and alcohol intake can also increase the synthesis of triglyceride. Therefore, restricting alcohol intake to one or two servings per week and adhering to a low-fat, high-fiber diet will improve hypertriglyceridemia.

Exercise has been shown to increase LPL activity. Even a single exercise session can reduce triglycerides and increase HDL. The impact of exercise on LDL is less clear. With low to moderate exercise regimens, clearance of VLDL particles increases LDL production. However, this effect is not seen with high-intensity exercise programs. A decrease in LDL cholesterol occurs with high-intensity exercise, and this effect is independent of weight loss.

PHARMACOTHERAPY

If diet and exercise modifications do not sustain a normal lipid profile, drug therapy is appropriate. Likely benefit needs to be balanced with potential adverse effects when

Table 63-5 **Pharmacologic Agents Commonly Used for the Treatment of Hyperlipidemia**				
Drug Class	**LDL**	**HDL**	**Triglycerides**	**Side Effects**
HMG-CoA inhibitors	↓ 20%-60%	↑ 5%-10%	↓ 10%-30%	Liver toxicity, myositis, rhabdomyolysis, enhanced warfarin effect
Cholesterol absorption inhibitors	↓ 17%	No effect	No effect	Abnormal liver enzymes in combination with an HMG-CoA inhibitor, potential increase in cancer risk and cancer death
Bile acid sequestrants	↓ 15%-30%	Slight increase	No effect	Nausea, bloating, cramping, abnormal liver function, interference with the absorption of other drugs such as warfarin and thyroxine
Fibric acids	↓ 5%-20%	↑ 15%-35%	↓ 35%-50%	Nausea, cramping, myalgias, liver toxicity, enhanced warfarin effect
Nicotinic acid	↓ 10%-25%	↑ 15%-35%	↓ 25%-30%	Hepatotoxicity, hyperuricemia, hyperglycemia, flushing, pruritus, nausea, vomiting, diarrhea

↓, Decreased; ↑, increased; HMG-CoA, 3-hydroxy-3-methylglutaryl-coenzyme A.

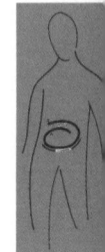

determining drug therapy. Many patients require two or three agents to achieve adequate control.

HMG-CoA reductase is the rate-limiting enzyme involved in cholesterol biosynthesis. Inhibition of this enzyme decreases cellular cholesterol pools and subsequently increases uptake of LDL cholesterol from the circulation. HMG-CoA reductase inhibitors (e.g., lovastatin, pravastatin, simvastatin, fluvastatin, atorvastatin, and rosuvastatin) increase cholesterol utilization, decrease VLDL synthesis, and increase HDL synthesis. As a result, lower LDL and triglyceride levels and higher HDL levels are noted with treatment. Meta-analysis of primary and secondary CHD prevention trials has shown reductions in all-cause and cardiovascular mortality rates with statin therapy. These agents limit progression and may even cause regression of coronary atherosclerosis. Therefore, they are first line in the management of abnormal LDL cholesterol. Elevated liver enzymes and muscle toxicity are potential dose-related complications. Myositis can occur with statins alone but is a higher risk when statins are used in combination with nicotinic acid or fibric acid derivatives. Some of these agents can also potentiate the effect of warfarin.

Cholesterol absorption inhibitors (e.g., ezetimibe) function by interfering with the transport of cholesterol at the intestinal brush border. They increase cholesterol utilization and decrease LDL cholesterol levels. Although there is a reduction in LDL cholesterol, improvements in cardiovascular events and mortality with treatment have not been confirmed. Ezetimibe can be used as a single agent or in combination with an HMG-CoA reductase inhibitor to lower LDL cholesterol levels. In combination, this agent can increase serum transaminase levels and potentially increase the risk for cancer and cancer death. The evidence linking ezetimibe to cancer risk is limited, and more studies are needed to confirm this association.

Drugs that interfere with the absorption of cholesterol from the intestinal lumen will increase cholesterol utilization and decrease circulating levels. Bile acid sequestrants (e.g., cholestyramine, colestipol, and colesevelam) bind bile acids in the intestinal lumen and increase fecal excretion. Subsequently, more LDL cholesterol is utilized by the liver to synthesize bile acids. The decrease in cellular cholesterol pools upregulates LDL receptors and decreases the amount of LDL in the circulation. Mild increases in HDL cholesterol are also noted with this agent as a result of increased intes-

tinal HDL formation. Treatment is associated with a reduction in the incidence of CHD. Bile acid sequestrants can be used alone for mild lipid dysfunction or combined with another lipid-lowering agent such as an HMG-CoA reductase inhibitor. Abnormal liver function and gastrointestinal symptoms (nausea, bloating, and cramping) are common side effects that limit the use of bile acid sequestrants. They can interfere with the absorption of other drugs such as warfarin and thyroxin; therefore, it is important to time the intake of such medications away from the bile acid sequestrant.

Fibric acid derivatives such as gemfibrozil and fenofibrate activate peroxisome proliferator-activated receptor alpha (PPARa) and increase FFA oxidation in muscle and liver. A consequent decrease in net hepatic lipogenesis leads to diminished VLDL and subsequent LDL production. Fibric acid derivatives also enhance LPL activity and HDL synthesis. As a result, treatment is usually associated with not only lower triglyceride and LDL levels but also higher HDL levels. An increase in LDL sometimes occurs with the initiation of fibric acid derivatives. This derives from increased VLDL conversion to LDL as a consequence of enhanced LPL activity. The impact of fibric acid derivatives on LDL levels needs to be balanced with their benefits. Reduced cardiovascular events have been demonstrated in a subset of individuals with high triglyceride (>200 mg/dL) and low HDL (<40 mg/dL) levels, but improvements in cardiovascular or all-cause mortality otherwise has not been confirmed with these agents. Liver toxicity and myositis are potential side effects of fibric acid derivatives, and these changes also interfere with the metabolism of warfarin, leading to a need for its dose adjustment.

Nicotinic acid has an antilipolytic effect and thus decreases the influx of FFA to the liver. As a result, hepatic VLDL synthesis and LDL production are reduced. Nicotinic acid also decreases HDL catabolism and prevents the transfer of cholesterol from HDL to VLDL particles. Lower triglyceride and LDL levels and higher HDL levels are noted with treatment. In addition, nicotinic acid stimulates tissue plasminogen activator and prevents thrombosis. It is the preferred agent for the reduction of lipoprotein(a) [Lp(a); discussed later in this chapter]. The cardioprotective effect of nicotinic acid may be linked to its effect on Lp(a) and HDL. Side effects include hepatotoxicity, hyperuricemia, hyperglycemia, and flushing.

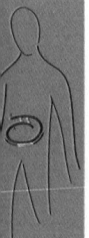

Table 63-6 **Secondary Causes of Hyperlipidemia**		
Clinical	**Elevated Lipoprotein**	**Mechanism**
Diabetes	Chylomicron, VLDL, LDL	Increase in VLDL production and decrease in VLDL/LDL clearance
Obesity	Chylomicron, VLDL, LDL	Increase in VLDL production and decrease in VLDL/LDL clearance
Lipodystrophy	VLDL	Increase in VLDL production
Hypothyroidism	LDL, VLDL	Decrease in LDL/LDL clearance
Estrogen	VLDL	Increase in VLDL production
Glucocorticoids	VLDL, LDL	Increase in VLDL production and conversion to LDL
Alcohol	VLDL	Increase in VLDL production
Nephrotic Syndrome	VLDL, LDL	Increase in VLDL production and conversion to LDL

LDL, low-density lipoprotein; VLDL, very-low-density lipoprotein.

Specific Disorders of Lipid Metabolism

A number of specific disorders of overproduction or impaired removal of lipoproteins result in dyslipidemia. These disorders are often familial, but secondary causes also need to be considered. Comorbid conditions (diabetes, hypothyroidism), medications (estrogen, glucocorticoids, β blockers), and lifestyle factors (diet, alcohol) can increase the production and clearance of lipoproteins (Table 63-6). Addressing these factors can often normalize lipid levels. If abnormalities persist, evaluation of genetic causes and treatment with pharmacologic therapy should be considered.

FAMILIAL HYPERCHOLESTEROLEMIA

Mutations in the gene that encodes the LDL (apo B/E) receptor results in familial hypercholesterolemia (FH). Impairment in LDL receptor synthesis or function decreases the clearance of LDL and increases circulating LDL levels. Excess LDL then enters macrophages through scavenger receptors resulting in foam cell and cholesterol plaque formation. These plaques deposit in arteries (atheroma), skin or tendons (xanthoma), eyelids (xanthelasma), and iris (corneal arcus). The homozygous (HM) form of this autosomal dominant disorder is rare. Affected individuals present early in life with elevated total cholesterol (600 to 1000 mg/dL) and LDL (550 to 950 mg/dL). Triglyceride and HDL levels are normal. They develop CHD, aortic stenosis due to atherosclerosis of the aortic root, and tendon xanthomas. These xanthomas commonly involve the Achilles tendon and present as tendonitis. If untreated, patients with HM FH typically die from myocardial infarction before age 20 years. The heterozygous (HZ) form of FH affects 1 in 500 individuals, with the partial receptor defect resulting in cells displaying half the normal number of fully functional LDL receptors. These individuals have lower elevated total cholesterol (>300 to 600 mg/dL) and LDL (250 to 500 mg/dL) levels than those with the HM form. Premature CHD (<45 years of age in men and <55 years of age in women) and tendon xanthomas are characteristic clinical findings.

Although FH can be established by identifying one of the many known gene mutations in the LDL receptor or by demonstrating diminished LDL receptor function, the diagnosis of FH usually is made on the basis of clinical features. Elevated total cholesterol (>300 mg/dL) and LDL (>250 mg/dL) in an individual with personal or family history of premature CHD and tendon xanthomas identifies individuals at risk for FH. Treatment requires a low-fat (<20% of total calories), low cholesterol (<100 mg per day) diet in combination with drug therapy. Usually FH patients require multiple agents to lower cholesterol levels to target range. Bile acid sequestrants are considered in younger individuals because of their limited side-effect profile, but more potent agents such as statins, cholesterol absorption inhibitors, and niacin are necessary in high-risk older individuals. In patients who do not tolerate medications or who have limited receptor function, ileal bypass surgery to decrease gastrointestinal absorption of bile acids or LDL apheresis to remove excess LDL can be considered.

FAMILIAL DEFECTIVE APOLIPOPROTEIN B-100

In this autosomal dominant disorder, a defect in the apo B-100 protein results in impaired binding of LDL particles to the LDL receptor. Most cases are linked to a single mutation (glutamine for arginine substitution) in the apo B-100 gene, but other mutations in the apo B-100 gene have also been identified in recent years. The disorder affects as many as 1 in 750 Caucasians with hypercholesterolemia. The clinical presentation is similar to FH, with elevated total cholesterol and LDL levels associated with premature CHD and tendon xanthomas. However, the HM and HZ clinical forms are milder than in FH because apo E–mediated clearance of remnant particles is still functional. Total cholesterol ranges from 350 to 550 mg/dL in HM and 200 to 350 mg/dL in HZ. DNA analysis can identify the apo B-100 gene mutation and confirm the diagnosis, but genetic diagnosis is not necessary to initiate therapy. A low-cholesterol, low-fat diet in combination with a statin, bile acid resin, or niacin is recommended to lower cholesterol levels to target ranges.

ELEVATED PLASMA LIPOPROTEIN(a)

Lp(a) is a specialized form of LDL assembled extracellularly from apolipoprotein(a) and LDL. Disulfide bridges link apo(a) to apo B-100 located on the surface of LDL particles. Apo(a) has sequence homologous with the fibrin-binding domains of plasminogen and, when present at elevated levels, interferes with fibrinolysis by competing with plasminogen. This leads to decreased thrombolysis and increased clot formation. Lp(a) also binds macrophages, promoting foam cell formation and atherosclerotic plaques. Genetic predisposition, African American heritage, and conditions associated with elevated LDL levels such as FH influence serum Lp(a) levels. Screening should be considered in individuals with family or personal history of premature CHD without dyslipidemia or in individuals refractory to cholesterol lowering therapy. The diagnosis can be made by documenting an Lp(a) level of more than 30 mg/dL in a patient with premature CHD. The primary goal of therapy is to lower LDL levels with agents such as statins. If LDL goals cannot be achieved, then Lp(a)-lowering therapy with niacin can be considered. Niacin decreases Lp(a) by as much as 38%, and it also stimulates tissue plasminogen activator and prevents thrombosis.

POLYGENIC HYPERCHOLESTEROLEMIA

Hypercholesterolemia in most individuals is thought to reflect small influences of many different genes. The exact nature of these genetic defects is poorly defined, but apo E may play a role in the pathogenesis. Apo E4 on chylomicron and VLDL remnants has a high affinity for the LDL receptor. Elevated binding of apo E4–containing lipoproteins to LDL receptors may downregulate LDL receptor synthesis and increase circulating LDL levels. Environmental factors such as diet can influence chylomicron and VLDL production, resulting in downregulation of the LDL receptor in high apo E4 conditions. This leads to an increased propensity for CHD, and treatment with LDL-lowering agents is recommended based on risk factors (see Table 63-5).

FAMILIAL COMBINED HYPERLIPOPROTEINEMIA

Familial combined hyperlipoproteinemia (FCHL) is an autosomal dominant polygenic disorder affecting 1% to 2% of the population. Factors such as diet, glucose intolerance, and medications can influence the phenotypic presentation. In FCHL, excess VLDL is synthesized in the liver. VLDL is hydrolyzed by LPL to produce LDL. Mutations in the LPL gene affecting its expression or function can decrease the efficiency of VLDL catabolism. Dysfunction of LPL is noted in one third of patients with FCHL. Diminished LPL activity increases circulating VLDL triglyceride. Furthermore, fewer VLDL remnant particles are available for HDL synthesis. Therefore, FCHL needs to be considered in all patients with total cholesterol level higher than 250 mg/dL, triglycerides higher than 175 mg/dL, or HDL lower than 35 mg/dL. There are no definitive diagnostic tests, but family screening can help confirm the diagnosis. The phenotype of FCHL is variable, with individuals displaying high LDL cholesterol, high VLDL triglyceride, or both based on the genetic defect and environmental factors. Patients also typically have high apo B (>120 mg/dL) and a low LDL cholesterol–to–apo B-100 ratio (<1.2). They accumulate small dense LDL particles, which are thought to be atherogenic and contribute to premature coronary artery disease. Xanthomas or xanthelasmas are not a feature of this disorder. Affected individuals require a low-fat, low-cholesterol diet plus multiple lipid-lowering drugs to achieve target goals. Fibric acid derivatives, which hydrolyze the triglyceride core of VLDL particles and increase LDL production, are recommended for treatment of the hypertriglyceridemia. Patients with FCHL often additionally require a statin or niacin to lower LDL cholesterol.

FAMILIAL DYSBETALIPOPROTEINEMIA

Apo E on the surface of lipoprotein particles binds LDL receptors and facilitates clearance of remnant particles from the circulation. The apo E2 allele has a lower affinity for LDL receptors than the E3 and E4 alleles. In individuals homozygous for apo E2, LPL hydrolyzes the triglyceride core, and the resulting cholesterol-rich lipoproteins (chylomicrons, VLDL, and IDL remnant particles) accumulate in the circulation. Expression of this phenotype usually requires a precipitating condition that increases lipoprotein production (e.g., diabetes, alcohol consumption) or decreases clearance (e.g., hypothyroidism). In addition to the more common autosomal recessive mutation of apo E described previously, several apo E mutations have been described that result in an autosomal dominant phenotype presenting in childhood and not requiring a secondary factor to express the phenotype. Premature CHD, peripheral vascular disease, and xanthomas involving the palmer crease are characteristic clinical features. Individuals with familial dysbetalipoproteinemia have elevated total cholesterol (300 to 400 mg/dL) and triglycerides (300 to 400 mg/dL). The ratio of total cholesterol to triglyceride in VLDL particles is elevated (>0.2), and the remnant VLDL (β-VLDL or IDL) particles can be detected with agarose gel electrophoresis. Definitive diagnosis requires genetic testing to identify apo E2 homozygosity or mutation. Treatment of coexisting conditions such as diabetes and hypothyroidism can normalize lipid levels in apo E2 homozygotes. If target levels are not achieved, dietary therapy and lipid-lowering drugs such as fibric acid derivatives and HMG-CoA reductase inhibitors should also be considered.

LIPOPROTEIN LIPASE DEFICIENCY

Mutations in the LPL gene resulting in deficiency of LPL synthesis or function lead to increased circulating chylomicron and VLDL particles and severe hypertriglyceridemia. Homozygous LPL deficiency is rare. It presents in childhood with triglycerides higher than 1000 mg/dL. Heterozygous LPL deficiency occurs in 2% to 4% of the population and usually requires a precipitating factor such as uncontrolled diabetes to manifest the phenotype. These individuals have moderate hypertriglyceridemia (250 to 750 mg/dL) that can increase to levels above 1000 mg/dL with secondary factors, such as insulin resistance or estrogen therapy. This can result in the chylomicronemia syndrome, characterized by marked hypertriglyceridemia (>1000 to 2000 mg/dL), pancreatitis, eruptive xanthomas, lipemia retinalis, and hepatosplenomegaly. Visual inspection demonstrates lipemic plasma. After refrigeration for 12 hours, a creamy top layer (increased chylomicrons) or turbid plasma infranatant (increased VLDL), or both, can be demonstrated. Documentation of diminished LPL activity confirms the diagnosis. A diet low in fat (<10% of total calories or <20 to 25 g per day) is the primary treatment. Secondary factors such as uncontrolled diabetes and alcohol use should be addressed, and VLDL-lowering agents (e.g., fibric acid

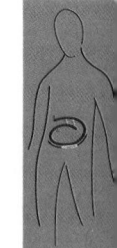

derivatives and niacin) may be needed to prevent severe hypertriglyceridemia.

APOLIPOPROTEIN C-II DEFICIENCY

Apo C-II is an activating cofactor for lipoprotein lipase. Deficiency of apo C-II is a rare autosomal recessive disorder that leads to increased chylomicrons and VLDL particles in the circulation, resulting in severe hypertriglyceridemia. Clinical manifestations are similar to LPL deficiency, including hypertriglyceridemia (>1000 mg/dL) and symptoms of pancreatitis, eruptive xanthomas, lipemia retinalis, and hepatosplenomegaly. Documenting the absence of apo C-II by plasma electrophoresis or demonstrating improvement in LPL activity with the addition of apo C-II confirms the diagnosis. Treatment of mild to moderate hypertriglyceridemia is similar to LPL deficiency. Recommendations include appropriate management of secondary factors such as diabetes and hypothyroidism, dietary fat restriction (<10% of calories), and drug therapy (e.g. fibric acid derivatives). For severe hypertriglyceridemia, plasma transfusion (with apo C-II) can be considered to lower triglyceride levels by activating LPL.

FAMILIAL HYPERTRIGLYCERIDEMIA

Familial hypertriglyceridemia is an autosomal dominant disorder characterized by overproduction of hepatic VLDL. The exact defect or mutation is unknown. Secondary factors that increase VLDL, such as diabetes, alcohol ingestion, and estrogen therapy, appear to exacerbate this condition. Low HDL associated with familial hypertriglyceridemia is related to increased catabolism. Individuals with this condition present with hypertriglyceridemia (200 to 500 mg/dL) and low HDL (<35 mg/dL). The decrease in HDL increases the risk for CHD. Secondary factors can exacerbate the problem by raising triglyceride levels above 1000 mg/dL and increasing the risk for pancreatitis and xanthomas. This diagnosis is considered in individuals with a family and personal history of hypertriglyceridemia, CHD, and normal LDL levels. A cloudy infranant noted after overnight refrigeration of plasma identifies a disorder of VLDL metabolism. Treatment starts with management of secondary factors that may exacerbate the condition. Dietary fat restriction (<10% of calories) and drug therapy with niacin and fibric acid derivates should be initiated if target goals are not achieved.

Prospectus for the Future

- Target goals for LDL treatment are continuously debated. More aggressive LDL management may be recommended as more evidence supporting lower LDL levels becomes available.
- The long-term risks of various drugs will need to be balanced with the potential benefit of achieving treatment goals. Further studies evaluating potential complications will guide therapeutic decisions. The potential cancer risk associated with ezetimibe will need to be clarified.

- Disorders of lipid metabolism result from defects in the production and removal of lipoproteins. A better understanding of these defects may lead to the development of drug therapy aimed at specific genetic mutations or enzyme dysfunction.
- Development of agents targeting HDL metabolism may play a role in CHD prevention.

References

Cobb MM, Teitelbaum HS, Breslow JL: Lovastatin efficacy in reducing low-density lipoprotein cholesterol levels on high- vs low-fat diet. JAMA 265:997-1001, 1991.

Gordon T, Castelli WP, Hjortland MC, et al: High density lipoprotein as a protective factor against coronary artery disease. The Framingham Study. Am J Med 62:707-715, 1997.

Gould AL, Rossouw JE, Santanello NC, et al: Cholesterol reduction yields clinical benefit: Impact of statin trials. Circulation 97:946-958, 1998.

Grundy SM, Cleeman JI, Merz CN, et al: Implications of recent clinical trials for the National Cholesterol Education Program (NCEP) Adult Treatment Panel III Guidelines. Circulation 110:227-239, 2004.

Hokanson JE, Austin MA: Plasma triglyceride level is a risk factor for cardiovascular disease independent of high-density lipoprotein cholesterol: A meta-analysis of population-based prospective studies. J Cardiovasc Risk 3:213-224, 1996.

Kraus WE, Houmard JA, Duscha BD, et al: Effect of the amount and intensity of exercise on plasma lipoproteins. N Engl J Med 347:1483-1489, 2002.

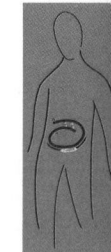

Disorders of Metals and Metalloproteins

David G. Brooks

Wilson Disease

Wilson disease, or hepatolenticular degeneration, is the result of the defective excretion of copper. Accumulation of this metal produces damage to multiple organs, with the liver and brain prominently affected. Wilson disease is an autosomal recessive genetic disorder that affects people worldwide with a frequency approximating 1 in 30,000.

NORMAL COPPER METABOLISM

Copper is an essential dietary trace element. A balance of dietary intake and hepatobiliary excretion meets physiologic requirements. Humans ingest 1 to 5 mg/day, and an adult body contains 100 to 150 mg copper. Copper is absorbed in the proximal small intestine. The liver, which is the main organ for copper homeostasis, rapidly takes up absorbed copper. The liver plays important roles in transport, storage, and excretion of copper. Copper is normally excreted into bile canaliculi in a regulated fashion that is dependent on copper concentration in hepatocytes. Up to 95% of plasma copper is bound to ceruloplasmin, an abundant plasma protein produced by the liver. The putative role of ceruloplasmin as a copper transporter to extrahepatic tissues has been called into question by the absence of copper deficiency in aceruloplasminemia, a genetic disease featuring the absence of apoceruloplasmin. Rather, ceruloplasmin is more likely to play a critical role in recycling iron, highlighting an interaction of iron and copper homeostasis.

PATHOGENESIS

Mutations in patients with Wilson disease occur in a gene, *ATP7B,* which encodes a copper-transporting adenosine triphosphatase (ATPase). This protein transports copper across cell membranes and is essential for exporting copper from hepatocytes into the bile canaliculi. Wilson disease protein also transports cytosolic copper into membrane-bound compartments of hepatocytes containing newly synthesized apoceruloplasmin. In the absence of ATP7B transporter,

copper is not transported, and apoceruloplasmin is secreted into the blood, where it has a rapid turnover. Thus, low plasma ceruloplasmin levels are a helpful diagnostic sign of Wilson disease (Table 64-1). Copper accumulates slowly in liver (see Table 64-1) and later in other organs. High levels of copper are a risk factor for generating reactive oxygen species, which contribute to end-organ damage. Liver dysfunction, the most common presentation in childhood, usually appears after 6 years of age but has been reported as young as 3 years of age. Presentations vary from acute hemolysis or fulminant liver failure to chronic, progressive liver failure or neuropsychiatric disease. Most patients have liver biopsy evidence of some cirrhosis resulting from copper-mediated damage. Hepatocellular carcinoma occurs rarely but has been reported in men long after treatment was initiated so that surveillance is indicated. Neurologic symptoms, in particular as a result of basal ganglia dysfunction, are the initial presentation in up to 40% to 50% of patients. Parkinsonian symptoms predominate with dystonia, choreoathetosis, and tremor. A minority of patients experience psychiatric symptoms, including personality change, depression, or cognitive impairment, all of which indicate that the cerebral cortex is affected by copper deposition. Associated findings include *hemolytic anemia* (negative Coombs test) and kidney damage (*nephrolithiasis* and *Fanconi syndrome* with amino aciduria and glucosuria). Cardiac dysrhythmia, osteoporosis, rhabdomyolysis, arthralgia, and endocrine dysfunction have also been reported.

DIAGNOSIS

A combination of laboratory tests strongly supports the diagnosis of Wilson disease (see Table 64-1). About 95% of patients have a low ceruloplasmin level (<0.2 g/L), with some having normal levels because ceruloplasmin is an acute-phase reactant that is high during inflammation such as fulminant liver failure. Serum copper is slightly decreased and non–ceruloplasmin-bound serum copper is usually elevated. A significant increase in urinary copper excretion (>100 mcg per 24 hours) is almost always present, which

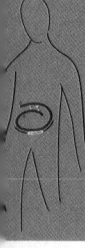

Table 64-1 **Diagnostic Copper Testing in Wilson Disease**		
Test	Levels in Healthy Persons	Levels in Wilson Disease
Liver copper content (mcg Cu/g dry weight)	10-50	100-2000
Serum ceruloplasmin (mg/dL)	20-45	0-20
Serum copper (mcg/dL)	70-160	25-70
Urinary copper (mcg/day)	3-35	100-1000

should increase further with chelator therapy. Liver biopsy often reveals micronodular cirrhosis with nodular regeneration, copper deposition, and elevated copper content (>250 mcg/g dry weight), which remains the gold standard of diagnosis. Sunflower cataracts and Kayser-Fleischer rings, which are yellow-brown to green deposits at the periphery of the cornea, strongly support the diagnosis. Magnetic resonance imaging (MRI) of basal ganglia may show degeneration or evidence suggestive of copper deposition. Genetic testing is available; however, hundreds of mutations are known, which means that only specialized laboratories offer this service. In defined ethnic groups, identifying genetic mutations that confirm Wilson disease may be practical and have important genetic counseling implications for family members. For example, the H1069Q mutation is found in up to 50% of Caucasian patients and, when present in the homozygous state, is reported to predict later onset disease with a higher frequency of neurologic complications.

TREATMENT

Wilson disease is a treatable genetic disorder. Therefore, this diagnosis is an important consideration in anyone with unexplained hemolysis or liver, basal ganglia, or psychiatric signs or symptoms. The goal of therapy is to reduce total-body copper burden without inducing copper deficiency. The mainstays of therapy to induce negative copper balance are chelation to remove excess copper already in the body and inhibiting absorption of dietary copper. Two copper chelators are approved for clinical use: trientine (Syprine) and D-penicillamine (Cuprimine). Historically, penicillamine was the treatment of choice. However, 10% to 20% of patients develop side effects of this therapy that can be treatment limiting and severe, including bone marrow aplasia. For D-penicillamine, treatment can be initiated with 1 to 3 g per day divided into two to four doses, although titrating the dose up from 250 to 500 mg per day may improve tolerance. Pyridoxine (vitamin B$_6$) should be supplemented while taking penicillamine. Twenty-four hour urine copper excretion should increase from 1 to 5 mg per day with symptomatic improvement on average after 4 months of therapy. Complete blood counts and urinary protein are important to monitor during penicillamine therapy. Further, under no circumstances should D-penicillamine be abruptly stopped; doing so increases the risk for acute hepatic decompensation. Trientine is reported to have a lower incidence of side effects than penicillamine. It can be started at 1200 to 1800 mg per day divided into three doses but reduced to 900 to 1200 mg per day for maintenance therapy. Both chelators should be given before or after but not with food. Copper reduction therapies should be expected to take 6 to 8 weeks to begin to show evidence of efficacy and may require a couple years to reach maximal effect.

A novel dietary strategy, high-dose zinc (150 mg per day divided in three doses), can significantly decrease copper absorption. Zinc inhibits net copper absorption by inducing the small intestine to produce the copper-chelating protein, metallothionein. Metallothionein-bound copper is sloughed with small intestinal absorptive cells. Zinc can cause dyspepsia, and changing the formulation (acetate, sulfate, or gluconate) may improve this side effect. As an essential nutrient, zinc is generally well tolerated and is increasingly appreciated as a cornerstone of therapy in Wilson disease. Starting acutely ill patients on combination therapy with chelator and zinc is indicated, whereas maintenance therapy with zinc alone is possible after an acute "de-coppering" stage. Monitoring 24-hour urine copper during therapy is important to ensure compliance. The level should reach 3 to 8 μmol per day, which is about 200 to 500 mcg copper per day lost in urine. With zinc supplementation, the goal is to reach 24-hour urinary copper below 2 μmol per day, whereas concurrent quantitation of urinary zinc monitors compliance with oral zinc therapy. It is important to monitor blood non–ceruloplasmin-bound copper for the target range of 50 to 150 mcg/L during therapy, so that overtreatment does not result in copper deficiency and secondary sideroblastic anemia and hemosiderosis. Supplementation with the antioxidant vitamin E taken with meals or N-acetyl cysteine may offset some of the organ damage induced by reactive oxygen species. A diet low in copper minimizing shellfish, nuts, mushrooms, and chocolate can be an adjunct to therapy. Urinalysis and blood counts should be followed closely during penicillamine therapy. Giving a test dose of penicillamine is important because it triggers hypersensitivity reactions strong enough to prevent its use in up to 10% of patients. Fever, lymphadenopathy, cytopenias, lupus erythematosus-like reactions, and nephrotic syndrome can result. Trientine is an alternative treatment for those with hypersensitivity reactions to penicillamine. Liver transplantation, even from living related donors who carry a single defective gene for Wilson disease, has been a successful treatment for those with progressive liver failure.

Hemochromatosis

Hemochromatosis is the condition of excessive iron storage causing dysfunction of a characteristic pattern of organs. It is important for physicians to detect hemochromatosis because it is a fatal disease that is entirely preventable if diagnosed early. Hemochromatosis may be primary, or it may develop secondary to multiple transfusions, when it is sometimes referred to as *hemosiderosis*. The primary form, which is known as *hereditary hemochromatosis* (HH), is the focus of this section.

NORMAL IRON METABOLISM

The adult male body contains 4 g of iron, over half of which is in the form of hemoglobin. To meet the daily iron require-

Table 64-2 Iron Indices in Healthy Persons and in Patients with Symptomatic Hemochromatosis		
Index	**Levels in Healthy Persons**	**Levels in Hemochromatosis**
Plasma iron (mcg/dL)	50-150	180-300
Total iron-binding capacity (mcg/dL)	250-375	200-300
Percent transferring saturation	20-40	80-100
Serum ferritin (ng/mL)	10-200	900-6000
Urinary iron after 0.5 g desferrioxamine	0-2	9-23
Liver iron (mcg/100 mg dry weight)	30-140	600-1800

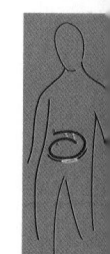

ment for erythropoiesis, iron is recycled from the reticulo-endothelial system. Iron is absorbed in the duodenum, and the efficiency of absorption is tightly regulated. Thus, the duodenum responds to bodily iron requirements and can significantly increase absorption of iron in response to iron deficiency. Iron is not actively excreted, although about 1 mg of iron is lost daily through sloughed cells. Iron loss is significantly increased by menstrual bleeding and pregnancy; hence, women are less susceptible to HH than men. These losses are offset by absorption of 1 to 3 mg of iron daily in normal individuals (and abnormally high iron absorption in patients with hemochromatosis).

The liver is critical for iron storage and transport (as well as pathology of HH). Iron stored in *ferritin* protein in the liver is less prone to form reactive oxygen species. Ferritin secretion from the liver is positively correlated with hepatic iron stores. Hepatocytes secrete the iron bound to the transport protein (apo) transferrin, which circulates about 20% to 40% saturated with iron (Table 64-2). Transferrin-bound iron is the major source of iron for extrahepatic tissues that have transferrin receptors. After transferrin receptor–mediated endocytosis, iron may be released in the acidic environment of an intracellular vesicle (endosome), and transferrin is recycled to be released at the cell surface.

Recent discovery of *hepcidin*, a polypeptide hormone, has shed new light on iron physiology. Hepcidin is produced by the liver in response to iron stores and is believed to signal the need for iron absorption to the duodenum and reticuloendothelial system. Hepcidin may be upregulated in anemia of chronic disease causing abnormal iron distribution and absorption.

PATHOGENESIS OF HEREDITARY HEMOCHROMATOSIS

Four types of hereditary hemochromatosis are known. The genetic bases of these disorders are known in three of the four types, and all defective gene products have a role in cellular iron trafficking. In two of the types, the defective genes encode ferritin or transferrin receptors. In the third type, which is the common form of hereditary hemochro-

matosis, discovery of the gene has generated new insight into the basis of iron homeostasis. Only the common form of hereditary hemochromatosis is discussed in this chapter.

The common form of hereditary hemochromatosis is the result of defects in a gene and protein called HFE, hence the name HFE-linked hemochromatosis. This gene is near the major histocompatibility complex (MHC) locus on chromosome 6, in keeping with the longstanding observation that certain MHC isotypes (e.g., human leuko-cyte-associated antigen [HLA-A3]) are co-inherited with hemochromatosis. The HFE protein is an MHC class I–like molecule that requires association with β_2-microglobulin to function. In the absence of either HFE or β_2-microglobulin, mice develop iron overload reminiscent of human hemochromatosis. HFE binds tightly to the transferrin receptor and regulates its affinity for transferrin ligand. More than 85% of hemochromatosis in patients of northern European ancestry is attributable to two specific HFE mutations that interfere with its function. The most common mutation in patients results in the substitution of tyrosine for the normal cysteine at position 282 (C282Y). This mutation is most concentrated in people of northern European ancestry, a finding that accounts for the Caucasian predilection for HH. The C282Y mutation is found in 1 in 10 Caucasians in the United States. By mendelian genetics, 1 in 400 Caucasians carries two of these mutations. However, the observed prevalence of hemochromatosis associated with end-organ damage is at least an order of magnitude less common than this genetic prevalence. In Australia, 28% of male and 1.4% of female homozygotes for C282Y mutation developed iron overload disease, indicating that a minority of individuals with two mutations will develop HH. Put another way, the positive predictive value of a genetic test is low. This phenomenon, called *reduced penetrance,* explains why genetic testing has limited utility as a screening tool for this disorder. However, testing for C282Y or another common mutant allele, H63D, is useful in patients with iron overload to confirm the diagnosis of hemochromatosis and for counseling family members of a confirmed case.

The essential defect in hereditary hemochromatosis is increased absorption of dietary iron. A slight increase in the efficiency of iron absorption, coupled with the inability to excrete iron, leads to increasing hepatic iron storage as a function of time. With increasing iron stores, the liver secretes more ferritin, and serum transferrin becomes increasingly saturated with iron. Initially, a patient may have general signs such as fatigue. Later, signs of liver disease, such as increased serum transaminases, are apparent. Liver biopsy shows increased iron stores in hepatocytes with sparing of Kupffer cells; a specimen should be analyzed to quantitate the amount of iron. High iron stores can lead to a generation of toxic reactive oxygen species, fibrosis, cirrhosis, hepatocellular carcinoma, and death.

The earliest symptoms of hemochromatosis include fatigue, lethargy, arthralgia, and right upper quadrant discomfort. As the capacity of liver to store iron safely is exceeded, particularly after transferrin saturation reaches 100%, iron is deposited in other tissues. Deposition in the synovium produces iron-induced arthritis, which is particularly evident in the second and third metacarpophalangeal joints. In the pancreatic islets, β cells are damaged, with decreased insulin secretion culminating in diabetes mellitus.

Iron can cause restrictive cardiomyopathy and a predisposition to conduction system abnormalities, resulting in arrhythmias. Hypogonadism, secondary to hypopituitarism, can result in impotence, menstrual irregularities, or premature menopause. Discoloration of the skin, often a gray-brown color referred to as *bronzing*, is characteristic of late hemochromatosis. The classic triad of *bronze diabetes with liver failure* is a late manifestation that is rarely observed today. Physicians should strive to recognize the early, more general symptoms of fatigue and arthralgia because treatment can prevent permanent organ damage.

DIAGNOSIS

In its earliest stages, hyperferritinemia and transferrin saturation above 50% are the only signs of hemochromatosis (see Table 64-2). Serum ferritin levels above 200 ng/mL in women or 300 ng/mL in men are frequently used to define iron overload. Transferrin saturation is calculated as serum iron ÷ total iron-binding capacity (TIBC). Modern laboratory measurements are usually of serum transferrin, and the TIBC is calculated as 1.4 × serum transferrin. If these values are marginally elevated on a random sample, a repeat measure on a fasting blood sample is indicated. If the transferrin saturation is maintained greater than 50%, evaluation for liver disease is indicated. Serum ferritin greater than 1000 ng/mL has been reported to carry a significantly increased risk for cirrhosis. As the disease progresses, hepatomegaly with abnormal liver function tests may develop. Liver biopsy is the only method to ascertain whether fibrosis is present and to prove increased hepatic iron content (see Table 64-2), the gold standard for the diagnosis of HH. A useful diagnostic test of iron overload is the concept of "mobilizable iron" defined as the mass of iron that can be safely removed by phlebotomy without inducing anemia. A unit of blood is estimated to contain 250 mg iron from a man and 200 mg from a woman. If a prospective patient can donate more than 8 to 10 U or 2 g of iron in less than a year without anemia, they have iron overload. Genetic testing in an individual with elevated serum iron indices can confirm the diagnosis of hemochromatosis. MRI has potential for detecting hepatic iron overload, and future research will be aimed at making this noninvasive test more quantitative.

TREATMENT

Symptomatic patients without treatment have a 5-year survival rate of 10%. Early diagnosis is crucial in hemochromatosis because treatment may prevent serious complications such as cirrhosis and hepatocellular carcinoma. Established arthritis, hypogonadism, and liver fibrosis remain resistant to treatment, although proper treatment will slow progression. Therapy consists of phlebotomy to remove iron from the body; this can increase the 10-year survival rate to 75% in patients with cirrhosis. Because the source of excess iron is dietary, removing iron supplements from the diet of a patient with hemochromatosis is imperative. Because vitamin C aids absorption of iron, recommending avoidance of vitamin C supplements is prudent. Iron is typically limiting for erythropoiesis so that blood can be removed at more frequent intervals from patients with hemochroma-

tosis than from normal individuals. Patients with severe iron loading can tolerate weekly or biweekly phlebotomy without anemia for months. A running total of units of blood removed and corresponding hemoglobin should be maintained. Serum iron indices should be checked periodically during phlebotomy therapy. Goals include maintaining ferritin below 50 ng/mL and transferrin saturation below 30%. After these goals have been reached, maintenance phlebotomy 2 to 5 times each year is required to prevent reaccumulation of iron. It is important for patients with evidence of liver disease to avoid other hepatotoxins such as alcohol.

SCREENING

As a common, genetic disease associated with well-tolerated preventive and treatment measures, HH has been a frequent topic of discussion about screening. Repeated investigation of the issue has led to the conclusion that widespread public health screening is not justified at this time. However, screening within targeted populations should be considered. These include males of Northern European ancestry, individuals with a positive family history of iron overload, and patients with unexplained related conditions such as fatigue, arthralgia, diabetes, liver disease, cardiomyopathy, and hypogonadism. Serum ferritin and transferrin saturation are an appropriate initial screening test. If elevated, the algorithm outlined earlier under "Diagnosis" should be followed. As previously discussed, genetic testing should not be used to screen patients with unknown liver disease because it has limited positive predictive value, and the existing genetic tests do not detect all causes of HH particularly outside Caucasian ethnic backgrounds.

Porphyrias

Porphyria is the name given to a group of genetic or acquired diseases associated with deficient synthesis of heme. Heme is an essential cofactor for the structure and function of hemoglobin and proteins such as cytochrome P-450. Bone marrow produces more than 80% of body heme at a steady state to support erythropoiesis. Liver produces about 15% of total heme, but its synthesis can be increased 10-fold. For example, heme synthesis will be induced by ingestion of a drug that relies on a heme-containing enzyme for detoxification. This induction of hepatic heme synthesis underlies the important observation that certain drugs trigger porphyria attacks (Table 64-3). Porphyrias result from partial deficiency of one of seven enzymes involved in biosynthesis of heme (Fig. 64-1). Attacks of porphyria are associated with the accumulation of the biochemical intermediates in the heme synthesis pathway that precede the deficient enzyme (see Fig. 64-1). Some of these intermediates are toxic and can lead to the observable sign of dark, reddish urine. The two major classes of porphyria, bone marrow and hepatic, derive from the organ accounting for the overproduction of heme synthesis intermediates (Table 64-4).

Four of the five hepatic porphyrias have acute onset of neurovisceral pain as a result of the accumulation of early intermediates of heme synthesis such as δ-aminolevulinic acid (ALA) and porphobilinogen (see Fig. 64-1). Named *acute* for their hallmark abrupt presentation (and sometimes resolution), these porphyrias also have chronic features, including pain, neuropathy, and depression. Excess porphyrins, produced in bone marrow porphyrias, deposit in skin and absorb light, which confers photosensitivity and results in cutaneous manifestations such as blistering of sun-exposed skin. This section describes three porphyrias that are the most common and encompass the cardinal biochemical and clinical features of these disorders.

ACUTE INTERMITTENT PORPHYRIA

Acute intermittent porphyria (AIP) is an autosomal dominant disorder due to half or less normal activity of porphobilinogen (PBG) deaminase. Under most circumstances, half-normal activity of this enzyme is sufficient to prevent porphyria; indeed, up to 90% of people with half-normal enzyme activity never experience attacks. PBG deaminase is the third enzyme in the pathway of heme biosynthesis (see Fig. 64-1). When it is limiting, there is accumulation of the two intermediates of the pathway before this enzyme (ALA and PBG) (see Fig. 64-1). A high urinary PBG level during an attack is a critical diagnostic feature, although the level is often normal between attacks. Finding deficient PBG deaminase enzyme activity in red blood cells confirms the diagnosis.

As the names *acute* and *intermittent* imply, acute attacks punctuate prolonged well periods in patients with AIP. The acute presentation of AIP can be dramatic and life-threatening. Abdominal pain, largely thought to be the result of neurotoxicity, is present in more than 90% of patients with acute attacks. Abdominal pain may be severe enough to prompt surgical evaluation for an acute abdomen and can be associated with nausea, vomiting, and bowel dysmotility. Neuropathy is evidenced by decreased sensation or muscle weakness that may involve cranial and respiratory nerves.

Table 64-3 **Partial List of Drugs Precipitating Attacks of Acute Intermittent Porphyria**
Barbiturates
Carbamazepine
Chlorpropamide
Chlordiazepoxide
Danazol
Dapsone
Ergot preparations
Estrogens
Ethanol
Glutethimide
Griseofulvin
Meprobamate
Oral contraceptives
Phenytoin
Progestins
Pyrazinamide
Sulfonamide antibiotics
Theophylline
Tolbutamide
Valproic acid

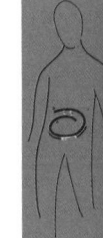

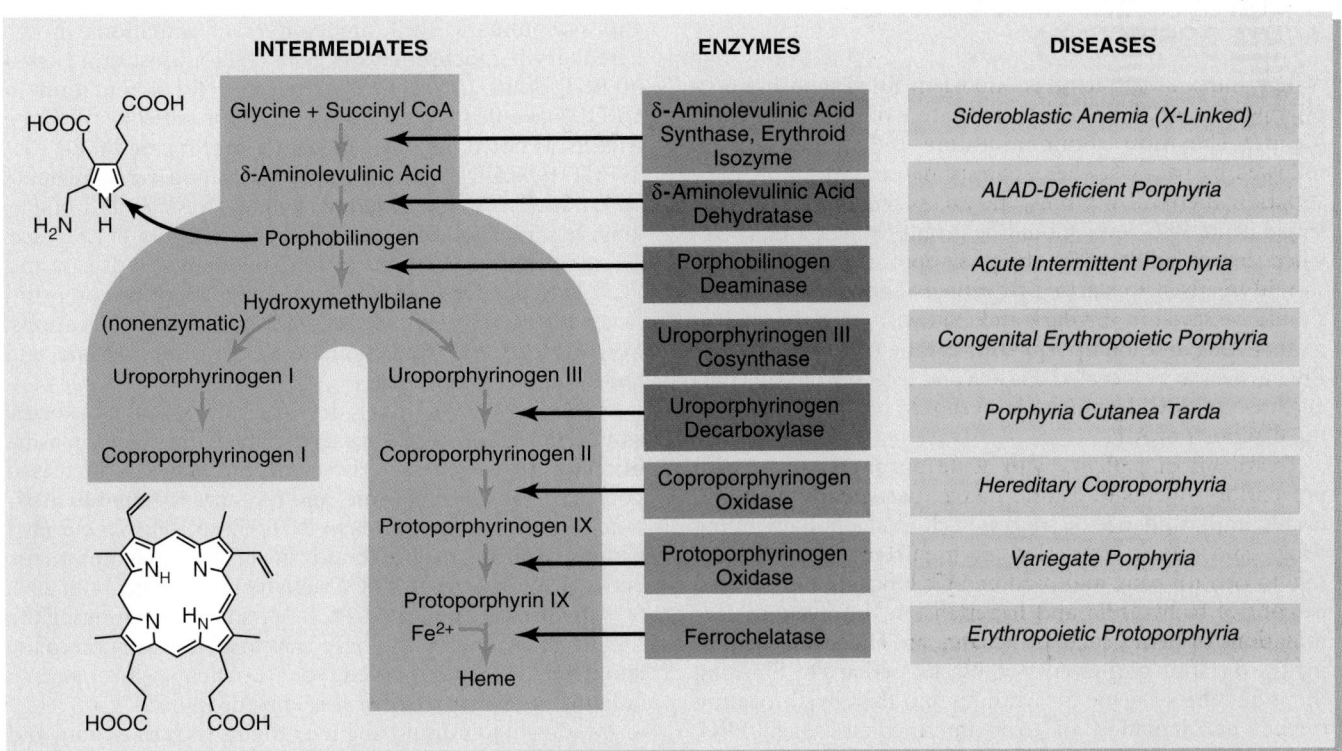

Figure 64-1 The heme biosynthetic pathway and the major diseases of porphyrin metabolism. The initial and last three enzymes *(in red)* are mitochondrial, and the other four *(in blue)* are cytosolic. X-linked sideroblastic anemia is not classically considered a porphyria. ALAD, aminolevulinic acid dehydratase. (From Anderson KE: The porphyrias. In Goldman L, Bennett JC [eds]: Cecil Textbook of Medicine, 21st ed. Philadelphia, WB Saunders, 2000, p 1124.)

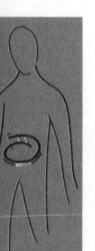

Table 64-4 Porphyrias Grouped by Organ Source of Excess Heme Precursors

Organ Source	Porphyria	Prevalence	Neurologic Symptoms	Skin Drug Photosensitivity	Inducible
Liver	ALA dehydratase porphyria	Very rare	+	–	+
	Acute intermittent porphyria	5-10/100,000	+	–	+
	Porphyria cutanea tarda	Uncertain, but most common porphyria	+	+	+
	Hereditary coporphyria	Rare	+	+	+
	Variegate porphyria	Not rare	+	+	+
Bone marrow	Congenital erythropoietic porphyria	Rare	–	+	–
	Erythropoietic protoporphyria	Several hundred known worldwide	–	+	–

ALA, δ-aminolevulinic acid.

Sympathetic tone is high with hypertension and tachycardia. Central nervous system manifestations include anxiety, paranoia, depression, and seizures, which may result in part from hyponatremia due to inappropriate secretion of antidiuretic hormone.

Most patients suffer their initial attack after puberty. Triggers of attacks include drugs, particularly those that induce the mitochondrial cytochrome P-450 system such as barbiturates, carbamazepine, and sulfonamides (see Table 64-3). Caloric restriction, fasting, surgery, states of high progesterone, infections, and in particular the interaction of more than one of these triggers have precipitated attacks.

DIAGNOSIS AND TREATMENT OF ACUTE PORPHYRIAS

A high index of suspicion is important for diagnosing porphyrias because of the nonspecific nature of presenting complaints. The most common feature is abdominal pain, followed by pain elsewhere, paresis, nausea, vomiting, constipation, mental symptoms, and excess sympathetic tone. A single urine PBG level should be promptly sent and, if elevated in an adult with above symptoms, consideration should be given to starting treatment. The urine specimen should be saved in the dark and cold without preservatives so that ALA and total porphyrins can be quantitated if the PBG proves to be elevated. Plasma and fecal porphyrins plus erythrocyte PBC deaminase level should be sent to confirm the diagnosis of AIP.

Treatment of patients with acute porphyria starts with prevention. Adequate caloric intake, particularly carbohydrates, and avoidance of triggers such as alcohol, offending drugs, and caloric restriction are important. Narcotics are safe to control pain, and β-adrenergic blockers can be used to control tachycardia and hypertension. Intravenous formulations of heme, such as hematin, are effective in reducing the duration and severity of attacks, perhaps by blunting the induction of heme biosynthesis and thereby abrogating further accumulation of toxic intermediates (e.g., PBG, ALA). Indeed, prompt institution of intravenous hematin therapy is pivotal because rare episodes of acute porphyria are life-threatening or associated with permanent neurologic impairment such as paresis.

PORPHYRIA CUTANEA TARDA

Porphyria cutanea tarda (PCT) is the most common porphyria and shows the cardinal feature of bullous involvement of sun-exposed skin. This results from accumulation of uroporphyrinogen and related heme-synthetic intermediates, which absorb light and confer photosensitivity. PCT is due to decreased activity of the hepatic enzyme uroporphyrinogen decarboxylase. More than 75% of patients have type I or *sporadic* disease, in which the family history is negative for affected relatives, and there is no mutation in the gene (*UROD*) encoding the enzyme. Triggers of attacks include supplemental estrogen, alcohol, iron overload, hepatitis C virus (HCV), and AIDS. Many patients with iron overload and symptomatic PCT are carriers of mutations in the hereditary hemochromatosis gene (*HFE*). Most other cases of PCT occur in people heterozygous for a mutation in *UROD*, so-called type II disease. In these patients, the same triggers as noted for AIP can elicit symptomatic PCT.

PCT typically begins in early adulthood with subacute appearance of fragile skin and includes vesicles and bullae, grayish skin discoloration, and hypertrichosis of the face. There is a complicated relationship between liver disease and PCT: liver involvement may be a cause, effect, or comorbid factor for PCT. There may be mild transaminase elevations, iron overload, HCV infection, liver cirrhosis, hepatoma, and hepatocellular carcinoma.

Diagnosis of PCT includes skin and family histories, consideration of recently started medicines, and plasma fluorescence for characteristic porphyrin peaks. Increased porphyrins in plasma, urine, and feces are required to attribute clinical manifestations to PCT. Up to 100-fold elevated uroporphyrins can be found in urine of symptomatic patients. A low level of *UROD* activity is found in about 25% of patients with inherited PCT. Mutation screening of the *UROD* gene may be the only way to detect asymptomatic family members of so-called type III patients who appear to only manifest deficiency of this enzyme in liver.

Avoiding and minimizing liver toxins such as alcohol and excess iron is a mainstay of therapy. Treatment includes avoiding triggers or removing any excess iron by phlebotomy and chloroquine, or sometimes both of these measures. It is important to lower the burden of porphyrins, and chloroquine is useful by forming a complex with porphyrin that has improved excretion. Chloroquine is given at low dose (125 mg and no more than 250 mg twice weekly), with up to 2 months required for demonstrable biochemical improvement and 1 year for remission. Dialysis does not remove plasma porphyrins, and this contributes to an increased incidence of type I PCT in end-stage renal failure patients. PCT in the setting of dialysis is a therapeutic challenge because chloroquine does not work; low-volume phlebotomy and desferrioxamine, an iron chelator, have been tried.

ERYTHROPOIETIC PORPHYRIA

Erythropoietic porphyria (EPP) results from deficiency of the last enzyme in heme biosynthesis, ferrochelatase. As a result of this late block in the pathway, large amounts of protoporphyrin accumulate (see Fig. 64-1) and produce serious cutaneous damage through a photodynamic reaction as observed in patients with PCT. A brief exposure to sunlight can produce burning, redness, and edema suggestive of angio-edema developing within hours and resolving over several days after sun exposure. Vesicles and bullae are less common than in patients with PCT. Unlike PCT, manifestations of EPP typically occur in childhood and can even have severe congenital forms. A reddish urine in diapers is sometimes the initial clue in congenital forms. About one fourth of EPP patients will have liver involvement, with gallstones found in up to 10% of patients.

A massive increase in erythrocyte protoporphyrin levels is the diagnostic hallmark of EPP, so much so that fluorescent red blood cells can sometimes be visualized on a blood smear. Fecal protoporphyrins are usually elevated in symptomatic patients, whereas high urinary protoporphyrins are not as elevated and may indicate hepatic involvement. Avoidance of sun or use of potent sunscreens is the mainstay of prevention. Avoiding alcohol and drugs known to induce heme synthesis can be helpful. β-carotene is a useful adjunct therapy that may limit oxidative damage to sun-exposed skin, although it takes weeks to fully penetrate the skin where it has its effect. Liver transplantation has been performed for severe liver disease.

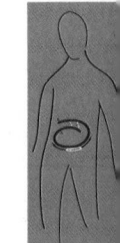

Prospectus for the Future

- Identification of factors that will protect a person with a deleterious genotype from developing hemochromatosis, Wilson disease, or a porphyria. Development of drugs and other therapeutic approaches will be based on this knowledge.

- Effective screening strategies will be expanded, based on biochemical indices for hemochromatosis, with more people entering therapy at earlier stages of the disease.

References

Adams PC: Hemochromatosis. Clin Liver Dis 8:735-753, 2004.

Ala A, Walker AP, Ashkan K, et al: Wilson's disease. Lancet 369:397-408, 2007.

Anderson KE, Bloomer JR, Bonkovsky HL, et al: Recommendations for the diagnosis and treatment of the acute porphyrias. Ann Intern Med 142:439-450, 2005.

Andrews NC: Forging a field: The golden age of iron biology. Blood 112:219-230, 2008.

Brewer GJ, Askari FK: Wilson's disease: Clinical management and therapy. J Hepatol 42(Suppl 1):S13-S21, 2005.

Beutler E, Felitti VJ, Koziol JA, et al: Penetrance of 845G→A (C282Y) HFE hereditary haemochromatosis mutation in the USA. Lancet 359:211-218, 2002.

Cizewski Culotta V, Gitlin JD: Disorders of copper transport. In Scriver CR, Beaudet AL, Valle D, et al (eds): The Metabolic and Molecular Basis of Inherited Disease, 8th ed. New York, McGraw-Hill, 2001, pp 3105-3126.

Kauppinen R: Porphyrias. Lancet 365:241-252, 2005.

Neimark E, Shilsky ML, Schneider BL: Wilson's disease and hemochromatosis. Adolesc Med Clin 15:175-194, 2004.

Qaseem A, Aronson M, Fitterman N, et al: for the Clinical Efficacy Assessment Subcommittee of the American College of Physicians: Screening for hereditary hemochromatosis: A clinical practice guideline from the American College of Physicians. Ann Intern Med 143:517-521, 2005.

Schmitt B, Golub RM, Green R: Screening primary care patients for hereditary hemochromatosis with transferrin saturation and serum ferritin level: Systematic review for the American College of Physicians. Ann Intern Med 143:522-536, 2005.

Steinberg KK, Cogswell ME, Chang JC, et al: Prevalence of C282Y and H63D mutations in the hemochromatosis (*HFE*) gene in the United States. JAMA 285:2216-2222, 2001.

Section XII

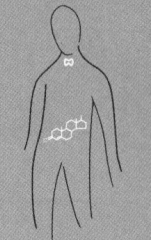

Endocrine Disease

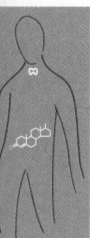

Hypothalamic-Pituitary Axis

Vivien S. Herman-Bonert

Anatomy and Physiology

The pituitary gland, weighing 500 to 900 mg, lies at the base of the skull in the sella turcica within the sphenoid bone. The cavernous sinus borders laterally on the pituitary gland. The optic chiasm courses over the superior aspect. Two thirds of the pituitary gland is composed of the anterior lobe, and one third is the posterior lobe.

The anterior pituitary gland receives a rich vascular supply, largely from the hypothalamus via a hypothalamic-pituitary portal circulation. Hypothalamic stimulatory and inhibitory hormones are directly transported via the hypothalamic-pituitary portal circulation to specific cells of the anterior pituitary gland, where they regulate synthesis and secretion of pituitary trophic hormones (Fig. 65-1; **Web Figs. 65-1 and 65-2**).

A specific pituitary cell type secretes each of the anterior pituitary hormones: adrenocorticotropic hormone (ACTH), growth hormone (GH), prolactin (PRL), and thyroid-stimulating hormone (TSH). In addition, the same cell secretes the gonadotropins luteinizing hormone (LH) and follicle-stimulating hormone (FSH). Arginine vasopressin (AVP), also known as *antidiuretic hormone* (ADH), is synthesized in the hypothalamus and transported through the pituitary stalk to the posterior lobe of the pituitary gland (Table 65-1), where it is stored and available to be secreted when stimulated. Oxytocin is also stored and secreted by the posterior pituitary lobe.

Pituitary Tumors

Each of the five pituitary cell types, either singly or in combination, can give rise to benign pituitary adenomas, which secrete hormones characteristic of the particular cell type. Prolactinomas are the most common secretory pituitary tumors. Isolated reports of pituitary carcinomas with distant metastases have been described.

The earliest clinical manifestations of pituitary tumors are usually the characteristic signs and symptoms caused by the hormone hypersecretion. Subsequently, if the tumor is large, local manifestations of tumor enlargement may develop. Pressure on surrounding structures can cause signs and symptoms of large pituitary adenomas (secretory or nonsecretory). Headache is a frequent symptom. If the tumor extends into the suprasellar space, the optic chiasm may be compressed, which classically results in bitemporal hemianopia. Lateral extension into the cavernous sinus can result in ophthalmoplegia, diplopia, or ptosis as a result of dysfunction of the third, fourth, and sixth cranial nerves. Compression of surrounding normal pituitary tissue by an enlarging tumor mass can cause hyposecretion of one or several pituitary trophic hormones, resulting in signs and symptoms of hypopituitarism. Destructive pituitary lesions result in hormone loss, which follows a particular pattern: initially GH secretion is reduced, followed by LH and FSH, then TSH, and lastly ACTH.

The presence of a pituitary tumor is confirmed by pituitary magnetic resonance imaging (MRI) (**Web Fig. 65-3**). The contrast agent gadolinium is used to help differentiate small pituitary lesions from normal anterior pituitary tissue. Microadenomas are defined as pituitary lesions less than 10 mm in diameter. Macroadenomas are pituitary lesions more than 10 mm in diameter. They may cause significant deviation of the pituitary stalk to the opposite side. Adenomas exceeding 15 mm frequently have suprasellar extension with compression and displacement of the optic chiasm. An MRI may also show lateral extension of large adenomas into the cavernous sinus. A primary congenital defect or herniation of the arachnoid membrane through an incompetent diaphragma sella, either after pituitary surgery or radiation, can cause empty sella syndrome, the most common cause of an enlarged sella.

Endocrine evaluation should precede imaging studies because about 10% to 20% of the normal population harbors

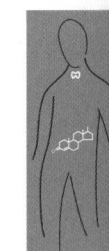

nonfunctional asymptomatic pituitary microadenomas that are incidentally detected by MRI (Table 65-2).

Disorders of Anterior Pituitary Hormones

GROWTH HORMONE

GH is a 191–amino acid peptide with a molecular weight of 22,000 Da. Secretion is stimulated by the 40– and 44–amino acid hypothalamic growth hormone–releasing hormone (GHRH) and inhibited by the hypothalamic tetradecapeptide somatostatin. These hypothalamic factors bind to pituitary somatotroph cells and regulate GH secretion. GH binds to receptors in the liver and induces secretion of insulin-like growth factor I (IGF-I), which circulates in the blood bound to binding proteins (BPs), the most important of which is IGF-BP3. IGF-I mediates most of the growth-promoting effects of GH. GH also affects carbohydrate metabolism.

Evaluation of Growth Hormone Reserve

Provocative tests that stimulate the somatotroph are necessary to assess GH deficiency (GHD) because basal GH levels are frequently very low even in normal individuals. Insulin-induced hypoglycemia (insulin tolerance test [ITT]) is the gold standard test for assessing GH reserve. Insulin (0.05 to 0.15 U/kg) is administered intravenously to reduce the patient's blood glucose levels to 50% of initial blood glucose or to 40 mg/dL with serial sampling of serum GH and glucose. Hypoglycemia is a potent stimulus for GH secretion, and a normal response is a peak GH level in excess of 5 ng/mL at 60 minutes in adults and 10 ng/mL in children. Combined infusion of GHRH and arginine is as sensitive and specific as insulin-induced hypoglycemia in stimulating GH secretion in adulthood and is recommended in elderly patients and in patients with ischemic heart disease or seizures. Alternate tests validated for the evaluation of adult GHD include glucagon and arginine plus growth hormone–releasing peptide (GHRP) stimulation tests.

A single GH stimulation test is sufficient for the diagnosis of adult GHD. However, patients with a low serum IGF level and three or more pituitary hormone deficiencies have more than a 97% chance of having GHD and do not need to undergo GH stimulation testing. The GH cutoff for the diagnosis of GHD varies with age, body mass index, and the GH stimulation test employed. IGF-I levels can be used as a screening test for GH deficiency because GH regulates IGF-I levels. GH deficiency is associated with low IGF-I and low IGF-BP3. A low serum IGF-I level is suggestive of GHD; however, a normal IGF-I level does not rule out GHD.

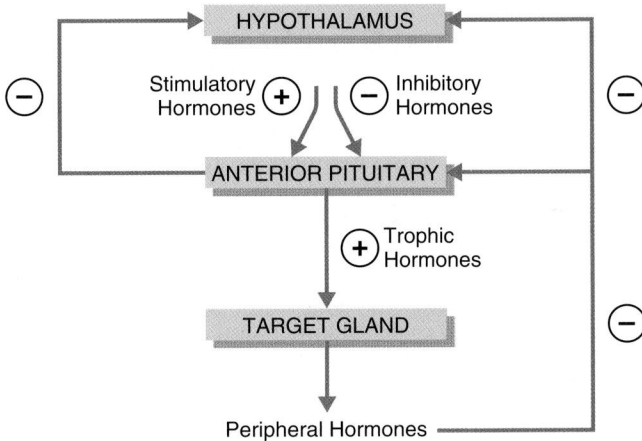

Figure 65-1 Feedback control of the hypothalamic-pituitary target gland axis.

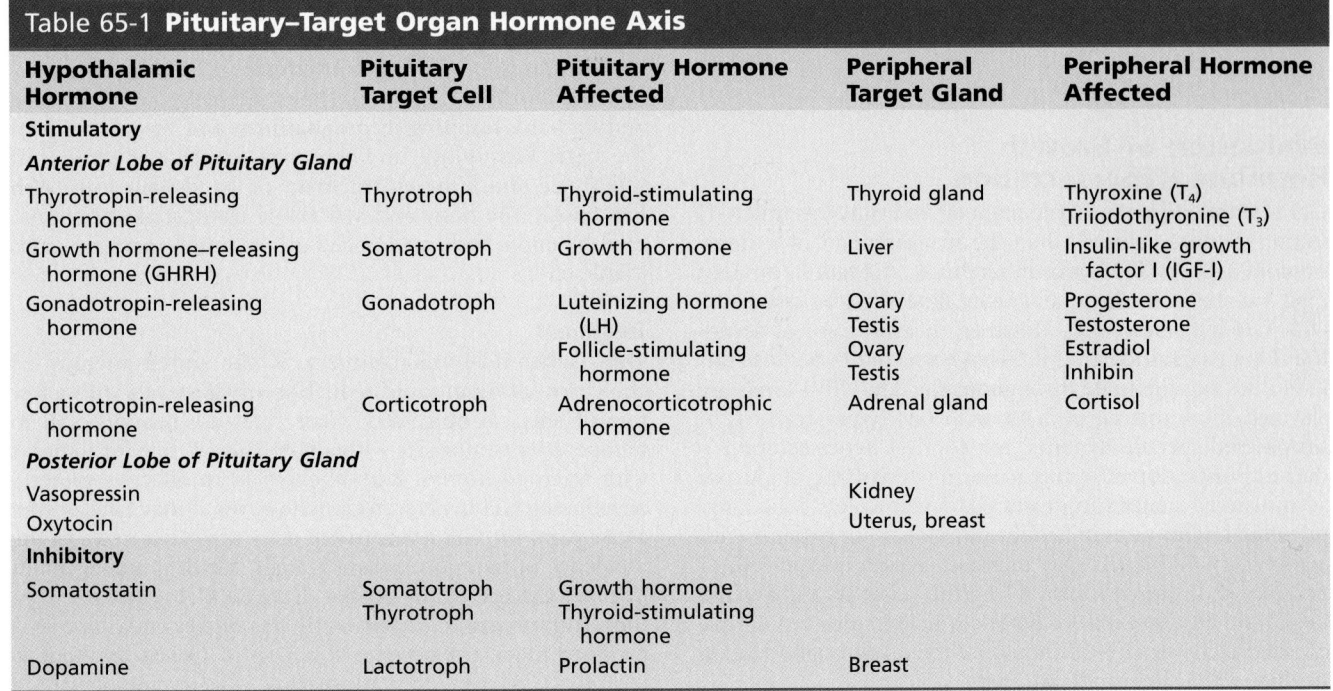

Table 65-1 **Pituitary–Target Organ Hormone Axis**				
Hypothalamic Hormone	**Pituitary Target Cell**	**Pituitary Hormone Affected**	**Peripheral Target Gland**	**Peripheral Hormone Affected**
Stimulatory				
Anterior Lobe of Pituitary Gland				
Thyrotropin-releasing hormone	Thyrotroph	Thyroid-stimulating hormone	Thyroid gland	Thyroxine (T$_4$) Triiodothyronine (T$_3$)
Growth hormone–releasing hormone (GHRH)	Somatotroph	Growth hormone	Liver	Insulin-like growth factor I (IGF-I)
Gonadotropin-releasing hormone	Gonadotroph	Luteinizing hormone (LH) Follicle-stimulating hormone	Ovary Testis Ovary Testis	Progesterone Testosterone Estradiol Inhibin
Corticotropin-releasing hormone	Corticotroph	Adrenocorticotrophic hormone	Adrenal gland	Cortisol
Posterior Lobe of Pituitary Gland				
Vasopressin			Kidney	
Oxytocin			Uterus, breast	
Inhibitory				
Somatostatin	Somatotroph Thyrotroph	Growth hormone Thyroid-stimulating hormone		
Dopamine	Lactotroph	Prolactin	Breast	

Table 65-2 Screening Tests for Pituitary Disorders

Disorder	Tests
Pituitary Tumor	
Acromegaly	IGF-I
	OGTT: Measure BS and GH (0, 60, 120 min)
Prolactinoma	Basal serum prolactin
ACTH-secreting tumor	24-hr urine-free cortisol and creatinine level
	1 mg overnight dexamethasone suppression test
	2 mg and 8 mg dexamethasone suppression tests
	Serum ACTH
	Dexamethasone-CRH test
	Bilateral inferior petrosal sinus sampling
TSH-secreting tumor	Serum TSH, TFT
Gonadotropin-secreting tumor	FSH, LH, α subunit
Hypopituitarism	
Growth hormone deficiency	IGF-I
	GH provocative test: ITT Arginine-GHRH
Gonadotropin deficiency	Women: basal estradiol, LH, FSH
	Men: testosterone (total; free), LH, FSH
TSH Deficiency	Serum TSH, free T₄
ACTH Deficiency	ACTH
	Provocative test: ITT
	Metyrapone test
	Cortrosyn-stimulation test (1 mcg and 250 mcg)

ACTH, adrenocorticotropic hormone; BS, blood sugar; CRH, corticotropin-releasing hormone; FSH, follicle-stimulating hormone; GH, growth hormone; GHRH, growth hormone–releasing hormone; IGF-I, insulin-like growth factor I; ITT, insulin tolerance test; LH, luteinizing hormone; OGTT, oral glucose tolerance test; T₄, thyroxine; TSH, thyroid-stimulating hormone; TFT, thyroid function test.

Evaluation of Growth Hormone Hypersecretion

GH is secreted in a pulsatile manner, and thus dynamic GH testing is more valuable than the measurement of a single random GH level. Moreover, cirrhosis, starvation, anxiety, type 1 diabetes mellitus, and acute illness can be associated with GH hypersecretion. However, measurement of serum IGF-I is a useful indicator of GH hypersecretion because this level does not fluctuate throughout the day. IGF-I levels are elevated in almost all patients with GH hypersecretion. A simple and specific dynamic test for GH hypersecretion is the administration of oral glucose, in which 100 g of glucose administered orally suppresses GH levels to less than 1 ng/mL after 120 minutes in healthy individuals. In patients with acromegaly, GH levels may increase, remain unchanged, or decrease (however, not below 1 ng/mL) after an oral glucose load. If no pituitary mass is detected, an extrapituitary source of ectopic GH or GHRH should be sought through imaging studies of the chest and abdomen.

Adult Growth Hormone Deficiency

GH deficiency during infancy and childhood is exhibited as growth retardation, short stature, and fasting hypoglycemia. Adult GH deficiency manifests as increased abdominal adiposity, reduced muscle strength and exercise capacity, decreased lean body mass and increased fat mass, reduced bone mineral density, glucose intolerance and insulin resistance, abnormal lipid profile, and impaired psychosocial well-being. Adult GH deficiency is frequently accompanied by other symptoms of panhypopituitarism.

Treatment

GH is administered in adulthood as a subcutaneous daily injection (0.1 to 0.3 mg per day). GH replacement therapy in adults decreases fat mass, increases lean body mass and bone mineral density, and is associated with improved cardiovascular risk factors (e.g., lipid profile, waist-to-hip ratio, central obesity).

Acromegaly and Gigantism

In childhood, GH hypersecretion leads to gigantism; in adults whose long bone epiphyses are fused, GH excess causes acromegaly with local overgrowth of bone in the acral areas. GH hypersecretion is almost always caused by a GH-secreting pituitary adenoma. About 70% of patients with acromegaly have macroadenomas. Ectopic GHRH secretion can occur with pancreatic islet cell tumors and bronchial or intestinal carcinoids. Ectopic GH secretion occurs rarely with pancreas, breast, and lung tumors. Both ectopic GH and GHRH are clinically exhibited with acromegaly but are extremely rare.

Clinical Features

The clinical features of acromegaly are insidious, and it may take several years for the disfiguring features to be diagnosed. Untreated, acromegaly causes increased rates of morbidity and mortality late in the course of the disorder. The most classic clinical feature is acral enlargement, exhibited as a widening of the hands and feet and a coarsening of the facial features; the frontal sinuses enlarge, leading to prominent supraorbital ridges, and the mandible grows downward and forward, resulting in prognathism and wide spacing of the teeth. Ring, glove, and shoe sizes increase as a result of soft tissue and bony enlargement of hands and feet (**Web Fig. 65-4**). The bony and soft tissue changes are accompanied by endocrine, metabolic, and systemic manifestations (Table 65-3).

Treatment

Trans-sphenoidal microsurgery is the initial therapy of choice, resulting in rapid reduction of GH levels with a low rate of surgical morbidity. Cure rates are proportional to preoperative tumor size with a 90% success rate for patients with microadenomas. Radiotherapy is an effective method of reducing GH hypersecretion; however, it may take as long as 20 years for GH levels to fall after radiotherapy, and the incidence of hypopituitarism is high. Medical management involves the use of drugs that decrease GH secretion from the pituitary tumor (somatostatin analogues, dopamine agonists) or block the peripheral action of GH at the hepatic receptor (GH receptor antagonists). Octreotide acetate, a

Table 65-3 **Clinical Features of Acromegaly**	
Change	**Manifestations**
Somatic Changes	
Acral changes	Enlarged hands and feet
Musculoskeletal changes	Arthralgias
	Prognathism
	Malocclusion
	Carpal tunnel syndrome
	Proximal myopathy
Skin changes	Sweating
Colon changes	Polyps
	Carcinoma
Cardiovascular symptoms	Cardiomegaly
	Hypertension
Visceromegaly	Tongue
	Thyroid
	Liver
Endocrine-Metabolic Changes	
Reproduction	Menstrual abnormalities
	Galactorrhea
	Decreased libido
Carbohydrate metabolism	Impaired glucose tolerance
	Diabetes mellitus
Lipids	Hypertriglyceridemia

long-acting somatostatin analogue, is effective in reducing GH and IGF-I levels to normal in 40% to 65% of patients and shrinks tumor mass in about 50% of cases. A long-acting, slow-releasing depot preparation of octreotide administered once monthly is as effective as short-acting subcutaneous octreotide preparations. Side effects of octreotide include diarrhea, abdominal cramps, flatulence, and gallstone formation. Bromocriptine, a dopamine agonist, is effective in suppressing GH in only a minority of patients with acromegaly. The GH receptor antagonist, pegvisomant, binds to the GH receptor on the hepatic surface and thus blocks the normal physiologic action of GH. The mechanism of normal GH action at the liver involves binding of the GH to its hepatic receptor, followed by receptor dimerization, which then activates signaling pathways that result in IGF-I generation. Pegvisomant blocks GH receptor dimerization and subsequent IGF-1 generation and normalizes IGF-1 levels in 97% of patients with acromegaly. Liver function tests and pituitary adenoma size must be monitored on a long-term basis.

PROLACTIN

Prolactin (PRL), a 198–amino acid, 22,000-Da polypeptide, is synthesized and secreted by pituitary lactotrophs. Hypothalamic dopamine provides predominantly inhibitory control of PRL secretion, allowing only a low basal rate of secretion. Thyrotropin-releasing hormone (TRH) and vasoactive intestinal polypeptide are putative PRL-releasing factors. PRL secretion is episodic. Estrogens increase basal and stimulated PRL secretion; glucocorticoids and TSH blunt TRH-induced PRL secretion. PRL levels increase during pregnancy. After childbirth, PRL stimulates milk production. However, elevated PRL levels are not needed to maintain lactation, and basal PRL secretion falls as the infant's suckling reflex maintains lactation.

Prolactinomas

Microprolactinomas are more common in women, whereas macroadenomas occur more frequently in men. PRL inhibits pulsatile gonadotropin secretion and suppresses the midcycle LH surge with consequent menstrual irregularities. Hyperprolactinemia in women can cause hypogonadotropic hypogonadism, resulting in estrogen deficiency. In men who have hyperprolactinemia, testosterone levels are usually suppressed.

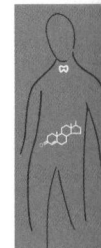

Clinical Features
Prolactinomas are often recognized earlier in women, who have menstrual irregularities and infertility, as opposed to men, who exhibit decreased libido and erectile dysfunction.

About 90% of women who have hyperprolactinemia have amenorrhea, galactorrhea, or infertility. If the prolactinoma occurs in adolescents before the onset of menarche, they may have primary amenorrhea. Prolactinomas account for 15% to 20% of secondary amenorrhea. Anovulation is associated with infertility. Galactorrhea may not be clinically obvious and may be discovered only during breast examination.

Estrogen deficiency may cause osteopenia, vaginal dryness, hot flashes, and irritability. PRL stimulates adrenal androgen production, and androgen excess can result in weight gain and hirsutism. Hyperprolactinemia may be associated with anxiety and depression.

Men usually exhibit a loss of libido and erectile dysfunction as a result of hypogonadism. These symptoms are often attributed to causes other than prolactinoma, which results in frequent delay in diagnosis until visual impairment, headache, and hypopituitarism develop.

Diagnosis
Several physiologic conditions (e.g., pregnancy, stress, nipple stimulation), as well as certain medications (e.g., phenothiazines, methyldopa, cimetidine, metoclopramide) and pathologic states (e.g., hypothyroidism, chronic renal failure, chest wall lesions), increase PRL secretion. These conditions may be associated with mildly elevated PRL levels; however, basal PRL levels in excess of 200 ng/mL usually imply prolactinoma. MRI confirms the diagnosis of prolactinoma.

Treatment
Medical management with a dopamine agonist (e.g., bromocriptine, cabergoline) restores gonadal function and fertility in most patients. Dopamine agonists cause tumor shrinkage in a significant number of patients with macroadenomas. Side effects of dopamine agonists, which occur more frequently with bromocriptine than cabergoline, include dizziness, nausea, vomiting, nasal stuffiness, and orthostatic hypotension. Cabergoline-related cardiac valvulopathy was recently reported in patients with Parkinson disease receiving doses of cabergoline far greater than used for the treatment of prolactinoma. However, valvulopathy is of concern in young patients requiring long-term dopamine agonist therapy, and bromocriptine, if tolerable, is the preferred therapy, until well-controlled prospective clinical studies are available. Trans-sphenoidal surgery is indicated in patients who are intolerant or resistant to medical treatment.

THYROID-STIMULATING HORMONE

TSH, a 28,000-Da glycoprotein hormone, is synthesized and secreted by the pituitary thyrotroph cells. TSH secretion is stimulated by the hypothalamic tripeptide TRH. The inhibitory effect of hypothalamic somatostatin augments the negative feedback inhibition of TSH secretion by peripheral thyroid hormones. TSH attaches to receptors on the thyroid gland and activates adenylyl cyclase, stimulating iodine uptake and the synthesis and release of the thyroid hormones thyroxine (T_4) and triiodothyronine (T_3). T_4 and T_3, in turn, exert negative feedback inhibition on pituitary TSH and hypothalamic TRH secretion.

Evaluation of TSH Secretion

TSH is measured by ultrasensitive assays (immunoradiometric assays), which can accurately distinguish low, normal, and high TSH levels. The ultrasensitive TSH assay has largely replaced the need for any further tests. The presence of low circulating TSH levels in the presence of low thyroid hormone levels differentiates secondary (central) hypothyroidism as a result of hypothalamic-pituitary dysfunction from primary hypothyroidism, which manifests low thyroid hormone levels, with concomitant high TSH levels.

TSH Deficiency

TSH deficiency causes thyroid gland involution, hypofunction, and clinical hypothyroidism. Clinical features of hypothyroidism include lethargy, constipation, cold intolerance, bradycardia, weight gain, poor appetite, dry skin, and delayed relaxation time of peripheral reflexes.

Treatment

Patients with central hypothyroidism are treated with thyroxine. Measuring the serum FT4 level, which should be in the mid to normal range, assesses the adequacy of thyroid replacement. TSH levels are low to normal in central hypopituitarism; thus, TSH levels cannot be used to monitor thyroid hormone replacement dosage in secondary hypothyroidism.

Thyrotropin-Secreting Pituitary Tumors

Thyrotropin-secreting pituitary tumors are extremely rare, exhibiting hyperthyroidism, goiter, and inappropriately elevated (or normal) TSH levels in the presence of elevated serum thyroid hormone levels. TSH-secreting tumors are usually plurihormonal, secreting GH, PRL, and the glycoprotein hormone α subunit, as well as TSH. These tumors are often resistant to removal, which necessitates several surgical procedures or radiotherapy. Octreotide acetate, a somatostatin analogue, has been found to be useful in decreasing TSH secretion in patients with these tumors and has been shown to shrink the tumor in some cases. Iodine-131 thyroid ablation or thyroid surgery may be needed to control thyrotoxicosis.

ADRENOCORTICOTROPIC HORMONE

ACTH, a 39–amino acid peptide, is synthesized as part of a larger 241–amino acid precursor molecule, proopiomelanocortin, which is subsequently cleaved enzymatically into β-lipotropin (β-LPH), ACTH, joining peptide, and an amino-terminal peptide in the anterior lobe of the pituitary gland. ACTH is then cleaved into β-melanocyte–stimulating hormone and corticotropin-like peptide (ACTH [18-39]), whereas β-LPH is split into LPH and β-endorphin.

Hypothalamic corticotropin-releasing hormone (CRH) and to a lesser extent ADH stimulate ACTH secretion by pituitary corticotroph cells. ACTH stimulates cortisol synthesis and secretion from the adrenal gland. Cortisol exerts a negative feedback on ACTH and CRH secretion. ACTH is secreted in pulses and is under circadian control, reaching maximal levels in the last hours before awakening, followed by a steady decline to a nadir in the evening. Both psychological and physical stresses increase ACTH and cortisol secretion, whereas glucocorticoids inhibit ACTH secretion as well as CRH and ADH synthesis and release. ACTH also maintains adrenal size by increasing protein synthesis.

Evaluation of ACTH Secretion

Excess ACTH secretion results in hypercortisolemia, which may be caused by an ACTH-secreting pituitary adenoma (Cushing disease) or by ectopic ACTH secretion. ACTH deficiency results in adrenocortical insufficiency, with decreased secretion of cortisol. Aldosterone secretion is largely regulated by the renin-angiotensin axis; therefore, aldosterone secretion remains intact (see Chapter 67).

Basal ACTH Levels

Random basal ACTH measurements are unreliable because of the short plasma half-life and pulsatile secretion of the hormone. Interpretation of plasma ACTH levels requires concomitant assessment of plasma cortisol levels. Because ACTH regulates cortisol secretion, plasma cortisol levels better reflect hypothalamic-pituitary-adrenal function. An 8:00 AM cortisol less than 3 mcg/dL suggests adrenal insufficiency. ACTH levels can be used to differentiate primary from secondary adrenal insufficiency. Plasma ACTH levels are normal to high in adrenal insufficiency because of a primary adrenal disorder and are low to absent in adrenal insufficiency secondary to hypothalamic-pituitary hypofunction (see Chapter 67).

Evaluation of ACTH Reserve

To assess the adequacy of ACTH reserve under conditions of stress, provocative testing is performed. The insulin-induced hypoglycemia test previously described as a stimulus for pituitary GH release also stimulates the hypothalamic-pituitary-adrenal axis. A peak cortisol level of at least 18 mcg/dL confirms normal ACTH reserve. Insulin-induced hypoglycemia is the most reliable test of the ACTH secretory response to stress. The test is contraindicated in older patients and in patients with cerebrovascular disorders, seizure disorders, or cardiovascular disease. Metyrapone (30 mg/kg orally at midnight) inhibits the 11-β-hydroxylase enzyme in the adrenal gland, which converts 11-deoxycortisol to cortisol. Low cortisol stimulates CRH and ACTH. An 11-deoxycortisol level greater than 7 mg/dL, with a simultaneous serum cortisol level less than 5 mcg/dL, the morning after metyrapone administration, indicates an adequate response. If compromised adrenal function is suggested, the ITT and metyrapone tests are potentially hazardous, and a physician should closely monitor patients.

Prolonged ACTH deficiency results in adrenal atrophy, and thus ACTH status can be assessed indirectly by measuring adrenal cortisol reserve. Cortrosyn-stimulation testing correlates well with the ITT. About 250 mcg cosyntropin (Cortrosyn; synthetic ACTH [1-24]) administered intravenously or intramuscularly results in a peak cortisol level of more than 20 mcg/dL within 60 minutes in normal individuals. An inadequate response implies either impaired pituitary ACTH secretion or primary adrenal failure. Numerous recent studies suggest that low-dose (1 mcg) ACTH stimulation provides a more sensitive test than the supraphysiologic 250-mcg dose.

Evaluation of ACTH Hypersecretion

Pituitary corticotroph adenomas in Cushing disease or ectopic ACTH-secreting tumors result in ACTH hypersecretion and hypercortisolemia.

Initially, a diagnosis of hypercortisolemia must first be confirmed by measuring 24-hour urinary-free cortisol levels, midnight plasma or salivary cortisol levels, or lack of suppression of an 8:00 AM serum cortisol after 1 mg of dexamethasone administered at 11:00 PM on the evening before (1 mg overnight dexamethasone suppression).

After confirming Cushing syndrome and hypercortisolemia, plasma ACTH levels are measured to differentiate between ACTH-dependent Cushing syndrome (pituitary or ectopic ACTH secretion) and ACTH-independent Cushing syndrome (adrenal adenoma or hyperplasia). This differential diagnosis is discussed in Chapter 67.

ACTH Deficiency

ACTH deficiency results in adrenal failure, causing lethargy, weakness, nausea, vomiting, dehydration, orthostatic hypotension, coma, and, if untreated, death.

Treatment

Patients with adrenal insufficiency should be treated with hydrocortisone, 15 to 25 mg per day in two or three divided doses; cortisone acetate, 25 to 37.5 mg per day; or prednisone, 5 to 7.5 mg per day. The dose should be increased 5- to 10-fold in times of stress. Stress doses of steroid should be administered if the patient undergoes surgery with rapid tapering of the dose postoperatively. The dose of steroid should be doubled when the patient has minor illnesses.

Mineralocorticoid replacement is not required with central adrenal insufficiency because the renin-aldosterone system is intact.

ACTH-Secreting Pituitary Tumors

ACTH-secreting pituitary tumors result in hypercortisolemia associated with obesity, moon facies, cervicodorsal dysplasia, striae, thinning of the skin, hirsutism, hypertension, menstrual irregularities, glucose intolerance, mood changes, proximal myopathy, and osteopenia (Fig. 65-2). The differential diagnosis of hypercortisolemia is discussed in Chapter 67.

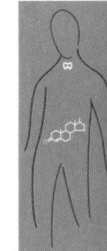

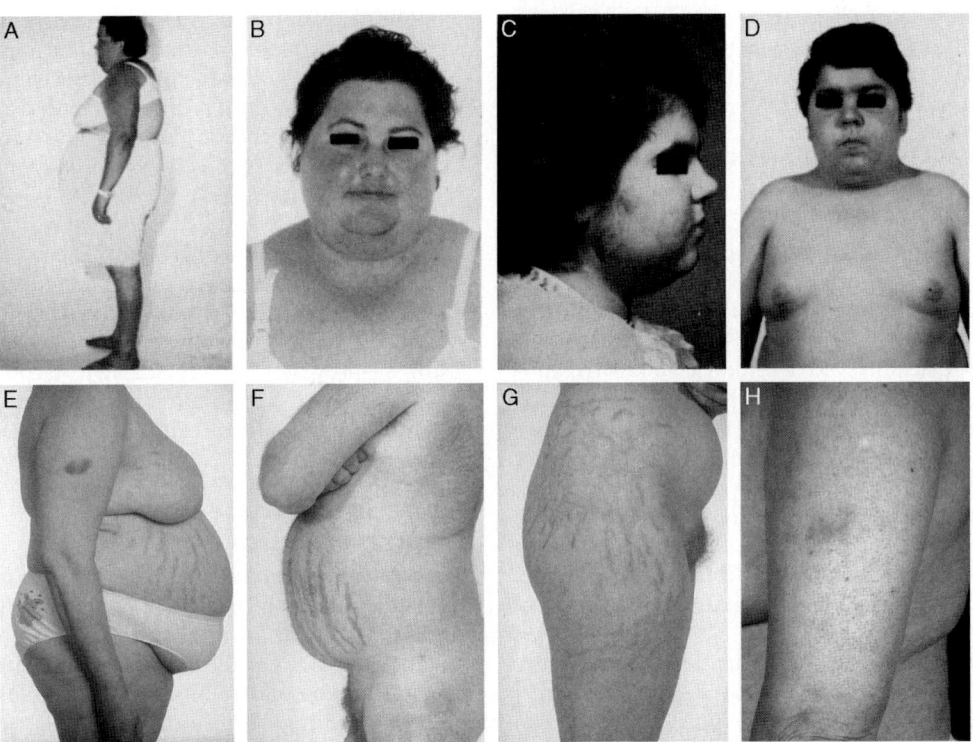

Figure 65-2 Clinical features of Cushing syndrome. **A,** Centripetal and some generalized obesity and dorsal kyphosis in a 30-year-old woman with Cushing disease. **B,** Same woman as shown in **A,** depicting moon facies, plethora, hirsutism, and enlarged supraclavicular fat pads. **C,** Facial rounding, hirsutism, and acne in a 14-year-old girl with Cushing disease. **D,** Central and generalized obesity and moon facies in a 14-year-old boy with Cushing disease. **E, F,** Typical centripetal obesity with livid abdominal striae observed in a 41-year-old woman (**E**) and a 40-year-old man (**F**) with Cushing disease. **G,** Striae in a 24-year-old patient with congenital adrenal hyperplasia treated with excessive doses of dexamethasone as replacement therapy. **H,** Typical bruising and thin skin of a patient with Cushing disease. In this case, the bruising has occurred without obvious injury. (From Larsen PR, Kronenberg H, Melmed S, et al: Williams Textbook of Endocrinology, 10th ed. Philadelphia, WB Saunders, 2003.)

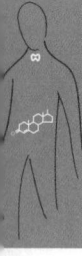

Treatment

Treatment modalities used to control ACTH hypersecretion in Cushing disease include trans-sphenoidal resection, radiation therapy, and medical therapy. Drugs that block steroid synthesis include ketoconazole, metyrapone and aminoglutethimide, mifepristone, and trilostane.

Treatment of ectopic ACTH syndrome is designed to remove the ectopic tumor if possible.

GONADOTROPINS (LUTEINIZING HORMONE AND FOLLICLE-STIMULATING HORMONE)

Gonadotroph secretion of LH and FSH is regulated by hypothalamic gonadotropin-releasing hormone (GnRH), a 10–amino acid peptide secreted in a pulsatile manner. Gonadal steroids (estrogen and testosterone) and peptides (inhibin and activin) regulate negative feedback inhibition. Basal LH and FSH are secreted in a pulsatile manner, concordantly with the pulsatile release of GnRH. GnRH release determines the onset of puberty and generates the midcycle gonadotropin surges necessary for ovulation. Gonadal steroids exert both positive and negative feedback effects on gonadotroph secretion. In addition, the gonadal polypeptide inhibin, produced by ovarian granulosa cells and testicular Sertoli cells, negatively inhibits FSH secretion, whereas activins stimulate FSH secretion. LH and FSH bind to receptors in the ovaries and testes and stimulate sex steroid secretion (predominantly LH) as well as gametogenesis (predominantly FSH). LH stimulates gonadal steroid secretion by testicular Leydig cells and by the ovarian follicles. In women, the ovulatory LH surge results in rupture of the follicle and then luteinization. FSH stimulates Sertoli cell spermatogenesis in men and follicular development in women.

Evaluation of Hypothalamic-Pituitary-Gonadal Axis

LH and FSH levels vary with age, and with the menstrual cycle in women. Prepubertal gonadotropin levels are low, and postmenopausal women have elevated levels. Male FSH and LH levels are pulsatile but fluctuate less than those in women. During the follicular phase of the menstrual cycle, LH levels rise steadily, with a midcycle spike that stimulates ovulation. FSH rises during the early follicular phase, falls in the late follicular phase, and peaks at midcycle, concurrent with the LH surge. Both LH and FSH levels fall after ovulation.

Basal testosterone and FSH levels are measured in men. Low basal testosterone and FSH levels, indicative of hypogonadism, are confirmed by measuring three pooled samples drawn 20 minutes apart, which compensates for the normal pulsatile gonadotropin secretion.

Gonadotropin and sex steroid estimation in women is more complex. However, women with regular menstrual cycles and a documented normal luteal-phase serum progesterone concentration are unlikely to have significant gonadotropin dysfunction. In women with amenorrhea, measurement of serum LH, FSH, estradiol, PRL, and human chorionic gonadotropin (hCG) can differentiate among (1) primary ovarian failure, with elevated FSH and LH levels and normal PRL levels; (2) hyperprolactinemia, with elevated PRL and normal to low follicular-phase LH, FSH, and estra-diol levels; and (3) pregnancy, with a positive hCG, normal to high PRL, normal LH, and high estradiol.

Gonadotropin deficiency is best diagnosed by concurrent measurement of serum gonadotropins and gonadal steroid concentrations. Low or normal FSH and LH levels in the presence of a low testosterone level (in men) or a low estradiol level (in women) confirm the diagnosis of gonadotropin deficiency. Low levels of gonadal steroids in the presence of elevated gonadotropin levels suggest primary gonadal failure.

Gonadotropin Deficiency

Central hypogonadism during childhood results in failure to enter normal puberty. Girls have delayed breast development, scant pubic and axillary hair, and primary amenorrhea. In boys, the phallus and testes remain small, and body hair is sparse. Sex steroids are required for closure of the epiphyses of the long bones; thus, in isolated gonadotropin deficiency, growth continues (as GH is intact) because epiphyseal fusion fails, resulting in tall adolescents with eunuchoid proportions (upper segment–to–lower segment ratio < 1:1). In adult women, hypogonadism is exhibited as breast atrophy, loss of pubic and axillary hair, and secondary amenorrhea. Hypogonadal men develop testicular atrophy, decreased libido, erectile dysfunction, decreased muscle mass and bone mineral density, loss of body hair, and elevated low-density lipoprotein (LDL) cholesterol levels.

Treatment

Androgen replacement therapy is recommended in men with central hypogonadism. Testosterone can be administered as an intramuscular injection (testosterone enanthate, 200 to 300 mg every 2 or 3 weeks) or as a transdermal patch (2.5 to 5 mg per day) or gel (2.5 to 10 mg per day). Adequate replacement results in a mid-normal serum testosterone level.

Premenopausal women with central hypogonadism should receive estrogen replacement therapy, and, if they have a uterus, they should receive progesterone either continuously or cyclically to protect the uterine lining. Estrogen-progesterone replacement recommendations for postmenopausal hypopituitary women are the same as for postmenopausal women without hypopituitarism.

Gonadotropin-Secreting Pituitary Tumors

Gonadotropin-secreting pituitary tumors are rare and have been reported mainly in men. Most tumors are large at the time of presentation and hypersecrete only FSH. Patients usually have signs and symptoms of local pressure, such as visual impairment. Patients may also exhibit hypogonadism with low or normal testosterone levels or low or normal sperm counts. This results from inhibitory effects of chronically high levels of gonadotropins (LH and FSH) on the testicles. In rare cases, excess LH may stimulate testosterone levels.

Surgical removal of gonadotropin-secreting adenomas is the usual primary treatment; however, patients may require subsequent radiotherapy.

Hypothalamic Dysfunction

In children and young adults, craniopharyngioma is the most frequent cause of hypothalamic dysfunction. Primary central nervous system tumors, pinealomas, and dermoid and epidermoid tumors also cause hypothalamic dysfunction in adulthood. Clinical manifestations of tumors that can cause hypothalamic dysfunction include visual loss, symptoms of raised intracranial pressure (headache and vomiting), hypopituitarism (including growth failure), and diabetes insipidus. Hypothalamic disturbances include disorders of thirst (e.g., polydipsia, polyuria, dehydration), appetite (e.g., hyperphagia, obesity), temperature regulation, and consciousness (e.g., somnolence, emotional lability). Diabetes insipidus is a common manifestation of hypothalamic lesions but rarely occurs with primary pituitary lesions. An MRI can confirm the diagnosis. Because hypopituitarism occurs frequently with hypothalamic lesions, anterior pituitary function should be assessed.

Craniopharyngioma is treated by surgical resection and may require subsequent radiotherapy. Biopsy of other types of hypothalamic tumors is usually required for histologic diagnosis before surgical resection because some, such as dysgerminoma, may be radiosensitive.

Hypopituitarism

Hypopituitarism results from diminished secretion of one or more pituitary hormones. The syndrome results either from anterior pituitary gland destruction or dysfunction secondary to deficient hypothalamic stimulatory-inhibitory factors that normally regulate pituitary function. Congenital or acquired lesions can also cause hypopituitarism (Table 65-4). Pituitary insufficiency is usually a slow, insidious disorder. Pituitary lesions may result in single or multiple hormone losses.

DIAGNOSIS

The diagnosis of pituitary hormone deficiency has been previously discussed in relation to the individual hormones.

TREATMENT

Patients with panhypopituitarism must have adequate replacement of growth hormone, T_4, glucocorticoids, and appropriate sex steroids. Children with short stature resulting from GH deficiency should receive GH replacement therapy. The safety and efficacy of GH replacement therapy for adults who develop GH deficiency is being evaluated. Testosterone therapy in men restores libido and potency, growth of body hair, and muscle strength. Estrogen replacement therapy in women maintains secondary sex characteristics and prevents hot flashes. Both testosterone and estrogen may protect bone from osteoporosis. Hypogonadotropic female patients may require ovulation induction and in vitro fertilization to treat infertility. In patients with combined TSH and ACTH deficiency, glucocorticoids should be replaced before T_4 because T_4 may aggravate adrenal insufficiency and may precipitate acute adrenal failure.

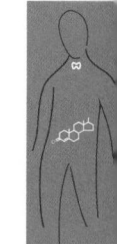

Table 65-4 **Causes of Hypopituitarism**	
Type of Disorder	**Cause**
Congenital	Septo-optic dysplasia Prader-Willi syndrome Laurence-Moon-Biedl syndrome Isolated anterior pituitary hormone; releasing factor deficiency

Tumors	Pituitary tumors
	  Secretory adenomas
	  Nonsecretory adenomas
	Hypothalamic tumors
	Craniopharyngioma
	Hamartoma
	Pinealoma
	Dermoid
	Epidermoid
	Glioma
	Lymphoma
	Meningioma
	Metastatic cancers

Infiltrative	Hemochromatosis Langerhans cell histiocytosis Sarcoidosis Metastatic carcinoma (breast and bronchus) Amyloidosis
Infectious	Tuberculosis Mycoses Syphilis
Physical trauma	Cranial trauma and hemorrhage Ionizing radiation Stalk section Surgery
Vascular	Postpartum pituitary necrosis (Sheehan syndrome) Pituitary apoplexy Carotid aneurysm

Posterior Pituitary Gland

The posterior pituitary gland secretes ADH and oxytocin. These hormones are synthesized in the hypothalamic nuclei in neuronal cell bodies that extend from the hypothalamus to the posterior pituitary. ADH binds to receptors on the renal tubule, increasing the water permeability of the luminal membrane of the collecting duct epithelium, thus facilitating reabsorption of water and concentration of the urine. Maximal ADH effect results in a small volume of concentrated urine with a high osmolarity (as high as 1200 mOsm/kg). Deficiency of ADH results in a large volume of very dilute urine (as low as 100 mOsm/kg). In addition to the renal tubular effects, ADH also binds to peripheral arteriolar receptors, causing vasoconstriction and resultant increase in blood pressure. However, a countereffect to the hypertensive effect of ADH is that ADH also causes bradycardia and the inhibition of sympathetic nerve activity.

Deficiency of ADH or insensitivity of the kidneys to ADH results in diabetes insipidus, which is exhibited as polyuria and polydipsia. Inappropriate secretion of ADH in excess amounts results in the syndrome of inappropriate antidiuretic hormone production (SIADH) and causes a hyponatremic state.

Oxytocin causes uterine smooth muscle contraction.

DIABETES INSIPIDUS

Vasopressin deficiency occurs with posterior pituitary dysfunction and leads to diabetes insipidus with polyuria, polydipsia, and nocturia. Diabetes insipidus can be of a central (neurogenic) origin where the posterior lobe of the pituitary fails to secrete adequate amounts of ADH; or it can be of nephrogenic origin, caused by failure of the kidney to respond to adequate amounts of circulating ADH. Regardless of the cause, patients are polyuric, secreting large volumes of dilute urine. This causes cellular and extracellular dehydration, stimulating thirst, which results in polydipsia. The causes of central diabetes insipidus are entirely different from those of nephrogenic diabetes insipidus (Table 65-5).

Differential Diagnosis

Diabetes insipidus (central or nephrogenic) must be distinguished from primary polydipsia, a compulsive disorder of thirst in which patients drink in excess of 5 to 10 L per day of water, resulting in decreased ADH secretion and subsequent diuresis. One possible distinguishing clinical feature is that patients with diabetes insipidus prefer cold beverages. Several tests can be performed to confirm the diagnosis of diabetes insipidus and differentiate the syndrome from primary polydipsia. Initially, random simultaneous samples of plasma and urine for evaluation of sodium and osmolarity are obtained. In diabetes insipidus (central or nephrogenic), inappropriate diuresis results in a urine osmolarity that is less than that of plasma osmolarity. Plasma osmolarity may be elevated, depending on the patient's state of hydration. However, in primary polydipsia, both plasma and urine are dilute.

Table 65-5 Causes of Diabetes Insipidus

Central Diabetes Insipidus

Idiopathic
Familial
Hypophysectomy
Infiltration of hypothalamus and posterior pituitary
  Langerhans cell histiocytosis
  Granulomas
Infection
Tumors (intrasellar and suprasellar)
Autoimmune

Nephrogenic Diabetes Insipidus

Idiopathic
Familial
  V_2 receptor gene mutation
  Aquaporin-2 gene mutation
Chronic renal disease (e.g., chronic pyelonephritis, polycystic kidney disease, or medullary cystic disease)
Hypokalemia
Hypercalcemia
Sickle cell anemia
Drugs
Lithium
Fluoride
Demeclocycline
Colchicine

The primary test used to differentiate the causes of polyuria is the water deprivation test (**Web Fig. 65-5**). The patient is denied fluids for 12 to 18 hours, and body weight, blood pressure, urine volume, urine specific gravity, and plasma and urine osmolarity are measured every 2 hours. Careful supervision is required because patients with diabetes insipidus may become rapidly dehydrated and hypotensive if denied access to water, in which case the test is stopped. A normal response is a decrease in urine output to 0.5 mL per minute, as well as an increase in urine concentration to greater than that of plasma. Patients with diabetes insipidus (either central or nephrogenic) maintain a high urine output, which continues to be dilute (specific gravity 1.005) despite water deprivation. In patients with primary polydipsia, urine osmolarity increases to values greater than plasma osmolarity. Water deprivation is continued until the urine osmolarity plateaus (an hourly increase of <30 mOsm/kg for 3 successive hours). At that point, 5 units of aqueous vasopressin are administered subcutaneously, and the urine osmolarity is measured after 1 hour. In patients with complete central diabetes insipidus, urine osmolarity increases above plasma osmolarity, whereas in nephrogenic diabetes insipidus, the urine osmolarity increases less than 50% in response to ADH. Patients with partial central diabetes insipidus also show an increase in urine osmolarity, but it is less than 50%, whereas patients with primary polydipsia have increases of less than 10%. ADH levels should be measured during the water deprivation test. Patients with nephrogenic diabetes insipidus have normal or increased levels of ADH during water deprivation, in contrast to those with complete central diabetes insipidus, who have suppressed levels. Patients with partial central diabetes insipidus show a smaller than normal increase in plasma ADH during water deprivation. Patients should be cautioned not to drink large amounts of fluid until the effects of the aqueous vasopressin have worn off (4 to 8 hours) to avoid symptomatic hyponatremia.

Treatment
Central Diabetes Insipidus

Desmopressin acetate (DDAVP), a synthetic analogue of ADH, is usually administered intranasally or orally in the treatment of diabetes insipidus. Frequency of administration is determined by the severity of the disease. Adequacy of replacement is monitored by regular measurement of serum sodium and urine output.

Nephrogenic Diabetes Insipidus

As far as possible, the underlying disease process should be reversed. Specific treatment of nephrogenic diabetes insipidus is designed to maintain a state of mild sodium depletion with reduction in the solute load on the kidneys and subsequent increased proximal tubular reabsorption. Diuretics coupled with dietary salt restriction can be used to achieve this goal.

SYNDROME OF INAPPROPRIATE ANTIDIURETIC HORMONE PRODUCTION

See Chapter 28.

Prospectus for the Future

- U.S. Food and Drug Administration approval and clinical use of several novel therapies for secretory pituitary tumors (e.g., somatostatin receptor subtype and selective analogue therapy, universal somatostatin receptor ligand for acromegaly)
- Long-term studies to define indications, safety, and efficacy of GH replacement therapy in adulthood
- Development of novel methods of GH administration including long-acting depot and intranasal preparations

- Clear understanding of the relative roles of surgery, radiation therapy, and novel medical therapies for the treatment of pituitary tumors
- Definition of the role of primary medical therapy in the treatment algorithms for pituitary tumors
- Controlled, prospective clinical studies to evaluate the long-term effects of low-dose dopamine agonist therapy on cardiac valve integrity

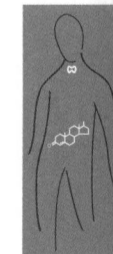

References

Arnaldi G, Angeli A, Atkinson AB, et al: Diagnosis and complications of Cushing's syndrome: A consensus statement. J Clin Endocrinol Metab 88:5593-5602, 2003.

Biller BM, Grossman AB, Stewart PM, et al: Treatment of adrenocorticotropin-dependent Cushing's syndrome: A consensus statement. J Clin Endocrinol Metab 93:2454-2462, 2008.

Biller BM, Samuels MH, Zagar A, et al: Sensitivity and specificity of six tests for the diagnosis of adult GH deficiency. J Clin Endocrinol Metab 87:2067-2079, 2002.

Boscaro M, Barzon L, Fallo F, Sonino N: Cushing's syndrome. Lancet 357:783-791, 2001.

Clemmons DR, Chihara K, Freda PU, et al: Optimizing control of acromegaly: Integrating a growth hormone receptor antagonist into the treatment algorithm. J Clin Endocrinol Metab 88:4759-4767, 2003.

Growth Hormone Research Society: Consensus guidelines for the diagnosis and treatment of adults with GH deficiency. Summary statement of the GH Research Society Workshop on Adult GH Deficiency. J Clin Endocrinol Metab 83:379-381, 1998.

Ho KK, for the 2007 GH Deficiency Consensus Workshop Participants: Consensus guidelines for the diagnosis and treatment of adults with GH deficiency II: A statement of the GH Research Society in association with the European Society for Pediatric Endocrinology, Lawson Wilkins Society, European Society of Endocrinology, Japan Endocrine Society, and Endocrine Society of Australia. Eur J Endocrinol 157:695-700, 2007.

Melmed S: Medical progress: Acromegaly. N Engl J Med. 355:2558-2573, 2006.

Melmed S, Casanueva FF, Cavagnini F, et al: Acromegaly treatment consensus workshop participants. Guidelines for acromegaly management. J Clin Endocrinol Metab 87:4054-4058, 2002.

Schlechte JA: Clinical practice. Prolactinoma. N Engl J Med 349:2035-2041, 2003.

Chapter 66

Thyroid Gland

Vivien S. Herman-Bonert and Theodore C. Friedman

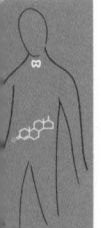

The thyroid gland secretes thyroxine (T_4) and triiodothyronine (T_3), both of which modulate energy utilization and heat production and facilitate growth. The gland consists of two lateral lobes joined by an isthmus. The weight of the adult gland is 10 to 20 g. Microscopically, the thyroid is composed of several follicles that contain colloid surrounded by a single layer of thyroid epithelium. The follicular cells synthesize thyroglobulin, which is then stored as colloid. Biosynthesis of T_4 and T_3 occurs by iodination of tyrosine molecules in thyroglobulin.

Thyroid Hormone Physiology

THYROID HORMONE SYNTHESIS

Dietary iodine is essential for synthesis of thyroid hormones. Iodine, after conversion to iodide in the stomach, is rapidly absorbed from the gastrointestinal tract and distributed in the extracellular fluids. After active transport from the bloodstream across the follicular cell basement membrane, iodide is enzymatically oxidized by thyroid peroxidase, which also mediates the iodination of the tyrosine residues in thyroglobulin to form monoiodotyrosine and diiodotyrosine. The iodotyrosine molecules couple to form T_4 (3,5,3′,5-tetraiodothyronine) or T_3 (3,5,3-triiodothyronine). Once iodinated, thyroglobulin containing newly formed T_4 and T_3 is stored in the follicles. Secretion of free T_4 and T_3 into the circulation occurs after proteolytic digestion of thyroglobulin, which is stimulated by thyroid-stimulating hormone (TSH). Deiodination of monoiodotyrosine and diiodotyrosine by iodotyrosine deiodinase releases iodine, which then reenters the thyroid iodine pool (**Web Fig. 66-1**).

THYROID HORMONE TRANSPORT

T_4 and T_3 are tightly bound to serum carrier proteins: thyroxine-binding globulin (TBG), thyroxine-binding prealbu-min, and albumin. The unbound or free fractions are the biologically active fractions and represent only 0.04% of the total T_4 and 0.4% of the total T_3.

PERIPHERAL METABOLISM OF THYROID HORMONES

The normal thyroid gland secretes T_4, T_3, and reverse T_3, a biologically inactive form of T_3. Most of the circulating T_3 is derived from 5′-deiodination of circulating T_4 in the peripheral tissues. Deiodination of T_4 can occur at the outer ring (5′-deiodination), producing T_3 (3,5,3′-triiodothyronine), or at the inner ring, producing reverse T_3 (3,3,5′-triiodothyronine).

CONTROL OF THYROID FUNCTION

Hypothalamic thyrotropin-releasing hormone (TRH) is transported through the hypothalamic-hypophysial portal system to the thyrotrophs of the anterior pituitary gland, stimulating synthesis and release of TSH (Fig. 66-1). TSH, in turn, increases thyroidal iodide uptake and iodination of thyroglobulin, releases T_3 and T_4 from the thyroid gland by increasing hydrolysis of thyroglobulin, and stimulates thyroid cell growth. Hypersecretion of TSH results in thyroid enlargement (goiter). Circulating T_3 exerts negative feedback inhibition of TRH and TSH release.

PHYSIOLOGIC EFFECTS OF THYROID HORMONES

Thyroid hormones increase basal metabolic rate by increasing oxygen consumption and heat production in several body tissues. Thyroid hormones also have specific effects on several organ systems (Table 66-1). These effects are exaggerated in hyperthyroidism and lacking in hypothyroidism, accounting for the well-recognized signs and symptoms of these two disorders.

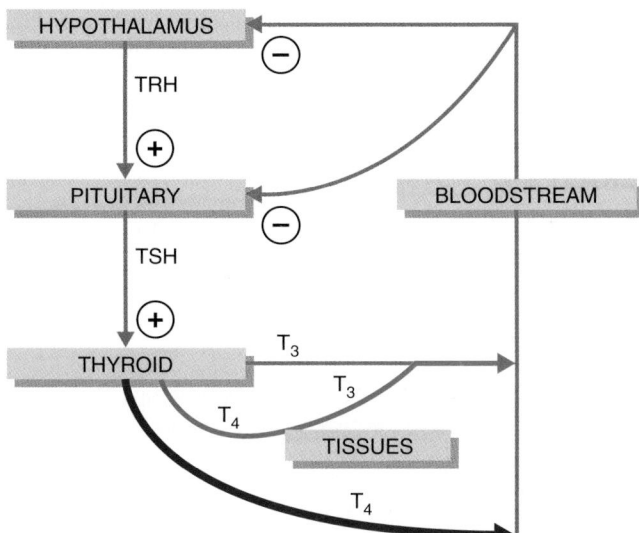

Figure 66-1 Hypothalamic-pituitary-thyroid axis. T_3, triiodothyronine; T_4, thyroxine; TRH, thyrotropin-releasing hormone; TSH, thyroid-stimulating hormone.

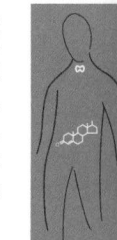

Table 66-1 **Physiologic Effects of Thyroid Hormone**
Cardiovascular Effects
Increased heart rate and cardiac output
Gastrointestinal Effects
Increased gut motility
Skeletal Effects
Increased bone turnover and resorption
Pulmonary Effects
Maintenance of normal hypoxic and hypercapnic drive in the respiratory center
Neuromuscular Effects
Increased muscle protein turnover and increased speed of muscle contraction and relaxation
Lipids and Carbohydrate Metabolism Effects
Increased hepatic gluconeogenesis and glycogenolysis, as well as intestinal glucose absorption
Increased cholesterol synthesis and degradation
Increased lipolysis
Sympathetic Nervous System Effects
Increased numbers of β-adrenergic receptors in the heart, skeletal muscle, lymphocytes, and adipose cells
Decreased cardiac α-adrenergic receptors
Increased catecholamine sensitivity
Hematopoietic Effects
Increased red blood cell 2,3-diphosphoglycerate, facilitating oxygen dissociation from hemoglobin with increased oxygen available to tissues

Thyroid Evaluation

Thyroid gland function and structure can be evaluated by (1) determining serum thyroid hormone levels, (2) imaging thyroid gland size and architecture, (3) measuring thyroid autoantibodies, and (4) performing a thyroid gland biopsy by fine-needle aspiration (FNA).

TESTS OF SERUM THYROID HORMONE LEVELS

Total serum T_4 and T_3 measure the total amount of hormone bound to thyroid-binding proteins by radioimmunoassay. Total T_4 and total T_3 levels are elevated in hyperthyroidism and are low in hypothyroidism. Increase in TBG (as with pregnancy or estrogen therapy) increases the total T_4 and T_3 without actual hyperthyroidism. Similarly, total T_4 and T_3 are low despite euthyroidism in conditions associated with low thyroid-binding proteins (e.g., congenital decrease, protein-losing enteropathy, cirrhosis, nephrotic syndrome). Thus, further tests to assess the free hormone level that reflects biologic activity must be performed. Free T_4 level is usually measured directly or by dialysis or ultrafiltration.

Serum TSH is measured by a third-generation immuno-metric assay, which uses at least two different monoclonal antibodies against different regions of the TSH molecule, resulting in accurate discrimination between normal TSH levels and levels below the normal range. Thus, the TSH assay can diagnose clinical hyperthyroidism (elevated free T_4 and suppressed TSH) and subclinical hyperthyroidism (normal free T_4 and suppressed TSH). In primary (thyroidal) hypothyroidism, serum TSH is supranormal because of diminished feedback inhibition. The TSH is usually low but may be normal in secondary (pituitary) or tertiary (hypothalamic) hypothyroidism.

Serum thyroglobulin measurements are useful in the follow-up of patients with papillary or follicular carcinoma. After thyroidectomy and iodine-131 (^{131}I) ablation therapy, thyroglobulin levels should be less than 0.5 mcg/L while the patient is on suppressive levothyroxine treatment. Levels in excess of this value indicate the possibility of persistent or metastatic disease.

Calcitonin is produced by the C-cells of the thyroid and has a minor role in calcium homeostasis. Calcitonin measurements are invaluable in the diagnosis of medullary carcinoma of the thyroid and for monitoring the effects of therapy for this entity.

THYROID IMAGING

Technetium-99m (^{99m}Tc) pertechnetate is concentrated in the thyroid gland and can be scanned with a gamma camera, yielding information about the size and shape of the gland and the location of the functional activity in the gland (thyroid scan). The thyroid scan is often performed in conjunction with a quantitative assessment of radioactive iodine uptake by the thyroid with ^{123}I, which quantitates thyroid uptake. Functioning thyroid nodules are called *warm* or *hot* nodules; *cold* nodules are nonfunctioning. Malignancy is usually associated with a cold nodule; 16% of surgically removed cold nodules are malignant.

Thyroid ultrasound evaluation is useful in the differentiation of solid nodules from cystic nodules. It also may be used to guide the clinician during FNA of a nodule (**Web Fig. 66-2**).

THYROID ANTIBODIES

Autoantibodies to several different antigenic components in the thyroid gland, including thyroglobulin (TgAb), thyroid peroxidase (TPO Ab, formerly called *antimicrosomal antibodies*), and the TSH receptor, can be measured in the serum. A strongly positive test for TPO Ab indicates autoimmune thyroid disease. Elevated thyroid receptor–stimulating antibody occurs in Graves disease (see the discussion under "Pathogenesis" later in this chapter).

THYROID BIOPSY

FNA of a nodule to obtain thyroid cells for cytologic evaluation is the best way to differentiate benign from malignant disease. FNA requires adequate tissue samples and interpretation by an experienced cytologist.

Hyperthyroidism

Thyrotoxicosis is the clinical syndrome that results from elevated circulating thyroid hormones. Clinical manifestations of thyrotoxicosis are due to the direct physiologic effects of the thyroid hormones as well as to the increased sensitivity to catecholamines. Tachycardia, tremor, stare, sweating, and lid lag are all due to catecholamine hypersensitivity.

SIGNS AND SYMPTOMS

Table 66-2 lists the signs and symptoms of hyperthyroidism. Thyrotoxic crisis, or *thyroid storm*, is a life-threatening complication of hyperthyroidism that can be precipitated by surgery, radioactive iodine therapy, or severe stress (e.g., uncontrolled diabetes mellitus, myocardial infarction, acute infection). Patients develop fever, flushing, sweating, significant tachycardia, atrial fibrillation, and cardiac failure. Significant agitation, restlessness, delirium, and coma frequently occur. Gastrointestinal manifestations may include nausea, vomiting, and diarrhea. Hyperpyrexia out of proportion to other clinical findings is the hallmark of thyroid storm.

DIFFERENTIAL DIAGNOSIS

Thyrotoxicosis usually reflects excess secretion of thyroid hormones resulting from Graves disease, toxic adenoma,

Table 66-2 **Signs and Symptoms of Hyperthyroidism**
Symptoms
Nervousness
Heat intolerance
Fatigue and weakness
Palpitations
Increased appetite
Weight loss
Oligomenorrhea
Signs
Tachycardia
Atrial fibrillation
Wide pulse pressure
Brisk reflexes
Fine tremor
Proximal limb-girdle myopathy
Chemosis

multinodular goiter, or thyroiditis (Table 66-3 and Fig. 66-2). However, it may be the result of excessive ingestion of thyroid hormone or, rarely, thyroid hormone production from an ectopic site as observed in struma ovarii.

GRAVES DISEASE

Graves disease, the most common cause of thyrotoxicosis, is an autoimmune disease that is more common in women, with a peak age incidence of 20 to 40 years. One or more of the following features are present: (1) goiter; (2)

Table 66-3 **Causes of Thyrotoxicosis**
Common Causes
Graves disease
Toxic adenoma (solitary)
Toxic multinodular goiter
Less Common Causes
Subacute thyroiditis (de Quervain or granulomatous thyroiditis)
Hashimoto thyroiditis with transient hyperthyroid phase
Thyrotoxicosis factitia
Postpartum (probably variant of silent thyroiditis)
Rare Causes
Struma ovarii
Metastatic thyroid carcinoma
Hydatidiform mole
Thyroid-stimulating hormone-secreting pituitary tumor

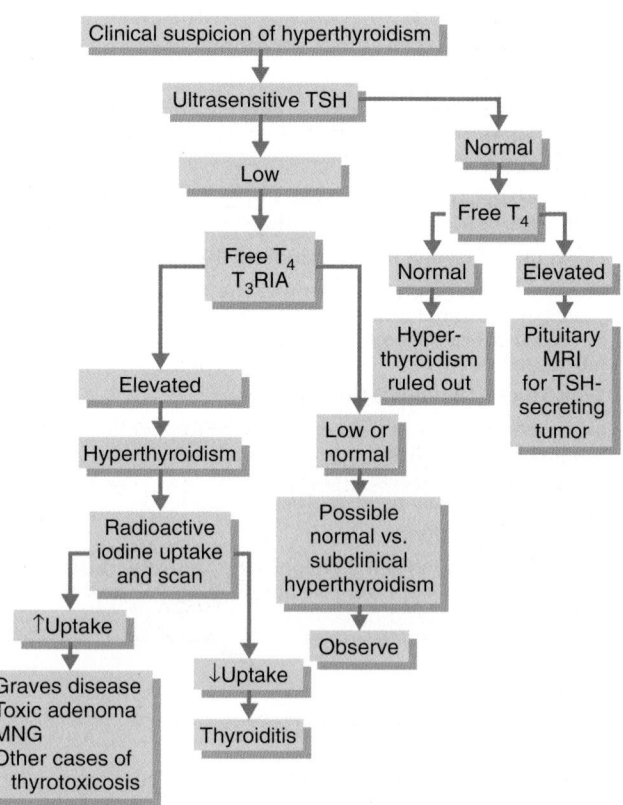

Figure 66-2 Algorithm for differential diagnosis of hyperthyroidism. MNG, multinodular goiter; MRI, magnetic resonance imaging; T₃RIA, triiodothyronine radioimmunoassay; T₄, thyroxine; TSH, thyroid-stimulating hormone.

thyrotoxicosis; (3) eye disease ranging from tearing to proptosis, extraocular muscle paralysis, and loss of sight as a result of optic nerve involvement; and (4) thyroid dermopathy, usually observed as significant skin thickening without pitting in a pretibial distribution (pretibial myxedema).

Pathogenesis

Thyrotoxicosis in Graves disease is due to the overproduction of an antibody that binds to the TSH receptor. These thyroid-stimulating immunoglobulins increase thyroid cell growth and thyroid hormone secretion. Ophthalmopathy is due to inflammatory infiltration of the extraocular eye muscles by lymphocytes, with mucopolysaccharide deposition. The inflammatory reaction that contributes to the eye signs in Graves disease may be caused by lymphocytes sensitized to antigens common to the orbital muscles and thyroid.

Clinical Features

The common manifestations of thyrotoxicosis (see Table 66-2) are characteristic features of younger patients with Graves disease. In addition, patients may exhibit a diffuse goiter or the eye signs characteristic of Graves disease. Older patients often do not have the florid clinical features of thyrotoxicosis, and the condition termed *apathetic hyperthyroidism* is exhibited as flat affect, emotional lability, weight loss, muscle weakness, congestive heart failure, and atrial fibrillation resistant to standard therapy.

Eye signs of Graves disease may be either a nonspecific manifestation of hyperthyroidism from any cause (e.g., thyroid stare) or may result from Graves disease as a result of a specific inflammatory infiltrate of the orbital tissues leading to periorbital edema, conjunctival congestion and swelling, proptosis, extraocular muscle weakness, or optic nerve damage with visual impairment (**Web Fig. 66-3**).

Pretibial myxedema (thyroid dermopathy) occurs in 2% to 3% of patients with Graves disease and exhibits a thickening of the skin over the lower tibia without pitting. Onycholysis, characterized by separation of the fingernails from their beds, often occurs in patients with Graves disease. Thyroid acropachy, or clubbing, may also occur in Graves disease.

Laboratory Findings

Elevated T_4 and/or T_3 and a suppressed TSH confirm the clinical diagnosis of thyrotoxicosis. Thyroid-stimulating immunoglobulin is usually elevated and may be useful in patients with eye signs who do not have other characteristic clinical features. Increased uptake of ^{123}I differentiates Graves disease from early subacute or Hashimoto thyroiditis, in which uptake is low in the presence of hyperthyroidism. Magnetic resonance imaging or ultrasonography of the orbit usually shows orbital muscle enlargement, whether or not clinical signs of ophthalmopathy are observed.

Treatment

Three treatment modalities are used to control the hyperthyroidism of Graves disease. They are antithyroid drugs, radioactive iodine, and surgery.

Antithyroid Drugs

The thiocarbamide drugs propylthiouracil, methimazole, and carbimazole block thyroid hormone synthesis by inhibiting thyroid peroxidase. Propylthiouracil also partially inhibits peripheral conversion of T_4 to T_3. Medical therapy must be administered for a prolonged period (1 to 2 years) until the disease undergoes spontaneous remission. On cessation of medication, 40% to 50% of patients remain in remission, and the patients who experience relapse usually then undergo definitive surgery or radioactive iodine treatment. Side effects of the thiocarbamide regimen include pruritus and rash (in about 5% of patients), cholestatic jaundice, acute arthralgias, and, rarely, agranulocytosis (in 0.5% of patients). Patients must be instructed to discontinue the medication and consult a physician if they develop fever or sore throat because these symptoms may indicate agranulocytosis. At the onset of treatment during the acute phase of thyrotoxicosis, β-adrenergic blocking drugs help alleviate tachycardia, hypertension, and atrial fibrillation. As the thyroid hormone levels return to normal, treatment with β blockers is tapered.

Radioactive Iodine

In terms of cost, efficacy, ease, and short-term side effects, radioactive iodine has benefits that exceed both surgery and antithyroid drugs; however, most patients become hypothyroid following its use. ^{131}I is often the treatment of choice in adults with Graves disease. It is contraindicated in women who are pregnant, but it does not increase the risk for birth defects in offspring conceived after ^{131}I therapy. Patients with severe thyrotoxicosis, very large glands, or underlying heart disease should be rendered euthyroid with antithyroid medication before receiving radioactive iodine because ^{131}I treatment can cause a release of preformed thyroid hormone from the thyroid gland into the circulation; this release can precipitate cardiac arrhythmias and exacerbate symptoms of thyrotoxicosis. After administering radioactive iodine, the thyroid gland shrinks, and patients become euthyroid over a period of 6 weeks to 3 months. About 80% of patients become hypothyroid after radioactive iodine treatment. Serum-free T_4 and TSH levels should be monitored and replacement with levothyroxine instituted if hypothyroidism occurs. Hypothyroidism always occurs after surgical total thyroidectomy, frequently after subtotal thyroidectomy, and in a smaller percentage of patients after antithyroid medication, mandating lifelong monitoring of all patients with Graves disease.

Surgery

Either subtotal or total thyroidectomy is the treatment of choice for patients with very large glands and obstructive symptoms or multinodular glands, or for patients desiring pregnancy within the next year. It is essential that the surgeon be experienced in thyroid surgery. Preoperatively, patients receive 6 weeks of treatment with antithyroid drugs to ensure that they are euthyroid at the time of surgery. Two weeks before surgery, oral-saturated solution of potassium iodide is administered daily to decrease the vascularity of the gland. Permanent hypoparathyroidism and recurrent laryngeal nerve palsy occur postoperatively in less than 2% of patients.

TOXIC ADENOMA

Solitary toxic nodules, which are usually benign, occur more frequently in older patients. Clinical manifestations are

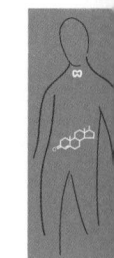

those of thyrotoxicosis. Physical examination shows a distinct solitary nodule. Laboratory investigation shows suppressed TSH and significantly elevated T_3 levels, often with only moderately elevated T_4. Thyroid scan shows a hot nodule of the affected lobe with complete suppression of the unaffected lobe. Solitary toxic nodules are treated with radioactive iodine. However, unilateral lobectomy after the administration of antithyroid drugs to render the patient euthyroid may be required for large nodules.

TOXIC MULTINODULAR GOITER

Toxic multinodular goiter occurs in older patients with long-standing multinodular goiter, especially in patients from iodine-deficient regions who are exposed to increased dietary iodine or receive iodine-containing radiocontrast dyes. The presenting clinical features are frequently tachycardia, heart failure, and arrhythmias.

Physical examination shows a multinodular goiter. The diagnosis is confirmed by laboratory features of suppressed TSH, elevated T_3 and T_4, and a thyroid scan with multiple functioning nodules. The treatment of choice is often ^{131}I ablation. It is especially effective in patients with small glands and a high radioactive uptake.

SUBCLINICAL HYPERTHYROIDISM

In subclinical hyperthyroidism, T_4 and T_3 levels are normal with a suppressed TSH. The causes of this condition include early presentation of all forms of hyperthyroidism, including Graves disease, toxic adenoma, and toxic multinodular goiter. Because these patients, especially those who are older, are at an increased risk for developing cardiac dysrhythmias, many patients with a persistently suppressed TSH should be treated with thiocarbamide drugs or radioactive iodine. A decreased bone mineral density is another indication for treatment.

THYROIDITIS

Thyroiditis may be classified as acute, subacute, or chronic. Although thyroiditis may eventually result in clinical hypothyroidism, the initial presentation is often that of hyperthyroidism as a result of acute release of T_4 and T_3. Hyperthyroidism caused by thyroiditis can be readily differentiated from other causes of hyperthyroidism by suppressed uptake of radioactive iodine, reflecting decreased hormone production by damaged cells.

A rare disorder, acute suppurative thyroiditis, exhibits high fever, a redness of the overlying skin, and thyroid gland tenderness; it may be confused with subacute thyroiditis. If blood cultures are negative, needle aspiration should identify the organism. Intensive antibiotic treatment and, occasionally, incision and drainage are required.

Subacute Thyroiditis

Subacute thyroiditis (de Quervain or granulomatous thyroiditis) is an acute inflammatory disorder of the thyroid gland, probably secondary to viral infection, which resolves completely in 90% of cases. Patients with subacute thyroiditis complain of fever and anterior neck pain. The patient may have symptoms and signs of hyperthyroidism. The classic feature on physical examination is an exquisitely tender thyroid gland. Laboratory findings vary with the course of the disease. Initially, the patient may be symptomatically thyrotoxic with elevated serum T_4, depressed serum TSH, and low radioactive iodine uptake on scan. Subsequently, the thyroid status will fluctuate through euthyroid and hypothyroid phases and may return to euthyroidism. An increase in radioactive iodine uptake on the scan reflects recovery of the gland. Treatment usually includes nonsteroidal anti-inflammatory drugs, but a short course of prednisone may be required if pain and fever are severe. During the hypothyroid phase, replacement therapy with levothyroxine may be indicated.

Postpartum thyroiditis resembles subacute thyroiditis in its clinical course. It usually occurs within the first 6 months after delivery and goes through the triphasic course of hyperthyroidism, hypothyroidism, and then euthyroidism, or it may develop with only hypothyroidism. Some patients have an underlying chronic thyroiditis.

Chronic Thyroiditis

Chronic thyroiditis (Hashimoto or lymphocytic thyroiditis) from destruction of normal thyroidal architecture by lymphocytic infiltration results in hypothyroidism and goiter. Riedel struma is probably a variant of Hashimoto thyroiditis, characterized by extensive thyroid fibrosis resulting in a rock-hard thyroid mass. Hashimoto thyroiditis is more common in women and is the most common cause of goiter and hypothyroidism in the United States. Occasionally, patients with Hashimoto thyroiditis may have transient hyperthyroidism with low radioactive iodine uptake, owing to the release of T_4 and T_3 into the circulation. Chronic thyroiditis can be differentiated from subacute thyroiditis in that the gland is nontender to palpation and antithyroid antibodies are present in high titer. Early in the disease, TgAb is significantly elevated, but it may disappear later. TPO Ab is usually present early and generally remains present for years. Radioactive iodine uptake may be high, normal, or low. Serum T_3 and T_4 levels are either normal or low; when low, the TSH is elevated. FNA of the thyroid shows lymphocytes and Hürthle cells (enlarged basophilic follicular cells). Hypothyroidism and significant glandular enlargement (goiter) are indications for levothyroxine therapy. Adequate doses of levothyroxine are administered to normalize TSH levels and shrink the goiter.

Thyrotoxicosis Factitia

Thyrotoxicosis factitia exhibits typical features of thyrotoxicosis from ingestion of excessive amounts of thyroxine, often in an attempt to lose weight. Serum T_3 and T_4 levels are elevated and TSH is suppressed, as is the serum thyroglobulin concentration. Radioactive iodine uptake is absent. Patients may require psychotherapy.

Rare Causes of Thyrotoxicosis

Struma ovarii occurs when an ovarian teratoma contains thyroid tissue, which secretes thyroid hormone. A body scan

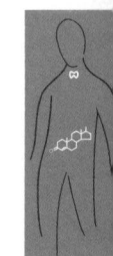

confirms the diagnosis by demonstrating uptake of radioactive iodine in the pelvis.

Hydatidiform mole is due to proliferation and swelling of the trophoblast during pregnancy, with excess production of chorionic gonadotropin, which has intrinsic TSH-like activity. The hyperthyroidism remits with surgical and medical treatment of the molar pregnancy.

Hypothyroidism

Hypothyroidism is a clinical syndrome caused by deficiency of thyroid hormones. In infants and children, hypothyroidism causes retardation of growth and development and may result in permanent motor and mental retardation. Congenital causes of hypothyroidism include agenesis (complete absence of thyroid tissue), dysgenesis (ectopic or lingual thyroid gland), hypoplastic thyroid, thyroid dyshormogenesis, and congenital pituitary diseases. Adult-onset hypothyroidism results in a slowing of metabolic processes and is reversible with treatment. Hypothyroidism is usually primary (thyroid failure), but it may be secondary (hypothalamic or pituitary deficiency) or the result of resistance at the thyroid hormone receptor (Table 66-4). In adults, autoimmune thyroiditis (Hashimoto thyroiditis) is the most common cause of hypothyroidism. This condition may be isolated or part of the polyglandular failure syndrome type II (Schmidt syndrome), which also includes insulin-dependent diabetes mellitus, adrenal insufficiency, pernicious anemia, vitiligo, gonadal failure, hypophysitis, celiac disease, myasthenia gravis, and primary biliary cirrhosis. Iatrogenic causes of hypothyroidism include ^{131}I therapy, thyroidectomy, and treatment with lithium or amiodarone. Iodine deficiency or excess can also cause hypothyroidism.

CLINICAL MANIFESTATIONS

The clinical presentation of hypothyroidism (Table 66-5) depends on the age of onset and severity of thyroid deficiency. Infants with congenital hypothyroidism (also called *cretinism*) may exhibit feeding problems, hypotonia, inactivity, an open posterior fontanelle, and edematous face and hands. Mental retardation, short stature, and delayed puberty occur if treatment is delayed.

Hypothyroidism in adults usually develops insidiously. Patients often complain of fatigue, lethargy, and gradual weight gain for years before the diagnosis is established. A delayed relaxation phase of deep tendon reflexes (*hung-up reflexes*) is a valuable clinical sign characteristic of severe hypothyroidism. Subcutaneous infiltration by mucopolysaccharides, which bind water, causes the edema (termed *myxedema*) and is responsible for the thickened features and puffy appearance of patients with severe hypothyroidism (**Web Fig. 66-4**).

Severe untreated hypothyroidism can result in myxedema coma, characterized by hypothermia, extreme weakness, stupor, hypoventilation, hypoglycemia, and hyponatremia, and is often precipitated by cold exposure, infection, or psychoactive drugs.

LABORATORY TESTS

Laboratory abnormalities in patients with primary hypothyroidism include elevated serum TSH and low total and free T_4. A low or low-normal morning serum TSH in the setting of hypothalamic or pituitary dysfunction characterizes secondary hypothyroidism. Often, the serum total and free T_4 levels are at the lower limits of normal.

Table 66-4 **Causes of Hypothyroidism**
Primary Hypothyroidism
Autoimmune
Hashimoto thyroiditis
Part of polyglandular failure syndrome, type II
Iatrogenic
[131]I therapy
Thyroidectomy
Drug Induced
Iodine deficiency
Iodine excess
Lithium
Amiodarone
Antithyroid drugs
Congenital
Thyroid agenesis
Thyroid dysgenesis
Hypoplastic thyroid
Biosynthetic defect
Secondary Hypothyroidism
Hypothalamic Dysfunction
Neoplasms
Tuberculosis
Sarcoidosis
Langerhans cell histiocytosis
Hemochromatosis
Radiation treatment
Pituitary Dysfunction
Neoplasms
Pituitary surgery
Postpartum pituitary necrosis
Idiopathic hypopituitarism
Glucocorticoid excess (Cushing syndrome)
Radiation treatment

Table 66-5 **Clinical Features of Hypothyroidism**
Children
Learning disabilities
Mental retardation
Short stature
Delayed bone age
Delayed puberty
Adults
Fatigue
Cold intolerance
Weight gain
Constipation
Menstrual irregularities
Dry, coarse, cold skin
Periorbital, peripheral edema
Delayed reflexes
Bradycardia

Hypothyroidism is often associated with hypercholesterolemia and elevated creatine phosphokinase skeletal muscle (MM) fraction (the fraction representative of skeletal muscle). Anemia is usually normocytic, normochromic but may be macrocytic (vitamin B_{12} deficiency resulting from associated pernicious anemia) or microcytic (caused by nutritional deficiencies or menstrual blood loss in women). Because TPO Ab is usually positive in Hashimoto thyroiditis, the major cause of hypothyroidism in adults, its measurement is helpful in deciding whether L-thyroxine treatment is appropriate in patients with subclinical hypothyroidism (discussed later).

DIFFERENTIAL DIAGNOSIS

Because the initial manifestations of hypothyroidism are subtle, the early diagnosis of hypothyroidism demands a high index of suggestion in patients with one or more of the signs or symptoms (see Table 66-5). Early symptoms that are often overlooked include menstrual irregularities (usually menorrhagia), arthralgias, and myalgias.

Laboratory diagnosis may be complicated by the finding of a low total T_4 in euthyroid states associated with low TBG, such as nephrotic syndrome, cirrhosis, or TBG deficiency. TSH and free T_4 levels are normal in these instances. A low total T_4 may also be found with nonthyroidal illness (*euthyroid sick syndrome*), a condition occurring in acutely ill patients. In such patients, total and occasionally free T_4 levels are low, and the serum TSH level is usually normal but may be mildly elevated. This condition may be differentiated from primary hypothyroidism by absence of a goiter, negative antithyroid antibodies, and elevated serum reverse T_3 levels as well as by clinical presentation. The thyroid hormone levels return to normal with resolution of the acute illness, and the patients do not require levothyroxine therapy.

TREATMENT

Patients with hypothyroidism should be initially treated with synthetic levothyroxine. Although T_3 is the more bioactive thyroid hormone, peripheral tissues convert T_4 to T_3 to maintain physiologic levels of the latter. Thus, administration of levothyroxine results in bioavailable T_3 and T_4. Levothyroxine has a half-life of 8 days; consequently, it needs to be given only once a day. The average replacement dose of levothyroxine for adults is 75 to 150 μg per day. In healthy adults, 1.6 μg/kg per day is an appropriate starting dose. In some older patients and patients with cardiac disease, levothyroxine should be increased gradually, starting at 25 μg daily and increasing this dose by 25 μg every 2 weeks, although most patients can safely be started on a full replacement dose. The therapeutic response to levothyroxine therapy should be monitored clinically and with serum TSH levels, which should be measured 6 weeks after a dose adjustment. TSH levels between 0.5 and 2 mU/L are optimal. Patients with secondary hypothyroidism (pituitary or hypothalamic dysfunction) should be treated with levothyroxine until their free T_4 is in the mid-normal range because TSH measurements are not useful to guide therapy in this condition.

In patients with myxedema coma, 300 to 400 mg of levothyroxine is administered intravenously as a loading dose, followed by 50 mg daily and hydrocortisone (100 mg intravenously 3 times a day) and intravenous fluids. Steroids should be given before thyroxine in autoimmune conditions. The underlying precipitating event should be corrected. Respiratory assistance and treatment of hypothermia with warming blankets may be required. Although myxedema coma carries a high mortality rate despite appropriate treatment, many patients improve in 1 to 3 days.

Subclinical Hypothyroidism

In subclinical hypothyroidism, T_4 and T_3 levels are normal or low normal, with a mildly elevated TSH. Some of these patients will develop overt hypothyroidism. The decision about when to treat patients with a mildly elevated TSH is controversial; it is frequently recommended that patients should be treated with levothyroxine if they have a TSH greater than 5 mU/L on two occasions and either positive anti–TPO Ab test results or a goiter. If the patient does not have an appreciable goiter and has negative anti–TPO Ab results, the patient should be treated with levothyroxine only if he or she has a TSH greater than 10 mU/L on two occasions.

Goiter

Enlargement of the thyroid gland is called *goiter*. Patients with goiter may be euthyroid (simple goiter), hyperthyroid (toxic nodular goiter or Graves disease), or hypothyroid (nontoxic goiter or Hashimoto thyroiditis). Thyroid enlargement (often focal) may also be the result of a thyroid adenoma or carcinoma. In nontoxic goiter, inadequate thyroid hormone synthesis leads to TSH stimulation with resultant enlargement of the thyroid gland. Iodine deficiency (endemic goiter) was once the most common cause of nontoxic goiter. With the use of iodized salt, it is now almost nonexistent in North America.

Dietary goitrogens can cause goiter, and iodine is the most common goitrogen. Other goitrogens include lithium and vegetable products such as thioglucosides found in cabbage. Thyroid hormone biosynthetic defects can cause goiter associated with hypothyroidism or, with adequate compensation, euthyroidism.

A careful thyroid examination coupled with thyroid hormone tests can delineate the cause of the goiter. A smooth, symmetrical gland, often with a bruit, and hyperthyroidism are suggestive of Graves disease. A nodular thyroid gland with hypothyroidism and positive antithyroid antibodies is consistent with Hashimoto thyroiditis. A diffuse, smooth goiter with hypothyroidism and negative antithyroid antibodies may be indicative of iodine deficiency or a biosynthetic defect. Goiters may become very large, extend substernally, and cause dysphagia, respiratory distress, or hoarseness. An ultrasound evaluation or radioactive iodine scan delineates the thyroid gland, and a TSH level can determine the functional activity of the goiter.

Hypothyroid goiters are treated with thyroid hormone at a dose that normalizes TSH. Euthyroid goiters may be treated with levothyroxine therapy; however, in most cases, especially with long-standing goiters, regression is unlikely. Surgery is indicated for nontoxic goiter only if obstructive symptoms develop or substantial substernal extension is present.

Solitary Thyroid Nodules

Thyroid nodules are common. They can be detected clinically in about 4% of the population and are found in about 50% of the population at autopsy. Benign thyroid nodules are usually follicular adenomas, colloid nodules, benign cysts, or nodular thyroiditis. Patients may have one prominent nodule on clinical examination, but thyroid ultrasound evaluation may reveal multiple nodules. Although most nodules are benign, a small percentage are malignant. In addition, most thyroid cancers are low-grade malignancies. History, physical examination, and laboratory tests can be helpful in differentiating benign from malignant lesions (Table 66-6). For example, lymph node involvement or hoarseness is strongly suggestive of a malignant tumor.

The major etiologic factor for thyroid cancer is childhood or adolescent exposure to head and neck radiation. Previously, radiation was used to treat an enlarged thymus, tonsillar disease, hemangioma, or acne. Recently, exposure to radiation from nuclear plants (e.g., Chernobyl, Ukraine) has contributed to an increased incidence of thyroid cancer. Patients with a history of irradiation should have a baseline thyroid ultrasound and their thyroid carefully palpated every 1 to 2 years.

A dominant nodule (>1–1.5 cm) or nodules with ultrasound features compatible with neoplasia should undergo FNA, which is a safe procedure that has reduced the need for surgical excision. An expert cytologist can identify most benign lesions (75% of all biopsies). In addition, malignant lesions (5% of biopsies), such as papillary, anaplastic, and medullary carcinoma, can be specifically identified. Follicular neoplasms, however, cannot be diagnosed as benign or malignant by FNA; a cytology report of follicular neoplasia, along with "suspicious" cytology, requires surgical excision. However, if the patient has a follicular lesion and a suppressed TSH, a thyroid scan should be performed because hot nodules are rarely malignant.

Although in the past benign thyroid nodules were treated with levothyroxine suppression, this is no longer recommended because it is uncommon for thyroid nodules to shrink substantially with levothyroxine.

Thyroid Carcinoma

The types and characteristics of thyroid carcinomas are presented in Table 66-7. Papillary carcinoma is associated with local invasion and lymph node spread. Poor prognosis is associated with thyroid capsule invasion, size greater than 2.5 cm, age at onset older than 45 years, tall cell variant, and lymph node involvement. Follicular carcinoma is slightly more aggressive than papillary carcinoma and can spread by local invasion of lymph nodes or hematogenously to bone, brain, or lung. Many tumors show both papillary and follicular cell types. Patients may exhibit metastases before diagnosis of the primary thyroid lesion. Anaplastic carcinoma tends to occur in older individuals, is very aggressive, and rapidly causes pain, dysphagia, and hoarseness.

Medullary thyroid carcinoma is derived from calcitonin-producing parafollicular cells and is more malignant than papillary or follicular carcinoma. It is multifocal and spreads both locally and distally. It may be either sporadic or familial. When familial, it is inherited in an autosomal dominant

---

Table 66-6 High-Risk Factors for Malignancy in a Thyroid Nodule

History

Head and neck irradiation
Exposure to nuclear radiation
Rapid growth
Recent onset
Young age
Male sex
Familial incidence (medullary and about 5% of papillary)

Physical Examination

Hard consistency of nodule
Fixation of nodule
Lymphadenopathy
Vocal cord paralysis
Distant metastasis

Laboratory and Imaging

Elevated serum calcitonin
Cold nodule on technetium scan
Solid lesion with microcalcifications on ultrasonography

Table 66-7 Characteristics of Thyroid Cancers

Type of Cancer	Percentage of Thyroid Cancers	Age of Onset (yr)	Treatment	Prognosis
Papillary	80	40-80	Thyroidectomy, followed by radioactive iodine ablation	Good
Follicular	15	45-80	Thyroidectomy, followed by radioactive iodine ablation	Fair to good
Medullary	3	20-50	Thyroidectomy and central compartment lymph node dissection	Fair
Anaplastic	1	50-80	Isthmusectomy followed by palliative x-ray treatment	Poor
Lymphoma	1	25-70	X-ray therapy and/or chemotherapy	Fair

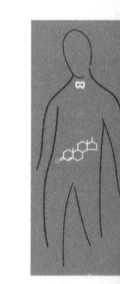

pattern and is part of multiple endocrine neoplasia type IIA (medullary carcinoma of the thyroid, pheochromocytoma, and hyperparathyroidism) or multiple endocrine neoplasia type IIB (medullary carcinoma of the thyroid, mucosal neuromas, intestinal ganglioneuromas, marfanoid habitus, and pheochromocytoma). Elevated basal serum calcitonin levels confirm the diagnosis. Evaluation for *RET* proto-oncogene mutations should be performed in patients with medullary carcinoma, and, if present, all first-degree relatives of the patients should be examined.

TREATMENT

Lobectomy may be performed for isolated papillary microcarcinoma. However, most papillary or follicular tumors require thyroidectomy with a central compartment lymph node dissection, as well as a modified neck dissection if evidence of lateral lymph node metastases is found. After surgery, patients with low-risk, small carcinomas may be administered doses of levothyroxine sufficient to keep the TSH level in the low-normal or slightly suppressed range and monitored with serum thyroglobulin determinations and neck ultrasound examinations. Patients with large lesions and those at high risk for persistence or metastatic disease should be treated with radioactive iodine. Sufficient levothyroxine is then administered to suppress serum TSH to subnormal levels. Frequent clinical and ultrasound neck examinations for masses should be accompanied by measurement of serum thyroglobulin levels. Thyroid cancer patients are considered to have no residual disease if neck ultrasound imaging studies are negative and there is no rise in serum thyroglobulin after TSH stimulation. Recurrence and metastases are also evaluated by ^{131}I whole-body scans carried out under conditions of TSH stimulation, which increase ^{131}I uptake by the thyroid tissue. Elevated TSH levels can be achieved by withdrawal of thyroxine supplementation for 6 weeks. As an alternative, to avoid the resultant symptomatic hypothyroidism, recombinant human TSH can be administered while the patient remains on thyroid hormone replacement. A rise in serum thyroglobulin levels suggests recurrence of thyroid cancer. Local or metastatic lesions that take up ^{131}I (whole-body scan) can be treated with radioactive iodine after the patient has stopped thyroid hormone replacement, whereas those that do not take up ^{131}I can be treated with surgical excision or local x-ray therapy.

Medullary carcinoma of the thyroid requires total thyroidectomy with removal of the central lymph nodes in the neck. Completeness of the procedure is determined by measurement of serum calcitonin, which is also used in monitoring for recurrence.

Anaplastic carcinoma is treated with isthmusectomy to confirm the diagnosis and to prevent tracheal compression, followed by palliative x-ray treatment. Thyroid lymphomas are also treated with x-ray therapy or chemotherapy, or both.

The prognosis for well-differentiated thyroid carcinomas is good. The patient's age at the time of diagnosis and sex are the most important prognostic factors. Men older than 40 years of age and women older than 50 years of age have higher recurrence and death rates than do younger patients. The 5-year survival rate for invasive medullary carcinoma is 50%, whereas the mean survival for anaplastic carcinoma is 6 months.

Prospectus for the Future

- Use of recombinant TSH in combination with radioactive iodine to treat euthyroid goiters and recurrences and metastases of thyroid cancers
- Genetic identification of patients at risk for autoimmune thyroid disease
- Differentiation of benign from malignant follicular neoplasms on FNA tissue by immunogenetic methodology
- Development of effective targeted chemotherapies for thyroid cancer

References

Brent GA: Clinical practice. Graves' disease. N Engl J Med 358:2594-2605, 2008.
Cooper DS, Doherty GM, Haugen BR, et al: Management guidelines for patients with thyroid nodules and differentiated thyroid cancer. Thyroid 16:109-142, 2006.

Hegedus L: Clinical practice: The thyroid nodule. N Engl J Med 351:1764-1771, 2004.
Roberts CGP, Ladenson PW: Hypothyroidism. Lancet 363:793-803, 2004.
Sherman SI: Thyroid carcinoma. Lancet 361:501-511, 2003.
Surks MI, Ortiz E, Daniels GH, et al: Subclinical thyroid disease: Scientific review and guidelines for diagnosis and management. JAMA 291:228-238, 2004.

Adrenal Gland

Theodore C. Friedman

Physiology

The adrenal glands (Fig. 67-1) lie at the superior pole of each kidney and are composed of two distinct regions: the cortex and the medulla. The adrenal cortex consists of three anatomic zones: the outer *zona glomerulosa,* which secretes the mineralocorticoid aldosterone; the intermediate *zona fasciculata,* which secretes cortisol; and the inner *zona reticularis,* which secretes adrenal androgens. The adrenal medulla, lying in the center of the adrenal gland, is functionally related to the sympathetic nervous system and secretes the catecholamines epinephrine and norepinephrine in response to stress.

The synthesis of all steroid hormones begins with cholesterol and is catalyzed by a series of regulated, enzyme-mediated reactions (Fig. 67-2). Glucocorticoids affect the metabolism, cardiovascular function, behavior, and inflammatory and immune response (Table 67-1). Cortisol, the natural human glucocorticoid, is secreted by the adrenal glands in response to ultradian, circadian, and stress-induced hormonal stimulation by adrenocorticotropic hormone (ACTH). Plasma cortisol has significant circadian rhythm; levels are highest in the morning. ACTH, a 39–amino acid neuropeptide, is part of the pro-opiomelanocortin (POMC) precursor molecule, which also contains β-endorphin, β-lipotropin, corticotropin-like intermediate-lobe peptide (CLIP), and various melanocyte-stimulating hormones (MSHs). The secretion of ACTH by the pituitary gland is regulated primarily by two hypothalamic polypeptides: the 41–amino acid corticotropin-releasing hormone (CRH) and the decapeptide vasopressin. Glucocorticoids exert negative feedback on CRH and ACTH secretion. The brain hypothalamic-pituitary-adrenal (HPA) axis (Fig. 67-3) interacts with and influences the function of the reproductive, growth, and thyroid axes at multiple levels, with major participation of glucocorticoids at all levels.

The renin-angiotensin-aldosterone system (Fig. 67-4) is the major regulator of aldosterone secretion. Renal juxtaglomerular cells secrete renin in response to a decrease in circulating volume or a reduction in renal perfusion pressure, or both. Renin is the rate-limiting enzyme that cleaves the 60-kD angiotensinogen, synthesized by the liver, to the bioinactive decapeptide angiotensin I. Angiotensin I is rapidly converted to the octapeptide angiotensin II by angiotensin-converting enzyme in the lungs and other tissues. Angiotensin II is a potent vasopressor and stimulates aldosterone production but does not stimulate cortisol production. Angiotensin II is the predominant regulator of aldosterone secretion, but plasma potassium concentration, plasma volume, and ACTH levels also influence aldosterone secretion. ACTH also mediates the circadian

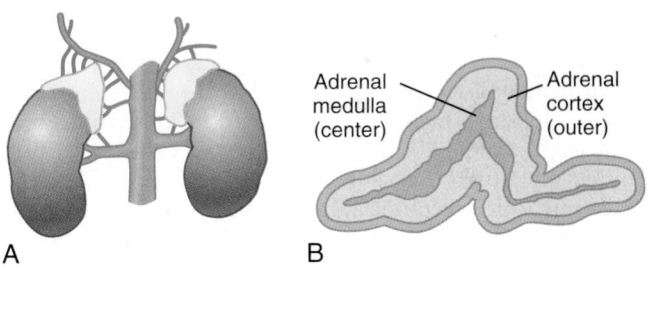

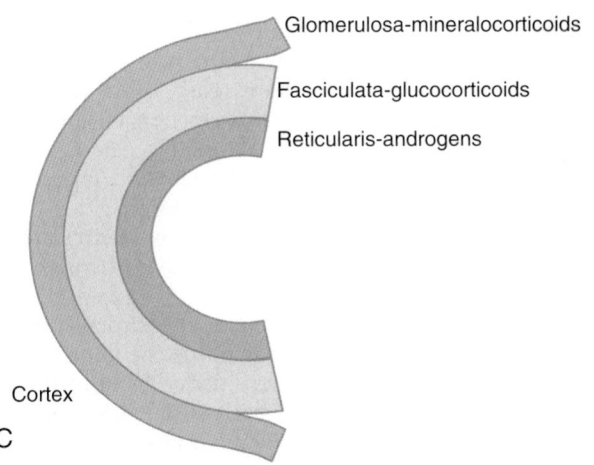

Figure 67-1 A, Anatomic location of the adrenal glands. **B,** Distribution of adrenal cortex and medulla. **C,** Zones of the adrenal cortex.

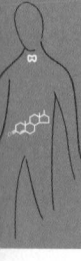

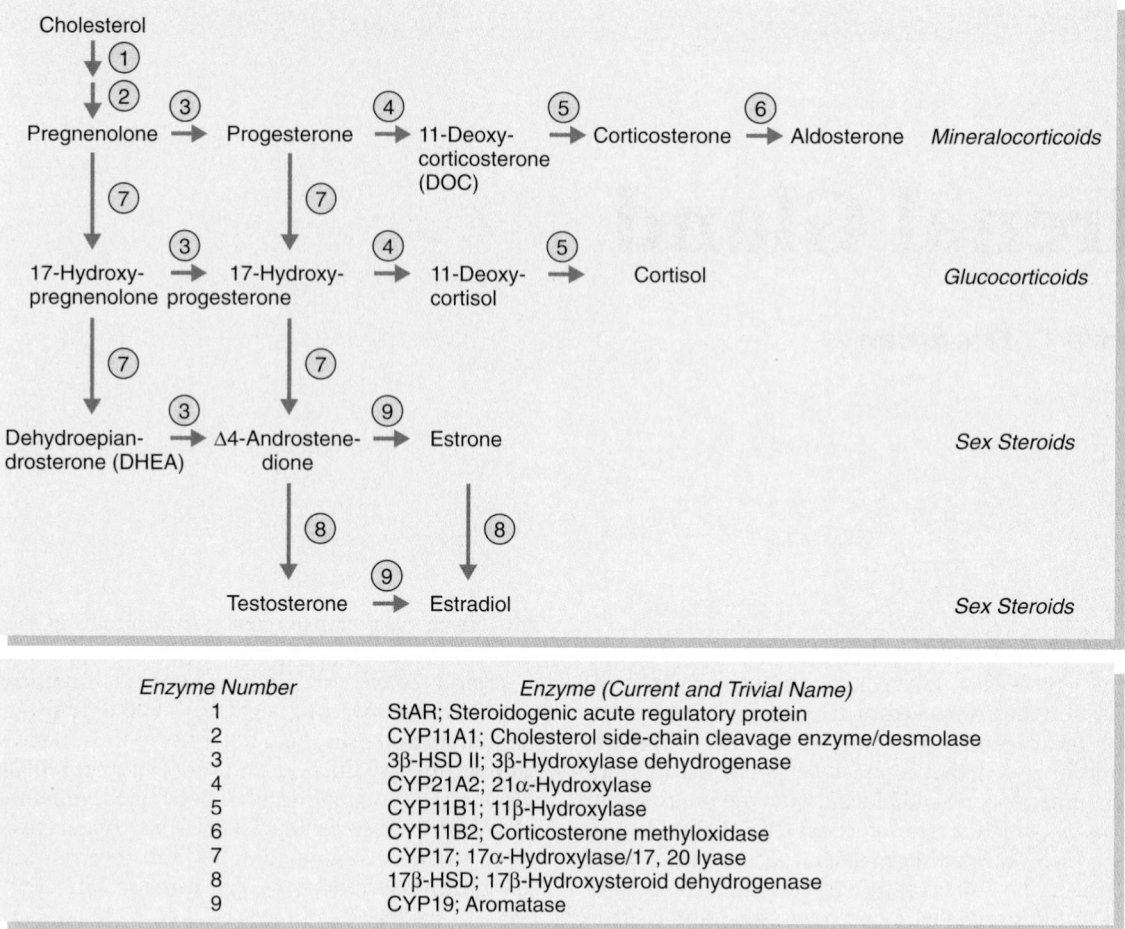

Enzyme Number	Enzyme (Current and Trivial Name)
1	StAR; Steroidogenic acute regulatory protein
2	CYP11A1; Cholesterol side-chain cleavage enzyme/desmolase
3	3β-HSD II; 3β-Hydroxylase dehydrogenase
4	CYP21A2; 21α-Hydroxylase
5	CYP11B1; 11β-Hydroxylase
6	CYP11B2; Corticosterone methyloxidase
7	CYP17; 17α-Hydroxylase/17, 20 lyase
8	17β-HSD; 17β-Hydroxysteroid dehydrogenase
9	CYP19; Aromatase

Figure 67-2 Pathways of steroid biosynthesis.

rhythm of aldosterone; as a result, the plasma concentration of aldosterone is highest in the morning. Aldosterone binds to the type I mineralocorticoid receptor. In contrast, cortisol binds to both the type I mineralocorticoid and type II glucocorticoid receptors, although the intracellular enzyme 11β-hydroxysteroid dehydrogenase (11β-HSD) type II, which catabolizes cortisol to inactive cortisone, limits the functional binding to the former receptor. The availability of cortisol to bind to the glucocorticoid receptor is modulated by 11β-HSD type I, which interconverts cortisol and cortisone. Binding of aldosterone to the cytosol mineralocorticoid receptor leads to sodium (Na^+) absorption and potassium (K^+) and hydrogen (H^+) secretion by the renal tubules. The resultant increase in plasma Na^+ and decrease in plasma K^+ provide a feedback mechanism for suppressing renin and, subsequently, aldosterone secretion.

About 5% of cortisol and 40% of aldosterone circulate in the free form; the remainder is bound to corticosteroid-binding globulin and albumin.

Adrenal androgen precursors include dehydroepiandrosterone (DHEA) and its sulfate and androstenedione. These are synthesized in the zona reticularis under the influence of ACTH and other adrenal androgen-stimulating factors. Although they have minimal intrinsic androgenic activity, they contribute to androgenicity by their peripheral conversion to testosterone and dihydrotestosterone. In men, excessive adrenal androgens have no clinical consequences; however, peripheral conversion of excess adrenal androgen precursor secretion in women results in acne, hirsutism, and virilization. Because of gonadal production of androgens and estrogens and the secretion of norepinephrine by sympathetic ganglia, deficiencies of adrenal androgens and catecholamines are not clinically recognized.

Adrenal Insufficiency

Glucocorticoid insufficiency can be primary, resulting from the destruction or dysfunction of the adrenal cortex, or secondary, resulting from ACTH hyposecretion (Table 67-2). Autoimmune destruction of the adrenal glands (Addison disease) is the most common cause of primary adrenal insufficiency in the industrialized world, accounting for about 65% of cases. Usually both glucocorticoid and mineralocorticoid secretions are diminished in this condition and, if untreated, may be fatal. Isolated glucocorticoid or mineralocorticoid deficiency may also occur, and it is becoming apparent that mild adrenal insufficiency (similar to subclinical hypothyroidism, discussed in Chapter 66) should also be diagnosed and treated. Adrenal medulla function is usually spared. About 70% of patients with Addison disease have antiadrenal antibodies.

Tuberculosis used to be the most common cause of adrenal insufficiency. However, its incidence in the

Table 67-1 **Actions of Glucocorticoids**

Metabolic Homeostasis

Regulate blood glucose level (permissive effects on gluconeogenesis)
Increase glycogen synthesis
Raise insulin levels (permissive effects on lipolytic hormones)
Increase catabolism, decrease anabolism (except fat), inhibit growth hormone axis
Inhibit reproductive axis
Stimulate mineralocorticoid receptor by cortisol

Connective Tissues

Cause loss of collagen and connective tissue

Calcium Homeostasis

Stimulate osteoclasts, inhibit osteoblasts
Reduce intestinal calcium absorption, stimulate parathyroid hormone release, increase urinary calcium excretion, decrease reabsorption of phosphate

Cardiovascular Function

Increase cardiac output
Increase vascular tone (permissive effects on pressor hormones)
Increase sodium retention

Behavior and Cognitive Function

Immune System

Increase intravascular leukocyte concentration
Decrease migration of inflammatory cells to sites of injury
Suppress immune system (thymolysis; suppression of cytokines, prostanoids, kinins, serotonin, histamine, collagenase, and plasminogen activator)

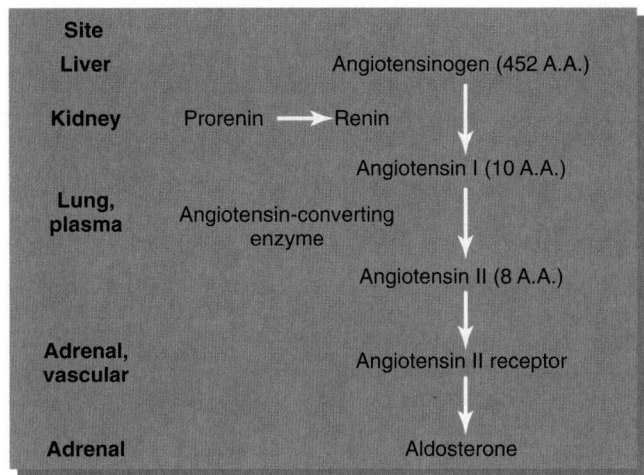

Figure 67-4 Renin-angiotensin-aldosterone axis. A.A., amino acids.

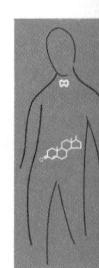

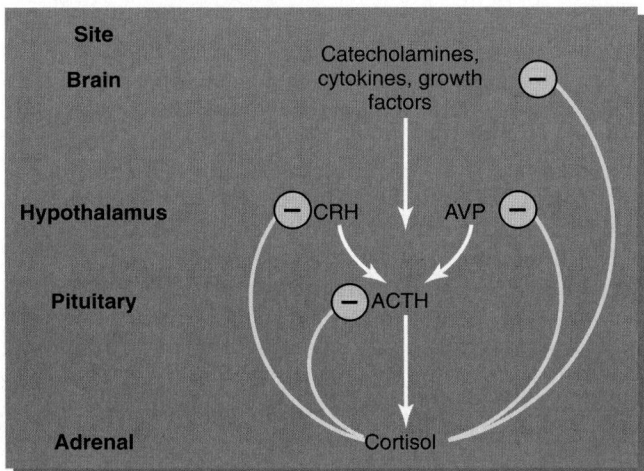

Figure 67-3 Brain hypothalamic-pituitary-adrenal axis. ACTH, adrenocorticotropic hormone; AVP, arginine vasopressin; CRH, corticotropin-releasing hormone.

industrialized world has decreased since the 1960s, and it now accounts for only 15% to 20% of patients with adrenal insufficiency; calcified adrenal glands can be observed in 50% of these patients. Rare causes of adrenal insufficiency are provided in Table 67-2. Many patients with HIV infection have decreased adrenal reserve without overt adrenal insufficiency.

Addison disease may be part of two distinct autoimmune polyglandular syndromes. The triad of hypoparathyroidism, adrenal insufficiency, and mucocutaneous candidiasis char-acterize type I polyglandular autoimmune syndrome, also termed *autoimmune polyendocrine-candidiasis-ectodermal dystrophy* or *autoimmune polyglandular failure syndrome.* Other, less common manifestations include hypothyroidism, gonadal failure, gastrointestinal malabsorption, insulin-dependent diabetes mellitus, alopecia areata and totalis, pernicious anemia, vitiligo, chronic active hepatitis, kera-topathy, hypoplasia of dental enamel and nails, hypophysitis, asplenism, and cholelithiasis. This syndrome develops in childhood. Type II polyglandular autoimmune syndrome, also called *Schmidt syndrome*, is characterized by Addison disease, autoimmune thyroid disease (Graves disease or Hashimoto thyroiditis), and insulin-dependent diabetes mellitus. Other associated diseases include pernicious anemia, vitiligo, gonadal failure, hypophysitis, celiac disease, myasthenia gravis, primary biliary cirrhosis, Sjögren syndrome, lupus erythematosus, and Parkinson disease. This syndrome usually develops in adults.

Common manifestations of adrenal insufficiency are anorexia, weight loss, increasing fatigue, occasional vomiting, diarrhea, and salt craving. Muscle and joint pain, abdominal pain, and postural dizziness may also occur. Signs of increased pigmentation (initially most significantly on the extensor surfaces, palmar creases, and buccal mucosa) often occur secondary to the increased production of ACTH and other POMC-related peptides by the pituitary gland (**Web Fig. 67-1**). Laboratory abnormalities may include hyponatremia, hyperkalemia, mild metabolic acidosis, azotemia, hypercalcemia, anemia, lymphocytosis, and eosinophilia. Hypoglycemia may also occur, especially in children.

Acute adrenal insufficiency is a medical emergency, and treatment should not be delayed pending laboratory results. In a critically ill patient with hypovolemia, a plasma sample for cortisol, ACTH, aldosterone, and renin should be obtained, and then treatment with an intravenous bolus of 100 mg of hydrocortisone and parenteral saline administration should be initiated. A plasma cortisol concentration of more than 34 µg/dL rules out the diagnosis of adrenal crisis, whereas a value of less than 20 µg/dL in the setting of shock is consistent with adrenal insufficiency. A plasma cortisol value between 20 µg/dL and 34 µg/dL in the

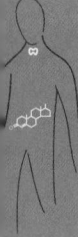

Table 67-2 Syndromes of Adrenocortical Hypofunction

Primary Adrenal Disorders

Combined Glucocorticoid and Mineralocorticoid Deficiency

Autoimmune

Isolated autoimmune disease (Addison disease)
Polyglandular autoimmune syndrome, type I
Polyglandular autoimmune syndrome, type II

Infectious

Tuberculosis
Fungal
Cytomegalovirus
Human immunodeficiency virus

Vascular

Bilateral adrenal hemorrhage
Sepsis
Coagulopathy
Thrombosis; embolism
Adrenal infarction

Infiltration

Metastatic carcinoma and lymphoma
Sarcoidosis
Amyloidosis
Hemochromatosis

Congenital

Congenital adrenal hyperplasia
 21-hydroxylase deficiency
 3β-ol dehydrogenase deficiency
 20,22-desmolase deficiency
Adrenal unresponsiveness to ACTH
Congenital adrenal hypoplasia
Adrenoleukodystrophy
Adrenomyeloneuropathy

Iatrogenic

Bilateral adrenalectomy
Drugs: metyrapone, aminoglutethimide, trilostane,
 ketoconazole, o,p'-DDD, mifepristone

Mineralocorticoid Deficiency without Glucocorticoid Deficiency

Corticosterone methyl oxidase deficiency
Isolated zona glomerulosa defect
Heparin therapy
Critical illness
Converting-enzyme inhibitors

Secondary Adrenal Disorders

Secondary Adrenal Insufficiency

Hypothalamic-pituitary dysfunction
Exogenous glucocorticoids
After removal of an ACTH-secreting tumor

Hyporeninemic Hypoaldosteronism

Diabetic nephropathy
Tubulointerstitial diseases
Obstructive uropathy
Autonomic neuropathy
Nonsteroidal anti-inflammatory drugs
β-Adrenergic drugs

ACTH, adrenocorticotropic hormone.

In a patient with chronic symptoms suggestive of adrenal insufficiency, a basal morning plasma cortisol measurement or a 1-hour cosyntropin test, or both, should be performed. In the later test, 0.25 mg ACTH (1-24) (cosyntropin) is given intravenously, and plasma cortisol is measured 0, 30, and 60 minutes later. A normal response is a plasma cortisol concentration higher than 20 μg/dL at any time during the test. A patient with a basal morning plasma cortisol concentration of less than 5 μg/dL and a stimulated cortisol concentration below 18 μg/dL probably has evident adrenal insufficiency and should receive treatment. A basal plasma morning cortisol concentration between 10 and 18 μg/dL in association with a stimulated cortisol concentration lower than 18 μg/dL probably indicates impaired adrenal reserve and a requirement for receiving cortisol replacement under stress conditions (as described in a later discussion under "Treatment" in this chapter). Recently, a 1-mcg cosyntropin test to assess partial adrenal insufficiency has been described. This test may identify more patients who need cortisol replacement under stress conditions but should not be used to determine which patients need daily cortisol replacement.

Once the diagnosis of adrenal insufficiency is made, the distinction between primary and secondary adrenal insufficiency needs to be established. Secondary adrenal insufficiency results from inadequate stimulation of the adrenal cortex by ACTH. This can result from lesions anywhere along the hypothalamic-pituitary axis or as a sequela of prolonged suppression of the HPA axis by exogenous glucocorticoids. The presentation of secondary adrenal insufficiency is similar to that of primary adrenal insufficiency with a few important differences. Because ACTH and other POMC-related peptides are reduced in secondary adrenal insufficiency, hyperpigmentation does not occur. In addition, because mineralocorticoid levels are normal in secondary adrenal insufficiency, symptoms of salt craving, as well as the laboratory abnormalities of hyperkalemia and metabolic acidosis, are not present. However, hyponatremia is often observed as a result of increased secretion of the antidiuretic hormone (ADH) (resulting from volume depletion and ADH cosecretion with CRH), which accompanies glucocorticoid insufficiency, resulting in impaired water excretion. Because corticotropin is the most preserved of the pituitary hormones, a patient with secondary adrenal insufficiency caused by a pituitary lesion usually has symptoms or laboratory abnormalities consistent with hypothyroidism, hypogonadism, or growth hormone deficiency. To distinguish primary from secondary adrenal insufficiency, a basal morning plasma ACTH value and a standing (upright for at least 2 hours) serum aldosterone level and plasma renin activity should be measured. A plasma ACTH value of more than 20 pg/mL (normal value is 5 to 30 pg/mL) is consistent with primary adrenal insufficiency, whereas a value less than 20 pg/mL probably represents secondary adrenal insufficiency. An upright plasma renin activity of more than 3 ng/mL per hour in the setting of a suppressed aldosterone level is consistent with primary adrenal insufficiency, whereas a value less than 3 ng/mL per hour probably represents secondary adrenal insufficiency. The 1-hour cosyntropin test is suppressed in both secondary and primary adrenal insufficiency.

Secondary adrenal insufficiency occurs commonly after the discontinuation of glucocorticoids. Alternate-day

setting of a severely ill patient may indicate partial adrenal insufficiency. In severe illness, albumin and cortisol-binding globulin (CBG) are low, resulting in a low total but not free cortisol level; thus, a low total cortisol level may not be diagnostic of adrenal insufficiency in this setting.

glucocorticoid treatment, if feasible, results in less suppression of the HPA axis than does daily glucocorticoid therapy. The natural history of recovery from adrenal suppression is first a gradual increase in ACTH levels, followed by the normalization of plasma cortisol levels and then normalization of the cortisol response to ACTH. Complete recovery of the HPA axis can take up to 1 year, and the rate-limiting step appears to be recovery of the CRH neurons.

TREATMENT

After stabilization of acute adrenal insufficiency, patients with Addison disease require lifelong replacement therapy with both glucocorticoids and mineralocorticoids. Many patients are overtreated with glucocorticoids and undertreated with mineralocorticoids. Because overtreatment with glucocorticoids results in insidious weight gain and osteoporosis, the minimal cortisol dose tolerated without symptoms of glucocorticoid insufficiency (usually joint pain) is recommended. An initial regimen of 15 to 20 mg hydrocortisone first thing in the morning and 5 mg hydrocortisone at around 4:00 PM mimics the physiologic dose and is recommended. Whereas glucocorticoid replacement is fairly uniform in most patients, mineralocorticoid replacement varies greatly. The initial dose of the synthetic mineralocorticoid fludrocortisone should be 100 μg per day, and dosage should be adjusted to keep the standing plasma renin activity between 1 and 3 ng/mL per hour. A standing plasma renin activity higher than 3 ng/mL per hour, while the patient is taking the correct glucocorticoid dosage, is suggestive of undertreatment with fludrocortisone.

Under the stress of a minor illness (e.g., nausea, vomiting, fever higher than 100.5° F), the hydrocortisone dose should be doubled for as short a period as possible. The inability to ingest hydrocortisone pills may necessitate parenteral hydrocortisone administration. Patients undergoing a major stressful event (i.e., surgery necessitating general anesthesia, major trauma) should receive 150 to 300 mg parenteral hydrocortisone daily (in three divided doses) with a rapid taper to normal replacement during recovery. All patients should wear a medical information bracelet and should be instructed in the use of intramuscular emergency hydrocortisone injections.

Hyporeninemic Hypoaldosteronism

Mineralocorticoid deficiency can result from decreased renin secretion by the kidneys. Resultant hypoangiotensinemia leads to hypoaldosteronism with hyperkalemia and hyperchloremic metabolic acidosis. Plasma sodium concentration is usually normal, but total plasma volume is often deficient. Plasma renin and aldosterone levels are low and unresponsive to stimuli, including hypokalemia. Diabetes mellitus and chronic tubulointerstitial diseases of the kidney are the most common underlying conditions leading to the impairment of the juxtaglomerular apparatus. A subset of hyporeninemic hypoaldosteronism is caused by autonomic insufficiency and is a frequent cause of orthostatic hypotension. Stimuli such as upright posture or volume depletion,

mediated by baroreceptors, do not cause a normal renin response. Administration of pharmacologic agents such as nonsteroidal anti-inflammatory agents, angiotensin-converting enzyme inhibitors, and β-adrenergic antagonists can also produce conditions of hypoaldosteronism. Fludrocortisone and the α_1 agonist midodrine are effective in correcting the orthostatic hypotension and electrolyte abnormalities caused by hypoaldosteronism.

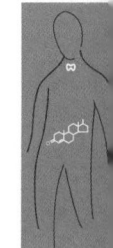

Congenital Adrenal Hyperplasia

Congenital adrenal hyperplasia (CAH) refers to disorders of adrenal steroid biosynthesis that result in glucocorticoid and mineralocorticoid deficiencies. Because of deficient cortisol biosynthesis, a compensatory increase in ACTH occurs, inducing adrenal hyperplasia and overproduction of the steroids that precede blockage of enzyme production (see Fig. 67-2). Five major types of CAH exist, and the clinical manifestations of each type depend on which steroids are in excess and which are deficient. All these syndromes are transmitted in an autosomal recessive pattern. 21-Hydroxylase (CYP21) deficiency is the most common of these disorders and accounts for about 95% of patients of CAH. In this condition, there is a failure of 21-hydroxylation of 17-hydroxyprogesterone and progesterone to 11-deoxycortisol and 11-deoxycorticosterone, respectively, with deficient cortisol and aldosterone production. Cortisol deficiency leads to increased ACTH release, causing overproduction of 17-hydroxyprogesterone and progesterone. Increased ACTH production also leads to increased biosynthesis of androstenedione and DHEA, which can be converted to testosterone. Patients with 21-hydroxylase deficiencies can be divided into two clinical phenotypes: classic 21-hydroxylase deficiency, usually diagnosed at birth or during childhood, and late-onset 21-hydroxylase deficiency, which develops during or after puberty. Two thirds of the patients with classic 21-hydroxylase deficiency have various degrees of mineralocorticoid deficiency (salt-losing form); the remaining one third is not the salt-losing form (simple virilizing form). Both decreased aldosterone production and increased concentrations of precursors that are mineralocorticoid antagonists (progesterone and 17-hydroxyprogesterone) contribute to salt loss in the salt-losing form, in which the enzymatic block is more severe.

The most useful measurement for the diagnosis of classic 21-hydroxylase deficiency is that of plasma 17-hydroxyprogesterone. A value greater than 200 ng/dL is consistent with the diagnosis. Late-onset 21-hydroxylase deficiency represents an allelic variant of classic 21-hydroxylase deficiency and is characterized by a mild enzymatic defect. This deficiency is the most frequent autosomal recessive disorder in humans and is present especially in Ashkenazi Jews. The syndrome usually develops around the time of puberty with signs of virilization (hirsutism and acne) and amenorrhea or oligomenorrhea. This diagnosis should be considered in women with unexplained hirsutism and menstrual abnormalities or infertility. The diagnosis is made from the finding of an elevated level of plasma 17-hydroxyprogesterone (>1500 ng/dL) 30 minutes after administration of 0.25 mg of synthetic ACTH (1-24).

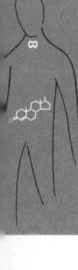

The aim of treatment for classic 21-hydroxylase deficiency is to replace glucocorticoids and mineralocorticoids, suppress ACTH and androgen overproduction, and allow for normal growth and sexual maturation in children. A proposed approach to treating classic 21-hydroxylase deficiency recommends physiologic replacement with hydrocortisone and fludrocortisone in all affected patients, including those with the simple virilizing form. The deleterious effects of excess androgens can then be prevented by the use of an antiandrogen agent (flutamide) and an aromatase inhibitor (testolactone) that blocks the conversion of testosterone to estrogen.

Although the traditional treatment for late-onset 21-hydroxylase deficiency is dexamethasone (0.5 mg per day), the use of an antiandrogen such as spironolactone (100 to 200 mg per day) or flutamide (125 mg per day) is probably more effective and has fewer side effects. Mineralocorticoid replacement is not needed in late-onset 21-hydroxylase deficiency.

11β-Hydroxylase (CYP11B1) deficiency accounts for about 5% of the patients with CAH. In this syndrome, the conversions of 11-deoxycortisol to cortisol and 11-deoxycorticosterone to corticosterone (the precursor to aldosterone) are blocked. Affected patients usually have hypertension and hypokalemia because of increased amounts of precursors with mineralocorticoid activity. Virilization occurs, as with 21-hydroxylase deficiency, and a late-onset form exhibiting as androgen excess also occurs. The diagnosis is made from the finding of elevated plasma 11-deoxycortisol levels, either basally or after ACTH stimulation.

Rare forms of CAH are 3β-HSD type II, 17α-hydroxylase (CYP17), and steroidogenic acute regulatory protein deficiencies.

Syndromes of Adrenocorticoid Hyperfunction

Hypersecretion of the glucocorticoid hormone cortisol results in Cushing syndrome, a metabolic disorder affecting carbohydrate, protein, and lipid metabolism. Hypersecretion of mineralocorticoids such as aldosterone results in a syndrome of hypertension and electrolyte disturbances.

CUSHING SYNDROME

Pathophysiology

Increased production of cortisol is seen in both physiologic and pathologic states (Table 67-3). Physiologic hypercortisolism occurs in stress, during the last trimester of pregnancy, and in persons who regularly perform strenuous exercise. Pathologic conditions of elevated cortisol levels include exogenous or endogenous Cushing syndrome and several psychiatric states, including depression, alcoholism, anorexia nervosa, panic disorder, and alcohol or narcotic withdrawal.

Cushing syndrome may be caused by exogenous ACTH or glucocorticoid administration or by endogenous overproduction of these hormones. Endogenous Cushing syndrome

Table 67-3 **Syndromes of Adrenocortical Hyperfunction**
States of Glucocorticoid Excess
Physiologic States
Stress
Strenuous exercise
Last trimester of pregnancy
Pathologic States
Psychiatric conditions (pseudo-Cushing disorders)
Depression
Alcoholism
Anorexia nervosa
Panic disorders
Alcohol and drug withdrawal
ACTH-dependent states
Pituitary adenoma (Cushing disease)
Ectopic ACTH syndrome
Bronchial carcinoid
Thymic carcinoid
Islet cell tumor
Small cell lung carcinoma
Ectopic CRH secretion
ACTH-independent states
Adrenal adenoma
Adrenal carcinoma
Micronodular adrenal disease
Exogenous Sources
Glucocorticoid intake
ACTH intake
States of Mineralocorticoid Excess
Primary Aldosteronism
Aldosterone-secreting adenoma
Bilateral adrenal hyperplasia
Aldosterone-secreting carcinoma
Glucocorticoid-suppressible hyperaldosteronism
Adrenal Enzyme Deficiencies
11β-hydroxylase deficiency
17α-hydroxylase deficiency
11β-hydroxysteroid dehydrogenase, type II
Exogenous Mineralocorticoids
Licorice
Carbenoxolone
Fludrocortisone
Secondary Hyperaldosteronism
Associated with hypertension
Accelerated hypertension
Renovascular hypertension
Estrogen administration
Renin-secreting tumors
Without hypertension
Bartter syndrome
Sodium-wasting nephropathy
Renal tubular acidosis
Diuretic and laxative abuse
Edematous states (cirrhosis, nephrosis, congestive heart failure)

ACTH, adrenocorticotropin hormone; CRH, corticotropin-releasing hormone.

is either ACTH dependent or ACTH independent. ACTH dependency accounts for 85% of patients and includes pituitary sources of ACTH (Cushing disease), ectopic sources of ACTH, and, in rare instances, ectopic sources of CRH. Pituitary Cushing disease accounts for 80% of patients with ACTH-dependent Cushing syndrome. Ectopic secretion of ACTH occurs most commonly in patients with small cell lung carcinoma. These patients are older, usually have a history of smoking, and primarily exhibit signs and symptoms of lung cancer rather than those of Cushing syndrome. Patients with the clinically apparent ectopic ACTH syndrome, in contrast, have mostly intrathoracic (lung and thymic) carcinoids. The remaining patients have pancreatic, adrenal, or thyroid tumors that secrete ACTH. ACTH-independent causes account for 15% of patients with Cushing syndrome and include adrenal adenomas, adrenal carcinomas, micronodular adrenal disease, and autonomous macronodular adrenal disease. The female-to-male ratio for noncancerous forms of Cushing syndrome is 4:1.

Clinical Manifestations

The clinical signs, symptoms, and common laboratory findings of hypercortisolism observed in patients with Cushing syndrome are listed in Table 67-4 (see also Fig. 65-2). Typically, the obesity is centripetal, with a wasting of the arms and legs, which is distinct from the generalized weight gain observed in idiopathic obesity. Rounding of the face (called *moon facies*) and a dorsocervical fat pad *(buffalo hump)* may occur in obesity that is not related to Cushing syndrome, whereas facial plethora and supraclavicular filling are more specific for Cushing syndrome. Patients with Cushing syndrome may have proximal muscle weakness; consequently, the physical finding of the inability to stand up from a squat or out of a car seat can be quite revealing. Sleep disturbances, mood swings, and other psychological abnormalities are frequently seen. Cognitive dysfunction and severe fatigue

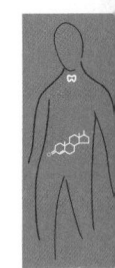

are often found. Menstrual irregularities often precede other cushingoid symptoms in affected women. Patients of both sexes complain of a loss of libido, whereas affected men frequently complain of erectile dysfunction. Adult-onset acne or hirsutism in women should also suggest Cushing syndrome. The skin striae observed in patients with Cushing syndrome are violaceous (i.e., purple, dark red), with a width of at least 1 cm. Thinning of the skin on the top of the hands is a specific sign in younger adults with Cushing syndrome. Old pictures of patients are extremely helpful for evaluating the progression of the physical stigmata of Cushing syndrome.

Associated laboratory findings in Cushing syndrome include elevated plasma alkaline phosphatase levels, granulocytosis, thrombocytosis, hypercholesterolemia, hypertriglyceridemia, and glucose intolerance, diabetes mellitus, or both. Hypokalemia or alkalosis usually occurs in patients with severe hypercortisolism as a result of the ectopic ACTH syndrome.

Diagnosis

If the history and physical examination findings are suggestive of hypercortisolism, then the diagnosis of Cushing syndrome can usually be established by collecting urine for 24 hours and measuring urinary-free cortisol (UFC). UFC excretion reflects plasma-unbound cortisol that is filtered and excreted by the kidney. This test is extremely sensitive for the diagnosis of Cushing syndrome because in 90% of affected patients, the initial UFC level is greater than 50 μg per 24 hours when measured by high-pressure liquid chromatography (HPLC) or mass spectroscopy cortisol assays. Patients with Cushing disease usually have UFC levels between 50 and 200 μg per 24 hours, whereas patients with the ectopic ACTH syndrome and cortisol-secreting adrenal adenomas or carcinomas frequently have UFC levels greater than 200 μg per 24 hours (Fig. 67-5).

Cortisol is normally secreted in a diurnal manner; the plasma concentration is highest in the early morning (between 6:00 and 8:00 AM) and lowest around midnight. The normal 8:00 AM plasma cortisol level ranges between 8 and 25 μg/dL and declines throughout the day. By 11:00 PM, the values are usually less than 5 μg/dL. Most patients with Cushing syndrome lack this diurnal variation. Thus, although their morning cortisol levels may be normal, their evening concentrations are significantly higher. Evening or night values greater than 50% of the morning values are consistent with Cushing syndrome. Measurement of random morning cortisol levels is not particularly helpful.

The overnight dexamethasone suppression test has been widely used as a screening test to evaluate patients who may have hypercortisolism. Dexamethasone, 1 mg, is given orally at 11:00 PM, and plasma cortisol is measured the following morning at 8:00 AM. A morning plasma cortisol level greater than 3 mcg/dL suggests hypercortisolism. This test produces a significant number of both false-positive and false-negative results, but is still recommended by the 2008 Endocrine Society consensus guidelines.

Because of the difficulty of obtaining nighttime plasma cortisol levels, measurement of late-night salivary cortisol has been developed to assess hypercortisolism. Late-night salivary cortisol reflects circulating free cortisol and can be obtained by the patient on one or more occasions and mailed

Table 67-4 **Signs, Symptoms, and Laboratory Abnormalities of Hypercortisolism**
Fat redistribution (dorsocervical and supraclavicular fat pads, temporal wasting, centripetal obesity, weight gain) (95%)
Menstrual irregularities (80% of affected women)
Thin skin and plethora (80%)
Moon facies (75%)
Increased appetite (75%)
Sleep disturbances (75%)
Hypertension (75%)
Hypercholesterolemia and hypertriglyceridemia (70%)
Altered mentation (poor concentration, decreased memory, euphoria) (70%)
Diabetes mellitus and glucose intolerance (65%)
Striae (65%)
Hirsutism (65%)
Proximal muscle weakness (60%)
Psychological disturbances (emotional lability, depression, mania, psychosis) (50%)
Decreased libido and impotence (50%)
Acne (45%)
Osteoporosis and pathologic fractures (40%)
Virilization (in women) (40%)
Easy bruisability (40%)
Poor wound healing (40%)
Edema (20%)
Increased infections (10%)
Cataracts (5%)

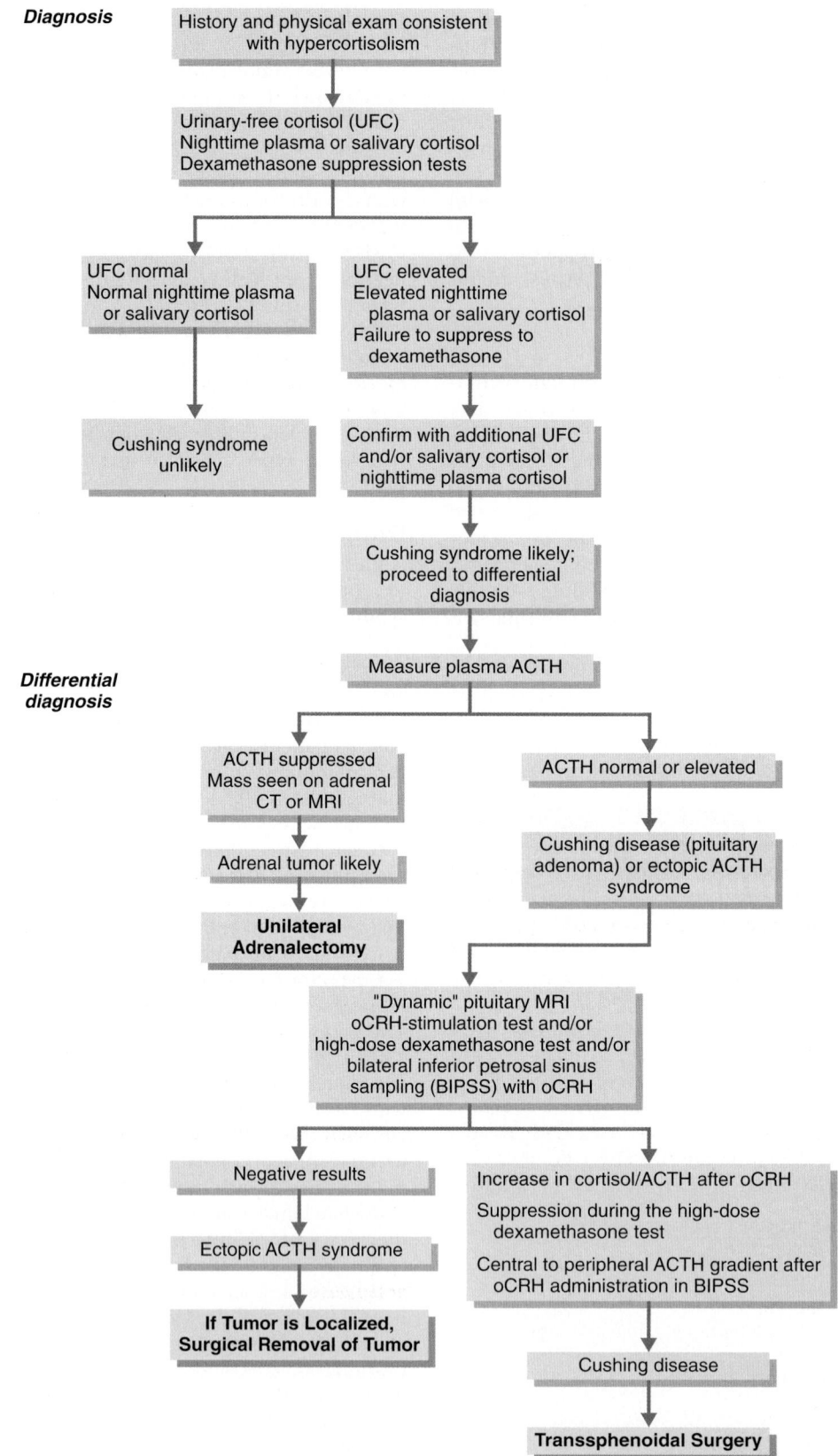

Figure 67-5 Flowchart for evaluating a patient with probable Cushing syndrome. ACTH, adrenocorticotropic hormone; CT, computed tomography; MRI, magnetic resonance imaging; oCRH, ovine corticotropin-releasing hormone.

to a reference laboratory. This test appears to have a high degree of sensitivity and specificity for the diagnosis of Cushing syndrome. Growing evidence suggests that a large number of patients found to have Cushing syndrome have cortisol levels that are elevated on some occasions but not on all occasions. For this reason, multiple measurements of UFC or salivary cortisol may be needed to both diagnose and exclude Cushing syndrome, especially in subjects with suggestive signs and symptoms of hypercortisolism. Thus, both positive and negative tests of hypercortisolism need confirmation before proceeding to the differential diagnosis of Cushing syndrome.

Differential Diagnosis

Once the diagnosis of Cushing syndrome is established, the cause of the hypercortisolism needs to be ascertained, which is accomplished by biochemical studies that evaluate the feedback regulation of the HPA axis, by venous sampling techniques, and by imaging procedures. The initial approach is to measure basal ACTH levels that are normal or elevated in Cushing disease and the ectopic ACTH syndrome but are suppressed in primary adrenal Cushing syndrome. Patients with a suppressed ACTH level can proceed to adrenal imaging studies. To distinguish between Cushing disease and the ectopic ACTH syndrome, the high dose or 8-mg overnight dexamethasone suppression test, ovine CRH (oCRH) test, and bilateral simultaneous inferior petrosal sinus sampling are used.

In the dexamethasone suppression test (Liddle test), 0.5 mg of dexamethasone is given orally every 6 hours for 2 days, followed by 2 mg of dexamethasone every 6 hours for another 2 days. On the second day of the high dose of dexamethasone, UFC is suppressed to less than 10% of that of the baseline collection in patients with pituitary adenomas but not in patients with the ectopic ACTH syndrome or adrenal cortisol–secreted tumors. Although the Liddle test is often helpful in establishing the cause of Cushing syndrome, it has some disadvantages. The test requires accurate measurement of urine collections, often necessitating inpatient hospitalization. In about 50% of patients with bronchial carcinoids causing ectopic ACTH production, cortisol secretion is suppressible by high-dose dexamethasone, which yields a false-positive result. In addition, because patients with Cushing syndrome are often episodic secretors of corticosteroids, considerable variation in daily UFC excretion can occur, and false results can be obtained. Therefore, the Liddle test should be interpreted cautiously and other confirmatory tests should be performed before surgery is recommended.

An overnight high-dose dexamethasone suppression test is helpful in establishing the cause of Cushing syndrome. In this test a baseline 8:00 AM cortisol level is measured, and then 8 mg of dexamethasone is given orally at 11:00 PM. At 8:00 AM the following morning, a plasma cortisol measurement is obtained. Suppression, which would occur in patients with pituitary Cushing disease, is defined as a decrease in plasma cortisol to less than 50% of the baseline level. Few patients with bronchial carcinoid have been examined; as a result, the suppressibility of these tumors by high-dose overnight dexamethasone is not well established.

The oCRH test can also be used to establish the cause of Cushing syndrome. Pituitary corticotrophs of normal indi-

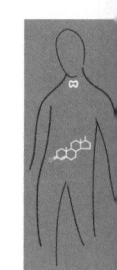

viduals and of patients with pituitary Cushing disease respond to oCRH by increasing the secretion of ACTH and therefore cortisol. Thus, the oCRH test cannot be used to distinguish normal persons from patients with pituitary Cushing disease. Patients with cortisol-secreting adrenal tumors have low or undetectable concentrations of ACTH that do not respond to the oCRH test. Patients with ectopic ACTH secretion have high basal ACTH levels that do not increase with the oCRH test. In patients with both the ectopic ACTH syndrome and primary adrenal hypercortisolism, cortisol levels do not change in response to the oCRH test. Discrepancies between the oCRH and dexamethasone tests necessitate further work-up to ascertain the diagnosis.

Bilateral inferior petrosal sinus sampling (BIPSS) is an accurate and safe procedure for distinguishing pituitary Cushing disease from the ectopic ACTH syndrome. Venous blood from the anterior lobe of the pituitary gland empties into the cavernous sinuses and then into the superior and inferior petrosal sinuses. Venous plasma samples for ACTH determination are obtained from both inferior petrosal sinuses, along with a simultaneous peripheral sample, both before and after intravenous bolus administration of CRH. In baseline measurements an ACTH concentration gradient of 1.6 or more between a sample from either of the petrosal sinuses and the peripheral sample is strongly suggestive of pituitary Cushing disease, whereas patients with the ectopic ACTH syndrome or adrenal adenomas have no ACTH gradient between their petrosal and peripheral samples. After CRH administration, a central-to-peripheral gradient of more than 3.2 is consistent with pituitary Cushing disease. The use of CRH has enabled complete distinction of pituitary Cushing disease from nonpituitary Cushing syndrome. An ACTH gradient ipsilateral to the side of the tumor is found in 70% to 80% of patients sampled. Although BIPSS requires an experienced radiologist in petrosal sinus sampling, this procedure is available at many tertiary care facilities.

Imaging of the pituitary gland by magnetic resonance imaging (MRI) with gadolinium is the preferred procedure for localizing a pituitary adenoma. In many centers, a *dynamic* MRI is performed, which visualizes the pituitary as the gadolinium enters and leaves the gland. This test detects about 60% to 90% of pituitary ACTH-secreting tumors and can detect many pituitary tumors as small as 2 mm in diameter. About 10% of normal individuals may have a nonfunctioning pituitary adenoma found on a pituitary MRI. It is therefore recommended that pituitary imaging not be the sole criterion for the diagnosis of pituitary Cushing disease.

Treatment

The preferred treatment for all forms of Cushing syndrome is appropriate surgery. Pituitary Cushing disease is best treated by trans-sphenoidal surgery. When the operation is performed by an experienced neurosurgeon, the cure rate is higher than 80%. Trans-sphenoidal surgery carries very low rates of morbidity and mortality. Growth hormone and androgen deficiency in both sexes are the most common complications of surgery. Other complications (e.g., meningitis, cerebrospinal fluid leakage, optic nerve damage, isolated thyrotropin deficiency) are uncommon. Patients who have failed initial pituitary surgery or have recurrent Cushing disease may be treated with either pituitary irradiation or bilateral adrenalectomy. Irradiation has more long-term complications than trans-sphenoidal surgery and results in curing about 60% of patients, but it may take up to 5 years to render a person eucortisolemic. Panhypopituitarism eventually develops in almost all these patients; consequently, growth hormone, thyroid, gonadal, and even steroid replacement may be needed. A more appealing option for patients with Cushing disease who remain hypercortisolemic after pituitary surgery is bilateral adrenalectomy, followed by lifelong glucocorticoid and mineralocorticoid replacement therapy. About 10% of patients with Cushing disease who undergo bilateral adrenalectomy develop Nelson syndrome, which is an ACTH-secreting macroadenoma that often causes visual field deficits and hyperpigmentation. The incidence of Nelson syndrome is reduced if patients undergo pituitary irradiation.

In patients with the ectopic ACTH syndrome, it is hoped that the tumor is localized by appropriate scans and can be removed surgically. A unilateral adrenalectomy is the treatment of choice in patients with a cortisol-secreting adrenal adenoma. Patients with cortisol-secreting adrenal carcinomas initially should also be managed surgically; however, they have a poor prognosis, with only 20% surviving more than 1 year after diagnosis.

Medical treatment for hypercortisolism may be needed to prepare those patients for surgery who are undergoing or have undergone pituitary irradiation and are awaiting its effects or who are not surgical candidates or who elect not to have surgery. Ketoconazole, o,p′-DDD, metyrapone, aminoglutethimide, mifepristone, and trilostane are the most commonly used agents for adrenal blockade and can be used alone or in combination.

PRIMARY MINERALOCORTICOID EXCESS

Pathophysiology

Increased mineralocorticoid activity is exhibited by salt retention, hypertension, hypokalemia, and metabolic alkalosis. The causes of primary aldosteronism (see Table 67-3) are aldosterone-producing adenoma (75%), bilateral adrenal hyperplasia (25%), adrenal carcinoma (1%), and glucocorticoid-remediable hyperaldosteronism (<1%). The adrenal enzyme defects-11β-HSD type II, 11β-hydroxylase, and 17α-hydroxylase deficiencies and apparent mineralocorticoid excess (from licorice or carbenoxolone ingestion, which inhibits 11β-HSD type II, or from a congenital defect in this enzyme) are also states of functional mineralocorticoid overactivity. Secondary aldosteronism (see Table 67-3) results from an overactive renin-angiotensin system.

Primary aldosteronism is usually recognized during evaluation of hypertension or hypokalemia and represents a potentially curable form of hypertension. Up to 5% of patients with hypertension have primary aldosteronism. These patients are usually between the ages of 30 and 50 years, and the female-to-male ratio is 2:1.

Clinical Manifestations

Hypertension, hypokalemia, and metabolic alkalosis are the main clinical manifestations of hyperaldosteronism; most of the presenting symptoms are related to hypokalemia. Symptoms in patients with mild hypokalemia are fatigue, muscle weakness, nocturia, lassitude, and headaches. If more severe

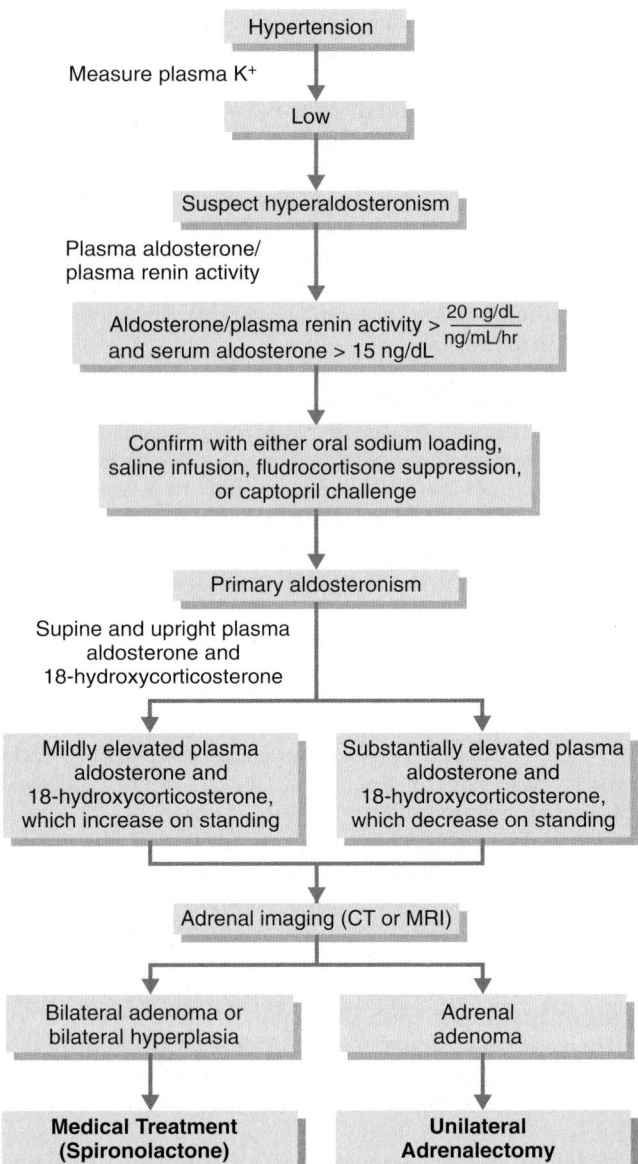

Figure 67-6 Flowchart for evaluating a patient with probable primary hyperaldosteronism. CT, computed tomography; MRI, magnetic resonance imaging.

hypokalemia exists, polydipsia, polyuria, paresthesias, and even intermittent paralysis and tetany can occur. Blood pressure can range from being minimally elevated to very high. A positive Trousseau or Chvostek sign may occur as a result of metabolic alkalosis.

Diagnosis and Treatment

Initially, hypokalemia in the presence of hypertension must be documented (Fig. 67-6). The patient must have adequate salt intake and discontinue diuretics before potassium measurement. If hypokalemia is found under these conditions and the patient is taking spironolactone, then it should be stopped, and a morning plasma aldosterone level and a plasma renin activity (PRA) should be measured. A serum aldosterone–to-PRA ratio greater than 20 ng/dL per hour and a serum aldosterone level greater than 15 ng/dL suggest the diagnosis of hyperaldosteronism. Following the finding of an elevated serum aldosterone/PRA ratio, confirmatory tests for hyperaldosteronism should be performed. These include oral sodium loading, saline infusion, fludrocortisone suppression or captopril challenge.

Once the diagnosis of primary aldosteronism has been demonstrated, distinguishing between an aldosterone-producing adenoma and a bilateral hyperplasia is important because the former is treated with surgery and the latter is treated medically. In the initial test (a postural challenge), an 8:00 AM supine blood sample is drawn for plasma aldosterone, 18-hydrocorticosterone, renin, and cortisol measurement. The patient then stands for 2 hours, and an upright sample is drawn for measurement of the same hormones. A basal plasma aldosterone level of less than 20 ng/dL is usually found in patients with bilateral hyperplasia, and a value greater than 20 ng/dL suggests the diagnosis of adrenal adenoma. In bilateral hyperplasia, plasma aldosterone often increases as a result of the increase in renin in response to the upright position, whereas in adenoma, plasma aldosterone levels usually fall as a result of decreased stimulation by ACTH at 10:00 AM in comparison with ACTH stimulation at 8:00 AM. At 8:00 AM, a plasma 18-hydroxycorticosterone level of greater than 50 ng/dL that falls with upright posture occurs in most patients with an adenoma, whereas an 8:00 AM level less than 50 ng/dL that rises with upright posture occurs in most patients with bilateral hyperplasia.

A computed tomography (CT) scan of the adrenal glands should be performed to localize the tumor. The patient should undergo unilateral adrenalectomy if a discrete adenoma is observed in one adrenal gland, if the contralateral gland is normal, and if biochemical test results are consistent with an adenoma. Patients in whom biochemical study findings are consistent with an adenoma but CT results are consistent with bilateral disease should undergo adrenal venous sampling for aldosterone and cortisol measurement. Patients in whom biochemical and localization study findings are consistent with bilateral hyperplasia should be treated medically, usually with eplerenone or spironolactone. Those in whom biochemical study results are consistent with bilateral hyperplasia should also be evaluated for dexamethasone-suppressible hyperaldosteronism by receiving a trial of dexamethasone, which reverses the hyperaldosteronism in this rare autosomal dominant disorder.

Hyperaldosteronism and hypertension secondary to activation of the renin-angiotensin system can occur in patients with accelerated hypertension, in those with renovascular hypertension, in those receiving estrogen therapy, and rarely in patients with renin-secreting tumors. Hyperaldosteronism without hypertension occurs in patients with Bartter syndrome, sodium-wasting nephropathy, and renal tubular acidosis, as well as those who abuse diuretics or laxatives.

Adrenal Medullary Hyperfunction

The adrenal medulla synthesizes the catecholamines norepinephrine, epinephrine, and dopamine from the amino acid tyrosine. Norepinephrine, the major catecholamine produced by the adrenal medulla, has predominantly α-agonist actions, causing vasoconstriction. Epinephrine acts primarily on the β receptors, having positive inotropic and chronotropic effects on the heart, causing peripheral vasodilation and increasing plasma glucose concentrations in response to

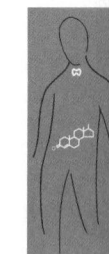

hypoglycemia. The action of circulating dopamine is unclear. Whereas norepinephrine is synthesized in the central nervous system and sympathetic postganglionic neurons, epinephrine is synthesized almost entirely in the adrenal medulla. The adrenal medullary contribution to norepinephrine secretion is relatively small. Bilateral adrenalectomy results in only minimal changes in circulating norepinephrine levels, although epinephrine levels are dramatically reduced. Thus, hypofunction of the adrenal medulla has little physiologic effect, whereas hypersecretion of catecholamines produces the clinical syndrome of pheochromocytoma.

PHEOCHROMOCYTOMA

Pathophysiology

Although pheochromocytomas can occur in any sympathetic ganglion in the body, more than 90% of pheochromocytomas arise from the adrenal medulla. Most extra-adrenal tumors occur in the mediastinum or abdomen. Bilateral adrenal pheochromocytomas occur in about 5% of the cases and may occur as part of familial syndromes. Pheochromocytoma occurs as part of multiple endocrine neoplasia type IIA or IIB. The former (Sipple syndrome) is marked by medullary carcinoma of the thyroid, hyperparathyroidism, and pheochromocytoma; the latter is characterized by medullary carcinoma of the thyroid, mucosal neuromas, intestinal ganglioneuromas, marfanoid habitus, and pheochromocytoma. Pheochromocytomas are also associated with neurofibromatosis, cerebelloretinal hemangioblastosis (von Hippel-Lindau disease), and tuberous sclerosis.

Clinical Manifestations

Because most pheochromocytomas secrete norepinephrine as the principal catecholamine, hypertension (often paroxysmal) is the most common finding. Other symptoms include the triad of headache, palpitations, and sweating, as well as skin blanching, anxiety, nausea, fatigue, weight loss, and abdominal and chest pain. Emotional stress, exercise, anesthesia, abdominal pressure, or intake of tyramine-containing foods may precipitate these symptoms. Orthostatic hypotension can also occur. Wide fluctuations in blood pressure are characteristic, and the hypertension associated with pheochromocytoma usually does not respond to standard antihypertensive medicines. Cardiac abnormalities, as well as idiosyncratic reactions to medications, may also occur.

Diagnosis and Treatment

Although measurements of fractionated catecholamine and metanephrine levels in the urine are the most used screening tests, plasma-free metanephrine and normetanephrine levels are the best tests for confirming or excluding pheochromocytoma because the metabolism of catecholamines to free metanephrines is independent of catecholamine release and can be performed in the absence of hypertension and other symptoms. A plasma-free metanephrine level greater than 0.61 nmol/L and a plasma-free normetanephrine level greater than 0.31 nmol/L are consistent with the diagnosis of a pheochromocytoma. If the values are only mildly elevated, a clonidine suppression test could be performed. In this test, clonidine (0.3 mg) is given orally, and plasma catecholamines (including free metanephrine and normetanephrine) are measured before and 3 hours after administration. In normal persons, catecholamine levels decrease into the normal range, whereas in patients with pheochromocytoma, levels are unchanged or increase. Once the diagnosis of pheochromocytoma is made, a CT scan of the adrenal glands should be performed. Most intra-adrenal pheochromocytomas are readily visible on this scan and enhance with contrast. If the CT scan is negative, then extra-adrenal pheochromocytomas can often be localized by iodine 131-labeled metaiodobenzylguanidine (^{131}I-MIBG), positron emission tomography, octreotide scan, or abdominal MRI. Pheochromocytomas show a high signal intensity on T2-weighted images.

The treatment of pheochromocytoma is surgical if the lesion can be localized. Patients should undergo preoperative α blockade with phenoxybenzamine 1 to 2 weeks before surgery. β-Adrenergic antagonists should be used before or during surgery. About 5% to 10% of pheochromocytomas are malignant. ^{131}I-MIBG or chemotherapy may be useful, but the prognosis is poor. α-Methyl-*p*-tyrosine, an inhibitor of tyrosine hydroxylase, the rate-limiting enzyme in catecholamine biosynthesis, may be used to decrease catecholamine secretion from the tumor.

INCIDENTAL ADRENAL MASS

Clinically inapparent adrenal masses are discovered inadvertently in the course of diagnostic testing or treatment for other clinical conditions that are not related to the suggestion of adrenal disease and thus are commonly known as *incidentalomas* (**Web Fig. 67-2**). Some of these tumors secrete a small amount of excess cortisol, leading to a condition called *subclinical Cushing syndrome*. A morning ACTH level and an overnight 1-mg dexamethasone test are recommended for patients with an adrenal incidentaloma. Patients with hypertension should also undergo measurement of serum potassium level, plasma aldosterone concentration or plasma renin activity ratio, and urine or plasma-free metanephrines. Surgery should be considered in all patients with functional adrenal cortical tumors that are hormonally active or larger than 4 cm. Tumors not associated with hormonal secretion of less than 4 cm can be monitored with repeat imaging and hormonal assessment.

PRIMARY ADRENAL CANCER

Primary adrenal carcinomas are rare, with an incidence of 1 to 5 per million persons. The female-to-male ratio is 2.5 : 1, and the mean age of onset is 40 to 50 years. About 25% of patients have symptoms, including abdominal pain, weight loss, anorexia, and fever. At presentation, metastatic spread is evident in 75% of cases. In an incidentally discovered adrenal mass, large size is more likely to be malignant. For tumors that are larger than 6 cm, 25% of these are adrenocortical carcinomas, and resection is definitely recommended for tumors larger than 6 cm and often recommended for tumors greater than 4 cm. In patients who do not have a known cancer, most adrenal masses that turn out to be malignant are primary adrenocortical carcinomas, whereas in patients with a known malignancy, an adrenal mass is likely to be a metastasis in about 75% of patients. Eighty percent of primary adrenal carcinomas are functional, with glucocorticoid alone (45%) or glucocorticoid plus androgens (45%) being the most common hormones secreted.

The treatment of adrenocortical carcinomas is surgery; this includes removing the primary tumor with an adrenalectomy followed by resection of metastasis (usually lung or liver) as they are detected. These cancers are usually resistant to radiation and chemotherapy, but the adrenolytic compound, mitotane, has been shown to improve survival in patients with this tumor. Adrenocortical carcinomas carry a poor prognosis, with overall 5-year survival rates of less than 20%.

Prospectus for the Future

- Appreciation of the role tissue-specific, intracellular glucocorticoid excess plays in common diseases such as osteoporosis, depression, cardiovascular disease, diabetes, and hypertension

- Selective adrenal adenomectomy, sparing normal adrenal tissue
- Appreciation of the importance of mild (subclinical) adrenal insufficiency and excess

References

Falorni A, Laureti S, DeBellis A, et al: Italian Addison network study: Update of diagnostic criteria for the etiological classification of primary adrenal insufficiency. J Clin Endocrinol Metab 89:1598-1604, 2004.

Grumbach MM, Biller BM, Braunstein GD, et al: Management of the clinically inapparent adrenal mass ("incidentaloma"). Ann Intern Med 138:424-429, 2003.

Nieman LK, Biller BM, Findling JW, et al: The diagnosis of Cushing's syndrome: An Endocrine Society Clinical Practice Guideline. J Clin Endocrinol Metab 93:1526-1540, 2008

Pacak K, Ilias I, Adams KT, Eisenhofer G: Biochemical diagnosis, localization and management of pheochromocytoma: Focus on multiple endocrine neoplasia type 2 in relation to other hereditary syndromes and sporadic forms of the tumour. J Intern Med 257:60-68, 2005.

Vaughan ED Jr: Diseases of the adrenal gland. Med Clin N Am 88:443-466, 2004.

Young WF Jr: Clinical practice: The incidentally discovered adrenal mass. N Engl J Med 356:601-610, 2007.

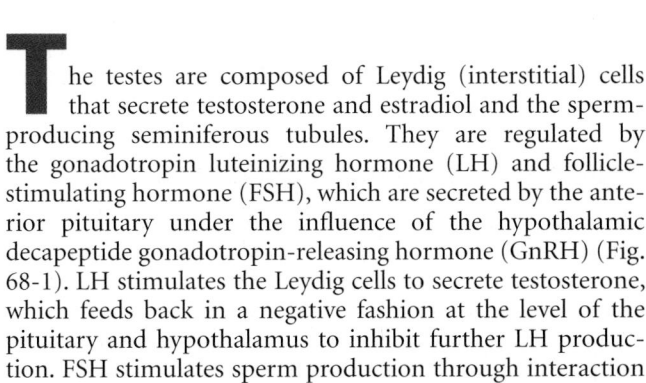

Male Reproductive Endocrinology

Glenn D. Braunstein

The testes are composed of Leydig (interstitial) cells that secrete testosterone and estradiol and the sperm-producing seminiferous tubules. They are regulated by the gonadotropin luteinizing hormone (LH) and follicle-stimulating hormone (FSH), which are secreted by the anterior pituitary under the influence of the hypothalamic decapeptide gonadotropin-releasing hormone (GnRH) (Fig. 68-1). LH stimulates the Leydig cells to secrete testosterone, which feeds back in a negative fashion at the level of the pituitary and hypothalamus to inhibit further LH production. FSH stimulates sperm production through interaction with the Sertoli cells in the seminiferous tubules. Feedback inhibition of FSH is through gonadal steroids, as well as through inhibin, a glycoprotein produced by Sertoli cells.

Biochemical evaluation of the hypothalamic-pituitary-Leydig axis is carried out by the measurement of serum LH and testosterone concentrations, whereas a semen analysis and a serum FSH determination provide an assessment of the hypothalamic-pituitary-seminiferous tubular axis. The ability of the pituitary to release gonadotropins can be tested dynamically through GnRH stimulation, and the ability of the testes to secrete testosterone can be evaluated through injections of human chorionic gonadotropin (hCG), a glycoprotein hormone that has biologic activity similar to that of LH.

Hypogonadism

Either testosterone deficiency or defective spermatogenesis constitutes *hypogonadism*. Often both disorders coexist. The clinical manifestations of androgen deficiency depend on the time of onset and the degree of deficiency. Because testosterone is required for wolffian duct development into the epididymis, vas deferens, seminal vesicles, and ejaculatory ducts, as well as for virilization of the external genitalia through the major intracellular testosterone metabolite, dihydrotestosterone, early prenatal androgen deficiency leads to the formation of ambiguous genitalia and to male

pseudohermaphroditism. Androgen deficiency occurring later during gestation may result in micropenis or *cryptorchidism,* the unilateral or bilateral absence of testes in the scrotum resulting from the failure of normal testicular descent. During puberty, androgens are responsible for male sexual differentiation, which includes growth of the scrotum, epididymis, vas deferens, seminal vesicles, prostate, penis, skeletal muscle, and larynx. Additionally, androgens stimulate the growth of axillary, pubic, facial, and body hair, as well as increased sebaceous gland activity, and they are responsible through conversion to estrogens for the growth and fusion of the epiphyseal cartilaginous plates clinically seen as the *pubertal growth spurt.* Thus, prepubertal androgen deficiency leads to poor muscle development, decreased strength and endurance, a high-pitched voice, sparse axillary and pubic hair, and the absence of facial and body hair. The long bones of the lower extremities and arms may continue to grow under the influence of growth hormone, a condition leading to eunuchoid proportions in which the arm span exceeds the total height by 5 cm or more, and growth of the lower extremities is greater relative to total height. Postpubertal androgen deficiency may result in a decrease in libido, impotence, low energy, fine wrinkling around the corners of the eyes and mouth, and diminished facial and body hair.

Male hypogonadism may be classified into three categories according to the level of the defect (Table 68-1). Diseases directly affecting the testes result in *primary* or *hypergonadotropic hypogonadism,* characterized by oligospermia or azoospermia and low testosterone levels but with elevations of LH and FSH because of a decrease of the negative feedback regulation on the pituitary and hypothalamus by androgens, estrogens, and inhibin. In contrast, hypogonadism from lesions in the hypothalamus or pituitary gives rise to *secondary* or *hypogonadotropic hypogonadism* because the low testosterone level or ineffective spermatogenesis is a result of inadequate stimulation of the testes by insufficient or inadequate concentrations of the gonadotropins. The third category of hypogonadism is the result of defects in androgen action.

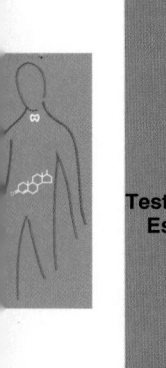

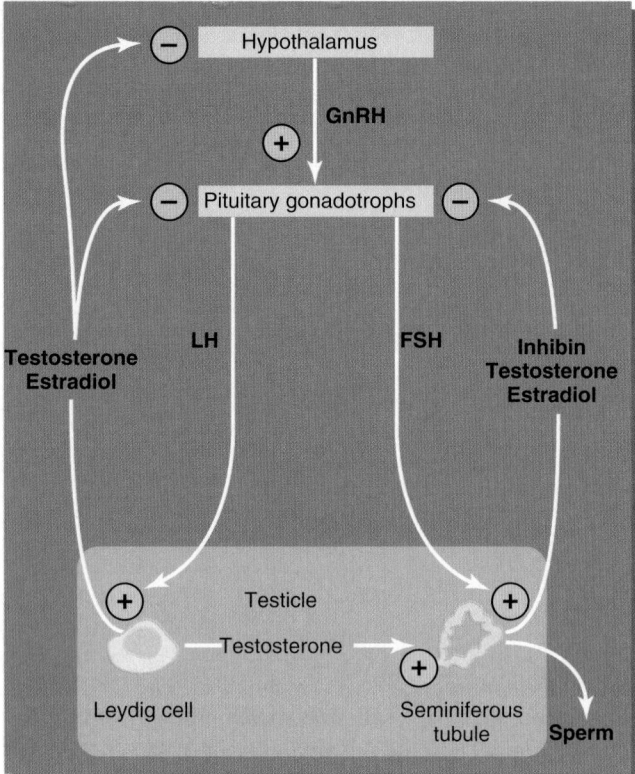

Figure 68-1 Regulation of the hypothalamic-pituitary-testicular axis. +, Positive feedback; −, negative feedback; FSH, follicle-stimulating hormone; GnRH, gonadotropin-releasing hormone; LH, luteinizing hormone.

Table 68-1 **Classification of Male Hypogonadism**
Hypothalamic-Pituitary Disorders (Secondary Hypogonadism)
Panhypopituitarism
Isolated gonadotropin deficiency
Complex congenital syndromes
Hyperprolactinemia
Hypothalamic dysfunction
Gonadal Disorders (Primary Hypogonadism)
Klinefelter syndrome and associated chromosomal defects
Myotonic dystrophy
Cryptorchidism
Bilateral anorchia
Seminiferous tubular failure
Adult Leydig cell failure
Androgen biosynthesis enzyme deficiency
Defects in Androgen Action
Testicular feminization (complete androgen insensitivity)
Incomplete androgen insensitivity
5α-reductase deficiency

HYPOTHALAMIC-PITUITARY DISORDERS

Panhypopituitarism occurs congenitally from structural defects or from inadequate production or the release of the hypothalamic-releasing factors. The condition may also be acquired through replacement by tumors, infarction from vascular insufficiency, infiltrative disorders, autoimmune diseases, trauma, and infections.

Kallmann syndrome is a form of hypogonadotropic hypogonadism associated with problems in the ability to discriminate odors, either incompletely (*hyposmia*) or completely (*anosmia*). This syndrome results from a defect in the migration of the GnRH neurons from the olfactory placode into the hypothalamus. Thus, it represents a GnRH deficiency. Patients remain prepubertal, with small, rubbery testes, and they develop eunuchoidism (**Web Fig. 68-1**).

Hyperprolactinemia may result in hypogonadotropic hypogonadism because prolactin elevation inhibits normal GnRH release, decreases the effectiveness of LH at the Leydig cell level, and also inhibits some of the action of testosterone at the target organ level. Normalization of prolactin levels through withdrawal of an offending drug, by surgical removal of the pituitary adenoma, or with the use of dopamine agonists reverses this form of hypogonadism.

Weight loss or systemic illness in male patients can cause another form of secondary hypogonadism, *hypothalamic dysfunction*. This weight loss or illness induces a defect in the hypothalamic release of GnRH and results in low gonadotropin and testosterone levels. This condition is commonly observed in patients with cancer, AIDS, and chronic inflammatory processes.

PRIMARY GONADAL ABNORMALITIES

The most common congenital cause of primary testicular failure is *Klinefelter syndrome*, which occurs in about 1 of every 600 live male births and is usually caused by a maternal meiotic chromosomal nondisjunction that results in an XXY genotype. At puberty, clinical findings include the following: varying degrees of hypogonadism; gynecomastia; small, firm testes measuring less than 2 cm in the longest axis (normal testes measure 3.5 cm or greater); azoospermia; eunuchoid skeletal proportions; and elevations of FSH and LH (**Web Fig. 68-2**). Primary gonadal failure is also found in patients with another congenital condition, *myotonic dystrophy*, which is characterized by progressive weakness; atrophy of the facial, neck, hand, and lower extremity muscles; frontal baldness; and myotonia.

About 3% of full-term male infants have *cryptorchidism,* which spontaneously corrects during the first year of life in most of these children; consequently, by 1 year of age, the incidence of this condition is about 0.75%. When the testes are maintained in the intra-abdominal position, the increased temperature leads to defective spermatogenesis and oligospermia. Leydig cell function generally remains normal, and therefore adult testosterone levels are normal. *Bilateral anorchia,* also known as the vanishing testicle syndrome, is a rare condition in which the external genitalia are fully formed, thus indicating that ample quantities of testosterone and dihydrotestosterone were produced during early embryogenesis. However, the testicular tissue disappears before or shortly after birth, and the result is an empty scrotum. Differentiation from cryptorchidism can be made through an hCG stimulation test. Patients with cryptorchidism have an increase in serum testosterone after an injection of hCG, whereas patients with bilateral anorchia do not.

Acquired gonadal failure has numerous causes. The adult seminiferous tubules are susceptible to a variety of

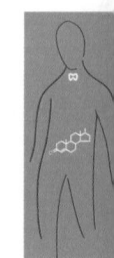

injuries, and seminiferous tubular failure is found after infections such as mumps, gonococcal or lepromatous orchitis, irradiation, vascular injury, trauma, alcohol ingestion, and use of chemotherapeutic drugs, especially alkylating agents. The serum FSH concentrations may be normal or elevated, depending on the degree of damage to the seminiferous tubules. The Leydig cell compartment may also be damaged by these same conditions. In addition, some men experience a gradual decline in testicular function as they age, possibly because of microvascular insufficiency. The decreased testosterone production may clinically exhibit lowered libido and potency, emotional lability, fatigue, and vasomotor symptoms such as hot flushes. The serum LH concentration is usually elevated in this situation.

DEFECTS IN ANDROGEN ACTION

When either testosterone or its metabolite, dihydrotestosterone, binds to the androgen receptor in target cells, the receptor is activated and binds DNA with resulting stimulation of transcription, protein synthesis, and cell growth, which collectively constitutes androgen action. An absence of androgen receptors causes the syndrome of *testicular feminization,* a form of male pseudohermaphroditism. These genetic males have cryptorchid testes but appear to be phenotypic females. Because androgens are inactive during embryogenesis, the labial-scrotal folds fail to fuse, and a short vagina results. The fallopian tubes, uterus, and upper portion of the vagina are absent because the testes secrete müllerian duct inhibitory factor during early fetal development. At puberty, these patients have breast enlargement because the testes secrete a small amount of estradiol, and the peripheral tissues convert testosterone and adrenal androgens to estrogens. Axillary and pubic hair does not grow because androgen action is required for development. The serum testosterone concentrations are elevated as a result of continuous stimulation by LH, the concentrations of which are raised because of the inability of the testosterone to act in a negative feedback fashion at the hypothalamic level. Patients may have incomplete forms of androgen insensitivity caused by point mutations affecting the androgen receptor gene, and clinically these patients show varying degrees of male pseudohermaphroditism.

Patients who lack the 5α-reductase enzyme required to convert testosterone to dihydrotestosterone are born with a *bifid scrotum,* which reflects abnormal fusion of the labial-scrotal folds, and *hypospadias,* in which the urethral opening is in the perineal area or in the shaft of the penis. At puberty, androgen production is sufficient to partially overcome the defect; the scrotum, phallus, and muscle mass enlarge, and these patients appear to develop into physiologically normal men.

DIAGNOSIS

Figure 68-2 illustrates an algorithm for the laboratory evaluation of hypogonadism in a phenotypic man. Serum concentrations of LH, FSH, and testosterone should be obtained, and a semen analysis should be performed. A low testosterone level with low concentrations of gonadotropins indicates a hypothalamic-pituitary abnormality, which needs to be evaluated with serum prolactin determination and radiographic examination. Elevated concentrations of gonadotropins with a normal or low testosterone level reflect a primary testicular abnormality. If no testes are palpable in the scrotum and careful *milking* of the patient's lower abdomen does not bring retractile testes into the scrotum, an hCG stimulation test should be performed. A rise in serum testosterone concentrations indicates the presence of functional testicular tissue, and a diagnosis of cryptorchidism can be made. An absence of a rise in testosterone levels suggests bilateral anorchia. Small, firm testes in the scrotum are highly suggestive of Klinefelter syndrome; this diagnosis needs to be confirmed with a chromosomal karyotype. Testes more than 3.5 cm in the longest diameter that are of normal consistency or are soft indicate postpubertal acquired primary hypogonadism. If the major abnormality is a deficient sperm count with or without an elevation of FSH, differentiation between a ductal problem and acquired primary hypogonadism must be made. When spermatozoa are present, at least the ducts emanating from one testicle are patent; this condition indicates an acquired testicular defect. If the patient has no sperm in the ejaculate, a primary testicular or ductal problem may cause this condition. The seminal vesicles secrete fructose into the seminal fluid. Therefore, the presence of fructose in the ejaculate should be followed by a testicular biopsy to determine whether the defect results from spermatogenic failure or from an obstruction of the ducts leading from the testes to the seminal vesicles. Absence of seminal fluid fructose indicates a congenital absence of the seminal vesicles and vas deferens.

MALE INFERTILITY

Infertility affects about 15% of couples, and male factors appear to be responsible in about 40% of cases. Female factors account for another 40%, whereas a couple factor is present in about 20% of cases. In addition to the defects in spermatogenesis that occur in patients with hypothalamic, pituitary, testicular, or androgen action disorders, hyperthyroidism, hypothyroidism, adrenal abnormalities, and systemic illnesses may also result in defective spermatogenesis, as can microdeletions of genetic material on the Y chromosome. Disorders of the vas deferens, seminal vesicles, and prostate may also lead to infertility, as can diseases affecting the bladder sphincter that may result in *retrograde ejaculation,* in which the sperm passes into the bladder rather than through the penis. Anatomic defects of the penis as observed in patients with hypospadias, poor coital technique, and the presence of antisperm antibodies in the male or female genital tract also are associated with infertility.

THERAPY FOR HYPOGONADISM AND INFERTILITY

Treatment of androgen deficiency in patients who have hypothalamic-pituitary or primary testicular abnormalities is best accomplished with exogenous testosterone administration, either through intramuscular injection of intermediate-acting testosterone esters or with transdermal testosterone patches or gel. Testosterone therapy increases libido, potency, muscle mass, strength, athletic endurance, and hair growth on the face and body. Side effects include

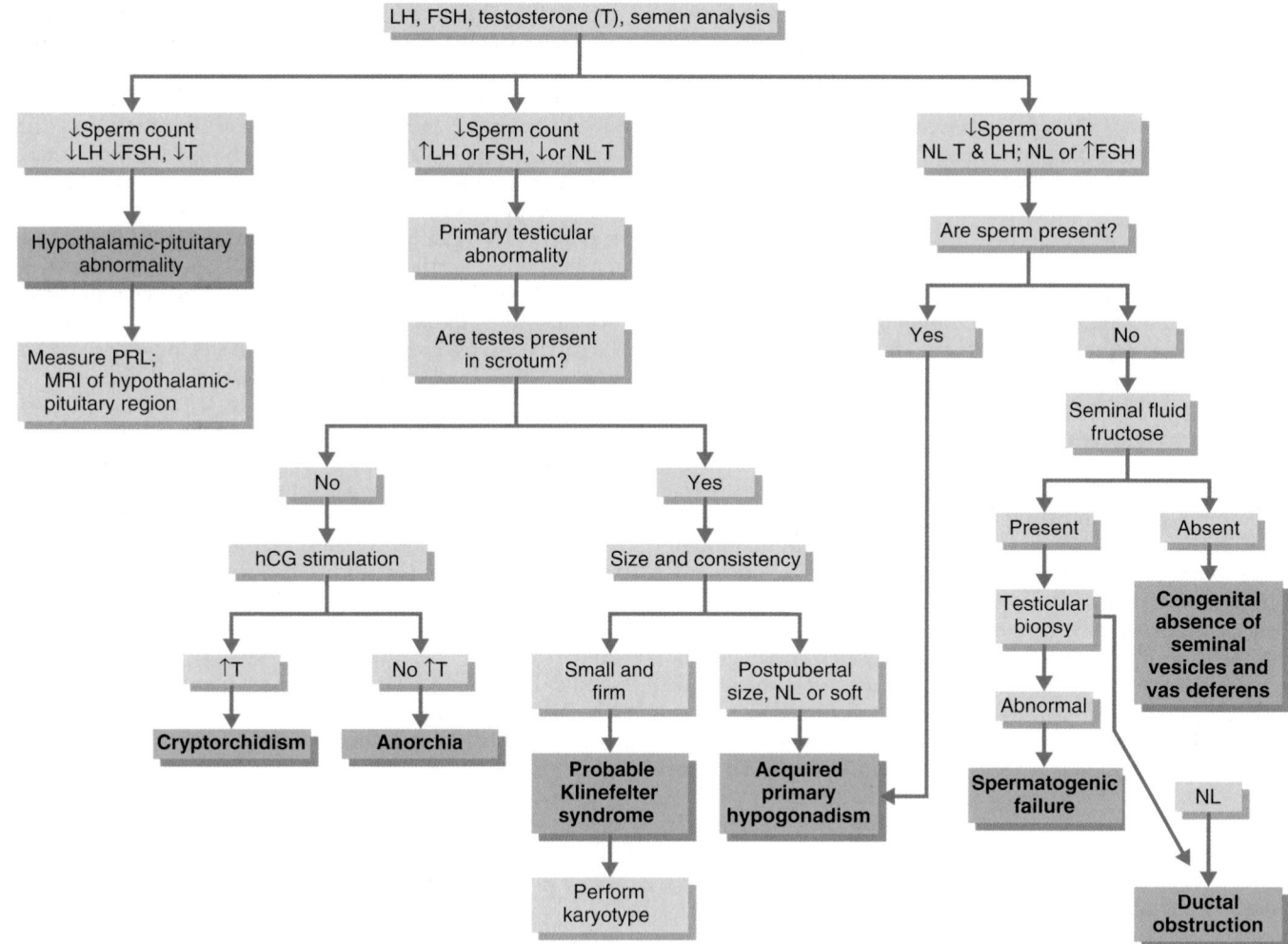

Figure 68-2 Laboratory evaluation of hypogonadism. ↑, Elevated; ↓, decreased or low; FSH, follicle-stimulating hormone; hCG, human chorionic gonadotropin; LH, luteinizing hormone; MRI, magnetic resonance imaging; NL, normal; PRL, prolactin.

acne, fluid retention, erythrocytosis, BPH, and, rarely, sleep apnea. This therapy is contraindicated in patients with cancer of the prostate.

If fertility is desired, patients with hypothalamic abnormalities may develop virilization and spermatogenesis with the use of GnRH given in a pulsatile fashion subcutaneously with an external pump. Direct stimulation of the testes in patients with hypothalamic or pituitary abnormalities may be accomplished with the use of exogenous gonadotropins, which increase testosterone and sperm production. If primary testicular failure is present and the patient has oligospermia, an attempt can be made to concentrate the sperm for intrauterine insemination or in vitro fertilization. If the azoospermia is due to ductal obstruction, repair of the obstruction may be undertaken, or aspiration of sperm from the epididymis may be accomplished for in vitro fertilization.

Gynecomastia

Gynecomastia refers to a benign enlargement of the male breast resulting from proliferation of the glandular component. This common condition is found in as many as 70% of pubertal boys and in about one third of adults 50 to 80 years old. Estrogens stimulate and androgens inhibit breast glandular development. Thus, gynecomastia is the result of an imbalance between estrogen and androgen action at the breast tissue level. This condition may result from an absolute increase in free estrogens, a decrease in endogenous free androgens, androgen insensitivity of the tissues, or enhanced sensitivity of the breast tissue to estrogens. Table 68-2 lists the common conditions associated with gynecomastia.

Gynecomastia must be differentiated by mammogram from fatty enlargement of the breasts without glandular proliferation and other disorders of the breasts, especially breast carcinoma. *Male breast cancer* is usually seen as a unilateral, eccentric, hard or firm mass that is fixed to the underlying tissues. It may be associated with skin dimpling or retraction, as well as crusting of the nipple or nipple discharge. In contrast, gynecomastia occurs concentrically around the nipple and is not fixed to the underlying structures.

Painful and tender gynecomastia in a pubertal adolescent should be monitored with periodic examinations because, in most patients, pubertal gynecomastia disappears within 1

Table 68-2 Conditions Associated with Gynecomastia

Physiologic Conditions

Neonatal
Pubertal
Involutional

Pathologic Conditions

Neoplasms
Testicular
Adrenal
Ectopic production of human chorionic gonadotropin
Primary gonadal failure
Secondary hypogonadism
Enzyme defects in testosterone production
Androgen insensitivity syndromes
Liver disease
Malnutrition with refeeding
Dialysis
Hyperthyroidism
Excessive extraglandular aromatase activity
Drugs
Estrogens and estrogen agonists
Gonadotropins
Antiandrogens or inhibitors of androgen synthesis
Cytotoxic agents
Efavirenz
Alcohol
HIV
Idiopathic

year. Incidentally discovered, asymptomatic gynecomastia in an adult requires a careful assessment for the following: alcohol, drug, or medication use; liver, lung, or kidney dysfunction; and signs and symptoms of hypogonadism or hyperthyroidism. If these conditions are not present, only follow-up is required. In contrast, in an adult with recent onset of progressive painful gynecomastia, thyroid, liver, and renal function should be determined. If test results are normal, serum concentrations of hCG, LH, testosterone, and estradiol should be measured. Further evaluation should be carried out according to the scheme outlined in Figure 68-3.

Removal of the offending drug or correction of the underlying condition causing the gynecomastia may result in regression of the breast glandular tissue. If the gynecomastia persists, a trial of antiestrogens, such as tamoxifen, may be given for 3 months to see whether regression occurs. Gynecomastia that has been present for more than 1 year usually contains a fibrotic component that does not respond to medications. Therefore, correction usually requires surgical removal of the tissue.

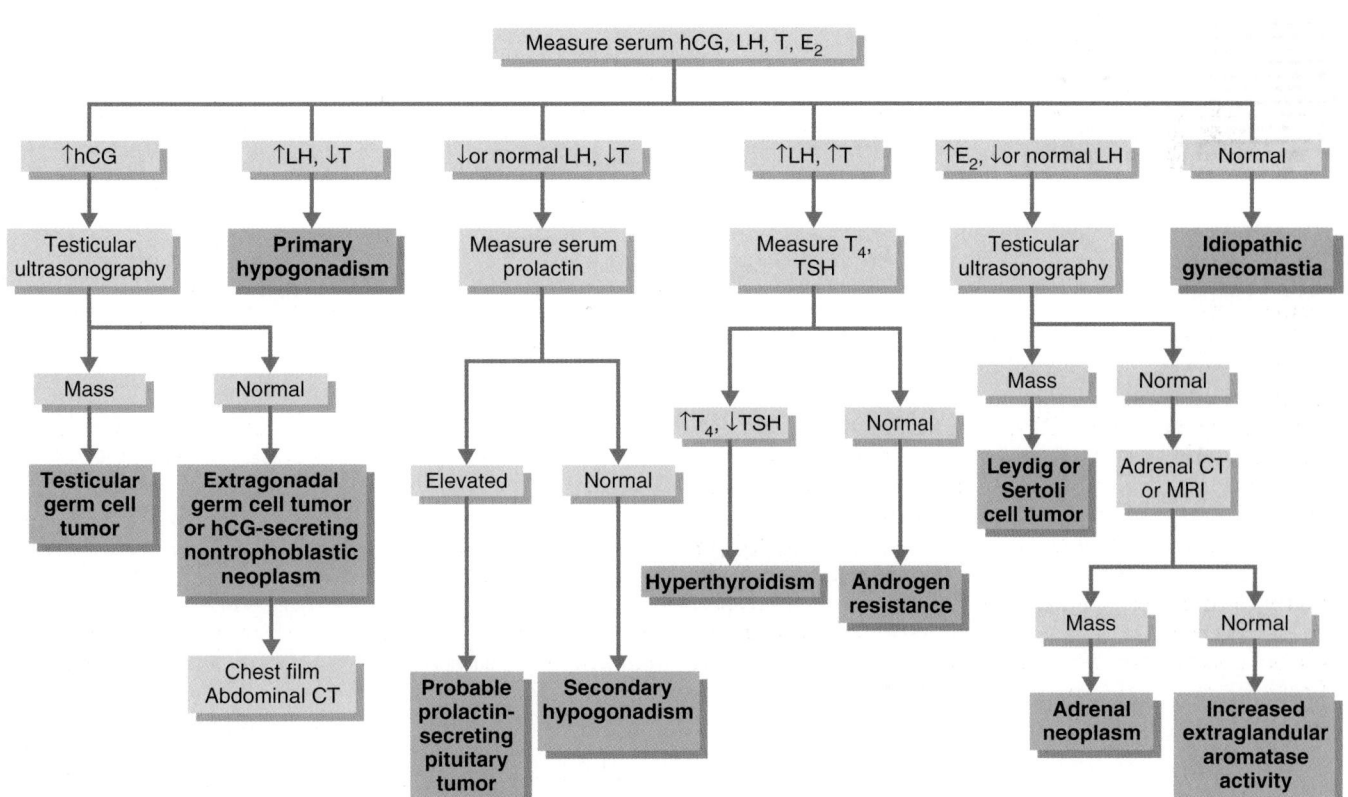

Figure 68-3 Diagnostic evaluation for causes of gynecomastia based on measurements of serum human chorionic gonadotropin (hCG), luteinizing hormone (LH), testosterone (T), and estradiol (E$_2$). ↑, Increased; ↓, decreased; CT, computed tomography; MRI, magnetic resonance imaging; T$_4$, thyroxine; TSH, thyroid-stimulating hormone. (From Braunstein GD: Gynecomastia. N Engl J Med 328:490-495, 1993. Copyright © 1993, Massachusetts Medical Society.)

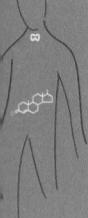

Prospectus for the Future

- Prospective, randomized, double-blind studies that examine the risks and benefits of testosterone replacement in aging men with a low level of testosterone
- Improved definition of the molecular basis for unexplained infertility
- New genetic tools for evaluating the androgen receptor
- Improved gonadotropin assays to differentiate hypogonadotropic hypogonadism from the low

serum gonadotropin concentrations found at times in normal men
- Elucidation of the roles of inhibin and leptin in gonadal function and fertility
- Improved definition of environmental toxins that affect testicular function

References

Barthold JS, Gonzalez R: The epidemiology of congenital cryptorchidism, testicular ascent and orchiopexy. J Urol 170:2396-2401, 2003.

Bhasin S, Cunningham GR, Hayes FJ, et al: Testosterone therapy in adult men with androgen deficiency syndromes: An Endocrine Society Clinical Practice Guideline. J Clin Endocrinol Metab 91:1995-2010, 2006.

Braunstein GD: Gynecomastia. N Engl J Med 357:1229-1237, 2007.

Khorram O, Patrizio P, Wang C, Swerdloff R: Reproductive technologies for male infertility. J Clin Endocrinol Metab 86:2373-2379, 2001.

Lanfranco F, Kamischke A, Zitzmann M, Nieschlag E: Klinefelter's syndrome. Lancet 364:273-283, 2004.

McVary KT: Erectile dysfunction. N Engl J Med 357:2472-2481, 2007.

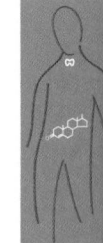

Diabetes Mellitus

Philip S. Barnett and Glenn D. Braunstein

Abbreviations

ACEI—angiotensin II–converting enzyme inhibitor
ARB—angiotensin II receptor blocker
BG—blood glucose
BMI—body mass index
BP—blood pressure
CDE—certified diabetes educator
Cr—creatinine (serum)
CSII—continuous subcutaneous insulin infusion
CVD—cardiovascular disease
DKA—diabetic ketoacidosis
DPP-4—dipeptidyl peptidase-4
ESRD—end-stage renal disease
FFA—free fatty acid
FPG—fasting plasma glucose
GDM—gestational diabetes mellitus
GFR—glomerular filtration rate
GIP—glucose-dependent insulinotropic polypeptide
GLP-1—glucagon-like peptide-1
HbA_{1c}—glycosylated hemoglobin
HDL—high-density lipoprotein
HGP—hepatic glucose production
HLA—human leukocyte antigen
HNKS—hyperosmolar nonketotic syndrome
hs-CRP—highly selective creatine phosphokinase
IFG—impaired fasting glucose
IGT—impaired glucose tolerance
IMT—intima medial thickness
IR—insulin resistance
LDL—low-density lipoprotein
MI—myocardial infarction
NYHA—New York Heart Association
OGTT—oral glucose tolerance test
PAI-1—plasminogen activator inhibitor-1
PCOS—polycystic ovarian syndrome
PPAR—peroxisome proliferator activated receptor
PPG—postprandial glucose
RN—registered nurse
SMBG—self-monitoring of blood glucose
TC—total cholesterol

T1DM—type 1 diabetes mellitus
TZD—thiazolidinedione
T2DM—type 2 diabetes mellitus
TG—triglyceride
VLDL—very low-density lipoprotein
USDA—U.S. Department of Agriculture

Definition

Diabetes mellitus comprises a heterogeneous group of metabolic diseases that are characterized by chronic hyperglycemia and disturbances in carbohydrate, lipid, and protein metabolism resulting from defects in insulin secretion, insulin action, or both. Fasting (chronic) and postprandial hyperglycemia are mainly responsible for the acute, short-term, and late complications, which affect all body organs and systems.

U.S. population statistics for 2007 show that the total prevalence of diabetes in all ages was an estimated 23.6 million people (8% of the population; 12.0 million men, 11.5 million women 20 years or older); 17.9 million diagnosed, 5.7 million undiagnosed, and 57 million with prediabetes. In people 20 years or older, the prevalence was 23.5 million (10.7%), and in those 60 years or older, the prevalence rose to 12.2 million (23.1% of all people in this age group). The incidence of diabetes in people 20 years or older was 1.6 million. The total cost of diabetes in the United States in 2007 was estimated to be $174 billion (direct medical costs $116 billion, and indirect costs $58 billion), with a per capita annual health care cost of $11,744, 3 times more than in people without diabetes. Diabetes, the sixth leading cause of death by disease in the United States, accounts for almost 18% of all deaths in people over 25 years of age, and it is the leading cause of end-stage renal disease (ESRD), new cases of blindness, and nontraumatic lower limb amputations in the United States. Cardiovascular disease is the major cause of diabetes-related death and is 2 to 5 times more common in patients with diabetes than in the general population. Life expectancy in middle-aged patients is reduced by 5 to 10 years. The prevalence of

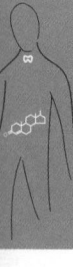

diabetes worldwide is reaching pandemic proportions; currently, more than 150 million (300 million people by 2025), in large part because of increased obesity (65% of U.S. adults are overweight or obese), poor nutrition, and sedentary lifestyles in both adults and children.

Diagnosis

Presentation of patients with diabetes depends on the type of diabetes and the stage of the pathologic process. Patients with *type 1 diabetes mellitus* (T1DM) commonly present with classic acute symptoms of hyperglycemia: polydipsia, polyuria, weight loss, and, less frequently, polyphagia, blurred vision, and pruritus, 25% for the first time in diabetic ketoacidosis (DKA). In patients with *type 2 diabetes mellitus* (T2DM), the disease is often present for many years (average 4 to 7 years) before diagnosis, and as many as 50% have an established cardiovascular complication at the time of diagnosis. The symptoms are usually less acute than those in T1DM, and they may be accompanied by lethargy and fatigue in what was, until recently, a generally older population. With the current epidemic of obesity, there is a concomitant increase in the incidence and prevalence of T2DM in childhood and adolescence; 2 million adolescents (12 to 19 years of age) have *prediabetes*. Chronic hyperglycemia may be associated with impairment of growth, susceptibility to infections (e.g., balanitis, vaginitis), and slow wound healing. Risk factors for T2DM are listed in Table 69-1 and include sedentary lifestyle, poor nutrition, and overweight and obesity.

Diagnostic criteria for diabetes are listed in Table 69-2. Any of the three serum glucose measurements may be used for diagnosis and must be confirmed, on a subsequent day, by any one of the three. The diagnostic *fasting plasma glucose* (FPG) correlates with the 2-hour postchallenge glucose cutpoint, resulting in fewer people with undiagnosed and misdiagnosed diabetes. These low cut-off diagnostic values identify critical levels at which the prevalence of microvascular complications increases dramatically, and set new levels for earlier and aggressive diabetes therapy, in an attempt to prevent these complications.

Although the *oral glucose tolerance test* (OGTT) remains the standard for diagnostic purposes, measurement of FPG by comparison, which is simpler, cheaper, equally accurate, faster to perform, more reproducible, and convenient, is used for routine diagnosis. Measurement of *glycosylated hemoglobin* (HbA$_{1c}$) is a useful tool for monitoring glycemic control and for making therapeutic decisions but is not recommended for diagnostic purposes. The OGTT is still used for diagnosing gestational diabetes (Table 69-3).

In the United States, estimates indicate that at least 57 million people have blood glucose levels greater than normal but less than those diagnostic for diabetes, a state referred to as *prediabetes*. These people are generally euglycemic and have abnormal glucose responses only when challenged with an OGTT. Depending on the diagnostic test, this group or metabolic stage is referred to as having either *impaired fasting glucose* (IFG) or *impaired glucose tolerance* (IGT) (see Table 69-2). This category of people may be considered to have *subclinical diabetes*, in a similar fashion to other subclinical hormone conditions (e.g., subclinical hypothyroid-

Table 69-1 Screening Criteria for Diabetes in Asymptomatic, High-Risk Adults

1. Testing for diabetes should be considered in all persons ≥45 years and, if normal, should be repeated at 3-year intervals.
2. Testing should be considered at a younger age (<30 years) or performed more frequently in individuals who:
   a. Are overweight (BMI > 25) or who have central obesity with normal BMI (18.5-24.9)
   b. Have a habitually sedentary lifestyle
   c. Have a first-degree relative with diabetes (i.e., parent or sibling, 45%-80% in T2DM, 5% in T1DM; equates to a 40% risk)
   d. Are members of a high-risk ethnic population (e.g., African American, Latino, Hispanic American, Native American, Asian American, Pacific Islander)
   e. Have delivered a baby weighing >9 lb (4 kg), have experienced unexplained perinatal death, or have been diagnosed with gestational diabetes
   f. Are hypertensive (≥140/90 mm Hg)
   g. Have an HDL cholesterol level ≤35 mg/dL (0.9 mmol/L) and/or a triglyceride level ≥250 mg/dL (2.82 mmol/L)
   h. Had, on previous testing, impaired glucose tolerance (plasma glucose ≥140 mg/dL [7.8 mmol/L] but <200 mg/dL [11.1 mmol/L] during 2 hr after 75-g oral glucose tolerance test) or impaired fasting glucose (plasma glucose 100-125 mg/dL [5.6-6.9 mmol/L])
   i. Have other clinical conditions associated with insulin resistance (e.g., PCOS, acanthosis nigricans [60%-90% in T2DM])
   j. Have a history of vascular disease, particularly cardiovascular and cerebrovascular

BMI, body mass index (weight [kg]/height [m²]); HDL, high-density lipoprotein; PCOS, polycystic ovary syndrome; T1DM, type 1 diabetes mellitus; T2DM, type 2 diabetes mellitus.
Adapted from the American Diabetes Association: Clinical Practice Recommendations 2008. Diabetes Care 31(Suppl 1), 2008.

ism or hyperthyroidism) or *preclinical* conditions (e.g., pre-hypertension). These people are at increased risk for developing T2DM (7% per year) and its complications, particularly cardiovascular (50% increased risk), and need to be identified for early counseling and treatment, which includes lifestyle modification with weight loss and increased physical activity. Obese patients younger than 60 years and at very high risk may benefit from the addition of metformin.

Screening for Diabetes

Screening for T1DM involves the measurement of autoantibody markers (antibodies to islet cells, insulin, glutamic acid decarboxylase, and tyrosine phosphatase). Several reasons mitigate against the routine screening of both healthy children in the general population and those at high risk for developing T1DM (siblings of patients with T1DM); these include lack of established cut-off values for immune markers, lack of consensus regarding effective therapy for patients with positive test results, and lack of cost-effectiveness.

Screening of certain high-risk populations for T2DM (see Table 69-1) is considered cost-effective. More than one third of people with T2DM are undiagnosed. Twenty-five to 33% of patients with T2DM have family members with diabetes. Because of the insidious nature of T2DM, patients have a

Table 69-2 Criteria for the Diagnosis of Diabetes Mellitus

Plasma Glucose	Normal	Impaired Fasting Glucose§	Impaired Glucose Tolerance§	Diabetes Mellitus
Fasting*	<100 (5.6)	≥100 and <126	—	≥126 (7.0)
2-hour postload	<140 (7.8)	—	≥140 and <200	≥200 (11.1)
Random†	—	—	—	≥200 with symptoms

*Fasting; no caloric intake for at least 8 hours.
　†Random; refers to any time of day, unrelated to meals. The classic symptoms of hyperglycemia include polyuria, polydipsia, and weight loss.
　§Prediabetes refers to impaired fasting glucose and/or impaired glucose tolerance.
　The standard oral glucose tolerance test, defined by the World Health Organization, requires a 75-g anhydrous glucose load.
　Numbers represent venous plasma glucose values in mg/dL. Numbers in parentheses represent venous plasma glucose values in mmol/L.
　To definitively make the diagnosis of diabetes, these criteria should be confirmed on another day using any of the three tests.
　Data from the American Diabetes Association: Clinical Practice Recommendations 2008. Diabetes Care 31(Suppl 1), 2008.

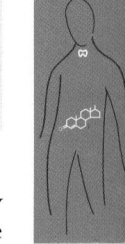

Table 69-3 Screening and Diagnostic Criteria for Gestational Diabetes Mellitus

Plasma Glucose	50-g Screening Test	75-g Diagnostic Test	100-g Diagnostic Test
Fasting	—	≥95	≥95 (5.3)
1 hr	≥140	≥180	≥180 (10.0)
2 hr	—	≥155	≥155 (8.6)
3 hr	—	—	≥140 (7.8)

50-g, 75-g, and 100-g refer to oral glucose loads.
　Numbers represent venous plasma glucose values in mg/dL. Numbers in parentheses represent venous plasma glucose values in mmol/L.
　Data from the American Diabetes Association: Clinical Practice Recommendations 2008. Diabetes Care 31(Suppl 1), 2008.

high risk for developing complications by the time of clinical diagnosis (see "Complications," later in this chapter). Early diagnosis and treatment may reduce the burden of this disease, its complications (particularly microvascular and macrovascular disease), and associated comorbidities, such as dyslipidemia, hypertension, and obesity.

Gestational diabetes mellitus (GDM) refers to the presence of glucose intolerance that develops during pregnancy and usually returns to normal after delivery. GDM occurs in 2% to 5% of all pregnancies, but it may complicate as many as 14% in certain populations (see Table 69-1, criterion 2d) and accounts for about 90% of diabetes during pregnancy. If this condition is not diagnosed, or left untreated, the consequences for both mother and fetus may be severe. Screening for GDM is routinely performed between 24 and 28 weeks of gestation in women older than 25 years and in younger women who fulfill one or more of the criteria in Table 69-1 (2a through 2d and 2g). Women at high risk (obese, personal history of GDM, glycosuria, first-degree relative with diabetes) should be screened at their initial obstetric or prenatal visit. A positive screening test (plasma glucose ≥140 mg/dL [7.8 mmol/L] 1 hour after a 50-g glucose challenge administered to a nonfasting patient) dictates the need for diagnostic testing with a 3-hour, 100-g OGTT performed in the fasting state (≥8 hours without caloric intake). Meeting or exceeding any two or more of the plasma glucose values listed in Table 69-3 is diagnostic of GDM. Women with GDM should be reclassified 6 or more weeks postpartum (see Table 69-2). About 25% of lean women and up to 50% of obese women will go on to develop overt diabetes

(types 1 or 2), IFG, or IGT over a 20-year period. Pregnancy serves as a provocative test and not as a risk factor for the future development of diabetes.

Classification

Improved understanding of the origins and pathogenesis of diabetes has facilitated revision of the classification of diabetes mellitus (Table 69-4) from one based mainly on therapeutic considerations, such as insulin dependence or independence, to one based on etiology. Any patient with diabetes may require insulin therapy at some stage of the disease, irrespective of the classification.

TYPES 1 AND 2 DIABETES

The underlying pathologic process in most patients with T1DM (5% to 10% of people with diabetes) is autoimmune destruction of the pancreatic islet β cells with absolute loss of insulin secretion. The disease has strong human leukocyte antigen (HLA) associations and numerous antibody markers of immune destruction (Table 69-5). In a few patients with T1DM, the pathogenesis remains idiopathic. Patients with β-cell destruction or failure resulting from identifiable nonautoimmune causes are not included in this class. T2DM (90% to 95% of people with diabetes) results from variable combinations of insulin resistance and insulin secretory defects (β-cell dysfunction), with one or the other abnormality predominating in a given patient.

Distinguishing between T1DM and T2DM is not always a simple process. T2DM is diagnosed in children as young as 6 years and may account for as many as 25% to 33% of all new cases of diabetes diagnosed in adolescents 9 to 19 years of age, often associated with an increase in weight and parallel decrease in physical activity. These adolescents may even present in DKA before they ultimately achieve control of their disease with diet and oral antihyperglycemic agents. T1DM can also occur in elderly patients. This condition has been described as *latent autoimmune diabetes of adulthood* [LADA] (also known as late-onset autoimmune diabetes, or *type 1.5DM*) and may account for many insulin-requiring patients previously misclassified as T2DM. Patients with T1DM who later develop obesity, insulin resistance, and possibly metabolic syndrome and T2DM are said to have *double-double, hybrid,* or *type 3* diabetes.

Hyperglycemia, the metabolic hallmark of diabetes, changes in degree over time, which reflects the severity and

700 **Section XII**—Endocrine Disease

stage of the underlying pathologic process, which may progress, regress, or remain static, and the effectiveness of its treatment, but does not signal an alteration in the *nature* of the process.

Prediabetes is a condition (defined previously) that warrants close attention and treatment to prevent progression to T2DM and the significant cardiovascular diseases that develop in this prodromal period.

OTHER SPECIFIC TYPES OF DIABETES

These groups together account for 1% to 2% of patients with diabetes. Inheritance of *maturity-onset diabetes of the young*

Table 69-4 Etiologic Classification of Diabetes Mellitus

Type 1 Diabetes Mellitus
Immune mediated
Idiopathic
LADA

Type 2 Diabetes Mellitus

Other specific types
Genetic defects of β-cell function
Genetic defects in insulin action
Diseases of the exocrine pancreas
Endocrinopathies
Drug or chemical induced
Infections
Uncommon forms of immune-mediated diabetes
Other genetic syndromes sometimes associated with diabetes
Gestational diabetes mellitus

LADA, latent autoimmune diabetes of adults.
Data from the American Diabetes Association: Clinical Practice Recommendations 2008. Diabetes Care 31(Suppl 1), 2008.

(MODY types 1 to 5) is autosomal dominant, and hyperglycemia appears before the age of 25 years.

Within the small group of *genetic insulin-resistance states,* impaired insulin action is the result of either a defective insulin receptor molecule (type A insulin resistance, leprechaunism, or Rabson-Mendenhall syndrome) or abnormalities in postreceptor signal transduction pathways (lipoatrophic diabetes).

Destruction of the pancreas results in reduced insulin secretion, with subsequent development of diabetes.

Several *insulin counter-regulatory hormones* (glucagon, catecholamines, cortisol, and growth hormone) that antagonize insulin action and increase insulin resistance precipitate diabetes when they are produced in excess. Excess *aldosterone* production by a tumor, through induction of hypokalemia and increased production of *somatostatin,* may impair insulin secretion and cause diabetes. The hyperglycemia in these cases resolves after successful removal of the responsible tumor.

The mechanism of *drug-* or *chemical-induced diabetes* depends on the offending agent: β-cell destruction (by the rodenticide Vacor, intravenous pentamidine, or α-interferon with autoantibodies), impaired insulin action (nicotinic acid and glucocorticoids), or peripheral insulin resistance and impaired conversion of proinsulin to insulin (protease inhibitors). In some forms of immune-mediated diabetes, anti-insulin receptor antibodies may cause insulin resistance.

METABOLIC SYNDROME

Also known as the *insulin resistance syndrome, Reaven syndrome, dysmetabolic syndrome,* and *syndrome X,* the metabolic syndrome is not a subclass of diabetes mellitus,

Table 69-5 General Comparison of the Two Most Common Types of Diabetes Mellitus

	Type 1	Type 2
Previous terminology	Insulin-dependent diabetes mellitus, type I, juvenile-onset diabetes	Non–insulin-dependent diabetes mellitus, type II, adult-onset diabetes
Age of onset	Usually <30 yr, particularly childhood and adolescence, but any age	Usually >40 yr, but increasingly at younger ages
Genetic predisposition	Moderate; environmental factors required for expression; 35%-50% concordance in monozygotic twins; several candidate genes proposed	Strong; 60%-90% concordance in monozygotic twins; many candidate genes proposed; some genes identified in maturity-onset diabetes of the young
Human leukocyte antigen associations	Linkage to DQA and DQB, influenced by DRB3 and DRB4 (DR2 protective)	None known
Other associations	Autoimmune; Graves disease, Hashimoto thyroiditis, vitiligo, Addison disease, pernicious anemia	Heterogeneous group, ongoing subclassification based on identification of specific pathogenic processes and genetic defects
Precipitating and risk factors	Largely unknown; microbial, chemical, dietary, other	Age, obesity (central), sedentary lifestyle, previous gestational diabetes (see Table 69-1)
Findings at diagnosis	85%-90% of patients have one and usually more autoantibodies to ICA512, IA-2, IA-2β, GAD$_{65}$, IAA	Possibly complications (microvascular and macrovascular) caused by significant hyperglycemia in the preceding asymptomatic period
Endogenous insulin levels	Low or absent	Usually present (relative deficiency), early hyperinsulinemia
Insulin resistance	Only with hyperglycemia	Mostly present
Prolonged fast	Hyperglycemia, ketoacidosis	Euglycemia
Stress, withdrawal of insulin	Ketoacidosis	Nonketotic hyperglycemia, occasionally ketoacidosis

GAD, glutamic acid decarboxylase; IA-2, IA-2β, insuloma-associated protein 2 and 2β (tyrosine phosphatases); IAA, insulin autoantibodies; ICA, islet cell antibody; ICA512, islet cell autoantigen 512 (fragment of IA-2).

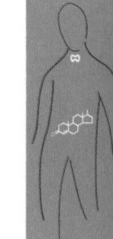

although it is extremely common in patients with diabetes and affects at least 50 million people in the United States (one in three to four adults). It consists of a cluster of clinical findings and laboratory abnormalities that include obesity (central, abdominal, or visceral), increased sympathetic nervous system activity, hypertension, glucose intolerance, insulin resistance (the common etiologic factor), hyperinsulinemia (compensatory), T2DM, dyslipidemia (hypertriglyceridemia, increased small dense low-density lipoprotein [LDL$_3$], and decreased high-density lipoprotein [HDL]), fatty liver, enhanced postprandial lipemia, disordered fibrinolysis (elevated plasminogen activator inhibitor-1 [PAI-1], tissue-type plasminogen activator, clotting factors VII and XII, and fibrinogen, with decreased levels of antithrombotic factors C and S and antithrombin III), hyperuricemia, systemic inflammation (especially vascular), and endothelial dysfunction (**Web Table 69-1**). To date, no national or international agreement exists on the cut-points for these various components, nor a consensus regarding the definition or actual existence of a *syndrome*. Abdominal adiposity, regarded by most authorities as a prerequisite for the diagnosis, is associated with increased lipolysis, increased free fatty acids (FFAs), and tumor necrosis factor-α (TNF-α), with decreased adiponectin. This syndrome is associated with a greatly increased risk for atherosclerotic vascular disease, specifically coronary artery disease, diabetes, and polycystic ovarian syndrome (PCOS).

CARDIOMETABOLIC RISK

Obesity, insulin resistance, metabolic syndrome, T2DM, and cardiovascular disease are all interconnected through the clusters of cardiometabolic risk factors, which include abdominal obesity, fasting hyperglycemia, hypertension, dyslipidemia (elevated LDL and triglycerides, low HDL), endothelial dysfunction, intravascular inflammation, and thrombotic tendency. Seventy to 80% of these patients will die from cardiovascular disease. To be effective, treatment needs to be initiated as early as possible and target each individual risk factor. Treatment includes lifestyle modifications, such as healthy calorie restricted diet, exercise, and weight reduction and smoking cessation. Achieving a 10% weight loss from baseline leads to improvements in lipids, blood pressure and peripheral insulin sensitivity.

Pathogenesis

TYPE 1 DIABETES

Generally, T1DM is an autoimmune disease in which some environmental insult (microbial, chemical, or dietary) triggers an autoimmune reaction in a genetically susceptible individual. HLA-DR3 or HLA-DR4 is present in 90% to 95% of patients with T1DM compared with 45% to 50% in the general population. Predominantly cell-mediated (mononuclear cells; mainly macrophages and CD8$^+$ T lymphocytes) destruction of the β cells of the islets of Langerhans is associated with several autoantibodies to islet cell constituents (see Table 69-5). These antibodies, some of which may occur secondary to release of antigens following β-cell death, serve as markers of the immune destruction. Figure 69-1 illustrates how the autoimmune process may be present for several years, with competing destruction and regeneration of β cells, before the disease becomes clinically apparent. At

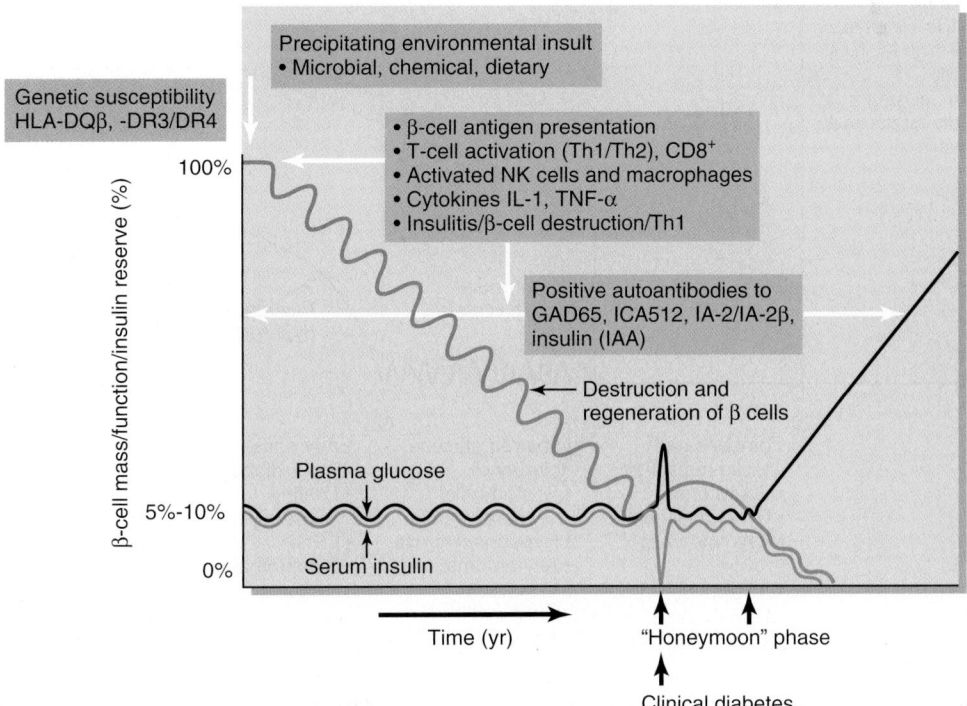

Figure 69-1 Natural history of type 1 diabetes mellitus. The *honeymoon* period with temporary improvement in β-cell function occurs with the initiation of insulin therapy at the time of clinical diagnosis. ICA512, islet cell autoantigen 512 (fragment of IA-2); IA-2, IA-2β, tyrosine phosphatases; GAD, glutamic acid decarboxylase; HLA, human leukocyte antigen; ICA, islet cell antibody; IL-1, interleukin-1; NK, natural killer; Th1, subset of CD4$^+$ helper T cells responsible for cell-mediated immunity; Th2, subset of CD4$^+$ helper T cells responsible for humoral immunity; TNF-α, tumor necrosis factor-α.

this time, the critical mass of remaining β cells (10% to 20%) is unable to sustain compensatory insulin secretion at a level sufficient to maintain normal blood glucose values. After diagnosis and institution of insulin therapy, patients usually have some degree of recovery of β-cell function to the extent that exogenous insulin requirements drop to extremely low levels (*honeymoon* period). This period usually lasts for a couple of months but may be as long as a year. Patients should continue insulin administration throughout this time, even at these low doses. β-cell insulin secretion eventually fails completely, and, at this point, patients become insulin dependent, with DKA developing in the absence of insulin replacement.

TYPE 2 DIABETES

There is a significant but poorly defined genetic predisposition to the development of T2DM, complicated by the heterogeneous nature of the disease and the influence of acquired factors. Five main elements characterize the pathophysiology: (1) insulin resistance, (2) β-cell dysfunction, (3) dysregulated hepatic glucose production (HGP), (4) abnormal intestinal glucose absorption, and (5) obesity.

Insulin resistance results from defective intracellular signaling following binding of insulin to its receptor. This defect results in decreased intracellular glucose transporter activity. In the preclinical phase, the pancreatic β cells compensate for a genetically predetermined peripheral (skeletal muscle, adipose tissue, and liver) *insulin resistance* by producing more insulin (hyperinsulinemia) to maintain euglycemia. Some patients are identified at this stage while they are clinically asymptomatic.

With time, the β cells gradually fail to compensate for the progressive increase in insulin resistance (stage of IGT or IFG; 40% reduction of β-cell mass), and eventually hyperglycemia becomes clinically manifest as diabetes mellitus (80% to 90% reduction of β-cell mass) (Fig. 69-2). Insulin secretion continues, albeit not in the hyperinsulinemic range, with resultant relative insulin deficiency. Classically, early loss of the first phase of glucose-stimulated insulin secretion occurs (peaking at 10 minutes), with subsequent gradual loss of the second phase (starting 30 minutes after glucose stimulus and peaking at 60 minutes). Other features of *β-cell dysfunction* include dysrhythmic pulsatile insulin secretion, defective glucose potentiation of nonglucose insulin secretagogues (the incretins: glucose-

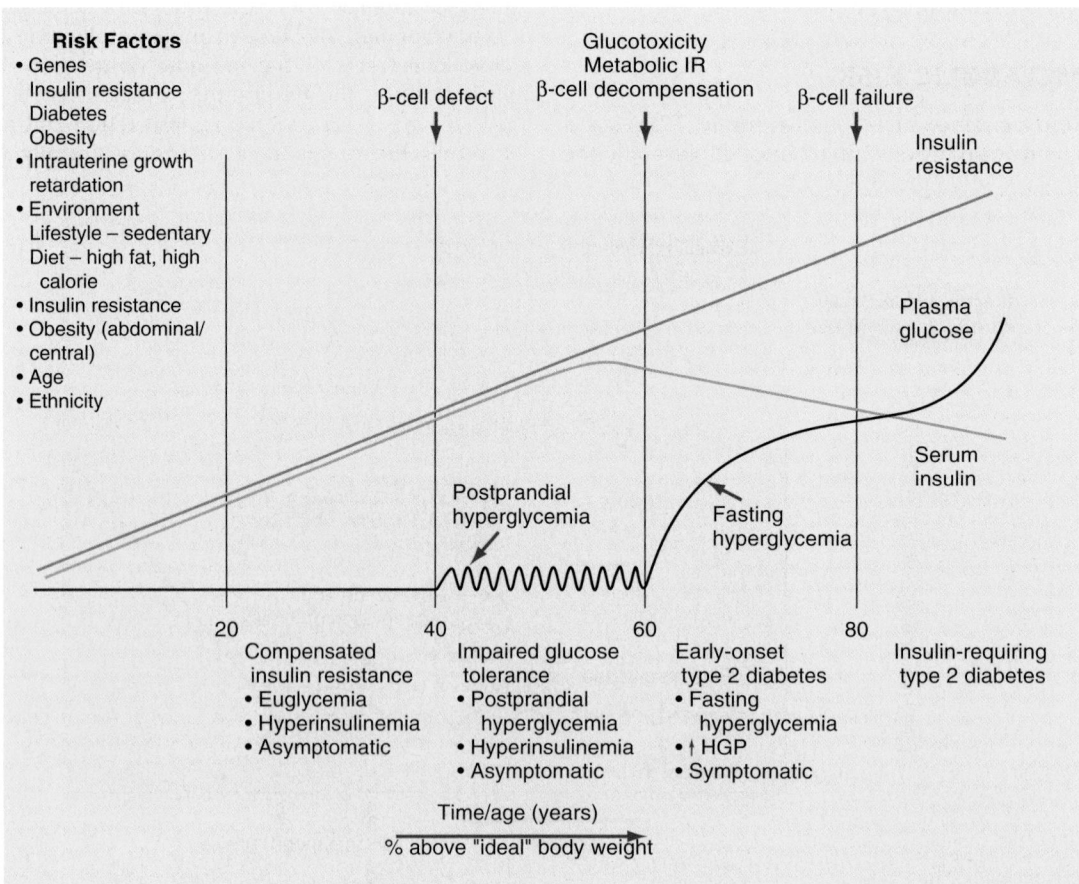

Figure 69-2 Natural history of type 2 diabetes mellitus. The numbers for percentage greater than *ideal* body weight are only approximate. Similarly, the age markers for the different phases of β-cell decompensation toward overt diabetes and an insulin-requiring state are approximate guides. Certain groups are more insulin sensitive and require a greater loss of β-cell function to precipitate diabetes than do obese insulin-resistant people, who develop diabetes after small declines in β-cell function. Use of insulin in patients with type 2 diabetes varies considerably and is not age dependent. Insulin resistance increases proportionately to adiposity, represented here by weight. HGP, hepatic glucose production; IR, insulin resistance.

dependent insulinotropic polypeptide [GIP] and glucagon-like peptide-1 [GLP-1]), increased proinsulin-to-insulin ratio (from defective protease activity), accumulation of islet amyloid polypeptide, increased glucagon secretion from islet α cells, and *glucotoxicity.* Glucotoxicity refers to the effect of chronic hyperglycemia in decreasing insulin secretion (through impaired β-cell sensitivity) and insulin activity (by increasing insulin resistance and insulin receptor tyrosine kinase activity). Glucotoxicity is a function of the duration and magnitude of the hyperglycemia and contributes to the progressive worsening of hyperglycemia. Elevated FFA levels, the result of unrestrained adipose tissue lipolysis in the relative absence of insulin, also have a toxic effect on β cells *(lipotoxicity)* and, together with intracellular protein glycation, contribute further to the failure of these cells. FFAs exacerbate hyperglycemia through increased oxidation in skeletal muscle and liver, where they decrease glucose utilization and increase gluconeogenesis, respectively. In obesity, the increased FFAs released from visceral fat stimulate increased hepatic synthesis of triglycerides and may impair first-pass hepatic metabolism of insulin, contributing to hyperinsulinemia.

Before the appearance of fasting hyperglycemia (elevated FPG), in the latter stages of compensatory hyperinsulinemia, it is possible to demonstrate *abnormal postprandial glucose* (PPG) *metabolism,* IGT, that is not evident clinically. Therapeutic intervention at this point may prevent or delay the onset of T2DM. The relative contributions of insulin resistance and insulin secretory defect to the pathogenesis in individual patients vary, with insulin resistance playing a dominant role in most patients who are obese (about 80% to 90% of patients in the United States) and failure of insulin secretion being more important in patients of normal weight.

Excessive HGP (25% to 50% higher than normal) results from inadequate suppression of hepatic gluconeogenesis, the result of hepatic insulin resistance, exacerbated by waning insulin secretion from failing β cells. Postprandial HGP is markedly increased, with a variable increase in the basal rate. Within the diabetic liver, decreased glycogen synthesis and increased fat synthesis also occur.

Hyperglycemia, with or without autonomic nerve involvement, may contribute to *gastric dysmotility* (symptomatic or not) and alterations in the rate and timing of glucose absorption (usually increased), with consequent exacerbation of hyperglycemia, resulting in a vicious cycle.

Endothelial dysfunction is the precursor of the extensive vasculopathy seen in patients with diabetes. FFAs that are increased in T2DM acutely impair endothelial function as well as raise blood pressure. Insulin improves endothelium-dependent vasodilation, but with insulin resistance and hyperinsulinemia, impairment of vascular nitric oxide production and insulin-induced vasodilation occur, with proliferation of vascular smooth muscle cells. Several markers of acute *inflammation* (including interleukin-6 [IL-6], C-reactive protein, and TNF-α) have been demonstrated in people with IGT, newly diagnosed diabetes, and atherosclerosis. Low-grade chronic inflammation in this group of patients is associated with insulin resistance through interference with insulin signal transduction.

Other endocrine associations in people with T2DM are subclinical hypercortisolism (7%), mainly adrenal in origin, and lowered levels of testosterone in males.

Management

GOALS

The goals of management can be divided into three stages: (1) short term, involving immediate treatment to relieve symptoms such as polydipsia, polyuria, or acute infections; (2) intermediate term, to return the patient to a physiologic state and social life that are as normal as possible; and (3) long term, to prevent the development, or delay the progression, of the complications of diabetes. People diagnosed with this chronic disease experience a range of emotions, including denial, anger, guilt, and depression, and most require some form of psychological support.

The cornerstones of a comprehensive diabetes management plan include patient education, healthy nutrition, weight control, physical activity, self-monitoring of blood glucose (SMBG), and antihyperglycemic agents when necessary. Patient education aims to *empower patients* by equipping them with the necessary knowledge about diabetes and self-management skills with which to make meaningful decisions about their health on a daily basis. Treatments need to be individualized, addressing medical, psychosocial, and lifestyle issues.

With the rapidly growing therapeutic armamentarium for the management of patients with diabetes, there are innumerable treatment algorithms. It is now possible to prescribe drugs that actually have disease modifying potentials. Certain previously automatically prescribed medications (e.g., sulfonylureas) are now giving way to drugs such as the incretins and amylin mimetics as first-line agents. The early use of insulin in T2DM patients still lags behind the early use of oral agents. Of prime importance is the need to manage each patient individually. It is now possible to fit the diabetes into the patient and not the patient into the diabetes.

BLOOD GLUCOSE MONITORING

Control of blood glucose levels is a crucial component of the diabetes management plan because hypoglycemia and hyperglycemia are major contributors to the complications of diabetes. *SMBG* with blood glucose meters, by all patients, facilitates adjustments in treatment and also acts as an educational tool for the patient. Ideally, SMBG should be performed as frequently as practicable—fasting, preprandial, 2 hours postprandial (especially in GDM; measure at 1 hour postprandial), at bedtime, and occasionally at 2:00 AM to 3:00 AM—and values should be recorded. Continuous glucose monitoring systems (measurement of interstitial fluid, or intravenous, glucose levels at 5-minute intervals for 72 hours) detect trends in glucose levels not possible with regular SMBG. This approach facilitates fine-tuning of diabetes treatments.

The *HbA_{1c}* value (nonenzymatic irreversible glycosylation of the hemoglobin molecule, HbA_{1c}, depends on ambient plasma glucose levels; the average life span of a red blood cell, and hence its HbA_{1c}, is 120 days), by providing a measure of the average blood glucose level (**Web Table 69-2; Web Fig. 69-1**) over the preceding 2 to 3 months, serves as an indicator of diabetes control (Table 69-6). Testing frequency is 2 or more times per year in patients with T2DM with stable glycemic control and meeting treatment goals, and 4

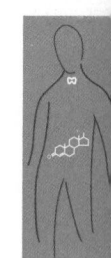

Table 69-6 Blood Glucose Goals for Glycemic Control in Patients with Diabetes*

Biochemical Index	Normal	Goal	Action Suggested
Preprandial fasting glucose (mg/dL)[†]	60-100 (3.3-5.6)	<100 (6.1)	<80 or >140 (<4.4 or >7.8)
Postprandial glucose (mg/dL)[†]	<140	<140	>180 (10.0)
Bedtime glucose (mg/dL)[†]	<110	100-140	<100 or >160 (<5.6 or >8.9)
HbA₁c (%)	<6	<6.5	>8

*These values are generalized to the entire population of nonpregnant adults with diabetes. Glycosylated hemoglobin (HbA$_{1c}$) is referenced to a nondiabetic range of 4.0% to 6.0% (mean, 5.0%; standard deviation, 0.5%).

[†]Measurement of capillary blood glucose. Postprandial blood glucose refers to the level 2 hours after the beginning of a meal.

Numbers represent venous plasma glucose values in mg/dL. Numbers in parentheses represent venous plasma glucose values in mmol/L.

Data from American Diabetes Association: Clinical Practice Recommendations 2008. Diabetes Care 31(Suppl 1): 2008, and American College of Endocrinology consensus statement on guidelines for glycemic control. Endocr Pract 8(Suppl 1):5-11, 2002.

or more times per year for patients with T1DM, those with poor glycemic control, or those after therapy change. Caution must be exercised in using HbA$_{1c}$ as the only gauge of diabetes control. Patients with wide fluctuations in blood glucose levels may sometimes have normal, average blood glucose levels and HbA$_{1c}$. Elevated HbA$_{1c}$ despite normal FPG *(good control)* is frequently the result of elevated PPG (>200 mg/dL in 75% of patients with T2DM with HbA$_{1c}$ values ≥7%; HbA$_{1c}$ = FPG + PPG) (see "Tight Control," later in this chapter). Records of SMBG are usually more informative and useful for making therapeutic decisions than HbA$_{1c}$. The HbA$_{1c}$ in measuring the average blood glucose level over the preceding 2 to 3 months may be close to goal while actual daily blood glucose levels fluctuate between hyperglycemia and hypoglycemia. The importance of PPG cannot be overestimated. Elevated PPG, not FPG, is an independent risk factor for cardiovascular disease and all-cause mortality (**Web Fig. 69-2**). This graph demonstrates the relative contributions of the FPG and PPG to hyperglycemia depending on HbA$_{1c}$ quintiles.

Spuriously low levels of HbA$_{1c}$ may be seen in patients with hemoglobinopathies such as homozygous or heterozygous HbS, C, G, or H. Variable levels of HbA$_{1c}$ may be noted with HbE or persistent HbF. β-thalassemia and sickle cell trait, with increased frequency of hemolysis, result in shortened red blood cell life span, reduced time available for glycosylation of hemoglobin, and thus falsely low HbA$_{1c}$ levels.

Measurement of serum *fructosamine* may be a useful marker for shorter-term assessment of integrated glucose concentrations (2 to 4 weeks), for example, during pregnancy.

STANDARDS OF CARE AND SPECIFIC TREATMENT GOALS

Regular patient assessment includes weight, blood pressure, pulse, SMBG records, foot examination, and discussion about smoking cessation at every office visit, with quarterly assessment of HbA$_{1c}$ (**Web Table 69-3**). Determination of microalbuminuria, serum creatinine levels, dilated retinal examination, general physical, neurologic (with autonomic testing), cardiac, nephrology, and dental examinations, with comprehensive foot evaluation, should be performed yearly, provided all are normal. Influenza vaccine should be administered yearly and Pneumovax every 5 years. Following the initial measurement of serum lipids, the frequency of reevaluation is dictated by results and treatment and should be done at least yearly. **Web Table 69-3** lists the optimal clinical and biochemical evaluation frequencies in people with diabetes. Regular diabetes education should be an integral part of every patient's management plan. Patients should be advised to carry some documentation regarding their diabetes status (e.g., Medic Alert bracelet).

Blood glucose goals for glycemic control are listed in Table 69-6.

Aspirin therapy should be considered in every patient with diabetes, provided that no contraindications exist.

Goals for lipid levels are influenced by cardiovascular risk factors (see Chapter 9). Optimal values are LDL cholesterol under 100 mg/dL (2.6 mmol/L) or less than 70 mg/dL in patients with established cardiovascular disease, HDL cholesterol over 45 mg/dL (1.15 mmol/L) for men and over 55 mg/dL (1.4 mmol/L) for women, and triglycerides under 150 mg/dL (1.7 mmol/L). Hydroxymethylglutaryl coenzyme A reductase inhibitors, or *statins,* are highly effective in the management of diabetic dyslipidemia and, together with their anti-inflammatory actions and improvement in endothelial function, may reduce the risk for cardiovascular events by about 30%. Fibrates or niacin (used with caution in patients with T2DM) may be required for lowering triglycerides or elevating HDL, respectively (see Chapter 62). Combined use of several classes of agents may be necessary for lipid control. Combination tablets of ezetimibe and simvastatin, fibrates with statins, and niacin with statins facilitate compliance and efficacy at lower doses than if used separately.

Normal urinary albumin-to-creatinine ratio is less than 30 mcg/mg. Microalbuminuria refers to an albumin-to-creatinine ratio of 30 to 299 mcg/mg and macroalbuminuria greater than 300 mcg/mg.

Blood pressure management is discussed under "Macrovascular Complications."

The previous paragraphs address the problems of β-cell failure, insulin resistance, and comorbidities. The other major contributors to the modern epidemic of T2DM are excess weight, obesity, and a sedentary lifestyle. These conditions are managed through lifestyle changes including weight loss, healthy nutrition, and exercise (see later discussion).

MEDICAL NUTRITION THERAPY

Medical nutrition therapy should be individualized to the patient's lifestyle, exercise regimen, eating habits, culture, and financial resources. A prescription for a *diabetic diet* no longer exists, nor is there a need to purchase *diabetic foods.* Be wary of foods that state "*no sugar added*"; that means that there already is more than enough sugar in that particular food. Patients can now have their cake and eat it. Current medications allow patients that freedom. Moderation is important, and for most patients there are no absolute inhibited foods, besides possibly juices and sodas (liquid sugar). In treating hypoglycemia when the patient can take orally, a set amount of juice (usually initially 4 ounces) may be drunk, being aware that this is a treatment and not a treat, in having too much. Dietary recommendations are generally in line with those for the general population: increased intake of fruit and vegetables, whole grains and fish, and maintaining moderate calorie restriction. Daily energy requirements include consumption of a balanced, healthy diet composed of 10% to 20% protein (1 g/kg body weight, provided no nephropathy exists), less than 35% total fat (<10% saturated, ≤10% polyunsaturated, 10% to 20% monounsaturated and transunsaturated, and <200 to 300 mg cholesterol), and 45% to 60% carbohydrate (see Chapter 61).

Soluble fiber (>15 g/1000 kcal) in the diet delays carbohydrate absorption (dampening the PPG peak) and improves serum lipid profiles. Insoluble fiber contributes to satiety (especially important if overweight) and *gastrointestinal homeostasis.*

Salt (NaCl) intake should be restricted to less than 6 g per day. Partial substitution of potassium chloride or magnesium chloride may be beneficial.

In addition to dietary counseling, reference to the food pyramid, generated by the U.S. Department of Agriculture (USDA), will provide general guidance for all individuals on daily nutritional requirements and the foods that provide these requirements.

Dietary adjustments are based on nutritional assessment, blood pressure, renal function, and HbA_{1c}, as well as on diabetic treatment goals. The *glycemic index* refers to the increase in blood glucose after ingestion of a particular food, expressed as a percentage of the increase in blood glucose following ingestion of the equivalent amount of glucose. For a given food, the glycemic index will vary according to the method of preparation and the concurrently ingested foods. Current recommendations encourage consumption of foods with a low glycemic index. *Carbohydrate counting* involves using either a simple system of exchanges, or *carbs* (15-g carbohydrate portions), or the more precise carbohydrate gram counting. This method allows for fine-tuning of insulin dosing during mealtimes. Training in nutrition self-management empowers patients to make correct food choices, plan meals, exercise, and calculate bolus doses of insulin.

Alcohol is allowed in moderation (≤2 drinks for men and ≤1 drink for women per day [21 units per week for men, 14 units per week for women]; one alcoholic beverage is equivalent to 12 oz beer, 5 oz wine, or 1.5 oz spirits) and should always be taken with food. Alcohol is not metabolized to glucose, and inhibits gluconeogenesis, an effect that may result in hypoglycemia as late as 8 to 16 hours after consumption. Alcohol should not be substituted for food, but, when alcohol calorie content needs to be calculated as part of a meal plan, it should be counted as fat calories (one alcoholic beverage = two fat exchanges).

WEIGHT-MANAGEMENT THERAPY

Overweight (body mass index [BMI] of 25.0 to 29.9) and obesity (BMI >30) are major risk factors for T2DM and cardiovascular disease. (BMI = weight [kg]/height [m^2]). *Healthy, reasonable, achievable,* and *sustainable* body weights

are more realistic terms than *desirable* or *ideal* body weight. A strong correlation exists between increasing BMI and the risk for T2DM. As little as 5% to 10% weight loss in overweight and obese patients reduces the risk for diabetes and leads to increased insulin sensitivity, with improvement in glycemic control, and the possibility of a reduction or cessation of antihyperglycemic therapy. This degree of weight loss also leads to significant improvements in dyslipidemia and blood pressure, as well as an increase in longevity. Behavioral modification and meal replacements, including low- or very-low-calorie diets, in a structured weight-reduction or maintenance program, are of proven efficacy in patients who are unable to lose weight on their own or with the support of a qualified nutritionist. Portion control and self-monitoring are necessary behavioral adjuncts.

The pharmaceutical agents approved by the U.S. Food and Drug Administration (FDA) for adjuvant use in weight reduction, with close medical supervision, are sibutramine (1 year; longer at physician discretion), orlistat (unrestricted long term), phentermine (limited to 3 months), and diethylpropion, benzphetamine, and phendimetrazine (short term).

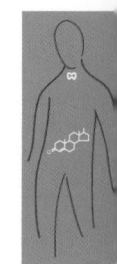

BARIATRIC SURGERY

An increasingly recognized therapeutic modality in the diabetes treatment armamentarium is bariatric surgery. These procedures are either *restrictive,* reducing bowel lumen circumference (e.g., lap-band procedure), or *bypass,* usually circumventing stomach and upper small bowel (e.g., Roux-en-Y gastric bypass). This is highly effective in T2DM patients with morbid obesity (BMI > 40 kg/m^2) and in obese individuals (BMI > 35 kg/m^2), with obesity-associated comorbidities, including hypertension, coronary artery disease, sleep apnea, and visceral obesity. Claims of "cure" of diabetes in T2DM patients who lose between 50% and 75% of their baseline weight are being increasingly recognized. The sooner bariatric surgery is performed following the diagnosis of T2DM, the greater the preservation of β–cell mass and improved resolution of T2DM with recovery of first-phase insulin response.

In addition to weight loss due to the restrictive or malabsorptive nature of the operative procedure, there is a hormonal component that is still being elucidated. Gastric bypass and biliopancreatic diversion-duodenal switch operations specifically stimulate incretin (GLP-1) and postprandial peptide YY (PYY) secretion (both synthesized in the L cells of the terminal ileum) through earlier presentation of food to the ileum, bypassing the foregut. GLP-1 stimulates insulin secretion, inhibits glucagon secretion, and delays gastric emptying. Both these hormones are responsible for early satiety. Diminished ghrelin levels and loss of diurnal variation occur following gastric bypass operations. Gastric bypass patients are in a state of negative energy balance with reduced glucose toxicity and improved β-cell function.

EXERCISE THERAPY

As with nutrition and weight management, physical activity is recognized as a specific therapy for patients with diabetes and is an independent risk factor for death. Benefits, many independent of associated weight loss, include

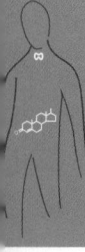

improvements in the sense of well-being, blood pressure, endothelial function, insulin sensitivity, lipid profile (consistent reduction in very-low-density lipoprotein [VLDL]), cardiorespiratory fitness, and glycemic control, with reduction in HbA$_{1c}$.

Notably, exercise itself, unless extreme, will not contribute to significant weight loss, but will, however, help in weight maintenance and prevention of weight gain. Ideally, this regimen involves moderate aerobic exercise (e.g., walking) for 60 to 90 minutes per day or vigorous exercise for 35 minutes per day (Specifically, the USDA advocates that everyone should be physically active for at least 30 minutes most days of the week; 60 minutes per day of physical activity to prevent weight gain; 60 to 90 minutes per day of physical activity to sustain weight loss). Resistance exercises do not burn as many calories as an equivalent time of aerobic exercise, and how effective this form of exercise is compared with aerobic exercise is unknown at present. Physical activity can be measured by duration, distance, and intensity. Using a pedometer, recommendations are that 8000 to 10,000 steps per day are necessary for weight maintenance. Medical evaluation is advised to determine the target level of fitness and appropriate exercise based on the presence and degree of microvascular or cardiovascular complications. Blood glucose levels should be measured before any exercise activity is initiated. Exercise should not be undertaken in patients with FPG greater than 250 mg/dL (13.8 mmol/L) with ketones, or greater than 300 mg/dL (16.6 mmol/L) without ketones, because this may paradoxically precipitate DKA. If FPG is less than 100 mg/dL (5.5 mmol/L), exercise may result in hypoglycemia, and carbohydrate should be consumed in advance. With the initiation of an exercise program, SMBG should be performed every 30 minutes during exercise lasting longer than 30 to 45 minutes; glucose or carbohydrate may need to be consumed, depending on glucose levels.

TIGHT CONTROL

With few exceptions, the aim of achieving euglycemia, or *tight control* (see Table 69-6, "Goal" column) in all patients with diabetes is now supported by several large studies. In patients with T1DM, when compared with patients receiving standard care, intensive treatment prevented or slowed the onset or progression of the microvascular complications of diabetes: retinopathy by 76%, neuropathy by 60%, and proteinuria by 54%. The threefold increase in the incidence of significant hypoglycemia should not deter attempts to achieve euglycemia. In patients with T2DM, an overall reduction in microvascular complications of 25% occurs with tight control. Tight glycemic control in several other studies has been associated with statistically significant reductions in macrovascular morbidity and mortality in patients with T2DM.

A continuum of risk for complications and the level of glycemia exists, with no glycemic threshold for complications within or above the normal glucose range. Every percentage point reduction in HbA$_{1c}$ is associated with a 40% reduction in the risk for complications in patients with T1DM and a 35% reduction in patients with T2DM. A target HbA$_{1c}$ value of less than 6.5% is recommended. Pregnant women with diabetes should aim for an HbA$_{1c}$ value of 6%.

Tight control of blood pressure significantly reduces the incidence of stroke, heart failure, microvascular complications, loss of vision, and diabetes-related deaths, supporting the aggressive treatment of even mild to moderate hypertension in patients with diabetes in an attempt to reduce blood pressure to less than 130/80 mm Hg (or 125/75 mm Hg in patients with renal insufficiency and proteinuria >1 g per 24-hour period). The reduction in microvascular complications with improved blood pressure control is independent of glycemic control.

Achieving tight control through intensive therapy of all metabolic derangements and comorbidities, including blood pressure and serum lipids, requires regular, close follow-up with a comprehensive diabetes health care team. In patients with T1DM, the use of multiple daily insulin injections (*basal* [long-acting insulin delivered subcutaneously once or twice daily], *bolus* [regular or rapid-acting insulin administered subcutaneously at mealtimes), or the use of a programmable insulin infusion pump (continuous subcutaneous insulin infusion [CSII]) is necessary to achieve glycemic control. In patients with T2DM, exercise, medical nutrition therapy, weight reduction, and combination oral antihyperglycemic agents may suffice, although failure to achieve glucose targets necessitates the use of insulin in combination with oral agents or alone (about 58% of patients) (basal-bolus insulin delivery). This regimen should be started sooner rather than later. Seventy-six percent of all patients taking insulin have T2DM. In women with gestational diabetes, when proper diet and exercise fail to achieve acceptable blood glucose control, insulin is required. Until recently, oral antihyperglycemic agents have been contraindicated in pregnancy. New data suggest that use of metformin in women with gestational diabetes is safe and effective. Insulin may be required temporarily in some patients during serious infections or surgery. CSII reduces the frequency and severity of hypoglycemia, especially nocturnal, and allows greater freedom of lifestyle (with exclusion of fixed mealtimes), and its use is equally applicable in patients with T2DM.

Normalization of FPG has been the focus of tight control. Studies now confirm that elevated PPG levels are associated with increased cardiovascular morbidity and mortality, and all-cause mortality in patients with T2DM, and may have greater predictive power than FPG levels. Correction of PPG values may reduce cardiovascular disease and mortality in these patients. Several therapies specifically target PPG and include the rapid-acting insulin analogues (lispro, aspart, glulisine), meglitinides, D-phenylalanine derivatives, α-glucosidase inhibitors, and dietary fiber.

It is now well-established that tight control of blood glucose, by means of intensive insulin therapy (intravenous or subcutaneous [constant or basal-bolus]), in patients with *stress hyperglycemia* undergoing surgery, or in intensive care units, significantly reduces morbidity (e.g., septicemia, acute renal failure requiring dialysis, red blood cell transfusions, critical illness polyneuropathy, wound infections, time on ventilator) and mortality by 30% to 50%, as well as reducing length and cost of hospital stay. This benefit of tight blood glucose control in acute situations is not limited to people with diabetes; it has also been documented in all patients with stress-induced hyperglycemia who do not have diabetes (and return to euglycemia following hospital discharge), or in people not previously known to have diabetes (newly discovered diabetes).

Tight control may be inappropriate in infants and children younger than 13 years (no long-term studies have been conducted); in patients with a shortened life expectancy, severe cardiovascular disease (in whom hypoglycemia may be deleterious), end-stage microvascular disease, or minimal complications of diabetes after 20 to 25 years; and in those with recurrent hypoglycemia or hypoglycemia, or both, unawareness.

INSULIN DOSING

Standard insulin therapy consists of one to two injections per day using intermediate- or long-acting insulin with or without short- or rapid-acting insulin. This approach provides simplicity, relative safety, and increased compliance. Premixed insulins such as 70/30 (70% neutral protamine Hagedorn [NPH]/30% regular), 75/25 (75% neutral protamine lispro [NPL]/25% lispro or aspart or glulisine), or 50/50 (50% NPH/50% regular), usually administered twice daily, provide ease of use but are less likely to achieve good glycemic control. A split or mixed regimen of NPH/regular or NPL/lispro (or aspart or glulisine) twice daily (two thirds of the calculated total daily dose before breakfast and one third before dinner; at each time two-thirds NPH or NPL and one-third regular or lispro or aspart or glulisine) dictates regular mealtimes and insulin injections.

Intensive insulin therapy refers to multiple (three or more) daily injections (MDIs) or CSII. Multiple-injection regimens include use of regular or rapid-acting insulins 3 times daily (adjusted before meals) in combination with NPH twice daily or at bedtime, or glargine insulin once daily, called *basal-bolus therapy.* By approximating normal physiologic timing of insulin delivery, patients are able to achieve better glycemic control and improve lifestyle flexibility. NPH should be given at least 30 minutes before a meal and can be mixed with regular insulin in the same syringe. Relatively *peakless,* long-acting, once-daily glargine or detemir should be administered at the same time each day and should not be mixed with other insulins. Use of the insulin pump tends to yield significantly better blood glucose values than MDI, using less insulin than nonpump regimens. Use of the pump allows patients more freedom and versatility in their lifestyle with no fixed times for meals or any other activities. CSII compared with MDI is superior in numerous ways, including less severe hypoglycemic events and less DKA. The pump is the next best thing to an artificial pancreas or pancreatic or β-cell transplantation. Insulin absorption is more predictable than with other forms of insulin therapy and allows more flexibility and accuracy with basal rate and bolus dosing calculations.

Calculating insulin doses is still somewhat empirical but may be improved through carbohydrate counting, calculation of insulin-to-carbohydrate ratios, and insulin sensitivity. Starting doses of insulin vary from 0.4 to 1.0 μg/kg per day (T1DM) and from 0.2 to 1.5 μg/kg per day (T2DM), depending on patient size, degree of glycemia, and severity of insulin resistance. The calculated total daily insulin requirement is divided according to the administration regimen chosen. In general, 40% to 50% of the total daily dose provides basal requirements. The other 50% to 60% is divided between meals according to insulin sensitivity at each time of day using the approximate ratios of 0.5 to 1.2 U insulin to 10 g carbohydrate (slightly more at breakfast). This is referred to as *carbohydrate counting,* the approximate insulin requirement to maintain euglycemia following mealtime carbohydrate consumption, for example, before breakfast (rapid or regular insulin), 15% to 25%; before lunch (rapid-acting or regular insulin), 15%; and before dinner (rapid-acting or regular insulin), 15% to 20%. In addition to the insulin dose derived from carbohydrate counting, it is also necessary to add an amount of insulin calculated as the *insulin correction factor.* This is based on insulin sensitivity. Thus, the insulin administered at mealtime is referred to as *prandial* or *nutritional* insulin and consists of the sum of scheduled (above), prandial (I/CHO ratio), and correction dose (amount of insulin calculated to bring blood glucose down to ideal mealtime value of 100 mg/dL (e.g., 1 U for every 50 mg/dL above 100 mg/dL).

Calculating insulin dosing for pump users (**Web Table 69-4**) is done as follows. Starting doses of insulin for total daily dosing (TDD):

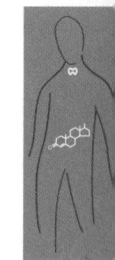

i. Based on prepump TDD: reduce TDD by 25% to 30% for pump TDD, *or*
ii. Calculated based on weight: 0.24 × weight (lb), or 0.53 × weight (kg)

Basal rate is usually 45% to 50% of pump TDD: total basal/24 hours = hourly basal rate. The number of basal rates can be increased with time and data. The initial basal rate may need to be supplemented by other rates to cover different tissue sensitivities at different times of the day. The basal rates stabilize blood glucose levels between meals and during the night (increased hepatic glucose production).

The "other half" of the TDD is used for mealtime bolus dosing. The dose is dependent on (a) premeal blood glucose (correction bolus for high blood glucose values above an ideal of 100 mg/dL), (b) the insulin-to-carbohydrate (I/CHO) ratios; and (c) the level of activity. The following calculations apply:

$$I/CHO\ ratio = 2.8 \times weight\ (lb)/TDD$$

500 Rule for estimating the I/CHO ratio: 500/TDD = *x* g; therefore, the ratio is 1 U to *x* g (e.g., 500/50 = 10; 1 U = 10 g

Correction bolus: Determine how much glucose is lowered by 1 unit of rapid acting insulin; the insulin sensitivity factor (ISF). Use the 1700 rule to estimate ISF. ISF = 1700/ TDD.

Correction bolus calculation: Current blood glucose (BG) − ideal BG/ISF.

Bolus insulin may be given as a routine push, as a square wave (extending insulin delivery over a longer period of time than normal), or as a dual wave (also extending insulin delivery over a longer period of time than normal, with a certain percentage being delivered as normal).

Insulin requirements are increased during intercurrent illness, pregnancy, and the adolescent growth spurt. On average, insulin dose adjustments are made every 2 to 3 days, and increments can be by as much as 10% to 20% of the total daily dose. When blood glucose values rise to greater than 250 mg/dL, patients should check for ketones, which are readily detected in the urine.

ELEVATIONS OF FASTING PLASMA GLUCOSE

The *Somogyi effect* refers to rebound hyperglycemia that follows undetected hypoglycemia, commonly nocturnal, in the early hours of the morning. The elevated FPG in this situation is treated by decreasing the preceding evening dose of insulin or by altering the timing of administration (from predinner to bedtime), or altering the type of insulin used, based on the expected time to maximal effect of the insulin. This approach reduces hypoglycemia and prevents the rebound. In the *dawn phenomenon*, the nocturnal secretion of growth hormone is responsible for a nighttime-to-morning rise in blood glucose. This condition is treated by increasing the evening dose of insulin or by altering the timing of administration or the type of insulin used. In both these situations, meal composition and quantity should also be evaluated. Poor insulin injection technique is an extremely common reason for increasing insulin requirements or unexplained fluctuations in blood glucose values, despite adherence to a strict exercise and nutrition program. Rotating use of different anatomic sites for injection may be responsible for variable and erratic insulin absorption, and repeated injection into a single site leads to local *resistance* through lipohypertrophy and tissue fibrosis. Rotation of injection sites exclusively into the abdominal subcutaneous tissue is optimal.

TYPE 1 DIABETES MELLITUS

Prevention of T1DM, using immune modulation or dietary manipulation, in people at high risk or in newly diagnosed patients is not yet possible.

Patients with T1DM have an absolute requirement of *insulin* for survival. This requirement also applies to patients with diabetes resulting from total or near-total β-cell depletion, as in chronic pancreatitis or pancreatic resection. Most insulin preparations are manufactured enzymatically or by recombinant DNA technology (including insulin analogues), and most are available at a concentration of 100 U/mL (U-100). Based on pharmacodynamic properties, the types of insulins currently available are rapid-acting (ultrashort), regular (short-acting) intermediate-acting, and long-acting preparations (Table 69-7; **Web Fig. 69-3**). Insulin therapy is usually started in the outpatient setting unless DKA with hospital admission is the initial presentation. Multiple different insulin regimens exist.

TYPE 2 DIABETES MELLITUS

Prevention of T2DM has been achieved through *lifestyle changes* (healthy diet, weight reduction, and regular exercise) in people at high risk (e.g., IGT), with the incidence of T2DM reduced by as much as 58%, whereas the use of *metformin* reduced the incidence by only 31%.

The aim of treatment in T2DM is to reverse insulin resistance, control intestinal glucose absorption, normalize HGP, improve β-cell glucose sensing and insulin secretion, and ultimately prevent the occurrence of long-term complications. Provided that pharmacologic therapy is not required immediately (FPG < 250 mg/dL), all newly diagnosed patients should be given at least a 1-month trial of diet, exercise, and weight management. If this regimen does not lead to adequate blood glucose control, the physician will need to prescribe oral or subcutaneous antihyperglycemic agents or insulin, or both. After FPG is controlled, substituting a noninsulin agent in patients who were initiated on insulin may be possible. Maximal-dose sulfonylurea therapy has been used effectively as initial treatment in patients with marked hyperglycemia, with doses decreasing as control improves. The regimen of *bedtime insulin, NPH, and daytime sulfonylurea therapy* (BIDS) has been successful in patients with T2DM as regular therapy or as a transition stage from noninsulin antihyperglycemic therapy to total insulin therapy. Metformin could be substituted for the sulfonylurea in BIDS.

The eight classes of *noninsulin antidiabetic agents* currently available are listed in Table 69-8. The insulin secretagogues (sulfonylureas, meglitinides, and D-phenylalanine derivatives) have similar mechanisms of action and may cause hypoglycemia, hence the term *oral hypoglycemic agents*. The other classes of noninsulin agents each target a different pathologic process and are referred to as *antihyperglycemic agents*. T2DM is a progressive disease, and monotherapy is seldom permanently successful.

Combination drug therapy using submaximal doses of two or more agents, including insulin, each targeting a different metabolic abnormality, has synergistic effects that may be far greater than the effects of any agent used alone at maximal dose. The incidence and severity of adverse events are also reduced with combination therapy, and, in addition, improved compliance and, in many instances, a cost savings takes place. Although some physicians still use a stepped-care approach, many now initiate therapy with drugs from more than one class of antihyperglycemic agents, depending on the patient's profile and the predominant pathologic defects (see Table 69-8). Additional agents are added (not substituted) if adequate glycemic control is not achieved at 25% to 75% of the maximal dose. Only one agent from each class should be used in an individual patient at any one time. Regular blood glucose estimations allow timely increases in drug doses and the addition of other agents as necessary. Comprehensive combination therapy requires a multipronged approach to the treatment of hyperglycemia, dyslipidemia, obesity, hypertension, and the associated comorbidities, with proactive preventive measures when appropriate.

Sulfonylureas

For many years, the only class of oral hypoglycemic (antihyperglycemic) agents available has as its principal action the stimulation of endogenous insulin secretion from the pancreatic β cells. The drugs in this class also increase β-cell sensitivity to glucose and exert some influence in diminishing insulin resistance. These agents have vasoconstrictive properties, raise blood pressure (chlorpropamide), prevent

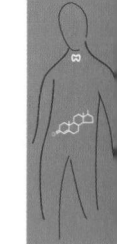

Table 69-7 **Types of Insulin**

Insulin Type	Generic Name	Preprandial Injection Timing* (hr)	Onset* (hr)	Peak* (hr)	Duration* (hr)	Blood Glucose (BG) Nadir* (hr)
Rapid acting	Lispro[†]	0-0.2	0.1-0.5	0.5-2	<5	2-4
	Aspart[‡]	0-0.2	0.1-0.3	0.6-3	3-5	1-3
	Glulisine¶	0-0.25 (15 min before a meal or within 20 min of starting a meal)	0.15-0.3	0.5-1.5	1-5.3	2-4
Short acting	Regular	0.5-(1)	0.3-1	2-6	4-8	3-7
Intermediate acting	Lente	0.5-(1)	1-2	4-12	(≤16)	Before next meal
	NPH	0.5-(1)	1-3	6-15	16-26	6-13
Long acting	Ultralente	0.5-(1)	4-6	8-30	24-36	10-28
	Glargine[§]	‖Once daily; evening meal or bedtime: twice daily; 12 hourly	1.1-4	No peak	10.8->24	Before next dose
	Detemir	‖Once daily; evening meal or bedtime: twice daily; 12 hourly	1.1-4	No peak	12-24	Before next dose
Human Premixed						
NPH/regular	70/30	0.5-(1)	0.5-1	2-12	14-24	3-12
NPH/regular	50/50	0.5-(1)	0.5-1	2-5	14-24	3-12
Insulin Analogue Premixed						
Lispro protamine/lispro	75/25	0.25	0.15-0.25	1	14-24	—
Aspart protamine/aspart	70/30	0.25	0.15-0.3	2-4	24	—

*Time profiles depend on several factors, including dose, anatomic site of injection, method (subcutaneous, intramuscular, or intravenous; above profiles are for subcutaneous injections), duration of diabetes, type of diabetes, degree of insulin resistance, level of physical activity, presence of obesity, and body temperature. Some time ranges are wide to include data from several separate studies. Preprandial injection timing depends on premeal blood glucose (BG) values and insulin type. If BG is low, it may be necessary to inject insulin and eat immediately (carbohydrate portion of meal first). If BG is high, it may be necessary to delay meal after insulin injection and eat carbohydrate portion last.

[†]Insulin analogue with reversal of lysine and proline at positions 28 and 29 on the B chain of the insulin molecule.

[‡]Insulin analogue with substitution of aspartic acid for proline at position 28 on the B chain of the insulin molecule.

[§]Insulin analogue with substitution of glycine for asparagine at position 21 on the A chain and addition of two arginines to the carboxyl terminus of the B chain of the insulin molecule.

¶Insulin analogue with substitution of lysine for asparagine at position 3 on the B chain and glutamic acid for lysine at position 29 on the B chain of the insulin molecule.

‖Administer at same time each day, unrelated to meals. Morning administration may result in greater glucose lowering and less nocturnal hypoglycemia.

Do not mix glargine, detemir, or Ultralente insulins with other insulins.

70/30, 70% NPH, 30% regular or 70% NPL/30% aspart; 50/50, 50% NPH, 50% regular; 75/25, 75% NPL, 25% lispro; 70/30, 70% NPA, 30% aspart; NPH, neutral protamine Hagedorn; NPL, neutral protamine lispro; NPA, neutral protamine aspart.

ischemic preconditioning in the heart, and increase plasma levels of PAI-1. The drugs differ in potency, time of onset, duration of action, plasma protein binding, absorption characteristics, and route of metabolism and excretion. Some involve novel delivery systems. At maximal dose, these drugs are all equally effective (except tolbutamide) in lowering blood glucose levels. Primary failure to respond to sulfonylureas occurs in 20% to 25% of patients. Secondary failure occurs at the rate of 10% to 15% per year, in part because of progressive β-cell failure and insulin resistance and in part because of poor patient compliance. Replacing one agent with another in this class is unlikely to produce a substantially different effect and is not recommended unless for reasons of patient compliance. The risk for hypoglycemia, the major adverse effect, increases with increasing patient age, use of a preparation with a long half-life (e.g., chlorpropamide), and renal dysfunction. Weight gain is also a recognized side effect. Characteristics of patients best suited for sulfonylurea therapy include diagnosis at greater than 30 years of age, disease presence for less than 5 years, residual β-cell function, relative lack of obesity, and FPG less than 300 mg/dL (see Table 69-8).

Biguanides (Metformin)

The major mechanism of action of this insulin sensitizer is in reducing HGP by inhibiting gluconeogenesis. This drug also increases anaerobic glycolysis with resultant increased lactate production, enhances glucose uptake and utilization by muscle, and decreases intestinal glucose absorption. In addition to its glucose-lowering effect, this drug is associated with weight loss (5 to 10 lb), possibly related to mild nausea and anorexia, a decrease in plasma insulin levels, and significant lipid-lowering effects (decreasing total cholesterol, LDL, and triglyceride by 10% to 20% and increasing HDL). Metformin improves endothelial function, lowers PAI-1 levels, and reduces cardiovascular events. It is well suited for use in obese, hyperlipidemic

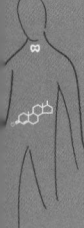

Table 69-8 **Noninsulin Antidiabetic Agents**

	Sulfonylureas	Biguanides	α-Glucosidase Inhibitors	Thiazolidinediones	Meglitinides	D-Phenyl Alanine Derivatives
Generic name	Glimepiride	Metformin	Acarbose	Rosiglitazone	Repaglinide	Nateglinide
	Glyburide: micronized, nonmicronized Glipizide, glipizide XL Chlorpropamide Tolbutamide	Metformin XR	Miglitol	Pioglitazone		
Mode of action	↑↑ Pancreatic insulin secretion chronically ↑ Tissue insulin sensitivity	↓↓ HGP ↓ peripheral IR ↓ intestinal glucose absorption	Delays PP digestion of carbohydrates and absorption of glucose leading to ↓↓ PP hyperglycemia	↓↓ Peripheral IR ↑↑ Glucose disposal ↓ HGP	↑↑ Pancreatic insulin secretion acutely	↑↑ Pancreatic insulin secretion acutely
Preferred patient type	Diagnosis age >30 yr, lean, diabetes <5 yr, insulinopenic	Overweight, IR, fasting hyperglycemia, dyslipidemia	PP hyperglycemia	Overweight, IR, dyslipidemia, renal dysfunction	PP hyperglycemia, insulinopenic	PP hyperglycemia, insulinopenic
Therapeutic Effects						
↓ HbA$_{1c}$† (%)	1-2	1-2	0.5-1	0.8-1.6 (2.6 with 45 mg pioglitazone monotherapy, in newly diagnosed)	1-2	1-2
↓ FPG* (mg/dL)	50-70	50-80	15-30	25-50	40-80	40-80
↓ PPG* (mg/dL)	~90	80	40-50	—	30	30
Insulin levels	↑	—	—	—	↑	↑
Weight	↑	↓	—	↑	↑	↑
Lipids		↓ LDL ↓↓ TG	↓ TG	LDL$_3$, TC (rosi) ↓↓ TG (pio) ↑ HDL (both)		
Side effects	Hypoglycemia, weight gain, GI side effects	Diarrhea, abdominal discomfort, lactic acidosis Contraindicated: Cr >1.5 mg/dL (men), >1.4 mg/dL (women), hepatic disease, CHF, alcoholism	Abdominal pain, bloating, flatulence, diarrhea Contraindicated: inflammatory bowel disease, bowel obstruction, cirrhosis Cr >2.0 mg/dL	Edema, anemia, weight gain Contraindicated: ALT >2.5 upper limit of normal, NYHA class 3 or 4, hepatic disease, alcoholism	Hypoglycemia (low risk), caution if moderate/ severe liver disease, slight weight gain	Hypoglycemia (low risk), caution if moderate/ severe liver disease
Route of administration	Oral	Oral	Oral	Oral	Oral	Oral
Dose(s)/day	1-3	2-3	1-3	1-2	1-4+	1-4+
Maximum daily	Depends on agent	2550	150 (>60 kg BW)	45 (pioglitazone)	16	360
Dose (mg)			300 (>60 kg BW)	8 (rosiglitazone)		

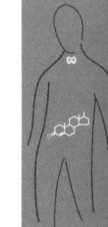

DPP-4 Inhibitors	Amylin Mimetics	Incretin Mimetics	Combination Preparations			
			Glyburide/ metformin	Glipizide/ metformin	Rosiglitazone/ metformin	Rosiglitazone/ glimepiride
itagliptin phosphate	Pramlintide	Exenatide (GLP-1 agonist)				
nhibits DPP-4 resulting in ↑ levels of incretins (GLP-1, GIP)	↓ Glycemic surges ↓ PP glucagon secretion ↓ TG fluxes Delays gastric emptying Inhibits ghrelin	↑ Glucose dependent pancreatic β-cell insulin synthesis and secretion ↓ Glucagon secretion Restores first-phase insulin release ↓ FPG ↓ Gastric emptying ↓ PPG β-cell preservation (induction of β-cell neogenesis → Anti apoptosis → β-cell mass)	As for individual agents	As for individual agents	As for individual agents	As for individual agents
n combination with diet and exercise, metformin or TZD	Insulin-treated DM (as adjunctive therapy) wide glycemic fluctuations, insulin resistant, predominant PPG, obese	Advanced T2DM Obese Inadequate response to metformin and/or sulfonylurea Adjunct to oral medications				
0.6-1.4	0.6-0.9	0.8-1.3				
25 51 ↑	— ↓ ↓ ↓ ↓ TG	14-25 (at 1 yr) 63-71 ↓ ↓	1.5	2.1	1.2	1.6
Nasopharyngitis Upper respiratory tract infections Headache	Nausea, headache, anorexia, early satiety, weight loss (↓ calorie intake; ↓ fat, protein, CHO), vomiting, indigestion, abdominal pain, tiredness, dizziness, hypoglycemia (in combination with insulin and/or sulfonylurea) More common in T1DM	Nausea, vomiting, diarrhea, headache, dose dependent anorexia, ↓ food intake, weight loss Hypoglycemia when in combination with sulfonylurea (dose dependent) DO NOT use in T1DM or DKA	As for individual agents (may be reduced because of lower individual component doses)	As for individual agents (may be reduced because of lower individual component doses)	As for individual agents (may be reduced because of lower individual component doses)	As for individual agents (may be reduced because of lower individual component doses)
Oral	Subcutaneous injection (abdomen, thigh)	Subcutaneous injection (abdomen, thigh, arm)				
1	1-3	1-2	1-2	2	2	1
100	Type 1 (180 mcg) Type 2 (360 mcg)	10 mcg	20/2000	20/2000	8/2000	8/8

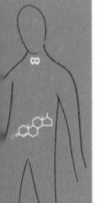

Table 69-8 **Noninsulin Antidiabetic Agents—Cont'd**

	Sulfonylureas	**Biguanides**	**α-Glucosidase Inhibitors**	**Thiazolidinediones**	**Meglitinides**	**D-Phenyl Alanine Derivatives**
Range/dose (mg)	Depends on agent	500-1000	25-50 (>60 kg BW) 25-100 (>60 kg BW), slow titration of dose	15-45 (pioglitazone) 4-8 (rosiglitazone)	0.5-4	60-120
Optimal administration time	~30 min premeal (some with food, others on empty stomach)	With meal	With first bite of meal	With/without meal (breakfast)	Preferably <15 min premeal; (omit if no meal)	Preferably <15 min premeal (omit if no meal)
Main site of metabolism/ excretion	Hepatic/renal, fecal	Not metabolized/ renal excretion	2% of acarbose absorbed/fecal, 50%-100% of migitol absorbed/not metabolized renal	Hepatic/fecal	Hepatic/fecal, renal	Renal 80%, hepatic/fecal 10%

*Not yet FDA approved.
†Values combined from numerous studies; values are also dose dependent.
↑, Increased; ↓, decreased; —, unchanged; ALT, alanine aminotransferase; BW, body weight; CHF, congestive heart failure; CHO, carbohydrate; Cr, creatinine; DKA, diabetic ketoacidosis; FPG, fasting plasma glucose; GLP-1, glucagon-like peptide-1; HbA$_{1c}$, glycosylated hemoglobin; HDL, high-density lipoprotein; HGP, hepatic glucose production; IR, insulin resistance; LDL, low-density lipoprotein; LDL$_3$, large buoyant LDL; NYHA, New York Heart Association; PP, postprandial; PPAR, peroxisome proliferator activated receptor; PPG, postprandial plasma glucose; T1DM, type 1 diabetes mellitus; T2DM, type 2 diabetes mellitus; TG, triglyceride; XR, XL, extended release.

patients with T2DM. Metformin's use in patients with IGT and the metabolic syndrome, as prophylaxis against development of diabetes, has proved successful. Primary failure rates are about 12%, and secondary failure rates are between 5% and 10%. Strong evidence-based support can be found for using metformin as initial therapy, especially in overweight or obese individuals, and often in combination with an agent or agents from another class.

Major adverse effects are gastrointestinal and metabolic. Gastrointestinal side effects include metallic taste, anorexia, nausea, abdominal discomfort, and diarrhea; these are usually mild and transient and improve with temporary reduction in dose and administration with meals. The major metabolic side effect is lactic acidosis, which occurs most often in patients with renal disease (creatinine, ≥ 1.5 mg/dL in men and ≥1.4 mg/dL in women), low cardiac output, impaired hepatic function, excessive alcohol intake, or concomitant use of radiographic contrast.

α-Glucosidase Inhibitors (Acarbose and Miglitol)

Within the small bowel lumen, α-glucosidase inhibitors competitively inhibit the breakdown of complex carbohydrates by antagonizing pancreatic α-amylase and the microvillar brush border α-glucosidase enzymes, thereby delaying glucose absorption and dampening the PPG (and insulin) peaks, with modest effect on FPG levels. When acarbose is taken with the first bite of a carbohydrate-containing meal, only 1% to 2% of the drug is absorbed. Major common side effects are gastrointestinal, including bloating, abdominal discomfort, diarrhea, and flatulence. These effects occur at the initiation of therapy and with dose increases, but they

commonly disappear with continued use. The side effects can be minimized by starting with a low dose (12.5 to 25 mg once daily) and increasing it gradually over several weeks to a maintenance dose of 50 to 100 mg 3 times daily, depending on the patient's body weight (see Table 69-8). These agents do not cause hypoglycemia when used alone, but hypoglycemia may occur when they are used in combination with insulin, a sulfonylurea, a meglitinide, or a D-phenylalanine derivative. Oral treatment of hypoglycemia during therapy with these agents requires administration of pure glucose, fructose, or lactose (not sucrose, maltose, or starch).

Thiazolidinediones (Rosiglitazone and Pioglitazone)

Thiazolidinediones, which are peroxisome proliferator activated receptor-γ (PPAR-γ) agonists, reduce insulin resistance, improve the peripheral action of insulin (*insulin sensitizers*), and reduce hyperglycemia by increasing glucose uptake and utilization in peripheral tissues and reducing HGP. These agents increase the differentiation of preadipocytes to adipocytes and may cause an increase in total-body fat mass, with remodeling (increased number of small, insulin-sensitive adipocytes) and redistribution (visceral to subcutaneous) of body fat. Improvements in serum lipids (decrease in triglycerides [TGs] and free fatty acids (FFAs), increase in HDL, and increase in large buoyant LDL [LDL$_1$]) depend on each particular agent and may occur through nuclear PPAR-γ activation. Thiazolidinediones have little effect in the presence of euglycemia and thus tend not to produce hypoglycemia when used as monotherapy. They bind to PPAR-γ to induce transcription of several genes involved in glucose and lipid metabolism. Because of their

DPP-4 Inhibitors	Amylin Mimetics	Incretin Mimetics	Combination Preparations			
25-100 dependent on renal function	Type 1 (15-60 mcg) Type 2 (60-120 mcg)	5-10 mcg (start with 5 mcg; ↑ to 10 mcg after 1 month if necessary)	1.25/250-20/2000	2.5/250-20/2000	1/500-8/2000	4/1-8/8
Daily with or without food	Immediately before major meals (≥250 cal or ≥30 g CHO) Do not mix with insulin Halve dose of rapid/short- acting or fixed-mixed insulin	Within 60 min of breakfast and dinner	With meals	With meals	With meals	With first meal of the day
	Renal	Renal excretion (proteolytic degradation)	As for individual agents	As for individual agents	As for individual agents	As for individual agents

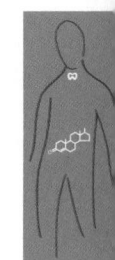

mechanism of action on receptors in the cell nucleus, 3 to 4 weeks may be required to produce a clinical effect and 10 to 12 weeks for a full effect. Dosage adjustments should therefore only be made every 3 months.

Activation of PPAR-γ, found predominantly in fat, results in a decrease in FFAs and an increase in insulin sensitivity and glucose uptake, resulting in lowering of plasma glucose levels. Activation of PPAR-α, in liver and muscle, lowers plasma TG levels and raises HDL levels by stimulating fatty acid oxidation and lowering apolipoprotein (apo) CIII and apo AI. In addition to their glucose-lowering properties, their actions include anti-inflammatory effects (especially on the vasculature, with reduction in macrophage migration, macrophage foam cell formation, IL-6, highly sensitive C-reactive protein [hs-CRP], monocyte chemotactic protein-1, and white blood cell count), mild blood pressure reduction, increased thrombolysis (reduction in PAI-1 activity as well as antigen levels), reduced vascular smooth muscle proliferation (improvement in carotid intima medial wall thickness [IMT], a useful index for monitoring atherosclerosis progress), improved endothelial function and vascular activity, reduced urinary albumin excretion, and preservation of β-cell function (partly through a reduction in the rate of β-cell apoptosis). These agents increase adipose-derived adiponectin levels, thereby enhancing liver and muscle insulin sensitivity and fat oxidation and inhibiting endothelial inflammation. The anti-inflammatory action helps restore insulin sensitivity and reverse the atherosclerotic process. Restoration of endothelial integrity is demonstrated by improvement in endothelium-mediated brachial vasodilation.

Severity of cardiovascular disease is often assessed by determination of IMT, as already mentioned. Some of the therapies used in the management of diabetes are responsible for a reduction in IMT and may in fact act synergistically, namely exercise, thiazolidinediones, and hydroxymethylglutaryl–coenzyme A (HMG-CoA) reductase inhibitors. They may also improve cardiovascular risk markers.

Pioglitazone, when part of standard therapy, has been shown to reduce the combined risk for heart attacks, strokes, and death by 16% in high-risk patients with T2DM.

Thiazolidinediones (TZD) do not have to be taken with food. Combination with insulin therapy may facilitate a reduction in insulin dose or even its discontinuation. A 25% primary failure rate is probably caused by inappropriate use in patients with minimal endogenous insulin secretion. Rosiglitazone may be given as monotherapy or in combination with metformin or a sulfonylurea. Pioglitazone may be used as monotherapy or with insulin, sulfonylureas, or metformin. Side effects include dilutional anemia, edema, and mild weight gain. These drugs should be used with caution in patients at risk for heart failure. Hypoglycemia is a risk when these drugs are used in combination with oral hypoglycemia agents, amylin, or incretin mimetics. Therapy with this class of drugs should be initiated early while reasonable β-cell function still exists.

Although pioglitazone and rosiglitazone do not appear to cause liver dysfunction, as did their predecessor troglitazone, the FDA recommends that therapy with TZDs should not be initiated if the serum alanine aminotransferase level is greater than 2.5 times the upper limit of normal. Patients should have liver function tests performed every 2 months for the first year and periodically thereafter. No restrictions in renal insufficiency are recommended.

Meglitinides (Repaglinide) and D-Phenylalanine Derivatives (Nateglinide)

The mechanism of action of meglitinides and D-phenylalanine derivatives is similar to that of the sulfonylureas in stimulating insulin secretion from the pancreas. The advantages of these classes over the sulfonylureas are the rapid onset and short duration of action, which suppress postprandial hyperglycemia. They should be taken with meals and omitted in the absence of a meal, a feature that permits flexibility of lifestyle. The stimulation of prandial insulin secretion avoids chronic stimulation of β cells and results in reduced between-meal and nocturnal hyperinsulinemia, a feature of sulfonylurea therapy. The insulin secretagogue action is glucose dependent, sensitizing β cells to secrete more insulin in response to elevated glucose levels. For this reason, hypoglycemia is seen less often than with sulfonylureas. Clinical response to these agents is seen within about 1 week. These drugs may be prescribed in the presence of renal dysfunction. Combination therapy of a sulfonylurea with either of these agents is not FDA approved.

Combination Preparations of Antihyperglycemic Agents

Increasingly, pharmaceutical companies are manufacturing combinations of oral agents (e.g., glyburide and metformin, glipizide and metformin, rosiglitazone and metformin, rosiglitazone and glimepiride, sitagliptin and metformin), which, although in fixed doses, may help improve patient compliance when faced with increasing numbers of drugs to swallow each day (see Table 69-8). Combination therapy, while promoting synergistic effects, also allows for lower doses of each agent with a reduced risk for side effects.

To further enhance patient compliance, certain oral agents are formulated as long-acting, slow, or extended-release preparations (e.g., glipizide XL, metformin XR) and in solution (e.g., metformin) for children.

Currently available antihyperglycemic therapeutic agents, other than insulin, each treat separate metabolic problems in patients with diabetes. Combinations of these drugs target some of the dysfunctions in the spectrum of actions performed by insulin. Research is directed at manipulating endogenous compounds to produce agents able to approximate normal physiologic homeostatic control of hyperglycemia as closely as possible.

Incretin Mimetics

Incretin mimetics constitute a novel class of antidiabetic agents that mimic the actions of naturally occurring incretins (gut hormones) involved in the enteroinsular axis. The importance of this class of hormones with respect to plasma glucose levels following food ingestion is noted in the *incretin effect:* a greater insulin secretory response after similar increases in plasma glucose concentrations following oral, compared with intravenous, routes of glucose administration. **Web Fig. 69-4** demonstrates the incretin effect in normal individuals and its diminution in T2DM. The hormones GLP-1 (accounting for 70% to 80% of the incretin effect), GLP-2, and the gastric inhibitory peptide, GIP, are secreted from the small intestine (GLP-1 from enteroendocrine L cells of the distal ileum, GIP from enteroendocrine K cells of the proximal jejunum) following nutrient ingestion. Serum GLP-1 levels are generally lower in people with diabetes. GLP-1 regulates blood glucose through several mechanisms: (1) enhancing glucose-dependent pancreatic β-cell insulin secretion with subsequent promotion of insulin-mediated tissue glucose uptake; (2) inhibition of glucagon secretion from pancreatic α cells during hyperglycemia, or the fed state (leading to reduced HGP, insulin requirements, and PPG excursions); (3) restoration of first-phase insulin release (lost early in T2DM); (4) increased second-phase insulin secretion; and (5) insulin-sensitizing effect and delayed gastric emptying (limiting PPG excursions). GLP-1 also protects and preserves β cells from damage by FFAs and cytokines. It does not impair the glucagon response to hypoglycemia. Other effects include depressed appetite and increased satiety, resulting in reduced food intake with subsequent weight loss. Prevention of pancreatic β-cell deterioration (a central feature of T2DM) and increasing β-cell mass involves regeneration through proliferation and differentiation, neogenesis, and antiapoptosis of β cells by GLP-1.

The incretin mimetic available for therapeutic use at present is exenatide (structurally identical to exendin-4, derived from the saliva of the Gila monster lizard), the naturally occurring GLP-1 analogue. This preparation is resistant to inactivation by dipeptidyl peptidase-4 (DPP-4). Used as an adjunct in T2DM when sulfonylureas and metformin do not adequately control blood glucose, exenatide is administered subcutaneously before breakfast and dinner (see Table 69-8). A long-acting GLP-1 analogue, liraglutide, is currently in clinical trials. Compared with a sulfonylurea, this agent, given subcutaneously once daily, produced less hypoglycemia.

Amylin Mimetics

Amylin, a peptide hormone, is synthesized in pancreatic β cells and stored with insulin within secretory granules. It is co-secreted with insulin, in equimolar amounts, in response to nutrient stimuli. Biochemical characteristics are similar to insulin except that it is metabolized and excreted mainly by the kidneys. The main functions of amylin are (1) to control postprandial glucose levels through inhibition of postprandial glucagon secretion, with subsequently decreased HGP; (2) delayed gastric emptying and thus carbohydrate absorption, and (3) reduced food intake through centrally mediated early satiety. Amylin also acts in an autocrine fashion to inhibit pancreatic β-cell insulin secretion.

With β-cell destruction (T1DM), or atrophy and *exhaustion* (T2DM), the secretion of insulin and amylin is absent and reduced, respectively.

Pramlintide, a stable analogue of amylin, is approved for use in both T1DM and T2DM as adjunctive therapy. Concurrent insulin doses should be halved at the initiation of pramlintide therapy. In addition to dampening PPG peaks, pramlintide is also effective in reducing glucose fluctuations throughout the day. It is given subcutaneously and at lower doses in patients with T1DM than those with T2DM (see Table 69-8). Side effects include nausea, vomiting, and transient headaches. Hypoglycemia may result when used in combination with sulfonylureas.

Dipeptidyl Peptidase-4 Inhibitors

DPP-4 inhibitors selectively (no effect on DPP-8 or DPP-9) and reversibly block GLP-1 and other incretin degradation, thereby prolonging the activity of natural incretins. They increase insulin synthesis and release, while suppressing the release of glucagon in a glucose-dependent manner, lowering the potential for hypoglycemia. In patients with T2DM, there is an improvement in β-cell function and insulin sensitivity.

TREATMENT OF THE METABOLIC SYNDROME

Lifestyle modification, including weight reduction and enhanced physical activity, are the most important aspects of treatment in this group of patients. Obviously, each of the dysmetabolic factors present needs to be managed in its own right. All treatments are greatly facilitated by weight reduction, a 10% weight loss being associated with major metabolic improvements. Useful adjunctive pharmacotherapy includes the insulin sensitizers, metformin, and TZDs, with beneficial elevation of adipose tissue-specific adiponectin.

Complications

ACUTE COMPLICATIONS

Hypoglycemia

Hypoglycemia is discussed in Chapter 70.

Lactic Acidosis

A rare event, lactic acidosis is discussed in Chapter 28.

Diabetic Ketoacidosis

Although DKA develops most commonly in patients with T1DM, it can be seen in patients with T2DM, especially during acute illness. DKA is defined as being present in patients with absolute or relative insulin deficiency when the following criteria are met:

1. *Hyperglycemia:* plasma glucose levels greater than 250 mg/dL
2. *Ketosis:* moderate to severe ketonemia (ketone levels positive at a serum dilution of ≥1:2, or serum β-hydroxybutyrate concentration >0.5 mmol/L) and moderate ketonuria (2+ to 3+ by the nitroprusside method). The nitroprusside reagent reacts primarily to acetoacetate and, to a lesser extent, acetone, but does not detect β-hydroxybutyrate. When lactic acidosis coexists with DKA, there is a shift toward more β-hydroxybutyrate production, which decreases the reactivity with the nitroprusside reagent.
3. *Acidosis:* pH less than or equal to 7.3 or bicarbonate less than or equal to 15 mEq/L

Associated metabolic and plasma abnormalities include dehydration, increased osmolality (usually >320 mOsm/kg), increased anion gap (>12 mEq/L), increased serum amylase, elevated white blood cell count, and hypertriglyceridemia.

Precipitating factors for DKA are infection (30%), often minor (respiratory or urinary tract) new-onset diabetes (25%), problems with insulin administration (20%), *stress,* and many less frequent causes. Insulin deficiency and raised insulin counter-regulatory hormones result in increased HGP and decreased peripheral glucose utilization, leading to hyperglycemia and hyperosmolality with consequent osmotic diuresis, electrolyte loss (sodium, potassium, phosphate, magnesium, calcium, and chloride), and dehydration. Activation of insulin-sensitive lipase stimulates release of FFAs from adipose tissues, which are oxidized in the liver to produce ketone bodies. Diminished peripheral utilization of ketones during insulin deficiency results in ketosis and metabolic acidosis.

DKA develops within hours to days. The ill feeling associated with the metabolic acidosis leads patients to seek early medical attention, a feature that accounts for the lower levels of glucose and osmolality compared with those in hyperosmolar nonketotic syndrome (HNKS) (Table 69-9). DKA may not always be obvious at the time of presentation because early signs and symptoms are subtle. Symptoms include nausea, vomiting, thirst, polydipsia, polyuria, abdominal pain, weakness, fatigue, and anorexia. Signs include tachycardia, orthostatic hypotension, poor skin turgor, warm or dry skin and mucous membranes, hyperventilation or Kussmaul respiration,

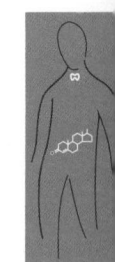

Table 69-9 Hyperglycemic Crises: A Comparison of Diabetic Ketoacidosis and Hyperosmolar Nonketotic Syndrome		
Feature	**Diabetic Ketoacidosis**	**Hyperosmolar Nonketotic Syndrome**
Age of patient	Usually <40 yr	Usually >60 yr
Duration of symptoms	Usually <2 days	Usually >5 days
Plasma glucose	Usually <600 mg/dL	Usually >600 mg/dL
Serum sodium	Normal or low (130-140 mEq/L)	Normal or high (145-155 mEq/L)
Serum potassium	Normal or high (5-6 mEq/L)	Normal (4-5 mEq/L)
Serum bicarbonate	<15 mEq/L	>15 mEq/L
Ketone bodies	Positive at ≥1:2 dilution	Negative at 1:2 dilution
pH	<7.35	>7.3
Serum osmolality	Usually <320 mOsm/kg	Usually >320 mOsm/kg
Fluid deficit	≤10% body weight	≤15% body weight
Cerebral edema	Subclinical asymptomatic, rare clinically	Very rare
Prognosis	3%-10% mortality rate (>20% for people >65 yr)	10%-20% mortality rate
Subsequent course	Insulin therapy required in most cases	Insulin therapy not usually required

hypothermia or normothermia, ketones on the breath, weight loss, and altered mental status or coma.

Initial assessment includes mental status, presence of gag or cough reflex, abdominal succussion splash (requiring a nasogastric tube), and urinary output. The search for a precipitating cause (e.g., infection or sepsis, myocardial infarction, pregnancy, cerebrovascular accident, trauma, psychosocial factor) is crucial, both to treating the underlying disorders and to facilitating resolution of the DKA. Baseline investigations should include plasma glucose, plasma acetone, serum electrolytes, serum lipid profile, serum amylase and lipase, full blood count with differential, arterial blood gas determination, blood cultures, culture of abscess or infected site, urine glucose and ketones, urine microscopy and culture, chest radiograph, abdominal radiograph (with abdominal pain), electrocardiogram, cardiac enzymes (if appropriate), CT scan of the brain if appropriate, lumbar puncture (if appropriate), serum osmolality, and anion gap. (Calculation of serum osmolality: $2[Na^+ (mEq/L)] + 2[K^+ (mEq/L)] + glucose [mg/dL]/18 + BUN [mg/dL]/2.8$. Calculation of anion gap: $Na^+ - [Cl^- + HCO_3^-]$).

Most important in the therapy of DKA is the restoration of circulating plasma volume, with maintenance of cardiac output and renal function (**Web Table 69-4**). Intravenous fluid lowers blood glucose through serum dilution and enhanced urinary glucose loss, lowers osmolality and ketones, and improves the peripheral utilization of ketones and glucose. Insulin administration facilitates the peripheral uptake of ketones and glucose, thereby decreasing urinary glucose loss, and, significantly, inhibits hepatic glucose production. Electrolyte imbalances should be corrected concurrently with fluid and insulin replacement and treatment of the precipitating cause. To track the course of treatment, several parameters require regular monitoring:

1. Hourly: Vital signs (temperature, pulse rate, respiratory rate, blood pressure), mental status, fluid intake and output, plasma glucose, insulin infusion rate, arterial blood gases, electrocardiogram (initially, and if in the intensive care unit, preferably continuous monitoring)
2. Every 1 to 2 hours: Serum electrolytes (sodium, potassium, chloride, and bicarbonate), electrocardiogram until stable
3. Every 6 hours: Serum phosphate, magnesium, calcium, blood urea nitrogen, and creatinine

With correction of the metabolic abnormalities, the frequency of their measurements should be reduced appropriately. Weight should be measured initially and then daily. Note that ketones are only measured to help confirm the diagnosis of DKA and subsequently to establish its resolution. With changes in the ratios of the different serum ketones, the routine methods used to measure these may falsely suggest transient elevation in ketones. Tracking the decrease in the anion gap will provide information regarding control of DKA.

Hyperosmolar Nonketotic Syndrome (Hyperglycemic Hyperosmolar State)

HNKS occurs almost exclusively in patients with T2DM, who are usually elderly and physically impaired, with limited access to free water. The pathogenesis of HNKS is similar to

that of DKA but may be distinguished from it by the more marked hyperglycemia, the relative absence of acidosis and ketonemia, and the greater degree of dehydration (see Table 69-9). Low FFA levels result in the absence of ketone bodies, with reduced nausea and vomiting. Increased lactic acid levels result from poor tissue perfusion and are more marked than in DKA. Insulin resistance is usually present, with normal or elevated levels of serum insulin. As many as 30% to 40% of patients over 65 years of age with HNKS may have previously undiagnosed diabetes. HNKS usually develops insidiously over days to weeks. Precipitating and complicating factors may include infection, intestinal obstruction, mesenteric thrombosis, pulmonary embolism, peritoneal dialysis, heat stroke, hypothermia, subdural hematoma, severe burns, and an extensive list of drugs. Some of these conditions may themselves result from the severe dehydration and poor tissue perfusion of HNKS.

Therapy of HNKS follows the same general principles as that of DKA, with particular emphasis on intravenous fluid therapy and potassium replacement. Fluid replacement should follow the same pattern as in DKA, but a greater total volume is usually required. Careful monitoring is necessary because patients often have cardiac and other comorbid conditions. Restoration of the fluid deficit should proceed more slowly than in DKA, ideally over 36 to 72 hours. Insulin therapy should only be started after rehydration is in progress. These patients may be sensitive to insulin and may require reduced doses. In view of the severe dehydration and predisposition to vascular thrombosis, these patients should receive heparin (unfractionated or low molecular weight) prophylaxis (5000 U heparin subcutaneously, usually twice daily).

CHRONIC COMPLICATIONS

Chronic complications include microvascular complications (nephropathy, retinopathy, and neuropathy) and macrovascular or cardiovascular complications (hypertension, coronary artery disease, peripheral vascular disease, and cerebrovascular disease). Several different mechanisms are responsible for the development of chronic complications and include activation of the polyol pathway (with accumulation of sorbitol), formation of glycated proteins and advanced glycation end products (cross-linked glycated proteins), abnormalities in lipid metabolism, increased oxidative damage, hyperinsulinemia, hyperperfusion of certain tissues, hyperviscosity, platelet dysfunction (increased aggregation), endothelial dysfunction, and activation of various growth factors.

MICROVASCULAR COMPLICATIONS

The incidence of microvascular complications is significantly higher in patients with T1DM than in those with T2DM.

Nephropathy

Diabetic nephropathy is the most common cause of ESRD in developed countries (about 30% of cases). About 20% to 30% of people with T1DM and T2DM develop nephropathy, and the incidence increases with duration of diabetes. Fewer people with T2DM than with T1DM progress to ESRD (20%

versus 75%, respectively, after 20 years). Certain ethnic and racial groups have high prevalence rates of severe nephropathy (Native Americans, Mexican Americans, and African Americans).

Initially, increased glomerular filtration rate (GFR) and renal blood flow occur in all patients and are not associated with any histologic changes. This condition progresses to glomerular hypertrophy, renal enlargement, expansion of the mesangial matrix, and thickening of the glomerular basement membrane, resulting in glomerulosclerosis (**Web Figs. 69-5, 69-6, and 69-7**). Subsequently, the GFR returns to normal, with an associated increase in intraglomerular pressure and the appearance of microalbuminuria (20 to 200 mcg per minute, 30 to 300 mg per 24 hours) 10 to 15 years after the diagnosis of diabetes (present in 30% of middle-aged patients with T1DM or T2DM). This *incipient* or *preclinical diabetic nephropathy* is followed by a decline in GFR as the albumin excretion rate increases.

Microalbuminuria is a risk factor for cardiovascular events and is associated with a 10- to 20-fold increased risk for progression to diabetic nephropathy. Rigorous control of blood glucose and blood pressure (using angiotensin II–converting enzyme [ACE] inhibitors or angiotensin II–receptor blockers [ARBs]) or use of ACE inhibitors or ARBs in nonhypertensive patients with microalbuminuria can prevent or even reverse the progression toward renal failure. β-blockers and nondihydropyridine calcium-channel antagonists, effective in reducing cardiovascular events, may also be considered, as may thiazide diuretics.

By about 15 years after the onset of diabetes, macroalbuminuria (>200 mcg per minute, >300 mg per 24 hours; dipstick positive) is generally present. Continued blood pressure control is essential, and some dietary protein restriction (0.6 to 0.8 g/kg per day) is probably helpful, but meticulous blood glucose control is unlikely to prevent the inexorable progression of overt diabetic nephropathy to ESRD. The rate of decline in GFR, however, may be slowed, but not halted, by blood pressure and glucose control with protein restriction. Measurement of serum creatinine is an inaccurate guide to the degree of GFR impairment. Within 5 years of the appearance of macroalbuminuria, GFR will have declined by 50% in about 50% of patients; within a further 3 to 4 years, one half of these patients will have ESRD. Dialysis (hemoperitoneal or peritoneal) or renal transplantation is initiated when the GFR is less than 15 mL per minute (serum creatinine ≥10 mg/dL) (see Chapter 28).

Screening for proteinuria should be performed annually in all patients, starting at the time of diagnosis in patients with T2DM and 5 years after the diagnosis in patients with T1DM. The simplest method of screening for microalbuminuria is measurement of the ratio of protein (albumin) to creatinine in a random spot urine specimen. This measurement correlates closely with 24-hour urinary protein estimations.

Retinopathy

The presence and severity of diabetic retinopathy are related to age at diagnosis and the duration of diabetes; 100% of patients with T1DM and 60% to 80% of those with T2DM are affected by 20 years. Retinopathy is the most common cause of blindness in persons between the ages of 20 and 74 years in the developed world. About 25% of patients with

T2DM may already have evidence of retinopathy at the time of diagnosis. The incidence of this complication is increased in Mexican Americans and African Americans.

Diabetic retinopathy is a progressive condition of increasing severity, accelerated by poor glycemic control (**Web Fig. 69-8**). *Background,* or *nonproliferative, retinopathy* consists of increased capillary permeability, dilation of venules, and the presence of microaneurysms (focal, saccular, and fusiform dilations of capillary walls as sequelae of loss of supporting pericytes and ischemic occlusion of retinal capillaries). At this stage, hemorrhages deep in the retina appear as dots, whereas more superficial nerve fiber layer hemorrhages are linear or resemble flames or *blots.* Leakage of plasma through permeable and ischemic capillary walls leads to the formation of hard exudates as the water is reabsorbed, leaving behind deep, intraretinal yellow deposits of proteins and lipids. These deposits may be present at any stage of diabetic retinopathy. Collections of hard exudates in a circular pattern *(circinates)* reflect the presence of retinal edema that pushes these exudates peripherally. When these exudates surround the macula, they highlight macular edema *(maculopathy),* a sight-threatening condition requiring urgent attention.

Retinal venous occlusion results in beading, reduplication, and venous loops. *Intraretinal microvascular abnormalities,* which are abnormal dilated capillaries within the retina, result from widespread capillary occlusion. Superficial retinal microinfarcts result in hypoxic necrosis of retinal nerve fibers and appear as white, *cotton-wool spots* with irregular margins. These changes signify a worsening of the retinopathy into the *preproliferative stage.* The widespread retinal ischemia and hypoxia represented by these changes result in the release of several angiogenic growth factors, which lead to the development of new vessels *(neovascularization)* on the retina, optic disc, or iris *(rubeosis iridis).* Inhibitors of protein kinase C, which block the production of vascular endothelial growth factor, are potentially beneficial. This stage is referred to as *proliferative retinopathy* and is also characterized by scarring. The new vessels are extremely fragile, extending through the internal limiting membrane, where they lie between the retina and vitreous, or attaching to the vitreous and extending into it. Bleeding into the preretinal (subhyaloid) space results in a boat-shaped hemorrhage. Hemorrhage from new vessels in the vitreous may cause sudden loss of vision. Neovascularization and fibrosis at the angle of the anterior chamber prevent normal drainage of aqueous and lead to *neovascular glaucoma* and a blind, painful eye. Shrinkage and retraction of the vitreous from the retina, which occurs with age, may result in hemorrhage from neovascularization, and traction on the retina from associated fibrous tissue. Further proliferation of fibrous tissue may lead to a traction retinal detachment with visual loss, most marked with macular involvement.

Premature development of *senile cataracts* occurs in patients with diabetes. *Snowflake lens opacities* develop in younger patients, particularly during periods of poor glycemic control. Referral to an ophthalmologist for urgent argon laser therapy is mandatory in patients with proliferative retinopathy, diabetic maculopathy, and possibly preproliferative retinopathy. This therapy can be sight-saving. *Vitrectomy* may be performed in patients with extensive, long-standing,

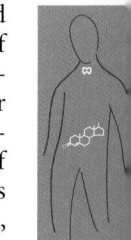

unresolving vitreal hemorrhage or when new traction retinal detachment affects the macula or is associated with a retinal tear.

Annual dilated funduscopic examination by an ophthalmologist should be performed in all patients with diabetes, starting 5 years after diagnosis in patients with T1DM. Improvement of glycemic control may transiently worsen retinopathy, before ultimately improving it over a longer period.

Neuropathy

The likelihood of involvement of the nervous system by diabetes increases with duration of disease and is influenced by the degree of glycemic control (occurring in up to 70% of people with diabetes). Any part of the peripheral or autonomic nervous system may be affected. *Peripheral polyneuropathy* occurs most commonly, which usually presents as a bilaterally symmetrical, distal, primarily sensory (with or without motor) polyneuropathy, with a *glove-and-stocking* distribution. Pain, numbness, hyperesthesias, and paresthesias progress to sensory loss. This condition, together with loss of proprioception, leads to an abnormal gait, with repeated trauma and fractures of the tarsal bones, sometimes resulting in the development of Charcot joints. These changes lead to abnormal pressures in the feet that, together with the soft tissue atrophy related to peripheral arterial insufficiency, result in foot ulcers that may progress to osteomyelitis and gangrene. Detailed, regular neurologic examination of all patients is essential, to elicit the early loss of light touch (using a 5.07/10 g monofilament), reflexes, and vibratory sensation. Painful neuropathies are difficult to treat, and, although they are self-limited, they may persist for years. Improvement in glycemic control should be the primary therapeutic goal. Analgesia should start with aspirin, acetaminophen, and nonsteroidal anti-inflammatory agents before codeine and addictive drugs such as pentazocine or narcotics are prescribed. Anticonvulsants, including phenytoin, carbamazepine, gabapentin, and pregabalin, as well as the antidepressant amitriptyline, may provide moderate relief. Burning pain may respond to the topical application of capsaicin cream. Use of plastic skin (e.g., OpSite film), transcutaneous nerve stimulation, and nerve block are sometimes effective for chronic pain.

Mononeuropathies usually present acutely, may involve any nerve in the body, and are generally self-limiting. The cranial nerves most commonly involved are the third, sixth, and fourth, in that order. *Radiculopathies* are self-limited painful sensory syndromes of one or more spinal nerves, usually of the chest or abdomen. *Diabetic amyotrophy* causing muscle atrophy and weakness commonly involves the anterior thigh muscles and pelvic girdle and may also be self-limited, resolving after several months.

Potential new therapies for diabetic peripheral neuropathy include aldose reductase inhibitors (inhibit excessive activity of the polyol pathway), aminoguanidine (inhibit formation of AGES), γ-linoleic acid (replacement is needed because of impaired production), antioxidants (e.g., α-lipoic acid), vasodilators, and recombinant human nerve growth factor.

Autonomic neuropathy of the sympathetic and/or parasympathetic systems has numerous presentations. Most commonly involved is the gastrointestinal tract, with gastric dysmotility (30% to 50%), gastroparesis, and small bowel bacterial overgrowth, responsible for delayed gastric emptying, early satiety, postprandial nausea, abdominal fullness, bloating and discomfort, constipation, and diarrhea (usually nocturnal). Gastropathy is frequently responsible for erratic and unpredictable blood glucose levels, with hyperglycemia itself exacerbating the dysmotility, even in people without diabetes. *Gastroparesis* may respond to treatment with metoclopramide or domperidone (dopamine D2 antagonists), erythromycin (motilin agonist) for bacterial overgrowth, cisapride (cholinergic agonist), or mosapride (selective serotonin 5-HT4 receptor agonist). *Diarrhea* may respond to loperamide or diphenoxylate and atropine. *Orthostatic hypotension* can be treated by attention to mechanical factors such as elevation of the head of the bed, gradual rising from a lying to standing position, use of support stockings, and sometimes use of fludrocortisone. *Cardiac rhythm disturbances* can result in syncope and cardiorespiratory arrest. *Bladder involvement* may result in urinary retention or incontinence. In men, *erectile dysfunction* is multifactorial and may also be related to vascular insufficiency or venous leaks. Arousal is the main problem in the sexual dysfunction of women with diabetes.

DIABETIC FOOT

Care of the feet of patients with diabetes is extremely important to prevent foot ulcers and amputations. Risk factors include distal symmetrical polyneuropathy, peripheral arterial insufficiency, areas of increased pressure, limited joint mobility and bony deformities, obesity, and chronic hyperglycemia. Patient education about foot care includes advice on daily foot inspection, appropriate footwear, drying and nail cutting, and referral to a podiatrist when necessary. Early detection and treatment of blisters, ulcers, trauma, and cellulitis may prevent progression to osteomyelitis and amputation. Treatment of ulcers may include débridement, antibiotics, growth-stimulating factors, reduction of weight bearing (elevation, casting), and improvement in arterial supply (surgical or medical).

MACROVASCULAR COMPLICATIONS

Cardiovascular and cerebrovascular diseases include hypertension, myocardial ischemia and infarction, transient ischemic attacks and strokes, and peripheral vascular disease. Seventy to 80% of people with diabetes die from a macrovascular event. The risk for such an event (2 to 4 times increased in patients with T2DM or >20% over 7 years) in people with diabetes is equivalent to that of nondiabetic patients with established cardiovascular disease (i.e., those who have already had a macrovascular event, e.g., postmyocardial infarction). Thus, all patients with diabetes and no prior cardiovascular event are considered *coronary heart disease,* or *cardiovascular disease, risk equivalents* (**Web Fig. 69-9**). Following a first cardiac event in people with diabetes, the chance of a second event increases dramatically to 45%. The pathogenesis of *atherosclerosis* (increasingly recognized as an inflammatory disease) and *vascular thrombosis* in people with diabetes is similar to that in people without diabetes, albeit markedly accelerated in the former. Tight glucose control, including acutely

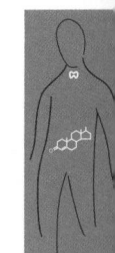

postmyocardial infarction, results in improvement in cardiovascular disease. Women with diabetes have the same risk profile as men at all ages. *Hypertension* (50% of patients with T2DM), dyslipidemia (40% of patients with T2DM at diagnosis), obesity, hyperglycemia, and smoking are major risk factors.

In people with diabetes, the risk for death from hypertension is greater than from hyperglycemia. Aggressive treatment of hypertension, to less than 130/80 mm Hg, reduces both macrovascular and microvascular complications and should preferably start with an ACE inhibitor or ARB, for added renal protection. All other classes of antihypertensive agents may be used, including selective β_1-blocking drugs, which are also used in the secondary prevention of myocardial infarction. β blockers may increase the severity of hypoglycemia by inhibiting glycogenolysis and gluconeogenesis and may mask the warning symptoms and signs of hypoglycemia by blunting the adrenergic response to hypoglycemia. However, the potential adverse effects of β blockers in patients with diabetes have not been consistently observed in the clinical setting. Most hypertensive patients require combination antihypertensive therapy, using, on average, three different classes of agents, including diuretics. In hypertensive patients with microalbuminuria or macroalbuminuria, nondihydropyridine calcium channel blockers may be added to the list of other drugs.

The procoagulant state of the blood in patients with diabetes is caused by *platelet hypersensitivity* to the aggregating properties of thromboxane (synthesized in excess), as well as disordered fibrinolysis and increased levels of the prothrombotic mediator, PAI-1 (see "Metabolic Syndrome," earlier in this chapter). Low-dose aspirin (81 to 162 mg per day) is recommended as primary prevention in patients with diabetes who are at high risk for cardiovascular disease, as well as secondary prevention in those with evidence of large vessel disease. Additionally, smoking cessation and management of obesity, dyslipidemia, hypertension, and hyperglycemia, together with initiation of safe exercise, all decrease the risk and severity of macrovascular disease. Lifestyle modification is the single most important therapeutic intervention in addressing insulin resistance, glucose control, and overall cardiovascular risk. Glycemic control is a stronger risk factor for microvascular disease than for macrovascular.

CURE AND PREVENTION OF DIABETES

The concepts of prevention, cure, and treatment of diabetes are all part of a continuum without absolute borders. The influence of any intervention will depend on what point in time action is taken.

Metabolic control of diabetes is possible through replacement of insulin. Insulin replacement may be in the form of exogenous insulin (injections, insulin pump; open or closed loop [artificial pancreas]), endogenous insulin (transplantation of pancreas, islets of Langerhans, or β cells), or insulin gene therapy. Besides the insulin pump and insulin injections, none of these modalities has achieved adequate independence as a viable long term therapy.

Primary prevention of diabetes is the holy grail of diabetes research. Although still limited, the improved ability to predict the development of types 1 and 2 diabetes in certain select high-risk groups has resulted in several separate national and international clinical trials to study whether certain therapies administered to asymptomatic high-risk individuals, or newly diagnosed patients, may prevent the appearance of either type of diabetes. In people at high risk for developing T1DM, preventing or altering the autoimmune process has included avoidance of intact dairy proteins, use of nicotinamide, immune modulators, monoclonal antibody preparations, and administration of intravenous and oral insulins. To date, none of these approaches has proved successful. Several clinical trials are still ongoing. Prevention of T2DM in high-risk individuals (e.g., prediabetes, prior GDM, PCOS [see Table 69-1]) has focused on lifestyle modifications to increase exercise, improve healthy nutrition, and control weight. This approach has proved highly successful in reducing the incidence of T2DM by as much as 58%, compared with a 31% reduction in incidence using pharmacotherapy (specifically metformin). Pharmacotherapy to reduce insulin resistance and improve β-cell function, including use of currently available oral antidiabetic agents, is also being investigated.

Secondary prevention of the development of complications of diabetes and tertiary prevention of progression of established complications to end-stage disease was discussed previously.

Prospectus for the Future

The pathogeneses of diabetes and its complications continue to be elucidated, opening original avenues for targeted therapy. New approaches to controlling and modifying this disease, using endogenous physiologic pathways, include use of amylin and incretin mimetics. The glitazars constitute a group of combination preparations of PPAR agonists: α (target of T2DMs) with γ (target of fibrates), and α with γ and δ. The combination of PPAR-α and -γ in a single compound delivers dual management of hyperlipidemia (dose-dependent decrease in TG, increase in HDL, and decrease in apo B) and improved tissue insulin sensitivity, with additional benefits in the metabolic syndrome. They are also responsible for reductions in albumin-to-creatinine ratio, hs-CRP, PAI-1, and fibrinogen. The improvements in plasma lipid and glucose levels, particularly in the postprandial state, hold promise for cardiovascular risk reduction. The list of additional benefits proposed for these combination agents includes an *antiproliferative* role, angiotensin II antagonism, antioxidant, antihypertensive, correction of endothelial dysfunction, reduction in hypertensive and postmyocardial infarction cardiac fibrosis, reduction in visceral, hepatic, and myocellular adipose accumulation, and upregulation of macrophage lipoprotein lipase. These agents may be responsible for weight gain or dyspnea and should not be used in patients with New York Heart Association (NYHA) class III or IV heart failure or in those already taking TZDs and fibrates. At this time, no member of this class has received FDA approval.

Prospectus for the Future—Cont'd

The endocannabinoid system (ECS) is an endogenous signaling system comprising two types of receptors, CB1 and CB2, and several endogenous ligands, endocannabinoids. This system is tonically overactive in human obesity, leading to weight gain, hepatic lipogenesis, insulin resistance, dyslipidemia, and impaired glucose homeostasis. This system potentially provides novel therapeutic targets to control the host of cardiometabolic risk factors so rife in T2DM.

Ninety percent of the renal filtered glucose is reabsorbed by the low-affinity/high-capacity Na$^+$ glucose co-transporter 2 (SGLT-2) and facilitated diffusion glucose transporter 2 (GLUT-2) in the renal proximal tubular cells. Several selective inhibitors of SGLT-2 are being developed. They exhibit glucose-lowering effects independently of insulin secretion and increase urinary glucose excretion by inhibiting renal glucose reabsorption. These drugs may provide a new and unique approach to the treatment of diabetes mellitus.

In the evolving pharmacotherapeutic approaches to treating disease, diabetes, hyperlipidemia, and cardiovascular diseases in particular, the concept of a *polypill* to manage several separate but connected metabolic problems is taking hold (e.g., a combination of antihypertensive, antilipid, antioxidant, antihyperglycemic, antiplatelet, and possibly anti-inflammatory agents).

Adipose cell-derived adiponectin and adipokines will play increasingly important roles in the management of T2DM.

Algorithms that dictate the order of prescribing therapeutic agents for blood glucose control, is changing in the light of new therapies such that drugs responsible for β-cell preservation and regeneration will be advocated as first-line treatments before β-cell secretagogues and the other currently available antihyperglycemic agents.

Evaluation of alternate insulin formulations and analogues, delivery routes, and devices includes oral, buccal, nasal, pulmonary, dermal, rectal, and conjunctival. A long-acting polyethylene glycol (pegylated) inhaled insulin is currently under development. Exubera is the first recombinant human inhaled insulin powder to be marketed to the public. It is taken before meals and appears to achieve blood glucose levels comparable to levels achieved with injected insulins. This drug has been withdrawn by the manufacturing pharmaceutical company apparently as a result of poor patient and physician acceptance.

Research proceeds on mechanical devices such as an implantable artificial pancreas, continuous glucose monitoring and sensing, and noninvasive glucose sensors.

Inflammatory markers in diabetes are now well established. The role of anti-inflammatory therapy is still a matter for discussion and clinical trial evaluation.

Cure of this multifaceted chronic disease grows closer. Improvements in islet cell transplantation technology and antirejection protocols are improving prognosis in these patients. β-cell preservation, regeneration, and proliferation, as well as pancreatic ductal cell differentiation to restore pancreatic β-cell mass with the aid of incretins and islet neogenesis gene-associated protein, are promising lines of investigation. Stem cell and gene therapy, too, hold the potential prospects of cure. Anti-CD3 monoclonal antibody alone and in combination with proinsulin peptide is being tested in human phase III studies in patients with newly diagnosed T1DM. A short course of anti-CD3 in phase II studies of patients with recently diagnosed T1DM has demonstrated preserved β-cell function and reduced insulin need for up to 18 months after treatment. Studies in mice have demonstrated reversal of recent-onset T1DM with no recurrence during their lifetimes.

The status of bariatric surgery in the management algorithm of diabetes is currently under review. Successful, minimally invasive laparoscopic techniques are yielding promising results in morbidly obese individuals.

Prediction and ultimately prevention still depend on elucidation of the exact genetic, constitutional, and environmental factors responsible for the group of diseases called diabetes mellitus.

References

American Diabetes Association: Clinical practice recommendations 2008. Diabetes Care 31(Suppl 1):S1-S85, 2008.

American Diabetes Association: Economic costs of Diabetes in the U.S. in 2007. Diabetes Care 31:1-20, 2008.

Diabetes Control and Complications Trial Research Group: The effect of intensive treatment of diabetes on the development and progression of long-term complications in insulin-dependent diabetes mellitus. N Engl J Med 329:977-986, 1993.

Diabetes Prevention Research Group: Reduction in the evidence of type 2 diabetes with life-style intervention or metformin. N Engl J Med 346:393-403, 2002.

Einhorn D, Rosenstock J (eds): Type 2 diabetes and cardiovascular disease. Endocrinol Metab Clin North Am 34:1-235, 2005.

Keymeulen B, Vandemeulebroucke E, Ziegler AG, et al: Insulin needs after CD3-antibody therapy in new-onset Type 1 diabetes. N Engl J Med 352:2598-2608, 2005.

U.K. Prospective Diabetes Study (UKPDS) Group: Intensive blood-glucose control with sulfonylureas or insulin compared with conventional treatment and risk of complications in patients with type 2 diabetes (UKPDS 33). Lancet 352:854-865, 1998.

U.K. Prospective Diabetes Study (UKPDS) Group: Effect of intensive blood-glucose control with metformin on complications in overweight patients with type 2 diabetes (UKPDS 34). Lancet 352:837-853, 1998.

Van den Berghe G, Wouters P, Weekers F, et al: Intensive insulin therapy in critically ill patients. N Engl J Med 345:1359-1367, 2001.

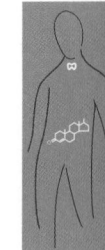

Hypoglycemia

Philip S. Barnett

Definition

Hypoglycemia is defined as a recorded blood glucose concentration lower than normal. Plasma glucose is maintained on a day-to-day basis within a narrow range of 72 to 144 mg/dL (4 to 8 mmol/L) by several hormonal and neural factors. Failure of any of these glucoregulatory mechanisms may result in hypoglycemia. Clinically significant hypoglycemia is rare and is based on the demonstration of Whipple triad: signs and symptoms of hypoglycemia, in the presence of a low plasma glucose concentration (<45 mg/dL), that are relieved by restoration of plasma glucose to normal concentrations. Low plasma glucose values without signs and symptoms, or vice versa, do not constitute clinical hypoglycemia.

Physiology of Glucose Homeostasis

Normal fasting and preprandial plasma glucose values are less than 110 mg/dL (6.1 mmol/L). Postprandially, increases in blood glucose and insulin concentrations, influenced by meal composition, size, and time of day, peak at 1 hour and return to normal after 3 to 4 hours. Two-hour postprandial glucose values do not exceed 140 mg/dL (7.8 mmol/L). The postprandial state comprises the first 4 to 5 hours after a meal. Insulin is the predominant hormone, suppressing hepatic glucose production, promoting glycogen storage, and stimulating extrahepatic glucose utilization. As plasma glucose levels decline (<80 mg/dL), so does insulin secretion. Peripheral glucose utilization declines, whereas there is an increase in glycogenolysis, gluconeogenesis, lipolysis, and proteolysis, resulting in the synthesis of gluconeogenic precursors: lactate, pyruvate, amino acids, and fatty acids. The postabsorptive state begins 4 to 5 hours after a meal.

The response to low plasma glucose levels, *glucose counter-regulation*, occurs on several levels. Central nervous system detection of low glucose levels stimulates the hypothalamus and pituitary to release growth hormone and adrenocorticotropin. Catecholamines, particularly epinephrine, are released from the adrenal medulla, and cortisol is released from the adrenal cortex. Insulin secretion is reduced, and glucagon secretion is augmented as a direct effect of low blood glucose concentration on pancreatic islets and in response to central neurogenic stimulation. Of the four counter-regulatory hormones (glucagon, epinephrine, growth hormone, and cortisol), glucagon is the most important in the acute response to hypoglycemia, 65 to 70 mg/dL. It acts rapidly to increase hepatic glucose production through *glycogenolysis,* the major source of fasting glucose, and *gluconeogenesis,* which becomes increasingly important as glycogen stores are depleted. Hepatic glycogen stores are usually sufficient to maintain glucose levels for about 8 hours. In patients with type 1 diabetes mellitus (T1DM) of more than 3 to 5 years' duration, the glucagon response is lost. Epinephrine is also part of the rapid counter-regulatory hormone response to hypoglycemia and plays a major role when it replaces the lost glucagon response in patients with T1DM. Epinephrine is also subsequently lost as a response to hypoglycemia 10 to 15 years after diagnosis in about 25% of patients with diabetes. Epinephrine inhibits insulin secretion and thereby inhibits glucose uptake by muscle. It stimulates glycogenolysis and lipolysis, and the resultant increase in free fatty acids (FFAs) acts as a stimulus for hepatic gluconeogenesis. Growth hormone and cortisol characterize the delayed response to hypoglycemia (2 to 3 hours), enhancing glucagon's effect and antagonizing the action of insulin by accelerating hepatic gluconeogenesis, suppressing muscle glucose utilization, and stimulating lipolysis, ketogenesis, and proteolysis. With prolonged hypoglycemia, the liver responds through autoregulation with an increase in glucose production. For growth hormone, these defense mechanisms start at a blood glucose level of 60 to 65 mg/dL, and less than 60 mg/dL for cortisol.

SIGNS AND SYMPTOMS OF HYPOGLYCEMIA

The various signs and symptoms of hypoglycemia appear at different glycemic thresholds and in response to different

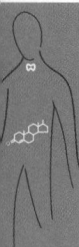

Table 70-1 Signs and Symptoms of Hypoglycemia

Neuroglycopenic

Warmth, weakness
Headache
Tiredness, drowsiness
Fainting, dizziness
Blurred vision
Mental dullness, confusion
Abnormal behavior
Amnesia
Seizures
Loss of consciousness
Coma
Death

Neurogenic

Sweating
Pallor
Hunger
Tachycardia or hypertension
Palpitations
Tremor, shaking
Nervousness, anxiety
Irritability
Tingling, paresthesias (mouth and fingers)
Nausea, vomiting

mechanisms. They can be divided into *neurogenic* (increased autonomic nervous system activity) and *neuroglycopenic* (depressed activity of the central nervous system) (Table 70-1). Signs and symptoms may vary among patients but are fairly constant for a given person. Accommodation to hypoglycemia results from a resetting of glycemic thresholds. As many as 25% of patients with diabetes, mainly type 1, may suffer from *hypoglycemic unawareness,* with serious consequences. Loss of warning symptoms and signs results from progressive loss of glucagon and epinephrine responses over time, lowering of the glycemic threshold by intensive therapy or repeated hypoglycemic episodes, and autonomic dysfunction resulting from the diabetic process. The delayed counter-regulatory responses of growth hormone and cortisol are usually too late to prevent neuroglycopenia. A prior episode of hypoglycemia often impairs detection of a subsequent one, especially if it occurs soon after the first. In some patients, hypoglycemia awareness may be restored if hypoglycemia is rigorously prevented.

The definition of a normal blood glucose level depends on the circumstances, the sex of the patient, and the sample tested: arterial, venous, or capillary blood, and whole blood versus plasma or serum. Venous plasma is the usual sample measured, and its glucose concentration is about 15% higher than that of whole blood. Patients with diabetes use capillary whole blood for daily self-monitoring purposes. Some newer glucose-sensing devices sample interstitial fluid. Normal plasma glucose values during a fast are different in men and women; in men, the fasting plasma glucose concentration is 55 mg/dL (3.1 mmol/L) at 24 hours and 50 mg/dL (2.8 mmol/L) at 48 and 72 hours, whereas, in premenopausal women, it may be as low as 35 mg/dL (1.9 mmol/L) at 24 hours without symptoms of hypoglycemia. Exercise in healthy persons generally does not lead to a fall in glucose levels.

Concern about hypoglycemia stems from its possible devastating effects on the brain. The central nervous system cannot synthesize glucose or store enough glycogen for more than a few minutes' glucose supply. The brain cannot use FFAs as an energy source, and ketone bodies, which are generated late, are not useful in acute hypoglycemia. Medium-chain triglycerides appear to protect the brain from injury during acute hypoglycemia. Because glucose is the predominant metabolic fuel for the central nervous system, significant hypoglycemia can cause acute and permanent brain dysfunction, and, if prolonged, it may result in brain death.

Acute hypoglycemia causes cognitive dysfunction, which does not appear to be permanent in most patients with T2DM. Elderly patients do appear, however, to develop a permanent subtle form of cognitive dysfunction. T2DM is associated with an increased risk for dementia. Repeated hypoglycemic episodes appear to modify cognitive responses and reduce hypoglycemic awareness through some form of cerebral adaptation.

GLYCEMIC THRESHOLDS

Despite the ranges of normality discussed previously, the glycemic thresholds discussed in this paragraph apply to the general population. Falling plasma glucose concentrations trigger a set sequence of events. Within the physiologic plasma glucose range, a drop in glucose to less than 80 mg/dL (4.5 to 4.6 mmol/L) results in decreased insulin secretion. At levels slightly lower than the normal range, 70 mg/dL (3.6 to 3.8 mmol/L), secretion of the insulin counter-regulatory hormones occurs: glucagon and epinephrine at 68 mg/dL, growth hormone at 60 mg/dL, and cortisol at 60 mg/dL (3.2 mmol/L). The glycemic threshold for symptoms of hypoglycemia is about 54 mg/dL (3 mmol/L) and, for cognitive dysfunction, about 47 mg/dL (2.6 mmol/L). These glycemic thresholds vary in response to the level of glucose control, particularly in patients with diabetes; poorly controlled diabetes with persistent hyperglycemia results in higher glucose thresholds, whereas lower glucose thresholds are reset after single or repeated hypoglycemic episodes. In some people, major symptoms of central nervous system dysfunction may not occur until the plasma glucose concentration reaches 20 mg/dL because these people have a compensatory increase in cerebral blood flow.

Clinical Classification of Hypoglycemia

Hypoglycemia occurs most commonly as a side effect of the treatment of diabetes mellitus, usually associated with impairment of insulin counter-regulatory responses. Severe hypoglycemia occurs in as many as 25% of patients with diabetes. It is more frequently associated with young patients and older adults, especially if the patient is fasting, has erratic meal times, has alcohol on an empty stomach (decreased endogenous glucose production), has recently engaged in strenuous exercise (up to 12 hours), has renal impairment (reducing insulin excretion), has low glycosylated hemoglobin (HbA$_{1c}$), has had a short duration of diabetes, or has had a prior severe hypoglycemic episode, and is more common during sleep. The incidence increases with attempts to achieve euglycemia through tight control of glucose concentrations; 65% of patients with T1DM in the Diabetes Control and Complications Trial and 11% of patients with type 2 diabetes mellitus (T2DM) in the United Kingdom Prospective Diabetes Study had episodes of hypoglycemia that required assistance of a second party to administer therapy with either intramuscular or subcutaneous glucagon or intravenous glucose. Men tend to suffer from hypoglycemia more commonly than women. Patients with T1DM have longer hypoglycemic episodes and greater frequency than patients with T2DM treated with insulin or oral hypoglycemic agents. Two to 4% of T1DM patients will die of a hypoglycemic episode. In patients with T2DM, duration of hypoglycemia is greater at night, especially after midnight, than during the day.

Other causes of hypoglycemia in patients with diabetes include overdose of insulin or oral insulin secretagogues, missed or delayed meals, and uncompensated (without supplemental calories or a decrease in insulin dose) exercise (immediate or delayed, up to 24 hours). Increased insulin sensitivity may also be responsible. *Nocturnal hypoglycemia,* exhibited by night sweats, snoring, vivid dreams, and deep sleep, occurs in as many as 50% of patients receiving insulin. Maximal insulin sensitivity at 2:00 or 3:00 AM may coincide with peak exogenous insulin action. Treatment usually includes changing one or more of the following: timing of intermediate-acting insulin from dinner to bedtime, insulin dose, type of insulin (e.g., glargine), type of insulin delivery (e.g., insulin pump), time of meal, and meal composition. In addition, adding a snack and using uncooked cornstarch can be considered.

The following discussion addresses the separate causes of hypoglycemia listed in Table 70-2.

FASTING (POSTABSORPTIVE) HYPOGLYCEMIA

Fasting (postabsorptive) hypoglycemia results from an imbalance between hepatic glucose production (decreased) and peripheral glucose utilization (increased).

Drugs

Insulin, sulfonylureas, meglitinides, and alcohol are the most common causes of fasting hypoglycemia. Insulin is a well-recognized cause of hypoglycemia in the treatment of diabetes. Elevated serum insulin levels in the absence of elevated C-peptide levels can detect *factitious hypoglycemia* resulting from the covert use of insulin by persons with and without diabetes.

Overdose with sulfonylureas occurs commonly in elderly patients taking long-acting and highly potent agents such as chlorpropamide or glyburide. This overdose is usually inadvertent but occasionally intentional (factitious), and it may be determined by measuring serum or urine sulfonylurea levels. Because of the mechanism of sulfonylurea action (insulin secretagogue), insulin and C-peptide levels are elevated. Patients with sulfonylurea-induced hypoglycemia should not be discharged from the emergency room after

---

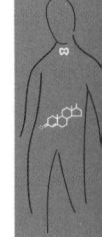

Table 70-2 **Clinical Classification of Hypoglycemia**
Fasting (Postabsorptive) Hypoglycemia
Drugs
Insulin, sulfonylureas,* meglitinides,* alcohol
β-adrenergic antagonists (nonselective)
Quinine, pentamidine*
Salicylates, sulfonamides, phenylbutazone, bishydroxycoumarin, ranitidine, doxepin, imipramine, cimetidine
Others
Critical illness
Hepatic, renal, and cardiac dysfunction
Adrenal insufficiency†
Sepsis or shock
Malnutrition or anorexia nervosa
Hormone deficiencies
Hypopituitarism (growth hormone)
Catecholamine deficiency (epinephrine)
Glucagon deficiency
Endogenous hyperinsulinemia
Pancreatic β-cell disorders
Tumor (insulinoma)
Nontumor
β-cell secretagogue (e.g., sulfonylurea, meglitinide)
Autoimmune hypoglycemia
Insulin autoantibodies
Insulin receptor autoantibodies
Islet β-cell antibodies
Addison's disease†
Ectopic insulin secretion (rare)
Exogenous hyperinsulinemia
Hypoglycemia of infancy and childhood
Non–β-cell tumors
Reactive (Postprandial) Hypoglycemia
Alimentary hypoglycemia
Idiopathic (functional) hypoglycemia
Congenital enzyme deficiencies in adults
Hereditary fructose intolerance
Galactosemia

*Responsible for endogenous hyperinsulinemia.
†Cortisol deficiency may result from adrenal insufficiency from numerous causes, including infection, hemorrhagic destruction, and autoimmune disease.
Adapted from Cryer PE: Hypoglycemia: Pathophysiology, Diagnosis and Management. New York, Oxford University Press, 1997.

---

initial normalization of plasma glucose concentrations because hypoglycemia recurs soon afterward as a result of the long half-life of many of these agents, which may be even longer in patients with comorbid conditions such as renal dysfunction. Several days of continuous glucose treatment may be required before the hypoglycemia resolves. Hypoglycemia related to meglitinide, or D-phenylalanine derivative therapy or overdose, would not be expected to be as severe as that caused by sulfonylureas because of its short duration of action.

Excessive alcohol consumption is a common cause of hypoglycemia. In patients with diabetes treated with oral agents or insulin, the combination with alcohol can be dangerous. Hypoglycemia may occur many hours after ingestion of alcohol (*morning after the night before*). Alcohol suppresses hepatic gluconeogenesis, not glycogenolysis, and hypoglycemia occurs in malnourished patients with chronic alcoholism or following a several-day binge of alcohol consumption with minimal food intake (depleted hepatic glycogen reserves).

Nonselective β_2-adrenergic antagonists may cause hypoglycemia in patients with diabetes (especially type 1) who do not have a normal glucagon counter-regulatory response and depend on the adrenergic response to hypoglycemia. β_2-Adrenergic antagonists mask the adrenergic symptoms and impair recovery from hypoglycemia. These agents also reduce the glycogenolytic response to epinephrine in muscle. Low doses of β_1-selective adrenergic antagonists do not produce these effects, although their selectivity is incomplete in high doses.

Pentamidine (particularly parenteral), through β-cell destruction, causes acute insulin release with hypoglycemia. Following this acute phase, the destroyed β cells fail to produce insulin, and hyperglycemia ensues. In children, salicylates may lead to increased insulin secretion through prostaglandin inhibition. Quinine can cause excessive pancreatic insulin release. Sulfonamides may rarely be responsible.

Critical Illness

In hospitalized patients, the most common cause of hypoglycemia is use of drugs, especially insulin. Single- or multiple-organ system failures (particularly hepatic, renal, cardiac, and adrenal), malnutrition, sepsis, and shock are next. The mechanism of hypoglycemia in each setting is multifactorial and not always entirely clear. Disease or failure of one organ system may affect another system, resulting in hypoglycemia, such as that seen in right ventricular cardiac failure causing hepatic congestion. Hepatic failure results in impaired gluconeogenesis as well as an inability to store and release glycogen. Renal failure may lead to prolongation of the half-life of hypoglycemia-inducing agents (sulfonylureas, meglitinides, and insulin). Malnutrition also plays a major role in renal failure as a cause of hypoglycemia. In starvation, there is loss of adipose tissue and gluconeogenic precursors. Insulin antibodies and hypothyroidism may delay insulin clearance and increase the risk for hypoglycemia. In adrenal insufficiency, lack of cortisol, which normally supports gluconeogenesis, may result in hypoglycemia. Sepsis is associated with increased glucose utilization in excess of glucose production. Severe malaria may be associated with hypoglycemia resulting from increased glucose utilization by parasitized red blood cells.

Insulinoma

Insulinoma is a rare pancreatic β-cell tumor that has an incidence of 1 in 250,000 patient-years and is more common in women (60%) than in men. It occurs at all ages; the median age at diagnosis is 50 years in sporadic instances and 23 years in patients with multiple endocrine neoplasia type I syndrome (8% to 10% of patients). Most of these tumors are benign (90% to 95%), solitary (93%), confined to the pancreas (99%), and small (average, 1 to 2 cm). Characteristically, insulinomas remain undiagnosed or misdiagnosed (20%) as psychiatric or neurologic disorders for several years. Long-term excessive insulin secretion, or *hyperinsulinemia*, which is not responsive to falling glucose concentrations in the fasting state, results in persistent hypoglycemia. Patients eat frequently to stave off the hypoglycemia and may gain weight (20%). Adaptation to the hypoglycemia

Table 70-3 **Protocol for Performing a 72-Hour Fast**
1. Patient admitted to hospital. Stop all nonessential medications. Calorie- and caffeine-free drinks are permitted. Start fast after evening meal at 1800 hr.
2. Blood glucose level monitored by bedside reflectance glucose meter every 4 hr and when symptoms of hypoglycemia develop. The presence of urinary ketones confirms that the patient is fasting.
3. When symptoms of hypoglycemia develop accompanied by a blood glucose level of ≤50 mg/dL (plasma glucose of ≤45 mg/dL), draw *diagnostic labs*, consisting of a fasting plasma glucose concentration; β-hydroxybutyrate serum insulin, C-peptide, and proinsulin levels; and a serum sample for sulfonylurea agents and insulin-like growth factor I (IGF-I) and IGF-II levels (the latter three to be sent only once per fast). The fast is terminated at this time.
4. In the absence of documented hypoglycemia at the end of 72 hr, the fast is terminated. Vigorous exercise for 2 hr may result in a fall in blood glucose. If the patient is symptomatic, give 1 mg of glucagon, intravenously or intramuscularly.
5. The patient is fed a meal and is discharged from the hospital.
6. If severe, persistent hypoglycemia is documented, the patient may need to be started on medication, such as diazoxide, to prevent further episodes of hypoglycemia while the work-up is proceeding.

over time results in manifestation of neuroglycopenic symptoms far more commonly than neurogenic symptoms. Most patients have fasting hypoglycemia (plasma glucose <45 mg/dL), demonstrated by a 72-hour fast (Table 70-3), and inappropriately elevated serum insulin, C-peptide, and proinsulin levels (>20% of total insulin). Some patients have reactive hypoglycemia as well. A C-peptide suppression test, in which endogenous insulin and C-peptide are normally suppressed during an insulin infusion, is impaired in the presence of an insulinoma. This test is not routinely performed.

After the biochemical diagnosis of an insulinoma, surgical resection by an experienced surgeon is generally recommended, irrespective of negative tumor localization studies. Localization of insulinomas using computed tomography, ultrasound (including endoscopic), magnetic resonance imaging, celiac axis angiography, aortography, or transhepatic portal venous sampling may be unsuccessful because of the generally small size of these tumors. An octreotide scan may prove useful. At operation, tumors are often found by intraoperative ultrasound or palpation of the pancreas. Distal pancreatectomy is sometimes performed if no tumor is found during the surgical procedure.

In patients who are unwilling to undergo surgical treatment, in patients awaiting surgery, or in those in whom surgical treatment has failed, medical therapy using diazoxide, which inhibits insulin secretion, or octreotide is indicated. Continuous subcutaneous infusion of glucagon prevents hypoglycemia. In patients with malignant insulinoma, streptozotocin, with or without doxorubicin or fluorouracil, has been used.

Non–β-Cell Tumors

Fasting hypoglycemia may be caused by a wide variety of rare, non–β-cell tumors. Many (about 50%) are large, slow-growing mesenchymal tumors, which are often malignant. More than one third of these tumors are retroperitoneal, one third intra-abdominal, and the rest intrathoracic. Epithelial tumors include hepatocellular carcinomas (about 25%), adrenocortical carcinomas (5% to 10%), and gastrointestinal (carcinoid) tumors (5% to 10%). Lymphomas account for 5% to 10%. In most patients, overproduction of insulin-like growth factor II (IGF-II) and, more particularly, the incompletely processed form, *big* IGF-II, is responsible for hypoglycemia as a result of their direct insulin-like actions as well as their suppression of glucagon and growth hormone and hence IGF-I levels.

Diagnosis is made based on hypoglycemia in a patient with a known tumor or elevated IGF-II levels. A 72-hour fast reveals hypoglycemia with appropriately suppressed serum insulin, C-peptide, and proinsulin levels. Treatment involves tumor resection. If surgical treatment is not completely successful, glucocorticoids may be beneficial.

Insulin and Insulin Receptor Autoantibodies

Hypoglycemia may result from production of insulin autoantibodies and insulin receptor autoantibodies, which are extremely rare and may be associated with other autoimmune disorders. Antibody binding to insulin may result in hypoglycemia by releasing insulin at an inappropriate time or by preventing its degradation. Insulin receptor antibodies may be *blocking*, causing insulin resistance. Alternatively, antibodies with receptor-agonist activity may produce hypoglycemia with elevated C-peptide levels.

REACTIVE (POSTPRANDIAL) HYPOGLYCEMIA

Reactive (postprandial) hypoglycemia typically occurs within 4 hours of food consumption; glucose levels fall more rapidly than insulin levels. Some people with impaired glucose tolerance initially have a delayed excessive insulin response to a meal that results in reactive hypoglycemia. In all forms of fasting hypoglycemia, patients may also demonstrate reactive hypoglycemia.

Alimentary Hypoglycemia

Alimentary hypoglycemia occurs in people who have undergone gastric surgery (gastrectomy, gastrojejunostomy, pyloroplasty, gastric bypass, or vagotomy) and consists of postprandial vasomotor symptoms: palpitations, tachycardia, lightheadedness, sweating, postural hypotension, and sometimes abdominal discomfort and vomiting. This *early dumping syndrome* occurs within 30 minutes of eating and is caused by rapid emptying of food from the stomach into the duodenum, associated with a large fluid shift into the gut lumen. The *late dumping syndrome* occurs between 90 and 180 minutes after eating, resulting in dizziness, lightheadedness, palpitations, sweating, confusion, and rarely syncope. Rapid emptying into the upper small bowel of a meal rich in simple carbohydrates results in abrupt hyperglycemia, enhanced secretion of insulinotropic incretins,

early marked hyperinsulinemia, and subsequent hypoglycemia. Treatment of both syndromes includes frequent small meals and elimination of simple sugars and liquids at mealtime.

Idiopathic Hypoglycemia

The existence of idiopathic hypoglycemia, an overdiagnosed condition, is still in dispute. In most patients, adrenergic symptoms, which are usually vague, do not occur simultaneously with biochemical hypoglycemia and are not relieved by consuming food. Occasionally, artificial testing situations (5-hour oral glucose tolerance test [OGTT]; 72-hour fast) may suggest the diagnosis, but these findings are not borne out following consumption of a mixed meal.

Diagnostic Work-Up of Hypoglycemia

A thorough history and physical examination are crucial. Hypoglycemia occurs most commonly in patients with drug-treated diabetes mellitus. Confirmation of hypoglycemia is essential before any work-up. Ambulatory patients can be trained in self-monitoring of blood glucose (SMBG), particularly during symptomatic episodes. However, frequent SMBG may miss as many as 50% of hypoglycemic episodes. Use of a continuous glucose monitoring system (CGMS) may be helpful in this setting, with the patient recording symptoms. If blood glucose levels are low (<50 mg/dL) and the symptoms resolve after carbohydrate ingestion, the patient probably has true hypoglycemia. If symptoms are present without documentation of hypoglycemia, an alternate explanation must be sought. If hypoglycemia occurs in the fed state, after excluding a history of gastric surgery, the likely cause is impaired glucose tolerance (confirmed by OGTT) or, in rare cases, idiopathic reactive hypoglycemia (diagnosis by exclusion). If reactive hypoglycemia is diagnosed, the patient should consult a dietitian for a diet plan designed to ameliorate these episodes (e.g., frequent low-carbohydrate meals).

Fasting hypoglycemia is more likely to be caused by an organic medical problem, although some of the underlying disorders (such as insulinoma and adrenal insufficiency) can produce both fasting and reactive hypoglycemia (see Table 70-2). Adrenal insufficiency should be ruled out with a cosyntropin test. When patients are hospitalized and are acutely ill, the distinction between fasting and reactive hypoglycemia is less clear; the work-up is then based on an understanding of the patient's underlying medical problems and therapies and the influence of these factors on blood glucose homeostasis.

The standard evaluation of hypoglycemia attributable to any other underlying cause includes hospital admission for a supervised 72-hour fast (see Table 70-3). During the fast, patients are only allowed noncaloric, noncaffeinated beverages and essential medications. These patients should be active during the day. About 75% of patients with an insulinoma develop symptomatic hypoglycemia within the first 24 hours, 10% in the next 24 hours, and only 5% in the final 24 hours. Difficulties in performing the fast arise when blood glucose levels fall to less than 50 mg/dL and the patient has no symptoms of hypoglycemia or when the patient develops

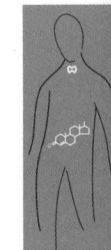

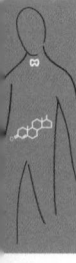

Table 70-4 Interpretation of Results from a 72-Hour Fast

Condition	Plasma Glucose (mg/dL)	Insulin (mcU/mL)	C-Peptide (nmol/L)	Proinsulin (pmol/L)	Plasma Sulfonylurea Level (nmol/L)	Insulin-like Growth Factor II
Normal*	≥45 in men, >36 in women	<6	<0.2	<5	—	—
Insulinoma	≤45	>6	>0.2	>5	—	—
Exogenous insulin	≤45	≥6†	<0.2	<5	—	—
Sulfonylurea agents	≤45	≥6	≥0.2	≥5	>0.2	—
Tumor secreting	≤45	≤6	<0.2	<5	—	+(↓ IGF-I)

*Normal insulin, C-peptide, and proinsulin levels may be higher if blood glucose levels are not less than 60 mg/dL.
†Insulin levels may be very high (100 mcU/mL) in these patients.
IGF, insulin-like growth factor; —, present; + elevated.
Adapted from Service FJ: Hypoglycemic disorders. N Engl J Med 332:1144-1152, 1995.

symptoms with normal blood glucose levels. In the former situation, continued measuring blood glucose levels should be performed, with the patient under close medical observation, until the concentration falls to less than 50 mg/dL. In the latter instance, the fast can be continued as long as is clinically warranted to convince both patient and physician that the symptoms are not associated with hypoglycemia. Table 70-4 summarizes the expected findings in various conditions at the completion of the fast.

Artifactual or pseudo hypoglycemia is a test-tube phenomenon caused by excessive glucose utilization by elevated leukocytes in certain chronic leukemias, hemolytic anemia, and polycythemia. Concern about technical problems with sample collection, storage, and analysis warrants repeat testing.

Factitious fasting hypoglycemia may be seen most commonly in health care workers, patients with diabetes, and their relatives. These patients will have low C-peptide and low proinsulin serum levels.

Treatment

The diagnosis of hypoglycemia should be considered in every unconscious patient. The initial treatment of a confused or comatose patient is to infuse a 50-mL intravenous bolus of 50% glucose, preferably after obtaining a blood sample for laboratory analysis. If hypoglycemia is documented, blood should then be tested for electrolytes, blood urea nitrogen and creatinine, ketones (urine and plasma), insulin (<6 mU/mL), C-peptide, cortisol, drugs, toxins, hypoglycemic agents (e.g., sulfonylurea [<0.2 nmol/L] or meglitinide), and alcohol. A plasma insulin-to-glucose ratio of greater than 0.4 is significant. A portion of the sample should be kept for later analysis of proinsulin, insulin antibodies, and lactate, when necessary.

Intravenous, intramuscular, or subcutaneous glucagon (1 mg) can be used in the absence of an intravenous glucose preparation. The bolus of glucose should be followed by the continuous infusion of 5% to 10% glucose (rarely, 20% to 30%) at a rate sufficient to keep the plasma glucose level greater than 100 mg/dL (starting at 100 mL per hour). The requirement of 8 to 10 g of glucose per hour to prevent recurrent hypoglycemia suggests diminished glucose production as a cause of the hypoglycemia, with higher requirements reflecting increased peripheral glucose utilization. When the patient is capable of eating, a diet with a minimum of 300 g of carbohydrate per day should be supplied. In many situations, especially after administration of long-acting insulin or oral hypoglycemic agents, hypoglycemia persists for an extended time. Treatment and close observation should continue during this time to prevent a relapse. Mild hypoglycemia can be managed with oral glucose tablets (4 or 5 g), fruit juice, or the equivalent, followed by a snack containing carbohydrate and protein, if the patient has to wait more than 30 minutes for the next meal. Thiamine should be administered when alcohol consumption is suggested.

Long-term therapy depends on the cause of the hypoglycemia. If the hypoglycemia is a secondary process, such as from hepatic or renal failure, or sepsis, treatment of the underlying disorder will resolve the hypoglycemia. If the hypoglycemia results from an insulinoma, surgical removal of the tumor is the treatment of choice.

Recurrent hypoglycemia in patients with diabetes requires a multidisciplinary intervention with attention to detail at every level of management, including education, nutritional advice, frequent glucose monitoring (including CGMS), and physiologic insulin and oral agent therapy (including administration technique).

Dietary therapy is the cornerstone of the management of all types of reactive hypoglycemia. Patients should avoid simple and refined carbohydrates. Some patients also benefit from frequent, small meals or snacks that contain a mixture of carbohydrate, fat, and protein. If a regimen of avoidance of simple carbohydrates and eating more frequently is ineffective, restricting the daily carbohydrate intake to 35% to 40% of total calories and increasing protein intake can be helpful. Drug therapy with propantheline bromide or phenytoin may sometimes be helpful, but it should be reserved for severe cases. If the disorder results from alimentary hypoglycemia, dietary therapy is usually helpful; in refractory instances (rare), surgical treatment to slow gastric transit time may be successful.

Prospectus for the Future

Successful islet transplantation, β-cell regeneration, or implantable artificial pancreas will result in *physiologic* insulin levels and eliminate the curse of hypoglycemia related to mismatches between insulin and serum glucose levels in patients with diabetes mellitus.

New therapeutic approaches in the management of diabetes should reduce the frequency and severity of hypoglycemic episodes (see Chapter 69), especially as we aim for tight glycemic control.

Heightened awareness of the causes, sequelae, and treatment of hypoglycemia should reduce its frequency and severity.

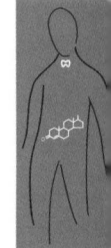

References

American Diabetes Association Workgroup on Hypoglycemia: Defining and reporting hypoglycemia in diabetes: A report from the American Diabetes Workgroup on Hypoglycemia. Diabetes Care 28:1245-1249, 2005.

American Diabetes Association: Hypoglycemia and employment/licensure. Diabetes Care 31:1:94, 2008.

Banarer S, Cryer PE: Hypoglycemia in type 2 diabetes. Med Clin North Am 88:1107-1116, 2004.

Cryer PE, Davis SN, Shamoon H: Hypoglycemia in diabetes. Diabetes Care 26:1902-1912, 2003.

Marks V, Teale JD: Investigation of hypoglycemia. Clin Endocrinol 44:133-136, 1996.

Saleh M, Grunberger G: Hypoglycemia: An excuse for poor glycemic control? Clin Diabetes 19:161-167, 2001.

Service FJ: Hypoglycemic disorders. N Engl J Med 332:1144-1152, 1995.

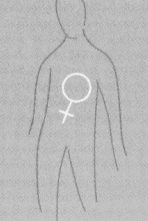

Section XIII

Women's Health

Women's Health Topics

Deborah Ehrenthal, Patricia Carney, Renee Kottenhahn, and Pamela Charney

A. Introduction

Over the past few decades, there has been increasing exploration of how a patient's individual characteristics, such as sex and age, affect physiology, health, disease presentation, and management. Science inquiry has gradually expanded to other potential differences such as ethnic and racial background, and the impact of socioeconomic factors and geographic location. At this point, there is adequate information about differences between males and females to alter medical care in many areas. This chapter will review some of the known sex differences, highlighting diseases unique to women and some key areas in which differences between women and men alter health and medical care.

What Is Women's Health?

Women's health is defined currently as a multidisciplinary approach to the health and care of women patients. Specialists in this area come from a wide range of disciplines and often enjoy collaborating. The conceptual growth of women's health beyond gynecologic and obstetrical issues coincided with an increase in the number of women becoming physicians in the United States as well as curiosity among clinicians and researchers in how women and men differ.

Health, both physical and psychological, is affected by biologic, cultural, societal, and economic issues throughout the age spectrum. As the interaction of these factors has been explored, new insights have emerged. For example, tobacco use, as well as the success of smoking cessation, is affected by many factors. Generally, men smoke more than women in America, but there are wide differences between racial-ethnic and educational groups. Among women, Native Americans have the highest tobacco use rates (and represent the only group in which women smoke at higher rates than men), whereas women self-identified as Asian have the lowest rates of tobacco use. Lower educational level correlates with greater tobacco use, and 1 in 3 high school graduates but only 1 in 10 college graduates smokes. This is one reason why tobacco companies advertise more prominently on billboards in poor neighborhoods. As the price of cigarettes increase, there are lower rates of initiation among teenagers. Similarly, there are important differences in tobacco cessation. Women tend to have more difficulty stopping cigarette consumption both initially and long term than men. Women are more likely to stop smoking in response to social pressure, especially from their children, whereas men are more likely to stop smoking as the result of peer pressure at work. A major barrier to tobacco cessation for women is fear of weight gain. Repeatedly when surveyed, women smokers are not willing to gain *any* weight while stopping tobacco use. However, the average smoker who stops cigarette use gains 10 pounds, and as many as 20% while stopping use gain 20 pounds or more. Black smokers also have more trouble stopping. This difference has been linked to that the finding that black smokers lack an enzyme that breaks down tobacco products and therefore obtain higher levels of nicotine in their bloodstream after smoking than white or Mexican American smokers. This effect is even found after smoking only two cigarettes daily. All smokers, regardless of age or sex, will reap the benefits of smoking cessation, even older smokers and those with tobacco-related diseases. Specific cessation therapies are discussed in Chapter 17.

Women's health focuses on conditions unique in women (pregnancy), conditions that are more common in women (breast cancer, osteoporosis, rape, and hypertension), and conditions that have different presentations, natural history, risk factors, prevention, or treatments in women and men (heart disease, urinary tract infections, sexually transmitted diseases). As more is known, the specific topic areas included within the field of women's health has expanded. For example, post-traumatic stress was initially identified among returning war veterans, predominantly male, who had seen extensive combat. Only as successful therapeutic approaches developed was it realized that this syndrome was also present among survivors of non–war-related trauma, especially among many women. In addition, as the number of women in the military has increased and medical care has begun to focus on this group, it has become more common knowledge that women veterans may also experience post-traumatic stress from their experiences in the armed forces. Several women's health topics are reviewed in detail in other chapters, including osteoporosis, eating disorders, urinary tract infections, and sexually transmitted diseases.

Knowledge expands as critical questions are defined and answered. There have been several important ongoing studies that have dramatically increased knowledge in women's health. Each study has defined a group of individuals, a cohort, and follows them prospectively over time. As new scientific questions have evolved, it has been possible to use these cohorts to provide preliminary results. One limitation of the earlier studies was the lack of diversity in the participants in the cohort. Results from a more diverse cohort group have broader population implications.

Perhaps the most important cohort studies that have improved our ability to explore sex differences are the Framingham Study, the Nurses Health Study, and the Women's Health Initiative (WHI). The first was the Framingham Study, a longitudinal prospective cohort of adults living in Framingham, Massachusetts. The initial goal of the study was to identify risk factors for heart disease by following this large and stable cohort of men and women in their 40s. In the initial reports, men with chest pain were more likely to die of heart disease than women who reported chest pain. This supported the perception at the time that heart disease was a disease of men. It wasn't until women were observed into their 50s that women began developing symptoms and dying of heart disease. When researchers looked back and further defined chest symptoms from the earlier reports, it was found women and men with typical angina symptoms had similar outcomes. However, women were more likely to report any symptoms than men, including some type of chest pain. In fact, angina is the most common presenting symptom of coronary artery disease in women, whereas for men, it is most likely an acute myocardial infarction. The Framingham data set also revealed that silent myocardial infarctions are more common in women than men. The Framingham study is now multigenerational and has been expanded to include the greater diversity of individuals living in Framingham.

The Nurse's Health Study is a national ongoing survey of a cohort of female nurses that has provided detailed information about risk factors, disease presentation, and outcomes for decades. Participants complete extensive questionnaires regularly and have occasionally provided specimens for analysis. Because it is a prospective cohort group, it has been possible to evaluate many risk factors. Among tobacco smokers, the adverse health effects are dose related, and those smoking one or two cigarettes daily have less health problems than those smoking a pack of cigarettes daily but more problems than nonsmokers. Higher levels of physical activity have correlated with less weight gain with aging and lower rates of cancer and cardiovascular disease. Detailed dietary information has allowed comparison of fat (olive oil was better than margarine and butter) and other dietary impacts on health outcomes. Limitations of the study include the population and the self-report nature of the data.

Finally, the WHI enrolled women 50 to 79 years of age in three clinical trials and an observational arm. The population of the WHI is the most ethnically and racially diverse of the three studies. The clinical trials were all randomized, double-blinded with placebo control. Two were designed to resolve questions about the impact of estrogens and estrogens plus progesterone on the risk for a variety of important health outcomes for women during the postmenopausal period. These included cardiovascular risk, maintenance of bone density, risk for breast cancer, and development of dementia. Although these pharmaceutical trials have ended, the observational study continues. The WHI clinical trials of hormonal therapy have dramatically changed the therapeutic approach to menopause. Whereas earlier observational studies, including the Nurses Health Study, had suggested that hormonal therapy decreased cardiovascular events after menopause, this careful prospective trial found that there was no substantial cardiovascular benefit with either estrogen alone or estrogen and progesterone. This trial is discussed later in this chapter in more detail.

Biology and Physiology

There are substantial biologic and physiologic differences between males and females. Some differences have been long acknowledged, whereas other areas are just beginning to be explored.

BIOLOGY

Women are generally smaller physically than men—about 5 inches shorter. Renal mass is less, and in the past decade, this has been acknowledged in defining normal renal function. The shorter urethral distance places women at much higher risk for urinary tract infections than men. Physically, an individual's volume of muscle and fat varies by sex and age. Because of the pelvis requirements needed to allow childbirth, the hip and knee angles from the pelvis are different by sex. This leads to different stresses and lower extremity injuries in women than generally occur in men. Women's anatomically smaller blood vessels are finally becoming less of a barrier to invasive therapies as smaller catheters have been developed.

Both women and men are most likely to die of cardiovascular disease. Cancer is the second most common cause of death for women and men. However, the most likely new cancer diagnosis and cause of death is breast cancer for women (and prostate cancer for men). The third most common cause of death is stroke. Interestingly for middle-aged women younger than 65 years, white women are most likely to die of chronic obstructive pulmonary disease (of these groups, white women have the highest rate of tobacco use), black women are most likely to suffer a stroke (in a

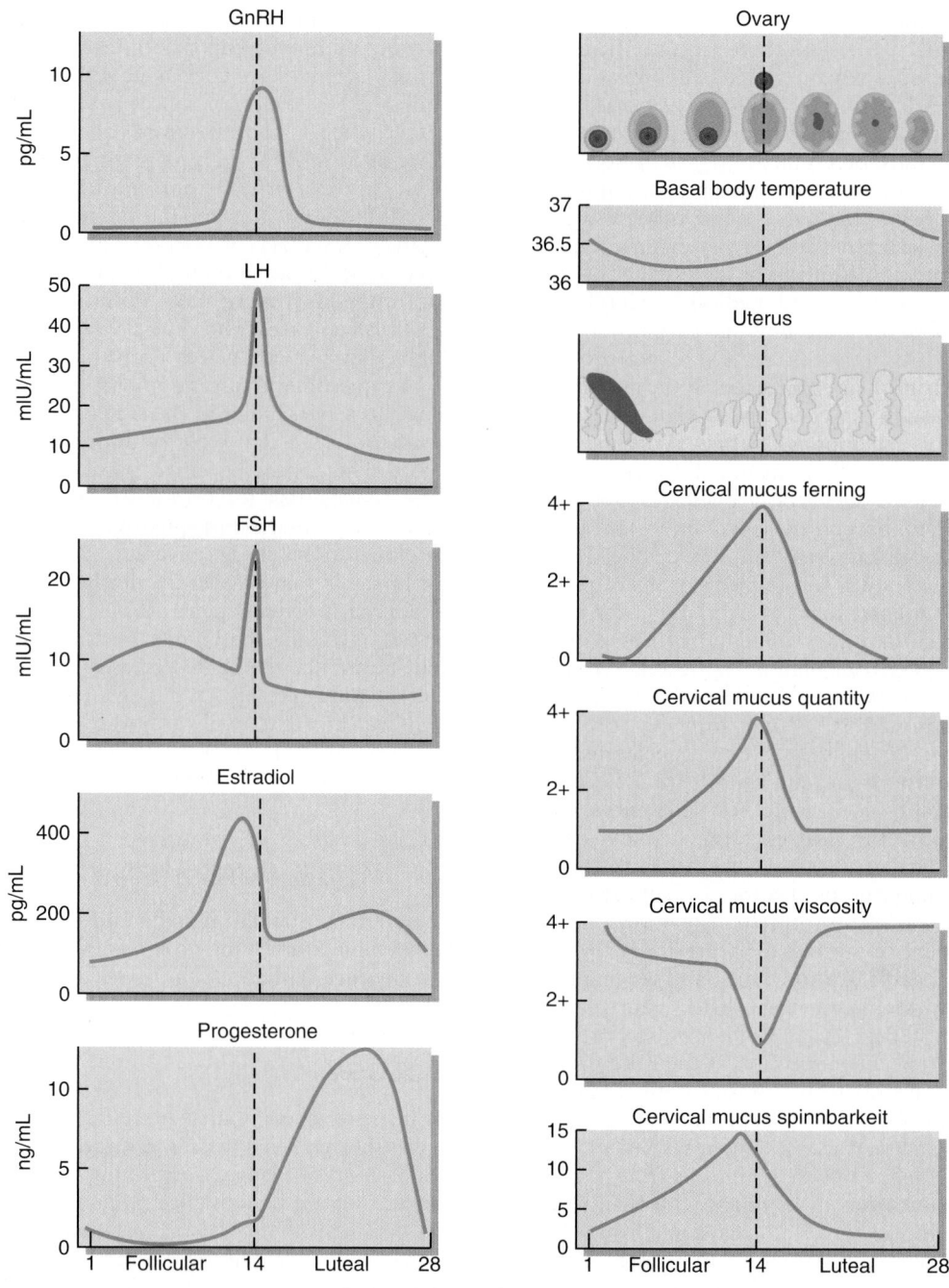

Figure 71-1 Schematic representation of the normal menstrual cycle. FSH, follicle-stimulating hormone; GnRH, gonadotropin-releasing hormone; LH, luteinizing hormone. (From Braunstein GD: Female reproductive disorders. In Hershman JD [ed]: Endocrine Pathophysiology: A Patient-Oriented Approach. Philadelphia, Lea & Febiger, 1988, p 153.)

population with early onset of hypertension), and Hispanic women are most likely to die of diabetes and its complications (high rates of obesity and diabetes).

PHYSIOLOGY

Comparative Physiology

This section focuses predominantly on reproductive physiology. However, the most interesting and provocative findings have occurred through exploring sex differences in physiology. Substantial cardiovascular physiologic differ-

ences have been documented. For example, in order to increase cardiac output, females increase heart rate, whereas men increase stroke volume. Because increases in stroke volume are limited by the need for relaxation so that the cardiac chambers can refill, there is a greater physiologic cap for increases in cardiac output in women. Sympathetic tone also appears to vary by sex and may be one reason that premenopausal women tend to have lower blood pressure than age-matched men. Gastrointestinal physiologic differences have also been highlighted. Gastric alcohol absorption is faster in women. Hepatic drug clearance varies by sex, ethnicity, and race, depending on the enzyme studied. Females are more likely to develop gallstones.

Reproductive Physiology

Estrogen levels vary substantially throughout life. Estrogen levels are low in childhood. At the time of puberty, the hypothalamus begins releasing gonadotropin-releasing hormone (GnRH), leading to ovarian stimulation. Eventually, most women develop a regular menstrual cycle with associated periodic increases in estrogen and then progesterone in response to the luteinizing hormone (LH) and follicular-stimulating hormone (FSH) released by the pituitary gland. Increasing numbers of estrogen receptors have been identified in both reproductive and nonreproductive organs, including brain, arterial vessel wall, bone, smooth muscle, and urethra. During pregnancy, hormonal levels further increase. With perimenopause, the time close to the development of menopause, estrogen and progesterone levels become more erratic. These fluctuating levels are often associated with hot flashes, weight gain, and irritability. Finally, with menopause, estrogen levels are generally low. In addition to estrogens, the ovary produces androgens, such as testosterone and androstenedione, which are peripherally converted to estrogen, especially in fat cells. Obese women are exposed to higher circulating estrogen levels after menopause than thinner women.

The *menstrual cycle* consists of three distinct phases: the follicular or proliferative phase; ovulation; and the luteal or secretory phase. The physiologic changes that are a part of the menstrual cycle, including variations in hormones, the uterine lining, cervical mucus, and changes in basal body temperature (when taken upon first awakening), are graphically represented in Figure 71-1. The menstrual cycle duration tends to become consistent for most young women, lasting between 21 and 35 days. Often in perimenopause, the duration will decrease.

During the *follicular phase*, the hypothalamus secretes GnRH, which stimulates the pituitary to release FSH and LH. These hormones in turn stimulate estrogen secretion by a cohort of ovarian follicles. The estrogen secretion simultaneously facilitates proliferation of the endometrium. Eventually, one follicle becomes dominant and is destined for ovulation. *Ovulation* occurs soon after the LH surge.

With ovulation, the oocyte leaves the dominant follicle and migrates toward the fallopian tubes. At this time, the cervical mucus covering the cervical os become less viscous, thus facilitating passage of sperm at the uterine entrance.

The remaining cells in the follicle become the *corpus luteum,* which produces progesterone during this *luteal phase.* If fertilization does not occur, progesterone is secreted for about 14 days, and then the follicle involutes. This is associated with decreasing levels of estrogen and progesterone. The endometrium sheds in response to the falling estrogen and progesterone levels and results in menstruation. If fertilization occurs, progesterone continues to be secreted to support early pregnancy.

Menstrual bleeding is variable, but usually lasts less than 7 days. Bleeding disorders may be associated with heavier menstrual bleeding. Menstrual bleeding may be associated with cramping that is often better relieved with nonsteroidal anti-inflammatory drugs (NSAIDs) than acetaminophen. A menstrual cycle will be *anovulatory* if an oocyte is not released and thus does not create a luteal phase. This may result in a missed period. Women with chronic anovulation will experience irregular bleeding due to an unstable endometrium resulting from unopposed estrogen. Hormonal contraception use tends to produce lighter menstrual bleeding over time owing to the progesterone dominance of the preparation.

Sex Differences in Socialization and Economics

As children grow up, their self-esteem, behaviors, and self-expectations are shaped by those around them—both immediate family and community. Often, expectations vary by sex. Throughout much of the world, girls and women have lower rates of literacy than boys and men. Age of first pregnancy is later in those who have more years of education. Income is generally higher for men than women in both the industrialized and agricultural world. Similarly, poverty rates are higher for women throughout the world.

B. Preventive Health Recommendations for Women

Many organizations put forth recommendations and guidelines for preventive care for women, including specialty organizations such as the American College of Obstetrics and Gynecology, the American Cancer Society, the American Diabetes Association, and the U.S. Preventive Services Task Force. Table 71-1 highlights evidence-based

recommendations for preventive care for women at average risk, including screening recommendations during pregnancy. Additional screening is often recommended for women with specific risk factors, and this list represents the interventions with the best evidence for impact on health outcomes.

Table 71-1 Preventive Health Recommendations for Women

	Recommendation	Age and Interval
Screening		
Obesity	Blood pressure, height and weight, body mass index	Every 1-2 yr
Hyperlipidemia	Lipid panel	Start age 45 yr
Cancer	Mammogram	Start age 40 yr, then annually
	Papanicolaou test	Every 1-3 yr for women with a cervix
	Fecal occult blood testing, sigmoidoscopy, or colonoscopy	Start at age 50 yr
Infectious diseases	Chlamydia	Annual to age 25 yr, then if patient remains high risk
Osteoporosis	Bone densitometry	Begin by age 65 yr
Mental health	Depression	All adults
Other		
Immunizations		
	Influenza	Yearly
	Rubella	Check titer or vaccinate
	Tetanus-diphtheria—(pertussis)	dT every 10 yr (TdAP booster at least once after age 11 yr)
	Human papillomavirus	To age 26 yr
	Varicella	Susceptible women
Chemoprophylaxis		
	Folic acid supplement	400 mcg daily
	Calcium intake/supplement	Periodically
Counseling		
	Tobacco and alcohol misuse	Periodically
	Promote healthy diet; promote breastfeeding; counsel regarding sexually transmitted infections, avoiding unintentional injuries, seat belt use	Periodically
Additional screening and counseling during pregnancy	Rh(D) incompatibility screening, iron deficiency anemia, asymptomatic bacteriuria	Testing in the first trimester
	Rubella	Check titer, vaccinate postpartum if negative
	Hepatitis B	HBsAg
	HIV, syphilis, gonorrhea	Testing in the first trimester
	Gestational hypertensive disorders	Ongoing
	Depression	Postpartum

C. Health Issues Across the Life Course

Adolescence

APPROACH TO THE ADOLESCENT

Providing health care to adolescents requires specific skills of the medical provider. Adolescent patients are naïve health consumers and often do not express their needs clearly because they have yet to develop sophisticated communication skills and often have a very limited knowledge of their own physiology, including what is "normal" and what is not. Many young women are reluctant to engage in the medical encounter because of embarrassment or fear. It is incumbent on the medical provider to acknowledge these issues and engage the adolescent using developmentally appropriate language and a compassionate manner.

CONFIDENTIALITY

Most adolescents come to office appointments accompanied by an adult. Although parental involvement in minors' health care decisions is desirable, many adolescents will not disclose their social or health history unless they are interviewed alone and with the assurance of confidentiality. Time spent alone with the patient is critical to discovering hidden agendas. Because statutes for the care of minors vary from state to state, the medical provider must be familiar with what legal rights young patients have to accessing reproductive health services without the involvement of a parent. Online resources from the Alan Guttmacher Institute (http://www.guttmacher.org) can provide state-specific policies regarding a minor's rights to accessing contraception, sexually transmitted infection (STI) services, prenatal care, and abortions, and what rights minors have as parents.

Proactive discussion with patient and parent together detailing office confidentiality policies, including how privacy is maintained and when it must be broken (e.g., abuse and suicidality, STI reporting to health departments), is critical to facilitating effective health care encounters. It is not uncommon, however, for adolescents to underestimate their parent's understanding of their circumstance. Many dyads share the same but unvoiced concerns (e.g., the need for contraception), in which case the clinician can help facilitate disclosure and open discussions of health care delivery.

SEXUAL HISTORY

Gender and number of past and present partners should be tactfully elicited as part of the sexual history along with history of sexual abuse, assault, date rape, or physically abusive partner. It is also important to know whether the patient is intoxicated during sex because intercourse may not be voluntary or protected. Young women need to be encouraged to be safe and selective in their relationships and encouraged either to abstain from sex (i.e., oral, vaginal, or anal sex) or to be in a long-term, mutually monogamous relationship with an uninfected partner. Health providers may need to teach young patients strategies in self-advocacy and "how not to have sex," as well as helping young women understand what constitutes a "healthy" relationship. Risk for pregnancy and contraceptive options are also important topics for discussion (see below).

SEXUALLY TRANSMITTED INFECTIONS AND HUMAN PAPILLOMAVIRUS

Adolescents who are sexually active are at particular risk for sexually transmitted diseases. Younger women have relative biologic susceptibility to some diseases, such as chlamydia, because of cervical ectopy. Adolescents frequently have unprotected intercourse because they cannot access, do not like, or cannot negotiate appropriate use of condoms. Many teenagers have sexual partnerships of short duration (serial monogamy) or "primary" and "secondary" (concurrent) sexual relationships further compounding their risk for acquiring disease. Some adolescents have partners of either sex regardless of whether they define themselves as "hetero" or "homo" sexual. Some adolescents, aware of potential infection, cannot access testing because of transportation, lack of insurance, or confidentiality concerns and thus continue to put themselves and others at risk.

Among females, the highest rates of reported chlamydia infection in 2006 occurred among adolescent and young women (2863 cases and 2797 cases per 100,000 females for those aged 15 to 19 and 20 to 24 years, respectively) Because many adolescents with sexually transmitted infections are asymptomatic, young patients will not appreciate their risk

for acquiring, transmitting, or needing treatment for disease. For this reason, it is recommended that any adolescent who has engaged in sexual intimacy be screened for gonorrhea and chlamydia. Patients with confirmed disease should complete therapy, notify their partners to be treated, and abstain from sex until all partners are tested and complete treatment. Because of the risk for reinfection subsequent to treatment, patients with confirmed disease should be rescreened in 3 months.

Many girls acquire human papillomavirus (HPV) infection during their adolescent years. The availability of a quadrivalent HPV vaccine offers an opportunity to decrease the burden of vaccine HPV-type–related cervical cancer, cervical cancer precursors, vaginal and vulvar cancer precursors, and anogenital warts. In 2006, the U.S. Food and Drug Administration (FDA) approved an HPV vaccine, Gardasil, and the Advisory Committee on Immunization Practices (ACIP) has recommended routine vaccination of females aged 11 to 12 years with three doses of the quadrivalent HPV vaccine. Catch-up vaccination is recommended for females aged 13 to 26 years. Papanicolaou (Pap) smear screening is recommended in sexually active adolescents about 3 years after initiation of sexual intercourse regardless of HPV vaccination status.

In addition to appreciating the importance of HPV vaccination, medical providers undertaking women's health issues are also afforded the opportunity to counsel or provide other vaccinations scheduled during the adolescent years, including the meningococcal vaccination and Tdap (conferring added protection against pertussis), and to confirm that childhood vaccinations for hepatitis A and B and varicella have been completed.

PRIMARY AMENORRHEA

By age 14 years, more than 95% of girls have reached menarche. Some girls will quickly establish a regular menstrual cycle; however, early cycles tend to be irregular, and more than half of the cycles are anovulatory owing to an immature hypothalamic-pituitary axis. In general, as the adolescent matures, there is a progression to more regular cycles, but up to one third will still have anovulatory cycles after 5 years. *Primary amenorrhea* is defined as the absence of a first menses by age 16 years. However, when evaluating an adolescent for amenorrhea, it is important to consider other developmental milestones. Figure 71-2 illustrates Tanner staging of breast maturation for girls and adolescents. Menarche is usually seen 2 years after the start of breast development and by the time Tanner stage 4 is reached. Therefore, a girl who has not begun menses by age 14 years or within 2 years of obtaining Tanner stage 4 breast development should be further evaluated.

There is a broad differential diagnosis that must be considered, and pregnancy must always be excluded. The most common cause of primary amenorrhea is ovarian failure, hypergonadotropic hypogonadism. This occurs when there is a failure of the ovary to respond to the signals from the pituitary gland and can be caused by Turner syndrome or other genetic abnormalities, or be a sequelae of chemotherapy or radiation therapy received in the past. The next most common cause of primary amenorrhea is müllerian agenesis, or congenital absence of the female genital tract.

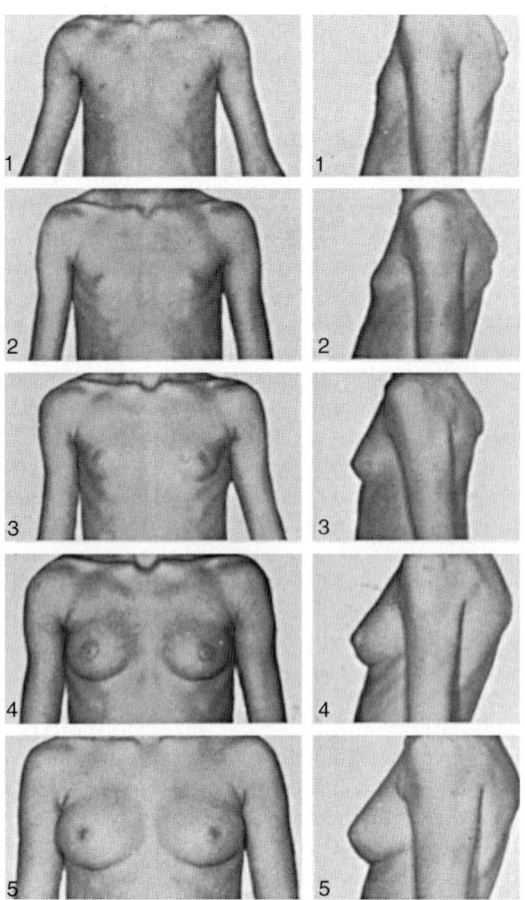

Figure 71-2 Sex maturity ratings of breast changes in adolescent. (From Kliegman, Robert M. et al. Nelson Textbook of Pediatrics, 18th ed. Philadelphia, WB Saunders, 2007. Courtesy of JM Tanner, MD, Institute of Child Health, Department of Growth and Development, University of London, London, England.)

In addition, other outflow tract abnormalities, including imperforate hymen, transverse vaginal septum, and androgen insensitivity, may all present in the adolescent girl who has failed to menstruate. Finally, chronic anovulation may be the underlying abnormality.

A detailed history and physical examination will suggest the cause of amenorrhea. As above, developmental milestones should be obtained. Girls with outflow tract obstruction, such as an imperforate hymen, may present with cyclic pelvic pain. A thorough history may uncover evidence of excessive exercise or an eating disorder, often referred to as the *female athlete triad* (amenorrhea, osteopenia, eating disorder). Alternatively, there may be signs and symptoms of androgen excess, such as acne, hirsutism, or obesity, to suggest polycystic ovary syndrome (PCOS) as a cause of chronic anovulation. The physical examination should include inspection of the external genitalia as well as imaging with pelvic ultrasound to further define anatomy. Pregnancy should always be excluded with a sensitive urine human chorionic gonadotropin (hCG) level tested in the office. Further laboratory testing should include FSH, LH, prolactin, and thyroid-stimulating hormone (TSH) to evaluate pituitary and thyroid function. If there are signs of androgen excess, a free and total testosterone level should be measured; if there is a suggestion of hypothalamic hypogo-

nadism, an estradiol level can be helpful to identify hypoestrogenemia. If the FSH and LH are elevated, premature ovarian failure is present, and a karyotype should be obtained to identify androgen insensitivity and other chromosomal abnormalities such as Turner syndrome.

Reproductive Age

Women during their childbearing years are generally free from chronic health problems and often receive their health care episodically from a gynecologist, a primary care physician, or both. They commonly defer their own health care needs while caring for their family. Most women do present nearly annually for cervical cancer screening or for prenatal care. Although women seek care for primarily reproductive needs, perhaps the most important role for the health care provider is to work with women to identify their short- and long-term health risks and support their effort to change behaviors that could affect current reproductive health, as well as future risk for cardiovascular disease and cancer.

Establishment of healthy lifestyles and avoidance of unhealthy behaviors is an important focus for this age group and can have long-term effects. Women should be counseled to continue or begin regular physical activity, increase dietary intake of fruits and vegetables, maintain adequate intake of calcium, and avoid unhealthy behaviors, including tobacco use. Although the health care provider can be key in identifying risk factors and initiating the process of addressing these risks, behavior change is difficult and often requires the ongoing support of the provider as well as a partnership with resources that may be available in the community. This may include referral to smoking cessation programs, weight loss and exercise programs, and programs targeting other risk factors such as substance abuse and mental health.

This section discusses several important health issues that are unique to women in this age group and that reflect areas in which health care for women must be tailored to address important needs. These include pregnancy planning and preconception health, including contraception; the use of medications for women who are pregnant, breastfeeding, or have childbearing potential; the postpartum follow-up of pregnancy complications; and assessment of infertility. In addition, menstrual disorders, often the presenting symptom for important underlying medical problems, are reviewed. Finally, screening for cervical cancer and the management recommendations for the abnormal Pap smear are described.

PRECONCEPTION, PREGNANCY PLANNING, AND POSTPARTUM CONSIDERATIONS

Preconception Health Care and Pregnancy Planning as a Part of Routine Care for Women

The health of a woman at the time of conception can have a major impact on the course of her pregnancy and the health of her child. Because nearly half of all pregnancies in the United States are unplanned, preconception health care must be provided on an ongoing basis for all women regardless of whether they are actively planning to conceive.

As discussed below, pharmaceutical use must be carefully reviewed because there are commonly used medications that are known teratogens that should not be used by women with pregnancy potential. In addition, many common health risks and behaviors are known to increase the risk for fetal anomalies, premature birth, and other adverse pregnancy outcomes. Before pregnancy, the preconception period, is the best time to address these and other risk factors to improve outcomes. Care management before conception and during the prenatal period improves outcomes for women with many common health risks, including obesity, tobacco use, diabetes, seizure disorders, and HIV infection.

Preconception care must be incorporated into routine preventive health care for women of childbearing age by all providers. This includes working with women to develop a reproductive plan, to support their efforts to implement that plan, and to identify important health risks and recommendations to improve their health and therefore improve the odds for a healthy pregnancy if and when they choose to conceive. All women should be advised to take daily supplemental folic acid, in the form of a multivitamin containing at least 400 μg of folic acid, in order to prevent neural tube defects should they conceive. Adequate folic acid levels are critical very early in embryogenesis, and supplementation must begin during the months before conception. This is one of the few public health measures proved to have a meaningful impact on outcomes, but studies show only 30% of women in the United States follow this recommendation. It is also important to verify immunity to rubella, hepatitis B, and varicella before pregnancy and to vaccinate as needed, remembering that women should avoid conception within 1 month of receiving an MMR or varicella vaccine. In addition, screening for risks such as HIV and other STIs should be considered, and women should be advised about the potential risks associated with herbs, over-the-counter medications, and some prescription medications. Finally, as discussed later, contraceptive options should be presented and discussed.

Taking a Sexual History

When obtaining a sexual history, it is important to use concrete and nonjudgmental language that will be familiar to the patient and provide the information needed in making decisions about risk for conception, STIs, and need for contraception. Confidentiality must be assured. If asked "are you sexually active?" an answer "no" does not assure a period of abstinence. The history should include questions about sexual practices, including number of partners, gender of partners, and steps taken to protect against transmission of infections as well as pregnancy prevention. Prior history of STIs, as well as specific risks for HIV and hepatitis, should be elicited. Exploration about safety, especially in relation to sexual activity, should be pursued. Finally, condom use and risk reduction strategies should be discussed.

Contraception

There are currently a variety of contraceptive options available to women with varying levels of effectiveness, as described in Table 71-2. The most common method used by women in the United States is the oral contraceptive pill (31%), followed by tubal sterilization (27%), the male condom (18%), and vasectomy (9%). Younger women rely

Table 71-2 Contraceptive Effectiveness

	Method
Always very effective (0%-1% failure)	Vasectomy, female sterilization, etonogestrel subdermal implant 68 mg, copper-bearing intrauterine device, levonorgestrel intrauterine device
Very effective when used correctly and consistently Effective as commonly used (2%-12% failure)	Combined oral contraceptive pills, patches, vaginal rings, depot medroxyprogesterone acetate injection, progesterone-only pills while breastfeeding
Effective when used correctly and consistently Only somewhat effective as commonly used (15%-30% failure)	Condom, diaphragm, coitus interruptus, spermicide, cervical cap

more often on the oral contraceptive pill, older women on sterilization. The choice of a contraceptive method must be individualized and include careful consideration of the risks and benefits of the method as well as the acceptability of the method and the risks associated with an unplanned pregnancy. In general, most methods are very safe for use by most women; however, the use of hormonal contraception can carry unacceptable risks for women with medical problems, and the decision about optimal contraceptive choice can be complex. The World Health Organization's *Medical Eligibility Criteria for Contraceptive Use* is an excellent resource, is frequently updated, is available online, and can help the provider balance the risks and the benefits.

Combined Hormonal Contraceptives

These contraceptives contain both estrogen and a progestin and are available in multiple delivery systems in addition to the traditional oral contraceptive pill (OCP). They act to prevent pregnancy through multiple mechanisms, including suppression of ovulation, as well as effects on the uterine lining, tubal function, and cervical mucus. Oral formulations contain estradiol in doses of 20 to 50 μg and various progestins with varying levels of androgen activity. The OCP may be monophasic or triphasic, although triphasic OCPs may be associated with higher rates of breakthrough bleeding. There are two new methods for delivery of combination hormonal contraceptives that do not require daily dosing and therefore are preferred by some women. The Nuvaring is a small plastic ring that is placed in the vaginal vault for continuous absorption of hormones for 3 weeks and then removed for a week, inducing a withdrawal bleed. The estrogen patch is placed on the skin weekly for 3 weeks, followed by a patch-free week, and provides cutaneous absorption of combined estrogen and progestin.

Combined hormonal contraceptives are effective as commonly used and are safe for use by most women and carry noncontraceptive benefits, including a reduced risk for anemia, ovarian cancer, functional ovarian cysts, endometrial cancer, and dysmenorrhea. Use of all combination hormonal contraceptives is *contraindicated* for women older than 35 years who smoke; women with a history of heart disease or cerebrovascular disease; women with significantly impaired liver function; women with a history of thromboembolic disorders; and those with known or suspected breast or endometrial cancer, severe hyperlipidemia, migraine with aura, uncontrolled hypertension, symptomatic gallbladder disease, undiagnosed vaginal bleeding, or known or suspected pregnancy. The contraceptive patch is approved for use in women weighing up to 199 lbs owing to diminished efficacy for women with higher weight. There is some evidence that women who use the patch may have an increase risk for thromboembolic complications.

Progestin-Only Methods

These methods include the medroxyprogesterone acetate depot injection Depot-Provera and the progestin-only pill and work by inhibiting ovulation as well as impairing transport of sperm and implantation. Both methods can be used by most women with contraindications to estrogens. The long-acting Depo-Provera is administered by an intramuscular injection every 12 weeks and is a highly effective method of contraception. The major side effects and risks associated with its use are breakthrough bleeding, weight gain, and loss of bone density. Loss of bone density appears to be reversible, but consideration should be given to long-term use by women with other risk factors for osteoporosis. Depo-Provera is an excellent choice for women who have contraindications to estrogens. The progestin-only "mini" pill has a lesser degree of effectiveness. This method is less popular and tends to be used in settings in which there is a lower fecundity, such as women in their 40s and women during the postpartum period.

Intrauterine Methods

The intrauterine devices (IUDs) have become popular methods of contraception owing to their high level of reliability, longevity, and favorable side-effect profile. They work by preventing fertilization and implantation, and their effects are rapidly reversible upon withdrawal of the device. The copper IUD is highly effective and can be left in place for up to 10 years. It can be associated with increased menstrual cramping and heavier menstrual flow. The Mirena IUS is a levonorgestrel-releasing intrauterine system that works to prevent pregnancy through multiple pathways. Mirena generally creates a thinner endometrial lining and is better tolerated by some women. The IUD and IUS are typically used by parous women who are in a mutually monogamous relationship. They are contraindicated for use by women with an active cervical infection or with a history of pelvic inflammatory disease (PID). This method can be an excellent choice for women with contraindications to hormonal methods who require highly reliable contraception. One barrier to use of this method is a high cost up front; however, the cost over the lifetime of the device is less than the cost of hormonal methods.

Emergency Contraception

Plan B is an oral progestin-only preparation approved by the FDA to prevent pregnancy after unprotected sexual intercourse or a contraceptive failure. The method does nothing to interfere with an already established pregnancy. The over-the-counter method is most effective if begun within 24 hours, but effectiveness with use within 72 hours is up to 89%. Counseling before use is undertaken to ensure that the patient understands that this method is not appropriate for use as an ongoing contraceptive, but should be used in the case of emergency or failure of another method of contraception.

PRESCRIBING MEDICATION DURING THE REPRODUCTIVE YEARS

Childbearing potential must be considered when prescribing medications for prevention or to treat chronic and acute conditions. The provider must be aware of a woman's sexual history, her current and future plans for reproduction, and the reliability of her current contraceptive method before choosing to recommend a medication or an immunization, or give advice about the use of herbs or other complementary strategies. It is important to remember that benefits may outweigh the risks associated with the use of some medications needed to manage serious health risks during pregnancy. There are therefore few medications whose use is absolutely contraindicated in this setting. The concern over the potential adverse effects of medications on a growing fetus has often led providers to underutilize or underdose medications in women because of a current pregnancy or lactation. However, decisions about medication use during pregnancy and lactation are complex and often involve striking a balance between benefit and risk.

The FDA requires that drug labeling include information about drug use during pregnancy and lactation, and the FDA pregnancy categories shown in Table 71-3 were designed

Table 71-3	**Food and Drug Administration Categories of Drug Safety During Pregnancy**
Category	**Interpretation**
A	Adequate, well-controlled studies in pregnant women have not shown an increased risk to the fetus in any trimester of pregnancy.
B	Animal studies have revealed no evidence of harm to the fetus; however, there are no adequate and well-controlled studies in pregnant women. *Or:* Animal studies have shown an adverse effect, but adequate and well-controlled studies in pregnant women have failed to demonstrate a risk to the fetus in any trimester.
C	Animal studies have shown an adverse effect, and there are no adequate and well-controlled studies in pregnant women. *Or:* No animal studies have been conducted, and there are no adequate and well-controlled studies in pregnant women.
D	Adequate, well-controlled or observational studies in pregnant women have demonstrated a risk to the fetus. However, the benefits of therapy may outweigh the potential risk.
X	Adequate, well-controlled or observational studies in animals or pregnant women have demonstrated positive evidence of fetal abnormalities or risks, and the use of the product is contraindicated in women who are or may become pregnant.

to convey the fetal risks based on animal or human data, or both. However, these categories can be misleading and are often misused by health care practitioners. The FDA is currently revising the required content and format for pregnancy and lactation labeling to enable providers to make more informed decisions with their patients.

The shortcoming of the current FDA labeling system has led some experts to develop other categorization systems. One useful system categorizes medications as generally justifiable, justifiable under certain circumstances, and almost never justifiable. For a more detailed discussion, the reader is referred to *Medical Care of the Pregnant Patient*. A good example of a medication that should never be used when there is a possibility of pregnancy is radioactive iodine, whose use will lead to destruction of the fetal thyroid. On the other hand, decision making about the use of other medications can be more complex (Table 71-4).

Pregnancy potential is also important to consider, especially for medications whose adverse effects are known to occur in the first trimester when pregnancy is often not yet recognized. An interesting dilemma is the use of angiotensin-converting enzyme inhibitors by women in this age group. Their use should be avoided by women with pregnancy potential because of their effects on the fetal renal system throughout pregnancy. On the other hand, they play an important role in the prevention of diabetic nephropathy. Preconception care of diabetic women should weigh the risk against the benefits in diabetic women and develop an individualized approach. This may include discontinuation of the medication or, alternatively, continuation with a vigilant plan to identify pregnancy and discontinue the medication immediately after conception. Antiepileptic medications are another example of medications whose use must be considered carefully during the preconception period. Although these are known teratogens, a woman may require them to control a seizure disorder. Tailoring of these medications in anticipation of pregnancy to as few as possible has been shown to diminish the risk for fetal anomalies.

PREGNANCY COMPLICATIONS AND POSTPARTUM CARE

Women with prior problem pregnancies should receive postpartum care and pregnancy planning advice based on their obstetrical history. Women with a history of *gestational diabetes* are at increased risk for developing adult-onset diabetes later in life. It is recommended that these women have an oral glucose tolerance or fasting plasma glucose testing at the 6-week postpartum visit and then be followed with periodic testing if this test is normal. Because gestational diabetes identifies women who are at high risk for later diabetes, advice should focus on lifestyle changes, including exercise and weight loss. Women whose pregnancies were complicated by a *gestational hypertensive disorder*, such as preeclampsia or gestational hypertension, are at increased risk for hypertension later in life and should have their cardiovascular risk evaluated, lifestyle modification recommended, and blood pressure followed. It is recommended that women with a history of a prior *neural tube defect* take 4 g of folic acid daily, women with a personal or family history of genetic disorders may benefit from genetic counseling before conception. Women with a history of *preterm labor* should

Table 71-4 Medications that Require Consideration of Risks and Benefits

Medication	Associated Risk
Angiotensin-converting enzyme inhibitors/angiotensin receptor blockers	Renal failures, renal tubular dysgenesis, decreased skull ossification
Antiepileptic drugs (e.g., phenytoin, carbamazepine, phenobarbital, valproic acid)	Neural tube defects, congenital heart disease, facial changes, developmental delay
Coumadin	Skeletal and central nervous system defects, Dandy Walker syndrome
Methimazole	Various congenital anomalies
Cytotoxic chemotherapeutic agents (e.g., cyclophosphamide)	Central nervous system malformations
Penicillamine	
Diethylstilbestrol (DES)	Female: genital tract abnormalities, adenosis, increased risk for clear cell cancer and breast cancer Male: anatomic abnormalities, infertility, increased risk for testicular cancer
Isotretinoin	Severe congenital malformations
Methotrexate	Fetal anomalies
Others: tetracyclines, statins, androgens, live-attenuated vaccines, lithium, herbs	Various

plan to see an obstetrical provider who takes advantage of state-of-the-art methods to affect recurrence.

Two important conditions to recognize during the postpartum period are *postpartum depression* and *postpartum thyroiditis*. Although most mothers experience mood fluctuations after delivery, these symptoms do not interfere with their ability to care for themselves or their infants. Women whose symptoms persist for 2 weeks or more should be screened for postpartum depression. Postpartum depression is experienced by 10% to 15% of women, and the symptoms are those of a clinical depression. The two greatest risk factors for postpartum depression are a history of depression before pregnancy and depression during the current pregnancy. Dual diagnoses are found to be common in many high-risk populations, and tobacco use, binge drinking, and adolescent age are associated risk factors. There are several tools that can be used to screen for depression, including the CES-D and PHQ-9. Postpartum psychosis is rare, seen in 1 or 2 per 1000 mothers, can present 2 to 3 days after delivery, and is associated with a high risk for suicide or infanticide if not treated.

Postpartum thyroiditis is an autoimmune thyroiditis that can be seen in 5% to 10% of women during the first postpartum year. The syndrome presents most often 6 months postpartum and is characterized by transient, often unrecognized, thyroiditis followed by hypothyroidism, and ending with resolution. About 20% to 30% of women will remain hypothyroid. Management focuses on management of symptoms during the hyperthyroid stage, often with β blockers, as well as support with thyroid replacement hormone during the hypothyroid phase. Those women who do return to a euthyroid state are at increased risk for postpartum hypothyroidism during a subsequent pregnancy and at increased risk for hypothyroidism over time. All women will require long-term follow-up with annual thyroid testing.

GYNECOLOGIC COMPLAINTS

Abnormal Menses

For women of reproductive age, a normal menstrual cycle is a marker of general good health. Menstrual disorders are common and generally fall into two main categories: *amenorrhea* and *abnormal uterine bleeding*. When the menstrual cycle is found to be abnormal, the underlying cause must be sought. Abnormalities may indicate problems related to the reproductive system, such as premature ovarian failure, or may be an early sign of an important underlying systemic illness. Management of menstrual cycle abnormalities focuses on addressing the underlying pathology, supporting the consequential anemia, protecting the uterus from endometrial hyperplasia due to unopposed estrogen, and minimizing osteoporosis risk for women with a hypothalamic etiology. Details are discussed below.

Amenorrhea

Amenorrhea occurs in 5% of women each year and is defined as the absence of menses for at least 3 to 6 months outside of the setting of pregnancy or lactation. Primary amenorrhea is generally recognized during the teenage years when menses fail to begin by age 16 years and was discussed earlier. Women who have had a previously established menstrual pattern are considered to have *secondary amenorrhea*. *Oligomenorrhea* occurs when menses are irregular or infrequent, with cycle length usually greater than 35 to 40 days, and is often associated with *chronic anovulation* or oligo-ovulation.

As shown in Table 71-5, pathologic causes of amenorrhea and oligomenorrhea may occur at any point in the endometrial-ovarian-pituitary-hypothalamic axis. The differential diagnosis is broad and can be organized into five main categories: (1) ovarian failure, (2) anovulation, (3) medication induced, (4) uterine outflow tract abnormalities, and (5) physiologic. The most common cause of secondary amenorrhea is pregnancy, which is easily identified by a sensitive urine pregnancy test in the office. Lactation causes amenorrhea as well and may be expected for up to 6 months in a woman who is exclusively breastfeeding her infant. Prolonged amenorrhea can follow cessation of some hormonal contraceptives, especially depot medroxyprogesterone acetate, as well as other medications. Finally, menopause should be suspected in the woman older than 45 years, and this explanation should be considered before an extensive evaluation of amenorrhea is undertaken.

Evaluation should begin with history, physical examination to assess comorbidities and anatomy, and an office test of urine hCG. Further evaluation should include testing of serum TSH, prolactin, and FSH. These tests will identify

Table 71-5 **Abnormal Menstrual Cycle**

Secondary Amenorrhea	Causes
Physiologic	Pregnancy, lactation, menopause
Ovarian	Radiation- or chemotherapy-induced ovarian failure, chromosomal abnormalities, autoimmune or idiopathic premature ovarian failure
Anovulation	Hyperandrogenism (polycystic ovary syndrome, congenital adrenal hyperplasia), hyperprolactinemia (prolactinoma, phenothiazines, narcotics, and other medications), hyperthyroidism, hypothyroidism, hypopituitarism, pituitary adenoma, Cushing syndrome, hypothalamic hypogonadism (eating disorder, athletic triad, stress)
Medications	Hormonal, cytotoxic, others
Uterine outflow tract abnormalities	Surgery
Abnormal Bleeding	
Structural	Uterine fibroids, endometrial or endocervical polyp, cervical cancer, endometrial hyperplasia, endometrial cancer
Hormonal	Chronic anovulation, hypothyroidism, waning ovarian function, estrogen secreting tumors
Coagulopathies	Thrombocytopenia, platelet dysfunction

women with hypothyroidism, prolactinoma, and ovarian failure. Women who show signs of androgen excess or a history consistent with PCOS should have total or free testosterone and 17-α-hydroxyprogesterone measured at 8:00 AM to rule out testosterone-secreting tumors and congenital adrenal hyperplasia.

Assessment of adequate estrogen can be done by measuring a serum estradiol level or with a progesterone challenge. The progesterone challenge involves administration of oral medroxyprogesterone for 10 days and watching for the expected "withdrawal bleed" after completion. Women who bleed have normal estrogen levels and are likely to have chronic anovulation, most often due to PCOS. Women who fail to have a withdrawal bleed are suspected to have low levels of estrogen, and amenorrhea may be due to anovulation and failure of the hypothalamic-pituitary axis. However, women with a history of uterine instrumentation or other gynecologic surgery may have an outflow tract abnormality and therefore fail to show a withdrawal bleed. This can be identified by creating an artificial cycle with combined estrogen and progestin administration and looking for a bleed after a few months when the uterine lining has had the opportunity to develop. Failure to bleed to combined hormonal cycling suggests a uterine or outflow tract abnormality.

Management of amenorrhea will depend on the underlying abnormality identified. Women with chronic anovulation are at risk for endometrial hyperplasia because of the unopposed estrogens and should be cycled using oral progesterone to induce a monthly withdrawal bleed. Those with hypoestrogenic states should be evaluated for potential estrogen replacement; women with an endometrial abnormality should be referred to a gynecologist.

Abnormal Bleeding

Abnormal bleeding can be the presenting symptom of a wide variety of abnormalities, including anovulation, endometrial pathology, or a coagulopathy. Evaluation begins with assessment of the pattern of bleeding through a detailed menstrual history. This should include information about the onset, duration, pattern, and quantity of bleeding. Women with *polymenorrhea* have a cycle less than 21 days in length; women with oligomenorrhea have an interval greater than 40 days. Women with excessive bleeding in duration or quantity have *menorrhagia*. Women with bleeding between menses are said to have *menometrorrhagia*. Prior menstrual history should be assessed to determine whether the patient has ever established a normal ovulatory cycle.

Key in the evaluation is to elicit evidence of ovulatory cycles by inquiring about *moliminal* symptoms, such as breast tenderness, cramping, or fluid retention, before the onset of bleeding. Identification of anovulatory bleeding focuses the differential diagnosis quickly to hormonal causes. Anovulatory bleeding is the result of failed ovulation and the absence of a luteal phase. The ovary secretes estrogen unopposed by progesterone and leads to a continued proliferation of the endometrium. This endometrium is unstable, which results in periodic, irregular, and often heavy bleeding. Bleeding due to coagulopathy will follow a typically ovulatory pattern and is experienced as heavy regular bleeding. A personal or family history of bleeding disorders should be sought because even in this age group, a large fraction of women with coagulopathies, such as von Willebrand disease, have not yet been diagnosed.

Physical examination will identify evidence of chronic or acute blood loss, verify the source of bleeding, and suggest a systemic etiology such as thyroid disease or PCOS. Genitourinary examination may identify a cervical polyp, typically associated with postcoital bleeding, or an enlarged uterus suggesting uterine fibroids. Pregnancy must always be excluded with a sensitive office urine pregnancy test; a Pap smear and cervical cultures should be obtained to assess for cervical disease or infection as the cause of abnormal bleeding. Laboratory testing should include a complete blood count and thyroid studies; testing for von Willebrand disease should be considered. In women at risk for endometrial hyperplasia or endometrial cancer, including women older than 35 years, and women with obesity or a history of chronic anovulation, evaluation of the endometrium should be pursued. The office endometrial biopsy using a piston-suction device, an ultrasound evaluating endometrial stripe, or a sonohysterogram should be considered to identify women with hyperplasia.

If the evaluation fails to identify an underlying abnormality, a woman is considered to have *dysfunctional uterine bleeding*. Management of abnormal bleeding will depend on the underlying pathology identified and the degree of anemia caused by the bleeding. Control of bleeding is generally achieved through the use of combination of estrogen and progestin preparations such as OCPs.

INFERTILITY

According to the Centers for Disease Control and Prevention, 12% of U.S. women have trouble conceiving or carrying a pregnancy to term. Infertility is generally considered when a couple fails to conceive after 1 year of intercourse without contraception. Infertility is more common with increasing age and is becoming a more frequent cause of infertility as women are deferring pregnancy and attempting to conceive at older ages. Infertility may be due to either female factors or male factors. The most common female factor is anovulation, which is often related to metabolic abnormalities as discussed in the sections above. Other factors are pelvic factors, such as adhesions due to a prior infection, surgery, or endometriosis, and cervical and uterine factors. Male factors include abnormal sperm number, motility, or morphology as well as erectile or ejaculatory dysfunction.

Evaluation should include a complete reproductive, medical, and gynecologic history and a physical examination to help identify any metabolic or structural gynecologic abnormalities. Testing will follow and includes basal body temperature charting for a month to confirm ovulation, an FSH on cycle day 3 to measure ovarian reserve, and prolactin and TSH levels to identify hormonal abnormalities in women with menstrual disorders. Male evaluation begins with a semen analysis. Finally, a hysterosalpingogram will establish patency of the fallopian tubes if the semen analysis is normal. Once this evaluation is complete, the underlying abnormality should be treated. Referral to infertility specialists or urologists is warranted based on findings.

CERVICAL CANCER SCREENING AND THE ABNORMAL PAPANICOLAOU TEST

HPV is highly prevalent in the United States, and it is estimated that 50% of sexually active men and women acquire HPV at some point during their life. Low-risk strains of HPV are associated with genital warts; high-risk strains are associated with cervical cancer. HPV infection can clear spontaneously, but in about 10% of women, the infection remains, putting the host at an increased risk for cervical cancer. The slow and predictable progression from cervical dysplasia to carcinoma has allowed routine cervical cancer screening to successfully reduce the incidence of cervical cancer in the United States. Recommendations on the frequency of testing as well as the management of the abnormal Pap smear have evolved with the utilization of HPV testing to triage Pap tests as well as an improved understanding of the progression and regression of abnormalities.

Screening for cervical cancer screening is strongly recommended for all women in this age group who have been sexually active and who have a cervix. Screening should start within 3 years of a sexual debut and continue annually. Women who are considered to be at low risk for cervical cancer and have had three consecutive normal findings can be screened every 2 to 3 years. Women who have had a hysterectomy with removal of the cervix for benign disease do not require screening for cervical cancer.

A Pap smear is collected by scraping the endocervical canal and is considered *adequate for evaluation* if there are endocervical cells present. Current recommendations for the management of the abnormal test are age specific. For women in this age group, a Pap reading of atypical squamous cells of uncertain significance (ASC-US) requires follow-up: if the cytologist cannot rule out a high-grade squamous intraepithelial lesion (ASC-H), if testing is positive for high-risk HPV strains, or if repeat testing done at 6 months is abnormal, colposcopy should be recommended. All women with a Pap test showing low-grade squamous intraepithelial lesion (LGSIL) or high-grade squamous intraepithelial lesion (HGSIL) should undergo colposcopy. Pap tests that show atypical glandular cells (AGCs) or endometrial cells should undergo colposcopy or endometrial biopsy, or both.

Women with HIV infection represent a special case because of the increased prevalence of squamous intraepithelial lesions and the more aggressive course of cervical changes. Pap testing twice in the first year is recommended, followed by annual testing if these tests are normal. Women with any testing that shows ASC-US should proceed directly to colposcopy rather than waiting for HPV typing or repeat testing.

Perimenopause and Menopause

Although *menopause* can be explicitly defined (when a woman has not had a menstrual cycle for 12 consecutive months or when her ovaries have been removed), the transition toward menopause can be erratic and prolonged over a 5- to 10-year period. It is characterized by ovarian and endocrine changes that ultimately result in the depletion of primordial oocyte stores and the cessation of ovarian estrogen production. It is a common time for women to present to their physicians with a number of specific complaints and offers an excellent opportunity not only for education but also for counseling on a number of important lifestyle issues.

Even before birth, follicular atresia results in a linear decline in the number of ovarian follicles available for ovulation. At birth, 1 to 2 million follicles remain; by puberty, this number decreases to 300,000 to 500,000. A more accelerated loss of follicles begins at about 37 years of age and is correlated with a small increase in FSH and decrease in inhibin. As FSH increases, the follicular phase of the cycle decreases, and one of the earliest clinical signs of the menopausal transition is the shortening of the menstrual cycle from a mean length of 30 days in the early reproductive years to 25 days in the early menopause transition. Increased levels of FSH may also promote an increase in the number of follicles recruited per cycle, resulting in increased, not decreased, levels of estrogen. This would explain some of the common complaints of perimenopausal women of breast pain, bloating, and heavy menses.

Later in the menopausal transition, the few remaining follicles respond poorly to FSH, and anovulation may occur. Menstrual cycles may become erratic with prolonged periods of oligomenorrhea. Ovulation may still occur, and women in this time period are advised to continue effective contraception until 12 months of amenorrhea have occurred.

Table 71-6	**Abnormal Uterine Bleeding Patterns in Perimenopausal Women**

Heavy menstrual bleeding (>80 mL), especially with clots
Menstrual bleeding lasting >7 days or ≥2 days longer than usual
Intervals of <21 days from the onset of one menstrual period to the onset of the next period
Any spotting or bleeding between periods
Uterine bleeding after sexual intercourse

Data from North American Menopause Society (NAMS). Menopause Practice: A Clinician's Guide, 3rd ed. Cleveland, OH, 2007.

SYMPTOMS IN THE PERIMENOPAUSE

Fluctuations in ovarian hormones can result in a number of symptoms. Changes to the menstrual flow are to be expected. The clinician needs to be aware, however, of bleeding patterns that may represent underlying pathology and not normal, perimenopausal changes. These patterns are summarized in Table 71-6.

The link to hormonal fluctuations for other symptoms is less clear. These include insomnia, mood disturbances, and cognitive changes. Sleep disturbances in perimenopausal women compared with premenopausal women are a well-documented phenomenon. Women experiencing nighttime hot flashes or sweats can have significantly disturbed sleep patterns resulting in a number of daytime complaints, including fatigue, irritability, and difficulty concentrating. Not all women reporting insomnia, however, report vasomotor symptoms. Potentially, hot flashes may not wake a woman from sleep but may interfere with the quality of her sleep. It is also important to investigate other factors in these women, including significant life stresses. Sleep apnea and use of medications that disturb the normal sleep cycle (including alcohol) should also be investigated.

Women experience higher rates of depression than men. The peak incidence for depression for women is in their 30s; most epidemiologic studies do not demonstrate an increased risk for depression during the menopausal transition. Women who do experience significant depression at this time are more likely to have experienced depression earlier in their lives, particularly at times of hormonal change (e.g., postpartum depression, premenstrual dysphoric disorder (PMDD)). Nevertheless, many women during the menopausal transition report symptoms of irritability, fatigue, and general moodiness. Sleep deprivation due to vasomotor symptoms may be one cause. A clear link to hormone levels has not been established; some women may be more sensitive to the changes in their previous cycles. Women in midlife may also experience stressors related to changing relationships with children, parents, and spouses. Issues related to self-concept and body image may emerge or be exacerbated. Mood issues during the perimenopausal transition should be approached in the same multifactorial way as at other ages.

Many women in the perimenopause complain of difficulties with concentration and memory. Sleep deprivation or ongoing stressors and distractions may be contributing factors. Evidence is lacking for a link between hormone levels and a decline in cognitive skills.

MENOPAUSE

The average age for menopause in the Western world is 51.4 years, with a range of 40 to 58 years. Women who smoke experience an earlier menopause in a dose-dependent fashion, an average of 1.5 years sooner. Evidence suggests that the age of menopause has remained unchanged over the past few centuries. What has changed, however, is the number of women who survive into the menopausal years. In the United States, the average life expectancy for a woman is almost 80 years. This means that many women will spend at least one third of their lifetime in the postmenopausal years.

In the 1960s, menopause was considered an estrogen deficiency "disease" in need of treatment. Although symptoms such as hot flashes and vaginal dryness may develop during menopause, the process itself is a normal part of the life cycle. In addition to the physical changes experienced by women, many consider the menopause transition to also be an important psychosocial passage. This transition offers clinicians the opportunity to help women focus on important preventive health measures and detect major chronic diseases as early as possible. Although menopause itself is not a disease, the postmenopausal years are associated with an increased risk for certain disease processes, most notably cardiovascular disease and osteoporosis.

Vasomotor Symptoms and the Use of Estrogen

The "hot flash" is the hallmark symptom of menopause. In the United States, up to 75% of women who experience a natural menopause and 90% of women who experience a surgical menopause will experience hot flashes. About 10% to 15% of women will experience hot flashes that are very frequent or severe. For most women, vasomotor symptoms are self-limited, lasting an average of 1 to 2 years; a significant minority of women, however (up to 25%), may experience symptoms for greater than 5 years.

The exact etiology of a hot flash is not understood, although we do know it is related to a disturbance of hypothalamic thermoregulation and that hot flashes are essentially a vascular phenomenon. During the period of time immediately before the onset of a hot flash, there is an increase in heart rate and cutaneous blood flow. A measurable rise in skin temperature occurs owing to increased vasodilation with a concomitant decrease in core body temperature. The woman experiences the sudden onset of warmth, ranging from noticeable to markedly uncomfortable, especially over the face and upper body. This may be accompanied by significant perspiration. Hot flashes may occur a few times a year or several times a day.

In the 1950s, it was discovered that estrogen could relieve hot flashes. In the 1960s, estrogen use increased not only for the relief of vasomotor symptoms, but as a way of treating "estrogen deficiency." In 1975, a study published in the *New England Journal of Medicine* showed that women who used estrogen for more than seven years had a 14-fold increase in uterine cancer. In the 1980s, it was discovered that the addition of a progestin significantly decreased this risk. Endometrial hyperplasia is reduced to essentially zero when low-dose progestin is continued for 12 to 13 days per month. Women with an intact uterus must use combination estrogen-progestin therapy to prevent endometrial hyperplasia and cancer.

Estrogen remains the only FDA-approved medication for the treatment of menopausal vasomotor symptoms as well as the most effective. It is also FDA approved for the treatment of urogenital atrophy and the prevention of osteoporosis. In the 1980s and 1990s, several large observational studies found that estrogen therapy was associated with a 50% decrease in cardiovascular disease among postmenopausal women. The potential benefit of such a decrease was so significant that many clinicians began prescribing estrogen for the sole purpose of cardiovascular protection. This assumption was not subjected to rigorous scientific study until the 1990s, when the results of the HERS trial (Heart and Estrogen/Progestin Replacement Study) found that women with preexisting heart disease developed increased cardiac events when placed on estrogen, not decreased.

The WHI was designed to look at various hormone regimens and their effects on disease prevention in postmenopausal women, particularly cardiovascular disease. More than 16,000 women participated in the trials, which ran for 5.6 years in the combined estrogen-progestin arm and 6.8 years in the estrogen-only arm. In the combined-therapy group, there was an absolute excess risk for events in the global index of 19 per 10,000 person years. Most importantly, the investigators saw an increased risk for *coronary heart disease* (CHD) (heart rate [HR] 1.29, 95% confidence interval [CI] 1.02 to 1.63), an increased risk for stroke (HR 1.41, 95% CI 1.07 to 1.85), an increased risk for pulmonary embolism (HR 2.13, 95% CI 1.39 to 3.25), and a trend toward increased risk for breast cancer (HR 1.26, 95% CI 1.0 to 1.59). The combined trial was discontinued because of this excess risk. The conclusion from the combined-therapy trial was that combination estrogen-progestin therapy should not be initiated or continued for the prevention of CHD.

The estrogen-only trial did not find a significant difference in CHD (HR .91, CI 95% 0.75 to 1.12) or for breast cancer (HR 0.77, 95% CI 0.59 to 1.01). They did, however, see the same increased risk for stroke (HR 1.39, 95% CI 1.10 to 1.77), and this trial was also discontinued early. Overall, the estimated excess risk in the global index was two events per 10,000 person-years (nonsignificant), and the conclusion was that estrogen alone should not be recommended for the prevention of chronic disease in postmenopausal women.

Although much has been written on the findings of the WHI and whether or not it was truly a trial of primary prevention (average age of subjects was 63.2 years), the results did not support the idea that estrogen therapy prevents cardiovascular disease. Additional trials are underway to address this issue in younger postmenopausal women, but until their completion, hormone therapy should not be used in this way.

Current Recommendations for Estrogen

After the WHI, several large societies put together guidelines for the use of postmenopausal hormone therapy, including the American College of Obstetricians and Gynecologists (ACOG) and the North American Menopause Society (NAMS). The general tenor of the guidelines is that estrogen and estrogen-progestin therapy are appropriate for the treatment of vasomotor symptoms and for urogenital atrophy in women who have been appropriately counseled. Hormone therapy should not be used for the prevention of cardiovascular disease. Estrogen therapy and estrogen-progestin therapy may increase the risk for stroke in post-menopausal women. It is also likely estrogen-progestin therapy increases the risk for breast cancer with use beyond 5 years; the effect with estrogen therapy is less clear. Estrogen therapy and estrogen-progestin therapy significantly reduce the risk for osteoporotic fractures in postmenopausal women; however, other medications are also effective in this regard. Finally, the concepts of "lowest dose" and "shortest period of time" have been incorporated into most guidelines.

Additional research with regard to ultralow doses, route of use (transdermal versus oral), and use in younger post-menopausal women are underway. Until that time, thorough discussion with patients on the benefits and potential risks of therapy is important.

Alternative Therapies

Interest in nonhormonal and "natural" alternatives in the treatment of menopausal symptoms is extremely high. It is estimated that as many as 75% of menopausal women have used some form of alternative or complementary treatment to relieve menopausal symptoms. Many women do not inform their physicians which products they are using, thus creating the risk for serious interactions with prescribed medications or ongoing medical conditions.

Behavioral options such as dressing in layers, regular exercise, stress reduction techniques, and avoidance of known triggers are safe and helpful for a number of women. Some of the more common herbal remedies include isoflavones (soy, red clover), black cohosh, dong quai, ginkgo, ginseng, kava, Vitex, and valerian. Many of these alternatives appear to be effective in the short term, possibly owing to the high placebo effect known to exist in studies of vasomotor symptoms. Others may legitimately improve menopause-related symptoms. A few of the products can result in significant harm (e.g., use of Kava and liver damage). Even if the clinician does not actively promote the use of alternative therapies, it is imperative to be aware of use by patients and to know which products can cause serious side effects.

SEXUALITY

Sexual concerns are often an issue for women at menopause, although a woman may be hesitant to share these concerns with her health care provider. As estrogen levels decline, there is thinning of the vaginal epithelium, which results in decreased vaginal elasticity. Decreased vaginal blood flow results in decreased vaginal secretions and decreased lubrication during sexual activity. Intercourse may become painful. Symptomatic vaginal atrophy can occur in up to 40% of postmenopausal women, but only about 25% will seek treatment for their symptoms. Other causes of vaginal pain, such as infection, should be ruled out.

For some women, vaginal lubricants (used at the time of intercourse) may be sufficient. Vaginal moisturizers (used on a regular basis to retain vaginal moisture) are also available. Topical vaginal estrogen is very effective in relieving the symptoms of vaginal atrophy with very little systemic

Table 71-7	**Factors that May Influence Sexual Functioning in Women**	
Biological	Medications (e.g., antidepressants, antihypertensives)	
	Vaginal atrophy, pain with intercourse	
	Low testosterone levels (e.g., bilateral oophorectomy)	
	Illness (e.g., diabetes, hypothyroidism, cerebrovascular accident)	
	Sleep disturbances, fatigue	
	Disability or pain from illness (e.g., arthritis)	
	Incontinence	
Psychological	Depression	
	Body image	
Interpersonal	Marital Issues	
	Poor communication	
	Partner's sexual problems (e.g., erectile dysfunction)	
	Partner's health problems (e.g., myocardial infarction)	
Sociocultural	Ageism ("too old" to want sex)	
	Multiple other obligations and commitments	
	Lack of partner	

absorption and should be considered in women who do not obtain relief from over-the-counter measures and have no other contraindications.

Decreased interest in sex is one of the most common sexual complaints of women in midlife (up to 40% in one survey). A large, population-based trial, however, showed that menopausal status had a smaller impact on sexual desire than other factors, such as overall health, partner's health, and other lifestyle issues. Biologic, psychological, interpersonal, and sociocultural factors all affect sexual functioning in women (Table 71-7). It is important for the clinician to be aware of the high prevalence of sexual issues in this population and to inquire about any sexual concerns. Having appropriate referral resources and patient literature available is helpful.

CARDIOVASCULAR DISEASE

The risk for cardiovascular disease increases for women at the time of menopause. It is estimated that one in eight women aged 45 to 65 years has some form of heart disease. This increases to one in three above the age of 65 years. A woman who has gone through menopause is twice as likely to develop heart disease as a woman of the same age who has not gone through menopause. An early, surgical menopause carries the most risk.

During the premenopausal years, it is thought that estrogen increases levels of high-density lipoprotein (HDL), which promotes the removal of cholesterol from the arteries. Estrogen also appears to exert a vasodilatory effect on blood vessels. Although women enjoy a protection against cardiovascular disease compared with men during their premenopausal years, with diabetes or increasing age, this protection disappears. Counseling women in the early postmenopausal years on the common high risk factors associated with heart disease (such as smoking, obesity, and elevated blood sugar) may help to ameliorate some of the negative effects that occur with decreasing estrogen levels.

OSTEOPOROSIS

A clear link exists between the loss of estrogen production at the time of menopause and the development of osteoporosis. With the onset of menopause, bone loss temporarily accelerates, and women may lose up to 5% of their bone mass per year over the next 5 years. About 20% of white women aged 50 years or older have osteoporosis; this number increases to 52% over the age of 80 years. Up to 90% of all hip and spine fractures in white women aged 65 to 84 years can be attributed to osteoporosis. Women who experience an early menopause are at greater risk. Screening for osteoporosis, education, counseling, and treatment are important aspects in the care of postmenopausal women.

Estrogen therapy is FDA approved for the prevention but not the treatment of osteoporosis. Alternate therapies have become more popular since the results of the WHI. These include bisphonates, calcium, and vitamin D. The pathophysiology as well as diagnosis and treatment of osteoporosis are covered elsewhere in this book. Estrogen therapy and estrogen-progestin therapy work best if started within 5 to 10 years of menopause. Estrogen use produces substantial gains in bone mass with reduction in both vertebral and hip fractures. When the medication is discontinued, bone loss once again accelerates. Effects are also diminished in women older than 75 years.

GENITOURINARY SYMPTOMS

Urinary incontinence rates increase with aging. Urinary incontinence is common after menopause, with about 25% of women affected. Urinary incontinence is often multifactorial. The endothelium of the urethra and bladder becomes more fragile and less elastic with menopause. The tone that maintains the urethra also decreases with aging. Uterine prolapse and the development of a cystocele and rectocele also increase the risk for incontinence. The risk for urinary incontinence is greater as body weight increases and abdominal weight places additional pressure on the urinary bladder. Uterine prolapse, if it occurs, also increases pressure on the bladder. Urinary incontinence and its treatment are discussed in detail in Chapter 133. The number of behavioral and pharmacologic treatment options has dramatically increased.

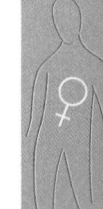

D. Special Topics

Cardiovascular Disease

Cardiovascular disease includes hypertension, coronary artery disease (CAD), cardiomyopathy, stroke, and sudden death. For all women and men, increasing age is the greatest risk factor for cardiovascular disease. It is estimated that one in eight women aged 45 to 65 years has some form of heart disease. This increases to one in three above the age of 65 years. Black women are at greater risk for death from CAD and stroke than white women. Over the past few decades, CAD mortality has been decreasing among American women less than men. Many experts believe this is probably related to less attention to cardiac risk reduction in women. In a recent telephone survey, the most frequent reason women had not discussed heart health with their physician was that their provider did not bring up this issue.

During adolescence and young adult years, the avoidance of tobacco exposure is key. Individuals should be encouraged to avoid weight gain and to be physically active. Special preventive efforts and screening should occur with families with early-onset hypertension, diabetes, or heart disease. In cohort studies, even adolescent black women have higher blood pressure, weight, and insulin resistance than adolescent white women from the same area.

It is not clear why angina is most often the first symptom of coronary disease in women, whereas myocardial infarction is the most common first symptom is men, or why the onset of clinical heart disease is about 10 years later in women than men. There is controversy about the reasons for this long-observed difference in age of onset. Some observational data suggest that a woman who has gone through menopause is twice as likely to develop heart disease as a woman of the same age who has not gone through menopause. An early, surgical menopause carries the most risk. However, the early observational studies of women with surgical menopause often did not analyze for tobacco use, and the role of hormonal therapy for these women after early menopause is not clear. Tobacco consumption lowers the age of natural menopause in a dose-related fashion—heavier exposure to tobacco more substantially leads to earlier onset of menopause.

Once diagnosed with CAD, specific medications and treatments improve outcomes for both women and men. At least among women after myocardial infarction, there has been limited improvement in assuring that women also receive best therapy (aspirin, β blockers, angiotensin-converting enzyme inhibitor, and lipid treatment) to reach goal levels. Cardiac rehabilitation improves outcomes after myocardial infarction, but women are less likely to attend. It is not clear whether this is an issue of referral or patient preference.

Sex differences in congestive heart failure have received increased attention. Both with an acute myocardial infarction and afterward women are more likely to experience congestive heart failure symptoms than men. Women are at higher risk for diastolic dysfunction, and its natural history is still being defined. Systolic dysfunction may occur after ischemia, viral illness, or alcoholism. Regardless of etiology, patients with a low ejection fraction are at risk for fatal arrhythmia. Because implantable cardioverter-defibrillators (ICDs) decrease this risk, they are recommended. Unfortunately, less devices are currently implanted in women than men meeting ICD criteria.

Stroke is the third most common cause of death in the United States (after heart disease and cancer). Stroke rates vary by sex, age, race-ethnicity, educational level, and geographic location. At younger ages, stroke is more common in men, but more older women die from stroke. Increasing age correlates with higher risk for stroke. Native and black Americans have higher rates of stroke than whites and Asian Americans; this may be related to higher rates of hypertension, diabetes, and hyperlipidemia. The risk for stroke is greatest in the Southeast.

Hypertension is perhaps the most common cardiovascular disease. The prevalence increases with age and is most common in black women. Framingham data revealed that with a systolic blood pressure higher than 180 mm Hg, the annual incidence of CHD (angina, coronary insufficiency, myocardial infarction, or death from these diagnoses) in women older than 65 years is more than 30%, whereas for men older than age 65 years, it is about 50%. If medication is required, drug side effects aid the choice of medication.

Obesity, Metabolic Syndrome, Polycystic Ovary Syndrome, and Diabetes

The prevalence of obesity has been steadily increasing, with a doubling among Americans older than 20 years from 1980 to 2002. Similarly, the prevalence of diabetes has increased dramatically, and these trends are expected to continue in adults because the metabolic syndrome is becoming more prevalent among children.

Obesity is not only linked to multiple cardiac risk factors but also independently associated with coronary artery event rates. The pattern of weight distribution is also predictive of coronary events, with more events among women with the apple shape, with a greater central or abdominal girth, than among those with the pear shape, with more weight on the hips and buttocks. A greater waist circumference increases health risk regardless of body mass index (BMI). In obesity, loss of even 10% of body weight has very positive metabolic effects.

During the past several years, the metabolic effects associated with obesity have been viewed as a spectrum disorder. Greater weight increases insulin resistance and the incidence of diabetes and hypertension. With more lipid screening, the relationship of obesity and diabetes to lipid levels has been elucidated. A subset of obese individuals have the *metabolic syndrome*, defined in the Third Report of the National Cholesterol Education Program Expert Panel on Detection, Evaluation, and Treatment of High Blood Cholesterol to include obesity, glucose intolerance, hypertension, and lipid abnormalities.

PCOS is a common metabolic disorder unique to women. Seen in a least 5% to 10% of women, it is characterized by oligo-ovulation or anovulation, evidence of androgen excess, and polycystic ovaries on ultrasound. Reproductive symptoms include irregular menses, acne, hirsutism, infertility, and increased risk for uterine cancer. Metabolic complications are associated with PCOS, including insulin resistance, diabetes, hypertension, and hyperlipidemia, as are higher rates of CAD. Pharmacologic and lifestyle interventions may improve prognosis, including aggressive management of tobacco use, lipoprotein abnormalities, and hypertension. Regular exercise can also improve glucose and blood pressure control as well as insulin resistance.

Diabetes is a growing health epidemic. In the past decade, cardiac mortality rates have increased by 23% for diabetic women yet decreased by 27% for nondiabetic women. In comparison, CAD mortality rates have declined for diabetic (13%) and nondiabetic (36%) men. Black and Hispanic women have especially high prevalence rates of diabetes.

Once a woman is diagnosed with diabetes, her "female advantage" in relation to CAD risk is lost. There is a higher risk for first myocardial infarction as well as more congestive heart failure complications and hospital mortality. It may be that less frequent identification and treatment of cardiovascular risks may be responsible for the differences in outcomes trends for women compared with men. For diabetic women, the dose-response hazards of tobacco use have been documented in the Nurses Health Study with 20 years of follow-up. The relative risk for a CAD event was 2.68 for current diabetic smokers of more than 15 cigarettes daily, 1.66 for current diabetic smokers of less than 15 cigarettes daily, and 1.21 for past diabetic smokers. Diabetic women who had not smoked for 10 years had a cardiovascular risk similar to that of nonsmoking diabetic women. Lipid abnormalities commonly occur in diabetic patients. At the time of diagnosis of type II diabetes, women have substantially lower HDL cholesterol than age-matched nondiabetic women, as well as higher low-density lipoprotein (LDL) and triglyceride levels.

Breast Complaints

Breast complaints can include a variety of symptoms, including pain, nipple discharge, and palpable mass. The risk for breast cancer increases with age, and women in younger age groups are more likely to experience symptoms related to benign breast disease. Regardless of age, women with breast complaints are generally most concerned about the possibility of breast cancer. A sensitive discussion should take place about the difference between benign and malignant disease and the difficulty in differentiating some symptoms based simply on physical examination. Women should be assured that most breast masses are benign. Prompt evaluation and a discussion about the importance of a careful follow-up are essential.

A *palpable mass* may be a cystic or a solid lesion, and these cannot be distinguished accurately by physical examination. A solid lesion may be a benign fibroadenoma or a malignant lesion, but again the characteristics of the physical examination cannot reliably distinguish the two. Some providers will perform a fine-needle aspirate in the office and, if the mass disappears completely and the fluid is not bloody, will follow-up to ensure resolution before completing a mammograph or ultrasound. Alternatively, a mammograph and targeted ultrasound will provide a more definitive evaluation. All palpable lesions that cannot be identified by breast ultrasound as a simple cyst or other benign lesion will require biopsy for tissue diagnosis. This is true for lesions that cannot be visualized by mammography or ultrasound. The role of mammography in this setting is to look for other coincident lesions, not to establish a diagnosis.

Breast pain, *mastalgia*, is a common complaint but often leads to concern and anxiety about an underlying malignancy. Although it rarely results from cancer, this must be carefully ruled out by physical examination and mammography as well as a careful follow-up after one or two menstrual cycles to ensure a stable examination. Breast pain is usually cyclic in nature and is thought to be associated with hormonal changes. It may be triggered by the use of combined hormonal contraceptives or the initiation of estrogen replacement therapy for the treatment of menopausal symptoms. There is some evidence that reducing intake of caffeine can improve symptoms.

Nipple discharge may be expressed from most women, but *spontaneous* nipple discharge always requires a further evaluation. Bilateral, guaiac-negative, milky discharge, or *galactorrhea*, is typically the result of a hormonal abnormality, most often a prolactinoma. Women with a prolactinoma will typically present with amenorrhea. Galactorrhea can also be seen with other pituitary tumors, caused by a hypothalamic or pituitary stalk lesion, chest wall trauma, hypothyroidism, and host of medications. Evaluation should include serum TSH and prolactin levels followed by magnetic resonance imaging of the head if the prolactin level is elevated. Unilateral bloody discharge is suggestive of a papilloma or other benign lesion; malignancy must always be carefully excluded.

Mastitis is a breast infection that can occur in the postpartum setting as the result of bacterial infection. It will present as the acute onset of a localized pain and erythema and is associated with fever and influenza-like symptoms. Mastitis is most often unilateral and is generally caused by *Staphylococcus* species or *Escherichia coli* and is treated with oral antibiotics and continued breastfeeding to empty the involved breast. It may be complicated by recurrent mastitis or formation of a breast abscess. Nonlactational infection may also occur as a chronic subareolar infection known as *periductal mastitis*. This is treated with oral antibiotics and warm soaks. These may also be complicated by abscess formation or require surgical excision to treat recurrent infection.

Pelvic Pain

Pelvic pain may be acute or chronic and is a common and challenging problem for both the clinician and the patient. Acute pelvic pain can present over hours or days and may be the result of gynecologic, gastrointestinal, or urinary pathology. Gynecologic causes will include complications of pregnancy, acute pelvic infection, or pain related to ovarian processes, including cyst and torsion. The possibility of a ruptured ectopic pregnancy must be quickly assessed by history and pregnancy testing because of its potentially life-threatening course. Ectopic pregnancy can be excluded by the presence of an intrauterine pregnancy on vaginal ultrasound examination. Other causes of acute pelvic pain include urinary tract infection and acute appendicitis. The evaluation of acute pelvic pain includes a thorough general and reproductive history and a physical examination, including a pelvic examination. Diagnostic testing should include basic laboratory tests, including a complete blood count, a pregnancy test, cervical cultures for chlamydia and gonorrhea, a urinalysis, and a pelvic ultrasound.

Chronic pelvic pain is considered when a woman has noncyclic pelvic pain for at least 6 months. It is highly prevalent, affecting one in seven women in the United States, and is most common among women of reproductive age. The causes of chronic pelvic pain include gynecologic, urologic, gastrointestinal, musculoskeletal, and psychological. The four most commonly diagnosed etiologies are endometriosis, adhesions, irritable bowel syndrome, and interstitial cystitis. It is common for more than one cause to be identified. Important gynecologic causes of chronic pain include endometriosis, adenomyosis, adhesions, and uterine fibroids. A history of physical or sexual abuse is associated with chronic pain and should be investigated sensitively, and safety should be established. In addition to a complete history and physical examination, including a pelvic examination, evaluation of chronic pelvic pain includes basic laboratory tests, including complete blood count, an erythrocyte sedimentation rate, a pregnancy test, cervical cultures for chlamydia and gonorrhea, a urinalysis, and a pelvic ultrasound.

A gastrointestinal evaluation should be considered for women with symptoms suggestive of irritable bowel syndrome. If initial evaluation has failed to lead to a diagnosis, laparoscopy will identify a pelvic abnormality in most cases. Interstitial cystitis should be considered for women with chronic urgency, frequency, nocturia or dysuria, and negative urine cultures. Evaluation must exclude other forms of infectious cystitis, neoplasm, and stones. Urodynamic testing and cystoscopy are often recommended.

Management of chronic pelvic pain will be determined by the underlying etiology identified and will often involve input from subspecialists. For those women who have not had a specific diagnosis, medical therapy includes the use of hormones and NSAIDs. A multidisciplinary approach, which includes medications and addresses dietary and psychosocial factors, has been shown to be superior to medical treatment alone.

Intimate or Domestic Violence

Violence and its impact frequently affect the health of patients and their providers. Interpersonal violence occurs more often between individuals who know each other, rather than among strangers. Intimate partner violence is described by the American Medical Association as "characterized as a pattern of coercive behaviors that may include repeated battering and injury, psychological/emotional abuse, sexual assault, progressive social isolation, deprivation, and intimidation. These behaviors are perpetrated by someone who is or was involved in an intimate relationship with the victim." Women are more often in the role of being battered than initiating violence. Surveys of health professionals reveal a higher prevalence of a past history of intimate partner violence than in the general public.

Interpersonal violence occurs at all ages, among all racial and ethnic groups, and regardless of educational or socioeconomic level. Intimate partner violence occurs throughout the world, including within one in four American families. About 25% of American women experience intimate violence sometime during their life. When violence occurs between adults, often the children in these homes also personally experience violence. Although in most states it is not required to report violence between adults, it is always required to report to the appropriate protective services agency if there is a concern that violence is affecting children, disabled individuals, or elderly people.

Sexual assault or being forced to engage in sexual activity can occur as part of intimate partner violence, but also occurs among individuals who are less intimate. Rape implies forced entry with oral, vaginal, or rectal penetration. Multiple surveys have found that the risk for rape is greatest among teenagers and young women. About 20% of American high school women report rape, with 10% reporting that the attack was by an intimate partner.

Women who are battered are at the greatest risk for death at the time they leave their abusive partner. Therefore, it is essential that the woman herself determine the timing of this step to maximize safety. Providers play an essential role by being a witness, treating the woman with respect as the adult she is, and documenting evidence of trauma to be available in the future.

There are several important long-term medical sequelae of interpersonal violence. Victims tend to use more ambulatory and inpatient care. Homicide by an intimate partner was reported as the cause of death in 33% of women killed compared with 4% of men. Psychological complications include post-traumatic stress disorder, depression, substance abuse, and sexual dysfunction. Acute problems include rape, leading to 5% of pregnancies annually, STIs, and other trauma complications. Chronic health problems can include headaches, irritable bowel syndrome, and pelvic pain.

Screening for interpersonal violence is essential. In contrast, many specialists suggest all patients be screened, whereas others suggest screening when certain diagnoses are being considered. Women who have been battered report that nonjudgmental inquiry made by a provider has opened the door for consideration of options besides accepting continued abuse. It is essential that screening for interpersonal violence be completed when the patient has privacy and is separate from friends and family. It is especially important to separate patients from overbearing partners before asking these types of questions. Examples of appropriate screening questions are listed in Table 71-8.

Table 71-8 **Potential Screening Questions for Interpersonal Violence: SAFE Questions**
Introduce the question:
"I ask all my patients about their experiences with violence."
"Because violence is so common, I ask my patients if they have been hurt by someone close to them."
S—Stress/Safety: "Do you feel safe in your relationship?"
A—Afraid/Abused: "Have you ever been in a relationship in which you were threatened, hurt, or afraid?"
F—Friends/Family—"Are your friends or family aware that you have been hurt? Could you tell them, and would they be able to give you support?"
E—Emergency Plan—"Do you have a safe place to go and the resources you need in an emergency?"

Patients who present with trauma should always be screened directly as well as acquiring details of how the specific injury occurred and when the decision to obtain medical care was made. Women are at higher risk if there are multiple injuries, especially at different stages of healing, or injuries that occur more often with intimate trauma, such as a perforated tympanic membrane, facial fractures, and vulvar or rectal abrasions or wounds. Pregnancy and the postpartum period is a high-risk time for abuse. Women who are abused may have a delay in seeking medical care because they often need to seek permission before presenting for medical care. Women with multiple somatic complaints, especially when many are nonanatomic, should be screened, as well as women with depression, anxiety, chronic sleep disorders, or pelvic pain.

The physician's response to the disclosure of intimate partner violence can have an immediate positive therapeutic impact. It is key to acknowledge that it took courage to share this information and that no one deserves to be treated as described. By treating the victim respectfully as a competent adult, the physician can create an environment that facilitates problem exploration. The first immediate concern is whether the victim and children, if present, will be safe leaving the office. If not, there is a national network of safe houses, and emergency departments often can provide information. The second task is to set up regular follow-up with the option for the patient to receive psychological counseling. Often, coming to a doctor is one of the few places a victim may safely go. There are multiple national as well as local resources available. National hotlines with toll-free numbers listed in phone directories provide access to support as well as information about local resources. In addition, most emergency departments have specially trained staffs that are aware of local resources. Most victims need time and emotional healing to determine a long-term safe plan.

Prospectus for the Future

Current research focusing on the actions of sex hormones throughout the body and in different parts of the life cycle will affect our understanding of physiology and biology. Exploration of cultural factors has the potential to improve communication between providers and patients and improve the effectiveness of health interventions. Over the next decade, it is expected that clinically important sex differences will be elucidated that will change our approach to the care of individual patients in both health and disease.

References

Briggs GG, Freeman RK, Yaffe SJ: Drugs in Pregnancy and Lactation: A Reference Guide to Fetal and Neonatal Risk. Philadelphia, Lippincott Williams & Wilkins, 2005.

Carlson KJ, Eisenstat SA, Frigoletto FD Jr, Schiff I: Primary Care of Women, 2nd ed. Philadelphia, Mosby, 2002.

Hatcher RA, Trussell J, Nelson AL, et al: Contraceptive Technology, 19th ed. New York, Ardent Media, 2007.

Liebschutz JM, Frayne S, Saxe GN: Violence against women: A physician's guide to identification and management. Philadelphia, ACP Press, 2003.

North American Menopause Society: Menopause Practice: A Clinician's Guide, 3rd ed. Cleveland, OH, North American Menopause Society, 2007.

Rosene-Montella K, Keely E, Barbour LA, Lee RV: Medical Care of the Pregnant Patient, 2nd ed. Philadelphia, ACP Press, 2008.

Speroff L, Fritz MA: Clinical Gynecologic Endocrinology and Infertility, 7th ed. Philadelphia, Lippincott Williams & Wilkins, 2005.

World Health Organization: Medical Eligibility for Contraceptive Use, 3rd ed. Geneva, World Health Organization, 2004. This and other materials are available at http://www.who.int/reproductive-health/publications/mec/.

Section XIV

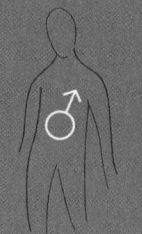

Men's Health

Men's Health Topics

Jonathan S. Starkman, Douglas F. Milam, and Joseph A. Smith, Jr.

T his chapter addresses disorders unique to men because of involvement of the male genitalia and reproductive system. It incorporates aspects of voiding, oncology, reproductive function, and infection.

A. Benign Prostatic Hyperplasia

Benign prostatic hyperplasia (BPH), a nonmalignant enlargement of the prostate gland, is a common condition in the aging male patient. It is estimated that more than 90% of all men will develop histologic evidence of BPH during the course of their lifetime; of those, greater than or equal to 50% will develop lower urinary tract symptoms (LUTS) that prompt them to seek medical care. Broadly speaking, LUTS can be divided into two groups: obstructive voiding symptoms and irritative voiding symptoms (Table 72-1).

Although most patients who seek medical care for BPH do so because of the associated LUTS, it is important to realize that these same symptoms can be the result of several different factors, including systemic illnesses such as diabetes mellitus, as well as neurologic conditions including spine disease, parkinsonism, multiple sclerosis, and cerebrovascular disease (Fig. 72-1). It is important to evaluate the patient for these non–BPH-related conditions to ensure optimal management. It is also important to pay close attention to medication use because a number of medications used in the elderly population can result in various urologic symptoms, including both obstructive and irritative voiding symptoms.

Pathophysiology

Prostate growth and the subsequent development of BPH occur under the influence of testosterone and the more metabolically active dihydrotestosterone. Testosterone, which is produced by the testes and controlled through the hypothalamic-pituitary gonadal axis, is converted to dihydrotestosterone by the action of the enzyme 5α-reductase. Dihydrotestosterone is the major intracellular androgen and is believed to be responsible for the development and maintenance of the hyperplastic cell growth characteristic of BPH.

The development of BPH occurs predominantly in the periurethral prostatic tissue referred to as the *transition zone* (Fig. 72-2). Tissue growth in this area leads to the phenomenon of bladder outlet obstruction (BOO), which leads to LUTS. BOO occurs as a result of two mechanisms: (1) mechanical obstruction, resulting from an increased tissue volume in the periurethral zone of the prostate; and (2) dynamic obstruction, which is the result of decreased bladder neck relaxation during voiding and increased smooth muscle tone in the bladder neck and prostate gland. Also important, but less well characterized, is the response of the bladder muscle to the increase in outlet resistance provided by the combination of mechanical obstruction and increased prostatic and bladder neck smooth muscle tone. As bladder outlet resistance increases, the bladder responds by increasing the force of contraction. This added work results in physical and mechanical changes in bladder function.

Early in the course of the development of BOO, the bladder is able to compensate; however, with persistent obstruction, the patient will typically develop LUTS, particularly irritative voiding symptoms such as nocturia, frequency, and urgency. These symptoms frequently drive patients to seek medical care. Later during the course of the obstructive process, the bladder wall becomes thickened and loses compliance. The subsequent loss of compliance results in a decrease in the functional capacity of the bladder, which exacerbates the patient's irritative voiding symptoms.

Diagnosis

The initial evaluation of a patient presenting with LUTS suggestive of BPH should include a detailed medical history,

focusing on the patient's urinary symptoms, as well as the patient's past medical history, including comorbid conditions and any previous surgical procedures, general health conditions, and history of alcohol and tobacco use. The assessment of a patient's symptoms can be facilitated with the use of the American Urological Association (AUA) symptom index (also known as the *international prostate symptom score*, IPSS). This is a self-administered validated questionnaire consisting of seven questions related to the symptoms of BPH and BOO. Using the AUA symptom index, symptoms can be classified as mild (0 to 7), moderate (8 to 19), or severe (20 to 35). Validated instruments such as the AUA symptom index are useful during the initial evaluation as an overall assessment of symptom severity and during follow-up visits to assess the effectiveness of any interventions, medical or surgical.

A general physical examination should also be performed that includes a digital rectal examination (DRE) and a focused neurologic examination. Urinalysis, either by dipstick or microscopic examination of urine sediment, is also mandatory to rule out hematuria or evidence of urinary tract infection. Glycosuria can also be a significant finding, particularly if not previously identified. The initial clinical practice guidelines for the diagnosis of BPH recommended a serum creatinine to assess renal function in all patients presenting with signs or symptoms suggestive of BPH. However, this recommendation has come under some scrutiny as a result of its low yield for the detection of renal insufficiency secondary to obstructive uropathy. Serum creatinine is no longer a routine part of the BPH work-up. According to the same clinical practice guidelines, measurement of prostate-specific antigen (PSA) is optional during the initial evaluation. PSA can function as a surrogate for prostate volume measurement in addition to being a screening test for prostate cancer. The National Institutes of Health (NIH)–sponsored study, MTOPS, demonstrated that PSA increases linearly with prostate volume and that PSA greater than 4 ng/mL conveys a 9% risk for requiring surgical therapy for benign disease over a 4.5-year period.

The following additional diagnostic tests are also considered optional; however, they may be useful, particularly in

Table 72-1 **Lower Urinary Tract Symptoms**	
Irritative	**Obstructive**
Frequency	Hesitancy
Nocturia	Slow stream
Urgency	Stop-and-start voiding
Urge incontinence	Sensation of incomplete emptying

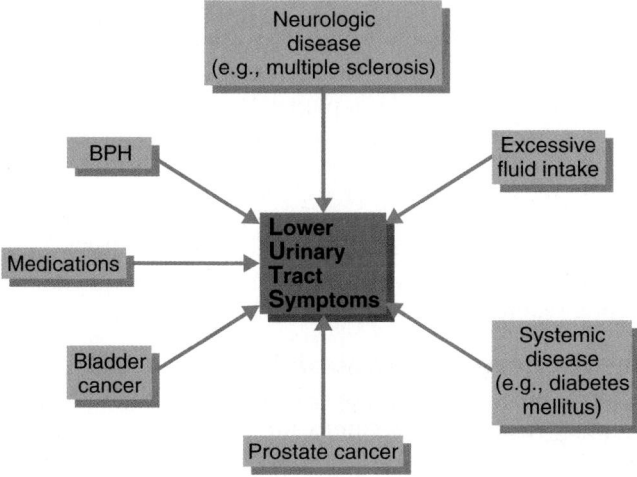

Figure 72-1 Causes of lower urinary tract symptoms. BPH, benign prostatic hyperplasia.

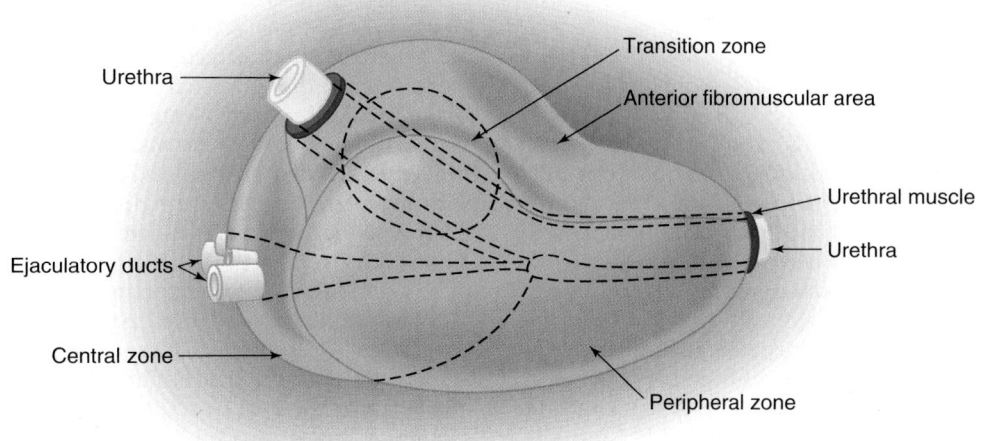

Figure 72-2 Zonal anatomy of the prostate gland.

patients with moderate to severe AUA symptom scores, in determining whether the patient's symptoms are compatible with obstruction from BPH. Uroflowmetry is a noninvasive method of measuring urinary flow rate. The maximal urinary flow rate, Qm, is generally considered the most useful method for identifying patients with BOO. However, patients with diminished flow rates may also have impaired bladder contraction. Typical values range from 25 mL per second in a young man without BOO to 10 mL per second or lower in a man with significant BOO. Measurement of postvoid residual (PVR) urine may be accomplished by urethral catheterization or, preferably, ultrasonography. Elevated PVR volumes indicate an increased risk for acute urinary retention and eventual need for surgical intervention. The NIH-sponsored MTOPS study demonstrated that 7% of men with PVR greater than 39 mL required surgical intervention over a 4.5-year period. Elevation of PVR greater than 200 mL raises the question of functional impairment of the bladder and warrants further evaluation with urodynamic testing.

Urodynamic evaluation involves the introduction of pressure monitoring transducers into the bladder and rectum and subsequent measurement of intravesical and intra-abdominal pressures. These relationships, particularly those relating intravesical pressure and flow rate while voiding (pressure-flow studies), can provide significant information about the nature of the patient's symptoms and the presence or absence of BOO. Pressure-flow studies are most useful in distinguishing BOO caused by BPH from impaired bladder contraction (hyper or hypo). However, this is an invasive modality that requires specific urologic expertise for its optimal use. Routine cystoscopic examination is optional in the evaluation of the patient with BPH. It is most frequently performed either in the course of evaluating the patient for a potentially invasive therapy, such as surgical resection, or for the evaluation of a coexisting condition, such as hematuria.

Routine evaluation of the upper tracts (kidneys and ureters) with excretory urography or ultrasonography is not recommended for the average BPH patient unless there is concomitant urinary pathology (i.e., hematuria, urinary tract infection, renal insufficiency, a history of prior urologic surgery, or a history of nephrolithiasis). Likewise, transrectal ultrasonography (TRUS) is not routinely recommended unless it is used for preoperative assessment of prostate gland size while planning surgical intervention.

Differential Diagnosis

Many conditions can cause LUTS in the aging male. DRE and PSA testing are helpful in distinguishing between BPH and prostate cancer. Typically, early-stage prostate cancer is asymptomatic. Therefore, patients may have both conditions concurrently. Although PSA testing is not sufficiently sensitive or specific to reliably differentiate BPH from prostate cancer, it is a useful tool to stratify a patient's risk for the presence of prostate cancer. Prostatitis is another condition that can cause LUTS. It may result from bacterial infection or from a nonbacterial inflammatory process, and the symptoms may substantially overlap those of BPH, particularly in the older male. Diabetes mellitus, neurologic diseases such as Parkinson disease or cerebrovascular disease, or

other conditions of the urinary tract, such as urethral strictures, may result in LUTS seen in patients with BPH. Finally, many medications, particularly those with significant anticholinergic side effects, may mimic the symptoms associated with BPH.

Management

MEDICAL THERAPY

Medical management is the preferred first-line treatment option for patients diagnosed with LUTS from BPH. Most patients can be managed effectively with a minimum of side effects using the medications discussed below. The NIH MTOPS study conclusively demonstrated that combination therapy with both a long-acting α blocker and a 5α-reductase inhibitor was more effective than single-agent therapy alone. In general, medical management is initiated for patients with moderate to severe AUA symptom scores. However, it is important to note that, in the absence of indications for surgery (refractory urinary retention, hydronephrosis with or without renal impairment, recurrent urinary tract infections, recurrent gross hematuria, or bladder calculi), the decision to embark on any course of therapy, medical or otherwise, is principally driven by the degree of bother caused by the patient's symptoms. Every patient has a different perception of his symptoms; therefore, nocturia twice nightly, while a minor nuisance to some, may represent a significant problem for others. There is no absolute AUA symptom score or other objective measure that dictates the need for initiation of therapy for symptomatic BPH. Each patient must be evaluated individually and his treatment course tailored to his individual situation.

α-adrenergic Antagonists

α-adrenergic antagonists, or α blockers, are the most commonly prescribed medications for the treatment of LUTS associated with BPH. The bladder neck and prostate are richly innervated with α-adrenergic receptors, specifically α_{1a} receptors, which constitute about 70% to 80% of the total number of α receptors in these areas. α_{1b} receptors modulate vascular smooth muscle contraction and are located in the bladder neck and prostate to a lesser degree.

Doxazosin, terazosin, tamsulosin, and extended-release alfuzosin are long acting α-receptor antagonists. They are generally administered once daily, usually at bedtime to minimize the potential for orthostatic hypotension. These medications act through α_1 receptors and can cause vasodilation resulting in transient hypotension and lightheadedness. Blood pressure reduction is greater in patients with hypertension (average reduction of 10 to 15 mm Hg) relative to normotensive patients (average reduction 1 to 4 mm Hg). Overall, 10% to 20% of patients experience some often transient side effects from these medications, including dizziness, asthenia, headaches, peripheral edema, and nasal congestion. Dose titration is recommended for doxazosin and terazosin to minimize occurrence of these adverse effects and optimize therapeutic response. Doxazosin and terazosin require at least 4 or 5 mg, respectively, to achieve a therapeutic effect. Maximal response is usually seen within 1 to 2 weeks with doxazosin and 3 to 6 weeks with terazosin.

Overall, these drugs reduce symptom scores by 40% to 50% and improve urinary flow rates by 40% to 50% in about 60% to 65% of patients treated.

Tamsulosin is a selective α_{1a} receptor antagonist with a long half-life. It has a significantly lower degree of nonspecific α-receptor binding compared with other α-receptor antagonists. Therefore, side effects such as postural hypotension and dizziness are less common. This drug does not appreciably affect blood pressure in hypertensive or normotensive patients. Maximal response is usually seen within 1 to 2 weeks of the initiation of therapy.

5α-reductase Inhibition (Finasteride and Dutasteride)

Finasteride and dutasteride block the intracellular conversion of testosterone to 5-dihydrotestosterone by inhibiting the action of the enzyme 5α-reductase. This results in an approximate 18% to 25% reduction in prostate gland size over 6 to 12 months. It is most effective in reducing symptoms and preventing disease progression in patients with large prostate glands (>40 mL), although recent evidence suggests that symptomatic improvement and stabilization of disease progression may occur in treated men with prostatic size down to 30 mL. 5α-reductase inhibition has also been shown to decrease the risk for urinary retention and the risk for subsequent surgical intervention, again, predominantly in those patients with larger glands. Initial response is seen within 6 months, and maximal effect occurs 12 to 18 months after the initiation of therapy.

Finasteride and dutasteride reduce serum PSA by about 50%. This must be taken into consideration when interpreting PSA values in men taking these agents. After 6 months of therapy, the effective PSA level in a patient taking finasteride or dutasteride may be calculated by multiplying the measured PSA by 2. Free PSA (the percentage of non–protein-bound PSA) is also reduced by about 50%. Use of finasteride or dutasteride may result in sexual dysfunction, including decreased erectile rigidity, decreased libido, and decreased ejaculate volume. Erectile dysfunction (ED) caused by 5α-reductase inhibitor therapy is reversible and returns to baseline within 2 to 6 months after discontinuation of therapy.

Phytotherapy

There is a growing body of evidence to suggest that various plant extracts may have a therapeutic effect in the treatment of LUTS associated with BPH. Saw palmetto berry (*Serenoa repens*) extracts are the most widely used and studied. Use of saw palmetto has been shown to improve symptom scores in randomized trials in Europe. The extent of therapeutic improvement is at this point unclear but appears to be substantially less than the U.S. Food and Drug Administration (FDA)–approved medications described previously. *Africanum* (African plum) extract has also been used to treat symptoms associated with BPH. However, less is known about its overall efficacy and mechanism of action.

Use of herbal or plant extracts for the therapeutic management of symptomatic BPH remains somewhat controversial in the United States, despite their widespread use in Europe, particularly Germany. There is, however, growing interest in the evaluation of these compounds in the United States. Clinical trials are currently ongoing; however, results will not be available for several years.

SURGICAL MANAGEMENT

Minimally Invasive Therapy

Although transurethral resection of the prostate (TURP) remains the gold standard for the surgical treatment of BPH, substantial effort has been devoted to the development of less invasive and less morbid methods of treating patients with symptomatic BPH. This has led to a proliferation of minimally invasive therapies, primarily using different methods of generating heat within the prostate gland, resulting in tissue destruction. The office-based heat techniques described below transiently increase bladder outlet obstruction for 1 to 2 weeks because of postprocedure swelling. Maximal tissue reduction and treatment effect occur within 12 weeks.

Transurethral microwave thermotherapy (TUMT) is one of the most widely studied minimally invasive methods of treating patients with symptomatic BPH. Catheter-mounted transducers use microwave energy (30 to 300 Hz) to heat prostatic tissue, resulting in coagulative necrosis and shrinkage of the prostate gland. The subsequent reduction in prostate transition zone volume results in an improvement in flow rates and symptom scores. Transurethral needle ablation (TUNA) uses low-level radio frequency energy to effect similar changes within the prostate gland. Other therapies currently available or in development include interstitial lasers and high-intensity focused ultrasound. All these therapies are designed to deliver sufficient energy to the prostate to cause tissue destruction, resulting in smaller prostate glands and an attendant improvement in patient symptoms.

The most common side effects of these treatments are temporary increases in irritative voiding symptoms, transient urinary retention (TUR), hematuria, and ejaculatory dysfunction (primarily retrograde ejaculation). Late complications, such as urethral strictures and ED, have been reported but are significantly less common than with traditional surgical approaches. The major benefits of these less invasive therapies are the reduction in traditional surgical morbidities such as bleeding, fluid absorption (TUR syndrome), and the risks associated with general or spinal anesthesia, as well as decreased rates of long-term complications such as incontinence, ED, bladder neck contractures, and urethral strictures. Additional important advantages include decreased anesthetic requirements and potential elimination of hospitalization resulting from the fact that most of these procedures can be accomplished safely on an outpatient basis, either in the office or in an ambulatory surgical setting.

Success rates for the heat-based minimally invasive therapies are intermediate between those achieved with medical management and with traditional surgical therapy, with 65% to 75% of patients experiencing symptomatic improvement and improved flow rates. The long-term durability of these therapies appears good but is presently being evaluated.

Traditional Surgical Management

TURP remains the gold standard for the surgical management of symptomatic BPH. This procedure involves endoscopic removal of periurethral prostate tissue. Improvements

Table 72-2 **Success in Medical versus Surgical Management of Benign Prostatic Hyperplasia**					
	α₁ **Blockers**	**Finasteride**	**TURP**	**TUIP**	**Open Surgery**
Percentage of symptom improvement	48	31	82	73	79
Percentage of flow rate improvement	40-50	17	120	100	185
Mean probability of achieving the above improvement (%)	74	67	88	80	98

TUIP, transurethral incision of the prostate; TURP, transurethral resection of the prostate.

in the conventional technique have included using bipolar electrosurgical cutting, which allows saline irrigant and eliminates the chance of TUR syndrome. Newer competitive operating room–based therapies have evolved that produce a similar end result as TURP. These include holmium laser enucleation (HOLEP) and potassium titanyl phosphate (KTP) laser treatment, which use high-energy laser light to remove transition zone tissue. These operating room procedures, all of which produce similar results, produce the greatest improvement in both urinary flow rate, bladder emptying, and symptom score. TURP, HOLEP, and KTP are useful for all but the largest prostate glands (>100 g), which are best managed with open surgical enucleation. Although they are most effective, complications following the operating room–based therapies are higher than those caused by minimally invasive office-based approaches. Urinary incontinence, retrograde ejaculation, and urethral stricture rates are all higher after operating room procedures than office-based therapies. Perioperative morbidity, including the need for blood transfusion, although substantially decreased by technical improvements, is likewise higher after TURP and similar procedures. However, standard electrosurgical resection of the prostate, TURP, is the most effective surgical treatment for symptomatic BPH, short of open surgical enucleation. Success rates, as measured by improvements in symptom score and increases in urinary flow rates, are 80% to 90% following TURP.

Transurethral incision of the prostate (TUIP) is another more limited surgical procedure consisting of incision of the bladder neck and proximal prostatic urethra. Although more invasive than the heat-based therapies, in properly selected patients (i.e., those with prostate glands less than 30 g in size), success rates approach those seen following TURP. Morbidity following TUIP is significantly less than that following TURP, but long-term durability of symptom relief is less than that seen with TURP.

Open surgical enucleation, or simple prostatectomy, is reserved for patients with very large glands. Success rates are high following this approach; however, the rate of complications following open surgical resection is highest of all the traditional surgical approaches (Table 72-2).

The management of LUTS resulting from BPH has undergone a dramatic shift from principally a surgical approach to a medical approach. Most patients presenting with LUTS believed to be secondary to BPH are initially managed medically as discussed above. This, coupled with the aging of the U.S. population, has resulted in a shift of the care of these patients from the urologist to the primary care physician. In the absence of severe LUTS or indications for early surgical intervention, the primary care physician can now successfully manage most patients with mild to moderate BPH. Patients not responding to medical therapy are often offered office-based minimally invasive surgical therapy.

References

Blute ML, Larson T: Minimally invasive therapies for benign prostatic hyperplasia. Urology 58 (6 Suppl 1):33-40, discussion 40-41, 2001.

Fagelman E, Lowe FC: Herbal medications in the treatment of benign prostatic hyperplasia (BPH). Urol Clin North Am 29:23-29, vii, 2002.

Lepor H, Lowe FC: Evaluation and nonsurgical management of benign prostatic hyperplasia. In Walsh PC, Retik AB, Vaughan ED Jr. et al (eds): Campbell's Urology, 8th ed. Philadelphia, WB Saunders, 2002, pp 1337-1378.

Lowe FC, McConnell JD, Hudson PB, et al, for the Finasteride Study Group: Long-term 6-year experience with finasteride in patients with benign prostatic hyperplasia. Urology 61:791-796, 2003.

Lummus WE, Thompson I: Prostatitis. Emerg Med Clin North Am 19:691-707, 2001.

McConnell JD, Roehrborn CG, Bautista OM, et al, for the Medical Therapy of Prostatic Symptoms (MTOPS) Research Group: The long-term effect of doxazosin, finasteride, and combination therapy on the clinical progression of benign prostatic hyperplasia. N Engl J Med 349:2387-2398, 2003.

Roehrborn CG, Bartsch G, Kirby R, et al: Guidelines for the diagnosis and treatment of benign prostatic hyperplasia: A comparative, international overview. Urology 58:642-650, 2001.

Roehrborn CG, Bruskewitz R, Nickel JC, et al, for the Proscar Long-Term Efficacy and Safety Study Group: Sustained decrease in incidence of acute urinary retention and surgery with finasteride for 6 years in men with benign prostatic hyperplasia [clinical trial]. J Urol 171:1194-1198, 2004.

Sarma AV, Jacobson DJ, McGree ME, et al: A population based study of incidence and treatment of benign prostatic hyperplasia among residents of Olmsted County, Minnesota: 1987 to 1997 [see comment]. J Urol 173:2048-2053, 2005.

Trock BJ, Brotzman M, Utz WJ, et al: Long-term pooled analysis of multicenter studies of cooled thermotherapy for benign prostatic hyperplasia results at three months through four years. Urology 63:716-721, 2004.

B. Prostatitis

Prostatitis is an extremely common clinical condition, estimated to account for one in four office visits to urologists. It is the most common urologic diagnosis in men less than 50 years old and is the third most common diagnosis in men older than 50 years. It is associated with a multitude of symptoms ranging from pelvic pain to voiding dysfunction. Until recently, the diagnosis of prostatitis was poorly defined and based primarily on clinical history. Treatment of the prostatitis syndromes remains equally problematic, with the efficacy of the most common therapies lacking evidence-based guidelines. Recently, the NIH developed a standardized classification of prostatitis syndromes:

NIH category I: acute bacterial prostatitis (ABP)
NIH category II: chronic bacterial prostatitis (CBP)
NIH category III: chronic pelvic pain syndrome (CPPS)
NIH category IIIa: inflammatory CPPS
NIH category IIIb: noninflammatory CPPS
NIH category IV: asymptomatic prostatitis

Chronic nonbacterial prostatitis or CPPS (categories IIIa and IIIb) is the most common symptomatic type of prostatitis and may be the most prevalent of all prostate disorders, including BPH. Despite this, chronic nonbacterial prostatitis or CPPS remains enigmatic and has not been conclusively demonstrated to be primarily a disease of the prostate or the result of a defined inflammatory process.

Acute Bacterial Prostatitis

Acute bacterial prostatitis is a relatively uncommon serious systemic illness requiring aggressive treatment with intravenous antibiotics. Patients typically present with fevers, chills, dysuria, and perineal and low back pain. Advanced cases may present with signs of sepsis. Physical examination may reveal a distended bladder, and DRE usually reveals a warm, boggy, and tender prostate. Rectal examination should be performed with caution to minimize the risk for inducing bacteremia as a result of overaggressive manipulation of the gland. Some urologists recommend deferring a rectal examination if the clinical presentation is highly suggestive of acute prostatitis.

Laboratory analysis typically reveals an elevated white blood cell count and a positive urine culture. Localization examination is contraindicated because the pathogen is identified in the midstream urine. If the patient has evidence of urinary retention, a suprapubic cystostomy tube should be considered for bladder drainage to minimize transurethral instrumentation. Those not acutely septic can be managed with an indwelling urethral catheter. Acutely ill patients are typically hospitalized for parenteral antibiotics and supportive care. Patients should be treated for a total of 30 days with combined parenteral and oral antibiotics to reduce the risk for development of chronic prostatitis. Fluoroquinolones are recommended because they achieve excellent tissue levels within prostate tissue. Although bacterial persistence or conversion to chronic bacterial prostatitis is low, follow-up urine cultures should be obtained to document clearance of the infection. In rare cases, a prostatic abscess may form, especially in immunocompromised patients (i.e., those with diabetes or HIV). This can be evaluated with TRUS or contrast-enhanced pelvic computed tomography (CT) and is treated with surgical transurethral unroofing of the abscess cavity and supplementary antibiotics.

Chronic Bacterial Prostatitis

Chronic bacterial prostatitis is associated with inflammation of the prostate gland and recurrent urinary tract infections with bacteria localized to the prostate through standardized localization testing. Etiologic agents range from common uropathogens to cryptic organisms difficult to culture. The differential diagnosis includes cystitis, urethritis, and CPPS (categories IIIa and IIIb). Symptoms are nonspecific and include LUTS, pelvic pain, and sexual dysfunction, either alone or in combination. Physical examination may reveal abdominal tenderness, testicular or epididymal tenderness, prostate tenderness, or tenderness associated with DRE. The prostate is often normal to palpation, although it may be enlarged secondary to concomitant BPH.

Traditional testing of the urine in this patient population is accomplished by evaluation of urine in the following manner. The first voided urine (VB-1) is collected, followed by collection of midstream urine (VB-2). Following this, a DRE is performed, and the prostate is massaged. Expressed prostatic secretions (EPS) are then collected. The patient is then asked to void again, and the post–prostatic massage urine (VB-3) is collected. Evaluation of each of these fractions can provide evidence of the source of any infection. Chronic bacterial prostatitis is diagnosed when there are 10 times the number of white blood cells in the EPS or VB-3 relative to the VB-1 or VB-2. Alternatively, culture of the EPS or VB-3 must grow 10-fold more organisms than the VB-1 or VB-2. One may also compare preprostatic and post–prostatic massage urine for the presence of white blood cells and uropathogenic organisms. Although these measures are commonly described for the accurate diagnosis of prostatitis, a presumptive diagnosis is often made based on clinical symptoms, EPS, and urinalysis findings.

Treatment involves a 4- to 8-week course of antimicrobial therapy. This can be extended to 12 weeks in those who respond initially but fail to eradicate the organism from the genitourinary tract. Broad-spectrum antibiotics such as trimethoprim-sulfamethoxazole (TMP-SMX) or a fluoroquinolone are indicated for the treatment of chronic bacterial prostatitis and must be tailored to the suspected pathogen. Studies have shown excellent tissue levels of these drugs within the prostate. Typically, between 60% and 80% of patients are cured with 1- to 3-month treatment courses. One third of patients will relapse with recurrent symptoms and bacteriuria. For patients who have relapsing infections, long-term suppressive therapy may be indicated, whereas patients who have recurrent infections with different organisms are best treated with low-dose prophylactic antibiotics. Surgery is rarely indicated in patients with chronic bacterial prostatitis because cure rates of only 33% are achieved with aggressive TURP, probably because most of the infected tissue lies in the peripheral zone of the prostate, as opposed to the transition zone. Treatment endpoints are the clearance of appropriate cultures and the resolution of the patient's symptoms.

Chronic Nonbacterial Prostatitis or Chronic Pelvic Pain Syndrome

The NIH category III CPPS makes up the largest percentage of patients with clinical prostatitis. These syndromes are the most difficult to diagnose and treat and are the most poorly understood pathophysiologically. In addition, there is a substantial economic impact associated with CPPS, which warrants further research to determine more effective treatment strategies. Patients with CPPS typically present with a combination of pain (perineal, low back, suprapubic, groin, or scrotal), voiding dysfunction (dysuria, weak stream, frequency, urgency, or nocturia), and sexual dysfunction (painful ejaculation or low libido). The presence of pelvic pain, regardless of the degree of associated symptoms, is mandatory for the diagnosis of category III prostatitis. Because of the varied symptoms among patients, the NIH created a validated symptom index that is now available for the initial assessment and subsequent follow-up of patients with chronic prostatitis (NIH-CPSI). It is a 13-item questionnaire with three domain scores: (1) pain, (2) urinary symptoms, and (3) quality of life. The clinical evaluation of patients with CPPS often includes clinical history and examination, administration of the NIH-CPSI, urinary tract localization studies, and urinary flow rate with PVR.

Inflammatory CPPS (NIH category IIIa) is associated with the same symptoms seen in CBP; however, no causative organism is typically identified. Pelvic pain is a frequent symptom that may be exacerbated by stress, certain dietary factors, or vigorous physical exercise. The etiology of the symptoms is unclear, but patients' quality of life is significantly affected by the presence of this disorder. Rectal examination typically reveals nonspecific findings, and the prostate may be tender or indurated, although, more frequently, the examination results are within normal limits. Urinalysis should be normal, and urine cultures should be sterile. The EPS often reveal significant numbers of white blood cells but, again, should be sterile. Treatment can be frustrating

for both patients and providers and includes measures such as warm baths and nonsteroidal anti-inflammatory drugs (NSAIDs), with some urologists recommending prostatic massage for patients who ejaculate infrequently. The routine use of antibiotics is common, but controversial. Generally, antibiotic therapy should be limited to an empirical 2-week course of an appropriate antibiotic and terminated if there is no clinical response to treatment. If the patient responds, extension to a full 6-week course may be indicated.

Noninflammatory Chronic Pelvic Pain Syndrome

Noninflammatory CPPS, also known as *prostatodynia*, is typically seen in younger male patients (20 to 50 years). They typically present with symptoms suggestive of prostatitis, including pelvic pain and voiding symptoms, but have negative urine cultures, normal EPS, and a normal prostate on DRE. Stress is a frequent component of the symptom complex.

Treatment in this population again includes the same supportive measures mentioned previously. α-adrenergic antagonists are the primary pharmacologic agent used to treat this condition, although efficacy data are scant. NSAIDs are also useful and may be used in conjunction with tricyclic antidepressants for the management of chronic pain. The anticholinergic side effects of the tricyclics can also help with the associated frequency and urgency often experienced by these patients. Biofeedback and other stress management techniques have been used with limited success.

Recently, small studies have suggested that the heat-based minimally invasive methods used to treat BPH may have some role in the treatment of noninflammatory CPPS. TUMT has been shown to decrease pain and voiding symptoms in small series of patients. Larger studies are needed to confirm the utility and safety of this approach.

This is a difficult and demanding problem for both patients and physicians. Patients have frequently seen multiple physicians, and some have chronic pain and other psychiatric problems, such as depression or anxiety disorders. It is important to remember that, despite our poor understanding of the pathophysiology of this condition, it is common and has a major impact on quality of life. Appropriate clinical concern, coupled with good patient communication and rational treatment strategies, is the foundation for the successful management of this challenging group of patients.

References

Calhoun EA, Collins MM, Pontari MA, et al: The economic impact of chronic prostatitis. Arch Intern Med 164:1231-1236, 2004.
Carver BS, Bozeman CB, Williams BJ, Venable DD: The prevalence of men with National Institutes of Health category IV prostatitis and association with serum prostate specific antigen. J Urol 169:589-591, 2003.
Cheah PY, Liong ML, Yuen KH, et al: Terazosin therapy for chronic prostatitis/chronic pelvic pain syndrome: A randomized, placebo controlled trial. J Urol 169:592-596, 2003.
Hau VN, Schaeffer AJ: Acute and chronic prostatitis. Med Clin North Am 88:483-494, 2004.
Lummus WE, Thompson I: Prostatitis. Emerg Med Clin North Am 19:691-707, 2001.

Nickel JC: Prostatitis syndromes: An update for urologic practice. Can J Urol 7:1091-1098, 2000.

Nickel JC: The three A's of chronic prostatitis therapy: Antibiotics, alpha blockers, and anti-inflammatories. What is the evidence? BJU Int 94:1230-1233, 2004.

Nickel JC, Downey J, Ardern D, et al: Failure of monotherapy strategy for the treatment of difficult chronic prostatitis/chronic pelvic pain syndrome patients. J Urol 172:551-554, 2004.

Nickel JC, Pontari M, Moon T, et al: A randomized, placebo controlled, multicenter study to evaluate the safety and efficacy of rofecoxib in the treatment of chronic nonbacterial prostatitis. J Urol 169:1401-1405, 2003.

Schaeffer AJ: Etiology and management of chronic pelvic pain syndrome in men. Urology 63:75-84, 2004.

Schaeffer AJ: NIDDK-sponsored chronic prostatitis collaborative research network (CPCRN) 5 year data and treatment guidelines for bacterial prostatitis. Inter J Antimicrob Agents 24S:S49-S52, 2004.

Shoskes DA, Hakim L, Ghoniem G, et al: Long-term results of multimodal therapy for chronic prostatitis/chronic pelvic pain syndrome. J Urol 169:1406-1410, 2003.

Turner JA, Ciol MA, Von Korff M, Berger R: Validity and responsiveness of the national institutes of health chronic prostatitis symptom index. J Urol 169:580-583, 2003.

C. Erectile Dysfunction

Impotence is a condition defined by inability to attain or maintain adequate penile rigidity sufficient for intercourse. Impotence is the most common cause of ED in the United States. Other important, although less common, causes of ED include Peyronie disease, trauma, and rapid ejaculation. About 10 million Americans are affected by ED. Table 72-3 illustrates the prevalence of ED measured in the Massachusetts Male Aging Study. As one can see, at age 40 years, about 5% of men never have penile rigidity sufficient for vaginal penetration. By age 70 years, at least 15% of men experience complete ED, whereas about 50% have varying degrees of ED. Age and physical health are the most important predictors of the onset of ED. Smoking was the most important lifestyle variable, and ED did not correlate with male hormone levels.

Mechanism of Erection

Psychogenic or tactile sexual stimulation, or both, is the initial point in the pathway leading to penile erection. Nerve signals are carried through the pelvic plexus, a portion of which condenses into the cavernous nerves of the penile corpora cavernosa. The pelvic plexus receives input from both the sympathetic and parasympathetic nervous system. Sympathetic fibers originate in the thoracolumbar spinal cord, condense into the hypogastric plexus located immediately below the aortic bifurcation, and course into the pelvic plexus. Parasympathetic fibers originate in sacral spinal cord segments 2 through 4 and join the pelvic plexus. Discrete nerves carrying both sympathetic and parasympathetic fibers innervate the organs of the pelvis. In 1982, Walsh and Donker demonstrated that nerves coursing immediately lateral to the urethra continue on to innervate the corpora cavernosa. It is now known that branches of those nerves are the principle innervation of the neuromuscular junction, where arterial smooth muscle controls penile blood flow.

Sexual stimulation causes the release of nitric oxide (NO) by the cavernous nerves into the neuromuscular junction (Fig. 72-3). NO activates guanylyl cyclase, which converts guanosine triphosphate (GTP) into cyclic guanosine monophosphate (cGMP). Protein kinase G is activated by cGMP and in turn activates several proteins that decrease intracellular calcium (Ca^{2+}) concentration. Decreased smooth muscle Ca^{2+} concentration causes muscular relaxation, cavernosal artery dilation, increased blood flow, and subsequent penile erection. The control of blood flow on the venous outflow side is less well understood.

Table 72-3 **Relationship of Risk Factors to Erectile Dysfunction: Prevalence (%) of Complete Erectile Dysfunction**				
			Risk Factor Plus Smoking Status	
Risk Factor	**Prevalence**	**Smoker**	**Former Smoker**	**Nonsmoker**
Age 40 yr	5.1			
Age 70 yr	15			
Diabetes*	28			
Heart disease*	39	56	21	8.5
Hypertension*	15	20		
All patients	9.6			

*Patients diagnosed with and undergoing treatment for these conditions.
   Data from Feldman HA, Goldstein I, Hatzichristou DG, et al: Impotence and its medical and psychosocial correlates: Results of the Massachusetts Male Aging Study. J Urol 151:54-61, 1994.

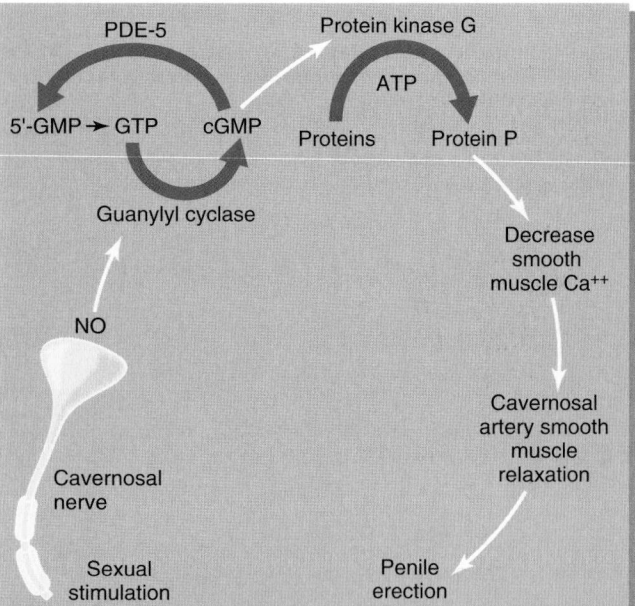

Figure 72-3 Sexual stimulation causes the release of nitric oxide (NO) by the cavernous nerve into the neuromuscular junction. ATP, adenosine triphosphate; cGMP, cyclic guanosine monophosphate; GMP, guanosine monophosphate; GTP, guanosine triphosphate; PDE-5, phosphodiesterase type 5.

Causes of Erectile Dysfunction

Psychogenic ED was formerly thought to be the most common etiology of ED. Progressive advances in understanding of the mechanics and neurophysiology of erectile function have identified other more common causes of ED. Psychogenic ED is now thought to represent less than 15% of patients seen by ED specialists. The anatomic site now believed to be the most common cause of ED is the neuromuscular junction, where the cavernosal nerves meet the smooth muscle and endothelium of the deep cavernous penile arteries. This is where NO and cGMP play a critical role in regulating penile blood flow. This so-called endothelial dysfunction may be an early tipoff of evolving systemic arterial disease. Other less common causes of decreased erectile rigidity include endocrine disorders, vascular disease, central and peripheral nerve disorders, drug-induced ED, and venogenic ED.

NEUROMUSCULAR JUNCTION DISORDERS

NO is released from cavernosal nerves, causing activation of guanylyl cyclase within the corpus cavernosum. Figure 72-3 illustrates that there are several steps that, if not functioning properly, could impede erectile function. Most research at this time is focused on generation of NO by the cavernous nerves. Further understanding of all the steps in the erectile pathway will likely implicate other biochemical reactions as causing ED. The fact that at least 60% of patients with ED from all causes other than trauma or medical treatment respond to phosphodiesterase type 5 (PDE-5) inhibition is strong evidence supporting the inference that biochemical

dysfunction at the neuromuscular junction is by far the most common cause of ED.

ENDOCRINE DISORDERS

Testosterone plays a permissive role in erectile function. Endocrine disorders may directly or indirectly decrease plasma free or bound testosterone. The most obvious, but one of the least prevalent, causes of ED is hypogonadism. Erectile ability is partially androgen dependent. These patients present with decreased or absent libido in addition to loss of erectile rigidity. Physical examination of the testes in patients afflicted with primary or secondary hypogonadism often demonstrates soft, atrophic gonads. Androgen replacement (testosterone cypionate, 200 mg every 2 to 3 weeks, or daily topical testosterone gel or patch preparations) is expected to induce return of erectile function in patients with very low or undetectable serum testosterone concentrations resulting from hypogonadism. These patients are relatively uncommon, however. More commonly, the impotent patient will have normal or mildly decreased levels of circulating androgens. Testosterone replacement rarely restores erectile function in those with mildly decreased serum testosterone levels and should not be routinely given for that indication. Testosterone supplementation is never indicated for patients with normal circulating androgen levels.

The most common endocrine disorder affecting erectile ability is diabetes mellitus. Diabetes affects both the autonomic and somatic nervous system in addition to causing atherosclerotic vascular disease. The most important effect diabetes has on erectile ability appears to relate to loss of function of long autonomic nerves. Erection is partially mediated by efferent parasympathetic cholinergic neural stimuli. Loss of long cholinergic neurons results in interruption of the efferent side of the erectile reflex arc. Diabetes also appears to produce dysfunction of the neuromuscular junction at the level of arterial smooth muscle in the penile corpora cavernosa. Studies have indicated markedly decreased acetylcholine and NO concentrations in the trabeculae of the corpora cavernosa in diabetic patients. These findings probably represent a combination of neural loss and neuromuscular junction dysfunction.

Other endocrine disorders, including hypothyroidism, hyperthyroidism, and adrenal dysfunction, may uncommonly cause ED. Because of the uncommon occurrence of thyroid and adrenal conditions in those presenting for treatment of ED, testing of those axes is not a part of the routine work-up of ED.

VASCULAR DISEASE

Vascular disease is a frequent cause of ED in the United States. This is primarily due to the high prevalence and often severe nature of peripheral vascular disease. Penile erection is obtained by a combination of relaxation of arteriolar smooth muscle and increasing venous resistance of channels penetrating the wall of the corpora cavernosa. Arterial disease may decrease erectile ability either by mechanical obstruction of the vascular lumen or more commonly by endothelial dysfunction, which as discussed previously interrupts to neural control mechanism of vascular smooth muscle function. This process leads to complete filling of the corpora cavernosa with blood at systemic blood pressure. The principle blood vessels supplying the corpora cavernosa are the cavernosal arteries. These vessels are terminal branches of the pudendal artery, which is the terminal branch of the internal iliac artery. Either large or small vessel arterial disease may decrease corporal blood pressure, leading to failure to achieve penile lengthening and rigidity.

Normal penile erection requires a functioning vascular tree upstream from the cavernosal arteries. Many cases of ED were formerly attributed to anatomic vascular disease when the problem actually was with control of cavernosal artery smooth muscle. Pharmacologic injection therapy involves injecting vasodilator agents (prostaglandin E_1 [PGE_1], papaverine, phentolamine, or combinations of those) into the corpora cavernosa to produce erection by dilating the corporal artery smooth muscle. More than 90% of patients with ED respond to this type of therapy, indicating that atherosclerotic arterial narrowing is not the etiology of most cases of ED.

Veno-occlusive disease in the penis is also a significant cause of ED. These patients often experience normal initial rigidity, but quickly, and before ejaculation, lose their erection.

NEUROGENIC ERECTILE DYSFUNCTION

Pure neurogenic ED is a frequent cause of erectile failure. Interruption of either somatic or autonomic nerves or their end units may cause ED. These nerves control the flow of blood into and likely out of the corpora cavernosa. Afferent somatic sensory signals are carried from the penis through the pudendal nerve to S2 through S4. This information is routed both to the brain and to spinal cord autonomic centers. Parasympathetic autonomic nerves originate in the intermediolateral gray matter of S2 through S4. These preganglionic fibers exit the anterior nerve roots to join with the sympathetic fibers of the hypogastric nerve to form the pelvic plexus and cavernosal nerves. The paired cavernosal nerves penetrate the corpora cavernosa and innervate the cavernous artery and veins. Parasympathetic ganglia are located distally near the end organ.

Sympathetic innervation also originates in the intermediolateral gray matter but at thoracolumbar levels T10 through L2. Sympathetic efferents course through the retroperitoneum and condense into the hypogastric plexus located anterior and slightly caudal to the aortic bifurcation. A concentration of postganglionic sympathetic fibers forms the hypogastric nerve, which is joined by parasympathetic efferents. Adrenergic innervation appears to play a role in the process of detumescence. High concentrations of norepinephrine have been demonstrated in the tissue of the corpora cavernosa and tributary arterioles. Additionally, the α-adrenergic antagonist phentolamine is routinely used for intracorporal injection therapy to produce erection.

Afferent signals capable of initiating erection can either originate within the brain, as is the case with psychogenic erections, or result from tactile stimulation. Patients with spinal cord injury often respond to tactile sensation but usually require medical therapy to maintain the erection

Medication Class	Decreased Erectile Rigidity	Ejaculatory Dysfunction
β-adrenergic antagonists	Common	Less common
Sympatholytics	Expected	Common
α$_1$ agonists	Uncommon	Uncommon
α$_2$ agonists	Common	Less common
α$_1$ antagonists	Uncommon	Less common*
Angiotensin-converting enzyme inhibitors	Uncommon	Uncommon
Diuretics	Less common	Uncommon
Antidepressants	Common†	Uncommon‡
Antipsychotics	Common	Common
Anticholinergics	Less common	Uncommon

Table 72-4 **Frequency of Decreased Erectile Rigidity and Ejaculatory Dysfunction by Medication Class**

*Patients able to ejaculate, but retrograde ejaculation is seen in 5% to 30%.
†Uncommon with serotonin reuptake inhibitors.
‡Delayed or inhibited ejaculation with serotonin reuptake inhibitors.

through intercourse. There is no discreet center for psychogenic erections. The temporal lobe appears to be important; however, other locations such as the gyrus rectus, the cingulate gyrus, the hypothalamus, and the mammillary bodies also appear to be important.

MEDICATION-INDUCED ERECTILE DYSFUNCTION

Commonly prescribed medications often cause or contribute to decreased erectile function. A complete list of these agents and their mechanisms of action is beyond the purview of this text. Table 72-4 lists the major classes of medications implicated in ED and suggests how commonly these medications interfere with erectile function. Often in clinical practice one finds that patients are on specific classes of medications for important reasons. For that reason, substituting a different medication is usually unsuccessful in restoring erectile function in patients who often have several risk factors for ED. Proceeding directly to treatment of ED is usually the preferred option in all but the most straightforward cases.

Medical and Surgical Treatment

Since the introduction of sildenafil in 1998, the Process of Care Model for the Evaluation and Treatment of ED has been adopted and targets the primary care provider as the initial source of care for patients with ED. Currently available therapies for ED include oral PDE-5 inhibitors, intraurethral alprostadil, intracavernous vasoactive injection therapy, vacuum constriction devices, and penile prosthesis implantation. A stepwise treatment approach is adopted, starting with oral agents and progressing to more invasive therapeutic interventions as indicated (Fig. 72-4). Informed

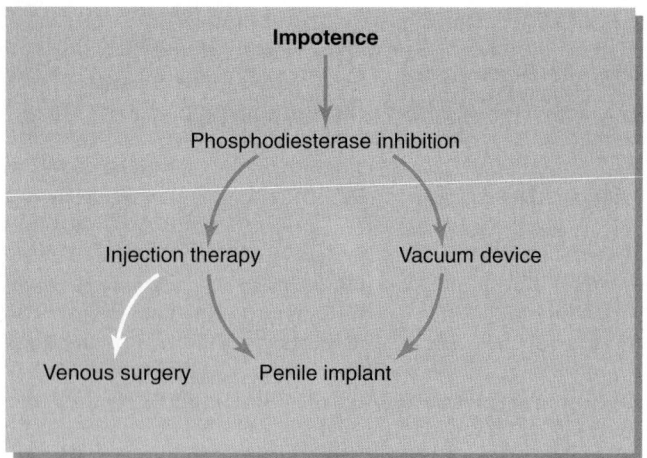

Figure 72-4 A logical treatment algorithm for impotence.

patient decision making is critical toward successful progression through the plan of care pathway. Patient referral is primarily based on failure of specific medical therapy as well as the need or desire for specialized diagnostic testing and management. As a result, most prescriptions for oral PDE-5 inhibitors are written by primary care providers, and specialized diagnostics such as Doppler ultrasound of the penile arteries and nocturnal penile tumescence (NPT) testing are used by urologists to work up select cases.

ORAL PHOSPHODIESTERASE TYPE 5 INHIBITORS

Current medical therapy is based on inhibition of PDE-5. Figure 72-3 illustrates that cGMP is broken down to inactive 5'-GMP by PDE-5. Sildenafil, vardenafil, and tadalafil competitively inhibit PDE-5 breakdown of cGMP by binding to the catalytic domain of PDE-5. Use of a PDE-5 inhibitor results in improved erectile rigidity even in patients with decreased NO or cGMP synthesis. Not all patients respond to PDE-5 inhibition, however. Adequate sexual stimulation and intact neural and vascular pathways are necessary to produce an adequate amount of NO and cGMP to increase deep penile artery blood flow. PDE-5 inhibitors are effective in men with organic, psychogenic, neurogenic, and mixed cases of ED. The overall response rate is 70%, with placebo response rates of 20% to 30%. In terms of disease-specific response to oral agents, improved erections were observed in 70% of hypertensive patients, 80% of spinal cord injury patients, 56% of diabetic patients, and 42% of radical prostatectomy patients.

PDE-5 inhibition should be considered first-line therapy, unless contraindicated. At the present time, there are no evidence-based data or randomized trials supporting superior efficacy of one drug over another. All the agents are hepatically metabolized. Initial concerns about concomitant use of PDE-5 inhibitors and α blockers have been resolved. Phosphodiesterase inhibitors should not be used concurrently with nitrate medications because a large (>25 mm Hg) synergistic drop in blood pressure is observed in many patients. Periodic follow-up is necessary to determine therapeutic efficacy, side effects related to PDE-5 inhibition, and a change in health status, including medications.

PHARMACOLOGIC INJECTION THERAPY

Several vasoactive agents can be safely injected directly into the corpora cavernosa to produce penile erection. Commonly used agents include PGE$_1$, papaverine, and phentolamine. These agents can be either used alone or in combination. As monotherapy, PGE$_1$ is most commonly used, and of the three, only PGE$_1$ has been evaluated in rigorous clinical trials and has specific marketing approval from the FDA for the treatment of ED. PGE$_1$ and papaverine are often used alone. Phentolamine, in contrast, is used to potentiate the action of papaverine or is used in combination with both PGE$_1$ and papaverine. These vasoactive drugs are frequently combined (bimix and trimix) to achieve increased efficacy and decreased side effects.

Injection therapy has two principal risks, priapism and corporal scarring causing penile curvature. Priapism has been reported to occur in 1% to 4% of patients. Prolonged erections occur more commonly in patients with neurogenic ED, especially young males with spinal cord injury. Significant acquired penile curvature is seen uncommonly and usually follows several years of injection therapy. Penile curvature appears to be less common with use of PGE$_1$ than papaverine. The most common problem with pharmacologic injection therapy is not complications from therapy but rather that 50% to 60% of patients stop using the technique by 1 year.

INTRAURETHRAL DRUG THERAPY

PGE$_1$ can be inserted into the urethra using a pellet applicator. This method of delivery assumes substantial venous communications between the corpus spongiosum surrounding the urethra and the corpus cavernosum. As a consequence, the technique is considerably less effective than intracavernous injection.

VACUUM CONSTRICTION DEVICES

These devices enclose the penis in a plastic tube with an airtight seal at the penile base. Air is pumped out of the cylinder, creating a vacuum. Blood flows into the corporal bodies, leading to penile erection. A constriction band remains on the base of the penis to maintain erection. Simultaneous use of a vacuum device and a phosphodiesterase inhibitor is safe. Many patients couple the two techniques to achieve satisfactory results.

PENILE PROSTHESIS

A penile prosthesis is implanted in the operating room. Two general types of devices can be implanted: semirigid and inflatable. Most patients prefer the inflatable devices because they provide a more natural erection when inflated and a flaccid penis when deflated. Although more invasive than the other techniques, a penile prosthesis is the most effective long-term option for impotence treatment. Ninety percent of patients and partners are satisfied with the result.

FUTURE TREATMENTS

We have just completed a period of rapid expansion in the understanding and treatment of ED. Much of the biochemical pathway leading to erection has been elucidated, and several effective oral medications have been introduced. Future medical treatments will depend on identification of specific biochemical events in the erection pathway that are unique to penile function. PDE-5 was a good example of this. To this point, other biochemical events such as production of cGMP are ubiquitous in other important systems of the body and do not make good targets for drugs designed to enhance erectile function. We anticipate that other classes of oral medications will have to await further advances in the basic understanding of erectile function.

Important interval improvements have been made in the design of implantable penile prostheses that made the devices more durable and resistant to infection. Improvements in the connection between tubing and corporal cylinders have cut the mechanical failure rate to less than 5% in 5 years. Components also have special coatings that either contain antibiotics or absorb antibiotics applied topically at the time of implantation. These improvements have cut the rate of postoperative infection in half.

References

Cappelleri JC, Rosen RC: The Sexual Health Inventory for Men (SHIM): A 5-year review of research and clinical experience. Int J Impotence Res 17:307-319, 2005.

Carson CC, Lue TF: Phosphodiesterase type 5 inhibitors for erectile dysfunction. Br J Urol Int 96:257-280, 2005.

Feldman HA, Goldstein I, Hatzichristou DG, et al: Impotence and its medical and psychosocial correlates: Results of the Massachusetts Male Aging Study. J Urol 151:54-61, 1994.

Kostis JB, Jackson G, Rosen R, et al: Sexual dysfunction and cardiac risk (the Second Princeton Consensus Conference). Am J Cardiol 96:313-321, 2005.

Milbank AJ, Montague DK: Surgical management of erectile dysfunction [review]. Endocrine 23:161-165, 2004.

Montague DK, Jarow JP, Broderick GA, et al, for the Erectile Dysfunction Guideline Update Panel. Chapter 1: The management of erectile dysfunction. An AUA update. J Urol 174:230-239, 2005.

D. Carcinomas of Men

Prostate Cancer

Carcinoma of the prostate is the most common cancer that occurs in men and the second leading cause of cancer death. Prostate cancer incidence increases with advancing age. Clinical diagnosis of prostate cancer is unusual before the latter half of the fifth decade of life but increases progressively thereafter.

Risk factors for prostate cancer are poorly understood (Table 72-5). There is some racial correlation because prostate cancer is more common in African American men than in whites. A high-fat diet has been implicated in some studies. An NIH-sponsored trial evaluating the role of selenium and vitamin E for prostate cancer prevention was terminated early because of apparent lack of effect. There is no demonstrated association between prostate cancer and cigarette smoking, sexual activity, or a prior history of prostatitis or BPH.

There is considerable disparity between the autopsy incidence of prostate cancer and clinical detection of the disease. Pathologic examination of step-sectioned prostate specimens shows histologic evidence of prostate cancer in more than 50% of men older than 60 years. The overwhelming majority of these "autopsy" or "latent" cancers are less than 0.2 mL in volume and of a low pathologic grade. These tumors are distinctly different from their clinically diagnosed counterparts. The reason for this disparity and the factors that may trigger development of clinically aggressive disease are unknown.

DETECTION AND DIAGNOSIS

There is ongoing controversy about the value of prostate cancer screening. Much of this is fueled by the failure to take into account age and comorbidity. Whereas men with a less than 10-year life expectancy may not benefit from prostate cancer screening, those younger than 70 to 75 years who are otherwise in good health have a substantial risk for morbidity or mortality from untreated prostate cancer. Most experts recommend routine screening in this group.

Both the DRE and serum PSA determination have a role in the early diagnosis of prostate cancer. Prostate cancer typically arises from the peripheral portion of the prostate, which can be palpated on DRE. Induration or nodularity of the prostate on DRE should be considered suspicious for prostate cancer.

PSA is a protein produced by both benign and malignant prostate cells. Serum PSA may be elevated in the face of prostate enlargement, inflammation, or cancer (Table 72-6). Although an elevated PSA is not diagnostic of prostate cancer, it may lead to a prostate biopsy to exclude cancer. Probably because of progressive enlargement in prostate size, serum PSA values increase as men age. The historical view of a value of less than 4 ng/mL as a "normal" PSA has been abandoned with the recognition that PSA represents a continuum of risk with no lower threshold. The comparative rate of change for PSA over time, sometimes termed *PSA*

Table 72-5 **Possible Risk Factors for Prostate Cancer**
Age (increasing incidence with advancing age)
Race (highest incidence in African Americans)
Family history
Diet (possible link to high-fat diet)
Genetic (inherited genetic pattern more complex than with some other tumors)

Table 72-6 **Causes of Increased Prostate-Specific Antigen**
Benign prostatic hyperplasia
Prostatitis
Urinary tract infection
Prostatic trauma (urethral catheterization or prostatic massage)
Carcinoma

Table 72-7 **Treatment Options for Localized Prostate Cancer**
Radical prostatectomy (robotic or open)
Brachytherapy (iodine-125, etc., seeds)
External-beam irradiation
Cryotherapy
Hormonal therapy
Active surveillance

velocity, can be informative. In general, a change in PSA of greater than 0.75 ng/mL is considered worrisome and may prompt a prostate biopsy.

Whenever prostate cancer is suspected, either because of an abnormality in DRE or PSA rise, prostate biopsy is performed. TRUS imaging of the prostate is used to guide prostate biopsy. Prostate cancers typically have a hypoechoic appearance. However, TRUS is of limited value for diagnosis and is used primarily to direct biopsies. Transrectal cores of prostate tissue are obtained. This is an office-based procedure, and local infiltration of lidocaine (Xylocaine) around the prostate minimizes discomfort. Usually 12 or more tissue cores are taken systematically from the entire prostate.

Prostate cancer most often is graded according to the Gleason system. This scoring system uses two numbers based on the primary and secondary histologic pattern. Gleason sums of 2, 3, or 4 are uncommon with clinically detected cancers. Gleason 5 or 6 tumors are most common, whereas sums of 8, 9, and 10 imply an aggressive tumor behavior.

DRE is the most useful test for determining local tumor extent. CT scanning is of limited value and usually not indicated clinically for determining either local extent or nodal metastasis. Magnetic resonance imaging (MRI) of the prostate using an endorectal coil is used in some centers, but the ultimate value of the procedure for either detection or staging is uncertain. In patients with high-grade tumors or a substantially elevated PSA, a bone scan is indicated because bone is the most common site of distant spread. Soft tissue metastasis is unusual in the face of a normal bone scan.

TREATMENT OF LOCALIZED DISEASE

There is considerable controversy about the best management approach for clinically localized prostate cancer, and patients should enter in to an informed decision making process (Table 72-7). In men with less than 10-year life expectancy otherwise, active treatment often is unnecessary. The risk for progression and death within 10 years is sufficiently low that observation alone is appropriate. Increasingly, some men with a greater than 10-year life expectancy but a tumor with apparently favorable features pursue a program of active surveillance. In general, active surveillance should be restricted to men with a PSA of less than 10 ng/mL, no palpable prostate nodules, a Gleason sum of 6 or less, and fewer than 2 or 3 positive biopsy cores. Typically, repeat prostate biopsy is recommended every 1 to 3 years in men on active surveillance to ensure that higher-volume or higher-grade tumor is not evident. PSA and DRE are performed every 6 months. The underlying premise of active surveillance (i.e., that treatment can be safely deferred until there is some evidence of disease progression) is unproved, but it is known that many men with favorable features of the primary tumor do not develop progressive disease in their lifetime.

For men with a greater than 10-year life expectancy otherwise, curative therapy usually is indicated. Surgical removal of the prostate (radical prostatectomy) is the treatment with the most proven ability for long-term cure of prostate cancer. Contemporary radical prostatectomy is an operation with limited perioperative morbidity. The greatest drawbacks to the procedure are the risks for long-term consequences. Significant incontinence occurs in only around 2% of men, but up to 10% may have at least some degree of mild stress incontinence. The cavernosal nerves, which are responsible for dilation of the blood vessels that lead to penile tumescence, lie immediately adjacent to the prostate. Dissection of these nerves from the prostate (nerve-sparing radical prostatectomy) is appropriate in patients with tumors localized to the prostate. The success of nerve-sparing prostatectomy is related to patient age and preoperative erectile function. Preservation of potency can be achieved in up to 60% to 80% of patients. Increasingly, robotic-assisted laparoscopic prostatectomy is becoming the preferred surgical approach for radical prostatectomy. The less invasive surgical approach permits quicker patient recovery, less bleeding, and shorter hospital stay compared with open surgery with no distinct differences in continence, potency, or tumor control between the two approaches.

After radical prostatectomy, serum PSA should decline to an undetectable range. No measurable PSA is produced from any source other than prostate cells. Metastatic foci of cancer continue to produce PSA, so an undetectable value is an excellent prognostic sign. Furthermore, an increase in PSA to a detectable range precedes other signs or symptoms of prostate cancer recurrence after radical prostatectomy almost 99% of the time. Thus, PSA is an extremely sensitive and specific marker for following men after radical prostatectomy. PSA values greater than 0.2 ng/mL are considered diagnostic of tumor recurrence after radical prostatectomy.

Radiation therapy is the primary alternative to surgery for localized prostate cancer. Radiation can be administered by external-beam therapy using intensity-modulated radiation treatment (IMRT) or using proton-beam therapy. No significant difference in outcomes has been shown between proton-beam treatment and conventional radiation. Each is delivered over a 7- to 8-week time frame. Brachytherapy is an alternative method of radiation that can be performed with different isotopes, but iodine-125 is used most commonly. Supplementation of brachytherapy with external-beam irradiation is used in some centers.

PSA typically declines after radiation treatment but may not reach nadir levels for 2 years. Determination of treatment failure is more problematic than after surgery. An increase in PSA over nadir levels may prompt a prostate biopsy to rule out residual disease.

Side effects of radiation treatment occur most commonly because of radiation damage to the bladder or rectum. Patients may experience frequency of voiding or bowel movements or blood in the urine or stool. ED appears to occur at about the same frequency as after surgical treatments.

Focal therapy using either freezing of the prostate (cryotherapy) and high-intensity focused ultrasound (HIFU) are being explored. Limitations of this approach include the known multifocal nature of prostate cancer as well as difficulty in adequate imaging of the tumor for localization. Currently, focal therapy is considered highly experimental.

TREATMENT OF ADVANCED DISEASE

Endocrine manipulation remains the primary form of treatment for patients with advanced or metastatic carcinoma of the prostate. The goal of therapy is to deprive the prostate cancer cells of serum androgens. This can be accomplished by either surgical or medical castration. Surgical orchiectomy removes both testes, the source of testosterone production. Luteinizing hormone–releasing hormone (LHRH) analogues are administered by a slow-release depot injection, with formulations lasting from 3 to 12 months. These drugs have the paradoxical effect of decreasing serum luteinizing hormone release from the pituitary gland and, consequently, diminishing testosterone production from the testis. Testosterone declines to castrate values within a few days after surgical orchiectomy and a few weeks after administration of an LHRH analogue.

In response to androgen deprivation, prostate cancer typically undergoes rapid regression. This is manifested by a decrease in prostate size, improvement in any disease symptoms such as bone pain, and a rapid decline in serum PSA. The duration of response varies but is usually on the order of a couple of years for patients who present with metastatic disease. Hormonal therapy generally is well tolerated but frequently causes hot flushes and is associated with some degree of osteoporosis, weight gain, and loss of muscle mass with long-term use (Table 72-8).

Antiandrogens may also be used in hormonal therapy of patients with prostate cancer. These oral medications exert their effect by blocking the metabolism of androgens at the cellular level rather than by decreasing serum values. Antiandrogens may be used in combination with LHRH

Table 72-8 **Long-Term Side Effects of Androgen Deprivation Therapy**
Hot flashes
Loss of libido
Impotence
Osteoporosis
Decreased facial hair
Loss of muscle mass
Weight gain

analogues to block the effect of adrenal androgens in addition to testosterone. Despite multiple randomized studies, the value of combination treatment compared with LHRH analogues alone is still a matter of debate.

Once prostate cancer shows evidence of progression despite hormonal therapy, the prognosis for patients is poor. Bone pain is managed with appropriate analgesics and irradiation. Chemotherapy using docetaxel in combination with steroids has been shown to provide some quality-of-life benefit as well as extend survival but for only a limited period of time.

Penile Carcinoma

Squamous cell carcinoma of the penis is an uncommon tumor in the United States and the rest of the developed world, with a rate of less than 1 case per 100,000 men and an estimated 1470 cases in the United States for 2005. It is diagnosed almost exclusively in uncircumcised men. Neonatal circumcision appears to have a protective effect. Circumcision in adulthood or late childhood does not appear to confer the same level of protection. Chronic irritation and inflammation are key etiologic factors because most men have poor hygiene leading to phimosis of the foreskin. There is further evidence linking the development of penile cancer with some serotypes of the human papillomavirus (HPV types 16 and 18). Smoking and other forms of tobacco use have also been a consistent finding in several epidemiologic studies of penile cancer risk factors.

Squamous cell carcinoma typically presents as a painless, nonindurated, ulcerated mass involving the glans penis and coronal sulcus. Infection of the primary lesion is common and may produce foul-smelling, purulent discharge and reactive inguinal lymphadenopathy. Delay in diagnosis is common because patients often do not seek immediate treatment secondary to fear and embarrassment, whereas prolonged treatment with antibiotics may delay confirmatory biopsy of the lesion.

DIAGNOSIS AND TREATMENT

Evaluation of suspicious lesions begins with clinical assessment of both the tumor and inguinal lymph nodes. Imaging studies are not routinely recommended because physical examination has proved the most accurate predictor of tumor stage. A diagnosis of carcinoma of the penis is confirmed by histologic evaluation of an excisional biopsy. Prognosis is directly correlated with grade of the tumor and extent of invasion. Adverse prognostic factors include high histopathologic grade, vascular invasion, and advanced pathologic stage ($\geq$T2).

The classic operation for squamous cell carcinoma of the penis is partial penectomy with a 2-cm negative margin. If the tumor is confined to the distal penis, a sufficient length of proximal penile shaft can be preserved so that the patient can still void in a standing position.

Larger tumors that invade the more proximal penile shaft require total penectomy. The entire corpora cavernosa are excised back to the ischial tuberosity. A perineal urethrostomy is created that allows voiding in a sitting position.

Contemporary studies are now attempting to stratify patients who would benefit from organ-preserving therapies with improved functional and cosmetic results. These treatment approaches include topical treatments (5-fluorouracil), external-beam radiation therapy, Moh microsurgery, laser ablation (carbon dioxide and Nd:YAG), and complete tumor excision with phallic reconstruction. Patients with Tis, Ta, and T1 (grade 1 and 2) tumors at low risk for metastasis appear to be ideal candidates for this approach. The main drawback is the increased risk for local tumor recurrence.

Inguinal lymph node dissection is indicated in patients with palpable inguinal nodes that persist after antibiotic therapy or in those with nonpalpable nodes with risk factors for regional metastasis (histopathologic grade 3, vascular invasion, and ≥T2). Traditionally, there has been significant morbidity associated with inguinal lymph node dissection (lymphedema, skin necrosis, deep vein thrombosis). However, several contemporary studies have shown a decreased incidence and severity of complications. Modified lymphadenectomy and sentinel node biopsy aim to detect occult metastases while minimizing patient morbidity.

The prognosis for patients with distant metastatic disease or nodal metastasis above the inguinal ligament is poor. Squamous cell carcinoma of the penis is moderately chemosensitive, and numerous regimens have been studied, reflecting the lack of superior efficacy of one combination over another. A durable response to chemotherapy is unusual, and further studies with novel agents and multimodal therapy are currently being investigated.

Testis Cancer

The management of patients with testicular carcinoma has become a model for the multidisciplinary approach to solid tumors. As a result of effective surgery, radiation therapy, and combination chemotherapy, survival approaches 99% for low-risk disease and 80% for high-risk disease. Testicular tumors are the most common solid malignancy in men aged 15 to 34 years. The incidence of testis cancer appears to be increasing over the past 25 years.

Cryptorchidism (undescended testicle) is a well-accepted risk factor for subsequent development of carcinoma. Abnormalities in spermatogenesis are well documented (thought to be a primary effect of the tumor), and up to 15% of patients are diagnosed with testicular cancer during a work-up for male factor infertility. Two to 3% of patients present with bilateral tumors, and 5% to 10% of patients develop cancer in the normal contralateral testicle. Despite impairments in spermatogenesis, most men with testicular cancer are capable of fathering children, and a discussion of fertility issues is extremely important, especially in patients who may require adjuvant therapies such as external-beam radiation and systemic chemotherapy.

The most common presenting sign or symptom of testis cancer is a firm, painless mass arising from the testis. Patients may present with an acute scrotum as a result of tumor hemorrhage, and up to 33% of patients are treated for presumed epididymitis. Scrotal ultrasonography is diagnostic because testis cancer is usually distinguishable from benign scrotal disease because of the clear involvement of the testicular parenchyma rather than the paratesticular tissues. Signs and symptoms of advanced disease include cough, gastrointestinal symptoms (mass), back pain (retroperitoneal metastasis), neurologic symptoms (brain metastasis), lower extremity swelling (iliac or inferior vena cava thrombus), and supraclavicular lymphadenopathy.

DIAGNOSIS AND STAGING

Initial management of the primary tumor is inguinal orchiectomy with high ligation of the spermatic cord. Histopathology distinguishes germ cell tumors (GCTs) from stromal tumors. Seminoma is the most common GCT occurring in pure form. Teratoma, yolk sac tumors, embryonal carcinoma, and choriocarcinoma are classified as nonseminomatous GCT and frequently occur as mixed GCT (more than one histologic pattern within the primary tumor).

Testicular cancer is unique in that serum tumor markers (STMs) play an important role in tumor staging. STMs include β-human chorionic gonadotropin (β-hCG), α-fetoprotein (AFP), and serum lactate dehydrogenase. Elevations of the serum hCG may be seen in choriocarcinoma, embryonal carcinoma, and 15% of seminomas. Elevated AFP can be seen in yolk sac tumors and embryonal carcinoma, and excludes a diagnosis of seminoma. These markers may be secreted either by the primary tumor or by metastatic foci (Table 72-9).

The retroperitoneal lymph nodes are the most common initial site of metastasis. Therefore, staging of the retroperitoneum with an abdominal CT scan is important in evaluating the extent of disease. However, accurate staging of the retroperitoneum remains problematic, with the literature quoting a 20% to 30% false-negative and false-positive rate with CT scanning. Common landing zones for lymph node metastasis include the precaval, inter-aortocaval, and preaortic lymph nodes below the renal hilum and above the aortic bifurcation. Chest x-ray or thoracic CT completes the clinical staging because the lungs and posterior mediastinum are the most common sites of distant metastatic disease.

TREATMENT

Histopathology, pathologic stage, and serum tumor marker status are used to determine subsequent treatment following inguinal orchiectomy. All patients with elevated serum tumor markers after orchiectomy receive cisplatin-based chemotherapy, regardless of histology. Radiation therapy and retroperitoneal lymph node dissection (RPLND) have a

Table 72-9 **Testis Cancer Staging Studies**
Tumor markers
AFP—elevated only with nonseminomatous tumors
β-hCG—may be increased with either seminoma or nonseminomatous tumor
Abdominal CT scan—retroperitoneal nodes most common site of regional nodal metastasis
Chest radiograph or CT scan—lung is most frequent site of distant metastasis
AFP, α-fetoprotein; β-hCG, β-human chorionic gonadotropin; CT, computed tomography.

high likelihood of failure in the face of elevated serum markers.

Seminoma presents as clinical stage I in 70%, stage II in 20%, and stage III in 10% of cases. Although surveillance and single-agent carboplatin are options in patients with stage I seminoma, most experts recommend radiation therapy to the retroperitoneum in patients with stage I and II disease due to the radiosensitivity of seminomas. Patients with bulky stage II (lymph node >5 cm) and stage III disease receive combination chemotherapy.

Nonseminomatous GCT present more frequently with advanced stage (stage I, 30%; stage II, 40%; and stage III, 30%). RPLND is frequently recommended in patients with clinical stage I or low-volume stage II disease. Reasons for recommending RPLND include accurate pathologic staging of the retroperitoneum, low relapse rate (< 2%) after properly performed RPLND, curative potential in the face of viable GCT, and the potential for retroperitoneal teratoma, which is resistant to chemotherapy. Side effects associated with RPLND include lymphocele, chylous ascites (0.4%), and small bowel obstruction (1% to 2%). Nerve-sparing RPLND is able to preserve antegrade ejaculation in greater than 80% of patients. Primary chemotherapy is sometimes recommended to patients with stage I or II nonseminomatous testis cancers. Also, some men may choose surveillance alone for a stage I tumor, which implies normal serum markers and abdominal CT scan. Up to 25% may be expected to develop recurrence, usually within 2 years, and chemotherapy is used upon evidence of recurrence.

Platinum-based chemotherapy is the standard for patients with advanced disease. Cure rates of 70% to 80% are achieved even in patients who present with relatively bulky metastatic disease. Side effects of chemotherapy include renal dysfunction, neuropathy, Raynaud phenomenon, hematologic toxicity, cardiovascular toxicity, and 0.5% risk for secondary leukemias.

References

Amato RJ, Ro JY, Ayala AG, Swanson DA: Risk adapted treatment for patients with clinical stage I nonseminomatous germ cell tumors of the testis. Urology 63:144, 2004

Atsu N, Eskicorapci S, Uner A, et al: A novel surveillance protocol for stage I nonseminomatous germ cell testicular tumors. Br J Urol Int 92:32-35, 2003.

Bostwick DG, Qian J, Civantos F, et al: Does finasteride alter the pathology of the prostate and cancer grading? [review]. Clin Prostate Cancer 2:228-235, 2004.

Busby JE, Pettaway CA: What's new in the management of penile cancer? Curr Opin Urol 15:350-357, 2005.

Classen J, Schmidberger H, Meisner C, et al: Radiotherapy for stages IIA/B testicular seminoma: Final report of a prospective multicenter clinical trial. J Clin Oncol 21:1101-1106, 2003.

D'Amico AV, Chen MH, Roehl KA, Catalona WJ: Preoperative PSA velocity and the risk of death from prostate cancer after radical prostatectomy. N Engl J Med 351:125-135, 2004.

d'Ancona CA, de Lucena RG, Querne FA, et al: Long term follow up of penile carcinoma treated with penectomy and bilateral modified inguinal lymphadenectomy. J Urol 172:498-501, 2004.

Eggener SE, Roehl KA, Catalona WJ: Predictors of subsequent prostate cancer in men with a prostate specific antigen of 2.6 to 4.0 ng/ml and an initially negative biopsy. J Urol 174:500-504, 2005.

Holmberg L, Bill-Axelson A, Helgesen F, et al: A randomized trial comparing radical prostatectomy with watchful waiting in early prostate cancer. N Eng J Med 347:781-789, 2002.

Joerger M, Warzinek T, Klaeser B, et al: Major tumor regression after paclitaxel and carboplatin polychemotherapy in a patient with advanced penile cancer. Urology 63:778-780, 2004.

Klein EA, Thompson IM, Lippman SM, et al: SELECT: The next prostate cancer prevention trial. J Urol 166:1311-1315, 2001.

Klotz L: Active surveillance for prostate cancer: For whom? J Clin Oncol 23:8165-8169, 2005.

Kroon BK, Horenblas S, Lont AP, et al: Patients with penile carcinoma benefit from immediate resection of clinically occult lymph node metastases. J Urol 173:816-819, 2005.

Llein EA, Tangen CM, Goodman PJ, et al: Assessing benefit and risk in the prevention of prostate cancer: The prostate cancer prevention trial revisited. J Clin Oncol 23:7460-7466, 2005.

MacVicar GR, Pienta KJ: Testicular cancer. Curr Opin Oncol 16:253-256, 2004.

Nelson BA, Cookson MS, Smith JA Jr, Chang SS: Complications of inguinal and pelvic lymphadenectomy for squamous cell carcinoma of the penis: A contemporary series. J Urol 172:494-497, 2004.

Oldenburg J, Alfsen GC, Lien HH, et al: Postchemotherapy retroperitoneal surgery remains necessary in patients with nonseminomatous testicular cancer and minimal residual tumor masses. J Clin Oncol 17:3310-3317, 2003.

Rippentrop JM, Joslyn SA, Konety BR: Squamous cell carcinoma of the penis: Evaluation of data from the Surveillance, Epidemiology, and End Results Program. Cancer 101:1357-1363, 2004.

Roehl KA, Han M, Ramos CG, et al: Cancer progression and survival rates following anatomical radical retropubic prostatectomy in 3,478 consecutive patients: Long-term results. J Urol 172:910-914, 2004.

Sanchez-Ortiz RF, Pettaway CA: The role of lymphadenectomy in penile cancer. Urol Oncol 22:236-244, 2004.

Sanda MG, Dunn RL, Michalski J, et al: Quality of life and satisfaction with outcome among prostate cancer survivors. N Engl J Med 358:1250-1261, 2008.

Schmoll HJ, Kollmannsberger C, Metzner B, et al: Long term results of first line sequential high dose etoposide, ifosfamide, and cisplatin chemotherapy plus autologous stem cell support for patients with advanced metastatic germ cell cancer: An extended phase I/II study of the German Testicular Cancer Study Group. J Clin Oncol 15:4083-4091, 2003.

Smith JA Jr, Herrell SD: Robotic-assisted laparoscopic prostatectomy. Do minimally invasive approaches offer significant advantages? J Clin Oncol 23:8170-8175, 2005.

Stephenson AJ, Scardino PT, Eastham JA, et al: Postoperative nomogram predicting the 10-year probability of prostate cancer recurrence after radical prostatectomy. J Clin Oncol 23:7005-7012, 2005.

Stephenson AJ, Sheinfeld J: The role of retroperitoneal lymph node dissection in the management of testicular cancer. Urol Oncol 22:225-235, 2004.

Tannock IF, deWit R, Berry WR, et al: Docetaxel plus prednisone or mitoxantrone plus prednisone for advanced prostate cancer. N Engl J Med 351:1502-1512, 2004.

Thompson IM, Pauler DK, Goodman PJ, et al: Prevalence of prostate cancer among men with a prostate specific antigen level < or = 4.0 ng/ml [erratum appears in N Engl J Med 14:1470, 2004]. N Engl J Med 350:2239-2246, 2004.

Zhou P, Chen MH, McLeod D, et al: Predictors of prostate cancer-specific mortality after radical prostatectomy or radiation therapy. J Clin Oncol 23:6992-6998, 2005.

E. Benign Scrotal Diseases

Varicocele

Varicoceles are classically described as abnormal dilation of the veins of the pampiniform plexus. Subclinical varicocele can be present in up to 15% of the male population, whereas the prevalence increases to 30% to 50% of men presenting with primary infertility, and as high as 70% to 80% of patients with secondary infertility. Varicoceles are diagnosed during work-up for male factor infertility, scrotal pain syndromes, and asymptomatic testicular atrophy. Physical examination can reveal the classic "bag of worms": testicular atrophy and tender scrotal contents. Semen analysis reveals multiple abnormalities reflecting a characteristic "stress pattern," although this is not pathognomonic. The diagnosis of varicocele remains a clinical one, although scrotal ultrasound with Doppler is helpful in certain situations. The presence of two or three veins with diameter larger than 3 mm and retrograde flow with Valsalva maneuver is consistent with clinical varicocele. Surgical intervention for subclinical varicoceles is not indicated. Pathophysiology of varicocele has historically been poorly understood. Regardless, there is dilation of the internal spermatic vein and transmission of increased hydrostatic pressure across dysfunctional venous valves. Stasis of blood in the venous system disturbs countercurrent heat exchange responsible for maintaining testicular temperature and results in testicular parenchymal damage and impaired spermatogenesis. Because of anatomic considerations, varicoceles are more commonly left sided. However, unilateral varicoceles have a bilateral effect on spermatogenesis and local testicular steroidogenesis. Indications for surgical correction of a clinical varicocele include male factor infertility, testicular atrophy in adolescents with ipsilateral varicocele, and intractable pain attributed to the varicocele. It should be noted that pain is rarely caused by clinical varicoceles, and surgical varicocelectomy often does not produce symptomatic relief for the patient. Common surgical techniques include high retroperitoneal ligation of the internal spermatic vein, microsurgical inguinal and subinguinal varicocelectomy, and laparoscopic varicocelectomy. The inguinal approach using surgical magnification has the highest success and lowest complication and recurrence rates. Semen parameters improve in 60% to 80% of men with pregnancy rates of 20% to 60%. The most common complication is hydrocele formation, whereas a rare complication is inadvertent ligation of the testicular artery resulting in testicular atrophy and loss.

Epididymitis

Acute epididymitis is a clinical syndrome that presents with fever, acute scrotal pain, and swelling as a result of inflammation and infection of the epididymis. Pathophysiologically, epididymitis is caused by retrograde bacterial spread from the bladder or urethra. In men younger than 35 years of age, the most common causes are organisms associated with urethritis, namely gonococcus and *Chlamydia trachomatis*. In older men, *Escherichia coli* and other coliform bacteria are the causative organisms, usually in association with lower urinary tract infection associated with symptoms of bladder outlet obstruction. Patients with acute epididymitis have significant inflammation, and the causative organism can be determined by Gram stain and culture of a urethral swab or midstream urine specimen. Interestingly, the antiarrhythmic amiodarone is associated with a noninfectious cause of epididymitis secondary to concentration of the drug in the epididymis. The most important consideration in diagnosing acute epididymitis is differentiating this disease from acute testicular torsion. Physical examination can be nonspecific, although focal epididymal swelling and tenderness are suggestive, and the presence of white cells in the urine or urethral swab is indicative of an infectious etiology. Scrotal ultrasound with Doppler flow can be extremely helpful in differentiating acute epididymitis from torsion in difficult cases. Treatment is generally supportive, including narcotic analgesics, NSAIDs, scrotal support with an athletic supporter, cold ice packs, and targeted antimicrobial therapy. In general, patients younger than 35 years should be treated with ceftriaxone (Rocephin) and doxycycline, or a single dose of azithromycin (Zithromax). Older patients are empirically treated with a fluoroquinolone or TMP-SMX for 2 to 4 weeks. Complications associated with acute epididymitis include abscess formation, testicular infarction, infertility, and chronic epididymitis or orchalgia. Surgical intervention is rarely necessary, although in select cases, orchiectomy and epididymectomy can be therapeutic when solid indications are present.

Hydrocele

A hydrocele is a serous fluid collection within the parietal and visceral layers of the tunica vaginalis of the scrotum. Hydroceles may surround the testicle or the testicle and spermatic cord, or communicate with the peritoneal cavity through a patent processus vaginalis. These communicating hydroceles are uncommon in the adult population and are more commonly identified in the pediatric age group in association with an indirect hernia. Patients usually present to the physician with complaints of heaviness in the scrotum, scrotal pain, and an enlarging scrotal mass. Diagnosis is easily made with physical examination and transillumination of the hydrocele. If the testis is not easily palpable in a young patient, ultrasound can rule out an occult testicular tumor with secondary or reactive hydrocele. Hydroceles are caused by increased secretion or decreased reabsorption of serous fluid by the tunica vaginalis. Infection, trauma, neoplastic disease, and lymphatic disease are causative in most adults, whereas the remainder of cases are idiopathic. Treatment of symptomatic hydroceles is surgical. Although the recurrence rate is significantly higher with aspiration and sclerotherapy, this can be a good option in patients who are considered poor surgical candidates. Hydrocelectomy procedures involve either some form of excision of the redundant tunica vaginalis versus a plication of the sac without excision. Overall complications occur in up to 20% of patients, with hematoma seen in 15%, infection or abscess and hydrocele recurrence in 9%, and chronic pain in 1%.

Testicular Torsion

Testicular torsion is considered a true urologic emergency. The testicular blood supply is through the testicular artery (aorta), the vasal artery (inferior vesicle artery), and the cremasteric artery (inferior epigastric artery). All three vessels are transmitted to the testicle through the spermatic cord. Torsion of the spermatic cord impairs arterial inflow as well as venous outflow producing the characteristic symptoms of acute scrotal pain, swelling, and nausea and vomiting. If detorsion is not performed within 6 to 8 hours, testicular infarction and hemorrhagic necrosis are likely to occur. Typically, patients are younger than 21 years, although testicular torsion can occur into early adulthood. Symptoms usually include the acute onset of testicular and scrotal pain, scrotal swelling, and nausea and vomiting. Ecchymosis and involvement of the scrotal skin occur in more advanced cases, but the testis has infracted by that point. Delay in presentation and diagnosis is more common in the adult patient population and is related to patient and physician factors. Often there is an antecedent history of trauma or physical activity. The diagnosis of testicular torsion remains a clinical one, and surgical exploration is undertaken when the index of suspicion is high. Doppler ultrasonography is extremely useful in differentiating testicular torsion from other causes of the acute scrotum, such as acute epididymitis, torsion of the appendix testis, and trauma. Important surgical principles include surgical detorsion and assessment of testicular viability in the operating room. If the testis is determined to be viable, bilateral orchiopexy is performed using the technique of three-point fixation (sutures placed medially, laterally, and inferiorly). Otherwise, in the presence of infarction, orchiectomy is recommended. Orchiopexy of the contralateral testicle is always performed simultaneously. When diagnosis and surgery occur in a timely fashion, testicular salvage rates approach 70%. Delayed surgical therapy, for whatever reason, results in the salvage rate dropping off to 40%.

Prospectus for the Future

- Improved basic science understanding of the molecular biology of benign prostate growth
- Improved understanding of the neurophysiology of detrusor function associated with bladder outlet obstruction
- Refined methods for the minimally invasive management of symptomatic BPH
- Improved outcomes research regarding long-term benefits of less invasive therapy for BPH, both medical and surgical
- Improved understanding of the immunourologic characteristics and mechanisms of the prostate and urethra
- Enhanced understanding of the neuroanatomy and neurophysiology of the prostate and bladder, with an emphasis on pain and sensory mechanisms in the prostate, bladder, and surrounding tissues
- Better standardized protocols for therapeutic intervention trials for the treatment of noninflammatory chronic pelvic pain syndrome
- Novel therapies for noninflammatory chronic pelvic pain syndrome (e.g., thermotherapy, phytotherapy)
- Better markers of tumor aggressiveness for men with localized prostate cancer
- Improved specificity of prostate cancer screening methods
- Understanding of the cause and prevention of testis cancer

References

Hopps CV, Goldstein M: Varicocele: Unified theory of pathophysiology and treatment. AUA Update Series 23:12, 2004.
Karmazyn B, Steinberg R, Kurareid L, et al: Clinical and radiographic criteria of the acute scrotum in children: A retrospective study in 172 boys. Pediatr Radiol 35:302-310, 2005.
Kiddoo DA, Wollin TA, Mador DR: A population based assessment of complications following outpatient hydrocelectomy and spermatocelectomy. J Urol 171:746-748, 2004.
Kruska JD, Culkin DJ: Outpatient scrotal surgery: Management of benign scrotal diseases. AUA Update Series 24:11, 2005.
Lavallee ME, Cash J: Testicular Torsion: Evaluation and Management. Curr Sports Med Rep 4:102-104, 2005.
Neiderberger C: Microsurgical treatment of persistent or recurrent varicocele. J Urol 173:2079-2080, 2005.
Raman JD, Walmsley K, Goldstein M: Inheritance of varicoceles. Urology 65:1186-1189, 2005.

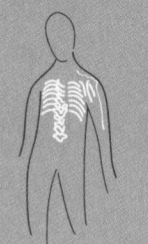

Section XV

Diseases of Bone and Bone Mineral Metabolism

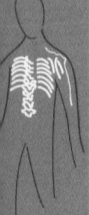

Normal Physiology of Bone and Mineral Homeostasis

Andrew F. Stewart

Calcium Homeostasis

The maintenance of normal calcium homeostasis is critical to survival for at least three reasons. First, serum calcium concentrations regulate the degree of membrane excitability in muscle and nervous tissue. Increases in serum calcium lead to refractoriness to stimulation of neurons and muscle cells, which translates clinically into coma and muscular weakness. Conversely, reductions in serum calcium lead to increases in neuromuscular excitability that translate clinically into convulsions and spontaneous muscle cramps and contractions referred to as *carpopedal spasm* or *tetany*. Second, terrestrial life requires the existence of a skeleton, and calcium is the major structural cation in the skeleton. Specifically, the mineral phase of the skeleton is composed of a calcium salt called *hydroxyapatite,* and reductions in bone mineral content lead to spontaneous fractures. Third, intracellular calcium has a major intracellular signaling role, and control of intracellular calcium is essential to the survival of all cells. This mechanism is used to advantage pharmacologically through the widespread clinical use of drugs that regulate intracellular calcium concentrations and calcium-channel activity for the treatment of a wide variety of human diseases. Thus, physicians, regardless of their specialty, will encounter disorders of calcium homeostasis on a regular basis.

The serum total calcium concentration is normally maintained at about 9.5 mg/dL. Of this amount, about 4.5 mg/dL is bound to serum proteins, principally albumin, and about 0.5 mg/dL circulates as insoluble complexes such as calcium sulfate, phosphate, and citrate. The remaining about 4.5 mg/dL circulates as free or unbound or ionized calcium. This free, ionized serum calcium is important clinically and physiologically. This calcium is available (1) to be filtered at the glomerulus, (2) to interact with cell membranes to regulate their electrical potential or excitability, and (3) to enter and exit the skeletal hydroxyapatite crystal lattice. Thus, it is important to maintain a normal ionized serum calcium, although total serum calcium is customarily measured in most clinical laboratories. From a clinical standpoint, recognizing that, in some instances, total serum calcium can change without a change in the ionized calcium is also important. For example, if a decline in serum albumin occurs as a result of hepatic cirrhosis or the nephrotic syndrome, a corresponding decline in the total serum calcium will ensue, but the ionized serum calcium concentration will remain normal. Thus, at times, measuring the ionized serum calcium directly is important.

Given the central importance of calcium homeostasis to terrestrial life, the fact that a complex group of regulatory processes have evolved to protect the integrity of this system is not surprising. A corollary of this concept is that, when a physician encounters patients in whom hypercalcemia, hypocalcemia, or disorders of skeletal mineralization have occurred, multiple safety control points have been breached. These control points are discussed here.

From a homeostatic control point of view, the calcium ion interfaces with three important compartments, as shown in the calcium *physiologic black box* in Figure 73-1. An important point to recall is that, although intracellular calcium is important in intracellular signaling, it is quantitatively unimportant in overall systemic calcium homeostasis, largely because intracellular calcium concentrations are tiny (nanomolar) compared with extracellular calcium concentrations (millimolar). Thus, the three critical regulatory fluxes that maintain normal serum calcium concentration are with the intestine, the kidney, and the skeleton.

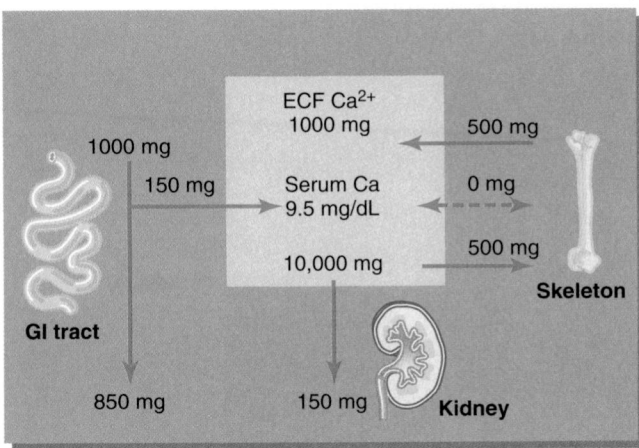

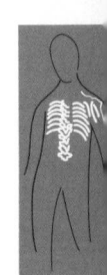

Figure 73-1 The calcium *physiologic black box*. The central box represents extracellular fluid (ECF), which contains a total of about 1000 mg of calcium. This black box has three interfaces with the gastrointestinal (GI) tract, the skeleton, and the kidney, as discussed in detail in the text. The fluxes into and out of the ECF are measured in milligrams per day.

CALCIUM FLUXES INTO AND OUT OF EXTRACELLULAR FLUID

Intestinal Calcium Absorption

The normal dietary calcium intake for an adult human is about 1000 mg per day. Of this amount, about 300 mg is absorbed (i.e., unidirectional absorption is about 30%), and this absorption occurs in the duodenum and proximal jejunum. Interestingly, about 150 mg per day of calcium is secreted by the liver (in bile), the pancreas (in pancreatic secretions), and the intestinal glands such that net absorption (called *fractional absorption*) of calcium is about 15% of intake. The mechanisms that regulate the 150 mg per day of calcium secreted by the gastrointestinal (GI) tract have not been well studied, despite their obvious quantitative importance. The efficiency of calcium absorption is regulated at the level of the small intestinal epithelial cell, the enterocyte, by the active form of vitamin D, 1,25-dihydroxyvitamin D (1,25[OH]$_2$D, also called *calcitriol*), with increases in 1,25(OH)$_2$D leading to enhanced calcium absorption and decreases in 1,25(OH)$_2$D causing reduced absorption of dietary calcium. Thus, dietary calcium absorption can be increased, at least over the short term, by increasing calcium intake, by increasing plasma 1,25(OH)$_2$D concentrations, or by both measures. Pathologic increases in serum calcium (hypercalcemia) can be caused by increases in circulating 1,25(OH)$_2$D (as in sarcoidosis) or by excessive calcium intake (the milk-alkali syndrome). Conversely, hypocalcemia can occur as a result of a decline in 1,25(OH)$_2$D (chronic renal failure and hypoparathyroidism are examples). An overall view of the impact of the GI tract can be summarized as follows: If an individual consumes 1000 mg of calcium per day, and if net absorption is 150 mg per day, then he or she will excrete 850 mg of calcium in feces per day.

Renal Calcium Handling

The normal ionized serum calcium concentration, as noted previously, is about 4.5 mg/dL. The normal glomerular filtration rate is 120 mL per minute. Multiplying these two numbers produces the filtered load of calcium, which proves to be about 10,000 mg per day. In terms of overall regulation of calcium homeostasis, this number is very large, making the point that the kidney is the most important moment-to-moment regulator of the serum calcium concentration. The amount also emphasizes that disorders of renal calcium handling (e.g., thiazide diuretic use, hypoparathyroidism) can be expected to lead to significant abnormalities in serum calcium homeostasis.

Of the 10,000 mg filtered at the glomerulus each day, about 9000 mg (90%) is reabsorbed *proximally*, meaning in the proximal convoluted tubule, the pars recta, and the thick ascending limb of Henle loop. This 90% is absorbed in conjunction with sodium and chloride reabsorption and is not subject to regulation by parathyroid hormone (PTH). In contrast, the remaining 10%, or 1000 mg, that arrives at the distal tubule on a daily basis is subject to regulation, with PTH stimulating renal calcium reabsorption. This anticalciuric effect of PTH can be extremely efficient, and elevated PTH concentrations can essentially eliminate calcium excretion into the urine. This action is a potent mechanism for retaining calcium under conditions of calcium deprivation (e.g., a low-calcium diet, vitamin D deficiency, intestinal malabsorption) and can contribute to hypercalcemia under pathologic conditions, as in primary hyperparathyroidism.

About 150 mg of calcium is excreted by the kidney in the final urine on a daily basis in a healthy individual. If the kidney filters 10,000 mg of calcium each day, and if 150 mg is excreted in the final urine, 9850 mg is reabsorbed at proximal and distal sites. Thus, 98.5% of filtered calcium is reabsorbed by the nephron. Conversely, the normal *fractional excretion of calcium* is about 1.5%.

Viewed from a whole-organism standpoint, a healthy person is in zero calcium balance with respect to the outside world: intake (1000 mg per day) − output [(850 mg in feces per day) + (150 mg in urine per day)] = 0.

Skeletal Biology and Calcium Homeostasis

The skeletal compartment contains about 1.2 kg of calcium in a male adult and 1.0 kg in a female adult. As noted earlier, most of this calcium is in the crystal hydroxyapatite, a calcium phosphate salt. Although calcium contributes in an important way to the structural integrity of the skeleton, as noted previously, the skeleton also serves as a quantitatively large reservoir, as well as a sink, for adding and removing calcium to and from the extracellular fluid (ECF) compartment at appropriate times.

The adult skeleton is composed of two fundamental types of bone: (1) cortical (or lamellar) bone and (2) trabecular (or cancellous) bone (Fig. 73-2). Cortical bone predominates in the skull and the shafts of long bones, and trabecular bone predominates at other sites, such as the distal radius, the vertebral bodies, and the trochanters of the hip. Bone is not an inert tissue, as might be imagined from visiting the dinosaur room at a natural history museum; instead, bone is a vital tissue that is continually turning over. The adult skeleton is completely remodeled every 3 to 10 years. This remodeling is perhaps best appreciated by recalling that orthopedic surgeons routinely and intentionally set fractures imperfectly, knowing that the normal processes of bone

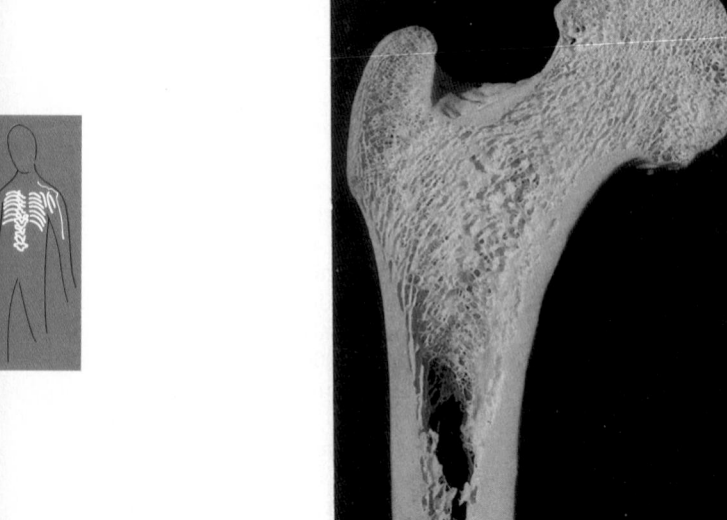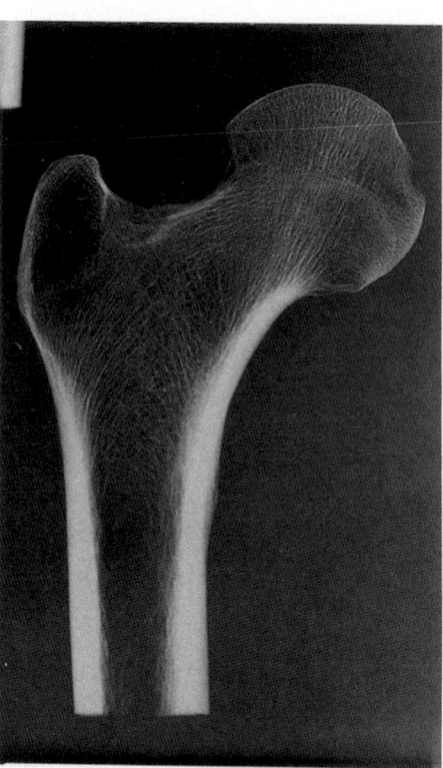

Figure 73-2 The structure of human bone. This figure depicts a human proximal femur examined using a gross pathologic specimen *(left panel)* and a radiograph of the same section *(right panel)*. Note that two different types of bone are represented. One type is called *cortical bone* (also called *lamellar bone*) and the other *cancellous bone* (also called *trabecular bone*). Note that the proportion of trabecular and cortical bone differs by location. For example, the shaft of the femur contains mostly cortical bone, whereas the proximal end of the femoral neck and the greater trochanter contain little cortical bone and almost exclusively trabecular bone. This distinction is important because most osteoporotic fractures occur at sites in which trabecular bone predominates, including the greater trochanter, the femoral neck, the vertebrae, and the distal radius. (Courtesy of Webster S. S. Jee, MD, University of Utah.)

remodeling will lead to restoration of the original shape of a given bone with the passage of time.

The cells that regulate bone turnover can be divided into those that remove old bone, those that provide new bone (Fig. 73-3; see also Chapter 75), and those that regulate these two processes. Cells that remove (or *resorb*) old bone are *osteoclasts*. These cells are large, metabolically active, multinucleated cells derived from the fusion of circulating macrophages. They deposit themselves on the surface of bone and form a *sealing zone* over the bone surface into which they secrete protons (acid), proteases (such as collagenase), and proteoglycan-digesting enzymes (such as hyaluronidase). The acid solubilizes hydroxyapatite crystals, releasing calcium, and the enzymes digest bone proteins and proteoglycans (e.g., collagen, osteocalcin, osteopontin), which constitute the nonmineral or *osteoid* component of bone. Osteoclasts literally move along the surface of trabecular bone plates and drill tunnels in cortical bone, periodically releasing the digested contents within their sealed zones into the bone marrow space and thereby creating resorption lacunae, called *Howship lacunae*, on the trabecular bone surface. The released calcium contributes to the ECF calcium pool, and the released proteolytic products, such as deoxypyridinoline cross-links (collagen fragments and hydroxyproline) can be used clinically as indices of bone resorption.

On the other side of the bone turnover equation is new bone formation. This task is accomplished by *osteoblasts*, which, in turn, are derived from marrow stromal cells or bone surface lining cells. Osteoblasts synthesize and secrete the components of the nonmineral phase of bone, called *osteoid*. These components are mostly proteins and include collagen, osteopontin, osteonectin, osteocalcin, and a plethora of growth factors, including transforming growth factor-β and insulin-like growth factor I, as well as proteoglycans. This complex serves as the scaffolding into which the mineral crystal hydroxyapatite forms its lattices.

In the past decade, attention has focused on a third, previously underappreciated, bone cell type: the *osteocyte*. These cells are descendents of osteoblasts and are embedded into the mineralized phase of bone. Osteocytes physically connect with one another, as well as cells at the mineral surface, through long dendritic processes. These dendritic processes extensively permeate the mineralized phase of bone through an elaborate canalicular network. Osteocytes serve a critical role in sensing biomechanical strain within bone, and through their cellular extensions to the cell surface, also communicate signals that attract, activate, or repress osteoclasts and osteoblasts. That is, they determine which areas of the skeleton require new bone formation and which need to be targets of osteoclastic bone remodeling.

Through this process of bone turnover, or bone remodeling, osteoclasts continually remove old bone, and osteoblasts continually produce new osteoid that mineralizes, in the end, replacing the old bone removed by osteoclasts with new bone. Teleologically, this process is viewed as serving to

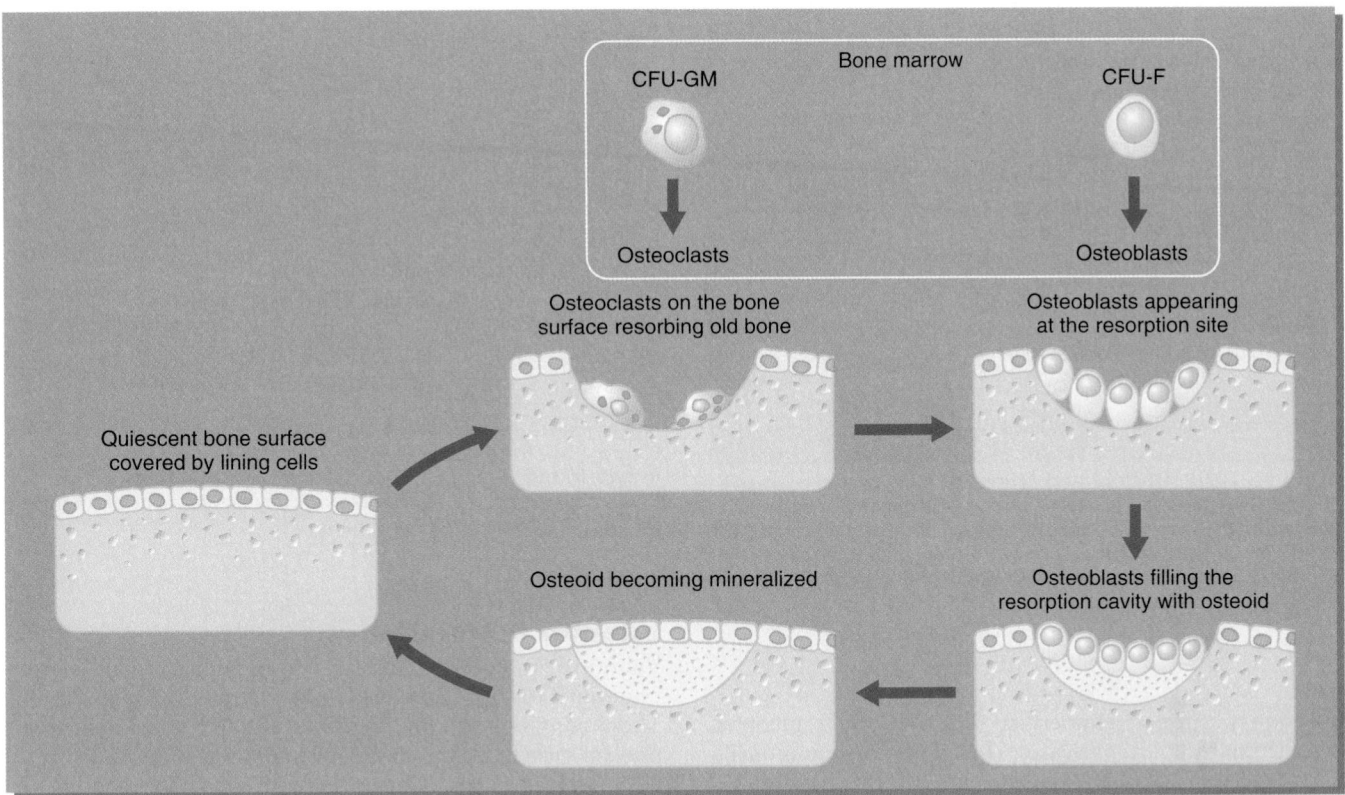

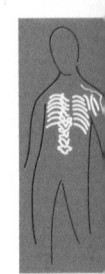

Figure 73-3 The cellular components of bone remodeling. As described in the text in detail, bone remodeling is a continuous process that involves the activation of osteoclast precursors in the macrophage lineage (abbreviated here as CFU-GM) to become actively resorbing osteoclasts, which literally tunnel into the bone surface to dig *resorption lacunae*. Osteoblast precursors in the fibroblast–bone marrow stromal cell lineage (abbreviated here as CFU-F) then appear and become active at the sites of prior resorption, and secrete new osteoid, which later mineralizes to *fill* the lacunae created by osteoclastic bone resorption. (From Manolagas SC, Jilka RL: Bone marrow, cytokines, and bone remodeling: Emerging insights into the pathophysiology of osteoporosis. N Engl J Med 332:305-311, 1995.)

replace old bone (and by implication defective or damaged bone with microfractures and reduced mechanical strength) with new, mechanically strong bone, although the evidence for this action is limited. Indeed, the principal therapy for osteoporosis at present is with so-called antiresorptives such as estrogens, estrogen-like drugs, and bisphosphonates, which dramatically reduce bone turnover and yet appear to improve not only bone mass but also bone mechanical properties.

From a systemic calcium homeostatic standpoint, however, this process is important. Osteoclasts can be used to access calcium from the skeleton in times of need to maintain a normal serum calcium concentration. Conversely, unmineralized osteoid produced by osteoblasts can be used at appropriate times as a sink into which excess serum calcium can be deposited. Under normal circumstances, estimates are that osteoclasts resorb bone at a rate such that about 500 mg of calcium is removed per day from the skeleton and delivered into the ECF compartment. At the same time, osteoblasts produce osteoid that mineralizes at a rate such that about 500 mg of calcium leaves the ECF and enters the skeleton at new sites. Seen from the perspective of the *black box* in Figure 73-1, the skeleton is in zero calcium balance with the ECF, and the whole organism is in zero calcium balance with the external world, as described previously.

Considering the complexity of this calcium homeostatic system and the importance of maintaining tight control over serum calcium, an obvious need exists for systemic regulation and integration of the fluxes across the GI tract, the skeletal compartment, and the kidney. The two key metabolic regulatory hormones that coordinate these activities are PTH and the active form of vitamin D, 1,25(OH)$_2$D.

REGULATORY HORMONES

Parathyroid Hormone

PTH is a peptide hormone produced by the four parathyroid glands (Fig. 73-4). These glands are located behind the normal thyroid lobes, two on the right, and two on the left. Through the calcium sensor—a G-protein–coupled receptor for calcium that is located on the surface of the parathyroid cell—the serum ionized calcium concentration is continuously monitored. This exquisitely sensitive system functions such that minor (e.g., 0.1 mg/dL) reductions in serum ionized calcium lead to PTH secretion and, similarly, minor increments in serum calcium lead to suppression of PTH secretion.

PTH is secreted as an 84–amino acid peptide hormone and is rapidly (half-life of about 3 to 5 minutes) cleaved by the Kupffer cells in the liver into amino-terminal and carboxy-terminal species. Of these forms, the intact 84–amino acid peptide and the amino-terminal species are biologically active. The amino-terminal form of PTH is also cleared rapidly (half-life of about 5 minutes) in this case in

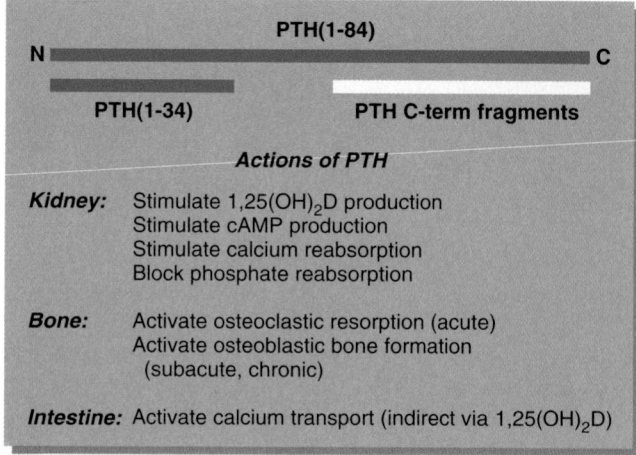

Figure 73-4 The structure and actions of parathyroid hormone (PTH). PTH is secreted as an 84–amino acid protein, which is cleaved in the liver to derivative amino- and carboxy-terminal forms. The actions of the amino-terminally intact forms of PTH are listed here and discussed in detail in the text. cAMP, cyclic adenosine monophosphate.

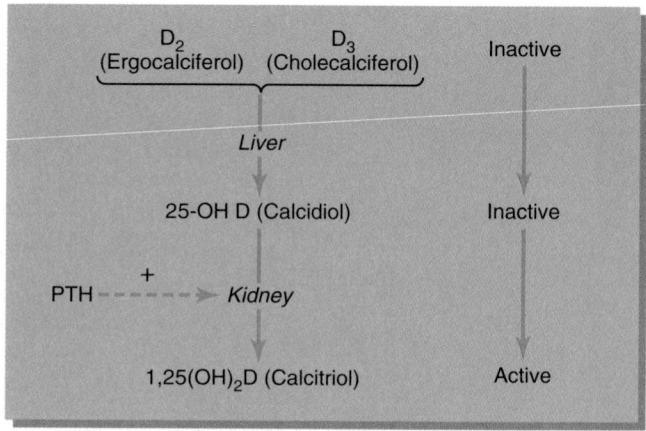

Figure 73-5 The vitamin D metabolic pathway. Vitamin D exists in two forms, D_2 and D_3, that pass through two steps in the liver and kidney to yield the biologically active form of vitamin D, $1,25(OH)_2D$. See text for details.

the kidney through glomerular filtration and proteolytic destruction by apical proteases. The continuous monitoring of the serum calcium concentration by the parathyroid glands, the immediate secretion of PTH in response to hypocalcemia, and the rapid clearance of PTH after secretion allow the parathyroid gland and PTH to act as critical, moment-to-moment regulators of the serum calcium. This tight regulatory control maintains the serum calcium at a normal level with rather remarkable precision.

PTH has three target organs, two direct and one indirect. The first direct target organ is the kidney, where renal calcium excretion is inhibited. Additional renal effects of PTH are to inhibit phosphate and bicarbonate reabsorption, which produce phosphaturia and hypophosphatemia, as well as a proximal renal tubular acidosis, respectively. These renal actions of PTH are essentially immediate. PTH has an additional direct effect on the proximal tubule to stimulate the production of the active form of vitamin D, $1,25(OH)_2D$, as described later. The second direct target organ of PTH is the skeleton. Here, PTH has the ability to mobilize calcium immediately from the skeleton through activation of osteoclastic bone resorption. Over the longer term (days to weeks), PTH also stimulates the activity of osteoblasts to produce new bone and thereby removes calcium from the circulation. The skeletal effects of PTH are discussed in more detail later. The ability to stimulate osteoclasts acutely without activating bone formation is important for the rapid delivery of calcium to the ECF. Finally, PTH has the indirect effect of increasing intestinal calcium absorption through its ability to increase renal synthesis of $1,25(OH)_2D$. This action, too, is described in more detail in the following section on vitamin D absorption. Seen in concert, PTH is secreted in response to hypocalcemia, and the actions of PTH combine to restore a low serum calcium to normal by preventing renal calcium losses, by adding calcium to the ECF from the skeleton, and by stimulating, indirectly through $1,25(OH)_2D$, increases in intestinal calcium absorption.

Vitamin D Metabolism

Vitamin D is really two different compounds, ergocalciferol (vitamin D_2) and cholecalciferol (vitamin D_3) (Fig. 73-5). These compounds were identified through their ability to prevent rickets in humans and laboratory animals. In fact, both substances are actually inactive precursors, one (D_3) derived principally from skin exposed to sunlight, and the other (D_2) derived from plant sterols. Both D_2 and D_3 are present in multivitamins and commercial dietary supplements. These two precursors are converted passively by the enzyme vitamin D-25-hydroxylase in the liver to the respective 25-hydroxyvitamin D (25-OH D) derivatives. These derivatives, too, are inactive precursors, but they have clinical significance of two types. First, severe liver disease such as cirrhosis prevents this essential step and leads to vitamin D–deficient syndromes collectively called *hepatic osteodystrophy*. Second, 25-OH D is the standard clinical laboratory measure of the vitamin D status (repletion versus deficiency) in a patient with hypocalcemia, osteomalacia or rickets, osteoporosis or intestinal malabsorption, and other similar conditions.

25-OH D is next converted, or activated, in the renal proximal tubule by the enzyme 25-hydroxyvitamin D 1-α-hydroxylase to the active form of the vitamin, $1,25(OH)_2D$. This substance is also called *calcitriol*, in contrast to 25-OH D, which some call *calcidiol*. Because $1,25(OH)_2D$ is the active form of vitamin D, its production is necessarily regulated, and this is accomplished primarily by PTH, with increases in PTH-stimulating $1,25(OH)_2D$ production and decreases in PTH-diminishing $1,25(OH)_2D$ synthesis. As noted previously, the primary action of $1,25(OH)_2D$ is to regulate intestinal calcium absorption. Thus, PTH, through $1,25(OH)_2D$, indirectly regulates calcium absorption from the diet by the intestine. This action has importance clinically because the hypocalcemia of hypoparathyroidism is, in an important way, a result of inadequate intestinal calcium absorption. Conversely, hyperparathyroidism is associated with hypercalciuria and nephrolithiasis, both of which are direct results of increases in circulating $1,25(OH)_2D$. Finally, as should be clear from the previous discussion, measurement of $1,25(OH)_2D$ can be used as an index of both parathyroid function and intestinal calcium absorption.

Calcitonin

Calcitonin is produced by the parafollicular or C cells of the thyroid gland in response to hypercalcemia. It was once viewed as an essential calcium-regulating hormone. Clearly, pharmacologic doses of calcitonin may reduce the serum calcium, and although everyone agrees that it is secreted in response to hypercalcemia, little evidence exists that calcitonin has homeostatic relevance in humans. Indeed, compelling evidence suggests that calcitonin is unimportant in human physiology. First, malignant tumors of the parafollicular cell (medullary carcinomas of the thyroid) routinely overproduce calcitonin and lead to enormous, long-term (years or decades) elevations in circulating calcitonin concentrations. This has no effect on serum calcium or any apparent skeletal effect. Conversely, thyroidectomy, whether achieved surgically or medically using radioiodine ablation, removes calcitonin, but this, too, has no apparent adverse effect on serum calcium or skeletal homeostasis. Thus, calcitonin is a hormone in search of a function, at least in humans.

INTEGRATION OF CALCIUM HOMEOSTASIS

The foregoing regulatory system would be all that is needed to control calcium homeostasis if humans received continuous GI infusions of calcium. Of course, all normal people experience periods of high calcium intake (e.g., diets including cheese, milk, ice cream, yogurt) as well as periods of low calcium intake (diets without these dairy products). Even on a daily basis, normal people eat at times and fast at other times between meals. Given the importance of maintaining the serum calcium concentration in a very narrow range, all these regulatory processes must be, and are, coordinated during periods of high calcium intake and of low calcium intake.

Ingestion of a greater than normal dietary calcium load (Fig. 73-6A) leads to a mild rise in serum calcium followed by immediate suppression of PTH. This action leads to an immediate *opening* of the renal distal tubular calcium *floodgates*. It also leads to an immediate reduction in osteoclastic activity. This latter effect not only prevents continued bone resorption but also allows continuation of calcium entry from ECF to an unmineralized osteoid *sink*. These two effects lead to a rapid and short-term reduction in serum calcium to normal. However, if the high-calcium diet is maintained over the long term, these adaptations are insufficient; continued renal calcium wasting would lead to hypercalciuria (with nephrolithiasis and nephrocalcinosis) and to excessive skeletal mineralization (osteopetrosis). Hence, two additional responses (see Fig. 73-6B) are required to prevent these potential long-term adverse effects of a high-calcium diet. First, subacute or chronic suppression of PTH results in a reduction in circulating 1,25(OH)$_2$D. This action, in turn, leads to a reduction in the efficiency of calcium absorption from the intestine and a reduction of calcium entry into the ECF and hence a reduction of urinary calcium excretion. Second, a chronic decrement in PTH leads to a chronic decline in osteoblastic activity such that no osteoid is formed, and the ability to deposit calcium into the skeletal sink is lost.

Conversely, during brief periods of dietary calcium deficiency (Fig. 73-7A), as occurs between meals, for example, the serum calcium declines almost imperceptibly, the PTH rises, and this increase immediately prevents renal calcium losses from continuing. At the same time, an acute activation of osteoclasts occurs, and this action delivers calcium into the ECF. Thus, the acute response to low calcium intake is the appropriate elimination of renal calcium losses and the development of a new source of calcium entry into the ECF. Over the longer term, however, this response is inadequate and would lead to skeletal demineralization. Hence, a longer-term solution is required. This adaptation is again twofold (see Fig. 73-7B). First, a chronic low calcium intake, as would occur in a person with lactose intolerance, for example, leads to a chronic elevation in PTH, and this, over a matter of days to weeks, leads to an increase in 1,25(OH)$_2$D. This increase, in turn, leads to an increase in the efficiency of calcium absorption from the intestine (an increase in the

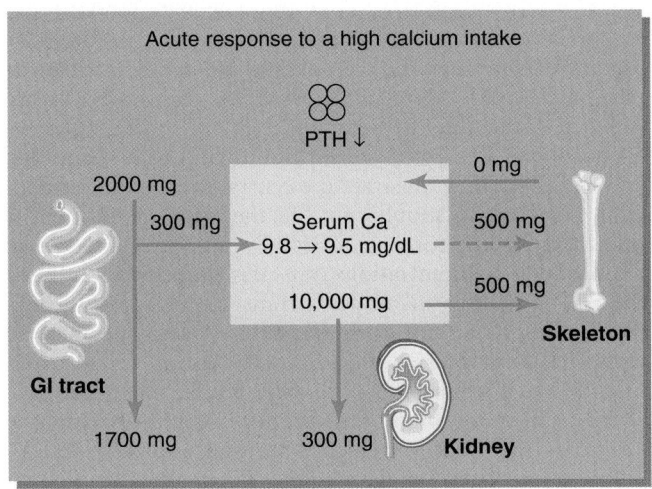

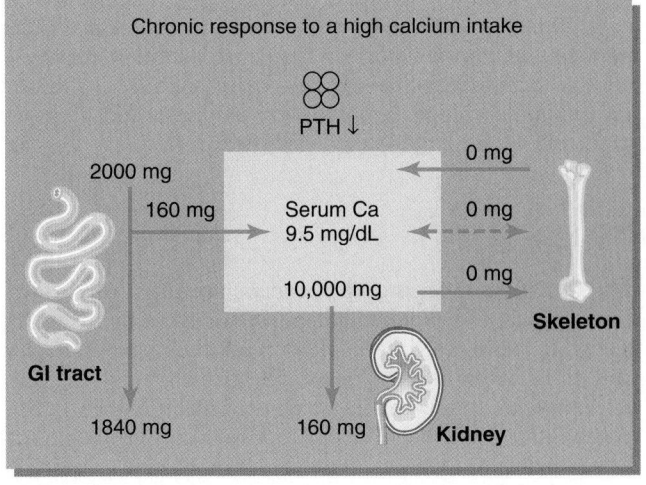

A   **B**

Figure 73-6 The response to increases in calcium intake. **A,** The acute response. **B,** The chronic response. Details are provided in the text. GI, gastrointestinal; PTH, parathyroid hormone.

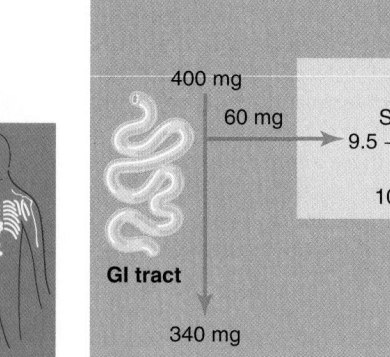
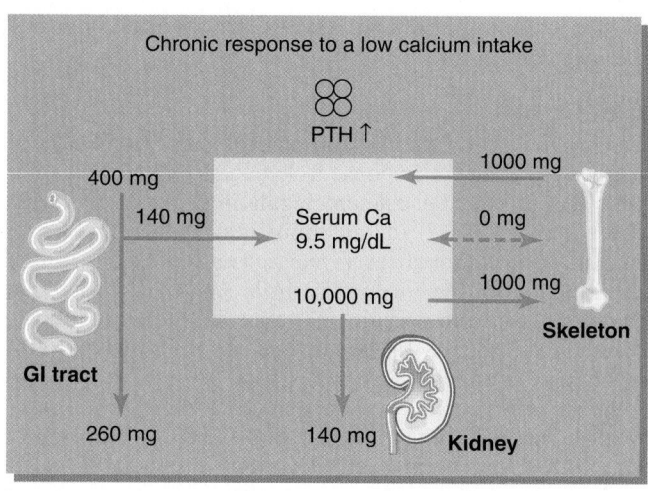

Figure 73-7 The response to decreases in calcium intake. **A,** The acute response. **B,** The chronic response. Details are provided in the text. GI, gastrointestinal; PTH, parathyroid hormone.

fractional absorption of calcium) to compensate for the reduction in dietary intake. Second, a chronic elevation in PTH will lead to an increase in osteoblast activity and osteoid synthesis, with resultant increases in skeletal calcium deposition. In this new steady-state adaptation to a low-calcium diet, PTH will be elevated, and coupled increases in both osteoclastic and osteoblastic activities will take place (i.e., an increase in bone turnover), but net skeletal calcium losses will be negligible or normal.

In summary, from an evolutionary standpoint, as life moved from a calcium-rich marine environment to terrestrial life, in which calcium availability is variable and unpredictable, a complex, but rather beautiful, regulatory mechanism has evolved that permits survival without requiring intentional behavioral adaptations for the vagaries of calcium availability. This evolution was essential in evolutionary terms because calcium is so essential for all aspects of mammalian, indeed all eukaryotic, life. As discussed in Chapter 74, disorders that cause hypercalcemia or hypocalcemia are always caused by abnormalities at the interface of the ECF with the intestine, the kidney, or the skeleton, and in several of these interfaces. Moreover, given the robustness of these homeostatic adaptive processes, disorders that cause hypocalcemia or hypercalcemia are rarely subtle: The physician need only recall these homeostatic premises to dissect the pathophysiologic process with precision and accuracy and treat the underlying disorder effectively.

Phosphate Homeostasis

The terms *phosphorus* and *phosphate* are often used interchangeably. To be parochial, phosphorus is an inorganic element, abbreviated as P in physical chemistry literature and as Pi in physiologic usage. Of course, the biologically relevant molecule is the negatively charged, trivalent phosphate ion PO_4. Phosphorus is the form that most clinical laboratories measure rather than the more biologically relevant phosphate ion. To make matters more complex, phosphate is an important physiologic buffer, and, at neutral pH in blood, phosphate is apportioned between HPO_4 (diva-

lent) and H_2PO_4 (monovalent). The practical effect of this dichotomy is that, whereas physicians receive phosphorus measurements in milligram per deciliter (mg/dL) units, pharmaceutical preparations contain phosphorus in millimoles (mmol). Many physicians are unable to convert milligrams to millimoles, and dosing errors are common. An example is the replacement of potassium-using K-Phos, in which relatively standard amounts of potassium ion (e.g., 40 mEq) given intravenously are coupled with potentially life-threatening amounts of phosphate (30 mmol, or 900 mg). A chart converting milligrams to millimoles in common phosphate-containing preparations is provided in Table 73-1.

Phosphate regulates or participates in the regulation of an enormous number of biologic processes. These actions of phosphate are fundamental to life itself and range from (1) being an integral component of the DNA double helix, to (2) shuttling oxygen from hemoglobin to cells and vice versa using 2,3-diphosphoglycerate (2,3-DPG), to (3) intracellular signaling through kinases that attach phosphate groups to other molecules, to (4) facilitating critical intracellular messenger systems such as cyclic monophosphate (cAMP) and inositol phosphates, to (5) maintaining basic intracellular redox status through the nicotinamide adenine dinucleotide phosphate (NADP-NADPH) system, to (6) serving as the gateway to the glucose metabolic pathway through glucose 6-phosphate. These actions are but a handful of examples, and, although they illustrate the central importance of adequate phosphorus supplies for life, they also underscore the point that phosphorus is primarily an intracellular ion. Extracellular concentrations are less important because the ECF functions mainly as a transport conduit through which phosphorus must travel from the skeleton or intestine to reach the cell interior. In addition to these critical intracellular roles, phosphate does have a key extracellular role as well: The anion pairs with calcium in the hydroxyapatite crystal lattice that provides structural integrity to the skeleton (see previous discussion). Thus, as with calcium, phosphate is critical to skeletal strength, and disorders of phosphorus homeostasis, such as hypophosphatemic rickets, lead to pathologic skeletal fractures. Also in parallel

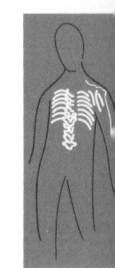

Table 73-1 Examples of Therapeutic Phosphorus Preparations

Preparations	Composition* (per mL)	pH	mOsm/ kg H_2O	Phosphate (mmol/mL)	Phosphorus (mg/mL)	Sodium (mEq/mL)	Potassium (mEq/mL)
Oral							
Cow's milk (whole)	—	—	288	0.029	0.9	0.025	0.035
Neutra-Phos[†]	Na_2HPO_4, NaH_2PO_4, K_2HPO_4, KH_2PO_4	7.3	—	0.107	3.33	0.095	0.095
Phospho-Soda[†]	180 mg $Na_2HPO_4 \cdot 7H_2O$ + 480 mg $NaH_2PO_4 \cdot H_2O$	4.8	8240	4.150	128.65	4.822	0
Acid sodium phosphate	136 mg $Na_2HPO_4 \cdot 7H_2O$ + 58.8 mg H_3PO_4 (NF 85%)	4.9	1740	1.018	35.54	1.015	0
Neutral sodium phosphate	145 mg $Na_2HPO_4 \cdot 7H_2O$ + 18.2 mg $NaH_2PO_4 \cdot H_2O$	7.0	1390	0.673	20.86	1.214	0
Parenteral							
Neutral sodium phosphate	10.07 mg Na_2HPO_4 + 2.66 mg $NaH_2PO_4 \cdot H_2O$	7.35	202	0.090	2.80	0.161	0
Neutral sodium, potassium phosphate	11.5 mg Na_2HPO_4 + 2.58 mg KH_2PO_4	7.4	223	0.100	3.10	0.162	0.019
Na Phosphate[†]	142 mg Na_2HPO_4 + 276 mg $NaH_2PO_4 \cdot H_2O$	5.7	5580	3.000	93.00	4.000	0
K Phosphate[†]	236 mg K_2HPO_4 + 224 mg KH_2PO_4	6.6	5840	3.003	93.11	0	4.360

*Hydration states are important. For example, 268 mg $Na_2HPO_4 \cdot 7H_2O$ (molecular weight 268) equals 1.00 mmol, whereas 268 mg Na_2HPO_4 (molecular weight 142) equals 1.89 mmol.

[†]Commercial preparations: Neutra-Phos, Willen Drug Company, Baltimore (Neutra-Phos K has twice as much potassium and no sodium); Phospho-Soda, C. B. Fleet Company, Lynchburg, Virginia (enema is one third the strength of Phospho-Soda and can be used orally); Na Phosphate, Abbott Laboratories, North Chicago, Illinois; K Phosphate, Invenex Pharmaceuticals, Grand Island, New York, or Abbott Laboratories. Because Neutra-Phos was not readily dissolved and its specific composition is unknown, data shown are those provided by the manufacturer.

H_2O, water; K_2HPO_4, dipotassium hydrogen phosphate; KH_2PO_4, potassium dihydrogen phosphate; Na_2HPO_4, disodium hydrogen phosphate; NaH_2PO_4, sodium dihydrogen phosphate.

From Lentz RD, Brown DM, Kjellstrand CM: Treatment of severe hypophosphatemia. Ann Intern Med 89:941-944, 1978.

with calcium, the skeleton serves as a major storage site for phosphate that can be, and is, accessed in times of severe phosphate deficiency.

Two corollaries of these broad and critical intracellular roles for phosphate are that: (1) clinically significant intracellular phosphate deficiency may exist without marked hypophosphatemia (ideally, assessing intracellular phosphorus concentrations would be preferred, but this is not clinically possible); and (2) importantly, severe, life-threatening phosphate deficiency is often unrecognized because its manifestations are so completely nonspecific yet common in intensive care unit settings (reduced levels of consciousness, hypotension, respirator dependence, and weakness). Astute clinicians learn to recognize general debility as a potential sign of phosphorus deficiency. Phosphate repletion in this setting may produce dramatic results.

In contrast to the regulation of serum calcium concentration, which is very tight, the regulation of serum phosphate concentrations is relatively lax. The serum phosphorus is maintained in a broad range between about 3.0 and 4.5 mg/dL. At least two reasons for this lax maintenance exist. First, as noted previously, in contrast to extracellular calcium concentrations, the precise maintenance of which are critically important to survival, extracellular phosphate concentrations are not critically important. Thus, room can be found for laxity in the system. Second, because phosphate is so abundant inside plant and animal cells, phosphate is abundant in almost any diet such that evolutionary pressure has not been intense to develop a systemic regulatory mechanism for phosphate.

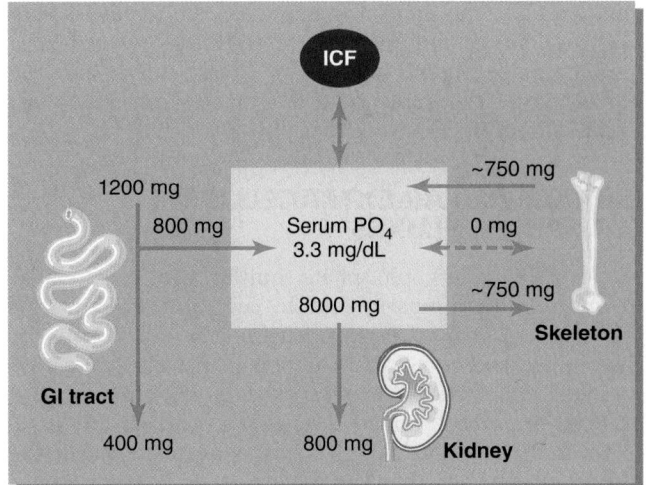

Figure 73-8 The phosphate *physiologic black box*. See Figure 73-1 for nomenclature and the text for details. GI, gastrointestinal; ICF, intracellular fluid.

As with calcium, a *black box* can be developed for phosphate metabolism as well (Fig. 73-8). This black box represents ECF and, as with calcium, has interfaces with the GI tract, the kidney, and the skeleton. In addition, because most phosphate is contained within cells, the phosphate black box has a quantitatively significant interface with the intracellular compartment.

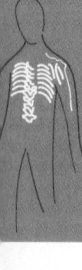

INTESTINAL PHOSPHATE ABSORPTION

A normal diet contains about 1200 to 1600 mg of phosphorus, and about two thirds of this amount, or 800 to 1200 mg, is absorbed each day. Absorption occurs in the duodenum and jejunum. Although vitamin D compounds can increase the intestinal absorption of phosphorus, this effect is modest, and phosphate absorption in the intestine can be considered as occurring with a fixed fractional absorption of about 67%. In the normal world of phosphate abundance, this amount is more than ample. Conversely, under conditions of dietary phosphorus deficiency, as occurs in chronic alcoholism (alcoholic beverages generally do not contain phosphorus), intensive care units (without adequate oral or parenteral alimentation), intestinal malabsorption, or phosphate-binding antacid use, failure to provide this amount of phosphorus presents a physiologic challenge for which no physiologic remedy exists.

SKELETAL PHOSPHATE FLUXES

As with calcium, osteoclastic bone resorption and osteoblastic new bone formation (see Figs. 73-1 and 73-3) lead to phosphate exit and entry, respectively, from the skeleton. Although the skeleton can thus be used as a source of phosphorus, in general, phosphorus can be viewed as a passive passenger with calcium in the calcium regulatory process described previously in the section on calcium. Again, however, under pathophysiologic conditions, skeletal calcium fluxes may become important. Skeletal destruction in multiple myeloma or severe immobilization syndromes leads not only to hypercalcemia but also to hyperphosphatemia, which, with the concomitant hypercalcemia, leads to nephrocalcinosis and renal failure. Conversely, osteoblastic metastases in prostate cancer and breast cancer and the hungry bone syndrome following parathyroidectomy all lead to clinically significant hypophosphatemia.

INTRACELLULAR-EXTRACELLULAR PHOSPHATE FLUXES

As noted previously, phosphate shuttles from extracellular to intracellular compartments. In general, the control of these fluxes can best be envisioned as being performed at the cellular level by as yet incompletely understood cellular mechanisms. From a clinical standpoint, these issues become important under certain settings. For example, in the setting of metabolic acidosis, phosphate leaves the intracellular compartment and may lead to hyperphosphatemia, whereas, under conditions of alkalosis, serum phosphate concentrations decline, and hypophosphatemia develops as phosphate enters the intracellular compartment. Other clinical situations in which intracellular phosphate has important clinical implications are in the settings of crush injury (rhabdomyolysis) and the tumor lysis syndrome, in both of which large intracellular loads of phosphate are delivered into the ECF and result in hypocalcemia, seizures, nephrocalcinosis, and renal failure. Finally, glucose shifts phosphate into cells as glucose 6-phosphate, and overzealous intravenous or oral caloric restitution in the undernourished patient can result in severe hypophosphatemia and sudden death.

RENAL PHOSPHATE HANDLING

By far the most important mechanism for maintaining a normal serum phosphorus concentration is renal phosphorus handling. As with calcium, phosphate is filtered by the glomerulus. *Tubular reabsorption of filtered phosphate* (TRP) occurs at a rate such that about 90% of phosphate is reabsorbed (i.e., the TRP is normally about 90%), and the remaining 10% is excreted. This 10% represents the *fractional excretion of phosphorus* (Fe_{Pi}). The Fe_{Pi} can be calculated in a spot urine sample as follows:

$$Fe_{Pi} = (\text{urine Pi [in mg/dL]/urine creatinine [in mg/dL]}) \times \\ (\text{serum creatinine [in mg/dL]/} \\ \text{serum phosphorus [in mg/dL]})$$

The TRP is simple to calculate:

$$TRP = 1 - Fe_{Pi}$$

The renal handling of phosphorus is best considered as a tubular maximum (Tm)-regulated process. For example, a renal Tm for glucose exists and is set at about 180 mg/dL. When the serum glucose rises above 180 mg/dL, glycosuria occurs. Of course, the serum glucose normally does not rise above 180 mg/dL; therefore, glucose does not normally appear in the urine. A similar process occurs with the Tm for phosphorus (TmP), with one exception. The TmP is normally identical to a normal serum phosphorus concentration in blood, about 3.3 mg/dL. If the serum phosphate concentration rises above this level, phosphaturia occurs, and the serum phosphorus declines to 3.3 mg/dL. If the serum phosphate concentration declines below 3.3 mg/dL, then filtered phosphate is entirely reabsorbed, and urinary phosphate excretion declines to zero. Thus, the TmP can be considered as a *dam* in the *phosphate reservoir,* over which excess phosphate *spills,* and whose level controls the *level* or concentration of serum phosphorus.

The one exception to this concept is that, unlike the glucose Tm, which is fixed at 180 mg/dL, the TmP is not fixed but can be moved upward or downward, depending on metabolic needs and prevailing metabolic conditions, as described in the following section.

The TRP or Fe_{Pi}, as described previously, can be readily calculated, and then the TmP can be derived from the nomogram of Bijvoet, shown in Figure 73-9. This process proves enormously useful in clinical practice because it is the central starting point for determining whether hypophosphatemia is principally renal or nonrenal in origin.

PARATHYROID HORMONE AND PHOSPHATONINS

PTH has long been appreciated to be phosphaturic, that is, to lower the TmP or, more accurately, to inhibit proximal renal tubular phosphate reabsorption. Indeed, the initial bioassay for PTH action in humans, the Ellsworth-Howard test, assessed the responsiveness of the TRP to infusion of bovine parathyroid gland extract. This characteristic also explains the hypophosphatemia associated with primary and secondary hyperparathyroidism and, conversely, the hyperphosphatemia associated with hypoparathyroid states. Thus,

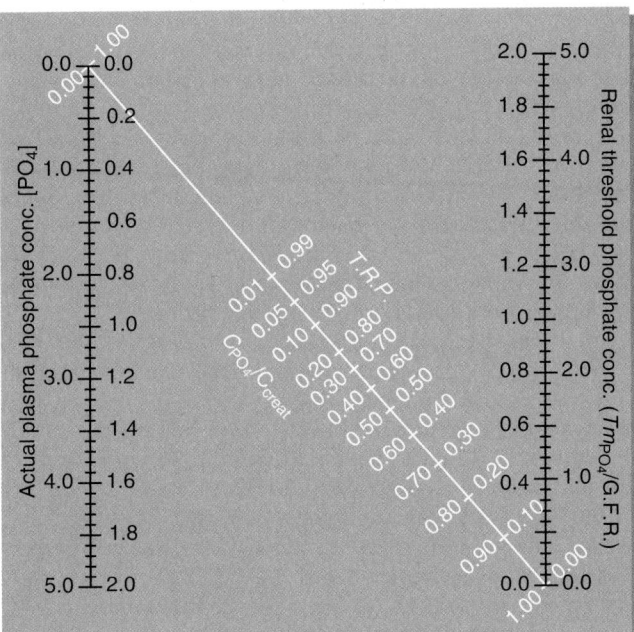

Figure 73-9 The tubular maximum for phosphorus-glomerular filtration rate (TmP-GFR) nomogram. This nomogram allows the conversion of the fractional excretion of phosphorus (or its inverse, the tubular reabsorption of filtered phosphate [TRP]) into the TmP-GFR. The TRP is calculated, as described in the text, and a line is drawn extending from the serum phosphorus *(leftmost line)*, through the TRP *(middle, diagonal line)*, to the left line, which represents the TmP/GFR. TmP values are provided in both millimolar (mmol) and milligram per deciliter (mg/dL) units. TmP values below 1.0 mmol or 2.5 mg/dL are abnormal and indicate phosphaturia. (From Walton RJ, Bijvoet OLM: Nomogram for derivation of renal threshold phosphate concentration. Lancet 2:309-310, 1975.)

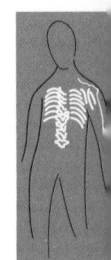

in TmP terms, excessive PTH lowers the TmP, whereas low PTH values allow the TmP to rise to supranormal levels.

It has been clear for many years, however, that other factors regulate the level of the TmP. For example, experimental dietary phosphorus deprivation in laboratory animals and humans leads to a PTH-independent increase in the TmP, and high-phosphate feeding results in a PTH-independent decline in the TmP. Thus, for decades, investigators in this area have postulated the existence of a phosphaturic hormone that has been called *phosphatonin*. Despite decades of research, phosphatonin has remained elusive. This area has become one of intense focus recently with the discovery of the cause of three disorders. In one of these disorders, X-linked hypophosphatemic rickets, also known as *vitamin D–resistant rickets*, causative inactivating mutations have been identified in the *PHEX* enzyme. Current models suggest that mutant *PHEX* fails to inactivate normal amounts of phosphatonin, and this failure leads to phosphaturia and hypophosphatemia. In two other disorders, autosomal-dominant hypophosphatemic rickets and oncogenic osteomalacia, overproduction of fibroblast growth factor-23 (FGF-23) has been demonstrated, and many clinicians believe that FGF-23 is the long-sought phosphatonin. Other investigators have suggested that matrix extracellular phosphoglycoprotein *(MEPE)* or secreted frizzled-related protein 4 *(sFRP4)* may serve as phosphatonins as well. Much remains to be worked out in this arena, but clearly, a hormonal system that regulates renal phosphorus handling exists, and the kidney is the prime regulatory organ for phosphate homeostasis.

Regulation of Serum Magnesium

Magnesium is a divalent cation, as is calcium. With this exception, magnesium homeostasis has closer parallels with phosphorus homeostasis. Both magnesium and phosphate are principally intracellular, with concentrations inside the cell that far exceed those outside the cell. Both substances govern key intracellular regulatory processes. In the case of magnesium, these processes include such fundamental events as DNA replication and transcription, translation of RNA, the use of adenosine triphosphate as an energy source, and regulated peptide hormone secretion. Both magnesium and phosphate are abundant in the marine environment and therefore became incorporated into basic life processes early in the evolution of single-celled organisms. Both substances are abundant in terrestrial diets, whether vegetarian or carnivorous, given their abundance inside all kinds of cells. Given this abundance, little evolutionary pressure to develop a complex regulatory network exists. As with phosphate, because the important site of magnesium availability is within the cell, ECF serves only as a conduit for magnesium, and serum magnesium concentrations are not tightly regulated. As with phosphate, because magnesium is principally intracellular, measurement of serum magnesium may provide false estimates of actual total-body and intracellular magnesium status. Finally, as with phosphate, because magnesium is so essential for fundamental processes such as gene transcription and cellular energy use, life-threatening magnesium deficiency is often unrecognized because its symptoms are frustratingly nonspecific: weakness, respirator dependence, diffuse neurologic syndromes including seizures, and cardiovascular collapse.

Magnesium, as noted previously, is a divalent cation. Its molecular weight is 24, which is to say that 1 mole is 24 g, and, because it is divalent, one equivalent is 12 g. These considerations are significant clinically because magnesium measurements in blood are often provided in mg/dL or milliequivalents per liter (mEq/L), oral magnesium supplements in milligrams per tablet or milliequivalents per vial, and urinary magnesium excretion in milliequivalents or milligrams per 24 hours. Quantitative perspective in this clinical world of variable units can easily be lost. Constructing a *black box* for magnesium is helpful, as shown in Figure 73-10, in which magnesium is provided in both milligram and milliequivalent units.

As with phosphorus, magnesium has quantitatively important interfaces with the intestine, the skeleton, intracellular supplies, and the kidney. At the level of the intestine, as noted previously, magnesium is widely available in normal diets, and regulation here is limited: the body absorbs about one third of what is ingested. Under normal circumstances, dietary magnesium is abundant, absorption is ample, and magnesium deficiency does not occur. However, with alcoholism (a pure alcohol diet contains no magnesium), in intensive care unit settings in which adequate nutrition often

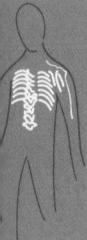

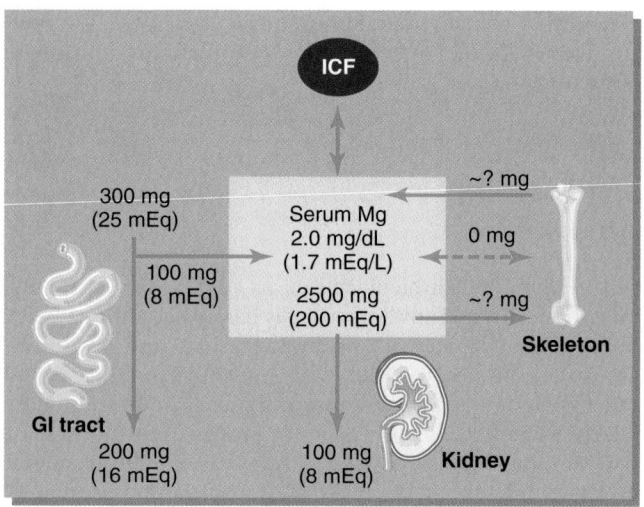

Figure 73-10 The magnesium *physiologic black box*. See Figure 73-1 for nomenclature and the text for details. Magnesium values are provided in both milligram (mg) and milliequivalent (mEq) units. GI, gastrointestinal; ICF, intracellular fluid.

is not provided, or with intestinal malabsorption, magnesium deficiency may occur.

At the level of the skeleton, magnesium is incorporated into the hydroxyapatite crystal as mineralization of osteoid occurs, and it is released by osteoclastic bone resorption (see Figs. 73-1 and 73-3). In quantitative terms, these fluxes are small.

Many instances of magnesium deficiency are caused by excessive renal losses. Examples include the magnesuria that accompanies saline infusions, diuretic use, alcohol use, and secondary hyperaldosteronism states such as cirrhosis and ascites. As with calcium and phosphorus, the fractional excretion of magnesium (FeMg) can be calculated, and this should be used as an index as to whether the kidney is appropriately conserving magnesium in states of hypomagnesemia or whether renal magnesium wasting is the cause of the hypomagnesemia. The normal FeMg is 2% to 4%. Hypomagnesemic individuals should display FeMg values below 1% to 2%.

With regard to homeostatic regulation, magnesium homeostasis can best be viewed as a renal Tm-regulated process (see the general principles described previously for the TmP under "Renal Phosphate Handling"), with the renal Tm for magnesium set at a fixed level of about 2.2 mg/dL. In this scenario, abundant dietary magnesium exists, and excessive magnesium intake is managed by spillage of excess magnesium, over the Tm set at 2.2 mg/dL, into the urine. Conversely, in settings of dietary magnesium deficiency, which equate evolutionarily with caloric deficiency, short-term magnesium deficiency is prevented when serum levels fall below the renal Tm of 2.0 mg/dL, and long-term deficiency is associated with, and becomes of lesser importance than, death by starvation. With regard to hormonal regulation, no known independent regulatory system for magnesium exists.

Prospectus for the Future

Although it may seem from this chapter that calcium, PTH, vitamin D, magnesium and phosphorus homeostasis, and skeletal biology are well understood, it should be clear that many of the details of the physiology as described in this chapter have been elucidated over the past 10 to 15 years, and indeed, new hormones (e.g., FGF-23) and diseases continue to accumulate at a rapid rate. The truth is that this area of research is dynamic, with many central unanswered questions. For example, although we know that the GI tract (pancreas, biliary system, and intestinal glands) secretes calcium and that this action is important quantitatively (150 mg per day), we know nothing about how this process is regulated or whether daily losses can be prevented. Similarly, although we now appreciate that phosphate has direct effects on the parathyroid gland and that these effects may be important in chronic renal failure, we do not know precisely what constitutes the parathyroid phosphorus sensor. Moreover, we know that hypomagnesemia and hypophosphatemia result in substantial intensive care unit morbidity and mortality, yet we remain inadequate at recognizing the nonspecific signs and symptoms of these diseases.

We know that bone density is a critical determinant of osteoporotic fracture, but we also know that *bone mass* accounts for only about 50% of fracture risk, with the other 50% representing issues of *bone quality*. Yet we have little understanding of what, at a molecular or structural level, determines or defines *bone quality*. In osteoporosis, most of the currently available pharmacologic agents inhibit osteoclast activity and are therefore *antiresorptives* or *anticatabolic agents*. What we really need for osteoporosis are agents that can potently stimulate osteoblasts to synthesize new bone, called *skeletal anabolic agents*. One agent, recombinant PTH, has recently been approved, and others are in the pharmaceutical pipeline. Another example of the limitations of our current understanding is a debate over the pulsatile secretion of PTH. Is the secretion pulsatile, and if so, how frequent are the pulses? Is pulsatile secretion important for PTH physiology as it obviously is for gonadotropin-releasing hormone biology, and is it important in pathophysiology? Whereas to the new initiate in mineral and bone physiology, everything has seemingly been discovered already, this assumption is far from the truth!

References

Berndt T, Kumar R: Phosphatonins and the regulation of phosphate homeostasis. Annu Rev Physiol 69:341-359, 2007.

DeGroot L, Jameson LJ (eds): Endocrinology, 5th ed. Philadelphia, WB Saunders, 2006.

Favus MF (ed): The American Society for Bone and Mineral Research Primer on Metabolic Bone Diseases and Disorders of Mineral Metabolism, 6th ed. Washington DC, American Society for Bone and Mineral Research, 2006.

Kronenberg HM, Melmed S, Polonsky KS, Larsen PR (eds): Williams Textbook of Endocrinology, 11th ed. Philadelphia, WB Saunders, 2008.

Lentz RD, Brown DM, Kjellstrand CM: Treatment of severe hypophosphatemia. Ann Intern Med 89:941-944, 1978.

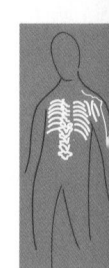

Disorders of Serum Minerals

Steven P. Hodak and Andrew F. Stewart

In this chapter, disorders that lead to increases or decreases in the circulating concentrations of calcium, phosphorus, and magnesium are considered. The reader is urged, in considering these disorders, to review the appropriate section in Chapter 73 describing the normal physiology of calcium, phosphorus, and magnesium metabolism. The optimal approach to diagnosing and treating these disorders is to understand their underlying physiology and pathophysiology. Beginning here, coherent diagnostic and successful therapeutic plans can best be developed. Although obvious at one level, years of experience suggests a common and persistent propensity to jump to the common items on the differential diagnosis list without fully considering the other options, and, in so doing, to overlook the correct, and often easily treatable, diagnosis. For example, hypercalcemia in the setting of a pulmonary nodule may indicate the presence of humoral hypercalcemia of malignancy, and many physicians will jump to this diagnosis with its grim prognosis. However, this complex might also represent hypercalcemia in a patient with treatable tuberculosis (TB) or primary hyperparathyroidism (HPT) in a person with a long-standing and inactive pulmonary scar.

Complete differential diagnoses are provided in the tables that follow. My practice is to consider every diagnosis in the appropriate table in every patient with a disorder of mineral metabolism. Hypercalcemia attributed by some physicians to *cancer* has proved in many instances to be due to sarcoid, HPT, hyperthyroidism, milk-alkali syndrome, and a host of other conditions, and hypocalcemia attributed by some physicians to *hypoparathyroidism* has proved to be due to easily treatable causes such as hypomagnesemia resulting from sprue or chemotherapy with cisplatin in some cases and in others to reductions in albumin in patients with the nephrotic syndrome. Each of these examples was incorrectly diagnosed initially but became obvious with appropriate consideration and testing.

Hypercalcemia

SYMPTOMS AND SIGNS

Hypercalcemia causes hyperpolarization of neuromuscular cell membranes and therefore refractoriness to stimulation (see Chapter 73). This condition presents clinically as skeletal muscular weakness, smooth muscle hypoactivity with constipation and ileus, and the full spectrum of mental dysfunction, progressing from lassitude to mild confusion to deep coma. Hypercalcemia also leads to renal failure. It causes a reduction in the glomerular filtration rate (GFR) through afferent arteriolar vasoconstriction and, through activation of the calcium receptor in the distal nephron, causes a form of nephrogenic diabetes insipidus, associated with polydipsia and polyuria. These events lower the extracellular fluid (ECF) volume and lower the GFR as well. Hypercalcemia may lead to interstitial calcium phosphate crystal deposition in the kidney (nephrocalcinosis or interstitial nephritis) and nephrolithiasis with obstructive uropathy. Hypercalcemia may also lead to shortening of the QTc interval on the electrocardiogram. Frequently, however, hypercalcemia is discovered on routine laboratory testing.

Whether a person develops symptoms depends on several factors. One of these factors is the degree of hypercalcemia. People with serum calcium values above 13 mg/dL are generally symptomatic. Also important is the duration of hypercalcemia. A gradual increase in serum calcium, even into the severe 15- to 17-mg/dL range, may cause little in the way of symptoms if it occurs slowly enough. Finally, the overall health, age, and general status of the person in whom hypercalcemia occurs will influence the severity of symptoms. For example, a child with severe immobilization-induced hypercalcemia in the 15-mg/dL range may be completely alert, whereas an elderly person with underlying

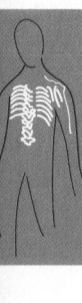

Alzheimer disease and narcotic use may become comatose with a serum calcium of 11.5 mg/dL.

PATHOPHYSIOLOGY

The physiologic *black box* described in Chapter 73 can and should be considered when attempting to diagnose or treat hypercalcemia. These disorders can be grouped into factitious disorders (e.g., caused by abnormalities in serum proteins), renal disorders (e.g., thiazide diuretic or lithium use), gastrointestinal disorders (e.g., sarcoid or the milk-alkali syndrome), skeletal disorders (e.g., hypercalcemia of malignancy, immobilization hypercalcemia), and combined disorders (primary HPT is a good example, with important gastrointestinal [GI] and renal components). Considering each diagnosis in Table 74-1 in the context of the mechanism that might be operative in a given patient brings clarity of diagnosis and corresponding appropriateness to therapy.

DIFFERENTIAL DIAGNOSIS

Malignancy-Associated Hypercalcemia

The most common cause of hypercalcemia among hospitalized patients is cancer. Hypercalcemia occurs late in the course of cancer, and rapid progression to more severe hypercalcemia and rapid death is the rule. The 50% survival rate among patients with cancer following the development of hypercalcemia is about 30 days. In general, hypercalcemia is only encountered in patients with large tumor burdens. Conversely, small, occult cancers rarely cause hypercalcemia. The exceptions to this rule are small tumors of the neuroendocrine variety, such as islet cell tumors and bronchial carcinoids. Certain tumors are common causes of hypercalcemia, including breast, renal, squamous, and ovarian carcinomas, as well as multiple myeloma and lymphoma. Conversely, certain other common cancers are not commonly associated with hypercalcemia, exemplified by colon, prostate, and gastric carcinoma. The occurrence of hypercalcemia should always provoke a complete search for the entities described in Table 74-1, particularly in patients with these latter types of cancer, given the likelihood that a vigorous search will reveal a second, more treatable form of hypercalcemia.

Cancer may lead to hypercalcemia through several mechanisms, the most common of which is *humoral hypercalcemia of malignancy* (HHM). HHM accounts for about 80% of patients with malignancy-associated hypercalcemia (MAHC) and is the result of secretion by tumors of parathyroid hormone–related protein (PTHrP). PTHrP mimics the actions of parathyroid hormone (PTH) on the kidney to prevent calcium excretion and on the skeleton to activate osteoclasts and induce bone resorption. PTHrP is the product of many normal cell types and is normally produced at low levels. The cause of the increase in PTHrP synthesis in cancer is most often not known but has been demonstrated to be due to PTHrP gene duplication or transcriptional upregulation of the PTHrP gene in some patients. Tumors classically associated with the HHM mechanism are squamous carcinomas of any site (including larynx, lung, cervix, and esophagus), renal carcinomas, ovarian carcinomas, and lymphomas associated with human T-cell lymphotropic virus type I (HTLV-I). More recently, the fact that

Table 74-1 Disorders Associated with Hypercalcemia

Malignancy-Associated Hypercalcemia

Humoral hypercalcemia of malignancy
Hypercalcemia caused by 1,25(OH)$_2$D-secreting lymphomas
Hypercalcemia caused by direct skeletal invasion
True ectopic hyperparathyroidism

Primary and Tertiary Hyperparathyroidism

Familial Hypocalciuric Hypercalcemia or Familial Benign Hypercalcemia

Granulomatous Disorders

Sarcoid
Berylliosis
Foreign body
Tuberculosis
Coccidioidomycosis
Blastomycosis
Histoplasmosis
Granulomatous leprosy
Eosinophilic granuloma
Histiocytosis
Inflammatory bowel disease

Endocrine Disorders Other than Hyperparathyroidism

Hyperthyroidism
Pheochromocytoma
Addisonian crisis
VIPoma (WDHA syndrome)

Medications

Thiazides
Aminophylline
Lithium
Estrogen/antiestrogen in breast cancer with bone metastases *(estrogen flare)*
Vitamin D and derivatives (calcitriol, dihydrotachysterol)
Vitamin A (including retinoic acid derivatives)
Foscarnet

Milk-Alkali Syndrome

Immobilization plus High Bone Turnover

Juvenile skeleton
Paget disease
Myeloma and breast cancer with bone metastases
Prehumoral hypercalcemia of malignancy
Mild primary hyperparathyroidism
Secondary hyperparathyroidism (e.g., from continuous ambulatory peritoneal dialysis)
Chronic and acute renal failure
Recovery phase of rhabdomyolysis-induced acute renal failure
Chronic hemodialysis
Calcitriol
Immobilization
Decreased calcium clearance
Calcium carbonate

Total Parenteral Nutrition (TPN)

Calcium-containing TPN in patients with decreased glomerular filtration rate
Chronic TPN in patients with short bowel syndrome

Hyperproteinemia

Volume contraction with hyperalbuminemia
Myeloma with calcium-binding immunoglobulin

End-Stage Liver Disease

Manganese Intoxication

1,25(OH)$_2$D, 1,25-dihydroxyvitamin D; VIPoma, vasoactive intestinal peptide–producing tumor; WDHA, watery diarrhea, hypokalemia, and achlorhydria.

breast cancer commonly produces hypercalcemia through this mechanism, as well, has become known. In general, hypercalcemia in HHM occurs in the absence of skeletal metastases or in the presence of a limited number of skeletal metastases, and, if tumor resection or ablation is possible, hypercalcemia reverses. These observations, together with histologic evidence for aggressive bone resorption at sites within the skeleton not involved by tumor, make clear that HHM is indeed the result of a tumor-derived *humor* or hormone. This example is perhaps the only one in which PTHrP acts in an *endocrine* fashion, more typically behaving as a paracrine, autocrine, or intracrine growth and developmental factor. In addition to hypercalcemia, these patients display reductions in PTH, reductions in 1,25-dihydroxyvitamin D (1,25[OH]$_2$D), elevations in PTHrP, and reductions in serum phosphorus and the tubular maximum for phosphorus (TmP) (see Chapter 73).

A second form of MAHC is that caused by local tumor invasion of the skeleton, a process referred to as *local osteolytic hypercalcemia* (LOH). LOH accounts for about 20% of patients with MAHC. In these patients, in contrast to those with HHM, the skeletal metastatic or primary tumor burden is large, and the offending tumor is most often a breast cancer or a hematologic neoplasm such as multiple myeloma, leukemia, or lymphoma. The local factors within the skeleton that are secreted by tumors to induce osteoclastic bone resorption include PTHrP, macrophage inflammatory protein-1-α (MIP1α), receptor-activating nuclear factor kappa B ligand (RANKL), interleukin-6, interleukin-1, and likely others as well. These patients display reductions in both PTH and PTHrP, as well as 1,25(OH)$_2$D, and generally have normal to elevated serum phosphorus values.

A third form of MAHC is due to *secretion of 1,25(OH)$_2$D by lymphomas and dysgerminomas*. These instances are unusual and are interesting from a mechanistic standpoint. Although direct bone involvement may occur and may contribute to hypercalcemia, the increase in 1,25(OH)$_2$D leads to intestinal calcium hyperabsorption as well as to systemically driven bone resorption. Thus, this condition is in essence a malignant version of the hypercalcemia that occurs in sarcoidosis (see "Granulomatous Disorders," later). The fact that macrophages produce 1,25(OH)$_2$D and that overproduction of 1,25(OH)$_2$D occurs in some lymphomas is now well documented. Under normal circumstances, 1,25(OH)$_2$D behaves as an immunomodulatory cytokine, produced locally in small amounts by lymphoreticular cells but not contributing significantly to systemic concentrations of 1,25(OH)$_2$D. However, under certain conditions, large amounts of 1,25(OH)$_2$D are produced by a given lymphoma, and hypercalcemia ensues. Thus, lymphomas are particularly interesting in that they may cause hypercalcemia through an HHM mechanism with systemic PTHrP secretion through a local skeletal invasion mechanism and through systemic production of 1,25(OH)$_2$D. Recently, the syndrome has been observed in association with ovarian dysgerminomas.

Finally, although most instances of HHM are due to PTHrP, several well-documented case reports of *ectopic secretion of authentic PTH* have come to light. These case reports have included a colon carcinoma, a squamous carcinoma of the lung, a small cell carcinoma of the ovary, and a neuroendocrine tumor.

Primary and Tertiary Hyperparathyroidism

Although MAHC is the most common cause of hypercalcemia among inpatients, primary HPT is by far the most common cause among healthy outpatients. Together, MAHC and HPT account for about 90% of cases of hypercalcemia. Most often, the hypercalcemia is mild, with serum calcium values in the 10.6- to 11.5-mg/dL range. However, HPT can occasionally produce spectacular hypercalcemia in the 20-mg/dL range. About 85% of the time, hypercalcemia results from a single parathyroid adenoma that overproduces PTH, and in about 15% of patients, it is due to multiple-gland hyperplasia. In less than 1% of patients, HPT may result from parathyroid carcinoma. The diagnosis is made by the discovery of an elevated serum PTH in a patient with hypercalcemia. Hypophosphatemia, a reduction in the TmP, increased plasma 1,25(OH)$_2$D, an increase in serum chloride, and a reduction in serum bicarbonate are also typical features.

Most often, primary HPT is asymptomatic. However, some patients develop hypercalciuria and calcium nephrolithiasis, most often as a result of calcium oxalate and, less commonly, calcium phosphate stones. In addition, some patients with HPT, especially those with more severe HPT, experience a reduction in bone mineral density characterized histologically as hyperparathyroid bone disease or *osteitis fibrosa cystica* (see Chapter 75). Other patients may develop mild to severe renal failure as a result of the considerations described under "Symptoms and Signs" of hypercalcemia earlier. Each of the previously mentioned conditions—significant osteopenia, hypercalciuria, kidney stones, reduced renal function, and a serum calcium greater than 1 mg/dL above normal—is considered an indication for parathyroidectomy. Other patients may be monitored conservatively. Some authors believe that cognitive dysfunction, peptic ulcers, and hypertension may result from HPT, but many disagree. Most people would regard these indications as *soft* indications for surgery at best.

The cause of parathyroid adenomas is most often not known, but mutations of the cyclin D1 and parafibromin genes have been described in some patients, and mutations in other genes have been identified in the adenomas of others. Mutations in *pRb*, the retinoblastoma gene, and in the parafibromin gene, have been identified in some parathyroid carcinomas.

HPT can occur as part of one of the multiple endocrine neoplasia (MEN) syndromes, in association with pituitary and islet tumors (MEN-I) or with pheochromocytomas and medullary carcinoma of the thyroid (MEN-II).

Secondary HPT, by definition, is an appropriate increase in circulating PTH associated with eucalcemia or hypocalcemia, occurring in an attempt to correct hypocalcemia resulting for example from vitamin D deficiency or chronic renal failure. *Tertiary* HPT refers to HPT associated with hypercalcemia that appears in the setting of prolonged stimulation of the parathyroid glands, such as chronic renal failure with hypocalcemia or chronic vitamin D deficiency resulting from malabsorption. Chronic parathyroid stimulation leads to parathyroid hyperplasia and at times adenomas, and these may, if they fail to suppress with the development of hypercalcemia, cause hypercalcemia. The classic example is

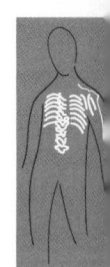

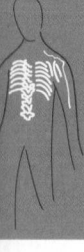

the development of PTH-dependent hypercalcemia following successful renal transplantation.

Familial Hypocalciuric Hypercalcemia

Familial hypocalciuric hypercalcemia (also known as *familial benign hypercalcemia*) is an autosomal dominant, inherited disorder that is due to heterozygous inactivating mutations in the calcium receptor. Thus, parathyroid glands that bear this receptor on their surface (see Chapter 73) inappropriately perceive circulating calcium concentrations to be low, therefore behaving as though the patient is hypocalcemic, and appropriately secrete additional PTH. This action causes the serum calcium to rise, and, with an elevated calcium, the PTH returns to a high-normal level. The hypercalcemia is usually mild, in the 11- to 12-mg/dL range, but may be higher. Importantly, because the calcium receptor is also expressed in the kidney, the kidney inappropriately conserves calcium, leading to hypocalciuria and contributing to hypercalcemia. Urine calcium excretion is in the 20- to 100-mg per day range. Finally, because the defective calcium receptor is also expressed in the central nervous system (CNS), the hypercalcemia goes unperceived by the CNS, and affected individuals are therefore asymptomatic. Thus, the two names of this syndrome describe it accurately.

With the exception of the hypocalciuria and the autosomal dominant pattern of inheritance, these individuals are similar to patients with primary HPT; they have mildly elevated calcium concentrations in the setting of a high-normal to mildly elevated PTH. Because affected individuals are asymptomatic and do not develop adverse sequelae from the syndrome, its primary importance is that affected individuals be properly identified and protected from unnecessary parathyroidectomy. Partial or subtotal parathyroidectomy has no effect on these individuals, and total parathyroidectomy causes hypoparathyroidism.

In some patients, two defective alleles of the calcium sensor are inherited. These individuals may have complete inability to sense calcium and therefore develop severe and symptomatic hypercalcemia, with serum calcium values in the 15- to 20-mg/dL range. Because of the severity of this disorder, homozygous individuals usually present in infancy with so-called neonatal severe hyperparathyroidism. In contrast to the mild heterozygous condition described previously, homozygous individuals require urgent total parathyroidectomy in infancy.

Granulomatous Disorders

Almost all granulomatous disorders can lead to hypercalcemia, as noted in Table 74-1. The prototypes are sarcoidosis, TB, and the fungal diseases listed. Briefly, as previously described for lymphomas, granulomas, as with the kidney, have the ability to convert inactive 25-hydroxyvitamin D to the active metabolite, $1,25(OH)_2D$. Thus, individuals with these disorders, when exposed to sunlight, ultraviolet radiation, or relatively trivial quantities of dietary vitamin D, may develop mild to severe hypercalcemia. Examples include sunlight-induced (i.e., summertime) hypercalcemia in patients with sarcoidosis and hypercalcemic flares in patients with TB given dietary supplements with multivitamins after hospitalization. Hypercalcemia results from components of both intestinal calcium hyperabsorption and $1,25(OH)_2D$-induced bone resorption, with the former being the most important in most cases. Because of the hypercalcemia, PTH is suppressed, and serum phosphorus is elevated. The combination of hypercalcemia and hyperphosphatemia may lead to nephrocalcinosis and renal failure. The treatment is a low dietary calcium intake, a low vitamin D intake, limiting sun exposure, hydration and loop diuretics to accelerate calcium clearance, and, if the hypercalcemia is severe, glucocorticoids. Of course, treatment of the underlying granulomatous disorder is the most effective and prudent long-term therapy.

Endocrine Disorders Other than Hyperparathyroidism

In addition to HPT, four other endocrine disorders have been associated with the development of hypercalcemia. One of these disorders is *hyperthyroidism*. As many as 50% of people with hyperthyroidism have been described as having at least mild hypercalcemia. The hypercalcemia is only rarely greater than 11 mg/dL but may be as high as 13 mg/dL. The mechanism is believed to be an increase in osteoclast activation by thyroid hormone. A second disorder is *pheochromocytoma*. Some of these individuals are hypercalcemic as a result of primary HPT occurring as part of the MEN-II syndrome (discussed previously under "Primary and Tertiary Hyperparathyroidism"), but others have been reported to become hypercalcemic as a result of PTHrP secretion by their pheochromocytoma. Severe *hypoadrenalism* with hypotension, so-called addisonian crisis, has been reported to lead to hypercalcemia that responds to volume replacement and glucocorticoids. The mechanism is not known. Finally, islet cell tumors that produce vasoactive intestinal polypeptide (VIP), called *VIPomas*, although rare, are regularly associated with hypercalcemia. VIPomas lead to the watery diarrhea, hypokalemia, achlorhydria (WDHA) syndrome, also referred to as pancreatic cholera.

Medications

Certain medications may cause hypercalcemia. These drugs include thiazide diuretics and lithium, which appear to increase renal tubular calcium reabsorption, and the phosphodiesterase inhibitors aminophylline and theophylline, for which the hypercalcemic mechanism is unknown. Both vitamins D and A and their more active congeners, such as $1,25(OH)_2D$ and *cis*-retinoic acid, respectively, may also cause hypercalcemia. Vitamin D causes hypercalcemia primarily by stimulating intestinal calcium absorption but can also stimulate osteoclastic bone resorption. Vitamin A stimulates bone resorption. The antiviral agent, foscarnet, has been reported to cause hypercalcemia by unknown mechanisms. Finally, estrogens and tamoxifen have been described to cause hypercalcemia in the setting of breast cancer with extensive skeletal metastases, the so-called estrogen flare.

Milk-Alkali Syndrome

The normal intake of calcium is in the range of 600 to 1200 mg per day for most people, and, as reviewed in Chapter 73, absorption of calcium from the diet is tightly controlled. However, ingestion of very large quantities of calcium may overwhelm this system and lead to hypercalcemia. This condition was originally described in the 1940s in patients ingesting enormous quantities of milk, cream, and antacids but is still encountered today with some regularity in patients ingesting large quantities of calcium carbonate or other calcium-containing antacids for peptic disease. In general, for hypercalcemia to occur, calcium intake must exceed 4 g per day and is often in the 10- to 20-g per day range. Severe hypercalcemia is common and may lead to renal failure.

Immobilization

Beginning with the polio epidemic in the 1950s, continuing with space missions in the 1970s, and now most commonly observed in the setting of quadriplegia in young adults or children, immobilization hypercalcemia is common and often severe. Development of the syndrome requires two conditions: essentially *complete immobilization* or weightlessness for a period of at least weeks and occurring on a *background of high bone turnover,* as occurs in young adults or children, mild primary or secondary HPT, Paget disease, and malignant skeletal disease such as breast cancer with bone metastases or multiple myeloma. The basis for the syndrome is that immobilization or weightlessness activates osteoclastic bone resorption and at the same time inhibits osteoblastic activity, producing a severe uncoupling of bone resorption from formation, with rapid and enormous net losses of calcium from the skeleton into the ECF. Left untreated, the condition results in severe demineralization. The syndrome is associated with hypercalciuria as well, and this, together with chronic urinary catheterization, leads to urinary tract infection and severe calcium nephrolithiasis. The most effective treatment for the hypercalcemia is active weight bearing. Hydration and antiresorptive drugs such as the bisphosphonates may be used.

Chronic and Acute Renal Failure

Chronic and acute renal failure has been associated with hypercalcemia. The more common initial abnormality is hypocalcemia induced by a reduction in kidney-derived $1,25(OH)_2D$ and an increase in serum phosphate as a result of diminished glomerular filtration. However, hypercalcemia may occur in patients with chronic renal failure as a result of calcium antacid use or as a result of $1,25(OH)_2D$ or paracalcitol treatment to prevent renal osteodystrophy. Moreover, immobilization in the setting of chronic renal failure—for example, for peritonitis in the setting of peritoneal dialysis—may also lead to hypercalcemia. In the setting of acute renal failure resulting from rhabdomyolysis (crush injury), transient rebound hypercalcemia has been described as renal failure resolves and serum phosphate concentrations decline.

Parenteral Nutrition

Enteric and parenteral nutrition have both been associated with hypercalcemia. Large doses of oral calcium provided in hypercaloric enteric feeding regimens, particularly in the setting of reduced renal function, may lead to what is in essence a form of the milk-alkali syndrome. More mysterious is the well-described hypercalcemic syndrome occurring in patients treated with total parenteral nutrition (TPN). These patients typically have short bowel syndrome and are on long-term TPN. In some patients, the hypercalcemia can be traced to large amounts of calcium, vitamin D, or aluminum in the TPN solution. In other patients, however, these factors do not appear to be operative, and the pathophysiologic mechanisms remain unexplained.

Hyperproteinemia

About 50% of circulating calcium is bound to serum albumin and other proteins. Thus, increases in serum proteins will naturally lead to an increase in total, but not ionized, serum calcium concentrations. This increase is commonly observed in settings of volume depletion and dehydration and may account for the hypercalcemia observed in patients with addisonian crisis described previously under "Hypercalcemia." A more unusual form of this syndrome occurs in patients with myeloma or Waldenström macroglobulinemia, whose abnormal immunoglobulin specifically binds calcium and leads to an increase in total, but not ionized, serum calcium. This scenario, of course, is not the norm in patients with myeloma and hypercalcemia, who have increases in the ionized component of serum calcium. Patients with this syndrome do not display features typical of authentic hypercalcemia: reduced mental status, prolonged QTc interval on electrocardiogram, and hypercalciuria.

End-Stage Liver Disease

Patients with end-stage liver disease awaiting transplantation have been described as being hypercalcemic. The pathophysiologic mechanism underlying this syndrome is not known.

Manganese Intoxication

Manganese intoxication in individuals who drink water from contaminated wells has been described. Again, the pathophysiologic mechanism is not understood.

TREATMENT OF HYPERCALCEMIA

Therapy for hypercalcemia is optimally directed at reversing the underlying pathophysiologic abnormality. Although this principle may seem obvious, it is often overlooked in practice. Thus, reversal of hypercalcemia associated with cancer is most effectively treated over the long term by antineoplastic therapy; correction of hypercalcemia in sarcoidosis is best treated using effective antisarcoid therapy. Seen from this perspective, all other therapies are temporizing, intended to lower calcium while waiting for a response to more definitive therapy. In general, disorders associated with increased intestinal calcium absorption (e.g., sarcoid, milk-alkali syndrome, $1,25[OH]_2D$-secreting lymphomas) are best treated by consuming a low-calcium diet and avoiding vitamin D. Hypercalcemia in the setting of volume depletion and diminished renal function is best treated by expanding the ECF volume and GFR with saline and encouraging diuresis with loop diuretics. Medication-induced hypercalcemia, such as thiazide-induced hypercalcemia, is best treated by discontinuation of the offending medication. Disorders associated with increased osteoclastic bone resorption, such as MAHC and immobilization hypercalcemia, are best treated using inhibitors of bone resorption such as the bisphosphonates, pamidronate or zoledronate. Disorders with multiple abnormalities will require combinations of these measures. Resection of parathyroid tissue in patients with parathyroid disease is effective. A point worth emphasizing is that not everyone requires treatment for hypercalcemia: Patients with mild HPT with borderline serum

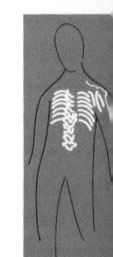

calcium values and without other complications may be observed. Patents with end-stage refractory cancer with severe hypercalcemia may arguably be best served by withholding therapy. Familial hypocalciuric hypercalcemia is best left untreated.

Hypocalcemia

SYMPTOMS AND SIGNS

As described in Chapter 73, hypocalcemia leads to a reduction in the potential difference across cell membranes, which leads to hyperexcitability, particularly of cells of the neuromuscular class. Hence neuromuscular cells spontaneously fire and produce spontaneous seizures, paresthesias, and skeletal muscle contractions (referred to as *carpal spasm*, *pedal spasm*, or *tetany*). Two physical signs are observed on examination: Trousseau sign, which is spontaneous contraction of the forearm muscles in response to application of a blood pressure cuff around the upper arm and inflation to above systolic pressure, and Chvostek sign, which is twitching of the facial muscles with gentle tapping of the facial nerve as it exits the parotid gland. An electrocardiographic sign is a prolonged QTc interval. Rarely, severe hypocalcemia has been reported to cause hypocontractility of the myocardium and congestive heart failure because calcium is required for muscle contraction. Finally, prolonged hypoparathyroidism may be associated with basal ganglia calcification, which is asymptomatic but impressive on computed tomography scans and plain x-ray films of the skull.

PATHOPHYSIOLOGY

Hypocalcemia may result from five general mechanisms: (1) a reduction in serum binding proteins (albumin), (2) an increase in serum phosphate with a resultant increase in the calcium-phosphate solubility product, (3) an increase in renal calcium excretion, (4) a reduction in intestinal calcium absorption, or (5) a loss of calcium from the ECF into the skeleton. The reader is referred to Chapter 73 for more details regarding normal calcium homeostasis. In practice, several of these factors are operative in several disorders. For example, in hypoparathyroidism, a reduction in intestinal calcium absorption combines with an inability to reabsorb calcium from the distal tubule to cause hypocalcemia; or, in breast cancer with extensive osteoblastic metastases, increases in osteoblast activity remove calcium from the ECF, and anorexia leads to a reduction in intestinal calcium intake. From a diagnostic perspective, understanding pathophysiologic mechanisms is important because the clinical setting and routine biochemistry analyses will help include or exclude certain diagnoses. From a therapeutic standpoint, this knowledge is important as well because effective therapy requires that the underlying disorder be appropriately managed. Thus, giving oral vitamin D supplements to a patient with sprue may not be effective unless the underlying malabsorption is treated; parenteral vitamin D may be more effective.

DIFFERENTIAL DIAGNOSIS

The disorders that may lead to hypocalcemia are summarized here and in Table 74-2.

Table 74-2 Differential Diagnosis of Hypocalcemia

Hypoparathyroidism

Surgical
Idiopathic and autoimmune
Infiltrative diseases
Wilson disease (copper)
Hemochromatosis
Sarcoidosis
Metastatic (breast) cancer
Congenital
Isolated, sporadic
DiGeorge syndrome
Infant of mother with hyperparathyroidism
Hereditary
X-linked
Parathyroid gland calcium receptor–activating mutations
PTH signal peptide mutation
GCMB mutation

Pseudohypoparathyroidism

Type Ia—multiple hormone resistance, Albright hereditary
  osteodystrophy
Type Ib—PTH resistance without other abnormalities
Type Ic—specific PTH resistance, resulting from defect in
  catalytic subunit of PTH-receptor complex
Type II—specific PTH resistance, postreceptor–adenylyl
  cyclase defect, undefined

Vitamin D Disorders

Absent ultraviolet exposure
Vitamin D deficiency
Fat malabsorption
Vitamin D–dependent rickets, renal 1-α-hydroxylase
  deficiency, 1,25-dihydroxyvitamin D–receptor defects
Chronic renal failure
Hepatic failure

Hypoalbuminemia

Sepsis

Hypermagnesemia and Hypomagnesemia

Rapid Bone Formation

Hungry bone syndrome after parathyroidectomy or
  thyroidectomy
Osteoblastic metastases
Vitamin D therapy of osteomalacia, rickets

Hyperphosphatemia

Crush injury, rhabdomyolysis
Renal failure
Tumor lysis
Excessive PO_4 administration (PO, IV, PR)

Medications

Mithramycin, plicamycin
Bisphosphonates
Calcitonin
Fluoride
EDTA
Citrate
Intravenous contrast
Foscarnet

Pancreatitis

Hypoalbuminemia
Hypomagnesemia
Calcium soap formation

EDTA, ethylenediaminetetraacetic acid; IV, intravenous; PO, by mouth; PO_4, phosphate; PR, per rectum; PTH, parathyroid hormone.

Hypoparathyroidism

Hypoparathyroidism causes hypocalcemia as a result of a decrease in intestinal calcium absorption (a result of low circulating 1,25[OH]$_2$D concentrations, which are a result of low circulating PTH), combined with reduced renal calcium reabsorption in the distal tubule (as a result of decreased circulating PTH). Hypoparathyroidism may be idiopathic or autoimmune, occurring either in isolation or as part of the polyglandular failure syndrome in association with Graves hyperthyroidism, Hashimoto thyroiditis, Addison disease, type 1 diabetes, vitiligo, mucocutaneous candidiasis, and other autoimmune disorders. Hypoparathyroidism may also be commonly encountered as surgical hypoparathyroidism in patients who have undergone thyroid, parathyroid, or laryngeal surgery for multinodular goiter or Graves disease, for parathyroid hyperplasia, or for carcinoma of the larynx or esophagus. Surgical and autoimmune hypoparathyroidism together account for most patients with hypoparathyroidism. Less common causes include congenital hypoparathyroidism caused by DiGeorge syndrome, isolated parathyroid failure, or activating mutations in the calcium receptor gene (autosomal dominant hypoparathyroidism), the PTH gene, or the glial cell missing-B *(GCMB)* gene. Finally, rarely, tissue infiltrative diseases such as breast cancer, Wilson disease (copper deposition), hemochromatosis (iron deposition), or sarcoidosis may destroy or replace normal parathyroid tissue.

The diagnosis is made by finding a low serum ionized calcium level in a patient with an inappropriately reduced serum PTH concentration. In general, the phosphorus concentration is high normal or frankly elevated, and plasma 1,25(OH)$_2$D concentrations are reduced (see Chapter 73 for the underlying physiologic factors).

One potential treatment for hypoparathyroidism is subcutaneous injection of PTH. Although this treatment has been accomplished successfully in clinical trials, PTH is not approved for this indication. Thus, treatment is normally directed at increasing intestinal calcium absorption through the use of large doses of calcium (about 2000 mg per day) and the active form of vitamin D, 1,25(OH)$_2$D, in normal replacement amounts (0.25 to 1.0 μg per day). The goal is to induce sufficient intestinal calcium hyperabsorption to overwhelm the ability of the kidney to excrete it. Although this method is the only tenable therapy, it carries the risk for inducing significant hypercalciuria and therefore nephrocalcinosis and nephrolithiasis. Accordingly, 24-hour urinary calcium must be measured regularly, and hypercalciuria minimized, which generally means maintaining the serum calcium in the low-normal range, about 8.5 to 9.0 mg/dL. In some instances, calcium and vitamin D alone may be ineffective or may induce severe hypercalciuria. In such cases, addition of a thiazide diuretic such as hydrochlorothiazide, which stimulates renal calcium reabsorption, may be effective in preventing hypercalciuria and at the same time raising the serum calcium.

Pseudohypoparathyroidism

Pseudohypoparathyroidism refers to a group of disorders that have in common resistance to the actions of PTH. In most cases, the resistance is due to different types of inactivating mutations in the signal-transducing protein Gs-α. Patients may be resistant only to PTH, or they may be resistant to multiple peptide hormones, including thyroid-stimulating hormone (with hypothyroidism) and follicle-stimulating hormone and luteinizing hormone (with hypogonadism). The most common form of the syndrome, type Ia, is associated with multiple hormone resistance and a phenotype referred to as *Albright hereditary osteodystrophy*, which includes short stature, shortened fourth and fifth metacarpals and metatarsals, obesity, mental retardation, subcutaneous calcifications, and café-au-lait spots. Because the disorder is hereditary, a clear family history of this phenotype is often present, as well as a family history of hypocalcemia or seizures.

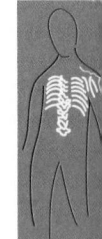

Biochemically, these patients resemble those with hypoparathyroidism; they are hypocalcemic and have hyperphosphatemia. The diagnosis is made by the finding of an elevated circulating PTH in a patient with hypocalcemia and hyperphosphatemia in whom other causes of hypocalcemia and secondary hypoparathyroidism have been excluded. The diagnosis can be confirmed by infusing PTH and failing to observe the normal phosphaturic, cyclic adenosine monophosphate, and calcemic responses.

The treatment is similar to that of hypoparathyroidism.

Vitamin D Disorders

Active vitamin D, 1,25(OH)$_2$D, is required to absorb calcium from the intestine. Activation of vitamin D requires adequate exposure to vitamin D from diet or by sunlight exposure, an intact intestine through which to absorb calcium and vitamin D, an intact liver with which to convert vitamin D to 25-hydroxyvitamin D, and an intact kidney to convert 25-hydroxyvitamin D to 1,25(OH)$_2$D (see Chapter 73). Therefore, developing hypocalcemia and osteomalacia or rickets (see Chapter 75) in settings in which one or more of these steps is disrupted is common. Specifically, malabsorption syndromes, such as short bowel syndrome and celiac sprue, lead to hypocalcemia as a result of calcium and vitamin D malabsorption. Chronic liver diseases, particularly primary biliary cirrhosis, lead to hypocalcemia and osteomalacia. Chronic renal insufficiency leads to failure to produce 1,25(OH)$_2$D, with reductions in serum calcium and inefficient absorption of intestinal calcium. Normal diets contain little in the way of vitamin D. Although Western diets are supplemented with vitamin D in milk and multivitamins, diets composed of no milk, human milk, or unsupplemented bovine milk are vitamin D deficient. Relatively trivial exposure to sunlight can provide ample vitamin D and replace dietary needs for vitamin D. However, in settings in which both sun exposure and dietary intake of vitamin D are poor (cloudy climates, excessive clothing or body covering, prolonged nursing in infants, and the standard *tea and toast* diet of older adults), vitamin D deficiency is the rule rather than the exception.

Certain genetic syndromes occur in which the enzyme vitamin D 1-α-hydroxylase is mutated (vitamin D–dependent rickets type I) or in which the vitamin D receptor is mutated (vitamin D–dependent rickets type II). Affected individuals have severe hypocalcemia, alopecia, severe rickets, and dental abnormalities, and are easy to recognize and confirm if the diagnosis is considered.

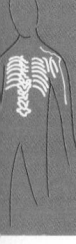

Finally, long-term, high-dose treatment with anticonvulsants such as phenytoin or phenobarbital or their derivatives may lead to hypocalcemia and osteomalacia.

Hypoalbuminemia

Reductions in serum albumin, as occur in burn patients, the nephrotic syndrome, malnutrition, and cirrhosis, lead to reductions in serum total calcium without a reduction in the ionized serum calcium. Of course, these disorders may also be associated with other conditions that lead to bona fide reductions in the ionized serum calcium as well. Several formulas exist for correcting total calcium for albumin, but none is entirely accurate. Therefore, measuring ionized calcium directly is important if the authentic ionized serum calcium concentration level is needed.

Sepsis

Gram-positive and gram-negative sepsis has been associated with hypocalcemia that is generally mild. The mechanisms are poorly understood. Hypocalcemia occurring in the setting of sepsis appears to confer a particularly adverse prognosis.

Hypermagnesemia

Magnesium is a divalent cation, as is calcium, and in very high concentrations may therefore mimic the actions of calcium to suppress PTH and, in so doing, lead to a functional type of hypoparathyroidism and hypocalcemia. In practice, this condition is uncommon and is seen typically in patents with severe hypermagnesemia (serum magnesium concentrations in the 10-mg/dL range) caused by renal failure accompanied by magnesium antacid ingestion or following the treatment of eclampsia with large doses of intravenous magnesium.

Hypomagnesemia

Hypomagnesemia is one of the most common causes of hypocalcemia. It is encountered often in patients with alcoholism, malnutrition, cisplatin therapy for cancer, and intestinal malabsorption syndromes. Hypomagnesemia both inhibits PTH secretion (a magnesium adenosine triphosphatase is required for PTH secretion) and prevents the calcemic actions of PTH on the kidney and skeleton. Thus, magnesium deficiency causes a functional form of hypoparathyroidism as well as resistance to PTH. The treatment is straightforward: magnesium replacement (see "Hypomagnesemia," later). This treatment corrects the syndrome in minutes to hours. The clinical reality, however, is that this common syndrome is often overlooked and mistreated with intravenous calcium or vitamin D, which are unnecessary and, unless the hypomagnesemia is corrected, ineffective.

Rapid Bone Formation

Increased rates of bone mineralization, out of proportion to the rate of bone resorption, will lead to net calcium entry into the skeleton and, if these rates are large, hypocalcemia. This state occurs in several clinical settings. One condition is the *hungry bone* syndrome that may follow parathyroidectomy. In this syndrome, a patient, usually with severe primary or secondary HPT, undergoes parathyroidectomy. Preoperatively, the rates of bone turnover, both resorption and formation, are very high but are approximately coupled.

Postoperatively, the rate of osteoclastic bone resorption abruptly declines with the decline in PTH, but the elevated rate of mineralization of previously formed osteoid remains the same as it was preoperatively for days to a week or more (see Chapter 73 for mechanisms). Because of this acute postoperative imbalance, the skeleton becomes a *sink* for calcium, and hypocalcemia ensues. Another example of this phenomenon may occur in patients with vitamin D deficiency who have severe osteomalacia or rickets and large amounts of unmineralized osteoid. When these patients are treated with vitamin D, rapid mineralization of unmineralized osteoid occurs, and, again, the skeleton becomes a *sink* for calcium, and hypocalcemia ensues. A final example of rapid bone formation leading to hypocalcemia occurs in the setting of extensive osteoblastic bone metastases, as may occur in prostate cancer or breast cancer and occasionally other types of malignancy.

Hyperphosphatemia

Disorders that lead to hyperphosphatemia (see the later section on "Hyperphosphatemia") may cause hypocalcemia as a result of exceeding the calcium-phosphate solubility product in serum. Examples of disorders that may cause the kind of severe hyperphosphatemia required include rhabdomyolysis (from crush injuries), renal failure, and the tumor lysis syndrome. Severe hyperphosphatemia may also be seen following the ingestion of large amounts of phosphate-containing purgatives in preparation for colonoscopy, by the inadvertent perforation of the rectum during the administration of phosphate enemas, and with overzealous administration of intravenous phosphate. In all these examples, the onset of hyperphosphatemia is relatively abrupt, and the hypocalcemia is immediate and severe. Commonly, the first sign of this sequence of events is a seizure. The treatment involves reducing the serum phosphorus by whatever means necessary. Giving intravenous calcium should be avoided because it will simply be precipitated into soft tissues.

Medications

Certain medications may cause hypocalcemia, including those used to treat hypercalcemia, such as mithramycin (plicamycin), the bisphosphonates (e.g., pamidronate, zoledronate), and calcitonin. Hypocalcemia induced by these agents is rare but has been reported. Fluoride intoxication from ingestion of sodium fluoride, inhalation of fluoride-containing anesthetic gases, or drinking of fluoride-contaminated water may cause hypocalcemia. Ethylenediaminetetraacetic acid is a calcium chelator that causes hypocalcemia if infused intravenously. Citrate, as is used in citrated blood for transfusion, is also a calcium chelator and may cause hypocalcemia in the setting of large-volume transfusions. Radiographic intravenous contrast agents may also cause hypocalcemia, as may the antiviral drug foscarnet.

Pancreatitis

Pancreatitis commonly causes hypocalcemia. The classic mechanism is the formation of calcium–free fatty acid soaps, according to the following scenario. Pancreatitis occurs and releases lipase into the retroperitoneum and peritoneum, which leads to the autodigestion of retroperitoneal and omental fat. This action releases free fatty acids such as palmitate, linoleate, and stearate from triglyceride fat stores, and these negatively charged ions tightly bind (chelate) calcium in ECF. This binding leads to the formation of insoluble calcium–free fatty acid salts in the retroperitoneum and rapidly depletes the extracellular calcium, causing hypocalcemia. The hypocalcemia is reversible by calcium infusion and will self-terminate when the pancreatitis improves. Hypocalcemia is a poor prognostic sign among patients with pancreatitis. An important point to remember is that other causes of hypocalcemia occur in patients with pancreatitis, including hypoalbuminemia, hypomagnesemia, and vitamin D deficiency, and these causes should be specifically excluded.

Hyperphosphatemia

SYMPTOMS AND SIGNS

Hyperphosphatemia produces no specific signs per se. It is usually identified incidentally on routine chemical screens or as a result of the induction of hypocalcemia, as described in the preceding section.

PATHOPHYSIOLOGY

Hyperphosphatemia develops as a result of two general mechanisms. One mechanism is a large load of phosphate into the ECF, delivered through the GI tract, intravenous medications, or endogenous sources such as muscle or tumor. The second mechanism is the inability to excrete phosphate, as occurs in renal failure (acute or chronic). As noted in Chapter 73, essentially all natural foods contain phosphate, and therefore almost any diet will contain substantial quantities of phosphate. Normally, this phosphate is easily cleared by the healthy kidney, but this ability is lost as the GFR declines below about 20 to 30 mg/dL.

DIFFERENTIAL DIAGNOSIS

Differential diagnosis of hyperphosphatemia is listed here and in Table 74-3.

Table 74-3 **Causes of Hyperphosphatemia**
Artifactual
Hemolysis
Increased Gastrointestinal Intake
Rectal enemas
Oral Phospho-Soda purgatives
Gastrointestinal bleeding
Intravenous Phosphate Loads
K-Phos
Blood transfusions
Endogenous Phosphate Loads
Tumor lysis syndrome
Rhabdomyolysis (crush injury)
Hemolysis
Reduced Renal Clearance
Chronic or acute renal failure
Hypoparathyroidism
Acromegaly
Tumoral calcinosis

Artifactual

Hyperphosphatemia may occur artifactually as a result of hemolysis in blood collection tubes. Erythrocytes, as with all cells, are rich in phosphate, and, if they are allowed to remain for prolonged periods at room temperature or if blood is obtained too rapidly or through too narrow a needle, they will lyse and release their contents into serum, which will then be reported as being hyperphosphatemic. One clue is that the same phenomenon occurs with potassium. Thus, the occurrence of unexplained hyperkalemia and hyperphosphatemia should trigger the collection of a fresh sample and immediate repeat determination of serum phosphate.

Increased Gastrointestinal Intake

Hyperphosphatemia may occur in patients receiving large oral phosphate loads. In a recent literature review, most cases of phosphate-induced hypocalcemia were caused by the administration of phosphate-containing purgatives as preparation for colonoscopy. Another underappreciated cause of this phenomenon is the inadvertent perforation of the rectum during the administration of a rectal Phospho-Soda enema, with delivery of large amounts of phosphate directly into the peritoneal cavity, from which it is rapidly absorbed. Finally, upper GI tract bleeding from ulcers of gastritis provides a large GI phosphate load and may be associated with hyperphosphatemia.

Intravenous Phosphate Loads

Large amounts of phosphate may be administered as part of a means to replete potassium using potassium phosphate preparations. What appear to be trivial quantities of potassium preparation (e.g., 20 to 40 mEq of K-Phos) actually contain large amounts of phosphate and may lead to severe hyperphosphatemia and hypocalcemia (see Chapter 73). A second vehicle for delivering phosphate intravenously is transfusions of red blood cells, which ultimately hemolyze and release their copious phosphate stores.

Endogenous Phosphate Loads

Hyperphosphatemia may result from the destruction of large amounts of tissue. This destruction is encountered in three situations. Tumor lysis syndrome is one such situation, typified by a large Burkitt lymphoma responding promptly to chemotherapy with massive cell death. A second phenomenon is acute rhabdomyolysis resulting from a crush injury or drug overdose, which leads to massive release of phosphate from within skeletal muscle cells. A third example is severe hemolysis resulting from autoimmune causes or blood group mismatch. In each of these cases, a large phosphate load is delivered into the ECF, and, in addition, other nephrotoxic molecules such as hemoglobin, myoglobin, and uric acid are released, which reduces the ability of the kidney to clear the large phosphate load. This combination is potentially lethal, resulting in renal failure, severe hypocalcemia, seizures, and sometimes death.

Reduced Renal Clearance

As noted in Chapter 73, renal clearance of phosphate is the main mechanism for maintaining phosphate homeostasis. Thus, the fact that disorders of the kidney lead to hyperphosphatemia is not surprising. These disorders include

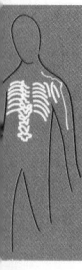

both acute and chronic forms of renal failure. In addition, functional renal abnormalities occur that may lead to hyperphosphatemia. First, because PTH prevents phosphate reabsorption in the proximal nephron, hypoparathyroidism is typically associated with high-normal to frankly elevated serum phosphorus values. Second, acromegaly is associated with hyperphosphatemia. The mechanisms for this association are not well understood, but it appears to be renal in origin. A condition called *tumoral calcinosis*, in which the ability of the kidney to clear phosphate is specifically defective, leads to chronic hyperphosphatemia and accumulation of calcium-phosphate salts around large joints of the appendicular skeleton. Recently, this syndrome has been shown to be due to inactivating mutations in the *FGF-23* or *GALNT3* genes. Finally, children, particularly adolescents, have higher serum phosphate concentrations than adults.

Hypophosphatemia
SYMPTOMS AND SIGNS

As noted in Chapter 73, phosphate participates in a vast array of key cellular processes, from DNA synthesis and replication, to energy generation and use, to oxygen uptake and delivery by erythrocytes, to maintaining the redox state of every cell in the body. The signs of phosphate depletion are therefore nonspecific, diffuse, and often life threatening. These signs may include respirator dependence, congestive heart failure, coma, hypotension, and generalized weakness and malaise. Because the signs and symptoms are so nonspecific, they are frequently attributed to other causes and are left untreated. They typically occur in intensive care unit (ICU) settings, in which oral nutrition is nonexistent and intravenous phosphate repletion inadequate and in which diuretics and saline infusion accelerate renal phosphate losses. Appropriate therapy can produce startling results, with patients suddenly returning from being moribund to being ambulatory, extubated, and conversant.

Chronic hypophosphatemia leads to defects in skeletal mineralization, a phenomenon called *rickets* in children or *osteomalacia* in adults. These syndromes produce weakness, bone pain, bowing of the long bones, and fractures or pseudofractures (see Chapter 75).

DIFFERENTIAL DIAGNOSIS

Disorders can be divided into hypophosphatemia resulting from inadequate intake, from excessive renal losses, from excessive skeletal uptake, or from shifts of phosphate from the ECF into cells (Table 74-4). These abnormalities are discussed individually later. From a diagnostic standpoint, measuring the TmP, as described in Chapter 73, is important because it provides rapid determination of which class of hypophosphatemia the patient is confronting.

Inadequate Phosphate Intake

Disorders that involve inadequate phosphate intake are associated with a high TmP. Because essentially all foods are rich in phosphate, becoming phosphate depleted based on inadequate dietary intake is difficult. However, in settings of severe caloric deprivation, inadequacies can occur. Examples include anorexia nervosa, prisoner-of-war camps, prolonged

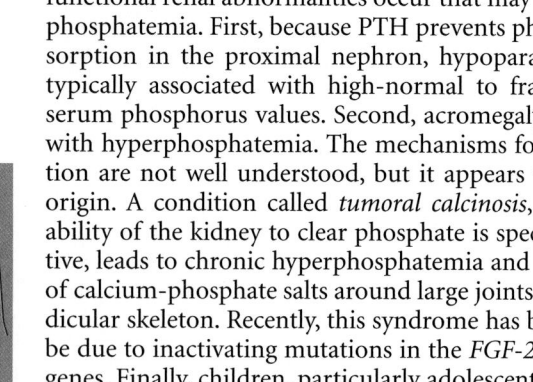

Table 74-4 **Causes of Hypophosphatemia**

Inadequate PO$_4$ Intake
Starvation
Malabsorption
PO$_4$-binding antacid use
Alcoholism

Renal PO$_4$ Losses
Primary, secondary, or tertiary hyperparathyroidism
Humoral hypercalcemia of malignancy (parathyroid hormone–related protein)
Diuretics, calcitonin
X-linked hypophosphatemic rickets
Autosomal dominant hypophosphatemic rickets
Oncogenic osteomalacia
Fanconi syndrome
Alcoholism

Excessive Skeletal Mineralization
Hungry bone syndrome after parathyroidectomy
Osteoblastic metastases
Healing osteomalacia, rickets

PO$_4$ Shifts into Extracellular Fluid
Recovery from metabolic acidosis
Respiratory alkalosis
Starvation refeeding, intravenous glucose

PO$_4$, phosphate.

ICU care, malabsorption syndromes, and chronic alcoholism. In the first three disorders, caloric intake is scant, and therefore little phosphate is consumed. In alcoholism, caloric intake may be high, but alcohol is devoid of phosphate. Finally, the use of phosphate-binding antacids such as aluminum hydroxide gels may lead to severe phosphate deficiency, hypophosphatemia, and osteomalacia.

Excessive Renal Phosphate Losses

Disorders involving excessive losses are associated with a low TmP. PTH is phosphaturic, and therefore all types of HPT are associated with hypophosphatemia, as long as renal function is normal. This state is widely appreciated for primary HPT but is less well appreciated for secondary HPT, particularly occurring in the setting of vitamin D and calcium malabsorption. Indeed, a low serum phosphate may be the first and only noticeable clue to severe vitamin D deficiency. In my experience, this fact has led to the diagnosis of celiac sprue in unsuspected cases on many occasions.

PTH-related protein (PTHrP, see earlier section on "Malignancy-Associated Hypercalcemia") is also phosphaturic, as is PTH, and patients with humoral hypercalcemia of malignancy are commonly hypophosphatemic for this reason, as long as their renal function is intact. They frequently become more hypophosphatemic during hospitalization as a result of saline infusion, diuretics, and inadequate oral or intravenous phosphate nutrition.

Medications such as calcitonin, as well as thiazide and loop diuretics, are potent phosphaturic agents, and their use without phosphate replacement therapy will lead to hypophosphatemia. Ethanol is also in this category.

Certain genetic disorders may lead to severe renal phosphate wasting (see Chapter 75). These disorders include X-linked hypophosphatemia (XLH), also referred to as *vitamin D–resistant rickets*, and autosomal dominant hypophosphatemic rickets (ADHR). In ADHR, the disorder appears to be due to the overproduction of fibroblast growth factor-23 (FGF-23), one of the long-sought *phosphatonins* (see Chapter 73), and, in XLH, the cause is an inactivating mutation in the *PHEX* gene, which encodes an extracellular protease. Another renal phosphate-wasting syndrome is oncogenic osteomalacia, also referred to as *tumor-induced osteomalacia*. Now appreciated is that this disorder, as in ADHR, is due to overproduction by small, often occult, mesenchymal tumors such as hemangiopericytomas of FGF-23, secreted frizzled-related protein 4 (sFRP4), or matrix extracellular phosphoglycoprotein (MEPE) (see Chapter 73).

Acquired or inherited diffuse renal proximal tubular disorders, such as Fanconi syndrome, may lead to hypophosphatemia as a result of renal phosphate wasting.

Excessive Skeletal Mineralization

In metabolic situations under which the rate of bone formation, or more specifically bone mineralization, is increased with respect to the rate of bone resorption by osteoclasts, large amounts of phosphate may enter the skeleton, leading to hypophosphatemia. One example is the hungry bone syndrome that occurs following parathyroidectomy, as described in the previous section on "Hypocalcemia." Other examples are osteoblastic metastases and the treatment of vitamin D–deficient rickets of osteomalacia with vitamin D (see the previous section on "Hypocalcemia" for additional details). In each of these settings, phosphate enters the mineralizing phase of osteoid as calcium phosphate (hydroxyapatite) and does so at rates such that hypophosphatemia ensues.

Phosphate Shifts into Extracellular Fluid

Phosphate can be shifted from serum into the intracellular compartment by a rise in ECF pH from low to normal or from normal to high. Thus, recovery from a metabolic acidosis, such as diabetic ketoacidosis, and the development of a respiratory alkalosis both lead to hypophosphatemia. One of the most stunning examples of this phenomenon is the shift of phosphate into cells following the administration of oral carbohydrate or parenteral glucose to victims of starvation or anorexia nervosa. Insulin increases the rate of glucose uptake into cells and its subsequent phosphorylation to glucose 6-phosphate. A person with no phosphate reserves so treated will abruptly become more severely hypophosphatemic and may die suddenly of respiratory or circulatory failure. Hence, refeeding of starvation victims should be accomplished slowly and with attention to phosphate repletion.

TREATMENT

Phosphorus replacement is best accomplished through the oral route and is generally given in divided doses 2 to 4 times per day in the range of 2000 to 4000 g per day. Doses above 1000 to 2000 mg per day will often cause diarrhea initially (phosphate is used as a purgative), but, with gradual increments, larger doses may be well tolerated. Intravenous phosphate should only be given with a clear understanding of the quantities involved (see Chapter 73) and in patients in whom oral administration is not an option. Frequent monitoring of serum phosphorus, calcium, and creatinine are

Table 74-5 **Causes of Hypermagnesemia and Hypomagnesemia**
Hypermagnesemia
Renal failure accompanied by magnesium antacid use
Parenteral magnesium sulfate administration for eclampsia
Hypomagnesemia
Inadequate intake
Starvation
Malabsorption
Alcoholism
Vomiting, nasogastric suction
Excessive renal losses
Diuretics
Saline infusion
Secondary aldosteronism
Cirrhosis
Congestive heart failure
Osmotic diuresis, hyperglycemia
Cisplatin, aminoglycoside antibiotics, amphotericin
Hypokalemia
Hypercalcemia, hypercalciuria
Proximal tubular diseases
Genetic defects

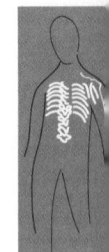

required. Doses up to 500 to 800 mg per day intravenously may be required.

Hypermagnesemia
SYMPTOMS AND SIGNS

Clinically significant hypermagnesemia is uncommon. The symptoms are drowsiness, and the signs are hyporeflexia and eventually neuromuscular, respiratory, and cardiovascular collapse. It may also lead to hypocalcemia (see the previous section on "Hypocalcemia"). Hypermagnesemia is seen in essentially two settings: (1) severe renal failure accompanied by the administration of magnesium-containing antacids, and (2) following the intravenous administration of large doses of magnesium sulfate for eclampsia or preeclampsia.

DIFFERENTIAL DIAGNOSIS

The differential diagnosis of hypermagnesemia is brief and is limited to the two disorders noted previously (Table 74-5). Mild hypermagnesemia is common in patients on dialysis, but severe hypermagnesemia is less common in renal failure and occurs in the settings of renal failure accompanied by parenteral or oral magnesium salt administration, such as the use of magnesium-containing antacids or phosphate binders. Hypermagnesemia still occurs commonly, but in a controlled fashion, in the treatment of eclampsia, wherein obstetricians administer large doses of intravenous magnesium sulfate, while observing the blood pressure and reflexes, to pregnant women with eclampsia. Indeed, a therapeutic endpoint is when the reflexes diminish or disappear.

Hypomagnesemia
SYMPTOMS AND SIGNS

Hypomagnesemia is common but, as with hypophosphatemia, is often overlooked or ignored. Magnesium is essential

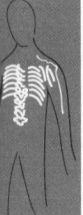

for a broad range of biologic processes, and thus hypomagnesemia may cause a broad array of systemic abnormalities (see Chapter 73 for details). Hypomagnesemia may cause hypocalcemia, seizures, and paresthesias independent of hypocalcemia and may cause a broad array of neuromuscular, cardiovascular, or respiratory symptoms. Commonly, hypomagnesemia occurs in an ICU setting in which magnesium administration and diet are inadequate, magnesuric intravenous saline is administered along with diuretics, and serum magnesium is never measured. It responds rapidly and dramatically to parenteral magnesium replacement.

DIFFERENTIAL DIAGNOSIS

Differential diagnoses are listed here and in Table 74-5.

Inadequate Intake

Inadequate intake of magnesium is common among alcoholics and the generally undernourished. It may occur as part of an intestinal malabsorption syndrome and may result from continuous vomiting or nasogastric suctioning. Again, these situations are all common in ICU settings and are often overlooked.

Excessive Renal Losses

Excessive renal losses of magnesium are also common in clinical practice; thiazide and loop diuretics both cause renal magnesium losses, and saline infusion has a similar effect. Magnesium is also lost by the kidney in response to aldosterone in primary hyperaldosteronism but more commonly in the secondary hyperaldosteronism associated with cirrhosis, volume depletion, congestive heart failure, and other common disorders. Osmotic diuresis, as occurs, for example, with poorly controlled diabetes mellitus, causes renal magnesium loss. Certain nephrotoxic drugs such as cisplatin, aminoglycoside antibiotics, and amphotericin induce proximal tubular injury and a severe form of renal magnesium wasting. Hypokalemia may lead to magnesium wasting by the kidney, and the reverse is true as well. Hypercalcemia and hypercalciuria lead to renal magnesium excretion as well, although the cellular basis for this excretion is not fully understood. Genetic or inherited causes of renal magnesium wasting such as mutations in the paracellin-1 gene also occur but are rare. Finally, many diseases that lead to proximal tubular injury, such as Fanconi syndrome and interstitial nephritis, may lead to magnesium wasting.

TREATMENT

Magnesium can be replaced intramuscularly or intravenously. In general, 24 to 48 mEq per 24 hours as magnesium sulfate is provided (see Chapter 73 for unit conversion). Oral magnesium salts such as magnesium oxide are also available, but administering large doses of magnesium orally is difficult because of the cathartic effects of magnesium.

Prospectus for the Future

As is the case with normal mineral and bone physiology, much remains to be learned regarding disorders of serum minerals. What are the genetic defects that underlie most parathyroid adenomas? What additional disease of the calcium-sensing receptor remains to be defined? Will novel calcium receptor agonists and antagonists be useful to better repress or stimulate PTH secretion on primary and secondary hyperparathyroidism and hypoparathyroidism? Can we develop a long-term regimen for treating hypoparathyroidism that does not result in hypercalciuria, kidney stones, nephrocalcinosis, and renal failure over time? What will prove to be the most clinically effective and cost-effective agents in treating hypercalcemia of malignancy: the current round of intravenous bisphosphonates or monoclonal antibodies being developed against osteoclasts or their developmental pathways? Finally, what are the real *phosphatonins,* how do they work, and how can we best diagnose and treat rickets and osteomalacia resulting from renal phosphorus losses in disorders such as XLH? These questions and many more will occupy researchers in this area for decades to come.

References

DeGroot L, Jameson LJ (eds): Endocrinology, 5th ed. Philadelphia, WB Saunders, 2006.

Favus MF (ed): The American Society for Bone and Mineral Research Primer on Metabolic Bone Diseases and Disorders of Mineral Metabolism, 6th ed. Washington DC, American Society for Bone and Mineral Research, 2006.

Ichikawa S, Lyles KW, Econs MJ: A novel GALNT3 mutation in a pseudoautosomal dominant form of tumoral calcinosis: Evidence that the disorder is autosomal recessive. J Clin Endocrinol Metab 90:2469-2471, 2005.

Nazeri ASA, Reilly RF: Hereditary etiologies of hypomagnesemia. Nat Clin Pract Nephrol 4:80-89, 2008.

Silverberg SJ, Bilezikian JP: The diagnosis and management of asymptomatic primary hyperparathyroidism. Nat Clin Pract Endocrinol 2:494-503, 2006.

Stewart AF: Hypercalcemia associated with cancer. N Engl J Med 352:373-379, 2005.

Stewart AF: Translational Implications of the parathyroid calcium receptor. N Engl J Med 351:324-326, 2004.

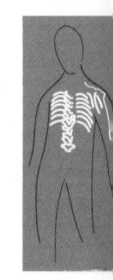

Metabolic Bone Diseases

Shane O. LeBeau and Andrew F. Stewart

Metabolic bone disease is a term used to describe a host of skeletal diseases (Table 75-1). Most of these disorders are associated with low bone mass, but some, such as the osteosclerotic and osteopetrotic disorders, are not. In a sense, the term is misleading because many of these disorders are not *metabolic* at all; rather, they have genetic, viral, or other causes. Still, *metabolic bone disease* is useful as an umbrella term for all diffuse skeletal disorders. The term in its broadest sense also includes osteoporosis and Paget disease of bone, which are discussed in Chapters 76 and 77, respectively. The term also includes osteosclerotic disorders such as fluoride intoxication and genetic disorders that lead to osteopetrosis. It may also include focal skeletal diseases such as polyostotic fibrous dysplasia. In general, these are rare diseases. In this chapter, the focus is on the other common members of this family, as listed in Table 75-1, that might be encountered by an internist. To be sure, many additional rare "metabolic" bone diseases exist and, depending on the context, should be sought. Perhaps the most important message to be gleaned from this chapter, in this era of widespread access to bone density measurements using dual-energy x-ray absorptiometry (DXA), is the concept that low bone mass identified by DXA is not equivalent to a diagnosis of osteoporosis (see Chapter 76). This concept is not broadly appreciated among internists or even among radiologists who may perform DXA measurements. For example, DXA cannot determine whether a patient has low bone mass as a result of osteoporosis, as opposed to osteomalacia or multiple myeloma, yet commonly, DXA reports refer to *osteoporosis*. Every patient assigned a diagnosis of osteoporosis by DXA warrants full consideration for one of the other diagnoses in Table 75-1. Thus, the primary physician must determine whether a patient with a low bone mass revealed by DXA actually has *osteoporosis* or might actually have a distinct metabolic bone disease.

Differential Diagnosis

HYPERPARATHYROID BONE DISEASE (OSTEITIS FIBROSA CYSTICA)

Hyperparathyroid bone disease, or osteitis fibrosa cystica (OFC), results from chronically elevated parathyroid hormone (PTH) concentrations. Elevated PTH concentrations, in turn, may result from primary hyperparathyroidism that is due, for example, to a parathyroid adenoma, carcinoma, or hyperplasia; to secondary hyperparathyroidism caused by malabsorption, vitamin D deficiency, or chronic renal failure; or to tertiary hyperparathyroidism in the setting of renal failure (see Chapter 74 for details). Patients with primary and tertiary hyperparathyroidism are characterized by hypercalcemia, whereas those with secondary hyperparathyroidism by definition are eucalcemic or hypocalcemic. PTH elevations are commonly severe.

Patients may complain of bone pain or diffuse aches and pains. The skeletal disease is characterized by *high turnover*, meaning coupled increases in both osteoclastic bone resorption and osteoblastic synthesis of osteoid and accelerated rates of bone mineralization (Fig. 75-1). Markers of bone

Table 75-1 **Metabolic Bone Disease**
Osteoporosis (see Chapter 76)
Paget Disease of Bone (see Chapter 77)
Hyperparathyroid Bone Disease (Osteitis Fibrosa Cystica)
Osteomalacia and Rickets
Hypophosphatemic syndromes Vitamin D syndromes Anticonvulsants Aluminum Metabolic acidosis
Renal Osteodystrophy
Genetic Diseases
Osteogenesis imperfecta Hypophosphatasia Osteoporosis-pseudoglioma syndrome Miscellaneous
Infiltrative Diseases
Multiple myeloma Lymphoma, leukemia Sarcoid Malignant histiocytosis Mastocytosis Gaucher disease Hemolytic diseases (thalassemia, sickle cell)
Transplant Osteodystrophy

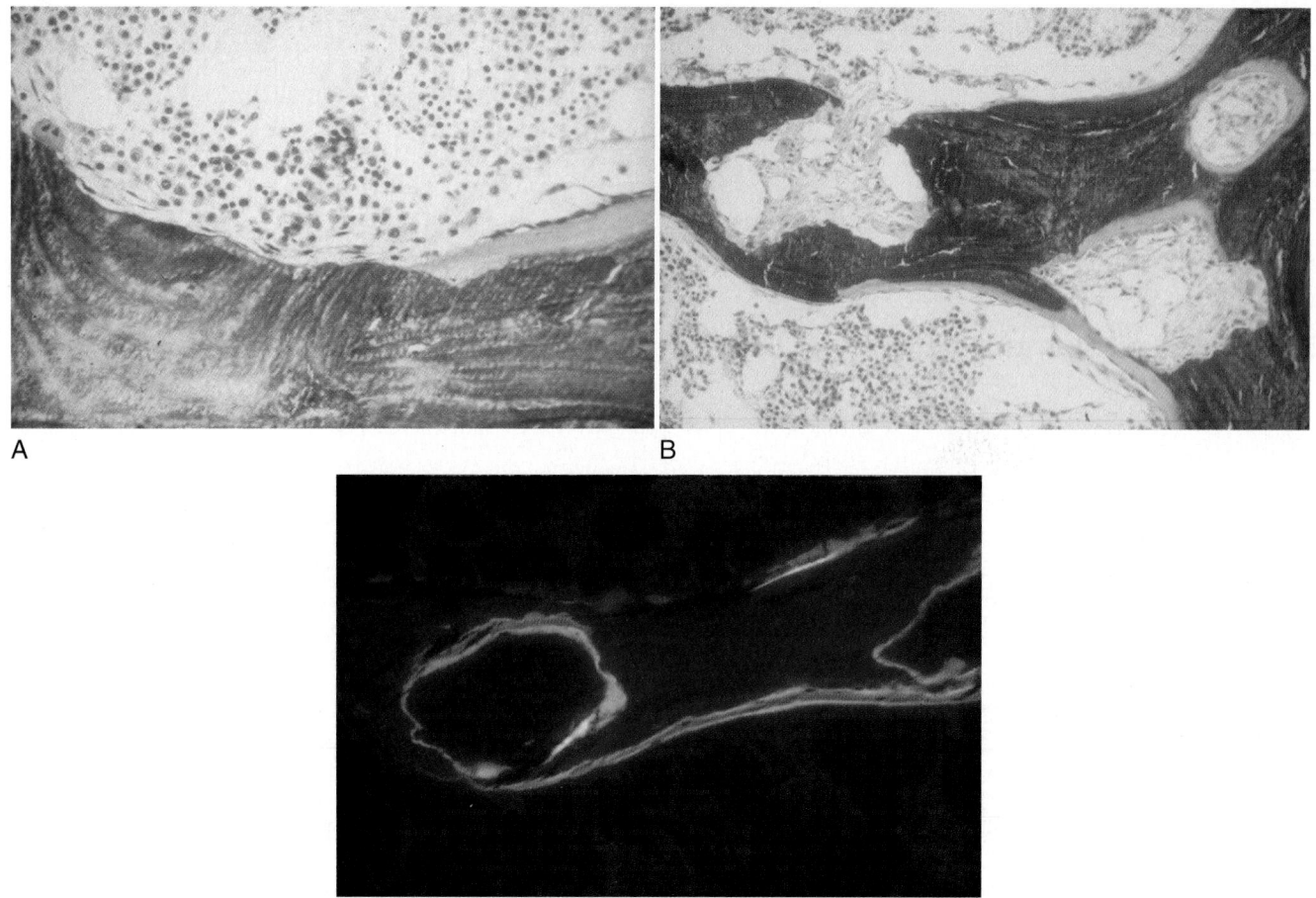

Figure 75-1 A, A normal bone-remodeling unit (see Chapter 73) provides an example of normal bone histologic mechanisms. At the bottom half of the figure is a normal mineralized trabecular bone surface *(dark blue)*. The top half of the slide shows normal bone marrow. In between is the trabecular bone surface. On the bone surface on the extreme left is a binucleated osteoclast that has moved across the bone surface over the previous week or two, resorbing (removing) old bone. On the extreme right surface, the bone surface is covered by osteoid *(light blue)* secreted by the overlying osteoblasts. In between the osteoclast- and osteoblast-covered surfaces of the trabecular bone are a large number of flat, fibroblastoid cells referred to as *lining cells.* **B,** Bone histologic display in a patient with primary hyperparathyroidism showing the classic features of *osteitis fibrosa cystica*. Note that far more osteoid and far more osteoblasts and osteoclasts exist than in the normal example **(A)**. Note also that three large microcysts are present that have been created by aggressive osteoclastic bone resorption. These microcysts account for the *cystica* component of osteitis fibrosa cystica. Finally, note that the marrow space, particularly within the microcysts, is filled with fibroblasts. These fibroblasts make up the *fibrosa* component of osteitis fibrosa cystica. **C,** Tetracycline labeling of a bone biopsy from a patient with hyperparathyroid bone disease. Note the bright-yellow parallel lines on the trabecular bone surface. These lines represent the two sets of tetracycline labeling, which occurred 14 days apart. From these sets, the mineralization rate can actually be described in microns per day, the so-called *mineral apposition rate,* and is increased dramatically in this example, as is typical of hyperparathyroid bone disease. Contrast with Figure 75-3B, in which no tetracycline labeling is present.

formation, such as alkaline phosphatase and osteocalcin, are increased, as are markers of bone resorption, such as *N*-telopeptide, hydroxyproline, and deoxypyridinolines. These changes are reflected on undecalcified bone biopsy, which reveals increases in the number and activity of osteoclasts and osteoblasts, increased quantities of unmineralized osteoid, accelerated rates of osteoid mineralization (determined using tetracycline labeling), microcysts in cortex and trabeculae (the *cystica* of OFC), and increased numbers of fibroblasts and marrow stroma (the *fibrosa* of OFC).

Bone density may be normal, as assessed using DXA, or it may be low. The pathognomonic radiologic signs of severe hyperparathyroid bone disease are a *salt-and-pepper* appearance of the calvarium, resorption of the tufts of the terminal phalanges and distal clavicles, subperiosteal resorption of the radial aspect of the cortex of the second phalanges, and

brown tumors (actually collections of osteoclasts that produce gross lytic lesions) of the pelvis and long bones (Fig. 75-2). All these radiologic signs disappear with parathyroidectomy, and bone mass, assessed by DXA, typically increases rapidly and markedly after parathyroidectomy.

The treatment of hyperparathyroid bone disease involves remediation of the chronically elevated PTH concentrations, either through parathyroidectomy in primary or tertiary hyperparathyroidism or through correction of the underlying cause of secondary hyperparathyroidism. If mild and if bone mass is normal, then no treatment may be required. Recently, reduction of serum calcium using the parathyroid calcium receptor mimetic drug cinacalcet has been added to this armamentarium. Cinacalcet is indicated in patients with chronic renal failure with secondary hyperparathyroidism and in patients with parathyroid carcinoma who have failed

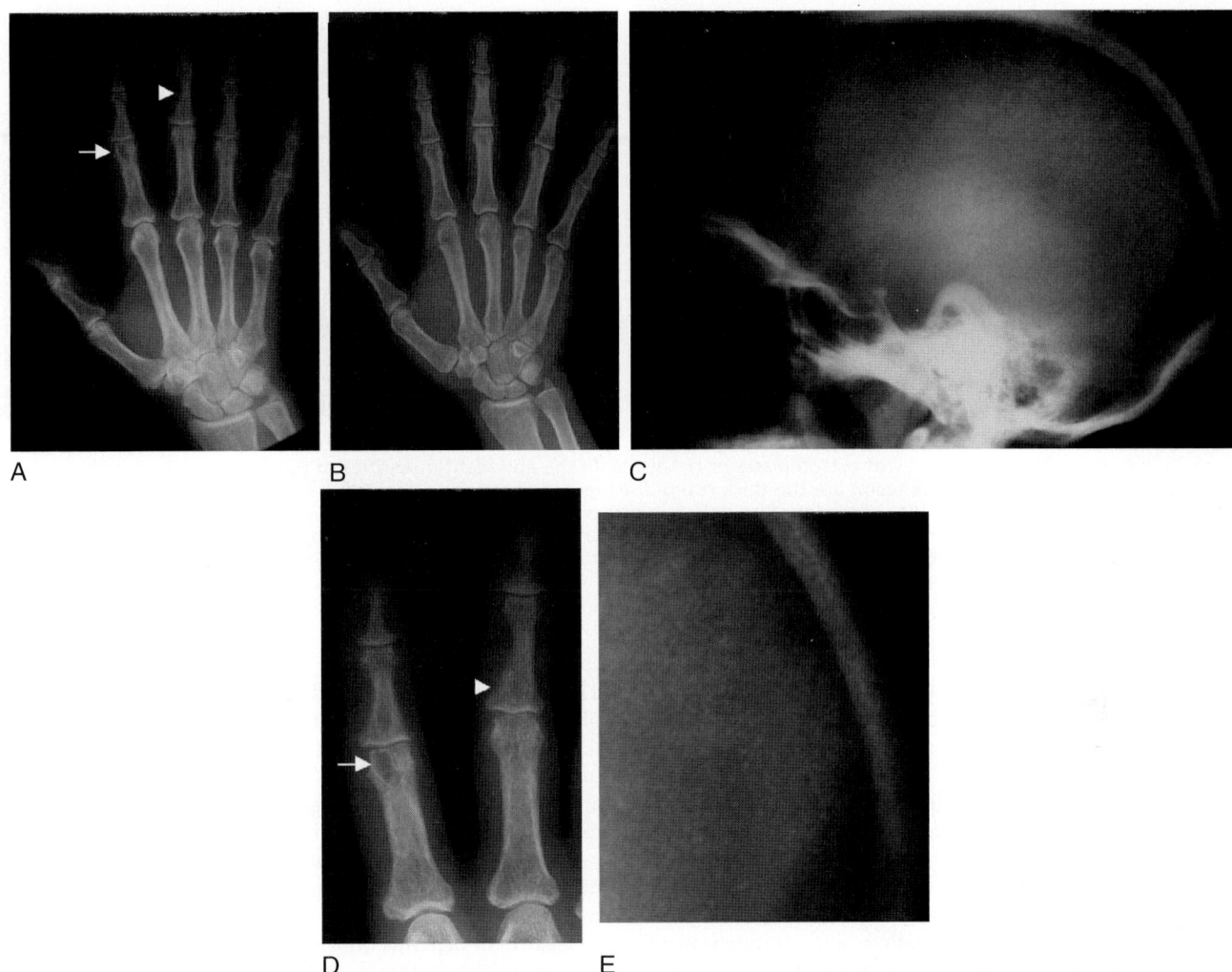

Figure 75-2 Skeletal radiographic changes of hyperparathyroidism. **A,** A hand film from a patient with primary hyperparathyroidism. The *arrow* indicates a typical Brown tumor, or giant cell tumor, which is a collection of osteoclasts that lead to macrocystic changes in bone. The *arrowhead* indicates the irregular radial surface of a phalanx resulting from subperiosteal bone resorption, also typical of hyperparathyroidism. Both the Brown tumor and the subperiosteal resorption refill and disappear when the offending parathyroid tumor or hyperplasia is resected. **B,** A normal hand film for comparison. No Brown tumors are present, and the phalangeal periosteal surfaces are smooth. **C,** The classic *salt-and-pepper* appearance of the skull observed in hyperparathyroidism. The periosteal surfaces of the inner and outer cortices or tables of the calvarium are indistinct as a result of subperiosteal bone resorption. In addition, the lateral view of the calvarium is hazy and indistinct, with micropunctations. **D** and **E,** Expanded views of **A** and **C** for greater detail. (Courtesy of Drs. J. Towers and D. Armfield, University of Pittsburgh.)

surgical resection. Although cinacalcet is effective in lowering the serum calcium in primary hyperparathyroidism, evidence of its efficacy in correcting skeletal abnormalities is lacking, and it is not approved for this indication.

Moderate to severe hypocalcemia may postoperatively accompany parathyroidectomy. This condition is referred to as the *hungry bone syndrome* and results from the sudden removal of the stimulus to osteoclastic activity by removing excess PTH in the setting of increased osteoblastic activity with unmineralized, but continuously mineralizing, osteoid. The syndrome abates when the osteoid mineralizes. Of course, postoperative hypocalcemia may also be due to intentional or inadvertent surgical hypoparathyroidism.

Finally, hyperparathyroid bone disease may be *pure,* as in a patient with severe primary hyperparathyroidism caused by a parathyroid adenoma, or it may be *mixed,* occurring as a component of the bone disease in vitamin D–deficient osteomalacia, in immunosuppressant-induced

transplant bone disease, or in renal osteodystrophy (see later discussion).

OSTEOMALACIA AND RICKETS

Osteomalacia and rickets are common both in the United States and in the rest of the world and are commonly overlooked. Two definitions are important. First, osteomalacia and rickets are essentially the same disorders, with the difference being semantic; by definition, rickets occurs in children with open growth plates (epiphyses), whereas osteomalacia occurs in adults with closed epiphyses. Second, the fundamental abnormality in these disorders is an inability to mineralize (i.e., form hydroxylapatite crystals within) *osteoid seams* (see Chapter 73); these patients have osteoblasts and can synthesize osteoid, but they mineralize it inefficiently or not at all. This fundamental inability to mineralize osteoid results in the accumulation of the characteristic thick

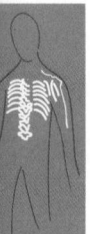

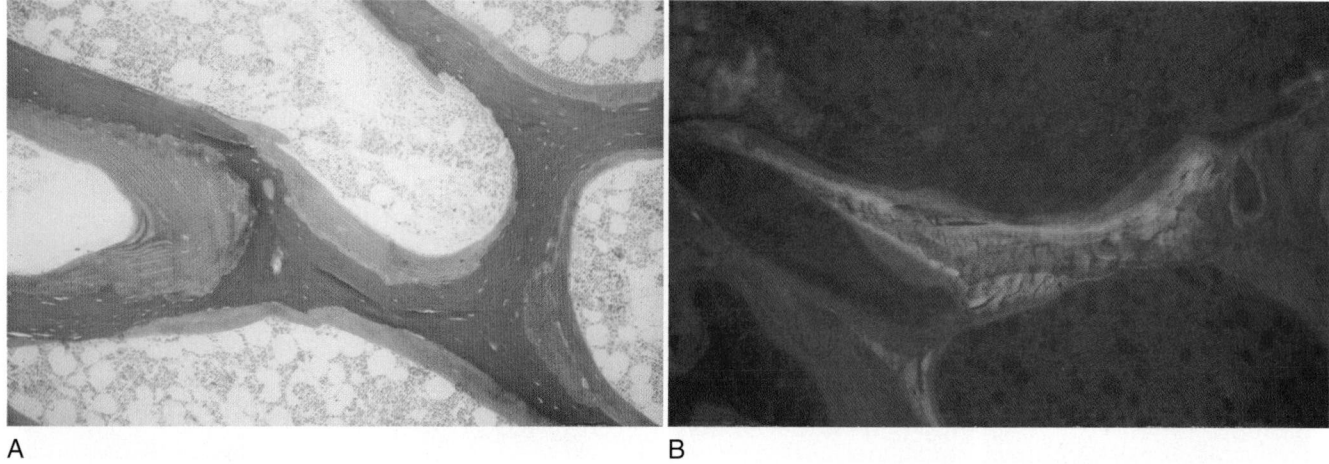

A   B

Figure 75-3 **A,** Bone histologic display of osteomalacia or rickets. Note the abundant quantities of partially and chaotically mineralized osteoid *(orange)*. These seams are the thick *osteoid seams* and represent osteoid that has been produced by osteoblasts but that cannot mineralize—the signature defect in osteomalacia and rickets. **B,** To confirm that the increase in osteoid seen in **A** is due to a defect in mineralization, tetracycline labeling can be performed. In this example, only very weak tetracycline labeling occurs. Compare with the rapid and aggressive mineralization observed in Figure 75-1C. This confirms the presence of a mineralization defect.

osteoid seams seen on bone biopsy (Fig. 75-3) and a reduction in the mineral component of bone so that it is deficient mechanically, which leads to bone pain, pseudofractures, fractures, bowing of the long bones, and other skeletal deformities (Fig. 75-4). In children (i.e., in rickets), the inability to mineralize the growth plate leads, in addition, to bulbous knobby deformities of the knees, ankles, and costochondral junctions (the *rachitic rosary*) and dental abnormalities. The characteristic radiologic signs of osteomalacia are Looser zones or Milkman pseudofractures. Rickets also shows gross defects in epiphyseal mineralization and compensatory increases in size of the joints and periarticular bone.

Understanding that the disorder is caused by a failure of mineralization, the underlying pathophysiologic mechanism can clearly be understood. These disorders result from an inability to form hydroxyapatite (calcium phosphate) crystals in osteoid, the nonmineralized phase of bone (see Chapter 73). This inability may result from hypophosphatemia (a common cause), a deficiency of calcium (an extremely rare cause), a deficiency of vitamin D (a common cause), or the presence of toxins that interfere with mineralization, such as aluminum, incompletely defined inhibitors of mineralization in uremic plasma, and long-term high-dose anticonvulsant use. Finally, because calcium salts are acid soluble, chronic metabolic acidoses (e.g., as occurs with the chronic bicarbonate wasting seen in patients with ureteral implants into ileal conduits) can result in osteomalacia or rickets. Thus, the causes of these mineralization disorders are, in essence, *vitamin D disorders* (malabsorption, liver disease), *hypophosphatemic disorders* (X-linked hypophosphatemic rickets, autosomal dominant hypophosphatemia, and oncogenic osteomalacia), *metabolic acidoses, drug-related disorders,* and *genetic conditions* (vitamin D–dependent rickets types I and II, and hypophosphatasia) (see Chapter 73).

The diagnosis is suggested in the setting of low bone mass, the characteristic radiologic signs noted previously, or unexplained bone pain or weakness. Of course, all these signs are late signs, and the disorder is optimally considered early in the course of the diseases described previously. The diagnosis is supported by demonstrating reductions of plasma 25-hydroxyvitamin D or its active form, 1,25-dihydroxyvitamin D (1,25[OH]$_2$D), hypophosphatemia, or increases in alkaline phosphatase, occurring in an appropriate clinical setting. The diagnosis can often be made clinically but can also be confirmed using undecalcified bone biopsy following oral double tetracycline labeling techniques, which are used to quantitate the degree of failure of mineralization.

Treatment depends on the underlying cause and includes an appropriate vitamin D compound, calcium, or phosphate, or a combination, as appropriate, and removal of the inhibitor of mineralization, when appropriate and possible. These diseases are gratifying to treat because the responses are often dramatic, and patients change rapidly from being chronically ill to feeling robust and healthy.

RENAL OSTEODYSTROPHY

Renal osteodystrophy is actually a collection of disorders that in moderate to severe forms leads to bone pain, pathologic fractures, and demineralization, all occurring in the setting of end-stage renal disease or dialysis. Subclinical renal osteodystrophy is common. The syndrome includes pure secondary hyperparathyroidism (see Fig. 75-1B), occurring as a result of defective renal production of 1,25(OH)$_2$D combined with an increase in serum phosphate, which lead to hypocalcemia as a result of reduced intestinal calcium absorption and calcium phosphate precipitation into soft tissues, respectively (see Chapter 73). This circumstance, in turn, evokes a severe increase in PTH secretion that then causes dramatic increases in bone turnover, demineralization, and fracture. These patients may respond dramatically to oral or parenteral replacement of 1,25(OH)$_2$D and the calcium receptor agonist cinacalcet. Other patients with *renal osteodystrophy* have adequately controlled serum calcium and phosphate, and therefore PTH, as a result of adequate oral calcium supplementation and phosphate

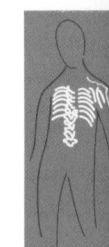

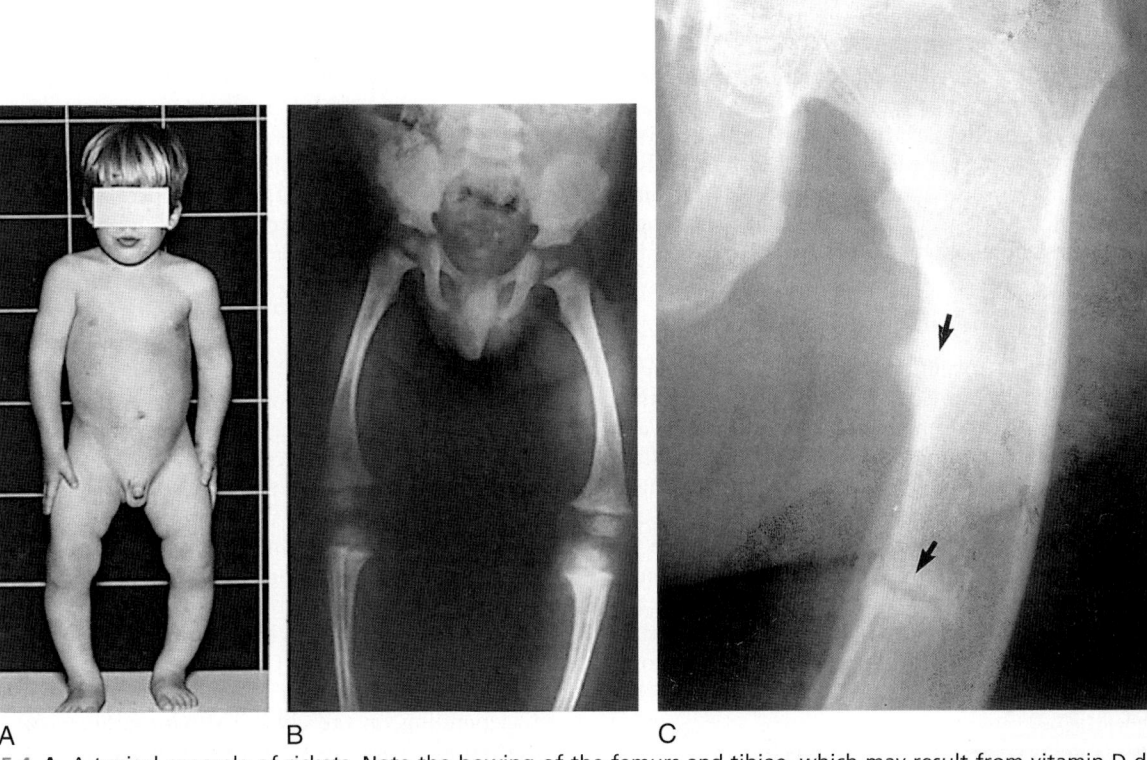

A   B   C

Figure 75-4 **A,** A typical example of rickets. Note the bowing of the femurs and tibiae, which may result from vitamin D deficiency, phosphate deficiency, or other causes. **B,** A skeletal radiograph of a child with rickets. Note that the weight-bearing bones of the lower extremities are bowed and that the epiphyses are open, mottled, and overgrown. **C,** Looser zones or pseudofractures characteristic of osteomalacia or rickets. Because the epiphyses are closed, the patient is an adult. This radiograph is diagnostic of osteomalacia.

binders, but they display severe osteomalacia (bone pain, reduced bone mineral density on DXA or bone biopsy, and thickened osteoid seams on bone biopsy with a mineralization defect apparent from tetracycline labeling) (see Fig. 75-3). The precise cause of the mineralization defect is uncertain. These patients, too, may respond dramatically to vitamin D replacement. Other patients with *renal osteodystrophy* have combinations of secondary hyperparathyroidism and osteomalacia (Fig. 75-5); still others have *low turnover* or *aplastic bone disease.* These terms are intended to describe patients on dialysis who have the opposite of secondary hyperparathyroidism and osteomalacia: little or no osteoblastic activity, osteoid, or osteoclastic activity. The condition may result from inhibitors of bone turnover, such as aluminum intoxication in the past; from excessive treatment with 1,25(OH)$_2$D, with suppression of PTH, causing low bone turnover; or from as yet unidentified causes. As with other bone diseases, understanding the cause is critical for effective treatment. Being aware of the syndrome so that it is recognized early and treated before bone pain and fractures occur is optimal.

GENETIC DISEASES

Genetic diseases that lead to reductions in bone mass are not common but are seen with some frequency in practices devoted to skeletal disease. Perhaps the most common

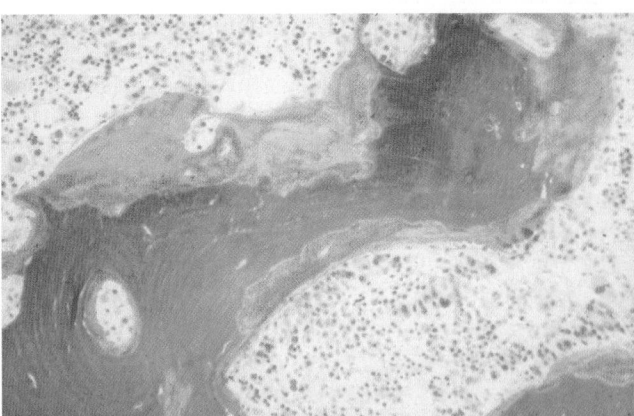

Figure 75-5 Renal osteodystrophy. This photomicrograph of a biopsy from a patient on dialysis demonstrates many of the classic features of renal osteodystrophy. These features include evidence of aggressive osteoclastic bone resorption (see numerous osteoclastic lacunae on the bone surface, as compared with the smooth surfaces in Figure 75-1A) and abundant partially and chaotically mineralized areas of osteoid (*orange*).

among these uncommon disorders is *osteogenesis imperfecta,* which may be mild or severe and may be present in neonates or older people, depending on the severity and the mutation involved. Mutations in the collagen I gene most often cause these disorders. *Hypophosphatasia* is due to a mutation

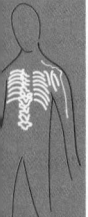

in the tissue-nonspecific alkaline phosphatase gene. These patients also display demineralization, fracture, and bone pain and have little or no measurable alkaline phosphatase. In the past several years, a new genetic disorder has been defined, called the *osteoporosis-pseudoglioma syndrome* (severe autosomal dominant osteoporosis with blindness). This disorder is due to inactivating mutations in the low-density lipoprotein-related protein 5 *(LRP5)* gene and, although very rare, is particularly interesting because activating mutations in the same gene have been shown recently to lead to an autosomal dominant form of very high bone mass. Myriad other genetic disorders exist that lead to low bone mass; some are treatable, others less so.

INFILTRATIVE DISEASES

Patients with multiple myeloma or Waldenström macroglobulinemia classically develop skeletal demineralization, and this is true as well for some patients with leukemia and marrow lymphomas. Other disorders associated with diffuse marrow infiltration by benign, or at least less malignant, processes can also lead to diffuse osteopenia, bone pain, and fracture, and all these disorders should be considered in the setting of unexplained *osteoporosis*. Examples include hemolytic anemias such as thalassemia or sickle cell disease, sarcoidosis with diffuse marrow involvement, Gaucher disease with lipid-laden marrow giant cells, malignant mastocytosis, and diffuse histiocytosis.

TRANSPLANT OSTEODYSTROPHY

Patients who have undergone or are undergoing organ transplantation commonly have severe *osteoporosis*. In some patients, this condition is due to treatment with immunosuppressive drugs such as glucocorticoids, tacrolimus, or cyclosporine, all of which are potent inhibitors of bone formation and regularly lead to reductions in bone mass. Some evidence indicates that they may activate osteoclastic bone resorption as well. In other patients, decreased bone mineral density exists before transplantation as a result of their organ failure or treatment thereof. In still other patients—for example, those with primary biliary cirrhosis—components of osteoblast failure, as well as calcium or vitamin D deficiency, may exist. In patients, such as those with end-stage lung or cardiac disease, contributing components of physical inactivity and generalized malnutrition may be present as well. In yet other patients with end-stage renal disease, all the components of renal osteodystrophy, as discussed previously, may be operative. This group of patients is particularly vexing because they often have severe, but retrospectively preventable, disease by the time they see an expert in metabolic bone disease, and therapy in late stages is incompletely effective. In addition, these patients may be in the "Catch-22" situation of being denied organ transplantation because of *severe osteoporosis* that, in retrospect, was preventable. This disorder can be expected to become increasingly common as organ transplantation becomes more common.

Treatment

Treatment of all these conditions depends on the underlying disorder. Primary and tertiary hyperparathyroidism are treated, if clinically indicated, with surgical resection of the affected parathyroid tissue. Osteomalacia and rickets improve when either the appropriate replacement drug is administered (e.g., vitamin D, calcium, or phosphate, or a combination) or the offending agent (e.g., anticonvulsants) is removed. Secondary hyperparathyroidism in a patient on dialysis can be treated with a combination of the active form of vitamin D (1,25[OH]$_2$D [calcitriol] or analogues), calcium supplementation, phosphate binders, and cinacalcet, depending on the clinical situation. Secondary hyperparathyroidism due to vitamin D deficiency can be treated with oral or intramuscular injections of the much less expensive parent compound, vitamin D. Other items in Table 75-1 require attention to the underlying disorder.

The most important therapeutic point is that these disorders are commonly amenable to treatment and can have dramatic and satisfying responses to therapy, both for the physician and for the patient. The main stumbling block is that these diagnoses are commonly never considered, and the DXA report of *osteoporosis* is passively accepted and never investigated. The key clinical message, then, is that, whenever a patient is designated as having *osteoporosis,* the physician should mentally run through the checklist in Table 75-1 and eliminate, or investigate, these disorders as appropriate.

Prospectus for the Future

Better understanding of metabolic bone diseases, including but not limited to osteoporosis, represents one of the largest challenges facing researchers as the population ages. We know so little about how bone is made (we do not even know how it mineralizes) or why some people develop osteoporosis while others with identical risk factors do not. We recognize that postmenopausal women with osteoporotic fracture have bone densities some 50% of normal, yet the current generation of osteoporosis drugs increases bone density by only 2% to 9%. Clearly, we have a long way to go in this arena. Moreover, what is the cause of *low turnover renal osteodystrophy* or *adynamic bone disease* in patients on dialysis? Why do some of these patients get this disorder while others do not, what are the additional cytokines that cause bone resorption in breast cancer and myeloma, and what drugs can be developed to block these events? Why is rickets still so prevalent in the Third World and in U.S. cities as well, and what can we do at a public health level to prevent this unnecessary disease? How can we teach physicians that, just because low bone density found in a bone density study is interpreted to mean *osteoporosis,* that it might equally well represent multiple myeloma, OFC, or osteomalacia? Thus, basic, clinical, and public health issues abound in this area, and the coming decade will see answers to at least some of these questions.

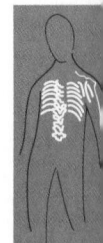

References

DeGroot L, Jameson LJ (eds): Endocrinology, 5th ed. Philadelphia, WB Saunders, 2006.

Favus MF (ed): The American Society for Bone and Mineral Research Primer on Metabolic Bone Diseases and Disorders of Mineral Metabolism, 6th ed. Washington DC, American Society for Bone and Mineral Research, 2006.

Khosla S, Westendorf JJ, Oursler MJ: Building bone to reverse osteoporosis and repair fractures. J Clin Invest 118:421-428, 2008.

Lindsay R, Cosman F, Zhao H, Bostrom MP, et al: A novel tetracycline labeling strategy for longitudinal evaluation of the short term effects of anabolic therapy with a single iliac crest bone biopsy. J Bone Min Res 21:366-373, 2006.

Moe S, Drueke T, Cunningham J, et al: Definition, evaluation and classification of renal osteodystrophy: A position statement from Kidney Disease: Improving Global Outcomes (KIDIGO). Kidney Int 69:1945-1953, 2006.

Stewart AF: Translational implications of the parathyroid calcium receptor. N Engl J Med 351:324-326, 2004.

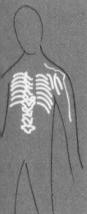

Osteoporosis

Susan L. Greenspan

Osteoporosis, the most common disorder of bone and mineral metabolism, affects about 50% of women older than 50 years. The National Institutes of Health Consensus Development Panel on Osteoporosis Prevention defines osteoporosis as a skeletal disorder characterized by compromised bone strength, predisposing a person to an increased risk for fracture. Bone strength reflects primarily the integration of two main features: (1) bone density and (2) bone quality. Bone density reflects the peak adult bone mass and the amount of bone lost in adulthood. Bone quality is determined by bone architecture, bone geometry, bone turnover, mineralization, and damage accumulation (i.e., microfractures) (Fig. 76-1).

Epidemiologic Factors

In the United States, 1.5 million osteoporotic fractures occur each year, comprising 700,000 vertebral fractures, 250,000 radial fractures, 250,000 hip fractures, and 300,000 other fractures. Hip fractures have the most serious consequences by far, with a mortality rate of more than 20% within the first year. More than 50% of patients with hip fracture will be unable to return to their previous ambulatory state, and about 10% of them will be placed in long-term care facilities. Three fourths of all hip fractures occur in women. After the age of 50 years, the lifetime risk for hip fracture is 17% for white women, compared with 6% for white men. When defined by bone mineral densitometry, 13 to 17 million women have *low bone mass* at the hip, and 4 to 6 million postmenopausal white women have osteoporosis. Although morbidity is decreased with vertebral fractures, mortality is increased as a result of the risk for cardiovascular and pulmonary disease that is associated with an escalating number of vertebral fractures. Only one third of radiologically diagnosed vertebral fractures receive medical attention.

Risk Factors

The major risk factors for osteoporosis have been previously outlined by the National Osteoporosis Foundation (NOF)

and include personal history of fracture in adulthood, fracture history in a first-degree relative, low body weight (<127 lb), current smoking, and use of oral corticosteroid therapy for longer than 3 months. Additional risk factors include impaired vision, early estrogen deficiency (<45 years of age), dementia, poor health or frailty, recent falls, low calcium intake (lifelong), low physical activity, and alcohol consumption (>2 drinks per day). Risk factors specific to hip fracture were identified by the Study of Osteoporotic Fractures, an epidemiologic trial that prospectively monitored 9704 postmenopausal women older than 65 years. Risk factors for hip fracture included age, history of maternal hip fracture, weight, height, poor health, previous hyperthyroidism, current use of long-acting benzodiazepines, poor depth perception, tachycardia, previous fracture, and low bone mineral density. Investigators found that the more risk factors a woman had, the greater was her risk for fracture.

Peak Bone Mass and Bone Loss

Peak bone mass is determined primarily by genetic factors. Men have a higher bone mass than women, and African Americans and Hispanics have a higher bone mass than whites. Multiple genes, including vitamin D–receptor alleles, estrogen receptor genes, and the *high bone mass* gene, are thought to be associated with bone mass, but studies are ongoing. Other factors that contribute to the development of peak bone mass are the use of gonadal steroids, timing of puberty, calcium intake, exercise, and growth hormone.

The causes of bone loss in adults are multifactorial. The pattern of bone loss differs in women compared with men, and bone loss is greater in sites rich in trabecular bone (e.g., spine) than cortical bone (e.g., femoral neck) (Fig. 76-2). Estrogen deficiency during menopause contributes significantly to bone loss in women because they may lose 1% to 5% of bone mass per year in the first few years after menopause. Women continue to lose bone mass throughout the remainder of their lives, with another acceleration of bone loss occurring after age 75 years. The mechanism of this

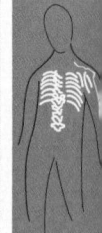

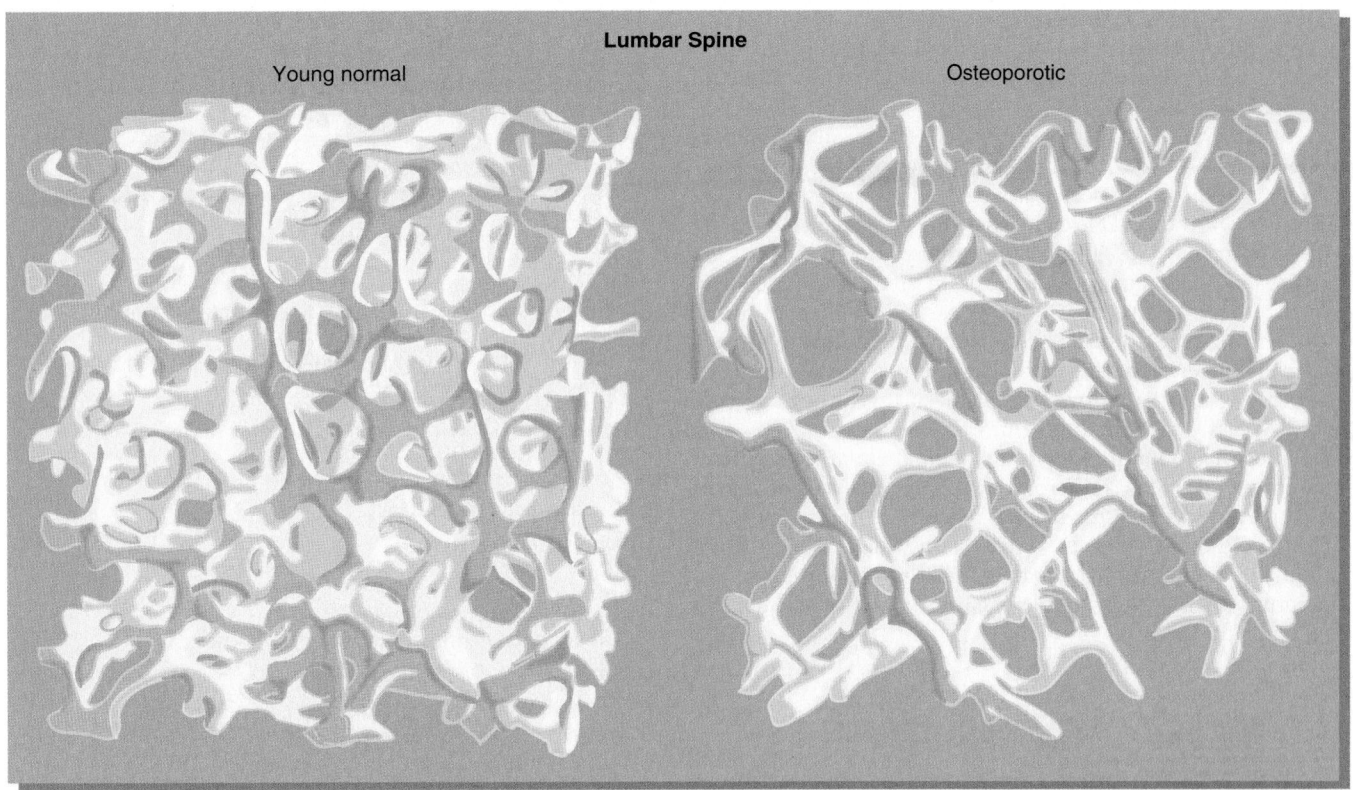

Figure 76-1 Three-dimensional reconstruction by microcomputed tomography of a lumbar spine sample from a young adult normal woman and from a woman with postmenopausal osteoporosis. In the osteoporotic woman, not only is bone mass reduced, but also microarchitectural deterioration of bone structure occurs. Whereas the platelike structure in the normal case is very isotropic, the structure in the osteoporotic case shows preferential loss of horizontal struts; the plates have become rods that are thin and farther apart, and there is a concomitant loss of trabecular connectivity. These changes lead to a reduction in bone strength that is more than would be predicted by the decrease in bone mineral density. (From Riggs BL, Khosla S, Melton LJ 3rd: Sex steroids and the construction and conservation of the adult skeleton. Endocr Rev 23:279-302, 2002. Images courtesy of Ralph Mueller, PhD, Swiss Federal Institute of Technology [ETH] and University of Zurich, Zurich, Switzerland.)

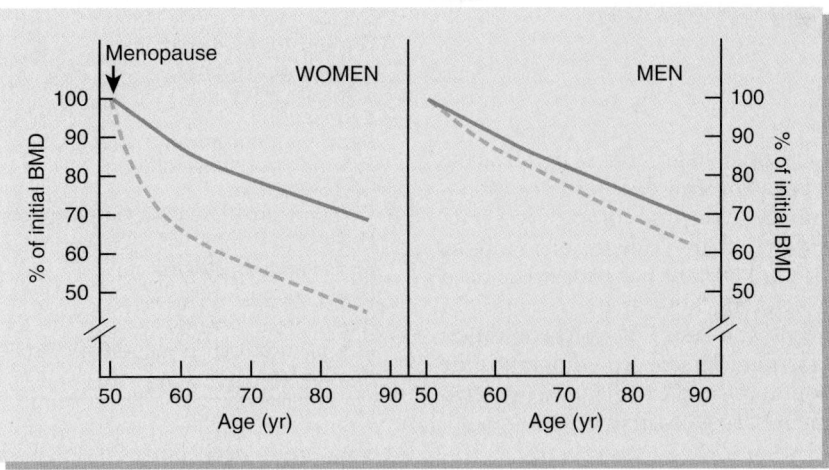

Figure 76-2 Patterns of age-related bone loss in women and in men. *Dashed line* represents trabecular bone and *solid lines,* cortical bone. The figure is based on multiple cross-sectional and longitudinal studies using dual-energy x-ray absorptiometry. BMD, bone mineral density. (Reproduced with permission from Khosla S, Riggs BL: Pathophysiology of age-related bone loss and osteoporosis. Endocrinol Metab Clin N Am 34:1015-1030, 2005.)

accelerated loss in old age is not clear. Estrogen deficiency influences a host of local cytokines, which affect osteoblastic and osteoclastic activity as well as bone turnover. In an adult, skeletal integrity is further influenced by calcium intake, vitamin D intake, physical activity, and body weight. Finally, multiple causes of secondary bone loss have been found.

Medications that commonly cause bone loss include excess thyroid hormone, glucocorticoids, antiseizure medications, heparin, gonadotropin-releasing hormone agonists, aromatase inhibitors, and depo-medroxyprogesterone. Endocrine diseases resulting in female or male hypogonadism also lead to bone loss. Hyperparathyroidism, hyperthyroidism, and

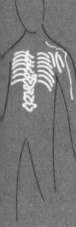

hypercortisolism also commonly cause bone loss, as can vitamin D deficiency. Gastrointestinal problems can contribute to decreased absorption of calcium and vitamin D (Table 76-1).

All patients should have a work-up for secondary causes of bone loss. This would include a serum calcium (albumin) level to rule out hyperparathyroidism or malnutrition; a 25-hydroxyvitamin D level to assess for vitamin D deficiency or insufficiency; alkaline phosphatase level to assess for Paget disease, malignancy, cirrhosis, or vitamin D deficiency; liver and renal function tests to assess for liver or renal abnormalities; 24-hour urine calcium and creatinine to evaluate for hypercalciuria or malabsorption; a test for sprue in patients with anemia or hypocalciuria; thyrotropin to rule out hyperthyroidism; and serum protein electrophoresis to rule out myeloma in older adults with anemia. Often, measurement of the parathyroid hormone level is needed to interpret calcium and vitamin D levels. A more extensive work-up can be done in severe or unusual cases. A bone biopsy is rarely needed. Markers of bone turnover may be helpful but are quite variable in clinical practice and usually reserved for research.

Clinical Manifestations

Unlike many other chronic diseases with multiple signs and symptoms, osteoporosis is considered a *silent* disease until fractures occur. Whereas 90% of hip fractures occur after a fall, two thirds of vertebral fractures are silent and occur with minimal stress such as lifting, sneezing, and bending. An acute vertebral fracture may result in significant back pain, which decreases gradually over several weeks with analgesics and physical therapy. Patients with significant vertebral osteoporosis may have height loss, kyphosis, and severe cervical lordosis (known as a *dowager's hump*).

Diagnosis

The diagnosis of osteoporosis is made following an acute clinical fracture or with bone mineral densitometry assessment. Radiographs can reveal a vertebral compression fracture (Fig. 76-3); however, radiologic evidence of low bone mass may not be present until 30% of bone mass has been lost. In addition, when assessing bone mass, radiographs may be read inappropriately as a result of overpenetration or underpenetration of the film. Therefore, radiographs are a poor indicator of osteoporosis, and the diagnosis is often made based on bone mineral densitometry.

BONE MINERAL DENSITY

Bone mineral density can be assessed through a variety of techniques. In 1994, the World Health Organization (WHO) developed a classification system for osteoporosis and low bone mass (osteopenia) based on data from white postmenopausal women (Table 76-2). Osteoporosis was defined as a bone mineral density less than or equal to 2.5 standard deviations below young adult peak bone mass (T-score ≤−2.5 SD). Low bone mass (osteopenia) is defined as a bone mass measurement between 1.0 and 2.5 standard deviations

Table 76-1 **Secondary Causes of Low Bone Mass**
Endocrine Diseases
Female hypogonadism
Hyperprolactinemia
Hypothalamic amenorrhea
Anorexia nervosa
Premature and primary ovarian failure
Female athlete triad
Male hypogonadism
Primary gonadal failure (e.g., Klinefelter syndrome)
Secondary gonadal failure (e.g., idiopathic hypogonadotropic hypogonadism, androgen deprivation therapy for prostate cancer)
Hyperthyroidism
Hyperparathyroidism
Hypercortisolism
Vitamin D insufficiency or deficiency
Gastrointestinal Diseases
Subtotal gastrectomy
Gastric bypass surgery
Malabsorption syndromes
Chronic obstructive jaundice
Primary biliary cirrhosis and other cirrhoses
Bone Marrow Disorders
Multiple myeloma
Monoclonal gammopathy of unknown significance (MGUS)
Lymphoma
Leukemia
Hemolytic anemias
Systemic mastocytosis
Disseminated carcinoma
Connective Tissue Diseases
Osteogenesis imperfecta
Ehlers-Danlos syndrome
Marfan syndrome
Homocystinuria
Drugs
Alcohol
Antiseizure medications
Aromatase inhibitors
Chemotherapy
Cyclosporine
Depo-medroxyprogesterone
Excess thyroid hormone
Glucocorticoids
Gonadotropin-releasing hormone agonists
Heparin
Miscellaneous Causes
Immobilization
Rheumatoid arthritis
Chronic obstructive pulmonary disease
Weight loss

below adult peak bone mass (T-score between −1.0 and −2.5 SD). Normal bone mineral density is defined as assessments above 1.0 standard deviation below adult peak bone mass (T-score ≥−1.0 SD). The *gold standard* for assessing bone mineral density is dual-energy x-ray absorptiometry (DXA), which has excellent precision and accuracy. Measurements are made of the hip and spine, and about 30% of the time, discordance is found between these measurements (Fig. 76-4). Therefore, classification is based on the lowest value (total spine, total hip, or femoral neck). Bone mineral density can also be measured by hip or spine quantitative computed tomography (QCT). However, few normative

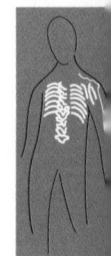

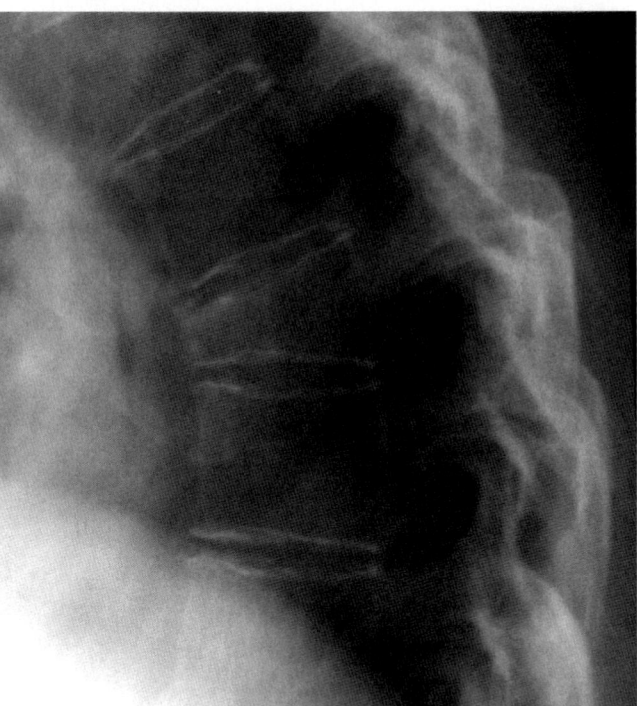

Figure 76-3 Lateral spine radiograph demonstrating a thoracic anterior wedge compression fracture.

Table 76-2 World Health Organization Classifications for Osteoporosis

Classification	Criteria for Bone Mineral Density
Normal	Above −1.0 SD of young adult peak mean value
Low bone mass (osteopenia)	Between −1.0 and −2.5 SD of young adult peak mean value
Osteoporosis	Below −2.5 SD of young adult peak mean value

SD, standard deviation.

data are available for hip QCT, vertebral precision is inferior to that of DXA, and radiation doses are significantly higher than those of DXA. Finally, single-photon absorptiometry of the forearm and peripheral measures, such as finger DXA and heel ultrasound, have also been used to assess bone mass (Table 76-3).

Classification can vary significantly by the skeletal site and the device used for assessment. For example, the average woman would be diagnosed with osteoporosis at age 60 years when assessing the lateral spine but not until she is older than 100 years if heel ultrasound is used. Although all these measurements have an accuracy of 1% to 3%, precision is best with forearm or spine DXA (about 1%). Furthermore, the WHO classification should only be used with DXA.

Experts recommend that bone mineral density be monitored after 2 years, depending on the site to be assessed and the type of therapy prescribed. For example, trabecular bone, which is more metabolically active than cortical bone, is more likely to show improvements with stronger-acting antiresorptive agents. Changes in bone mass with potent antiresorptive therapy are more prominent in the spine compared with other areas. Seeing no changes in forearm bone mineral density over time is common, despite good precision. Although the heel has a high percentage of trabecular bone, precision is poor, and monitoring should not be done at this site.

The NOF recommends obtaining a bone mineral density assessment in all women older than 65 years, postmenopausal women younger than 65 years with one risk factor, and women who have had a fracture (Table 76-4). The U.S. Preventive Services Task Force recommends bone density tests in all women older than 65 years and women between 60 and 64 years with a risk factor. The NOF recommends obtaining a bone mineral density in men 70 years and older. Currently, databases are available for white, African American, and Hispanic men and women.

In general, bone mass measurements by DXA examine the spine and hip. However, in patients with hyperparathyroidism, in which cortical bone loss is often seen, forearm DXA should also be assessed. Older patients with osteoporosis often have falsely elevated bone mineral density measurements at the spine as a result of atypical calcifications from degenerative joint disease, sclerosis, or aortic calcifications. Although lateral bone mineral density measurements eliminate these artifacts, they are often difficult to perform because of overlap of the ribs on L2 and overlap of the pelvic brim on L4. Classification should only be made if two or more vertebrae are available for analysis because of the high error rate when only one vertebra is assessed. QCT is recommended less often than DXA because of the former's high radiation exposure and cost.

The WHO has developed an assessment to predict the 10-year risk for hip or any major osteoporotic fracture for postmenopausal women and men aged 50 years and older. The "FRAX," fracture risk assessment tool, incorporates femoral neck T-score, age, gender, height, weight, and specific risk factors, including history of adult fracture, parental hip fracture, current smoking, glucocorticoids, rheumatoid arthritis, alcohol (≥3 drinks per day), and secondary osteoporosis. The fracture risk prediction is specific for race and country and should only be used in patients not on therapy.

Prevention

General preventive measures for all patients include calcium and vitamin D supplementation, exercise, and fall prevention techniques. The recommended daily allowance of calcium was recently reviewed by the National Academy of Science and increased to 1200 mg daily for postmenopausal women. Calcium intake can be accomplished by dietary consumption or supplementation. The supplements should generally be pure calcium carbonate or pure calcium citrate, taken in divided doses of about 500 to 600 mg twice daily. Calcium carbonate must be taken with meals for best absorption, whereas calcium citrate may be taken with or without food. Calcium supplements are currently available as tablets and in chewable and liquid forms. Many foods, such as orange juice and some cereals, are now calcium fortified.

Vitamin D is important for calcium absorption and bone mineralization. Vitamin D has nonskeletal benefits and

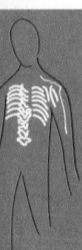

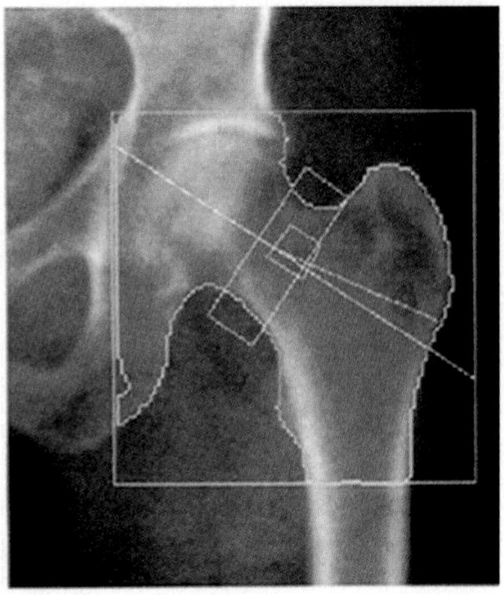

k = 1.145, d0 = 53.2
93 × 97

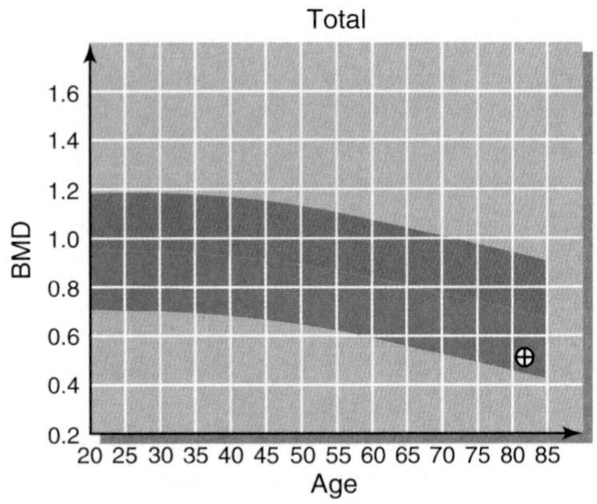

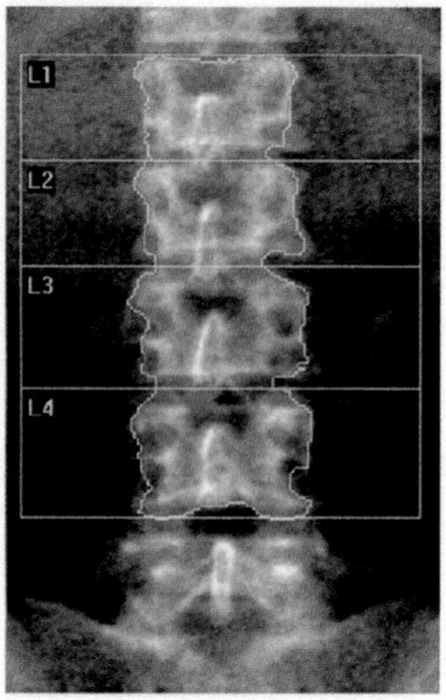

k = 1.135, d0 = 48.6
116 × 137

Region	Area (cm²)	BMC (g)	BMD (g/cm²)	T-Score	PR (%)	Z-Score	AM (%)
Neck	4.68	1.89	0.404	−4.0	48	−1.6	69
Troch	10.63	4.13	0.388	−3.1	55	−1.3	75
Inter	16.59	9.90	0.597	−3.2	54	−1.3	74
Total	31.89	15.91	0.499	−3.6	53	−1.5	74
Ward's	1.19	0.32	0.268	−4.0	37	−0.9	72

Total BMD CV 1.0%, ACF = 1.028, BCF = 1.006, TH = 5.163
WHO Classification: Osteoporosis
Fracture Risk: High

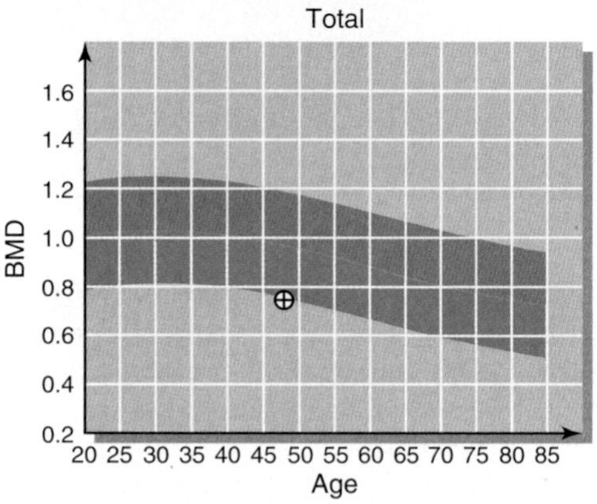

Region	Area (cm²)	BMC (g)	BMD (g/cm²)	T-Score	PR (%)	Z-Score	AM (%)
L1	12.52	8.04	0.642	−2.6	69	−2.0	74
L2	13.41	9.74	0.726	−2.7	71	−2.1	76
L3	16.21	11.96	0.738	−3.1	68	−2.5	73
L4	17.42	13.94	0.800	−2.9	72	−2.2	77
Total	59.56	43.68	0.733	−2.9	70	−2.2	75

Total BMD CV 1.0%, ACF = 1.028, BCF = 1.006, TH = 5.848
WHO Classification: Osteoporosis
Fracture Risk: High

Figure 76-4 Right, This patient has a lumbar spine (L1 through L4) bone mineral density (BMD) of 0.733 g/cm² *(white circle with cross)* as measured by dual-energy x-ray absorptiometry (DXA) and a T-score of −2.9. The reference database graph displays age- and sex-matched mean BMD levels ±2 standard deviations (SDs) *(shaded areas)* derived from a normative database from the manufacturer (Hologic, Inc., Bedford, Mass). The T-score indicates the difference in SD between the patient's BMD and the predicted sex-matched mean peak young adult BMD; z-value, the difference in SD between the patient's BMD and the sex- and age-matched mean BMD; and percentage of mean, the patient's BMD as a percentage of the mean peak young adult BMD or age-matched BMD level. **Left,** This patient has a total hip BMD of 0.499 g/cm² *(white circle with cross)* as measured by DXA, a femoral neck T-score of −4.0, and a total hip T-score of −3.6. The reference database graph displays age- and sex-matched mean BMD levels ±2 SDs *(shaded areas)* derived from the third National Health and Nutrition Examination Survey. The T-score indicates the difference in SD between the patient's BMD and the predicted sex-matched mean peak young adult BMD; z-score, the difference in SD between the patient's BMD and the sex- and age-matched mean BMD; and percentage of mean, the patient's BMD as a percentage of the mean peak young adult BMD or age-matched BMD level. (Adapted from bone densitometry report, QDR-4500A bone densitometer, Hologic, Inc., Bedford, Mass.)

has been associated with improvement in muscle strength, prevention of falls, and decrease in prostate, colon, and breast cancer. Vitamin D comes from two sources: diet and photosynthesis. Because dietary sources of vitamin D are limited (e.g., fortified milk), and patients are often advised to avoid sun exposure for prevention of skin cancer and wrinkles, many studies have now documented vitamin

D deficiency and insufficiency in older adults. In addition, older patients have reduced ability to synthesize vitamin D in the skin. Low vitamin D levels can lead to secondary hyperparathyroidism.

Vitamin D can be taken in a multivitamin, in a calcium supplement, or in pure form. In pure form, cholecalciferol (D_3) is preferable to ergocalciferol (D_2). Most multivitamins

Table 76-3 Techniques for Measuring Bone Mass

Sites Measured	Precision (%)	Accuracy (%)	Scan Time	Radiation Dose Entrance Exposure (mrem)
Quantitative computed tomography Lumbar spine Total hip Total radius	2-10	5-20	10-15 min	100-2000
Single-photon absorptiometry Proximal radius Distal radius Calcaneus	1-3	4-6	3-5 min	10-20
Dual-photon absorptiometry Posteroanterior lumbar spine Lateral lumbar spine Proximal femur Total body	2-6	4-10	20-40 min	10-15
Dual-energy x-ray absorptiometry Posteroanterior lumbar spine Lateral lumbar spine Proximal femur Total body	1-3	3-15	2-5 min	1-35
Calcaneal ultrasound	1.4	3	10 sec	N/A

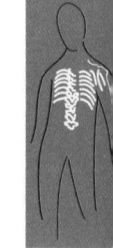

Table 76-4 National Osteoporosis Foundation Recommendations for Bone Mineral Density Testing

1. All postmenopausal women younger than 65 years who have one or more additional risk factors for osteoporosis (besides menopause)
2. All women aged 65 years and older regardless of additional risk factors
3. Postmenopausal women who present with fractures (to confirm diagnosis and determine disease severity)
4. All men aged 70 years and older

contain 400 IU to 800 IU of vitamin D. The current recommended dose is up to 1000 IU for adults. Older patients with severe vitamin D deficiency may be given 50,000 IU of vitamin D once per week for 3 months to bring serum vitamin D into the normal range. Activated vitamin D is rarely needed and should not be given on a regular basis for postmenopausal osteoporosis.

Weight-bearing exercise is important for maintaining skeletal integrity. Results are controversial concerning studies on different types and duration of exercise in postmenopausal women and men. In general, however, weight-bearing or resistance training exercises are suggested and have been shown to improve bone mass or maintain skeletal integrity. In patients with new vertebral fractures, physical therapy is important for improving posture and increasing strength in back muscles.

Because 90% of hip fractures and a significant number of vertebral fractures occur during a fall, fall prevention modalities are suggested for frail older patients. Fall-proofing the household includes installing grab bars in the bathroom and hand rails on stairways, avoiding loose throw rugs and cords, ensuring good lighting by the bedside, and moving objects within easy reach in the kitchen. Other fall prevention modalities include eliminating medications that cause dizziness or postural hypotension (if possible), assessing the need for assistive devices (e.g., canes, walkers), and ensuring appropriate footwear and good vision. In addition, several studies have now demonstrated that hip protectors significantly reduce hip fractures in residents in nursing homes. However, compliance is often poor with these products.

Treatment

The NOF developed treatment guidelines that incorporate the 10-year fracture risk prediction. The NOF suggests treatment for postmenopausal women and men 50 years and older as follows:

1. An adult fragility fracture at the hip or spine
2. Osteoporosis by bone mineral density T-score of less than or equal to 2.5 at the spine, total hip, or femoral neck after appropriate evaluation
3. Other prior fractures and low bone mass (T-score between −1.0 and −2.5 SD)
4. Low bone mass (T-score between −1.0 and −2.5 SD) and a 10-year hip fracture risk of 3% or higher or a 10-year all-major osteoporosis-related fracture risk of 20% or higher based on U.S. adapted model
5. Low bone mass (T-score between −1.0 and −2.5 SD) and secondary causes associated with high risk of fracture (glucocorticoids, total immobilization)

Patients taking glucocorticoids can fracture with a normal bone density. The American College of Rheumatology suggests patients starting glucocorticoids, who will be treated for 3 months or longer, have a bone density and start antiresorptive therapy. This is especially true for postmenopausal women and men.

BISPHOSPHONATES

Bisphosphonates are the mainstay of osteoporosis prevention and treatment. They inhibit the cholesterol synthesis

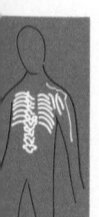

Table 76-5 U.S. Food and Drug Administration–Approved Therapies for Prevention and Treatment of Osteoporosis

Agent	Prevention	Treatment	Dose	Vertebral Fracture Reduction	Hip Fracture Reduction	Cost Per Year
Alendronate	Yes	Yes	Prevention: 5 mg PO daily, 35 mg PO weekly Treatment: 10 mg PO daily, 70 mg PO weekly	Yes	Yes	$965 (but is now generic)
Risedronate	Yes	Yes	Prevention and treatment: 5 mg PO daily, 35 mg PO weekly, 150 mg PO monthly	Yes	Yes	$965
Ibandronate	Yes	Yes	2.5 mg PO daily, 150 mg PO monthly, 3 mg IV every 3 mo	Yes	No	$1043 ~$2000
Zoledronic acid	No	Yes	5 mg IV yearly	Yes	Yes	~$1000
Raloxifene	Yes	Yes	60 mg PO daily	Yes	No	$1082
Hormone replacement therapy	Yes	*Management*	0.625 mg PO daily conjugated estrogen or equivalent (0.45, 0.3 mg also available)	Yes	Yes	$65-$522
Calcitonin	No	Yes	200 IU daily intranasal	Yes	No	$1148
Teriparatide (PTH [1-34])	No	Yes	20 mcg SC daily	Yes	No	$8528

PO, orally; PTH, parathyroid hormone; SC, subcutaneously.

pathway in the osteoclasts, thereby causing early apoptosis and inhibiting osteoclast migration and attachment. In the United States, the bisphosphonates alendronate, risedronate, ibandronate, and zoledronic acid have been approved for the prevention and treatment of osteoporosis. Alendronate has been shown to increase bone mass by about 8% at the spine and 4% at the hip over 3 years. This increase has been associated with approximately a 50% reduction in spine, hip, and forearm fractures (Table 76-5). Alendronate is prescribed at 5 mg daily or 35 mg once weekly for osteoporosis prevention and 10 mg daily or 70 mg once weekly (with or without vitamin D 2800 IU/tablet or 5600 IU/tablet) for the treatment of osteoporosis. Alendronate has been approved for use in men and patients with glucocorticoid-induced osteoporosis.

Risedronate is approved for the prevention and treatment of osteoporosis at a dose of 5 mg per day, 35 mg per week, 75 mg in two consecutive doses per month, or 150 mg per month. Large-scale, multicenter studies have shown improvements in bone mass of about 6% to 7% at the spine and 3% at the hip over 3 years. In addition, these studies revealed a 50% reduction in vertebral fractures, 40% reduction in nonvertebral fractures, and 40% reduction in hip fractures (see Table 76-5). Risedronate is approved for treatment of osteoporosis in men and for the prevention and treatment of patients with glucocorticoid-induced osteoporosis.

Ibandronate is approved for the prevention and treatment of postmenopausal osteoporosis. After 3 years of treatment, ibandronate increased bone density by 6.5% at the spine and 3.4% at the hip, and reduced new vertebral fractures by 62%. No reductions in nonvertebral or hip fractures were noted. Ibandronate is approved at an oral dose of 2.5 mg daily, or 150 mg monthly. Ibandronate is approved for treatment at an intravenous dose of 3 mg every 3 months.

Zoledronic acid is approved for the treatment of postmenopausal osteoporosis. The pivotal trial demonstrated increases of 6.9% of bone density at the spine and 6.0% at the hip and reduced spine fractures by 70%, nonvertebral fractures by 25%, and hip fractures by 41% after 3 years. Zoledronic acid is given at a dose of 5 mg intravenously once a year.

Because oral bisphosphonates are poorly absorbed, they must be taken first thing in the morning on an empty stomach with a full glass of water. Patients must wait 30 minutes (when taking alendronate and risedronate) to 60 minutes (when taking ibandronate) before eating and must not lie down. Potential side effects of bisphosphonates include epigastric distress, heartburn, and esophagitis. Intravenous bisphosphonates have been associated with an influenza-like syndrome following the infusion. Bisphosphonates can also cause arthralgias and myalgias. Osteonecrosis of the jaw is a rare adverse event of abnormal bone growth in the jaw, more often associated with high-dose intravenous bisphosphonates in patients with cancer. Atrial fibrillation has been reported with intravenous zoledronic acid, but studies are trying to determine whether this is a class event.

The cost of most bisphosphonate therapy averages about $1000 per year (see Table 76-5). However, generic forms of alendronate are now available.

ESTROGEN AGONISTS-ANTAGONISTS

Estrogen agonists-antagonists were previously called selective estrogen-receptor modulators (SERMs) because they have some estrogen-like and anti–estrogen-like benefits. Raloxifene is currently approved for the prevention and treatment of osteoporosis. The Multiple Outcomes of Raloxifene Evaluation (MORE) trial found that bone mass was increased by 4% at the spine and 2.5% at the femoral neck over 3 years. This increase was associated with a 50% reduction in vertebral fractures. No change in nonvertebral or hip fractures was seen (see Table 76-5). Treatment was also associated with improved lipid status, as shown by decreased total and low-density lipoprotein cholesterol. Raloxifene is not associated with endometrial hyperplasia, thus patients do not have bleeding or spotting, nor do they have breast tenderness or swelling. Raloxifene also reduces the risk for invasive breast cancer in postmenopausal women with osteoporosis and in women at high risk for invasive breast cancer. Patients do have the same small risk of deep vein thrombosis or pulmonary embolus that is found with hormone replacement therapy (HRT). Raloxifene will not relieve postmenopausal symptoms and may exacerbate hot flushes. Raloxifene can be given with or without food in a daily oral form at 60 mg per day. Studies have not found a significant impact on cardiovascular disease.

HORMONE REPLACEMENT THERAPY

Investigators of the Women's Health Initiative, a large, randomized, placebo-controlled, multicenter trial evaluating HRT, reported a 36% reduction in hip and vertebral fractures after 5.2 years. In addition to improvements in bone mass, other benefits include improved lipid profile, decreased colon cancer, and decreased menopausal symptoms. However, because of the potential risks of HRT (cardiovascular events, breast cancer, deep vein thrombosis, pulmonary embolus, and gallbladder problems), it should only be used for relief of menopausal symptoms, and other agents should be used for the prevention or treatment of osteoporosis.

CALCITONIN

Calcitonin is a 32–amino acid peptide produced by the parafollicular cells of the thyroid gland. It is currently approved in a subcutaneous dose but is rarely used. The U.S. Food and Drug Administration (FDA) approved the use of calcitonin for the treatment of postmenopausal osteoporosis in a nasal form at a dose of 200 IU per day, taken in alternating nostrils. The Prevent Recurrence of Osteoporotic Fractures (PROOF) study, a large, multicenter trial, did not show any significant changes in bone mineral density after 3 years of treatment. However, the 200-IU dose was associated with a 50% reduction in vertebral fractures (see Table 76-5). No effect on nonvertebral or hip fractures was noted.

PARATHYROID HORMONE

Parathyroid hormone (PTH), an anabolic agent, has been shown to significantly increase bone mineral density and reduce both vertebral and nonvertebral fractures over 18 months. In a large study of postmenopausal women, teriparatide (PTH amino acid sequence 1 through 34), 20 μg, increased spinal bone mineral density by 9.7% and hip bone mineral density by 2.6%, and was associated with a 65% reduction in vertebral fractures and a 53% reduction in nonvertebral fractures. Teriparatide is taken as a sub-

cutaneous, daily dose and is approved by the FDA for postmenopausal women and men at high risk for fracture. PTH (1-84) is approved for use in Europe. Other forms of PTH and parathyroid hormone–related protein (PTHrP) are under investigation. Teriparatide is often prescribed for patients who fail, cannot tolerate, or have a contraindication for bisphosphonate therapy. Teriparatide, the only available anabolic agent in the United States, costs roughly $8500 per year.

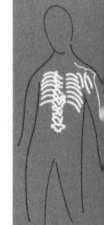

FUTURE THERAPIES

The receptor activator of nuclear factor kappa B (RANK) and its ligand (RANKL) are mediators of osteoclast activity. An antibody to RANKL has been shown to reduce osteoclast activity, decrease bone resorption, and improve bone mass. Strontium is an approved agent for the treatment of osteoporosis in Europe. The exact mechanism of action is not fully understood, but strontium is thought to stimulate osteoblast proliferation and inhibit osteoclast formation. Cathepsin K inhibition appears to inhibit bone resorption with no major impact on bone formation. Another anabolic therapeutic target includes inhibition of sclerostin (antibody to sclerostin). Studies are ongoing.

Combination therapy has been examined with two antiresorptive agents or antiresorptive and anabolic agents together. Studies examining two antiresorptive agents have included HRT plus alendronate, HRT plus risedronate, and alendronate plus raloxifene. Overall, studies with combination therapy have suggested greater improvements in bone mass over therapy with single agents. Although dual treatment with antiresorptive agents appears to be safe and well tolerated, studies have not shown greater fracture reduction, so this type of combination therapy with two antiresorptive agents is generally not given to patients. Studies have suggested greater improvements in bone mineral density with PTH plus raloxifene than with PTH alone. The combination of PTH plus alendronate provides no greater benefit than monotherapy with PTH. However, following PTH therapy, patients benefit from antiresorptive therapy with alendronate rather than calcium supplementation alone.

VERTEBROPLASTY AND KYPHOPLASTY

Vertebroplasty involves injection of cement (polymethylmethacrylate) into a compressed vertebra to prevent the vertebral body from further collapse. Alternatively, kyphoplasty introduces a balloon into the vertebral body to expand it, followed by cement placement inside the balloon. This approach not only expands the vertebral body but also increases some of the height. Although no controlled trials of these procedures have been conducted, studies suggest that they result in significant reductions in pain. Ongoing studies are needed to determine whether differences in outcomes can be found between vertebroplasty and kyphoplasty or whether potential risks exist to adjacent vertebrae after the procedure. Currently, these procedures are only recommended for patients with significant pain from vertebral fractures and are not routinely performed in asymptomatic patients with vertebral osteoporosis.

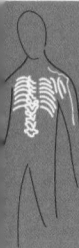

Prospectus for the Future

Osteoporosis affects about 50% of women older than 50 years. Although many risk factors exist for low bone mass, the major risk factors for osteoporosis include a personal history of fracture in adulthood, fracture history in a first-degree relative, low body weight, current smoking, and use of oral corticosteroid therapy. Because osteoporosis is largely a silent disease until manifestation of fracture, bone mineral density can be used to assess bone mass before a clinical fracture and is also used to monitor the disease. Osteoporosis is classified as a bone mineral density measurement of the hip or spine of equal to or less than −2.5 standard deviations below young adult peak bone mass. National guidelines suggest that all women older than 65 years have a bone mass measurement, and those younger than 65 years have a bone mass measurement if they have additional risk factors. General preventive measures for all patients include calcium of about 1200 mg daily in divided doses, vitamin D supplementation of up to 1000 IU per day, weight-bearing exercise, and fall prevention for older adults. The mainstays of prevention and treatment include daily, once-weekly, or once-monthly oral bisphosphonates or intravenous bisphosphonates every 3 or 12 months. Raloxifene, an estrogen agonist-antagonist, and calcitonin have also been approved as therapy for osteoporosis. Teriparatide (PTH [1-34]), an anabolic agent, is approved for treatment of patients at high risk for osteoporosis. Future therapies include other forms of PTH, other anabolic agents, an antibody to RANKL (a mediator of osteoclast activity), and cathepsin K. Monotherapy with PTH appears to be of greater benefit than combination therapy with an antiresorptive.

References

Kanis JA: Diagnosis of osteoporosis and assessment of fracture risk. Lancet 359:1929-1936, 2002.

National Osteoporosis Foundation: Clinician's Guide to Prevention and Treatment of Osteoporosis. Washington DC, The Foundation, 2008.

U.S. Department of Health and Human Services: Bone Health and Osteoporosis (USHHS): A Report of the Surgeon General. Rockville, MD, USHHS, Office of the Surgeon General, 2004.

U.S. Preventive Services Task Force: Screening for osteoporosis in postmenopausal women: Recommendations and rationale. Ann Intern Med 137:526-528, 2002.

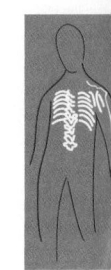

Paget Disease of Bone

Mara J. Horwitz and G. David Roodman

Paget disease is one of the more common bone diseases in adults. In contrast to most other metabolic bone diseases (discussed in previous chapters), which are diffuse and involve the entire skeleton, Paget disease is a focal bone disorder. It can be monostotic (involving a single bone) or polyostotic (involving multiple bones). Although Paget disease is a chronic condition, over the long course of the disease, new lesions rarely develop. The clinical description of Paget disease by Sir James Paget over 100 years ago is still accurate today. The primary cellular abnormality of Paget disease is increased osteoclastic bone resorption. This intense bone resorption is followed by exuberant formation of new bone that is of poor quality. Most patients with Paget disease are asymptomatic, and the disorder is detected by an increased serum alkaline phosphatase level or unexpectedly on a routine radiograph. However, a significant proportion of patients can have bone pain, skeletal deformity, fractures, high-output cardiac failure, or nerve compression syndromes. The most dreaded complication of Paget disease is development of osteosarcoma in the pagetic lesion. Although this development is extremely rare (<1%), the incidence of osteosarcoma in patients with Paget disease is about 1000-fold greater than in age-matched normal controls.

Incidence and Prevalence

Paget disease affects about 2% of the population older than 45 years in the United States. It is common in Great Britain, Germany, France, Australia, and New Zealand but is extremely rare in Scandinavia, Asia, sub-Saharan Africa, and the Arab Middle East. In some areas of Great Britain, the incidence of Paget disease may reach 5% to 6%. However, the incidence of Paget disease appears to have decreased during the past 20 years for unknown reasons. Paget disease is most commonly diagnosed in patients older than 50 years and has only rarely been reported in patients younger than 40 years. Estimates are that the incidence nearly doubles with every decade past the age of 50 years. Both men and women are affected, but it has a slight male predominance.

Etiologic Factors

The cause of Paget disease is unknown. Studies over the past 30 years, including immunohistochemical, ultrastructural, and in situ hybridization studies, have suggested a possible viral origin for Paget disease. Osteoclasts in pagetic lesions are markedly increased in number and size. A striking feature of osteoclasts from patients with Paget disease is the characteristic nuclear inclusions that are similar to nucleocapsids of paramyxoviruses. Several groups have demonstrated that these nuclear inclusions cross-react with antibodies against respiratory syncytial virus, measles virus, and canine distemper virus. Furthermore, in situ hybridization studies have shown the presence of measles virus nucleocapsid transcripts in pagetic osteoclasts. Friedrichs and associates have reported the full-length sequence of the measles virus nucleocapsid protein from a patient with Paget disease. Further supporting a potential role of paramyxoviruses in Paget disease, Kurihara and colleagues transfected normal osteoclast precursors with the measles virus nucleocapsid gene and reported that the osteoclasts that formed were very similar to pagetic osteoclasts. Recently, Kurihara and colleagues have targeted the measles virus nucleocapsid gene to cells in the osteoclast lineage in transgenic mice and shown that these mice develop bone lesions and osteoclast that are characteristic of pagetic lesions in patients. Other groups in Great Britain have reported that canine distemper virus is present in pagetic osteoclasts. However, other investigators have failed to detect paramyxovirus transcripts in pagetic osteoclasts or their precursors. Thus, the role that paramyxovirus plays in the cause of Paget disease is controversial.

In addition to a viral origin for Paget disease, a strong genetic component exists. Multiple families have been identified that demonstrate vertical transmission of Paget disease in an autosomal dominant fashion with variable penetrance. These large kindred links have led to the identification of several chromosomal loci for Paget disease, including chromosomes 18, 5, 6, and 2. The most common locus that is linked to Paget disease has been identified on chromosome 5. This gene encodes sequestosome 1, an adapter protein that may be involved in the receptor activator of nuclear factor kappa B ligand (RANKL)–signaling pathway. Mutations in this gene occur in almost 30% of patients with familial Paget disease and have also been reported in a small proportion of patients with sporadic rather than familial Paget disease. In one family from Japan with very-early-onset Paget disease, a mutation in the *RANK* gene on chromosome 18 has been reported. RANKL and its receptor, RANK, are critical factors involved in osteoclast formation and survival. However, the role that mutations in sequestosome 1 play in the development of Paget disease is still unclear. Kurihara and colleagues have recently targeted the mutant sequestosome 1 gene to human osteoclasts in vitro and to osteoclasts in transgenic mice and have shown that the osteoclasts that form do not express the characteristics of pagetic osteoclasts and the mice harboring the mutant gene do not develop pagetic bone lesions.

Pathologic and Pathophysiologic Factors

In pagetic lesions, osteoclasts are increased in number and size and have increased rough endoplasmic reticulum and mitochondria, consistent with their increased metabolic activity. Osteoblasts, which are morphologically normal, are also increased in number in the lesions. Initially, osteoclastic bone resorption is increased, followed by increased numbers of osteoblasts that form large amounts of woven bone (Fig. 77-1). This marked increase in osteoblasts accounts for the sclerotic lesions so typical on radiographic examination (Fig. 77-2), for the increase uptake of radionuclide on bone scan (Fig. 77-3), and for the increase in serum alkaline phosphatase, the biochemical hallmark of Paget disease. Ultimately, the pagetic lesions become sclerotic. The vascularity of the abnormal bone is increased.

The increased bone resorption probably results from increased production of cytokines that enhance osteoclast formation. For example, levels of interleukin-6, a potent stimulator of osteoclast formation, are increased in pagetic lesions but not in normal bone. In addition, RANKL levels also are increased in the bones involved with Paget disease but not in the uninvolved bones from the same patients. The factors that enhance bone formation have not been clearly identified but may include transforming growth factor-β, insulin-like growth factor, and fibroblast growth factor, which are present in large quantities in bone and can be released by osteoclastic bone resorption.

Clinical Presentation

Paget disease may affect any skeletal site. It most commonly involves the pelvis, vertebrae, skull, tibia, and femur. It may be monostotic (affecting only one bone) or more commonly polyostotic (affecting two or more bones) and is often asymmetrical in its distribution. Although progression of the disease may occur at a given site, the appearance of new lesions is rare. As noted previously, most patients with Paget disease are asymptomatic, and the disease is detected by an increased serum alkaline phosphatase level or discovered unexpectedly on a routine radiograph. Among patients

who are symptomatic, bone pain is the most common complaint (Table 77-1). Bone pain in Paget disease can be due to the pagetic lesion itself but more often results from the joint distortion and nerve compression caused by adjacent pagetic bone.

Arthritis is often found in joints near areas involved with Paget disease, particularly when subchondral bone is affected or when the integrity of the joint is compromised by enlarged or distorted bones. Skeletal deformities occur most frequently in affected sites in the skull and long bones of the lower extremities. The skull can become enlarged, and temporal bone involvement may affect hearing and cause other cranial nerve palsies or headaches. Softening of the base of the skull may produce flattening (*platybasia*) with the development of basilar invagination and may lead to cranial nerve and spinal cord compression syndromes. Affected long bones of the lower extremity can become bowed. Fissure fractures along the convex surface of long bones and pathologic fractures in weight-bearing bones are not uncommon. Spinal cord or nerve root compression with associated radicular pain and weakness may result from expanding pagetic lesions in the spine. Because pagetic lesions tend to be highly vascular, increased warmth in the skin over affected areas is often present.

Complications and Associated Conditions

Secondary arthritis is a common and often debilitating complication of periarticular Paget disease. Hyperuricemia and gout may occur with increased frequency in affected persons. Highly vascularized pagetic lesions have been reported to cause a *vascular steal* syndrome, and high-output cardiac failure has been described in severe disease. The most serious complication of Paget disease is sarcomatous degeneration. This situation occurs most often in the setting of severe polyostotic disease and may be heralded by a sudden increase in pain, a soft tissue mass, an abrupt increase in serum alkaline phosphatase, or a pathologic fracture. Although extremely rare (<1%), osteosarcoma in Paget patients is about 1000-fold greater than in age-matched normal controls. Sarcomatous degeneration is the main cause of death caused by Paget disease. Although most Paget-associated tumors are osteosarcomas, fibrosarcomas, and chondrosarcomas may also be seen.

Diagnostic Evaluation

Paget disease is most often diagnosed using a combination of biochemical markers of bone turnover and radiologic abnormalities. Biochemical markers of bone formation (such as serum alkaline phosphatase) and bone resorption (such as N-telopeptide cross-links [NTX], C-telopeptide cross-links [CTX], and phenazopyridine [Pyridium] cross-links) are usually increased in patients with active disease. For most patients with Paget disease, serum total alkaline phosphatase is an adequate and sensitive indicator of disease activity. However, serum bone-specific alkaline phosphatase may be a more sensitive marker than serum total alkaline

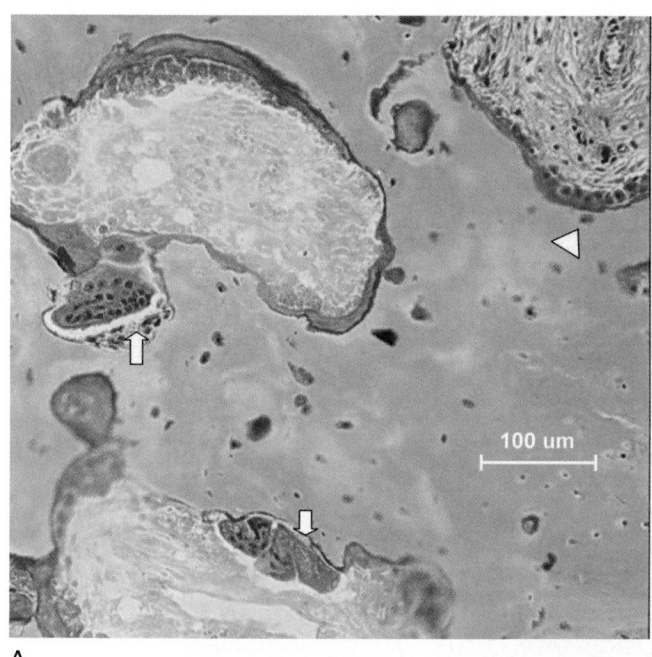

A

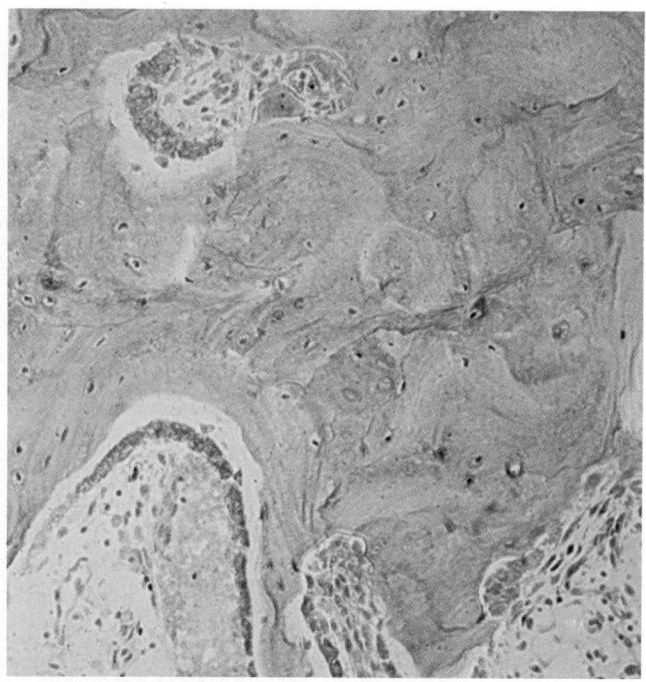

B

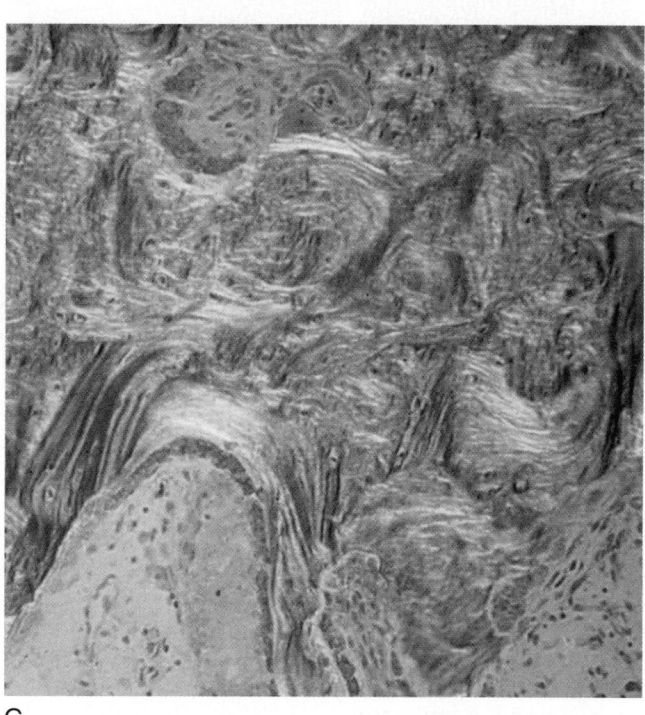

C

Figure 77-1 Typical histologic abnormalities present in bone biopsies from patients with Paget disease. **A,** Increased numbers of abnormal osteoclasts *(arrows)* and increased numbers of osteoblasts are seen *(arrowhead).* **B,** Increased numbers of osteoblasts are shown forming large amounts of woven bone. **C,** Polarized light view of the specimen shown in **B** demonstrating the mosaic pattern of highly disorganized woven bone formed by osteoblasts in Paget disease. Large amounts of sclerotic bone are present. (Photomicrographs courtesy of Dr. David Dempster, Helen Hayes Hospital, Columbia University.)

phosphatase for assessing disease in patients with low levels of disease activity. Serum osteocalcin, another marker of bone formation, is often in the normal range and is not a clinically useful marker of disease activity.

A bone scan at the time of diagnosis is the most useful test to define the location and extent of lesions (see Fig. 77-3). Radiographs of the affected areas confirm the presence of

Paget disease and are useful for evaluating complications and local disease progression (see Fig. 77-2). The radiologic abnormalities seen on standard radiographs may reflect one of the three distinctive stages of pagetic lesions. The earliest lesions are osteolytic lesions, which are often observed as *osteoporosis circumscripta* in the skull (see Fig. 77-2A) or as an advancing *blade of grass* in long bones (see Fig. 77-2B).

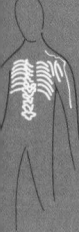

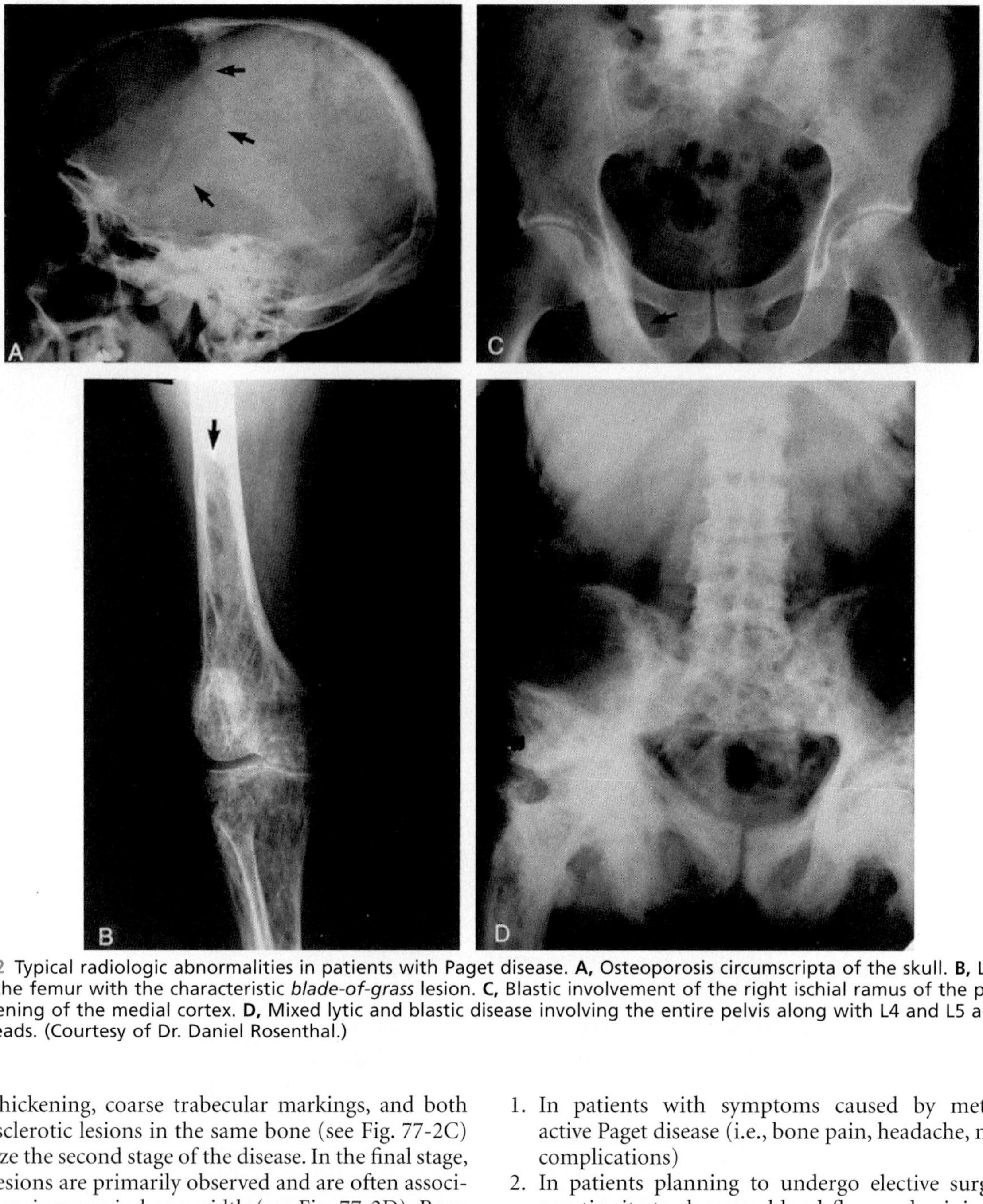

Figure 77-2 Typical radiologic abnormalities in patients with Paget disease. **A,** Osteoporosis circumscripta of the skull. **B,** Lytic lesions in the femur with the characteristic *blade-of-grass* lesion. **C,** Blastic involvement of the right ischial ramus of the pelvis with thickening of the medial cortex. **D,** Mixed lytic and blastic disease involving the entire pelvis along with L4 and L5 and both femoral heads. (Courtesy of Dr. Daniel Rosenthal.)

Cortical thickening, coarse trabecular markings, and both lytic and sclerotic lesions in the same bone (see Fig. 77-2C) characterize the second stage of the disease. In the final stage, sclerotic lesions are primarily observed and are often associated with an increase in bone width (see Fig. 77-2D). Bone biopsy is rarely needed to diagnose Paget disease and should be avoided in weight-bearing areas. However, it is important to distinguish Paget disease of bone from other disorders associated with osteoblastic lesions such as metastatic prostate cancer, fibrous dysplasia, focal osteosclerosis, a poorly healing fracture, and giant cell tumors. In addition to radiologic evaluation, formal audiometry to assess hearing loss is indicated in patients with skull involvement.

Treatment

The two major goals of therapy are to relieve symptoms and to prevent complications. Potential indications for treatment include the following four situations:

1. In patients with symptoms caused by metabolically active Paget disease (i.e., bone pain, headache, neurologic complications)
2. In patients planning to undergo elective surgery on a pagetic site to decrease blood flow and minimize intraoperative blood loss
3. In the management of hypercalcemia, which is a rare complication that can occur when a patient with severe Paget disease is immobilized for a prolonged period
4. In patients who may be at high risk for complications if disease progresses locally, such as those at risk for bowing deformities in long bones, for hearing loss as a result of skull enlargement, for neurologic complications resulting from vertebral involvement, and for secondary arthritis where a pagetic lesion is located next to a major joint

Treatment of Paget disease usually involves a combination of nonpharmacologic therapy (i.e., physical therapy) and pharmacologic therapy. Pharmacologic therapy includes antiresorptive agents (Table 77-2) and analgesics for pain

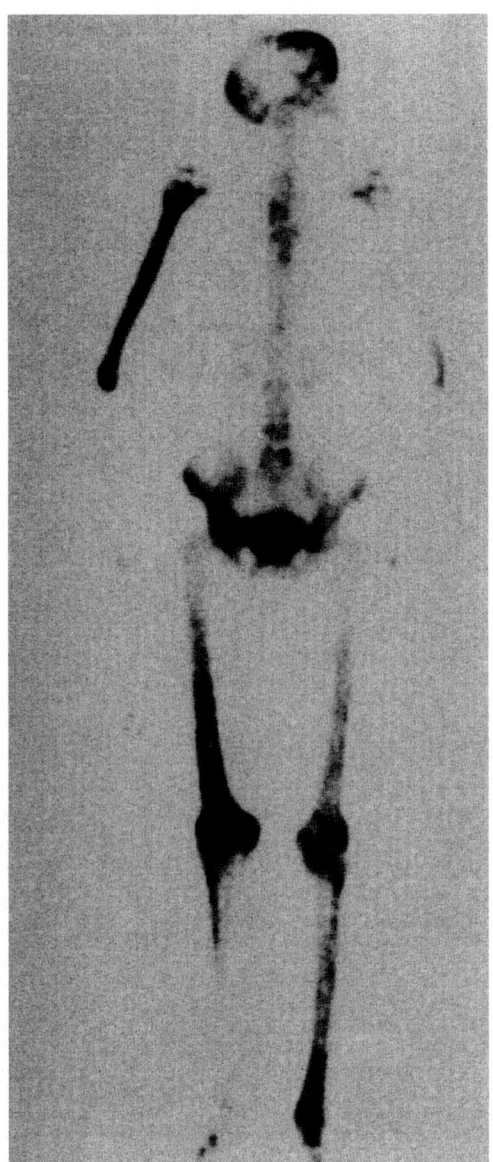

Figure 77-3 Whole-body bone scan demonstrating abnormalities in a patient with polyostotic Paget disease. Increased radionuclide uptake is seen in the skull, right humerus, pelvis, right femur, and left tibia. (Courtesy of The Paget's Foundation.)

management. The second-generation bisphosphonates form the mainstay of therapy for Paget disease. The bisphosphonates decrease bone resorption at pagetic sites by inhibiting osteoclasts both directly and indirectly. The aim of therapy is to decrease the biochemical markers of bone metabolism (i.e., total alkaline phosphatase) well into the normal range. Currently six bisphosphonates have been approved by the U.S. Food and Drug Administration for treating Paget disease: intravenous zoledronate and pamidronate and oral etidronate, tiludronate, alendronate, and risedronate. Etidronate and tiludronate are less potent than the other bisphosphonates and therefore rarely used in the United States today. Previously, etidronate sodium was the only bisphosphonate available, and although effective, its use was limited because of a tendency to induce mineralization disorders when given at higher doses or for a longer period.

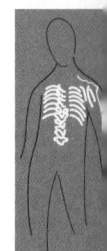

Table 77-1 Clinical Manifestations of Paget Disease

Musculoskeletal pain
Degenerative arthritis in joints near affected areas
Headaches
Skeletal deformity
Pathologic fractures
Enlarged skull
Erythema and warmth over pagetic bones
Hearing loss
Platybasia with or without basilar invagination
Neurologic compression syndromes
Angioid streaks in retina
Increased cardiac output; rarely congestive heart failure
Bone tumors
  Osteogenic sarcoma
  Fibrosarcoma
  Chrondrosarcoma
  Reparative granuloma
  Giant cell tumor
Laboratory abnormalities
  Increased serum alkaline phosphatase (bone fraction)
  Increased urinary hydroxyproline
  Hypercalciuria and hypercalcemia during immobilization
  Hyperuricemia
Characteristic radiographs
Increased uptake on bone scan

Table 77-2 Treatment of Paget Disease

Drug	Route	Dose
Bisphosphonates		
Alendronate (Fosamax)	Oral	40 mg/day for 6 months
Risedronate (Actonel)	Oral	30 mg/day for 2 months
Pamidronate (Aredia)	Intravenous	30-60 mg/day for 3 days
Zoledronate (Zometa)	Intravenous	5 mg single infusion
Etidronate (Didronel)	Oral	400 mg/day for 6 months
Tiludronate (Skelid)	Oral	400 mg/day for 3 months
Other		
Calcitonin (Miacalcin)	Subcutaneous injection	50-100 U/day

The introduction of the more potent amino-bisphosphonates—pamidronate, alendronate, risedronate, and zoledronate—represents a significant advance in the treatment of Paget disease. These agents often induce a biochemical remission in patients with Paget disease without producing mineralization defects at the recommended doses. Intravenous pamidronate can be given as two or three 30- to 60-mg infusions in patients with mild disease. More severe disease may require 60 to 90 mg on a weekly or twice-weekly basis. Cumulative doses of 240 to 480 mg may be required in some patients. Alendronate normalizes markers of bone turnover in most patients with Paget disease when

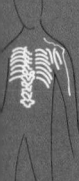

given in an oral dose of 40 mg per day for 6 months. Fewer than 10% of patients treated with alendronate have a biochemical recurrence within 12 months. Risedronate has similar effects on biochemical indices for bone turnover and is recommended at 30 mg per day for 2 months. Intravenous zoledronate is the most potent of the bisphosphonates and may be an alternative in patients with refractory disease. It has been shown to normalize alkaline phosphatase levels in more than 88% of patients with sustained remissions lasting at least 24 months after a single dose. It is given as a 5-mg single intravenous infusion. Calcium and vitamin D supplementation therapy is recommended for patients taking the more potent bisphosphonates to prevent hypocalcemia or secondary hyperparathyroidism. Resistance to individual bisphosphonates can occur. However, patients often respond to an alternate bisphosphonate. Therefore, some patients may require the use of more than one medication in the long-term management of the disease. Serum alkaline phosphatase should be measured at baseline and 2 to 3 months after the treatment is completed.

Salmon calcitonin was, at one time, the agent of choice for the treatment of Paget disease. The usual dose of 50 to 100 U per day by subcutaneous injection has been shown to reduce markers of bone turnover by up to 50%, decrease bone pain, and decrease many of the vascular and neurologic complications associated with Paget disease. However, secondary resistance to salmon calcitonin is not uncommon. It is not as potent as the bisphosphonates. Use of salmon calcitonin today is limited primarily to patients who are unable to receive either oral or intravenous bisphosphonates (i.e., creatinine clearance < 35).

Pain caused by bone deformity or arthritic changes is often relieved with acetaminophen or nonsteroidal anti-inflammatory drugs.

Orthopedic surgery may be indicated in the management of pagetic lesions when a complete fracture through pagetic bone occurs, to realign a severely arthritic knee, and for total joint arthroplasty in a severely affected hip or knee. Preoperative treatment with a bisphosphonate is recommended when possible in an attempt to decrease the vascularity of the lesion and minimize intraoperative bleeding. Surgical decompression may also be indicated if cranial nerve involvement or spinal nerve root compression is not relieved with medical therapy.

Prospectus for the Future

Although Paget disease is the second most common bone disease after osteoporosis, for unknown reasons, the incidence appears to be decreasing. Some experts believe this decline may be related to a decrease in the frequency of measles or other paramyxoviral infections with widespread vaccination. The reasons for this decline remain one principal unanswered question in Paget disease. The second major area of controversy in Paget disease continues to surround its cause. The contribution of a genetic component versus a viral component remains the largest area of ongoing Paget research. On the viral side of the argument, although studies during the past 30 years—immunohistochemical, ultrastructural, and in situ hybridization studies—have suggested a paramyxoviral origin for Paget disease, other investigators have failed to detect paramyxovirus transcripts in pagetic osteoclasts or their precursors. On the genetic side, mutations in the gene that encodes an adaptor protein in the RANKL-signaling pathway occur in almost 30% of patients with familial Paget disease. In addition, genetic linkage of Paget disease with chromosomal loci on chromosomes 18, 5, 6, and 2 also exists. Obviously, combined genetic and viral causes are possible and probably likely. Ongoing research in these areas will continue to shed light on this disease of complex origin.

References

Altman RD, Bloch DA, Hochberg MC, et al: Prevalence of Paget's disease of bone in the United States. J Bone Miner Res 15:461-465, 2000.

Kurihara N, Hiruma Y, Zhou H, et al: Mutation of the sequestosome 1 (*p62*) gene increases osteoclastogenesis but does not induce Paget disease. J Clin Invest 117:133-142, 2007.

Kurihara N, Zhou H, Reddy SV, et al: Expression of measles virus nucleocapsid protein in osteoclasts induces Paget's disease-like bone lesions in mice. J Bone Miner Res 21:446-455, 2006.

The Paget Foundation and the NIH Osteoporosis and Related Bone Diseases National Resource Center: A Physician's Guide to The Management of Paget's Disease of Bone: An Educational Outreach Project of the Paget Foundation for Paget's Disease of Bone and Related Disorders and NIH Osteoporosis and Related Bone Diseases National Resource Center. New York, The Paget Foundation, 2007.

Proceeding of the 3rd International Symposium on Paget's Disease, Napa, California. J Bone Miner Res 14(Suppl 2):1-104, 1998.

Roodman GD, Windle JJ: Paget disease of bone. J Clin Invest 115:200-208, 2005.

Selby PL, Davie MWJ, Ralston SH: Guidelines on the management of Paget's disease of bone. Bone 31:366-373, 2002.

Siris ES, Roodman GD: Paget's disease of bone. In Favus MJ (ed): Primer on the Metabolic Bone Diseases and Disorders of Mineral Metabolism, 6th ed. Washington DC, American Society for Bone and Mineral Research, 2006, pp 320-329.

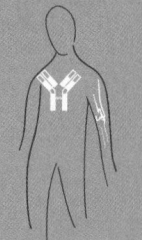

Section XVI

Musculoskeletal and Connective Tissue Disease

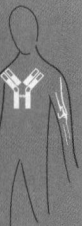

Approach to the Patient with Rheumatic Disease

Niveditha Mohan

Rheumatic diseases encompass a range of musculo-skeletal and systemic disorders that often involve joints and periarticular tissues and include diseases that are thought to be autoimmune in cause. The causes of arthritis range from local trauma to infection, gout, osteoarthritis, and autoimmune connective tissue diseases, such as rheumatoid arthritis and systemic lupus erythematosus (SLE). Distinguishing localized processes from those that are systemic, executing logical diagnostic procedures, and embarking on appropriate therapeutic courses depend on careful clinical evaluation. As in other areas of medicine, history and physical examination are paramount, and laboratory tests are more confirmatory than diagnostic. The *connective tissue screen* is performed at the bedside, not in the laboratory. The practice of either including or excluding systemic connective tissue disease on the basis of laboratory panels is unreliable and therefore unwise.

Musculoskeletal History and Examination

Features in the medical history that are useful in distinguishing different types of arthritis are listed in Tables 78-1 and 78-2. When a patient has a musculoskeletal complaint, a thorough history and physical examination will provide the diagnosis in the majority of patients. Further investigations are necessary to confirm or support the clinical diagnosis. A logical approach to musculoskeletal complaints is indispensable to arriving at the correct diagnosis.

The first step is to confirm that the complaint is truly originating from the musculoskeletal system and not referred pain relating to other organ system pathology (e.g., left shoulder pain secondary to cardiac disease). The next question would be to define whether the problem is articular or extra-articular based on the history of the presenting illness. Appreciating the demographics of different illnesses provides useful information for diagnostic evaluation. Spondyloarthropathies are more commonly diagnosed in pre-dominantly young men, SLE in young women, gout in middle-aged men and postmenopausal women, and osteoarthritis in the older adult population. The age of the patient can be a clue to specific rheumatic disorders. Asymmetrical pain and swelling in the knees have different connotations in a 70-year-old patient than they do in a 20-year-old patient. Other host characteristics that may have a bearing on the cause of disease include immune status.

Immunocompromised patients should always be evaluated for infectious arthritis; patients with HIV may have a severe form of Reiter syndrome or a sudden flare of psoriasis or psoriatic arthritis. The patient's history provides the basis for distinguishing inflammatory from noninflammatory arthropathies. *Inflammatory arthritis* is characterized by pain at rest, morning stiffness, gelling, joint swelling, and joint tenderness. In *osteoarthritis* and *nonarthritic musculoskeletal problems,* pain is generally not present at rest and is precipitated by activity. Occasionally, however, osteoarthritic joints are stiff and are initially improved with activity. In *crystal-induced arthritis* the onset is abrupt, in *septic arthritis* it is less so, and in most other disorders it is slow and insidious. Patterns of joint involvement—monoarthritis (1, septic or crystal-induced arthritis), pauciarthritis or oligoarthritis (2 to 4, Reiter or psoriatic arthritis), or polyarthritis (5 and above, rheumatoid arthritis or lupus)—can be typical of certain disorders. Symmetry, migratory features, large versus small joints, and locations (axial versus appendicular) characteristic of specific diseases are also key items in the patient's history. Presence of enthesopathy can be a clue to the presence of a spondyloarthropathy. Constitutional features such as fatigue, weight loss, and fever are seen in systemic autoimmune disease and infection but not in localized conditions. It is also important to do a thorough review of systems to identify the "company it keeps" that will provide clues to defining associated systemic syndromes. Many exceptions can be found to these basic demographic and clinical generalizations, but they are often helpful starting points when a patient is being evaluated for the first time.

On physical examination, active and passive range of motion in all joints should be carefully assessed, and the

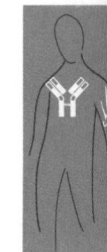

presence of tenderness, swelling, warmth, erythema, deformity, and joint effusions should be evaluated (Fig. 78-1). Patients are frequently unaware of detectable joint abnormalities, including deformity and effusion, and the presence of either is a sign of joint disease. Reported pain may be referred from another site, and this feature can be elucidated by examination. Thus pain in the knee is often a sign of hip disease and may be reproduced on examination of the hip. The presence of palpable synovitis, or a thickening of the synovial membrane, is helpful in diagnosing inflammatory arthritides such as rheumatoid arthritis. Different diseases have distinctive patterns of joint involvement, which provides critical diagnostic information. For example, prominent disease of distal interphalangeal joints is seen in psoriasis and in inflammatory osteoarthritis. Wrist and metacarpophalangeal involvement are almost universal in rheumatoid arthritis but rare in osteoarthritis. Examination of the axial skeleton may reveal diminished lumbar flexion, decreased rotational motion of the spine, and decreased chest expansion, as well as features of ankylosing spondylitis and other spondyloarthropathies. Patients may report symptoms in only a single joint, but finding additional affected joints on physical examination could change the entire evaluation of a patient.

Rheumatic diseases may involve any organ system, and a full physical examination should be performed on all patients. Alopecia (SLE), funduscopic changes (SLE), uveitis (spondyloarthropathy and juvenile arthritis), conjunctivitis (reactive arthritis), sicca symptoms (Sjögren syndrome), oral and other mucous membrane ulcers (reactive arthritis, SLE, and Behçet syndrome), lymphadenopathy (SLE and Sjögren syndrome), and cutaneous lesions (psoriasis, dermatomyositis, scleroderma, SLE, and vasculitides) should be considerations. Recurrent otorhinolaryngolic complaints, such as sinusitis, should be suspected for Wegener's granulomatosis. Lesions of psoriasis in the scalp, umbilicus, and anal crease; thickening of the skin on the fingers in scleroderma; and mucous membrane ulcers are often overlooked. The lung examination may show evidence of interstitial fibrosis (scleroderma, SLE, rheumatoid arthritis, and myositis), and a cardiac evaluation may reveal aortic insufficiency (SLE and spondyloarthropathy), pulmonary hypertension (systemic sclerosis), or evidence of cardiomyopathy (systemic sclerosis, myositis, and amyloidosis). Pleural and pericardial rubs may be present in SLE, rheumatoid arthritis, and scleroderma. Hepatosplenomegaly (SLE and rheumatoid arthritis) and abdominal distention (scleroderma) are also valuable clinical clues. Muscular examination may reveal weakness from myositis, neuropathy (vasculitis and SLE), or myopathy (steroid myopathy) or synovitis (rheumatoid arthritis, SLE, spondyloarthropathy). A complete neurologic examination is critical and may reveal carpal tunnel syndrome, peripheral neuropathy such as mononeuritis multiplex (an asymmetrical sensory and/or a motor

---

Table 78-1 Clinical Features Helpful in Evaluation of Arthritis

Age, sex, ethnicity, family history
Pattern of joint involvement
Monoarticular, oligoarticular, polyarticular
Large versus small joints
Symmetry
Insidious versus rapid onset
Inflammatory versus noninflammatory pain (e.g., morning stiffness, gelling, night pain)
Presence of constitutional symptoms and signs (e.g., fever, fatigue, weight loss)
Presence of synovitis, bursitis, tendinitis
Involvement of other organ systems (e.g., rash, mucous membrane lesions, nail lesions)
Presence of arthritis-associated diseases (e.g., psoriasis, inflammatory bowel disease)
Anemia, proteinuria, azotemia
Presence of erosive joint disease

Table 78-2 Differentiating Features of Common Arthritides

Disease	Demographics	Joints Involved	Special Features	Laboratory Findings
Gout	Men, postmenopausal women	Monoarticular or oligoarticular	Podagra, rapid onset of attack, polyarticular gout, tophi	SF: Crystals, high WBC, >80% PMN
Septic arthritis	Any age	Usually large joints	Fever, chills	SF: High WBC, >90% PMN, culture
Osteoarthritis	Increases with age	Weight-bearing, hands		Noninflammatory SF
Rheumatoid arthritis	Any age, predominantly women ages 20-50 yr	Symmetrical, small joints disease	Rheumatoid nodules, extra-articular	SF: High WBC, >70% PMN
Reactive arthritis (Reiter syndrome)	Young males	Oligoarticular, asymmetrical	Urethritis, conjunctivitis, skin and mucous membranes	SF: Moderate WBC, >50% PMN
Spondyloarthropathy	Young to middle-aged men	Axial skeleton, pelvis (sacroiliac joints)	Uveitis, aortic insufficiency, enthesopathy	
Systemic lupus erythematosus	Women in childbearing years	Hands, knees	Nonerosive joint disease, autoantibodies, mostly mononuclear; multi-organ disease	SF: Low-to-moderate WBC, almost 100% have antinuclear antibodies

PMN, neutrophils; SF, synovial fluid; WBC, white blood cells.

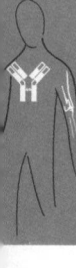

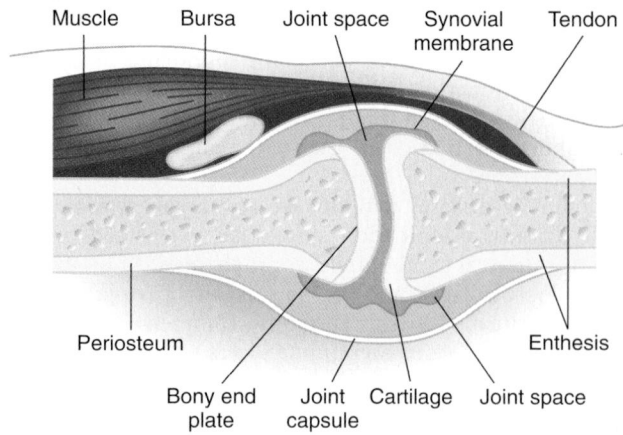

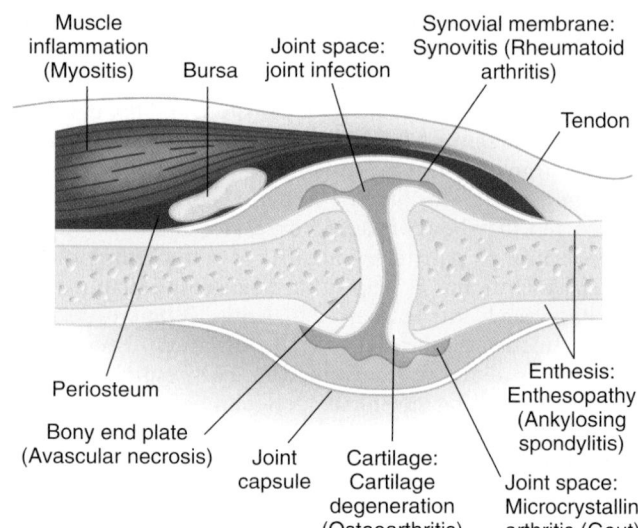

Figure 78-1 Anatomic structures of the musculoskeletal system *(left)*. Location of musculoskeletal disease processes *(right)*. (From Gordon DA: Approach to the patient with musculoskeletal disease. In Bennett JC, Plum F [eds]: Cecil Textbook of Medicine, 20th ed. Philadelphia, WB Saunders, 1996, p 1440.)

neuropathy as seen in many vasculitides), and central nervous system disease (SLE and vasculitis). Recurrent miscarriages, livedo reticularis, Raynaud phenomenon, and recurrent thrombotic events are suspicious for antiphospholipid antibody syndrome (primary or secondary to SLE).

At the initial evaluation, one important question is whether diagnosis and treatment of the patient's problem require urgent attention. Infectious processes obviously belong in this category. The presence of acute joint inflammation, fever, and systemic signs such as chills, night sweats, and leukocytosis all provide supporting evidence for infection. Gouty arthritis may share some or all of these clinical features, but its onset tends to be more abrupt. Inflammation extending beyond the margins of the joint is characteristic of septic arthritis and is otherwise seen only in crystal disease and rheumatoid arthritis. Nonarticular processes—cellulitis, septic bursitis, tenosynovitis, and phlebitis—may mimic infectious arthritis. Analysis of synovial fluid is the key to diagnosis.

Acute nerve entrapment or spinal cord compression, tendon rupture, and fractures may all occur in the absence of obvious trauma. Spinal cord compression may be the result of a herniated disk or vertebral subluxation. Tendon rupture may occur in inflammatory arthritides, particularly in the wrist in rheumatoid arthritis. Pelvic and other *insufficiency* fractures may be seen in patients with osteoporosis or osteomalacia. Careful musculoskeletal and neurologic examinations help in the detection of these disorders, each of which requires urgent treatment.

In systemic rheumatic diseases, the onset is usually more insidious, and the clinical course is prolonged. Treatment is usually less urgent and can be safely deferred, particularly if the diagnosis is uncertain. However, potential threats to life or the possibility of serious and/or irreversible organ damage may exist in some disorders. In SLE and systemic vasculitis, patients may have central or peripheral nervous system disease, including brain and peripheral nerve infarcts, glomerulonephritis, inflammatory or hemorrhagic lung disease, coronary artery involvement, intestinal infarcts, and digital infarcts. Threatened digital loss may also be seen in sclero-

derma and Raynaud's disease. Renal crisis may occur in scleroderma, with vasculopathy leading to renal infarcts, azotemia, micro-angiopathy, and severe hypertension. Urgent therapy to ameliorate or prevent damage may be indicated in these disorders. In giant-cell arteritis, acute blindness is a potential complication, and the diagnosis requires urgent therapy even before confirmatory biopsy. Acute inflammatory myositis should be promptly treated because it may progress rapidly to the involvement of the respiratory musculature. In some cases, major organ involvement may be occult. When systemic disease is suggested, the patient's lung and kidneys should be carefully evaluated.

Laboratory Testing

As noted earlier, *synovial fluid analysis* is an important part of the evaluation of arthritis (Table 78-3). It helps distinguish inflammatory from noninflammatory arthritis and can be diagnostic of infectious arthritis or crystal disease. Synovial fluid consists of an ultrafiltrate of plasma into which synovial lining cells secrete hyaluronic acid, which is responsible for the high viscosity of synovial fluid. Evaluation of synovial fluid should include the following: (1) cell count and differential, (2) crystal examination for sodium urate and calcium phosphate dehydrate crystals, and (3) Gram stain and culture. Synovial fluid glucose and protein are not diagnostically useful tests. Synovial fluid examination should be performed in the evaluation of all acute arthritides and all situations in which joint infection is probable and ideally should be performed on at least one occasion in the evaluation of chronic inflammatory arthritis. Aspiration and analysis of fluid before therapy are critical to appropriate decision making.

Although autoantibodies are often considered the hallmark of rheumatic diseases, their diagnostic utility in individual patients is actually much less than commonly believed. Although almost 100% of patients with SLE have antinuclear antibodies, as do most patients with scleroderma and autoimmune myositis, the proportion of patients with positive

Table 78-3 Classification of Synovial Effusions by Synovial White Cell Count

Group	Diagnosis (Examples)	Appearance	Synovial Fluid White Cell Count (mm³)*	Polymorphonuclear Cells (%)
Normal		Clear, pale yellow	0-200	<10
I. Noninflammatory	Osteoarthritis; trauma	Clear to slightly turbid	50-2000 (600)	<30
II. Mildly inflammatory	Systemic lupus erythematosus	Clear to slightly turbid	100-9000 (3000)	<20
III. Severely inflammatory (noninfectious)	Gout	Turbid	2000-160,000 (21,000)	~70
	Pseudogout	Turbid	500-75,000 (14,000)	~70
	Rheumatoid arthritis	Turbid	2000-80,000 (19,000)	~70
IV. Severely inflammatory (infectious)	Bacterial infections	Very turbid	5000-250,000 (80,000)	~90
	Tuberculosis	Turbid	2500-100,000 (20,000)	~60

*Mean values in parentheses.

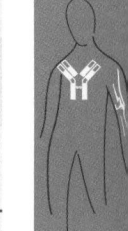

test results in other rheumatic diseases is much lower. Conversely, 15% to 25% of healthy persons have antinuclear antibodies when commercial test kits are used, sometimes in high titers. Older persons and patients with nonrheumatic systemic diseases such as malignant disease and nonrheumatic autoimmune diseases such as thyroiditis or hypothyroidism have even higher frequencies. Other specific autoantibodies may be more useful and are discussed in subsequent chapters. *Rheumatoid factor* is found in approximately 80% to 90% of patients with rheumatoid arthritis but also in a variety of other rheumatic diseases, in chronic infection, in neoplasia, and in almost any state that can cause chronic hyperglobulinemia. Neither a positive nor a negative test result is diagnostic, and results should be interpreted only in clinical context. Antibodies to cyclic citrullinated peptides are helpful in diagnosing rheumatoid arthritis. Antibody tests should be ordered and repeated only if they can be of help in making the diagnosis, assessing the prognosis, or altering treatment plans.

Tests for acute phase proteins, C-reactive protein, and erythrocyte sedimentation rate are nonspecific, but positive results suggest the presence of inflammatory disease. In some cases, such as in patients with giant-cell arteritis and polymyalgia rheumatica, these tests may be useful both in diagnosis and in monitoring the course of disease and therapy. The presence of anemia may suggest chronic disease or hemolytic anemia. Leukopenia, especially lymphopenia, suggests SLE, and thrombocytosis indicates active inflammation. Leukocytosis may also reflect inflammation or infection, and glucocorticoid therapy also elevates the white blood cell count, often dramatically. Urinalysis should always be performed in patients with systemic disease, and proteinuria, red blood cells, and casts should be considered as evidence of occult renal disease. Laboratory tests should always be considered within the context of the clinical presentation.

Radiographic Studies

Radiographic evaluation often shows changes characteristic of particular diseases. In established rheumatoid arthritis, patients often have classically erosive disease of the small joints of the wrists, the ulnar styloid, the metacarpophalangeal and proximal interphalangeal joints, and the small joints in the foot. The erosions are bland and nonreactive. In contrast, erosive psoriatic arthritis causes a sclerotic reaction, and the patient may have characteristic telescoping of joints, the so-called *pencil-in-cup lesions.* Large erosions with overhanging sclerotic margins and even juxta-articular tophi may be seen in gout. In ankylosing spondylitis, sacroiliitis is observed on pelvic films and has high diagnostic specificity. *Syndesmophytes* (calcification of the outer rim of the annulus fibrosis), bridging osteophytes, calcification of spinal ligaments, and a typical bamboo spine in late stages are seen on lumbar and chest radiographs. Joint space narrowing, bony spurs, and sclerosis are seen in osteoarthritis. *Chondrocalcinosis* is a common finding and may be asymptomatic or may lead to crystal arthritis (pseudogout). In acute arthritis, radiographs are much less helpful because bony changes take time to develop; only in septic joint disease is destruction observed in the early stages.

Imaging modalities such as magnetic resonance imaging (MRI), radionuclide scans, ultrasound, and computed tomography are often useful in assessing diseases of bones, joints, muscle, and soft tissues. Ultrasound may be used to detect synovial cysts, especially Baker cysts of the knee. MRI is the procedure of choice for evaluating early avascular necrosis of bone, especially the hips, as well as suggested meniscal or rotator cuff disease. MRI is also the preferred procedure for evaluating intervertebral disk disease with suggested radiculopathy and spinal stenosis. MRI is also very useful in evaluating solid lesions of bone and joints, including neoplastic lesions. The sensitivity of MRI for detecting edema (water) makes it useful in evaluating inflammatory muscle disease of both infectious and noninfectious causes. An MRI is a sensitive but not a specific modality for evaluating osteomyelitis, properties shared with radionuclide imaging. MRI should not supplant clinical evaluation or plain radiography.

In many instances, diagnosis can be made with certainty only by pathologic examination of tissue. Muscle biopsy may be necessary to establish a diagnosis of inflammatory muscle disease, and nerve biopsy may be needed to detect vasculitis. Skin biopsy is often quite useful in differentiating the many causes of skin disease in rheumatology. Renal biopsy is often needed for diagnosis, as well as for treatment decisions and prognosis.

Summary

The evaluation of arthritis begins with a careful assessment of the location and pattern of joint involvement, the differentiation of inflammatory from mechanical and other causes, and the consideration of nonarticular systemic features. The patient's age and sex, family history, and medication history, as well as the presence of other medical conditions, are also important; they are often key features. Laboratory and radiographic studies, in particular synovial fluid analysis, provide confirmatory and sometimes diagnostic information.

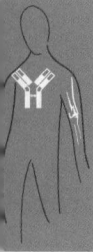

Prospectus for the Future

- A thorough history and physical examination will remain the basis of rheumatic disease diagnosis.

- Improvements in key laboratory studies, including serologic tests and imaging techniques, are useful in confirming or supporting the clinical diagnosis in most patients.

References

Felson DT: Epidemiology of the rheumatic diseases. In Koopman WJ (ed): Arthritis and Allied Conditions, 13th ed. Baltimore, Williams & Wilkins, 1997, p 3.

Gordon DA: Approach to the patient with musculoskeletal disease. In Goldman L, Bennett JC (eds): Cecil Textbook of Medicine, 21st ed. Philadelphia, WB Saunders, 2000, pp 1472-1475.

Sergent JS: Approach to the patient with pain in more than one joint. In Kelley WN, Harris ED Jr, Ruddy S, et al (eds): Textbook of Rheumatology, 5th ed. Philadelphia, WB Saunders, 1997, p 381.

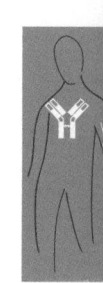

Rheumatoid Arthritis

Larry W. Moreland

Rheumatoid arthritis (RA) is a chronic, systemic, inflammatory disorder of unknown cause. It is characterized by symmetrical, polyarticular pain and swelling, morning stiffness, and fatigue. RA has a variable course, often with periods of exacerbations and, less frequently, true remissions. Outcomes are also variable, ranging from the rarely seen remitting disease to severe disease that brings disability and even, in some patients, premature death. Without treatment, the majority of patients will experience progressive joint damage. In some patients this results in significant disability within just a few years. The past decade has seen an unprecedented change in the treatment paradigm for this disease. Several targeted biologic therapies are available; the most notable are the anti–tumor necrosis factor (TNF) therapies.

Epidemiologic Features and Genetics

RA is a worldwide problem, with a prevalence of 0.5% to 1% of the adult population and an annual incidence of 0.03% with substantial variation across different studies and time periods. Overall, RA appears to be less common in Asia and Africa than in the United States and Europe, and it has been suggested that the incidence of RA decreases from northern to more southern European countries. The disease affects individuals at any age, including infants and the elderly; however, it occurs most commonly in women aged 40 to 50 years. RA is not very common in men under 45 years of age, but the incidence rises steeply with increasing age. In women, the incidence rises to age 45, plateaus until age 75, and then declines. Numerous studies have demonstrated increased mortality in patients with RA compared with the general population. There are reports of increased risk of death from gastrointestinal (GI), cardiovascular, respiratory, hematologic, and infectious diseases.

The pathophysiology of RA has undergone intensive investigation over the past 25 years. It is well known that an individual's genetic background plays a critical role in the susceptibility to and severity of RA. Careful studies have revealed a 15% concordance in monozygotic twins, which is approximately 4 times greater than the rate in dizygotic twins, which supports a genetic component. Disease transmission is complex and likely involves many genes. The genes with the greatest impact lie in the class II major histocompatibility (MHC) locus. There is a strong association of RA with a specific sequence on the beta chains of select human leukocyte antigen (HLA)–DR haplotypes. This "shared epitope" contains amino acids 70 to 74 (glutamine-leucine-arginine-alanine-alanine) and is also known as *QKRAA*.

The underlying cause of the disease—that is, the triggers in the susceptible host—are unknown. It is possible that RA may consist of multiple diseases now defined by some common clinical manifestations, and there may not be a single predominant mechanism of initiation or perpetuation.

Pathologic Features

A current concept is that inflammation and tissue destruction in the rheumatoid synovium result from complex cell-cell interactions. The process may be initiated by an interaction between antigen-presenting cells (APCs) and CD4$^+$ T cells. APCs display complexes of class II MHC molecules and peptide antigens that bind to specific receptors on the T cells. With an appropriate "second signal" or costimulation delivered by the APC to the T cell, a clonal expansion of T-cell subsets occurs. This stimulates synovial macrophages to secrete proinflammatory cytokines, such as interleukin-1 (IL-1), TNF-α, and IL-6 to activate multiple inflammatory and destructive pathways.

Joint damage in RA results from proliferation of the synovial intimal layer to form a pannus that overgrows, invades, and destroys adjacent cartilage and bone, evident on radiographs as loss of joint space and juxta-articular bone erosion. Fibroblast-like synoviocytes and macrophages are the predominant cellular components of the invading pannus. Extracellular matrix damage resulting from synovial expansion is caused by several families of enzymes, including serine proteases and cathepsins. Matrix metalloproteinases, produced mostly by synoviocytes in the intimal lining, are also important mediators of tissue destruction.

Pathophysiologic Features

The pathogenesis of RA is complex, and the disease is heterogeneous. Multiple pathways independently contribute, as demonstrated by the similar and non-overlapping response rates to cytokine-, T-cell–, and B-cell–targeted therapies (Table 79-1 and Fig. 79-1). It is reasonable to hypothesize that the disease can be divided into multiple stages. An induction phase can provide an environment in the joint that permits recruitment of inflammatory cells. Cigarette smoke, bacterial products, viral components, and other environmental stimuli may enhance and amplify this process. A genetic propensity for autoreactivity might initiate an irreversible pathway to RA. Specific genes are probably part of this process, including MHC class II genes, protein tyrosine phosphatase, non-receptor type 22 (*PTPN22*), and cytokine promoter polymorphisms. The destructive phase then may occur, which can be antigen dependent and independent, involving mesenchymal elements such as fibroblasts and synoviocytes. Bone erosions result from local differentiation and activation of osteoclasts, whereas cartilage damage appears to be caused by proteolytic enzymes produced by synoviocytes, macrophages, and synovial fluid neutrophils. Counter-regulatory mechanisms (e.g., soluble TNF receptors, suppressive cytokines, protease inhibitors, natural cytokine antagonists) are not produced in high enough levels to offset the inflammatory and destructive process. However, therapeutic interventions that modulate any of these pathogenic processes have been shown to have significant impact on both clinical signs of RA and the destructive component of the disease.

Cytokines, which are hormone-like proteins that regulate many immune cell functions, have been implicated in critical components of RA synovial inflammation. The inflammatory milieu of the joint is dominated by proinflammatory factors produced by macrophages and fibroblasts, especially in the synovial intimal lining. These (and other) cytokines, which include IL-1, IL-6, TNF, granulocyte-macrophage colony-stimulating factor [GM-CSF], IL-15, IL-18, IL-32, and most members of the chemokine family, have been identified at both the protein and the mRNA levels.

The autoantibodies found most frequently in patients with RA are antibodies against IgM (lgM rheumatoid factor [IgM-RF] and anticyclic citrullinated peptide [anti-CCP]). There has been a large body of literature recently on the diagnostic, prognostic, and pathogenic significance of anti-CCP antibodies. Although the research has just begun into the pathophysiologic significance of anti-CCP antibodies, there is emerging data that the presence of these antibodies predicts a less favorable disease course and radiologic progression.

Clinical Features

RA is a symmetrical polyarthritis typically involving the small joints of the hands and feet, the wrists, and the ankles. Other joints frequently involved include the cervical spine, shoulders, elbows, hips, and knees. Any diarthrodial (synovial) joint may be involved, including the apophyseal, temporomandibular, and cricoarytenoid joints. Involved joints are swollen, warm, and tender, and they may have effusions. The synovium, normally a few cell layers thick, becomes palpable on examination (*synovitis*). Prolonged *morning stiffness*, usually lasting more than 1 hour and often many hours, is a classic feature in RA, and symptoms are generally improved with moderate activity (Table 79-2).

Over time, RA progresses to joint destruction and deformity. Erosive lesions of bone and cartilage are radiographically and pathologically visible at the margins of bone and cartilage, the site of synovial attachment. *Tenosynovitis*, or inflammation of tendon sheaths, leads to tendon malalignment, stretching, and/or shortening. Among common deformities are ulnar deviation at the metacarpophalangeal joints and volar subluxation at these joints, volar subluxation at the wrists, and flexion and extension contractures in the proximal and distal interphalangeal (DIP) joints of the fingers that lead to characteristic *swan-neck deformity* (flexion contracture at the DIP joint and hyperextension at the proximal interphalangeal joint) or *boutonnière deformity* (flexion contracture at the proximal interphalangeal joint and hyperextension at the DIP joint). Erosions of the ulnar styloid can lead to sharp bony prominences and rupture of extensor tendons. Synovitis at the wrists can lead to median nerve compression and carpal tunnel syndrome. Cervical spine disease may lead to C1-C2 subluxation and spinal cord compression; caution should be taken in moving the neck when the patient is being anesthetized for a surgical procedure. The degree of subluxation can be monitored by looking at the distance between C1 and the odontoid in flexion-extension films. Rupture of synovial fluid from the knee into the calf (Baker cyst) may mimic deep-venous thrombosis or, occasionally, cellulitis.

Table 79-1 **Pathogenesis of Rheumatoid Arthritis**

Tissue Phase

Immune cell localization to synovial tissue
T- and B-cell and monocyte recruitment
T-cell activation and proliferation and cytokine release
B-cell elaboration of rheumatoid factor and other antibodies
Monocyte elaboration of inflammatory cytokines: IL-1, TNF-α, IL-6
Synovial cell proliferation and activation by IL-1 and TNF-α
Release of inflammatory eicosanoids (PGE$_2$)
Synthesis of collagenase and other matrix metalloproteinases
Erosions of bone and cartilage
Osteoclast and chondrocyte activation
Release of proteases
Resorption of bone and cartilage

Fluid Phase

Immune complexes in synovial fluid
Complement activation and release of C3a, C5a
Neutrophil recruitment and activation
Release of prostaglandins, leukotrienes, and reactive oxygen species
Release of lysosomal enzymes
Vasodilation, development of joint effusions, pain, and swelling
Superficial cartilage erosions

IL-1, interleukin-1; IL-6, interleukin-6; PGE$_2$, prostaglandin E$_2$; TNF-α, tumor necrosis factor-α.

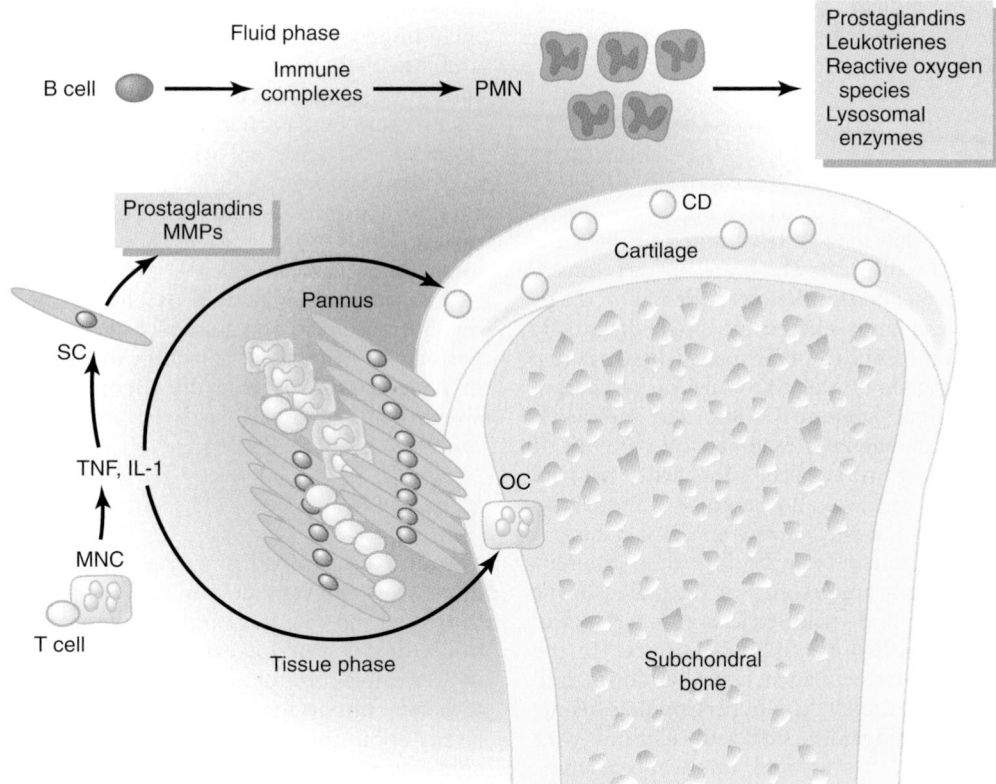

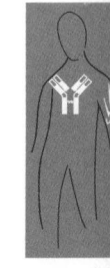

Figure 79-1 Pathogenetic events in rheumatoid arthritis. The proliferative synovial pannus invades at the bone-cartilage interface. Interleukin-1 (IL-1) and tumor necrosis factor–α (TNF) activate synovial cells (SC) to produce prostaglandins and matrix metalloproteinases (MMPs). In the synovial fluid, polymorphonuclear leukocytes (PMN), activated by immune complexes and complement, produce mediators of inflammation and destruction. CD, chondrocyte; MNC, mononuclear cell; OC, osteoclast.

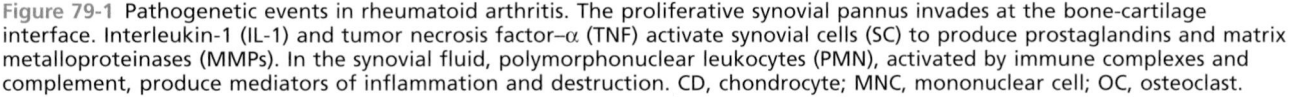

Table 79-2 **Clinical Characteristics of Rheumatoid Arthritis**

Articular

Morning stiffness, "gelling"
Symmetrical joint swelling
Predilection for wrists and proximal interphalangeal, metacarpophalangeal, and metatarsophalangeal joints
Erosions of bone and cartilage
Joint subluxation and ulnar deviation
Inflammatory joint fluid
Carpal tunnel syndrome
Baker cyst

Nonarticular

Rheumatoid nodules: subcutaneous, pulmonary, scleral
Lung disease
Vasculitis, especially skin, and peripheral nerves
Pleuropericarditis
Scleritis and episcleritis
Leg ulcers
Felty syndrome

The clinical course and severity of the arthritis are variable. Some patients have mild, slowly progressive disease with few deformities and little bony destructive change. At the opposite extreme are patients who have a rapidly progressive course that, if left untreated, leads to crippling and deforming arthritis. Most patients fall in between these extremes with various levels of disability; some have a waxing and waning course over a period of years with acute episodes of single- or multiple-joint exacerbations.

RA is a systemic disease with constitutional symptoms: fatigue, low-grade fever, weight loss, and myalgia. Anemia is also common. Specific organs other than the musculoskeletal system may be involved (see Table 79-2). Grossly palpable subcutaneous *rheumatoid nodules* can occur almost anywhere but are common along other extensor tendon surfaces, especially at the elbows, and less commonly in the lungs, pleura, pericardium, sclerae, and other sites, including the heart in rare cases. The occurrence of multiple pulmonary nodules in patients with RA and pneumoconiosis is known as *Caplan syndrome*. Pleuritis, pericarditis, and interstitial lung fibrosis occur in a few patients; pericarditis can be severe, and acute interstitial lung disease can be associated with pulmonary hemorrhage. Vasculitis, associated with circulating complexes of immunoglobulin G (IgG) and rheumatoid factor (RF), leads to cutaneous lesions, including ulcers and skin necrosis, and mononeuritis multiplex. Secondary *Sjögren syndrome* (sicca complex) is often present (see Chapter 85). *Felty syndrome* (splenomegaly, leukopenia, and recurrent pulmonary infections) is a rare complication and is often accompanied by leg ulcers and vasculitis. Extra-articular manifestations of RA are more commonly seen among patients who test positive for RF. Even in patients without vasculitis or pulmonary or pleuropericardial disease, the mortality rate in RA is increased by a variety of causes, including side effects of therapy and infection. Premature and accelerated atherosclerosis is an increasingly recognized problem among patients with RA and is thought, at least, to be partially a result of the effects of chronic inflammation.

Diagnosis

Diagnosing a chronic illness, such as RA, and separating it from other conditions that may be self-limited or have different outcomes can be difficult. There are no early-onset, disease-specific features, and the characteristic hallmarks of the disease develop over time. There is no single diagnostic test that enables a diagnosis of RA to be made with certainty. Instead, diagnosis depends on the accumulation of characteristic symptoms, signs, laboratory data, and radiologic findings. RA is a clinical diagnosis. Symmetrical synovitis of small joints—that is, warm, swollen joints with synovial hypertrophy, morning stiffness, and fatigue—is the classic symptom. *Systemic lupus erythematosus* (SLE) can have a similar clinical presentation and may be difficult to differentiate unless other features are present. In rare cases, *Lyme disease* is polyarticular and symmetrical at onset. *Viral arthritis* is best distinguished by its limited course. In the older patient, polymyalgia rheumatica, hypothyroidism, and paraneoplastic syndromes, including hypertrophic osteoarthropathy, should be considered. Crystal arthropathies (gout and pseudogout) can, if left untreated, rarely appear clinically as chronic polyarthritis.

No test is necessary to establish a diagnosis of RA, and all laboratory results may be normal in certain patients. Routine tests are often not characteristic and lack specificity; however, certain data may contribute to the diagnosis and assessment of the severity of RA in an individual.

RF was identified as an antibody (typically IgM but also IgG or others) that binds to the Fc fragment of IgG. It is detectable in the serum of 70% to 80% of patients with RA but may not be present in early disease. It is unclear whether the production of RF is of pathologic relevance to RA, because RF production also frequently occurs in patients with SLE; Sjögren syndrome; endocarditis; sarcoidosis; liver and lung diseases, including hepatitis B and C infection; and other conditions. In addition, RF may be detected in the serum of apparently healthy individuals, especially people older than 50 and in smokers. In an individual patient, the titer does not correlate with disease activity, but it does appear that patients with severe erosive arthritis or with extra-articular disease are likely to have relatively high titers. The presence of a positive serum RF does not establish a diagnosis of RA, but when combined with a typical clinical picture, it does help to confirm the clinical impression.

Anti-CCPs have been identified as a more specific marker for RA. Anti-CCP antibodies, detected using enzyme-linked immunosorbent assay, have a much higher specificity (>95%) than RF, with similar sensitivity (68% to 80%). These antibodies, which can be detected several years before the development of clinical RA (and before the development of RF), can be helpful in diagnosing RA in patients with RF-negative (seronegative) arthritis. They also appear to mark more severe outcomes, such as radiographic joint damage and poor prognosis. Because of their higher specificity for RA, anti-CCP antibodies may be useful in differentiating RA

from other conditions with positive rheumatoid factors, including Sjögren syndrome, infection, and hepatitis.

Acute phase reactants, such as erythrocyte sedimentation rate and C-reactive protein, are usually elevated in the presence of active inflammation but are not specific for the diagnosis of RA. They are useful in distinguishing RA from noninflammatory conditions such as osteoarthritis or fibromyalgia. However, a significant number of RA patients have normal levels of these reactants, despite clinical evidence of joint inflammation.

Synovial fluid analysis is usually not necessary when the diagnosis is already established, but arthrocentesis should be performed to rule out infection or crystalline arthropathy in patients who develop disproportionate discomfort and swelling of one joint.

Treatment

The ultimate goals of RA management are to reduce pain and discomfort; prevent deformities and loss of normal joint function, and maintain normal physical, social, and emotional function and capacity to work. Management begins with effective communication between physician and patient. It is very important to educate the patient and his or her family about the nature and course of the disease—the specific causes of the discomfort and the goals, problems, and expectations of treatment. Misunderstandings about the disease may lead to frustration, depression, and withdrawal.

Nonpharmacologic therapeutic options include reduction of joint stress, and physical and occupational therapy. Local rest of an inflamed joint can reduce joint stress, as can weight reduction, splinting, and use of walking aids and specially designed assistive devices. Vigorous activity should be avoided during disease flares, although full range of motion of joints should be maintained by a graded exercise program to prevent contractures and muscle atrophy.

The former pharmacologic approach to the treatment of RA was to begin with symptomatic treatment of inflammation using nonsteroidal anti-inflammatory drugs (NSAIDs) in addition to rest and corticosteroid injections. If the disease did not significantly improve, more potent disease-modifying antirheumatic drugs (DMARDs) were started. This is no longer the recommended approach for the treatment of RA. Maintaining normal joint structure and anatomy can be achieved only by controlling the disease before any irreversible damage has occurred. Studies have revealed that DMARD therapy early in the course of RA slowed disease progression more effectively than did delayed use. Effective, aggressive treatment can improve both signs and symptoms, and radiographic progression, even in long-standing disease. This has led to a general agreement that the inflammation of RA should be controlled as completely as possible, as soon as possible, and that this control should be maintained for as long as possible.

NSAIDs are probably the most frequently used drugs in the treatment of RA, at least early in the disease process. They reduce joint pain and swelling and improve function, but they have no effect on the underlying disease process, and exacerbation of symptoms occurs quickly after metabolic elimination of the drugs. They are rarely, if ever, used alone for treatment of RA.

The major therapeutic effect of NSAIDs relates to their ability to suppress the synthesis of prostaglandins by inhibiting the enzyme cyclo-oxygenase (COX), which exists in two isoforms: COX-1 and COX-2. COX-1 is expressed in many tissues and is primarily responsible for the production of prostaglandins by endothelium and gastric mucosa, leading to homeostatic and cytoprotective effects. COX-2 is undetectable in most tissues; its expression increases during development and inflammation and can be induced by several proinflammatory stimuli. It is hypothesized that the anti-inflammatory effects of NSAIDs are mainly the result of COX-2 inhibition and that inhibition of COX-1 is responsible for most of the GI toxicity.

Glucocorticoids remain important in the treatment of RA, especially for acute exacerbations of disease. These agents are usually used sparingly, in low-to-medium doses, and optimally for short periods. Although glucocorticoids are useful for brief exacerbations of the disease or to bide time while waiting for DMARDs to work, many patients require more prolonged use of low doses for optimal control of disease activity, even when other immunomodulatory drugs are also prescribed. The long-term side effects of glucocorticoids can be substantial and particularly devastating in a disease such as RA that is already marked by relative immobility. Side effects include osteoporosis and pathologic fractures, avascular necrosis of bone, obesity, glucose intolerance, and many other problems. Screening, prevention, and treatment for osteoporosis should be considered in all patients who receive long-term therapy with glucocorticoids. Intra-articular glucocorticoids are extremely useful and efficacious in exacerbations involving only a few joints, and intra-articular delivery of these agents is associated with almost no side effects.

Although NSAIDs and glucocorticoids are important for the treatment of RA, they do not control symptoms or alter the disease course for the majority of patients. Current practice is to place most patients with RA on DMARDs (Table 79-3). Previously, many of these drugs were given only late in the course of disease to patients with severe disease. Recognition of the extent of disability resulting from RA and growing evidence that DMARD use inhibits the progression of erosive disease and disability have led to earlier and more widespread use of these agents.

A wide variety of DMARDs is now available for use in treating RA. Methotrexate remains the most widely used DMARD for RA; its popularity is a result of its high degree of efficacy combined with good tolerability. Table 79-3 includes several agents of historical interest but almost no current use, including D-penicillamine and gold preparations. Similarly, azathioprine and cyclosporine are now less commonly used, whereas cyclophosphamide is used almost only in extremely severe disease, especially with extra-articular manifestations such as vasculitis. Hydroxychloroquine and sulfasalazine are frequently prescribed for patients with mild-to-moderate disease and/or in combination with other agents. Leflunomide is a relatively new immunosuppressive drug that is used for moderate-to-severe RA and shares several potential toxicities with methotrexate.

BIOLOGIC THERAPIES

The newest and seemingly most effective therapeutic agents for RA are DMARDs that are *anticytokine-directed therapies*

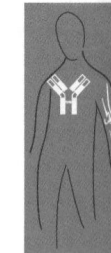

Table 79-3 **Treatment of Rheumatoid Arthritis**
Glucocorticoids
Systemic (oral, intravenous, intramuscular)
Intra-articular
Nonsteroidal Anti-Inflammatory Drugs
Aspirin
Nonacetylated salicylates
Nonsalicylate nonselective prostaglandin inhibitors
Selective cyclo-oxygenase-2 inhibitors
Disease-Modifying Antirheumatic Drugs
Hydroxychloroquine
Sulfasalazine
Azathioprine
Cyclosporine
Cyclophosphamide
Methotrexate
Leflunomide
Disease-Modifying Antirheumatic Drugs—Biologic Agents
Etanercept (soluble TNF receptor)
Infliximab (chimeric anti-TNF antibody)
Adalimumab (fully human anti-TNF antibody)
Anakinra (IL-1–receptor antagonist)
Abatacept (T-cell–costimulation inhibitor)
Rituximab (anti-CD20 B-cell–depleting agent)

IL, interleukin; TNF, tumor necrosis factor.

and commonly referred to as *biologics*. In the past few years, three biologic response modifiers capable of neutralizing TNF have been developed, tested, and approved for patients with RA. The anti-TNF drugs etanercept, infliximab, and adalimumab inhibit inflammation by binding TNF before it reaches its cell-bound receptor. Infliximab and adalimumab also bind to cell-bound TNF. Blockers of TNF have demonstrated remarkable benefit for many patients and have set a new standard for efficacy for DMARDs. All of the available TNF blockers are given by intravenous or subcutaneous injection, are quite expensive, and carry risks of reactivation of tuberculosis and increased risk for some other infections; otherwise, they are well tolerated. Other biologic agents now available for treatment of RA include an IL-1 receptor antagonist, anakinra; an inhibitor of T-cell costimulation, abatacept; and a B-cell–depleting agent, rituximab. Antagonists or modulators of many other cytokines are under development for RA.

Although methotrexate and the biologic drugs have brought about a remarkable overall improvement in the ability to treat RA, it is important to recognize that many patients still have active disease despite using these drugs, even in combination, and the need for different, safer, and more efficacious treatment options for RA still exists.

Joint replacement surgery plays an extremely important role in patients who have had severe destructive joint disease, particularly in the knee and hip. Early reconstructive surgery in the hand and foot can improve function and sometimes can prevent deformity and tendon rupture. Total joint arthroplasty can have life-changing benefits for patients with RA with destructive joint disease.

Physical therapy and *occupational therapy* also continue to play important roles for many patients with RA. Physical therapy improves muscle strength and conditioning and maintains joint mobility. Splints for the wrists, used at night, may help prevent deformity. Various appliances are available that help protect joints and make daily activities easier, ranging from Velcro "buttons" to special grips for keys and writing implements to raised chairs and toilet seats.

Summary

In summary, considerable strides have been made in understanding the pathogenesis and clinical outcomes of RA.

Although the underlying cause of RA is unknown, advances in cell biology, immunology, and molecular biology have led to dramatic alterations in therapies available to treat this disease. The development of novel effective biologic agents and the earlier introduction of aggressive therapy should prevent joint deformity and destruction and should improve short- and long-term outcomes. Assessment of efficacy in long-term studies and evaluation of long-term risks and toxicities will determine whether these drugs become the new paradigms for the treatment of RA.

Prospectus for the Future

- As the immune abnormalities in individual RA patients are defined, personalized medicine approaches will be developed.
- It is of importance to gain an understanding of the pathology involved with the increased prevalence of accelerated atherosclerosis in RA patients.

- The expense of current biologic therapies often limits their availability. Economic and political considerations will be essential if they are to be made available to all patients.

References

Fox DA: Etiology and pathogenesis of rheumatoid arthritis. In Koopman WJ, Moreland LW (eds): Arthritis and Allied Conditions, 15th ed. Philadelphia: Lippincott Williams & Wilkins, 2004.

Klareskog L, van der Heijde D, de Jager JP, et al: Therapeutic effect of the combination of etanercept and methotrexate compared with each treatment alone in patients with rheumatoid arthritis: double-blind randomised controlled trial. Lancet 363:675-681, 2004.

O'Dell JR, Haire CE, Erikson N, et al: Treatment of rheumatoid arthritis with methotrexate alone, sulfasalazine and hydroxychloroquine, or a combination of all three medications. N Engl J Med 334:1287-1291, 1996.

Saag KG, Teng GG, Moreland LW, et al: American College of Rheumatology 2008 recommendations for the use of nonbiologic and biologic disease-modifying antirheumatic drugs in rheumatoid arthritis. Arthritis Rheum 59:762-784, 2008.

Shanahan J, Moreland LW: Investigational biologic therapies for the treatment of rheumatic diseases. In: Koopman WJ, Moreland LW (eds): Arthritis and Allied Conditions, 15th ed. Philadelphia: Lippincott Williams & Wilkins, 2004.

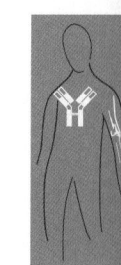

Spondyloarthropathies

Douglas W. Lienesch

The *spondyloarthropathies* are a related group of inflammatory disorders with clinical features unique among rheumatic diseases. The five types of spondyloarthropathy in adults are ankylosing spondylitis, reactive arthritis (Reiter syndrome), arthritis of inflammatory bowel disease (Crohn disease and ulcerative colitis), psoriatic arthritis, and undifferentiated spondyloarthropathy. A juvenile form of spondyloarthropathy exists that is similar to ankylosing spondylitis and generally persists into adulthood. The cardinal clinical feature of the spondyloarthropathies is inflammation of the sacroiliac joints (sacroiliitis) and the spine (spondylitis). Inflammation of tendon insertion sites (enthesitis), inflammation of entire digits (dactylitis), and inflammation of one to four lower extremity joints (oligoarthritis) are typical extraspinal skeletal findings. A positive family history, eye inflammation (anterior uveitis or conjunctivitis), and the absence of rheumatoid factor and subcutaneous nodules are common. Further classification of these disorders is based on the presence of psoriatic skin or nail changes, inflammatory bowel disease, or a history of preceding gastrointestinal or genitourinary infection.

Epidemiologic Features

One of the most fascinating aspects of the spondyloarthropathies is the strong associations with human leukocyte antigen (HLA) B27, a specific allele of the B locus of the HLA-encoding class I major histocompatibility complex genes. The frequency of HLA-B27 among whites is approximately 6% to 8%. However, up to 90% of white patients with ankylosing spondylitis and 80% of white patients with reactive arthritis or juvenile spondyloarthropathy are HLA-B27 positive; these percentages are even higher among those patients with uveitis. The rate of HLA-B27 positivity among patients with inflammatory bowel disease or psoriasis with peripheral arthritis is not markedly increased unless spondylitis is present, in which case the frequency of HLA-B27 is 50%. The frequency of HLA-B27 varies widely among other ethnic groups and accounts for the wide variation of the prevalence of ankylosing spondylitis in different populations.

Ankylosing spondylitis is much more common among adolescent boys and young men, but this finding may reflect underdiagnosis in women, in whom disease manifestations may be milder than they are in men. *Reactive arthritis* is more common among men when it follows genitourinary *Chlamydia trachomatis* infection, but the sex distribution is even among patients after dysentery. *Inflammatory arthritis* including spondylitis affects approximately 5% to 8% of patients with psoriasis and 10% to 25% of patients with ulcerative colitis or Crohn disease. Men and women are affected equally. The prevalence of spondyloarthropathy, particularly psoriatic and reactive arthritis, is increased in populations with high human immunodeficiency virus (HIV) infection rates.

Pathogenesis and Pathophysiology

Although the strong association of HLA-B27 and the spondylarthropathies is well established, a specific role in the pathogenesis of these disorders has not been elucidated. Animal models in which rodents transgenic for HLA-B27 develop inflammatory abnormalities strikingly similar to those seen in HLA-B27–associated human diseases provide compelling indirect evidence for a pathogenic role. When raised in a germ-free environment, these animals remain disease free, suggesting a key additional environmental factor.

In addition to the strong genetic links to the spondyloarthropathies, important associations exist between specific bacterial agents and disease pathogenesis. Genitourinary infection with *C. trachomatis* or diarrheal illness with *Shigella, Salmonella, Campylobacter,* and *Yersinia* species, as well as *Klebsiella pneumoniae* infection, can induce reactive arthritis. These infections appear to trigger an inflammatory response, possibly as a result of persistence of bacterial antigens. However, no one theory of pathogenesis of spondyloarthropathies explains the clinical spectrum of these disorders, and more research is clearly needed to solidify an understanding of their origin. The complex role of the

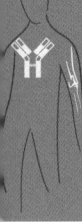

immune system in the spondyloarthropathies is highlighted by the observation that patients infected with HIV appear more likely to have severe disease, especially psoriatic arthritis. It is interesting to note that when HIV infection is treated with antiviral agents, the incidence of spondyloarthropathy declines.

Although there has been a dramatic increase in our understanding of the cellular and molecular mechanisms in inflammatory joint disease, the pathophysiology of spondyloarthropathies remains incompletely understood. Inflammation of the sacroiliac joints, spine, and entheses is a unique feature of these disorders. Pathophysiologic studies show that the inflammation originates at the interface of bone and cartilage in the sacroiliac joint, and bone and fibrocartilage in the enthesis. Macrophages and CD4$^+$ and CD8$^+$ T cells are present, and the proinflammatory cytokine *tumor necrosis factor-α* (TNF-α) is abundant. Synovial tissue becomes inflamed and osteoclasts are activated, leading to bone resorption, reminiscent of rheumatoid arthritis (RA) joint inflammation. Unlike in RA, this early bone resorption is followed by a secondary phase during which osteoblast activity predominates, leading to new bone formation in periarticular bone (hyperostosis) and around joints (osteophytosis) or vertebral bodies (syndesmophytes). Ultimately, bony fusion of joints (ankylosis) occurs. The relationship between these paradoxical phases of bone resorption and proliferation is an area of active investigation.

Clinical Features

COMMON CLINICAL FEATURES AMONG THE SPONDYLOARTHROPATHIES

The spondyloarthropathies have considerable clinical overlap with one another and are most easily considered as a group of related disorders. Table 80-1 outlines the clinical features of these disorders. The cardinal clinical features common to all of these disorders are inflammatory spine pain or an asymmetrical predominantly lower extremity oligoarthritis. Inflammatory spine pain should be suspected in young patients (younger than age 40) who have an insidious onset of chronic low back pain or buttock pain associated with prolonged morning stiffness and relieved by exercise. The characteristic peripheral joint disease typically involves one to four joints, usually in the lower extremities, and may be associated with tendon insertion inflammation (enthesitis) or sausage digits (dactylitis). Symmetrical polyarthropathy involving the upper extremities and clinically similar to RA is seen in some forms of psoriatic and inflammatory bowel disease–related arthritis. The presence of anterior uveitis, enthesitis, dactylitis, psoriatic skin or nail changes, inflammatory bowel disease, a family history of spondyloarthropathy, or a history of a preceding gastrointestinal or genitourinary infection is suggestive of spondyloarthropathy. Subcutaneous nodules, rheumatoid factor, and antinuclear antibodies are usually absent. In a given patient the clinical features of these disorders may accumulate over a prolonged period of time. Some patients will not initially demonstrate the typical findings of a specific disorder. These patients are considered to have *undifferentiated spondyloarthropathy;* many will later manifest clinical findings consistent with one of the specific subtypes of spondyloarthropathy.

Inflammatory spine pain is caused by *sacroiliitis* and *spondylitis.* Sacroiliitis may develop in a subtle fashion with low back or gluteal area pain, but it can also cause severe pain. Patients generally have significant morning stiffness, sometimes of many hours' duration, and pain after periods of inactivity. Spondylitis may occur at any area of the spine, but it often begins in the lumbar spine and subsequently progresses to the cervical and thoracic regions. The sacroiliac joints and spine become painful and stiff with increasingly reduced range of motion as bony fusion of the vertebral column and facet joints occurs over time. Involvement of

Table 80-1 Comparison of the Spondyloarthropathies

	Ankylosing Spondylitis	Posturethral Reactive Arthritis	Postdysenteric Reactive Arthritis	Enteropathic Arthritis	Psoriatic Arthritis
Sacroiliitis	+++++	+++	++	+	++
Spondylitis	++++	+++	++	++	++
Peripheral arthritis	+	++++	++++	+++	++++
Articular course	Chronic	Acute or chronic	Acute or chronic	Acute or chronic	Chronic
HLA-B27	95%	60%	30%	20%	20%
Enthesopathy	++	++++	+++	++	++
Common extra-articular manifestations	Eye	Eye	GU	GI	Skin
	Heart	GU	Eye	Eye	Eye
		Oral and/or GI			
		Heart			
Other names	Bekhterev arthritis	Reiter syndrome	Reiter syndrome	Crohn disease	
				Ulcerative colitis	
	Marie-Strümpell disease	SARA			
		NGU			
		Chlamydial arthritis			

GI, gastrointestinal; GU, genitourinary; HLA, human leukocyte antigen; NGU, nongonococcal urethritis; SARA, sexually acquired reactive arthritis; + = relative prevalence of a specific feature.
Data from Cush JJ, Lipsky PE: The spondyloarthropathies. In Goldman L, Bennett JC (eds): Cecil Textbook of Medicine, 21st ed. Philadelphia, WB Saunders, 2000, pp 1499-1507.

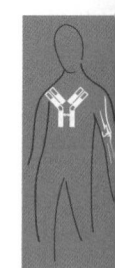

the thoracic spine and costovertebral joints may result in a restrictive lung physiologic condition. Fusion of the spine increases the risk of vertebral fractures in patients with spondyloarthropathies and, depending on the angle of fusion, may cause significant kyphosis and reduced line of sight. When bony fusion is complete, the pain may be significantly reduced.

Enthesitis may occur in many different anatomic locations. These include spinous processes, costosternal junctions, ischial tuberosities, plantar aponeuroses, and Achilles tendons.

The *peripheral arthritis* of the spondyloarthropathies, when it occurs, begins as an episodic, asymmetrical, oligoarticular process often involving the lower extremities. The arthritis can progress and may become chronic and disabling. A unique feature of spondyloarthropathies is the appearance of fusiform swelling of an entire finger or toe, referred to as *dactylitis* or *sausage digits.*

Uveitis, or inflammatory disease of the anterior chamber of the eye, is a common extra-articular manifestation of the spondyloarthropathies, especially among patients who are HLA-B27 positive. Bouts of uveitis are usually monocular, acute at onset, painful, and accompanied by eye redness and blurred vision. Recurrent attacks are common. Uveitis may be serious and lead to blindness. Anterior uveitis may be the presenting symptom of spondyloarthropathy; thus all patients with anterior uveitis should be screened for signs and symptoms of these disorders.

Spondyloarthropathies may occasionally involve other organ systems and may cause significant morbidity and mortality. *Aortitis,* especially occurring in the ascending segment, can result in aortic insufficiency from aortic root dilation, aortic dissection, and cardiac conduction system abnormalities. Pulmonary fibrosis of the apical regions can occur, often in an insidious fashion. Spinal cord compression can result from atlantoaxial joint subluxation, cauda equina syndrome, or vertebral fractures. In rare cases, long-standing spondyloarthropathy is associated with secondary amyloidosis.

SPECIFIC CLINICAL FEATURES OF THE SPONDYLOARTHROPATHIES

Ankylosing Spondylitis
The cardinal clinical feature of ankylosing spondylitis is inflammatory spine pain. Over time, spine involvement ascends from the sacroiliac joints to involve all levels of the spine. There is progressive loss of motion owing to ankylosis of the vertebral column and apophyseal joints. Costovertebral involvement leads to decreased chest expansion and restrictive lung physiology. There is a high risk of traumatic spine fracture because of loss of mobility and secondary osteoporosis of the vertebral bodies. Axial involvement of the shoulders and hips is common and associated with a worse prognosis. Peripheral oligoarthritis, enthesitis, and dactylitis are more common in females. Diagnosis requires demonstration of radiographic sacroiliitis (sacroiliac joint erosions, sclerosis, and/or ankylosis). Anterior uveitis is common. Aortitis, upper lobe pulmonary fibrosis, cauda equina syndrome, and amyloidosis are less common and seen in late disease.

Reactive Arthritis
Among the unique clinical features of reactive arthritis (Reiter syndrome) are *urethritis, conjunctivitis,* and certain dermatologic problems. The urethritis may be secondary to the chlamydial infection that triggers the disease, or it may be a sterile inflammatory discharge also seen in diarrhea-associated disease. Conjunctivitis may be mild in reactive arthritis and is distinct from uveitis. *Keratoderma blennorrhagicum* is a distinct papulosquamous rash usually found on the palms or soles. *Circinate balanitis* is a rash that may appear on the penile glans or shaft of men with reactive arthritis. Nonpitting *nail thickening* and *oral ulcers* may also occur in patients with reactive arthritis. These lesions can be confused with similar findings in patients with psoriasis and inflammatory bowel disease, respectively.

Reactive arthritis usually manifests with oligoarthritis, *without* the classic triad of Reiter syndrome. Therefore this term is no longer preferred. Most cases will be self-limited. Chronic or relapsing arthritis and chronic spondylitis is associated with HLA-B27 and *Chlamydia* infection.

Psoriatic Arthritis
Five identifiable clinical patterns of psoriatic arthritis are recognized: (1) *distal interphalangeal joint involvement with nail pitting;* (2) *asymmetrical oligoarthropathy* of both large and small joints; (3) *arthritis mutilans,* a severe, destructive arthritis; (4) *symmetrical polyarthritis,* identical to RA; and (5) *spondyloarthropathy.* These patterns are not exclusive, and clinical overlap is significant. Spondylitis or sacroiliitis may occur along with any of the other four patterns. The prevalence of HLA-B27 is increased among the patients with spondylitis or sacroiliitis but not among patients with the other patterns. Psoriatic skin or nail disease predates arthritis in most cases, but both may occur concomitantly or joint disease may precede skin involvement. Rarely, joint disease indistinguishable from psoriatic arthritis is present in patients with a family history but no personal history of psoriatic skin disease.

Enteropathic Arthritis (Inflammatory Bowel Disease)
Crohn disease and ulcerative colitis (see also Chapter 38) are frequently associated with both spondyloarthropathy and peripheral arthritis. The peripheral arthritis is typically nonerosive, oligoarticular, and episodic, and degree of joint involvement fluctuates with gut activity. In addition, a more chronic, symmetrical polyarthritis may occur in Crohn disease.

Radiographic Features
The radiographic features of the spondylarthropathies are highly specific and, in the correct clinical setting, virtually diagnostic of these diseases. Sacroiliitis is usually the earliest radiographic sign of spine disease and results in sclerosis and erosions of the sacroiliac joints with eventual bony fusion (Fig. 80-1A). Many different radiographic changes occur secondary to chronic spondylitis, including ossification of the annulus fibrosus, calcification of spinal ligaments, bony sclerosis and *squaring* of vertebral bodies, and ankylosis of apophyseal joints. These changes can lead to vertebral fusion and a bamboo spine appearance (Fig. 80-1B). Radiographic findings progress over many

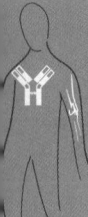

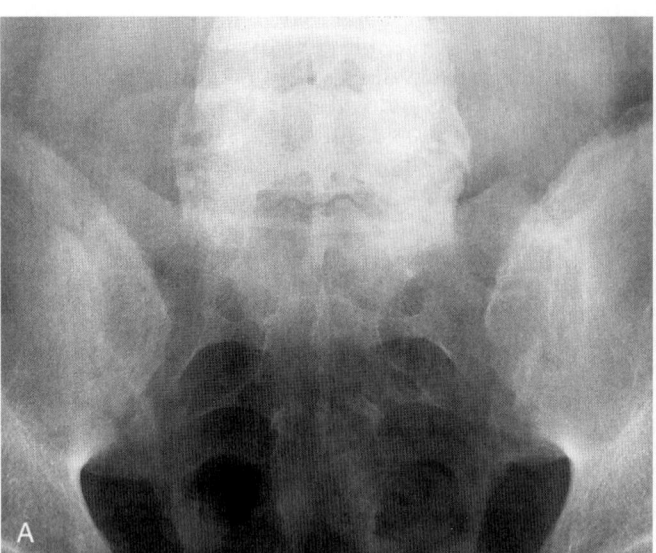

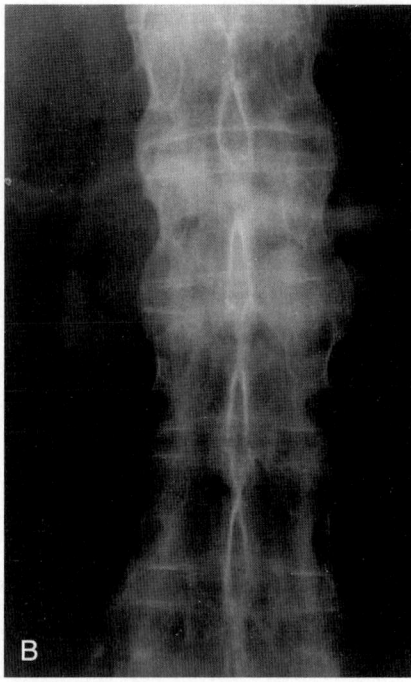

Figure 80-1 **A,** Bilaterally symmetrical sacroiliitis in ankylosing spondylitis. **B,** Lumbar spondylitis in ankylosing spondylitis with symmetrical, marginal bridging syndesmophytes and calcification of the spinal ligament. (From Cush JJ, Lipsky PE: The spondyloarthropathies. In Goldman L, Bennett JC [eds]: Cecil Textbook of Medicine, 21st ed. Philadelphia, WB Saunders, 2000, pp 1499-1507.)

years of illness and may not be apparent in early disease. However, during this "preradiographic period," magnetic resonance imaging (MRI) demonstrates bone inflammation (osteitis) and erosion at the sacroiliac joints and vertebral bodies, and computed tomography (CT) shows bony sclerosis and joint erosions.

Bone erosions, sclerosis, and new bone formation may occur at sites of enthesitis. Erosions at bone-cartilage interface (subchondral erosions), sclerosis, and bone proliferation are hallmarks of reactive and psoriatic arthritis. In severe cases such as the arthritis mutilans form of psoriatic arthritis, total or subtotal bone resorption (osteolysis) of a phalange may occur.

Treatment

No cure has yet been found for any of the spondyloarthropathies, but effective treatment for many of the manifestations is available. *Patient education* regarding the disease is essential and allows for identification of affected family members and early presentation of urgent clinical features such as uveitis. *Physical therapy,* including a daily stretching program, postural adjustments, and strengthening, can be useful in maintaining proper bony alignment, reducing deformities, and maximizing function. Selective use of *orthopedic surgery* may be highly effective in correcting significant spinal deformities or instability.

Nonsteroidal anti-inflammatory drugs (NSAIDs) can provide significant relief of spinal pain and stiffness, and many patients take these drugs continually for years. No clear evidence indicates that systemic glucocorticoids benefit patients with spondyloarthropathies, and these agents are generally avoided. *Intra-articular glucocorticoid injection* into the sacroiliac or other involved joints may provide temporary relief. Similarly, the role and efficacy of older immuno-

suppressive agents in the treatment of the axial manifestations of the spondyloarthropathies have not been established. In contrast, the peripheral arthritis of spondyloarthropathies has been shown in clinical trials to improve with *sulfasalazine. Methotrexate* is also regularly used for the peripheral arthritis, but no large clinical trials have been performed with this agent in these diseases.

TNF blockers (infliximab, etanercept, and adalimumab) represent a substantial breakthrough in treatment of the spondyloarthropathies. The efficacy of these agents is now well established, and these drugs have rapidly become the treatment of choice for patients with ankylosing spondylitis who do not satisfactorily or fully respond to NSAIDs and physical therapy. TNF blockers can significantly reduce pain, improve function, and improve quality of life and may prevent or slow disease progression and structural damage. These drugs are effective in psoriatic arthritis and have been demonstrated to retard radiographic progression in the peripheral joints. Infliximab and adalimumab reduce gut inflammation in ulcerative colitis and Crohn disease, with concomitant reduction in symptoms of joint and spine inflammation.

Flares of *uveitis* require care by an ophthalmologist experienced in treating inflammatory eye diseases. Topical or intraocular glucocorticoids may suffice, but systemic therapy with glucocorticoids or immunosuppressive medications may be necessary to control the inflammation and prevent permanent visual loss. The role of TNF blockers in uveitis is under study.

Reactive arthritis is usually self-limited, and joint symptoms are managed with NSAIDs or intra-articular corticosteroid injections. When chronic arthritis or spondylitis develops, interventions are similar to those employed in ankylosing spondylitis. Evaluation and treatment for *C.*

trachomatis and associated sexually transmitted diseases in patients with reactive arthritis and their sex partners are essential. Early treatment reduces the frequency of reactive arthritis. Long term antibiotics are ineffective for treatment of gastroenteritis-associated reactive arthritis. In reactive arthritis after *C. trachomatis,* clinical trials of long-term antibiotics have had mixed results, and this practice will require further study before it can be adopted.

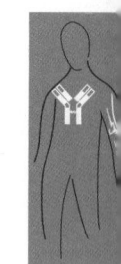

Prospectus for the Future

- Increased insights into the immunogenetics of the spondyloarthropathies may lead to greater understanding of the pathophysiologic features of these diseases.
- Further research on the use of biologic agents, especially antitumor necrosis-α products, in the treatment of

spondyloarthropathies may help determine whether the structural and functional deterioration these diseases often cause can be prevented with long-term therapy.

References

Arnett FC: Seronegative spondyloarthropathies: B. Reactive arthritis (Reiter's syndrome) and enteropathic arthritis. In Klippel JH (ed): Primer of the Rheumatic Diseases, 12th ed. Atlanta, Arthritis Foundation, 2001, pp 245-250.

Boumpas DT, Illei GG, Tassiulas IO: Psoriatic arthritis. In Klippel JH (ed): Primer of the Rheumatic Diseases, 12th ed. Atlanta, Arthritis Foundation, 2001, pp 233-238.

Cush JJ, Lipsky PE: The spondyloarthropathies. In Goldman L, Bennett JC (eds): Cecil Textbook of Medicine, 21st ed. Philadelphia, WB Saunders, 2000, pp 1499-1507.

Inman RD: Seronegative spondyloarthropathies: D. Treatment. In Klippel JH (ed): Primer of the Rheumatic Diseases, 12th ed. Atlanta, Arthritis Foundation, 2001, pp 255-258.

Keat A: Seronegative spondyloarthropathies: C. Ankylosing spondylitis. In Klippel JH (ed): Primer of the Rheumatic Diseases, 12th ed. Atlanta, Arthritis Foundation, 2001, pp 255-258.

Khan MA: Update on spondyloarthropathies. Ann Intern Med 136:896-907, 2002.

Mansour M, Cheema JS, Naguwa SM, et al: Ankylosing Spondylitis: A Contemporary Perspective on Diagnosis and Treatment. Semin Arthritis Rheum 36:210-223, 2007.

Mease PJ: Psoriatic arthritis therapy advances. Curr Opin Rheumatol 17:426-432, 2005.

Rihl M, Klos A, Köhler L, Kuipers JG: Reactive arthritis. Best Pract Res Clin Rheumatol 20:1119-1137, 2006.

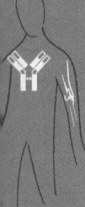

Systemic Lupus Erythematosus

Jennifer Rae Elliott

Systemic lupus erythematosus (SLE, lupus) is the classic systemic autoimmune disease and is of unknown cause. Lupus predominantly affects young women of childbearing age but can also afflict young men and older individuals of either sex. The clinical manifestations are protean, ranging from fatigue and oral ulcerations to life-threatening renal and neurologic disease. Typically the disease fluctuates with periods of flares and clinical quiescence. In the long term this leads to damage to internal organs from inflammation and medication use. Lupus is diagnosed via a thorough history and physical examination combined with laboratory testing. Although there is no cure for SLE, patients are treated aggressively with a variety of medications, including immunosuppressants. Unique considerations must be given to patients with SLE regarding pregnancy, cardiovascular disease (CVD), malignancy, and bone health.

Epidemiology

The reported incidence and prevalence of SLE vary greatly, reflecting the heterogeneity of the disease. The incidence of SLE is estimated at 1.8 to 7.6 cases per 100,000 per year and appears to have increased over time. Prevalence rates range widely from 14.6 to 149.5 per 100,000 persons.

Lupus is a disease of women, the majority of whom are diagnosed between the ages of 15 and 45. During these childbearing years, the female to male ratio is 10 to 15:1. This discrepancy is less distinct (2:1) in young children and older patients.

Lupus also has a predilection for non-white groups. The prevalence rates of lupus in blacks (3×), Caribbean blacks (5×), Asians (2×), and Hispanics are greater than in whites. Blacks and Hispanics also have more severe disease and an overall worse prognosis than whites.

In 1955, lupus patients had a 50% 5-year survival rate. Since then, landmark advances have been made in the diagnosis (antinuclear antibody testing and classification criteria for SLE) and care (antibiotics, corticosteroids, and hemo-dialysis) of lupus patients. Current 5- and 10-year survival rates are >90%. In addition to ethnicity (described earlier), renal and neurologic disease are poor prognostic markers for mortality.

A bimodal pattern of mortality is seen in lupus. Early (<5 years) deaths are attributed to active lupus disease and infections; later deaths (>5 years) are sequelae of chronic SLE complications and medications, as well as of CVD and infections. Recent data suggest that malignancy-associated morbidity and mortality are lifelong risks, but are greatest early in the disease.

Pathogenesis

Although the pathogenesis of SLE is not completely known, persons who develop lupus likely have a genetic predisposition, in the setting of immune system dysregulation, environmental triggers, and hormonal milieu. The genetic contribution to SLE is emphasized by the high concordance rate in monozygotic twins (>20%) as opposed to the lower concordance among other siblings (<5%). The search for potential genes in lupus is an active area of research. Genes coding for certain human leukocyte antigens, complement system components, immunoglobulin receptors, and various other specific proteins have all been considered possible candidate genes associated with SLE. Many different immune abnormalities have been noted in patients with SLE, a finding implicating dysregulation of both the humoral and cellular immune systems in the pathogenesis of the disease. This dysregulation leads to loss of tolerance and autoimmune destruction of healthy tissues, hallmarked by the production of autoantibodies and immune complexes. Various environmental triggers, including microorganisms and ultraviolet light exposure, may influence the development of lupus and lupus activity itself. In addition, the striking differences in disease prevalence between men and women, as well as the effect of pregnancy on lupus disease activity, suggest a role for hormones in the pathogenesis of SLE.

Clinical Manifestations

Virtually any organ system may be involved in SLE, often in many different ways. Table 81-1 outlines the many clinical manifestations of SLE.

CONSTITUTIONAL

Fatigue, fever, lymphadenopathy, and generalized arthralgias and myalgias are common is lupus patients. The most common symptom, fatigue (>90%), can also be the most debilitating. One should exclude other reasons for fatigue, including anemia, hypothyroidism, and fibromyalgia. Malignancy should also be suspected if lymphadenopathy persists (see later).

MUCOCUTANEOUS

Oral ulcerations may be painful or painless and are classically located on the tongue or palate. Skin manifestations of SLE are protean and include the classic malar (butterfly) rash, discoid lesions (permanent scarring and disfigurement), alopecia, and photosensitivity.

MUSCULOSKELETAL

Arthralgias and inflammatory arthritis are common manifestations in lupus (>75%). The arthritis of lupus is usually nonerosive (as opposed to rheumatoid arthritis), but a subset of patients (10%) have *Jaccoud arthropathy* with reversible hand deformities secondary to inflammation and joint laxity.

CARDIOPULMONARY

More than 60% of lupus patients have pericarditis and pleuritis during their disease course. Subsequent pericardial or pleural effusions are typically exudative, with low normal glucose levels. Valvular thickening and noninfective Libman-Sacks endocarditis are frequently observed on echocardiography and autopsy studies. Myocarditis should be suspected in patients with cardiopulmonary symptoms and fever. Pulmonary hemorrhage is a rare and potentially catastrophic manifestation of SLE that may result in fulminant hemoptysis and respiratory failure. Premature CVD in lupus is described later.

RENAL

Nephritis is a major cause of morbidity and mortality in lupus patients. It can manifest with hematuria and/or proteinuria, and the clinical spectrum of glomerulopathies is classified by the World Health Organization (Class I to VI). Class IV (diffuse, proliferative) lupus nephritis has the worst prognosis but is also the most amenable to aggressive systemic therapy

NEUROPSYCHIATRIC

Neuropsychiatric symptoms are broad, including sensorimotor neuropathy, headache, cognitive dysfunction, anxiety, and psychosis, as well as life-threatening cerebrovascular, vasculitis, and transverse myelopathy.

HEMATOLOGIC

Leukopenia, primarily lymphopenia, anemia, and thrombocytopenia are very common in SLE patients. Anemia is secondary to hemolysis or chronic disease. Antiphospholipid and anticardiolipin antibodies are present in one third of lupus patients and are associated with multiple thromboses, thrombocytopenia, and recurrent spontaneous miscarriages (see Chapter 78).

VASCULAR

Over 40% of all lupus patients have Raynaud phenomenon. Venous (pulmonary emboli, deep venous thrombosis) and arterial clots are typically secondary to antiphospholipid and anticardiolipin antibodies. Small vessel vasculopathy or vasculitis can occur in any organ system (neurologic, gastrointestinal) and can be life threatening.

OCULAR

Keratoconjunctivitis sicca from secondary Sjögren syndrome (see Chapter 86) is the most common ocular manifestation of SLE. Episcleritis, scleritis, and retinal vasculitis are rare.

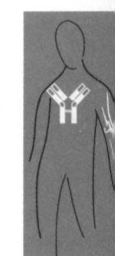

Diagnosis

SLE is a clinical diagnosis; no single test or feature is definitively diagnostic of the disease. Many patients' clinical disease evolves over time, and only after several years (and several different visits to physicians) are patients recognized as having SLE.

Criteria for the classification of SLE were established to more accurately conduct lupus research studies (Table 81-2). Although these classification criteria are not meant to be diagnostic, practicing clinicians can use them, with a comprehensive examination, as a guide to help diagnose SLE. One must always consider other rheumatic diseases (rheumatoid arthritis, Sjögren syndrome), infections (endocarditis, hepatitis), and malignancy in the differential diagnosis of SLE.

Various autoantibodies are found in patients with SLE and are the hallmark laboratory feature of the disease (Table 81-3). These autoantibodies are often present before the onset of SLE clinical manifestations. Virtually all patients with SLE (>95%) test positive for antinuclear antibodies. Although many of the specific antigens to which these antinuclear antibodies are directed have been determined and are useful both diagnostically and clinically in SLE, some antibodies are also seen in other autoimmune diseases. Antibodies to double-stranded DNA and the Smith antigen are highly specific for lupus, whereas antibodies to SSA/Ro and SSB/La antigens are also commonly found in patients with Sjögren syndrome and rheumatoid arthritis. Certain antibodies are associated with specific clinical manifestations of disease, particularly anti–double-stranded DNA antibodies with lupus nephritis. Autoantibodies alone are not

Table 81-1 Clinical Manifestations of Systemic Lupus Erythematosus

Cardiac

Pericarditis*
Pericardial effusion
Myocarditis
Valvular thickening
Libman-Sacks endocarditis
Atherosclerotic heart disease

Constitutional

Fatigue
Fever
Lymphadenopathy
Weight loss
Anorexia

Gastrointestinal

Hypomotility
Mesenteric vasculitis
Malabsorption
Protein-losing gastroenteropathy
Lupus enteropathy
Thrombosis of mesenteric and hepatic vasculature
Hepatitis
Hepatomegaly
Splenomegaly
Pancreatitis
Acalculous cholecystitis
Peritonitis

Hematologic

Leukopenia*
Lymphopenia*
Hemolytic anemia*
Nonhemolytic anemia (anemia of chronic disease, iron-deficiency anemia)
Thrombocytopenia*
Antiphospholipid antibody syndrome

Mucocutaneous

Oral, genital, nasal ulcers*
Angioedema
Alopecia
Photosensitivity*
Malar (butterfly) rash*
Discoid lesions*
Subacute cutaneous lupus
Tumidus
Panniculitis
Vasculitis
Chilblain
Urticaria
Periungual erythema

Musculoskeletal

Arthritis*
Arthralgias
Jaccoud arthropathy
Avascular necrosis
Myositis

Table 81-1 Clinical Manifestations of Systemic Lupus Erythematosus —cont'd

Neuropsychiatric

Seizures*
Cerebritis, aseptic meningitis
Cerebrovascular disease
Transverse myelitis
Chorea
Headache
Cognitive impairment
Autonomic dysfunction
Cranial neuropathy
Peripheral neuropathy
Psychosis*
Anxiety
Depression
Mood disorder

Ocular

Keratoconjunctivitis sicca
Episcleritis
Scleritis
Retinal vasculitis
Arterial and venous occlusions
Optic neuritis

Pulmonary

Pleuritis*
Pleural effusion
Pneumonitis
Alveolar hemorrhage
Interstitial lung disease
Bronchiolitis obliterans
Pulmonary hypertension
Pulmonary emboli
Vasculitis
Acute reversible hypoxemic syndrome
Shrinking lung syndrome

Renal

Cellular casts or glomerulonephritis*
Proteinuria or membranous nephropathy or nephrotic syndrome*

Reproductive

Recurrent spontaneous abortions
Premature fetal delivery
Neonatal lupus

Serologic Abnormalities

Autoantibodies*
Hypocomplementemia
Elevated acute phase reactants

Vascular

Raynaud phenomenon
Livedo reticularis
Arterial or venous thrombosis
Vasculitis (almost any location)

*An item in the American College of Rheumatology diagnostic criteria.

diagnostic for any autoimmune disease but must be interpreted in the clinical context.

Clinical Subsets

Some patients with autoimmune symptoms have clinical and laboratory features of two or more specific autoimmune diseases and are considered to have an overlap syndrome. Mixed connective tissue disease is characterized by overlaps among SLE, scleroderma, and myositis with a high titer of anti-U1 RNP antibody levels. For patients who have a few autoimmune manifestations but do not yet meet criteria of a specific autoimmune disease, the term *undifferentiated connective tissue disease* is used. These patients typically are

Table 81-2 **Updated Criteria for Classification of Systemic Lupus Erythematosus***

Criterion	Definition
1. Malar rash	Fixed erythema, flat or raised, is observed over the malar eminences, tending to spare the nasolabial folds.
2. Discoid rash	Erythematous raised patches develop with adherent keratotic scaling and follicular plugging; atrophic scarring may occur in older lesions.
3. Photosensitivity	Skin rash occurs as a result of unusual reaction to sunlight by patient history or physician observation.
4. Oral ulcers	Oral or nasopharyngeal ulceration, usually painless, is observed by the physician.
5. Arthritis	Nonerosive arthritis involves two or more peripheral joints, characterized by tenderness, swelling, or effusion.
6. Serositis	a. Pleuritis: Convincing history of pleuritic pain exists, or rub is heard by a physician, or pleural effusion is in evidence. OR b. Pericarditis: Is documented by electrocardiogram or rub or evidence of pericardial effusion.
7. Renal disorder	a. Persistent proteinuria is >0.5 g/day or >3+ if quantitation is not performed. OR b. Cellular casts: May be red cell, hemoglobin, granular, tubular, or mixed.
8. Neurologic disorder	a. Seizures: Occur in the absence of offending drugs or known metabolic derangements (e.g., uremia, ketoacidosis, electrolyte imbalance) OR b. Psychosis: Occurs in the absence of offending drugs or known metabolic derangements (e.g., uremia, ketoacidosis, electrolyte imbalance)
9. Hematologic disorder	a. Hemolytic anemia: Develops with reticulocytosis. b. Leukopenia: <4000/mm^3 total is documented on two or more occasions. c. Lymphopenia: <1500/mm^3 is documented on two or more occasions. OR d. Thrombocytopenia: <100,000/mm^3 develops in the absence of offending drugs.
10. Immunologic disorder	a. Anti-DNA: Antibody to native DNA in abnormal titer. b. Anti-Sm: Presence of antibody to Sm nuclear antigen. OR c. Positive finding of antiphospholipid antibodies is based on (1) an abnormal serum level of immunoglobulin G (IgG) or IgM anticardiolipin antibodies, (2) a positive test result for lupus anticoagulant using a standard method, or (3) a false-positive result from a serologic test for syphilis is known to be positive for at least 6 months and is confirmed by *Treponema pallidum* immobilization or fluorescent treponemal antibody absorption test.
11. Antinuclear antibody	An abnormal titer of antinuclear antibody is documented by immunofluorescence or an equivalent assay at any point in time and in the absence of drugs known to be associated with drug-induced lupus syndrome.

*The classification is based on 11 criteria. For the purpose of identifying patients in clinical studies, a person shall be said to have SLE if any four or more of the 11 criteria are present, serially or simultaneously, during any interval of observation.

Data from Tan EM, Cohen AS, Fries JF, et al: The 1982 revised criteria of the classification of systemic lupus erythematosus. Arthritis Rheum 25:1271, 1982; and Hochberg MC: Updating the American College of Rheumatology Revised Criteria for the Classification of Systemic Lupus Erythematosus. Arthritis Rheum 40:1725, 1997.

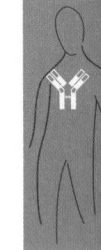

Table 81-3 **Autoantibodies Associated with Systemic Lupus Erythematosus**

Target Antigen	Approximate Frequency
Nuclear Antigens	99
dsDNA	70
Sm	38
RNP (U1-RNP)	33
Ro (SSA)	49
La (SSB)	35
Phospholipids	21
Ribosomal P	10

From Crow M. Systemic lupus erythematosus. In Goldman L, Ausiello DA, Arend W, et al (eds): Cecil Textbook of Medicine, 23rd ed. Philadelphia, WB Saunders, 2008, p 2029.

early in their disease course and will eventually develop a specific autoimmune disease.

Treatment

No cure for lupus has yet been identified, and treatment is aimed at educating patients, reducing inflammation, suppressing the immune system, and closely monitoring patients to identify disease manifestations as early as possible. Treatment with glucocorticoids and immunosuppressive agents has reduced both the morbidity and the mortality of patients with SLE, although these treatments themselves are associated with extensive toxicity. Physicians caring for lupus patients must carefully weigh the benefits of therapy against the known risks of treatment.

Patient education and prophylactic measures to prevent disease flares are key in the care of patients with lupus. Sunscreens (high sun protection factor [SPF]) and ultraviolet ray protective clothing are very effective in avoiding photosensitivity skin rashes and systemic flares. Protective or warm clothing is helpful in treating Raynaud phenomenon in SLE, and these patients may also benefit from vasodilator therapy. Low-dose aspirin is frequently prescribed for patients with positive antiphospholipid and anticardiolipin antibodies to prevent thrombotic events. Other treatments for antiphospholipid antibody syndrome are discussed in Chapter 82. Routine (non-live) immunizations, such as those for influenza and pneumococcus, are recommended for all patients. Psychological support is essential for patients with SLE because this chronic disease may lead to depression and feelings of being overwhelmed.

Nonsteroidal anti-inflammatory medications may be used for mild arthralgias, but glucocorticoids remain the main anti-inflammatory agent and one of the most effective medications for lupus. Glucocorticoids are used for almost all manifestations of lupus in doses ranging from low alternate-day doses to large intravenous (IV) doses. Given the chronic nature of the disease, glucocorticoids are often used over many years and may lead to extensive toxicity, including obesity, diabetes mellitus, accelerated atherosclerosis, osteoporosis, avascular necrosis, cataracts, and increased risk of infections. To avoid such toxicities, different immunomodulating or immunosuppressant agents (described later) are used to provide a steroid-sparing effect, as well as for greater disease control.

Antimalarial medications (hydroxychloroquine and chloroquine) are very effective agents in SLE and are considered standard of care for lupus. Antimalarials are especially beneficial for fatigue, mild arthritis, and mucocutaneous manifestations of SLE. These medications are often chronic therapies and are safe to use in pregnancy. The most serious side effect of antimalarials is retinal toxicity, although it is extremely uncommon. Risk factors for retinal toxicity are therapy >5 years, renal or hepatic disease, age >60 years, dose >6.5 mg/kg, and obesity. Patients should have baseline and annual ophthalmologic examinations with visual field testing.

Azathioprine and methotrexate are both immunosuppressive agents prescribed in patients with lupus either when glucocorticoids alone are not fully effective or to allow for a reduction in the glucocorticoid dose. Toxicities of azathioprine include cytopenias, increased infection risk, and potential association of hematologic malignant disease (controversial). Azathioprine may be used during pregnancy for severe internal organ lupus (especially nephritis). Methotrexate is particularly effective with inflammatory arthritis associated with lupus. In addition to cytopenias and infections, liver function abnormalities, alopecia, nausea, and pneumonitis are potentially seen with methotrexate. Because it is teratogenic, methotrexate should be stopped 3 to 6 months before pregnancy. Both drugs require monthly laboratory monitoring.

Mycophenolate mofetil (MMF) is increasingly used to treat patients with internal organ involvement of lupus, particularly nephritis. MMF inhibits purine synthesis of lymphocytes and has been standard treatment in the prevention of solid-organ transplant rejection. Recent clinical trials have shown that MMF is as efficacious as intravenous (IV) cyclophosphamide (described later) for inducing remission of active lupus nephritis. Toxicity of MMF includes gastrointestinal disturbance and leukopenia; it also has a category D rating in pregnancy.

Patients with neurologic lupus, rapidly progressive nephritis, or vasculitis of internal organ systems are often treated with cyclophosphamide, the most potent immunosuppressive agent (alkylating agent) used to treat SLE. Because it is extremely toxic, this drug is generally reserved for the most severe disease manifestations of lupus. In a series of studies, primarily conducted at the National Institutes of Health, monthly IV cyclophosphamide was effective in reducing the rate of progression of lupus nephritis to end-stage renal disease. Acute toxicities of cyclophosphamide include pancytopenia, alopecia, mucositis, and hemorrhagic cystitis. Long-term cyclophosphamide use may lead to transitional cell carcinoma, hematologic malignant disease, sterility, premature menopause, and opportunistic infections.

Many other treatments have been used in SLE, although extensive clinical trials demonstrating efficacy are lacking. Among these drugs, intravenous immunoglobulin may be effective for SLE-related thrombocytopenia and catastrophic antiphospholipid syndrome. Thrombotic thrombocytopenic purpura secondary to SLE may be treated with plasmapheresis. Immunoablation with high-dose cyclophosphamide with or without autologous stem cell transplant has been tried in a small number of patients with progressive active disease that is refractory to conventional immunosuppressive therapy; unfortunately mortality is high, and data are preliminary.

Great potential and optimism exist for "biologic" immunomodulating agents that focus on various aspects of the immune system, including B cells, interactions between B and T cells, and cytokines. The most promising current therapeutic agents are those that deplete B cells, producers of autoantibodies. Among these, rituximab has been successfully used in refractory lupus patients with hematologic and renal disease manifestations.

Special Issues in the Care of Patients with Systemic Lupus Erythematosus

PREGNANCY

Pregnant women with lupus have higher rates of both pregnancy loss (miscarriage and stillbirth) and preterm delivery (premature rupture of membranes, preeclampsia, and intrauterine growth restriction). Lupus activity preceding conception, especially nephritis, hypertension, and antiphospholipid antibody syndrome, are clear risk factors for pregnancy complications in SLE. Pregnancy itself may place women with lupus at greater risk for a flare, particularly if the disease, specifically nephritis, was active before conception.

Neonatal lupus is a rare disorder in which maternal anti-SSA/Ro-SSB/La antibodies cross the placenta and injure the fetus. Mothers with these autoantibodies have a 2% risk of having a child with congenital heart block (CHB). These mothers are screened with fetal heart tones and fetal echocardiography between weeks 16 and 34 of gestation. Treatment with a fluorinated corticosteroid (dexamethasone)

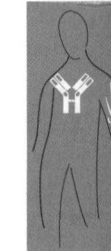

may be beneficial; however, a considerable number of children with CHB do not survive (30%) or experience morbidity, with over 60% requiring pacemakers. More common manifestations of neonatal lupus are skin rashes, cytopenias, and hepatosplenomegaly, all of which resolve within 6 to 8 months (after maternal autoantibodies are removed from the child's circulation). Mothers of children with neonatal lupus do not necessarily have SLE or Sjögren syndrome; however, some of these women eventually are diagnosed with an autoimmune disease.

With careful prenatal screening and planning, women with lupus can successfully have a healthy child. Prenatal monitoring of anti-SSA/Ro-SSB/La antibodies and antiphospholipid and anticardiolipin antibodies and a prepregnancy high-risk obstetric consultation are critical. Ideally, women with lupus should have clinical quiescence for 6 months before considering a planned pregnancy. Special consideration must also be given to medications, as the majority of immunosuppressants (methotrexate, mycophenolate mofetil, and cyclophosphamide) are teratogenic.

HORMONAL THERAPY

Hormones are thought to play a role in the development of SLE, given its female predominance. Consequently, rheumatologists have historically been hesitant to prescribe estrogen therapy for fear of inducing a flare. Recently, randomized, placebo-controlled clinical trials, described in the next paragraphs, have helped to guide hormonal therapy in women with lupus.

A multicenter randomized trial revealed that oral contraceptive therapy does not appear to increase the risk of SLE flares in women with mild or stable SLE disease activity. However, this is not generalizable to all women with SLE, in particular those whose disease is active or severe and those with prior thrombotic events or antiphospholipid and anticardiolipin antibodies. Clearly, an effective form of birth control is necessary for young sexually active women with SLE, especially those taking teratogenic medications. Physicians must carefully discuss the risks and benefits of birth control with lupus patients.

Hormone replacement therapy (HRT) is a controversial topic, regardless of lupus status. However, it is of particular interest in SLE because some women with lupus reach menopause prematurely. In a recent clinical trial of HRT in SLE patients with mild or stable disease, with no prior thrombotic events, antiphospholipid and anticardiolipin antibodies, or malignancies of women, no lupus patients had severe clinical flares, but 20% did have mild to moderate flares. These findings suggest that brief (1 year) HRT may have a role in alleviating menopausal symptoms or in treating osteoporosis in a certain subset of women with SLE.

CARDIOVASCULAR DISEASE

As survival and therapies for lupus have improved, CVD has emerged as a leading cause of morbidity and mortality. Lupus patients are 5 to 10 times more likely than healthy individuals to have a coronary event. More striking, premenopausal women aged 35 to 44 are more than 50 times as likely as healthy women to experience a myocardial infarc-

tion. Autopsy series have revealed atherosclerotic heart disease as the underlying mechanism of CVD in SLE. The cause of this premature atherosclerosis in lupus is multifactorial and includes inflammatory mediators, lupus-related factors (premature menopause, corticosteroid therapy, disease activity), and traditional cardiovascular risk factors.

Prevention of CVD is a critical aspect of the care of lupus patients. Although no firm CV management guidelines exist for SLE patients, many argue that lupus patients should be considered and treated as coronary heart disease risk-equivalents. Cardiac disease must be thought of and aggressively evaluated in SLE patients with both typical and atypical cardiac symptoms, regardless of age.

MALIGNANCY

Recently, a multicenter international cohort of nearly 10,000 lupus patients reported an increased risk of malignancy in SLE compared with the general population. Most striking was a threefold to fourfold increased risk of non-Hodgkin lymphoma. Other hematologic, lung, and hepatobiliary cancers were also described with increased frequency in SLE patients. Malignancy risk appears to be highest early in the disease course, but malignancy is clearly a risk throughout a patient's life span. Older age, tobacco use, SLE disease damage, and immunosuppressant use appear to be associated with cancers in SLE; however, the exact mechanism of malignancy in SLE is not yet fully elucidated.

Although lymph node enlargement is a common manifestation in lupus patients, physicians must have a high index of suspicion for malignancy if the lymphadenopathy does not resolve with lupus treatment, is tender or nonmobile, or occurs without other lupus symptoms.

BONE HEALTH

Lupus patients have higher rates of low bone mineral density (BMD), osteoporosis, and fractures, than do healthy age-matched subjects. The increased risk is accounted for by both traditional risk factors, such as female sex, white race, older age, and low body weight, and lupus-associated factors. Fatigue and articular symptoms secondary to SLE may limit physical activity, leading to loss of bone strength. Furthermore, therapies commonly used in lupus contribute to overall loss of bone health. Corticosteroids reduce bone mass and are an independent risk factor for fractures in women with SLE. Cyclophosphamide use can lead to premature ovarian failure, another risk factor for osteoporosis. In addition, lupus disease damage, regardless of steroid use, leads to low BMD, suggesting that SLE itself is a risk factor for low BMD. Another contributing factor may be that lupus patients are commonly asked to avoid sun exposure, which can lead to low vitamin D levels and insufficient absorption of calcium.

Given these SLE-specific risk factors for low BMD, prevention of osteoporosis is extremely important. Although osteoporosis screening guidelines for SLE patients are the same as for the general population, bone density scans should also be considered in patients with premature menopause and those who are or who will be on chronic (>3 months) corticosteroids.

Prospectus for the Future

- Advances in the understanding of the immunopathologic features of SLE, providing a logical framework for specific targeting and testing of new biologic therapies.
- Clinical trial data to evaluate the efficacy of new biologic agents for the treatment of SLE.

- Development of formal management guidelines for osteoporosis and cardiovascular care in patients with SLE.

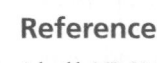

References

Arbuckle MR, McClain MT, Rubertone MV, et al: Development of autoantibodies before the clinical onset of systemic lupus erythematosus. N Engl J Med 349:1526-1533, 2003.

Austin HA 3rd, Klippel JH, Balow JE, et al: Therapy of lupus nephritis. Controlled trial of prednisone and cytotoxic drugs. N Engl J Med 314:614-619, 1986.

Bernatsky S, Boivin JF, Joseph L, et al: An international cohort study of cancer in systemic lupus erythematosus. Arthritis Rheum 52:1481-1490, 2005.

Buyon J, Petri, MA, Kim MY, et al: The effect of combined estrogen and progesterone hormone replacement therapy on disease activity in systemic lupus erythematosus: a randomized trial. Ann Intern Med 142:953-962, 2005.

Domsic RT, Ramsey-Goldman R, Manzi S: Epidemiology and classification of SLE. In: Hochberg MC, Silman AJ, Smolen JS, et al (eds): Rheumatology, 4th ed. Philadelphia, Mosby, 2008.

Ginzler EM, Dooley MA, Aranow C, et al: Mycophenolate mofetil or intravenous cyclophosphamide for lupus nephritis. N Engl J Med 353:2219-2228, 2005.

Lee C, Almagor O, Dunlop DD, et al: Disease damage and low bone mineral density: An analysis of women with systemic lupus erythematosus ever and never receiving corticosteroids. Rheumatology (Oxford) 45:53-60, 2006.

Lee C, Ramsey-Goldman R: Bone health and systemic lupus erythematosus. Curr Rheumatol Rep 7:482-489, 2005.

Manzi S, Meilahn EN, Rairie JE, et al: Age-specific incidence rates of myocardial infarction and angina in women with systemic lupus erythematosus: comparison with the Framingham Study. Am J Epidemiol 145:408-415, 1997.

Petri M, Kim MY, Kalunian KC, et al: Combined contraceptives in women with systemic lupus erythematosus. N Engl J Med 353:2550-2558, 2005.

Antiphospholipid Antibody Syndrome

Surabhi Agarwal and Amy H. Kao

Antiphospholipid antibody syndrome (APS) is a disorder characterized by recurrent vascular thrombosis and/or recurrent pregnancy loss in the presence of positive antiphospholipid (aPL) antibodies. The aPL antibodies were initially identified in patients with false-positive syphilis screening test results (positive result in the absence of syphilis). Lupus anticoagulant (LAC) was later described in patients with systemic lupus erythematosus (SLE), which was also frequently associated with a false-positive result of a screening test for syphilis and was paradoxically associated with thrombosis and recurrent pregnancy loss. LAC is a misnomer because this in vitro anticoagulant effect reflects the prolonged activated partial thromboplastin time (aPTT), and the presence of LAC does not indicate a diagnosis of lupus. Furthermore, both LAC and anticardiolipin (aCL) antibodies were shown to bind to phospholipid-binding plasma proteins and not directly to phospholipids.

Pathogenesis

Animal studies suggest that aPL may be directly pathogenic. The linear correlation between antibody levels and risk of thrombosis further supports their pathogenic role. aPL can cause β_2-glycoprotein I (β_2-GPI)–dependent endothelial activation by upregulation of expression of adhesion molecules and secretion of proinflammatory cytokines. β_2-GPI interferes with Von Willebrand factor–dependent platelet activation; neutralization of this effect by β_2-GPI antibodies may also potentiate the risk of thrombosis. aPL also induces platelet activation, leading to increased platelet adhesion and thromboxane synthesis. In addition, aPL may confer acquired resistance to the anticoagulant properties of protein C and annexin A5, further contributing to the increased risk of thrombosis. aPL displaces annexin A5 from the trophoblastic surface, which may contribute to pregnancy loss. Important to note, aPL-mediated thrombosis and fetal loss are complement-dependent, and heparin therapy acts via complement inhibition rather than as an anticoagulant as previously believed.

Clinical Features

A subset of people with aPL antibodies eventually exhibit manifestations of APS. Both arterial and venous thrombosis may occur in vessels of any size. Venous thrombosis, especially of the lower extremities, is by far the most common manifestation. Up to half of affected patients develop associated pulmonary embolism. The most common site of arterial thrombosis is the central nervous system, with manifestations including seizures, stroke, dementia, and psychosis. Transverse myelitis, chorea, and Guillain-Barré syndrome have also been reported. In addition, *microthrombotic* disease is being recognized as a manifestation of APS. Renal failure may occur as a result of microthrombosis and renal artery thrombosis.

Cardiac valve thickening (Libman-Sacks endocarditis) is frequently found in patients with APS. These noninfectious vegetations may be a source of embolism. Any valve can be affected, with mitral regurgitation being the most frequent hemodynamic abnormality, followed by aortic regurgitation. This is frequently asymptomatic; and the need for surgery is uncommon. Unlike rheumatic heart disease and bacterial endocarditis, valvular thickening is diffuse and rarely causes rupture.

A major feature of APS is recurrent pregnancy loss, especially after the 10th week of gestation. Fetal distress, intrauterine growth retardation, premature births, uteroplacental insufficiency, and oligohydramnios contribute to major pregnancy morbidity. Preeclampsia and HELLP syndrome (hemolysis, elevated liver enzymes, and low platelet count) are also frequent complications.

Other prominent manifestations of APS include mild thrombocytopenia, with platelet count usually above 50,000/mL; APS seldom causes hemorrhage. Hemolytic anemia is relatively uncommon and may occur simultaneously with thrombocytopenia (Evans syndrome). Livedo reticularis may often be noted on physical examination of patients with APS. Leg ulcers, gangrene, thrombophlebitis, nailfold infarcts, cutaneous necrosis, and necrotizing purpura may be seen.

The term *catastrophic APS* (CAPS) has been coined to describe patients who exhibit multiple microthromboses, positive aPL antibodies, and often a life-threatening illness resulting in multi-organ failure that can be clinically indistinguishable from sepsis or thrombotic thrombocytopenic purpura. Although the precise cause of CAPS remains unclear, preceding infection has been reported in multiple cases and is thought to be a precipitating factor.

Diagnosis

The classification criteria of APS are shown in Table 82-1. The presence of clinical features with laboratory evidence of aPL antibodies is necessary to establish the diagnosis of APS. In addition, the patient should repeat testing for aPL antibodies at least 12 weeks apart using the same laboratory because transient elevation can be seen with

infections, malignancies, medications, and other autoimmune diseases.

APS is considered *primary* if it occurs in isolation and *secondary* if it occurs in conjunction with other autoimmune diseases such as SLE. There are no major differences in severity or clinical consequences between primary and secondary APS. Progression from primary APS to SLE is unusual. The reported prevalence of various aPL antibodies in SLE ranges from 16% to 55%. Patients with SLE who have aPL antibodies not only have an increased risk of thromboembolism and pregnancy complications but are also found to have a higher prevalence of pulmonary hypertension, Libman-Sacks endocarditis, and neurologic complications (seizures, strokes, and transverse myelitis).

As mentioned previously in this chapter, aPL antibody assays detect a heterogeneous group of antibodies that bind serum proteins such as β_2-GPI, prothrombin, cardiolipin, annexin A5, and other negatively charged phospholipids. The assays that are useful clinically include LAC, aCL, and β_2-GPI antibodies. Various methods, such as the Russell viper venom time, aPTT, kaolin clotting time, and hexagonal lipid neutralization test, are used to test for LAC. Anticoagulation therapy may interfere with these assays. The presence of LAC is the strongest predictor of thrombosis among aPL antibodies. The immunoglobulin (Ig) isotypes of aCL antibodies may be IgG, IgM, or IgA. The specificity of these antibodies for APS increases with higher titer and is the highest with the IgG isotype.

Management

Currently, treatment for APS is tailored to the patient and the associated clinical manifestations. For patients with vascular thrombosis, indefinite anticoagulation is usually prescribed as prophylaxis against recurrence. Warfarin is the usual drug of choice for long-term therapy, with a target of international normalized ratio (INR) between 2 and 3. Higher INR level (3 to 4) is not more effective and is associated with bleeding complications. Unfractionated and low–molecular-weight heparin is also an effective anticoagulant for APS patients and is used in patients who experience recurrent events while on warfarin therapy or in patients who are or plan to become pregnant.

Treatment in patients with persistently elevated aPL antibody levels without thrombosis has not been well established and is not clearly indicated. Low-dose aspirin (75 to 100 mg) has been considered a logical option, but its efficacy has not been substantiated by prospective studies. Hydroxychloroquine, an antimalarial drug commonly used in SLE, may be protective against the development of thrombosis by reducing the binding of aPL–β_2-GPI complexes to phospholipid bilayers. Risk factor modification, including avoidance of oral contraceptives and hormonal therapy, smoking cessation, and aggressive management of dyslipidemia, hypertension, and diabetes, should always be considered in these patients. Anticoagulation prophylaxis should be also considered in high-risk situations, such as surgery and prolonged immobilization.

Risk of recurrent pregnancy loss in APS can be reduced with combination treatment of low-dose aspirin and heparin. Intravenous immunoglobulin (IVIG) and plasmapheresis

---

Table 82-1 Revised Classification Criteria of Antiphospholipid Syndrome

Antiphospholipid antibody syndrome (APS) is present if at least one clinical criterion and one laboratory criterion are met.

Clinical Criteria

1. Vascular thrombosis: One or more clinical episodes of arterial, venous, or small vessel thrombosis, in any tissue or organ. Thrombosis must be confirmed by objective validated criteria (i.e., unequivocal findings of appropriate imaging studies or histopathology). For histopathologic confirmation, thrombosis should be present without significant evidence of inflammation in the vessel wall.
2. Pregnancy morbidity
   (a) One or more unexplained deaths of a morphologically normal fetus at or beyond the 10th week of gestation, with normal fetal morphology documented by ultrasound or by direct examination of the fetus OR
   (b) One or more premature births of a morphologically normal neonate before the 34th week of gestation because of (i) eclampsia or severe preeclampsia; (ii) recognized features of placental insufficiency OR
   (c) Three or more unexplained consecutive spontaneous abortions before the 10th week of gestation, with maternal anatomic or hormonal abnormalities and paternal and maternal chromosomal causes excluded.

Laboratory Criteria

1. Lupus anticoagulant (LAC) present in plasma on two or more occasions at least 12 weeks apart.
2. Anticardiolipin (aCL) antibody of immunoglobulin G (IgG) and/or IgM isotype in serum or plasma, present in medium or high titer (i.e., >40 GPL or greater than the 99th percentile), on two or more occasions at least 12 weeks apart, measured by a standardized enzyme-linked immunosorbent assay (ELISA).
3. Anti–β_2-glycoprotein I antibody of IgG and/or IgM isotype in serum or plasma (in titer greater than the 99th percentile) present on two or more occasions at least 12 weeks apart, measured by a standardized ELISA.

have been used with mixed results in refractory cases. Warfarin should be switched to therapeutic doses of heparin before and during pregnancy because of the teratogenic effects of warfarin. Pregnancy in APS patients is considered high risk and requires a team approach with careful monitoring by the obstetrician and hematologist.

Corticosteroids and immunosuppression have a minimal role in management of thrombosis in APS except in CAPS.

Although there are no randomized controlled trials for treatment of CAPS, combinations of corticosteroids, anticoagulation, and/or plasmapheresis have been used. Evidence to support the use of cyclophosphamide has been documented mainly in patients with SLE with CAPS. Infections have been identified as a major precipitating factor for initiation of CAPS cascade; hence infection must be treated aggressively in these patients.

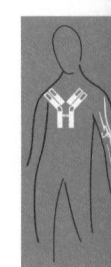

Prospectus for the Future

- Large cohort studies may provide data for better risk stratification and targeted prophylactic therapy.

- Complement inhibition may be a potential novel therapy in the treatment of recurrent pregnancy loss in patients with APS. However, further studies are warranted.

References

Asherson RA, Cervera R, Piette JC, et al: Catastrophic antiphospholipid syndrome: Clues to the pathogenesis from a series of 80 patients. Medicine (Baltimore) 80:355-377, 2001.

Del Papa N, Guidali L, Sala A, et al: Endothelial cells as target for antiphospholipid antibodies. Human polyclonal and monoclonal anti-beta 2-glycoprotein I antibodies react in vitro with endothelial cells through adherent beta 2-glycoprotein I and induce endothelial activation. Arthritis Rheum 40:551-561, 1997.

Finazzi G, Marchioli R, Brancaccio V, et al: A randomized clinical trial of high-intensity warfarin vs. conventional antithrombotic therapy for the prevention of recurrent thrombosis in patients with the antiphospholipid syndrome (WAPS). J Thromb Haemost 3:848-853, 2005.

Galli M, Luciani D, Bertolini G, Barbui T: Lupus anticoagulants are stronger risk factors for thrombosis than anticardiolipin antibodies in the antiphospholipid syndrome: A systematic review of the literature. Blood 101:1827-1832, 2003.

Holers VM, Girardi G, Mo L, et al: Complement C3 activation is required for antiphospholipid antibody-induced fetal loss. J Exp Med 195:211-220, 2002.

Lellouche F, Martinuzzo M, Said P, et al: Imbalance of thromboxane/prostacyclin biosynthesis in patients with lupus anticoagulant. Blood 78:2894-2899, 1991.

Merkel PA, Chang Y, Pierangeli SS, et al: The prevalence and clinical associations of anticardiolipin antibodies in a large inception cohort of patients with connective tissue diseases. Am J Med 101:576-583, 1996.

Miyakis S, Lockshin MD, Atsumi T, et al: International consensus statement on an update of the classification criteria for definite antiphospholipid syndrome (APS). J Thromb Haemost 4:295-306, 2006.

Nojima J, Kuratsune H, Suehisa E, et al: Acquired activated protein C resistance associated with IgG antibodies against beta2-glycoprotein I and prothrombin as a strong risk factor for venous thromboembolism. Clin Chem. 51:545-552, 2005.

Rand JH, Wu XX, Quinn AS, et al: Hydroxychloroquine directly reduces the binding of antiphospholipid antibody-beta2-glycoprotein I complexes to phospholipid bilayers. Blood 112:1687-1695, 2008.

Chapter **83**

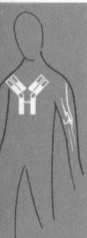

Systemic Sclerosis (Scleroderma)

Robyn T. Domsic and Thomas A. Medsger, Jr.

The hallmark of systemic sclerosis (SSc) is cutaneous and visceral fibrosis, which is reflected in the other common term for the disease, *scleroderma*, which derives from the Greek *scleros*, meaning thick, and *derma*, referring to skin. The disorder can range from a relatively benign condition to a rapidly progressive disease leading to significant morbidity or death. Although cutaneous manifestations are the most obvious, it is the visceral involvement that can be the most severe or disabling. Awareness of and monitoring for potential organ complications are essential in caring for patients with SSc, as early detection and treatment of complications minimize morbidity and mortality.

Epidemiology

The annual incidence of SSc in the United States is approximately 20 cases per million persons. As many patients with SSc live for many years, the prevalence is 240 cases per million. The incidence and prevalence varies somewhat throughout the world and is generally lower in Europe and Asia.

SSc more commonly affects women, with a 3 : 1 female:male ratio. It occurs in individuals of all ages, from childhood to the elderly, but is most frequent in the fourth through seventh decades. The familial pattern of inheritance is not as evident in SSc as in other rheumatic diseases, although many patients with SSc have family histories of autoimmune thyroid disease, rheumatoid arthritis, and lupus. Twin studies have demonstrated a 5% rate of concordance in both monozygotic and dizygotic twins, suggesting that both genetics and environment contribute to its occurrence.

Pathologic Considerations

The pathogenesis of SSc is complex and has not been fully elucidated. However, there are three clear components: (1) fibrosis with overproduction of collagen and other connective tissue matrix proteins, (2) vascular injury and obliteration, and (3) immune system activation (Fig. 83-1). The involvement of all three of these systems initially became evident from autopsy examinations. Examination of the skin reveals thickening of the dermis with excessive deposition of collagen fibrils, and fibrous replacement of subcutaneous fat and secondary skin appendages such as hair follicles and sebaceous glands. Vascular changes include endothelial cell injury and subintimal thickening leading to luminal narrowing with occasional vascular occlusion. Periadventitial fibrosis is frequent. The vascular changes are seen in the skin but also may occur in the pulmonary, cardiac, and renal systems and involve arteries, arterioles, and capillaries. Cutaneous inflammatory infiltrates consist of activated mononuclear cells, T lymphocytes, and monocytes in the dermis, often in a perivascular distribution. True vasculitis is conspicuously absent.

The interplay among the vascular, connective tissue, and immunologic changes is complex. Fibroblasts are found in increased numbers in the skin and other tissues, live longer, and produce an overabundance of collagen. Although fibroblasts can be activated by the immune system in normal skin repair, cultured skin fibroblasts have a persistent SSc phenotype, suggesting an abnormality not requiring continued immune stimulation. Other potential factors may contribute to fibrosis, including hypoxia and local cytokine changes. Endothelial cell activation with resultant leukocyte migration, smooth muscle cell proliferation, and matrix deposition have been implicated in the vascular changes. In the serum, increased levels of inflammatory markers (sedimentation rate) and circulating cytokines are seen. More than 95% of patients with SSc have one of nine serum autoantibodies relatively specific to scleroderma, all of which are directed at distinct antigens. These antibodies are helpful in classifying patients, but to date, their pathogenic role has not been elucidated.

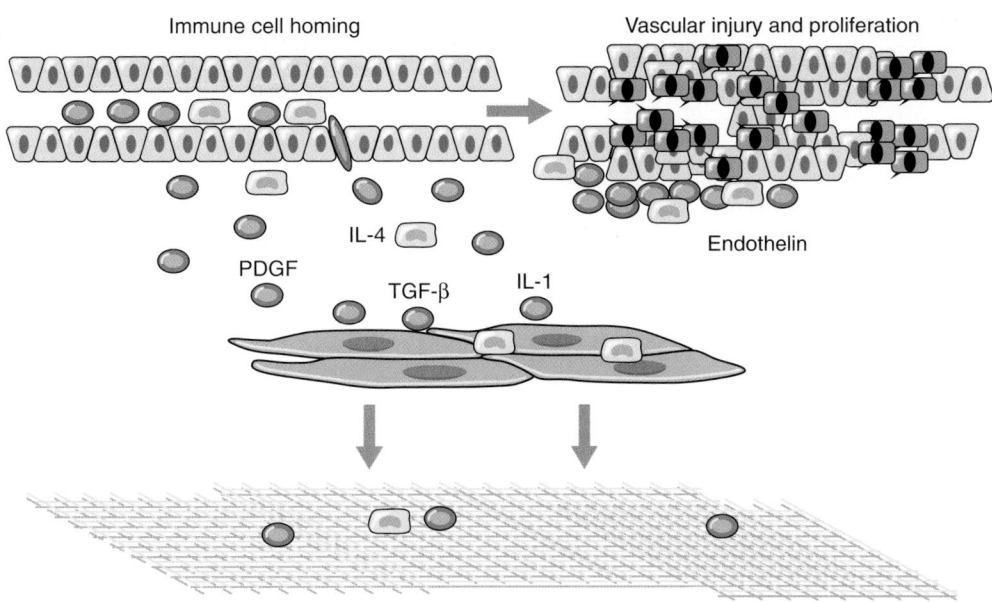
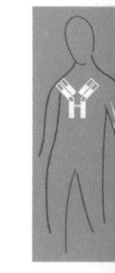

Immune cell homing

Vascular injury and proliferation

IL-4

PDGF

TGF-β

IL-1

Endothelin

Accumulation of interstitial matrix

Figure 83-1 Pathogenetic processes in systemic sclerosis. Vascular injury leads to intimal proliferation of both endothelial cells *(red)* and smooth muscle cells *(blue)*. Fibroblasts are activated to deposit increased amounts of interstitial matrix. IL, interleukin; PDGF, platelet-derived growth factor; TGF-β, transforming growth factor-β.

Clinical Features

SKIN CLASSIFICATION

SSc is separated into two major clinical subsets, diffuse cutaneous and limited cutaneous sclerosis, defined by the degree and extent of skin involvement. Patients with limited cutaneous involvement experience skin thickening limited to the extremities (below the elbows and knees). Patients with diffuse cutaneous SSc have similar distal changes and also involvement of the upper arms, thighs, or trunk at some time during the disease course. A small proportion of patients (<1%) have no skin thickening but have one or more typical SSc visceral manifestations. The term *SSc sine scleroderma* has been used to describe these patients whose disease behaves like that in individuals with limited skin disease. This distinction is important, as patients with diffuse disease are more likely to develop certain complications such as renal crisis, whereas those with limited disease are more predisposed to other problems such as pulmonary arterial hypertension (Table 83-1).

SEROLOGIC CLASSIFICATION

Serologic classification is also important, as autoantibodies define patients with SSc with similar clinical manifestations. For example, patients with anticentromere antibody almost always have limited skin disease and are at risk for pulmonary hypertension during follow-up. Individuals with anti-topoisomerase (also termed *anti–Scl-70*) or anti–RNA polymerase III antibody are likely to have diffuse disease. Those with anti–RNA polymerase III antibody have an increased risk of "renal crisis," whereas those with anti–Scl-70 have a higher frequency of interstitial lung disease (ILD).

RAYNAUD PHENOMENON AND PERIPHERAL VASCULAR INVOLVEMENT

Nearly all patients with SSc experience Raynaud phenomenon, which is defined as a triphasic vascular response to cold consisting of pallor, cyanosis, and reactive hyperemia. The onset of Raynaud phenomenon can precede the development of skin changes by years in some patients. Severe involvement may result in ischemia with loss of digital tip tissue including digital pitting scars, ulcers, and, rarely, gangrene. A frequent finding in late-stage disease is visibly dilated capillaries and venules of the hands, face, and lips.

INTERSTITIAL LUNG DISEASE

ILD can be one of the most serious complications of SSc and needs to be monitored for routinely. The initial presentation is often a nonproductive cough and gradual onset of dyspnea on exertion (often over several months to years). High-resolution chest computed tomography (CT) typically shows bibasilar fibrotic changes, which can be progressive, and pulmonary function tests show reduced forced vital capacity (FVC). On pathology, the most frequently seen pattern is nonspecific interstitial pneumonitis. Patients with anti–Scl-70 are at highest risk for development of ILD.

PULMONARY ARTERIAL HYPERTENSION

Pulmonary arterial hypertension not associated with ILD is detected in 10% to 25% of patients with SSc, more commonly in those with limited disease, although it can occur in those with long-standing diffuse disease. Presentation is generally with rapidly progressive dyspnea (over several months). Pulmonary function tests reveal a reduced diffusion capacity for carbon monoxide (D_{LCO}) out of

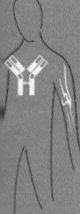

Table 83-1 **Clinical Features of Systemic Sclerosis**		
	Diffuse	**Limited**
Skin induration	Widespread; extremities, trunk, face	Face and extremities distal to the elbow or knee
Raynaud phenomenon	80%-90%; ischemia, digital ulcers	95%-100%; ischemia, digital ulcers
Telangiectasia	Common	May be extensive
Calcinosis	Occurs, more frequent in limited	Common
Esophageal hypomotility and reflux	80% may be severe; strictures	90%; may be severe
Intestinal hypomotility or malabsorption	Common, may be severe	Less common, not usually severe
Interstitial lung disease	Common, major cause of death	Frequent
Pulmonary hypertension	Often secondary to pulmonary fibrosis; primary type less common	10%; primary type
Cardiac fibrosis, cardiomyopathy	Common	Less common
Renal disease	Renal crisis and vasculopathy	Very rarely seen
Myositis	<20%; may be severe	<20%; may be severe
Tendon friction rubs	Common with active skin disease	Rarely—indicate likely progression to diffuse disease if present
Antinuclear antibodies	98%	98%
Anti–SCL-70	30%-40%	10%-15%
Anti–RNA polymerase III	Up to 50%	
Anti-centromere	3%	40%-50%

proportion to any concomitant reduction in FVC. Screening is generally performed by echocardiogram and should be confirmed by right heart cardiac catheterization. Both left ventricular diastolic dysfunction and associated ILD should be considered as causes of pulmonary arterial hypertension in patients with SSc.

SCLERODERMA RENAL CRISIS

Renal crisis generally manifests as the abrupt onset of accelerated hypertension accompanied by a rise in serum creatinine and microscopic hematuria and proteinuria on urinalysis. Microangiopathic hemolytic anemia and thrombocytopenia are frequent. Although once the major contributor to mortality, renal crisis can now be easily managed with an angiotensin-converting enzyme (ACE) inhibitor. The typical setting for renal crisis is early diffuse disease. During this time patients should check their blood pressure once weekly, reporting a rise in systolic blood pressure of >30 mm Hg from baseline.

CARDIAC INVOLVEMENT

Patients with SSc experience three primary types of cardiac involvement. These include pericarditis, myocarditis, and myocardial fibrosis leading to congestive heart failure and arrhythmias because of fibrosis of the conduction system. These complications can be underrecognized in patients with SSc but are frequently found at autopsy.

GASTROINTESTINAL MANIFESTATIONS

At least one gastrointestinal manifestation will affect 80% or more of patients with SSc. Gastrointestinal manifestations are a significant cause of morbidity. All areas of the gastrointestinal tract may be affected. Patients experience heartburn and distal dysphagia of solid foods owing to relaxation of the esophageal sphincter and esophageal dysmotility,

respectively. Neuropathic changes and fibrosis of the muscularis of the small intestine can lead to hypomotility and symptoms of postprandial abdominal distention. The hypomotility can lead to bacterial overgrowth and ultimately to malabsorption, as the bacteria may digest pancreatic enzymes. Signs and symptoms include abdominal pain and distention, along with watery diarrhea or steatorrhea. Occasionally, when severe atony of the small intestine develops, patients will develop a functional ileus, or intestinal pseudoobstruction. Similar to the small bowel, the colon may develop impaired motor function, resulting in constipation, and occasionally "overflow" diarrhea. Wide-mouthed diverticula can be seen. The internal anal sphincter may become fibrotic, resulting in fecal incontinence.

MUSCULOSKELETAL MANIFESTATIONS

Musculoskeletal manifestations are common. Tendons can become inflamed and fibrotic, particularly in early diffuse disease. Palpable tendon or bursal friction rubs are virtually pathognomonic of SSc and often are a harbinger of diffuse disease before widespread skin thickening has occurred. Destructive arthropathy is occasionally seen. Some patients develop a bland myopathy that manifests as nonprogressive, mild proximal muscle weakness and wasting. Other patients, particularly if they have overlapping features with other connective tissue diseases, can develop myositis.

Differential and Diagnosis

Raynaud disease, or "primary" Raynaud, is prominent in the differential for SSc. Two features that identify patients with Raynaud who have or may later develop SSc or another connective tissue disease are abnormal nailfold capillaries (dilation or dropout) and a positive antinuclear antibody

(ANA) test result. Neither of these features is found in Raynaud disease, which is more often familial.

When initially evaluating a patient with SSc features, it is important to determine whether she or he has SSc alone or overlapping with another connective tissue disease, such as systemic lupus erythematosus or polymyositis. Although these disorders are covered elsewhere, patients with these conditions (also referred to as *mixed connective tissue disease*) often will demonstrate SSc-like findings including scleroderma skin changes, Raynaud phenomenon, and esophageal dysmotility.

There are a number of scleroderma "mimics," which at times can be confusing to distinguish from SSc (Table 83-2). These include eosinophilic fasciitis (EF), morphea, and the localized forms of scleroderma, such as linear scleroderma (more frequently seen in children). Nephrogenic systemic fibrosis (NSF) is a recently described disorder now recognized to be a complication of gadolinium administration for radiographic studies in the setting of renal failure. EF is distinguished by peripheral blood eosinophilia with thickening of the forearm fascia leading to clawing of the hands, but lack of skin thickening of the fingers. Morphea reveals isolated patches of induration followed by atrophic skin, often in a dermatomal pattern. Linear scleroderma more frequently affects children. NSF manifests as symmetrical, bilateral fibrotic indurated papules, plaques, or subcutaneous nodules, which can be erythematosus, on the lower legs or hands. The lesions are often preceded by edema and may initially be misdiagnosed as cellulitis. This diagnosis should be considered in any patient being evaluated for a fibrotic disorder who has renal failure, regardless of the cause of renal disease. All SSc mimics lack Raynaud phenomenon, characteristic SSc internal organ involvement, and SSc-associated serum antibodies.

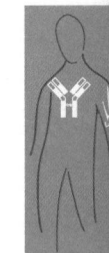

Patient Care and Treatment

As no single therapy exists for SSc, it is vital that patients with SSc be appropriately monitored for organ manifestations, thereby allowing for early identification and therapy targeted at specific organ complications (Table 83-3). Consultation with a rheumatologist is helpful in this respect. In general, all patients should undergo screening evaluation for ILD and pulmonary hypertension at the time of diagnosis and every 2 to 3 years thereafter. Patients with active diffuse cutaneous disease should undergo weekly monitoring of blood pressure, evaluating for increases suggestive of renal crisis. These patients should also have skin thickness scores assessed for progression or regression of cutaneous disease. Both patients with diffuse disease and those with limited disease can develop gastrointestinal manifestations as noted previously, and objective studies can be ordered as warranted by symptoms. Education of patients and family members regarding the disease and the patient's classification (early or late diffuse or limited disease) can be helpful in alleviating patient anxiety.

RAYNAUD PHENOMENON

Calcium channel blockers have been widely used for decades and are generally well tolerated by patients. Long-acting nifedipine is effective in over half of patients, and newer agents such as amlodipine are also frequently prescribed. The angiotensin receptor blocking agent losartan has been shown to reduce the severity and frequency of Raynaud attacks in a placebo-controlled trial. In patients who experience digital ulcerations, more aggressive therapy may be warranted. Sildenafil has been studied and found to be helpful in uncontrolled studies. Topical nitroglycerin administered to the hand may be a useful adjunct. Bosentan has been shown in randomized placebo-controlled trials to prevent the formation of new digital ulcerations in patients with SSc and Raynaud, although it has not yet been approved by the U.S. Food and Drug Administration (FDA) for this indication. Although used more frequently in Europe, monthly intravenous (IV) prostacyclins have also been used to treat and prevent digital ulcerations. Surgical interventions include sympathectomy of the digital, radial, or ulnar artery and venous bypass for ulnar or radial artery occlusion.

Table 83-2 **Scleroderma-like Syndromes**	
Other Diseases	**Distinguishing Features**
Morphea	Patchy or linear distribution
Eosinophilic fasciitis	Sparing of hands
	Biopsy shows involvement extending to fascia and muscle
Scleredema (of Buschke)	Prominent involvement of neck, shoulders, and upper arms; hands spared
	Associated with diabetes
Scleromyxedema	Association with gammopathy; skin lichenoid and thickened but not tethered
	May have Raynaud phenomenon
Graft-versus-host disease	Skin changes similar to scleroderma; vasculopathy
Nephrogenic-fibrosing dermopathy	Indurated plaques or nodules on the legs or arms, sparing the face, often preceded by edema
Environmental Agents and Drugs	
Bleomycin	Skin and lung fibrosis similar to scleroderma
L-Tryptophan	Eosinophilia-myalgia; from contaminant or metabolite (described in the 1980s)
	Fever, eosinophilia, neurologic manifestations, pulmonary hypertension
Organic solvents	Trichloroethylene and others implicated
	Clinically indistinguishable from idiopathic systemic sclerosis
Pentazocine	Localized lesions at injection sites
Toxic oil syndrome	Contaminated rapeseed oil (Spanish epidemic, 1981)
	Similar to eosinophilia myalgia syndrome
Vinyl chloride disease	Vascular lesions, acro-osteolysis, sclerodactyly
	No visceral disease
Gadolinium	Nephrogenic systemic fibrosis

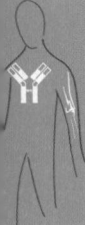

Table 83-3 **Therapeutic Approaches to Systemic Sclerosis**

Manifestation	Pathophysiologic Features	Treatment
Raynaud phenomenon	Vascular hyperreactivity and obliteration	Calcium channel blocker
		Angiotensin receptor blockers, vasodilators, and smoking cessation
Digital ulcers	Vascular changes leading to ischemia	Raynaud treatment as above or treatment with sildenafil or monthly prostanoids.
		Bosentan may reduce new digital ulcerations.
		Digital sympathectomy or vascular bypass when there is evidence of radial or ulnar vasculopathy.
Esophageal reflux	Loss of lower esophageal sphincter function	Proton-pump inhibitors; H$_2$-blockers
Intestinal hypomotility	Damage to the myenteric plexus; intestinal fibrosis and atrophy	Promotility agents
Malabsorption	Bacterial overgrowth	Rotating antibiotics
		Monitoring and supplementation of fat-soluble vitamins and iron
Interstitial lung disease	Inflammation; fibrosis	Cyclophosphamide, mycophenolate mofetil corticosteroids
Pulmonary hypertension	Vascular obliteration	Prostacyclin analogs, endothelin-receptor antagonists, sildenafil
Cardiac arrhythmia	Myocardial ischemia and fibrosis	Anti-arrhythmic agents
Renal crisis	Vasculopathy with upregulated renin-angiotensin system	Angiotensin-converting enzyme (ACE) inhibitors
Myositis	Inflammation	Corticosteroids; methotrexate or other immunosuppressive agents
Skin thickening	Inflammation, Fibrosis	D-Penicillamine, mycophenolate, mofetil, or other investigational drugs

In patients with SSc with recurrent digital ulcerations or other thrombotic events with Raynaud disease, evaluation for a hypercoagulable state, particularly for lupus anticoagulant, should be performed. If a hypercoagulable state is present, the use of aspirin or other anticoagulants should be considered.

CUTANEOUS DISEASE

No therapeutic agent has been found to improve skin thickening in diffuse scleroderma patients in a randomized, placebo-controlled trial. There are several methodologic issues that may have contributed to the negative findings, including the drugs chosen, patient populations, and trial designs. In the past, considerable attention was given to methotrexate and D-penicillamine. Methotrexate provided conflicting results, and D-penicillamine, unfortunately, was never studied in a placebo-controlled fashion. Currently several drugs are undergoing clinical trials. These agents act by either reducing collagen synthesis or increasing collagen breakdown. Several reports on the benefit of autologous stem cell transplantation have been published, and two multicenter randomized, controlled trials of cyclophosphamide versus stem cell transplantation are currently enrolling patients.

SCLERODERMA RENAL CRISIS

Early identification and treatment with ACE inhibitors have dramatically improved survival and outcomes of scleroderma renal crisis. ACE inhibitors should be titrated to maintain a "normal" blood pressure, preferably <125/75. Even if a patient with renal crisis becomes dialysis-dependent initially, if ACE inhibitor therapy is maintained, some patients may experience a slow reversal of renal vascular damage and can discontinue dialysis during the first 2 years after the onset of this complication.

INTERSTITIAL LUNG DISEASE

Early recognition of inflammatory ILD is important if treatment is to prevent progression to distortion of lung architecture and irreversible fibrosis. A recent large U.S. randomized, placebo-controlled trial demonstrated statistically significant but modest benefit with the use of cyclophosphamide at 1 year. However, after an additional year off therapy, cyclophosphamide-treated patients lost their benefit, suggesting other treatment options are needed. Small case series suggest potential benefit of mycophenolate mofetil, but this drug has not been tested in a randomized trial. Lung transplantation can be considered for end-stage ILD.

PULMONARY ARTERIAL HYPERTENSION

In recent years, several agents have been approved for the treatment of pulmonary arterial hypertension in patients with SSc. Subset analyses of several placebo-controlled drug trials have shown improvement in established SSc or connective tissue disease–related pulmonary hypertension. These have included sildenafil, bosentan, ambrisentan, treprostenil, and epoprostenol. Theoretically, treatment of patients with early, less severe disease would improve outcomes, but such studies are only beginning to be reported. Because patients with SSc-related pulmonary hypertension have a worse prognosis than those with primary pulmonary hypertension, we strongly recommend referring patients with SSc with pulmonary hypertension to a tertiary care facility with a dedicated pulmonary hypertension clinic.

CARDIAC MANIFESTATIONS

Diastolic dysfunction, which is often underrecognized in SSc, can be evaluated on echocardiogram when performed for pulmonary hypertension screening. Many SSc deaths occur suddenly, possibly because of ventricular arrhythmias. Therefore it is prudent to obtain a resting electrocardiogram early in the disease course. Palpitations noted by the patient should be addressed with a formal cardiac arrhythmia evaluation.

GASTROINTESTINAL MANIFESTATIONS

Gastroesophageal reflux, which is present in nearly all patients with SSc, can be treated with proton pump inhibitors and conservative measures including elevation of the bed and avoidance of alcohol and caffeine. If untreated, reflux esophagitis can progress to stricture. Patients experiencing severe esophageal, gastric, or small bowel dysmotility may improve with the use of prokinetic drugs, such as

metoclopramide, erythromycin, or octreotide. If bacterial overgrowth is present, rotating antibiotics may be of assistance. In advanced small bowel involvement with malabsorption, supplementation of iron, calcium, and fat-soluble vitamins may be required. Occasionally, total parenteral nutrition is necessary. Unexplained iron deficiency anemia in patients with SSc should suggest the possibility of gastric antral vascular ectasias, which are treated with laser photocoagulation, and requires initial surveillance. Patients with this particular condition should be routinely monitored for iron deficiency anemia.

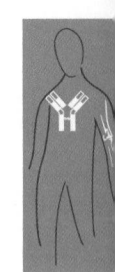

SKELETAL MUSCLE, JOINT, AND TENDON

Bland myopathy is generally nonprogressive and is treated with physical therapy. If myositis is suspected, as evidenced by elevation of serum muscle enzymes, abnormal electromyogram, or muscle biopsy, steroids and immunosuppressive therapy (such as methotrexate or azathioprine) may be helpful. Of note, both patients with limited disease and those with diffuse disease can develop contractures of the hands owing to tendon involvement. Physical therapy with daily stretching exercises directed at the finger joints should be instituted.

Prospectus for the Future

Effective therapy for both vascular and skin disease in scleroderma has been lacking. A multitude of potential reasons include lack of specific identified molecular targets, inadequate trial design, and difficulty in patient recruitment. An important clinical research emphasis should be defining and understanding clinical and serologic disease subsets. The SSc research community is working toward this. In the last few years, additional potential molecular targets have been identified. Many of these are involved with the fibrotic process, which affects virtually all organ systems in the disease. Clinical trial consortia in both the United States and Europe are now working together to develop trials to test potential agents, increasing hope that important treatment advances will be made in the future.

References

Mayes MD: The scleroderma book: A guide for patients and families. New York, Oxford University Press, 1999.

Medsger TA: Natural history of systemic sclerosis and the assessment of disease activity, severity, functional status, and psychologic well-being. Rheum Dis Clin North Am 29:255-275, 2003.

Ong VH, Brough G, Denton CP: Management of systemic sclerosis. Clin Med 5:214-219, 2005.

Varga J: Raynaud phenomenon, scleroderma, overlap syndromes and other fibrosing syndromes. Curr Opin Rheumatol 17:735-767, 2005.

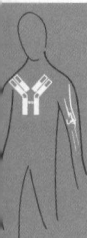

Idiopathic Inflammatory Myopathies

Larry W. Moreland

The idiopathic inflammatory myopathies (IIMs) include polymyositis, dermatomyositis, myositis associated with malignancy, myositis associated with other connective tissue disease, and inclusion body myositis. These conditions have in common the clinical features of progressive symmetrical proximal weakness, elevation of muscle enzymes, muscle histologic features demonstrating mononuclear inflammatory cell infiltrates and muscle fiber necrosis, and characteristic electromyographic abnormalities. The IIMs differ in their association with extramuscular manifestations and with certain autoantibody profiles (Tables 84-1 and 84-2). The presence of mononuclear cell infiltration in muscle and frequent immune abnormalities, including autoantibodies, in patients with IIM has resulted in most of these disorders being thought of as autoimmune or immune-mediated diseases. This has also been the basis for the major therapeutic approaches for IIM that have been directed toward decreasing inflammation in the many organs that may be affected in these diseases.

The IIMs as a group and individually are relatively rare conditions, with estimated prevalence rates of 2 to 10 cases per million and incidence rates of 0.5 to 8.4 cases per million. The male-to-female ratio is approximately 2:1 for polymyositis and dermatomyositis; inclusion body myositis predominates in men. The age distribution of IIMs is bimodal, with a peak at ages 10 to 15 years in children with dermatomyositis and another peak at ages 40 to 60 years. Both myositis associated with malignancy and inclusion body myositis are more common after the age of 50 years.

Pathologic and Pathophysiologic Features

The hallmark of the IIMs is inflammatory infiltrate within muscle tissue. The infiltrate is primarily lymphocytic, but macrophages, plasma cells, and sometimes eosinophils,

basophils, and neutrophils are present. In polymyositis the infiltrate typically clusters in the endomysial area around muscle fibers, whereas in dermatomyositis the infiltrate predominates in the perimysial area around the fascicles and small blood vessels. Perifascicular atrophy occurs more frequently in dermatomyositis (Fig. 84-1). Necrotizing vasculitis is uncommon. Inclusion body myositis is characterized by the presence of intracellular vacuoles, which under electron microscopy appear as intracytoplasmic, intranuclear tubular, or filamentous inclusions.

The association of IIMs with other autoimmune disorders (including Hashimoto's thyroiditis, myasthenia gravis, primary biliary cirrhosis, and connective tissue diseases), in some cases with autoantibodies (see Table 84-2), and the response to corticosteroids suggest an autoimmune pathogenesis. This hypothesis is also supported by the identification of T cells cytotoxic to muscle in biopsy specimens and in the peripheral blood of patients with polymyositis and dermatomyositis. Autoimmunity is also suggested by the finding of immunoglobulin deposition and complement components in the capillaries and small arterioles in dermatomyositis. In addition, antibodies to autoantigens have been associated with IIMs and their complications. For example, antibodies to Mi2 (a nuclear helicase) are found in patients with dermatomyositis and skin rash, and antibodies to Jo-1 (a histidine transfer RNA [tRNA] synthetase) are found in patients with polymyositis and interstitial lung disease. Inclusion body myositis probably represents a special case, given its distinctive pathologic features, because amyloid deposits have been identified in the vacuoles that characterize this condition. A wide variety of proinflammatory cytokines (e.g., interferon-γ, interleukin-1, tissue necrosis factor–α), chemokines (e.g., monocyte chemotactic protein), and cell adhesion molecules (e.g., platelet endothelial cell adhesion molecule–1, vascular cellular adhesion molecule) appear to be upregulated in the inflammatory myopathies. However, the sequence of events involved in the production of these molecules, their targets, and their precise role in muscle fiber damage and repair remain uncertain.

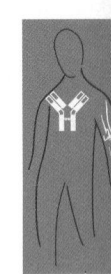

Table 84-1 Classification of the Idiopathic Inflammatory Myopathies

Primary idiopathic polymyositis

Primary idiopathic dermatomyositis

Polymyositis or dermatomyositis associated with malignancy

Juvenile dermatomyositis (or polymyositis)

Overlap syndrome of polymyositis or dermatomyositis with another autoimmune rheumatic disease

Inclusion body myositis

Table 84-2 Myositis Syndromes and Associated Autoantibodies

Autoantibody	Clinical Features	Treatment Response
Anti-Jo 1 (also known as antisynthetase)*	Polymyositis or dermatomyositis	Moderate with persistent disease
	Acute interstitial lung disease	
	Fever	
	Arthritis	
	Raynaud phenomenon	
Anti-SRP†	Polymyositis	Poor
	Abrupt onset	
	Severe weakness	
	Palpitations	
Anti-Mi2‡	Dermatomyositis	Good
	V sign and shawl sign	
	Cuticular overgrowth	

*Anti-Jo 1 is the most common myositis-specific autoantibody. It is known as *antisynthetase* because the putative antibody target is an RNA synthetase. The prevalence of anti-Jo 1 is approximately 20%. Other antisynthetase antibodies include anti-PL-7, anti-PL-12, anti-EJ, and anti-OJ, each of which has a prevalence of less than 3%.
†Prevalence is approximately 5%.
‡Prevalence is approximately 10%.
SRP, signal recognition particle.

Clinical Presentation

Patients with polymyositis are representative of the IIMs in their presentation and clinical features. The onset of the disease is typically insidious over a period of months, with proximal muscle weakness; in rare cases the presentation is more fulminant, with both proximal and distal muscle weakness. A more indolent onset over years with both proximal and distal involvement suggests inclusion body myositis. The symmetrical proximal muscle weakness often impairs performance of specific tasks such as getting up from a sitting position, getting out of a car, and reaching overhead or combing the hair, and it should be distinguished from conditions that produce a generalized fatigue or loss of energy that rarely interferes with these functions. Approximately one third of patients with polymyositis have upper esophageal involvement, which produces dysphagia and, occasionally, aspiration of oral contents. Myalgia occurs in approximately one half of patients, but it is generally mild, although it may cause confusion with polymyalgia rheumatica in older patients.

The assessment of muscle strength should include active resistive testing; the physician should keep in mind that this testing should also be supplemented by asking the patient to perform specific tasks such as getting up from a low chair without using his or her arms, raising the arms over the head, and lifting the head from the examining table when in the supine position. The examiner should be aware that assessment of motor power may be confounded by the fatigue or pain of arthritis or myalgia.

In dermatomyositis, a characteristic skin eruption occurs, usually preceding the development of myositis. In rare cases, patients have the classic skin manifestations without the myositis (*dermatomyositis sine myositis* or *amyopathic dermatomyositis*). The rash has several distinctive varieties: Gottron lesions, the erythematous or poikilodermatous rash, and the heliotrope rash. *Gottron papules* consist of erythematous, sometimes scaly papules, plaques, or macules (Gottron sign) over the metacarpophalangeal and proximal interphalangeal joints. The *poikilodermatous eruption* of dermatomyositis consists of an erythematous or violaceous rash on the face, trunk, neck, extremities, or scalp. Occasionally, a characteristic distribution in the shape of a V appears on the anterior chest, or the so-called *shawl sign* (back of neck, upper torso, and shoulders). The *heliotrope (lilac-colored) rash* occurs in 30% to 60% of patients with dermatomyositis and is located characteristically on the upper eyelids, but it may be difficult to detect in dark-skinned patients.

Various nonmuscular and nondermatologic manifestations of the IIM may occur (Table 84-3). Pulmonary involvement in polymyositis and dermatomyositis may take several forms, including respiratory muscle weakness, interstitial lung disease, pulmonary hypertension, pulmonary vasculitis, and aspiration pneumonia. Respiratory muscle involvement may include the chest wall musculature and the diaphragm and is clinically significant in approximately 5% of patients. Respiratory failure necessitating ventilatory assistance is fortunately rare. Esophageal and tongue involvement appears to be a risk factor for this complication. Interstitial lung disease occurs in approximately 10% to 30% of patients with either polymyositis or dermatomyositis and in the case of polymyositis is frequently associated with the presence of antisynthetase (Jo-1) antibodies, fever, Raynaud phenomenon, and arthritis (*antisynthetase syndrome*) (see Table 84-2). Curiously, the severity of the interstitial lung disease may be independent of the severity of myositis.

Cardiac involvement in IIM may include conduction blocks, arrhythmias, and myocarditis; it appears to be more common than previously estimated (up to 70% in one series) and, as in interstitial lung disease, may be independent of the severity of myositis. Dysphagia, the result of myositis of striated muscle in the upper one third of the esophagus, occurs in up to 30% of patients with IIM. Less common involvement includes cricopharyngeal muscle dysfunction and, in children with dermatomyositis, intestinal vasculitis.

The relationship of IIM with malignant disease has been clarified by population-based studies showing a modest increase in risk (approximate twofold relative risk) within 1 to 2 years of the diagnosis of dermatomyositis and possibly polymyositis. The malignancies associated with dermatomyositis include those that occur most commonly in the general population. They include cancers of the lung, breast,

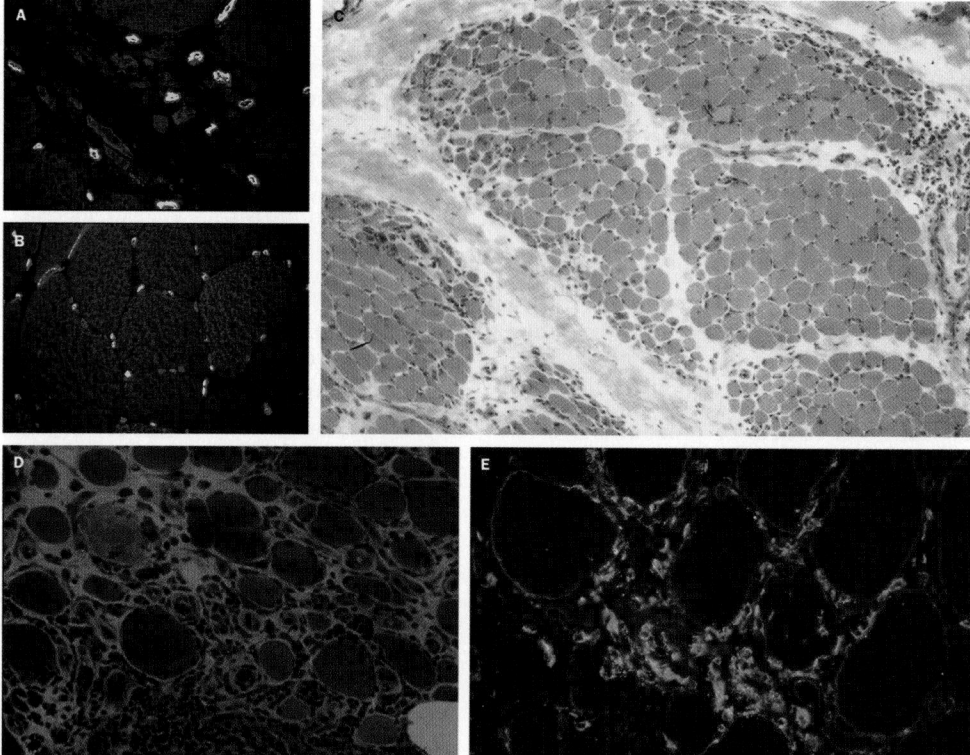

Figure 84-1 Histologic findings in polymyositis and dermatomyositis. Depletion of capillaries in dermatomyositis **(A)** with dilation of the lumen of the remaining capillaries, compared with a normal muscle **(B)**. **C,** Perifascicular atrophy in dermatomyositis. **D,** Endomysial inflammation in polymyositis and inclusion-body myositis with lymphocytic cells invading healthy fibers. **E,** MHC-I/ CD8 complex in polymyositis and inclusion-body myositis. MHC-I *(green)* is upregulated on all the muscle fibers, and CD8+ T cells *(orange),* which also express MHC-I, invade the fibers. (From Dalakas M, Hohlfeld R. Polymyositis and dermatomyositis. Lancet 362:971-982, 2003.)

Table 84-3 **Extramuscular Manifestations of Polymyositis and Dermatomyositis**
Pulmonary
Respiratory muscle weakness
Aspiration
Interstitial lung disease
Pulmonary vasculitis
Cardiac
Heart block
Arrhythmias
Cardiomyopathy
Gastrointestinal
Esophageal dysmotility
Stomach, small or large bowel dysmotility
Arthritis
Nonerosive, symmetrical, small joint

Diagnosis

When most of the known causes of myopathy are excluded by the clinical context and nature of the symptoms, the physical examination and laboratory testing should be directed at narrowing further the diagnostic possibilities and determining if more invasive procedures are needed. Muscle weakness needs to be distinguished from fatigability or pain that might limit function. The distribution of skeletal muscle tenderness or atrophy should be noted. Involvement of other muscles, including the heart, oropharynx, gastrointestinal tract, or ocular and respiratory muscles, as well as any other nonmuscle abnormalities, should be documented. Rashes need to be carefully evaluated and, in some cases, biopsied. The diagnosis of IIM is suggested by the typical history and physical examination. Muscle enzymes such as creatine phosphokinase and aldolase are significantly elevated. The diagnosis is confirmed by muscle biopsy, ideally an open biopsy to allow the optimal assessment of muscle architecture, although needle biopsy may be adequate for the diagnosis of polymyositis or dermatomyositis in many cases. The ideal muscle to sample for biopsy is one that is involved but not atrophic. Most commonly, the quadriceps or deltoid muscle is examined by biopsy. Magnetic resonance imaging (MRI) can detect muscle inflammation and damage and may improve the yield of biopsy diagnosis by directing the site of biopsy. Electron microscopy is helpful to establish the diagnosis of inclusion body myositis, and special stains to

colon, prostate, and ovary. Experts recommend a thorough history, examination, and screening rectal examination; Papanicolaou stain in women; urinalysis; blood chemistry studies; chest radiograph; and prostate-specific antigen measurement in men. Serial gynecologic examinations, transvaginal ultrasonography, and serial CA-125 determinations to screen fully for ovarian cancer in women with recently diagnosed dermatomyositis may also be reasonable.

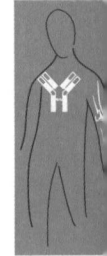

Table 84-4 **Typical Electromyographic Features of Polymyositis and Dermatomyositis**
Low-amplitude, short-duration motor unit action potentials
Typical myopathic pattern
Polyphasic potentials
Resulting from asynchronous firing of fibers
Increased insertional activity and fibrillation
Attributed to damage to nerve endings or motor end plates
Complex repetitive discharges
Thought to be the result of inflammatory damage to the sarcolemma

Table 84-5 **Differential Diagnosis of Idiopathic Inflammatory Myositis**
Infectious
Viral Myositis
Retroviruses (HIV, HTLV-1)
Enteroviruses (echovirus, coxsackievirus)
Other viruses (influenza, hepatitis A and B, Epstein-Barr virus)
Bacterial
Pyomyositis
Parasites
Trichinosis, cysticercosis
Fungi
Candidiasis
Idiopathic
Granulomatous myositis (sarcoid, giant cell)
Eosinophilic myositis
Graft-versus-host disease
Myositis associated with vasculitides
Endocrine and Metabolic Disorders
Hypothyroidism
Hyperthyroidism
Hypercortisolism
Hyperparathyroidism
Hypoparathyroidism
Hypocalcemia
Hypokalemia
Metabolic Myopathies
Myophosphorylase deficiency (McArdle disease)
Phosphofructokinase deficiency
Myoadenylate deaminase deficiency
Acid maltase deficiency
Lipid storage diseases
Acute rhabdomyolysis
Drug-Induced Myopathies
Alcohol
D-Penicillamine
Zidovudine
Colchicine
Chloroquine, hydroxychloroquine
Lipid-lowering agents
Cyclosporine
Cocaine, heroin, barbiturates
Corticosteroids
L-Tryptophan (eosinophilia myalgia syndrome)
Neurologic Disorders
Muscular dystrophies
Congenital myopathies
Motor neuron disease
Guillain-Barré syndrome
Myasthenia gravis
Autoimmune polyneuropathy
Eaton-Lambert syndrome
Paraneoplastic syndrome

HIV, human immunodeficiency virus; HTLV-1, human T-cell lymphotropic virus type 1.

identify excess glycogen or lipid are useful to exclude metabolic myopathies. With the possible exception of Jo-1 antibodies and the identification of the antisynthetase syndrome (see Table 84-2), the role of myositis-specific antibodies remains limited because they lack sensitivity, and not all are commercially available.

Electromyography alone cannot enable one to establish the diagnosis, but it can indicate muscle involvement in patients with dermatologic or nonmuscular features. Typical electromyographic features are listed in Table 84-4.

Differential Diagnosis

Patients with complaints of weakness or muscle pain are very common in clinical practice. Many different conditions should be considered in the differential diagnosis of myositis (Table 84-5). These include other myopathies (infectious myositis, drug-induced disorders, muscular dystrophies, metabolic myopathies, and endocrine disorders) and/or neurologic conditions (e.g., myasthenia gravis, Guillain-Barré syndrome).

Treatment

The mainstay of treatment for the IIMs consists of the corticosteroids. Initially, prednisone is begun at a high dose (e.g., 60 mg/day) until the creatine phosphokinase level has returned to normal or muscle strength has significantly improved. Occasionally, extremely high doses of intravenous corticosteroids are used for severely ill patients. Subsequently, corticosteroids are gradually tapered, depending on the clinical response. Approximately one third to one fourth of patients require additional immunosuppressive agents such as methotrexate or azathioprine because of steroid resistance, intolerable side effects, or inability to taper corticosteroids without inducing a flare-up in disease. Cyclophosphamide and cyclosporine have proved effective in patients who are resistant to steroid therapy; however, the toxicity of these agents limits widespread use. Mycophenolate mofetil is emerging as a promising and well-tolerated agent. Clinical trials have established the efficacy and low toxicity of intravenous gamma globulin in dermatomyositis. This therapy appears to work by blocking deposition of activated complement fragments and thereby protecting muscle capillaries from complement-mediated injury. Although intravenous gamma globulin is attractive because of its low toxicity, its long-term efficacy is unknown, and its long-term use is limited by its expense.

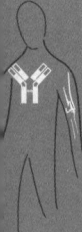

Prospectus for the Future

- The genetic factors that predispose individuals to develop dermatomyositis and polymyositis must be identified.
- The environmental triggers of myositis must be determined.

- Genetic, serologic, and other markers must be identified to predict treatment responses.

References

Baer AN: Advances in the therapy of idiopathic inflammatory myopathies. Curr Opin Rheumatol 18:236-241, 2006.

Callen JP: Immunomodulatory treatment for dermatomyositis. Curr Allergy Asthma Rep 8:348-353, 2008.

Greenberg SA: Inflammatory myopathies: Evaluation and management. Semin Neurol 28:241-249, 2008.

Koopman WJ, Moreland LW (eds): Arthritis and Allied Conditions: A Textbook of Rheumatology, 15th ed. Philadelphia, Lippincott Williams & Wilkins, 2004.

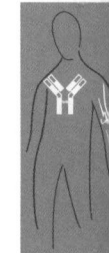

Sjögren Syndrome

Fotios Koumpouras

Sjögren syndrome is a chronic immune-mediated, inflammatory disorder of exocrine gland dysfunction. The syndrome can occur as a primary disorder or secondary to another connective tissue disease. The main exocrine glands that are affected include the lacrimal gland and the salivary glands, which can lead to dry eyes (keratoconjunctivitis sicca or xerophthalmia) and dry mouth (xerostomia). In addition, Sjögren syndrome can have systemic features including fatigue, fever, weight loss, and lymphadenopathy. The most common manifestations include inflammation of the exocrine glands by infiltration of mononuclear cells, resulting in gland destruction. Infiltration of visceral organs and skin can result in hepatitis, interstitial lung disease, vasculitis, and lymphoma, among others. Sjögren syndrome is associated with various autoantibodies, particularly antinuclear antibodies.

Patients are considered to have *secondary* Sjögren syndrome if they have another immunologic disorder, such as systemic lupus erythematosus, rheumatoid arthritis, systemic sclerosis (scleroderma), or primary biliary cirrhosis, and to have *primary* Sjögren syndrome if no underlying immunologic disorder is present. Although more common among women, Sjögren syndrome does affect men and is found among people of all ages, races, and ethnicities.

Clinical Features

The clinical features of Sjögren syndrome can be divided into those associated with exocrine gland dysfunction (Table 85-1) and those associated with extraglandular manifestations (Table 85-2). Dry eyes and mouth are by far the most common problems and can be very troubling to patients. Severe xerostomia can lead to tooth loss. Severe dry eyes can lead to corneal lesions and vision impairment. Many of the extraglandular manifestations, although often rare, can be life or organ threatening. The most common extraglandular feature is articular and the presence of Raynaud phenomenon.

The clinical association with Sjögren syndrome with lymphoma is well described. These lymphomas (usually B-cell types) may involve malignant transformation of clinically involved exocrine glands or may involve sites not clinically apparent, such as cervical lymph nodes. Maintaining a low threshold in considering the diagnosis of lymphoma is prudent in patients with Sjögren syndrome who develop new masses, exhibit constitutional features, or experience persistent glandular swelling that is either resistant to treatment or changes in character.

Neurologic involvement in Sjögren syndrome can be overlooked. Five percent to 25% of patients with Sjögren syndrome have neurologic involvement, and it can be a presenting symptom. Sjögren syndrome can affect the central nervous system, but more commonly it affects the peripheral nervous system. The most common central nervous system manifestation is focal or multifocal brain involvement, which can mimic multiple sclerosis. Spinal cord involvement also can occur. Less common is the presence of optic neuritis. Peripheral nervous system involvement most commonly manifests as neuropathy with dysesthesias. Traditional electromyogram and nerve conduction velocity studies can identify about half of these patients. However, identification of small sensory fiber involvement requires quantitative sudomotor autonomic testing and should be pursued if traditional nerve conduction velocities and electromyogram studies are negative.

Diagnosis

A number of different diagnostic criteria sets have been proposed for Sjögren syndrome without consensus on any one set. Common to each set of criteria is the requirement to demonstrate the following:

1. Subjective and objective evidence of both keratoconjunctivitis sicca and xerostomia
2. Presence of at least one of the following four autoantibodies: antinuclear antibodies, rheumatoid factor, anti-Ro antibodies, or anti-La antibodies (these last two types of autoantibodies are also known as *SS-A* and *SS-B*

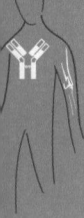

antibodies, respectively, and are so named for Sjögren syndrome)

3. Exclusion of underlying diseases that may mimic Sjögren syndrome

Leukopenia is common. Biopsy specimens from salivary glands, which are easily obtainable from the lower lip, may demonstrate characteristic findings of focal lymphocytic infiltration of predominantly CD4 T cells. These histologic features imply that cell-mediated processes are essential in the pathogenesis of Sjögren syndrome, although the precise antigenic target is unknown.

Keratoconjunctivitis sicca can be objectively documented by either measuring decreased tear production with the Schirmer filter paper test (>5 mm of wetting in 5 minutes after placement in the lower eyelid) or viewing corneal abrasions by rose-bengal staining and slit-lamp examination. Reduced salivary production can be demonstrated by provocative sialometry.

The differential diagnosis of Sjögren syndrome includes a variety of infectious and infiltrative diseases that may cause keratoconjunctivitis sicca symptoms and/or lacrimal and salivary gland enlargement. Human immunodeficiency virus causes diffuse infiltrative lymphadenopathy syndrome (DILS), which closely mimics Sjögren syndrome. DILS, however, involves predominantly CD8 T cells and tends to cause more xerostomia instead of keratoconjunctivitis sicca. Both conditions can cause bilateral parotitis and parotid gland swelling. Additional infections to consider in patients with sicca symptoms include hepatitis B and C, human T-cell leukemia virus, syphilis, and infection with mycobacteria. Infiltrative diseases may involve lacrimal and salivary glands and appear in a fashion similar to Sjögren syndrome. These infiltrative diseases include sarcoidosis, the amyloidoses, and hemochromatosis. Diseases that result in abnormal

Table 85-1 Clinical Features of Sjögren Syndrome Associated with Exocrine Gland Dysfunction

Problems Secondary to Lacrimal Gland Dysfunction

Dry, irritated eyes with foreign-body sensation
Corneal abrasions
Erythematous eyes

Problems Secondary to Salivary Gland Dysfunction

Dry mouth
Oral sores
Dental caries
Thrush
Lingual and labial fissures
Dysphagia
Gastroesophageal reflux
Parotid and/or submandibular gland swelling

Problems Secondary to Other Exocrine Dysfunction

Dyspareunia
Pancreatic malabsorption

Table 85-2 Extraglandular Clinical Features of Sjögren Syndrome

Skin and Mucous Membranes	Central Nervous System
Lower extremity purpura, associated with hyperglobulinemia and/or leukocytoclastic vasculitis on biopsy	Focal defects including multiple sclerosis, stroke
Photosensitive lesions, indistinguishable from those of subacute cutaneous lupus erythematosus	Diffuse deficits including dementia, cognitive dysfunction
	Spinal cord involvement including transverse myelitis
Pulmonary	**Peripheral Nervous System**
Chronic bronchitis secondary to dryness of the tracheobronchial tree	Peripheral sensorimotor neuropathy
Lymphocytic interstitial pneumonitis, interstitial pulmonary fibrosis, chronic obstructive lung disease, bronchiolitis obliterans organizing pneumonia, pseudolymphoma with intrapulmonary nodules	Trigeminal sensory neuropathy
Musculoskeletal	**Reticuloendothelial System**
Polymyositis	Splenomegaly
Polyarthralgias, polyarthritis	Lymphadenopathy and development of pseudolymphoma
Renal	**Liver**
Tubulointerstitial nephritis, type 1 renal tubular acidosis	Hepatomegaly
	Primary biliary cirrhosis
	Vascular
	Raynaud phenomenon
	Small-vessel vasculitis, with either a mononuclear perivascular infiltrate or leukocytoclastic changes on biopsy
	Endocrine
	Hypothyroidism caused by Hashimoto thyroiditis
	Other autoimmune endocrinopathies

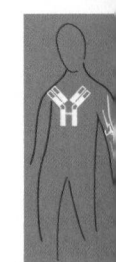

neural input to exocrine glands, such as multiple sclerosis, must also be considered in a patient with keratoconjunctivitis sicca symptoms.

Many drugs from various pharmaceutical classes have anticholinergic properties that result in clinically significant symptoms of dry eyes and dry mouth and mimic Sjögren syndrome. Such medication classes include antidepressants, decongestants, and antihypertensives. The list of medications with anticholinergic side effects is quite long, and all medications, including over-the-counter products, should be carefully reviewed in any patient with signs or symptoms of Sjögren syndrome. Alcohol and marijuana are common substances of abuse that can cause xerophthalmia and xerostomia.

Treatment

Treatment of Sjögren syndrome consists of either symptomatic care to ameliorate the exocrine deficiencies or systemic therapy for extraglandular involvement. Treatment options are outlined in Table 85-3. The interest in the potential therapeutic role of immunomodulatory biologic agents is increasing, especially B-cell–depleting agents. Patient education is important, and some measures outlined can be considered prophylactic.

Table 85-3 Treatment Options for Sjögren Syndrome

Local Treatment of Exocrine Dysfunction

Xerophthalmia

Artificial tears, preservative free
Eyeglasses and/or goggles
Punctal occlusion by means of plugs or electrocautery

Xerostomia

Artificial saliva
Salivary stimulators, either mechanical or electrical
Fluoride treatments and/or fastidious dental care
Avoid glucose lozenges and/or candies

Dyspareunia

Vaginal lubricants

Systemic Treatment of Exocrine Dysfunction

Pilocarpine or cevimeline
When possible, avoid or discontinue medications with anticholinergic effects

Treatment of Systemic Manifestations

Nonsteroidal anti-inflammatory drugs
Antimalarial agents: hydroxychloroquine or chloroquine
Glucocorticoids
Immunosuppressive agents, including methotrexate, azathioprine, mycophenolate mofetil, and gamma globulin

Prospectus for the Future

It is important to increase awareness of Sjögren syndrome, as it is often unrecognized. Atypical presentations of thrush, neuropathy, and multiple sclerosis–like disease all can occur with Sjögren syndrome.

Cytokine therapy, used in other rheumatic disorders such as rheumatoid arthritis and psoriatic arthritis, may be effective for Sjögren syndrome. Large placebo-controlled randomized trials will be necessary to further evaluate these therapies for Sjögren syndrome. In addition, cell-based therapies, such as the use of stem cells to replace depleted acinar tissue of salivary glands, lies in the future as a potential permanent therapy for patients with Sjögren syndrome.

References

Delalande S, de Seze J, Fauchais AL, et al: Neurologic manifestations in primary Sjögren syndrome: A study of 82 patients. Medicine 83:280-291, 2004.

Hansen A, Lipskey PE, Dörner T: Immunopathogenesis of primary Sjögren's syndrome: Implications for disease management and therapy. Curr Opin Rheumatol 17:558-565, 2005.

Pillimer SR: Sjögren's syndrome. In Klippel JH (ed): Primer of the Rheumatic Diseases, 12th ed. Atlanta, Arthritis Foundation, 2001, pp 377-384.

Chapter **86**

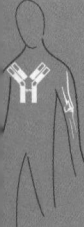

Systemic Vasculitis

Kathleen Maksimowicz-Mckinnon

The primary systemic vasculitides are a group of chronic inflammatory disorders characterized by immune-mediated injury of blood vessels. Inflammation leading to vessel necrosis, often accompanied by vessel thrombosis, results in subsequent ischemic tissue and organ injury. All organ systems are vulnerable to the vasculitides, although different preferential vessel and tissue targeting characterize each disorder. Although these disorders are rare, they can often be organ and life threatening. Because these consequences frequently can be averted by timely diagnosis and treatment, it is necessary for physicians to be able to promptly recognize these disorders. In this chapter, general concepts of classification and disease pathogenesis are reviewed, and disease features, diagnosis, and therapy for the more common vasculitides are outlined.

Classification

The classification and nomenclature of the vasculitides is based on the 1990 American College of Rheumatology Classification criteria and the Chapel Hill Consensus Conference definitions. These systems are based on affected vessel size, preferential organ involvement, and, when applicable, the presence of characteristic autoantibodies.

Identifying criteria that are both sensitive and specific for the classification of the vasculitides remains an ongoing challenge. There is remarkable diversity in disease presentation, and, as demonstrated in Figure 86-1, significant overlap exists among diseases when considering vessel involvement. Despite these limitations, classification systems are necessary to conduct clinical research, design treatment strategies and protocols, and determine patient prognosis.

Pathogenesis

For the majority of the vasculitides, the cause and pathogenesis of disease are unknown. It has been proposed that a number of diverse mechanisms act in concert to result in

vascular inflammation and consequent injury, and that it is likely that a sequence of events initiates this cascade against a background of genetic vulnerability (Fig. 86-2). Proposed triggers of disease include infection and environmental exposures (chemicals, pollutants). The best example of this purported relationship is the association that has been demonstrated between hepatitis B and C infections and the development of polyarteritis nodosa (PAN). However, for the majority of the vasculitides, these associations remain speculative.

Current evidence suggests that both humeral and cellular immune responses, cytokine and chemokine activation, and immune complex deposition are important in disease pathogenesis. However, it has become clear that normal protective and repair processes in the vessel can also contribute to injury and ischemia. For example, after injury, cellular migration and proliferation occurring as part of vessel repair can result in intimal hyperplasia, and the procoagulant milieu that is protective against hemorrhage may lead to thrombosis. So rather than a unidirectional "attack" directed against an innocent bystander, vasculitis is instead a dialogue between the immune system and the vessel, where both parties participate and contribute to disease pathogenesis.

Clinical manifestations of the vasculitides result primarily from the impairment of blood flow in injured vessels, which results in tissue and organ ischemia and subsequent injury. Flow can be interrupted by obliteration from destructive processes, thrombosis, or remodeling after injury. These changes can occur along a broad spectrum of severity; vary depending on the type of vasculitis and type and location of vessels involved; and are unique in any individual patient.

Clinical Features

Manifestations of the vasculitides are diverse and differ not only among disorders but also among patients. Often disease features are influenced by the vessel size and location. Common associations between the size of the affected vessel

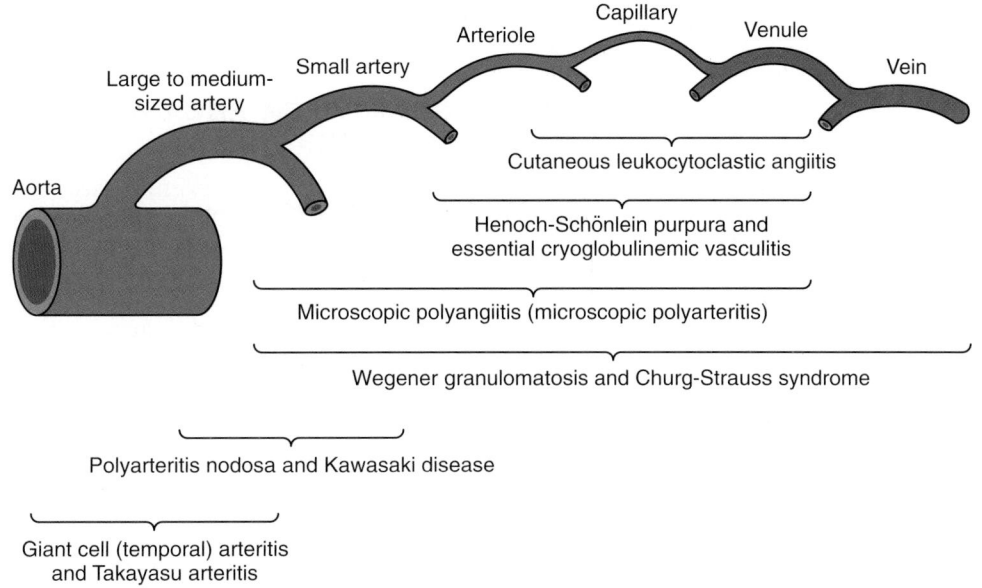
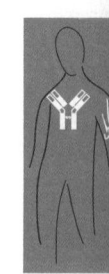

Figure 86-1 The vascular spectrum of the vasculitides. (From Jennette JC, Falk RJ, Andrassy K, et al: Nomenclature of systemic vasculitides. Proposal of an international consensus conference. Arthritis Rheum 37:187-192, 1994.)

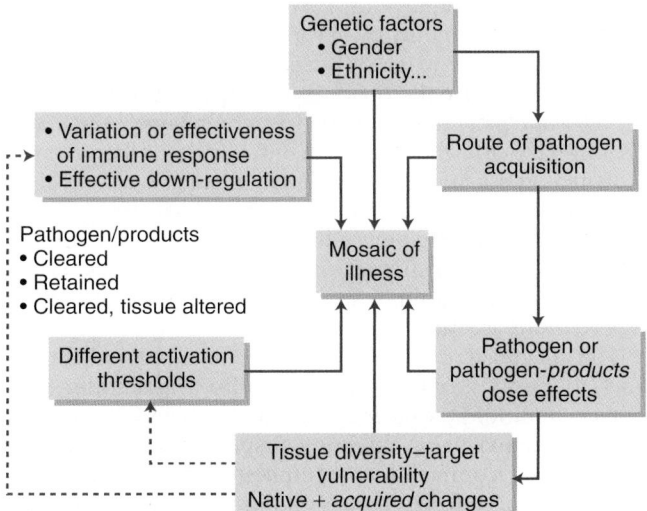

Figure 86-2 Factors affecting disease vulnerability and expression.

Table 86-1 **Typical Clinical Features Based on Vessel Size**		
Large	**Medium**	**Small**
Limb claudication	Cutaneous nodules	Purpura
Asymmetrical blood pressures	Ulcers	Vesiculobullous lesions
Absence of pulses	Livedo reticularis	Urticaria
Bruits	Digital gangrene	Glomerulonephritis
Aortic dilatation	Mononeuritis multiplex	Alveolar hemorrhage
	Microaneurysms	Cutaneous extravascular necrotizing granulomas
		Splinter hemorrhages
		Scleritis, episcleritis, uveitis
Constitutional symptoms in all: fever, weight loss, malaise, arthralgias		

and clinical manifestations are detailed in Table 86-1. It is important to be cognizant that patients generally do not manifest all of these features, and some patients may initially have only nonspecific constitutional signs and symptoms. The lack of specificity and diversity of signs and symptoms in any individual patient undoubtedly contribute to delays in diagnosis.

Small Vessel Vasculitis

ANTINEUTROPHIL CYTOPLASMIC ANTIBODY–ASSOCIATED VASCULITIDES

Wegener Granulomatosis

Wegener granulomatosis (WG) is a small to medium vessel granulomatous vasculitis that can affect nearly all organ systems. However, the most common sites affected are the sinuses and upper airway, the lungs, and the kidneys. Chronic refractory sinusitis, nasal crusting, and otitis media are common manifestations. Patients may also have cartilaginous inflammation and destruction, leading to the characteristic "saddle nose" deformity. Lung involvement in WG can include pulmonary nodules, often cavitary, infiltrates, or hemorrhage. Orbital pseudotumors are seen in WG and can cause optic nerve compression or proptosis and can impinge on extraocular muscles. In addition, neurologic, cutaneous and musculoskeletal signs and symptoms are common and encompass a wide variety of manifestations.

Patients can experience weeks to months of more subtle symptoms, such as sinusitis, arthralgias, or fatigue, before fulminant, organ-threatening disease occurs. However, presenting signs may be at the other end of the spectrum, with rapidly progressive glomerulonephritis or alveolar hemorrhage that may rapidly lead to organ damage, or even death.

The diagnosis of WG is most frequently established by tissue biopsy. Results of antineutrophil cytoplasmic antibody (ANCA) testing can be positive in nearly 90% of patients with renal disease but are less often positive in patients with limited involvement. Most patients with WG are found to have cytoplasmic ANCA (C-ANCA) anti–proteinase-3 type, but perinuclear ANCA (P-ANCA) anti-myeloperoxidase type has also been identified in WG patients. It is important to be cognizant that ANCA can be present in other conditions that can mimic WG, such as pulmonary infections (fungal, bacterial, or mycobacterial) and other autoimmune conditions. Hence, ANCA positivity is never adequate in itself to establish the diagnosis of WG or any other vasculitis. Conversely, patients with limited WG, which is generally described as disease restricted to the upper respiratory tract, are less likely to show ANCA positivity, so the absence of ANCA does not rule out the diagnosis of WG.

Churg-Strauss Syndrome

Churg-Strauss syndrome (CSS), also known as *allergic granulomatosis* and *angiitis,* is a small and medium vessel vasculitis differentiated from the other forms of small vessel vasculitis by its association with asthma and allergy. The majority of patients have asthma present for months to years before the onset of CSS, but some patients may manifest CSS and asthma simultaneously. In CSS patients with a preexisting asthma diagnosis, it is not infrequent for patients with stable, well-controlled asthma to note worsening or refractory asthma heralding the onset of CSS. Although patients with CSS often have sinusitis and pulmonary infiltrates, which are also seen in WG, in CSS the sinus disease is generally not destructive, and pulmonary infiltrates, unlike in WG, may be fleeting. CSS also often manifests with gastrointestinal, nervous system, and myocardial involvement.

As with WG, the diagnosis of CSS is made based on tissue biopsy in concert with appropriate history and clinical findings. Peripheral eosinophilia is a hallmark of CSS, and eosinophils are frequently seen in biopsy specimens of affected tissues. ANCA testing results are frequently positive in patients with CSS, but in contrast to WG, the majority of patients have P-ANCA anti-myeloperoxidase antibodies.

Microscopic Polyangiitis

Microscopic polyangiitis (MPA) is a predominantly small vessel vasculitis that preferentially affects the kidneys and lungs. Disease onset may be insidious, with constitutional symptoms such as fever, weight loss, and arthralgias present for months before diagnosis. Patients with renal involvement may have microscopic hematuria and proteinuria, or renal insufficiency resulting from glomerulonephritis. Alveolar hemorrhage is a characteristic manifestation of pulmonary involvement in MPA and may cause cough, dyspnea, and hemoptysis. Cutaneous and neurologic involvement are also frequent in MPA.

Diagnosis is established by tissue biopsy in the appropriate clinical scenario, similar to the other ANCA vasculitides.

ANCA are also frequent in MPA, and are most often P-ANCA/anti-myeloperoxidase type.

THERAPY FOR ANCA-ASSOCIATED VASCULITIS

Glucocorticoids are uniformly used in the treatment of ANCA-associated vasculitis. These disorders are characterized by relapsing disease, occurring in one third to one half of patients, so frequently a steroid-sparing immunosuppressive agent such as cyclophosphamide, azathioprine, or methotrexate is necessary to aid in maintaining disease remission. In general, daily oral cyclophosphamide is used in combination with glucocorticoid therapy in patients with fulminant organ- or life-threatening disease. Although the use of plasmapheresis remains controversial, it is often used as part of initial treatment in combination with immunosuppressive therapy in patients with alveolar hemorrhage or rapidly progressive glomerulonephritis, based on small studies suggesting potential benefit with regard to renal recovery and mortality.

HENOCH-SCHÖNLEIN PURPURA

Henoch-Schönlein purpura (HSP) is a small vessel vasculitis that occurs most frequently in young children, with a median age of onset of 4 years, but can develop at any age. HSP is characterized by the presence of palpable purpura (seen in 100% of patients), arthritis (generally large joint), and abdominal pain, which results from vascular inflammation, ischemia, and associated bowel wall edema. Renal involvement most often manifests as hematuria, with progression to clinically overt glomerulonephritis requiring directed therapy much less commonly noted. Central nervous system involvement and pulmonary hemorrhage have also been reported but are rare.

The diagnosis of HSP is most often made on clinical and laboratory grounds. Given that other vasculitides (and other conditions) can manifest with purpura, arthritis, and abdominal pain, obtaining tissue to aid in diagnosis is strongly recommended. Immunoglobulin A deposition can be seen in affected tissues and organs and is helpful in establishing the diagnosis of HSP in the appropriate clinical setting.

In the vast majority of patients, HSP is a self-limited condition, and treatment is supportive. Glucocorticoid therapy can aid in more rapid resolution of symptoms, but whether treatment can decrease the risk of relapsing disease or more serious manifestations remains controversial. Glucocorticoid therapy is generally used in patients who develop overt glomerulonephritis, with steroid-sparing immunosuppressive agents also considered in the setting of steroid-requiring or relapsing disease.

Medium Vessel Vasculitis

POLYARTERITIS NODOSA

PAN is a medium vessel vasculitis characterized by arterial aneurysmal and stenotic lesions of muscular arteries, often located at segmental and branch points. Although all organ

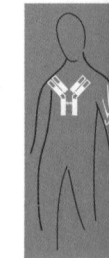

systems are vulnerable to PAN, the most common systems affected include the gastrointestinal, renal, and nervous systems. Unlike what is seen in small vessel vasculitis, renal involvement in PAN is not characterized by glomerulonephritis, but rather manifests with aneurysms and/or stenoses of renal arteries.

The diagnosis of PAN is made based on angiographic and/or biopsy findings in the appropriate clinical setting. Constitutional symptoms are frequent in PAN, including fever, fatigue, and weight loss. Anemia and hypertension are also common in PAN. ANCA generally are absent in PAN. PAN is frequently associated with hepatitis B and C and has also been documented in patients with human immunodeficiency virus (HIV) infection.

Glucocorticoid therapy and other immunosuppressive agents are used in the treatment of PAN. Although not all patients with PAN have chronic viral infection, testing for these infections when PAN is suspected is imperative, because antiviral therapy may be required not only for attaining control of the viral infection but also in the treatment of the associated vasculitis.

KAWASAKI DISEASE

Kawasaki disease (KD) is a medium vessel vasculitis most often seen in children under the age of 5. It is the most common cause of acquired heart disease in children in the United States and Japan. The diagnosis of KD is made based on the presence of four of the following characteristics plus fever >5 days: conjunctival injection, oropharyngeal changes (strawberry tongue, mucous membrane desquamation), peripheral extremity changes (cutaneous desquamation), polymorphous rash, and cervical lymphadenopathy. Arthralgias, abdominal pain, hepatitis, aseptic meningitis, and uveitis have also been reported in patients with KD. Coronary artery aneurysms, one of the most serious comorbidities of KD, generally appear within the first 4 weeks after onset of disease and are often detectable with echocardiography. Although areas of ectasia and small aneurysms may regress, larger aneurysms often persist and can result in coronary ischemia at any time after development, even into adulthood.

Intravenous immunoglobulin has significantly decreased the incidence of coronary artery aneurysms and is standard therapy for patients with KD. Because patients often manifest significant thrombocytosis, with platelet counts that can be over 1 million, aspirin is also used in the treatment of KD. Children with coronary aneurysms require long-term follow-up by a cardiologist even into adulthood for monitoring and sequential imaging because complications such as coronary stenosis or thrombosis may occur.

Large Vessel Vasculitis

TAKAYASU ARTERITIS

Takayasu arteritis (TA) is a rare large vessel vasculitis initially identified in East Asia but found worldwide. It preferentially affects young women of childbearing age but can be found in both sexes and encompasses a broader age range. TA affects the aorta and its primary branches and most often

results in stenotic lesions, although aneurysms are also seen. The most common sites of involvement in the United States include the subclavian and carotid arteries and the aorta. Hypertension can result from renal artery stenosis in TA and may be missed in patients who have bilateral upper extremity arterial stenoses. TA can manifest with mild nonspecific and self-limited constitutional symptoms, so the diagnosis may not be made until late in the disease course when vascular stenosis and subsequent claudicatory symptoms manifest. Patients can also have abrupt onset of fever, arthralgias, myalgias, weight loss, and fatigue. About 20% of patients have monophasic disease, whereas the remainder of patients have at least one relapse.

Diagnosis of TA is often based on vascular imaging studies, often demonstrating long, tapering stenotic lesions and/or aneurysmal lesions in the aorta and primary branches, after infectious and other causes of large vessel vasculitis have been eliminated. Some patients are diagnosed after vascular surgical procedures (e.g., aortic valve replacement) when vasculitis is detected on pathologic studies of the excised tissue. Detecting disease relapse in TA can be challenging, because patients may have active vasculitis even without clinical signs and symptoms and normal acute phase reactants. Generally, as part of disease surveillance, patients undergo sequential vascular imaging studies—magnetic resonance imaging (MR) or computed tomography (CT) angiography—to identify active disease. Because vascular injury often leads to progressive stenosis, disease activity is defined by identifying new vascular lesions in previously unaffected areas.

Because hypertension is an important factor contributing to disease-associated morbidity and mortality, it is imperative to obtain central arterial pressure measurements by catheter-directed angiography if patients demonstrate or develop arterial lesions affecting all four extremities; peripheral blood pressure measurements may be unreliable.

In most patients, glucocorticoid therapy is efficacious in attaining disease control. Patients with relapsing disease frequently require other immunosuppressive agents, such as methotrexate or azathioprine, to minimize steroid exposure and aid in maintaining disease remission. However, disease relapse often occurs even while patients are receiving these therapies. There are data suggesting that anti–tumor necrosis factor can aid in maintaining disease remission; however, larger prospective studies are needed to better define the role of such agents in the treatment of TA.

Surgical intervention is undertaken in TA when organ-threatening ischemia is present or peripheral claudicatory symptoms warrant operative intervention. Elective interventions should be performed when disease is quiescent, because restenosis occurs more frequently in patients with active disease at the time of surgery. Data from the National Institutes of Health (NIH) and Cleveland Clinic cohorts demonstrate better long-term outcomes in TA from arterial bypass surgery than from angioplasty with or without stent placement.

GIANT CELL ARTERITIS OF THE ELDERLY (TEMPORAL ARTERITIS)

Giant cell arteritis (GCA) is a large vessel vasculitis that primarily affects white patients over the age of 50, often

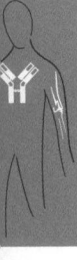

affecting the extracranial arteries. Patients frequently manifest new onset of headache, which is continuous, scalp or temporal artery tenderness, jaw claudication, visual disturbances, fatigue, and arthralgias. Patients can have an insidious or explosive onset of disease and can manifest primarily cranial or constitutional symptoms. Blindness occurs in about 15% of patients with GCA, even with appropriate therapy, and can occur at disease onset.

The diagnosis of GCA should be confirmed with a superficial temporal artery biopsy. Whether or not bilateral biopsies should be obtained initially remains an area of controversy, because a few cases have been reported in which the symptomatic temporal artery biopsy was negative but the asymptomatic contralateral artery demonstrated arteritis. Anemia and elevated acute phase reactants are commonly seen in patients with GCA.

Large vessel disease, similar to that seen in TA, has been reported in GCA. Aortitis is one of the most common manifestations of large vessel involvement in patients with GCA and leads to an increased risk of aortic aneurysm and subsequent dissection and rupture. Given this potential catastrophic complication, it has been suggested that GCA patients undergo yearly surveillance with chest radiography to look for aortic enlargement, but the potential impact of this intervention on outcomes in GCA remains speculative.

Glucocorticoids are the cornerstone of therapy in GCA. Patients often experience disease relapses with steroid tapering, but other immunosuppressive agents overall have not demonstrated steroid-sparing activity in GCA. Although many patients with relapsing disease are still given trials of other immunosuppressive agents, given the toxicities associated with long-term steroid use, most patients continue to require steroid therapy for maintaining disease remission.

Polymyalgia rheumatica (PMR), a syndrome characterized by pain and stiffness in the muscles of the neck, shoulder girdle, and hip girdle with other signs and symptoms of systemic inflammation, is associated with GCA. However, not all patients with GCA manifest PMR symptoms, and not all patients with PMR develop GCA. However, because the prevalence of GCA is higher in patients with PMR, they should be educated regarding signs and symptoms of GCA.

LEUKOCYTOCLASTIC VASCULITIS

Leukocytoclastic vasculitis (LCV) describes microscopic changes seen in a biopsy specimen of the skin including vessel wall infiltration, fibrin deposition, and necrosis. LCV can be noted in a variety of conditions, so although a diagnosis of systemic vasculitis should be entertained when LCV is found, other conditions should also be considered, based on the clinical scenario.

Primary vasculitic conditions that may manifest with LCV include HSP, the ANCA-associated vasculitides, and PAN. Secondary vasculitides, including those associated with other rheumatic diseases (systemic lupus erythematosus, Sjögren syndrome, rheumatoid arthritis), paraneoplastic syndromes, medications, and infections can also manifest with LCV.

As the definition implies, the diagnosis of LCV is established by tissue biopsy. The treatment of LCV depends on its underlying cause; hence, appropriate and thorough investigations to seek a cause should be undertaken when the diagnosis of LCV is made.

When no clear underlying cause is found, a variety of agents can be used to alleviate symptoms and rash including antihistamines, dapsone, colchicine, and glucocorticoids. These patients need be monitored carefully in case LCV is the initial manifestation of a systemic process in evolution, and the threshold for further evaluation and/or reevaluation for an underlying disorder in the setting of treatment failure or the emergence of new signs or symptoms should be low.

Differential Diagnosis

Many conditions can manifest similarly to the primary vasculitides, and misdiagnosis or delayed diagnosis is not uncommon when these disorders are being considered. Table 86-2 outlines general categories and examples of disorders that can mimic the primary systemic vasculitides.

Given that immunosuppressive therapy has significant associated risks and toxicities, and that it may be harmful in

Table 86-2 **Differential Diagnosis for Primary Systemic Vasculitis**
Infection
Endocarditis
Sepsis
Syphilis
Meningococcemia
Viral hepatitis
Tuberculosis
Disorders of Coagulation
Disseminated intravascular coagulation
Antiphospholipid antibody syndrome
Thrombotic thrombocytopenic purpura
Drug Toxicity
Sympathomimetic agents
Cocaine
Atherosclerotic and Embolic Disease
Peripheral vascular disease
Cholesterol embolization syndrome
Generalized atherosclerosis
Cardiac myxomas
Malignancy
Lymphoma
Disseminated carcinomatosis
Secondary Vasculitides Associated with Other Autoimmune Conditions
Systemic lupus erythematosus
Sjögren syndrome
Rheumatoid arthritis
Behçet disease
Sarcoidosis
Congenital Abnormalities and Anatomic Variants
Fibromuscular dysplasia
Ehlers-Danlos syndrome
Marfan syndrome
Other Disorders
Buerger disease
Calciphylaxis
Amyloidosis

other conditions that may mimic vasculitis (e.g., infection), it is critical that a thorough investigation be undertaken to exclude other diagnoses.

Additional Considerations in Treatment

Immunosuppressive therapy is associated with an increased risk of infection, with more intensive therapy leaving patients also vulnerable to opportunistic infections. Patients receiving combination therapy with moderate- to high-dose glucocorticoid therapy and another immunosuppressive agent generally are placed on prophylaxis for *Pneumocystis jiroveci* pneumonia (previously known as *PCP*). Furthermore, infectious conditions can often mimic or result in flares of systemic vasculitis. Careful evaluation is necessary to determine whether illness in a patient with known systemic vasculitis is caused by infection, active vasculitis, or both processes. Glucocorticoid therapy should never be abruptly discontinued, even in the setting of infection, because of the risk of adrenal crisis and also of disease relapse. In most cases, other immunosuppressive agents should be discontinued if infection is suspected or diagnosed and should not be resumed until antimicrobial therapy is completed and infection has

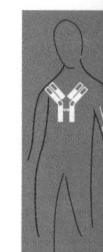

been eradicated. The dose of glucocorticoids may need to be adjusted to maintain disease control in this setting.

Glucocorticoid therapy is a common cause of bone loss in patients with systemic vasculitis and frequently results in osteopenia and osteoporosis. Studies have demonstrated that significant bone loss can occur even within the first 6 months of therapy, so calcium and vitamin D therapy should be initiated with the institution of glucocorticoid therapy, and a baseline bone density study obtained. Consideration should be given to additional preventative therapies in patients with decreased bone density at baseline, or those with other risk factors for bone loss.

Several immunosuppressive agents, including methotrexate and cyclophosphamide, used in the treatment of systemic vasculitis are teratogenic. Furthermore, cyclophosphamide therapy can result in premature ovarian failure. These factors need be considered when one chooses immunosuppressive therapy for the treatment of systemic vasculitis in women of childbearing age.

Immunosuppressive medications can be associated with additional long-term risks. One example of this is the known association between prolonged administration of cyclophosphamide and bladder hemorrhage and malignancy. Patients receiving immunosuppressive therapy should be under the care of physicians experienced in monitoring patients on these medications for associated risks and toxicities.

Prospectus for the Future

Understanding the cause and pathogenesis of the vasculitides is essential for scientific progress in the assessment and treatment of patients affected by these disorders. This knowledge will help generate:

- More precise diagnostic and classification criteria
- Diagnostic and monitoring studies with improved sensitivity and specificity
- Less toxic, better tolerated therapies
- Interventions for prevention of disease

References

Bloch DA, Michel BA, Hunder GG, et al: The American College of Rheumatology 1990 criteria for the classification of vasculitis. Patients and methods. Arthritis Rheum 33:1068-1073, 1990.

Fields C, Bower T, Cooper L, et al: Takayasu's arteritis: Operative results and influence of disease activity. J Vasc Surg 43:64-71, 2006.

Hoffman GS: Determinants of vessel targeting in vasculitis. Clin Dev Immunol 11:275-279, 2004.

Jennette JC, Falk RJ, Andrassy K, et al: Nomenclature of systemic vasculitides. Proposal of an international consensus conference. Arthritis Rheum 37:187-192, 1994.

Kerr GS, Hallahan CW, Giordano J, et al: Takayasu arteritis. Ann Intern Med 120:919-929, 1994.

Klemmer PJ, Chalermskulrat W, Reif MS, et al: Plasmapheresis therapy for diffuse alveolar hemorrhage in patients with small-vessel vasculitis. Am J Kidney Dis 42:1149-1153, 2003.

Maksimowicz-McKinnon K, Clark TM, Hoffman GS: Limitations of therapy and a guarded prognosis in an American cohort of Takayasu arteritis patients. Arthritis Rheum 56:1000-1009, 2007.

Mandel B: General approach to the diagnosis of vasculitis. In Hoffman GS, Weyand CM: Inflammatory Diseases of Blood Vessels. New York, Marcel Dekker, 2002, pp 239-254.

Molloy ES, Langford CA, Clark TM, et al: Anti-tumour necrosis factor therapy in patients with refractory Takayasu arteritis: long-term follow-up. Ann Rheum Dis 67:1567-1569, 2008.

Nakamura T, Matsuda T, Kawagoe Y, et al: Plasmapheresis with immunosuppressive therapy vs immunosuppressive therapy alone for rapidly progressive anti-neutrophil cytoplasmic autoantibody-associated glomerulonephritis. Nephrol Dial Transplant 19:1935-1937, 2004.

Nuenninghoff DM, Hunder GG, Christianson TJ, et al: Mortality of large-artery complication (aortic aneurysm, aortic dissection, and/or large artery stenosis) in patients with giant cell arteritis: a population-based study over 50 years. Arthritis Rheum 48:3532-3537, 2003.

Saleh A, Stone JH: Classification and diagnostic criteria in systemic vasculitis. Best Pract Res Clin Rheumatol 19:209-221, 2005.

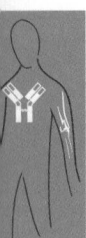

Crystal Arthropathies

Dana P. Ascherman

Gout

First described by Hippocrates approximately 2500 years ago, gout is a metabolic disorder that results from monosodium urate crystal formation after supersaturation of extracellular fluids. Clinical manifestations include acute and chronic arthritis, soft tissue deposits of monosodium urate (tophi), nephrolithiasis, and, rarely, urate nephropathy. Collectively, these abnormalities reflect overproduction or underexcretion of uric acid, a metabolic byproduct of purine metabolism. Working knowledge of purine synthesis and salvage pathways as well as predominantly renal clearance mechanisms affecting uric acid turnover is therefore critical in understanding the pathogenesis of gout.

EPIDEMIOLOGIC FACTORS

Gout is principally a disease of men over the age of 35 but clearly affects postmenopausal women as well as specialized populations that include organ transplant recipients. The prevalence of gout correlates with serum uric acid levels, which are typically low until puberty but increase thereafter in an age-dependent manner. Given the significant overlap in levels between patients with and without clinical manifestations of gout, however, serum uric acid remains a poor screening tool for this disorder. Despite this caveat, the risk of symptomatic gout increases from less than 1% in individuals with normal serum uric acid to 20% to 30% in those with levels 2 to 3 mg/dL above normal. For a given level of uric acid, the risk of developing gout appears similar between men and women; however, women typically have lower levels of serum uric acid than men (particularly before menopause, when estrogen appears to enhance urate excretion), explaining the gender discrepancy in this metabolic disorder. Overall, gout occurs in 2% to 3% of the adult male population, with a clear dependence on age. Whereas 0.24% of males with gout are younger than 44 years of age and 3.4% are in the 45- to 64-year-old age group, the prevalence increases to 5% in males older than 65 years of age. In contrast, prevalence rates are less than 0.1% in women younger than 44, increasing to 1.4% in women 45 to 64 years of age and 1.9% in those older than age 65.

URIC ACID METABOLISM AND PREDISPOSITION TO GOUT

Uric acid is the breakdown product of the purines adenine and guanine. The low solubility of uric acid, which at neutral pH is largely in the form of monosodium urate, allows for accumulation of monosodium urate crystals in the body of susceptible individuals possessing an imbalance of uric acid production and excretion. Total body uric acid stores are approximately 1800 mg, with a daily turnover of roughly 600 mg. Two thirds of daily input comes from de novo purine synthesis and/or salvage pathways, whereas one third comes from dietary sources. Two thirds of daily uric acid excretion occurs in the kidney, with the balance largely eliminated in the gastrointestinal tract.

Purine biosynthetic pathways have three basic features: (1) de novo synthesis driven by 5′-phosphoribosyl 1-pyrophosphate (PRPP) and glutamine, (2) purine interconversion (e.g., adenylic acid–inosinic acid–guanylic acid), and (3) reutilization pathways in which the intermediate breakdown products of adenine, guanine, and hypoxanthine are recaptured by reaction with PRPP rather than undergoing further degradation to xanthine and uric acid (Fig. 87-1). Recapture is catalyzed by the enzymes adenine phosphoribosyl transferase (APRT) and hypoxanthine-guanine phosphoribosyl-transferase (HGPRT). Abnormalities of these enzymes lead to an overaccumulation of PRPP that drives purine synthesis, resulting in increased serum levels of uric acid. Severe homozygous deficiency of HGPRT results in Lesch-Nyhan syndrome, a rare X-linked disorder characterized by self-mutilation, hyperuricemia, and gout. Heterozygous deficiency of HGPRT results in both hyperuricemia and gout at an early age without the neurologic complications of choreoathetosis, spasticity, dystonia, and developmental retardation observed in homozygotes. Some glycogen storage diseases and abnormalities of pentose shunt metabolism can also lead to the overproduction of uric acid.

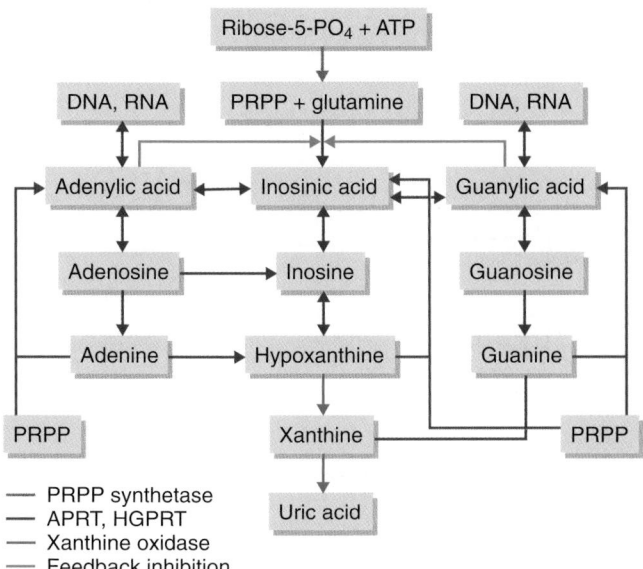

Figure 87-1 Biochemical pathways of purine synthesis, interconversion, and degradation. PRPP, 5′-phosphoribosyl 1-pyrophosphate; APRT, adenine phosphoribosyl transferase; HGPRT, hypoxanthine-guanine phosphoribosyltransferase.

Key:
— PRPP synthetase
— APRT, HGPRT
— Xanthine oxidase
— Feedback inhibition

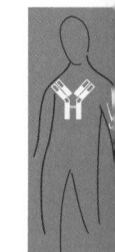

Table 87-1 **Causes of Hyperuricemia**	
Decreased Urate Excretion	**Increased Urate Production**
Impaired renal function	Ethanol
Dehydration	Myeloproliferative diseases
Acidosis	Ineffective erythropoiesis (sickle cell, thalassemia)
Low-dose salicylates	Widespread psoriasis
Diuretics	Cytotoxic drugs
Pyrazinamide	Glycogen storage diseases
Cyclosporine	G6PD deficiency
Levodopa	HGPRTase deficiency
Ethambutol	Increased PRPP synthetase activity
Nicotinic acid	
Lead	
Ethanol	
Many other drugs	
Hypothyroidism	

G6PD, glucose-6-phosphate dehydrogenase; HGPRTase, hypoxanthine-guanine phosphoribosyltransferase; PRPP, 5′-phosphoribosyl 1-pyrophosphate.

Overall, 10% to 20% of gout stems from increased uric acid production, of which less than 2% results from a defined enzyme deficiency. Secondary causes of uric acid overproduction include lymphoproliferative diseases (e.g., leukemias and lymphomas), disorders of hematopoiesis (e.g., sickle cell disease, thalassemia), and widespread psoriasis—each of which is associated with increased cell turnover and release of intracellular uric acid (Table 87-1). Clinically, however, the most significant stimulus to uric acid overproduction is alcohol, which can dramatically increase de novo synthesis through effects on adenosine triphosphate (ATP) metabolism.

Although these causes of uric acid overproduction are important, more than two thirds of individuals with gout (up to 90% in some series) have normal production levels of uric acid but have some impairment in renal clearance of uric acid (the primary route of uric acid excretion). Under normal circumstances, uric acid is filtered at the renal glomerulus, almost completely reabsorbed in the proximal tubule, and then actively secreted and reabsorbed in the distal and collecting tubules. Secondary gout may result from (1) any disorder leading to decreased renal blood flow and glomerular filtration; (2) diminished urine flow and acidosis, which favor urate reabsorption; or (3) drugs that compete for organic acid transport. Diuretics (including thiazides and furosemide), aspirin (which at low doses preferentially inhibits urate secretion), dehydration, and acidosis all lead to decreased urate clearance. Lead has long been associated with gout (saturnine gout), acting as a tubular toxin and thereby impairing urate clearance.

PATHOGENESIS OF ACUTE ARTHRITIS

When an imbalance between uric acid production and excretion leads to supersaturation of extracellular fluid and monosodium urate crystal deposition, an acute inflammatory monoarticular or oligoarticular arthritis may ensue.

Attacks of gouty arthritis can arise from de novo precipitation of microcrystals but often follow local trauma and shedding of crystals from previously formed intra-articular and periarticular deposits. Repetitive trauma to the first metatarsophalangeal (MTP) joint from weight-bearing activities may therefore underlie the predominant involvement of this joint. Beyond these physical factors, significant fluctuations in uric acid levels may also precipitate attacks. For example, dehydration, acidosis, alcohol ingestion, and extensive cell death from chemotherapy all lead to temporary increases in serum uric acid and are consequently linked with flares of gout. Alternatively, rapid lowering of uric acid levels likely leads to partial solubilization or breakdown of tophi and crystal shedding, potentially explaining the paradoxical association between gouty arthritis and the initiation of uric acid–lowering therapy with agents such as allopurinol.

Once formed and shed into the synovial fluid, monosodium urate crystals may activate complement (depending on the relative balance of proinflammatory and anti-inflammatory factors coating these crystals), leading to polymorphonuclear leukocyte (PMN) chemotaxis and crystal phagocytosis (Fig. 87-2). In turn, PMN activation triggers a cascade of intracellular events that ultimately lead to the release of degradative enzymes as well as an array of inflammatory mediators consisting of various cytokines, chemokines, prostaglandins, leukotrienes, and reactive-oxygen species. Specific chemotactic leukotrienes (leukotriene B$_4$) and chemokines (interleukin [IL]-8) promote further influx of PMNs in the setting of increased vascular permeability, perpetuating the local inflammatory response. This proinflammatory milieu persists until the synovial fluid cell profile shifts from PMNs to mature cells of monocyte and macrophage lineage.

CLINICAL PRESENTATION

Acute gouty arthritis is characterized by a rapid crescendo onset. Typically, affected patients go to sleep without

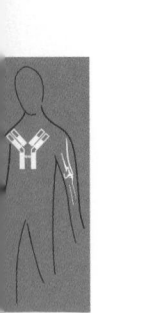

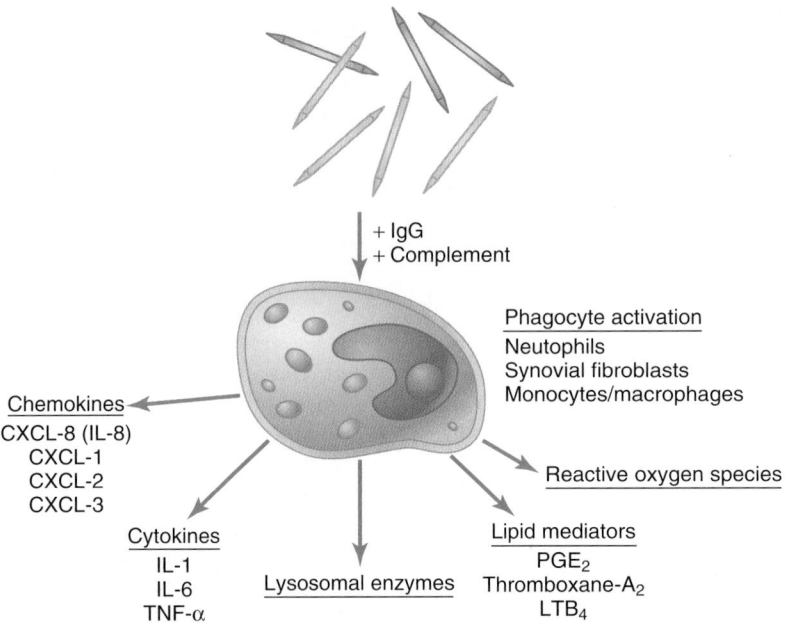

Figure 87-2 Pathogenesis of acute gout. Shedding of crystals leads to leukocyte activation and the release of inflammatory mediators. IgG, immunoglobulin G; PMN, polymorphonuclear leukocyte.

symptoms and subsequently awaken with severe pain, erythema, and swelling in the affected joint. The first MTP joint is the most commonly involved, resulting in an inflammatory condition termed *podagra*. Pain, warmth, and erythema often extend to the skin and surrounding soft tissue, producing a cellulitic appearance. As described by Sydenham in the 1800s, an inability to "bear the weight of bedclothes" develops, and patients frequently cannot put on a sock or cover the foot with a sheet. Although any joint may be affected in acute gout, the MTP, foot, ankle, and knee are most commonly involved. Inflammation of elbows, wrists, and small joints of the hands may also occur, but involvement of the hips, shoulders, and apophyseal joints is unusual. Hydrostatic factors may cause the predominant involvement of lower extremity joints. During the day when the legs are in a dependent position, transudation of plasma into the interstitial space occurs; at night, water is more quickly reabsorbed than uric acid, leading to higher concentrations of uric acid in the interstitial fluid and subsequent precipitation of crystals. The lower temperature in distal joints may also contribute to monosodium urate precipitation.

On examination, the skin overlying affected joints appears erythematous or even violaceous. The joint and surrounding soft tissue is warm or hot to touch and exquisitely tender, yielding extreme pain with passive as well as active range of motion. As indicated by the physical appearance of overlying skin and soft tissue, inflammation commonly extends beyond the confines of the joint. Occasionally, two or more joints are simultaneously involved. At times the process of gouty arthritis may be even more widespread, leading to a smoldering, chronic polyarthritis that can masquerade as rheumatoid arthritis or other inflammatory arthritides. Apart from the joints, an acute inflammatory process may occur in nonarticular structures such as bursae, sometimes causing confusion with septic bursitis.

DIAGNOSIS

The acute onset of inflammatory monoarthritis in a joint of the lower extremity is likely to be gout, particularly when the first MTP joint is affected in a middle-aged or older man. The differential diagnosis includes septic arthritis, pseudogout (calcium pyrophosphate dihydrate [CPPD] deposition disease), reactive arthritis (Reiter disease), monoarticular presentations of rheumatoid arthritis or other inflammatory arthritides, Lyme disease, viral arthritis, and sarcoidosis. Infectious arthritis is obviously the most important and usually the most difficult entity to differentiate at presentation. Both conditions, for example, can be associated with fever. Low-grade fever is relatively common in acute gout, but occasionally the patient's temperature may reach 39° C (102.2° F). Patients with septic arthritis may have a more insidious onset than patients with gout, are usually systemically ill with chills and sweats accompanying fever, and often develop peripheral leukocytosis with toxic granulation of peripheral blood PMNs. Nevertheless, none of these clinical features is pathognomonic for crystalline or septic arthritis, underscoring the importance of synovial fluid analysis.

The joint fluid in gout is classified as inflammatory, with more than 10,000 white blood cells (WBCs) per milliliter (sometimes >50,000 WBCs/mL) and more than 90% PMNs. Polarized light microscopic examination of synovial fluid is the key to diagnosis. Intracellular, needle-shaped, negatively birefringent crystals are both pathognomonic for, and essential to, the definitive diagnosis of acute gouty arthritis (Fig. 87-3). Viewed under polarized light with a red compensator, urate crystals are yellow when parallel to the compensator axis and blue when perpendicular. Crystals may range in length from 1 to 2 μm to 15 to 20 μm, appearing similar to a lance that has pierced the neutrophil (colloquially referred to as the "martini glass" sign). Extracellular crystals of typical size and shape are supportive, but not diagnostic,

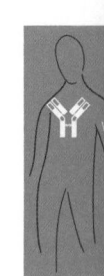

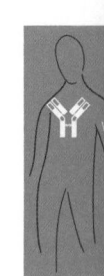

Figure 87-3 Polarized microscopy of **(A)** strongly negative birefringent monosodium urate crystals and **(B)** weakly positive CPPD crystals. Arrows indicate axis of polarization. **(A,** Adapted from the ACR Slide Collection on the Rheumatic Diseases; **B,** adapted from Saadeh C, Malacara JC: Calcium Pyrophosphate Deposition Disease. Available at: http://www.emedicine.com/med/topic1938. htm, May 4, 2006.)

of acute gouty arthritis. Urate crystals may also be seen in the white toothpaste-like material obtained from tophaceous deposits and occasionally from a joint into which a tophus has ruptured.

In 5% to 10% of gouty arthritis cases, crystals are not isolated from the affected joint. In other instances, particularly in small joints such as the MTP joint, synovial fluid may be difficult to aspirate. In a patient with known gout, a presumptive diagnosis is reasonable unless clinical features suggest septic arthritis. As previously indicated, serum uric acid is not a useful diagnostic screen, given that many patients have normal levels at the time of an acute attack and that elevated levels of uric acid are found in a high proportion of individuals lacking clinical manifestations of gout. Radiographs may show tophi or typical juxta-articular, "rat bite" erosions with sclerotic borders and overhanging edges (Martel sign). Mild peripheral blood leukocytosis, elevated erythrocyte sedimentation rate, and increased acute phase proteins may be seen but are entirely nonspecific.

CHRONIC POLYARTICULAR GOUT AND EXTRA-ARTICULAR MONOSODIUM URATE DEPOSITION

Gout may evolve into a chronic polyarthritis with or without acute attacks of arthritis. Patients with this form of gout often have multiple juxta-articular tophi and can develop destructive, erosive joint disease. Occasionally, polyarticular gout may appear similar to rheumatoid arthritis, and tophi may be mistaken for rheumatoid nodules. As indicated earlier, radiographs in chronic gout typically show sclerotic changes at erosive borders in a *juxta-articular* distribution, contrasting with the *peri-articular*, nonsclerotic, marginal erosions characteristic of rheumatoid arthritis. Synovial fluid analysis is diagnostic, justifying the examination of synovial fluid for crystals in patients with polyarthritis.

When significant monosodium urate crystal deposition does occur in the body, visible tophi may be present. Tophi most commonly form adjacent to joints, in bursae, on extensor surfaces of tendons, and, less commonly, on cartilaginous structures such as the pinnae of the ear. In severe cases, deposition may occur in other tissues, including the renal interstitium, where higher concentrations of uric acid are

Table 87-2 **Treatment of Acute Gout**		
Drug	**Route**	**Side Effects**
Colchicine	PO	Diarrhea, cramps
	IV	Bone marrow failure, neuromyopathy
NSAIDs	PO	Gastritis, bleeding, renal insufficiency
Glucocorticoids	PO, IV, IM	Increased blood sugar
	Intra-articular	Mask infection

IM, intramuscular; IV, intravenous; NSAIDs, nonsteroidal anti-inflammatory drugs; PO, oral.

achieved. Individuals who overproduce *and* overexcrete uric acid are at risk for developing renal stones; in general, those eliminating greater than 700 mg/day of urinary uric are at risk. Stones may be composed of uric acid, or uric acid may form a nidus for calcium and other types of stones.

TREATMENT

Acute Arthritis

A variety of treatments are effective for acute gouty arthritis (Table 87-2). Joint drainage per se has a therapeutic effect in removing degenerating PMNs and in relieving joint distension. Nonsteroidal anti-inflammatory drugs (NSAIDs) are highly effective when adequate anti-inflammatory doses are used and are often the first drug of choice; however, NSAIDs should be avoided in patients with renal insufficiency, a common association with gout. Colchicine prevents the release of PMN chemotactic factors and inhibits phospholipase activation, which is needed for prostaglandin synthesis. This medication is particularly effective early in a gout attack, resulting in rapid resolution of symptoms, but is much less effective after 24 hours. Colchicine can be given by repeated dosing every 1 to 2 hours with a strict total dose limit of 6 mg. However, the practice of using hourly administration until abdominal cramps or diarrhea supervene is to be discouraged. Intravenous colchicine is effective and rapid in onset of effect but must be used with extreme caution, particularly in the setting of hepatic or renal dysfunction. Given reported cases of fatal arrhythmia and bone marrow

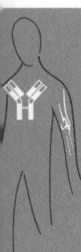

failure associated with use of intravenous colchicine, its use has been largely abandoned.

Alternatives to NSAIDs and colchicine include intra-articular glucocorticoids that have a rapid onset of action and are almost free of side effects. If the diagnosis of gout is fairly certain, various preparations of glucocorticoids may be instilled at the time of joint aspiration. Oral glucocorticoids in moderate-to-high doses may also be used; however, in patients with underlying diabetes or glucose intolerance, hyperglycemia may ensue. Nonetheless, in many patients with other comorbid medical conditions such as peptic ulcer disease and renal insufficiency, systemic glucocorticoids may be the best treatment option for acute gout. Parenteral adrenocorticotropic hormone and parenteral glucocorticoids are both effective treatments but are more costly. To prevent recurrent attacks after an acute attack of gout, colchicine prophylaxis for several weeks is a reasonable treatment option (see later discussion).

Intercritical and Chronic Gout

After a single attack of gout, the physician must decide whether to recommend long-term therapy. A substantial number of patients will have rare attacks, even if left untreated, leaving little rationale for immediate institution of lifelong therapy. On the other hand, patients with very high levels of serum uric acid or whose first attack occurs at a young age are at greatest risk of frequent attacks and subsequent development of chronic gouty arthritis, tophaceous gout, and/or destructive joint disease. If patients do have frequent recurrent attacks, then prophylactic treatment is advised (Table 87-3). In patients with mild gout and occasional attacks, prophylaxis with colchicine alone may be sufficient. However, in patients who have renal stones, tophi, erosive joint disease, polyarticular disease, or frequent, recurrent attacks of gout despite risk factor modification and prophylactic use of colchicine, long-term uric acid–lowering therapy is clearly indicated. The choice of agent depends (in part) on whether the patient overproduces uric acid or fails to efficiently eliminate this biochemical byproduct, a determination that rests on assessment of 24-hour urinary uric acid excretion occurring with a low-purine diet.

Uric acid–lowering agents fall into two general categories—uricosurics and xanthine oxidase inhibitors. Theoretically, uricosurics should be most commonly employed based on the distribution of uric acid underexcretion (90%) versus overproduction (10%) in the setting of gout. Probenecid, the prototypical uricosuric used in the United States, inhibits urate reabsorption in the distal tubule and promotes excretion. However, the effectiveness of probenecid hinges on intact renal function (glomerular filtration rate [GFR] >50 mL/min), and use of this medication may be impractical in many patients because of the requirement for increased fluid intake needed to prevent uric acid crystal formation in the renal tubules or urinary tract. Therefore, in patients who cannot tolerate probenecid or already have urate nephropathy or nephrolithiasis, allopurinol is a more appropriate choice. Allopurinol inhibits xanthine oxidase, the enzyme that catalyzes the formation of xanthine from hypoxanthine and uric acid from xanthine. It is effective in lowering the levels of uric acid whether they result from impaired clearance or from overproduction. Allopurinol, although generally safe, has greater toxicity than probenecid and has

Table 87-3	**Treatment of Intercritical Gout**	
Drug	**Mechanism of Action**	**Side Effects**
Colchicine	Destabilizes microtubules	Very safe (low dose); rare neuromyopathy
	Inhibits neutrophil chemotaxis, adhesion, and phagocytosis	
	No effect on uric acid	
NSAIDs	Inhibit cyclo-oxygenase	Peptic ulcer disease, renal insufficiency
	No effect on uric acid	
Probenecid	Uricosuric	Very safe
	No anti-inflammatory activity	
Allopurinol	Inhibits uric acid synthesis	Dermatitis, hepatitis, interstitial nephritis, marrow failure

NSAIDs, nonsteroidal anti-inflammatory drugs.

been associated with a severe hypersensitivity syndrome characterized by acute interstitial nephritis, hepatitis, and severe skin reactions. Recent studies suggest that febuxostat, a nonpurine inhibitor of xanthine oxidase, may be a potential alternative for patients with hyperuricemia and gout who are intolerant of allopurinol.

Once the decision is made to institute allopurinol or probenecid, concomitant colchicine prophylaxis should be initiated and continued for several months. Allopurinol, in particular, can precipitate gouty attacks when first administered, presumably because of the rapid lowering of uric acid levels that mobilizes tissue deposits and facilitates shedding of preformed crystals. For this reason, neither allopurinol nor probenecid should be started in the setting of an acute attack. In patients with persistent, chronic arthritis despite urate-lowering therapy, chronic use of nonsteroidal agents (other than aspirin) may be required for the control of pain and inflammation. Occasionally, surgical removal of tophi may be beneficial, particularly in locations where they become irritated, inflamed, or infected.

Although dietary modification is recommended as an adjunct to pharmacologic therapy, dietary purine intake accounts for a relatively small proportion of daily uric acid turnover. Therefore little clinical effect will likely occur from drastic dietary alterations. Nevertheless, anchovies, sweetbreads, organ meats, and cellular leafy vegetables such as spinach are particularly high in purines and should be excluded from the diet. Most importantly, alcohol should be avoided because of its dual impact on uric acid overproduction and impairment of renal tubular function.

Asymptomatic Hyperuricemia

In patients who are to receive chemotherapy, short-term prophylaxis with allopurinol may prevent both gout and renotubular precipitation of uric acid. Newer agents, including intravenous pegylated uricase, are also helpful in preventing the "tumor lysis" syndrome. Beyond this clinical situation, the significance of "asymptomatic" hyperuricemia has been the subject of detailed investigation based on associations with hypertension, renal dysfunction, cardiovascular disease, and the metabolic syndrome. Although a number of clinico-epidemiologic studies, animal models, and in vitro experimental systems collectively provide a compelling case that hyperuricemia is an independent risk factor for vascular endothelial and smooth muscle dysfunction, routine treatment of asymptomatic hyperuricemia is not currently recommended.

Calcium Pyrophosphate Dihydrate Deposition Disease

CPPD deposition disease results from the formation of CPPD crystals in articular cartilage and fibrocartilage as well as other periarticular structures. Such deposits are common and increase in incidence with advancing age, affecting over 30% of individuals older than 80 years of age. In most individuals with CPPD deposition, an asymptomatic radiographic finding termed *chondrocalcinosis* is observed. Typical areas of involvement include the menisci of the knee, the triangular fibrocartilage of the wrist, and the symphysis pubis. Articular cartilage may be involved anywhere, but the knee, wrist, and ankle are the most commonly affected sites.

Acute goutlike attacks of arthritis may result when crystals are shed from such deposits, particularly when these crystals are bound by opsonins such as immunoglobulin G (IgG); hence, the disease is often called *pseudogout*. In middle-aged women, a chronic, smoldering polyarthritis may be associated with CPPD deposition. Referred to as *chronic pyrophosphate arthropathy,* this entity has clinical and radiographic characteristics overlapping those of rheumatoid arthritis and osteoarthritis. For unknown reasons, chronic pyrophosphate arthropathy has a predilection for knees, wrists, shoulders, elbows, hips, ankles, midtarsal joints, and small joints of the hands—many of which are atypical sites for primary osteoarthritis. More rarely, chronic pyrophosphate arthropathy can be associated with hemorrhagic arthritis.

Although the vast majority of CPPD deposition disease is idiopathic, approximately 20% of cases are associated with underlying metabolic disorders such as hyperparathyroidism, hypomagnesemia, hypophosphatasia, and hemochromatosis. These associations undoubtedly stem from the roles of calcium, magnesium, alkaline phosphatase, and iron in chondrocyte-mediated pathways of ATP metabolism (magnesium, alkaline phosphatase) as well as crystal formation (calcium, iron). Of note, secondary forms of CPPD deposition disease may be the presenting clinical finding of the associated systemic disorder, typically occurring at an earlier age than idiopathic cases and often involving specific joints such as the second and third metacarpophalangeal joints.

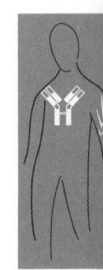

DIAGNOSIS AND TREATMENT

Detection of chondrocalcinosis on radiographs suggests, but does not establish, the diagnosis of CPPD arthropathy. Synovial fluid aspiration with demonstration of intracellular, positively birefringent, rhomboid-shaped crystals is therefore necessary to confirm the diagnosis of pseudogout or chronic pyrophosphate arthropathy (see Fig. 87-3). However, crystals may be small, fragmented, and difficult to detect, partly reflecting their susceptibility to degradation. Acute attacks of CPPD arthropathy are effectively treated with NSAIDs or with intra-articular glucocorticoids, although joint aspiration alone can be therapeutic. Low-dose colchicine may be effective in preventing recurrent attacks of pseudogout or managing persistent inflammation in chronic pyrophosphate arthropathy.

Other Crystal Disorders

Hydroxyapatite crystals are composed of basic calcium phosphates and deposit at soft tissue sites, particularly tendons and bursae. Although hydroxyapatite deposition in peri-articular structures such as the supraspinatus tendon and subacromial bursa can result in calcific tendinitis, shedding of crystals into the actual joint space can produce exuberant synovitis and a destructive arthropathy (including the "Milwaukee shoulder" syndrome). Oxalate crystals, on the other hand, may deposit in cartilage and intervertebral discs.

Prospectus for the Future

Future studies of long-term use will help define the role of new agents such as pegylated uricase and febuxostat in the prevention and management of gout.

References

Becker MA, Schumacher HR, Wortmann RL, et al: Febuxostat compared with allopurinol in patients with hyperuricemia and gout. N Engl J Med 353:2450-2461, 2005.

Doherty M: Calcium pyrophosphate dihydrate crystal-associated arthropathy. In Hochberg M, Silman A, Smolen J, et al (eds): Rheumatology, 3rd ed. Philadelphia, Mosby, 2003, pp 1937-1950.

Hershfield MS: Gout and uric acid metabolism. In Goldman L, Bennett JC (eds): Cecil Textbook of Medicine, 21st ed. Philadelphia, WB Saunders, 2000, pp 1541-1548.

Kanellis J, Feig DI, Johnson RJ: Does asymptomatic hyperuricemia contribute to the development of renal and cardiovascular disease? An old controversy renewed. Nephrology 9:394-399, 2004.

Kelley WN, Wortmann RL: Gout and hyperuricemia. In Kelley WN, Harris ED Jr, Ruddy S, Sledge CB (eds): Textbook of Rheumatology, 5th ed. Philadelphia, WB Saunders, 1997, p 1313.

McLean L: The pathogenesis of gout. In Hochberg, M, Silman A, Smolen J, et al (eds): Rheumatology, 3rd ed. Philadelphia, Mosby, 2003, pp 1903-1918.

Ryan LM, McCarty DJ: Calcium pyrophosphate crystal deposition disease, pseudogout and articular chondrocalcinosis. In Koopman WJ (ed): Arthritis and Allied Conditions, 13th ed. Baltimore, Williams & Wilkins, 1997, p 2103.

Schumacher HR Jr: Crystal deposition arthropathies. In Goldman L, Bennett JC (eds): Cecil Textbook of Medicine, 21st ed. Philadelphia, WB Saunders, 2000, pp 1548-1550.

Stamp LK, O'Donnell, JL, Chapman PT: Emerging therapies in the long-term management of hyperuricemia and gout. Intern Med J 37:258-266, 2007.

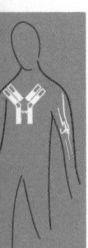

Osteoarthritis

C. Kent Kwoh

Epidemiology

Osteoarthritis (OA), also known as degenerative joint disease (DJD), is the most common arthritis and musculoskeletal disease. Over 26.9 million Americans over the age of 25 have some form of OA, and the prevalence of OA increases with age. The prevalence of radiographic OA varies by the joint involved, with 27.2% of all adults and over 80% of those over 65 having evidence of hand OA. With regard to knee OA, 37.4% of those over age 60 have radiographic evidence of disease. The prevalence of symptomatic OA is lower, with 6.8% of all adults having evidence of symptomatic hand OA and 16.7% of those over age 45 having evidence of symptomatic knee involvement. Hand and knee OA is more common among women, especially after age 50, and also is more common among African Americans. Nodal OA, involving the distal and proximal interphalangeal joints, is significantly more common in women and also is more common among female first-degree relatives.

OA is associated with major morbidity and is the leading cause of long-term disability in the United States. Lower extremity OA is the most common cause of difficulty with walking or climbing stairs, preventing an estimated 100,000 elderly Americans from independently walking from bed to bathroom. OA has a large economic impact as the result of both direct medical costs (e.g., physician visits, laboratory tests, medications, surgical procedures) and indirect costs (e.g., lost wages, home care, lost wage-earning opportunities). With the aging of the U.S. population, the burden of OA is expected to increase throughout the coming years.

Pathologic Factors

The causes of OA are complex and heterogeneous, and there is limited understanding of its pathophysiology. Its cardinal feature is progressive loss of articular cartilage with associated remodeling of subchondral bone. OA is best defined as joint failure, a disease process that involves the total joint including the subchondral bone, ligaments, joint capsule, synovial membrane, periarticular muscles, and articular car-

tilage. Joint failure may result from a variety of pathways subsequent to bone trauma and repetitive injury: joint instability caused by muscle weakness and ligamentous laxity; nerve injury and neuronal sensitization and/or hyperexcitability; low-grade systemic inflammation caused by subacute metabolic syndrome; or local inflammation resulting from synovitis.

OA is a complex disorder with one or more identifiable risk factors, which range from biomechanical, metabolic, or inflammatory processes, to congenital or developmental deformities of the joint, to genetic factors. As noted previously, age, sex, and race are prominent risk factors for OA. Biomechanical contributors include repetitive or isolated joint trauma related to certain occupations or physical activities that involve repeated joint stress and thus predispose an individual to early OA. Obesity may contribute from a biomechanical perspective or a systemic perspective related to a subacute metabolic syndrome. Certain metabolic disorders such as hemochromatosis and ochronosis are also associated with OA. High bone mineral density (BMD) has been shown to be associated with hip or knee OA. Estrogen deficiency may be a risk factor for hip or knee OA. Candidate gene studies and genome wide scans have identified a number of potential genetic markers of OA. Inflammatory joint diseases such as rheumatoid arthritis may result in cartilage degradation and biomechanical factors that lead to secondary OA. The destruction of the joint, including wearing away of articular cartilage, is therefore best viewed as the final product of a variety of possible etiologic factors.

The earliest finding in OA is fibrillation of the most superficial layer of the articular cartilage. With time, the disruption of the articular surface becomes deeper, with extension of the fibrillations to subchondral bone, fragmentation of cartilage with release into the joint, matrix degradation, and, eventually, complete loss of cartilage, leaving only exposed bone. Early in this process the cartilage matrix undergoes significant change, with increased water and decreased proteoglycan content. This progression is in contrast to the dehydration of cartilage that occurs with aging. The *tidemark* zone, separating the calcified cartilage from the radial zone, becomes invaded with capillaries. Chondrocytes initially are

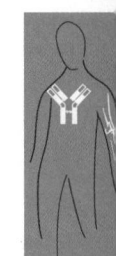

metabolically active and release a variety of cytokines and metalloproteinases, contributing to matrix degradation, which in the later stages results in the penetration of fissures to the subchondral bone and the release of fibrillated cartilage into the joint space. An imbalance between tissue inhibitors of metalloproteinases and the production of metalloproteinases may be operative in OA. Subchondral bone increases in density and cystlike bone cavities containing myxoid, fibrous, or cartilaginous tissue occur. Osteophytes, or bony proliferations at the margin of joints at the site of bone-cartilage interface, may also form at capsule insertions. Osteophytes contribute to joint-motion restriction and are thought to be the result of new bone formation in response to the degeneration of articular cartilage, but the precise mechanism for their production remains unknown.

A variety of crystals has been identified in synovial fluid and other tissues from osteoarthritic joints, most notably calcium pyrophosphate dihydrate and apatite. Although these crystals clearly have potent inflammatory potential, their role in the pathogenesis of OA remains unclear. Frequently these crystals are asymptomatic and do not correlate with extent or severity of disease.

The diversity of risk factors predisposing to OA suggests that a wide variety of insults to the joints, including biomechanical trauma, chronic articular inflammation, and genetic and metabolic factors, can contribute to or trigger the cascade of events that results in the characteristic pathologic features of OA described earlier. At some point, the cartilage degradative process becomes irreversible, perhaps the result of an imbalance of regulatory molecules such as tissue inhibitors of metalloproteinases. With progressive changes in articular cartilage, joint mechanics become altered, in turn perpetuating the degradative process.

Clinical Features and Diagnosis

Pain is the characteristic clinical feature of OA. Recent research has found that pain in OA may be reported as either a constant aching or as a more severe, intermittent pain. Pain is generally worse with activity and/or weight bearing and better with rest. In later stages pain may also occur at rest. Pain tends to be localized to the specific joint involved but may also be referred to a more distant site. The cause of the pain is unclear and is likely to be heterogeneous. Pain may be the result of an interaction among structural pathology; the motor, sensory, and autonomic innervation of the joint; and pain processing at both the spinal and cortical levels, as well as specific individual and environmental factors. Stiffness may be present, particularly after prolonged inactivity, but is not a major feature and is of short duration, usually lasting for <30 minutes. Examination of an involved joint may reveal joint-line tenderness and bony enlargement of the joint. Joint effusion and/or soft-tissue swelling may be present with knee involvement but tends to be intermittent. Persistent inflammation with joint warmth, effusion, and soft-tissue swelling is generally not seen. Crepitus with movement, limitation of joint motion, joint deformity, and/ or joint laxity are additional characteristic features that may be present. Several subtypes of generalized OA have

been identified. The nodal form of OA, involving primarily the distal interphalangeal joints, is most common in middle-aged women, typically with a strong family history among first-degree relatives. Erosive, inflammatory OA is associated with prominent erosive, destructive changes, especially in the finger joints, and may suggest rheumatoid arthritis, although systemic inflammatory signs and other typical features of rheumatoid arthritis (e.g., nodules, proliferative synovitis, extra-articular features, rheumatoid factor) are absent.

The diagnosis of OA is based on history, physical examination, and characteristic radiographic features. The physician must distinguish OA from other inflammatory joint diseases such as rheumatoid arthritis. Distinguishing OA from inflammatory joint diseases involves identifying the characteristic pattern of joint involvement and the nature of the individual joint deformity. Joints commonly involved in OA include the distal interphalangeal joints, proximal interphalangeal joints, first carpometacarpal joints, facet joints of the cervical and lumbar spine, hips, knees, and first metatarsophalangeal joints. Heberden and Bouchard nodes may be present in the hands. Involvement of the wrist, elbows, shoulders, and ankles is uncommon, except in the case of trauma, congenital disease, or endocrine or metabolic disease. The characteristic radiographic features of OA include subchondral sclerosis, joint-space narrowing, subchondral cysts, and osteophytes. The advent of magnetic resonance imaging (MRI) has demonstrated that additional morphologic abnormalities such as bone marrow lesions and meniscal degeneration may also be important features of OA.

Treatment

The natural history of OA is quite variable, with periods of relative stability interspersed with rapid deterioration. The management of OA should therefore be tailored to the individual patient and may include a combination of nonpharmacologic, pharmacologic, and surgical approaches. Patients should be educated regarding the objectives of treatment and the importance of changes in lifestyle, exercise, pacing of activities, and other measures to unload the damaged joint(s). The initial focus should be on self-help and patient-driven treatments rather than on passive therapies. Emphasis should be placed on encouraging adherence to both nonpharmacologic and pharmacologic therapies. Physical therapists may be helpful in providing instruction in appropriate exercises to reduce pain and preserve functional capacity. For knee and hip OA, assistive devices such as walking aids may be useful. Regular aerobic, muscle-strengthening and range-of-motion exercises may also be beneficial. Overweight patients with knee or hip OA should be encouraged to lose weight. A knee brace can reduce pain, improve stability, and diminish the risk of falling for patients with knee OA and mild or moderate varus or valgus instability. Advice concerning appropriate footwear is also important. For example, lateral wedged insoles can be of symptomatic benefit for some patients with medial tibiofemoral compartment OA. Spinal orthoses may provide benefit to patients with significant cervical or lumbar OA. Local applications of heat, ultrasound, or transcutaneous electrical nerve stimulation (TENS) may provide short-term benefit. Acupuncture may also be of symptomatic benefit in patients with knee OA.

Pharmacologic therapy for OA provides symptomatic relief but has not been shown to successfully alter the course of the disease. Pharmacologic therapy should therefore be selected based on its relative efficacy and safety. The use of concomitant medications and the presence of comorbidities also need to be taken into account. Acetaminophen (up to 4 g/day) may be an effective initial oral analgesic for treatment of mild to moderate pain in OA. In patients with symptomatic OA, nonsteroidal anti-inflammatory drugs (NSAIDs) should be used at the lowest effective dose, although their long-term use should be avoided if possible. If patients have risk factors for increased gastrointestinal toxicity, either a cyclo-oxygenase (COX)-2 selective agent or a nonselective NSAID with co-prescription of a proton pump inhibitor (PPI) or misoprostol for gastroprotection should be considered. It is important to note that all NSAIDs, including both nonselective and COX-2 selective agents, should be used with caution in patients with cardiovascular risk factors. Topical NSAIDs and capsaicin may be effective alternatives to oral analgesic or anti-inflammatory agents in knee OA and may also be use as adjunctive agents. Oral glucosamine and/or chondroitin sulfate may provide symptomatic benefit in patients with knee OA but may be slow acting, taking up to 6 months to show benefit. They should be discontinued if there has been no benefit after 6 months of therapy. If other interventions have been ineffective and/or contraindicated, weak opioids and narcotic analgesics may be considered for the treatment of refractory pain. Stronger opioids should be used for the management of severe pain only in exceptional circumstances. Injection of intra-articular corticosteroids may provide modest short-term symptomatic benefit with minimal toxicity, especially in the knee. Patients with moderate to severe pain and effusion and/or other local signs of inflammation may be more responsive. Intra-articular hyaluronate appears to have little if any benefit based on current evidence. Surgical management of OA includes total joint replacement, which has been shown to be extremely effective in relieving pain, decreasing disability, and improving function. With improvements in surgical technique and technology, the indications for total joint replacement have expanded to include both younger and older age groups. Other surgical options include osteotomy and unicompartmental knee replacement.

Prospectus for the Future

- Better understanding of the molecular events leading to cartilage loss in osteoarthritis will permit the development of novel therapies.

References

Dieppe PA, Lohmander S: Pathogenesis and management of pain in osteoarthritis. Lancet 365:965-973, 2005.

Helmick CG, Felson DT, Kwoh CK, et al: Estimates of the prevalence of arthritis and other rheumatic conditions in the United States. Part I. Arthritis Rheum 58:15-25, 2008

Zhang W, Moskowitz RW, Kwoh CK, et al: OARSI recommendations for the management of hip and knee osteoarthritis, Part I: Critical appraisal of existing treatment guidelines and systematic review of current research evidence. Osteoarthritis Cartilage 15:981-1000, 2007.

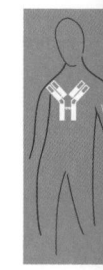

Nonarticular Soft Tissue Disorders

Niveditha Mohan

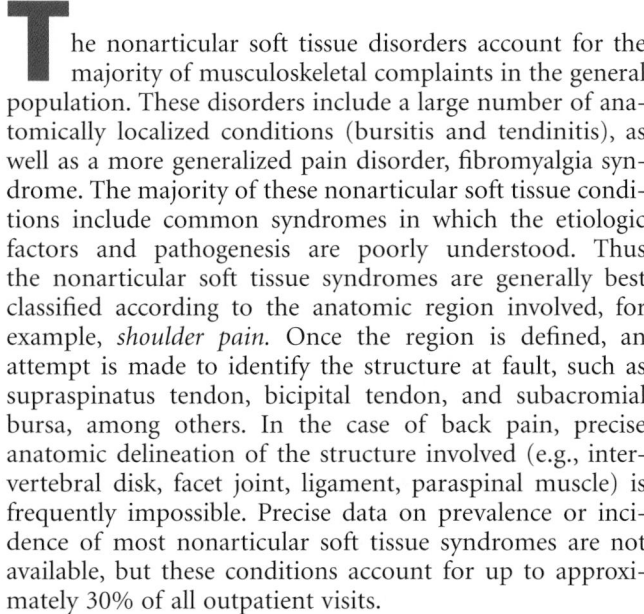

The nonarticular soft tissue disorders account for the majority of musculoskeletal complaints in the general population. These disorders include a large number of anatomically localized conditions (bursitis and tendinitis), as well as a more generalized pain disorder, fibromyalgia syndrome. The majority of these nonarticular soft tissue conditions include common syndromes in which the etiologic factors and pathogenesis are poorly understood. Thus the nonarticular soft tissue syndromes are generally best classified according to the anatomic region involved, for example, *shoulder pain*. Once the region is defined, an attempt is made to identify the structure at fault, such as supraspinatus tendon, bicipital tendon, and subacromial bursa, among others. In the case of back pain, precise anatomic delineation of the structure involved (e.g., intervertebral disk, facet joint, ligament, paraspinal muscle) is frequently impossible. Precise data on prevalence or incidence of most nonarticular soft tissue syndromes are not available, but these conditions account for up to approximately 30% of all outpatient visits.

Etiologic Factors and Pathogenesis

The precise pathophysiologic factors of most cases of nonarticular soft tissue disorders remain unknown, although in many cases predisposing factors can be identified, such as *overuse* or repetitive activities (e.g., *tennis elbow,* lateral epicondylitis) or biomechanical factors (e.g., leg-length discrepancy in trochanteric bursitis). The term *tendinitis* implies that an inflammatory process is present in the involved tendon sheath; however, small tendon tears, periostitis, and even nerve entrapment have been postulated as potential mechanisms. Similarly, although bursitis implies bursal inflammation, demonstrable inflammation is difficult to find. In some cases (e.g., acute bursitis of the olecranon or prepatellar bursa), the mechanism is an acute inflammatory response to sodium urate crystals deposited in the soft tissue, an extra-articular manifestation of gout. The favorable response of tendinitis and bursitis syndromes to anti-inflammatory agents, including corticosteroids, supports the view that at least one component of these syndromes is the result of an inflammatory process. In myofascial pain syndrome the causes are even more obscure. Frequently, overuse and trauma are cited as etiologic factors; however, many cases lack antedating mechanical considerations. In the case of fibromyalgia syndrome, recent research strongly suggests that alterations in central processing of sensory input contribute to the cardinal symptoms of persistent widespread pain and enhanced pain sensitivity. Exposure to psychosocial and environmental stressors, as well as altered autonomic nervous system and neuroendocrine responses, also may contribute to alterations in pain perception or pain inhibition.

Classification of Bursae

Many of the soft tissue rheumatic syndromes involve bursae. Bursae are closed sacs lined with mesenchymal cells that are similar to synovial cells; these sacs are strategically located to facilitate tissue gliding. Most bursae develop concurrently with synovial joints during embryogenesis, although new ones can develop in response to mechanical stress or inflammation (e.g., iliopsoas bursa, trochanteric bursa, semimembranous bursa). In general, bursae do not communicate with joints. An exception is the semimembranous or popliteal bursa in the knee, which communicates with the anterior knee in approximately 40% of individuals. The subacromial or subdeltoid bursa communicates with the glenohumeral joint only if a complete tear of the rotator cuff tendon occurs. Bursae are anatomically divided into the *superficial* bursae (e.g., suprapatellar, olecranon) and the *deep* bursae (e.g., subacromial, iliopsoas, trochanteric). Although most forms of bursitis involve isolated, local conditions, some may be the result of systemic conditions such as gout.

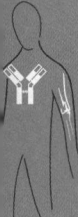

Table 89-1 **Differentiating Nonarticular Soft Tissue Disorders from Articular Disease**		
	Nonarticular Soft Tissue Disorders	**Articular Disease**
Limitation of motion	Active > passive	Active = passive
Crepitus of articular surfaces (structural damage)	0	+/0
Tenderness		
Synovial (fusiform)	0	+
Local	+	0
Swelling		
Synovial (fusiform)	0	+
Local	+/0	0

+, present; 0, absent.

Table 89-2 **Bursitis Syndromes**		
Location	**Symptom**	**Finding**
Subacromial	Shoulder pain	Tender subacromial space
Olecranon	Elbow pain	Tender olecranon swelling
Iliopectineal	Groin pain	Tender inguinal region
Trochanteric	Lateral hip pain	Tender at greater trochanter
Prepatellar	Anterior knee pain	Tender swelling over patella
Infrapatellar	Anterior knee pain	Tender swelling lateral or medial to patellar tendon
Anserine	Medial knee pain	Tender medioproximal tibia (below joint line of knee)
Ischiogluteal	Buttock pain	Tender ischial spine (at gluteal fold)
Retrocalcaneal	Heel pain	Tender swelling between Achilles tendon insertion and calcaneus
Calcaneal	Heel pain	Tender central heel pad

Diagnosis of Nonarticular Soft Tissue Disorders

Tendinitis, bursitis, and myofascial disorders should be distinguished from articular disorders. In most cases, this can be accomplished by a careful examination of the involved structure (Table 89-1). General principles of the musculoskeletal examination are as follows:

1. Observation: If deformity or soft tissue swelling is present, then is it fusiform (surrounding the entire joint in a symmetrical fashion) or is it localized? Local rather than fusiform deformity distinguishes nonarticular disorders from articular disorders.
2. Palpation: Is tenderness localized or in a fusiform distribution? Is an effusion present? Local, not fusiform or joint-line, tenderness distinguishes nonarticular disorders from articular disorders. The presence of an effusion almost always indicates an articular disorder.
3. Assessing range of motion: The musculoskeletal examination includes the assessment of both *active* range of motion (i.e., the patient attempts to move the symptomatic structure) and *passive* range of motion (i.e., the examiner moves the symptomatic structure). Articular disorders are generally characterized by equal impairment in both active and passive movements as a result of the mechanical limitation of joint motion resulting from proliferation of the synovial membrane, the presence of an effusion, or the derangement of intra-articular structures. Impairment of active movement characterizes nonarticular disorders to a much greater degree than passive movement.

Bursitis

CLINICAL PRESENTATION

Septic Bursitis

Superficial forms of bursitis, particularly olecranon bursitis and prepatellar and occasionally infrapatellar bursitis, are more frequently infected or involved with crystal deposition than are deep forms of bursitis. Presumably, these infections or involvements are the result of direct extension of organisms through subcutaneous tissues. Most commonly, *Staphylococcus aureus* is isolated from infected superficial bursae. Septic bursitis should be suspected where there is cellulitis, erythema, fever, and peripheral leukocytosis. Definitive diagnosis and especially exclusion of infection of subcutaneous bursae generally require aspiration of the distended bursa. The bursal fluid should be assessed for cell count, Gram stain, and culture and examined for crystals.

Nonseptic Bursitis

Nonseptic bursitis frequently appears as an overuse condition associated with sudden or unaccustomed repetitive activity of the associated extremity. The two most common types of bursitis are subacromial and trochanteric bursitis (Table 89-2). Subacromial bursitis is the most common overall cause of shoulder pain over the lateral upper arm or deltoid muscle that is exacerbated with abduction of the arm. Subacromial bursitis is the result of compression of the inflamed rotator cuff tendon between the acromion and humeral head. Because the rotator cuff forms the floor of the subacromial bursa, bursitis in this location often results from tendinitis of the rotator cuff. Occasionally, subacromial bursitis or rotator cuff tendinitis results from osteophyte compression of the rotator cuff tendon originating from the acromioclavicular joint. The differential diagnosis includes tears of the rotator cuff, intra-articular pathologic mechanisms of the glenohumeral joint, bicipital tendinitis, cervical radiculopathy, and referred pain from the chest.

Trochanteric bursitis is the result of inflammation at the insertion of the gluteal muscles at the greater trochanter and produces lateral thigh pain, which is often worse when the subject lies on the affected side. Women seem to be more prone to develop this condition, perhaps because of increased traction of the gluteal muscles as a result of the relatively broader female pelvis. Other potential risk factors include weight gain, local trauma, overuse activities such as jogging, and leg-length discrepancies (primarily on the side with the

Table 89-3 **Tendinitis Syndromes**

Location	Symptom	Finding
Extensor pollicis brevis and abductor pollicis longus (de Quervain tenosynovitis)	Wrist pain	Pain on ulnar deviation of the wrist, with the thumb grasped by the remaining four fingers (Finkelstein test)
Flexor tendons of fingers	Triggering or locking of fingers in flexion	Tender nodule on flexor tendon on palm over metacarpal joint
Medial epicondyle	Elbow pain	Tenderness of medial epicondyle
Lateral epicondyle	Elbow pain	Tenderness of lateral epicondyle
Bicipital tendon	Shoulder pain	Tenderness along bicipital groove
Patella	Knee pain	Tenderness at insertion of patellar tendon
Achilles	Heel pain	Tender Achilles tendon
Tibialis posterior	Medial ankle pain	Tenderness under medial malleolus with resisted inversion of the ankle
Peroneal	Lateral midfoot or ankle pain	Tenderness under lateral malleolus with passive inversion

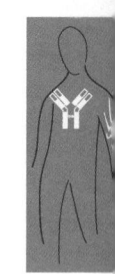

longer leg). These factors are thought to lead to increased tension of the gluteus maximus on the iliotibial band, producing bursal inflammation. The differential diagnosis of trochanteric bursitis includes lumbar radiculopathy (particularly of the L1 and L2 nerve roots), meralgia paresthetica (entrapment of the lateral cutaneous nerve of the thigh as it passes under the inguinal ligament), true hip joint disease, and intra-abdominal pathologic processes. Other bursitis syndromes are less common and listed in Table 89-2.

TREATMENT

Septic bursitis is treated with a combination of serial aspirations of the infected bursa and antibiotics, initially directed against *S. aureus* and then adjusted depending on the results of bursal fluid cultures. Recurrent septic bursitis may need surgical excision of the bursa in recalcitrant cases. The approach to nonseptic bursitis should include rest, local heat, and, unless contraindicated (e.g., by peptic ulcer disease, renal disease, advanced age), nonsteroidal anti-inflammatory drugs (NSAIDs). Usually, the most effective approach is a local injection of a corticosteroid. Superficial bursae with obvious swelling should be aspirated before the corticosteroid is injected. For deep bursae, such as the subacromial or trochanteric bursae, aspiration yields little if any fluid, and direct injection of a corticosteroid without attempted aspiration is reasonable. Caution is advised in attempted aspiration or injection of the iliopsoas bursa, the ischiogluteal bursa, and the gastrocnemius-semimembranosus bursa (Baker cyst). These bursae lie close to important neural and/or vascular structures, and aspiration under radiologic (ultrasound) guidance may be a safer option.

Tendinitis

CLINICAL PRESENTATION

Most tendinitis syndromes are the result of inflammation in the tendon sheath. Overuse with microscopic tearing of the tendon is the most common risk factor for tendinitis, but tendon compression by an osteophyte may occur, for example, in the rotator cuff tendon compressed by an osteophyte originating from the acromioclavicular joint.

One of the most common forms of tendinitis is lateral epicondylitis, also known as *tennis elbow* (Table 89-3). This is a common overuse syndrome among tennis players, but it can be seen in many other settings requiring repetitive extension of the forearm (e.g., painting overhead). The diagnosis is confirmed by exclusion of elbow joint pathology and the finding of local tenderness at the lateral epicondyle, which is typically exacerbated by forearm extension against resistance. Enthesopathies such as Achilles tendinitis and peroneal and posterior tibial tendinitis may occur in the setting of an underlying seronegative arthropathy such as Reiter disease or psoriatic arthritis. A history and clinical evaluation for these disorders should be pursued in the appropriate patient.

TREATMENT

Therapy for tendinitis—NSAIDs, local heat, and corticosteroid injection—is similar to that for bursitis. Rest, physical therapy, occupational therapy, and occasionally ergonomic modification are useful adjuncts. The goal of corticosteroid injection in tendinitis is to infiltrate the tendon sheath rather than the tendon itself, because direct injection into a tendon may result in rupture of the tendon. Corticosteroid injection of the Achilles tendon should be avoided because of the propensity of this tendon to rupture. Surgical management of tendinitis is indicated only with failures of conservative treatment. For example, chronic impingement of the supraspinatus tendon that is refractory to conservative treatment may require subacromial decompression.

Fibromyalgia Syndrome

Fibromyalgia syndrome, formerly known as *fibrositis,* is a controversial chronic pain condition characterized by persistent, widespread pain and tenderness to palpation at anatomically defined tender points located in soft tissue musculoskeletal structures. Associated systemic symptoms can include insomnia, cognitive dysfunction, depression, anxiety, recurrent headaches, dizziness, fatigue, morning stiffness, extremity dysesthesia, irritable bowel syndrome, and irritable bladder syndrome. Although the syndrome has only recently been the subject of investigation, descriptions of it exist far back in the medical literature. Controversy persists, however, because of the lack of objective diagnostic or pathologic findings.

PATHOPHYSIOLOGIC FEATURES

Fibromyalgia syndrome as defined by the American College of Rheumatology 1990 definition for clinical trials is a chronic widespread pain condition with characteristic tender points on physical examination, often associated with a constellation of symptoms such as fatigue, sleep disturbance, headache, irritable bowel syndrome, and mood disorders.

Investigators have examined diverse mechanisms in fibromyalgia syndrome, including studies of muscle, sleep physiologic processes, neurohormonal function, and psychological status. Although the pathophysiologic mechanisms remain unknown, an increasing body of literature points to central (central nervous system) rather than peripheral (muscle) mechanisms. Muscle tissue has been a focus of investigation for many years. Initial studies, including histologic and histochemical studies, suggested a possible metabolic myopathy; however, carefully controlled studies indicated that these abnormalities were simply the result of deconditioning. Sleep studies suggested that disruption of deep sleep (stage IV) by so-called *alpha-intrusion* (the normal awake electroencephalographic pattern) may play a causal role, but this finding was later observed in other disorders, more likely indicating effect rather than cause. In some cases, musculoskeletal injury has been implicated as a trigger for fibromyalgia, but social and legal issues cloud its causative role. Several studies have suggested that subtle hypothalamic-pituitary-adrenal axis hypofunction may occur in fibromyalgia syndrome, although it remains uncertain whether these changes are constitutive or are the result of fibromyalgia. A prevailing theory of pathogenesis is dysregulation of pain pathways leading to central sensitization and marked by neurotransmitter, neurohormone, and sleep physiology irregularities.

Fibromyalgia has long been linked to psychological disturbance. Most studies have confirmed high lifetime rates of major depression, which range from 34% to 71%, associated with fibromyalgia syndrome. High lifetime rates of migraine, irritable bowel syndrome, and panic disorder have also been associated with fibromyalgia syndrome, suggesting that fibromyalgia may be part of an *affective spectrum* group of disorders.

CLINICAL PRESENTATION AND DIFFERENTIAL DIAGNOSIS

The clinical presentation of fibromyalgia syndrome is generally that of the insidious onset of chronic, diffuse, poorly localized musculoskeletal pain, typically accompanied by fatigue and sleep disturbance. The physical examination shows a normal musculoskeletal examination, with no deformity or synovitis; however, widespread tenderness occurs, especially at tendon insertion sites, indicating a general reduction in pain threshold. The American College of Rheumatology has published the results of a multicenter

Table 89-4	**American College of Rheumatology Classification Criteria for Fibromyalgia Syndrome**

For classification purposes, patients are said to have fibromyalgia if both criteria are satisfied.

1. *History of chronic, widespread pain:* Pain is considered widespread when present above and below the waist on both sides of the body. *Chronic* is defined as greater than 3 months in duration.
2. *Pain in 11 of 18 tender points on digital palpation:* Points include occiput, low cervical, trapezius, supraspinatus, second rib, lateral epicondyle, gluteal, greater trochanter, knee.

study to identify clinical classification criteria for fibromyalgia syndrome, which were shown to have high sensitivity and specificity (Table 89-4). These criteria have facilitated population-based studies, which suggest that fibromyalgia syndrome affects approximately 2% of the population and up to 7% of women. Approximately 10% of surveyed patients are disabled to varying degrees by their symptoms; therefore the economic impact is large. The prevalence of fibromyalgia appears to be similar in most ethnic and racial groups.

Approximately one third of the patients identify antecedent trauma as a precipitant for their symptoms, one third of patients describe a viral prodrome, and one third have no clear precipitant. A variety of less typical presentations has been described, including a predominantly neuropathic presentation with paresthesias (numbness and tingling) in a nondermatomal distribution, an arthralgic rather than myalgic presentation, and an axial skeletal presentation (resembling degenerative disk disease). Many patients may have undergone invasive diagnostic tests and in some cases inappropriate procedures such as carpal tunnel release or cervical or lumbar laminectomies.

Conditions that should be considered in the differential diagnosis of fibromyalgia syndrome include polymyalgia rheumatica (in older patients), hypothyroidism, polymyositis, and early systemic lupus erythematosus or rheumatoid arthritis. In general, however, symptoms are exhibited for many months or years without evidence of other signs or symptoms of an underlying connective tissue disease, making other possible diagnoses unlikely. Laboratory and radiographic studies are usually normal in patients with fibromyalgia syndrome. Exclusion of other conditions, such as osteoarthritis, rheumatoid arthritis, and systemic lupus erythematosus, by radiography, erythrocyte sedimentation rate, assays for rheumatoid factor or antinuclear antibody, and other tests is no longer considered a necessary preliminary to the diagnosis of fibromyalgia syndrome, which should be diagnosed on the basis of positive criteria.

TREATMENT

The treatment of fibromyalgia includes reassurance that the condition is not a progressive, crippling, or life-threatening entity. A combination of treatment options, including medication and physical measures, is helpful in most patients. Medications shown to be helpful in short-term, double-blind, placebo-controlled trials include amitriptyline and cyclobenzaprine. Low doses of these medications (e.g., 10 to 30 mg of amitriptyline, 10 to 30 mg of cyclobenzaprine) are moderately effective and generally well tolerated. Studies have also shown that newer antidepressants of the serotonin-norepinephrine reuptake inhibitors (e.g., duloxetine, venlafaxine, bupropion) and $\alpha_2\delta$ ligands (gabapentin, pregabalin) are also effective, particularly in combination with low doses of tricyclic antidepressants. Patients should also be encouraged to take an active role in the management of their condition. They should, if possible, begin a progressive, low-level aerobic exercise program to improve muscular fitness and a sense of well-being. A combination approach is effective in most patients in alleviating symptoms, although a small minority of patients require more intensive treatment strategies, such as psychiatric treatment or referral to a pain center.

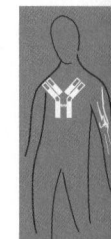

Prospectus for the Future

Better understanding of pathophysiology and improved trial design and outcome measures will facilitate the development of more effective therapies in soft tissue disorders.

References

Goldenberg DL, Burkhardt C, Crofford L: Management of fibromyalgia syndrome. JAMA 292:2388-2395, 2004.
Littlejohn GO: Balanced treatments for fibromyalgia. Arthritis Rheum 50:2725-2729, 2004.

Rheumatic Manifestations of Systemic Disorders

Fotios Koumpouras

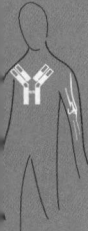

Many systemic disorders can express themselves through the musculoskeletal system. These often can be the presenting clue for the true nature of the underlying disorder (Table 90-1).

Rheumatic Syndromes Associated with Malignancy

HYPERTROPHIC OSTEOARTHROPATHY

Hypertrophic osteoarthropathy (HOA) is a syndrome that includes clubbing of fingers and toes, periostitis of the long bones, and arthritis. HOA can be primary, which is a hereditary form appearing in childhood and usually self-limited, or secondary. The secondary form can be either generalized or localized. Secondary generalized HOA is most often associated with neoplastic disease or infectious disease but can be seen in congenital heart disease, inflammatory bowel disease, cirrhosis, or Graves disease. Approximately 90% of cases are associated with lung cancer. Secondary localized HOA has been associated with hemiplegia, aneurysms, infective arteritis, and patent ductus arteriosus. In addition, isolated digital clubbing is associated with pleuropulmonary disease in approximately 80% of patients, but cancer is present in only a small minority of patients. Chronic digital clubbing does not appear to lead to the development of HOA. The long bones most commonly involved in HOA are the distal femur, tibia, and radius. The pathogenesis is unknown, although platelet-endothelial interactions with production of von Willebrand factor are thought to be important mechanisms.

HOA typically produces bone and joint pain with swelling that results from peri-articular periostitis. Joints appear swollen, but no proliferative synovium or inflammation develops, and joint fluid is noninflammatory. Radiographic features can be diagnostic and include periostitis with peri-osteal new bone formation, especially along the distal and/or proximal portion of long bones. Treatment of the underlying disorder ameliorates HOA.

LEUKEMIA AND LYMPHOMA

Leukemia may simulate various rheumatic syndromes by producing synovitis or bone pain resulting from direct invasion of the synovium or marrow expansion. Approximately 6% of adult patients with leukemia exhibit rheumatic manifestations, which precede the diagnosis of leukemia by an average of 3 months. The most common presentation is an asymmetric large-joint oligoarthritis, often accompanied by low back pain. Up to 60% of children with acute leukemia have been diagnosed with either monoarthritis or polyarthritis. Although lymphoma is frequently associated with bone lesions, arthritis is a rare presentation. The combination of nocturnal bone pain, hematologic abnormalities, and radiographic features such as periosteal elevation should suggest the possibility of leukemia. Treatment of the leukemia usually results in resolution of the musculoskeletal manifestations.

Vasculitis may also occur with leukemia, lymphoma, and other myelodysplastic disorders. Leukocytoclastic vasculitis is the most common clinical vasculitic paraneoplastic presentation. In addition, a polyarteritis nodosa–like vasculitis is the most common rheumatologic manifestation of hairy cell leukemia. The presentation of vasculitis may proceed or follow the malignancy diagnosis. The most common malignancies associated with vasculitis include hairy cell leukemia, leukemia, multiple myeloma, non-Hodgkin lymphoma, Hodgkin lymphoma, sarcoma, cervical carcinoma, breast carcinoma, prostate carcinoma, and colon cancer.

Sweet syndrome is an acute febrile neutrophilic dermatosis that mimics vasculitis and is associated with malignancy in approximately 15% of patients. It is most commonly seen with acute myelogenous leukemia but has been described with other types of malignancies. It can be associated with an acute, self-limited polyarthritis in 20% of the cases.

Table 90-1 **Systemic Conditions Associated with Rheumatic Manifestations**
Malignant Disorders
Hypertrophic osteoarthropathy
Lymphoma
Leukemia
Carcinoma polyarthritis
Hematologic Disorders
Hemophilia
Sickle cell disease
Thalassemia
Multiple myeloma
Amyloidosis
Gastrointestinal Disorders
Spondyloarthropathies
Whipple disease
Hemochromatosis
Primary biliary cirrhosis
Endocrinopathies
Diabetes
Hypothyroidism
Hyperthyroidism
Hyperparathyroidism
Acromegaly

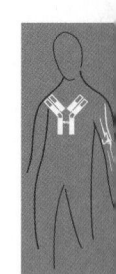

Hematologic Disorders

HEMOPHILIA

Hemarthrosis is the most common bleeding complication of either hemophilia A (factor VIII deficiency) or hemophilia B (factor IX deficiency) and occurs in up to two thirds of patients. Hemarthrosis may occur spontaneously or as the result of minor trauma, and the level of factor deficiency determines its frequency and age at onset. Acute, painful swelling of the knees, elbows, and ankles is the most common presentation. A chronic arthropathy with persistent synovitis may also occur, perhaps as a result of excessive iron deposition in synovial membrane and cartilage. Radiographic findings are those of degenerative joint disease, with joint space narrowing, subchondral sclerosis, and cyst formation. Widening of the femoral condylar notch is a late, diagnostic radiographic finding. Treatment consists of prompt administration of factor VIII or IX concentrate or recombinant forms, intra-articular corticosteroid injections, local ice application, rest, and later physical therapy. Aspiration is indicated only if concomitant sepsis is suggested or if the joint is unusually tense and only after factor replacement. No evidence suggests that prophylaxis for acute hemarthrosis may reduce the incidence of chronic synovitis and future joint damage.

SICKLE CELL DISEASE

Of the sickle cell hemoglobinopathies, sickle cell (SS) anemia, sickle cell–β-thalassemia, sickle cell–hemoglobin C (SC) disease, and sickle cell–hemoglobin D (SD) disease all produce musculoskeletal complications, which include painful crises, arthropathy, dactylitis, osteonecrosis, osteomyelitis, and gout. SS crises are the most common musculoskeletal features, producing pain in the chest, back, and joints. Involvement of joints may produce a painful arthritis, typically of the large joints. The mechanism of the arthropathy is thought to be an articular reaction to juxta-articular bone infarction or infarction of the synovial membrane by vascular occlusion from sickled erythrocytes. The synovial fluid is typically noninflammatory. Dactylitis resulting from vaso-occlusion in bone may occur in infants and young children, producing acute, painful, nonpitting edema of the hands and feet (hand-foot syndrome). This usually resolves spontaneously in a few weeks. Osteonecrosis of the femoral head, shoulder, and tibial plateau (in decreasing frequency) may also result from repeated crises and is most common in SS disease.

An increased incidence of septic arthritis and osteomyelitis has been associated with SS disease; *Salmonella* is the bacterial genus most frequently isolated in the patient with osteomyelitis (approximately 50%). Predisposition to *Salmonella* species is thought to be caused by functional asplenia. Osteomyelitis may be subtle and is often confused with sickle crisis. Bandemia is more suggestive of osteomyelitis. Combined technetium and gallium nuclear scans can be employed to help diagnosis.

In addition, hyperuricemia caused by renal tubular damage secondary to sickle cell disease can be seen in up to 40% of adult patients. Therefore gout can occur in patients with sickle cell disease, although it is uncommon. In children with sickle cell disease, hyperuricosuria without hyperuricemia occurs, presumably resulting from the increased marrow turnover and urate production.

Noninflammatory joint effusions adjacent to areas of bony crisis can occur, particularly at the knees and ankles. Focal muscle necroses as well as rhabdomyolysis are uncommon to rare manifestations.

MULTIPLE MYELOMA AND AMYLOIDOSIS

Multiple myeloma is one of the most common plasma cell dyscrasias and is frequently accompanied by musculoskeletal manifestations, which include bone pain resulting from lytic bone lesions, pathologic fractures, and osteoporosis. The diagnosis of multiple myeloma should be suggested in any of these clinical settings and is confirmed with the finding of a monoclonal gammopathy and sheets of immature neoplastic plasma cells on bone marrow biopsy. Primary (AL) amyloidosis accompanies approximately 15% of patients with myeloma. Alternatively, AL amyloidosis occurs without significant plasma cell proliferation on bone marrow biopsy, but patients have evidence of a plasma cell dyscrasia by virtue of the presence of a serum monoclonal gammopathy. AL amyloidosis results when amyloid protein, consisting of microscopic fibrils derived from monoclonal light chains, is deposited in organs such as the kidneys, heart, peripheral nerves, and gastrointestinal tract. It should be considered in the differential diagnosis of a patient older than 40 years of age who has nephritic syndrome, unexplained heart failure, idiopathic peripheral neuropathy, or hepatomegaly. Infrequently, amyloid joint infiltration produces a symmetrical, small-joint polyarthritis-simulating rheumatoid arthritis. Occasionally, significant infiltration of the shoulder joints with amyloid deposits produces an anterior glenohumeral soft tissue deformity known as the *shoulder pad sign*. Macroglossia and submandibular gland infiltration may also

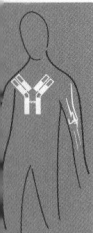

occur. The diagnosis of this form of amyloidosis is the most easily established, with the demonstration of apple-green birefringent fluorescence on Congo red staining of an abdominal fat pad aspirate, or rectal mucosal biopsy. Biopsy of affected areas, such as gastric mucosa in those with stomach involvement, also has a high yield. In addition, immunoelectrophoresis and immunofixation of serum and urine should be performed. Optimal treatment of AL amyloidosis now consists of high-dose chemotherapy with stem cell transplantation.

The three other principal systemic forms of amyloidosis are (1) secondary (AA) amyloidosis, (2) heredofamilial (familial amyloid polyneuropathy) amyloidosis, and (3) β_2-microglobulin–associated (β_2M) amyloidosis. AA amyloidosis is a rare complication of chronic inflammatory conditions such as rheumatoid arthritis, inflammatory bowel disease, and familial Mediterranean fever. Certain chronic infections such as leprosy, tuberculosis, and osteomyelitis are also associated with this form of amyloidosis. The amyloid fibrils are derived from the acute phase reactant, serum amyloid A protein. The disease usually causes proteinuria or gastrointestinal symptoms because of infiltration of the kidney or gastrointestinal tract. The diagnosis generally requires organ biopsy because the sensitivity of the abdominal fat pad aspirate is considerably lower in AA amyloidosis than it is in the AL form. Treatment consists of controlling the underlying disorder, producing the chronic inflammatory process.

Heredofamilial (familial amyloid polyneuropathy) amyloidosis is the least common form of amyloidosis. This rare autosomal dominant disease is the result of single-point mutations in the gene coding for transthyretin, a thyroid-transport protein. Transthyretin is synthesized principally in the liver. Amyloid fibrils in this disease are composed of fragments of mutant transthyretin that have a propensity to form amyloid fibrils. The condition typically causes an axonal and/or autonomic neuropathy late in life. Abdominal fat aspiration has high sensitivity in the diagnosis of this type of amyloidosis. Studies suggest that the optimal treatment is orthotopic liver transplantation, which prevents further production of the mutant transthyretin.

β_2M-associated amyloidosis occurs almost exclusively in patients on long-standing hemodialysis. This disease typically causes carpal tunnel syndrome and flexor tendon deposits in the hands or in the rotator cuff. Cystic bone deposits in the carpal bones, hips, shoulders, and cervical spine have also been described. The pathogenesis of β_2M-associated amyloidosis is not completely understood but may in part be the result of altered proteolysis of β_2-microglobulin in long-standing hemodialysis. Treatment includes physical measures such as splinting for carpal tunnel syndrome and physical therapy for shoulder involvement. Anti-inflammatory agents may provide additional symptomatic relief. Surgical removal of carpal or shoulder deposits may be required. Renal transplantation may be the most effective way to halt progression.

Gastrointestinal Diseases

WHIPPLE DISEASE

Whipple disease is a rare, multisystemic disease of late middle-aged to older men and is characterized by the presence of fever, abdominal pain, steatorrhea with weight loss, lymphadenopathy, and arthritis, the last of which is now known to be the result of infection with *Tropheryma whippleii*. Polyserositis, arterial hypotension, hyperpigmentation, and various central nervous system manifestations, such as personality changes, memory loss, dementia, and spastic paraparesis, may also occur. The organism's DNA can be detected in duodenal biopsy specimens. Biopsy has long been used to detect this unculturable organism in histiocytes of the lamina propria, which show intracytoplasmic inclusions of irregular granular material that is positive on periodic acid-Schiff staining. This last finding is not specific for Whipple disease, and therefore polymerase chain reaction assay to detect the organism's DNA is now the preferred technique for diagnosis.

The arthritis of Whipple disease occurs in 60% to 90% of patients and is the most common prodrome. Classically, the arthritis is an intermittent migratory oligoarthritis lasting from a few hours to days with spontaneous remission. Some patients have only arthralgia, whereas others have a florid polyarthritis. Synovial fluid findings are typically inflammatory with a high percentage of mononuclear cells. Treatment consists of antibiotic therapy with tetracycline, which results in complete resolution within 1 week to 1 month.

HEMOCHROMATOSIS

Hereditary hemochromatosis is an autosomal recessive disorder associated with increased iron absorption and deposition that, via hemosiderin, eventually produces multiorgan damage. Hemochromatosis is among the most common genetic diseases among Europeans, with a homozygous prevalence of 0.3% to 0.5% and a heterozygote frequency of 6.7% to 10%. Approximately 90% of white patients with hereditary hemochromatosis are homozygous for the same mutation (C282Y) in the *HFE* gene. HFE protein forms complexes with the transferrin receptor, which is important in iron transport, and mutations in *HFE* decrease the protein's affinity for the receptor, impairing iron transport and resulting in iron overload.

The classic clinical features of hemochromatosis include hepatic cirrhosis, cardiomyopathy, diabetes mellitus, pituitary dysfunction, hypogonadism, skin pigmentation, and sicca syndrome. Symmetrical arthropathy of the second and third metacarpal joints is a disabling complication that occurs in approximately 50% of patients. Radiographic manifestations are similar to those of osteoarthritis (see Chapter 88) and include characteristic "bird-beak" osteophytes arising from the radial side of the metacarpal. In addition, the presence of chondrocalcinosis can be seen in the wrists, as hemachromatosis is associated with calcium pyrophosphate deposition disease. Occasionally, superimposed attacks of pseudogout dominate the clinical picture. Osteoarthritis-like disease occurring in a middle-aged man with involvement of the metacarpophalangeal joints should indicate the possibility of hemochromatosis. Joint changes are irreversible. The diagnosis may be established with the identification of the mutated gene sequence in DNA obtained from peripheral blood.

PRIMARY BILIARY CIRRHOSIS

Primary biliary cirrhosis is an inflammatory disease of the intrahepatic bile ducts that is frequently associated with other disorders presumed to be autoimmune, including limited scleroderma (see Chapter 83), rheumatoid arthritis (see Chapter 79), Sjögren syndrome (see Chapter 85), autoimmune thyroiditis, and renotubular acidosis. Approximately 90% of patients have detectable immunoglobulin G–antimitochondrial antibodies, which are rare in other forms of liver disease. Up to 50% of patients with primary biliary cirrhosis have secondary Sjögren syndrome, which represents the most common rheumatic disorder associated with primary biliary cirrhosis. Other musculoskeletal complications include (1) osteomalacia caused by reduced vitamin D absorption and (2) accelerated osteoporosis. The diagnosis of primary biliary cirrhosis should be suggested in the patient with unexplained pruritus or elevated levels of serum alkaline phosphatase. A positive antimitochondrial antibody test provides strong evidence, which should then be confirmed with a liver biopsy.

Endocrine Disorders

DIABETES

Many musculoskeletal complications of diabetes exist (Table 90-2). One of the most common complications is the so-called *diabetic stiff-hand syndrome,* which is characterized by waxy thickening of the skin in long-standing type 1 or 2 diabetes. Occasionally, it may develop before the onset of overt diabetes and may create confusion because of the similarity of its appearance to that of scleroderma-like sclerodactyly. These changes are thought to be the result of excess sugar alcohols, such as sorbitol, producing excess water content in the skin and leading to increased stiffness. Joint contractures, flexor tendon contractures (including Dupuytren contractures), and joint thickening produce a condition known as *diabetic cheiroarthropathy* or the *syndrome of limited joint mobility;* these conditions appear to be related to the duration of diabetes. Although it is most common in the fingers, limited mobility may also occur in the shoulders. Diabetic periarthritis of the shoulders also referred to as *adhesive capsulitis* or *frozen shoulder.* It occurs in 10% to 30% of patients with diabetes mellitus and typically affects patients with non–insulin-requiring diabetes of long duration. About half the patients have bilateral involvement, although, curiously, the nondominant shoulders frequently are more severely involved. In many instances, adhesive capsulitis in diabetics can remit spontaneously in several weeks. When adhesive capsulitis is accompanied by vasomotor changes of the same upper extremity, this can be referred to as *shoulder-hand syndrome,* which is similar to reflex sympathetic dystrophy.

Charcot joints or neuropathic arthropathy may occur with any neuropathy but are most commonly associated with diabetes, although defects are present in less than 1% of all patients with diabetes. The condition affects men and women with equal frequency. Most patients are over age 40 years and have long-standing disease. Poorly controlled diabetes associated with diabetic peripheral neuropathy is the strongest risk factor. Tarsal and tarsometatarsal joints

Table 90-2 Musculoskeletal Manifestations of Endocrine Disease	
Endocrine Disease	**Musculoskeletal Manifestation**
Diabetes mellitus	Carpal tunnel syndrome Charcot arthropathy Adhesive capsulitis Syndrome of limited joint mobility (cheiroarthropathy) Diabetic amyotrophy Diabetic muscle infarction
Hypothyroidism	Proximal myopathy Arthralgias Joint effusions Carpal tunnel syndrome Chondrocalcinosis
Hyperthyroidism	Myopathy Osteoporosis Thyroid acropachy
Hyperparathyroidism	Myopathy Arthralgias Erosive arthritis Chondrocalcinosis
Hypoparathyroidism	Muscle cramps Soft tissue calcifications Spondyloarthropathy
Acromegaly	Carpal tunnel syndrome Myopathy Raynaud phenomenon Back pain Premature osteoarthritis
Cushing syndrome	Myopathy Osteoporosis Avascular necrosis

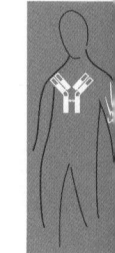

are most commonly involved, and trauma together with diminished pain perception, proprioception, and position sense are major factors in the genesis of this arthropathy. The most common presentation is swelling of the foot with little or no pain. Treatment consists of avoiding weight-bearing activities and application of a Charcot boot or soft cast. Prevention of skin oral ulceration over bony prominences is critical. End-stage Charcot deformity of the foot is referred to as "rocker-bottom feet."

Carpal tunnel syndrome is associated with diabetes. Up to 15% of all patients with carpal tunnel syndrome have diabetes. The condition causes typical paresthesias in median nerve distribution.

Diffuse idiopathic skeletal hyperostosis occurs in approximately 20% of non–insulin-requiring diabetic patients. Typically patients have neck and back stiffness associated with loss of motion. Pain tends not to be prominent. Spine radiographs demonstrating calcification of the anterior longitudinal ligament of four contiguous vertebrae are diagnostic. Lack of involvement of the apophyseal joints distinguishes this disorder from ankylosing spondylitis and osteoarthritis. Physical therapy and nonsteroidal anti-inflammatory medications are the mainstays of treatment.

HYPOTHYROIDISM

Almost one third of patients with frank hypothyroidism can exhibit objective musculoskeletal findings. Myxedematous arthropathy usually affects large joints. Patients may demonstrate swelling and stiffness, synovial membrane thickening, ligamentous laxity, and joint effusions. Synovial fluid is noninflammatory. In addition, hypothyroidism is associated with carpal tunnel syndrome, Raynaud phenomena, fibromyalgia-like muscle pain, and proximal muscle weakness with stiffness and increased creatinine kinase.

Pseudogout may also be a presenting manifestation of hypothyroidism. Myopathy, especially proximal, occurs in hypothyroidism and is often associated with elevated levels of creatine kinase. Muscle biopsy specimens show atrophy of type II fibers but no inflammation. Thyroid replacement results in gradual improvement of both the arthropathy and myopathy of hypothyroidism.

HYPERTHYROIDISM

Four principal rheumatic manifestations occur in thyrotoxicosis: proximal myopathy, shoulder periarthritis, thyroid acropachy (thickened skin with periosteal new bone formation), and osteoporosis. Myopathy is common, occurring in 70% of patients with hyperthyroidism, but it is seldom a presenting manifestation. Myopathy tends to be more common in elderly patients with apathetic hyperthyroidism. The concurrence of new onset atrial fibrillation should be a clue. Periarthritis of the shoulder (especially bilateral) occurs in up to 10% of patients. Thyroid acropachy is a rare complication of Graves disease and consists of clubbing and soft tissue swelling of the hands and feet. Radiographs show periosteal new bone formation, which is best seen on the radial aspect of the second and third metacarpals. It is strongly associated with ophthalmopathy and pretibial myxedema. The symptoms of thyroid acropachy occur as patients achieve euthyroidism. Osteoporosis is produced by increased bone turnover, which accompanies the hyperthyroid state.

HYPERPARATHYROIDISM

Musculoskeletal manifestations are common in hyperparathyroidism and are the initial manifestations in up to 15% of patients. Pseudogout is the most common rheumatic complication, occurring in up to 10% of patients with hyperparathyroidism, although radiographic chondrocalcinosis is seen in up to 40% of patients. A rheumatoid, arthritis-like disorder has also been described with involvement of the knees, wrists, hands, and shoulders, showing radiographic erosions. In contrast to rheumatoid arthritis, however, synovial proliferation is absent, the joint space is preserved, and erosions are characteristically on the ulnar side, as opposed to rheumatoid arthritis, in which the erosions are typically on the radial side.

Secondary hyperparathyroidism is common in patients with chronic renal failure and is a component of renal osteodystrophy. Musculoskeletal features are similar to those described earlier.

Sarcoidosis

Sarcoidosis is a multisystemic inflammatory disorder exhibited by the formation of noncaseating granulomas. It may be associated with both acute and chronic rheumatic manifestations. The acute syndrome is known as *Löfgren syndrome* and consists of the classic triad of hilar adenopathy, erythema nodosum, and arthritis. It occurs in approximately 15% of those patients with sarcoidosis. The arthritis is usually symmetrical and migratory; it frequently involves the ankles, although it may be difficult to distinguish from erythema nodosum and peri-arthritis of the ankle. Joint effusions are typically noninflammatory. The arthritis is nondeforming, nonerosive, and self-limiting, usually not lasting more than 3 to 4 months. Patients with the nonarticular manifestations of Löfgren syndrome have an excellent prognosis.

Chronic arthropathy involving the knees, ankles, wrists, and elbows occurs less frequently and is generally associated with active multisystemic disease. Synovial thickening and effusions are common; a synovial biopsy specimen may show the typical noncaseating granulomas. Treatment of acute sarcoid arthropathy includes the use of nonsteroidal anti-inflammatory drugs or, occasionally, a short course of corticosteroids. Treatment of the chronic arthropathy is dependent on the severity of the extra-articular manifestations that usually accompany it. Corticosteroids and other immunosuppressive agents are generally needed to control the systemic disease, which in turn can control the arthropathy. Bony involvement by sarcoidosis leads to lytic lesions, particularly over the phalanges, and can cause a pathologic fracture.

Prospectus for the Future

The future of recognizing rheumatic syndromes as part of systemic diseases relies on accurate diagnosis. With the employment of new cell-based assays, autoantibody tests, and physician recognition, the recognition of systemic disease with rheumatic manifestations can be facilitated. In addition, increasing the rheumatology workforce allows for rapid referral of patients who have rheumatic complaints that may be secondary to other systemic disorders, which in turn may lead to earlier diagnosis. Lastly, interdisciplinary care, such as in Centers of Excellence, allows for rapid referral among subspecialists when the diagnosis is in question.

References

Cagliero E, Apruzzese W, Perlmutter GS, Nathan DM: Musculoskeletal disorders of the hand and shoulder in patients with diabetes mellitus. Am J Med 112:487-490, 2002.

Gertz MA, Comenzo R, Falk RH, et al: Definition of organ involvement and treatment response in immunoglobulin light chain amyloidosis (AL): A consensus opinion from the 10th International Symposium on Amyloid and Amyloidosis, Tours, France, 18-22 April 2004. Am J Hematol 79:319-328, 2005

Simms RW: Less common arthropathies—hematologic and malignant disorders. In Klippel JH (ed): Primer on the Rheumatic Diseases, 12th ed. Atlanta, Arthritis Foundation, 2001, pp 431-434.

Section XVII

Infectious Disease

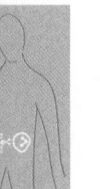

Organisms That Infect Humans

Benigno Rodríguez and Michael M. Lederman

Of diseases affecting humans, most that are curable and preventable are caused by infectious agents. The infectious diseases that capture the attention of physicians and the public periodically shift—for example, from syphilis to tuberculosis to acquired immunodeficiency syndrome (AIDS)—but the challenges of dealing with these processes endure. To the student, an understanding of infectious diseases offers insights into medicine as a whole. Osler's adage (with updating) remains relevant: "He [or she] who knows syphilis [AIDS], knows medicine."

Viruses

Viruses produce a wide variety of clinical illnesses. A virus consists of either DNA or RNA (in rare cases, both) wrapped within a protein nucleocapsid. The nucleocapsid may be covered by an envelope composed of glycoproteins and lipids; pathogenic viruses that lack an envelope tend to survive better in the environment and are more often transmitted by the fecal-oral route, whereas those that possess an envelope are more often transmitted by the parenteral route or through the genital or respiratory mucosae. Viral genes can code for only a limited number of proteins, and viruses possess no metabolic machinery. They are entirely dependent on host cells for protein synthesis and replication and are therefore obligate intracellular parasites. Some viruses are dependent on other viruses to replicate or produce active infection. Such is the case with the delta agent, which produces disease only in the presence of hepatitis B infection. All must attach to receptors on the host cell and achieve entry into the cell through mechanisms that include receptor-mediated endocytosis, fusion, pinocytosis, or, in the case of certain nonenveloped viruses, direct penetration of the cell membrane. Once within the cells, the virus uncoats, allowing its nucleic acid to use host cellular machinery to reproduce (productive infection) or to integrate into the host cell (latent infection). Some viruses, such as influenza virus, cause disease by lysis of infected cells. Others, such as hepatitis B virus, do not directly cause cell destruction but may involve the host immune responses in the pathogenesis of disease. Still others, such as the human T-lymphotropic virus type 1, promote neoplastic transformation of infected cells.

Viruses have developed several mechanisms for evading host defense mechanisms. By multiplying within host cells, viruses can avoid neutralizing antibodies and other extracellular host defenses. Some viruses can spread to uninfected cells by intercellular bridges. Others, especially the herpes group and human immunodeficiency virus (HIV), are capable of persisting latently without multiplication in a metabolically inactive form within host cells for prolonged periods. The influenza virus is capable of extensive gene rearrangements, resulting in significant changes in surface antigen structure. This allows new strains to evade host antibody responses directed at earlier strains.

Some viruses, as they exit the host cell during productive infection, may carry antigens of host cell origin, thus providing another potential mechanism for evading host defenses, whereas others block host immune defense mechanisms (such as expression of human leukocyte antigens). HIV induces both specific and nonspecific escape mechanisms by selectively deleting HIV-reactive T-cell clones and coating itself with a host-derived "glycan shield" that hinders neutralizing antibody attachment, while also causing profound global immune dysfunction that paralyzes host defenses.

Prions

Prions are a group of host-encoded transmissible proteins devoid of nucleic acid material that cause disease through accumulation of a pathogenic isoform of the prion protein. They are thought to be responsible for a number of progressive and ultimately fatal neurologic diseases in humans, including kuru, Creutzfeldt-Jakob disease (CJD), Gerstmann-Sträussler-Scheinker syndrome and familial fatal insomnia, and animal diseases such as scrapie and bovine spongiform encephalopathy ("mad cow disease"). Although some prion diseases (e.g., familial CJD) are inherited, others, including kuru and new variant CJD, are acquired through consumption of infected neural tissue. There is no known treatment for these disorders.

Bacteria

Bacteria comprise a tremendously varied group of organisms that are generally capable of cell-free growth, although some produce disease as intracellular parasites. There are numerous ways of classifying bacteria, including morphology, ability to retain certain dyes, growth in different physical conditions, ability to metabolize various substrates, and antibiotic sensitivities. Although combinations of these methods are used to identify bacteria in clinical bacteriology laboratories, relatedness for taxonomic purposes is established by DNA homology.

CHLAMYDIAE

Chlamydiae are obligate intracellular parasites; they always contain both DNA and RNA, divide by binary fission (rather than multiplying by assembly), can synthesize proteins, and contain ribosomes. Although classified as a unique family of bacteria, they are unable to synthesize adenosine triphosphate and thus depend on energy from the host cell to survive. The three chlamydial species known to cause disease in humans are *Chlamydia trachomatis, Chlamydophila pneumoniae,* and *Chlamydia psittaci. C. trachomatis* causes trachoma, the major cause of blindness in the developing world, and a variety of sexually transmitted genitourinary disorders, including urethritis, salpingitis, and lymphogranuloma venereum. *C. pneumoniae* is a common cause of atypical pneumonia, bronchitis, and sinusitis. *C. psittaci,* the cause of a common infectious disease of birds, can produce a serious systemic illness with prominent pulmonary manifestations in humans. Chlamydiae are susceptible to tetracyclines, rifampin, macrolides and related compounds, ketolides, and certain quinolones.

RICKETTSIAE AND EHRLICHIAE

Rickettsiae and ehrlichiae are also small bacterial organisms that, like chlamydiae, are obligate intracellular parasites. They are primarily animal pathogens that generally produce disease in humans through the bite of an insect vector, such as a tick, flea, louse, or mite. Most of these organisms specifically infect vascular endothelial cells. With the exception of Q fever and human ehrlichiosis, rash caused by vasculitis is a prominent manifestation of these often disabling febrile illnesses. These organisms are susceptible to tetracyclines and chloramphenicol.

MYCOPLASMAS

Mycoplasmas are the smallest free-living organisms. In contrast to viruses, chlamydiae, rickettsiae, and ehrlichiae, mycoplasmas can grow on cell-free media and produce disease without intracellular penetration. Like other bacteria, these organisms have a membrane, but unlike other bacteria, they have no cell walls. Thus antibiotics that are active against bacterial cell walls have no effect on mycoplas-

mas. At least 14 species of mycoplasma may cause disease in humans. *Mycoplasma pneumoniae* is an agent of pharyngitis and pneumonia. Although *Mycoplasma hominis, Ureaplasma urealyticum,* and the newly described *Mycoplasma genitalium* are primarily agents of genitourinary disease, they may also cause systemic infections, particularly in compromised hosts. Mycoplasmas are sensitive to erythromycin, tetracycline, a combined regimen of both, and most quinolones.

SPIROCHETES

Spirochetes are slender, motile, spiral organisms that are not readily seen under the microscope unless stained with silver or viewed under darkfield illumination. Many of these organisms cannot yet be cultured on artificial media or in cell culture. Four genera of spirochetes cause disease in humans. *Treponema* species include the pathogens of syphilis and the nonvenereal, endemic, syphilis-like illnesses of yaws, pinta, and bejel. The illnesses caused by these organisms are chronic and characterized by prolonged latency in the host. Penicillin is active against *Treponema. Leptospira* species are the causative agents of leptospirosis, an acute or subacute febrile illness occasionally resulting in aseptic meningitis, jaundice, and (in rare cases) renal insufficiency. *Borrelia* species are arthropod-borne spirochetes that are the causative agents of Lyme disease (see Chapter 95) and relapsing fever. During afebrile periods in relapsing fever, these organisms reside within host cells and emerge with modified cell surface antigens. These modifications may permit the bacterium to evade host immune responses and produce relapsing fever and recurrent bacteremia. *Spirillum minus* is one of the causative agents of rat-bite fever. *Helicobacter pylori* is a spirochete of the upper gastrointestinal tract that plays an important role in the pathogenesis of duodenal and gastric ulcers and also in certain neoplasms of the gastrointestinal tract.

ANAEROBIC BACTERIA

Anaerobes are organisms that cannot grow in atmospheric oxygen tensions. Some are killed by very low oxygen concentrations, whereas others are relatively aerotolerant. As a general rule, anaerobes that are pathogens for humans are not as sensitive to oxygen as nonpathogens. Anaerobic bacteria are primarily commensals. They inhabit the skin, gut, and mucosal surfaces of all healthy individuals. In fact, the presence of anaerobes may inhibit colonization of the gut by virulent, potentially pathogenic bacteria. Anaerobic infections generally occur in two circumstances:

- Contamination of otherwise sterile sites with anaerobe-laden contents. Examples include (1) aspiration of oral anaerobes into the bronchial tree, producing anaerobic necrotizing pneumonia; (2) peritonitis and intra-abdominal abscesses after bowel perforation; (3) fasciitis and osteomyelitis after odontogenic infections or oral surgery; and (4) some instances of pelvic inflammatory disease.
- Infections of tissue with lowered redox potential as the result of a compromised vascular supply. Examples include (1) foot infections in diabetic patients, in whom vascular disease may produce poor tissue oxygenation; and (2)

infections of pressure sores, in which fecal anaerobic flora gain access to tissue whose vascular supply is compromised by pressure.

The pathogenesis of anaerobic infections—that is, soilage by a complex flora—generally results in polymicrobial infections. Thus the demonstration of one anaerobe in an infected site generally implies the presence of others. Often, facultative organisms (organisms capable of anaerobic and aerobic growths) coexist with anaerobes. Certain anaerobes, such as *Clostridium*, produce toxins that cause well-defined systemic illnesses such as food poisoning, tetanus, and botulism. Other toxins may play a role in soft tissue infections (cellulitis, fasciitis, and myonecrosis) occasionally produced by *Clostridium* species. *Clostridium difficile* is the causative agent of pseudomembranous colitis, a diarrheal disease of varying severity (sometimes fatal) that has emerged as a major cause of morbidity in patients receiving antibiotic therapy and those in health care facilities. *Bacteroides fragilis,* the most numerous bacterial pathogen in the normal human colon, has a polysaccharide capsule that inhibits phagocytosis and promotes abscess formation. Clues to the presence of anaerobic infection include a foul odor; the presence of gas, which may be seen radiographically or manifested by crepitus on examination (although not all gas-forming infections are anaerobic); and the presence of mixed gram-positive and gram-negative flora on a Gram stain of purulent exudate, especially when there is little or no growth on plates cultured aerobically. Many pathogenic anaerobes are sensitive to penicillin. Exceptions are strains of *B. fragilis* (usually sensitive to metronidazole, clindamycin, or ampicillin-sulbactam) and *C. difficile* (which is almost always sensitive to metronidazole and vancomycin). Strains of *Fusobacterium* may also be relatively resistant to penicillin. As a general rule, infections caused by anaerobes originating from sites above the diaphragm are more often (but not always) penicillin sensitive, whereas infections below the diaphragm are often caused by penicillin-resistant organisms, notably *B. fragilis.*

GRAM-NEGATIVE BACTERIA

The cell walls of gram-negative bacteria, which appear pink on a properly prepared Gram stain, contain lipopolysaccharide, a potent inducer of cytokines such as tumor necrosis factor, and are associated with fever and septic shock. These organisms cause a wide variety of illnesses. Gram-negative bacteria are the most common cause of cystitis and pyelonephritis. *Haemophilus* species are common pathogens of the respiratory tract and cause otitis media, sinusitis, tracheobronchitis, and pneumonia. Lower respiratory tract infections with these organisms are particularly common in adults with chronic obstructive pulmonary disease. *Haemophilus* can be an important cause of meningitis, particularly in children. Except for *Haemophilus* and *Klebsiella* species, gram-negative bacteria are uncommon causes of community-acquired pneumonia but are common causes of nosocomial pneumonia.

Except for the peculiar risk of *Pseudomonas* infection in intravenous drug users, gram-negative organisms are rare causes of endocarditis on natural heart valves but are occasional pathogens on prosthetic valves. The Enterobacteria-ceae include *Escherichia coli, Klebsiella, Enterobacter, Serratia, Salmonella, Shigella,* and *Proteus.* These are large gram-negative rods. Except for the occasional presence of a clear space surrounding some *Klebsiella* representing a large capsule, these organisms are not readily distinguished from one another on Gram stain. The Enterobacteriaceae can be thought of as gut-related or genitourinary pathogens. *Salmonella,* a relatively common cause of enteritis, may occasionally infect atherosclerotic plaques or aneurysms. *Shigella* is an agent of bacterial dysentery. *Proteus* species, which split urea, are the agents associated with staghorn calculi of the urinary collecting system. Increasingly, gram-negative bacteria that are often resistant to multiple antibiotics are important causes of nosocomial infection. The genus *Bartonella* contains a group of emerging pathogens that cause uncommon, unique infections including bacillary angiomatosis, cat-scratch disease, and South American bartonellosis.

Gram-negative cocci that cause disease in humans include *Neisseria* and *Moraxella* species. These kidney bean–shaped diplococci are not distinguishable from one another on Gram stain. *Neisseria meningitidis* is an important cause of meningitis, and *Neisseria gonorrhoeae* causes gonorrhea. *Moraxella catarrhalis,* which is part of the normal oral flora, is a cause of lower respiratory tract infection.

GRAM-POSITIVE BACTERIA

Although these organisms (which appear deep purple on Gram stain) lack endotoxin, infections with gram-positive bacteria also produce fever and cannot be reliably distinguished on clinical grounds from infections caused by gram-negative bacteria.

Gram-Positive Rods

Infections caused by gram-positive rods are relatively uncommon outside certain specific settings. Diphtheria is rare (although epidemics have occurred in recent years), but other corynebacteria produce infections in the immunocompromised host and on prosthetic valves and shunts. Because corynebacteria are regular skin colonizers, they often contaminate blood cultures; in the appropriate setting, however, they must be considered potential pathogens. *Listeria monocytogenes* resembles *Corynebacterium* on initial isolation, and this food-borne pathogen is an increasingly important cause of meningitis and bacteremia in the immunocompromised patient. *Bacillus cereus* is a recognized cause of food poisoning. Serious infections with this and other *Bacillus* species occur among intravenous drug users. Infections with *Clostridium* species were discussed earlier.

Gram-Positive Cocci

Staphylococcus aureus is a common pathogen that can infect any organ system. It is a common cause of bacteremia and sepsis. The organism often colonizes the anterior nares, particularly among insulin-treated diabetics, hemodialysis patients, and injection drug users; these populations therefore have a greater frequency of infections with this organism. Hospital workers colonized with *S. aureus* have been responsible for hospital epidemics of staphylococcal disease.

Generally protected by an antiphagocytic polysaccharide capsule, staphylococci also possess catalase, which inactivates hydrogen peroxide—a mediator of bacterial killing by neutrophils. Staphylococci tend to form abscesses; the low pH within an abscess cavity also limits the effectiveness of host defense cells. Staphylococci elaborate several toxins that mediate specific manifestations of disease. A staphylococcal enterotoxin is responsible for staphylococcal food poisoning. Staphylococcal toxins also mediate the scalded skin syndrome and the multisystem manifestations of toxic shock syndrome. Most staphylococci are penicillinase producing, and an increasing proportion are resistant to penicillinase-resistant penicillin analogues. Although commonly referred to as *methicillin-resistant S. aureus* (MRSA), they are resistant to all β-lactams. Once found almost exclusively in hospitalized patients, MRSA strains that express novel pathogenic determinants, such as the Panton-Valentine leukocidin (PVL), and exhibit a distinctive antimicrobial resistance pattern have now become established in the community and are the cause of thousands of severe community-acquired infections each year. At the same time, the role of MRSA as a nosocomial pathogen continues, and MRSA has been responsible for widespread epidemics in health care institutions worldwide. Vancomycin remains active against most strains, but strains with reduced susceptibility and even complete resistance to this and other glycopeptides have recently been isolated from clinical cases. Resistance in these strains is the result of acquisition of mobile genetic elements from *Enterococcus* species, likely in the hospital setting. These strains are still uncommon but can cause severe disease, including bloodstream infections. Strains with decreased susceptibility to the oxazolidinone linezolid have now also been described.

Other staphylococci are distinguished from *S. aureus* primarily by their inability to produce coagulase. Some of these coagulase-negative staphylococci produce urinary tract infection (*Staphylococcus saprophyticus*). Another, *Staphylococcus epidermidis,* is part of the normal skin flora and an increasingly important cause of infection on foreign bodies such as prosthetic heart valves, ventriculoatrial shunts, and intravascular catheters. Like *Corynebacterium, S. epidermidis* may be a contaminant of blood cultures but in the appropriate setting should be considered a potential pathogen. *S. saprophyticus* is sensitive to a variety of antibiotics used in the treatment of urinary tract infection; *S. epidermidis* is usually resistant to all β-lactams but sensitive to vancomycin.

Streptococci are classified into groups according to the presence of serologically defined carbohydrate capsules (Lancefield typing). Group A streptococci produce skin infections, pharyngitis, and systemic infections. These organisms are also associated with the immunologically mediated poststreptococcal disorders—glomerulonephritis and acute rheumatic fever. Streptococci are further classified according to the pattern of hemolysis on blood agar—α for incomplete hemolysis (producing a green discoloration on the agar), β for complete hemolysis, and γ for nonhemolytic strains. An important α-hemolytic species is *Streptococcus pneumoniae* (pneumococcus), the most common cause of community-acquired pneumonia and an important cause of meningitis and otitis media. Penicillin resistance in pneumococcal isolates is an increasingly important problem and is often associated with concomitant resistance to other agents. Whereas pneumococcal pneumonia caused by

strains with intermediate penicillin resistance can still be successfully treated with very high doses of penicillin, other antimicrobial agents must now be used for pneumococcal meningitis (see Chapter 97). Penicillin-resistant *S. pneumoniae* generally remains susceptible to vancomycin. A heterogeneous group of streptococci, often improperly referred to as *viridans* (green) streptococci (these organisms may show α- or γ-hemolysis), includes several species of streptococcus that are common oral or gut flora and are important agents of bacterial endocarditis, abscesses, and odontogenic infections.

Formerly classified as members of the *Streptococcus* genus, enterococci are facultative anaerobes that, unlike the streptococci, exhibit variable degrees of resistance to penicillins and are uniformly resistant to cephalosporins. Vancomycin-resistant strains of enterococci are increasingly prevalent causes of serious hospital-acquired infections, particularly in immunocompromised and postsurgical patients, that are exceedingly difficult to treat.

MYCOBACTERIA

Mycobacteria comprise a group of rod-shaped bacilli that stain weakly gram positive. These organisms are rich in lipid content and are recognized in tissue specimens by their ability to retain dye after washing with acid alcohol (acid fast). These bacteria are generally slow-growing (some require up to 6 weeks to demonstrate growth on solid media), obligate aerobes. They generally produce chronic disease and survive for years as intracellular parasites of mononuclear phagocytes. Some escape intracellular killing mechanisms by blocking phagosome and lysosome fusion or by disrupting the phagosome. Almost all provoke cell-mediated immune responses in the host, and clinical disease expression may be related in large part to the nature of the host immune response. Tuberculosis is caused by *Mycobacterium tuberculosis*. Other mycobacteria (nontuberculous mycobacteria) can cause diseases resembling tuberculosis. Certain rapid-growing mycobacteria cause infections after surgery or implantations of prostheses, as well as epidemic and sporadic skin and soft tissue infections. *Mycobacterium avium* complex (MAC) is an important cause of disseminated infection among patients with AIDS. MAC is frequently resistant to drugs usually used in the treatment of tuberculosis. Leprosy is a mycobacterial disease of skin and peripheral nerves caused by the noncultivatable *Mycobacterium leprae*.

ACTINOMYCETALES

Nocardia and *Actinomyces* are weakly gram-positive filamentous bacteria. *Nocardia* is acid fast and aerobic; *Actinomyces* is anaerobic and not acid fast. *Actinomyces* inhabits the mouth, gut, and vagina and produces cervicofacial osteomyelitis and abscess, pneumonia with empyema, and intra-abdominal and pelvic abscess, the last often associated with intrauterine contraceptive devices. *Nocardia* most commonly produces pneumonia and brain abscess. Approximately half of patients with *Nocardia* infection have underlying impairments in cell-mediated immunity. Infections with either of these slow-growing organisms require long-term treatment. *Actinomyces* is relatively sensitive to many antibiotics; penicillin is the treatment of choice. *Nocardia* infections are treated with high doses of sulfonamides, but serious or resistant infections may require combinations of carbapenems, aminoglycosides, and cephalosporins.

Fungi

Fungi are larger than bacteria. Unlike bacteria, they have rigid cell walls that contain chitin as well as polysaccharides. They grow and proliferate by budding, by elongation of hyphal forms, and/or by spore formation. Except for *Candida* and related species, fungi are rarely visible on Gram-stained preparations but can be stained with Gomori methenamine silver stain. They are also resistant to potassium hydroxide and can often be seen on wet mounts of scrapings or secretions to which several drops of a 10% solution of potassium hydroxide have been added. Fungi are resistant to most antibiotics used in the treatment of bacterial infections and are typically treated with drugs active against their unusual cell wall. Most fungi can exist in a yeast form (round to ovoid cells that may reproduce by budding) and a mold form, a complex of tubular structures (hyphae) that grow by branching or extension.

Candida species are oval yeasts that often colonize the mouth, gastrointestinal tract, and vagina of healthy individuals. They may produce disease by overgrowth and/or invasion. *Candida* stomatitis (thrush) often occurs in individuals who are receiving antibiotic or corticosteroid therapy or who have impairments of cell-mediated immunity. Vulvovaginitis caused by *Candida* may occur in these same settings but can also occur in women with no apparent predisposing factors and more commonly in women with diabetes mellitus. *Candida* can also colonize and infect the urinary tract, particularly in the presence of an indwelling urinary catheter. *Candida* species may also gain entry into the bloodstream and produce fungemia with or without seeding of solid tissues, especially in hospitalized patients, in whom *Candida* species are now the fourth leading cause of intravascular infection. This most frequently occurs in the setting of neutropenia after chemotherapy, where the portal of entry is the gastrointestinal tract, or in individuals with intravascular catheters, which provide a route for cutaneous *Candida* to enter the systemic circulation (see Chapter 106). Largely as a consequence of widespread use of empiric and targeted antibiotic therapy, as well as more frequent immunosuppressive conditions, *Candida* species other than *Candida albicans* have become increasingly common causes of invasive disease in hospitals. These non–*C. albicans* species (e.g., *Candida glabrata*, *Candida krusei*, *Candida tropicalis*) are more often resistant to commonly used antifungals such as fluconazole and have therefore skewed the landscape of empiric antifungal therapy, especially in immunosuppressed patients, toward broader-spectrum agents such as amphotericin B and the echinocandins.

Histoplasma capsulatum is a dimorphic fungus endemic to the Ohio and Mississippi River valleys that produces asymptomatic infection or a mild febrile syndrome in most individuals and a self-limited pneumonia in some. In predisposed individuals, it can cause cavitary pulmonary disease and mediastinal fibrosis. Infants and immunosuppressed individuals, such as those with AIDS or neutropenia, are susceptible to the progressive disseminated form of the infection, which is potentially fatal (see Chapter 108). Systemic or progressive disease is treated with parenteral amphotericin B or itraconazole.

The dimorphic fungus *Coccidioides immitis* is endemic in the southwestern United States and, like *H. capsulatum*, produces a self-limited respiratory infection or pneumonia in most infected individuals. Immunocompromised individuals are at greatest risk for fatal systemic dissemination or meningitis. Fluconazole, itraconazole, or amphotericin B is used for progressive or extrapulmonary disease.

Cryptococcus neoformans is a yeast with a large polysaccharide capsule. It produces a self-limited or chronic pneumonia, but the most common clinical manifestation of infection with this fungus is a chronic meningitis. Although patients with impairment in cell-mediated immunity are at risk for cryptococcal meningitis, some patients with this syndrome have no identifiable immunodeficiency. Treatment is with amphotericin B combined with flucytosine. Long-term oral fluconazole therapy is effective in preventing relapse in persons with AIDS (see Chapter 108).

Blastomyces dermatitidis is a dimorphic organism also endemic in the Ohio and Mississippi River basins. Acute self-limited pulmonary infection is followed in rare instances by disseminated disease. Skin disease is most common, but bones, the central nervous system, and the genitourinary tract may be involved as well. Amphotericin B is used for treating systemic disease; itraconazole is appropriate for immunocompetent hosts.

Aspergillus is a mold that produces several clinical illnesses in humans. Acute bronchopulmonary aspergillosis is an immunoglobulin E–mediated hypersensitivity to *Aspergillus* colonization of the respiratory tract. This condition produces wheezing and fleeting pulmonary infiltrates in patients with asthma. Occasionally, *Aspergillus* will colonize a preexistent pulmonary cavity and produce a mycetoma or fungus ball. Hemoptysis is the most serious complication of such infection. Invasive pulmonary aspergillosis is a rare cause of chronic illness in marginally compromised hosts; more often, it is a cause of acute, life-threatening pneumonia or disseminated infection in patients with neutropenia or in recipients of organ transplants. Voriconazole is now the drug of choice for most cases of invasive aspergillosis; amphotericin B and the echinocandins remain important alternatives or concomitant agents.

The zygomycetes (Mucorales) are molds with ribbon-shaped hyphae that produce disease in patients with poorly controlled diabetes mellitus or hematologic malignancy or in recipients of organ transplantation. Invasive disease of the palate and nasal sinuses, which may extend intracranially, is the most common presentation, but pneumonia may be seen as well. These infections are generally treated with surgical excision plus high-dose amphotericin B.

Pneumocystis jiroveci (formerly Pneumocystis carinii) was once thought to be a protozoan; genetic analyses have classified *P. jiroveci* as a fungus. This organism causes life-threatening pneumonia in patients with impaired cell-mediated immunity; it is the most common major opportunistic pathogen in persons with AIDS (see Chapter 108).

Table 91-1 **Some Protozoal Diseases of Humans**

Protozoan	Clinical Illness	Transmission	Diagnosis
Plasmodium	Malaria: fever, hemolysis	Mosquito, transfusion	Peripheral blood smear
Babesia microti	Fever, hemolysis	Tick, transfusion	Peripheral blood smear
Trichomonas vaginalis	Vaginitis	Sexual contact	Vaginal smear
Toxoplasma gondii*	Fever, lymph node enlargement; encephalitis, brain abscess in compromised host	Raw meat, cat feces	Serologies, tissue biopsy
Entamoeba histolytica	Colitis, hepatic abscess	Fecal-oral	Stool smear, serologies
Giardia lamblia	Diarrhea, malabsorption	Fecal-oral	Stool smear, small bowel aspirate
Cryptosporidium*	Diarrhea	Fecal-oral	Sugar flotation, acid-fast stain of stool, biopsy
Isospora belli*	Diarrhea, malabsorption	Fecal-oral	Wet mount or acid-fast stain of stool
Microsporidium*	Diarrhea, malabsorption, dissemination	Fecal-oral	Small bowel biopsy Electron microscopy

*Important opportunistic pathogens in persons with acquired immunodeficiency syndrome (see Chapter 108).

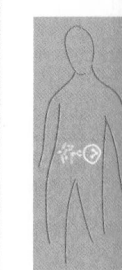

Protozoans

The protozoal pathogens listed in Table 91-1 are all important causes of disease within the United States. Infections caused by these organisms are diagnosed as indicated in Table 91-1 and are discussed in the relevant disease-oriented chapters.

Helminths

Diseases caused by helminths are among the most prevalent diseases in the developing world but are uncommon causes of illness in North America. In contrast to the pathogens discussed previously, helminths are multicellular parasites. Helminthic pathogens found in the United States include the roundworm *Ascaris* species (maldigestion and obstruction), the hookworm *Necator americanus* (intestinal blood loss), the pinworm *Enterobius vermicularis* (anal pruritus), and the threadworm *Strongyloides stercoralis* (gastroenteritis and dissemination in the immunocompromised host). It is important to recognize the risk of other helminthic diseases in travelers returning from endemic regions (see Chapter 110).

Prospectus for the Future

Clinicians should anticipate the identification of "novel" pathogens causing disease, as follows:
- Prevalent microbes not previously recognized as pathogenic
- "Discovery" of prevalent pathogens not previously identified

- Influx into new communities of pathogens prevalent elsewhere
- Increased frequency and distorted clinical presentation of uncommon pathogens as a consequence of immunosuppressive conditions and treatments
- Emergence of resistant strains of common pathogens

References

Bruckner DA, Colonna P: Nomenclature for aerobic and facultative bacteria. Clin Infect Dis 29:713-723, 1999.

Dermody TS, Tyler KL: Introduction to viruses and viral diseases. In Mandell GL, Bennett JE, Dolin R (eds): Principles and Practice of Infectious Diseases, 6th ed. Philadelphia, Elsevier, 2005, pp 1729-1742.

Summanen P: Microbiology terminology update: Clinically significant anaerobic gram-positive and gram-negative bacteria (excluding spirochetes). Clin Infect Dis 29:724-727, 1999.

Chapter **92**

Host Defenses Against Infection

Benigno Rodríguez and Michael M. Lederman

Host Defenses versus Mechanisms of Microbial Pathogenesis: The Struggle for Survival

As our experience suggests and as fossil records indicate, life is a continuous struggle for survival. Pathogenic and host defense evasive mechanisms of microbes are countered by multiple and overlapping host innate and adaptive immune defense mechanisms. In some cases, the pathogen "wins," with destruction of the host; in others, the host immune response prevails, with eradication of the microbe. Often there is a standoff characterized by latent infection or colonization without substantial morbidity to the host; sometimes the relationship is actually symbiotic, with both host and pathogen gaining from it. In settings of latent or colonizing pathogens, microbes have the capacity to activate and cause disease if host defenses become impaired. Much of our understanding of host defenses and their relationship to microbial pathogenesis has been derived from recognizing the spectrum of infections experienced by individuals with specific impairments of host defenses. Thus, persons with neutrophil depletion or defects in neutrophil function tend to experience bacterial and fungal infections, those with antibody defects are particularly at risk for infections caused by encapsulated bacteria, and persons with impairments in cell-mediated immunity tend to be at particular risk for infection with pathogens that replicate within host cells. Reflecting the importance of these insights, in the early days of the acquired immunodeficiency syndrome (AIDS) epidemic, astute clinicians recognized immediately that the kinds of infections seen in the first AIDS patients implicated an acquired impairment of cell-mediated adaptive immune defenses; this insight accelerated research on the pathogenesis and etiology of AIDS.

Evolutionary Advantage of Adaptable Organisms

Fundamental to our understanding of evolution is the concept that organisms most capable of adaptation to environmental stresses are most likely to survive, to propagate, and to persist. Thus, random mutations in the germline that confer survival advantage are passed on to adapting, succeeding generations. With this in mind, it is astounding that complex organisms such as humans can compete for survival with microbes much more capable of rapid genetic adaptation to challenge. The number of germline mutations over time is dependent on generation time, the number of offspring per generation, and the mistake rate of the DNA or RNA polymerase required for genomic replication. In each of these indices, microbes have the clear adaptive advantage. As an example, humans must survive at least 10 years or more before they are even capable of reproduction, and then they generate only a small number of offspring before dying. In contrast, bacteria can grow exponentially, with generation times measured in minutes to hours, and viruses express thousands of progeny with replication cycles that can be completed within hours to days. Human DNA polymerases have an error rate of approximately one base pair per 10^{12} per cellular division; bacterial DNA polymerases have an error rate of approximately one base pair per 10^6, and the reverse transcriptase of human immunodeficiency virus type 1 (HIV-1) has an error rate of approximately one base pair per 10^3 to 10^4 per replication. These mutations are to a large extent random, and most result in decreased function or are incompatible with survival. Because of the limited number of offspring humans produce, a faithful DNA polymerase that maximizes survival of an individual's descendants is important to our species. In contrast, microbes can generate many defective organisms with null mutations and still maintain a self-sustaining population of organisms arising from the small subset that harbor the rare mutations that confer a survival advantage. The rapid emergence of resistance to antimicrobials is reflective of the genetic flexibility of microbes. The ability to recognize and respond nonspecifically to foreign organisms has existed for millions of years and can be demonstrated even in relatively primitive life forms. But to survive in the struggle for the environment against microbes and their seemingly unending ability to replicate and evolve over short intervals of time, more complex species (including humans) with slow and infrequent germline evolution events require a system that can efficiently adjust to protect the individual against the constantly changing onslaught of microbial pathogens. Thus, with the appearance of the gnathostomes, or jawed vertebrates, an adaptable immune defense system emerged that for the first time permitted a rapid "evolution" of host defense to infectious agents without the need for reproduction or germline mutation. This "real-time evolution" is achieved through rearrangement (and, in the case of B lymphocytes, somatic mutation) of the genes encoding the receptors of T and B lymphocytes and the ability to expand clones of these microbe-specific cells—the directors of adaptive immune recognition.

Categories of Host Defenses and Risks for Infection

Over the course of species development, numerous mechanisms have evolved to protect larger organisms from infection or parasitization by another. These mechanisms can be categorized according to the primary defense mechanism as anatomic, humoral, or cellular, and according to their specificity and phylogenetics as innate or adaptive. Anatomic defenses are primarily innate or nonadaptive, whereas humoral and cellular defenses can be either innate or adaptive. Innate defenses, present in many primitive organisms, comprise a rapid, "already primed" response to microbial invasion, whereas adaptive responses may be more delayed in their onset but ultimately are both more specific in their targets and capable of providing "memory" of prior encounters to protect against recurrence of infection. Although it is important to distinguish between these two kinds of host defenses, both innate and adaptive immune mechanisms are intimately interactive, thereby providing, in most instances, remarkable synergistic protection against infection.

ANATOMIC DEFENSES

Anatomic defenses protect directly against microbial colonization and infection and are primarily located at sites with proximate environmental contact. Thus skin and mucosal surfaces are enriched with defenses ranging from the tightness of epithelial junctions to resist microbial penetration, to the presence of cough and gag reflexes to expel aspirated secretions, and to the presence of chemical agents such as acids and defensins with antimicrobial properties. Permissiveness to colonization of these surfaces by microbes of low pathogenicity prevents colonization and infection by more

virulent organisms. In some clinical settings, interference with anatomic defense mechanisms may increase the risk of infection. Therefore burns that denude the epithelial barrier, illnesses or intoxicants that suppress gag and cough reflexes, treatment with agents that decrease gastric pH, and treatment with antibiotics that disturb the commensal mucosal flora can increase the risks of microbial infection.

HUMORAL DEFENSES AGAINST INFECTION

Complement System

Humoral defenses, consisting of soluble compounds found in blood plasma and in other extracellular fluids, also play important roles in defense against microbes. One of the most important of these humoral defenses is the complement system. Complement activity results from the sequential interaction of a large number of plasma and cell membrane proteins. A simplified diagram of the most important steps in the complement cascade is shown in Figure 92-1. The *classic complement pathway* is activated by antibody-coated targets or antigen-antibody complexes through the interaction of the initial protein, C1, with the Fc receptor of the antigen-activated immunoglobulin (Ig) molecule The *alternative pathway* is activated in the absence of antibody by constituents of the microbial surface, including polysaccharides. Finally, the sugar-binding protein *mannose-binding lectin* can also activate the complement cascade after binding to surface mannose residues on viruses and other pathogens. All three pathways converge with the formation of C3 convertase, which leads to the production of the effector components of the complement system. C3b or iC3b deposited on the surface of microbes binds to complement receptors (CR1, CR3, and CR4) on neutrophils and macrophages and

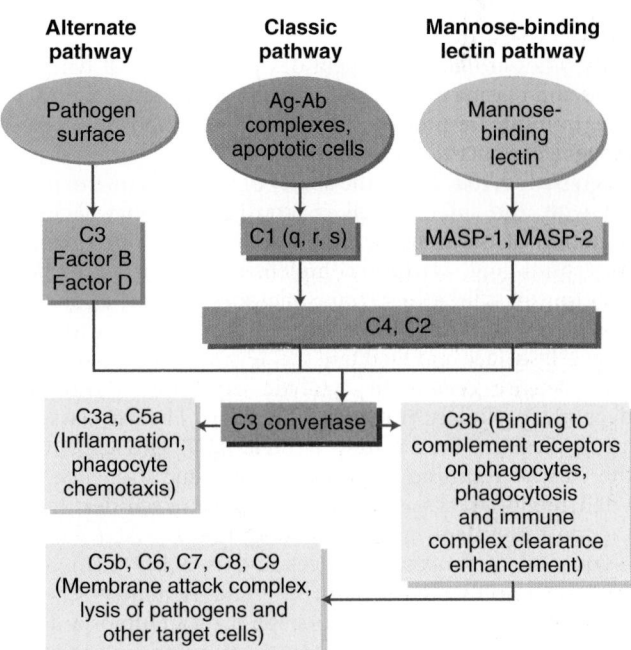

Figure 92-1 Simplified diagram of the complement system. The final effector components are shown in clear symbols at the bottom of the graphic, with a summary of their most important biologic activities. Not all molecular events leading to the final effector components are shown.

Table 92-1 **Properties of Human Immunoglobulins**

	IgG	IgA	IgM	IgD	IgE
H chain class	γ	α	μ	δ	ε
Molecular weight (approximate)	150,000	170,000	900,000	180,000	190,000
Complement fixation (classic)	++	0	++++	0	0
Opsonic activity (for binding)	++++	++	0	0	0
Reaginic activity	0	0	0	0	++++
Serum concentration (approximate mg/dL)	1500	150-350	100-150	2	2
Serum half-life (days)	23	6	5	3	2.5
Major functions	Recall response; opsonization; transplacental immunity	Secretory immunity	Primary response; complement fixation	?	Allergy; anthelmintic immunity

promotes phagocytosis. Moreover, C3b furthers clearance of immune complexes by linking them to CR1 on the erythrocyte surface. C5a is a chemotaxin for neutrophils and activates oxidative burst activity. C5a and C3a also stimulate histamine release from mast cells and thus promote inflammation. The ultimate effector element of the complement system is the membrane attack complex, which involves C5 to C9. This complex produces pores in the membrane of microbes and subjects them to osmotic lysis. Thus, the complement system can opsonize microbes, can directly damage them, and can also induce inflammation through liberation of chemotactically active fragments. Persons with complement deficiencies, particularly deficiencies in terminal components, are especially at risk for repeated infections with gram-negative encapsulated bacteria, especially *Neisseria* species.

Antibodies

Antibodies are large polypeptides produced by B lymphocytes and plasma cells that are key components of the adaptive immune response (Table 92-1). Antibody molecules recognize structural elements of microbial surfaces and, when bound, may block the ability of that structure to interact with and infect a cell (neutralization), may facilitate ingestion of the microbe by phagocytes (opsonization), or may bind and activate complement (discussed earlier), resulting in killing of certain microbes. Finally, antibodies may recognize microbial or other foreign antigens expressed on a cell surface and facilitate the destruction of that cell by host defense cells with cytolytic capabilities (antibody-dependent cellular cytotoxicity [ADCC]). The five classes of antibodies are summarized in Table 92-1. IgM constitutes the earliest immune response to antigenic challenge and often predominates in response to polysaccharides; IgG is the most prevalent Ig class in blood; IgA is present both in blood and at mucosal surfaces and is a key element in mucosal immune protection; IgD and IgM may serve as B-lymphocyte antigen receptors; IgE plays an important role in allergy by triggering mast cell activation and is also important in mediating responses to parasitic infestation. As components of the adaptive immune response, antibodies have great diversity in their recognition domains, and the generation of this diversity permits both targeted investment of

immune "energy" and the generation of immune memory. Antibodies provide protection against microbes primarily when these organisms are in the extracellular space. Once within cells that they infect, microbes are largely (but not always; see ADCC, earlier) invisible to antibody-mediated defenses. Persons with defects in antibody formation are at greatest risk for infection with encapsulated bacteria such as pneumococci.

CELLULAR DEFENSES AGAINST INFECTION

Phagocytic Cells

Phagocytic cells—neutrophils and macrophages—are rapidly recruited to sites of microbial invasion by chemoattractant cytokines called *chemokines,* among other mechanisms. These cells are able to ingest (phagocytose) microbes directly and, even more efficiently, when the microbes are opsonized (coated with antibody or complement), through attachment to specific receptors on the phagocyte cell surface. Once ingested, microbes are killed by a system of enzymes and other antimicrobial systems. These cells are efficient mediators of defense against many bacteria and fungi; decreases in the numbers or function of neutrophils place persons at risk for bacterial and fungal infection. Macrophages also serve as "professional antigen-presenting cells" (see later) and can activate cell-mediated immune defenses by presenting digested microbial peptides to T cells.

T Lymphocytes

T lymphocytes are critical effector and helper cells of the adaptive cell-mediated immune response that are generated through a complex process of selection in the thymus gland. In the thymus, the genes encoding the T-cell antigen receptor are rearranged, generating an enormous diversity of T-cell receptor (TCR) structures. T cells recognize peptide antigen bound by host cell surface human leukocyte antigens (HLAs). T cells with insufficient affinity or too great an affinity for host HLAs fail to survive thymic development. Thus the population of T cells with intermediate affinity for host HLA molecules that survive thymic maturation maintains a diverse yet selected repertoire of TCRs capable of recognizing a wide array of peptides when bound by cell surface HLA molecules. The TCR of CD4$^+$ T cells recognizes ingested peptides bound by class II HLA molecules, whereas class I HLA molecules bind peptides typically synthesized within the cell by invading pathogens for recognition by the TCRs of CD8$^+$ T cells. Not surprisingly, therefore, after TCR engagement, CD8$^+$ T cells destroy infected cells expressing the foreign peptides, whereas CD4$^+$ T cells are activated largely to express T-helper cytokines that enhance the function of other immune cells such as CD8$^+$ T cells, natural killer (NK) cells, macrophages, and B lymphocytes. On encountering antigen for the first time in lymph nodes, naive CD4$^+$ T cells proliferate and differentiate into effector cells with one of several functional phenotypes: T$_H$1 CD4$^+$ T cells produce predominantly interleukin (IL)-2 and interferon (IFN)-γ, tend to activate macrophages and induce B cells to produce opsonizing antibodies, and are central to an effective cellular immune response. T$_H$2 cells, on the other hand, produce mainly IL-4, IL-10, and IL-13, activate mast cells, induce IgM, IgE, and IgA production by B cells, and shift the system toward the humoral immune response. The balance between these two profiles is particularly important in infections caused by certain intracellular organisms, which require a vigorous T$_H$1 response to be eliminated, among other aspects of the immune response. A third functional phenotype is that of the T regulatory cell (Treg). T regulatory cells express high levels of the IL-2 receptor CD25 and the forkhead box transcription factor P3 (FOXP3) and typically serve to modulate immune responsiveness. A third differentiation subset of CD4$^+$ T cells, termed T$_H$17 because of its preferential expression of proinflammatory molecules of the IL-17 family (as well as IL-22), has recently been described and is important in protection against extracellular bacteria and fungi. Selective depletion of T$_H$17 cells in the intestinal mucosa may also play a role in the pathogenesis of progressive HIV-related immunodeficiency through interference with the epithelial barrier function against microorganisms in the intestinal lumen. Destruction of target cells by cytolytic CD8$^+$ T cells can be mediated by receptor-ligand interaction, whereby binding of receptors on the target cell (such as Fas) by ligand on the effector cell results in activation of programmed cell death (apoptosis) of the target. Perhaps more important, cytolytic cells are enriched for perforin, which, like the terminal components of complement, produces pores in the target cell membrane, and granzymes that gain entry to target cells through these pores and induce programmed cell death of the target. Impairments in T-cell numbers or function place persons at particular risk for infection with pathogens that replicate within host cells. Because of their central role in mediating immunologic help, decreases in CD4$^+$ T cells or their function also diminish many other aspects of host defense, such as antibody responses.

Natural Killer Cells

NK cells are large granular lymphocytes that, like CD8$^+$ T cells, have cytolytic function. These cells can kill tumor cells or normal cells infected by viruses. They are most active against target cells with low-level expression of class I HLA molecules, which, when present, activate inhibitory molecules on the NK cell surface. Because many viruses decrease host HLA class I expression as a means to evade host cytotoxic T-lymphocyte recognition, it is thought that NK cells may serve to identify and lyse cells resistant to antigen-specific T-cell–mediated cytotoxicity. As an effector of innate or nonadaptive host defense, NK cells are thought to be important also in early responses to viral infections and in defense against malignancy. NK cells also have receptors for IgG that, when binding the NK cells to target cells expressing viral antigens on the surface, can activate target cell lysis by the NK cell (ADCC). Rarely, persons with dramatic decreases in numbers of NK cells have been found to experience repeated and severe herpesvirus infections.

How Cells Communicate with Other Cells

Cellular interactions are critical for host defense against microbes. Cells need to signal other cells in order to attract them to sites of infection; cells can also arm and activate other cells to perform their function more effectively, and cellular interactions are essential to generate and amplify host adaptive immune responses. Cells establish these communications in two basic ways: by direct contact and by the expression of soluble factors—cytokines that bind to cellular receptors and result in the generation of intracellular signals that affect the function of the cell. Some cytokine receptors are very specific for a single cytokine (e.g., the high-affinity IL-2 receptor and IL-2), whereas others can be triggered by multiple cytokines (as is often the case for chemokine receptors). Chemokines are cytokines that induce cellular movement and play important roles in trafficking cells to appropriate sites. Different cell types may express the same cytokine, and one cytokine may target several cell types, resulting in different effects in each. Thus the network of cellular interactions in host defense can be quite complex.

INTERFERONS

IFNs are antiviral cytokines that can be induced as a response to viral infection; these cytokines also have potent effects on host defense cells and the priming of adaptive immune defenses. Type I IFNs (α and β) are produced by virus-infected cells, whereas type II IFN (IFN-γ) is produced by T cells and NK cells. The type I IFNs are induced by a variety of stimuli including double-stranded RNA that is not present in uninfected cells; therefore immediately after viral infection takes place, IFN is expressed by the infected cell and acts on IFN receptors to activate a number of host antiviral mechanisms, thereby rapidly attenuating viral replication. Hundreds of host genes can also be activated by type I IFNs, and thus IFNs not only activate antiviral defenses but also induce a complex array of cellular genes that prime and activate host defenses. IFN-γ also activates cytolytic activity of T cells and NK cells and activates monocytes.

How Enormous Diversity in Immune Recognition Is Possible

Because there is enormous diversity in the structure and sequence of microbial pathogens, host defenses must have

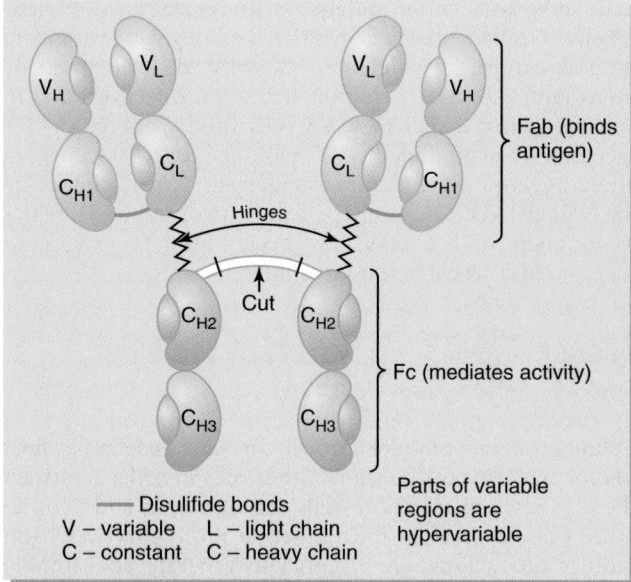

Figure 92-2 Diagram of the overall structure of immunoglobulin G, which is the basic structural pattern for all immunoglobulins (see text), drawn to highlight the various reactive areas and to emphasize the globular domain features of the immunoglobulin molecule. (From Bennett JC: Approach to the patient with immune diseases. In Bennett JC, Plum F [eds]: Cecil Textbook of Medicine, 20th ed. Philadelphia, WB Saunders, 1996, p 1394.)

the ability to generate and maintain a diverse repertoire of defenses against potential invaders. Both the humoral (B-cell driven) and cellular (T-cell driven) arms of the adaptive immune response are activated by the specific interaction of foreign antigen with cellular receptors. In the case of B cells, the receptor is a surface Ig (antibody) molecule that recognizes three-dimensional structures; in the case of the T cells, the receptor recognizes short foreign peptides from 8 to 20 amino acids in length that are bound to host HLA molecules. It is the flexibility of T-cell and B-cell receptor rearrangements that permits the adaptive immune system to respond to a large number of antigenic structures. B cells and T cells appear to use similar mechanisms to generate and express the diversity required for such a broad range of specific antigenic responses.

Five classes of antibodies (isotypes) are recognized (see Table 92-1). An *IgG antibody* (Fig. 92-2) consists of two light (κ or λ) chains and two heavy chains. Each antibody has constant regions, which are identical in structure to all antibodies of that class, and distinctive antigen recognition sites whose structures are variable. An IgG_1 molecule has two such antigen-combining sites. The antigen-combining sites of antibody molecules recognize the three-dimensional structure of an antigen and bind to it in a lock-and-key manner through multiple weak, noncovalent interactions. The variable regions consist of the approximately 110 amino-terminal amino acids of each chain. Three short, hypervariable regions are present in each of the light and heavy chains. The six hypervariable regions form the antigen-combining site.

Antibody diversity is generated as B lymphocytes mature and is understood at the molecular level. The variable portion of the heavy chain is encoded by three different genes: V, D, and J; investigators have identified 500 to 1000 different V genes, 10 D genes, and 4 J genes. The variable

portions of the light chains are encoded by V and J genes; investigators have identified 200 possible V genes and 6 J genes. During the differentiation of B cells in the bone marrow, somatic translocations randomly select the V, D, and J heavy chain genes and the V and J light chain genes that will be transcribed in that cell. The diversity achieved by this means is enormous. Somatic mutations in B cells as they divide after encountering antigen in lymphoid tissue (see later) allow the possibility of improving the fit between antibody and antigen; repeated or sustained exposure to antigen selects B cells capable of producing antibody with the highest binding affinity. These circulate as *memory cells.*

T lymphocytes can be divided into two subpopulations based on the polypeptide chains constituting the antigen receptor. The αβ *T cells*, constituting the larger population (approximately 95%), possess a receptor consisting of a heterodimer of α and β polypeptide chains. The variable portion of the αβ TCR is composed of the approximately 100 amino-terminal amino acids. The generation of diversity is by translocation of V, D, and J genes; this takes place as the cells mature within the thymus. During thymic maturation, T cells are selected for survival and exportation into the periphery according to their affinity for self-HLA molecules. Those with too great an affinity for self-peptides and HLA molecules and those with too low an affinity for self-HLA do not survive. Thus T cells that may have "autoimmune" reactivity and those with affinities too low to recognize any peptide bound to host HLA molecules are largely deleted from the circulating T-cell pool.

The TCR is directed at the foreign peptides bound by cell surface HLA molecules. αβ T cells can be divided by their surface expression of glycoproteins into CD4 and CD8 subpopulations. CD4 and CD8 cells also differ in their genetic restriction and function. Peptides bound by class I HLA are recognized by CD8+ T cells, whereas peptides bound by HLA class II molecules are recognized by CD4+ helper T cells. The TCR recognizes linear peptides of 8 to 20 amino acids in length. Importantly, in addition to their crucial role in recognizing antigens presented in this manner, T cells also provide costimulatory signals that enable the maturation and proliferation of naive B cells as they encounter antigen (discussed earlier), and thus link the humoral and cellular immune response (see discussion of the antibody response, later). Another subpopulation of T lymphocytes, γδ *T cells*, constitutes fewer than 5% of circulating and lymphoid T cells. These cells do not express CD4 or CD8; their TCRs contain heterodimers of γ and δ chains. Although there is diversity in the rearrangement of these chains, it is far less than that seen among αβ T cells. γδ T cells may not respond to peptides bound to major HLA molecules but instead tend to be activated directly by phospholipid antigens, by heat shock proteins, and by minor HLA molecules. Thus these cells comprise a defense intermediate between the intrinsic and adaptive host defenses.

Host-Microbe Interaction

THE PRIMARY ENCOUNTER AND ROLE OF INNATE DEFENSES

The skin and mucosal surfaces represent the primary interface with the external world and microbes. At these sites, anatomic barriers that also include certain intrinsic defenses and the normal microbial colonists as well as secretory antibody help to defend against the development of invasive disease. Mucosal colonization by pathogenic microbes, such as pneumococcal colonization of the oropharynx, can induce an adaptive immune response. If this response develops before tissue invasion takes place, colonization may result in acquisition of a protective antibody response. However, factors that disrupt normal host defenses, such as a depressed sensorium blocking gag and cough reflexes, cigarette smoking suppressing ciliary clearance, or intercurrent influenza virus infection denuding the tracheal epithelium, can increase the likelihood that colonization with a pathogenic microbe will result in invasive infection. Once anatomic barriers are breached and an invading microbe gains access to tissues, other intrinsic host defenses come into play rapidly. These rapid responders are phagocytic cells that express "toll-like" receptors for microbial elements such as cell wall lipopolysaccharide, other cell wall products, flagellins, or microbial nucleotide sequences. Phagocytic cells are then activated to ingest nearby microbes and to induce expression of chemotactic cytokines that facilitate entry of additional inflammatory cells to the site of microbial breach. Some microbes are armed to resist these defenses, as is the case for bacteria with capsules that resist phagocytosis. Host complement can be activated to bind to these capsules, helping to opsonize the bacterium to enhance phagocytosis and also to enhance ingress of inflammatory cells to the site. Because it generally takes several days to a few weeks for the adaptive immune system to mobilize and generate sufficient effector activity to protect the host, one key role of the innate immune system is to provide a method of limiting microbial replication and pathogenesis until the more potent and specific adaptive immune response can be mobilized. Activation of microbicidal phagocytic cells, complement and NK cell activation, and induction of antiviral IFNs all may play a role in the early innate defense against microbial invasion. It should be emphasized, however, that there are many collaborative interactions between innate and adaptive defense mechanisms to ensure optimal arming of host defenses.

GENERATION OF ADAPTIVE IMMUNE RESPONSES

Cell-Mediated (T-Cell) Responses

Skin and mucosal tissue contain large numbers of dendritic cells, such as Langerhans cells, that also express toll-like receptors. These cells ingest foreign antigens and foreign microbes and also may ingest dying inflammatory cells that have themselves ingested invading microbes. As they migrate to lymphoid tissues, these dendritic cells mature, degrading the ingested antigens and expressing these microbial peptides on cell surface HLA molecules. At the same time, these cells lose the ability to ingest additional material and begin to express numerous co-receptors that enhance their ability to interact with and activate T lymphocytes. In lymphoid tissues, these professional antigen-presenting cells encounter "naive" T cells that have undergone TCR gene rearrangement in the thymus, and a small number of these cells will (by chance) express a TCR configuration that recognizes an HLA-bound peptide. What largely restricts the breadth of immune recognition is the ability of peptide to bind to that

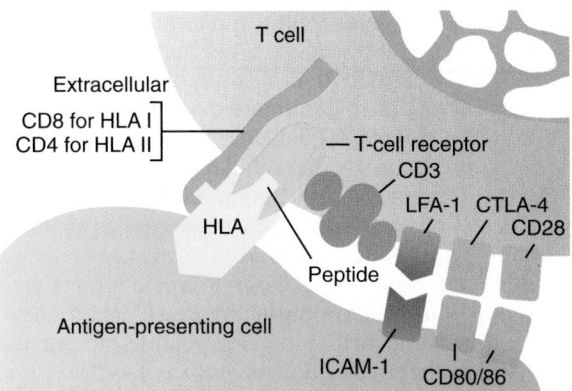

Figure 92-3 The molecular events in antigen presentation. Peptides within human leukocyte antigen (HLA) molecules on the antigen-presenting cell (APC) are bound weakly by T-cell receptor α and β chains. This interaction is stabilized and facilitated by interactions between the adhesion molecules LFA-1 on the T cell and its ligand ICAM-1 on the APC. T-cell and APC interactions between costimulatory molecules CD80 and CD86 on the APC and receptors such as CD28 or CTLA-4 on the T cell can result in T-cell activation or suppression, respectively.

particular HLA molecule. Thus different HLA molecules can bind different peptides, and this variable binding ability (and not so much the recognition by the T cell) determines an individual's ability to recognize a foreign peptide and mount an immune response to it. As discussed earlier, T cells with high affinity for self-peptides or too low an affinity for self-HLA molecules have already been deleted within the thymus. The relatively low-affinity interactions between TCR and HLA-bound peptide are supported by multiple co-receptor–ligand and adhesion molecule interactions between the T cell and antigen-presenting cell that also result in activation of the T cell (Fig. 92-3). The naive T cell is thus activated to divide time and time again, rapidly expanding the number of T cells with the same clonal antigenic specificity. T cells thus activated are no longer antigen "naive" but are now activated to express cytokines and/or to have cytolytic activity, and some will develop long-lived "memory" function. Cytokines expressed by CD4⁺ T-helper cells enhance the activity of other immune cells such as cytolytic CD8⁺ T cells and NK cells and are also critical to the development and maturation of B lymphocytes to result in the generation of antibody responses. T-helper cells also interact directly with dendritic cells, affecting their maturation and function.

Antibody Response

In lymphoid tissues, more complex antigens, including whole microbes, can be bound in an antigen-specific fashion by B lymphocytes, which have as their antigen receptor membrane-bound immunoglobulins (IgD and IgM). Thus bound, a particle can be ingested by the B cell and degraded, and then these microbial peptides are expressed on the B-cell surface HLA class II molecules. Thus, B lymphocytes may serve as professional antigen-presenting cells for recognition by CD4⁺ T cells. For most antigens, therefore, attraction of CD4⁺ T-cell help is essential to permit B lymphocyte expansion and ultimately antibody synthesis. As is the case for the interaction between the CD4⁺ T cell and other professional antigen-presenting cells, multiple receptor-ligand interactions stabilize the interaction between the TCR and the peptide HLA molecule that it recognizes on the B-cell surface. At the site of this intimate interaction, the CD4$^+$ T cell is activated to express T-helper cytokines that in turn activate the B cell, promoting cellular division and maturation. In this fashion microbial peptides that are recognized by CD4$^+$ T cells induce the "help" that is needed to result in generation and amplification of an antibody response to that microbe. Recognition of this basic principle has resulted in the development of "conjugate vaccines" that, through linkage of immune help inducing peptides to microbial sugars (which themselves do not induce T-cell responses) can enhance the antibody responses to these sugars. Conjugate vaccines are now used to prevent *Haemophilus* and pneumococcal infection.

The B lymphocytes thus activated by binding antigen to their surface receptors and helped by their interaction with CD4$^+$ T cells begin clonal replication and maturation. Replication amplifies the "mass" of antigen-reactive B cells, and maturation involves both transformation of B cells into antibody-secreting plasma cells and the induction of "class-switching," wherein the variable antigen-binding domains of the antibody are "switched" by gene rearrangements onto constant domains of different classes of antibody molecules. Thus an initial IgM response is followed later by an IgG response with the same specificity in terms of antigen recognition (hence the utility of a high-level IgM response to a microbial antigen as a clinically meaningful indicator of recent infection). These events take place largely in germinal centers within lymphoid tissue that is enriched also with follicular dendritic cells. These follicular dendritic cells can, for periods of years, trap and hold intact antigens on their surfaces and facilitate B-lymphocyte maturation. During the early course of antibody generation, the affinity of antibody molecules for their antigens can increase. This affinity maturation takes place during the rapid expansion of B lymphocytes and is the consequence of somatic hypermutation of sequences within the hypervariable regions of the antibody genes. Progeny B lymphocytes with greater surface immunoglobulin (receptor) affinity for antigen will be more rapidly activated to divide and will "outcompete" B lymphocytes with lower affinity receptors. The antibodies thereby secreted by progeny plasma cells become increasingly capable of binding microbial antigens with higher affinity. Thus the humoral immune response "evolves" in real time, selecting for B cells producing antibodies with progressively higher affinity for microbial pathogens.

Microbial Pathogenesis versus Host Defenses— the Continuing Drama

RESISTANCE TO EXTRACELLULAR BACTERIA: ENCAPSULATED ORGANISMS

Streptococcus pneumoniae

The type-specific polysaccharide capsule is a major virulence factor because of its antiphagocytic properties. Antibody to the polysaccharide is itself capable of preventing pneumo-

coccal disease, as reflected by experimental studies and the efficacy of pneumococcal polysaccharide vaccines.

In the absence of immunity, pneumococci reaching the alveoli are not effectively contained by the host. Their phagocytosis by neutrophils is inefficient, because organisms must be trapped against a surface to be ingested *(surface phagocytosis)*. The pneumococcus does, however, elicit a neutrophilic inflammatory response. The organism activates complement by the alternative pathway and interactions of C-reactive protein in serum with pneumococcal C-polysaccharide. Activated complement fragments (C3a, C5a, and C567) are chemotactic for neutrophils. Opsonic complement fragments (C3b) coating pneumococci favor their attachment to neutrophils but are less effective in promoting phagocytosis and killing than is specific antibody. Clinical observations also directly support the primal role of antibody in immunity. The development of specific antibody on days 5 to 9 of untreated pneumococcal pneumonia may produce a clinical "crisis," with dramatic resolution of symptoms. Opsonization of *S. pneumoniae* by type-specific anti-polysaccharide antibody promotes ingestion and oxidative burst activity, with destruction of the organism.

Neisseria meningitidis

Capsular polysaccharide also represents an important virulence factor for meningococci. In addition, pathogenic *Neisseria* species produce an IgA protease that dissociates the Fc fragment from the Fab portion of secretory and serum IgA and thus interferes with effector properties of the antibody molecule. Antibody-dependent, complement-mediated bacterial killing is the most critical host defense against meningococci. Therefore the presence of bactericidal antibody is associated with protection against the meningococcus. In epidemic situations, 40% of persons who become colonized with the epidemic strain but who lack bactericidal antibodies develop disease. Protective serum antibody is elicited by colonization with the following: (1) nonencapsulated and encapsulated strains of meningococci of low virulence, which elicit antibodies cross-reactive with virulent strains, and (2) *Escherichia coli* and *Bacillus* species with cross-reacting capsular polysaccharides. The lack of bactericidal activity in the serum of adolescents and adults manifesting susceptibility to *N. meningitidis* may be a result of blocking IgA antibody. Susceptibility of patients lacking C6, C7, or C8 to meningococcal infection provides important evidence that the dominant protective mechanism against this organism involves complement-mediated bacteriolysis.

RESISTANCE TO FACULTATIVE INTRACELLULAR PARASITES: MYCOBACTERIUM TUBERCULOSIS

Activation of host phagocytes provides the critical defense mechanism against *M. tuberculosis*. Primary infection progresses locally in the nonhypersensitive host, because ingested organisms persist and multiply within mononuclear phagocytes. The bacteria escape intracellular digestion by secreting products that inhibit phagolysosomal fusion. Antibody-coated mycobacteria do not evade phagolysosomal fusion but nonetheless resist degradation, probably because of shielding provided by their rich lipid content. The development of cellular immunity leads to T-lymphocyte–dependent macrophage activation and to the killing of the intracellular tubercle bacillus organism. The lesions of primary tuberculosis regress. However, latent foci persist, and delayed reactivation remains a threat throughout the lifetime of the host.

RESISTANCE TO OBLIGATE INTRACELLULAR PARASITES: VIRUSES

Host antiviral defense is characterized by overlap and redundancy, which allow an effective response to most viral agents. The key element of the response varies with the virus, the site, and the timing. Initially, infection is limited at the local site by type I IFNs, which increase the resistance of neighboring cells to spread of the infection. Complement directly neutralizes some enveloped viruses. NK cells destroy infected cells, a process enhanced by IFNs. As specific antibody is produced, IgA may neutralize the virus at mucosal surfaces; IgG may neutralize virus that has spread systemically to extracellular sites and also may allow uptake and destruction by FcR-bearing effector cells. Later, effector cytotoxic T lymphocytes are expanded and activated to lyse host cells expressing viral peptides in the context of HLA antigens. The host thus directs several defenses against viral infection. Humoral defenses are active against extracellular viruses and, if neutralizing antibody is present at high enough levels before infection, may prevent clinical infection entirely. Cell-mediated defenses largely play more critical roles in attenuating the magnitude of viral replication during chronic infection. Viruses at the same time have evolved numerous mechanisms to blunt or block host antiviral defenses. Many viruses can decrease the expression of class I HLA molecules on cells they infect, thereby limiting recognition of these cells by CD8[+] cytotoxic T lymphocytes. Many viruses that cause chronic infection, such as herpesviruses and HIV, can maintain a latent infection whereby, in the absence of viral protein synthesis, there are no viral peptide targets for recognition by cytotoxic T lymphocytes. Other viruses have acquired gene sequences that encode homologues of host cytokine or cytokine receptor genes that may help viruses escape from host immune surveillance or contribute to viral pathogenesis.

Prospectus for the Future

- Increased understanding of the molecular and cellular mechanisms responsible for the establishment and regulation of the immune response
- More accurate and reproducible techniques to quantify and evaluate the different components of the immune response
- Expanding role of genomics and proteomics as techniques to map the biochemical profiles that characterize the immune response to various pathogens, as well as prevalent antigens
- Innovative therapeutic interventions aimed at modulating specific components of the immune response selectively, and increased interest in clinically meaningful ways to evaluate the effectiveness of those interventions

References

Autran B, Molet L, Lederman MM: Host defenses against viral infection. In Boucher CAB, Galasso GJ (eds): Practical Guidelines in Antiviral Therapy. Amsterdam, Elsevier, 2002, pp 65-94.

Delves PJ, Roitt IM: The immune system (I). N Engl J Med 343:37-49, 108-117, 2000.

Goronzy JJ, Weyand CM: The innate and adaptive immune systems. In Goldman L, Ausiello D (eds): Cecil Textbook of Medicine, 22nd ed. Philadelphia, Elsevier, 2004, pp 208-217.

Holland SM, Gallin JI: Evaluation of the patient with suspected immunodeficiency. In Mandel GL, Bennett JE, Dolin R (eds): Principles and Practices of Infectious Diseases, 6th ed. Philadelphia, Elsevier, 2005, pp 149-160.

Janeway CA, Travers P, Walport M, Shlomchik M: Immunobiology: The Immune System in Health and Disease, 5th ed. New York, Garland Publishing, 2001.

Karp DR, Holer VM: Complement in health and disease. In Goldman L, Ausiello D (eds): Cecil Textbook of Medicine, 22nd ed. Philadelphia, Elsevier, 2004, pp 233-240.

Schwartz RS: Shattuck Lecture—Diversity of the immune repertoire and immunoregulation. N Engl J Med 348:1017-1026, 2003.

Von Andrian UH, Mackay CR: T-cell function and migration. Two sides of the same coin. N Engl J Med 334:1020-1034, 2000.

Laboratory Diagnosis of Infectious Diseases

Benigno Rodríguez and Michael M. Lederman

Five basic laboratory techniques can be used in the diagnosis of infectious diseases: (1) direct visualization of the organism, (2) detection of microbial antigen, (3) a search for "clues" produced by the host response to specific microorganisms, (4) detection of specific microbial nucleotide sequences, and (5) isolation of the organism in culture or propagation in cell culture. Each technique has its use and its pitfalls. The laboratory can usually provide the clinician with prompt, accurate, and, if the techniques are used judiciously, inexpensive diagnosis.

Diagnosis by Direct Visualization of the Organism

In many infectious diseases, pathogenic organisms can be directly visualized by microscopic examination of readily available tissue fluids. With the use of Gram or acid-fast stains, bacteria, mycobacteria, and *Candida* can be readily identified. An India ink preparation can often identify *Cryptococcus,* and potassium hydroxide (KOH) preparations can occasionally identify other fungal pathogens. Although antigen detection techniques are rapidly supplanting conventional staining and microscopy for identification of organisms such as *Giardia* in stool samples and *Cryptococcus* in cerebrospinal fluid (CSF) specimens (see later) because of their greater sensitivity and their decreased susceptibility to interobserver variation, the expediency of traditional direct visualization techniques in the presence of a large organism burden remains unmatched by these approaches. Examples of positive specimens prepared by conventional staining techniques are shown in Figures 93-1 and 93-2. Other techniques can also reveal clinically relevant pathogens. Silver staining using the Gomori methenamine technique can identify most fungi, including *Pneumocystis jirovecii.* Experienced pathologists can also identify *P. jirovecii* on Giemsa-stained specimens of induced sputum. Darkfield microscopy

can identify *Treponema pallidum,* and electron microscopy can sometimes detect viral particles in infected cells.

INDIA INK PREPARATION

A drop of centrifuged CSF is placed on a microscope slide next to a drop of artist's India ink. A coverslip is placed over the drops, and the area of mixing of CSF and India ink is examined at 100× magnification. Cryptococci are identified by their large capsules, which exclude the India ink (see Fig. 93-1).

Diagnosis by Detection of Microbial Antigens

Certain pathogens can be detected by examination of specimens for microbial antigens (Table 93-1). These studies can be performed rapidly—often within 1 hour. The diagnosis of meningitis caused by *Streptococcus pneumoniae, Cryptococcus neoformans,* some strains of *Haemophilus influenzae,* and *Neisseria meningitidis* can be made rapidly by detection of specific polysaccharide antigen in the CSF. Although these diagnoses may also be made by Gram stain or India ink preparation, antigen detection is especially helpful when attempts at direct visualization of the pathogen are not diagnostic (e.g., in the patient with partially treated bacterial meningitis). Immunofluorescence techniques (Fig. 93-3) using antibodies directed against the organisms identify pathogens such as *Legionella pneumophila* and *Bordetella pertussis* in respiratory secretions. Immunofluorescence can also be used to identify cells infected with influenza virus, respiratory syncytial virus, and adenovirus. Detection of urinary pneumococcal antigen can enhance the diagnostic capabilities of direct visualization and culture techniques in community-acquired pneumonia. Quantitation of cytomegalovirus (CMV) antigen in blood may help predict the development of active disease in immunocompromised patients.

The demonstration of hepatitis B surface antigen in blood establishes the presence of infection by this virus.

Diagnosis by Examination of Host Immune or Inflammatory Responses

Histopathologic examination of sampled or excised tissue often shows patterns of the host inflammatory response that

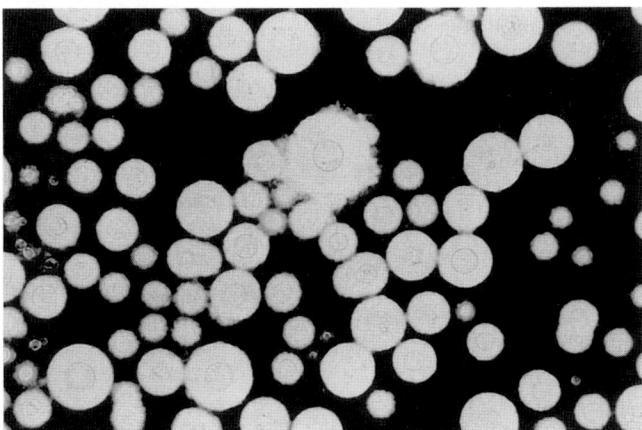

Figure 93-1 India ink preparation of cerebrospinal fluid revealing encapsulated cryptococci. Note the large capsules surrounding the smaller organisms.

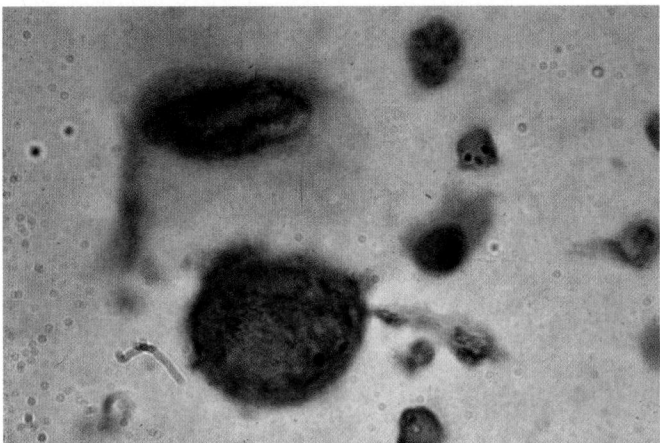

Figure 93-2 Tzanck preparation for diagnosis of herpesvirus infection. Note the multicolored giant cell *(bottom)* characteristic of herpes infection.

can narrow down diagnostic possibilities. As a general rule, a polymorphonuclear leukocytic infiltrate suggests an acute bacterial process. A lymphocytic infiltrate suggests a more chronic process and is characteristically seen in viral, mycobacterial, and fungal infections. Similarly, examination of infected fluids such as CSF may provide clues to possible causes. Bacterial infections generally provoke a polymorphonuclear leukocytosis with elevated protein and depressed glucose concentrations. Viral infections most often provoke a lymphocytic pleocytosis; protein elevations are less marked, and glucose levels are usually normal. Eosinophilia suggests helminthic infestations or certain fungal infections, such as coccidioidomycosis or aspergillosis, particularly the allergic forms of the latter. Granuloma formation suggests a mycobacterial cause. Certain parasites (such as *Schistosoma* species) and fungi (such as *Histoplasma, Cryptococcus,* and *Blastomyces* can also lead to granuloma formation. Some diseases, such as syphilis (obliterative endarteritis), cat-scratch disease (mixed granulomatous, suppurative, and lymphoid hyperplastic changes), and lymphogranuloma venereum (stellate abscesses), have fairly characteristic histologic features.

Several viral infections produce characteristic changes in host cells, which are detectable by cytologic examination. Skin or respiratory infection with herpesviruses, or pneumonia caused by CMV or measles virus, for example, can be diagnosed with reasonable accuracy by cytologic examination (e.g., Tzanck preparation for herpesvirus infection).

Host cell–mediated immune responses can be used to help make certain diagnoses. A positive skin test for delayed-type hypersensitivity to mycobacterial or fungal antigens indicates active or previous infection with these agents. A negative skin test may be seen despite active infection in individuals with depression of cell-mediated immunity (anergy). Control skin tests using commonly encountered antigens (e.g., *Candida*, mumps, *Trichophyton*) have been used in an attempt to exclude global anergy as the reason for a negative skin reaction, but their value as a diagnostic tool is questionable and they are therefore not routinely recommended. The QuantiFERON-TB test is an assay for detection of interferon-γ production by *Mycobacterium tuberculosis*–specific lymphocytes, and is an example of a clinically useful in vitro diagnostic procedure based on detection of the cellular immune response to a specific pathogen.

Host humoral responses may be used to diagnose certain infections, particularly those caused by organisms whose cultivation is difficult (e.g., *Ehrlichia chaffeensis*) or hazardous to laboratory personnel (e.g., *Francisella tularensis*). In general, two sera are obtained at intervals of at least 2

Table 93-1 **Diseases Often Diagnosed by Detection of Microbial Antigens**		
Disease	**Assay**	**Agent Detected**
Meningitis	Latex agglutination	*Streptococcus pneumoniae, Haemophilus influenzae, Neisseria meningitides, Cryptococcus*
Respiratory tract infection	Immunofluorescence Enzyme immunoassay	*Bordetella pertussis, Legionella pneumophila,* influenza virus, respiratory syncytial virus, adenovirus
Genitourinary tract infection	Enzyme immunoassay	*Chlamydia* species, herpes simplex viruses 1 and 2
Hepatitis B	Radioimmunoassay	Hepatitis B surface antigen

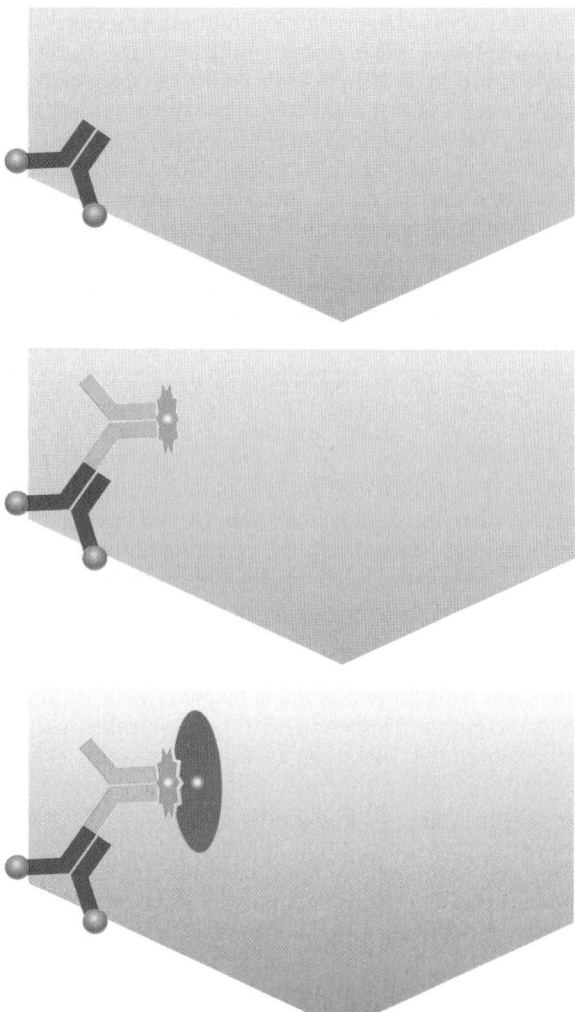

Figure 93-3 Diagram of the steps in the enzyme-linked immunosorbent assay (ELISA). Shown here is the form of ELISA used to detect antibodies (such as the test used to detect HIV infection); other forms of ELISA detect antigens. The process begins by adding the specimen to a well that has a purified antigen adsorbed to its inner surface, along with irrelevant proteins to cover the remaining well surface and prevent nonspecific binding. If specific antibodies are present in the sample, they will bind to the antigen; an antibody directed against human immunoglobulin labeled with an enzyme is then added. In the final step, the substrate for the enzyme is added; if there is attached antibody in the well, the linked enzyme will interact with the substrate and produce a color change that is proportional to the amount of antibody and can be read by a spectrophotometer.

weeks, and a fourfold or greater rise (or fall) in antibody titer generally suggests a recent infection. Antibodies of the immunoglobulin M class also suggest recent infection. Depending on the organism, assays may detect either specific (hepatitis viruses) or nonspecific, cross-reactive antibodies (syphilis non-treponemal tests). From another perspective, measurement of antibody levels in serum can determine if a person is likely protected from acquisition of infection or on the other hand might be a candidate for immunization. Measurement of serum antibodies to hepatitis A and hepatitis B virus is often used to determine if persons at risk are candidates for immunization.

Assays That Detect Microbial Nucleotide Sequences

Detection of microbial nucleotide sequences can provide a sensitive and specific means of identification of pathogens in clinical specimens. These genetic molecular diagnostic techniques can provide rapid speciation of slow-growing microbial isolates. In addition, these techniques can also provide rapid quantitation of pathogens that can establish the prognosis and also determine the effectiveness of modes of therapy. Finally, genetic analyses can identify genetic markers of antimicrobial resistance that can guide the selection of therapy.

The exquisite sensitivity and specificity of these techniques are consequences of the specificity of DNA base pairing and the dramatic amplifications of signals that can be provided by techniques such as the quantitative polymerase chain reaction (Fig. 93-4), nucleic acid sequence–based amplification, and branched-chain signal amplification analyses.

The sensitivity of these techniques has revolutionized laboratory diagnostics. For example, most standard techniques for detection of microbial antigens cannot reliably detect fewer than 100,000 molecules in clinical samples. In contrast, the genetic techniques discussed earlier are being routinely used now to identify as few as 20 to 50 molecules in clinical samples and can be modified to have even greater sensitivity. Table 93-2 lists some examples of diseases in which molecular diagnostic methods have represented a major advance in recent years.

Clinical Applications of Molecular Diagnostics

SPECIATION

The slow replication of mycobacteria limits rapid speciation of these organisms after their identification in clinical samples. In certain clinical settings, such as those that may occur in persons with human immunodeficiency virus (HIV) infection, the distinction between nontuberculous mycobacteria and *M. tuberculosis* may be particularly important. Genetic probes that distinguish among these organisms can provide rapid speciation after only limited growth.

DIAGNOSIS OF INFECTION

In acute HIV infection, detection of genomic HIV-1 RNA in plasma can provide diagnosis of this syndrome weeks before the development of diagnostic HIV specific antibodies (see Chapter 108). Nucleic acid amplification techniques are now routine for the diagnosis of gonorrhea and *Chlamydia* infections and can be performed on a single specimen, with a rapid turnaround time. Detection of herpes simplex virus sequences within CSF can provide a sensitive and specific diagnosis of herpes simplex encephalitis. Similar assays can be used for diagnosis of CMV, JC virus, Epstein-Barr virus, and *Bartonella henselae* infection. In certain anatomic

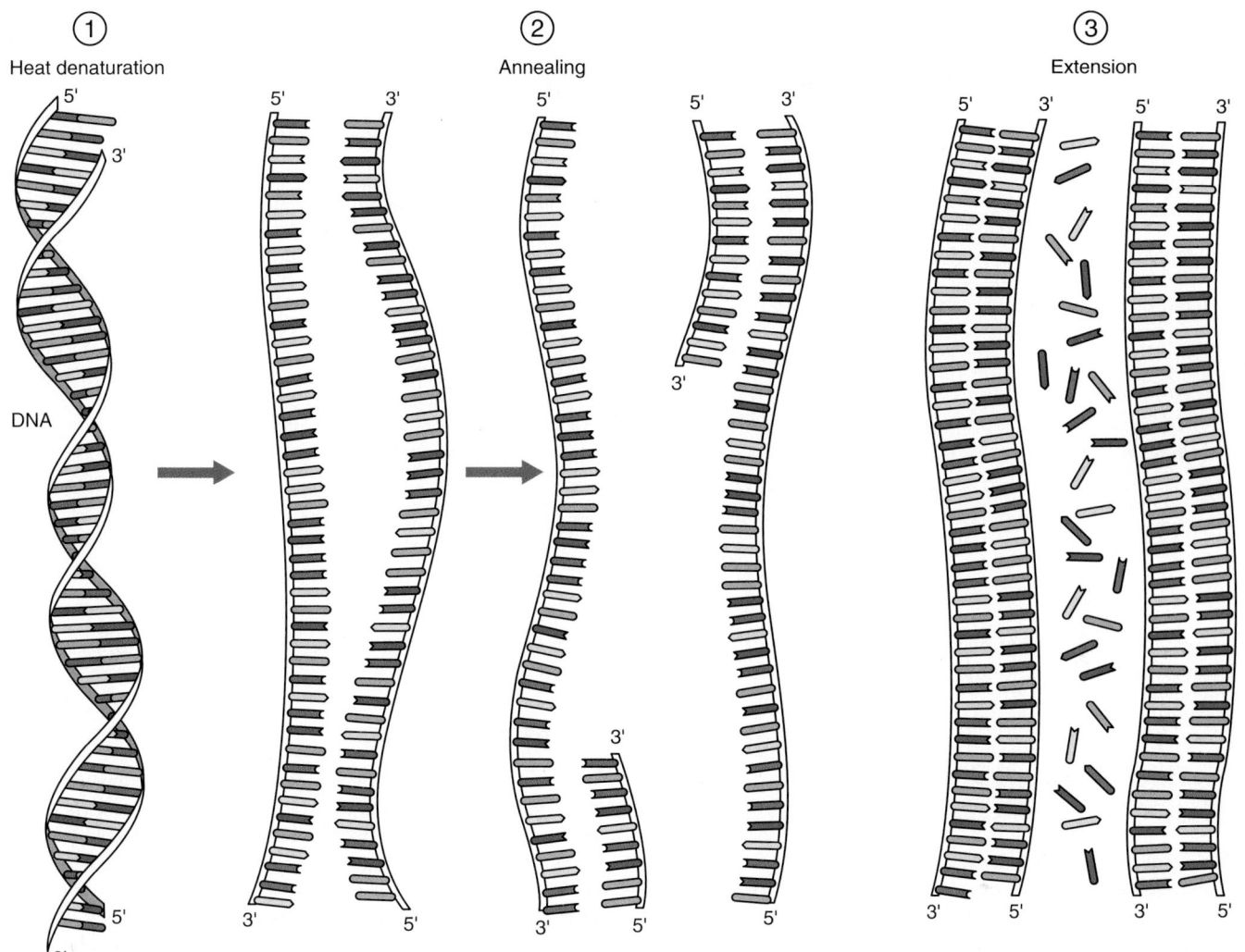

Figure 93-4 Schematic representation of polymerase chain reaction (PCR). The reaction solution contains the sample—presumably containing the target DNA, nucleotides, and primers, which will serve as building blocks for the amplified product, and polymerase enzymes that will catalyze the attachment of the nucleotides to the growing chain. (If the viral genome is composed of RNA, the genome must be first reverse transcribed to provide a complementary DNA template.) The first step in genomic amplification is denaturation, during which the solution is heated to 95°C to separate the two strands of DNA. The temperature is then lowered to allow the primers to attach to their complementary sequences on the single DNA strands, a process known as *annealing*. Finally, the mixture is heated again to a temperature at which the DNA polymerase catalyzes the attachment of further nucleotides to the primers (extension) until full double-stranded duplicates of the original DNA molecules are produced. If this process is repeated multiple times in a thermal cycler, a single DNA molecule can yield one million molecules after approximately 20 cycles.

locations such as the pericardium and the central nervous system, nucleic acid amplification may help in the diagnosis of tuberculosis. It is anticipated that numerous infectious diseases will soon be diagnosed with great sensitivity by means of these techniques. The exquisite sensitivity of this technique may, however, yield false-positive results unless the assays are carefully standardized.

QUANTIFICATION OF MICROBIAL BURDEN

Molecular diagnostic assays have been refined and standardized to permit reliable quantification of microbial genomic sequences in clinical samples. Quantification of CMV DNA, for example, has proven a useful tool in identifying individuals at risk for developing progressive CMV disease during chemotherapy-induced or organ transplantation–induced immunosuppression. These quantitative assays have also

provided evidence that the magnitude of microbial replication is predictive of disease progression in HIV infection, and sequential application of these techniques is now used routinely to monitor the activity of therapy for HIV and for hepatitis C virus infection.

DETECTING GENETIC MARKERS FOR ANTIMICROBIAL RESISTANCE

Microbial resistance to therapeutic interventions is an increasing problem in infectious diseases. When genetic sequences that confer resistance to therapies are known, assays to detect them can be applied rapidly to clinical samples, providing information that can be used to select treatment regimens. Direct analysis of plasma HIV sequences has provided genetic information that can predict the failure of specific modes of therapy; under certain circumstances, routine application of this information to the selection of

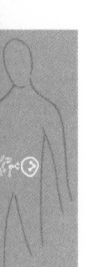

Table 93-2 **Diseases in Which Molecular Diagnosis Techniques Are Commonly Used**		
Pathogen	**Test**	**Clinical Situation**
Hepatitis C virus	Quantitative PCR	Confirmation of chronic infection; monitoring of the effectiveness of therapy; documentation of sustained virologic response
Cytomegalovirus	PCR Hybrid capture DNA test, CMV pp67 NASBA	Diagnosis of CMV encephalitis, myelitis on CSF specimens Prediction of development of clinical disease in seropositive immunocompromised patients
Chlamydia trachomatis, Neisseria gonorrhoeae	PCR, ligase chain reaction	Diagnosis of sexually transmitted diseases on a single specimen—now the standard of care in many centers
Hepatitis B virus	PCR	Quantification of viral burden; monitoring of response to therapy; determination of infectiousness
HIV	PCR, branched DNA amplification, NASBA	Quantification of viral replication; monitoring of response to therapy; confirmation of diagnosis in acute infection and mother-to-child transmission
Enteroviruses	Real-time PCR	Etiologic diagnosis of viral meningitis
Herpes simplex virus	PCR	Reliable diagnosis of HSV encephalitis, a life-threatening disease

HIV, human immunodeficiency virus; HSV, herpes simplex virus; NASBA, nucleic-acid-sequence–based amplification; PCR, polymerase chain reaction.

treatment regimens has been shown to improve the success rates of antiretroviral treatment.

Diagnosis by Isolation of the Organism in Culture

Isolation of a single microbial species from an infected site is generally considered evidence that the infection is caused by this organism. However, information obtained from the culture must be interpreted according to the clinical setting. For example, cultures obtained from ordinarily contaminated sites (e.g., vagina, pharynx) may be overgrown with nonpathogenic commensals, and fastidious organisms such as *Neisseria gonorrhoeae* are difficult to recognize unless cultured on a medium that selects for their growth. Similarly, cultures of expectorated "sputum" may also be uninterpretable if heavily contaminated with saliva. The culture of an organism from an ordinarily sterile site is reasonable evidence for infection with that organism. Conversely, the failure to culture an organism may simply result from inadequate culture conditions (e.g., "sterile" pus from a brain abscess cultured only on aerobic media). Most brain abscesses are caused by anaerobic bacteria that do not grow under aerobic conditions. Thus, when submitting samples for culture, the physician must alert the laboratory to likely pathogens.

Gram stains of specimens submitted for culture are often invaluable aids to the interpretation of culture results. A Gram stain of "sputum" will readily detect contamination by saliva if numerous squamous epithelial cells are seen. In contrast, a Gram stain revealing bacteria despite negative cultures suggests infection by fastidious organisms. The presence of an organism in high density and within neutrophils strongly suggests that the corresponding bacterial isolate is causing disease rather than colonizing the patient or contaminating the specimen. Gram staining of the initial clinical specimen may also help determine the relative importance of different isolates when cultures show mixed flora.

VIRAL ISOLATION

Because all viral pathogens that can be cultured require eukaryotic cells in which to grow, virus isolation is expensive and often laborious. Throat washings, rectal swabs, or cultures of infected sites should be transported immediately to the laboratory or, if this is not possible, placed in virus transport medium and refrigerated overnight until they can be cultured in the laboratory. Certain viruses such as HIV and CMV are often cultivated from whole blood samples. Notifying the laboratory of the suspected pathogens allows selection of the best cell lines or systems for culture. The clinician must be aware of the viruses that the hospital's laboratory can isolate, and consideration should be given to the clinical circumstances in which the specimen was obtained to properly interpret a positive result. This is particularly true in the case of viruses that can be shed intermittently in the absence of active disease, such as the herpes simplex viruses and CMV.

ISOLATION OF RICKETTSIAE, CHLAMYDIAE, AND MYCOPLASMAS

Rickettsiae are cultivated primarily in reference laboratories. Diagnosis of rickettsial illness is generally made on clinical grounds and confirmed serologically. Although chlamydiae can be propagated in cell cultures used in most hospital virology laboratories, chlamydial infection is most often diagnosed through antigen detection techniques. Mycoplasmas will grow on selective media; however, the prolonged period of incubation results in little advantage over serologic diagnosis.

BACTERIAL ISOLATION

Isolation of common bacterial pathogens is achieved readily by most hospital laboratories. Specimens should be carried promptly to the laboratory. In instances in which likely isolates may be fastidious (e.g., bacterial meningitis) and immediate processing cannot be ensured, the specimen should be placed directly onto the culture medium, with careful attention to sterile techniques. Widespread availability of transport media has minimized the need for this kind of approach. Blood culture is a special case of bacterial isolation technique, for which immediate inoculation into the culture medium is required. Blood culture samples are arguably some of the most critical specimen types processed by a microbiology laboratory, and errors in their collection and processing can have major clinical consequences. Common mistakes include insufficient blood volume (30 to 40 mL total is recommended for adults), collection of multiple specimens from the same venipuncture site or intravenous catheter (making it difficult to interpret the significance of normal skin colonizers and to estimate the persistence of the bacteremia), collection after antibiotic initiation, and less than meticulous aseptic technique (resulting in contaminant growth).

Isolation of anaerobic bacteria is often critically important for clinical diagnosis. When anaerobes are suspected, the specimen, if pus or liquid, can be drawn into a syringe, the air expelled, and the syringe capped before transport to the laboratory. Otherwise, specimens must be taken immediately to the laboratory or placed in an anaerobic transport medium appropriate for survival of pathogens. Because of contamination by oral anaerobes, sputum should not be cultured anaerobically unless the sample was obtained by transtracheal or percutaneous lung aspiration.

ISOLATION OF FUNGI AND MYCOBACTERIA

Specimens for fungal and mycobacterial culture must be processed and cultured by the microbiology laboratory. Although some fungi and rapidly growing mycobacteria grow readily on standard agars used for routine isolation of bacteria, others, such as *M. tuberculosis* and *Histoplasma capsulatum*, must be cultured on special media for as long as several weeks.

Prospectus for the Future

- Greater use of molecular methods for diagnosis and monitoring of infectious diseases

- Greater use of rapid bedside tests for the diagnosis of infectious diseases

References

Gill VJ, Fedorko DP, Witebsky FG: The clinician and the microbiology laboratory. In Mandell GL, Bennett JC, Dolin R (eds): Principles and Practice of Infectious Diseases, 6th ed. Philadelphia, Elsevier, 2005, pp 203-241.

Versalovic J, Lupski JR: Molecular detection and genotyping of pathogens: More accurate and rapid answers. Trends Microbiol 10:S15-S21, 2002.

Chapter **94**

Antimicrobial Therapy

Benigno Rodríguez and Michael M. Lederman

One of the most dramatic advances in medical practice in the twentieth century was the development of antimicrobial therapy. Antimicrobials are agents that interfere with microbial metabolism, resulting in inhibition of growth or death of bacteria, viruses, fungi, protozoa, or helminths. Some, like penicillin, are natural products of other microbes. Others, such as sulfa drugs, are chemical agents synthesized in the laboratory. Still others are semisynthetic, with chemical modifications of naturally occurring substances that result in enhanced activity (e.g., nafcillin) and/or diminished toxic effects.

The most effective antimicrobials are characterized by their relatively selective activity against microbes. Some, such as penicillins and amphotericin B, interfere with the synthesis of microbial cell walls that are absent in human cells. Others, such as trimethoprim and sulfa drugs, inhibit obligate microbial synthesis of essential nucleic acid intermediates, pathways not required by human cells. Still others, such as acyclovir, an antiviral agent, are relatively inactive until metabolized by pathogen-derived enzymes. Antiretroviral agents selectively inhibit viral elements that are essential for replication. More recently antiretroviral agents have been developed that inhibit host cellular factors necessary for viral replication. Antimicrobial agents, although typically selective in activity against microbes, have variable degrees of toxicity for human cells. Thus, monitoring for toxicity during antimicrobial therapy is always important.

Pathogen

If the pathogen has been clearly identified (see Chapter 93), a drug with a narrow spectrum of activity (i.e., highly selective for the particular pathogen) is usually the most reasonable choice. If the pathogen responsible for the patient's illness has not been identified, then the physician must choose a drug or combination of drugs active against the most likely pathogens in the specific setting. In either instance, the physician must be guided by patterns of antimicrobial resistance common in the community and in the specific hospital. Some pathogens (e.g., group A streptococci) are almost always sensitive to narrow-spectrum antimicrobials such as penicillin. Other pathogens, such as staphylococci, are variably resistant to penicillins but almost always susceptible to vancomycin. Resistance patterns, particularly among hospital-acquired bacteria, may vary widely and are important in devising antimicrobial strategies. Broad-spectrum antimicrobial coverage for all febrile patients ("shotgunning") must not be substituted for carefully evaluating the clinical problem and pinpointing therapy directed toward the most likely pathogen or pathogens. Widespread use of broad-spectrum antimicrobials almost invariably leads to emergence of resistant strains or the emergence of potentially fatal pathogens such as *Clostridium difficile*. However, the greater the severity of a patient's illness and the less certain the physician is of the responsible pathogen, the more important initial, empirical, broad-spectrum coverage becomes. Initial empirical treatment is also frequently indicated in the immunocompromised febrile patient (e.g., the patient with severe neutropenia secondary to chemotherapy). Once the pathogen is isolated and its antimicrobial sensitivities are known, empirical therapy must be scaled down to a definitive regimen with optimal activity against the specific microorganism.

Site of Infection

The location of the infection is also important in determining the selection and dosage of an antimicrobial. Deep-seated infections and bacteremic infections generally require higher doses of antimicrobials than, for example, superficial infections of the skin, upper respiratory tract, or lower urinary tract. Penetration of antimicrobials into sites such as the meninges, eye, and prostate is quite variable. Therefore treatment of infections at these sites involves selection of an antimicrobial agent that penetrates these tissues in concentrations sufficient to inhibit or kill the pathogen. The meninges are relatively resistant to penetration by most antimicrobials; inflammation renders them somewhat more permeable. High doses of antibiotics are therefore the rule when meningitis is treated. Bacterial infections of certain sites such as the heart valves or meninges must be treated with antibiotics that kill the microbe (bactericidal) as opposed to simply inhibiting growth (bacteriostatic). This is so because local host defenses at these sites are inadequate to rid the host of infecting organisms. Infections involving foreign bodies may be impossible to eradicate without removal of the foreign material.

Antimicrobials alone are often insufficient in the treatment of large abscesses. Although many drugs achieve reasonable concentrations in abscess walls, the low pH antagonizes the activity of some drugs (e.g., aminoglycosides), and some drugs bind to and are inactivated by the high concentrations of protein, white blood cells, and their products in these collections. The large number of organisms, their depressed metabolism in this unfavorable milieu, and the frequent polymicrobial nature of certain abscesses increase the likelihood that some organisms present may be resistant to antimicrobial therapy. Therefore most abscesses should be drained whenever anatomically possible.

Characteristics of the Antimicrobial

The physician must know the pharmacokinetics of the drug (i.e., its absorption, its penetration into various sites, and its metabolism and excretion) and its toxic effects, as well as its spectrum of antimicrobial activity, before selecting it for use (Table 94-1).

DISTRIBUTION AND EXCRETION

Lipid-soluble drugs, such as chloramphenicol and rifampin, penetrate most membranes, including the meninges, more readily than do more ionized compounds, such as the aminoglycosides. Understanding a drug's distribution, rate and site of metabolism, and route of excretion is essential in selecting the appropriate drug and dose. Drugs excreted unchanged in the urine may be particularly suitable for the treatment of lower urinary tract infection or for the treatment of systemic infection in the presence of renal insufficiency. Some antimicrobials are metabolized in the liver and must be adjusted appropriately in the presence of hepatic dysfunction.

ACTIVITY OF THE DRUG

The physician must understand the spectrum of activity of the drug against microbial isolates, the mechanism of activity of the agent, and whether it is bactericidal or bacteriostatic in achievable concentrations. It should be remembered, however, that the actual activity of an agent as bacteriostatic or bactericidal may depend on concentration at the anatomic site, the microorganism involved, or both. As a general rule, cell wall–active drugs are likely to be bactericidal. Bactericidal drugs are necessary for treatment of infections sequestered from effective host inflammatory responses, such as meningitis and endocarditis. With the exception of

aminoglycosides and certain azalide and macrolide antibiotics, agents inhibiting protein synthesis at ribosomal sites are generally bacteriostatic.

TOXIC EFFECTS OF THE DRUG

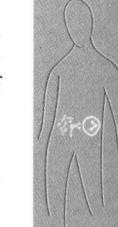

The physician must have a thorough understanding of the contraindications for use of the drug, as well as the major toxic effects and their general frequencies. This will help in evaluating the risks of treatment and will also assist in advising the patient about possible adverse reactions. History of drug hypersensitivity must be sought before any antimicrobial is prescribed. The presence or absence of previous reactions to penicillin should be documented for every patient. Patients with a history suggestive of immediate hypersensitivity to penicillin, such as hives, wheezing, hypotension, laryngospasm, or angioedema at any site, must be considered at risk for anaphylaxis. These patients should not receive penicillins or related drugs (cephalosporins or carbapenems) if adequate alternatives are available. Given the large number of currently available agents with activity against penicillin-susceptible organisms, the need for skin testing and desensitization is now much less common. In the rare cases when it is necessary, however, consultation with an experienced allergist is recommended. Examples of situations where desensitization using progressively larger doses of penicillin, either parenterally or orally, may be necessary include neurosyphilis and syphilis during pregnancy. Patients with a history of an uncomplicated morbilliform or delayed rash after penicillin therapy are not likely to be at risk for immediate hypersensitivity and may be treated with cephalosporins, for which the risk of cross-hypersensitivity to penicillins is likely to be in the range of 5%. Evidence suggests that cross-hypersensitivity to aztreonam is less common.

Route of Administration

Oral administration of antimicrobials can often prevent the morbidity and expense associated with parenteral (intravenous or intramuscular) administration. Although some antimicrobials (e.g., amoxicillin and the fluoroquinolones) are very well absorbed after oral administration, most patients hospitalized with severe infections should be treated, at least initially, with intravenous antibiotics. Gut absorption of antimicrobials can be unpredictable, and the intravenous route often permits administration of greater amounts of drug than can be tolerated orally. Intramuscular administration of some antimicrobials can result in excellent drug absorption but should be avoided in the presence of hypotension (erratic absorption) and coagulation disorders (hematomas). Repeated intramuscular injections are uncomfortable and for some drugs (e.g., pentamidine) can also result in the formation of sterile abscesses.

Duration of Therapy

Antimicrobial therapy should be initiated as part of a treatment plan of defined duration. In a few settings, the duration of optimal antimicrobial therapy is established (e.g., 10 days, but not 7 days, of oral penicillin will consistently prevent

Table 94-1 Characteristics of Commonly Used Antimicrobial Agents

Drug Class	Site of Action	Excretion/ Metabolism	Uses and Activity
Antibacterials			
β-Lactams			
Penicillins	Cell wall	Renal	Streptococci, *Neisseria,* oral anaerobes
β-lactamase–resistant penicillins (e.g., nafcillin)	Cell wall	Renal and/or hepatic	Methicillin-sensitive staphylococci
Amino penicillins (e.g., ampicillin)	Cell wall	Renal	Gram-positive organisms, not staphylococci, some gram-negative organisms
Extended-spectrum penicillins (e.g., piperacillin)	Cell wall	Renal	Broad-spectrum gram-positive organisms; gram-negative organisms, including *Pseudomonas,* not *Staphylococcus*
β-lactamase inhibitors (e.g., clavulanic acid)	Inactivate β-lactamase	Renal/metabolic	Used with ampicillin, amoxicillin, piperacillin, or ticarcillin; expand activity to include anaerobes, many gram-negative organisms, and methicillin-sensitive staphylococci
Cephalosporins[a]			
First generation (e.g., cefazolin)	Cell wall	Renal	Gram-positive organisms, many common gram-negative bacteria
Second generation (e.g., cefuroxime)		Renal	Some with anaerobic activity (e.g., cefoxitin)
Third generation (e.g., ceftriaxone)		Renal or hepatic	Some active against *Pseudomonas* (e.g., ceftazidime)
Fourth generation (e.g., cefepime)		Renal	Broadest spectrum including resistant nosocomial gram-negative organisms, and gram-positive cocci, including methicillin-sensitive staphylococci
Monobactams			
Aztreonam	Cell wall	Renal	Aerobic gram-negative bacilli
Carbapenems			
Imipenem-cilastatin, meropenem, ertapenem, doripenem	Cell wall	Renal	Very broad-spectrum, many gram-negative, including resistant nosocomial organisms, some enterococci, and methicillin-sensitive staphylococci, anaerobes
Glycopeptides			
Vancomycin	Cell wall	Renal	Coagulase-positive and coagulase-negative staphylococci, other gram-positive bacteria
Streptogramins			
Quinupristin-dalfopristin	Ribosome	Hepatic, fecal	Gram-positive organisms, including methicillin-resistant staphylococci and non-*faecalis* vancomycin-resistant enterococci
Lipopeptides			
Daptomycin	Cell membrane (?)	Renal	Coagulase-positive and coagulase-negative staphylococci, other gram-positive bacteria, including glycopeptide-resistant enterococci
Oxazolidinones			
Linezolid	Ribosome	Renal	Coagulase-positive and coagulase-negative staphylococci, other gram-positive bacteria, including glycopeptide-resistant enterococci, certain mycobacteria, *Nocardia*
Sulfonamides, trimethoprim	Inhibit nucleic acid synthesis	Renal	Gram-negative bacilli, *Salmonella, Pneumocystis jirovecii, Nocardia*
Fluoroquinolones (e.g., ciprofloxacin, levofloxacin, moxifloxacin)	DNA gyrase	Some hepatic metabolism	Broad spectrum, including *Legionella;* newer agents also active against streptococci or anaerobes
Metronidazole	DNA disruption	Hepatic metabolism	Anaerobes, *Clostridium difficile,* amebas, *Trichomonas*
Rifampin	Transcription	Hepatic metabolism/ renal	*Mycobacterium tuberculosis;* meningococcal and *Haemophilus influenzae* prophylaxis
Aminoglycosides	Ribosome	Renal	Gram-negative bacilli; no activity in anaerobic conditions

Table 94-1 **Characteristics of Commonly Used Antimicrobial Agents—Cont'd**

Drug Class	Site of Action	Excretion/ Metabolism	Uses and Activity
Chloramphenicol	Ribosome	Hepatic metabolism/ renal	Broad spectrum; active against *Salmonella*, anaerobes, *Rickettsia*, *Brucella*, *Bartonella*, but use limited by toxicity
Clindamycin	Ribosome	Hepatic metabolism/ renal	Anaerobes; gram-positive cocci
Tetracyclines	Ribosome	Renal/hepatic metabolism	Broad spectrum; especially useful for spirochetes, *Rickettsia*
Glycylcyclines			
Tigecycline	Ribosome	Renal/hepatic metabolism	Broad spectrum, including methicillin-resistant staphylococci, anaerobes, gram-negative organisms
Macrolides and Azalides			
Erythromycin	Ribosome	Hepatic	Gram-positive cocci, *Legionella*, *Mycoplasma*
Azithromycin, clarithromycin	Ribosome	Hepatic	High intracellular levels have enhanced activity against mycobacteria, *Toxoplasma*
Ketolides			
Telithromycin	Ribosome	Hepatic metabolism/ renal	Enhanced activity against gram-positive organisms, including methicillin-resistant staphylococci, intracellular respiratory pathogens, macrolide-resistant *Streptococcus pneumoniae*
Antifungals			
Polyenes			
Amphotericin B	Binds membrane ergosterol	Tissue breakdown	Most fungi; newer lipid formulations may be better tolerated
Flucytosine	Blocks DNA synthesis	Renal	Candidiasis; *Cryptococcus* with amphotericin B
Azoles	Block ergosterol biosynthesis		
Ketoconazole		Hepatic	Mucosal candidiasis, pulmonary histoplasmosis (nonmeningeal)
Itraconazole		Hepatic	Histoplasmosis, blastomycosis
Fluconazole		Renal	Candidiasis, cryptococcosis, coccidioidomycosis
Voriconazole		Hepatic	Invasive aspergillosis, *Fusarium* and *Scedosporium* infections, empiric for febrile neutropenia
Posaconazole		Hepatic	Prophylaxis of invasive fungal infections in immunosuppressed patients, zygomycosis (not FDA approved), refractory *Candida* infections
Echinocandins	Inhibit glucan synthesis		
Caspofungin		Chemical decay and degradation	*Candida* species, invasive aspergillosis
Micafungin			Esophageal candidiasis, prophylaxis of invasive *Candida* infections in bone marrow transplant recipients, empiric treatment in febrile neutropenia
Anidulafungin		Chemical decay and degradation	Candidemia, other systemic *Candida* infections, esophageal candidiasis
Antivirals			
Acyclovir	DNA polymerase	Renal	Herpes simplex, including encephalitis; herpes zoster
Famciclovir	DNA polymerase		Herpes simplex, zoster
Ganciclovir, valganciclovir	DNA polymerase	Renal	Cytomegalovirus, herpesviruses
Foscarnet	DNA polymerase	Renal	Cytomegalovirus, herpesviruses
Cidofovir	DNA polymerase	Renal	Cytomegalovirus, herpesviruses
Amantadine, rimantadine	Uncoating(?)	Renal	Influenza A treatment and prophylaxis
Zanamavir	Neuraminidase	Renal	Influenza A and B
Oseltamavir	Neuraminidase	Renal	Influenza A and B
Ribavirin	RNA synthesis(?)	Hepatic/renal	RSV, hepatitis C (together with interferon-α)
Interferon-α	Immunomodulator		Hepatitis B, C
Entecavir	DNA polymerase	Renal	Hepatitis B

Continued

Table 94-1 **Characteristics of Commonly Used Antimicrobial Agents—Cont'd**			
Drug Class	**Site of Action**	**Excretion/ Metabolism**	**Uses and Activity**
Antiretrovirals			
Nucleoside or nucleotide reverse transcriptase inhibitors[b]	HIV-1 reverse transcriptase	Renal and/or hepatic	HIV-1
Non-nucleoside reverse transcriptase inhibitors[c]	HIV-1 reverse transcriptase	Hepatic	HIV-1
Protease inhibitors[d]	HIV-1 protease	Hepatic	HIV-1
Fusion inhibitors[e]	HIV-1 viral entry	Catabolism	HIV-1
Chemokine receptor inhibitors[f]	Cellular CCR5	Hepatic/renal	HIV-1
Integrase inhibitors[g]	HIV-1 integrase	Hepatic	HIV-1

[a]As a rule. First-generation cephalosporins have better activity against gram-positive cocci and minimal CNS penetration. Second-generation cephalosporins have somewhat better activity against gram-negative bacteria and may penetrate the CNS. Third-generation cephalosporins have broader activity against gram-negative bacteria and generally penetrate the CNS, but they are relatively less active against gram-positive cocci. Fourth-generation cephalosporins have the broadest spectrum of activity, regaining activity against gram-positive organisms.
[b]These include zidovudine, stavudine, didanosine, zalcitabine, lamivudine, emtricitabine, tenofovir, and abacavir.
[c]These include efavirenz, nevirapine, etravirine, and delavirdine.
[d]These include indinavir, nelfinavir, ritonavir, saquinavir, amprenavir, fosamprenavir, tipranavir, atazanavir, darunavir, and lopinavir-ritonavir.
[e]The only currently approved agent is enfuvirtide.
[f]The only currently approved agent is maraviroc.
[g]The only currently approved agent is raltegravir.
CNS, central nervous system; FDA, U.S. Food and Drug Administration; HIV, human immunodeficiency virus; RSV, respiratory syncytial virus.

rheumatic fever after streptococcal pharyngitis); in many others the duration of treatment is empirical and sometimes can be based on the clinical and bacteriologic course. Bloodstream infections without endocarditis or other focal infections can generally be treated for 10 to 14 days. Pneumococcal pneumonia can be effectively treated in 7 to 10 days.

Combinations

Combinations of antimicrobials are indicated in serious infection when they provide more effective activity against a pathogen than any single agent. In some instances, combinations of drugs are used to prevent the emergence of resistance (e.g., infections caused by *Mycobacterium tuberculosis* and the human immunodeficiency virus). In others, combinations are used because they provide synergistic action against the pathogen (e.g., penicillin, a cell wall–active antibiotic, facilitates uptake of aminoglycosides by enterococci). In still other instances, drug combinations are used in empirical therapies to cover a wide spectrum of potential pathogens when the causative agent is unidentified or when infection is likely to be from a mixture of organisms (e.g., fecal soilage of the peritoneum). The use of more than one drug increases the likelihood of toxic effects, increases costs, and often increases the risk of superinfection.

Monitoring of Antimicrobial Therapy

The physician and patient should be alert to potential toxic effects and should be prepared to halt the drug in the event of serious toxic effects. Similarly, in vitro susceptibility is not necessarily synonymous with clinical effectiveness, and repeated clinical evaluation for resolution of both systemic and local signs of infection is the single most important monitoring tool available to the clinician treating an infectious process. For some antimicrobials, such as aminoglycosides, the ratio of effective to toxic drug levels is low, requiring

monitoring of serum levels of the drug to ensure safe and effective dosing. Vancomycin is another antimicrobial that often requires measurement of serum levels to optimize dosing, particularly with prolonged treatment or in the presence of renal failure.

Antiviral Agents

As obligate intracellular pathogens, viruses depend on interactions with host cellular machinery for completion of the life cycle. Thus many potential antiviral treatment strategies are limited by toxic effects on host cells. Specificity for viruses or virus-infected cells can be obtained by interfering with the function of unique viral elements (e.g., the M2 protein of influenza virus that is the target of amantadine and rimantadine) or by developing drugs such as acyclovir that must be processed by viral enzymes (in this instance, phosphorylated by herpesvirus thymidine kinase) before becoming active. In contrast to antibacterial drugs, however, antiviral agents generally have a limited spectrum of activity, each agent being useful against a small number of viruses. In the 1990s there was a dramatic increase in the numbers and types of drugs effective in the treatment of viral infections. This has been particularly striking in the field of antiretroviral therapies (see Chapter 108), and new agents against influenza, hepatitis B, and cytomegalovirus are now part of the therapeutic armamentarium. Additional developments in therapies for other viruses (e.g., hepatitis C) are anticipated.

Antifungal Agents

A number of drugs are useful when applied topically or systemically in the treatment of fungal diseases. Most target the ergosterol-containing cell membrane either by inhibiting ergosterol synthesis (azoles) or by aggregating in proximity to ergosterol and increasing membrane permeability (polyenes). Flucytosine inhibits fungal DNA synthesis. Echinocandins inhibit glucan synthesis. Increasing resistance to certain azoles and flucytosine among clinically relevant fungal isolates limits the utility of these agents in patients requiring chronic therapy.

Antimicrobial Resistance Testing

As treatment options expand, the emergence of antimicrobial resistance to therapies is predictable. Thus physicians must be prepared to evaluate the resistance patterns of specific microbial isolates. Resistance testing is now routinely provided for bacterial pathogens and in the design of antiretroviral treatment strategies (see Chapter 108). Certain resistance assays are not yet fully standardized, and all require some level of expertise to facilitate their interpretation. Thus interpretation of resistance assay results to guide treatment decisions, whether for serious bacterial, fungal, or viral infections, should generally involve discussion with an expert in infectious diseases.

Prospectus for the Future

- Newer classes of antiviral medications targeting hepatitis and other viruses
- Newer classes of antiretroviral medications targeting different phases of viral replication
- Newer classes of antibacterials targeting antibiotic-resistant organisms

- Newer, less toxic antifungal agents
- Antimicrobial peptides and other "designer" drugs with innovative mechanisms of action
- Improved agents for the treatment of parasitic and other diseases that are uncommon in Western developed countries (e.g., malaria, leishmania)

References

Craig WA: Antibacterial therapy. In Goldman L, Bennett JC (eds): Cecil Textbook of Medicine, 22nd ed. Philadelphia, Elsevier, 2005, pp 1753-1764.

Hayden FG: Antiviral drugs (other than antiretrovirals). In Mandell GL, Bennett JE, Dolin R (eds): Principles and Practice of Infectious Diseases, 6th ed. Philadelphia, Elsevier, 2005, pp 514-551.

Moellering RC, Eliopoulos GM: Principles of anti-infective therapy. In Mandell GL, Bennett JE, Dolin R (eds): Principles and Practice of Infectious Diseases, 6th ed. Philadelphia, Elsevier, 2005, pp 242-253.

Chapter **95**

Fever and Febrile Syndromes

Tracy L. Lemonovich and Robert A. Salata

Regulation of Body Temperature

Although normal body temperature ranges vary considerably, oral temperature readings in excess of 37.8° C (100.2° F) are generally abnormal. In healthy individuals, core body temperature is maintained within a narrow range, so that for each individual, daily temperature variations greater than 1° to 1.5° C are distinctly unusual. The hypothalamic nuclei that establish set points for body temperature control this homeostasis. Homeostasis is affected by a complex balance between heat-generating and heat-conserving mechanisms that raise or lower body temperature, respectively. Heat is regularly generated as a byproduct of obligate energy use (e.g., cellular metabolism, myocardial contractions, breathing). When an increase in body temperature is needed, shivering—nondirected muscular contractions—generates large amounts of heat. Cutaneous blood vessels constrict to diminish heat lost to the environment. At the same time, the person feels cold; this heat preference promotes heat-conserving behavior, such as wrapping up in a blanket.

Similarly, when a lower body temperature is needed, obligate heat loss to the environment occurs through the skin and by evaporation of water through sweat and respiration. Vasodilation flushes the skin capillaries, temporarily raising skin temperature but ultimately lowering core body temperature by increasing heat loss through the skin to the cooler environment. Sweating promotes rapid heat loss through evaporation, and at the same time the person feels warm and sheds blankets or initiates other activities to promote heat loss.

Fever and Hyperthermia

Fever is an elevated body temperature that is mediated by an increase in the hypothalamic heat-regulating set point. Although exogenous substances such as bacterial products may precipitate fever, the increase in body temperature is achieved through physiologic mechanisms. In contrast, hyperthermia is an increase in body temperature that overrides or bypasses the normal homeostatic mechanisms. As a general rule, body temperatures in excess of 41° C (105.8° F) are rarely physiologically mediated and suggest hyperthermia. Hyperthermia may occur after vigorous exercise, in patients with heat stroke, as a heritable reaction to anesthetics (malignant hyperthermia), as a response to phenothiazines (neuroleptic malignant syndrome), and occasionally in patients with central nervous system disorders such as paraplegia (see also Chapter 118). Some patients with severe dermatologic conditions are also unable to dissipate heat and therefore experience hyperthermia.

Fever is usually a physiologic response to infection or inflammation. Monocytes or tissue macrophages are activated by various stimuli to liberate various cytokines with pyrogenic activity (Fig. 95-1). Interleukin (IL)-1 is also an essential cofactor in initiating the immune response. Another pyrogenic cytokine, tumor necrosis factor (TNF)–α, activates lipoprotein lipase and may also play a role in immune cytolysis; TNF-β, or lymphotoxin, has similar properties. A fourth cytokine, interferon (IFN)-α, has antiviral activity (see Chapter 92). IL-6, a cytokine that potentiates B-cell immunoglobulin (Ig) synthesis, also has pyrogenic activity. Endogenous pyrogens activate the anterior preoptic nuclei of the hypothalamus to raise the set point for body temperature. Newer data suggest that there is also a more immediate stimulatory effect of exogenous pyrogens (e.g., bacterial lipopolysaccharide) in the production of fever. This occurs when exogenous pyrogens induce the release of prostaglandin E$_2$ (PGE$_2$), which either directly stimulates the anterior preoptic nuclei or causes excitation of vagal afferent nerves that transmit signals to these nuclei. Infection with all types of microorganisms can be associated with fever. Tissue injury with resulting inflammation, as observed in patients with myocardial or pulmonary infarction or after trauma, can produce fever. Certain malignancies such as lymphoma and leukemia, renal cell carcinoma, and hepatic carcinoma are also associated with fever. In some instances, fever is related to the liberation of endogenous pyrogens by monocytes in the inflammatory response surrounding the tumor; in other

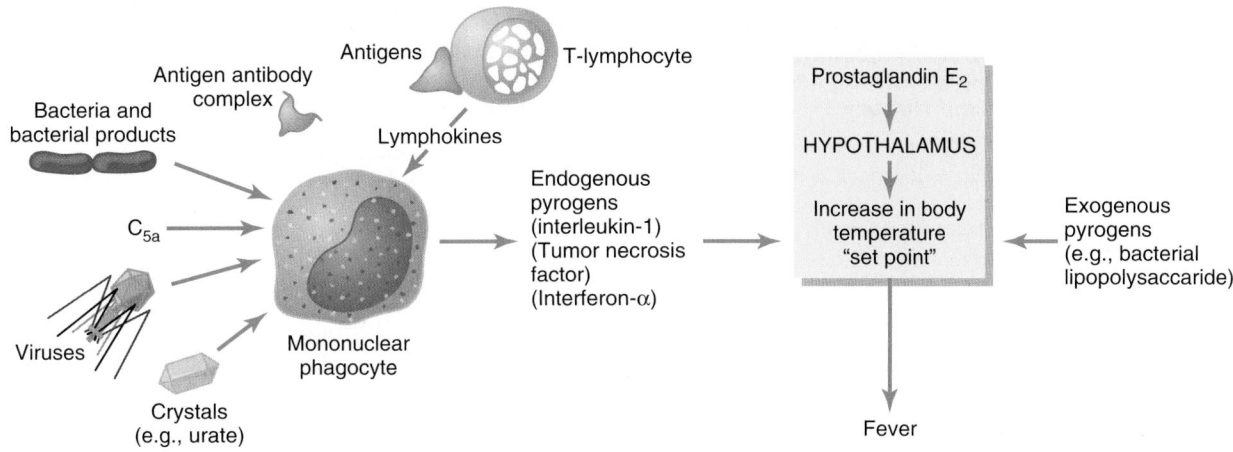

Figure 95-1 Pathogenesis of fever.

patients, the malignant cell may release an endogenous pyrogen. Many immunologically mediated disorders, such as connective tissue diseases, serum sickness, and some drug reactions, are characterized by fever. In most patients with drug-induced fevers, the mechanisms are unknown. Virtually any disorder associated with an inflammatory response (e.g., gouty arthritis) can be associated with fever. Certain endocrine disorders such as thyrotoxicosis, adrenal insufficiency, and pheochromocytoma can also produce fever.

The association of fever with infections or inflammatory disorders raises the question of whether fever is beneficial to the host. For example, IL-1 (an endogenous pyrogen) is critical for initiating the immune response, elevated temperatures marginally enhance certain in vitro immune responses, and some infectious organisms prefer cooler temperatures. It is not certain, however, that fever is helpful to humans in any infectious disease, with the possible exception of neurosyphilis. Fever is deleterious in certain situations. Among individuals with underlying brain disease and even in healthy older persons, fever can produce disorientation and confusion. Fever and the associated tachycardia may compromise patients, especially older individuals with significant cardiopulmonary disease. Fever should be controlled with antipyretics if the patient is particularly uncomfortable or whenever it poses a specific risk to the patient, such as with underlying severe congestive heart failure or myocardial infarction.

Heat stroke almost always results from prolonged exposure to high environmental temperatures and humidity, usually occurring in otherwise healthy individuals after strenuous exercise. Heat stroke is characterized by a body temperature greater than 40.6°C (105°F) and is associated with altered sensorium or coma and with cessation of sweating. Rapid cooling is critical to the patient's survival. Covering the patient with cold (11°C), wet compresses until the core temperature reaches 39°C is the most effective initial therapeutic approach and should be followed by intravenous infusions of fluids appropriate to correct the antecedent fluid and electrolyte losses.

FEVER PATTERNS

The normal diurnal variation in body temperatures results in a peak temperature in the late afternoon or early evening.

This variation often persists when patients have fever. In certain individuals, fever patterns may be helpful in suggesting the cause of fever. Rigors—true shaking chills—often herald a bacterial process (especially bloodstream infection), although they may occur in patients with viral infections, as well as in those with drug or transfusion reactions. Hectic fevers, which are characterized by wide swings in temperature, may indicate the presence of an abscess, disseminated tuberculosis, or collagen vascular diseases. Patients with non-*falciparum* malaria may have a relapsing fever with episodes of shaking chills and high fever, which are separated by 1 to 3 days of normal body temperatures and relative well-being. Medications that may have been recently initiated may cause high, constant fevers. Patients with tuberculosis may be relatively comfortable and unaware of a significantly elevated body temperature. Patients with uremia, diabetic ketoacidosis, or hepatic failure generally have a lower body temperature; thus, normal temperature readings in these settings may indicate infection. Similarly, older patients with infection often fail to mount a febrile response and may experience instead a loss of appetite, confusion, or even hypotension without fever. The administration of nonsteroidal anti-inflammatory drugs (NSAIDs) (e.g., aspirin, ibuprofen) or corticosteroids also blunts or ablates the febrile response.

Acute Febrile Syndromes

Fever is one of the most common complaints that bring patients to a physician. The challenge is in discerning the few individuals who require specific therapy from among the many with self-limited benign illness. The approach is simplified by considering patients in three groups: (1) those with fever without localizing symptoms and signs, (2) those with fever and rash, and (3) those with fever and lymphadenopathy. This chapter deals only with fever caused by microbial agents; however, autoimmune, neoplastic, and other disease processes are important causes of fever as well.

FEVER ONLY

Most patients with fever as their sole complaint defervesce spontaneously or exhibit localizing clinical or laboratory

Table 95-1 Infections Exhibiting Fever as the Sole or Dominant Feature

Infectious Agent	Epidemiologic Exposure and History	Distinctive Clinical and Laboratory Findings
Viral		
Rhinovirus, adenovirus, parainfluenza	None (adenovirus in epidemics)	Often URI symptoms; throat and rectal cultures, viral antigen testing
Enteroviruses	Summer, epidemic	Occasionally, aseptic meningitis, rash, pleurodynia, herpangina; serologic or nucleic acid testing
Influenza	Winter, epidemic	Headache, myalgias, arthralgias; nasopharyngeal culture, viral antigen testing
EBV, CMV	See text	See text; monospot test, quantitative nucleic acid testing
Colorado tick fever	Southwest and northwest tick exposure	Biphasic illness, leukopenia; blood, CSF cultures, serologic or nucleic acid testing
Bacterial		
Staphylococcus aureus	IV drug users, IV catheters, hemodialysis, dermatitis	Must exclude endocarditis; blood cultures
Listeria monocytogenes	Depressed cell-mediated immunity	Meningitis may also be present; blood, CSF cultures
Salmonella Typhi, Salmonella Paratyphi	Food or water contaminated by carrier or patient	Headache, myalgias, diarrhea or constipation, transient rose spots; blood, bone marrow, or stool cultures
Streptococci	Valvular heart disease	Low-grade fever, fatigue; blood cultures
After Animal Exposure		
Coxiella burnetii (Q fever)	Infected animals	Headache, occasionally pneumonitis, hepatitis, culture-negative endocarditis; serologic testing
Leptospira interrogans	Water contaminated by urine from dogs, cats, rodents, small mammals	Headache, myalgias, conjunctival suffusion, biphasic illness, aseptic meningitis; serologic testing
Brucella species	Exposure to cattle or contaminated dairy products	Occasionally epididymitis, sacroiliitis, endocarditis; blood cultures, serologic testing
Ehrlichia chaffeensis	South and southeast deer or dog tick exposure	Acute onset of headache, fever, myalgias; leukopenia and thrombocytopenia; blood smear, serologic or nucleic acid testing
Granulomatous Infection		
Mycobacterium tuberculosis	Exposure to patient with tuberculosis, known positive tuberculin skin test result	Back pain suggests vertebral infection; sterile pyuria or hematuria suggests renal infection; liver or bone marrow cultures, histology
Histoplasma capsulatum	Mississippi and Ohio River valleys	Pneumonitis, oropharyngeal lesions; culture and histology of bone marrow and oral lesions, serologic or antigen testing

CMV, cytomegalovirus; CSF, cerebrospinal fluid; EBV, Epstein-Barr virus; IV, intravenous; URI, upper respiratory infection.

findings within 2 to 3 weeks of the onset of illness (Table 95-1). Beyond 3 weeks, the patient can be considered to have a fever of unknown origin (FUO), a designation with its own circumscribed group of management considerations, as discussed later in this chapter.

Viral Infections

In young, healthy individuals, acute febrile illnesses generally represent viral infections. The causative agent is rarely established, largely because establishing the precise diagnosis seldom has major therapeutic implications. Rhinovirus, coronavirus, parainfluenza, and adenovirus infections are usually, but not invariably, associated with symptoms of coryza or upper respiratory tract infection (e.g., rhinorrhea, sore throat, cough, hoarseness). Respiratory syncytial virus (RSV) and human metapneumovirus (hMPV) infections can range from upper respiratory tract infection to bronchiolitis and severe pneumonia. Human bocavirus is a newly described cause of respiratory tract infections, primarily occurring in children. Enterovirus infections occur predominantly in the summer, usually in an epidemic setting.

Undifferentiated febrile syndromes account for the majority of enteroviral infections, but the etiologic features are more likely to be established definitively when a macular rash, aseptic meningitis, pericarditis, or a characteristic syndrome such as herpangina (vesicular pharyngitis caused by coxsackievirus A) or acute pleurodynia (fever, chest wall pain, and tenderness caused by coxsackievirus B) is present. Serologic surveys also indicate that many arthropod-borne viruses (California encephalitis virus; eastern, western, and Venezuelan equine encephalitis viruses; St Louis encephalitis virus) usually produce mild, self-limited febrile illnesses. West Nile virus, in particular, has recently become a common cause of febrile syndrome (less commonly associated with neurologic manifestations) during the summer months throughout the United States. Influenza causes sore throat, cough, myalgias, arthralgias, and headache in addition to fever; it most often occurs in an epidemic pattern during the winter months. It is unusual, however, for fever to persist beyond 5 days in uncomplicated influenza.

The mononucleosis syndromes caused by Epstein-Barr virus (EBV), primary human immunodeficiency virus (HIV) (see Chapter 108), cytomegalovirus (CMV), and (in rare cases) *Toxoplasma gondii* may sometimes manifest in a typhoidal manner—that is, with high fever but little or no detectable lymph node enlargement. Diagnosis and management are discussed later in the section on generalized lymphadenopathy and mononucleosis syndromes, in keeping with the more typical presentation of these processes. The mononucleosis syndromes are generally self-limited. The need to establish a specific diagnosis therefore is usually not urgent with the exception of acute HIV infection. Viral cultures of the throat and rectum and virus-specific antibodies in acute and convalescent serum samples may allow diagnosis of the specific viral cause. Acute retroviral syndrome (HIV) may require diagnosis through plasma p24 antigen or DNA or RNA polymerase chain reaction (PCR) assays because antibodies are frequently not detectable in the early stages (see Chapter 108).

The recognition of other viral syndromes, however, can be critically important. The outbreak of severe acute respiratory syndrome (SARS) in Southeast Asia highlights the importance of early recognition. In the spring of 2003, several people in local hospitals exhibited a variety of complaints that typically included fever and dry cough. Only through the combined efforts of the global medical community was the epidemic contained and the SARS coronavirus identified as the causative agent. Avian influenza is the latest in a series of emerging viruses to pose the threat of widespread infection. Fever is an important element in the early stages of this disease as well.

Bacterial Infections

Pathogenic bacteria most commonly cause sepsis or disseminated bloodstream infection (see Chapter 96). *Staphylococcus aureus* (**Web Fig. 95-1**) frequently causes sepsis without an obvious primary site of infection. Fever may be the predominant clinical manifestation of the illness. *S. aureus* sepsis should be considered in patients undergoing intravenous therapy with an indwelling catheter, patients on hemodialysis, intravenous drug users, and patients with severe chronic dermatoses. In the patient with *S. aureus* bacteremia, the question of whether intravascular infection exists is key in determining the length of therapy. The following risk factors are associated with infective endocarditis (IE): long duration of symptoms, underlying valvular disease, prior endocarditis, absence of removable focus of infection (e.g., intravenous catheter, soft tissue abscess), metastatic sites of infection (e.g., septic pulmonary emboli, arthritis), younger age, history of injection drug use, and new heart murmur. Transesophageal echocardiogram is frequently necessary to evaluate for an endovascular focus in *S. aureus* bacteremia, especially in patients at high risk for IE (see Chapter 100). *Listeria monocytogenes* bacteremia is seen predominantly in patients with depressed cell-mediated immunity and is the most common presentation of listeriosis in these hosts. Occasionally a relatively indolent clinical syndrome belies the bacterial cause of *S. aureus* and *L. monocytogenes* bacteremia.

Enteric fever—typhoid or paratyphoid fever—may also have fever alone as the primary clinical manifestation. The major species producing this syndrome are *Salmonella* Typhi and *Salmonella* Paratyphi, both of which have humans as their only reservoir. *Salmonella* Paratyphi usually produces less severe disease than *Salmonella* Typhi. Disease is acquired by ingesting food or water contaminated with fecal material from a chronic carrier or a patient with typhoid or paratyphoid fever. A large number of bacteria (10^6 to 10^8) must be ingested to cause disease in the normal host. Major host risk factors are achlorhydria, malnutrition, malignancy (particularly lymphomas), sickle cell anemia, and other defects in cellular and humoral immunity. *Salmonella* Typhi penetrates the gut wall and enters the lymphoid follicles (Peyer patches), where it multiplies within mononuclear phagocytes. Primary bacteremia occurs with spread to the reticuloendothelial system (liver, spleen, and bone marrow). After further multiplication at those sites, secondary bacteremia can occur and localize to lesions such as tumors, aneurysms, and bone infarcts. Infection of the gallbladder, particularly in the presence of gallstones, leads to a chronic carrier state. Approximately 2 weeks after exposure, patients develop prolonged fever with chills, headache, and myalgias. Diarrhea or constipation may be present but usually does not dominate the clinical picture. Occasionally, crops of rose spots (2- to 4-mm salmon-colored maculopapular lesions) appear on the upper abdomen but are evanescent. Typhoid fever usually resolves in about 1 month if left untreated. However, complication rates are high because of bowel perforation, metastatic infection, and the general debility of patients, which may last for months. *Salmonella* Typhi or Paratyphi may be isolated from blood, bone marrow, stool, or rose spots to confirm the diagnosis. Typhoid fever should be treated with third-generation cephalosporins or fluoroquinolones.

Localized bacterial infection can be clinically occult and can develop as an undifferentiated febrile syndrome. Intra-abdominal abscess, vertebral osteomyelitis, streptococcal pharyngitis, urinary tract infection, IE, and early pneumonia may all cause fever with surprisingly few clinical clues to the location of the infection. Therefore urinalysis, throat and blood cultures, and chest radiography should be performed in the patient who is febrile with features suggestive of a bacterial infection.

Eleven cases of inhalational anthrax in the United States in 2001 highlighted this bacterial infection as an important cause of fever without early localizing signs. The illness appeared biphasically with an initial influenza-like illness, followed by sepsis syndrome and severe respiratory distress. All patients had abnormal chest radiographs, with the majority demonstrating pleural effusions, mediastinal widening, and pulmonary infiltrates, with a high rate of positive blood cultures. Early recognition and initiation of appropriate antimicrobial therapy are essential to decreasing mortality. Antimicrobial prophylaxis for individuals with potential exposure is critical, combined with adjunctive postexposure vaccination.

Febrile Syndromes Associated with Animal Exposure

Q fever, brucellosis, and leptospirosis are diseases associated with exposure to fluids from infected animals and may have similar clinical presentations.

Q Fever

Q fever is an under-recognized cause of acute febrile illness. *Coxiella burnetii*, the causative agent, produces mild infection in livestock. Humans are infected by inhalation of aerosolized particles or by contact with hides, placenta, or amniotic fluids from infected animals. The source of animal exposure may go unnoticed.

A self-limited febrile illness is the most common presentation of Q fever. Other clinical syndromes include pneumonia, hepatitis, osteomyelitis, and neurologic manifestations. Pneumonia may be found incidentally during the initial febrile illness and is often accompanied by headache. Definitive diagnosis is usually based on a fourfold rise in titer of complement-fixing antibodies between acute and convalescent samples, as *C. burnetii* is difficult to isolate in culture. The treatment of choice for Q fever is doxycycline. Chronic Q fever may also cause endocarditis, often in the setting of underlying valvular disease or a prosthetic valve. The presence of hepatomegaly, splenomegaly, anemia, and purpuric rash caused by vasculitis in a patient with culture-negative endocarditis may be a clue to this diagnosis. Diagnosis is most often serologic; therapy usually involves prolonged combination antimicrobial therapy including doxycycline.

Leptospirosis

Humans are infected with *Leptospira* species, primarily *Leptospira interrogans*, by exposure to urine from infected animals, usually rodents, small mammals, livestock, dogs, and cats. Indirect exposure is most frequent, occurring by contact with contaminated wet soil or water. Direct contact also occurs in veterinarians, farm workers, hunters, and animal handlers. After an incubation period of approximately 1 week, patients develop chills, high fever, headache, and myalgias. The illness often follows a biphasic course. During the second phase of illness, fever is less prominent, but headache and myalgias are severe; aseptic meningitis is the most important manifestation of the second or immune phase of the illness. Suffusion of the bulbar conjunctivae with visible corkscrew vessels surrounding the limbus is a useful early sign of leptospirosis. Lymphadenopathy, hepatomegaly, and splenomegaly may also occur. Leptospirosis may also pursue a more severe clinical course characterized by renal and hepatic dysfunction and hemorrhagic diathesis (Weil syndrome). Laboratory studies in leptospirosis are often nonspecific but may reveal mild transaminase elevation and increase in serum creatine kinase. Darkfield examination can reveal leptospires in body fluids but has low sensitivity and specificity. Leptospires may also be isolated by culture of blood or cerebrospinal fluid (CSF). The diagnosis is most commonly made serologically by a fourfold rise in the microscopic agglutination test (MAT) antibody titer between acute and convalescent sera. Early antibiotic treatment shortens the duration of fever and may reduce complications. However, to be effective, antibiotics must be initiated presumptively, before serologic confirmation. Intravenous penicillin or ceftriaxone is used for severe disease, and oral doxycycline is effective for mild disease.

Brucellosis

Brucella species infect cattle (*Brucella abortus*), pigs (*Brucella suis*), sheep, and goats (*Brucella melitensis*). Humans are most commonly exposed occupationally via broken skin, aerosolized particles, or inoculation in the conjunctiva or by ingestion of unpasteurized dairy products. Acute disease is nonspecific and is often characterized by chills, fever, headache, and arthralgias and sometimes by lymphadenopathy, hepatomegaly, and splenomegaly. During the associated bacteremia, any organ may be seeded. Epididymo-orchitis, spondylitis (**Web Fig. 95-2**) or sacroiliitis, granulomatous hepatitis, and bone marrow involvement are characteristic localized findings. With or without antibiotic treatment of acute infection, brucellosis may relapse or enter a chronic phase, although treatment does reduce the incidence of complications and relapse. *Brucella* species can be isolated from blood or other normally sterile fluids; however, the diagnosis is often made serologically. Treatment consists of combination therapy with doxycycline plus either rifampin or streptomycin.

Granulomatous Infection
Tuberculosis

Extrapulmonary and miliary tuberculosis (**Web Fig. 95-3**) may cause a febrile syndrome. In disseminated tuberculosis, initial chest radiographs may be normal and tuberculin skin tests are often nonreactive. This finding is particularly true in older or immunocompromised patients. Protracted FUO should always suggest this possibility. Liver biopsy and bone marrow biopsy have a high yield in miliary disease. Genitourinary and vertebral tuberculosis may also develop as unexplained fever. However, careful history, urinalysis, intravenous pyelography, and radiographs of the spine should reveal the site of tissue involvement. Extrapulmonary tuberculosis should be treated for the first 2 months with four-drug therapy with isoniazid, rifampin, ethambutol, and pyrazinamide given orally. Thereafter, isoniazid and rifampin are continued for 7 months (longer in patients with skeletal tuberculosis). The ethambutol can be discontinued once the organism is shown to be sensitive to isoniazid. Corticosteroids may be a useful adjunctive measure in the patient with severe systemic toxicity or central nervous system involvement (see Chapter 97). The dose of corticosteroids should be tapered as soon as the patient shows symptomatic improvement.

Histoplasmosis

Most individuals living in endemic areas in the Mississippi and Ohio River valleys who become infected with *Histoplasma capsulatum* (**Web Fig. 95-4**) have a subclinical, self-limited febrile illness as a manifestation of acute pulmonary histoplasmosis (**Web Fig. 95-5**). Although patients may complain of chest pain or cough, physical examination of the chest is usually unremarkable despite radiographic findings of diffuse infiltrates and mediastinal or hilar adenopathy. Therefore, in the absence of chest radiographs, the lower respiratory tract component of the illness is easily overlooked. Cavitary pulmonary histoplasmosis occurs more insidiously with low-grade fever, productive cough, dyspnea, and weight loss. This syndrome is most likely to occur in older men with underlying chronic lung disease such as emphysema. Isolation of *H. capsulatum* in culture is variable and depends on specimen source and burden of disease. Serology is often used diagnostically, with a complement fixation (CF) antibody titer of at least 1:32 or a fourfold rise in titer being consistent with the diagnosis of acute histoplasmosis. Although spontaneous resolution of symptoms is normal in acute pulmonary histoplasmosis, unusually prolonged illness (more than 4 weeks) may require antifungal treatment with itraconazole or amphotericin B for more severe disease.

Progressive disseminated histoplasmosis may occur as a consequence of reactivation of latent infection in immunosuppressed individuals (e.g., those with acquired immunodeficiency syndrome [AIDS]) (see Chapter 108) or may reflect an uncontrolled primary infection. The febrile illness in such patients is protracted. Oropharyngeal nodules and ulcerative lesions are commonly found in disseminated histoplasmosis, biopsy of such lesions permits rapid diagnosis. Serologic studies are less helpful in disseminated histoplasmosis because they are positive in less than one half of patients. Cultures and Gomori-methenamine or Grocott silver stains of bone marrow biopsy specimens can establish the diagnosis. *Histoplasma* urine antigen detection is a sensitive predictor of disseminated infection. Disseminated histoplasmosis is initially treated with amphotericin B, but patients can often be switched to itraconazole to complete therapy once symptoms resolve. Duration of therapy is often 6 to 12 months, but immunosuppressed patients may require lifelong suppressive therapy.

Other Infections

Malaria characteristically produces febrile paroxysms that occur every 48 (*Plasmodium vivax*) to 72 (*Plasmodium malariae*) hours in some patients. However, during the first few days of illness, the fever may be low grade and sustained or intermittent. The diagnosis should therefore be suggested in all febrile travelers who have returned from endemic areas. Malaria may also occur, albeit rarely, in intravenous drug users and recipients of blood transfusions. *Plasmodium falciparum* (**Web Fig. 95-6**) causes a high level of parasitemia and is associated with a high mortality rate unless recognized and treated promptly. Daily fever often occurs in this form of malaria. Although *P. vivax* and *Plasmodium ovale* may cause relapsing infection long after primary infection because of latent extra-erythrocytic infection in the liver, the course is milder. Demonstration of parasites in blood smears establishes the diagnosis of malaria.

Many, if not most, infectious diseases may exhibit fever as an early finding with subclinical or eventual clinical involvement of specific organ systems. Examples include cryptococcosis, coccidioidomycosis, psittacosis, infection with *Legionella* species, and *Mycoplasma pneumoniae* infections. Pulmonary involvement by these infectious agents often produces few signs on physical examination; chest radiographs often reveal more prominent abnormalities than are clinically suggested.

FEVER AND RASH

Many of the febrile syndromes already discussed may occasionally be associated with a rash (Table 95-2). This section, however, considers diseases in which rash is a prominent feature of the presentation. The most life-threatening infections associated with fever and rash include meningococcemia, staphylococcal toxic shock syndrome (TSS), and Rocky Mountain spotted fever (RMSF).

Bacterial Diseases

Petechial lesions, purpura, and ecthyma gangrenosum are lesions associated with bacteremia (see Chapter 96). Dis-

Table 95-2 Differential Diagnosis of Infectious Agents Producing Fever and Rash

Maculopapular Erythematous

Enterovirus
EBV, CMV, *Toxoplasma gondii*
Acute HIV infection
Colorado tick fever virus
Salmonella Typhi
Leptospira interrogans
Measles virus
Rubella virus
Hepatitis B virus
Treponema pallidum
Parvovirus B19
Human herpesvirus 6

Vesicular

Varicella-zoster virus
Herpes simplex virus
Coxsackievirus A
Vibrio vulnificus

Cutaneous Petechiae

Neisseria gonorrhoeae
Neisseria meningitidis
Rickettsia rickettsii (Rocky Mountain spotted fever)
Rickettsia typhi (murine typhus)
Ehrlichia chaffeensis
Echoviruses
Viridans streptococci (endocarditis)

Diffuse Erythroderma

Group A streptococci (scarlet fever, toxic shock syndrome)
Staphylococcus aureus (toxic shock syndrome)

Distinctive Rash

Ecthyma gangrenosum—*Pseudomonas aeruginosa*
Erythema migrans—Lyme disease

Mucous Membrane Lesions

Vesicular pharyngitis—coxsackievirus A
Palatal petechiae—rubella, EBV, scarlet fever (group A streptococci)
Erythema—toxic shock syndrome (*Staphylococcus aureus* and group A streptococci)
Oral ulceronodular lesion—*Histoplasma capsulatum*
Koplik spots—measles virus

CMV, cytomegalovirus; EBV, Epstein-Barr virus; HIV, human immunodeficiency virus.

seminated gonococcemia (**Web Fig. 95-7**) causes sparse vesiculopustular, hemorrhagic, or necrotic lesions on an erythematous base, typically on the extremities and particularly their dorsal surfaces (see Chapter 107). Meningococcemia is also an important cause of fever and a rash that may range from a few petechiae to, in the most severe cases, purpura fulminans (**Web Fig. 95-8**).

Bacterial toxins produce characteristic clinical syndromes. Pharyngitis or other infections with an erythrogenic toxin-producing *Streptococcus* (**Web Fig. 95-9**) may lead to scarlet fever. Diffuse erythema begins on the upper part of the chest and spreads rapidly, although sparing palms and soles. Small red petechial lesions are found on the palate, and the skin has a sandpaper texture caused by occlusion of the sweat glands. The tongue at first shows a yellowish coating and then becomes beefy red. The rash of scarlet fever (**Web Fig. 95-10**) heals with desquamation. *Arcanobacterium haemolyticum* can also produce pharyngitis and rash.

Streptococcal TSS may also occur as a complication of group A streptococcal soft tissue infections. Major manifestations include cellulitis and/or fasciitis with shock, adult respiratory distress syndrome, renal failure, liver abnormalities, coagulopathy, and a generalized erythematous macular rash. Treatment consists of high-dose penicillin and clindamycin, early surgical intervention, supportive measures, and possibly intravenous immunoglobulin (IVIG). The mortality remains high (>30%) even with optimal current therapy.

Staphylococcal TSS (**Web Figs. 95-11 and 95-12**) was first recognized as a distinct clinical entity in 1978, with an increased number of cases seen in the early 1980s associated with the use of hyperabsorbable tampons. *S. aureus* strains producing TSS toxin (TSST-1) or other closely related exotoxins cause the syndrome. TSST-1 acts as a superantigen by directly binding T lymphocytes to antigen-presenting cells via MHC class II receptors, causing an immense cytokine release and ensuing inflammatory response. Previously, most patients have been 15- to 25-year-old girls and women who use tampons. Emerging settings in which nonmenstrual TSS occurs include use of contraceptive diaphragms, vaginal or cesarean deliveries, nasal surgery, influenza, and recalcitrant desquamative syndrome in patients with AIDS. Superficial staphylococcal infections and abscesses often cause TSS in men. Patients with TSS develop the abrupt onset of high fever (temperature >40°C [104°F]), hypotension, nausea and vomiting, severe watery diarrhea, and myalgias, followed in severe cases by confusion and oliguria. Characteristically, diffuse erythroderma (a sunburn-like rash) with erythematous mucosal surfaces is apparent. Later, intense scaling and desquamation of the skin occur, particularly on the palms and soles. Laboratory abnormalities include elevated levels of liver and muscle enzymes, thrombocytopenia, and hypocalcemia. Diagnosis is based on the clinical findings and requires specific exclusion of RMSF, leptospirosis, measles, and blood or CSF cultures negative for organisms other than *S. aureus*. Management of the patient consists of restoring an adequate circulatory blood volume by the administration of intravenous fluids, drainage of abscesses or débridement of affected tissues if necessary, and treatment of the staphylococcal infection with vancomycin or nafcillin. Vancomycin is the therapy of choice for known methicillin-resistant *S. aureus* (MRSA) or until susceptibilities are known. Prevention of recurrence targets avoidance of further tampon use and eliminating staphylococcal colonization of skin and mucosal sites. Decolonization regimens may include intranasal antibiotics such as mupirocin, antiseptic body washes, and systemic antibiotics such as rifampin along with other agents.

Rickettsial Diseases

In the United States, several rickettsial diseases are endemic including RMSF (**Web Fig. 95-13**), rickettsialpox, and murine typhus. Of these, RMSF is the most virulent, with a case-fatality rate of greater than 20% if early appropriate therapy is not given. Although originally described in the western United States, most cases occur in the South Atlantic south-central states. The causative organism, *Rickettsia rickettsii*, is transmitted from dogs or small wild animals to ticks and then to humans. Infection occurs primarily during warmer months, the periods of greatest tick activity. The tick transmits infection after 6 to 10 hours of feeding and may

be unnoticed. The fulminant onset of severe frontal headache, chills, fever, myalgias, and conjunctivitis occurs after 2 to 14 days; cough and shortness of breath develop in one fourth of patients. The diagnosis may be obscure at the onset. Rash characteristically begins on the third to fifth day of illness as 1- to 4-mm erythematous macules on the hands, wrists, feet, and ankles. Palms and soles may also be involved. The rash may be transient, but it usually spreads to the trunk and may become petechial. Intravascular coagulopathy develops in some patients who are severely ill. Diagnosis and the institution of appropriate therapy must be based on the clinical and epidemiologic findings; delay in treatment may be fatal. Confirmation of the diagnosis is usually retrospective by using an indirect immunofluorescence assay showing detectable serum antibodies during convalescence. Treatment is with doxycycline, given orally or parenterally, or oral tetracycline for 7 days.

Human Ehrlichiosis

Human ehrlichiosis is an acute, febrile illness caused most frequently by *Ehrlichia chaffeensis* (**Web Fig. 95-14**) (human monocytic ehrlichiosis [HME]) or *Anaplasma phagocytophilum* (human granulocytic anaplasmosis [HGA]). *E. chaffeensis* is transmitted by the dog tick *Amblyomma americanum* (the Lone Star tick) and causes illness with peak incidence in the summer months. Since the disease was first recognized in 1986, cases of HME have been identified most frequently in 21 contiguous southeastern states from Maryland to Texas, but have been documented in 47 states. The illness characteristically begins with fever, chills, headache, and myalgias, with a maculopapular rash occurring in less than one third of cases. Although a wide spectrum of illness exists, roughly one half of clinically recognized cases are associated with pulmonary infiltrates. Laboratory studies often reveal leukopenia, thrombocytopenia, and elevated liver transaminases. Acute respiratory distress syndrome often associated with renal failure may develop, most often occurring in older patients. If the disease is left untreated, the mortality rate may exceed 10% in hospitalized patients. More severe illness is usually associated with older age and immunocompromised status (e.g., from HIV, corticosteroid therapy, organ transplantation).

HGA peaks in July and occurs in areas where infected *Ixodes* ticks are found, including the Northeast, parts of the Midwest, and California. Nine percent of patients have concurrent Lyme disease or babesiosis because the same tick vector transmits these diseases. HGA usually exhibits a nonspecific influenza-like illness with fever, chills, malaise, headache, nausea, and vomiting. As in HME, leukopenia, thrombocytopenia, and elevations in hepatic transaminases are important laboratory features. Older patients tend to have more severe disease.

Presumptive diagnosis of HME or HGA is made on clinical grounds in patients with acute febrile illnesses, which are generally associated with decreasing leukocyte and platelet counts after tick exposure. Peripheral blood smears may show intracellular organisms called *morulae* in infected leukocytes, particularly in HGA. Serodiagnosis is sensitive but helpful only in retrospective confirmation of diagnosis. PCR methods for amplifying nucleic acids of *E. chaffeensis* and *A. phagocytophilum* appear to be effective for a timely diagnosis of active infection. Treatment with doxycycline or tetracycline is effective in decreasing both the duration and the severity of illness.

Major clinical distinctions between human ehrlichiosis and RMSF include the earlier, more frequent, and more severe cutaneous manifestations of RMSF and the more common pulmonary manifestations and characteristically decreasing leukocyte counts in ehrlichiosis.

Lyme Disease

Lyme disease is a common, multisystem spirochetal infection caused by *Borrelia burgdorferi* (**Web Fig. 95-15**) and is transmitted by the *Ixodes* species of ticks, *Ixodes scapularis* in the East and Midwest US and *Ixodes pacificus* in California. The largest number of cases are distributed in areas that correspond to distribution of the *Ixodes* vectors (the Northeast, Wisconsin, Minnesota, California, and Oregon); however, the infection is distributed broadly throughout North America and Western Europe. Between 3 days and 3 weeks after the tick bite, of which most individuals are unaware, patients develop a mild febrile illness, usually associated with headache, stiff neck, myalgias, arthralgias, and erythema migrans (EM) (**Web Fig. 95-16**). EM begins as a red macule or papule at the site of the tick bite; the surrounding bright red patch expands to a diameter of up to 15 cm. Partial central clearing is often seen. The centers of lesions may become indurated, vesicular, or necrotic, and several red rings may be found within the outer border. Smaller secondary lesions that are caused by disseminated spirochetes may appear within several days. Lesions are warm but nontender. Enlargement of regional lymph nodes is common. The rash usually fades in several weeks without treatment.

Several weeks after the onset of symptoms, important neurologic manifestations occur in more than 15% of patients. Most characteristic is meningoencephalitis with cranial nerve involvement and peripheral radiculoneuropathy. Bell palsy may occur as an isolated phenomenon; when associated with fever, this finding is strongly suggestive of Lyme disease. The CSF at this time shows a lymphocytic pleocytosis of approximately 100 cells/mL. Heart involvement may also exhibit as atrioventricular block, myopericarditis, or cardiomegaly.

Joint involvement eventually occurs in 60% of untreated patients. Early in the course, arthralgias and myalgias may be quite severe. Months later, arthritis often develops with significant swelling and little pain in one or two large joints, typically the knee. Episodes of arthritis may recur for months or years; in about 10% of patients the arthritis becomes chronic, and erosion of cartilage and bone occurs.

Diagnosis is usually based on a compatible clinical syndrome, potential exposure in an endemic area, and positive serologic testing. Serologic testing should not be performed in the setting of EM, as antibodies are likely to be negative in the first 1 to 2 weeks of disease. Serologic testing is performed in a two-step approach with an initial enzyme-linked immunosorbent assay (ELISA), followed by a confirmatory Western blot in those with positive or equivocal ELISA results. By 1 month of disease, essentially all patients with active infection have positive immunoglobulin G (IgG) titers. Antibody responses wane slowly after treatment but may remain present for years after infection. Antibodies to *B. burgdorferi* may also be detected in CSF in acute neu-

roborreliosis. In Lyme arthritis, synovial fluid contains an average of 25,000 cells/mL, mostly neutrophils. Synovial fluid PCR for *B. burgdorferi* DNA provides a moderately sensitive means of diagnosis before antibiotic treatment.

Treatment with doxycycline 200 mg orally within 72 hours of a deer tick bite in an endemic area appears to decrease the subsequent development of Lyme disease. Treatment of the early manifestations of Lyme disease with doxycycline or amoxicillin for 14 to 21 days usually prevents late complications. Neurologic and cardiac involvement should be treated with intravenous aqueous penicillin G or ceftriaxone for 14 to 28 days; first-degree atrioventricular block or an isolated facial palsy can usually be treated with an oral regimen. Arthritis can be treated with oral therapy for 30 to 60 days or intravenously for 14 to 28 days.

Viral Infections

The rashes associated with viral infections may be so typical as to establish unequivocally the cause of the febrile syndrome (**Web Table 95-1**). Varicella-zoster requires special consideration because of the availability of effective antiviral drugs. In normal children under the age of 12, antiviral therapy is not required for the treatment of chickenpox. However, for patients over age 12, those with chronic cutaneous or pulmonary disease, those receiving salicylate therapy, and immunocompromised hosts should receive antivirals because these patients are at higher risk for complications. Dermatomal herpes zoster should be treated in those older than age 50 to decrease the incidence, severity, and duration of post-herpetic neuralgia (PHN). Immunocompromised patients with herpes zoster should also be treated to prevent dissemination of infection. In addition, ophthalmic zoster demands antiviral treatment because of its association with vision loss related to the development of keratitis, iridocyclitis, or secondary glaucoma. In general, more severe disease with either chickenpox or herpes zoster requires intravenous acyclovir therapy, whereas milder disease may be treated orally with acyclovir or valacyclovir. Acute onset of high fever characterizes viral hemorrhagic fevers, along with, in some cases, bleeding complications and high mortality rates. Arthropod vectors usually transmit these infections; in some patients, they are acquired by direct contact with the reservoir animal or with infected persons and their body fluids. These illnesses include dengue, Marburg hemorrhagic, Ebola hemorrhagic, and Lassa fevers.

FEVER AND LYMPHADENOPATHY

Many infectious diseases are associated with some degree of lymph node enlargement. However, in some diseases, lymphadenopathy is a major manifestation. Lymph node enlargement can be further divided according to whether the enlargement is generalized or regional.

Generalized Lymphadenopathy: Mononucleosis Syndromes

The mononucleosis syndromes are important causes of fever and generalized lymph node enlargement.

Epstein-Barr Virus Infection

Approximately 90% of American adults have serologic evidence of EBV infection; most infections are subclinical and

Table 95-3	**Most Common Infectious Causes of Heterophil-Negative Atypical Lymphocytosis**
Babesiosis	
Chickenpox	
Cytomegalovirus	
Epstein-Barr virus (particularly in children)	
Human herpesvirus 6	
Human immunodeficiency virus (especially during acute seroconversion)	
Infectious mononucleosis	
Malaria	
Measles	
Toxoplasmosis	
Varicella	
Infectious hepatitis	

Table 95-4	**Differential Diagnosis of Monospot-Negative Mononucleosis**
Acute HIV infection	
EBV mononucleosis (particularly in children)	
Cytomegalovirus	
Acute toxoplasmosis	
Streptococcal pharyngitis	
Acute hepatitis B infection	

EBV, Epstein-Barr virus; HIV, human immunodeficiency virus.

occur before the age of 5 years or midway through adolescence. EBV causes approximately 80% of clinical cases of infectious mononucleosis. This acute illness usually develops late in adolescence after intimate contact with asymptomatic oropharyngeal shedders of EBV. Patients develop sore throat, fever, and generalized lymphadenopathy and sometimes experience headache and myalgias. From 5% to 10% of patients have a transient rash that may be macular, petechial, or urticarial. Palatal petechiae are often present, as is pharyngitis, which may be exudative. Cervical lymph node enlargement, particularly involving the posterior lymphatic chains, is prominent, although some involvement elsewhere is common. The spleen is palpably enlarged in about 50% of patients. Thrombocytopenia and hepatitis are common laboratory abnormalities. Autoimmune hemolytic anemia, encephalitis or aseptic meningitis, Guillain-Barré syndrome, and splenic rupture are rare but severe complications of EBV infection. The enlarged spleen may be very fragile, necessitating avoidance of contact sports and caution in splenic palpation. Three fourths of patients exhibit an absolute lymphocytosis. At least one third of their lymphocytes are atypical in appearance: large, with vacuolated basophilic cytoplasm, rolled edges often deformed by contact with other cells, and lobulated, eccentric nuclei. Immunologic studies indicate that some circulating B cells are infected with EBV and that the cells involved in the lymphocytosis are mainly reactive cytotoxic T cells. Atypical lymphocytes may also be seen in other viral illnesses (Table 95-3).

B-cell infection with EBV is a stimulus to the production of polyclonal antibodies. Heterophile antibody tests such as the Monospot rapid diagnostic test are sensitive and specific; false-positive results occur in rare cases in patients with lymphoma or hepatitis. Virus-specific antibodies also are produced in response to infection. The presence of IgM antibody to viral capsid antigen (VCA) is virtually diagnostic of acute infectious mononucleosis. The appearance of antibody to EBV nuclear antigen occurs late in the course of infection and is also indicative of recent EBV infection. These antibodies persist lifelong.

Infectious mononucleosis usually has a benign course with complete recovery even in patients with neurologic involvement, and fatalities are rare. The fever resolves after 1 to 2 weeks, although residual fatigue may be protracted. In general, patients should be managed symptomatically. Antibiotics, particularly ampicillin, should be avoided as the use of ampicillin causes a classic rash in almost all patients with EBV infection. This phenomenon can also be a diagnostic clue to the occurrence of EBV infection. Because EBV infection is predominantly latent, there is no role or available antiviral therapy directed against EBV. Corticosteroids are indicated in the rare individual with serious hematologic involvement (e.g., thrombocytopenia, hemolytic anemia) or impending airway obstruction as a result of massive tonsillar swelling. Acute bacterial superinfections of the pharynx and peritonsillar tissues should be considered when the course is unusually septic. Rarely, patients can have a persistent or recurrent syndrome with evidence of ongoing organ dysfunction including hemophagocytosis, lymphadenitis, hepatitis, and interstitial pneumonia with serologic evidence of chronic active EBV infection. In contrast to the majority of patients with acute infectious mononucleosis, these patients have a poor prognosis.

The differential diagnosis of Monospot-negative mononucleosis is shown in Table 95-4.

Cytomegalovirus

Serologic surveys indicate that by adulthood most people have been infected with CMV, but seroprevalence varies by country. In the United States, 60% to 70% of the population has been infected, and this approaches 100% in some parts of Africa. The ages of peak incidence of CMV infection are in the perinatal period (transmission via the birth canal or by breast milk) and during the second to fourth decades of life. Congenital CMV acquired in utero is usually a result of primary infection in the mother and can be fatal. Like other herpesviruses, CMV can establish latency after primary infection, leading to a potential for reactivation. This is often related to immune suppression.

There are several important modes of transmission in adults. CMV can be transmitted sexually, and virus can be isolated from both semen and the uterine cervix. The frequency of antibody to CMV and active viral excretion has been shown to correlate with number of sexual partners. Contact with oral secretions and fecal-oral transmission are the main sources of CMV infection within households and in child day-care workers. In addition, blood transfusions carry a risk of approximately 3% per unit of blood for transmitting CMV infection. This risk becomes substantial in the setting of open-heart surgery or multiple transfusions for other indications. The use of seronegative or

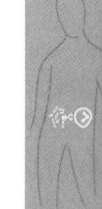

leukocyte-depleted blood products can minimize the risk of CMV transmission, particularly in high-risk CMV seronegative hematopoietic stem cell transplant recipients.

Primary infection with CMV causes a major proportion of cases of Monospot-negative mononucleosis (see Table 95-4). The distinction between CMV and EBV may be impossible on clinical grounds alone. However, CMV tends to involve older patients (mean age 29) and often produces milder disease, is less likely to cause pharyngitis, and often causes high fever with little or no peripheral lymph node enlargement. The infrequent but serious forms of neurologic and hematologic involvement that develop in EBV infection occur less commonly with CMV. As with EBV infection, hepatitis (which is usually mild and may be granulomatous) is common. Diagnosis of primary infection is usually made serologically by indirect fluorescent or CF antibody testing. The IgM antibody in particular is specific for primary infection. Isolation of CMV from body fluids or tissues can also be diagnostic in primary or reactivation of latent infection. CMV hybrid capture and PCR techniques have been developed to provide rapid laboratory diagnosis of CMV viremia and can be useful in certain patient groups such as solid organ or hematopoietic stem cell transplant recipients. CMV mononucleosis is usually a self-limited disease that does not require specific therapy. CMV infection in the immunocompromised host may be life threatening; in this setting it usually responds to therapy with ganciclovir, valganciclovir, or foscarnet.

Primary HIV Infection (Acute Retroviral Syndrome)

Typical presenting features of primary HIV infection overlap those of the mononucleosis syndrome (see Chapter 108). Although most patients with the acute retroviral syndrome seek medical attention, the correct diagnosis is missed in a large number of cases because of physician failure to consider HIV infection. Because it is of critical importance to both the patient and his or her sexual partners to establish this diagnosis (see Chapter 108), primary HIV infection must be considered in all patients with mononucleosis syndromes.

Toxoplasmosis

T. gondii is a parasite of cats and other felids. *T. gondii* is acquired in humans by ingestion of tissue cysts in undercooked meat, by ingestion of food or water contaminated by oocysts, or congenitally. Seroprevalence of *T. gondii* infection varies geographically, with rates in Western Europe and Africa being much higher than in the United States. Overall age-adjusted seroprevalence in the United States has been reported to be 22.5%. Seropositivity in HIV-infected patients in the United States is similar to that in the non–HIV-infected population. Only between 10% and 20% of infections in normal adults are symptomatic. Presentation may take the form of a mononucleosis-like syndrome, although maculopapular rash, abdominal pain caused by mesenteric and retroperitoneal lymphadenopathy, and chorioretinitis may also occur. Striking lymph node enlargement and involvement of unusual chains (occipital or lumbar) may necessitate lymph node biopsy to exclude lymphoma. More commonly, cervical adenopathy is observed in symptomatic patients. Overall, however, toxoplasmosis accounts for less than 1% of mononucleosis-like illnesses. Histologically,

focal distention of sinuses with mononuclear phagocytes, histiocytes blurring the margins of germinal centers, and reactive follicular hyperplasia indicate *Toxoplasma* infection. Acute acquired toxoplasmosis is suggested by the conversion of *T. gondii*–specific IgG and IgM antibodies from negative to positive; several different serologic tests are available including the Sabin-Feldman dye test, indirect fluorescent antibody test, and ELISA. Acute acquired toxoplasmosis is generally self-limited in the immunologically intact host and does not require specific therapy. Significant involvement of the eye or viscera is an indication for treatment with pyrimethamine plus sulfadiazine. Infection in immunocompromised hosts usually reflects reactivation of latent infection rather than acute acquired infection. Clinical manifestations are protean and often severe, the most common being encephalitis, pneumonitis, and myocarditis. Treatment with combination antimicrobial therapy is necessary.

Granulomatous Disease

Disseminated tuberculosis, histoplasmosis, and sarcoidosis may be associated with generalized lymphadenopathy, although involvement of certain lymph node chains can predominate. Lymph node biopsy shows granulomas or nonspecific hyperplasia.

Regional Lymphadenopathy
Pyogenic Infection

S. aureus and group A streptococcal infections produce acute suppurative lymphadenitis. The most frequently affected lymph nodes are submandibular, cervical, inguinal, and axillary, in that order. Involved nodes are large (>3 cm), tender, and firm or fluctuant. Pyoderma, pharyngitis, or periodontal infection may be present at the presumed primary site of infection. Patients are febrile and have leukocytosis. Fluctuant nodes should be aspirated. Otherwise, antibiotic therapy should be directed toward the most common pathogens. Penicillin G therapy is appropriate if pharyngeal or periodontal origin implicates a streptococcal or mixed anaerobic infection. Skin involvement suggests possible staphylococcal infection and is an indication for vancomycin or an oral antimicrobial with activity against MRSA (e.g., clindamycin, doxycycline, or trimethoprim-sulfamethoxazole) until susceptibilities are known. The dose and route of administration of the drug should be determined by the severity of the infection.

Tuberculosis

Scrofula, or tuberculous cervical adenitis, develops in a subacute to chronic fashion. Fever, if present, is low grade. A large mass of matted lymph nodes is palpable in the neck. In children, if *Mycobacterium tuberculosis* is the causative organism, then other sites of active infection are usually present from ongoing primary infection. In adults, extranodal disease is rare. The most common causative agent of lymphadenitis in children in the United States is *Mycobacterium avium* complex, followed by *Mycobacterium scrofulaceum.* Surgical excision is the treatment of choice and usually does not require chemotherapy.

Cat-Scratch Disease

Chronic regional lymphadenopathy after exposure to a cat scratch, lick, or bite should suggest the diagnosis. About 1 week after contact with the cat, a local papule or pustule may develop. One week later, regional adenopathy appears, usually of the head, neck, or upper extremity. Lymph nodes may be tender (sometimes exquisitely so) or just enlarged (1 to 7 cm). Fever is low grade if present at all. Lymph node enlargement usually persists for several months. The diagnosis can usually be established on clinical grounds. Lymph node biopsy shows necrotic granulomas with giant cells and stellate abscesses surrounded by epithelial cells. Pleomorphic gram-negative bacilli of *Bartonella henselae* can be identified in the lymph node biopsy specimens by a Warthin-Starry stain during the first 4 weeks of illness. Serologic testing can confirm the diagnosis. The course is usually self-limited and benign in immunocompetent individuals even without antimicrobial therapy but may be life threatening in persons with severe immunodeficiency. The best approach to the treatment of cat-scratch disease in the immunocompromised patient is not known, but erythromycin, azithromycin, or doxycycline may be helpful.

Ulceroglandular Fever

Tularemia is the classic cause of ulceroglandular fever. The syndrome is acquired by contact with tissues or fluids from an infected animal (including rabbits, beavers, squirrels, or birds) or the bite of an infected tick. Patients have chills, fever, an ulcerated skin lesion at the site of inoculation, and painful regional adenopathy. When infection is acquired by contact with animals, the skin lesion is usually on the fingers or hand, and lymph node involvement is epitrochlear or axillary. In tick-borne transmission, the ulcer is on the lower extremities, perianal region, trunk, head, or neck and the adenopathy is inguinal, femoral, occipital, or cervical. Most cases are diagnosed serologically, because Gram-stained preparations are usually negative; however, the causative organism, *Francisella tularensis,* may be isolated from blood, lymph nodes, and other body fluids if supportive media are used. *F. tularensis* is hazardous to laboratory personnel, who should be notified if this organism is suspected. A fourfold rise in agglutination titer between acute and convalescent serum confirms the diagnosis. PCR techniques for rapid diagnosis have also been developed and may be more sensitive than culture. Patients should be treated with streptomycin as the drug of choice for 7 to 14 days. Quinolones, doxycycline, and chloramphenicol are alternative agents with activity against *F. tularensis.*

Oculoglandular Fever

Conjunctivitis with preauricular lymphadenopathy can occur in tularemia, cat-scratch disease, sporotrichosis, lymphogranuloma venereum infection, listeriosis, and epidemic keratoconjunctivitis caused by adenovirus.

Inguinal Lymphadenopathy

Inguinal lymphadenopathy associated with sexually transmitted diseases (see Chapter 107) may be bilateral or unilateral. In primary syphilis, enlarged nodes are discrete, firm, and nontender. Early lymphogranuloma venereum causes tender lymphadenopathy with later matting of involved nodes and sometimes fixation to overlying skin, which assumes a purplish hue. The lymphadenopathy of chancroid is most often unilateral, is very painful, and is composed of fused lymph nodes. Tender inguinal lymphadenopathy

also occurs in primary genital herpes simplex virus infection.

Plague

Bubonic plague usually causes fever, headache, and a large mat of inguinal, axillary, or cervical regional lymph nodes near the site of the infected flea bite, which go on to suppurate and drain spontaneously. Plague, caused by *Yersinia pestis,* is an important consideration in the acutely ill patient in the southwestern United States with possible exposure to fleas and rodents. If plague is suggested, then blood cultures and aspirates of the buboes should be obtained, and streptomycin therapy should be instituted. Gram-stained preparations of the aspirate reveal gram-negative coccobacilli in two thirds of patients. A Wayson stain will reveal the characteristic safety-pin appearance of *Y. pestis* with dark blue staining polar bodies. Various serologic tests also allow for a rapid specific diagnosis as soon as 5 days after the onset of illness. Both plague and tularemia are potential bioterrorism agents.

Fever of Unknown Origin

Fever of unknown origin is the term applied to febrile illnesses with temperatures exceeding 38.3°C (101°F) that are of at least 3 weeks' duration and remain undiagnosed after 3 days in the hospital or after three outpatient visits. Improvements in noninvasive diagnostic testing have resulted in newly proposed categories of FUO (Table 95-5). They include (1) classic FUO, for which the common causes are infections, malignancy, rheumatologic or connective tissue diseases, and drug fever; (2) nosocomial FUO; (3) neutropenic (<500 neutrophils/mm³) FUO; and (4) HIV-associated FUO (see later discussion). The evaluation of FUO remains among the

---

Table 95-5 Fever of Unknown Origin—Definitions

Classic FUO

Fever ≥38.3°C (101°F) on multiple occasions
Duration ≤3 weeks
Uncertain diagnosis after investigations (3 hospital days or 3 outpatient visits)

Nosocomial FUO

Fever ≥38.3°C (101°F) on multiple occasions in hospitalized patient
Infection not incubating on admission
Uncertain diagnosis after 3-day evaluation, including 2-day microbiologic culture incubation

Neutropenic FUO

Fever ≥38.3°C (101°F) on multiple occasions
Absolute neutrophil count <500 cells/mm³
Uncertain diagnosis after 3-day evaluation, including 2-day microbiologic culture incubation

HIV-Associated FUO

Fever ≥38.3°C (101°F) on multiple occasions
Confirmed diagnosis of HIV infection
Fever 1 month (outpatients) or >3 days (inpatients)
Uncertain diagnosis after 3-day evaluation, including 2-day microbiologic culture incubation

FUO, fever of undetermined origin; HIV, human immunodeficiency virus.

most challenging problems facing the physician. Many illnesses that cause FUO are treatable, making the pursuit of the diagnosis particularly rewarding. No substitute for a meticulous history taking and physical examination exists; both should be repeated frequently during both the patient's hospital course and outpatient visits because recurrent questioning of the patient may reveal an important historical clue, and important physical findings may develop after the initial evaluation. These clues may direct the next series of diagnostic studies. Patients with FUO should always be offered HIV testing. Directed biopsy specimens of lesions should be stained and cultured for pathogenic microbes. In many instances, however, localizing clues are not present or fail to yield rewarding information. In these patients, bone marrow biopsy can reveal granulomatous or neoplastic disease, even in the absence of clinical evidence of bone marrow involvement. Similarly, liver biopsy may also reveal the cause of FUO but seldom in the absence of any clinical or laboratory evidence of liver disease. Exploratory laparotomy is rarely needed for diagnosis of FUO, as most anatomic abnormalities are able to be detected by computed tomography (CT) when used in combination with symptoms, signs, and laboratory abnormalities suggestive of an abdominal source of FUO. If tuberculosis remains a reasonable possibility after careful workup fails to establish a diagnosis, then an empiric trial of antituberculous therapy may be initiated while one awaits results of bone marrow, liver, and urine cultures.

Table 95-6 indicates the final diagnoses in a study of over 100 patients with FUO observed in the decade from 1970 to 1980. More recent studies have shown decreases over time in infections and malignancies as the causes of FUO, with increases in rheumatologic and connective tissue diseases and undiagnosed fevers. In general, infections and connective tissue diseases currently each cause approximately 15% to 25% of FUO cases, with malignancy usually causing less than 20% of cases. Undiagnosed FUO cases vary widely among studies; however, patients who remained undiagnosed after a thorough evaluation have an overall good prognosis. Table 95-6 emphasizes the range of diagnostic possibilities to be considered. Numbers of patients in each category are not presented because regional and temporal variations in the frequency of specific diagnoses are great.

CAUSES OF FEVERS OF UNKNOWN ORIGIN

Infections

Abscesses account for approximately one quarter to one third of infectious causes of FUO. Most of these abscesses are intra-abdominal or pelvic in origin because abscesses elsewhere (e.g., lung, brain, superficial abscesses) are more readily identifiable radiographically or as a result of the signs or symptoms they produce.

Intra-abdominal abscesses generally occur as a complication of surgery or leakage of visceral contents, as might occur with the perforation of a colonic diverticulum or appendicitis. Surprisingly, large abdominal abscesses may be present with few localizing symptoms. This development is especially true in the older or immunocompromised patient. Abscesses of the liver (see Chapter 102) occur most often as a consequence of inflammatory disease of the biliary tract or of the bowel; in the latter instance, bacteria reach the liver through portal blood flow. Liver abscesses can also be amebic in cause, especially in a traveler returning from an endemic area. Occasionally, blunt trauma predisposes the liver or spleen to abscesses, but splenic abscesses are often hematogenous in origin. Hepatic, splenic, or subdiaphragmatic abscesses are generally readily detected by ultrasonography or a CT scan. However, diagnosis of intra-abdominal abscess may be challenging because even large abscesses in the pericolonic spaces may be difficult to distinguish from fluid-filled loops of bowel on CT. Gallium or tagged white blood cell scanning, ultrasonography, or barium enemas may assist if the diagnosis is probable and a CT scan is not definitive.

Endovascular infections (IE, mycotic aneurysms, and infected atherosclerotic plaques) are uncommon causes of FUO because blood cultures are generally positive unless the patient has received antibiotics within the preceding 2 weeks. Infections of intravascular catheter sites are generally also associated with bacteremia unless the infection is limited to the insertion site. Diagnosis of endovascular infection is more difficult to make when blood cultures are negative because of infection with slow-growing or fastidious organisms, such as *Brucella* species, *C. burnetii* (Q fever), *Bartonella* species, or *Haemophilus* species. Diagnosis is especially difficult among patients who have been treated with antimicrobial agents. If endocarditis is suggested, then blood cultures should be repeated for at least 1 week after antimicrobial agents have been discontinued, the bacteriologic laboratory should be alerted to the possibility of infection with a fastidious organism, and evidence of valvular vegetations should be sought by transesophageal echocardiography (see Chapter 100). Occasionally, the suggestion of valvular infection is strong enough to warrant empiric antibiotic treatment of a presumed culture-negative endocarditis.

Table 95-6 **Fever of Unknown Origin: Possible Diagnoses**
Infections
Intra-abdominal abscesses
Subphrenic
Splenic
Diverticular
Liver and biliary tract
Pelvic
Mycobacterial
Cytomegalovirus
Infection of the urinary tract
Sinusitis
Osteomyelitis
Catheter infections
Other infections
Neoplastic diseases
Hematologic neoplasms
Non-Hodgkin lymphoma
Leukemia
Hodgkin disease
Solid tumors
Collagen diseases
Granulomatous diseases
Drug fever
Factitious fever

Data from Larson EB, Featherstone HJ, Petersdorf RG: Fever of undetermined origin: Diagnosis and follow-up of 105 cases, 1970-1980. Medicine 61:269-292, 1982.

Although most patients with osteomyelitis have pain at the site of infection, localizing symptoms are occasionally absent and patients have only fever. Technetium pyrophosphate bone scans and gallium scans demonstrate uptake at sites of osteomyelitis, but positive scans are not always specific for infection. Magnetic resonance imaging can be especially useful in differentiating between bone and soft tissue infections (see Chapter 101).

Mycobacterial infections, most frequently with *M. tuberculosis,* remain important causes of FUO. Patients with impaired cell-mediated immunity are at particular risk for disseminated tuberculosis, and occult infection with this organism is seen with particular frequency among older patients, AIDS patients, patients after organ transplantation, and those undergoing hemodialysis. Fever may be the only sign of this infection. Among both immunocompromised patients and previously healthy persons with disseminated tuberculosis, purified protein derivative skin test results are often negative. In some patients, careful review of chest radiographs reveals apical calcifications or upper lobe scars suggestive of remote tuberculous infection. A diffuse, often subtle radiographic pattern of *millet seed* densities, which is best visualized on the lateral chest views, is highly suggestive of disseminated tuberculosis. In this setting, transbronchial or open lung biopsy will establish the diagnosis, as sputum cultures may be positive in only 25%. Similar radiographic patterns may be seen in sarcoidosis, disseminated fungal infection (e.g., histoplasmosis), and some malignancies. Bone marrow or liver biopsy often reveals granulomas, and cultures of these samples are positive in 50% to 90% of patients with disseminated tuberculosis.

Viral infections, especially those caused by CMV or EBV, can produce prolonged fevers. Both infections may be seen in young, healthy adults. Recipients of blood are at risk for acute post-transfusion CMV infection. Recipients of solid organ or hematopoietic stem cell transplantation and other immunosuppressed patients may experience reactivation of latent CMV infection producing fever, leukopenia, and pulmonary and hepatic disease. Lymph nodes are often enlarged in EBV infection, and a peripheral blood smear usually reveals lymphocytosis with increased numbers of atypical lymphocytes. Occasionally, the atypical lymphocytosis is delayed several weeks after the onset of fever. A positive Monospot test result may clarify the diagnosis. Unexplained fever may be a complication of infection with HIV; most such fevers are attributable to concomitant opportunistic infections (see Chapter 108).

Simple lower urinary tract infections are readily diagnosed by symptoms and urinalysis. Complicated infections such as perinephric, renal, or prostatic abscess may be occult and result in FUO. In general, a history of antecedent urinary tract infection or disorder of the urinary tract is present. In prostatic abscess the prostate is usually tender on rectal examination. In suggested cases of perinephric, renal, or prostatic abscesses, the urinalysis should be repeated if it is initially normal because abnormalities of the sediment may be intermittent. Ultrasonography or a CT scan detects most of these lesions (see Chapter 105).

Although most patients with sinusitis have localizing symptoms, infections of the paranasal sinuses may occasionally exhibit fever only, particularly among hospitalized patients who have had nasotracheal and/or nasogastric intu-bation. Sinus films reveal fluid in the sinuses. Infection of the sphenoidal sinus may be difficult to detect unless special views or CT scans are obtained.

Neoplastic Diseases

Neoplasms account for less than 20% of FUOs. Some tumors, particularly those of hematologic origin and hypernephromas, release endogenous pyrogens. In others, the mechanism of fever is less clear but it may result from pyrogen release by infiltrating or surrounding inflammatory cells. Lymphomas can cause FUO; usually enlargement of lymph nodes or the spleen is found. The presentation of some lymphomas is with intra-abdominal disease only. CT scans may be helpful in detecting these tumors. Leukemia may also cause FUO, sometimes with a normal peripheral blood smear. Bone marrow examination reveals an increased number of blast forms. Solid tumors more typically associated with fevers include renal cell carcinoma, atrial myxoma, sarcoma, primary hepatocellular carcinoma, and tumor metastatic to the liver. Liver function abnormalities (predominantly alkaline phosphatase) are common in all these tumors except in atrial myxoma. Myxoma can be suggested in the presence of heart murmur and multisystem embolization (mimicking endocarditis) and is readily diagnosed by echocardiogram. Radiographic studies of the abdomen and retroperitoneum (CT or ultrasonography) generally detect the other tumors. Colon carcinoma must also be considered in the differential diagnosis, because one third or more of patients with this diagnosis may have low-grade fever; in some this is the only sign of disease.

Other Causes

Collagen vascular diseases account for approximately one quarter of FUOs, and this proportion has increased over time. Systemic lupus erythematosus is readily diagnosed clinically and serologically and thus accounts for a small proportion of patients with FUO. Vasculitis remains an important cause of FUO and should be suggested in febrile patients with embolization, infarctions, or multisystem disease. Giant cell arteritis should be considered in older patients with FUO, particularly in the presence of polymyalgia rheumatica symptoms (see Chapter 86). Systemic onset juvenile rheumatoid arthritis, or Still disease, can cause FUO with joint symptoms. An evanescent rash, sore throat, adenopathy, and leukocytosis may occur in this disorder, which is diagnosed on the basis of clinical criteria in the absence of other potential causes of fever.

Granulomatous diseases without a defined cause have been associated with FUO. Sarcoidosis often involves the lungs, skin, and lymph nodes. The majority of patients are anergic to skin test antigens. Diagnosis is based on the exclusion of an infectious cause and the demonstration of discrete, noncaseating granulomas on biopsy of bone marrow, liver, lung, or other tissues. Granulomatous hepatitis can exhibit prolonged fevers, occasionally lasting for years. Serum alkaline phosphatase levels are generally elevated; liver biopsy reveals granulomas, and no underlying cause can be demonstrated.

A number of miscellaneous disorders, including inflammatory bowel disease, hereditary periodic fever syndromes, hematoma, hyperthyroidism and other endocrinologic causes, disordered heat homeostasis, and hypertriglyceridemia make up the remainder of diagnosed FUO cases. Hereditary periodic fever syndromes include familial Mediterranean fever (FMF), TNF receptor-1 associated periodic syndrome (TRAPS), and hyper-IgD syndrome, as well as others. In the appropriate setting, drug-related fevers always demand consideration in the differential diagnosis. Fever may occur without other evidence of drug sensitivity such as rash or eosinophilia in more than 75% of cases. The fever may develop weeks to months after initiation of the drug. Although relatively more common with anticonvulsants (phenytoin and carbamazepine), antimicrobials (sulfonamides, penicillins, nitrofurantoin, and vancomycin), and antihypertensives (hydralazine and methyldopa), fever may occasionally result from any class of drug. A variable number of FUOs (10% to more than 50% in various studies) remains undiagnosed after careful evaluation. Most of these patients have experienced an indefinable but self-limited illness, with fewer than 10% developing an underlying serious disorder after several years of follow-up.

FEVER OF UNKNOWN ORIGIN IN SPECIAL GROUPS

Besides patients with *classic* FUO, several other groups of patients with fever in whom the diagnosis is not readily apparent deserve special attention. These special groups are encountered more frequently in clinical practice and include patients with nosocomial FUO (see Table 95-6).

Nosocomial Fever of Unknown Origin

Most patients with nosocomial FUO have significant underlying comorbidities that lead to hospitalization and complex treatment. The hospital environment, invasive procedures, foreign devices, antibiotic resistance, and alteration of host defenses by diseases or therapy set the stage for potentially unique infectious complications. Bacterial and fungal infections of the urinary tract, surgical wounds, respiratory tract, sinuses, bloodstream, and vascular catheter sites are significant concerns. A frequent cause of nosocomial FUO is *Clostridium difficile*–associated colitis, especially if diarrhea is minimal or absent. This disease is more often encountered in older patients, and a clue to the diagnosis can be an unexplained leukocytosis. Nosocomial FUO in the intensive care unit presents a unique challenge. Disorders to consider in this situation include cholesterol emboli syndrome or CMV postperfusion syndrome after open-heart surgery, nosocomial sinusitis related to nasotracheal or nasogastric intubation, intra-abdominal or pelvic abscess, invasive fungal infection (especially in patients on prolonged steroids), and nosocomial pneumonia. Patients with CMV postperfusion syndrome exhibit a mononucleosis-like syndrome several weeks after open-heart surgery. The risk of developing the condition is directly related to the number of blood units transfused during the procedure, and the diagnosis must be differentiated from Dressler syndrome, which is an autoimmune condition and more likely to occur 2 weeks after the procedure. Other causes of nosocomial FUO that are noninfectious in origin can be loosely divided into those in which the temperature exceeds 102° F and those in which the temperature is less than 102° F. Possible causes of nosocomial FUO with temperatures less than 102° F include tissue injury or infarction, thromboembolic disease, gastrointestinal hemorrhage, and acute pancreatitis. Noninfectious conditions associated with temperatures greater than 102° F include adrenal insufficiency and drug fever. Temperatures greater than 106° F are rarely from infectious causes. The most common causes of high fevers of this nature are neuroleptic malignant syndrome, malignant hyperthermia, disordered heat homeostasis caused by central nervous system trauma, and drug fevers. Most drug fevers are caused by common medications; consequently, a close review of a patient's active medication list is essential to make the diagnosis.

Immune-Deficient Fever of Unknown Origin

Patients who are immunosuppressed have a higher likelihood of infectious complications. Neutropenic FUO is undiagnosed fever in the context of persistent and severe neutropenia. In general, most patients in this category will have received cytotoxic and/or immunosuppressive therapy for their underlying disease. Regardless of the cause, complicating infections are frequently encountered when the absolute neutrophil count (mature neutrophils and bands) falls below 1000 cells/mm³ (and especially below 500 cells/mm³). Occult bacterial infections are the most frequent causes of fever, and deterioration may be rapid; empiric broad-spectrum antibiotics are mandated in patients with febrile neutropenia after appropriate cultures are obtained. If the cultures are negative and the patient remains febrile, then the patient is considered to have neutropenic FUO.

In patients with impaired cell-mediated immunity, FUO caused by agents other than bacteria is being increasingly recognized. Populations of patients who are receiving chronic steroids or who are using immunomodulatory agents to control underlying disease processes are growing. In these patients, occult fungal infections and reactivation of viral or mycobacterial diseases need to be considered when unexplained febrile episodes develop. For example, opportunistic infections in patients receiving anticytokine therapy such as TNF inhibitors for rheumatologic conditions and inflammatory bowel disease are being increasingly recognized, particularly mycobacterial infections such as tuberculosis. Other etiologic considerations in these patients should also always include perirectal or periodontal disease, drug-induced fever, relapse of underlying disease (especially hematologic malignancy), and thromboembolic conditions.

HIV-Associated Fever of Undetermined Origin

Fever is one of the most common symptoms in patients infected with HIV. With advanced HIV disease, more frequent causes of FUO include mycobacterial disease (especially disseminated *M. avium* complex), CMV (retinitis or colitis) infection, drug reactions, and bacterial line infections (see Chapter 108).

Factitious or Self-Induced Fever

Patients with factitious or self-induced illness present unique ethical and therapeutic problems. Once the possibility of factitious or self-induced illness is considered, the physician-patient relationship is changed. Typically the physician can rely on the good faith of the patient's history. In the case of factitious or self-induced illness, the physician must assume a more detached role to establish the diagnosis. Patients with factitious fever are typically young and often women. Many have been or are employed in health-related professions. Usually articulate and well educated, these patients are adept at manipulating their family, friends, and physicians. In these instances a consultant new to the patient may provide a detached and helpful perspective on the problem.

Clues to factitious fever include the absence of a toxic appearance despite high temperature readings, lack of an appropriate rise in pulse rate with fever, and absence of the physiologic diurnal variation in temperature. Suggested factitious readings can be evaluated by immediately repeating the reading with the nurse or physician in attendance. The use of electronic thermometers allows rapid and accurate recording of a patient's temperature (see also Chapter 118).

Self-injection of pyrogen-containing substances, usually bacteria-laden culture medium, urine, or feces, can produce bacteremia and high fever; usually these bacteremic episodes are polymicrobial and intermittent, often suggesting a diagnosis of intra-abdominal abscess. However, patients with self-induced bacteremia may appear remarkably well between episodes of fever. The occurrence of polymicrobial bacteremia in an otherwise healthy person should suggest the possibility of self-induced infection. Illicit ingestion of medications known by the patient to produce fever can also present a difficult diagnostic problem. Clues to the presence of self-induced illness are subtle. The patients are often emotionally immature. Some fabricate unrelated aspects of their history. The most extreme form of factitious or self-induced illness is called the Munchausen syndrome. Some patients are surprisingly stoic about the apparent seriousness of their illness and the procedures used to diagnose or treat them. In some instances, interviewing family members can elicit clues to the possibility of factitious or self-induced illness. Confirming the diagnosis is crucial and, in many instances, requires a search of the patient's hospital room. Although most will deny their role in inducing or feigning illness, the diagnosis must be explained, and psychiatric care is essential. These complicated patients are at risk for inducing life-threatening disease; some respond to psychiatric counseling.

Prospectus for the Future

Advances in medical technology will allow for faster and more accurate diagnosis and treatment of febrile syndromes. For example, new and sophisticated radiographic imaging techniques will provide more detailed identification of internal abnormalities. Highly specific molecular techniques, such as immunohistochemistry, in situ hybridization, and nucleic acid amplification will improve the ability to diagnose infectious causes of fever and FUO. In addition, the sequencing of human and microbial genomes and advances in functional genomics will significantly affect the development of new vaccines and therapies for pathogens associated with febrile syndromes.

Nevertheless, medical progress will also change the spectrum of febrile syndromes and FUO. For example, it is likely that the increased numbers and types of compromised hosts created by the expansion of transplantation programs and new immunosuppressive medications will add significant challenges for the diagnosis and management of febrile syndromes. In addition, the creation of new organisms by chance or through bioterrorism and the spread of old organisms to new parts of the world through increased global communication will shape the evolution of this area of medicine.

References

Beutler B, Beutler SM: Pathogenesis of fever. In Goldman L, Ausiello D (eds): Cecil Textbook of Medicine, 22nd ed. Philadelphia, Elsevier, 2004, pp 1730-1733.

Bleeker-Rovers CP, Vos FJ, de Kleijn EM, et al: A prospective multicenter study on fever of unknown origin: The yield of a structured diagnosis protocol. Medicine (Baltimore) 86:26-38, 2007.

Chang FY, Peacock JE Jr, Musher DM, et al: *Staphylococcus aureus* bacteremia: Recurrence and the impact of antibiotic treatment in a prospective multicenter study. Medicine (Baltimore) 82:333-339, 2003.

Corey L, Boeckh M: Persistent fever in patients with neutropenia. N Engl J Med 346:222-224, 2002.

Jones JL, Kruszon-Moran D, Wilson M, et al: *Toxoplasma gondii* infection in the United States: Seroprevalence and risk factors. Am J Epidemiol 154:357-365, 2001.

Knockaert DC, Dujardin KS, Bobbaers HJ: Long-term follow-up of patients with undiagnosed fever of unknown origin. Arch Intern Med 156:618-620, 1996.

Santos ES, Raez LE, Eckardt P, et al: The utility of a bone marrow biopsy in diagnosing the source of fever of unknown origin in patients with AIDS. J Acquir Immune Defic Syndr 37:1599-1603, 2004.

Vanderschueren S, Knockaert D, Adriaenssens T, et al: From prolonged febrile illness to fever of unknown origin: The challenge continues. Arch Intern Med 163:1033-1041, 2003.

Bacteremia and Sepsis Syndrome

Richard R. Watkins and Robert A. Salata

Sepsis syndrome is a leading cause of morbidity and mortality in hospitalized patients. There is a growing understanding of the pathophysiology of sepsis and recognition of the critical interdependence of the inflammatory and coagulation systems. Novel therapeutic approaches now being used and tested in sepsis syndrome are a direct result of the elucidation of the molecular mechanisms of sepsis and the practical applications of modern techniques of biochemistry and molecular biology to rational drug design.

The bases for current definitions of sepsis syndrome and related disorders are presented in Table 96-1 and Figure 96-1. Infection, defined by the presence of microbial pathogens in normally sterile sites, can be symptomatic or inapparent. Bloodstream infection (BSI) implies the presence of organisms that can be cultured from blood. Septicemia implies BSI with greater severity. Sepsis indicates clinical settings in which evidence of infection and a systemic response to infection exist (fever or hypothermia, tachycardia, tachypnea, leukocytosis or leukopenia). Sepsis syndrome emphasizes an even greater degree of severity, with evidence of altered organ perfusion with one of the following: hypoxemia, oliguria, altered mentation, or elevated serum lactate level. Severe sepsis represents a more advanced degree of organ dysfunction and is often associated with multi-organ failure. Septic shock indicates sepsis plus hypotension despite adequate intravenous fluid challenge. Refractory septic shock is defined as shock lasting more than 1 hour that is unresponsive to fluids and/or vasopressors. Noninfectious insults (e.g., thermal burns, severe trauma, severe pancreatitis, pulmonary contusion, certain toxins, therapy with monoclonal antibodies for solid organ transplant rejection) can also be associated with a severe systemic reaction simulating sepsis syndrome. The term *systemic inflammatory response syndrome* (SIRS) encompasses both infectious and noninfectious causes of a profound host inflammatory response with systemic symptoms and signs; sepsis syndrome is the predominant cause of SIRS.

Epidemiologic Factors

The incidence of sepsis and associated deaths has increased dramatically in the United States, and evidence suggests that this rise will continue. Septic shock is the most common cause of death in intensive care units and the thirteenth most common cause of death in the United States. More than 750,000 cases of sepsis occur in the United States each year, resulting in approximately 200,000 fatalities.

Historically, gram-negative organisms caused most cases of sepsis and septic shock. However, the National Nosocomial Infection Surveillance System indicates significant increases in the frequency of septicemia caused by gram-positive infections since 1985. Highest rates for hospital-acquired septicemias occur in patients with cancer and burn or trauma victims, as well as in high-risk nurseries. Hospital-acquired BSI is associated with 7.4 extra days of hospitalization and $4000 of extra hospital charges per occurrence. The most commonly identified bloodstream pathogens include staphylococci, streptococci, *Escherichia coli*, *Enterobacter* species, and *Pseudomonas aeruginosa*. Fungal bloodstream isolates are found less frequently, but their incidence increased over the last decade. In particular, fungemia from non-*albicans Candida*, with increasing resistance to azoles, has become more frequent, which has important implications for empiric antimicrobial therapy.

Major epidemiologic factors that have contributed to the increased occurrence of sepsis include the growing number of immunocompromised hosts resulting from more intense chemotherapy regimens, an aging population, and the aggressive employment of increasingly invasive procedures and complex surgery. The incidence of sepsis is greatest in the winter, suggesting an associated respiratory cause. Mortality varies among ethnic groups with African American men at highest risk. Also, age-adjusted sepsis mortality rates are highest at the extremes of age.

Table 96-2 lists organisms important in sepsis syndrome as they relate to host factors. Factors that have negatively

Table 96-1 **Definitions of Sepsis and Related Disorders**

Disorder	Definition
Infection	Microorganisms in a normally sterile site; subclinical or symptomatic
Bacteremia	Bacteria present in bloodstream; may be transient
Septicemia	Same as bacteremia but greater severity
Sepsis	Clinical evidence of infection plus systemic response to infection
Sepsis syndrome	Sepsis plus altered organ perfusion (hypoxemia, oliguria, altered mentation)
Severe sepsis	Sepsis syndrome plus hypotension and hypoperfusion
Septic shock	Sepsis with hypotension despite adequate fluid resuscitation; patients on vasopressors may not be hypotensive at the time hypoperfusion abnormalities are evident
Refractory septic shock	Shock lasting more than 1 hr that is unresponsive to fluid administration and/or vasopressors
Systemic inflammatory response syndrome (SIRS)	Wide variety of insults (infectious response syndrome and noninfectious) that initiate profound systemic responses; sepsis syndrome is a subset of SIRS Current definition includes two or more of the following: temperature >38°C or ≤36°C; tachycardia >90 beats/minute; respiratory rate >20 breaths/minute; $PaCO_2 \le 32$; white blood cell (WBC) count >12,000 cells/mm^3 or <4000 cells/mm^3, or >10% bands

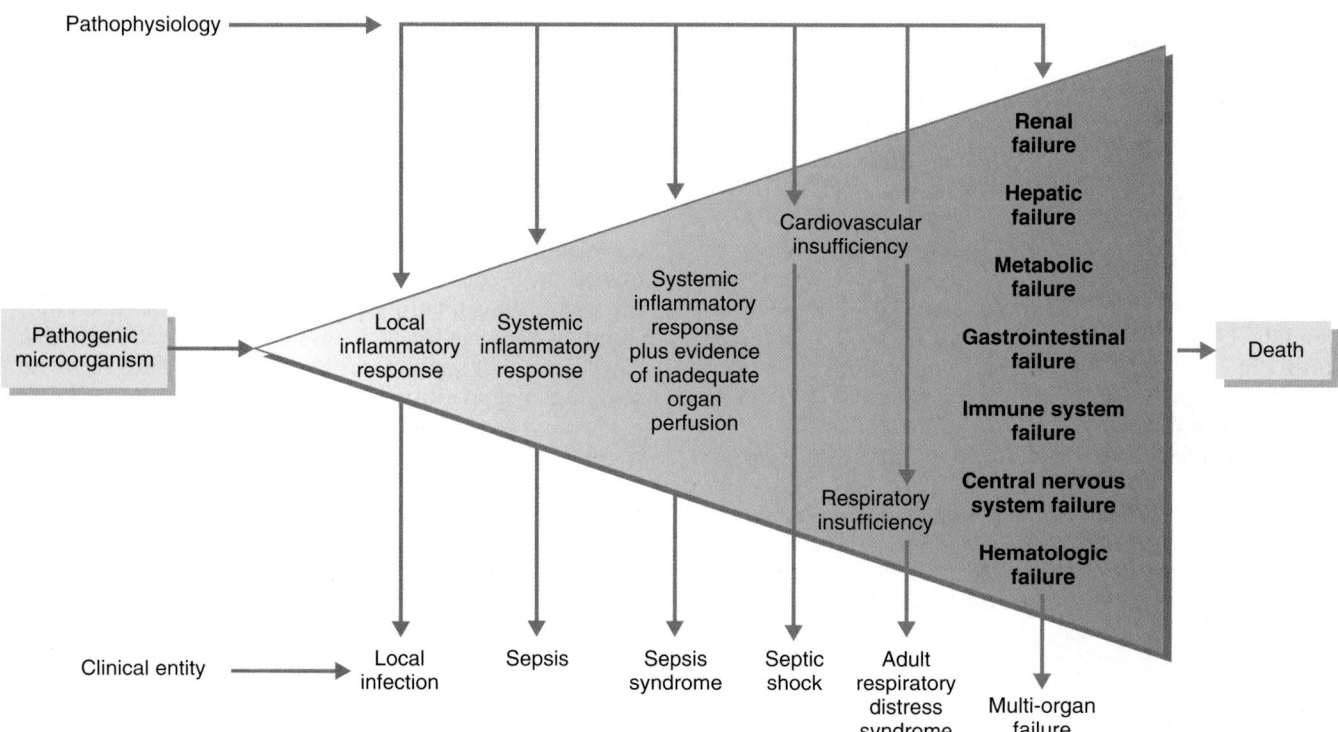

Figure 96-1 Natural history of the sepsis process.

influenced survival in the setting of BSI have included severity of underlying disease, delayed initiation of appropriate antimicrobial therapy, virulence of the pathogen (e.g., *P. aeruginosa*), extremes of age, site of infection (respiratory being more common than abdominal, which is more common than urinary), health care–associated infection, polymicrobial infection, and development of end-organ complications (acute respiratory distress syndrome, acute renal failure, disseminated intravascular coagulation [DIC], bowel ischemia or infarction, and coma). When evidence of dysfunction of two or more systems exists, the diagnosis of multi-organ system failure can be made. Mortality rises in proportion to the number of organ systems involved and is near 100% when four or more systems are dysfunctional.

Pathogenesis

The pathogenesis of sepsis is shaped largely by the infected host's complex response to the invading pathogen (Fig. 96-2). Sepsis with organ dysfunction occurs primarily when the host's responses to infection are inadequate. Gram-negative bacterial lipopolysaccharide (LPS), or endotoxin, is representative of a larger class of microbial products causally linked to septic shock syndrome. Cell wall products of gram-positive bacteria, such as teichoic acid and peptidoglycan, induce inflammatory responses similar to those produced by LPS. Sepsis syndrome may complicate infections with bacteria, viruses, fungi, rickettsiae, mycobacteria, and parasites. The pathogenesis of shock involves a series of events initiated by the invading pathogen or its products, and shock is produced through a causally related sequence of host responses.

The sepsis cascade begins when a pathogenic microorganism penetrates a host barrier. Local host defense cells (macrophages, mast cells, dendritic cells) detect molecules on the invader's cell wall by means of pattern-recognition receptors such as CD14 and toll-like receptors (TLRs). For example, TLR-2 recognizes the peptidoglycan of gram-positive bacteria, TLR-4 recognizes an LPS of gram-negative bacteria, and both TLR-2 and TLR-4 recognize the cell wall of *Aspergillus*. Binding of TLRs to epitopes on the microorganisms stimulates intracellular signaling and leads to the production of cytokines and inflammatory molecules such as tumor necrosis factor (TNF)–α and interleukin (IL)-1β. These molecules in turn activate neutrophils and endothelial cells, which results not only in killing of microorganisms but also damaging of endothelium by release of mediators that increase vascular permeability. Edema fluid then flows into the lungs and other organs, causing acute organ injury. Activated endothelial cells also release nitric oxide, a potent vasodilator.

Microorganisms stimulate adaptive immune responses in the course of sepsis. B cells release immunoglobulins that bind the microorganisms and promote their delivery by antigen-presenting cells to natural killer cells and neutrophils. Type 1 helper T cells (Th1 cells) secrete proinflammatory cytokines, whereas type 2 helper T cells (Th2 cells) release anti-inflammatory cytokines such as IL-4 and IL-10, depending on the infecting organism and other complex cell-cell interactions (Table 96-3).

Systemic inflammation influences activity of the coagulation system by directly and indirectly modulating production of procoagulant and anticoagulant molecules. In response to proinflammatory cytokines, tissue factor released by endothelium and associated thrombin formation, respectively, activate the extrinsic and intrinsic pathways of coagulation. Simultaneous depletion of endogenous anticoagulant molecules occurs, including proteins C and S, tissue factor pathway inhibitor, and antithrombin III, as well as

Table 96-2 Microorganisms Involved in Sepsis Syndrome in Relation to Host Factors

Host Factors	Organisms of Particular Importance
Asplenia	Encapsulated organisms: *Streptococcus pneumoniae, Haemophilus influenzae, Neisseria meningitidis, Capnocytophaga canimorsus*
Cirrhosis	*Vibrio, Yersinia,* and *Salmonella* species, other gram-negative rods, encapsulated organisms
Alcoholism	*Klebsiella* species, *Streptococcus pneumoniae*
Diabetes	Mucormycosis, *Pseudomonas* species, *Escherichia coli*
Steroids	Tuberculosis, fungi, herpesviruses
Neutropenia	Enteric gram-negative rods, *Pseudomonas, Aspergillus, Candida, Mucor* species, *Staphylococcus aureus, Streptococcal species*
T-cell dysfunction	*Listeria, Salmonella,* and *Mycobacterium* species, herpesvirus group (herpes simplex virus, cytomegalovirus, varicella-zoster virus)
AIDS	*Salmonella, Staphylococcus aureus* (including MRSA), *Mycobacterium avium* complex

MRSA, methicillin-resistant *Staphylococcus aureus.*

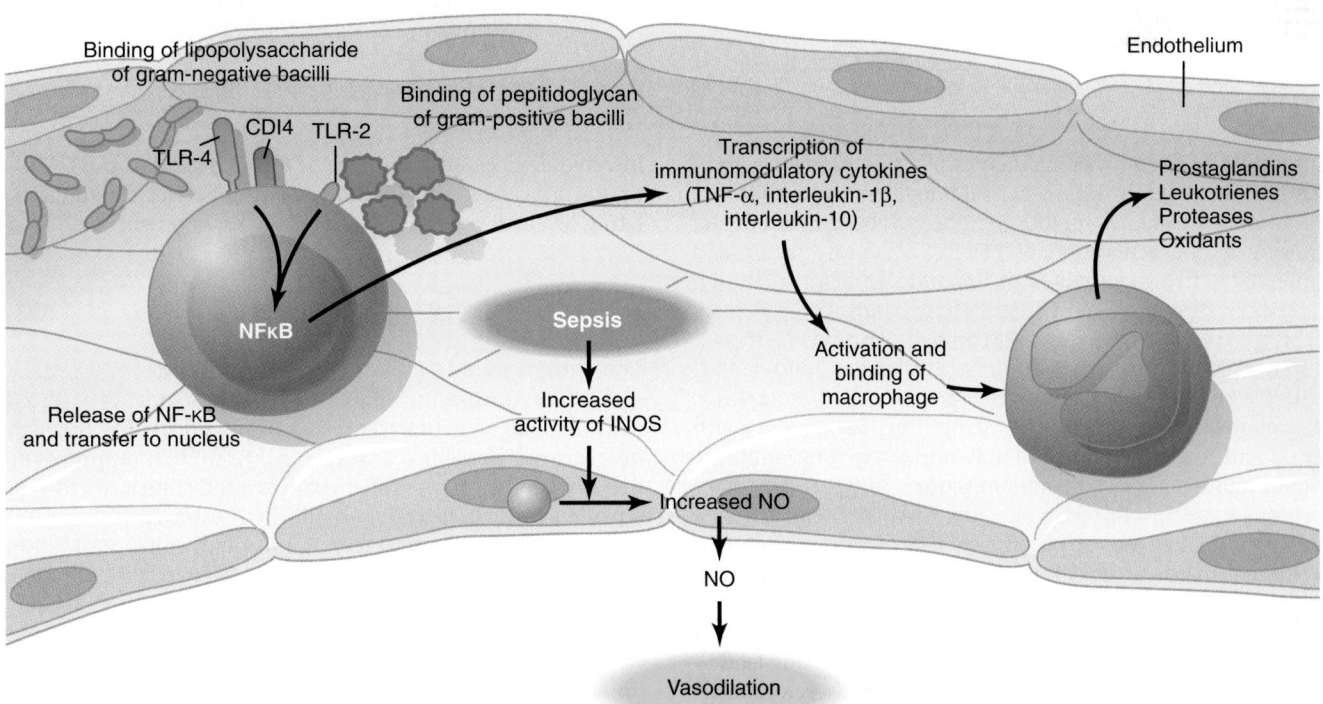

Figure 96-2 Inflammatory response to sepsis.

Table 96-3 Cytokines with a Potential Role in Systemic Inflammatory Response Syndrome

Cytokine	Source	Target Cell	Function
Granulocyte-macrophage colony-stimulating factor (GM-CSF)	T cells, macrophages, endothelial cells, fibroblasts	Myeloid precursor cells, neutrophils, eosinophils, macrophages	Proliferation of progenitor cells Differentiation and maturation of neutrophils and macrophages
Granulocyte colony-stimulating factor (G-CSF)	Monocytes, endothelial cells, fibroblasts, neutrophils	Neutrophils, promyelocytes	Proliferation of myeloid progenitor cells Enhanced neutrophil survival and function
IL-1 (α and β)	Macrophages, fibroblasts, T cells, endothelial cells, hepatocytes	Fibroblasts, T cells, monocytes, neutrophils	Induces cytokines (IL-2, IL-3, IL-6, TNF); induces B- and T-cell activation, growth, and differentiation Synthesis of acute phase reaction; induces fever, catabolism
IL-2	Activated T cells	Activated lymphoid cells	Enhances T- and B-cell immune responses Promotes cytotoxic T cells Induces IFN-γ and TNF
IL-4	Th2 T cells	B and T cells, macrophages, mast cells	Induces B-cell activation, proliferation, and differentiation and IgG$_1$ and IgE production Enhances MHC class I and II receptors
IL-6	Macrophages, fibroblasts, Th2 T cells	Lymphocytes, monocytes	Stimulates B-cell growth, differentiation, and activation Induces synthesis of acute phase reactants
IL-8	Monocytes, fibroblasts, endothelial cells	Neutrophils, monocytes	Enhanced neutrophil activity and histamine release
IL-12	Macrophages, B cells	T cells	Induces differentiation of Th1 cells Initiates production of IFN-α
IFN-γ	T cells	Macrophages, monocytes, T and B cells	Pronounced monocyte and macrophage activation Increased MHC class II expression
TNF-α (cachectin), TNF-β (lymphotoxin)	Monocytes, macrophages, lymphocytes, mast cells	Monocytes, macrophages, lymphocytes, neutrophils, fibroblasts	Induces cascade of inflammatory reactions (fever, catabolism, acute phase reactants) Induces multiple cytokines (IL-1, GM-CSF) Increases MHC class I expression Enhances B-cell proliferation and immunoglobulin production

IFN, interferon; IgE, immunoglobulin E; IgG$_1$, immunoglobulin G$_1$; IL, interleukin; MHC, major histocompatibility complex; TNF, tumor necrosis factor.

inhibition of fibrinolysis via increases in plasminogen activator inhibitor and thrombin-activatable fibrinolysis inhibitor. Endotoxin stimulates membrane phospholipid metabolism, leading to the generation of platelet-activating factor and other bioactive metabolites of arachidonic acid, including prostaglandins and leukotrienes. These compounds, in turn, exert a variety of synergistic and antagonistic effects on vascular endothelium, smooth muscle, platelets, and leukocytes. The resultant exaggerated procoagulant state leads to microvascular thrombosis (often in association with DIC) and tissue ischemia and may ultimately cause multiple organ failure. These proinflammatory and procoagulant responses are amplified by secondary ischemia and hypoxia through the release of plasminogen-activator inhibitor 1. Proinflammatory cytokines can also lead to host immunosuppression by causing apoptosis of circulating and tissue lymphocytes.

The altered signaling pathways in sepsis eventually lead to tissue injury and multiple organ failure. It is therefore critical to interrupt the sepsis cascade early by containing and eliminating the source (e.g., through antibiotics, removal of

infected devices, and drainage of infected fluid or pus). Multiple studies have shown an association between high circulating levels of proinflammatory markers and survival.

Clinical Manifestations

The clinical manifestations of sepsis syndrome are protean and often nonspecific (Table 96-4). The clinician is faced with the challenge of early recognition and sorting through the various possible causes of SIRS so that appropriate therapy can be initiated. Patients with the clinical picture of sepsis of uncertain origin should be presumed to have BSI and treated accordingly. Prompt, thorough cultures of blood and suspicious local sites should be followed immediately by initiation of antibiotics appropriate for the most likely pathogens as well as control of the source of infection (removal of infected devices and drainage of infected collections) if at all possible.

Fever and chills are usually present, but older or debilitated patients (especially those with renal or liver failure or

Table 96-4 Signs and Symptoms Indicative of Sepsis Syndrome

Fever (core temperature >38° C)

Hypothermia (core temperature ≤36°C)

Chills

Hyperventilation (mixed venous oxygen saturation >70%)

Mental status changes

Hypotension (systolic blood pressure ≤90 mm Hg or mean arterial pressure ≤70 mm Hg)

Leukopenia (white blood cell count <4000 cells/mm³)

Leukocytosis (white blood cell count >12,000 cells/mm³ or >10% bands)

Thrombocytopenia (platelet count ≤100,000/mm³)

End-organ failure: lung, kidney, liver, heart, disseminated intravascular coagulation, bowel

Hypoglycemia or hyperglycemia

Hyperlactatemia (>3 mmol/L)

those receiving systemic corticosteroids) may not develop fever. Hypothermia may occur and is associated with a poorer prognosis. One of the early clues to a systemic infectious process is the presence of hyperventilation and respiratory alkalosis.

Skin manifestations in sepsis can occur with any infectious agent and at times may represent the earliest signs of sepsis syndrome. Staphylococci and streptococci can be associated with cellulitis or diffuse erythroderma in association with toxin-producing strains. BSI with gram-negative bacteria can be associated with a skin lesion called *ecthyma gangrenosum* (round or oval 1- to 15-cm lesions with a halo of erythema and usually a vesicular or necrotic central area). Although ecthyma gangrenosum is most commonly associated with *P. aeruginosa,* other invaders such as *Aeromonas* organisms, *Klebsiella* organisms, *E. coli, Serratia* species, and fungal organisms may also cause ecthyma gangrenosum (see also Chapter 101). *Neisseria meningitidis* bacteremia is often heralded by petechial and hemorrhagic skin lesions and followed by rapidly progressive shock.

The sepsis syndrome is characteristically associated with hypotension and oliguria. In many patients, hypotension may initially respond to intravenous fluids. Other patients progress from an initial stage of hypotension, tachycardia, and vasodilation (warm shock) to deep pallor, vasoconstriction, and anuria (cold shock). Of all infectious causes of sepsis syndrome, gram-negative bacilli most often cause shock; up to 35% of patients with gram-negative sepsis develop shock, often with mortality rates between 40% and 70%.

As sepsis syndrome progresses, myocardial function can become profoundly depressed. This situation greatly complicates fluid management and necessitates continuous cardiopulmonary monitoring in an intensive care setting. Pulmonary complications of sepsis syndrome are frequent. Acute respiratory distress syndrome, characterized by arterial oxygen tension less than 50 mm Hg despite fractional inspired oxygen greater than 50%, diffuse alveolar infiltrates, and pulmonary capillary wedge pressure less than 18 mm Hg, occurs in 10% to 40% of patients with sepsis syndrome and is most frequently seen in conjunction with gram-negative

organisms. Increased pulmonary capillary permeability, resulting from inflammatory cytokines released during sepsis, is a major causative factor in acute respiratory distress syndrome and makes administration of intravenous fluids, often given in an attempt to improve cardiac output, extremely hazardous. Failure of respiratory muscles can also complicate sepsis and contribute significantly to morbidity and mortality.

Most patients with sepsis have a neutrophilic leukocytosis. Leukopenia may occur, most often with overwhelming bacteremias but also with severe systemic viral infections. Alcoholics and older adults are at increased risk for sepsis-associated neutropenia. A low platelet count and evidence of coagulopathy occur in up to 75% of patients with gram-negative bacillary bacteremia. DIC occurs in roughly 10% of patients with sepsis.

Renal insufficiency in sepsis syndrome is multifactorial and depends to varying degrees on the host, the microbe, and the therapy administered. Most often in sepsis, acute tubular necrosis is the basis for renal dysfunction and may be secondary to hypotension, volume depletion, or cytokines elaborated in sepsis syndrome. Acute renal failure associated with sepsis syndrome may be seen without overt hypotension. Tubulointerstitial disease caused by specific pathogens and/or antimicrobial therapy may also occur. Endocarditis may also be associated with immune complex–mediated glomerulonephritis.

Upper gastrointestinal tract bleeding may be a life-threatening complication in patients with sepsis who also have coagulopathy and thrombocytopenia. Liver dysfunction may occur with evidence of cholestatic jaundice or of hepatocellular injury. With bacteremia related to gram-negative bacilli, *hyperbilirubinemia of sepsis* often occurs, with little change in the other liver enzymes. Large increases in transaminase values usually indicate ischemia of the liver; these abnormalities usually resolve rapidly with restoration of blood pressure.

Increased serum lactate concentrations are seen in patients with severe sepsis and septic shock. Such increases occur as a consequence of increased glycolysis and pyruvate production. Impaired hepatic clearance of lactate and mitochondrial dysfunction also contribute to hyperlactatemia.

Hypoglycemia may complicate sepsis syndrome and can be a correctable cause of mental status change or seizures. Hypoglycemia occurs more frequently in individuals with underlying liver disease. Hyperglycemia may result during the body's acute metabolic response to infection, especially in diabetics or when glucose-containing intravenous fluids are given.

Diagnosis

The initial evaluation of the patient with possible sepsis syndrome ideally begins with a thorough history. However, in patients with fully developed sepsis syndrome, the working diagnosis is made on the basis of physical findings, and the detailed history must necessarily follow correction of hemodynamic problems, obtaining appropriate microbial culture samples, and empiric initiation of antimicrobial therapy. Attention should be focused on underlying diseases or predispositions to sepsis, previous infections and antimicrobial therapy, available microbiologic information, and symptoms suggesting localization of infection. A history of travel, environmental exposure, and any contact with infectious agents should be thoroughly explored. Information on the complications of previous treatment (e.g., toxic effects of drugs or drug allergies) can be critical in the selection of therapy.

Physical examination should focus on discovering clues to infection and localizing sites thereof. Appropriate specimens for microbiologic evaluation must be obtained. Two or three sets of blood cultures from patients with bacteremia yield the organism in 89% and 99% of patients, respectively.

The selection of additional laboratory studies should be based on the clinical manifestations. Patients with diarrhea should have a stool sample sent for a cytotoxic assay against *Clostridium difficile* toxins A and B. Obtaining appropriate diagnostic studies expeditiously is critical. These studies are usually aimed at delineating the focus of infection (e.g., cerebrospinal fluid examination, computed tomography scans) and determining whether adjunctive surgical therapy (e.g., abscess drainage, foreign body removal) is indicated. Patients whose condition is too unstable for transport to the radiology department may benefit from ultrasonography at the bedside.

Therapy

The key to managing sepsis is the early recognition of the systemic response and initiation of therapy before hypotension and complications ensue (Table 96-5). Patients with sepsis syndrome, especially if hypotensive, are best managed in the intensive care unit. The essential therapies of sepsis syndrome and septic shock include judicious fluid administration, oxygen, vasopressors, and antibiotics.

Early goal-directed therapy focused on optimal oxygen delivery to tissues is associated with improved survival. This therapy includes crystalloid fluid resuscitation, red blood cell transfusion to maintain a hematocrit of at least 30%, careful hemodynamic monitoring, and the use of inotropes in select persons. Antibiotic choices should reflect epidemiologic concerns (see Table 96-2), antibiotic resistance patterns, and potential sites of infection. Time does not allow withholding antimicrobial therapy until bacteremia or an infectious source is proved in patients with sepsis syndrome. Until culture results and other diagnostic studies are completed, empiric broad-spectrum antimicrobial therapy (covering both gram-positive and gram-negative pathogens, as well as antifungal therapy in select patients) is necessary in patients with sepsis (Table 96-6). Initiation of appropriate empiric antimicrobial therapy has a major impact on survival of these patients. As soon as a specific microbial cause has been established by culture, antibiotics should be changed, if necessary, to target the causative agent. Duration of antibiotics depends on the clinical response, infecting pathogen, and initial site of infection, with most courses lasting 7 to 14 days. Attention should also be directed to serum glucose control because maintenance of glucose at 80 to 110 mg/dL using intensive insulin therapy is associated with reduced mortality.

Table 96-5 **Recommended Management of Sepsis**
Start resuscitation immediately in patients with hypotension or serum lactate >4 mmol/L.
Obtain appropriate cultures before starting antibiotics, provided it does not significantly delay therapy.
Evaluate for a focus of infection amenable to source control (e.g., abscess drainage).
Remove intravascular catheters if potentially infected.
Begin broad-spectrum antibiotics within the first hour of severe sepsis and septic shock.
Fluid-resuscitate using crystalloids or colloids.
Give fluid challenges of 1L of crystalloids or 300 to 500 mL of colloids over 30 minutes.
Maintain mean arterial pressure ≥65 mm Hg.
Use norepinephrine and dopamine centrally administered as vasopressors of choice.
Use dobutamine in patients with myocardial dysfunction.
Give red blood cells when hemoglobin decreases to <7 g/dL to a target hemoglobin of 7 to 9 g/dL.
Target a tidal volume of 6 mL/kg in patients with acute respiratory distress syndrome.
Use intravenous insulin to keep blood glucose <150 mg/dL.
Give either low–molecular-weight heparin or unfractionated heparin for deep vein thrombosis prophylaxis.
Provide stress ulcer prophylaxis using H_2 blockers or a proton-pump inhibitor.

Data from Dellinger RP, Levy MM, Carlet JM, et al: Surviving Sepsis Campaign: International guidelines for management of severe sepsis and septic shock: 2008. Crit Care Med. 2008;36(1):296-327.

The limitations of currently available therapy for sepsis and septic shock are demonstrated by the continued high mortality rates associated with this disease, despite improvement in antibiotic therapy and critical care techniques. Standard approaches to therapy for sepsis and septic shock are crucial. Of the various steps in the pathogenesis of septic shock, beginning with tissue invasion by the offending organism and culminating in pathophysiologic phenomena associated with septic shock syndrome, current therapy addresses only the initial and final steps of this process (see Figs. 96-1 and 96-2). Few currently employed therapies target intermediate steps in the pathogenesis of septic shock, even though these steps dominate the disease process in fully developed sepsis syndrome. Newer strategies entail attempts to amplify selectively or modulate the host responses to the invading pathogen or its pathogenic products. Targets include the bacterium, endotoxin (or other bacterial products), host cells that respond to endotoxin, mediators produced by these cells in response to endotoxin, and cells injured by endotoxin-induced mediators (see Fig. 96-2).

Numerous studies have attempted to clarify the role of steroids in sepsis and septic shock. Recently a multicenter, randomized, double-blind, placebo-controlled trial found no improvement in survival or reversal of shock in patients who received hydrocortisone for shock or in those who did not have a response to corticotrophin. The benefit of treatment for adrenal insufficiency using corticosteroids now seems limited to patients with vasopressor-dependent septic shock. Trials targeting cytokines in sepsis have failed to demonstrate clinical efficacy. These studies have

Table 96-6 Initial Antibiotic Recommendations for Septic Patients*

Empiric coverage	Vancomycin 15 mg/kg q12h plus either piperacillin-tazobactam[†] 3.375 g IV q6h or imipenem 0.5 g IV q6h or meropenem 1.0 g IV q8h with or without an aminoglycoside (e.g., tobramycin 5 mg/kg IV q24).[‡]
Community-acquired pneumonia	Ceftriaxone 1 g IV q24h plus azithromycin 500 mg IV q24h or a fluoroquinolone (e.g., moxifloxacin 400 mg IV q24h or levofloxacin 750 mg IV q24h).[§]
Community-acquired urosepsis	Ciprofloxacin 400 mg IV q24h or ampicillin 2 g IV q6h plus gentamicin 5 mg/kg IV q24h.
Meningitis	Vancomycin 500-750 mg IV q6h plus ceftriaxone 2 g IV q12h plus dexamethasone 0.15 mg/kg IV q6h × 2-4 days preferably before antibiotics; add ampicillin 2 g IV q4h if *Listeria* is suspected.
Nosocomial pneumonia	Vancomycin 15 mg/kg q12h plus either piperacillin-tazobactam 4.5 g IV q6h or imipenem 0.5 g IV q6h or meropenem 1 g IV q8h or cefepime 2 g IV q12h plus either an aminoglycoside (e.g., amikacin 15 mg/kg IV q24h or tobramycin 7 mg/kg IV q24h) or levofloxacin (Levaquin) 750 mg IV q24h. Some authorities would substitute linezolid 600 mg IV q12h for vancomycin if MRSA is of significant concern or known to be the cause.
Neutropenia	Cefepime 2 g IV q8h; add vancomycin 15 mg/kg IV q12h if a central line is present and infection is a concern. Add antifungal coverage with liposomal amphotericin B 3-5 mg/kg q24h or caspofungin 70 mg IV × 1 then 50 mg IV q24h if fever persists ≥5 days. If invasive aspergillosis is highly suspected or proven, voriconazole 6 mg/kg IV q12h × 2 then 4 mg/kg IV q12h should be used.
Cellulitis and skin infections	Vancomycin 15 mg/kg IV q12h. Add piperacillin-tazobactam 4.5 g IV q6h in diabetics or immunocompromised patients. If necrotizing fasciitis is suspected, add clindamycin 900 mg IV; surgical débridement is crucial.

*Assumes normal renal function; dose adjustments required with impaired creatinine clearance.
[†]Substitute aztreonam 2 g IV q8h if penicillin allergic.
[‡]Monitor drug levels of aminoglycosides (i.e., peak and trough).
[§]Use ceftriaxone and azithromycin if the patient is admitted to the intensive care unit.
MRSA, methicillin-resistant *Staphylococcus aureus*.

emphasized that targeting a specific molecule as adjunctive therapy for sepsis may be inadequate, given the complex cascade and temporal relationships of factors involved in the pathophysiologic parameters of SIRS. Currently the only adjunctive therapeutic agent to clearly show significant reduction in mortality in sepsis syndrome is recombinant human activated protein C (rhAPC). In a multicenter, randomized, double-blind, placebo-controlled trial for severe sepsis, infusion of rhAPC resulted in a 6.1% absolute risk reduction for mortality. The major adverse effect in this trial was bleeding, occurring in 3.5% of patients receiving the drug. Although clinical experience with this agent is limited and optimal target populations have not been fully identified, rhAPC is currently the only medication approved by the U.S. Food and Drug Administration specifically for the treatment of severe sepsis in adults (Table 96-7). The Surviving Sepsis Campaign Guidelines are a comprehensive, up-to-date set of recommendations for treatment of sepsis.

Table 96-7 Exclusion Criteria for Recombinant Human Activated Protein C

Pregnancy or breastfeeding

Age <18 years or weight >135 kg

Platelet count <30,000/mm³

Conditions that increase the risk of bleeding:
  Surgery within 12 hours before the infusion
  A history of severe head trauma, stroke, or intracranial surgery within 3 months
  History of intracerebral arteriovenous malformation, cerebral aneurysm, or mass lesion
  History of congenital bleeding diathesis
  Gastrointestinal bleeding within 6 weeks
  Trauma considered to increase the risk of bleeding

A known hypercoagulable condition

Deep-vein thrombosis or pulmonary embolism within 3 months

Patient's family, physician, or both are not in favor of aggressive treatment or presence of an advance directive to withhold life-sustaining treatment

Prospectus for the Future

The evolving epidemiology of microbes causing bloodstream infection (BSI) and sepsis is a reflection of trends such as the increasing age of inpatients, higher numbers of immunocompromised individuals, and widespread antibiotic use. Technologic advances in microbe identification will therefore have an important role in the management of individuals with sepsis syndrome. The recent explosion in our understanding of microbial recognition by the immune system will lead to more rational immunomodulatory approaches to these patients.

Improved Diagnostics

Rapid diagnosis of the microbial cause of BSI and sepsis syndrome is essential to ensure both that antimicrobial therapy is directed against the appropriate pathogen and that coverage is not needlessly broad. Peptide nucleic acid–fluorescence in situ hybridization (PNA-FISH) can differentiate *Staphylococcus aureus* from the less pathogenic coagulase-negative staphylococci as well as different species of *Candida* sooner than

Prospectus for the Future—Cont'd

conventional methods. This may allow for earlier modification of antibiotics. Galactomannan and β-1,3-D-glucan testing may better identify fungi, such as *Aspergillus* and *Candida* species, respectively, than currently available techniques.

Immune-Based Therapies

Dysregulation of the immune response has long been the focus of novel therapies for sepsis syndrome. The identification of toll-like receptors and other pattern-recognition receptors as key players in host defense and the elucidation of subsequent intracellular signaling pathways have opened up new targets for potential pharmacologic intervention. Furthermore, the fact that immune dysregulation in critical illness exists across a spectrum is increasingly recognized, from heightened immune activation associated with systemic inflammatory response syndrome to severe immunodepression characterized by impairments in antigen presentation and proinflammatory cytokine production. Immunostimulatory approaches, including cytokines and growth factors, are under further study. Inhibition of apoptosis with anticaspases has been shown to improve survival in an animal model of sepsis. Lipids may modify innate immunity by binding lipopolysaccharide and are under investigation as well.

References

Dellinger RP, Levy MM, Carlet JM, et al: Surviving Sepsis Campaign: International guidelines for management of severe sepsis and septic shock: 2008. Crit Care Med 36:296-327, 2008.

DeMarco CE, MacArthur RD: Sepsis and septic shock. In Schlossberg D (ed): Clinical Infectious Disease. New York, Cambridge University Press, 2008, pp 9-19.

Martin GS, Mannino AM, Eaton S, Moss M: The epidemiology of sepsis in the United States from 1979 through 2000. N Engl J Med 348:1546-1554, 2003.

Munford RS: Sepsis, severe sepsis and septic shock. In Mandell GM, Bennett JE, Dolin R (eds): Principles and Practice of Infectious Diseases, 6th ed. New York, Elsevier, 2005, pp 906-926.

Russell JA: Management of sepsis. N Engl J Med 355:1699-1713, 2006.

Sprung CL, Annane D, Keh D: Hydrocortisone therapy for patients with septic shock. N Engl J Med 358:111-124, 2008.

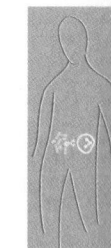

Infections of the Nervous System

Scott A. Fulton and Robert A. Salata

Infections of the central nervous system (CNS) range from fulminant, readily diagnosed septic processes to indolent illnesses requiring exhaustive investigation to identify their presence and define their causes. Neurologic outcome and survival depend largely on the extent of CNS damage before effective treatment begins. Accordingly, it is essential that the physician move quickly to achieve a specific diagnosis and institute appropriate therapy. The initial evaluation must, however, take into account both the urgency of beginning antibiotic treatment in bacterial meningitis and the potential hazard of performing a lumbar puncture in the presence of focal neurologic infection or mass lesions.

Patients with CNS infection usually exhibit some combination of fever, headache, altered mental status, depressed sensorium, seizures, focal neurologic signs, and stiff neck. The history and physical examination, the results of lumbar puncture when applicable (Table 97-1), and the neuroradiographic images provide the mainstays of diagnosis. The order in which the last two procedures are performed is critical. A subacute history, evolving over 7 days to 2 months, of unilateral headache with focal neurologic signs and/or seizures implies a mass lesion that may or may not be infectious in nature. A brain-imaging procedure should be performed first; lumbar puncture is potentially dangerous because it may precipitate cerebral herniation, even in the absence of overt papilledema. However, patients with acute symptoms of fever, headache, lethargy, confusion, and stiff neck should have an immediate lumbar puncture, and if this test proves abnormal, then antibiotics should be instituted rapidly for presumed bacterial meningitis. If the distinction between focal and diffuse CNS infection is unclear or adequate evaluation is not possible, as in the comatose patient, then cultures of blood, throat, and nasopharynx should be obtained, antibiotic therapy started, and an emergency scanning procedure performed. If the last is not possible, then lumbar puncture should be delayed pending evidence that no danger of herniation exists. Inevitably, this approach means that some patients will receive empiric parenteral antibiotics several hours before a lumbar puncture is performed. In acute bacterial meningitis, 50% of cerebrospinal fluid (CSF) cultures will be negative by 4 to 12 hours after antibiotics are instituted; negative CSF cultures are even more likely if the causative organism is a sensitive pneumococcus. Should the CNS infection actually represent acute bacterial meningitis, however, the characteristics of the CSF usually suggest the diagnosis because neutrophilic pleocytosis and some degree of hypoglycorrhachia (low CSF glucose) usually persist for at least 12 to 24 hours after antibiotics are instituted. Furthermore, Gram-stained preparation (or assay for microbial antigen in the CSF by latex agglutination) should indicate the causative organism even after antibiotics have rendered the CSF culture negative. Blood and nasopharyngeal cultures obtained before therapy are also likely to be positive in view of the high frequency of isolation of causative organisms from these sites. The approach of treating presumptive CNS infections promptly is often life saving and does not significantly compromise management. This approach to the use of scanning procedures is germane only for adults with community-acquired CNS infection. In children, technically adequate computed tomography (CT) requires heavy sedation; therefore scanning procedures must be reserved for more stringent indications.

Armed with the clinical presentation and the results of the lumbar puncture and CT scanning or magnetic resonance imaging, the clinician must decide on a probable cause and develop a plan for initial management and definitive evaluation. The task is simplified by addressing the following issues:

1. Is the host immunocompetent? The spectrum of CNS diseases and their causes shifts dramatically in the patient who is immunocompromised (**Web Table 97-1**). For example, the possibility of human immunodeficiency virus (HIV) infection must be determined expeditiously by serologic testing and polymerase chain reaction (PCR) if the likelihood is sufficiently high (see Chapter 108), because acute HIV infection may cause CNS signs and symptoms at seroconversion. Likewise, for patients who have been treated with immunosuppressive medications or immune response modifiers, cultures and PCR testing

Table 97-1 Typical Cerebrospinal Fluid Findings in Central Nervous System Infections

Infection	Cells	Neutrophils	Glucose	Protein
Bacterial meningitis	500-10,000/mcL	>90%	<40 mg/dL	>150 mg/dL
Aseptic meningitis	10-2000/mcL	Early >50%; late <20%	Normal	>100 mg/dL
Herpes simplex virus encephalitis	0-1000/mcL	>50%	Normal	<100 mg/dL
Tuberculous meningitis	50-500/mcL	Early >50%; late <50%	<30 mg/dL	>150 mg/dL
Syphilitic meningitis	50-500/mcL	<10%	<40 mg/dL	<100 mg/dL

for common and uncommon agents should be expedited if clinically indicated.

2. Are there relevant exposures? Exposure to persons with tuberculosis or HIV infection may be associated with the acquisition of these diseases. Ticks may transmit Lyme disease or spotted fever, and mosquitoes may transmit arboviral encephalitis. Exposure to livestock or unpasteurized dairy products suggests brucellosis. Residence in the Ohio and Mississippi River valleys increases the risk of histoplasmosis and blastomycosis; coccidioidomycosis is endemic to semi-arid regions of the Southwest. Travel and particularly residence in developing countries may suggest cysticercosis, echinococcal cyst disease, tuberculosis, and cerebral malaria.

3. Does the patient have meningitis, encephalitis, or meningoencephalitis? Is the disease acute, subacute, or chronic? These distinctions narrow and modify the differential diagnosis considerably and form the basis for the organization of the sections that follow. The meningitis syndrome consists of fever, headache, and stiff neck. Confusion and a depressed level of consciousness may occur as part of the encephalopathy in patients with acute bacterial meningitis. Seizures are rare and may indicate complicating processes such as cortical vein thrombosis. In contrast, encephalitis characteristically causes confusion, bizarre behavior, depressed levels of consciousness, focal neurologic signs, and seizures (generalized or focal). A presentation suggestive of encephalitis can raise a variety of issues quite different from those surrounding a patient with bacterial meningitis.

Meningitis

Meningitis is inflammation of the leptomeninges caused by infectious or noninfectious processes. The causes of infectious meningitis may be bacterial, viral, tuberculous, and fungal. The most common noninfectious causes are subarachnoid hemorrhage, cancer, and sarcoidosis. Infectious meningitis is considered in three categories: acute bacterial meningitis, aseptic meningitis, and subacute to chronic meningitis.

ACUTE BACTERIAL MENINGITIS

Epidemiologic Features

Three fourths of patients with acute bacterial meningitis are presented before the age of 15 years. *Neisseria meningitidis* causes sporadic disease or epidemics in closed populations. Closed population outbreaks often occur among students in primary and secondary schools and college students residing in dormitories. However, most cases occur in winter and spring and involve children younger than 5 years of age. *Haemophilus influenzae* meningitis is even more selectively a disease of childhood, with most cases developing by the age of 10 years. Infections are sporadic, although secondary cases may occur in close contacts. The incidence of *H. influenzae* meningitis has significantly declined with the widespread use of effective conjugated vaccines. In contrast, pneumococcal meningitis is a disease observed in all age groups. In addition, pneumococcus is becoming increasingly resistant to penicillin, making therapy more challenging (see later discussion). Recent clinical series of hospitalized adults show a relative frequency of 40% to 55% pneumococcal, 3% to 13% meningococcal, 10% to 13% listerial, and 4% to 8% *H. influenzae* for community-acquired meningitis. The use of the conjugated pneumococcal vaccine in early childhood should decrease the incidence of meningitis caused by *Streptococcus pneumoniae* in all age groups.

Vaccination is particularly important for persons with inherited (e.g., complement deficiency, sickle cell anemia) and acquired (e.g., HIV infection, splenectomy) immunodeficiency (see **Web Table 97-1**).

Close contact with a patient with *N. meningitidis* or *H. influenzae* disease increases the incidence of secondary cases of meningitis, sepsis, and epiglottitis. For example, the risk of meningococcal disease is 500 to 800 times greater in a close contact of a patient with meningococcal meningitis than it is with no contact. Asymptomatic pharyngeal carriers of *H. influenzae* can also spread infection to their contacts. Thus, prophylactic therapy for close contacts is critical to prevent secondary cases (see discussion of treatment and outcome).

Pathogenesis and Pathophysiologic Features

The bacteria that cause most community-acquired meningitis transiently colonize the oropharynx and nasopharynx of healthy individuals. Meningitis may occur in nonimmune hosts after bacteremia from an upper respiratory site (*N. meningitidis* or *H. influenzae*) or pneumonia and by the direct spread from contiguous foci of infection (nasal or mastoid sinuses).

The pathogenesis of acute bacterial meningitis is best understood for meningococcal disease. The carrier state occurs when meningococci adhere to pharyngeal epithelial cells by means of specialized filamentous structures termed *pili*. The production of immunoglobulin A (IgA) protease by pathogenic *Neisseria* species favors adherence by inactivating IgA, a major host barrier to mucosal colonization. Organisms enter and pass through epithelial cells to subepithelial tissues, where they multiply in nonimmune individuals and produce bacteremia. The localization of organisms to the CSF is not well understood but presumably depends on invasive properties of the capsular polysaccharide, which permit penetration of the blood-brain barrier. Immunity is conferred by bactericidal antibody and presumably is acquired by earlier colonization of the pharynx with non-pathogenic meningococci and other cross-reacting bacteria. The presence of blocking IgA antibody may increase susceptibility transiently in some individuals. Bacterial meningitis usually remains confined to the leptomeninges and does not spread to adjacent parenchymal tissue. Focal and global neurologic deficits develop because of involvement of blood vessels coursing in the meninges and through the subarachnoid space. In addition, cranial nerves and cerebral tissue can be damaged by the attendant inflammation, edema, and scarring, as well as by the development of obstructive hydrocephalus.

Gram-negative bacterial meningitis occurs mainly in severely debilitated persons or in individuals whose meninges have been breached or damaged by head trauma, a neurosurgical procedure, or a parameningeal infection or tumor.

Clinical Presentation

Patients with bacterial meningitis may exhibit fever, headache, lethargy, confusion, irritability, and stiff neck. One of three principal modes of onset can occur. (1) Approximately 25% of cases begin abruptly with fulminant illness; mortality is very high in this setting. (2) More often, meningeal symptoms progress over 1 to 7 days. (3) Meningitis may superimpose itself on 1 to 3 weeks of an upper respiratory–type illness; diagnosis is most difficult in this group. Occasionally, no more than a single additional neurologic symptom or sign hints at disease more serious than a routine upper respiratory tract infection. Stiff neck is absent in roughly one half of all patients with meningitis, notably in the very young, the old, and the comatose. A petechial or purpuric rash is found in one half of patients with meningococcemia; although not pathognomonic, palpable purpura is very suggestive of *N. meningitidis* infection. Approximately 20% of patients with acute bacterial meningitis have seizures, and a similar fraction has focal neurologic findings.

Laboratory Diagnosis

In acute bacterial meningitis the CSF usually contains 500 to 10,000 cells/mcL, mostly neutrophils (see Table 97-1). Glucose concentration falls below 40 mg/dL, and the protein level rises above 150 mg/dL in most patients. The Gram-stained preparation of CSF is positive in 80% to 88% of patients. However, certain cautionary notes are appropriate. Cell counts can be lower (occasionally zero) early in the course of meningococcal and pneumococcal meningitis or in patients with neutropenia. In addition, predominantly mononuclear cell pleocytosis may occur in patients who received antibiotics before the lumbar puncture. A similar mononuclear pleocytosis may be seen in meningitis caused by *Listeria monocytogenes, Mycobacterium tuberculosis,* and *Treponema pallidum* (secondary syphilis) (Table 97-2). Gram-stained preparations of CSF may be negative or misinterpreted when meningitis is caused by *H. influenzae, N. meningitidis,* or *L. monocytogenes* because gram-negative diplococci and coccobacilli may be difficult to visualize or

Table 97-2 Meningitis and Meningoencephalitis in the Immunocompromised Patient

Abnormality	Infectious Agent
Complement deficiencies (C6-C8)	*Neisseria meningitidis*
Splenectomy and/or antibody defects	*Streptococcus pneumoniae* *Haemophilus influenzae* Enterovirus *Neisseria meningitidis*
Sickle cell disease	*S. pneumoniae* *H. influenzae*
Impaired cellular immunity (e.g., HIV infection, chemotherapy, organ transplantation, and rheumatic diseases)	*Listeria monocytogenes* *Cryptococcus neoformans* *Toxoplasma gondii* *Histoplasma capsulatum* *Coccidioides immitis* *Mycobacterium tuberculosis* *Treponema pallidum* John Cunningham (JC) virus Cytomegalovirus Herpesviruses 1, 2, 6

discern. In addition, bacteria tend to be pleomorphic in CSF and may assume atypical forms. Compared with patients with acute meningitis caused by other bacterial pathogens, patients with *Listeria* infection have a significantly lower incidence of meningeal signs, and the CSF profile is significantly less likely to have a high white blood cell count or a high protein concentration. Gram stain is negative in two thirds of patients with listerial meningitis or meningoencephalitis. If interpretation of the Gram-stained CSF is not clear, then broad-spectrum antibiotics should be instituted while results of cultures are pending. If the initial Gram-stained preparation does not contain organisms, then examining the Gram-stained sediment prepared by concentrating up to 5 mL of CSF with a cytocentrifuge may reveal the causative organism.

Cultures of CSF, blood, fluid expressed from purpuric lesions, and nasopharyngeal swabs have a high yield. The last method is particularly valuable in patients who received antibiotic therapy before hospitalization because most antibiotics do not achieve substantial levels in nasopharyngeal secretions to eradicate the colonization state.

Recognition of meningitis may be difficult after head trauma or neurosurgery because the symptoms, signs, and laboratory findings of infection can be difficult to separate from those of trauma. A low level of CSF glucose usually indicates infection but can also be seen after subarachnoid hemorrhage. The causative organism, characteristically an enteric gram-negative bacillus (including *Pseudomonas aeruginosa*), may already have been cultured from an extraneural site such as a wound or urine. The known antibiotic sensitivities of such isolates therefore may provide a valuable guide to the initial treatment of meningitis in patients after neurosurgery.

All patients with meningitis caused by unusual agents or mixed infections and certain patients with meningitis caused by *S. pneumoniae* and *H. influenzae* should undergo radiography of nasal and mastoid sinuses to exclude a parameningeal focus of infection.

Differential Diagnosis

Classic acute bacterial meningitis resembles few other diseases. Ruptured brain abscess should be considered, particularly if the CSF white blood cell count is unusually high and focal neurologic signs are present or if there is an abrupt loss of consciousness. Parameningeal infections usually cause fever, headache, and local neurologic signs. CSF characteristically shows modest neutrophilic pleocytosis and moderately increased protein, but the CSF glucose level is usually normal. The CSF may be sterile in patients with bacterial meningitis who have already received antibiotics, but neutrophils commonly are present in CSF and the glucose level is depressed. Early in the evolution of viral or tuberculous meningitis, the pleocytosis may be predominantly neutrophilic. Serial CSF examinations, however, will show a progressive shift to mononuclear cell predominance. Similarly, acute viral meningoencephalitis may be difficult to distinguish clinically from bacterial meningitis, but the evolution of CSF findings and the clinical course usually decide the matter.

Treatment and Outcome

Bacterial meningitis requires prompt administration of appropriate antibiotics. If the Gram-stained smear of CSF indicates pneumococcal or meningococcal disease, then penicillin G or a third-generation cephalosporin (e.g., ceftriaxone, 1 g every 12 hours) should be administered intravenously. Because the frequency of intermediate and highly penicillin-resistant *S. pneumoniae* has increased significantly, additional therapy with vancomycin is recommended until the results of sensitivity testing are available. Alternative drugs for patients with severe penicillin allergy are vancomycin and meropenem. Patients with suggested *H. influenzae* meningitis should be treated with ceftriaxone (1 g given intravenously every 12 hours). In a patient with probable community-acquired meningitis, if the Gram-stained preparation of CSF is negative but clinical and laboratory findings suggest bacterial meningitis, then penicillin (or ampicillin) and ceftriaxone therapy should be started. Third-generation cephalosporins are the indicated choice for treating sensitive gram-negative enteric organisms causing meningitis. Agents such as ceftazidime (2 g given intravenously every 6 to 8 hours) may be effective against *P. aeruginosa*. If the organism is resistant to cephalosporins, then the patient should be treated with meropenem. Regardless of the results of sensitivity testing, chloramphenicol is not an adequate drug for the treatment of gram-negative bacillary meningitis; its use has been associated with unacceptably high mortality rates.

Experimental studies have suggested that the morbidity and mortality associated with acute bacterial meningitis results from the detrimental effects of the host inflammatory response. Conversely, inflammation also enhances penetration of antimicrobial agents into the CSF, and in this regard inflammation is considered beneficial. Treatment or modulation of host inflammatory responses during meningitis has evolved as therapeutic targets and adjunctive use of corticosteroids now are recognized as a standard of care in the initial treatment of suspected cases of bacterial meningitis in adults. However, corticosteroids have been shown to improve functional outcome and reduce mortality only in cases of acute pneumococcal meningitis. It is not known why corticosteroids do not offer similar benefits for infections caused by other encapsulated pathogens. Nonetheless, adjunctive use of corticosteroids (dexamethasone 10 mg administered with the first dose of antibiotic) should begin promptly in cases of suspected bacterial meningitis and should continue at 6-hour intervals for 4 days only when *S. pneumoniae* infection has been confirmed.

The management of bacterial meningitis extends beyond the patient. Contacts also must be protected because they are at substantial risk for developing meningococcal meningitis or serious *H. influenzae* disease. At the time when bacterial meningitis is first suggested, respiratory isolation procedures should be initiated. Antibiotic prophylaxis of contacts should begin when the clinical course or Gram-stained preparation of CSF suggests meningococcal or *H. influenzae* meningitis. The recommended drug for household and other intimate contacts of patients with meningococcal meningitis is rifampin, 10 mg/kg (up to 600 mg) twice daily for 2 days. The goal of prophylaxis of contacts of *H. influenzae* type B meningitis is to protect children younger than 4 years of age. Because the organism may be passed from patient to asymptomatic adults to an at-risk child, rifampin, 20 mg/kg (up to 600 mg) daily for 4 days, should be given to all members of the household and day care center of the index case who have contact with children younger than 4 years old. Alternatives to rifampin include intramuscular ceftriaxone or oral ciprofloxacin. Despite parenteral antibiotic therapy, patients with *N. meningitidis* or *H. influenzae* meningitis may have persistent nasopharyngeal carriage and should also receive rifampin treatment at the end of parenteral antibiotic therapy. Because *L. monocytogenes* is resistant to cephalosporins, ampicillin for a minimum of 15 to 21 days (with an aminoglycoside for the first 7 days) is the treatment of choice for *Listeria* meningitis.

Although hospital contacts of patients with meningococcal meningitis are at low risk for acquiring the carrier state and disease, secondary cases occasionally occur. Thus, personnel in close contact with the patient's respiratory secretions should receive prophylactic antibiotics. All persons receiving rifampin prophylaxis should be warned that their urine and tears will turn orange and that the antiestrogen effects of the drug will temporarily inactivate oral contraceptives.

Approximately 30% of adults with bacterial meningitis die of the infection. In survivors, deafness (6% to 10%) and other serious neurologic sequelae (1% to 18%) are common. The prognosis in individual cases depends largely on the level of consciousness and extent of CNS damage at the time of the first treatment. Misdiagnosis (50% of patients) and delays in starting antibiotics are factors in morbidity that physicians must try to avoid. Patients with suggested bacterial meningitis should be treated with antibiotics within 30 minutes of reaching medical care. Even after antibiotic therapy and presumed cure, bacterial meningitis may recur. The pattern of recurrence usually suggests a parameningeal infection or dural defect (Table 97-3).

Because more effective protein-conjugated vaccines are now available for some strains of *N. meningitidis*, *S.*

Table 97-3 **Three Rs of Central Nervous System Infection**		
R	**Deterioration**	**Possibilities**
Recrudescence	During therapy, same bacteria	Wrong therapy
Relapse	3-14 days after stopping treatment, same bacteria	Parameningeal focus
Recurrence	Delayed, same, or other bacteria	Congenital or acquired dural defects

Table 97-4 **Viral Etiologic Features of Encephalitis and Meningoencephalitis**
Herpes simplex virus (HSV-1, HSV-2, HHV-6)
Epstein-Barr virus
Varicella-zoster virus
Cytomegalovirus
Mumps
Measles
La Crosse virus
West Nile virus
St Louis encephalitis virus
Eastern equine encephalitis virus
Coxsackievirus
Echovirus
Rabies
Human immunodeficiency virus
JC (polyoma) virus
HHV, human herpesvirus; HSV, herpes simplex virus.

pneumoniae, and *H. influenzae* type B, vaccination of susceptible individuals can reduce these common types of bacterial meningitis.

ASEPTIC MENINGITIS

Leptomeningitis associated with negative Gram stains of CSF and negative cultures for bacteria has been designated aseptic meningitis, a somewhat unfortunate designation that often implies a benign illness that resolves spontaneously. However, assuming a high level of vigilance with this group of patients is important because they may have a potentially treatable but progressive illness.

Epidemiologic Features

Viral infections are the most frequent cause of aseptic meningitis (Table 97-4). Of those cases in which a specific causal agent can be established, 97% are caused by enteroviruses (particularly coxsackievirus B, echovirus, mumps virus, and lymphocytic choriomeningitis virus), herpes simplex virus (HSV) I and II, and *Leptospira*. Viral meningitis is most often a disease of children and young adults (70% of patients are younger than 20 years of age). Seasonal variation reflects the predominance of enteroviral infection; most cases occur in summer or early fall. Mumps usually occurs in winter, and lymphocytic choriomeningitis usually occurs in fall or winter.

Pathogenesis and Pathophysiologic Features

Localization to the meninges occurs during systemic viremia. The basis for the meningotropism of viruses that cause aseptic meningitis is not understood. HSV type 2 may cause meningitis during the course of primary genital herpes.

Clinical Presentation

The syndrome of aseptic meningitis of viral origin begins with the acute onset of headache, fever, photophobia, and meningismus associated with CSF pleocytosis. The headache is often described as the worst ever experienced and is exacerbated by sitting, standing, or coughing. In typical cases, the course is benign. The development of changes in sensorium, seizures, or focal neurologic signs shifts the diagnosis to encephalitis or meningoencephalitis. Additional clinical features may suggest a particular infectious agent. Patients with mumps may have concurrent parotitis or orchitis and usually give a history of appropriate contact. Lymphocytic choriomeningitis often follows exposure to mice, guinea pigs, or hamsters and causes severe myalgias; an infectious mononucleosis-like illness can ensue, with rash and orchitis. Leptospirosis often follows exposure to rats or mice or swimming in water contaminated by their urine; aseptic meningitis occurs in the second phase of the illness. Aseptic meningitis can also be seen in persons with HIV infection, either as a manifestation of the primary infection or as a later complication. The pleocytosis generally is modest, the protein level is only slightly elevated, and the glucose concentration is normal or slightly depressed. HIV serologic findings may be negative during acute HIV infection, but the diagnosis is readily established by detectable plasma HIV RNA (see Chapter 108).

Laboratory Diagnosis

In viral meningitis the CSF shows a pleocytosis of 10 to 2000 white blood cells/mL (see Table 97-1). Two thirds of patients have mainly neutrophils in the initial CSF specimen. However, serial lumbar punctures reveal a rapid shift (within 6 to 8 hours) in the CSF differential count toward mononuclear cell predominance. CSF protein is normal in one third of patients and almost always is less than 100 mg/dL. The level of CSF glucose is characteristically normal, although minimal depression occurs in mumps (30% of cases), in lymphocytic choriomeningitis (60%), and, less frequently, in echovirus and HSV meningitis. Serial lumbar punctures show a 95% reduction in cell count by 2 weeks. Stool cultures have the highest yield for enterovirus isolation (40% to 50%), whereas CSF and throat cultures are positive in approximately 15% of patients. Serologic studies also may indicate a specific causative agent; a fourfold rise in antibody titer is helpful in confirming the significance of a virus isolated from the throat or stool. Serologic studies are seldom useful in acute diagnosis, but PCR-based testing detects enteroviral RNA in CSF of approximately 70% of persons with aseptic meningitis.

Differential Diagnosis

Partially treated bacterial meningitis and a parameningeal focus of infection may be particularly difficult to distinguish from aseptic meningitis. Serial lumbar punctures may be helpful in establishing the former, and radiographs of the paranasal sinuses, mastoids, and spine may help confirm the latter. In addition, the differential diagnosis includes infectious agents that are not cultured on routine bacterial media and are considered to be causes of subacute meningitis (see the following discussion). Infective endocarditis may cause aseptic meningitis and is an important diagnostic consideration in the appropriate setting (see Chapter 100). Although less common, true noninfectious causes of meningitis (e.g., nonsteroidal anti-inflammatory drugs; immunoglobulin and immune response modifiers) should be included in the differential for aseptic meningitis.

Treatment and Course

Viral meningitis is generally benign and self-limited. HSV meningitis associated with primary genital herpes occasionally causes sufficient symptoms to warrant treatment with acyclovir. Medication-induced meningitis resolves with withdrawal of the offending agent.

SUBACUTE AND CHRONIC MENINGITIS

Certain infectious and noninfectious diseases can develop as subacute or chronic meningitis. *Chronic meningitis* refers to a clinical syndrome that develops over a course of several weeks, clinically takes the form of meningitis or meningoencephalitis, and is associated with a predominantly mononuclear pleocytosis in the CSF. The infectious causes of this syndrome may develop as a subacute to chronic meningitis (Table 97-5).

At the outset, considering the possible role of HIV as directly causing this syndrome or predisposing the patient to specific opportunistic infections such as cryptococcosis or toxoplasmosis is important; these may develop as subacute meningitis, although the latter most often develops as a mass lesion. However, the incidence of HIV-associated CNS cryptococcal and toxoplasmic infection has diminished greatly in the era of highly active antiretroviral therapy (HAART) (see Chapter 108).

Tuberculous meningitis results from the rupture of a parameningeal focus into the subarachnoid space. The presentation is generally one of subacute meningitis, with a neurologic syndrome being present for less than 2 weeks in over one half of the patients. Headache, fever, meningismus, and altered mental status are characteristic, with papilledema, cranial nerve palsies (II, III, IV, VI, or VII), and extensor plantar reflexes each occurring in about one fourth of patients. The initial CSF sample may show predominance of neutrophils, but the differential shifts to mononuclear cells within the next 7 to 10 days. Acid-fast bacilli are identified in the CSF sediment of 15% to 25% of patients. Because delayed treatment is associated with increased mortality, therapy is initiated before confirmation of the diagnosis by culture in most patients. More rapid diagnosis can be established by CSF PCR in the majority of patients. The clinical suggestion of tuberculous meningitis is heightened by a history of remote tuberculosis in one half of patients. Because concurrent pulmonary disease occurs in approximately one third of patients, smears or cultures of pulmonary secretions may support the diagnosis. Appropriate therapy consists of isoniazid, rifampin, ethambutol, and pyrazinamide. *Vascu-*

Table 97-5 Subacute to Chronic Meningitis

Causative Agent	Association
Human immunodeficiency virus	Direct involvement or opportunistic infection
Mycobacterium tuberculosis	May have extraneural tuberculosis
Cryptococcus neoformans	Compromised host
Coccidioides immitis	Southwestern United States
Histoplasma capsulatum	Ohio and Mississippi River valleys
Treponema pallidum	Acute syphilitic meningitis, secondary meningovascular syphilis
Lyme disease	Tick bite, rash, seasonal occurrence

litis related to entrapment of cerebral vessels in inflammatory exudate may lead to stroke syndromes. This rationale has been used for the use of corticosteroids as adjunctive therapy. Although strong evidence of improved outcome is not available, many authorities believe that corticosteroids should be given in tapering doses for 4 weeks when the diagnosis of tuberculosis is established, particularly if cranial palsies appear or stupor or coma supervenes.

Cryptococcal meningitis is the most common fungal meningitis and can occur in apparently normal, as well as immunocompromised, patients. The presentation is of insidious onset, followed by weeks to months of progressive meningoencephalitis, sometimes clinically indistinguishable from the course of tuberculous meningitis. Certain associations are useful in this differential diagnosis. The presence of immunosuppression suggests cryptococcosis, whereas chronic debilitating disease, miliary infiltrates on chest radiograph, or the syndrome of inappropriate secretion of antidiuretic hormone suggests tuberculosis. An India ink preparation of CSF reveals encapsulated yeast in 50% of patients with cryptococcal meningitis. More than 90% of patients have cryptococcal polysaccharide antigen in CSF or serum. Fungal cultures of urine, stool, sputum, and blood should be obtained; they may be positive in the absence of clinically apparent extraneural disease. Initial treatment of cryptococcal meningitis requires amphotericin B. Addition of flucytosine allows use of less amphotericin B. Fluconazole is also effective but causes less rapid sterilization of the CSF. Daily fluconazole is effective for maintenance therapy to prevent relapses in persons with acquired immunodeficiency syndrome (AIDS) and should continue until CD4 counts rise to over 200 cells/mcL after initiation of HAART.

Coccidioides immitis is a major cause of granulomatous meningitis in semi-arid areas of the southwestern United States; *Histoplasma capsulatum* may cause a similar syndrome in endemic areas (Ohio and Mississippi River valleys) (see Chapter 108).

Neurosyphilis reflects the fact that the spirochete causing syphilis *(T. pallidum)* invades the CNS in most instances of systemic infection. The organism then may either be cleared by host defenses or persist to produce a more chronic infection expressed symptomatically only years later. The most common form of neurosyphilis is asymptomatic; patients harbor a few white cells in the CSF and have a positive serologic test for syphilis. Symptomatic neurosyphilis can appear as acute or subacute meningitis (meningitic form), resembling other bacterial meningitis as discussed previously, and usually occurring during the stage of secondary syphilis when cutaneous findings are documented as well. Hydrocephalus and cranial nerve (VII and VIII) abnormalities may develop. CSF and serum serologic studies are usually strongly positive, and the disease is responsive to penicillin.

Meningovascular syphilis begins 2 to 10 years after the primary lesion. The disorder is characterized by both meningeal inflammation and a vasculitis of small arterial vessels, the latter leading to arterial occlusion. Clinically, the disorder produces few signs of meningitis but results in monofocal or multifocal cerebral or spinal infarction. The disorder may be mistaken for an autoimmune vasculitis or even arteriosclerotic cerebrovascular disease (stroke syndrome). The early and prominent spinal cord signs should lead the physician to expect syphilis, and the findings in the CSF of pleocytosis, elevated gamma globulin, and a positive serologic test for syphilis establish the diagnosis. Patients respond to antibiotic therapy, although recovery from focal abnormalities may be incomplete. Syphilis is more difficult to diagnose and may have an accelerated course in the HIV-infected individual. Meningovascular syphilis may develop within months of primary infection, despite treatment with intramuscular benzathine penicillin (see Chapter 107).

General paresis, once a common cause of admission to mental institutions, is now rare. The disorder results from syphilitic invasion of the parenchyma of the brain and begins clinically 10 to 20 years after the primary infection. Paresis is characterized by progressive dementia, sometimes with manic symptoms and megalomania and often with coarse tremors affecting facial muscles and tongue. The diagnostic clue is the presence of Argyll Robertson pupils. The CSF is always abnormal. The diagnosis is made by serologic tests. Early treatment with antibiotics usually leads to improvement but not complete recovery.

Tabes dorsalis is a chronic infective process of the dorsal nerve roots that appears 10 to 20 years after primary syphilitic infection. Lightning-like pains and a progressive sensory neuropathy affecting predominantly large fibers supplying the lower extremities characterize the disorder. A profound loss of vibration and position sense, as well as areflexia, occurs. Autonomic fibers are also affected, causing postural hypotension, trophic ulcers of the feet, traumatic arthropathy of the joints, and Argyll Robertson pupils. CSF serologic test results are usually positive. The disorder responds only partially to treatment with antibiotics.

Rare complications of syphilis include progressive optic atrophy, gumma (a mass lesion in the brain), congenital neurosyphilis, and syphilitic infection of the auditory and vestibular system.

Lyme disease, a tick-borne spirochetosis (see Chapter 95), is associated in 15% of clinically affected individuals with meningitis, encephalitis, or cranial or radicular neuropathies. Characteristically the neurologic disease begins several weeks after the typical rash of erythema chronicum migrans. Furthermore, the rash may have been so mild as to go unnoticed and usually has faded by the time neurologic manifestations appear. The diagnosis should be suggested when a patient develops subacute or chronic meningitis during late summer or early fall with CSF changes consisting of a modest mononuclear pleocytosis, protein values below 100 mg/dL,

and normal levels of glucose. The diagnosis is established serologically or by PCR analysis of CSF, which provides a sensitive approach to the diagnosis of CNS Lyme disease. Patients with early Lyme disease usually respond to oral doxycycline. Patients with late or disseminated Lyme disease respond less predictably to prolonged (14 to 21 days) courses of intravenous ceftriaxone.

Several noninfectious diseases may develop as subacute or chronic meningitis. Typical of this group is a CSF containing 10 to 100 lymphocytes, elevated protein levels, and a mildly to severely lower glucose level. Meningeal carcinomatosis represents diffuse involvement of the leptomeninges by metastatic adenocarcinoma, lymphoma, or melanoma. Cytologic analysis often identifies malignant cells. Sarcoidosis may cause basilar meningitis and asymmetrical cranial nerve involvement, as well as a low-grade pleocytosis, sometimes associated with borderline low levels of CSF glucose. Granulomatous angiitis and Behçet disease also belong in this category.

Approach to Diagnosis

Diagnosing the specific cause of subacute or chronic meningitis may be quite difficult. In patients with tuberculous or fungal meningitis, cultures may not become positive for 4 to 6 weeks or longer; moreover, meningitis caused by some fungi (e.g., *H. capsulatum*) is often associated with negative cultures of the CSF.

Because of the uncertainties involved in establishing the diagnosis of infectious diseases and even the question of whether a particular patient has an infectious or noninfectious disease, an organized approach must be taken. Routine laboratory tests (on multiple samples of CSF) should include an India ink preparation and cultures for bacteria, mycobacteria, and fungi. In addition, the patient with chronic meningitis of unknown cause should have the following: Venereal Disease Research Laboratories (VDRL) testing; cryptococcal antigens determined in blood and CSF samples; fluorescent treponemal antibody absorbed (FTA-ABS) and antinuclear antibody (and, when epidemiologically appropriate, antibody to *Borrelia burgdorferi*) in blood samples; *Histoplasma* antigen in urine and CSF samples; antibody to HIV and *H. capsulatum* in serum samples (and, when appropriate, *C. immitis*); and cytologic studies (three times) in CSF samples. A tuberculin skin test (intermediate strength, 5 TU) should be performed. Diagnosis by PCR of specific pathogens in CSF, when available, can expedite evaluation of patients with chronic meningitis.

The appropriate management is decided by the patient's clinical status and the results of these tests. If the CSF pleocytosis consists of more than 50 to 100 cells/mcL, then an infectious disease is likely. Empiric therapy for mycobacterial and/or fungal meningitis may be necessary. Repeated cytologic, microbiologic, and PCR studies of the CSF may reveal the diagnosis. If the pleocytosis is low grade (less than 50 cells/mcL), then a noninfectious cause is more likely; the condition may even be self-limited, the so-called "chronic benign lymphocytic meningitis." The approach to treating such patients must be individualized. Only rarely is brain or meningeal biopsy necessary or helpful. If all CSF studies are nondiagnostic and the patient's clinical condition is stable, then a period of careful observation is almost always preferable to an invasive diagnostic procedure.

Encephalitis

Acute viral and other infectious causes of encephalitis usually produce fever, headache, stiff neck, confusion, alterations in consciousness, focal neurologic signs, and seizures.

EPIDEMIOLOGIC FEATURES

A large number of viral and nonviral agents can cause encephalitis (see Table 97-5). Seasonal occurrence may help limit the differential diagnosis. Arthropod-borne viruses peak in the summer and fall (West Nile virus [WNV], California encephalitis [La Crosse virus], and western equine encephalitis peak in August; St Louis encephalitis peaks slightly later). The tick-borne infections (Rocky Mountain spotted fever [RMSF]) occur in early summer, enterovirus infections in late summer and fall, and mumps in the winter and spring. Geographic distribution is also helpful. Eastern equine encephalitis is confined to the coastal states. Serologic surveys indicate that infections by encephalitis viruses are most often subclinical. The reason so few among the many infected patients develop encephalitis is not clear.

HSV is the most frequent, treatable, and devastating cause of sporadic, severe focal encephalitis. Overall, it is implicated in 10% of all patients with encephalitis in North America. No age, sex, seasonal, or geographic preference exists.

PATHOGENESIS

Viruses reach the CNS via the bloodstream or peripheral nerves. HSV presumably reaches the brain by cell-to-cell spread along recurrent branches of the trigeminal nerve, which innervate the meninges of the anterior and middle fossae. Although this would explain the characteristic localization of necrotic lesions to the inferomedial portions of the temporal and frontal lobes, the reason why such spread is so rare is not clear, with one case of HSV encephalitis occurring per one million in the population per annum.

CLINICAL FEATURES

The course of HSV encephalitis is considered in this text in detail because of the importance of establishing the diagnosis of this treatable entity. Patients affected by HSV commonly describe a prodrome of 1 to 7 days of upper respiratory tract symptoms followed by the sudden onset of headache and fever. The headache and fever may be associated with acute loss of recent memory, behavioral abnormalities, delirium, difficulty with speech, and seizures (often focal). Disorders of the sensorium are not, however, always apparent at the time of presentation and are not essential for the working diagnosis of this eminently treatable but potentially lethal infection of the CNS.

LABORATORY DIAGNOSIS

In HSV encephalitis, the CSF can contain 0 to 1000 white blood cells/mcL, predominantly lymphocytes. Protein is moderately high (median 80 mg/dL). CSF glucose level is reduced in only 5% of individuals within 3 days of onset but becomes abnormal in additional patients later in the course of the disease. The CSF is normal in approximately 5% of patients. Other laboratory findings at onset are of little help, although focal abnormalities may be present in the electroencephalogram and appear on CT or magnetic resonance imaging brain scans by the third day in most patients. Acyclovir offers such high likelihood of therapeutic benefit in HSV encephalitis with so little risk in this highly fatal and neurologically damaging disease that brain biopsy should not be performed unless an alternative, treatable diagnosis seems very likely. A low level of CSF glucose should increase the suggestion that a granulomatous infection (e.g., tuberculosis, cryptococcosis) is present. If the initial CSF shows a low glucose level, then roughly one third of individuals will have an alternatively treatable infection. If CSF studies and brain imaging remain inconclusive in such circumstances, then biopsy may be appropriate.

Cerebral spinal fluid HSV DNA detection by PCR is highly sensitive and specific in HSV encephalitis. Additional PCR-based diagnostic tests are available for other viruses and should be considered in the appropriate clinical and epidemiologic settings. Viral cultures of stool, throat, buffy coat, CSF, and brain biopsy specimens, as well as indirect immunofluorescence or immunoperoxidase staining of tissues, may provide a specific diagnosis. However, viral isolation and serologic evidence of a rise in antibody titer usually come too late to guide initial treatment. In the case of HSV encephalitis, serologic studies are particularly helpful in 30% of individuals with a primary infection. In addition, CSF titers of antibody to HSV, which reflect intrathecal production of antibody, may show a diagnostic fourfold rise.

DIFFERENTIAL DIAGNOSIS

Acute (demyelinating) encephalomyelitis, infective endocarditis producing brain embolization, meningoencephalitis caused by *Cryptococcus neoformans, M. tuberculosis,* or the La Crosse virus, acute bacterial abscess, acute thrombotic thrombocytopenic purpura, cerebral venous thrombosis, vascular disease, and primary and metastatic tumors may all initially simulate HSV encephalitis.

TREATMENT AND OUTCOME

The course of viral encephalitis depends on the causative agent. Untreated HSV encephalitis has a high mortality rate (70%), and survival is associated with severe neurologic residua. Acyclovir therapy improves survival and greatly lessens morbidity in patients if initiated early, before deterioration to coma. Prognosis is particularly favorable in young patients (younger than 30 years old) with a preserved mental status at the time of presentation.

West Nile Virus

WNV was first identified in 1937 and recognized as a CNS pathogen as early as 1957 during an outbreak in Israel. Infections in the United States were heralded by an outbreak that occurred in New York City in 1999. WNV infection represents an emerging mosquito-borne infectious disease in the United States. Since the outbreak of WNV meningoencephalitis in New York City, WNV has spread to most states. Similar to most cases of viral meningitis and encephalitis,

WNV occurs primarily during the summer and early fall months. Culicine mosquitoes that have bitten infected birds (primarily crows and blue jays) transmit the disease. Although direct human-to-human transmission does not occur, WNV can be transmitted through blood products and organs donated from asymptomatic donors. Additional infections in children have resulted from transplacental transmission and through breastfeeding. Although most infections are asymptomatic, symptomatic patients often exhibit (within 3 to 15 days) a range of nonspecific signs and symptoms that include fever, headache, and myalgia, and in some patients acute flaccid paralysis. Seizures have been observed in less than one third of patients. A roseolar or maculopapular rash involving the face and trunk is seen in nearly 50% of patients. CSF fluid examination typically reveals a lymphocytic pleocytosis (3 to 100 cells/mcL, mild protein elevation, and a normal glucose level. Fatal cases of meningoencephalitis have been primarily limited to patients older than 65 years of age in whom autopsy studies reveal neuronal cell death and severe cerebral edema. The diagnosis is made based on clinical grounds and identification of WNV-specific IgM or RNA. Approximately 90% of patients will have positive WNV-specific IgM within 7 to 9 days of infection, whereas detection of viral RNA is more difficult because symptoms usually begin as the viremia wanes.

Recovery is the rule, although chronic fatigue, weakness, memory loss, and depression may follow WNV infections. Specific antiviral therapy is not available, and management is supportive. Both personal protective measures (e.g., insect repellents) and environmental control measures are important in controlling exposure to mosquitoes and limiting outbreaks and disease transmission.

Rabies

Rabies encephalitis is always fatal, requiring major attention on prevention. Currently, zero to six cases of rabies occur each year in the United States, and approximately 20,000 people receive postexposure prophylaxis.

The incubation period for rabies is generally 20 to 90 days, during which the rabies virus replicates locally and then migrates along nerves to the spinal cord and brain. Rabies begins with fever, headache, fatigue, and pain or paresthesias at the site of inoculation; confusion, seizures, paralysis, and stiff neck follow. Periods of violent agitation are characteristic of rabies encephalitis. Attempts at drinking produce laryngospasm, gagging, and apprehension. Paralysis, coma, and death supervene. When rabies is suggested, protective isolation procedures should be instituted to minimize additional exposure of the hospital staff to saliva and other infected secretions. Detecting rabies-neutralizing antibody or isolating the virus from saliva, CSF, and urine sediment confirm the diagnosis. Immunofluorescent rabies antibody staining of a skin biopsy specimen taken from the posterior neck is a rapid means of establishing the diagnosis.

Indications for prophylaxis are based on two central principles. First, the patient must have been exposed. Nonbite exposure is possible if mucous membranes or open wounds are contaminated with animal saliva; exposure to bat urine in heavily contaminated caves has been followed by rabies. Second, small rodents (rats, mice, chipmunks, and squirrels) and rabbits rarely are infected and have not been associated with human disease. Consultation with local or state health authorities is essential because certain areas of the United States are considered rabies free. In other areas, if rabies is present in wild animals, then dogs and cats have the potential to transmit rabies. Domestic dogs and cats should be quarantined for 10 days after biting someone; if they develop no signs of the illness, then no risk of transmission from their earlier bite is possible. Nondomestic animals should be destroyed and their brains examined for rabies virus by direct fluorescent antibody testing. Bites from bats, skunks, and raccoons always require treatment if the animal is not caught. Unusual behavior of animals and truly unprovoked attacks can be signs of rabies.

Currently, postexposure management consists of (1) thorough wound cleansing; (2) human rabies immune globulin, 20 IU/kg, one half infiltrated locally in the area of the bite and one half intramuscularly away from the site; and (3) human diploid cell rabies vaccine, 1.0 mL given intramuscularly four times for immunocompetent and five times for immunocompromised patients during a 1-month period. Individuals at high risk of exposure (e.g., veterinarians, spelunkers) should be vaccinated.

Spectrum of Tuberculous, Fungal, and Parasitic Infections

The spectrum of tuberculous, fungal, and parasitic infections of the CNS is briefly considered. Many, but not all, of these infections are increasing in incidence as the direct result of the increasing prevalence of HIV infection in the population (see Chapter 108).

TUBERCULOSIS

CNS tuberculosis can occur in several forms, sometimes without evidence of active infection elsewhere in the body. The most common form is *tuberculous meningitis*. This disorder is characterized by the subacute onset of headache, stiff neck, and fever. After a few days, affected patients become confused and disoriented. They often develop abnormalities of cranial nerve function, particularly hearing loss as a result of significant inflammation at the base of the brain. Most patients, if left untreated, lapse into coma and die within 3 to 4 weeks of onset. An accompanying arteritis may produce focal signs, including hemiplegia, during the course of the disorder. Tuberculous meningitis must be distinguished from other causes of acute and subacute meningeal infection, a process that is often not easy even after examination of the CSF. The pressure and cell counts are elevated with up to a few hundred cells, a mixture of leukocytes and lymphocytes. The protein level is elevated, usually above 100 mg/dL and often to very high levels, and the glucose concentration is depressed. Smears for acid-fast bacilli are positive in only 15% to 25% of CSF samples. Tuberculosis organisms grow on culture but only after several weeks. Thus, patients with subacutely developing meningitis consistent with tuberculosis should be treated with antituberculous agents before definitive diagnosis, if rapid PCR identification of mycobacterial antigens in CSF is not available. Large samples of CSF should be sent for culture, and a careful search should be made for tuberculosis elsewhere in the body.

Tuberculomas of the brain produce symptoms and signs either of the mass lesion or of meningitis with the tuberculomas being found incidentally. One or multiple lesions are identified on a CT scan, but the scan itself does not distinguish tuberculomas from brain tumor or other brain abscesses. Without evidence of meningeal or systemic tuberculosis, biopsy is necessary for diagnosis. Patients with tuberculomas usually respond well to antituberculous therapy, but brain lesions may remain visible on the CT scan long after the patient's condition has improved clinically; the clinical course, not the scan, predicts the outcome.

Less common manifestations of CNS tuberculosis include chronic arachnoiditis, characterized by a low-grade inflammatory response in the CSF and progressive pain with signs of either cauda equina or spinal cord dysfunction. The diagnosis of arachnoiditis is suggested by a myelogram showing evidence of fibrosis and compartmentalization instead of the usually smooth subarachnoid lining. The disorder responds poorly to treatment. Tuberculous myelopathy probably results from direct invasion of the organism from the subarachnoid space. Patients exhibit a subacutely developing myelopathy, characterized by sensory loss in either the legs or all four extremities, depending on the site of the spinal cord invasion. Many patients have additional signs of meningitis, including fever, headache, and stiff neck. The CSF usually contains cells and tuberculous organisms.

FUNGAL AND PARASITIC INFECTIONS

Fungal and parasitic infections of the CNS are less common than viral and bacterial infections and often affect patients who are immunosuppressed. Similar to bacterial infections, fungal and parasitic infections may cause either meningitis or parenchymal abscesses. These meningitides exhibit clinical symptoms that, although similar, are usually less severe and abrupt than those of acute bacterial meningitis. The common fungal causes of meningitis include cryptococcosis, coccidioidomycosis, and histoplasmosis. Cryptococcal meningitis is a sporadic infection that affects both patients who are immunosuppressed (>50%) and those who are nonimmunosuppressed. Headache and sometimes fever and stiff neck characterize the disorder. The clinical symptoms may evolve for periods as long as weeks or months; diagnosis can be made only by identifying the organism or its antigen in the CSF. *Histoplasma* and coccidioidal meningitides occur in endemic areas and often affect individuals who are nonimmunosuppressed. The diagnosis is suggested by a history of residence in appropriate geographic areas and is confirmed by CSF and serologic evaluation. Antifungal treatment, particularly in the nonimmunosuppressed patient, is usually effective.

Parasitic infections of the nervous system usually produce focal abscesses rather than diffuse meningitis. The most common infection to affect the patient who is nonimmunosuppressed is cysticercosis, a disorder caused by the larval form of the *Taenia solium* tapeworm and contracted by ingesting food or water contaminated with parasite eggs (see Chapter 110). The disorder is common in many resource-restricted regions, as well as in Southern California. The brain may be invaded in as many as 60% of infected persons.

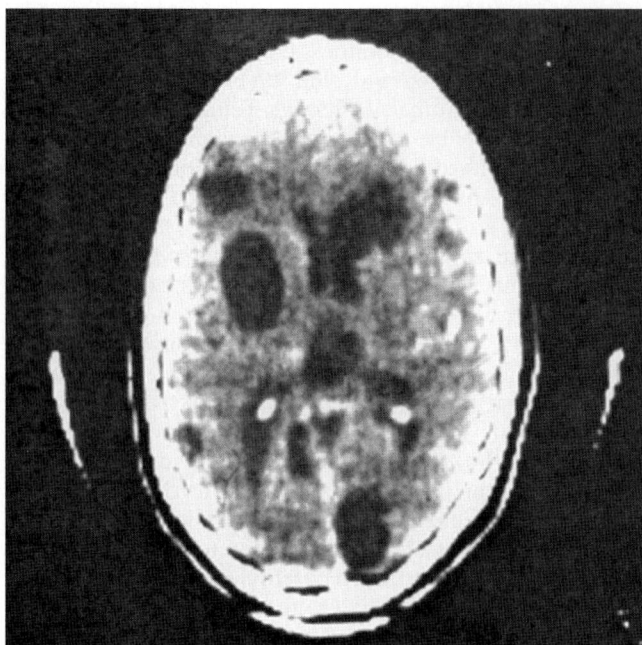

Figure 97-1 Neurocystercosis. A computed tomographic scan shows multiple confluent cysts.

Invasion of the brain leads to the formation of either single or multiple cysts, which often lie in the parenchyma but sometimes reside in the ventricles or subarachnoid space. Seizures and increased intracranial pressure are the most common clinical symptoms. A CT scan identifies small intracranial calcifications and hypodense cysts (Fig. 97-1). Serum indirect hemagglutination tests are usually positive and confirm the diagnosis. Where cysts obstruct the ventricular system to cause symptoms, shunting procedures may be necessary. The anthelmintic agent praziquantel may be effective therapy but has risks.

Toxoplasmosis of the brain, when it occurs in the adult, is a manifestation of immunosuppression. Patients with abnormal cellular immunity usually develop single or multiple abscesses, which generally appear as ring-enhancing lesions on a CT scan (Fig. 97-2). The management of CNS toxoplasmosis is discussed in Chapter 108.

Infection Risks Associated with Use of Emerging Immune Response Modifiers

Immune response modifiers have emerged as novel treatment modalities for patients with rheumatoid arthritis, psoriasis, multiple sclerosis, and Crohn disease that have been refractory to traditional disease-modifying agents (e.g., prednisone, methotrexate, cyclosporine, azathioprine). Many immune response modifiers are humanized monoclonal antibodies (e.g., infliximab [Remicade] and efalizumab [Raptiva]) or soluble receptor decoys that function as cytokine antagonists (e.g., etanercept [Enbrel]). In addition, humanized monoclonal antibodies have been used to condition donor hematopoietic cell allografts (alemtuzumab

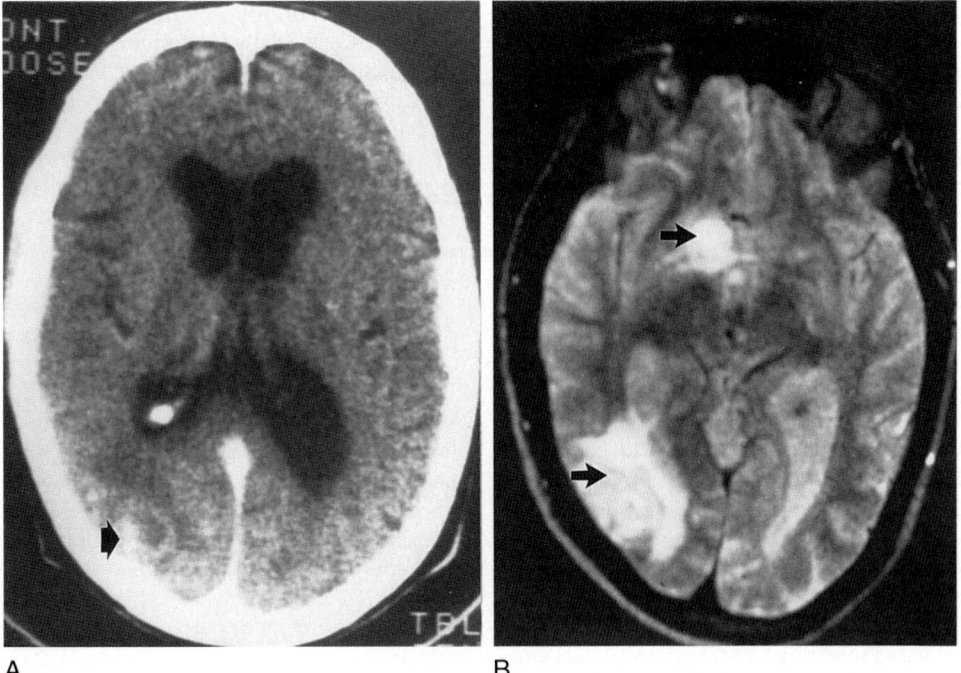

A   B

Figure 97-2 *Toxoplasma* abscesses in a patient with acquired immunodeficiency syndrome. **A,** Computed tomography (CT) scan shows a contrast medium–enhanced mass *(arrow)*. **B,** Magnetic resonance image reveals multiple masses *(arrows)* not visualized with CT scanning, leading physicians to suggest abscesses rather than tumor of mature T lymphocytes.

Table 97-6 Immune Response Modifiers Associated with Central Nervous System Infections

Immunotherapy	Mechanism of Action	Central Nervous System Infection
Infliximab	Inhibition of TNF-α	Aseptic meningitis
Adalimumab		West Nile virus encephalitis
Etanercept		*Aspergillus* brain abscess
		Mycobacterium tuberculosis meningitis
Efalizumab	Inhibition of CD11a-mediated cellular adhesion and migration	Aseptic meningitis
		Cryptococcal meningitis
Anti-thymocyte globulin	Inhibition of T cell immunity	Aseptic meningitis
Rituximab	Binding of CD20 and depletion of premature and mature B cells	PML (JC viral encephalitis)
Natalizumab	Inhibition of α4β1 integrin-mediated cellular adhesion and migration	PML (JC viral encephalitis)
Alemtuzumab	Binding of CD52 and depletion	HHV-6 encephalitis

HHV, Human herpesvirus; PML, progressive multifocal leukoencephalopathy; TNF, tumor necrosis factor.

[Campath]) and treat refractory cases of multiple sclerosis (rituximab [Rituxan]). Although immune response modifiers are frequently used in conjunction with traditional immunosuppressive medications that promote engraftment (e.g., prednisone, tacrolimus, and mycophenolate), immune response modifiers have a long half-life and extend the duration of profound immunosuppression. Thus, many immune response modifiers are associated with delayed appearance or reactivation of opportunistic or latent infections of the CNS, respectively.

The spectrum of infections associated with immune response modifiers includes many of the pathogens discussed previously (see Tables 97-2, 97-4, and 97-5) but fungal and mycobacterial organisms should be especially considered in the differential diagnosis of CNS infections. Some of the more commonly used agents deserve special

emphasis and are reviewed in Table 97-6. Infliximab and efalizumab administration has been implicated in cases of noninfectious aseptic meningitis, but these agents more commonly are associated with mycobacterial and fungal infections. Anti-thymocyte globulin also has been implicated in cases of aseptic meningitis. Reactivation of latent John Cunningham (JC) virus has been associated with natalizumab (Tysabri), which has been used to treat refractory multiple sclerosis, and with rituximab, which is used in patients with B-cell lymphomas or multiple sclerosis. Although JC virus causes an untreatable progressive multifocal leukoencephalopathy, it is important to raise awareness and recognition of this CNS infection promptly and reduce immunosuppression if possible. Alemtuzumab (Campath) has been used to reduce graft-versus-host disease (GVHD) in hematopoietic cell allografts, but it has been associated with human herpesvirus 6 (HHV-6) encephalitis. In addition, GVHD and its treatment (e.g., prednisone, tacrolimus, mycophenolate) represent independent risk factors for reactivation of HHV-6, which is treatable with ganciclovir or foscarnet.

The development and increased use of novel immune response modifiers pose additional risks for the development of less common viral, fungal, and mycobacterial CNS infections, especially in patients who have other immunosuppressive comorbidities. Therefore a thorough knowledge of a patient's current and past treatment history with immune response modifiers is essential for prompt diagnosis of uncommon opportunistic and latent infections of the CNS.

Prospectus for the Future

The expanded availability and use of immune response modifiers (e.g., infliximab, etanercept, rituximab, and efalizumab) for the treatment of several immune-mediated diseases (e.g., rheumatoid arthritis, Crohn disease, multiple sclerosis, and psoriasis) and for the conditioning of hematopoietic cell transplants may increase further the incidence and risk of less common central nervous system (CNS) infections, such as progressive multifocal leukoencephalopathy (PML), human herpesvirus 6 (HHV-6), and *Mycobacterium tuberculosis* infection.

CNS infections may result in permanent loss of cognitive and motor neuron function. Immunization can reduce the incidence and morbidity and mortality associated with select viral and bacterial infections of the CNS. This fact has been most evident from the near worldwide eradication of poliomyelitis. Recent development and use of newer protein-conjugated vaccines against *Haemophilus influenzae*, *Neisseria meningitidis*, and *Streptococcus pneumoniae* have dramatically reduced invasive CNS infections caused by these respiratory bacterial pathogens. Treatment of primary infections, prophylactic treatment of nonimmune contacts, and immunization of at-risk patients are important in controlling and preventing outbreaks.

Environmental control (e.g., insecticides) and personal protective measures (e.g., N,N-Diethyl-*meta*-toluamide [DEET]) are important measures that help reduce insect reservoirs and personal exposure to insect-borne CNS infections. However, transmission of new viruses (e.g., West Nile) through organ transplantation or blood transfusion mandates heightened awareness that often new asymptomatic infections may be transmitted unwittingly to others. Medical personnel must maintain a high index of suspicion for new and old CNS infections.

Sensitive molecular diagnostic tests (e.g., polymerase chain reaction [PCR] assays) will continue to evolve and will play a critical role in identifying both old and new emerging pathogens associated with CNS infections. Rapid identification of CNS pathogens may limit collateral exposure of high-risk patients such as older adults, who represent a large proportion of the general population.

References

General

Ziai WC, Lewin JJ: Update in the diagnosis and management of central nervous system infections. Neurol Clin 26:427-468, 2008.

Infections Associated with Immune Response Modifier Therapy

Boren EJ, Cheema GS, Naguwa SM, et al: The emergence of progressive multifocal leukoencephalopathy (PML) in rheumatic diseases. J Autoimmun 30:90-98, 2008.

Chan-Tak KM, Forrest G: West Nile virus meningoencephalitis and acute flaccid paralysis after infliximab treatment. J Rheum 33:191-192, 2006.

Crum NF, Lederman ER, Wallace MR: Infections associated with tumor necrosis factor-α antagonists. Medicine 84:291-302, 2005.

Kean J, Gershon S, Wise RP, et al: Tuberculosis associated with infliximab, a tumor necrosis factor alpha-neutralizing agent. N Engl J Med 345:1098-1104, 2001.

Kluger N, Girard C, Gonzalez V, et al: Efalizumab-induced aseptic meningitis. Br J Dermatol 156:189-191, 2007.

Langer-Gould A, Atlas SW, Green AJ, et al: Progressive multifocal leukoencephalopathy in a patient treated with natalizumab. N Engl J Med 353:375-381, 2005.

Marotte H, Charrin JE, Miossec P: Infliximab-induced aseptic meningitis. Lancet 358:1784, 2001.

Pelosini M, Focosi D, Rita F, et al: Progressive multifocal leukoencephalopathy: Report of three cases in HIV-negative hematological patients and review of literature. Ann Hematol 87:405-412, 2008.

Seeley WW, Marty FM, Holmes TM, et al: Post-transplant acute limbic encephalitis: Clinical features and relationship to HHV6. Neurology 69:156-165, 2007.

Singh N, Husain S: Infections of the central nervous system in transplant recipients. Transpl Infect Dis 2:101-111, 2000.

Tuxen AJ, Yong MK, Street AC, Dolianitis C: Disseminated cryptococcal infection in a patient with severe psoriasis treated with efalizumab, methotrexate and ciclosporin. Br J Dermatol 157:1067-1068, 2007.

Van Assche G, Van Ranst M, Sciot R, et al: Progressive multifocal leukoencephalopathy after natalizumab therapy for Crohn's disease. N Engl J Med 353:362-368, 2005.

Vu T, Carrum G, Hutton G, et al: Human herpesvirus-6 encephalitis following allogeneic hematopoietic stem cell transplantation. Bone Marrow Transplant 39:705-709, 2007.

Yousry T, Major EO, Ryschkewitsch C, et al: Evaluation of patients treated with natalizumab for progressive multifocal leukoencephalopathy. N Engl J Med 354:924-933, 2006.

Bacterial Meningitis

Behlau I, Ellner JJ: Chronic meningitis. In Mandell GL, Bennett JE, Dolin R (eds): Principles and Practice of Infectious Disease, 6th ed. Philadelphia, Elsevier, 2005, pp 1132-1143.

Bilukha OO, Rosenstein N: National Center for Infectious Diseases, Centers for Disease Control and Prevention (CDC): Prevention and control of meningococcal disease. Recommendations of the Advisory Committee on Immunization Practices (ACIP). MMWR Recomm Rep 54:1-21, 2005.

DeGans J, Van de Beek D: Dexamethasone in adults with bacterial meningitis. N Engl J Med 347:1549-1556, 2002.

Mace SE: Acute bacterial meningitis. Emerg Med Clin North Am 38:281-317; 2008.

Swartz MN: Bacterial meningitis. In Goldman L, Ausiello D (eds): Cecil Textbook of Medicine, 22nd ed. Philadelphia, WB Saunders, 2004, pp 1809-1824.

Tunkel AR, Hartman BJ, Kaplan SL, et al: Practice guidelines for the management of bacterial meningitis. Clin Infect Dis 39:1267-1284, 2004.

Aseptic Meningitis and Encephalitis

Baringer JR: Herpes simplex infections of the nervous system. Neurol Clin 26:657-674, 2008.

Hayes EB, Komar N, Nasci RS, et al: Epidemiology and transmission dynamics of West Nile virus disease. Emerg Infect Dis 11:1167-1173, 2005.

Hayes EB, Sejvar JJ, Zaki SR, et al: Virology, pathology and clinical manifestations of West Nile virus disease. Emerg Infect Dis 11:1174-1179, 2005.

Irani DN: Aseptic meningitis and viral myelitis. Neurol Clin 26:635-655, 2008.

Tunkel, AR, Glaser CA, Bloch KC, et al: The management of encephalitis: Clinical practice guidelines by the Infectious Diseases Society of America. Clin Infect Dis 47:303-437, 2008.

Molecular Diagnostics

Cinque P, Bossolasco S, Lundkvist A: Molecular analysis of cerebrospinal fluid in viral diseases of the central nervous system. J Clin Virol 26:1-28, 2003.

Speers DJ: Clinical applications of molecular biology for infectious diseases. Clin Biochem Rev 27:39-51, 2006.

Infections of the Head and Neck

Christoph Lange and Michael M. Lederman

Infections of the Ear

Otitis externa is an infection of the external auditory canal. The process may begin as a folliculitis or pustule within the canal. Staphylococci, streptococci, and other skin flora are the most common pathogens. Some cases of otitis externa have been associated with the use of hot tubs. This infection (swimmer's ear) is usually caused by *Pseudomonas aeruginosa*.

Patients with otitis externa complain of ear pain that is often quite severe, and they may also complain of itching. Pain and discomfort should be treated with analgesics. Obstructing debris or excess cerumen should be cleared from the canal, and the tympanic membrane should be inspected. Examination shows an inflamed external canal; the tympanic membrane may be uninvolved. (Patients with otitis media, in contrast, do not have involvement of the external canal unless the tympanic membrane is perforated.) Otitis externa with cellulitis can be treated with systemic antibiotics such as dicloxacillin or a macrolide and local heat. In the absence of cellulitis or perforation of the tympanic membrane, eardrops (0.3% ofloxacin solution *or* polymyxin B + neomycin + hydrocortisone) are sufficient. There are no randomized controlled trials that directly compare oral with topical antimicrobial therapy in otitis externa, and few that compare ototopicals. Higher tissue concentrations may be achieved with ototopicals compared with systemic antibiotic therapy.

Patients with diabetes mellitus are at risk for an invasive external otitis (malignant otitis) caused by *P. aeruginosa*. In malignant otitis externa, pain is a presenting complaint, and infection rapidly invades the bones of the skull and may result in cranial nerve palsies, invasion of the brain, and death. Computed tomography (CT) or magnetic resonance imaging of the cranial bones can establish the extent of disease. Treatment must include débridement of as much necrotic tissue as is feasible and at least 4 to 6 weeks of treatment with two different drugs active against *Pseudomonas* (a carbapenem, piperacillin, an antipseudomonal cephalosporin plus ciprofloxacin or aminoglycoside).

Otitis media is an infection of the middle ear seen primarily among preschool children but occasionally in adults as well. Infection caused by upper respiratory tract pathogens is promoted by obstruction to drainage through edematous, congested eustachian tubes. *Streptococcus pneumoniae, Haemophilus influenzae* (usually nontypable strains), and *Moraxella catarrhalis* are the most common bacterial pathogens, and viral infection from respiratory syncytial virus, influenza virus, enteroviruses, and rhinovirus may predispose to acute otitis media. Fever, ear pain, diminished hearing, vertigo, or tinnitus may occur. In young children, however, localizing symptoms may not be present. The tympanic membrane may appear inflamed, but for otitis media to be diagnosed with certainty, either fluid must be seen behind the membrane or diminished mobility of the membrane must be demonstrated by tympanometry or after air insufflation into the external canal.

Treatment with amoxicillin is recommended; however β-lactamase–producing strains of *H. influenzae* and *M. catarrhalis* are found in this setting, so the addition of a β-lactamase inhibitor may be preferred. Amoxicillin should be dosed at 80 mg/kg body weight to achieve high drug concentrations in the middle ear fluid. Addition of decongestants or corticosteroids is of no proven value. Complications of otitis media are uncommon but include infection of the mastoid air cells (mastoiditis), bacterial meningitis, brain abscess, and subdural empyema.

Infections of the Nose and Sinuses

Rhinitis is a common manifestation of numerous respiratory viral infections. It is characterized by a mucopurulent or watery nasal discharge that may be profuse. When rhinitis is caused by respiratory virus infection, pharyngitis, conjunctival suffusion, and fever may be present. Rhinitis can also be caused by hypersensitivity responses to airborne allergens. Patients with allergic rhinitis often have a history of atopy and often have a transverse skin crease on the bridge of the nose a few millimeters from the tip. The demonstration of eosinophils in a wet preparation of nasal secretions readily distinguishes allergic rhinitis from rhinitis of infectious origin (eosinophils can be identified in wet preparations by the presence of large refractile cytoplasmic granules). Occasionally, after head trauma or neurosurgery, cerebrospinal fluid (CSF) may leak through the nose. "CSF rhinorrhea" places patients at risk for bacterial meningitis. CSF is readily distinguished from nasal secretions by its low protein and relatively high glucose concentrations.

Sinusitis is an infection of the air-filled paranasal sinuses, which are thought to be sterile under normal conditions. Allergic rhinitis and structural abnormalities of the nose that interfere with sinus drainage also predispose to sinusitis. With chronic sinusitis, anaerobic bacteria play a more important role. Viral infections such as those caused by rhinovirus, influenza virus, parainfluenza virus, and adenovirus are frequently associated with sinusitis. Acute bacterial sinusitis is primarily caused by upper respiratory tract bacterial pathogens *S. pneumoniae* and *H. influenzae*, by *M. catarrhalis*, and less often by gram-negative bacteria, anaerobes, and staphylococci. Nosocomial sinusitis, to which patients are predisposed by nasal catheters, may be caused by *Staphylococcus aureus* or gram-negative bacteria.

Sinusitis may be difficult to distinguish from a viral upper respiratory tract illness, which in many instances precedes sinus infection. Patients may complain of persistent cough, headache, "stuffiness," a "toothache," or purulent nasal discharge. Headache may be exacerbated by bending over. Sinusitis should be suspected in a person with a febrile upper respiratory tract illness that lasts more than 7 to 10 days. There may be tenderness over the involved sinus, and pus may be seen in the turbinates of the nose.

Unfortunately, clinical signs and symptoms cannot identify patients with rhinosinusitis for whom treatment is clearly justified. Failure of a sinus to light up on transillumination may suggest the diagnosis, but not all sinuses transilluminate even in health. CT is more sensitive than sinus radiographs in establishing the diagnosis of sinusitis. Patients with bacterial sinusitis confirmed radiographically should be treated with a 10-day course of amoxicillin-clavulanate, cefuroxime, or levofloxacin along with nasal decongestants. Patients with high fever, facial swelling or erythema, or severe facial pain should also be treated for bacterial sinusitis, and the involved sinus should be identified by radiographs or CT scan. Patients who appear severely ill and those who do not respond quickly to antibiotic therapy should undergo sinus puncture for drainage and lavage and further microbiologic evaluation. Sinusitis may be complicated by bacterial meningitis, brain abscess, or subdural empyema. Therefore patients with sinusitis and neurologic abnormalities must be evaluated carefully for these complications, by CT if a space-occupying lesion is suspected or by CSF examination if meningitis is suspected (see Chapter 97).

Fungi also can produce disease of the nasal sinuses. Chronic indolent fungal sinusitis is most commonly associated with *Aspergillus fumigatus* or *Aspergillus flavus*. Treatment consists of surgery and systemic antifungal therapy. Fulminant (angioinvasive) sinusitis is mostly seen in immunocompromised patients, including those with diabetes mellitus and those with prolonged neutropenia secondary to chemotherapy. Clinical features include fever, cough, and nasal discharge and, with central nervous system (CNS) invasion, mental status changes. Causative fungi are *Aspergillus* species and organisms of the order Mucorales. Despite emergency surgery with sinus débridement and intravenous antifungal therapy, the prognosis is poor. *Aspergillus* species can cause fungus balls that typically produce nasal blockage as a symptom. Treatment in most cases is restricted to surgical débridement. Some instances of allergic sinusitis have been attributed to hypersensitivity to fungi. This syndrome occurs in immunocompetent patients with asthma; nasal polyps are found frequently. Medical therapy with topical and sometimes oral steroids is recommended. Polyps may require surgical intervention. Antifungal therapy is not used.

Infections of the Mouth and Pharynx

STOMATITIS

Stomatitis, or inflammation of the mouth, can be caused by a wide variety of processes. Patients with stomatitis may complain of diffuse or localized pain in the mouth, difficulty in swallowing, and difficulty in managing oral secretions. Various nutritional deficiencies (vitamins B_{12} and C, folic acid, and niacin), cytotoxic chemotherapies, and viral infections can produce stomatitis.

Thrush is an infection of the oral mucosa by *Candida* species. Thrush may be seen among infants and also in patients receiving broad-spectrum antibiotics or corticosteroids (systemic or inhaled), among patients with leukopenia (e.g., acute leukemia), among diabetics, and among patients with impairments in cell-mediated immunity (e.g., acquired immunodeficiency syndrome [AIDS]). In its milder form, thrush is manifested by an asymptomatic white, "cheesy" exudate on the buccal mucosa and pharynx that when scraped leaves a raw surface. In more severe cases there may be pain and also erythema surrounding the exudate. The diagnosis is suggested by the characteristic appearance of the lesions and is confirmed by microscopic examination of a potassium hydroxide preparation of the exudate, which reveals yeast and the pseudohyphae characteristic of *Candida*. Thrush related to administration of antibiotics and corticosteroids should resolve after the drugs are withdrawn. Otherwise, thrush can be managed with clotrimazole troches. Refractory thrush or candidal infection involving the esophagus should be treated with fluconazole, or rarely, when azole resistance has developed, it may require treatment with an echinocandin.

ORAL ULCERS AND VESICLES

Herpes Simplex Virus Infection

Although most recurrences of oral herpes simplex infections occur on or near the vermilion border of the lips, the primary infection usually involves the mouth and pharynx (Table 98-1). Generalized symptoms of fever, headache, and malaise often precede the appearance of oral lesions by as much as 24 to 48 hours. The involved regions are swollen and erythematous. Small vesicles soon appear; these rupture, leaving shallow, discrete ulcers that may coalesce. Autoinoculation

Table 98-1 **Oral Vesicles and Ulcers**
Primary herpes simplex infection
Aphthous stomatitis
Vincent stomatitis
Syphilis
Coxsackievirus A (herpangina)
Fungi (histoplasmosis)
Behçet syndrome
Systemic lupus erythematosus
Reiter syndrome
Crohn disease
Erythema multiforme
Pemphigus
Pemphigoid

may spread the infection; herpetic keratitis is one of the major infectious causes of blindness in the industrialized world. The diagnosis can be made by scraping the base of an ulcer. Wright or Giemsa stain of this material (Tzanck preparation) may reveal the intranuclear inclusions and multinucleated giant cells characteristic of herpes simplex infection. Viral cultures are more sensitive but more expensive. Diagnosis may also be established by immunoassay for viral antigen or by amplification of viral sequences in the scraping by polymerase chain reaction (PCR). Treatment of primary infection with acyclovir or valacyclovir will decrease the duration of symptoms but has no effect on the frequency of recurrence. Cytomegalovirus and varicella zoster virus are other herpesviruses that can cause oral ulcerations or vesicles, particularly in immunocompromised individuals.

Aphthous Stomatitis

Aphthae are discrete, shallow, painful ulcers on erythematous bases; they may be single or multiple and are usually present on the labial or buccal mucosa. Attacks of aphthous stomatitis may be recurrent and quite debilitating. The cause of the disease is uncertain, and many consider it an autoimmune disorder (see later). Symptoms may last for several days to 2 weeks. Treatment is symptomatic with saline mouthwash or topical anesthetics. Giant aphthous ulcers may occur in persons with AIDS and often respond to topical or systemic corticosteroids or to thalidomide.

Vincent Stomatitis

Vincent stomatitis is an ulcerative infection of the gingival mucosa caused by anaerobic fusobacteria and spirochetes. The patient's breath is often foul, and the ulcerations are covered with a purulent, dirty-appearing, gray exudate. Gram stain of the exudate reveals the characteristic gram-negative fusobacteria and spirochetes. Treatment with penicillin is curative. If not treated, the infection may extend to the peritonsillar space (quinsy) and even involve vascular structures in the lateral neck (see later).

Syphilis

Syphilis may produce a painless primary chancre in the mouth or a painful mucous patch that is a manifestation of secondary disease. The diagnosis should be considered in the sexually active patient with a large (>1 cm) oral ulceration and should be confirmed serologically, because darkfield

examination may be confounded by the presence of non-syphilitic oral spirochetes.

Herpangina

Herpangina is a childhood disease that causes painful, tiny, discrete ulcerations of the soft palate and is caused by infection with coxsackievirus A.

Fungal Disease

Occasionally an oral ulcer or nodule may be a manifestation of disseminated infection resulting from histoplasmosis. These ulcers are generally mildly or minimally symptomatic and are overshadowed by the constitutional symptoms of disseminated fungal illness.

Systemic Illnesses Causing Ulcerative or Vesicular Lesions of the Mouth

Recurrent aphthous oral ulcerations may be part of Behçet syndrome. Oral ulcerations have been associated with connective tissue diseases, such as systemic lupus erythematosus and Reiter syndrome, and with Crohn disease. Although isolated oral bullae and ulcerations may be seen in patients with erythema multiforme, pemphigus, and pemphigoid, almost all patients have an associated rash. The "iris" or "target" lesion of erythema multiforme is diagnostic. Otherwise, biopsy will establish the diagnosis. Corticosteroids may be life saving for patients with pemphigus. Corticosteroids are also used in the treatment of erythema multiforme major (Stevens-Johnson syndrome), although proof of their efficacy is not available.

PHARYNGITIS AND APPROACH TO THE PATIENT WITH SORE THROAT

When evaluating a patient with a sore throat, it is first important to distinguish between the relatively common and benign sore throat syndromes (viral or streptococcal pharyngitis) and the less common but more dangerous causes of sore throat. Patients with viral or streptococcal pharyngitis often give a history of exposure to persons with upper respiratory tract infections. Symptoms of cough, rhinitis, and hoarseness (indicating involvement of the larynx) suggest a viral upper respiratory tract infection, although it is important to remember that hoarseness may also be seen with more serious infections, such as epiglottitis.

Examination of the Throat

Two points regarding examination of the throat need emphasis. The first is that complete examination of the oral cavity is important. Not only will a thorough examination give clues to the cause of the complaint, but it may also provide early diagnosis of an asymptomatic malignancy at a time when cure is feasible. The second point is that the normal tonsils and mucosal rim of the anterior fauces are generally a deeper red than the rest of the pharynx in healthy subjects. This should not be mistaken for inflammation. Patients with pharyngitis often have a red, inflamed posterior pharynx. The tonsils are often enlarged and red and may be covered with a punctate or diffuse white exudate. Lymph nodes of the anterior neck are often enlarged.

If any of the seven *danger signs* listed in Table 98-2 is present, the clinician must suspect an illness other than

Table 98-2 Seven Danger Signs in Patients with Sore Throat

1. Persistence of symptoms longer than 1 week without improvement
2. Respiratory difficulty, particularly stridor
3. Difficulty in handling secretions
4. Difficulty in swallowing
5. Severe pain in the absence of erythema
6. A palpable mass
7. Blood, even in small amounts, in the pharynx or ear

Table 98-3 Causes of Pharyngitis

Viral

Human immunodeficiency virus
Respiratory viruses*
Adenovirus
Herpes simplex
Epstein-Barr virus
Coxsackievirus A (herpangina)
Cytomegalovirus
Mycoplasma pneumoniae

Bacterial

Group A *Streptococcus**
Group C *Streptococcus*
Mixed aerobic and anaerobic infections (Vincent, quinsy)
Corynebacterium diphtheriae
Arcanobacterium hemolyticum
Neisseria gonorrhoeae
Yersinia enterocolitica
Chlamydia pneumoniae
Mycoplasma pneumoniae

Fungal

Candida (thrush)

*Most frequent identifiable causes of pharyngitis.

viral or streptococcal pharyngitis. Symptoms persisting longer than 1 week are rarely caused by streptococci or viruses and should prompt consideration of other processes (see later section on persistent or penicillin-unresponsive pharyngitis). Respiratory difficulty, particularly stridor, difficulty in handling oral secretions, or difficulty in swallowing should suggest the possibility of epiglottitis or soft tissue space infection. Severe pain in the absence of erythema of the pharynx may be seen with some of the "extrarespiratory" causes of sore throat, as well as in some cases of epiglottitis or retropharyngeal abscess. A palpable mass in the pharynx or neck suggests a soft tissue space infection, and blood in the ear or pharynx may be an early indication of a lateral pharyngeal space abscess eroding into the carotid artery.

A good history and careful examination will distinguish between the common and benign causes of a sore throat and the unusual but often more serious causes.

Pharyngitis

Agents that have been associated with pharyngitis are presented in Table 98-3. More than half of all cases are caused by respiratory viruses or group A streptococci. Most of the remainder are without a defined cause. Most cases occur during the winter months. In practice, once a diagnosis of pharyngitis is established clinically, it is most important to distinguish between group A streptococcal infections, which should be treated with penicillin, and viral infections, which should be treated symptomatically (e.g., salicylates, saline gargles). Clinical criteria do not reliably predict streptococcal pharyngitis; however, the presence of fever, tonsillar exudates, and tender cervical lymphadenopathy and the absence of cough increase the likelihood of streptococcal infection. In patients with at least two of these findings, a positive rapid streptococcal antigen test will confirm the diagnosis. Some cases may be missed by this test, and for patients with three or four of these findings, clinicians may prefer to treat empirically with penicillin for 10 days.

Pharyngitis and Respiratory Virus Infections

Many patients with common colds caused by rhinovirus, coronavirus, adenovirus, or influenza virus have an associated pharyngitis. Other signs such as rhinorrhea, conjunctival suffusion, and cough suggest a cold virus; fever and myalgias suggest influenza. Symptoms generally resolve in a few days without treatment.

Infectious mononucleosis (IM) caused by Epstein-Barr virus is often associated with pharyngitis. Patients often also complain of malaise and fever. On examination, the pharynx may be inflamed and the tonsils hypertrophied and covered by a white exudate. Cervical lymph node enlargement is often prominent, and generalized lymph node enlargement and splenomegaly are common. Examination of a peripheral blood smear shows atypical lymphocytes, and the presence of heterophil antibodies (e.g., Monospot test) or a rise in antibodies to Epstein-Barr virus viral capsid antigen will confirm the diagnosis. Treatment is supportive. In instances when swelling threatens to compromise the airway, treatment with systemic corticosteroids may be considered. Patients with acute Epstein-Barr virus infection should be advised to abstain from contact sports, because traumatic rupture of the enlarged spleen may be fatal.

Primary human immunodeficiency virus (HIV) seroconversion illness is often manifested by fever, pharyngitis, and lymph node enlargement and is sometimes associated with a generalized maculopapular rash. A high index of suspicion is essential, because this diagnosis is often missed in clinical practice. Diagnosis is established by demonstration of HIV RNA in plasma (see Chapter 108).

Streptococcal Pharyngitis

Streptococcal pharyngitis may produce mild or severe symptoms. The pharynx is generally inflamed, and exudative tonsillitis is common but not universal. Fever may be present, and cervical lymph nodes may be enlarged and tender. Clinical distinction between streptococcal and nonstreptococcal pharyngitis is inaccurate, and patients with pharyngitis should therefore have a swab of the posterior pharynx tested for streptococcal infection. The growth of group A β-hemolytic streptococci or detection of group A streptococcal antigen is an indication for treatment with penicillin (or erythromycin if the patient is penicillin allergic). Antibiotics may shorten the duration of symptoms caused by this infection but are administered for 10 days primarily to decrease the frequency of rheumatic fever, which may follow untreated streptococcal pharyngitis.

Pharyngitis Caused by Other Bacteria

Diphtheria, caused by *Corynebacterium diphtheriae,* is not expected in the United States; the last case was reported in 2003 in an unvaccinated person who had traveled to Haiti. The gray pseudomembrane bleeds when removed and in rare cases may cause death by means of airway obstruction. Most morbidity and mortality in diphtheria are related to the elaboration of a toxin with neurologic and cardiac effects. Treatment consists of antitoxin plus erythromycin. A self-limited pharyngitis, often associated with a diffuse scarlatiniform rash, may be caused by *Arcanobacterium* (formerly *Corynebacterium*) *haemolyticum.* This infection, when recognized, can be treated with penicillin or erythromycin.

Epiglottitis

Epiglottitis, usually an aggressive disease of young children, occurs in adults as well. Early recognition of this entity is critical, because delay in diagnosis or treatment frequently results in death, which may occur abruptly, within hours after the onset of symptoms. This diagnosis must be considered in any patient with a sore throat and any of the following key symptoms or signs: (1) difficulty in swallowing; (2) copious oral secretions; (3) severe pain in the absence of pharyngeal erythema (the pharynx of patients with epiglottitis may be normal or inflamed); and (4) respiratory difficulty, particularly stridor.

Patients with epiglottitis often display a characteristic posture; they lean forward to prevent the swollen epiglottis from completely obstructing the airway and resist any attempt at placement in the supine position. The diagnosis can be confirmed by lateral radiographs of the neck or by indirect laryngoscopy with visualization of the swollen, erythematous epiglottis. This examination should be performed with the patient in the sitting position to minimize the risk of laryngeal spasm. Furthermore, the physician must be prepared to perform emergency tracheostomy should spasm occur. Therapy has two major objectives: protecting the airway and providing appropriate antimicrobial coverage. Because the most likely pathogen is *H. influenzae,* which may produce β-lactamase, a good antibiotic choice is a second- or third-generation cephalosporin or ampicillin-sulbactam. Corticosteroids may relieve some inflammatory edema; however, the role of this therapy remains unproven. Patients with respiratory difficulty should have the airway protected by endotracheal intubation or tracheostomy. Patients without respiratory complaints may be monitored continuously in an intensive care setting and intubated at the first sign of respiratory difficulty. Young children who are close contacts of patients with invasive disease caused by *H. influenzae* are themselves at particular risk for serious infection. Children younger than 4 years of age who have not received the complete *H. influenzae* vaccine series and are close contacts of the index patient, and all family members in a household with children younger than 4 years of age who have not been completely vaccinated, should receive prophylaxis with rifampin (20 mg/kg given orally, up to 600 mg twice daily for four doses).

Soft Tissue Space Infections

Quinsy

Quinsy is a unilateral peritonsillar abscess or phlegmon that is an unusual complication of tonsillitis. The patient has

Table 98-4 **Indications for Surgical Drainage: Parapharyngeal Soft Tissue Space Infections**	
Infection	**Indications for Surgery**
Quinsy	Abscess or respiratory compromise
Lateral pharyngeal space abscess	Abscess
Jugular vein septic thrombophlebitis	Febrile after 5-6 days of medical therapy
Retropharyngeal abscess	Abscess or respiratory compromise
Ludwig angina	Abscess or respiratory compromise

pain and difficulty in swallowing and often trouble in handling oral secretions. Trismus (inability to open the mouth because of muscle spasm) may be present. Examination shows swelling of the peritonsillar tissues and lateral displacement of the uvula. A mass may be felt on digital examination. In the phlegmon stage, penicillin therapy may be adequate; abscess can be identified by CT and requires surgical drainage (Table 98-4). If untreated, quinsy may result in glottic edema and respiratory compromise or lateral pharyngeal space abscess.

Septic Jugular Vein Thrombophlebitis

An uncommon complication of bacterial pharyngitis or quinsy is septic jugular vein thrombophlebitis (syndrome of postanginal sepsis). Several days after a "sore throat," the patient (in general, a teenager or young adult) will note increasing pain and tenderness in the neck. Often there is swelling at the angle of the jaw. The patient will have a high fever; bacteremia, usually with *Fusobacterium* species; and often septic pulmonary emboli. Treatment is intravenous penicillin, 24 million U/day, plus metronidazole, 500 mg every 6 hours. Patients with persistent fevers may require surgical excision of the jugular vein.

Lateral Pharyngeal Space Abscess

Lateral pharyngeal space abscess is a rare infection associated with serious morbidity because of the proximity of the lateral pharyngeal space to vascular structures. Extension to the jugular vein may result in thrombophlebitis with septic pulmonary emboli and bacteremia (syndrome of "postanginal sepsis," discussed earlier). Erosion of the carotid artery may also complicate this infection, with resultant exsanguination. This may be preceded by small amounts of blood in the ear or pharynx. This infection is generally associated with tenderness and a mass at the angle of the jaw. Prompt surgical intervention may be life saving.

Retropharyngeal Space Abscess

Retropharyngeal space abscess, a complication of tonsillitis, is rare in adults, because by adulthood the lymph nodes that give rise to this infection are generally atrophied. Most cases in adults are secondary to trauma (e.g., endoscopic) or to extension of a cervical osteomyelitis. The patient often has difficulty in swallowing and may complain of dyspnea, particularly when sitting upright. Diagnosis may be suspected by the presence of a posterior pharyngeal mass and confirmed by lateral neck films.

Ludwig Angina

Ludwig angina, a cellulitis or phlegmon of the floor of the mouth, is generally secondary to an odontogenic infection. The tongue is pushed upward, and there is often firm induration of the submandibular space and neck. Laryngeal edema and respiratory compromise may also occur and necessitate protection of the airway. Surgery may be necessary to decompress the infected space. Penicillin is the antibiotic of choice; protection of the airway is crucial in this setting, and endotracheal intubation should be provided if there is any suggestion of airway compromise.

Extrarespiratory Causes of Sore Throat

Several extrarespiratory causes of sore throat should be kept in mind. The older patient who complains of soreness in the throat when climbing stairs or when upset may be experiencing angina pectoris with an unusual radiation. The hypertensive patient with an abrupt onset of a "tearing pain" in the throat may have a dissecting aortic aneurysm. In these patients, swallowing is generally unaffected. Patients with de Quervain subacute thyroiditis may develop fever and pain in the neck radiating to the ears. In patients with thyroiditis, the thyroid is generally tender, and the sedimentation rate is markedly increased. Patients with vitamin deficiencies may complain of soreness in the mouth and throat (see discussion of stomatitis, earlier). Examination may reveal a red "beefy" tongue with flattened papillae, resulting in a smooth appearance.

Persistent or Penicillin-Unresponsive Pharyngitis

Most cases of viral or streptococcal pharyngitis are self-limited, and symptoms generally resolve within 3 to 4 days. In addition to acute HIV infection and IM, as discussed earlier, persistent sore throat should prompt consideration of the following possibilities.

Soft Tissue Abscess or Phlegmon

In rare cases tonsillitis extends to the soft tissues of the pharynx, producing a potentially life-threatening infection (see earlier discussion).

Pharyngeal Gonorrhea

Infection with *Neisseria gonorrhea* may affect almost any mucous membrane. In the head and neck, the most commonly affected areas include the pharynx and the conjunctiva, and the infection may occur without symptoms. This infection will not respond to doses of penicillin used for pharyngitis; moreover, the gonococcus is relatively resistant to phenoxymethyl penicillin (Pen-V). The gonococcus will not likely be identified on routine culture medium; isolation generally requires culture of a fresh throat swab on a selective medium such as Thayer-Martin (see Chapter 107).

Acute Lymphoblastic Leukemia

Persistent exudative tonsillitis may be a presentation of acute lymphoblastic leukemia (ALL). Diagnosis can be suspected after examination of the peripheral blood smear; however, some experience may be required to distinguish between the blasts of ALL and the atypical lymphocytes of IM.

Other Leukopenic States

Stomatitis or pharyngitis may be the presenting complaint of patients with *aplastic anemia* or *agranulocytosis*. Because some of these cases are drug induced (e.g., propylthiouracil, phenytoin), a complete medication history on initial presentation may suggest this possibility. Prompt discontinuation of the offending drug may be life saving.

Although sore throat is a common complaint of patients with relatively benign illness, it is sometimes the presenting complaint of a patient with a serious or life-threatening disease. Any of the key signs or symptoms shown in Table 98-2 should alert the clinician to the possibility of an extraordinary process.

Prospectus for the Future

- Simpler point of care assays for rapid diagnosis of bacterial and viral pharyngitis

- Broader use of imaging methods such as magnetic resonance imaging for accurate diagnosis of serious soft tissue infections of the neck

References

Alcaide M, Bisno AL: Pharyngitis and epiglottitis. Infect Dis Clin North Am 21:449-469, 2007.
Del Mar CB, Glasziou PP, Spinks AB: Antibiotics for sore throat. Cochrane Database Syst Rev 2:CD000023, 2004.
Montone KT: Infectious diseases of the head and neck. Am J Clin Pathol 128:35-67, 2007.
Oshuthorpe JD, Nielsen DR: Otitis externa: Review and clinical update. Am Fam Phys 74:1510-1516, 2006.
Young J, De Sutter A, Merenstein D, et al: Antibiotics for adults diagnosed with clinically acute rhinosinusitis. A meta-analysis of individual patient data. Lancet 371:908-914, 2008.

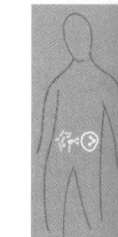

Infections of the Lower Respiratory Tract

Christoph Lange and Michael M. Lederman

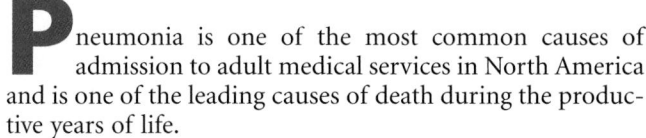neumonia is one of the most common causes of admission to adult medical services in North America and is one of the leading causes of death during the productive years of life.

Viruses, bacteria including chlamydia, rickettsia and mycoplasmas, fungi, protozoans, and parasites can all produce serious infection of the lower respiratory tract. A careful history and physical examination can provide clues to the likely cause of infection. The clinical spectra of pneumonias caused by different pathogens overlap considerably, however. Microscopic examination of respiratory secretions, although uncommonly applied now, can provide a rapid and useful step in the differential diagnosis of pneumonia.

Pathogenesis

Under normal circumstances the lower respiratory tract is generally sterile. Microbes can enter the lung to produce infection by hematogenous spread, by spread from a contiguous focus of infection, by inhalation of aerosolized particles, or, most commonly, by aspiration of oropharyngeal secretions. In the last instance, the organisms colonizing the oropharynx will determine the spectrum of microorganisms in the aspirated secretions and presumably the nature of the resultant pneumonia. Some organisms such as *Streptococcus pneumoniae* may transiently colonize the oropharynx in healthy individuals. Colonization often results in the development of protective antibodies to that strain. Aspiration of normal oropharyngeal flora may lead to necrotizing pneumonia caused by mixtures of oral anaerobic bacteria.

Inoculum size (the number of bacteria aspirated) is an important factor in the development of pneumonia. Studies using radioisotopes have shown that up to 45% of healthy men aspirate some oropharyngeal contents during sleep. In most instances, the bacteria aspirated are relatively avirulent, and backup defenses, including cough, mucociliary clearance, and other innate immune defenses, are adequate to prevent the development of pneumonia. Individuals with structural alterations of the oropharynx and lungs or patients with impaired cough reflexes or neuromuscular disease are at particular risk for the development of pneumonia as a result of aspiration. The specialized ciliated cells of the bronchial mucosa are covered by a layer of mucus that traps foreign particles, which are propelled upward by rhythmic beating of the cilia to a point where a cough can expel the particles. Impaired mucociliary transport, as seen in persons with chronic obstructive pulmonary disease, predisposes to bacterial infection. Denuding of the respiratory epithelium by infection with the influenza virus is one mechanism by which influenza predisposes to bacterial pneumonia. Within the alveoli and smaller airways, alveolar macrophages, granulocytes, lymphocytes, and small peptides such as defensins and humoral opsonins, including antibody and complement, serve as host defenses against infection.

Infection by *Mycobacterium tuberculosis* is usually acquired through inhalation of aerosolized contaminated droplet nuclei. A primary infection is established in the parenchyma of the lungs and in the draining lymph nodes, which may result in a progressive primary infection, but in most instances it remains clinically silent or produces a mild respiratory illness. The mycobacteria may remain alive, sequestered within host macrophages, and are contained by host cell-mediated defenses in granulomas. Reactivation of infection may never occur, may occur without apparent precipitating events, or may occur at times when host cell-mediated immune responses are impaired and granulomas break down. Examples of these impairments include starvation, intercurrent viral infections, administration of immunosuppressive drugs (including corticosteroids and therapies that block the activity of tumor necrosis factor [TNF]), and illnesses associated with immunosuppression, such as Hodgkin disease and human immunodeficiency virus (HIV) infection.

Epidemiology

Common pathogens of community-acquired and nosocomial pneumonia are shown in Table 99-1. As a general rule,

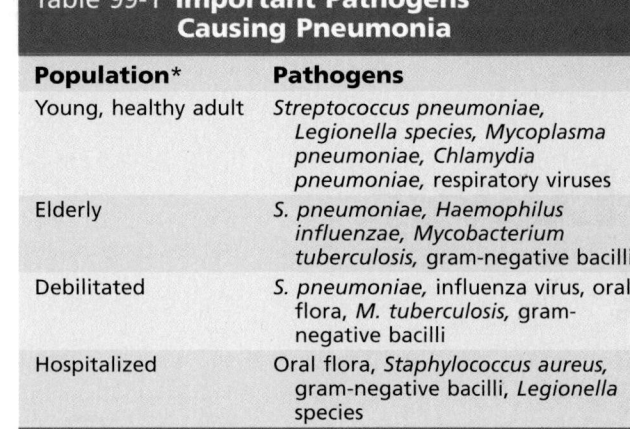

Table 99-1 Important Pathogens Causing Pneumonia

Population*	Pathogens
Young, healthy adult	*Streptococcus pneumoniae, Legionella* species, *Mycoplasma pneumoniae, Chlamydia pneumoniae,* respiratory viruses
Elderly	*S. pneumoniae, Haemophilus influenzae, Mycobacterium tuberculosis,* gram-negative bacilli
Debilitated	*S. pneumoniae,* influenza virus, oral flora, *M. tuberculosis,* gram-negative bacilli
Hospitalized	Oral flora, *Staphylococcus aureus,* gram-negative bacilli, *Legionella* species

*See also Chapters 108 and 109.

Table 99-2 Specific Disorders and Associated Pneumonias

Disorder	Pneumonia
Seizures	Aspiration (mixed anaerobes)
Alcoholism	Aspiration, *Streptococcus pneumoniae, Klebsiella pneumoniae* and other gram-negative bacilli
Diabetes mellitus	Gram-negative bacilli, *Mycobacterium tuberculosis*
Sickle cell disease	*S. pneumoniae, Mycoplasma pneumoniae*
Chronic lung disease	*S. pneumoniae, Haemophilus influenzae, Moraxella catarrhalis, Pseudomonas aeruginosa, Burkholderia cepacia* and other gram-negative bacilli
Chronic renal failure	*S. pneumoniae, M. tuberculosis, Legionella pneumophila*

Table 99-3 Exposures Associated with Pneumonia

Source or Location	Pneumonia
Cattle, goats, sheep	Q fever, brucellosis, tularemia
Rabbits	Tularemia
Birds	Psittacosis, avian-influenza, cryptococcosis, histoplasmosis*
Rodents	Hantavirus
Dog ticks	Ehrlichiosis
Southwestern United States	Coccidioidomycosis
Mississippi and Ohio River valleys	Histoplasmosis, blastomycosis
Developing countries	Tuberculosis

*Exposure to bird and bat droppings.

the pneumococcus is an important pathogen in all age groups, and influenza and tuberculosis become more frequent with increasing age. Although *Mycoplasma* occasionally produces pneumonia in the elderly, it is primarily a pathogen of the young. Certain systemic disorders appear to be associated with pneumonias caused by particular organisms (Table 99-2). The exposure history may be helpful in suggesting specific causative agents (Table 99-3). Pneumonias associated with bone marrow suppression and malignant disorders are discussed in Chapter 109.

Differential Diagnosis

A critical historical point in the differential diagnosis of pneumonia is the duration of symptoms. Pneumonia caused by pneumococci, *Mycoplasma,* or virus is usually an acute illness. Symptoms last for hours to a few days, although there may occasionally be a longer viral prodrome before bacterial superinfection. In contrast, symptoms of pneumonia lasting 10 days or more are rarely caused by the common bacterial pathogens and should raise suspicion of mycobac-

terial, fungal, or anaerobic pneumonia (anaerobes can produce acute or chronic infection) and/or the presence of an anatomic defect such as bronchiectasis or an endobronchial mass.

A history of an unusual exposure or the knowledge of the nature of an underlying immunodeficiency often provides clues to the cause of some less common pneumonias (see Table 99-3). Although these pneumonias are uncommon, they should be considered in the appropriate setting, because if improperly treated, some may be fatal.

A history of rhinitis or pharyngitis suggests respiratory virus or *Mycoplasma* or *Chlamydia* pneumonia. A persistent hacking, nonproductive cough characterizes some *Mycoplasma* infections; an abrupt onset of myalgia, arthralgia, headache, and fever is the typical clinical presentation of a patient with influenza virus infection and may also be seen with *Mycoplasma* pneumonia. A true rigor is very suggestive of a bacterial (often pneumococcal) pneumonia. Whereas small pleural effusions may be seen in nonbacterial pneumonias, severe pleuritic pain and/or empyema in a patient with pneumonia is highly suggestive of bacterial infection. Night sweats in the absence of rigors are seen in chronic pneumonias and suggest tuberculosis, fungal disease, or lung abscess.

Most patients with pneumonia have cough, fever, tachypnea, and tachycardia. Fever without a concomitant rise in pulse rate may be seen in legionellosis, *Mycoplasma* infections, and other "nonbacterial" pneumonias. Respirations may be shallow in the presence of pleurisy. Increasing tachypnea, cyanosis, and the use of accessory muscles for respiration indicate serious illness. Foul breath suggests anaerobic infection (e.g., lung abscess). Mental confusion in a patient with pneumonia should immediately raise the suspicion of meningeal involvement, which occurs most commonly in patients with pneumococcal pneumonia. Confusion may, however, be the most prominent clinical feature of pneumonia in elderly patients in the absence of associated meningitis. Nonetheless, patients with pneumonia who are confused must be evaluated by examination of cerebrospinal fluid.

Physical evidence of consolidation, dullness to percussion, bronchial breath sounds, crackles, increased fremitus, and whispered pectoriloquy suggest bacterial pneumonia. Early in the course of pneumonia, however, the physical examination findings may be normal.

RADIOGRAPHIC PATTERNS

No radiographic image is pathognomonic for a causative agent of pneumonia, but integration of radiographic and clinical findings may be useful in sorting through differential diagnostic possibilities.

As a rule of thumb, fever and malaise often help to differentiate the miliary pattern of tuberculosis from that of sarcoidosis, where patients may be without symptoms. A clinical-radiographic dissociation is a typical feature of *Mycoplasma* pneumonia, where the clinical suspicion of pneumonia is low but infiltrates are detected on the chest radiograph. The converse applies to patients with early *Pneumocystis jirovecii* pneumonia, in early miliary tuberculosis, or in hypersensitivity pneumonia wherein chest radiographs are often normal despite symptomatic clinical disease. Here, high-resolution computed tomography (CT) may demonstrate evidence of pathology. Likewise, early in the course of acute bacterial pneumonias, pleuritic chest pain, cough, purulent sputum, and inspiratory crackles may precede specific radiographic findings by many hours. A "negative" radiograph can never rule out the possibility of acute bacterial pneumonia when the patient's symptoms and signs point to this diagnosis; however, infiltrates should then appear within 24 hours. Common radiologic features of pneumonias are shown in Table 99-4. A lobar consolidation suggests a bacterial pneumonia; however, patients with chronic lung disease often do not manifest clinical or radiographic evidence of consolidation during the course of bacterial pneumonia. Interstitial infiltrates suggest a nonbacterial process but may also be seen in early staphylococcal pneumonia. Enlarged hilar lymph nodes suggest a concomitant lung tumor but may also be seen in primary tuberculous, viral, or fungal pneumonias. Large pleural effusions suggest streptococcal pneumonia or tuberculosis. Pneumatoceles are seen in patients after ventilator-mediated barotrauma but occur frequently in the evolution of staphylococcal pneumonia, particularly among children and also in patients with *P. jirovecii* pneumonia. The presence of cavitation identifies the pneumonia as necrotizing. This finding virtually excludes viruses and *Mycoplasma* and makes pneumococcal infection unlikely (see Table 99-4). Whenever possible, radiographs should be compared with older films.

OTHER LABORATORY FINDINGS

In patients with bacterial pneumonia, the white blood cell count is often (but not invariably) elevated. A left shift with immature forms is common. Patients with nonbacterial pneumonias tend to have lower white blood cell counts. The serum procalcitonin is a useful marker both for monitoring the severity of the bacterial infection as well as the treatment response. Modest elevations of serum bilirubin (conjugated) level may be noted in many bacterial infections but are particularly common in patients with pneumococcal pneumonia.

Diagnosis

When the patient exhibits abrupt onset of shaking chills, followed by cough, pleuritic chest pain, fever, rusty or yellow sputum, and shortness of breath, and the physical examination shows tachypnea and even minimal signs of alveolar inflammation (e.g., harsh breath sounds at one lung base), the presumptive diagnosis of bacterial pneumonia should be

Table 99-4 **Classical Radiologic Patterns of Pneumonia**

Radiologic Pattern	Clinical Situation	Predominant Microorganism
Lobar pneumonia	Community acquired Diabetes mellitus	*Streptococcus pneumoniae* *Mycoplasma pneumoniae* *Klebsiella pneumoniae* Gram-negative rods
Bronchopneumonia	Community acquired Nosocomial	*Legionella pneumophila* *Staphylococcus aureus* *Pseudomonas aeruginosa* *Stenotrophomonas maltophilia* Enterobacteriaceae
Interstitial pneumonia	Community acquired Immunosuppression	*M. pneumoniae* *Chlamydophila pneumoniae* Viruses *Pneumocystis jirovecii*
Cavitation and necrosis	Community acquired Tuberculosis risk factors Aspiration Bronchiectasis Preformed infected cavities Injection drug use, thrombophlebitis	*Mycobacterium tuberculosis* Anaerobic bacteria *or Streptococcus milleri* *P. aeruginosa* *Burkholderia cepacia* *Mycobacterium avium* *Aspergillus fumigatus* *S. aureus*
Large pleural effusions	Postpneumonia	*S. pneumoniae* *S. aureus* Group A streptococcus *M. tuberculosis*
Lymphadenopathy	Human immunodeficiency virus	*M. tuberculosis* Nontuberculous mycobacteria

Table 99-5 CRB-65 Score for the Risk Stratification in Community Acquired Pneumonia

Characteristics		Points
Mental confusion	Confusion regarding place and time	+1
Blood urea >19 mg/dL (>7 mmol/L)	Serum urea	+1
Respiratory rate >30/min	Respiratory rate	+1
Blood pressure: RR diastolic <60 mm Hg or systolic <90 mm Hg	Blood pressure	+1
>65	Age	+1

CRB-65 Risk Group	Fatality	Treatment Location
0	Low (1, 2%)	Outpatient
1 or 2	Moderate (8, 1%)	Consider admission
3 or 4	High (31%)	Admission, consider intensive care unit

RR, time duration between two consecutive R waves of an ECG.

made and appropriate therapy should be begun regardless of radiographic findings. The radiographic abnormalities in pneumonia may lag for several hours after the clinical onset of pneumonia, and when the clinical diagnosis of pneumonia is made, therapy should not be delayed while awaiting results of diagnostic procedures. When the diagnosis of pneumonia is made, heightened risks for mortality and hence decisions to treat as an outpatient, hospitalize, or place into an intensive care unit can be estimated according to the presence of confusion, serum urea >7 mmol/L (>19 mg/dL), respiration rate >30/min, blood pressure <90/60 mm Hg., and age >65 years (Table 99-5). Patients with one or more of these factors may benefit from hospitalization; those with three or more are often best managed in an intensive care unit. Decisions based on these scores must be made also in the context of good clinical judgment. For persons in whom outpatient treatment for pneumonia is recommended, a "second look" reevaluation should be performed 24 to 48 hours after the initial examination to ensure that good progress is being made and hospitalization is not needed.

Empirical antibiotic treatment without laboratory examination of sputum has been recommended for uncomplicated cases of community-acquired pneumonia, and in many instances a good sputum specimen is not readily provided by the patient. Nonetheless, in our view a pretreatment sputum examination helps guide management and is especially useful for review and guidance in instances of first treatment failure. Examination of respiratory secretions is especially valuable for prompt diagnosis and proper treatment of pneumonia in hospitalized patients or in outpatients with risk factors for infections with staphylococci or gram-negative rods; these risk factors include older age, recent hospitalizations, recent antibiotic therapy, underlying lung disease, or impairments of host defenses. The adequacy of a Gram-stained sputum specimen can be ascertained by

(1) the absence of squamous epithelial cells and (2) the presence of polymorphonuclear leukocytes (10 to 15 per high-power field). The presence of alveolar macrophages and bronchial epithelial cells confirms the lower respiratory tract origin of the specimen. The presence of a predominant organism, particularly if found within white blood cells in the absence of squamous cells, suggests that this is the likely pathogen. A specimen with many (>5 per high-power field) squamous epithelial cells is of no value for either culture or Gram stain, because it is contaminated with upper respiratory tract secretions.

In some cases the patient cannot produce an adequate sputum sample despite vigorous attempts at sputum induction using an aerosolized solution of 3% hypertonic saline. The sicker the patient and the greater the likelihood of a multidrug-resistant pathogen, the more important it is to get an adequate sample of sputum for examination and culture. In cases of aspiration of mouth flora, a mixture of oral streptococci, gram-positive rods, and gram-negative organisms is found. In some cases, there may be inflammatory cells and no organisms seen on Gram stain. This finding suggests a number of possibilities, many of which are "nonbacterial" pneumonias (Table 99-6). Unless the diagnosis of acute bacterial pneumonia is clear, an acid-fast stain or fluorescent auramine-rhodamine stain of sputum for mycobacteria should be performed. If legionellosis is suspected, immunofluorescence stains for *Legionella* can be used, although the yield on expectorated sputum is low. The demonstration of elastin fibers in a potassium hydroxide preparation of sputum establishes a diagnosis of necrotizing pneumonia (Table 99-7). Blood cultures should be obtained and may be positive in as many as 20% to 30% of patients with bacterial pneumonia.

Results of sputum cultures must be interpreted with caution, because pathogens causing pneumonia may fail to grow and sputum isolates may not be the pathogens responsible for infection. Careful screening of sputum specimens with Gram stain increases the accuracy of culture results. A tuberculin skin test or a blood test for interferon (IFN)-γ release in response to mycobacterial antigens should be applied in all cases of pneumonia of uncertain cause. A negative tuberculin test may occur despite active pulmonary and/or disseminated tuberculosis.

Specific Pathogenic Organisms

VIRAL AGENTS

Respiratory viral infection is usually limited to the upper respiratory tract, and only a small proportion of infected adults develop pneumonia. In children, viruses are the most common cause of pneumonia, and respiratory syncytial virus is the most frequent organism. In adults, viruses are estimated to account only for a minority of pneumonias, and the influenza virus is the most common organism. Patients at increased risk for influenzal pneumonia include the aged; patients with chronic disease of the heart, lung, or kidney; and women in the last trimester of pregnancy. Cytomegalovirus may cause severe pneumonia in immunosuppressed patients, especially in organ transplant recipients. When varicella occurs in adults, some 10% to 20% develop pneu-

Table 99-6 Sputum Gram Stain Showing Inflammatory Cells and No Organisms

Possibilities	Clinical Setting	Confirmation of Diagnosis	Treatment
Prior antibiotic treatment			
Viral pneumonia	Winter months influenza, may be mild or life threatening	Serologic studies, virus culture, antigen detection	Oseltamivir or zanamivir for influenza A or B, ribavirin for respiratory syncytial virus
Mycoplasma pneumoniae infection	Hacking, nonproductive cough	Cold agglutinins, serologic studies	Doxycycline or macrolide
Legionella pneumophila infection	Chronic lung disease, hospital acquired, summer predominance	DFA of sputum, bronchial brush biopsy, or pleural fluid, culture, serologic studies	Azithromycin or levofloxacin
Chlamydophila psittaci infection	Exposure to birds (e.g., parrots, turkeys)	Serologic studies	Tetracycline or doxycycline
Chlamydophila pneumoniae infection	Hacking cough, sinusitis	Serologic studies, antigen detection	Tetracycline or macrolides
Q fever	Exposure to cattle, South Africa	Serologic studies	Tetracycline or chloramphenicol

DFA, direct immunofluorescence assay.

Table 99-7 Necrotizing Pneumonias

Common

Tuberculosis
Staphylococcus
Gram-negative bacilli
Anaerobes
Fungi
Pneumocystis jirovecii

Rare

Streptococcus pneumoniae
Legionella
Viruses
Mycoplasma pneumoniae

monia, which commonly leaves a pattern of diffuse punctate calcification on chest radiographs. Measles is occasionally complicated by pneumonia. Cases of pneumonia and adult respiratory distress syndrome caused by hantavirus have been reported, primarily among persons residing in the southwestern United States. This severe, rapidly progressive, and often fatal infection occurs largely among otherwise healthy young adults who have been exposed to rodent droppings. Treatment is supportive.

Other viral pneumonias, of which influenza is the prototype in adults, typically occur in community epidemics and usually develop 1 to 2 days after the onset of flulike symptoms. Major features include a dry cough, dyspnea, generalized discomfort, unremarkable physical examination findings, and an interstitial pattern on the chest radiograph. Influenza-induced necrosis of respiratory epithelial cells predisposes to bacterial colonization. This may result in superimposed bacterial pneumonia, most often caused by *S. pneumoniae, Staphylococcus aureus,* or *Haemophilus influenzae.* A presumptive diagnosis may be made on the basis of the clinical presentation and the epidemiologic setting. Gram stain of sputum reveals inflammatory cells and rare bacteria. Detection of viral antigens in sputum can confirm the diagnosis rapidly. Viral isolation or serology also can establish the diagnosis, but not in time to guide management

decisions. Persons with laboratory-confirmed diagnosis of influenza B can benefit from treatment with the neuraminidase inhibitors oseltamivir or zanamivir for five days. If infection is caused by influenza A virus, zanamivir may be preferred or oseltamivir may be given together with rimantadine as influenza A viruses are increasingly resistant to oseltamivir. Treatment should be started within 48 hours of the onset of illness and is indicated for persons with influenza pneumonia or pneumonia complicated by bacterial superinfection and those who are very ill and at high risk for complications.

Recently, highly pathogenic influenza virus strains (H5N1) emerging from avian reservoirs have caused mortality in more than 65% of infected persons in some southeast Asian nations. If and when recombination with currently circulating strains occurs, avian influenza could potentially cause another devastating influenza pandemic. In the spring and summer of 2009, a new H1N1 strain of influenza caused disease worldwide. Younger patients were at most risk. The strain produced a typical flu-like syndrome. Fatalities were noted predominantly in patients with underlying conditions. Other viral agents that may cause pneumonia in adults include parainfluenza virus, respiratory syncytial virus, adenovirus, and newly described viruses such as metapneumovirus.

In 2003, pandemic spread of a newly identified coronavirus (SARS-CoV) caused morbidity in more than 8000 persons around the globe with a mortality of nearly 10%. To date, no effective antiviral treatment is available. Seasonal outbreaks of this severe acute respiratory syndrome and other emerging viral respiratory infections, such as Nipah virus and Hendra virus infections, may be anticipated.

BACTERIAL AGENTS

Streptococcus Pneumoniae

The pneumococcus is still the most common bacterial cause of pneumonia in the community. The organism colonizes the oropharynx in up to 25% of healthy adults. An increased predisposition to pneumococcal pneumonia is seen in persons with sickle cell disease, prior splenectomy, chronic lung disease, hematologic malignancy, alcoholism, HIV infection, and renal failure. Clinical features include fever, rigors, chills, cough, respiratory distress, signs of pulmonary consolidation, confusion, and herpes labialis. By the second or third day of illness, the chest radiograph typically shows lobar consolidation with air bronchograms, but a patchy bronchopneumonic pattern may also be found. Abscess or cavitation rarely occurs. Sterile pleural effusions occur in up to 25% of cases, and empyema occurs in 1%. Typically, a leukocytosis of 15,000 to 30,000 cells/μL with neutrophilia is found, but leukopenia may be observed with fulminant infection, particularly among alcoholics and persons with HIV infection. Gram-positive cocci in pairs can be seen on microscopic examination of expectorated sputum samples in >60% of cases in patients with pneumococcal pneumonia. Positive blood cultures are found in 20% to 25% of patients. In most regions of the world, penicillin G remains the treatment of choice. In regions with a higher frequency of penicillin-resistant pneumococci, or in persons who are severely ill, cephalosporins or vancomycin may be indicated, depending on regional antibiotic sensitivity patterns.

Staphylococcus Aureus

S. aureus infection accounts for 2% to 5% of community-acquired pneumonias, 11% of hospital-acquired pneumonias, and up to 26% of pneumonias after a viral infection. Persistent nasal colonization is observed in 15% to 30% of adults, and 90% of adults display intermittent colonization. Presentation is similar to that of pneumococcal pneumonia, but contrasting features include the development of parenchymal necrosis and abscess formation in up to 25% of patients and empyema in 10%. A hematogenous source of infection, such as septic thrombophlebitis, infective endocarditis, or an infected intravascular device, should be suspected in cases of staphylococcal pneumonia, particularly if the chest radiograph shows multiple or expanding nodular or wedge-shaped infiltrates. Early in staphylococcal pneumonia of hematogenous origin, sputum is rarely available. Blood cultures are usually positive, and associated skin lesions occur in 20% to 40% of cases. When sputum is available, Gram stain shows grapelike clusters of gram-positive cocci. *S. aureus* is recovered very easily from mixed culture samples, so its absence in a purulent specimen usually excludes it as a cause of the pneumonia.

An increasing proportion of community acquired *S. aureus* strains in the United States is now methicillin resistant (MRSA). In affected regions, initial treatment with vancomycin or linezolid is recommended until sensitivity studies indicate that the isolate is sensitive to semisynthetic penicillins or cephalosporins.

Haemophilus Influenzae

H. influenzae is a gram-negative coccobacillus often present in the upper respiratory tract, particularly among patients with chronic obstructive pulmonary disease. Its isolation from sputum in these patients is to be expected. Confirmation of its role in the pathogenesis of pneumonia depends on isolating the organism in the blood, pleural fluid, or lung tissue. Nevertheless, many cases of pneumonia caused by this organism will not be confirmed using these rigid criteria, and in a patient with pneumonia the demonstration

of gram-negative coccobacilli on Gram stain of sputum should prompt institution of treatment with ampicillin plus a β-lactamase inhibitor or a second- or third-generation cephalosporin.

Gram-Negative Bacilli

Gram-negative bacilli have emerged as pathogens of major importance with the introduction of potent antibiotics and the proliferation of intensive care units. They are frequently encountered in patients with structural abnormalities of the tracheobronchial tree, such as chronic obstructive pulmonary disease and cystic fibrosis in the setting of neutropenia, alcoholism, diabetes mellitus, malignancy, and chronic disease of the heart and kidney. They are ubiquitous throughout the hospital, contaminating equipment and instruments, and are the major source of nosocomial pneumonia.

Specific organisms have been associated with certain situations; for example, *Klebsiella pneumoniae* is particularly common in chronic alcoholics, *Escherichia coli* pneumonia is associated with bacteremias arising from the intestinal or urinary tract, and *Pseudomonas* species commonly infect the lungs of patients with cystic fibrosis. Precise etiologic diagnosis is confounded by the frequency with which these organisms colonize the upper airways in predisposed patients. Treatment of patients with *Pseudomonas aeruginosa* infection or seriously ill patients generally includes the use of two active agents, such as an extended spectrum penicillin, a carbapenem, or a third-generation cephalosporin plus a fluoroquinolone.

OTHER CAUSES OF ACUTE PNEUMONIA

Mycoplasma Pneumoniae

Not only is *Mycoplasma pneumoniae* a common cause of pneumonia in young adults, but it also produces a wide range of extrapulmonary features that may be the only findings. Fewer than 10% of infected patients develop symptoms of lower respiratory tract infection. Respiratory findings resemble those of viral pneumonia. Hacking, nonproductive cough is characteristic. Nonpulmonary features include myalgias, arthralgias, skin lesions (rashes, erythema nodosum and multiforme, or Stevens-Johnson syndrome), and neurologic complications (meningitis, encephalitis, transverse myelitis, cranial nerve, or peripheral neuritis). The occurrence of acute, multifocal neurologic abnormalities may be helpful in distinguishing *Mycoplasma* pneumonia from that caused by *Chlamydia* or *Legionella*. The neurologic abnormalities characteristically resolve completely as the acute illness subsides.

In some patients, cold agglutinins may be seen at the bedside by observing red blood cell clumping on the walls of a glass tube containing anticoagulated blood incubated on ice for at least 10 minutes; they are also occasionally positive in other respiratory infections. Complement fixation antibody testing can suggest the diagnosis. Treatment for 7 to 14 days with doxycycline or a macrolide decreases the duration of symptoms and hastens radiographic resolution but does not eradicate the organism from the respiratory tract.

Chlamydophila (Chlamydia) Pneumoniae

Five percent to 15% of cases of community-acquired pneumonia may be caused by *Chlamydophila pneumoniae* (formerly called the *TWAR* agent). Infection is spread presumably through the respiratory route, from person to person, and onset of disease is generally subacute, often manifested by pharyngitis, sinusitis, bronchitis, and pneumonia. The radiographic appearance of pneumonia caused by *C. pneumoniae* resembles that of *Mycoplasma* infection. Illness is relatively mild and often prolonged. Diagnosis of this infection is difficult and requires cultivation of the organism in special cell lines or testing of acute and convalescent sera for antibody levels. Although the organism is sensitive to macrolides and tetracyclines, treatment may have little effect on the course of disease.

Legionella

Legionella are fastidious gram-negative bacilli that were responsible for respiratory infections long before the well-publicized outbreak of legionnaires' disease in 1976, which led to the recognition of this distinct disease entity and to the identification of the responsible bacillus. (The high mortality rate from this outbreak of a hitherto unrecognized disease among participants at an American Legion convention destroyed the reputation of one of Philadelphia's finest hotels.) These organisms are distributed widely in water, and outbreaks have been related to their presence in water towers, air conditioners, condensers, potable water, and even hospital showerheads. Infection may occur sporadically or in outbreaks. Although healthy subjects can be affected, there is an increased risk in patients with chronic diseases of the heart, lungs, or kidneys; malignancy; and impairment of cell-mediated immunity. After an incubation period of 2 to 10 days, the illness usually begins gradually with a dry cough, respiratory distress, fever, rigors, malaise, weakness, headache, confusion, and gastrointestinal disturbance. The chest radiograph shows alveolar shadowing that may have a lobar or patchy distribution, with or without pleural effusions. Approximately half of patients have a mild disease course; in those with a more severe clinical course, the diagnosis is suggested clinically by the combination of a rapidly progressive pneumonia, dry cough, and multiorgan involvement. Microhematuria and a low serum sodium concentration are often present. Gram stain of sputum shows neutrophils and no organisms.

Diagnosis can be made by the following four methods:

- Indirect fluorescent antibody testing of serum is positive in 75% of patients, but up to 8 weeks is required for seroconversion.
- Direct fluorescence antibody testing of respiratory secretions is technically demanding and has a specificity of 95%. Sensitivity of this method is low when using expectorated sputum but greater in specimens obtained from bronchoscopy or transtracheal aspirate.
- *Legionella* antigen can be detected in urine with a sensitivity of 80% to 95% for *Legionella pneumophila* type 1.
- The organism can be cultured on charcoal yeast extract medium (the laboratory must be informed), but up to 10 days is required for growth.

Levofloxacin for 10 to 14 days or alternatively azithromycin for 7 to 10 days is effective therapy. Rifampin may be added in the gravely ill patient, but its value is unproven. Prompt treatment results in fourfold to fivefold reduction in mortality. Patients usually respond within 12 to 48 hours, and it is very unusual for fever, leukocytosis, and confusion to persist beyond 4 days of therapy.

COMMUNITY-ACQUIRED PNEUMONIA OF UNCERTAIN CAUSE

Although it is important to make the best effort to obtain specimens, there are many instances in which, because of difficulty in obtaining adequate sputum specimens or lack of laboratory facilities, empirical treatment of acute community-acquired pneumonia may be necessary. In such instances, initial therapy should be guided by the patient risk factors, comorbidities, and the severity of illness (Table 99-8).

TUBERCULOSIS

Approximately 25,000 new cases of tuberculosis occur in the United States each year, with a worldwide incidence of 7 to 10 million. In North America, a disproportionately high number of cases occurs among the foreign born, racial and ethnic minorities, and the poor. *M. tuberculosis* is transmitted by the respiratory route from an infected patient with pulmonary tuberculosis to a susceptible host. Primary infection may be documented by the development of a positive tuberculin skin test result or a positive blood test for IFN-γ release in response to mycobacterial antigens. Occasionally the patient develops sufficient symptoms of fever and nonproductive cough to visit a physician, and a chest radiograph is taken; patchy or lobular infiltrates are noted in the anterior segment of the upper lobes or in the middle or lower lobes, often with associated hilar adenopathy. Pleurisy with effusion is a less common manifestation of primary tuberculosis. Primary infection usually is self-limited, but hematogenous dissemination seeds multiple organs, and latent foci are established and become niduses for delayed reactivation. Overall, 5% to 10% of individuals with a positive tuberculin skin test result develop disease over their lifetime. Factors associated with progression to clinical disease are age (the periods of greatest biologic vulnerability to tuberculosis being infancy and old age); underlying diseases that depress the cellular immune response (see Chapter 109); diabetes mellitus, gastrectomy, silicosis, and sarcoidosis; and the interval since primary infection, with disease progression most likely in the first few years after infection. Anti–TNF-α therapy can lead to activation of latent tuberculosis infection. Early progression of infection to disease is known as *progressive primary tuberculosis* and may manifest as miliary tuberculosis, sometimes with meningitis, or as pulmonary disease of the apical and posterior segments of the upper lobes or lower lobe disease.

Most commonly, tuberculosis represents delayed reactivation. Symptoms begin insidiously with night sweats or chills and fatigue; fever is noted by fewer than 50% of patients, and hemoptysis by fewer than 25%. Physical examination findings may be unremarkable, or dullness and crackles may be present in the upper lung fields, occasionally with amphoric breath sounds. The chest radiograph may show cavitary disease with infiltrates in the posterior segment of the upper lobes or apical segments of the lower lobes; however, the radiographic findings in pulmonary tuberculosis can be quite variable.

Table 99-8 **Empirical Therapy for Treatment of Community-Acquired Pneumonia**	
Outpatient Treatment	
Previously healthy, no recent antibiotics	Azithromycin, doxycycline
Underlying comorbidities or recent (within 3 months) antibiotics or regions where macrolide-resistant *Pneumococcus* is prevalent	Levofloxacin, moxifloxacin, or gemifloxacin, 750 mg bid
Inpatient Treatment (Non-ICU)	Levofloxacin, moxifloxacin, or gemifloxacin (750 mg bid) *Or* A β-lactam (e.g., penicillin, ampicillin) plus azithromycin or azithromycin
Inpatient Treatment (ICU)	Cefotaxime, ceftriaxone, or ampicillin-sulbactam plus either azithromycin or (levofloxacin, moxifloxacin, or gemifloxacin)
Special Considerations	
If *Pseudomonas* is a concern	Piperacillin-tazobactam, cefepime, imipenem, or meropenem Plus ciprofloxacin or levofloxacin, 15 mg/kg every 12 hrs
If cMRSA is a concern	Add vancomycin or linezolid, 600 mg IV or PO every 12 hrs Azithromycin, 500 mg daily (IV, PO) Doxycycline, 100 mg bid PO Ciprofloxacin, 750 mg bid PO, 400 mg bid IV; levofloxacin, 750 mg daily (IV, PO); moxifloxacin, 400 mg daily (IV, PO); gemifloxacin, 320 mg daily PO Ampicillin-sulbactam, 500 mg q8h IV Piperacillin-tazobactam, 3.375 g IV q6h Ceftazidime, 2 g IV q8h; cefepime, 2 gm IV q12h Meropenem, 1 g IV q8h, imipenem, 1 g IV q8h

Data from Mandell LA, Wunderink RG, Anzueto A, et al: Infectious Diseases Society of America/American Thoracic Society consensus guidelines on the management of community-acquired pneumonia in adults. Clin Infect Dis 44(Suppl):S27-S72, 2007.
cMRSA, community-acquired methicillin-resistant *Staphylococcus aureus;* IV, intravenously; PO, orally.

Extrapulmonary tuberculosis also reflects reactivation of latent foci and accounts for approximately 15% of cases. Miliary tuberculosis is discussed in Chapter 95, meningeal tuberculosis in Chapter 97, and tuberculosis of bones and joints in Chapter 104.

The elderly and patients with diabetes mellitus are more likely to have lower lobe tuberculosis. Because of the growing proportion of elderly individuals in our society and the growing prevalence of HIV infection, "atypical" presentations of tuberculosis are increasingly common. In HIV-infected patients, involvement of the lower lobes is frequent and extrapulmonary tuberculosis, frequently involving lymph nodes, is almost as common as pulmonary involvement. Tuberculin skin tests are likely to be negative in patients with CD4+ T-cell counts <200 cells/μL. The index of suspicion must be high in these settings.

Before antituberculosis drug treatment is started, two or three sputum samples should be obtained for cultures; bronchoscopy and bronchial washing are indicated only if sputum smears are negative for acid-fast bacilli. Amplification of bacterial sequences by polymerase chain reaction (PCR) can distinguish between *M. tuberculosis* and nontuberculous mycobacteria. It is important to obtain baseline evaluation of liver function for individuals who are to receive potentially hepatotoxic drugs (isoniazid, rifampin, or pyrazinamide); color vision, visual fields, and acuity when ethambutol will be used; and audiometry for patients who are to receive streptomycin.

The main principle of chemotherapy for tuberculosis is to avoid resistance by treating with at least two drugs to which the organism is likely to be sensitive. Pulmonary tuberculosis should be treated with daily isoniazid (5 mg/kg, up to 300 mg), rifampin (10 mg/kg, up to 600 mg), ethambutol (15 to 25 mg/kg, up to 2.5 g), and pyrazinamide (15 to 30 mg/kg, up to 2.0 g) for 2 months, followed by isoniazid

and rifampin for 4 more months. A longer treatment duration (a total of 9 months) is suggested when cultures are still positive after 2 months of therapy. When *M. tuberculosis* is resistant to one or more antimycobacterial drugs, expert advice should be sought to design an alternative treatment regimen. Close monitoring during treatment is mandatory to maximize compliance and minimize side effects. Directly observed therapy is recommended by the World Health Organization (WHO) for all patients with tuberculosis.

Contact tracing is critical, because recent infection or additional cases of tuberculosis are likely in some household contacts. Preventive therapy should be considered for all young children and all adults with TST or IFN-γ release assay conversion or those with positive results of these studies who will receive immunosuppressive therapies (e.g., anti-TNF).

Treatment and Outcome

BACTERIAL PNEUMONIA

If the pathogen is readily identified on Gram stain, the antibiotic choices are straightforward (Table 99-9). Otherwise, empiric therapies are indicated (see Table 99-8). The decision as to whether a patient with pneumonia should be hospitalized can be aided by the results of the CRB-65/CURB scores (see Table 99-5). Patients who are treated at home must be able to take their medicines by mouth, should have others at home to attend to their needs, and should be seen again within 24 to 48 hours to ensure that there is an adequate clinical response.

Hospitalized patients should receive supplemental oxygen if hypoxemic. Patients at risk for the development of respiratory failure should be monitored in a critical care setting. Mechanical ventilation should be strongly considered in

Table 99-9 Targeted Initial Therapy for Pneumonia

Pathogen	Treatment
Streptococcus pneumoniae	Ceftriaxone, 2 g IV daily*
Mycoplasma pneumoniae	Azithromycin, 500 mg PO day 1, 250-500 mg PO days 2-7
Chlamydophila pneumoniae	Azithromycin, 500 mg PO day 1, 250-500 mg PO days 2-7
Haemophilus influenzae	Ampicillin-sulbactam, 500 mg q8h IV, or cefuroxime, 1 g q8h IV
Staphylococcus aureus	Vancomycin, 1 g IV q12h† or linezolid, 600 mg q12h IV
Legionella pneumophila	Levofloxacin, 500 mg IV or PO bid Azithromycin, 500 mg PO day 1, 250-500 mg PO days 2-7
Ehrlichia chaffeensis	Doxycycline, 100 mg PO bid
Mixed oral flora (anaerobes)	Ampicillin-sulbactam, 500 mg IV q8h, or clindamycin, 600 mg IV or PO q8h

Gram-negative rods
Double coverage against
  Pseudomonas aeruginosa
	Extended-spectrum penicillin (e.g., piperacillin-tazobactam, 3.375 g IV q6h) or third-generation
	  cephalosporin (e.g., ceftazidime, 2 g IV q8h)‡ or carbapenem (e.g., meropenem, 1 g IV q8h
	  plus fluoroquinolone (e.g., ciprofloxacin, 400 mg IV or 750 mg PO bid)

Tuberculosis	Isoniazid/vitamin B_6, 300/50 mg PO qd, plus rifampin, 600 mg PO qd, ethambutol, 15-25 mg/kg PO qd, and pyrazinamide, 30 mg/kg PO qd

*Levofloxacin, 500 mg daily, for penicillin-allergic patients. Vancomycin, 1 g IV twice daily, for penicillin-resistant isolates.
†Vancomycin or linezolid is preferred if methicillin-resistant *Staphylococcus aureus* (MRSA) is at all prevalent, and regimen can modified if the organism is found sensitive to nafcillin or cephalosporins.
‡Antibiotics can be adjusted when sensitivity data are available.
IV, intravenously; PO, orally.

those with a blood pH <7.25. Patients should be placed in a 45-degree sitting position to avoid aspiration. Meticulous attention must be paid to suctioning of oral secretions. Patients with suspected pulmonary tuberculosis should be placed in isolation rooms with negative pressure, frequent air exchange, and germicidal lamps to prevent nosocomial transmission of infection.

Patients treated for pneumococcal pneumonia should begin to improve within 48 hours after institution of antibiotics. Patients with pneumonia caused by gram-negative bacilli, staphylococci, *P. jirovecii*, and oral anaerobes may remain ill for longer periods after initiation of treatment. Several possibilities should be considered among patients who fail to improve or whose condition deteriorates during treatment.

ENDOBRONCHIAL OBSTRUCTION

Physical examination may fail to show sounds of consolidation, and radiographs may show evidence of lobar collapse. Bronchoscopy can establish the diagnosis.

UNDRAINED EMPYEMA

Radiographs may not always distinguish between fluid and consolidation; ultrasonography and CT can identify the fluid and provide direction for its drainage.

INCORRECT DIAGNOSIS OR TREATMENT

In cases in which clinical response is poor, the patient's hospital course and admission sputum stains should be reviewed by a clinician with expertise in the diagnosis and treatment of pneumonia. Pulmonary embolism with infarction, a treatable disease, can prove fatal if misdiagnosed as bacterial pneumonia. Misinterpretation of sputum gram-stained preparations with either failure to recognize an important pathogen or a treatment decision based on examination of an inadequate specimen is an avoidable pitfall of

medical practice. Bronchoscopy should be considered, both to obtain better specimens for diagnosis and to exclude underlying endobronchial obstruction.

THE PATIENT WITH PLEURAL EFFUSION AND FEVER

The approach to patients with pleural effusion and fever is quite straightforward: the fluid must be examined. If a bacterium other than *S. pneumoniae* is seen on Gram stain of pleural fluid or grown in culture, chest tube drainage is required. A pleural effusion infected with pneumococci can often be treated with simple needle aspiration and antibiotics. Among patients with pneumonia, fluids that have a pH of less than 7.2 and/or a glucose concentration below 40 mg/dL may require chest tube drainage for satisfactory resolution. Patients with empyema complicating an aggressive bacterial pneumonia such as that caused by group A streptococci may benefit from early surgical débridement of the pleural space (decortication).

Pleurisy caused by *M. tuberculosis* is often an acute illness. In most cases, pneumonia is not present or readily appreciated. Inflammatory cells—polymorphonuclear leukocytes, mononuclear leukocytes, or both—are present in the pleural fluid. Mesothelial cells are usually sparse (<0.5% of the total cell count). Pleural fluid glucose levels are often low but may be normal. Mycobacteria are rarely seen on stains of pleural fluid. As many as one third of these patients do not have positive tuberculin skin test results. Detection of M Tb antigen-specific IFN-γ– secreting T-cells in pleural fluid may help to establish a diagnosis of tuberculous pleuritis. Other causes of pleural effusion in this setting may be pulmonary infarction (fewer than half of patients produce a hemorrhagic exudate), malignancy (most do not have fever), and connective tissue diseases such as systemic lupus erythematosus and rheumatoid arthritis (the latter is typically associated with very low pleural fluid glucose levels). If the cause of the effusion is not evident, a biopsy of the pleura is needed.

Table 99-10 Prevention of Pneumonia: Candidates for Pneumococcal and Influenza Vaccines	
Factor	**Pneumococcal Vaccine (may be repeated after 5-7 yr)**
Patient ≥65 years	Yes
Chronic lung or heart disease	Yes
Sickle cell disease	Yes
Asplenic patients	Yes
Hodgkin disease	Yes
Multiple myeloma	Yes
Cirrhosis	Yes
Chronic alcoholism	Yes
Chronic renal failure	Yes
Cerebrospinal fluid leaks	Yes
Residents of chronic care facilities	Consider
Diabetes mellitus	Yes
Human immunodeficiency virus infection	Yes
Children receiving long-term aspirin therapy	No
Pregnant women in the second or third trimester during influenza season	No
Health care workers	No

Note that annual influenza immunization is now recommended for all persons over the age of 6 months. Trivalent inactivated vaccine (TIV) can be given to all persons who are not hypersensitive to its components. Live inactivated influenza vaccine can be given to healthy persons from 2 to 49 years of age. It should not be given to young children (<5 years old) with hyperactive airway disease or persons with underlying medical conditions placing them at higher risk for complications of influenza. TIV should be given to these persons instead.

Prevention

Pneumococcal pneumonia may be preventable by immunizing patients at high risk with polyvalent pneumococcal polysaccharide vaccine. The current polyvalent vaccine is 60% to 80% effective for a 5-year period in individuals with normal immune responses. Yearly immunization with influenza vaccine is also advised for many of these patients; by decreasing the attack rate of influenza, immunization also decreases morbidity and mortality resulting from secondary bacterial pneumonia (Table 99-10).

Patients without active tuberculosis but with skin test reactivity to purified protein derivative or a positive IFN-γ release assay in response to mycobacterial antigens are at risk for reactivation of infection. The development of active tuberculosis can be prevented in most instances by treatment for 9 to 12 months with isoniazid, 300 mg/day. Indications for prophylaxis are shown in Table 99-9.

Prospectus for the Future

- Preservation of clinical skills for diagnosis and treatment of pneumonia:
  - Development of better techniques for rapid etiologic diagnosis of pneumonia
  - Development of techniques for rapid evaluation of antimicrobial susceptibility

- An increasing incidence of drug resistance in bacteria causing pneumonia, including pneumococci, staphylococci, and gram-negative bacteria
- Preparation for outbreaks of life-threatening pneumonias such as those caused by organisms such as avian influenza

References

American Thoracic Society; Infectious Diseases Society of America: Guidelines for the management of adults with hospital-acquired, ventilator-associated, and healthcare-associated pneumonia. Am J Respir Crit Care Med 171:388-416, 2005.

Hansell DM, Armstrong P, Lynch DA, McAdams HP: Imaging of Diseases of the Chest. Philadelphia, Mosby, 2005.

Mandell LA, Wunderink RG, Anzueto A, et al: Infectious Diseases Society of America/American Thoracic Society consensus guidelines on the management of community-acquired pneumonia in adults. Clin Infect Dis 44 (Suppl):S27-S72, 2007.

Infections of the Heart and Blood Vessels

Benigno Rodríguez and Michael M. Lederman

Infective Endocarditis

Infective endocarditis (IE) ranges from an indolent illness with few systemic manifestations, readily responsive to antibiotic therapy, to a fulminant septicemic disease with malignant destruction of heart valves and life-threatening systemic embolization. The varied features of endocarditis relate in large measure to the different infecting organisms. Viridans group streptococci are prototypic bacteria that originate in the oral flora, infect previously abnormal heart valves, and may initially cause minimal symptoms despite progressive valvular damage. *Staphylococcus aureus,* in contrast, can invade previously normal valves and destroy them rapidly. Universally fatal in the preantibiotic era, endocarditis remains a life-threatening but potentially curable disorder.

EPIDEMIOLOGY

The average age of patients with endocarditis has increased in the antibiotic era to the current median of 58 years. This change can be attributed to the decreasing prevalence of rheumatic heart disease, the increasing prevalence of underlying degenerative heart disease, and the increasing frequency of procedures and practices predisposing older patients to bacteremia (genitourinary instrumentation, intravenous catheters, hemodialysis shunts). Rheumatic heart disease is now a predisposing factor in fewer than 25% of patients with IE in industrialized countries. Up to 24% of patients have congenital heart disease (exclusive of mitral valve prolapse). The propensity to develop endocarditis varies with the congenital lesion. For example, infection of a bicuspid aortic valve accounts for one fifth of cases of IE occurring in persons over the age of 60; a secundum atrial septal defect, however, rarely becomes infected. Mitral valve prolapse with valvular regurgitation also can predispose to endocarditis. Intravenous drug users have a unique propensity to develop IE of the tricuspid valve. On long-term follow-up, patients with prosthetic heart valves have a 4% to 17% lifetime risk of IE.

PATHOGENESIS

Endocarditis ensues when bacteria entering the bloodstream from an oral or other source lodge on heart valves, particularly those bearing platelet-fibrin thrombi as a consequence of prior valvular damage or turbulent blood flow. Bacteremia occurs frequently after dental extraction (18% to 85%) or periodontal surgery (32% to 88%), but also after everyday activities such as tooth brushing (0% to 26%) and chewing candy (17% to 51%). These episodes rarely result in endocarditis. The ability of certain organisms to adhere to platelet-fibrin thrombi, such as through production of extracellular dextran by some streptococcal strains, promotes occurrence of endocarditis after bacteremia caused by these organisms. The localization of infection is partly determined by the production of turbulent flow; therefore left-sided infection is much more common than right-sided infection, except among intravenous drug users. Vegetations usually are found on the valve surface facing the lower pressure chamber (e.g., atrial surface of the mitral valve), a relative haven for deposition of bacteria from the swift bloodstream. Occasionally, "jet lesions" develop in foci in which the regurgitant stream strikes the heart wall or the chordae tendineae. Once infection begins, bacteria proliferate freely within the interstices of the enlarging vegetation; in this relatively avascular site, they are protected from serum bactericidal factors and leukocytes.

The infection may cause rupture of the valve tissue itself or of its chordal structures, leading to either gradual or acute valvular regurgitation, with resultant congestive heart failure. Some virulent bacterial (e.g., *S. aureus, Haemophilus* species) or fungal vegetations may become large enough to obstruct the valve orifice or create a large embolus. Aneurysms of the sinus of Valsalva may occur and can rupture into the pericardial space. The conducting system may be affected by valve ring or myocardial abscesses. The infection may invade the interventricular septum, causing intramyocardial abscesses or septal rupture that can also damage the conduction system of the heart. Systemic septic emboli may occur with left-sided endocarditis, and septic pulmonary emboli may occur with right-sided endocarditis.

CLINICAL FEATURES

Some cases of endocarditis caused by oral streptococci become clinically manifest within 2 weeks of a precipitating event, such as dental extraction, but the diagnosis may be delayed an additional 4 to 5 weeks or more because of the paucity of symptoms. If the causative organism is slow growing and produces an indolent syndrome, symptoms may be extremely protracted (6 months or longer) before definitive diagnosis is made. The symptoms and signs of IE relate to systemic infection, emboli (bland or septic), metastatic infective foci, congestive heart failure, or immune complex–associated lesions. The most common complaints in patients with IE are fever, chills, weakness, shortness of breath, night sweats, loss of appetite, and weight loss. Musculoskeletal symptoms, particularly back pain, develop in nearly one half of patients and may dominate the presentation. Fever is present in 90% of patients. Fever is more often absent in elderly or debilitated patients or in the setting of underlying congestive heart failure, liver or renal dysfunction, or previous antibiotic treatment. Heart murmurs are frequent (85%); changing murmurs (5% to 10%) and new cardiac murmurs, when observed, suggest the diagnosis of IE. All too often, however, a soft new murmur heard during hospitalization is not new but rather newly noticed. With endocarditis involving the aortic or the mitral valve, congestive heart failure occurs in up to two thirds of patients; it may occur precipitously with perforation of a valve or rupture of chordae tendineae. The classical peripheral manifestations of endocarditis (Table 100-1) have become less common in recent years. Splenomegaly (25% to 60%) and clubbing (10% to 15%) are more likely when symptoms have been prolonged.

The clinical syndrome of IE differs in intravenous drug users. Fever remains the most common manifestation in this group, but the majority do not have an underlying cardiac lesion, and only one third of proven cases have audible murmurs on admission. Tricuspid valve infection is most common, probably because of scarring of the tricuspid valve by injected particulate matter. Some patients have pleuritic chest pain caused by septic pulmonary emboli, and round, cavitating infiltrates may be found on the chest radiograph. The infective foci are initially centered in blood vessels; only after they erode into the bronchial system does cough develop, which may be productive of bloody or purulent sputum.

Serious systemic emboli, associated with infection of the aortic or mitral valve, may cause dramatic findings, at times masking the systemic nature of IE. Stroke may be the initial manifestation of IE. Embolism to the splenic artery may lead to left upper quadrant pain, sometimes radiating to the left shoulder, a friction rub, and/or left pleural effusion. Renal, cerebral, coronary, and mesenteric arteries are frequent sites of clinically important emboli.

Neurologic manifestations occur in one third of patients with IE and may be the predominant clinical features in 10% of cases, sometimes delaying the diagnosis. Central nervous system (CNS) embolization is one of the most serious complications of IE, and acute neurologic deterioration is an ominous sign during IE, being associated with a twofold to fourfold increase in mortality. IE must always be considered in the differential diagnosis of stroke in young adults, as well as in all patients with valvular heart disease. Patients with IE may complain of headache or may develop seizures. The pathophysiologic explanation for these symptoms is not always apparent. In addition to stroke caused by vascular occlusion by an infected embolus, toxic encephalopathy, which may mimic psychosis, and meningoencephalitis also occur. The aseptic meningitis or meningoencephalitis seen in patients with IE is not always readily distinguished from viral causes of a similar syndrome.

The consequences of CNS embolization depend on the site of lodging and the bacterial pathogen, and clinical syndromes caused by CNS emboli may be distinctive. Organisms such as *Streptococcus viridans* initially produce a syndrome entirely attributable to the vascular occlusion; however, unnoticed damage to the blood vessel can result in formation of a mycotic aneurysm that may leak or rupture at a later date. Resolution of aneurysms may occur after antimicrobial therapy. In many patients, however, surgical clipping is necessary to prevent recurrent hemorrhage. Single aneurysms in accessible areas should be considered for prompt surgical clipping. *S. aureus,* in contrast, produces progressive infection extending from the site of embolization; brain abscess and purulent meningitis are common sequelae.

The kidney can be the site of abscess formation, multiple infarcts, or immune complex glomerulonephritis. When renal dysfunction develops during antibiotic therapy, drug toxicity is an additional consideration.

LABORATORY FINDINGS

Nonspecific laboratory abnormalities occur in IE and reflect chronic infection. These include anemia (typically normo-

Table 100-1 **Peripheral Manifestations of Infective Endocarditis**

Physical Finding (Frequency)	Pathogenesis	Most Common Organisms
Petechiae (20%-40%) (red, nonblanching lesions in crops on conjunctivae, buccal mucosa, palate, extremities)	Vasculitis or emboli	*Streptococcus, Staphylococcus*
Splinter hemorrhages (15%) (linear, red-brown streaks most suggestive of infective endocarditis when proximal in nail beds)	Vasculitis or emboli	*Staphylococcus, Streptococcus*
Osler nodes (10%-25%) (2- to 5-mm painful nodules on pads of fingers or toes)	Vasculitis	*Streptococcus*
Janeway lesions (<10%) (macular, red or hemorrhagic, painless patches on palms or soles)	Emboli	*Staphylococcus*
Roth spots (<5%) (oval, pale retinal lesions surrounded by hemorrhage)	Vasculitis	*Streptococcus*

cytic, normochromic in subacute cases), reticulocytopenia, increased erythrocyte sedimentation rate, hypergammaglobulinemia, circulating immune complexes, false-positive serologic test results for syphilis, and rheumatoid factor. The presence of rheumatoid factor may be a helpful clue to diagnosis in patients with culture-negative endocarditis. Urinalysis frequently shows proteinuria (50% to 60%) and microscopic hematuria (30% to 50%). The presence of red blood cell casts is indicative of immune complex–mediated glomerulonephritis. The finding of gram-positive cocci in the urine of a febrile patient with microscopic hematuria should prompt consideration of the possibility of IE.

The bacteremia of IE is continuous, but often low grade (often 1 to 100 bacteria per milliliter in subacute cases). Therefore, in most instances, all blood cultures are positive, and persistent bacteremia on multiple blood cultures may have diagnostic value in distinguishing IE from other causes of bacteremia. Three blood culture sets should be obtained 1 hour apart before the initiation of antibiotic therapy if possible; and two or three additional sets should be drawn if the patient has received antibiotic therapy in the preceding 1 to 2 weeks or if initial blood cultures are negative at 48 to 72 hours. Up to 14% of patients with IE may have negative blood cultures; half of these are patients who have received previous antibiotic therapy. Fastidious organisms, including *Legionella, Coxiella, Bartonella,* and *Chlamydia* and fungi account for the majority of the remaining cases. Cultures may be negative in as many as 50% of cases of fungal endocarditis. Although modern automated blood culture systems have improved detection of the HACEK group and nutritionally deficient streptococci that were previously difficult to cultivate, the fastidious organisms noted previously remain difficult to recover with conventional microbiologic techniques. Serologic tests and, more recently, nucleic acid target or signal amplification are necessary to diagnose infections from these pathogens.

Echocardiography is recommended in all cases of suspected IE. Although transthoracic echocardiography (TTE) may be sufficient when suspicion is low and the patient's body habitus and clinical condition allow for optimal imaging quality, transesophageal echocardiography (TEE) is considerably more sensitive, especially for small (<10 mm) vegetations, and is capable of identifying such complications of IE as ring abscesses and valvular perforation more readily than TTE. Valvular vegetations can be demonstrated in most (75% to 95%) cases of IE by TEE, but the enhanced detail provided by TEE also mandates caution in interpreting the findings in the presence of other structural abnormalities, such as prosthetic valves, which may produce nonspecific echoes that are easily mistaken for vegetations.

The clinical, microbiologic, and echocardiographic features discussed earlier, known as the Duke criteria, have been shown to be highly predictive of the likelihood of IE in various groups of patients, and recently proposed modifications have increased their diagnostic performance. The currently proposed Duke criteria are summarized in Table 100-2.

DIFFERENTIAL DIAGNOSIS

The diagnosis of IE usually is established on the basis of the clinical findings and the results of blood cultures. In some instances, the distinction between IE and nonendocarditis bacteremia may be difficult. Because the bacteremia is usually continuous in IE and intermittent in other bacteremias, the fraction of blood cultures that are positive may be helpful in distinguishing between these entities. The more frequent causative agents of IE are shown in Table 100-3. With increasing numbers of patients acquiring IE after invasive procedures or intravenous drug abuse, the relative importance of staphylococci has increased in recent years. In streptococcal infection, the speciation of the blood culture isolate may provide circumstantial evidence for or against infection of the heart valves (Table 100-4). The identity of the causative organism may be helpful for other bacteria as well; the ratio of IE to non-IE bacteremias is approximately 1:1 for *S. aureus,* 1:7 for group B streptococci, and 1:200 for *Escherichia coli. Streptococcus bovis* bacteremia and endocarditis are often (>50%) associated with colonic carcinomas or polyps. Hence, isolation of this organism warrants thorough evaluation of the lower gastrointestinal tract.

The initial presentation of IE can be misleading: the young adult may have a stroke, pneumonia, or meningitis; the elderly patient may have confusion or simply fatigue or malaise without fever. The index of suspicion for IE, therefore, must be high, and blood cultures should be obtained in these varied settings, particularly if antibiotic use is contemplated.

Major problems in diagnosis arise if antibiotics have been administered before blood is cultured or if blood cultures are negative. Attempts to culture slow-growing organisms, including those with particular nutritional requirements, should be done in consultation with a clinical microbiologist. The differential diagnosis of culture-negative endocarditis includes acute rheumatic fever, multiple pulmonary emboli, atrial myxoma, systemic vasculitis, and nonbacterial thrombotic endocarditis. Nonbacterial thrombotic endocarditis (sometimes called *marantic endocarditis*) occurs in patients with severe wasting, whether caused by malignancy or other conditions. Also, patients with systemic lupus erythematosus may develop sterile valvular vegetations, termed *Libman-Sacks lesions,* on the undersurfaces of the valve leaflets. These diagnoses should be considered and excluded, if possible, before a prolonged course of therapy for presumed culture-negative IE is begun. As noted earlier, the absence of vegetations on TEE makes a diagnosis of endocarditis unlikely.

MANAGEMENT AND OUTCOME

The outcome of endocarditis is determined by the extent of valvular destruction, the size and friability of vegetations, the presence and location of emboli, and the choice of antibiotics. These factors, in turn, are influenced by the nature of the causative organism and delays in diagnosis. The goal of antibiotic therapy is to halt further valvular damage and to cure the infection. Surgery may be necessary for hemodynamic stabilization, prevention of embolization, or control of drug-resistant infection.

Antibiotics should be selected on the basis of the clinical setting (Tables 100-5 and 100-6) and started as soon as blood cultures are obtained if the diagnosis of IE appears highly likely and the course is suggestive of active valvular destruction or systemic embolization. The antibiotics

Table 100-2 Modified Duke Criteria for the Diagnosis of Infective Endocarditis

Major Criteria

Blood culture positive for IE, defined as follows:

a. Typical microorganisms consistent with infective endocarditis (IE) from two separate blood cultures—viridans streptococci, *Streptococcus bovis,* HACEK group, *Staphylococcus aureus* or community-acquired enterococci in the absence of a primary focus *or*

b. Microorganisms consistent with IE from persistently positive blood cultures defined as follows: at least two positive cultures of blood samples drawn >12 hr apart; or all of three or a majority of four or more separate cultures of blood (with first and last sample drawn at least 1 hr apart) *or*

c. Single positive blood culture for *Coxiella burnetii* or anti–phase 1 IgG antibody titer >1:800

Evidence of endocardial involvement:

Echocardiogram positive for IE defined as follows: oscillating intracardiac mass on valve or supporting structures, in the path of regurgitant jets, or on implanted material in the absence of an alternative anatomic explanation; or abscess; or new partial dehiscence of prosthetic valve; new valvular regurgitation (worsening or changing or preexisting murmur not sufficient)

Minor Criteria

Predisposing heart condition or intravenous drug use

Fever, temperature >38° C

Vascular phenomena, major arterial emboli, septic pulmonary infarcts, mycotic aneurysm, intracranial hemorrhage, conjunctival hemorrhages, and Janeway lesions

Immunologic phenomena: glomerulonephritis, Osler nodes, Roth spots, and rheumatoid factor

Microbiologic evidence: positive blood culture but does not meet a major criterion as noted above (excluding single positive cultures for coagulase-negative staphylococci and organisms that do not cause endocarditis) or serologic evidence of active infection with organism consistent with IE

Interpretation

Definite Infective Endocarditis

Pathologic Criteria

Microorganisms demonstrated by culture or histologic examination of a vegetation, a vegetation that has embolized, or an intracardiac abscess specimen; *or*

Pathologic lesions; vegetation or intracardiac abscess confirmed by histologic examination showing active endocarditis

Clinical Criteria

Two major criteria *or*

One major criterion and three minor criteria *or*

Five minor criteria

Possible Infective Endocarditis

One major criterion and one minor criterion *or*

Three minor criteria

Infective Endocarditis Rejected

Firm alternative diagnosis explaining evidence of infective endocarditis or

Resolution of clinical syndrome with antibiotic therapy for <4 days *or*

No pathologic evidence of infective endocarditis at surgery or autopsy, with antibiotic therapy for <4 days *or*

Does not meet criteria for possible infective endocarditis as above

Data from Li JS, Sexton DJ, Mick N, et al: Proposed modifications to the Duke criteria for the diagnosis of infective endocarditis. Clin Infect Dis 30:633-638, 2000.
IgG, immunoglobulin G.

Table 100-3 Frequency of Infecting Microorganisms in Endocarditis

Native Valve	(%)	Prosthetic Valve Endocarditis (%)	Early	Late	Endocarditis in IVDU	(%)
Streptococci	50	Coagulase-negative staphylococci	33	29	*Staphylococcus aureus*	60
Enterococci	10	*S. aureus*	15	11	Streptococci	13
S. aureus	20	Gram-negative bacilli	17	11	Gram-negative bacilli	8
HACEK	5	Fungi	13	5	Enterococci	7
Culture negative	5	Streptococci	9	36	Fungi	5
		Diphtheroids	9	3	Polymicrobial	5
					Culture negative	5

Data from Levison ME: Infective endocarditis. In Bennett JC, Plum F (eds): Cecil Textbook of Medicine, 20th ed. Philadelphia, WB Saunders, 1996, pp 1596-1605.
HACEK, *Haemophilus, Actinobacillus, Cardiobacterium, Eikenella, Kingella;* IVDU, intravenous drug user.

Table 100-4 Relative Frequency of Infective Endocarditis (IE) and Non-IE Bacteremias for Various Gram-Positive Cocci

Species	IE: Non-IE
Streptococcus mutans	14:1
Streptococcus bovis	6:1
Enterococcus faecalis	1:1
Group B streptococci	1:7
Group A streptococci	1:32

Data from Parker MT, Ball LC: Streptococci and aerococci associated with systemic infection in man. J Med Microbiol 9:275, 1976.

Table 100-5 Syndromes Suggesting Specific Bacteria Causing Infective Endocarditis

Indolent Course (Subacute)

Viridans group streptococci
Streptococcus bovis
Enterococcus faecalis
Fastidious gram-negative rods

Aggressive Course (Acute)

Staphylococcus aureus
Streptococcus pneumoniae
Streptococcus pyogenes
Neisseria gonorrhoeae

Intravenous Drug Users

S. aureus and coagulase-negative staphylococci
Pseudomonas aeruginosa
E. faecalis
Candida species
Bacillus species

Intravenous Catheters

S. aureus and coagulase-negative staphylococci
Candida species
Aerobic gram-negative bacilli

Animal Contact

Bartonella species
Pasteurella species
Capnocytophaga species
Brucella species
Coxiella burnetii

Frequent Major Emboli

Haemophilus species
Bacteroides species

Table 100-6 Treatment of Endocarditis*

Staphylococcus aureus	Nafcillin or cefazolin or vancomycin ± gentamicin
Streptococcus pneumoniae	PCN G or ampicillin
Viridans group streptococci, Streptococcus bovis	PCN G or ampicillin or ceftriaxone + gentamicin
Enterococcus	Ampicillin or PCN G or vancomycin + gentamicin
Enterococcus, vancomycin-resistant	Linezolid or quinupristin-dalfopristin or imipenem ± ampicillin
HACEK organisms	Ceftriaxone or ampicillin-sulbactam or ciprofloxacin
Fungal	Amphotericin B + surgery
Pseudomonas	Antipseudomonal penicillin (e.g., piperacillin) or ceftazidime or cefepime + tobramycin

*See text for details. The choice among the various alternatives presented should be guided by sensitivity results. Therapy for prosthetic valve endocarditis may differ.
HACEK = Haemophilus, Actinobacillus, Cardiobacterium, Eikenella, Kingella; PCN G, penicillin G.

can be adjusted later on the basis of culture and sensitivity data.

Antibiotics

A number of different regimens have been advocated for the treatment of IE resulting from each of the causative organisms. Few, however, have been subjected to comparative trials. Both animal models and clinical data indicate that bactericidal regimens directed against the causative pathogen are associated with much greater rates of therapeutic success and are therefore the standard of therapy. The duration of treatment should be sufficient to sterilize the affected heart valves, usually 4 to 6 weeks in left-sided endocarditis.

Many but not all strains of viridans group streptococci and group D streptococci, such as S. bovis, are exquisitely sensitive to penicillin. The penicillin concentration inhibiting growth of such organisms is less than 0.1 mcg/mL, and they are killed by similar concentrations of penicillin. A variety of antibiotic regimens have been advocated to treat these forms of IE, and several appear to be equally effective. Aqueous penicillin G, 12 to 18 million U/day given intravenously (IV) for 4 weeks, is curative in almost all patients, as is a 2-week course of penicillin G plus gentamicin in younger patients with uncomplicated disease. In the stable patient at low risk for complications, some of the antibiotic course can be administered on an outpatient basis.

Treatment of enterococcal endocarditis and IE caused by other penicillin-resistant streptococci is much less satisfactory because of frequent relapses and high mortality. The recommended regimen for these strains is intravenous aqueous penicillin G, 18 to 30 million U/day, plus intravenous gentamicin, 3 mg/kg/day. This relatively low dose of aminoglycoside is associated with a lower incidence of nephrotoxicity. The aminoglycoside dose should be adjusted according to measured serum levels. In view of the high frequency of relapses, regimens to treat enterococcal infection should be continued for 6 weeks. Culture-negative endocarditis should be treated with the combination of a β-lactam and an aminoglycoside, with or without an agent active against intracellular pathogens (a tetracycline or a quinolone), depending on the level of suspicion for such organisms.

Determination of the minimum inhibitory concentration (MIC) and minimum bactericidal concentration (MBC) is important in the management of IE, as therapeutic success is largely dependent on the ability to achieve a bactericidal effect in the relative sanctuary of the vegetation. Serum bactericidal titers have been used in an attempt to translate these values to activity in vivo, but these assays have a limited role in current antimicrobial therapy of IE.

S. aureus endocarditis should be treated with intravenous nafcillin, 12 g/day, unless the isolate is penicillin sensitive, in which case penicillin, 12 million U/day, is the treatment of choice. Infection with a methicillin-resistant species of *Staphylococcus* necessitates the use of vancomycin. The lipopeptide daptomycin may be an alternative in certain patients, particularly those with right-sided endocarditis. The addition of an aminoglycoside hastens clearance of bacteremia and is indicated during the initial phases of therapy in very ill patients. The duration of antibiotic therapy for staphylococcal endocarditis of the mitral or aortic valve is a minimum of 6 weeks.

In the patient with streptococcal or staphylococcal IE and a history of serious penicillin allergy, vancomycin can be substituted for penicillin. Among patients at risk for complicated disease, consideration should be given to penicillin desensitization.

Pseudomonas endocarditis is a particular problem in intravenous drug users. Therapy should be initiated with tobramycin, 8 mg/kg/day IV, plus an extended-spectrum penicillin such as piperacillin, given IV every 4 hours, or a third- or forth-generation cephalosporin with antipseudomonal activity. The unusually high doses of aminoglycosides have improved the outcome of medical therapy of *Pseudomonas* infection of the tricuspid valve in younger patients with surprisingly little nephrotoxicity. Left-sided *Pseudomonas aeruginosa* infections, however, most often require surgery for cure. It is particularly important to measure serum drug levels and adjust dosages as appropriate when aminoglycosides are used. Quinolones may be of value in combined antibiotic treatment of *Pseudomonas* endocarditis, but experience with these agents is largely anecdotal.

Fungal endocarditis is refractory to antibiotics and almost always requires surgery for management. Amphotericin B generally is administered to such patients but is not in itself curative.

Surgery

The indications for early surgery in IE need to be individualized and forged by discussions with the cardiac surgeon. Refractory infection is a clear indication for surgery; as noted, the requirement for surgery is predictable in IE caused by certain organisms. Persistence of bacteremia for longer than 7 to 10 days, despite the administration of appropriate antibiotics, frequently reflects paravalvular extension of infection with development of valve ring abscess or myocardial abscesses. Medical cure is not likely in this setting. Intravenous drug users are more likely to have IE caused by organisms refractory to medical therapy (e.g., *Pseudomonas* species, fungi). Refractory tricuspid endocarditis may be amenable to valve débridement or excision without immediate placement of a prosthetic valve. Tricuspid valvulectomy may, however, be associated with the eventual onset of right-sided congestive heart failure.

Protracted fever is not unusual in patients undergoing treatment of endocarditis and should not automatically be equated with refractory infection. In fact, 10% of patients remain febrile for more than 2 weeks, and persistent fever is not an independent indication for surgery, particularly when tricuspid endocarditis is complicated by multiple septic pulmonary emboli with necrotizing pneumonia. Delayed defervescence also is common, despite appropriate antimicrobial therapy, with endocarditis caused by *S. aureus* and enteric bacteria.

Congestive heart failure refractory to medical therapy is the most frequent indication for early cardiac surgery. The extent of valvular dysfunction may be difficult to gauge clinically, particularly in patients with acute aortic regurgitation; in the absence of compensatory ventricular dilation, classic physical signs associated with aortic regurgitation, such as wide pulse pressure, may not be present. Echocardiography, fluoroscopy, and cardiac catheterization may be necessary to evaluate the extent of aortic regurgitation in some instances. However, when congestive heart failure develops in the patient with *S. aureus* IE, aortic valvular destruction usually is extensive, necessitating early surgery. Delaying surgery to prolong the course of antibiotic therapy is never appropriate if the patient is hemodynamically unstable or fulfills other criteria for surgical intervention. Prosthetic valve endocarditis (PVE) seldom occurs after cardiac valve replacement for IE, and its incidence is not influenced by duration of preoperative antibiotics.

Recurrent major systemic embolization is another indication for surgery. If valvular function is preserved, vegetations sometimes can be removed without valve replacement. Septal abscess, although often difficult to recognize clinically, and aneurysms of the sinus of Valsalva are absolute indications for surgery.

Prosthetic Valve Endocarditis

PVE complicates 3% to 6% of cardiac valve replacements within 5 years after surgery. Two separate clinical syndromes have been identified. Early PVE occurs within 60 days of surgery and most often is caused by *Staphylococcus epidermidis*, gram-negative enteric bacilli, *S. aureus*, or diphtheroids. The prosthesis may be contaminated at the time of surgery or seeded by bacteremia from extracardiac sites (e.g., intravenous cannula, indwelling urinary bladder catheter, wound infection, pneumonia). In addition to forming vegetations, which may be quite bulky and cause obstruction, particularly of mitral valve prostheses, circumferential spread of infection often causes dehiscence and paravalvular leak at the site of an aortic prosthesis. The combination of intravenous vancomycin, 2 g/day, and intravenous gentamicin, 3 mg/kg/day, plus oral rifampin, 900 mg/day, is indicated to treat *S. epidermidis* infection. Other infections should be treated with synergistic bactericidal combinations of antibiotics based on in vitro sensitivity testing. Surgery is mandatory in the presence of moderate to severe congestive heart failure. The rate of mortality from early PVE remains high.

Late PVE is most frequently caused by bacteremia from viridans group streptococci from an oral site that seeds a reendothelialized valve surface. Treatment with intravenous aqueous penicillin G, 12 to 20 million U/day, or ceftriaxone, 2 g/day, plus intravenous gentamicin, 3 mg/kg/day, is appropriate. The prognosis for cure with antibiotic therapy alone is better in patients infected with penicillin-sensitive streptococci. Moderate to severe congestive heart failure is the main indication for surgery. The rate of mortality from late PVE remains approximately 40%.

Table 100-7 **Prophylaxis of Infective Endocarditis**
Prophylaxis for Specific Procedures Recommended*
Prosthetic heart valves
Prior endocarditis
Cyanotic congenital heart disease (CHD), unrepaired; repaired CHD with prosthetic material or device (initial 6 months after the procedure only); partially repaired CHD with residual defects
Cardiac transplantation with ensuing cardiac valvulopathy
Prophylaxis *Not* Routinely Recommended
Most other congenital cardiac malformations
Acquired valvular dysfunction (e.g., rheumatic heart disease)
Hypertrophic cardiomyopathy
Mitral valve prolapse
Physiologic murmurs
Isolated secundum atrial septal defect
Surgically repaired atrial septal defect, ventricular septal defect, patent ductus arteriosus (after 6 mo)
Cardiac pacemakers, coronary artery stents, and defibrillators
History of rheumatic fever or Kawasaki disease without valvular dysfunction
Previous coronary artery bypass surgery
*For procedures that involve an area of established infection, the antimicrobial regimen used for treatment in high-risk patients should include the organisms likely to arise from that anatomic area that are commonly associated with endocarditis.

Table 100-8 **Procedures for Which Antimicrobial Prophylaxis Against Infective Endocarditis Is Recommended**
Dental Procedures
All procedures that involve manipulation of gingival tissue or the periapical region of teeth or perforation of the oral mucosa
Respiratory Tract Procedures
Tonsillectomy or adenoidectomy
Other invasive procedures involving incision or biopsy of the respiratory mucosa
Gastrointestinal and Genitourinary Tract Procedures
Prophylaxis no longer routinely recommended

Table 100-9 **Prophylactic Regimens Recommended for Dental, Oral, or Respiratory Tract Procedures in High-Risk Patients**
Amoxicillin, 2.0 g PO, 30 to 60 minutes before the procedure.
Allergic to penicillin: clindamycin, 600 mg PO, or cephalexin, 2.0 g PO, or azithromycin or clarithromycin, 500 mg PO, all given 30 to 60 minutes before the procedure
Unable to receive oral medication: ampicillin, 2.0 g, or cefazolin or ceftriaxone, 1.0 g, all given intramuscularly or intravenously 30 to 60 minutes before the procedure

Prophylaxis of Infective Endocarditis

Patients with prosthetic heart valves, patients with prior endocarditis, and persons with certain kinds of congenital heart lesions have an increased risk of IE. Other abnormalities of the aortic and mitral valve are also associated with an increased lifetime risk of IE, yet neither the value of nor the optimal regimens for antibiotic prophylaxis in this setting have been established definitively. Moreover, it is not clear that the overall risk of endocarditis as a result of dental procedures exceeds the risk of endocarditis as a result of other unrecognized bacteremias from oral sources. Thus only a small number of IE cases would be prevented with antibiotics for dental procedures, even if such prophylaxis were 100% effective. Revised recommendations by the American Heart Association indicate that prophylaxis may be reasonable for those patients at the highest risk for severe adverse outcomes only, and only for some specific procedures. Conditions that place patients at risk for endocarditis are presented in Table 100-7. Procedures for which prophylaxis is recommended are listed in Table 100-8, and appropriate prophylactic antibiotic regimens are presented in Table 100-9.

Administration of antibiotics has become an accepted practice for patients undergoing open heart surgery, including valve replacement. Intravenous cefazolin, 2 g at induction of anesthesia, repeated 8 and 16 hours later, or intravenous vancomycin, 1 g at induction and 0.5 g 8 and 16 hours later, is an appropriate regimen. Cardiac diagnostic procedures (catheterization), pacemaker placement, and coronary artery bypass do not pose sufficient risk to warrant the use of prophylactic antibiotics for IE or PVE.

Devices that are associated with high rates of infection and bacteremia (e.g., intravenous cannulas, indwelling urinary bladder catheters) should be avoided in hospitalized patients at risk for IE if at all possible; established local infections should be treated promptly and vigorously.

Bacterial Endarteritis and Suppurative Phlebitis

Bacterial endarteritis usually develops by one of three mechanisms: (1) arteries, particularly those with intimal abnormalities, may become infected as a consequence of transient bacteremia; (2) during the course of IE, septic emboli to vasa vasorum may lead to mycotic aneurysms; or (3) blood vessels also may be infected by direct extension from contiguous foci and trauma.

A septic presentation is characteristic of endarteritis caused by organisms such as *S. aureus.* Besides sepsis, the major problem caused by endarteritis is hemorrhage. Three percent to 4% of patients with IE develop intracranial mycotic aneurysms. Mycotic aneurysms in IE typically are situated peripherally and in the distribution of the middle cerebral artery. Focal seizures, focal neurologic signs, or aseptic meningitis may herald catastrophic rupture of such aneurysms. These premonitory findings therefore indicate the need for evaluation with arteriography; neurosurgical intervention should be contemplated if accessible lesions are demonstrated.

Infection of an atherosclerotic plaque can occur as a complication of bacteremia, particularly in elderly patients with bacteremia caused by *Salmonella* species. Traumatic endarteritis with pseudoaneurysm often complicates arterial injection of illicit drugs and rarely complicates arterial catheterizations. Treatment often requires combined medical and surgical management; antibiotic selection should be based on the results of in vitro sensitivity testing.

Suppurative thrombophlebitis usually is a complication of the use of intravenous plastic cannulas. Burn patients, especially those with lower extremity catheterization, are at particular risk. Typically, intravenous cannulas have been left in place 5 days or more. Often, the vein is sclerosed and tender, and the surrounding skin is erythematous. The vein should be milked to identify pus. If pus is present or if bacteremia and fever persist despite antibiotic therapy, involved segments of vein must be excised. Initial therapy should be selected to ensure coverage of the most common pathogens, *Staphylococcus* species (vancomycin, 15 mg/kg every 12 hours IV) and Enterobacteriaceae (e.g., piperacillin-tazobactam, 3.375 g every 6 hours IV).

Suppurative phlebitis is preventable. Peripheral intravenous cannulas should be inserted aseptically and replaced at least every 72 hours by well-trained personnel.

Prospectus for the Future

- Refinement in imaging techniques for the diagnosis and management of infectious endocarditis (IE) and its complications
- Increased use of molecular microbiology techniques for the diagnosis of culture-negative IE
- New biomaterials with increased resistance to microbial colonization

References

Baddour LM, Wilson WR, Bayer AS, et al: Infective endocarditis. Diagnosis, antimicrobial therapy, and management of complications. AHA scientific statement. Circulation 111:e394-e434, 2005.

Beynon RP, Bahl VK, Prendergast BD: Infective endocarditis. BMJ 333:334-339, 2006.

Chambers HF: Infective endocarditis. In Goldman L, Bennett JC (eds): Cecil Textbook of Medicine, 22nd ed. Philadelphia, Elsevier, 2005, pp 1794-1803.

Lederman MM, Sprague L, Wallis RS, Ellner JJ: Duration of fever during infective endocarditis. Medicine 71:52, 1992.

Mylonakis E, Calderwood SB: Infective endocarditis in adults. N Engl J Med 345:1318-1330, 2001.

Nishimura RA, Carabello BA, Faxon DP, et al: ACC/AHA 2008 guideline update on valvular heart disease: focused updated on infective endocarditis. J Am Coll Cardiol 52, 2008.

Skin and Soft Tissue Infections

Christoph Lange and Michael M. Lederman

Innate immune defense mechanisms render the normal skin remarkably resistant to infection. Most common infections of the skin are initiated by breaks in the epithelium. Hematogenous seeding of the skin by pathogens is less frequent.

Some superficial infections, such as folliculitis and furuncles, may be treated with local measures alone (e.g., incision and drainage). Other superficial infections (e.g., impetigo, cellulitis) necessitate systemic antibiotics. Deeper soft tissue infections, such as fasciitis and myonecrosis, necessitate emergency surgical débridement. As a general rule, infections of the face and hands should be treated particularly aggressively because of the risks of intracranial spread in the former and the potential loss of function as a result of closed-space infection in the latter.

Superficial Infections of the Skin

CIRCUMSCRIBED INFECTIONS OF THE SKIN

Vesicles, papules, pustules, nodules, and ulcerations are the lesions in the category of circumscribed infections of the skin (Table 101-1).

Folliculitis is a superficial infection of hair follicles. The lesions are crops of red papules or pustules that are often pruritic; careful examination using a hand lens shows hair in the center of most papules. Staphylococci, yeast, and, occasionally, *Pseudomonas* species are the most common pathogens. Local treatment with cleansing and hot compresses is usually sufficient. Topical antibacterial or antifungal agents also may be useful. The skin lesions of disseminated candidiasis seen in neutropenic patients may resemble folliculitis. In these ill patients, skin biopsy readily distinguishes the two processes; in disseminated disease, yeast is found within blood vessels and not simply surrounding the hair follicle.

Furuncles and carbuncles are subcutaneous abscesses caused by *Staphylococcus aureus*. Recently, community-associated methicillin-resistant *S. aureus* (cMRSA) has caused severe infections including those of skin and soft tissues such as cellulitis, necrotizing fasciitis, and myositis. Furuncles and carbuncles are red, tender nodules that may have a surrounding cellulitis and occur most prominently on the face and back of the neck. They often drain spontaneously. Furuncles may be treated with moist hot compresses. If fluctuant, the larger carbuncles necessitate incision and drainage. β-lactam antibiotics can no longer be considered to be reliable as empirical therapy for community-acquired skin and soft tissue infections. Antistaphylococcal antibiotics covering for MRSA (e.g., trimethoprim and sulfamethoxazole [TMP/SMX] or linezolid) should be given if the patient has systemic symptoms such as fever or malaise, if there is accompanying cellulitis, or if the lesions are on the head.

Impetigo is a superficial infection of the skin caused by group A streptococci, although *S. aureus* may also be found in the lesions. Impetigo is seen primarily among children, who initially develop a vesicle on the skin surface; this rapidly becomes pustular and breaks down, leaving the characteristic dry, golden crust. This pruritic lesion is highly contagious and spreads by the child's hands to other sites on the body or to other children. Gram stain shows gram-positive cocci in chains (streptococci); occasionally, clusters of staphylococci are also seen. Certain strains of streptococci causing impetigo have been associated with the later development of poststreptococcal glomerulonephritis. The differential diagnosis of impetigo includes herpes simplex infection and varicella. These viral lesions may become pustular; Gram stain of an unruptured viral vesicle or pustule should not, however, contain bacteria. A scraping of the pustule assayed for viral antigens can establish the diagnosis of herpes simplex or varicella if the differential diagnosis is uncertain. Topical mupirocin can be used to treat localized impetigo, but systemic antibiotics are recommended if the infection is extensive. Penicillin remains generally effective for treatment of impetigo; however, some authorities prefer penicillinase-resistant penicillins (e.g., dicloxacillin) because

Table 101-1 Circumscribed Cutaneous Infections (Predominant Organism)

Folliculitis (*Staphylococcus aureus*, *Candida* species)

Furuncles, carbuncles (*S. aureus*)

Impetigo (group A streptococci, *S. aureus*)

Ecthyma gangrenosum (gram-negative bacilli [systemic infection])

Anthrax

Vesicular or vesiculopustular lesions of the skin
  Impetigo
  Folliculitis
  Herpes simplex virus infection
  Varicella-zoster virus infection
  Rickettsialpox

Ulcerative lesions of the skin
  Pressure sores
  Stasis ulcerations
  Diabetic ulcerations
  Sickle cell ulcers
  Mycobacterial infection
  Fungal infection
  Ecthyma gangrenosum
  Syphilis
  Chancroid

penicillinase-producing staphylococci may also be present in these lesions. Large bullous lesions, particularly in children, suggest bullous impetigo caused by *S. aureus*. This should be treated initially with an antibiotic such as TMP/SMX or linezolid that is effective against MRSA. Antibiotics do not appear to affect the development of poststreptococcal glomerulonephritis but will prevent the spread of infection to others.

Ecthyma gangrenosum is a cutaneous manifestation of disseminated gram-negative rod infection, usually caused by *Pseudomonas aeruginosa* in neutropenic patients. The initial lesion is a vesicle or papule with an erythematous halo. Although generally small (<2 cm), the initial lesion may exceed 20 cm in diameter. In a short time the vesicle ulcerates, leaving a necrotic ulcer with surrounding erythema or a violaceous rim. Gram stain of an aspirate may show gram-negative rods; cultures of the aspirate are generally positive. Biopsy of the lesion shows venous thrombosis, often with bacteria demonstrable within the blood vessel walls. Because these lesions are manifestations of gram-negative rod bacteremia, treatment should be instituted immediately with ciprofloxacin or an aminoglycoside plus a third-generation cephalosporin, piperacillin, or a carbapenem to cover against *P. aeruginosa* until the results of culture and sensitivity studies are known (see also Chapter 96).

Herpes Simplex Virus

Oral infections caused by herpes simplex virus are discussed in Chapter 98, and genital infections are discussed in Chapter 107. On occasion, infection with this virus occurs on extra-oral or extragenital sites, usually on the hands. This is most often the case in health care workers but also may result from sexual contact or from autoinoculation. The virus may produce a painful erythema, usually at the junction of the nail bed and skin (whitlow). This progresses to a vesiculopustular lesion. At both stages of infection, herpetic whitlow

can resemble a bacterial infection (paronychia). When more than one digit is involved, herpes is much more likely. It is important to distinguish between herpetic and bacterial infections, because incision and drainage of a herpetic whitlow are contraindicated. Puncture of the purulent center of a paronychia and Gram stain of the exudate allow prompt and accurate diagnosis. In the case of herpetic whitlow, bacteria are not present unless the lesion has already drained and become superinfected. In the case of a bacterial paronychia, bacteria are readily seen. Recurrences of herpetic whitlow may be seen but are generally less severe than the primary infection. Treatment with oral acyclovir, famciclovir, or valacyclovir may shorten the duration of symptoms.

Varicella-Zoster Virus

Primary infection with varicella-zoster virus (chickenpox) is thought to occur through the respiratory route but may also occur through contact with infected skin lesions. Viremia results in crops of papules that progress to vesicles and then to pustules, followed by crusting. The lesions are most prominent on the trunk. This is almost always a disease of childhood. Systemic symptoms may precede development of the characteristic rash by 1 or 2 days but are mild except in the case of an immunocompromised patient or primary infection in the adult. In the immunocompromised patient, chickenpox can produce a fatal systemic illness. In otherwise healthy adults, chickenpox can be a serious illness with life-threatening pneumonia. Clinical diagnosis is based on the characteristic appearance of the rash. Impetigo and folliculitis are readily distinguished clinically by Gram stain of the pustule contents. Disseminated herpes simplex virus infection is seen only in the immunocompromised host or in patients with eczema. Viral culture or viral antigen detection will distinguish herpes simplex from herpes zoster in these settings. Most patients with rickettsialpox, which in rare cases is confused with chickenpox, also have an ulcer or eschar that precedes the generalized rash by 3 to 7 days and represents the bite of the infected mouse mite, which transmits the disease. Although officially eradicated, smallpox must be included in the differential diagnosis of chickenpox, when bioterrorism could be an issue. Lesions of smallpox are characteristically larger than those of varicella, are sometimes umbilicated, and tend to be more concentrated peripherally than the central lesions of varicella, and all tend to be at the same stage of development.

Immunocompromised children exposed to varicella should receive prophylaxis with zoster immune globulin. Immunocompromised persons and seriously ill patients with varicella should be treated with acyclovir. Prophylaxis within 96 hours of exposure with varicella-zoster immune globulin is recommended for adults at risk for complications (immunodeficiencies, malignancies, pregnancy). Active immunization against varicella-zoster virus is recommended for all children and susceptible adults in the United States.

After primary infection, the varicella-zoster virus persists in a latent state within sensory neurons of the dorsal root ganglia. The infection may reactivate, producing the syndrome of zoster (shingles). Pain in the distribution of the affected nerve root precedes the rash by a few days. Depending on the dermatome, the pain may mimic pleurisy, myocardial infarction, or gallbladder disease. A clue to the presence of early zoster infection is the finding of dysesthesia, an unpleasant sensation when the involved dermatome is gently stroked by the examiner's hand. The appearance of papules and vesicles in a unilateral dermatomal distribution confirms the diagnosis. Herpes zoster infections of certain dermatomes merit special attention. The Ramsay Hunt syndrome can be caused by infection involving the geniculate ganglia and causes painful eruption of the ear canal and tympanic membrane, often associated with an ipsilateral seventh cranial nerve (facial nerve) palsy. Infection involving the second branch of the fifth cranial nerve (trigeminal nerve) often produces lesions of the cornea. This infection should be treated promptly with systemic acyclovir to prevent loss of visual acuity. A clue to possible ophthalmic involvement is the presence of vesicles on the tip of the nose.

In most instances, dermatomal zoster is a disease of the otherwise healthy adult. However, immunocompromised patients (e.g., persons with human immunodeficiency virus [HIV] infection) and the elderly are at greater risk for reactivation of this virus. Patients with zoster should undergo a careful history taking and physical evaluation; in the absence of specific suggestive findings or recurrent episodes of zoster, these patients do not require an exhaustive evaluation for a malignancy or immunodeficiency.

In older, nonimmunocompromised patients, postherpetic neuralgia (severe, prolonged burning pain, with occasional lightning-like stabs in the involved dermatomes) may persist for 1 to 2 years and become disabling. A brief course of corticosteroids (40 to 60 mg of prednisone, tapered over 3 to 4 weeks) during the acute episode of zoster shortens the duration of acute neuritic pain but does not prevent postherpetic neuralgia. Initiation of treatment during the first 72 hours with antiviral drugs (e.g., valacyclovir, famciclovir) accelerates the healing of lesions and may decrease the occurrence of postherpetic neuralgia. Immunization with a high-titer attenuated virus vaccine (Zostavax) can protect against the occurrence of zoster and postherpetic neuralgia and is recommended for immunocompetent adults over the age of 60.

Cutaneous Mycobacterial and Fungal Diseases

Mycobacteria and fungi can produce cutaneous infection, manifesting generally as papules, nodules, ulcers, crusting lesions, or lesions with a combination of these features. *Mycobacterium marinum,* for example, can produce inflammatory nodules that ascend through lymphatic channels of the arm in individuals who keep or are exposed to fish; similar lesions caused by *Sporothrix schenckii* may be seen among gardeners. *Blastomyces dermatitidis* and *Coccidioides immitis* are other fungi that produce skin nodules or ulcerations.

As a general rule, a biopsy should be done on a chronic inflammatory nodule, crusted lesion, or nonhealing ulceration that is not readily attributable to pressure, vascular insufficiency, or venous stasis. Mycobacteria and fungi should be carefully sought, using acid-fast and silver stains and appropriate cultures. It is essential that biopsy samples for culture are not placed in formalin or other fixatives, as these will make cultivation for pathogens impossible. In specialized laboratories, gene amplification by polymerase chain reaction (PCR) may rapidly identify the causative microbe.

Ulcerative Lesions of the Skin

A common factor in the pathogenesis of many skin ulcers is the presence of vascular insufficiency. Microbial infection of these lesions is secondary but often extends into soft tissue and bone.

Pressure sores occur at weight-bearing sites in individuals incapable of moving. Patients with stroke, quadriplegia, or paraplegia, or patients in coma who remain supine, rapidly develop skin necrosis at the sacrum, spine, and heels, because pressures at these weight-bearing sites can exceed local perfusion pressure. Patients kept immobile on their sides will ulcerate over the greater trochanter of the femur. As the skin sloughs, bacteria colonize the necrotic tissues; abetted by further pressure-induced necrosis, the infection extends to deeper structures. Infected pressure sores are common causes of fever and occasional causes of bacteremia in debilitated patients. Not infrequently, a necrotic membrane hides a deep infection. The physician should probe the extent of a pressure sore with a sterile glove; potential sites of deeper infection should be probed with a sterile needle. Necrotic material must be débrided, and the ulceration may be treated with topical antiseptics and relief of pressure. Systemic antibiotics are indicated when bacteremia, osteomyelitis, or significant cellulitis is present. Anaerobes and gram-negative rods are the most frequent isolates. Skin grafting can be used to repair extensive ulceration in patients who can eventually be mobilized. Prevention of pressure sores by frequent turning and by inspection of pressure sites in immobilized patients is far more effective than treatment. The use of specialized beds that distribute pressure more evenly may be of particular value among immobilized patients.

Stasis Ulceration

Patients with lower extremity edema are at risk for skin breakdown and formation of stasis ulcers. These may become secondarily infected, but unless cellulitis is present, systemic antibiotics are not necessary and treatment is aimed at reducing the edema.

Diabetic Ulcers

Patients with diabetes mellitus often develop foot ulcers. Peripheral neuropathy may result in the distribution of stress to sites on the foot not suited to weight bearing and may also result in failure to sense foreign objects stepped on or caught within the shoe. The resulting ulceration heals poorly. This is related to microangiopathy, macroangiopathy, and poor metabolic control. Secondary infection with *S. aureus,* anaerobes, and gram-negative bacilli progresses rapidly to involve bone and soft tissue. Prevention of these events requires meticulous foot care, avoidance of walking barefoot, the use of properly fitting shoes, and checking the inside of the shoe before use. Once an ulcer develops, the physician should evaluate the patient promptly. Bed rest and topical antiseptics are always indicated. Systemic antibiotics active against anaerobes and gram-negative bacilli should be employed for all but the most superficial and clean wounds. In most instances, this treatment requires admission to the hospital. Aggressive management including optimization of the vascular supply, control of hyperglycemia, appropriate antibiotic treatment, immobilization, and state-of-the-art wound care (which may be enhanced by vacuum wound

Table 101-2 **Diffuse Cutaneous and Subcutaneous Bacterial Infections**	
Description	**Predominant Organisms**
Erysipelas	Group A streptococci
Cellulitis	Group A (B, C, and G) streptococci, *Staphylococcus aureus*, *Haemophilus influenzae*, *Clostridium perfringens*, other anaerobic organisms, gram-negative bacilli
Erythema migrans (expanding circular erythema after tick bite)	*Borrelia burgdorferi*
Fasciitis	Group A streptococci, *C. perfringens*, other anaerobic organisms, gram-negative bacilli
Myonecrosis	*C. perfringens*, streptococci, mixed anaerobes, gram-negative bacilli

Table 101-3 **Processes That May Resemble Cellulitis**	
Process	**Diagnosis**
Thrombophlebitis	Tender cord, no lymphangitis, ultrasound
Arthritis	Pain on passive joint movement, joint effusion, joint aspiration
Ruptured Baker cyst	History of arthritis, joint effusion, arthrogram, MRI
Brown recluse spider bite	Exposure history
Fasciitis	MRI, surgical exploration
Myositis	Muscle tenderness, less prominent skin involvement, MRI, surgical exploration

MRI, magnetic resonance imaging.

drainage) is indicated, because if the ulcer is left untreated or is improperly treated, the proximate bones and soft tissues of the entire foot may become involved. Once this involvement occurs, eradication of infection without amputation may be difficult.

Other Ulcerative Lesions of the Skin

Ulcerative lesions of the skin, particularly in the genital region, may be caused by *Treponema pallidum,* the agent of syphilis, or by *Haemophilus ducreyi,* the agent of chancroid (see Chapter 107).

DIFFUSE LESIONS OF SKIN

Erysipelas

Erysipelas is an infection of the superficial layers of the skin (Table 101-2); it is usually caused by group A streptococci. This infection, seen primarily among children and the elderly, most commonly occurs on the face. Erysipelas is a bright red to violaceous raised lesion with sharply demarcated edges. This sharp demarcation distinguishes erysipelas from the deeper tissue infection, cellulitis, the margins of which are not raised and merge more smoothly with uninvolved areas of skin. Fever is generally present in erysipelas, but bacteremia is uncommon; in rare cases, the pathogen can be isolated by aspiration or biopsy of the leading edge of the erythema (clysis culture). Penicillin, 2 to 6 million U/day, can be used if the diagnosis of streptococcal erysipelas can be made with confidence; defervescence is gradual. If distinction between erysipelas and cellulitis is not clear, treatment for staphylococcal infection with dicloxacillin is reasonable. If MRSA is common in the community, treatment with TMP/SMX or linezolid is indicated.

Cellulitis

Cellulitis is an infection of the deeper layers of the skin. Cellulitis has a particular predilection for the lower extremities, where venous stasis predisposes to infection. It predisposes to recurrent infection, perhaps by impairing lymphatic drainage. A breakdown in normal skin barriers almost always precedes this infection. Lacerations, small abscesses, tick bites (in the instance of erythema migrans caused by *Borrelia burgdorferi*), or particularly tiny fissures between the toes caused by minor fungal infection antedate the onset of pain, swelling, and fever. Although shaking chills often occur, bacteremia is infrequently documented. Linear streaks of erythema and tenderness indicate lymphatic spread. Regional lymph node enlargement and tenderness are common. Patches of erythema and tenderness may occur a few centimeters proximal to the edge of infection; they are probably caused by spread through subcutaneous lymphatics. Cellulitis of the calf is often difficult to distinguish from thrombophlebitis. Rupture of a Baker cyst or inflammatory arthritis may also mimic cellulitis (Table 101-3). Pain within the joint on passive motion suggests arthritis, whereas after a Baker cyst rupture, examination of the joint may yield relatively benign findings. Lymph node enlargement and lymphatic streaking virtually confirm the diagnosis of cellulitis. Most cases of lower extremity cellulitis are caused by group A β-hemolytic streptococci (less frequently group B, C, or G streptococci), but on occasion *S. aureus* is responsible. Purulence suggests that staphylococci and especially MRSA are likely present as MRSA often produces the Panton-Valentine leukocidin that is toxic to white blood cells. Gram-negative bacilli often cause cellulitis in neutropenic and other immunosuppressed patients. In patients with diabetes mellitus, streptococci and staphylococci are the predominant pathogens of cellulitis. However, if the cellulitis is associated with an infected ulceration of the skin, there is a good chance that anaerobic bacteria and gram-negative rods are also involved. After a cat or dog bite, cellulitis caused by *Pasteurella multocida* or other facultative anaerobes may develop.

Occupational exposures are often associated with painful cellulitis of the hands. Erysipeloid cellulitis (caused by *Erysipelothrix rhusiopathiae*) most often occurs in fish or meat handlers and responds to high doses of penicillin (12 to 20 million U/day). Freshwater exposures are associated with cellulitis caused by *Aeromonas* species, and saltwater exposures may result in aggressive cellulitis caused by *Vibrio* species; third-generation cephalosporins are usually effective in the treatment of these potentially lethal infections.

As in the case of erysipelas, cultures of blood and clysis cultures of the leading edge of infection rarely yield the pathogen. Patients with cellulitis whose condition appears toxic or who have underlying diseases causing impaired immune response should be hospitalized. Suitable oral agents for the treatment of cellulitis include dicloxacillin, clindamycin, or erythromycin, unless streptococci or staphylococci resistant to these agents are common in the community, in which instance TMP/SMX or linezolid is useful.

If *Haemophilus* infection is suspected, ampicillin-sulbactam is usually effective. Erythema migrans is treated with doxycycline, amoxicillin, or ceftriaxone.

Diabetics with foot ulcers complicated by cellulitis should be treated with agents active against anaerobes and enteric gram-negative rods. Only for the mildest of infections are oral antibiotics indicated (e.g., ampicillin-sulbactam; clindamycin plus levofloxacin). For more serious infections, hospitalization and parenteral therapy are warranted.

The control of diabetes should be optimized. Radiologic studies should be performed on patients with ulcers to determine if osteomyelitis is present (see Chapter 104). The affected limb should be elevated to enhance venous drainage. Prevention of cellulitis can be achieved by institution of measures aimed at reducing venous stasis and edema. Patients with recurrent cellulitis may benefit from antibiotic prophylaxis and resolution of venous stasis, if present.

Soft Tissue Gas

Crepitus on palpation of the skin indicates the presence of gas in the soft tissues. Although this often reflects anaerobic bacterial metabolism, subcutaneous gas can also be found after ventilator-induced barotrauma or after application of hydrogen peroxide to open wounds.

In the setting of soft tissue infection, crepitus suggests the presence of gas-forming anaerobes that may include clostridia or facultative bacteria such as streptococci or gram-negative rods. Roentgenograms will occasionally demonstrate gas before crepitus is detected (Fig. 101-1). Magnetic resonance imaging is more sensitive than other techniques in detecting soft tissue gas. The presence of gas in the setting of infection necessitates emergency surgery to determine the extent of necrosis and requirements for débridement. Involvement of the muscle establishes the diagnosis of myonecrosis (see later discussion) and mandates extensive débridement. Despite the often extensive crepitus seen in clostridial cellulitis, exploration shows the muscles to be

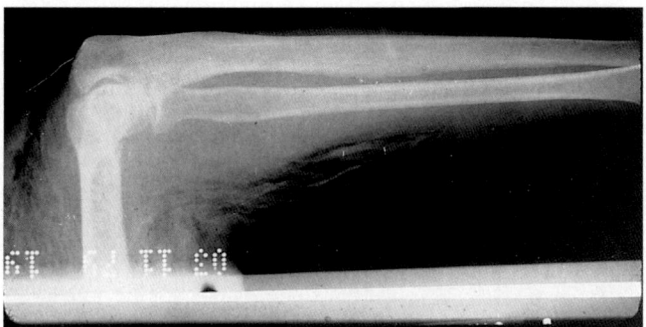

Figure 101-1 Radiograph of patient with clostridial myonecrosis shows gas within tissues. (Courtesy Dr. J. W. Tomford.)

uninvolved, and proper treatment is limited to débridement of necrotic tissue, open drainage, and antibiotics, usually penicillin G, 10 to 20 million U/day, and clindamycin, 900 mg every 8 hours. The principles of treatment for necrotizing soft tissue infections are (1) removal of necrotic tissue, (2) drainage, and (3) appropriate antibiotics. These apply to superficial necrotizing infections (clostridial cellulitis), deeper anaerobic infections (necrotizing fasciitis [see later discussion]), and deepest infections (necrotizing myonecrosis [see later discussion]).

Deeper Infections of the Skin and Soft Tissue

NECROTIZING FASCIITIS

Necrotizing fasciitis is a deep infection of the subcutaneous tissues that generally occurs after trauma (sometimes minor) or surgery but may occur spontaneously in previously healthy persons. Most cases are caused by β-hemolytic streptococci with or without staphylococci; some cases, especially in diabetics, are caused by mixtures of anaerobic organisms and gram-negative bacilli. Because fasciitis involves subcutaneous tissues, the skin may appear normal or may have a red or dusky hue. The clues to this diagnosis are pain and the presence of subcutaneous swelling, particularly in the absence of overlying cellulitis. In some instances, crepitus is present. In time, skin necrosis and dark bullae may develop. The patient's condition appears more toxic than one would expect from the superficial appearance of the skin. Radiographs may show gas within tissues; its absence does not exclude the diagnosis. Men with diabetes mellitus, urethral trauma, or obstruction may develop an aggressive fasciitis of the perineum called Fournier gangrene. Perineal pain and swelling may antedate the characteristic discoloration of the scrotum and perineum. Prompt débridement of all necrotic tissue is critical to the cure of these infections. Once the diagnosis is suspected, the patient must be taken immediately to the operating room, where incision and exploration will determine if fasciitis is present. Gram stain of necrotic material will guide antibiotic choice. Broad and repeated dissection with removal of infected tissue is required for cure.

INFECTIONS OF MUSCLE

Pyomyositis

Pyomyositis is a deep infection of muscle usually caused by *S. aureus* and occasionally by group A β-hemolytic streptococci or enteric bacilli. Most cases occur in warm or tropical regions, and most occur among children. Nonpenetrating trauma may antedate the onset of symptoms, suggesting that infection of a minor hematoma during incidental bacteremia may be causative. Patients have fever and tender swelling of the muscle; the skin is uninvolved or minimally involved. In older patients, myositis may mimic phlebitis. Diagnosis can be readily made, if suspected, by needle aspiration, ultrasonography, or computed tomography. Early aggressive débridement and appropriate antibiotics are usually curative.

Myonecrosis

Myonecrosis generally occurs after a contaminated injury to muscle. Within 1 or 2 days of injury, the involved extremity becomes painful and begins to swell. The patient's condition appears toxic, and he or she is often delirious. The skin may appear uninvolved at first but eventually may develop a bronzed-blue discoloration. Crepitus may be present but is not as prominent as in patients with necrotizing cellulitis (a less aggressive lesion). Most of these infections are caused by clostridial species (gas gangrene), but some are caused by streptococci, mixtures of anaerobes, or gram-negative rods. In rare cases, clostridial myonecrosis occurs spontaneously in the absence of trauma; most of these patients have an underlying malignancy, usually involving the bowel. Regardless of cause, this illness progresses rapidly, producing extensive necrosis of muscle. Hypotension, hemolytic anemia caused by clostridial lecithinase, and renal failure can complicate this illness. Gram stain of the thin and watery wound exudate reveals large gram-positive rods and very few inflammatory cells. Emergency surgery with wide débridement is essential. Large doses of penicillin (10 to 20 million U/day) plus clindamycin, 900 mg every 8 hours, may prevent further spread of the bacilli. Chloramphenicol may be used in patients with hypersensitivity to penicillin. If gram-negative rods are seen in the exudate, treatment with an extended-spectrum penicillin that also has excellent anaerobic activity (e.g., piperacillin-tazobactam) is indicated. Hyperbaric oxygen therapy is of uncertain value.

APPROACH TO THE PATIENT WITH "RED LEG"

Cellulitis of the leg is a common infection that is generally responsive to antibiotic therapy as discussed earlier. A willingness to accept this common diagnosis uncritically can result in missed diagnoses of other treatable diseases, which in some instances are life threatening (see Table 101-3).

The first key issue is to determine if the process is infectious. The presence of fever does not exclude inflammatory mimics of cellulitis that also may cause a red leg. The presence of ulcers or other wounds that provide entry to bacteria suggests infection; streaks of lymphangitis, tender lymph nodes, and skip areas of skin inflammation are highly suggestive of cellulitis. Thrombophlebitis may occasionally be distinguished by palpation of a tender, inflamed, and clotted vein; this diagnosis may be suggested by elevated fibrin degradation products in plasma (e.g., D-dimers) and confirmed by ultrasound. Septic or crystal-induced arthritis has findings most prominent around the affected joint, and even minimal passive joint motion is painful; aspiration of joint fluid is diagnostic.

For each patient in whom a diagnosis of cellulitis is presumed, the careful clinician must ask: Does this patient also have deeper infection, such as necrotizing fasciitis? Although this disorder is uncommon, it progresses at life-threatening speed, and clues to its presence are often subtle. To miss this diagnosis even for a few hours can place patients at risk for loss of limb or life. Clues to this diagnosis include pain and swelling out of proportion to degree of inflammation, particularly at sites where there is no erythema (alternatively, some patients may experience topical anesthesia as a sign of skin necrosis); a dusky or bluish appearance of the skin with development of hemorrhagic vesicles or bullae; clinical "toxicity" out of proportion to degree of fever; and history of rapid clinical progression. Magnetic resonance imaging sometimes will show gas in tissues. If the diagnosis of necrotizing fasciitis or of myonecrosis is suspected, emergent surgical exploration is required with repeated broad dissection to remove necrotic tissues. Antibiotic therapy plays a supplementary role.

Prospectus for the Future

- Improved methods of wound care management including use of recombinant growth factors
- Increased prevalence of drug-resistant bacteria in hospitals, extended care facilities, and the community
- Emphasis on better patient recognition of early signs of diabetic foot infections
- Improved treatment strategies for patients with recurring soft tissue infections

---

References

Lipsky BA: Medical treatment of diabetic foot infections. Clin Infect Dis 39(Suppl 2):S104-S114, 2004.

Moran GJ, Krishnadasan A, Gorwitz RJ, et al: Methicillin-resistant *S. aureus* infections among patients in the emergency department. N Engl J Med 355:666-674, 2006.

Stevens DL, Bisno AL, Chambers HF, et al: Practice guidelines for the diagnosis and management of skin and soft-tissue infections. Clin Infect Dis 41:1373-1406, 2005.

Stryjewski ME, Chambers HF: Skin and soft-tissue infections caused by community-acquired methicillin-resistant *Staphylococcus aureus*. Clin Infect Dis 46(Suppl 5):S368-S377, 2008.

Wilson ML, Winn W: Laboratory diagnosis of bone, joint, soft-tissue, and skin infections. Clin Infect Dis 46:453-457, 2008.

Intra-Abdominal Abscess and Peritonitis

Christoph Lange and Michael M. Lederman

Intra-Abdominal Abscess

There are two general categories of intra-abdominal abscess. The first is an infection of an intra-abdominal organ, generally arising as a consequence of hematogenous, lymphatic, or enteral spread. The second consists of extravisceral abscesses, which are localized collections of pus within the peritoneal or retroperitoneal space. These abscesses usually follow peritonitis or contamination by rupture or leakage from the bowel. Most patients with an intra-abdominal abscess are febrile; however, some patients (e.g., those with tuberculous abscesses) may not be. The fever may be recurrent and may be associated with rigors, suggesting intermittent bacteremia. Nausea, vomiting, and paralytic ileus are common with extravisceral abscesses. Clues to the presence of intra-abdominal abscess may be subtle and may include extravisceral gas or air-fluid levels on plain radiographs. Abdominal ultrasound, computed tomography (CT) and magnetic resonance imaging (MRI) have simplified both the diagnosis and the management of these potentially life-threatening infections.

With the exception of tuberculous and amebic abscess or multiple microabscesses of the liver, antibiotic therapy alone is rarely curative. Failure of the antibiotic to penetrate the abscess cavities, binding and inactivation of antibiotics within the abscess by proteins and bacterial enzymes, low pH, and low redox potential all contribute to the failure of medical management. Drainage is essential; antibiotics are important primarily to prevent bacteremia and seeding of other organs.

ABSCESSES OF SOLID ORGANS

Hepatic Abscess

Pyogenic liver abscess is a disease that occurs predominantly among individuals with other underlying disorders, most commonly biliary tract disease. Obstruction to biliary drainage allows infected bile to produce ascending infection of the liver. Inflammatory diseases of the bowel, such as appendicitis and diverticulitis, may also lead to hepatic abscess through spread of infection through portal veins

(Table 102-1). Hepatic abscesses are also recognized complications of liver transplantation. Penetrating or nonpenetrating trauma may also result in pyogenic liver abscess.

Clinical findings in patients with pyogenic hepatic abscess are often nonspecific. Most patients are febrile, but only about half have abdominal pain and tenderness. Two thirds have palpable hepatomegaly, but fewer than one in four is clinically jaundiced.

The chest roentgenogram may show an elevated right hemidiaphragm and atelectasis or effusion at the right lung base. The diagnosis is best achieved by contrast-enhanced CT of the abdomen or ultrasonography of the right upper quadrant. Pyogenic abscesses may be single or multiple; multiple abscesses often arise from a biliary source of infection.

Anaerobic bacilli, microaerophilic streptococci, and gram-negative bacilli are the predominant microorganisms in pyogenic liver abscess. Occasionally, *Staphylococcus aureus* causes hepatic abscesses during the course of bacteremic seeding of multiple organs. Positive blood cultures are obtained from about half the patients with pyogenic liver abscess.

Clinical laboratory studies generally show a moderate elevation of the alkaline phosphatase level, which is disproportionate to the modest elevation in bilirubin level that occurs in roughly half of patients. In contrast, patients with the nonspecific jaundice that occasionally accompanies bacterial infection at other sites generally have elevated bilirubin levels of as much as 5 to 10 mg/dL or more and only slightly elevated alkaline phosphatase levels. In patients with leukemia, multiple hepatic abscesses caused by Candida species may cause fever and poorly localized abdominal pain, and an elevated serum alkaline phosphatase level may be the only abnormality pointing to the hepatic origin. MRI is the most sensitive imaging technique for diagnosis.

Hepatic abscess caused by *Entamoeba histolytica* is rare in North America, although it should be suspected in a patient with fever and right upper quadrant pain who has traveled to or emigrated from the developing world. Amebic abscesses are generally single and are usually located in the right lobe of the liver. Only a minority of patients with amebic liver

Table 102-1 **Intra-Abdominal Abscesses**

Site	Predisposing Factors	Likely Pathogens	Diagnosis	Empirical Treatment*
Solid Organs				
Hepatic	Gastrointestinal or biliary sepsis, trauma	Gram-negative bacilli, anaerobes, streptococci, amebae	CT, MRI, ultrasonography	Drainage Vancomycin plus piperacillin-tazobactam or ampicillin-sulbactam
Splenic	Trauma, hemoglobinopathy, endocarditis, injection drug use	Staphylococci, streptococci, gram-negative bacilli	CT, MRI, ultrasonography	Vancomycin plus piperacillin-tazobactam or ampicillin-sulbactam Drainage and/or splenectomy
Pancreatic	Pancreatitis, pseudocyst	Gram-negative bacilli, streptococci	CT, MRI, ultrasonography	Drainage Piperacillin-tazobactam or ampicillin-sulbactam
Extravisceral				
Subphrenic	Abdominal surgery, peritonitis	Gram-negative bacilli, streptococci, anaerobes	CT	Piperacillin-tazobactam or ampicillin-sulbactam Drainage
Pelvic	Abdominal surgery, peritonitis, pelvic or gastrointestinal inflammatory disease	Gram-negative bacilli, streptococci, anaerobes	CT	Piperacillin-tazobactam or ampicillin-sulbactam Drainage
Perinephric	Renal infection or obstruction, hematogenous	Gram-negative bacilli, staphylococci	CT	Piperacillin-tazobactam or ampicillin-sulbactam plus vancomycin Drainage
Psoas	Vertebral osteomyelitis, hematogenous	Staphylococci, gram-negative bacilli, mycobacteria	CT	Piperacillin-tazobactam or ampicillin-sulbactam plus vancomycin (antituberculous therapy if indicated by histology or culture results) Drainage

*Dosages: ampicillin-sulbactam, 3 g IV every 6 hours; piperacillin-tazobactam, 3.375 g q6h IV.
CT, computed tomography; MRI, magnetic resonance imaging.

abscess have concurrent intestinal amebiasis. Antibody titers against *E. histolytica* are nearly always positive.

The Fitz-Hugh-Curtis syndrome, or gonococcal perihepatitis, may share some clinical manifestations suggestive of hepatic abscess and should be suspected in young, sexually active women with fever and right upper quadrant tenderness. Tumors involving the liver may produce fever and a clinical and radiologic picture that may mimic hepatic abscess. This is complicated by the occasional concurrence of malignancy and abscess. Patients with hepatic abscesses generally have a less acute illness than patients with cholecystitis or cholangitis. Ultrasonography, CT, and MRI are all useful in defining liver abscesses; MRI is most effective when the abscesses are less than 1 cm in diameter.

If pyogenic abscess is suggested, needle aspiration is indicated. With the guidance of ultrasonography or CT, a percutaneous catheter can be inserted into the abscess cavity for both diagnostic and therapeutic purposes. The pus should be Gram-stained and cultured aerobically and anaerobically. Unless the Gram stain indicates otherwise, initial therapy for pyogenic liver abscess should include drugs active against enteric aerobic and anaerobic bacteria (see Table 102-1). Antibiotics should be continued for at least 4 to 6 weeks. Surgery is required to relieve biliary tract obstruction and to drain abscesses that do not respond to percutaneous drainage and antibiotics. Patients with pyogenic liver abscess should be evaluated for a primary intra-abdominal source of infection.

Patients with hepatic abscesses caused by *Candida glabrata* require long-term therapy with an echinocandin, amphotericin B, or fluconazole, as determined by the microbiology of the fungus.

If epidemiologic features strongly suggest an amebic abscess, metronidazole is the drug of choice. Needle aspiration is necessary only to exclude pyogenic infection or, if the abscess is large or close to other viscera, to prevent rupture. In the case of amebic abscess, the "anchovy paste" material obtained by needle drainage is not pus but necrotic liver tissue. Trophozoites of *E. histolytica* are infrequently seen on aspiration of abscesses but are often seen on biopsy of the abscess capsule. Large numbers of white cells suggest pyogenic abscess or bacterial superinfection.

Splenic Abscess

Splenic abscesses are generally the result of hematogenous seeding of the spleen. In the preantibiotic era, splenic infarction and abscess were common complications of infective endocarditis. Now the most common predisposing factors are trauma and (in children) sickle cell disease. Patients with splenic abscess most often have left upper quadrant abdominal pain, which may be pleuritic. The left hemidiaphragm may be elevated, and there may be an associated pleural rub or effusion. The diagnostic approach, most likely causative agents, and initial antimicrobial therapy are outlined in Table 102-1. Splenectomy is usually the definitive treatment, but ultrasound- or CT-guided percutaneous drainage of large, solitary abscesses may also be successful in selected cases.

Pancreatic Abscess

Pancreatic abscess is an uncommon complication of pancreatitis. The symptoms of pancreatic abscess (fever, nausea, vomiting, and abdominal pain radiating to the back) resemble those of pancreatitis. Thus abscess should be suspected in cases of persistent or recurrent fever after pancreatitis. The inflamed organ becomes colonized and infected with microbes inhabiting the upper gastrointestinal tract. Enterobacteriaceae, anaerobes, and streptococci (including the pneumococci) are likely pathogens. The diagnosis may be made by abdominal ultrasound, CT, or MRI; however, radiographic definition of the pancreatic bed is often difficult. Initial antibiotic therapy (see Table 102-1) should be followed by drainage of the abscess as soon as the patient's condition is stable.

EXTRAVISCERAL ABSCESSES

Extravisceral abscesses most often arise after peritonitis, after intra-abdominal surgery, as a consequence of rupture of the bowel, or after extension of infection of a viscus, such as diverticulitis or appendicitis. Abscesses may occur in the subphrenic, pelvic, or retroperitoneal spaces. Fever, nausea, vomiting, and paralytic ileus are common. Although fever is almost always present, localizing symptoms may be very subtle, making the bedside diagnosis difficult. Predisposing factors, most likely causative pathogens, and appropriate initial antimicrobial therapy are outlined in Table 102-1.

When an abscess is suspected, CT, MRI, or ultrasound scans should be obtained. CT can identify abscesses in the retroperitoneal and abdominal spaces and guide percutaneous drainage. Ultrasonography may be more helpful in the identification of pelvic fluid collections. Fluid-filled abscesses may be difficult to distinguish from loops of viscera on CT or ultrasonography; review of such studies by an experienced radiologist is essential before they are considered negative. Radionuclide imaging using gallium-67– or indium-111–labeled leukocytes may be useful in localizing collections of pus when other studies are not diagnostic. Drainage of an abscess either by radiologic guidance or by surgery in conjunction with antibiotics is the mainstay of treatment.

Peritonitis

Peritonitis may occur spontaneously (primary peritonitis) or as a consequence of trauma, surgery, peritoneal dialysis, or peritoneal soilage by bowel contents (secondary peritonitis). Peritonitis also may be caused by chemical irritation. Patients with peritonitis generally complain of diffuse abdominal pain. They may have nausea and vomiting; some have diarrhea, and others have paralytic ileus. Patients are usually febrile and uncomfortable and prefer to lie quietly in the supine position. Physical examination may reveal diffuse tenderness, diminished bowel sounds, and evidence of peritoneal inflammation, including rebound tenderness and involuntary guarding. In patients with underlying ascites, the signs and symptoms of peritonitis may be more subtle, with fever as the only manifestation of infection.

PRIMARY PERITONITIS

Primary or spontaneous peritonitis occurs principally among persons with ascites associated with chronic liver disease or the nephrotic syndrome. Bacteria may infect ascitic fluid by means of bacteremic spread or transmural migration through the bowel or through the fallopian tubes. In cirrhotic patients, clearance of portal bacteremia by hepatic reticuloendothelial cells may be impaired by intrahepatic portosystemic shunting. Not surprisingly, therefore, gram-negative rods, especially *Escherichia coli*, are the predominant pathogens in spontaneous bacterial peritonitis; enteric streptococci are isolated in approximately one third of cases. Staphylococci, *Streptococcus pneumoniae*, or anaerobic bacilli are isolated in a smaller proportion of cases (Table 102-2).

In patients with ascites, the presenting symptoms may be nonspecific abdominal pain, nausea, vomiting, diarrhea, or altered mental status. Thus febrile patients with ascites should undergo paracentesis unless there is another certain explanation for fever. Inoculation of ascites fluid into blood culture bottles should be performed at the bedside. A leucocyte reagent strip (dipstick) is useful for a rapid diagnosis. A white blood cell count in the fluid that exceeds 250/µL is suggestive of infection. Gram stain may reveal the responsible pathogen. Antibiotic penetration into the peritoneum is excellent, and medical therapy is the treatment of choice (see Table 102-2) unless a mixture of bacterial isolates suggests soilage by bowel contents. Bacteria may be cultured from ascitic fluid in the absence of clinical findings of peritonitis (bacterascites), and as many as one third of patients with clinical and laboratory findings consistent with peritonitis have sterile ascitic fluid cultures. Treatment is indicated in these settings. Among patients with cirrhosis and ascites, or with a single episode of spontaneous bacterial peritonitis, prophylactic administration of norfloxacin or trimethoprim-sulfamethoxazole decreases the risk of spontaneous peritonitis.

SECONDARY PERITONITIS

If Gram stain or culture reveals a mixed flora or if anaerobes are suspected on stain or are cultured, secondary peritonitis caused by leakage of bowel contents should be suspected. Secondary peritonitis may follow penetrating abdominal trauma or surgery or may result from contamination of the peritoneum with bowel contents. This syndrome may be heralded by the sudden presentation of visceral rupture (e.g., perforated duodenal ulcer or appendix) or visceral infarction. In the postoperative setting, secondary peritonitis should be suspected in the patient whose abdominal discomfort and fever do not resolve, or even worsen, after the first few postoperative days. If peritonitis is secondary to the leakage of bowel contents, immediate surgical intervention is mandatory. Despite the use of appropriate antibiotics (see Table 102-2) and intensive support systems, mortality from generalized peritonitis in this setting approaches 50%.

Peritonitis is also a common complication of peritoneal dialysis. Most infections are caused by staphylococci, followed by gram-negative bacilli and yeast. Intraperitoneal antibiotics, administered via the dialysis catheter, are generally effective and may be preferred over intravenous

Table 102-2 Causes, Diagnosis, and Treatment of Peritonitis

Site	Predisposing Factors	Causative Agent	Clues to Diagnosis	Empirical Treatment*
Primary				
Spontaneous	Cirrhosis, nephrotic syndrome	Gram-negative bacilli, streptococci	>250 neutrophils/μL of ascites	Cefotaxime or piperacillin-tazobactam or ampicillin-sulbactam or if resistant *Escherichia coli* or *Klebsiella:* carbapenem or fluoroquinolone
Secondary				
Postoperative	Hemorrhage, visceral rupture	Gram-negative bacilli, streptococci, staphylococci, anaerobes	Postoperative fever, pain, prolonged ileus	Piperacillin-tazobactam or ampicillin-sulbactam or carbapenem
Chemical	Abdominal surgery	Bile, starch, talc	Postoperative fever, pain	Biliary drainage when indicated
Visceral rupture	Perforating ulcer, ruptured appendix, bowel infarction	Gram-negative bacilli, anaerobes, streptococci	Polymicrobial Gram stain or culture	Piperacillin-tazobactam or ampicillin-sulbactam or carbapenem Surgery
Peritoneal dialysis		Staphylococci, gram-negative bacilli	Pain, fever, neutrophilic pleocytosis	Vancomycin[†] + third-generation cephalosporin or piperacillin-tazobactam Consider catheter removal
Periodic peritonitis	Familial		Recurrent, familial	Colchicine prophylaxis, 0.6 mg two or three times daily
Tuberculosis	Infection of fallopian tubes or ileum	*Mycobacterium tuberculosis*	Lymphocytic pleocytosis, high protein level (>3g/dL) in ascitic fluid	Isoniazid, rifampin, pyrazinamide, ethambutol

*Dosages: ampicillin-sulbactam, 3 g IV every 6 hours; piperacillin-tazobactam, 3.375 g q6h IV; imipenem, 0.5 g q6h IV; metronidazole, 500 mg q6h IV; vancomycin, 1 g IV q12h; isoniazid, 300 mg/day; rifampin, 600 mg/day; ethambutol, 15-25 mg/kg/day; pyrazinamide, 25 mg/kg/day (maximum, 2.5 mg/kg/day); ceftazidime, 2 g q8h IV; moxifloxacin, 400 mg qd IV.
[†]Intraperitoneal vancomycin, initially 1 g/L dialysate, followed by 25 mg/L dialysate.

antibiotics. Refractory or recurrent peritonitis may necessitate dialysis catheter removal.

TUBERCULOUS PERITONITIS

Tuberculous peritonitis may occur as a result of hematogenous, lymphatic or local extension of tuberculous infection into the peritoneal cavity. Fever, abdominal pain, and weight loss are common. In patients with underlying ascites, a lymphocytic pleocytosis in the peritoneal fluid should suggest the diagnosis. Laparoscopy, with biopsy of the granulomatous peritoneal nodules, is the most effective approach to diagnosis. Standard antituberculous therapy over 6 months is generally curative (see Table 102-2).

Prospectus for the Future

- Increasing complexity of diagnostic and therapeutic challenges as more intra-abdominal infections are seen in the compromised, hospitalized patient

- Development of better imaging tools for the diagnosis of intra-abdominal infections

References

Cárdenas A, Ginès P: What's new in the treatment of ascites and spontaneous bacterial peritonitis. Curr Gastroenterol Rep 10:7-14, 2008.
Koulaouzidis A, Bhat S, Karagiannidis A, et al: Spontaneous bacterial peritonitis. Postgrad Med J 83:379-383, 2007.
Piraino B, Bender F: How should peritoneal-dialysis-associated peritonitis be treated? Nat Clin Pract Nephrol 4:356-357, 2008.

Wiggins KJ, Craig JC, Johnson DW, Strippoli GF: Treatment for peritoneal dialysis-associated peritonitis. Cochrane Database Syst Rev 1:CD005284, 2008.
Wong CL, Holroyd-Leduc J, Thorpe KE, Straus SE: Does this patient have bacterial peritonitis or portal hypertension? How do I perform a paracentesis and analyze the results? JAMA 299:1166-1178, 2008.

Infectious Diarrhea

Christoph Lange and Michael M. Lederman

Acute infectious diarrhea typically consists of an increased frequency of bowel movements of three or more times daily and at least 200 g of stool per day and lasting less than 14 days. Acute infectious diarrhea accounts for more than 2 million worldwide deaths annually. With the best techniques available, a specific causative agent can be identified in 70% to 80% of cases.

Pathogenesis and Pathophysiology: General Concepts

In general, pathogens or microbial toxins that produce acute diarrhea must be ingested. Therefore socioeconomic conditions that result in crowding, poor sanitation, and contaminated water sources lead to increased risk of diarrheal illnesses. Normally the low pH of the stomach, the rapid transit time of the small bowel, and antibody and innate host defense molecules produced by cells in the lamina propria of the small bowel are adequate to keep the jejunum and proximal ileum free of pathogenic microorganisms (although not sterile). Furthermore, the ileocecal valve inhibits retrograde migration of the huge numbers of bacteria that reside in the large bowel.

Pathogenic microorganisms can pass through the hostile environment of the stomach if (1) they are acid resistant (e.g., *Shigella*) or (2) they are ingested with food and are therefore partially protected in the neutralized environment. People with decreased gastric acidity are at increased risk for acute diarrheal disease.

In the small bowel, either the organisms colonize (e.g., *Vibrio cholerae, Escherichia coli*) or invade (e.g., rotavirus, noroviruses) the local mucosa, or they pass through to colonize and invade the mucosa of the terminal ileum (*V. cholerae, E. coli*) or colon (*Shigella*). Small bowel peristalsis deters colonization of most organisms. Special colonization factors such as fimbria (hairlike projections from the cell wall) or lectins (proteins that attach to mucosal cell surface carbohydrates) facilitate adherence of successful colonists to mucosal cell surfaces.

Organisms that do not have special colonization properties pass into the terminal ileum and colon, where they may compete with the naturally residing microorganisms. These resident intestinal bacteria produce substances that prevent intraluminal proliferation of most newly introduced bacterial species (*Bacteroides* produces inhibitory fatty acids; other enteric bacteria produce inhibitory colicins). The ability of the colonic enteropathogens (e.g., *Shigella dysenteriae*) to invade intestinal mucosa allows these microorganisms to multiply preferentially.

Types of Microbial Diarrheal Diseases

Microbes can cause diarrhea either directly by invasion of the gut mucosa or indirectly through elaboration of one of three classes of microbial toxins: secretory enterotoxins, cytotoxins, or neurotoxins. Toxins may be elaborated after microbial replication in the gut or, in some instances, are preformed and ingested directly.

SECRETORY TOXIN–INDUCED DIARRHEAS

Patients infected with secretory toxin–producing pathogens seldom have fever or other major systemic symptoms, and there is little or no inflammatory response. Characteristically, large numbers of bacteria (10^5 to 10^8) must be ingested with grossly contaminated food or water (although a small inoculum may produce disease in individuals with achlorhydria). The enterotoxin-producing bacteria then colonize, but do not invade, the small bowel. After multiplying to large numbers (10^8 to 10^9 organisms per milliliter of fluid), the bacteria produce enterotoxins that bind to mucosal cells, causing hypersecretion of isotonic fluid at a rate that overwhelms the reabsorptive capacity of the colon. The diarrhea is watery, with a low protein concentration and an electrolyte content that reflects its source. Rapid loss of this diarrheal fluid results in predictable saline depletion, base-deficit acidosis, and potassium deficiency. The amount and rate of fluid loss determine the severity of the illness. Certain of the secretory diarrheas, such as those caused by

V. cholerae or *E. coli* enterotoxins, can result in massive intestinal fluid losses, exceeding 1 L/hr in adults. The *V. cholerae* enterotoxin rapidly binds to monosialogangliosides of the gut mucosa and causes sustained stimulation of cell-bound adenylate cyclase. This results, through both increased secretion and decreased absorption of electrolytes, in net movement of large quantities of isotonic fluid into the gut lumen. The disease runs its course in 2 to 7 days, during which time continued fluid and electrolyte repletion is of critical importance.

Enterotoxigenic *E. coli* (ETEC), probably the major cause of traveler's diarrhea worldwide, produces two major types of plasmid-encoded bacterial enterotoxins. The labile toxin (LT) of *E. coli* is nearly identical in mode of action to cholera enterotoxin. The *E. coli* stable toxin (ST) causes gut fluid secretion through activation of guanylate cyclase. Secretory enterotoxins may also be produced by other enteropathogenic bacteria that cause diarrhea primarily through direct invasion (e.g., *Salmonella typhimurium, S. dysenteriae*).

CYTOTOXIN-INDUCED DIARRHEAS

Cytotoxins are soluble factors that directly destroy mucosal epithelial cells. *S. dysenteriae* elaborates a toxin (Shiga toxin) that causes the destructive colitis seen in patients with shigellosis. A closely related cytotoxin is produced by enterohemorrhagic *E. coli* strains that are associated with hemorrhagic colitis and hemolytic uremic syndrome. Other bacteria that can produce cytotoxins include *Clostridium perfringens* and *Vibrio parahaemolyticus*. *C. perfringens,* often ingested in contaminated meat or poultry, replicates within the small bowel and produces a secretory enterotoxin that also has cytotoxin activity. Toxin-induced diarrhea caused by *C. perfringens,* like that caused by *Staphylococcus aureus* and *Bacillus cereus,* has a short incubation period and brief (<36 hours) duration. *Clostridium difficile* can colonize the large bowel and, in the presence of antibiotic therapy that limits the growth of naturally occurring bacteria, can produce cytotoxins that can cause severe mucosal damage, producing a colitis that may have a pseudomembranous appearance or may resemble the diffuse colitis seen in shigellosis.

FOOD POISONING (CAUSED BY CYTOTOXINS, SECRETORY ENTEROTOXINS, AND/OR NEUROTOXINS)

Some toxins are ingested directly in food, as with *S. aureus* and *B. cereus* food poisoning. These organisms grow to a high concentration in the food, and ingestion of the toxins they produce causes the symptoms of food poisoning. Distinctive features of acute food poisoning include a short incubation period (2 to 6 hours), high attack rates (up to 75% of the population at risk), and prominent vomiting (probably caused by the effect of absorbed neurotoxins on the central nervous system).

Food poisoning syndromes of somewhat longer incubation (8 to 16 hours) can be caused by organisms ingested in food that produce toxins during replication in the bowel. In this setting, *B. cereus* produces a cytotoxin similar to *E. coli* LT. The longer-incubation food poisoning syndrome caused by some strains of *B. cereus* (often associated with ingestion of contaminated rice) may resemble the diarrhea caused by ETEC. *C. perfringens* can produce both secretory and cytotoxic enterotoxins after ingestion and replication in the bowel, also producing a longer-incubation food poisoning. Nausea and vomiting are less prominent than diarrhea in these food poisoning syndromes with longer incubation times.

DIARRHEAS CAUSED BY INVASIVE PATHOGENS

Diarrheas caused by invasive pathogens are usually accompanied by fever and other systemic symptoms, including headache and myalgia. Cramping abdominal pain may be prominent, and small amounts of stool are passed at frequent intervals, often associated with tenesmus. The invasive microorganisms often induce a marked inflammatory response, so that the stool contains pus cells, large amounts of protein, and often gross blood. Significant dehydration rarely results from this kind of diarrhea in adults, because the diarrheal fluid volume is small, seldom exceeding 750 mL/day, although critical dehydration may occur in children. Although certain clinical features are statistically more frequent in invasive diarrheas caused by specific enteropathogens (e.g., more severe myalgias with shigellosis, higher temperature spikes with salmonellosis), epidemiologic characteristics are more helpful than signs or symptoms in determining the causative agent in invasive diarrheal illnesses (Table 103-1).

Acute Shigellosis

Acute shigellosis occurs when susceptible individuals ingest fecally contaminated water or food. The bacteria are relatively resistant to killing by gastric acid; shigellosis can therefore occur after ingestion of only 10 to 100 microorganisms. Largely for this reason, direct person-to-person transmission (e.g., in day-care centers) is more common with shigellosis than with other bacterial enteric infections. The organism initially multiplies in the small intestine, producing watery, noninflammatory diarrhea. Later the organisms invade the colonic epithelium, causing the characteristic bloody stool. Unlike *Salmonella, Shigella* rarely causes bacteremia. The disease usually resolves spontaneously after 3 to 6 days, but the clinical course can be shortened by antimicrobial agents (see Table 103-1).

Acute Salmonellosis

Acute salmonellosis usually results from ingestion of contaminated meat, dairy, or poultry products. In the industrialized world, nontyphoidal *Salmonella* is often transmitted by means of commercially prepared dried and processed foodstuffs (e.g., spices). Unlike *Shigella, Salmonella* is remarkably resistant to desiccation. The nontyphoidal salmonellae invade primarily the distal ileum. The organism typically causes a short-lived (2 to 3 days) illness characterized by fever, nausea, vomiting, and diarrhea (This is in marked contrast to typhoid fever, a 3- to 4-week febrile illness, usually not associated with diarrhea, that is caused by *Salmonella typhi*).

Campylobacter jejuni Infection

C. jejuni may be responsible for up to a third of acute febrile diarrheal illnesses in North America. This organism may

Table 103-1 **Epidemiologic Characteristics of Common Invasive Enteric Pathogens**		
Microorganisms	**Epidemiologic Features**	**Recommended Treatment**
Shigella species	Outbreaks in child care centers or custodial institutions; person-to-person transmission	Fluoroquinolones (e.g., ciprofloxacin 500 mg bid) for 3 days Alt: TMP/SMZ
Nontyphoidal *Salmonella* species	Zoonosis; survives desiccation in processed foodstuff	Only when patient is severely ill, immunocompromised, >50 years old, has prosthesis, valvular heart disease, atherosclerosis, cancer, uremia: • Fluoroquinolones (e.g., ciprofloxacin 500 mg bid) for 5-7 days Alt: TMP/SMZ or ceftriaxone
Escherichia coli	Outbreaks caused by foodborne transmissions	None
E. coli (toxin producing)	Traveler's diarrhea	Levofloxacin 500 mg PO × 1, or azithromycin 1 g PO × 1 dose, or other fluoroquinolones for 3 days
Yersinia enterocolitica	Zoonosis; occasionally transmitted in dairy products	Only for severe infections: • Doxycycline and an aminoglycoside Alt: TMP/SMZ, a fluoroquinolone
Vibrio cholerae	Ingestion of seafood	O1 or O139: • Hydration plus azithromycin 1 g or doxycycline 300 mg Alt: single dose fluoroquinolone
Clostridium difficile	Follows antimicrobial therapy; nosocomial spread	Discontinuation of offending antimicrobial therapy Treatment with metronidazole (e.g., 500 mg tid for 10 days or vancomycin 500 mg to 1 g q 12 hrs)
Rotavirus	Outbreaks among children; worldwide distribution; unusual and mild in adults	No
Norovirus	Winter outbreaks; vomiting and diarrhea in families, nursing homes, schools, etc	No
Giardia lamblia	Day-care centers; waterborne transmission; IgA deficiency	Tinidazole 2 g × 1, or nitazoxanide 500 mg PO bid × 3 days, or metronidazole 500-750 mg tid for 7-10 days
Campylobacter jejuni	Consumption of undercooked poultry	Only if high fevers, bloody stools, and illness >1 wk: • Erythromycin 500 mg bid for 5 days Alt: fluoroquinolone
Cyclospora cayetanensis	Foodborne transmission; travel	TMP/SMZ 160/800 mg for 7-10 days
Cryptosporidium parvum	Waterborne transmission; travel; immunocompromised hosts	In HIV and AIDS: • Effective antiretroviral therapy plus nitazoxanide 500 mg PO bid for 14 days
Entamoeba histolytica	Person-to-person transmission; travel to or recent emigration from tropical regions	Metronidazole 750 mg tid for 5-10 days followed by either iodoquinol 650 mg tid for 20 days or paromomycin 500 mg tid for 7 days

AIDS, acquired immunodeficiency syndrome; HIV, human immunodeficiency virus; IgA, immunoglobulin A; TMP/SMZ, trimethoprim-sulfamethoxazole.

invade both the small intestine and the colon. Thus the range of symptoms is broad, ranging from an acute *Shigella*-type syndrome to a milder, but more protracted, diarrheal illness.

Other Invasive Enteropathogens

Three other organisms—*Yersinia enterocolitica, V. parahaemolyticus,* and enteroinvasive *E. coli*—also cause tissue invasion and acute diarrheal illnesses that may be clinically indistinguishable from those caused by the more commonly recognized invasive bacterial enteropathogens (see Table 103-1).

Another distinct *E. coli* strain—0157; H7 enterohemorrhagic *E. coli* (EHEC)—produces bloody diarrhea without evidence of mucosal inflammation (grossly bloody stool with few or no leukocytes), usually with little or no fever. The intestinal mucosal damage is caused by a Shiga-like toxin, which is also thought to be responsible for the hemolytic uremic syndrome, which develops in 2% to 5% of patients. In the past decade, EHEC has been responsible for several multistate outbreaks of acute diarrheal illness,

most often associated with ingestion of inadequately cooked hamburger meat.

Although most diarrhea-causing pathogens produce either invasive or enterotoxic diarrhea, both processes contribute to the illness in some situations. Certain strains of *Shigella*, nontyphoidal *Salmonella*, *Y. enterocolitica*, and *C. jejuni* both invade and produce secretory enterotoxins in vitro. Such enterotoxins may play a contributory role in the acute disease process. The invasive capacity of these organisms is, however, of paramount importance in their ability to produce disease.

Viral Causes of Diarrhea

Both rotavirus and norovirus invade and damage villous epithelial cells, with the degree of injury ranging from modest distortion of epithelial cells to sloughing of villi. Presumably, both rotavirus and norovirus cause diarrhea by interfering with the absorption of normal intestinal secretions. This may occur through selective destruction of absorptive villous tip cells with sparing of secretory crypt cells. Affected patients may have low-grade fever and mild to moderate cramping abdominal pain. The stool is usually watery, and its contents resemble those of a noninvasive process, with few inflammatory cells, probably because of lack of damage to the colon. Other viruses that can cause outbreaks of diarrhea include sapoviruses, astroviruses, and certain adenoviruses.

Protozoan Causes of Diarrhea

In North America, Rocky Mountain water sources are frequent origins of *Giardia lamblia* microepidemics. As is the case in shigellosis, ingestion of only a few organisms is required to establish infection. The organisms multiply in the small bowel, attach to and occasionally invade the mucosa, but do not cause gross damage to the mucosal cells. Clinical manifestations span the spectrum from an acute, febrile diarrheal illness to chronic diarrhea with associated malabsorption and weight loss. Diagnosis may be made by identification of the organism in either the stool or the duodenal mucus or by small bowel biopsy. *Entamoeba histolytica* may cause intestinal syndromes ranging from mild diarrhea to fulminant amebic colitis with multiple bloody stools, fever, and severe abdominal pain. Although *E. histolytica* has a worldwide distribution, it is an uncommon cause of diarrhea in the United States. Three other protozoa, *Cryptosporidium parvum, Isospora belli,* and *Cyclospora cayetanensis,* occasionally cause self-limited acute diarrheal illness in otherwise healthy individuals and may cause voluminous, life-threatening diarrheal disease in patients with immunodeficiencies. Stool examination will often distinguish *Giardia, Entamoeba, Isospora, Cryptosporidium, Microsporidia,* and *Cyclospora;* occasionally biopsy may be needed for diagnosis.

General Epidemiologic Considerations

In developing countries where sanitation is inadequate, young children (up to 2 years of age) contract multiple episodes of diarrhea, a process that engenders intestinal immunity to the majority of enteropathogens in their environment. Most of these diarrheal episodes are mild, but some are life threatening. In these areas, ETEC and rotavirus together cause the large majority of diarrheal illnesses. *Shigella* infections are far less common during this period.

Infants and small children in industrialized countries have fewer episodes of diarrhea than do those in developing countries, and the most common causative agent is the rotavirus. Most episodes are mild. ETEC and *Shigella* infections are infrequent except in a few defined population groups (e.g., individuals in custodial institutions).

Throughout the world, clinically significant diarrhea is relatively unusual in adults except in specific defined epidemics or common-source outbreaks caused by contaminated food or water. However, diarrhea is the most common illness to affect travelers. More than 20% of travelers to Latin America, Africa, South Asia, and the Middle East develop traveler's diarrhea. When immunologically inexperienced adults from the developed world visit developing countries, the organisms responsible are the same ones as those causing most childhood diarrhea in the country visited.

In addition to the pathogens listed earlier, certain sexually transmissible pathogens that may cause acute diarrheal illnesses among sexually active homosexual men (see Chapter 107) differ from those that most commonly occur in the general population.

Nosocomially acquired *C. difficile*–associated diarrhea, related to the use of broad-spectrum antibiotics such as fluoroquinolones and cephalosporins, has been increasingly observed in North America and Europe in the past decade, involving a more severe course, higher mortality, increased risk of relapse, and more complications than appreciated previously. This increased virulence is thought to be a result of greater toxin production by these emerging strains. Outbreaks of diarrhea with these strains are often difficult to control. Health care workers caring for persons with *C. difficile*–associated diarrhea should wash their hands with chlorhexidine solutions between all patient contacts, as spores of *C. difficile* are resistant to alcohol-based hand washing solutions.

Diagnosis

In managing life-threatening diarrheal illnesses, determining the specific causative agent is not as important as prompt repletion of lost electrolytes. Fluid losses represent the chief cause of serious morbidity and mortality in diarrheal illness. Moreover, antimicrobial therapy has proven of value in only a minority of cases (see Table 103-1). Discerning the epidemiology of the illness is often more helpful than are laboratory techniques in identifying cases in which antimicrobial therapy is likely to be helpful. Figure 103-1 provides a schematic approach to diagnosis and management.

The examination of a methylene blue–stained stool preparation for erythrocytes and white blood cells may be helpful in distinguishing between acute diarrheal illnesses caused by invasive pathogens and those caused by noninvasive pathogens. This is easily accomplished by adding one drop of methylene blue dye to one drop of liquid stool or mucus, allowing the preparation to air dry, and examining the specimen under the high dry microscope lens. Few, if any, leukocytes or erythrocytes are seen in the stools of patients with diarrhea caused by noninvasive organisms (e.g., ETEC). Variable numbers of leukocytes and erythrocytes are present in diarrheas secondary to invasive bacteria (e.g., *Shigella*) or cytopathic toxins (*C. difficile* toxin).

The precise diagnosis of any diarrheal illness lasting longer than 4 to 5 days is important because these illnesses (e.g., giardiasis) may be responsive to specific antimicrobial therapy. Furthermore, in patients with negative stool examinations and cultures, endoscopy may yield a diagnosis of a noninfectious disease (e.g., ulcerative colitis or Crohn disease).

Management: General Principles of Electrolyte Repletion Therapy

INTRAVENOUS FLUIDS

All acute diarrheal diseases respond to a similar fluid repletion regimen because voluminous infectious diarrhea in adults consistently produces the same pattern of electrolyte

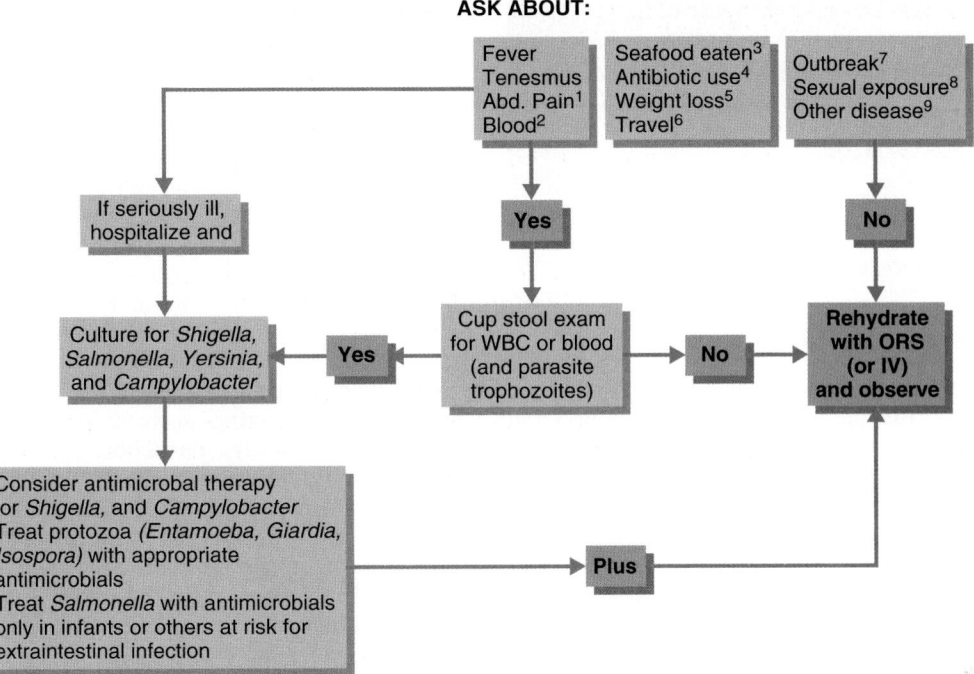

ASK ABOUT:

Figure 103-1 Approach to the diagnosis and management of acute infectious diarrhea.
1. If unexplained abdominal pain and fever suggest an appendicitis-like syndrome, culture for *Yersinia enterocolitica*.
2. Bloody diarrhea, in the absence of fecal leukocytes, suggests enterohemorrhagic *Escherichia coli* or amebiasis (where leukocytes are destroyed by the parasite).
3. Ingestion of inadequately cooked seafood prompts consideration of *Vibrio* infections or noroviruses.
4. Associated antibiotics should be stopped and *Clostridium difficile* considered.
5. Persistence of diarrhea (>10 days) with weight loss prompts consideration of giardiasis, cryptosporidiosis, or inflammatory bowel disease.
6. Travel to tropical areas increases the chance of enterotoxic *E. coli* (ETEC) as well as viral, protozoal *(Giardia, Entamoeba, Cryptosporidium)*, and, if fecal leukocytes are present, invasive bacterial pathogens.
7. Outbreaks should prompt consideration of *Staphylococcus aureus, Bacillus cereus, Clostridium perfringens*, ETEC, *Vibrio, Salmonella, Campylobacter,* or *Shigella* infection.
8. Sigmoidoscopy in symptomatic homosexual males should distinguish proctitis in the distal 15 cm (caused by herpesvirus, gonococcal, chlamydial, or syphilitic infection) from colitis (*Campylobacter, Shigella,* or *C. difficile* infection).
9. Immunocompromised hosts should have a wide range of viral (e.g., cytomegalovirus, herpes simplex virus, rotavirus), bacterial (e.g., *Salmonella, Mycobacterium avium* complex, *C. difficile*), protozoal (e.g., *Cryptosporidium, Isospora, Microsporidia, Entamoeba, Giardia*) and parasitic (*Strongyloides* hyperinfection syndrome) agents considered.
IV, intravenous; ORS, oral rehydration solution; WBC, white blood cell. (Adapted from Guerrant RL, Shields DS, Thorson SM, et al: Evaluation and diagnosis of acute infectious diarrhea. Am J Med 78:91-98, 1985.)

loss. The fluid losses of massive diarrhea can rapidly be corrected by infusing fluids intravenously that approximate those that have been lost. Lactated Ringer's solution is readily available and provides uniformly good results. With patients who are hypotensive, the intravenous fluids should initially be infused rapidly. Subsequent maintenance fluid administration can be guided by the patient's clinical appearance, including the vital signs, the appearance of neck veins, and skin turgor. Clinical evaluation alone provides an adequate guide to fluid replacement in most acute diarrheal illnesses. If intravenous fluids are administered in adequate quantities throughout the diarrheal illness, virtually every patient with diarrhea caused by toxigenic bacteria should be restored to health. Complications (e.g., acute renal failure secondary to hypotension) are exceedingly rare if these principles are followed.

ORAL FLUIDS

In most patients with acute diarrheal illness, fluid repletion can also be achieved through the oral route, using isotonic glucose-containing electrolyte solutions. A uniformly effective solution can easily be prepared by the addition of 2 tablespoons of sugar, a quarter teaspoon of salt (NaCl), and a quarter teaspoon of baking soda (NaHCO$_3$) into 1 L of boiled drinking water (Table 103-2). These fluids should be administered initially in large quantities, 250 mL every 15 minutes in adults, until clinical observations indicate that fluid balance has been restored. Thereafter, sufficient fluids are given to maintain normal balance; if stool output is measured, approximately 1.5 L of glucose-electrolyte solution should be given orally for each liter of stool. The oral glucose-electrolyte fluid does not decrease the volume of fluid lost through the intestinal tract but rather facilitates absorption of adequate fluid to counterbalance the toxin-induced fluid secretion.

Patients with fluid depletion caused by invasive microbial agents (e.g., rotavirus, *Salmonella*) also respond well to oral glucose-electrolyte therapy, although the pathogenesis of diarrheal disease caused by invasive microbes is quite different from that caused by enterotoxigenic bacteria.

Table 103-2 **Rehydration and Eating in Cases of Diarrhea**
Rehydration
1 L boiled (drinking) water 2 tablespoons sugar (or honey) $\frac{1}{4}$ teaspoon salt (NaCl) $\frac{1}{4}$ teaspoon baking soda (NaHCO$_3$)
"BRAT" Diet
Banana, rice, applesauce, toast

ANTIMICROBIAL THERAPY

Most acute infectious diarrheas do not require antibiotic therapy (see Table 103-1). In the noninvasive bacterial diarrheas, antibiotics dramatically decrease the volume of diarrhea only in cholera. Doxycycline, 300 mg in a single dose, is the drug of choice.

In the invasive bacterial diarrheas, short-term antimicrobial treatment significantly decreases the duration and severity of shigellosis. A quinolone such as ciprofloxacin, 500 mg twice daily for 5 days, is effective; trimethoprim-sulfamethoxazole, one double-strength tablet given twice daily, may be used if the organism is sensitive.

Antimicrobial therapy may also be helpful in decreasing the duration and severity of enteritis caused by *Yersinia* and *Campylobacter*. Ciprofloxacin, 500 mg twice daily for 5 days, is useful against these pathogens as well. Antimicrobial agents are of no known value in *V. parahaemolyticus* infections. In uncomplicated nontyphoidal *Salmonella* enteritis, antibiotics may prolong the fecal shedding of salmonellae. Treatment of nontyphoidal salmonella gastroenteritis is, however, indicated in certain settings to prevent bacteremia and its complications (e.g., meningitis, endovascular infection, or infections of joint or vascular prostheses). Treatment until defervescence with a third-generation cephalosporin or a quinolone is therefore indicated for patients with sepsis, those ill enough to be hospitalized, immunocompromised patients, patients with recognized atherosclerotic disease, patients with sickle cell disease, and patients with bone or vascular prostheses.

Antimicrobial therapy is indicated, paradoxically, for treatment of antibiotic-associated diarrhea. Antibiotic-associated diarrhea develops in 1% to 15% of patients who receive broad-spectrum antimicrobial agents and is caused by cytotoxins produced by *C. difficile*, which proliferate in the colonic mucosa when the colonization of bacteria that naturally live in the gut is disturbed. Peripheral leukocytosis is common. Although generally characterized by mild diarrhea, antibiotic-associated diarrhea may result in a potentially lethal pseudomembranous colitis. In all cases, the responsible antibiotic should be stopped. In moderately ill patients (fever, mucosal ulceration, and/or pseudomembranes), oral vancomycin (500 mg-1 g every 12 hours) or metronidazole (500 mg every 8 hours) should be started and continued for 10 days on the basis of strong clinical suspicion, before the diagnosis is confirmed by stool assay for *C. difficile* toxins. Empirical treatment with these agents should be avoided in patients with mild diarrhea that resolves with cessation of antibiotics because this may result in the emergence of antibiotic-resistant bacteria, such as vancomycin-resistant enterococci.

Antimicrobial agents decrease the duration and severity of giardiasis. In adults, metronidazole, 250 mg every 8 hours for 3 days, and quinacrine, 300 mg/day for 7 days, appear to be equally effective in adults. Acute intestinal amebiasis demands antimicrobial therapy. Metronidazole, 750 mg every 8 hours for 5 days, is the drug of choice in adults. The duration of diarrhea caused by *I. belli* is significantly shortened by administration of trimethoprim-sulfamethoxazole twice daily for 5 days.

ANTIMICROBIAL PROPHYLAXIS

Prophylactic antimicrobial agents are effective in preventing traveler's diarrhea, which is caused most often by ETEC. Doxycycline, trimethoprim-sulfamethoxazole, and a quinolone such as ciprofloxacin are each effective when taken once daily for up to 3 weeks. However, because of the rapid response of most patients to early treatment with any of these three agents, the advantages of prophylactic drugs are generally outweighed by their potential risks (adverse reactions).

SYMPTOMATIC THERAPY

Adjuvant symptomatic therapy is not essential but may provide modest symptomatic relief in acute infectious diarrheas associated with cramping abdominal pain. Bismuth subsalicylate, 0.6 g every 6 hours, may ameliorate symptoms of traveler's diarrhea. Agents that decrease intestinal motility (e.g., codeine, diphenoxylate, loperamide) also relieve the cramping abdominal pain associated with many acute diarrheal illnesses but are potentially hazardous because they may enhance the severity of illness in shigellosis, the prototype of invasive bacterial diarrheas.

Prospectus for the Future

- Continuing increase in the occurrence of diarrheal illness as populations migrate to urban areas in the developing world with inadequate clean water supply and waste disposal
- Increasing development of antibiotic resistance among pathogens causing acute diarrhea
- Development of better strategies to limit the nosocomial spread of *Clostridium difficile*

References

Access to toilets for all. Lancet 370:1590, 2007.

Gerding DN, Muto CA, Owens RC Jr: Treatment of *Clostridium difficile* infection. Clin Infect Dis 46(Suppl 1):S32-S42, 2008.

Hill DR, Ryan ET: Management of travellers' diarrhoea. BMJ 337:a1746, 2008.

Navaneethan U, Giannella RA: Mechanisms of infectious diarrhea. Nat Clin Pract Gastroenterol Hepatol 5:637-647, 2008.

Owens RC Jr, Donskey CJ, Gaynes RP, et al: Antimicrobial-associated risk factors for *Clostridium difficile* infection. Clin Infect Dis 46(Suppl 1):S19-S31, 2008.

Thielman NM, Guerrant RL: Clinical practice. Acute infectious diarrhea. N Engl J Med 350:38-47, 2004.

Infections Involving Bones and Joints

Christoph Lange and Michael M. Lederman

Arthritis

In adults, almost all cases of infective arthritis of natural joints occur through hematogenous seeding. Joint replacement surgery accounts for another significant proportion of septic arthritis cases. Causative agents for infective arthritis include bacteria (including mycobacteria), viruses, and fungi. In addition, certain viruses such as human parvovirus B19, rubella, and hepatitis B and C viruses can produce a polyarthritis by means of direct infection of joint synovial tissue or immune complex deposition. Immune mechanisms also underlie arthritis syndromes seen after diarrhea caused by *Salmonella, Shigella, Yersinia,* and *Clostridium difficile* infections; the majority of individuals with postdysentery arthritis syndrome share the human leukocyte antigen B27 (see Chapter 80).

ACUTE ARTHRITIS

Underlying joint disease, particularly rheumatoid arthritis, predisposes to septic arthritis. Many patients with septic arthritis give a history of joint trauma antedating symptoms of infection. Conceivably, disruption of capillaries during an unrecognized and transient bacteremia allows bacteria to spill into hemorrhagic and traumatized synovium or joint fluid, resulting in the initiation of infection. Joint replacement has a very low, although definite, incidence of septic arthritis.

Microbiology

Staphylococcus aureus is the most common cause of septic arthritis (Table 104-1). Patients with underlying joint disease and injection drug users are at particular risk for infection with this organism. *Pseudomonas aeruginosa* is another important cause of septic arthritis among injection drug users. Surgical cases are usually caused by staphylococcal species, both coagulase positive and coagulase negative.

Other gram-negative bacilli are infrequent causes of septic arthritis and are found primarily among elderly debilitated patients with chronic arthritis. In adults younger than age 30, *Neisseria gonorrhoeae* is the most likely pathogen. Isolates causing disseminated gonococcal infection with arthritis are generally resistant to killing by normal serum.

Clinical Presentation

Symptoms of septic arthritis are generally present for only a few days before the patient seeks medical attention. Fever is usual; shaking chills may occur. The knee is the most commonly affected joint and is generally painful and swollen. Fluid can be found in most infected joints, and limitation of motion is marked. In some cases, however, particularly among patients with underlying rheumatoid arthritis who are receiving corticosteroids, physical findings indicating infection may be subtle. In these individuals, who are at particular risk for septic arthritis, superimposed infection may be difficult to distinguish from a flare-up of underlying disease. Symmetrical symptoms in multiple joints are more indicative of a rheumatoid flare-up. Approximately 10% of cases of septic arthritis, however, involve more than one joint.

Differential Diagnosis of Acute Monoarticular or Oligoarticular Arthritis

Infections, crystal deposition (uric acid gout or calcium pyrophosphate pseudogout), trauma, osteoarthritis, ischemic necrosis, foreign bodies, tumors, and systemic diseases such as systemic lupus erythematosus can produce an acute monoarticular arthritis. Radiographs may show evidence of osteoarthritis, gouty tophi, or the linear densities of chondrocalcinosis, which are characteristic of pseudogout. All red, warm, tender joints must be aspirated. The synovial fluid should be cultured anaerobically and aerobically. A Gram-stained preparation should be examined, and a wet mount of fluid should be examined using a polarized microscope to look for crystals. Synovial fluid leukocyte counts and chemistries are of limited value in the differential diagnosis of a suspected septic joint. As a general rule, however, synovial fluid white blood cell counts in excess of 100,000/μL suggest either infection or crystal-induced disease (see Table 78-3). Blood cultures should be obtained in all cases of suspected septic arthritis.

Table 104-1 Infective Arthritis—Acute

	Causative Agent	Characteristics
Bacterial	*Staphylococcus aureus*	Most common overall; usually monarticular, large joint involvement
	Streptococcus species	Second most common overall
		Groups B, F, and G
		Associated with diabetes mellitus, malignancy, and genitourinary tract abnormalities
	Neisseria gonorrhoeae	Most common in young, sexually active adults; commonly polyarticular in onset; often associated with skin lesions
	Pseudomonas aeruginosa	Largely restricted to injection drug users; often involves sternoclavicular joint
Viral	Hepatitis B, rubella, mumps, parvovirus	Usually polyarticular, with minimal joint effusions, normal peripheral white blood cell count

Treatment

The two major modalities for treatment of acute septic arthritis are drainage and antibiotics. The first needle aspiration of a septic joint should remove as much fluid as possible. Initial antibiotic choice should be based on the clinical presentation and the results of the Gram stain. Staphylococcal infection should be treated with vancomycin, linezolid, or daptomycin until the results of in vitro antimicrobial resistance tests are available. A penicillinase-resistant penicillin may still be the best treatment option for drug-sensitive strains of staphylococci. Gonococcal infections should be treated with ceftriaxone, 1 g every 24 hours for 10 days. Arthritis caused by gram-negative rods should initially be treated with an aminoglycoside or a quinolone, such as ciprofloxacin, plus another drug active against *P. aeruginosa,* such as a third-generation cephalosporin or piperacillin. Arthritis caused by *S. aureus* or gram-negative bacilli should be treated with antibiotics for 4 to 6 weeks. Otherwise, 2 to 3 weeks of antibiotic treatment are usually sufficient to eradicate infection. The treatment for infected prosthetic joints is removal of the prosthesis plus antibodies.

Septic joints (with the notable exception of joints infected with gonococci) generally reaccumulate fluid after treatment is initiated. These reaccumulations must be removed by repeated needle aspirations as often as necessary. Indications for open surgical drainage of the joint include failure of the synovial fluid white blood cell count to fall after 5 days of antibiotic treatment and repeated needle aspirations, and the presence of loculated fluid within the joint. Septic arthritis of the hip is generally drained surgically because of the difficulty and potential hazard of repeated needle aspirations of this joint. Early surgical drainage also should be considered for joint infections with gram-negative rods or with *S. aureus.* Untreated or inadequately treated septic arthritis may be complicated by osteomyelitis. In instances in which the diagnosis and treatment have been delayed, radiographs of the involved joint should be obtained at the beginning and termination of treatment.

POLYARTICULAR ARTHRITIS

Arthritis involving multiple joints is generally a consequence of bacteremic seeding and is infrequently attributable to direct microbial invasion. In many instances, a polyarticular arthritis represents an immunologically mediated process. Acute rheumatic fever, a delayed immune-mediated response to group A streptococcal infection, may manifest as a migratory, asymmetrical arthritis of the knees, ankles, elbows, and wrists. Heart involvement, subcutaneous nodules, or erythema marginatum is present in a minority of cases. Most patients have serologic evidence of recent streptococcal infection. Anti-streptolysin O, anti-DNAse, and antihyaluronidase antibodies are usually present. The importance of making this diagnosis lies primarily in the requirement for long-term prophylaxis against streptococcal infection and the clinical response of this process to salicylates.

Viral infections including hepatitis B and C, rubella, parvovirus B19 infection, and mumps may be associated with polyarthritis. In mumps and rubella, the arthritis results from direct infection of articular tissue; with hepatitis viruses, the joint inflammation is a secondary result of the host immune response. Serum sickness, polyarticular gout, sarcoidosis, rheumatoid arthritis, and other connective tissue disorders must be considered in the differential diagnosis. Chronic essential mixed cryoglobulinemia induced by hepatitis B or C virus can cause arthralgias, although severe arthritis is rare. Because 10% of cases of septic arthritis involve more than one joint, acutely inflamed joints containing fluid should be tapped to exclude bacterial infection.

Disseminated gonococcal infection (see Chapter 107) may manifest with fever, tenosynovitis, or arthritis involving several joints and a characteristic rash. The rash may be petechial but usually consists of a few to a few dozen pustules on an erythematous base. Cultures of the joint fluid are usually negative at this stage, but blood cultures are often positive; Gram stain of a pustule may reveal the pathogen. Ceftriaxone, 1 g/day for 10 days, is curative.

CHRONIC ARTHRITIS

Mycobacteria and fungi may produce an indolent, slowly progressive arthritis, usually involving only one joint or contiguous joints, such as those of the wrist and hand (Table 104-2). Fever may be low grade or absent. Cultures of joint fluid may be negative. Some patients with tuberculous arthritis have no evidence of active disease in the lungs. As a general rule, patients with inflammatory chronic monoarticular arthritis should undergo synovial biopsy for mycobacterial and fungal cultures and histology. Granulomas indicate the likelihood of fungal or mycobacterial infection. Cultures should confirm the diagnosis.

Fungal osteoarticular infections are unusual and are typically a consequence of contiguous spread of local infection.

Table 104-2 Causes of Infective Arthritis—Chronic

Nontuberculous mycobacteria

Tuberculosis

Fungi

Lyme disease (oligoarticular)

Osteoarthritis caused by *Candida* species is relatively rare. Fungal arthritis should be treated surgically by arthroscopic débridement and drainage together with antifungal agents. Mycobacterial arthritis should be treated for 9 months with at least two drugs active against the isolate.

A spirochete, *Borrelia burgdorferi,* is the pathogen responsible for Lyme disease. Several months to years (mean 6 months) after the bite of the *Ixodes* tick and the characteristic expanding rash of erythema chronicum migrans, some patients develop an intermittent arthritis with large effusions involving one or more joints, usually including the knees. This chronic arthritis may result in joint destruction, but fever is unusual. Treatment with intravenous ceftriaxone, 4 g/day for 14 to 21 days, will halt the progression of disease in the majority of cases (see Chapter 95), but treatment during the rash stage with amoxicillin or doxycycline will prevent the later development of arthritis.

Septic Bursitis

In more than 80% of cases, septic bursitis is caused by *S. aureus* and involves predominantly the olecranon or the prepatellar bursa. In most instances there is a history of antecedent infection or irritation of the skin overlying the bursa. On examination, the skin over the bursa is red and often peeling. The bursa has a doughy consistency, and fluid may be found to be present on careful examination. Daily needle aspiration until sterile fluid is obtained and antibiotics that are selected according to the Gram-stain, culture, and sensitivity findings are generally curative. Occasionally, long courses of antibiotics (>2 to 3 weeks) may be required for cure.

Osteomyelitis

Infections of the bone occur either as a result of hematogenous spread or through extension of local infection.

HEMATOGENOUS OSTEOMYELITIS

This infection occurs most commonly in the long bones or vertebral bodies (Table 104-3). The peak age distributions are in childhood and old age. Individuals predisposed to hematogenous osteomyelitis include injection drug users, who are at risk for infections with *S. aureus* and *P. aeruginosa,* and patients with hemoglobinopathy, in whom nontyphoidal salmonellae often infect infarcted regions of bone. *Staphylococcus epidermidis* has emerged as an important nosocomial pathogen in patients with infected intravenous catheters. Like patients with septic arthritis, patients with hematogenous osteomyelitis often give a history of trauma antedating symptoms of infection, suggesting that transient, unrecognized bacteremia might result in infection of traumatized tissue.

Patients with acute hematogenous osteomyelitis generally manifest acute onset of pain, tenderness, and fever; there may also be soft tissue swelling over the affected bone. In most instances, physical examination distinguishes acute osteomyelitis from septic arthritis, because range of joint motion is preserved in osteomyelitis. In the first 2 weeks of illness, roentgenograms may be negative or show only soft tissue swelling; technetium scans or gallium scans are almost always positive, but technetium scans may also be positive in the setting of increased vascularity or increased bone formation of any cause. Magnetic resonance imaging (MRI) is the imaging technique of choice for diagnosis of osteomyelitis. Bone erosion, with decreased signal intensity on T1-weighted images and increased signal intensity on T2-weighted images, are seen on MRI before plain films are abnormal. After 2 weeks of infection, plain radiographs generally show some abnormality, and untreated osteomyelitis may produce areas of periosteal elevation or erosion followed by increased bone formation (sclerosis). The erythrocyte sedimentation rate is generally elevated, as is the white blood cell count.

A patient with back pain and fever must be considered to have a serious infection until proven otherwise. Spasm of the paravertebral muscles is common in patients with vertebral osteomyelitis but nonspecific. Point tenderness over bone suggests the presence of local infection. A good history should be obtained and a careful neurologic examination performed. Abnormalities of bowel or bladder or of strength or sensation in the lower extremities suggest the possibility of spinal cord involvement by means of spinal epidural abscess with or without osteomyelitis. Acute spinal epidural abscess is a surgical emergency. The challenge is to make the diagnosis before neurologic signs appear (see Chapter 128). MRI provides excellent definition of epidural or paravertebral abscess and is the diagnostic procedure of choice. Demonstration of an epidural abscess mandates immediate intervention, either by surgery or, in selected cases, by computed tomography–guided drainage. Although most cases of hematogenous osteomyelitis have an acute presentation, some cases may have an indolent course. These patients may have an illness of more than 1 year's duration characterized by pain and low-grade fever. Radiographs are abnormal but may show only collapse of a vertebral body. This most often occurs in infections with *P. aeruginosa,* but *Candida* species and *S. aureus* infections may also occasionally manifest in this manner.

Blood cultures are positive in about half of acute cases of osteomyelitis. Patients with acute osteomyelitis should have a needle biopsy and culture of the involved bone unless blood culture results are known beforehand. Antibiotic treatment directed against the causative pathogen for 4 to 6 weeks is usually sufficient for native bone and joint infections (in prosthetic joint infections rifampin is often added). In instances when a causative agent has not been identified after appropriate specimens have been cultivated for routine pathogens, a diagnosis of mycobacterial infection should be considered; if ordinary bacterial infection still remains the most likely diagnosis, treatment should include vancomycin for methicillin-resistant *S. aureus.*

Table 104-3 **Factors Predisposing to Hematogenous Osteomyelitis**	
Setting	**Likely Pathogens**
Injection drug use	*Staphylococcus aureus* *Pseudomonas aeruginosa*
Intravenous catheters	*S. aureus* *Staphylococcus epidermidis* *Candida* species
Urinary tract infection	Enterobacteriaceae

Table 104-4 Osteomyelitis Secondary to Contiguous Spread

Setting	Likely Microorganisms
Surgery, trauma	*Staphylococcus aureus* Aerobic gram-negative bacilli
Cat or dog bites	*Pasteurella multocida*
Human bites	Mixed anaerobic infections
Periodontal infections	Mixed anaerobic infections
Cutaneous ulcers	Mixed aerobic and anaerobic organisms

OSTEOMYELITIS SECONDARY TO EXTENSION OF LOCAL INFECTION

Local infection predisposes to osteomyelitis in several major settings (Table 104-4). The first is after penetrating trauma or surgery where local infection gains access to traumatized bone. In postsurgical infections, staphylococci and gram-negative bacilli predominate. Generally there is evidence of wound infection, with erythema, swelling, increased postoperative tenderness, and drainage. A traumatic incident often associated with osteomyelitis is either a human or an animal bite. Human bites, if deep enough, may result in osteomyelitis caused by anaerobic mouth bacteria. Cat bites notoriously result in the development of osteomyelitis because the cat's thin, sharp, long teeth often penetrate the periosteum. *Pasteurella multocida* is a frequent pathogen in this setting. A 4- to 6-week course of ampicillin-sulbactam 3 g q8h is recommended.

The intimate relationship of the teeth and periodontal tissues to the bones of the maxilla and mandible may predispose to osteomyelitis after local infection. Débridement of necrotic tissue and ampicillin-sulbactam 3 g q6h comprise an effective treatment, because mixed-anaerobic infections are usually present.

The third setting in which local infection predisposes to osteomyelitis is that of an infected sore or ulcer. Pressure sores of the sacrum or femoral region may erode into contiguous bone and produce an osteomyelitis (see Chapter 101) caused by several bacterial species including anaerobic organisms. Patients with diabetes mellitus often develop traumatic vascular ulcerations of their toes and feet, with eventual development of osteomyelitis. Anaerobes, streptococci, staphylococci, and gram-negative bacilli are often involved in these infections (see Chapter 101).

An ulcer area larger than 2 cm^2, probe patency through the ulcer to bone, an erythrocyte sedimentation rate of more than 70 mm/hr, and an abnormal plain radiograph are helpful in diagnosing the presence of lower extremity osteomyelitis in patients with diabetes. A negative MRI result makes the diagnosis much less likely when all of these findings are absent. Treatment involves débridement (often amputation in the case of diabetics) and antibiotics active against the pathogens involved for at least 6 weeks. Optimizing metabolic control and correction of macrovasculopathy if possible (e.g., by angioplasty) may improve wound healing; the benefits of vacuum-assisted drainage are controversial.

CHRONIC OSTEOMYELITIS

Untreated or inadequately treated osteomyelitis results in avascular necrosis of bone and the formation of islands of nonvascularized and infected bone called *sequestra*. Patients with chronic osteomyelitis may tolerate their infection reasonably well, with intermittent episodes of disease activity manifested by increased local pain and the drainage of infected material through a sinus tract. Some patients have tolerated chronic osteomyelitis for decades. A normochromic, normocytic anemia of chronic disease is common in this setting, and occasionally amyloidosis and, in rare cases, osteogenic sarcoma complicate this disorder. Fluorodeoxyglucose positron emission tomography may have the highest diagnostic accuracy for the diagnosis of chronic osteomyelitis.

S. aureus is responsible for the great majority of cases of chronic osteomyelitis; the major exception is among patients with sickle cell anemia, in whom nontyphoidal salmonellae may cause chronic infection of the long bones.

Cultures of sinus tract drainage do not reliably reflect the pathogens involved in the infection. Diagnosis and cure are best effected by surgical débridement of necrotic material followed by long-term administration of antibiotics active against the organism found in the surgical specimens.

Mycobacteria, most often *Mycobacterium tuberculosis*, can produce a chronic osteomyelitis. The anterior portions of vertebral bodies are the most common sites of infection. Hematogenous dissemination and lymphatic spread are the most likely routes of infection. Paravertebral abscess (often termed *cold abscess* because of lack of signs of acute inflammation) may complicate this infection. Diagnosis is usually confirmed by histologic examination and culture of biopsy material. Treatment against skeletal tuberculosis involves at least 9 months of standard therapy and often surgical débridement.

Prospectus for the Future

- Better limb sparing treatment modalities for diabetic osteomyelitis

- Improvement of multidisciplinary approaches in the treatment of chronic osteomyelitis

References

Butalia S, Palda VA, Sargeant RJ, et al: Does this patient with diabetes have osteomyelitis of the lower extremity? JAMA 299:806-813, 2008.

Kapoor A, Page S, Lavalley M, et al: Magnetic resonance imaging for diagnosing foot osteomyelitis: A meta-analysis. Arch Intern Med 167:125-132, 2007.

Lew DP, Waldvogel FA. Osteomyelitis. Lancet 364:369-379, 2004.

Margaretten ME, Kohlwes J, Moore D, Bent S: Does this adult patient have septic arthritis? JAMA 297:1478-1488, 2007.

Mathews CJ, Kingsley G, Field M, et al: Management of septic arthritis: A systematic review. Ann Rheum Dis 66:440-445, 2007.

Moran GJ, Krishnadasan A, Gorwitz RJ, et al: Methicillin-resistant *S. aureus* infections among patients in the emergency department. N Engl J Med 355:666-674, 2006.

Termaat MF, Raijmakers PG, Scholten HJ, et al: The accuracy of diagnostic imaging for the assessment of chronic osteomyelitis: a systematic review and meta-analysis. J Bone Joint Surg Am 87:2464-2471, 2005.

Infections of the Urinary Tract

Christoph Lange and Michael M. Lederman

The urethra, bladder, kidneys, and prostate are all susceptible to infection. Most urinary tract infections (UTIs) cause local symptoms, yet clinical manifestations do not always pinpoint the site of infection. The purpose of this chapter is to simplify the clinical and laboratory approach to diagnosis and treatment of UTIs. Infections associated with indwelling urinary catheters are discussed in Chapter 106.

Urethritis

Urethritis is predominantly an infection of sexually active individuals, usually men. The symptoms are pain and burning of the urethra during urination, and there is generally some discharge at the urethral meatus. Urethritis may be gonococcal in origin. However, nongonococcal urethritis is now more frequent in North America. Nongonococcal urethritis may be caused by *Chlamydia trachomatis* or *Ureaplasma urealyticum* and less commonly by *Trichomonas vaginalis* or herpesviruses. Diagnosis and management of urethritis are considered in Chapter 107.

Cystitis and Pyelonephritis

EPIDEMIOLOGY

Bacterial infection of the bladder (cystitis) and kidney (pyelonephritis) is more frequent in women, and the incidence of infection increases with age. Factors that predispose to UTI include instrumentation (e.g., catheterization, cystoscopy), pregnancy, anatomic abnormalities of the genitourinary tract, and diabetes mellitus.

PATHOGENESIS

Although some infections of the kidney may arise as the result of hematogenous dissemination, most UTIs ascend through a portal of entry in the urethra. Most pathogens responsible for community-acquired UTIs are bacterial species that naturally live in the human bowel. *Escherichia coli* is the most common isolate; in women, colonization of the vaginal and periurethral mucosa may antedate infection of the urinary tract. Bacteria with fimbriae capable of adherence to epithelial cells are more likely to cause UTIs, and persons whose epithelial cells bind these fimbriae may be at greater risk for infection. The longer and protected male urethra may account for the lower incidence of UTI in men. Motile bacteria may swim upstream, and reflux of urine from the bladder into the ureters may predispose to the development of kidney infection.

CLINICAL FEATURES

Suprapubic pain, discomfort, a burning sensation on urination, and frequency of urination are common symptoms of infection of the urinary tract. Back or flank pain or the occurrence of fever suggests that infection is not limited to the bladder (cystitis) but involves the kidney (pyelonephritis) or prostate as well. Clinical presentation, however, often fails to distinguish between simple cystitis and pyelonephritis. Approximately one half of infections that appear clinically to involve the bladder can be shown by instrumentation and other specialized techniques to affect the kidneys. Elderly or debilitated patients with infection of the urinary tract may have no symptoms referable to the urinary tract and may have only fever, altered mental status, or hypotension as a presenting sign.

LABORATORY DIAGNOSIS

Analysis of a midstream urine sample obtained from patients with infection of the bladder or kidney shows white blood cells (WBCs) and may also reveal red blood cells and slightly increased amounts of protein. The presence of at least 10 WBCs/mm^3 of midstream urine by counting chamber is defined as pyuria. The vast majority of patients with symptomatic or asymptomatic bacteriuria have pyuria. The presence of WBC casts in an infected urine sample indicates the presence of pyelonephritis. Bacteria may be seen in sedimented urine and can be readily identified by Gram stain. For asymptomatic women, bacteriuria is defined as two consecutive voided urine specimens with isolation of the same bacterial strain at levels of at least 105 colony-forming units (CFUs) per milliliter. In men a single, clean-catch, voided urine specimen with one bacterial species at concentrations >105 CFU/mL identifies bacteriuria. The diagnosis of bacteriuria is also established in both women and men from a single catheterized urine specimen (not from an indwelling catheter) with one bacterial species isolated at concentrations >102 CFU/mL.

A hazard in interpreting results of urine culture is that if the sample is allowed to stand at room temperature for a few hours before being cultured, bacteria can multiply. This results in spuriously high bacterial counts. For this reason, urine for culture should not be obtained from a catheter bag. Specimens that are not plated immediately should be refrigerated. Biochemical tests to detect bacteriuria are not reliable when numbers of bacteria are low.

TREATMENT AND OUTCOME

Asymptomatic bacteriuria has not been shown to be harmful in most adult populations. Antimicrobial treatment for asymptomatic bacteriuria is indicated only for pregnant women and for patients undergoing urologic instrumentation. These patients should be screened for asymptomatic bacteriuria and treated if test results are positive.

Pyuria accompanying asymptomatic bacteriuria is not an indication for antimicrobial treatment. On the other hand, all symptomatic patients with UTI should be treated with antimicrobials. Although most women with lower UTIs are cured by a single dose of antibiotic, such as a double-strength trimethoprim-sulfamethoxazole (TMP/SMZ 160/800 mg) tablet, a 3-day ("short course") treatment with ciprofloxacin 250 mg bid or TMP/SMZ 160/800 mg bid provides higher cure rates and is now generally recommended. (Note that in some regions, more than 20% of E. coli are resistant to TMP/SMZ.) β-lactams are not recommended for short-course therapy because of suboptimal clinical and bacteriologic results compared with those of other agents. Short-course therapy is not recommended for women with a history of UTI caused by a resistant bacterium, when the duration of symptoms is >1 week, or for men. In these patients 7 to 10 days of treatment are recommended. Cultures and results of sensitivity testing confirm the diagnosis and ascertain if the antibiotic is active against the pathogen, but these tests are not advocated in persons with uncomplicated cystitis unless treatment fails. Because of the difficulty in clinical distinction between cystitis and upper urinary tract disease, some patients treated for cystitis may experience relapse because of unrecognized upper tract disease. Recurrent UTIs in males should always raise the suspicion for an anatomic alteration of the urinary tract.

Occasionally, urine cultures obtained from a patient with symptoms of UTI and pyuria are reported as exhibiting "no growth" or "insignificant growth." This situation has been labeled the "urethral syndrome." Low numbers of bacteria (as few as 100/mL of urine) may produce such infections of the urinary tract. In other instances, the urethral syndrome may be caused by Chlamydia or Ureaplasma, which will not grow on routine culture media. Thus, if a patient with the urethral syndrome has responded to antibiotics, the course should be completed; otherwise, if symptoms and pyuria persist, the patient should receive a 7- to 10-day course of tetracycline, which is active against Chlamydia and Ureaplasma. Other considerations for patients with lower urinary tract symptoms and no or "insignificant" growth on cultures of urine include vaginitis, herpes simplex infection, and gonococcal infection (Neisseria gonorrhoeae will not grow on routine media used for urine culture). A pelvic examination and culture for gonococci may be indicated in this setting if the patient is sexually active. Men with urethral discomfort and discharge should be evaluated for urethritis (see Chapter 107). Men with suprapubic pain, frequency, and urgency should be evaluated for cystitis, as discussed earlier.

The presence of fever suggests that infection involves more than just the bladder. Young, otherwise healthy, febrile patients with UTI may be treated on an ambulatory basis with a fluoroquinolone for 2 weeks, provided that (1) their condition does not appear toxic, (2) they are able to take oral fluids and medications, (3) they have friends or family at home, (4) they have good provisions for follow-up, and (5) they have no potentially complicating features such as diabetes mellitus, history of renal stones, obstructive disease of the urinary tract, or sickle cell disease. In this setting, urine specimens should be sent for culture and antimicrobial susceptibility testing. Gram stain of urine in patients hospitalized for pyelonephritis will guide initial therapy. Initial therapy with TMP/SMZ for pyelonephritis can no longer be recommended in the United States because of high levels of resistance in E. coli and in other organisms that can cause urosepsis.

In ill patients with community-acquired pyelonephritis, parenteral treatment of a Gram-negative rod infection should be initiated with either a fluoroquinolone, piperacillin-tazobactam, or a third-generation cephalosporin. An aminoglycoside may be added if drug resistance is suspected or if the patient is very ill. The aminoglycoside should be promptly discontinued if antibiotic sensitivity studies indicate that it is not essential. The finding of gram-positive cocci in chains suggests that enterococci are the pathogens. This infection should be treated, at least initially, with vancomycin plus an aminoglycoside, until antimicrobial drug susceptibility of the enterococci is known. Gram-positive cocci in clusters may indicate staphylococci. Staphylococcus saprophyticus is a likely agent in otherwise healthy women and is sensitive to most antibiotics used in the treatment of UTI. In the older patient, Staphylococcus aureus should be considered, and this infection should initially be treated with vancomycin or linezolid, as methicillin-resistant S. aureus is increasingly prevalent even in the community. When antimicrobial resistance testing indicates susceptibility to a penicillinase-resistant penicillin, such as nafcillin or a cephalosporin, the regimen should be adjusted. Gram-positive cocci in the urine may represent endocarditis with septic embolization to the kidney.

Therapy should be simplified when reports of antimicrobial susceptibility are available. A repeat urine culture after 2 days of effective treatment should show sterilization or a marked decrease in the urinary bacterial count. If the patient fails to demonstrate some clinical improvement after 2 to 3 days of treatment, or if the clinical picture indicates sepsis and the patient has been febrile for more than 1 week, a complicating feature should be suspected. Intranephric or perinephric abscess or obstruction caused by a stone or an enlarged prostate may underlie this presentation. Ultrasonography is a good first diagnostic procedure in this setting. This will generally detect obstruction and collections of pus and will also detect stones greater than 3 mm in diameter. If ultrasonography is negative in this setting, computed tomography is indicated. Obstruction must be relieved and abscesses drained to result in cure. Computed tomography–guided percutaneous drainage is the procedure of choice whenever possible.

All patients with complicated UTI should have repeat urine cultures 1 to 2 weeks after treatment is completed to check for relapse. If relapse occurs, the patient may have pyelonephritis, prostatitis, or neuropathic or structural disease of the urinary tract. If a 6-week course of antibiotics active against the bacterial isolate is not effective in eradicating infection, the possibility of structural abnormalities or prostatic infection should be investigated. Urologic evaluation should be performed for all men with UTI (except urethritis) because of the high frequency of correctable anatomic lesions in this population.

Long-term antibiotic prophylaxis may benefit some persons who experience frequent UTI such as persons with obstructive uropathy or children with vesiculoureteral reflux. A single daily dose of nitrofurantoin 50 mg, TMP/SMZ 40/200, or ciprofloxacin 100 mg may suffice to prevent recurrence. Some women have frequent reinfections related to sexual activity. Prompt voiding and a single dose of an active antibiotic, such as 100 mg nitrofurantoin, 80/400 mg TMP/SMZ, or 100 mg ciprofloxacin just after sexual contact can decrease the reinfection rate in these women.

The occurrence of pyuria in the absence of bacterial growth on culture of urine ($<10^2$ colonies/mL) may be termed *sterile pyuria*. If this occurs in the patient with lower urinary tract symptoms, then chlamydial or gonococcal infection, vaginitis, or herpes simplex infection should be considered. In the absence of lower urinary tract symptoms, sterile pyuria may be seen in patients with interstitial nephritis of numerous causes or with tuberculosis of the urinary tract. Patients with renal tuberculosis often have nocturia, polyuria, and hematuria; more than half of male patients also have involvement of the genital tract, most commonly the epididymis. The diagnostic approach to urogenital tuberculosis includes the collection of three specimens of concentrated morning urine; the patient should avoid drinking for >12 hours, and the first-void portion of the urine is collected for mycobacterial cultures. Genital masses, when present, should be biopsied for microbiologic and histopathologic examination.

Prostatitis

Although prostatic fluid has antibacterial properties, the prostate can become infected, usually by direct invasion through the urethra. Symptoms of back or perineal pain and fever are common. Some patients have pain with ejaculation. Rectal examination usually shows a tender prostate. Patients with acute prostatitis generally have an abnormal urinary sediment and pathogenic bacteria in cultures of urine.

Acute prostatitis may be caused by the gonococcus but is most often caused by gram-negative bacilli. Treatment is directed against the pathogen observed on Gram stain of urine and is generally effective. Therapy should be continued for a minimum of 4 weeks. Parenteral therapy is required rarely. Prostatic abscesses can be drained with ultrasound guidance. Chronic prostatitis may be asymptomatic and should be suspected in men with recurrent UTIs. The urine sediment may be relatively benign in patients with chronic bacterial prostatitis. In this instance, comparison of the first part of the urine sample, midstream urine, excretions expressed by massage of the prostate, and postmassage urine should reveal bacterial counts more than 10-fold greater in the prostatic secretions and postmassage urine samples than in first-void and midstream samples. Treatment of chronic bacterial prostatitis is hampered by poor penetration of the prostate by most antimicrobial agents. Long-term (6 to 12 weeks) treatment with a fluoroquinolone or TMP/SMZ is indicated and is effective in 60% to 70% of cases.

Prospectus for the Future

- Better directed therapies to limit the spread of drug resistance
- Better assays to identify low level bacterial infection in symptomatic patients
- Better treatment for chronic infection of the prostate

References

Guay DR: Contemporary management of uncomplicated urinary tract infections. Drugs 68:1169-1205, 2008.

Lutters M, Vogt-Ferrier NB: Antibiotic duration for treating uncomplicated, symptomatic lower urinary tract infections in elderly women. Cochrane Database Syst Rev 3:CD001535, 2008.

Nicolle LE, Bradley S, Colgan R, et al: Infectious Diseases Society of America guidelines for the diagnosis and treatment of asymptomatic bacteriuria in adults. Clin Infect Dis 40:643-654, 2005.

Pohl A: Modes of administration of antibiotics for symptomatic severe urinary tract infections. Cochrane Database Syst Rev 4:CD003237, 2007.

Chapter **106**

Health Care–Associated Infections

Amy J. Ray, Michelle V. Lisgaris, and Robert A. Salata

A health care–associated or nosocomial infection is an infection that was not present or incubating at the time of admission to a health care facility. Although traditionally these infections have been described in the acute care setting, the proportion of such infections that occurs in long-term care and rehabilitation settings is increasing. Indeed, the risk of health care–associated infection (HAI) for such patient populations approaches that in the acute care setting. In most patients, infections appearing after 48 to 72 hours of hospitalization are considered to be nosocomially acquired.

In the United States a patient admitted to a health care facility has a 5% to 10% chance of developing an HAI. These infections result in significant morbidity and mortality, with 2 million infections and nearly 100,000 deaths annually. The medical costs of HAIs in the United States are estimated to be approximately $10 billion per year.

HAIs are unintended consequences of medical care. As with any infection, necessary elements for acquisition of infection are an infectious agent, a susceptible host, and a means of transmission. Pathogens in health care settings frequently include multidrug-resistant organisms such as methicillin-resistant *Staphylococcus aureus* (MRSA), vancomycin-resistant *Enterococcus*, highly resistant gram-negative bacilli, and *Clostridium difficile*. The increasing drug resistance of many of these pathogens makes treatment challenging. With regard to the host, some factors associated with increased risk are not avoidable, such as advancing age, immunosuppression, and severity of illness. Contributing factors that can be minimized by thoughtful patient management include prolonged duration of hospitalization, the inappropriate use of antibiotics, the prolonged use of indwelling urinary and bloodstream catheters, and the failure of health care personnel to wash their hands. It is important to note that the most common means of transmission of health care–associated pathogens is via the hands of health care workers.

Infection Control

Surveillance of HAIs and the implementation of practices to prevent and control them are the responsibility of infection-control personnel. Practices used to limit the spread of infection include isolating patients with potentially transmissible diseases (e.g., tuberculosis, influenza, MRSA infection), isolating patients at increased risk for acquiring infections (e.g., patients with neutropenia and cancer), and instituting mandatory hand washing and standard precautions with all patient contact. Standard precautions consider all blood and body fluids (e.g., cerebrospinal, amniotic, peritoneal, seminal, vaginal, blood-contaminated fluids) as potentially infectious. Gloves must be worn when exposure to these fluids is possible, especially with nonintact skin or mucosal surfaces. In addition, masks and gowns are worn when splashes are expected. Standard precautions are designed to reduce the risk of transmission of microorganism from both recognized and unrecognized sources of infection in hospitals and therefore must be used for every patient and every encounter.

Approach to the Hospitalized Patient with Possible Health Care–Associated Infection

The development of an HAI is often heralded by a rise in temperature. The only sign of infection, particularly in the older or demented patient, may be a change in mental status (Table 106-1). Confusion or alterations in vital signs may be the only sign of serious underlying infection. Respiratory alkalosis or metabolic acidosis (caused by lactate accumulation), either with or without hypoxia, may be present.

Table 106-1 **Signs of Infection in the Hospitalized Patient**
Fever or hypothermia
Change in mental status
Tachypnea and respiratory alkalosis
Hypotension
Oliguria
Leukocytosis

Table 106-2 **Factors That Contribute to Nosocomial Urinary Tract Infection**
Indwelling catheters
Extended duration of catheterization
Open drainage (versus closed-bag drainage)
Interruption of closed drainage system
Use of broad-spectrum antibiotics (Candida)

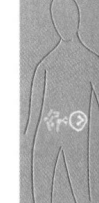

When evaluating a patient with a new fever or possible infection, the physician should first assess the stability of the patient's condition; hypotension, tachypnea, or new obtundation mandates rapid evaluation and treatment. The patient's comorbidities, medications, recent procedures, and hospital course must be reviewed. The physician should elicit a history directed at possible causes of the fever, given that the patient often has a specific complaint that helps identify the source. Possible causes for nosocomial infections by anatomic site are listed in **Web Table 106-1**. Special attention should be given to examination of the skin for rash (e.g., drug eruption, ecthyma gangrenosum, disseminated candidiasis), wounds, or pressure sores; in addition, the physician must examine the sinuses (especially with nasogastric or nasotracheal tubes in place), mouth (for candidiasis or herpes infections), lungs (for pneumonia or thromboembolism), abdomen (e.g., for *C. difficile*–associated colitis, postoperative abscess, biliary sepsis), catheters, joints (for septic arthritis, gout, and pseudogout), and extremities (for deep-venous thrombosis). The patient's medications should also be reviewed carefully for agents likely to produce fever (antibiotics and anticonvulsants especially). With drug fever, associated eosinophilia and/or rash is present in fewer than 25% of patients. Occasionally, a source of fever cannot be identified despite extensive evaluation. The classic definition of fever of unknown origin has recently been adapted to include the diagnosis of fever of unknown origin acquired nosocomially (see Chapter 95).

Catheter-Associated Urinary Tract Infections

Urinary tract infections are the most common HAI and result in 900,000 additional hospitalization days at a cost well over $615 million annually. Approximately 80% of nosocomial urinary tract infections are associated with the use of indwelling urinary catheters, and up to 16% of all patients in a health care setting will have a urinary catheter during their stay. Fifteen percent of nosocomial bacteremias originate from the catheterized urinary tract, and some studies have shown increased mortality in patients with a catheter-associated urinary tract infection (CAUTI).

Placement of an indwelling catheter into the urethra of a hospitalized patient facilitates access of pathogens to an ordinarily sterile site. Factors that predispose the patient to infection are shown in Table 106-2. The most common pathogens are enteric gram-negative rods; however, *Candida* and *Enterococcus* species are also important causes of infec-

tion. Prophylactic antibiotics, irrigation, urinary acidification, and use of antiseptics are of no value in preventing infection in this setting. Using indwelling catheters only when necessary can reduce CAUTI; studies have observed that 21% to 50% of all urinary catheters placed were for inappropriate indications. Urinary incontinence and routine fluid balance monitoring are not sufficient indications. Examples of situations in which catheterization is unavoidable may include the management of acute urinary retention or pressure wound healing in an incontinent patient. Thrice-daily straight (in-and-out) catheterization, with the use of aseptic technique, is less likely to produce infection than use of indwelling catheters, and many patients with dysfunctional bladders have used this technique for years without developing significant urinary tract infections.

If the use of an indwelling catheter is unavoidable, then the catheter drainage system should remain closed and unobstructed and kept securely fastened, with the collection bag remaining below the level of the bladder. The catheter should not be disconnected from the bag because specimens can be collected aseptically by inserting a needle through the distal catheter wall. Most important, the catheter should be removed as soon as possible. Additional strategies to reduce the incidence of urinary catheter–related infections have been the use of silver-coated or antibiotic-impregnated catheters; several studies have been performed and show either conflicting results or benefit only in select populations, respectively. Therefore implementation of their use as routine practice has not been widely recommended.

The clinical presentation of CAUTI is most commonly heralded by fever; localizing symptoms and signs may be absent in the catheterized patient. Microbiologic diagnosis usually requires the growth of at least 10^5 colony-forming units (CFU) of an organism per milliliter of a urine specimen collected aseptically from the catheter.

Asymptomatic bacterial colonization of the catheterized bladder is highly prevalent and need not be treated. *Candida* infection of the bladder often resolves once broad-spectrum antibiotics are discontinued and the indwelling catheter has been removed. If *Candida* infection persists, then oral fluconazole or single-dose intravenous amphotericin B will often eradicate the organism, although recurrence rates are high and the long-term benefit of this approach has not been demonstrated.

The best way to prevent CAUTI is to avoid catheterization unless absolutely necessary. For patients with indwelling urinary catheters, the most important risk factor of CAUTI is extended duration of catheterization; hence assessment for removal on a daily basis is encouraged.

Nosocomial Pneumonia

Pneumonia comprises 15% to 20% of all nosocomial infections, making it the second most frequent hospital-acquired infection. The vast majority of instances arise from aspiration of oropharyngeal contents. Aerobic gram-negative bacilli and often staphylococci, typically after the first 5 days of hospitalization, rapidly replace the normal oropharyngeal flora of the patient admitted to the hospital. The administration of broad-spectrum antibiotics, severe underlying illness (e.g., chronic lung disease), respiratory intubation, surgery, advanced age, and prolonged duration of hospitalization predispose individuals to colonization with these organisms.

Sedation, loss of consciousness, and factors that depress gag and cough reflexes place the colonized patient at increased risk for aspiration and the development of pneumonia. The development of a new pulmonary infiltrate in a hospitalized patient may represent pneumonia, atelectasis, aspiration of gastric contents, drug reaction, or pulmonary infarction. If pneumonia is suggested, then prompt identification of the pathogen and appropriate treatment are critical because nosocomial pneumonia carries a 20% to 50% risk of mortality. If the patient cannot produce a sputum specimen adequate for interpretation (<10 epithelial cells, >25 neutrophils per low-power [×100] field), then nasotracheal aspiration or bronchoscopic evaluation should be performed (see Chapter 99). Ventilator-associated pneumonia (VAP) accounts for up to 80% of nosocomially acquired respiratory infections; therefore the intubated patient in the intensive care unit should be monitored carefully for signs of pneumonia. Many patients are paralyzed to facilitate ventilator-dependent respiration. These patients have ineffective gag reflexes and often depressed cough as well and are therefore entirely dependent on suctioning to prevent aspiration. Patients whose airways are simply colonized but whose lower respiratory tracts are not infected should not be treated with antibiotics, despite positive sputum cultures. Premature treatment of colonization results in replacement of the initial colonists by more-resistant organisms, whereas delay in treatment of nosocomial pneumonia can result in death from overwhelming infection. The physician must therefore be able to accurately distinguish colonization from infection. The development of new fever, leukocytosis, pulmonary infiltrates, or deterioration of oxygenation suggests pneumonia rather than colonization. A Gram stain of sputum should be performed to identify the predominant organism or organisms, but initial antimicrobial therapy in these critically ill patients should include all likely pathogens because the high frequency of colonization makes interpretation of Gram stain results difficult. The use of clinical tools to assist in the distinction between colonization and infection, primarily in ventilated patients, is helpful in determining when antimicrobial treatment is needed (Fig. 106-1). The clinical pulmonary infection score (CPIS) assigns a numeric value to readily available clinical variables and assists in the determination of the presence of VAP. A CPIS of 6 has greater than 90% sensitivity in detecting pulmonary infection. Epidemics of nosocomial pneumonia are most often caused by transmission of pathogenic bacteria from the hands of medical personnel.

The results of Gram stain and culture of the sputum and aspirate or the results of bronchoscopy specimens guide

Diagnostic Criterion	Results	Points
Temperature (°C)	≥ 36.5 and ≤ 38.4	0
	≥ 38.5 and ≤ 38.9	1
	≤ 36.0 and ≤ 39.0	2
Leukocyte count (/μL)	≥ 4000 and ≤ 11,000	0
	< 4000 or > 11,000	1
	≥ 500 band forms	1
Tracheal secretions	Absent	0
	Nonpurulent	1
	Purulent	2
PaO_2/FiO_2 (mm/Hg)	> 240 or ARDS	0
	≤ 240 and no evidence of ARDs	2
Pulmonary radiographic findings	No infiltrate	0
	Diffuse or patchy infiltrate	1
	Localized infiltrate	2
Progression of pulmonary infiltrate	No radiographic progression	0
	Radiographic progression after excluding CHF/ARDS	2
Tracheal aspirate Gram stain and culture	No pathologic bacteria cultured	0
	Pathologic bacteria cultured	1
	Some pathologic bacteria on Gram stain	1

Figure 106-1 With use of these diagnostic criteria, a clinical pulmonary infection score of 6 or greater has better than 90% sensitivity in detecting pulmonary infection.

antibiotic therapy. Gram-negative rods have been the predominant pathogens in this setting over the past three decades; these infections should be treated with a fluoroquinolone or aminoglycoside plus an extended-spectrum penicillin or cephalosporin until results of culture and sensitivity testing are known. Recent data from the National Nosocomial Infection Surveillance System indicate that *S. aureus* is the most common cause of nosocomial pneumonia in critically ill patients in the United States and that the prevalence of methicillin resistance is on the rise among these organisms. Therefore if gram-positive cocci in clusters are seen, then vancomycin or linezolid should be administered until sensitivities are known. A mixed flora suggestive of aspiration of oral anaerobes should prompt treatment with clindamycin or a penicillin–β-lactamase inhibitor combination. In certain hospitals, nosocomial pneumonia caused by *Legionella* species is a consideration, and if suggested, then a fluoroquinolone or macrolide should be included in the initial treatment regimen until specific testing can be performed. Selection of an appropriate antimicrobial agent is critical because initial treatment with an antibiotic to which the causative organism is not sensitive is associated with a greater than twofold increase in mortality. Patients with nosocomial pneumonia should also receive aggressive respiratory therapy to promote coughing and expectoration of secretions.

Nosocomial pneumonias are best prevented in ventilated and nonventilated patients by (1) avoiding excessive sedation, (2) providing frequent suctioning and respiratory therapy, (3) positioning the patient in the semirecumbent position, (4) weaning the patient from mechanical respiratory support as soon as possible, (5) initiating early enteral nutrition with avoidance of gastric overdistention, (6) encouraging frequent hand washing by all health care personnel, and (7) avoiding injudicious use of broad-spectrum or high-dose antibiotics. In addition, for ventilated patients orotracheal intubation is preferred because of increased risk of sinusitis and possibly VAP when nasogastric intubation is performed. The use of a cuffed endotracheal tube with in-line or subglottic suctioning is encouraged to manage secretions and prevent aspiration.

Intravascular Catheter–Related Bloodstream Infections

More than 200,000 health care–associated bloodstream infections occur annually in the United States, the vast majority of which can be attributed to the presence of an intravascular catheter (catheter-related bloodstream infection [CRBSI]). Infections related to intravascular catheters may occur by means of bacteremic seeding or through infusion of contaminated material, but the vast majority of these infections occur through bacterial invasion at the site of catheter insertion. Catheters in frequent use today differ in their indications for use and their risk for CRBSI; therefore familiarization with appropriate selection may go a long way toward preventing CRBSI (Table 106-3; **Web Fig. 106-1**).

Bacteria migrating through the catheter insertion site may colonize the catheter and then produce a septic phlebitis or bacteremia without evidence of local infection. Factors associated with a greater risk of intravenous CRBSI are shown in Table 106-4. Coagulase-negative staphylococci are the predominant pathogen in this setting, followed in equal frequency by *S. aureus* and enterococci. *Candida* species have now surpassed individual gram-negative rods as the third leading cause of CRBSI. The rising incidence of candidemia and enterococcal bacteremia is a reflection of the increasing proportion of immunocompromised and severely ill patients being admitted to acute care facilities. As a group, gram-negative enteric bacilli are the fourth most common cause of nosocomial bacteremia. Patients receiving parenteral nutrition are at particular risk for systemic infection with *Candida* species and gram-negative bacilli.

If nosocomial bacteremia is suggested, then at least two sets of blood cultures should be obtained, one of which should be drawn from a peripheral vein and the other or others through the catheter of concern. Management of CRBSI varies according to the type of catheter involved and whether bacteremia-associated complications (e.g., septic thrombophlebitis, septic embolization, tunnel-site infection, endocarditis, osteomyelitis, metastatic seeding of bacteria) are present (see Table 106-3 and **Web Fig. 106-1**).

A peripheral catheter (and all readily removable foreign bodies) should be replaced if bacteremia develops and no other primary site of infection is found. The catheter should also be removed if fever without an obvious source or if local phlebitis develops. Once the catheter has been removed, the site should be compressed in an attempt to express pus from the catheter entry site. If septic thrombophlebitis is documented, then surgical exploration may be required. The value of culturing a peripheral catheter tip is limited unless semiquantitative techniques are used (e.g., isolation of >15 CFU of bacteria by the roll plate method). Routine replacement of peripheral indwelling intravascular catheters every 72 hours decreases the risk of CRBSI.

Central venous catheters are of the nontunneled, tunneled, or implanted device variety (**Web Fig. 106-1**). These catheters may be kept in place for prolonged periods with a lower infection risk than peripheral catheters. However, because they typically remain in place for prolonged periods of time, central venous catheters are associated with a greater overall rate of infection. Special microbiologic techniques can be employed to assist in the diagnosis of catheter-related bacteremia. When the diagnosis is confirmed, assessment for infection-related complications (e.g., port abscess, tunnel infection, endocarditis, septic thrombosis) should be performed to devise an appropriate management strategy. Consideration of catheter removal should be given with any nontunneled, central venous catheter–related bacteremia and is generally recommended. Removal of tunneled catheters or implanted devices is generally required when infectious complications occur. In situations in which the infected tunneled catheter or port cannot be removed, an *antibiotic lock* technique may be employed as an attempt to salvage the catheter. In cases of central venous catheter infections involving *Candida* species, other fungi, and *S. aureus*, attempts at catheter salvage have been largely unsuccessful.

Prevention of central line–related bloodstream infection (CLBSI) can be accomplished by practicing an evidence-based approach that includes avoidance of the femoral site for catheterization, hand hygiene before insertion, and maximum sterile barriers including full drape and cap, sterile gown, and gloves for the inserter. In addition, chlorhexidine gluconate (concentration ≥0.5%) is the preferred antiseptic for skin preparation for patients at least 2 months of age as it broadly inhibits microbial growth with a prolonged residual effect. Antiseptic-coated catheters such as those coated with silver sulfadiazine may also reduce infection rates in the adult patient population. A simple checklist of these insertion interventions combined with catheter removal as soon as possible has been shown to significantly reduce rates of CLBSI.

Clostridium difficile Infection

C. difficile infection (CDI) is the most clinically significant cause of hospital-acquired diarrheal disease and is often accompanied by fever and leukocytosis. It is a cause of significant morbidity and mortality and becoming increasingly difficult to control and eradicate. An epidemic strain of *C. difficile* associated with more severe disease, mortality, and frequent relapses has emerged in the United States, Canada, and Europe since 2003. *C. difficile* now rivals MRSA as the most common organism to cause HAIs in the United States. For full description of this important clinical condition, the reader is referred to Chapter 103.

Table 106-3 **Catheters Used for Vascular Access**

Catheter Type	Entry Location	Size	Replacement	Comments
Peripheral Catheters				The most commonly used short-term intravascular device
Venous catheter (IV)	Peripheral veins, usually of the forearm or the hand	<3 in	72 hr is recommended; 96 hr is safe if IV site is not indicative for thrombosis or phlebitis. Indicative for thrombosis or phlebitis.	Risk of phlebitis exists with prolonged use; CRBSI is rare.
Arterial catheter	Primarily used in radial artery	<3 in	Routine replacement is not supported unless malfunction or signs and symptoms of systemic complications exist.	For short-term use; commonly used to monitor hemodynamic status and to determine blood-gas levels of critically ill patients; risk of bloodstream infection may approach that of CVCs.
Midline catheter	Distal tip lies in proximal basilica or cephalic veins; does not enter central veins	3-8 in	Same as for arterial catheters.	Phlebitis occurs less often with midline catheters than with standard IV catheters; associated with lower rates of infection compared with CVCs.
Central Catheters (See **Web Fig. 106-1** for images)				
Nontunneled or short-term central venous catheter **(Web Fig. 106-1A and C)**	Subclavian, internal jugular, or femoral vein	≥8 cm*	Routine replacement is not supported unless malfunction or signs and symptoms of systemic complications are exhibited.	Accounts for the majority of all catheter-related bloodstream infections; placement in upper torso is preferred. Replacement of catheter over a guidewire is *only* acceptable in cases of catheter malfunction.
Peripherally inserted central venous catheter (PICC) **(Web Fig. 106-1B)**	Basilic, cephalic, or brachial vein into the SVC; provides an alternative to subclavian or jugular vein catheterization	≥20 cm*	Same as nontunneled venous catheters	Similar risk of infection as CVCs in patients hospitalized in intensive care units
Tunneled venous catheter (Broviac, Hickman) **(Web Fig. 106-1D)**	Subclavian, internal jugular, or femoral vein	≥8 cm*	Is the same as nontunneled venous catheters.	Lower rates of infection with tunneled venous catheters than with nontunneled catheters; cuff inhibits the migration of bacteria into the catheter tract or *tunnel*.
Implanted venous catheter (Mediport) **(Web Fig. 106-1E)**	Tunneled beneath skin into internal jugular or subclavian vein; accessed with needle placement into a subcutaneous port; needle may remain in place for up to 6 months, barring infection	≥8 cm*	Is the same as nontunneled venous catheters.	Carries lowest risk for CRBSI; no local care is required for maintenance; is a cosmetically appealing option for patients; requires surgery for removal.
Pulmonary artery catheter **(Web Fig. 106-1F)**	Enters central circulation through a Teflon-coated introducer placed in subclavian, internal jugular, or femoral vein	≥30 cm*	No recommendations for replacement of catheters that are required for >7 days.	Typically heparin bonded; carries same risk for CRBSI as central venous catheters; subclavian vein is insertion site of choice to reduce risk of CRBSI. Typically remains in place for an average duration of 3 days.

*Length depends on patient size.
 CRBSI, catheter-related bloodstream infection; IV, intravenous; SVC, superior vena cava; CVC, central venous catheter.
 Adapted from Mermel LA, Allon M, Bouza E, et al: Clinical practice guidelines for the diagnosis and management of intravascular catheter–related infections. 2009 update by the Infectious Diseases Society of America. Clin Infect Dis 49(1):1-45, 2009.

Table 106-4 **Factors Associated with Greater Risk of Intravenous Catheter–Related Infection**
Failure of staff to wash hands
Duration of catheterization >72 hr for peripheral intravenous catheters
Lower extremities and groin are at greater risk than upper extremities
Cutdown presents a greater risk than percutaneous insertion
Emergency insertion results in a greater risk than elective insertion
Breakdown in skin integrity (e.g., burns)
Insertion by physician is a greater risk than insertion by intravenous therapy teams

Surgical Site Infections

Surgical site infections (SSIs) occur in up to 5% of the inpatient surgical population in the United States. These infections increase length of hospital stay, are costly, and are associated with increased mortality. Infection at the surgical site usually occurs within the first 30 days postoperatively; however, in patients undergoing surgical placement of indwelling devices, surveillance for SSI continues up to 1 year postoperatively. The pathogenesis of these infections involves inoculation of skin bacteria at the time of the surgical incision. These infections can be classified as superficial, involving the skin and subcutaneous tissue; deep incisional, involving the fascia and muscles; or deep organ space. Prevention measures, such as minimizing preoperative length of stay, using nonirritative hair removal techniques, performing tight blood glucose control perioperatively, and using appropriate preoperative skin cleansing, are of great importance. If possible, preexisting infections must be treated before surgery to decrease the risk of bacterial seeding of the surgical site. Antibiotic therapy directed at staphylococci and streptococci, administered no later than 2 hours before the time of incision, markedly reduces but does not eliminate the risk of infection for select surgical procedures. Treatment of SSI should be directed by culture and may require débridement for cure.

Prospectus for the Future

Antimicrobial-resistant bacteria (methicillin-resistant *Staphylococcus aureus* [MRSA], vancomycin-resistant enterococci, extended-spectrum β-lactamase [ESBL]–producing gram-negative bacilli), produced by injudicious use of broad-spectrum antimicrobial agents, will continue to offer greater challenges in the treatment of nosocomially acquired infections. With continued medical advances, such as organ and bone marrow transplantations, the emergence of additional opportunistic nosocomial pathogens will undoubtedly occur. In addition, monitoring and controlling infections in chronic care facilities will be increasingly important because of the emergence and transmission of antibiotic-resistant bacteria in this patient population and the risk of introducing these strains into the hospital environment. As medical professionals, we must share with infection-control practitioners the burden of recognizing individuals who are at risk for developing HAIs and instituting appropriate measures to prevent these infections.

References

American Thoracic Society, Infectious Disease Society of America: Guidelines for the management of adults with hospital-acquired, ventilator-associated, and healthcare-associated pneumonia. Am J Respir Crit Care Med 162:505-511, 2005.

Anderson DJ, Kaye KS, Classen D, et al: Strategies to prevent surgical site infections in acute care hospitals. Infect Control Hosp Epidemiol 29:S51-S61, 2008.

Bartlett JG: Narrative review: The new epidemic of *Clostridium difficile*–associated enteric disease. Ann Intern Med 145:758-764, 2006.

Lo E, Nicolle L, Classen D, et al: Strategies to prevent catheter-associated urinary tract infections in acute care hospitals. Infect Control Hosp Epidemiol 29:S41-S50, 2008.

Marschall J, Mermel LA, Classen D, et al: Strategies to prevent central line–associated bloodstream infections in acute care hospitals. Infect Control Hosp Epidemiol 29:S22-S30, 2008.

Mermel LA, Allon M, Bouza E, et al: Clinical practice guidelines for the diagnosis and management of intravascular catheter-related infection. 2009 update by the Infectious Diseases Society of America. Clin Infect Dis 49(1):1-45, 2009.

Smith PW, Bennett G, Bradley S, et al: SHEA/APIC guideline: Infection prevention and control in the long-term care facility, July 2008. Infect Control Hosp Epidemiol 29:785-814, 2008.

Sexually Transmitted Infections

Corrilynn O. Hileman, Keith B. Armitage, and Robert A. Salata

Sexually transmitted infections (STIs) comprise a diverse group of infections caused by multiple microbial pathogens. These infections have common epidemiologic and clinical features. Since the mid 1980s, the field of STIs has evolved from one emphasizing the traditional venereal diseases of gonorrhea and syphilis to one concerned also with infections associated with *Chlamydia trachomatis*, herpes simplex virus (HSV), human papillomavirus (HPV), and human immunodeficiency virus (HIV).

Changes in sexual attitudes and practices have contributed to a resurgence of some, but not all, venereal infections. For example, after a decline in primary and secondary syphilis in the 1990s, between 2000 and 2006 the incidence of syphilis increased. Concurrently, rates of syphilis infection in men who have sex with men (MSM) also increased, suggesting that this at-risk group may in part be reason for the trend. Indeed, 64% of primary and secondary syphilis cases in 2006 occurred in MSM. Chlamydia, the most commonly reported STI in the United States, with over a million cases reported in 2006, has been increasing in prevalence as well. Rates in women are increasing more than men and most in women aged 15 to 19. This likely represents increased screening efforts; however, it may also reflect the trend toward earlier sexual debut.

At the outset, two common errors in approaching a patient with an STI should be avoided. The first error is failing to consider that an individual is at risk for an STI. All sexually active persons are at risk, not only because of their own sexual behavior, but because of their sexual partner's behavior as well. Failure to consider risk factors often results in mistakes in diagnosis, inappropriate treatment, poor follow-up of infected sexual contacts, and, ultimately, recurrent or persistent infection. A second error with STIs is failing to recognize and diagnose co-infection. The most serious co-infection is with HIV. The worldwide epidemic of STIs fuels the global spread of HIV. STIs, most of which can be readily diagnosed and treated, may greatly enhance the transmission of HIV infection. HIV, in turn, may alter the natural history of other STIs.

This chapter divides STIs into broad groups according to whether major initial manifestations are (1) genital ulcers; (2) urethritis, cervicitis, and pelvic inflammatory disease (PID); (3) vaginitis; or (4) warts. All patients with an STI should be strongly encouraged to undergo screening for HIV infection and other concurrent STIs (see Chapter 108). Updated information on STIs can be found on the Centers for Disease Control and Prevention website at *www.cdc.gov/std*.

Genital Ulcer Disease

Six infectious agents cause most genital ulcers (Table 107-1). The appearance of the lesions, natural history, and laboratory findings allow a clear-cut distinction among the possible causes in most instances. The two most common and significant infections in the United States are HSV-2 infection and syphilis.

HERPES SIMPLEX VIRUS INFECTION

Genital herpes infection has reached epidemic proportions, causing a corresponding increase in public awareness and concern. Genital herpes differs from other STIs in its tendency for spontaneous recurrence. Its importance stems from the morbidity, both physical and psychological, of the recurrent genital lesions; the danger of transmission of a fulminant, often fatal, disease to newborns; and an association with transmission of HIV-1 infection.

Epidemiologic Factors

HSV has a worldwide distribution. Humans are the only known reservoir of infection, which is spread by direct contact with infected secretions. Of the two types of HSV,

Table 107-1 Differentiation of Diseases Causing Genital Sores

Disease	Primary Lesion	Adenopathy	Systemic Features	Diagnosis and Treatment
Herpes genitalis (at least 50 million people have herpes genitalis in the United States; most caused by HSV-2)				
Primary	Incubation 2-7 days; multiple painful vesicles on erythematous base; persists 7-14 days	Tender, soft; often bilateral	Fever	Tzanck smear positive; tissue culture isolation, HSV-2 antigen; fourfold rise in antibodies to HSV-2 Rx: acyclovir, valacyclovir, or famciclovir for 7-10 days
Recurrent	Grouped vesicles on erythematous base; painful; lasts 3-10 days	None	None	Tzanck smear positive; tissue culture positive; HSV-2 antigen; titers not helpful Rx: same as above, except shorter duration required
Primary syphilis (90,000 cases in United States per year; caused by Treponema pallidum)	Incubation 10-90 days (mean, 21) Chancre: painless papule that ulcerates with firm, raised border and smooth base; usually single; may be genital or almost anywhere; persists 3-6 wk, leaving thin, atrophic scar	1 wk after chancre appears; bilateral or unilateral; firm, discrete, movable, no overlying skin changes, painless, nonsuppurative; may persist for months	Later stages	Cannot be cultured; positive darkfield; VDRL test positive, 77%; FTA-abs positive, 86% (see Table 107-2) Rx: see Table 107-3
Chancroid (2000 cases in United States per year; caused by Haemophilus ducreyi)	Incubation 3-5 days; vesicle or papule to pustule to ulcer; soft, not indurated; very painful	1 wk after primary in 50%; painful, unilateral in two thirds; suppurative	None	Organism in Gram stain of pus; can be cultured on special media (75%); direct yields highest from lymph node Rx: azithromycin, 1 g PO once, ceftriaxone, 250 mg IM once, ciprofloxacin, 500 mg PO twice daily for 3 days, or erythromycin base, 500 mg PO 3 times daily for 7 days; sexual partners should be treated
Lymphogranuloma venereum (600-1000 cases per year in United States; caused by Chlamydia trachomatis serovars L1, L2, L3)	Incubation 5-21 days; self-limited, painless papule, vesicle, or ulcer; lasts 2-3 days; noted in only 10%-40%	5-21 days after primary; one third bilateral, tender, matted iliac or femoral groove sign; multiple abscesses; coalescent, caseating, suppurative; thick yellow pus; sinus tracts; fistulas; strictures; genital ulcerations	Fever, arthritis, pericarditis, proctitis, meningoencephalitis, keratoconjunctivitis, preauricular adenopathy, edema of eyelids, erythema nodosum	Test genital or lymph node specimens for C. trachomatis by culture, direct immunofluorescence, or nucleic acid detection; LGV CF positive 85%-90% (1-3 wk); must have high titer (>1:16), cross-reacts with other Chlamydia; also positive STS, rheumatoid factor, cryoglobulins Rx: surgical drainage may be required; doxycycline, 100 mg PO twice daily for 21 days
Granuloma inguinale, or donovanosis (rare in United States; caused by Klebsiella granulomatis)	Incubation 9-50 days; at least one painless papule that gradually ulcerates; ulcers are large (1-4 cm), irregular, nontender, with thickened, rolled margins and beefy red tissue at base; older portions of ulcer show depigmented scarring, white; advancing edge contains new papules	No true adenopathy; in one fifth, subcutaneous spread through lymphatics leads to indurated swelling or abscesses of groin (pseudobuboes)	Metastatic infection of bones, joints, liver	Scraping or deep curetting at actively extending border; Wright or Giemsa stain reveals short, plump, bipolar staining; dark-staining Donovan bodies in macrophage vacuoles Rx: doxycycline, 100 mg PO twice daily for at least 21 days and until all lesions healed; may recur
Condyloma acuminatum (genital warts; caused by human papillomavirus)	Characteristic large, soft, fleshy, cauliflower-like excrescences around vulva, glans, urethral orifice, anus, perineum	None	None per se; association with cervical dysplasia or neoplasia	Chief importance is distinction from syphilis and chancroid Rx: topical podophyllin ± cryosurgery, laser resection

CF, complement fixation; FTA-abs, fluorescent treponemal antibody absorption; HSV, herpes simplex virus; IM, intramuscular; LGV, lymphogranuloma venereum; PO, orally; Rx, prescription; STS, serologic test for syphilis; VDRL, Venereal Disease Research Laboratory.

HSV-2 is the more frequent cause of genital infection. The major risk of infection is in the 14- to 29-year-old cohort and varies with sexual activity. Seroprevalence rates for HSV-2 infection are 22% in the general population and are as high as 40% to 50% in some North American populations. Many patients with serologic evidence of infection remain asymptomatic, and most transmission is thought to occur during periods of asymptomatic shedding of the virus.

Pathogenesis

After exposure, HSV replicates within epithelial cells and lyses them, producing a thin-walled vesicle. Multinucleated cells are formed with characteristic intranuclear inclusions. Regional lymph nodes become enlarged and tender. HSV also migrates along sensory neurons to sensory ganglia, where it assumes a latent state. Exactly how viral reactivation occurs is uncertain. During reactivation, the virus appears to migrate back to skin along sensory nerves.

Clinical Presentation

Genital lesions that develop 2 to 7 days after contact with infected secretions are the manifestation of the clinical illness. In men, painful vesicles usually appear on the glans or penile shaft; in women, they occur on the vulva, perineum, buttocks, cervix, or vagina. A vaginal discharge is frequently present. Primary infection is usually accompanied by inguinal adenopathy, fever, and malaise. Sacroradiculomyelitis or aseptic meningitis can complicate primary infection. Perianal and anal HSV-2 infections are especially common in MSM; tenesmus and rectal discharge often are the main complaints.

The precipitating events associated with genital relapse of HSV infection are poorly understood. In individual cases, stress or menstruation may be implicated. Overall, genital recurrences develop in approximately 60% of patients infected with HSV. However, the frequency of asymptomatic cervical recurrence in women is not known. Many patients describe a characteristic prodrome of tingling or burning for 18 to 36 hours before the appearance of lesions. Recurrent HSV genital lesions are decreased in number, are usually stereotyped in location, are often restricted to the genital region, heal more quickly, and are associated with fewer systemic complaints. Recurrences are much higher and disease is more severe and prolonged in HIV co-infected patients; particularly those with advanced acquired immunodeficiency syndrome (AIDS).

Laboratory Diagnosis

Although clinical features of HSV infection are suggestive diagnostically, these features are insensitive and not specific. Also, knowing the infection is caused by HSV-1 or -2 is helpful prognostically, as HSV-1 infections are less likely to recur and viral shedding is less. Diagnosis should be confirmed by laboratory testing. Isolation of HSV in cell culture is the gold standard for diagnosis, but sensitivity is low. Additional testing that may be performed includes Tzanck smear (66% sensitive) (see Chapter 93), Papanicolaou smear, immunofluorescent assay for viral antigen, and serologic testing. Direct antigen detection by means of an enzyme immunoassay test shows greater sensitivity than culture for later-stage HSV lesions and is equivalent to culture for early-stage infection. This is generally the diagnostic test of choice.

Serologic studies for HSV are generally useful only in the diagnosis of primary infection. Polymerase chain reaction (PCR) assays are available for the detection of HSV but are not currently approved by the U.S. Food and Drug Administration (FDA) for use on genital specimens.

Treatment

Antiviral therapy for herpes genitalis has been shown to be beneficial and is the mainstay of management. Oral acyclovir, valacyclovir, and famciclovir have all been shown to be effective in treatment of symptomatic HSV infection. Treatment of both primary and recurrent episodes can partially control signs and symptoms of the infection if initiated early in the course. After primary infection, treatment can follow one of two strategies (i.e., episodic or chronic daily suppressive treatment). Chronic daily suppressive therapy has been shown to decrease the number of recurrences by 70% to 80% in those with six or more episodes per year. This strategy has also been shown to decrease transmission of HSV from those infected, although viral shedding may still occur. Despite the benefits of chronic daily therapy, acquired resistance to acyclovir has been seen occasionally in HIV-infected persons and in other immunocompromised hosts (e.g., after bone marrow transplantation). HSV most commonly becomes acyclovir resistant through a mutation in the thymidine kinase gene. Acyclovir-resistant HSV infection is commonly characterized by chronic, progressive mucocutaneous ulcers.

In general, oral therapy is sufficient. It should be noted, however, that antiviral agents do not eradicate the latent stage of virus and do not affect the risk, frequency, or severity of recurrences once the medication is stopped. Hospitalization and administration of intravenous acyclovir are recommended for severe cases with fever, systemic symptoms, or extensive local or disseminated disease (e.g., pneumonia, meningitis, or hepatitis).

The greatest risk of neonatal HSV infection occurs in pregnant women who acquire herpes genitalis near term. This risk is as high as 30% to 50%. However, in those women with a history of recurrent HSV or if primary HSV infection occurs during the first half of pregnancy, the risk of neonatal acquisition is low (i.e., <1%). Regardless, if a woman has active cervical or vulvar lesions late in pregnancy, delivery by cesarean section should be considered. It should be noted, however, that even without active lesions, neonates exposed to asymptomatic shedding of HSV during parturition may also rarely acquire neonatal HSV. If HSV is acquired late in pregnancy or active lesions are present near term, some experts recommend administration of acyclovir. Consultation with an infectious diseases specialist also should be strongly considered.

SYPHILIS

Syphilis is of unique importance among the venereal diseases because early lesions heal without specific therapy; however, serious systemic sequelae of untreated syphilis pose a major risk to the patient, and transplacental infections can occur.

Epidemiologic Factors

Primary syphilis occurs mostly in sexually active 15- to 30-year-old individuals. The incidence of primary syphilis increased sharply in North America during the early 1990s but decreased in most risk groups in the early 2000s, with the exception of MSM. Approximately 50% of the sexual contacts of a patient with primary syphilis become infected. The long incubation period of syphilis becomes a key factor in designing strategies for contact tracing and management. Unless successful follow-up seems certain, contacts of proven cases must be treated with penicillin, the antibiotic of choice. HIV co-infection is increasing, which poses a serious problem because the mucosal lesions of primary syphilis facilitate transmission of HIV infection (see Chapter 108). Also, HIV appears to accelerate the course of syphilis, with more rapid and frequent involvement of the neurologic system.

Pathogenesis

Treponema pallidum penetrates intact mucous membranes or abraded skin, reaches the bloodstream by means of the lymphatics, and disseminates. The incubation period for the primary lesion depends on inoculum size, with a range of 3 to 90 days.

Natural History and Clinical Presentation

Primary syphilis is considered in Table 107-1. If the primary chancre is not treated, secondary syphilis may develop 6 to 8 weeks later. This time period can be accelerated in persons infected with HIV. With secondary syphilis, skin, mucous membranes, and lymph nodes are involved. A variety of skin manifestations may occur, including macular, papular, papulosquamous, pustular, follicular, or nodular lesions. Discrete, erythematous, macular lesions over the thorax or hyperpigmented macules on the palms and soles occur most commonly. In moist intertriginous areas, large, pale, flat-topped papules coalesce to form highly infectious plaques or condylomata lata; darkfield microscopy reveals that these lesions are teeming with spirochetes. Mucosal lesions are painless, dull, erythematous patches or grayish-white erosions. These lesions are infectious and darkfield positive as well.

Systemic manifestations of secondary syphilis include malaise, anorexia, weight loss, fever, sore throat, arthralgias, and generalized, nontender, discrete adenopathy. Specific organ involvement may develop and includes gastritis (superficial, erosive), hepatitis, renal involvement manifesting as nephritis or nephrotic syndrome (immune complex mediated), and symptomatic or asymptomatic meningitis. If secondary syphilis is not treated, one fourth of patients have relapses of the mucocutaneous syndrome within 2 years of onset. Thereafter, infected patients become asymptomatic and noninfectious except through blood transfusions or transplacental spread.

Latent syphilis, now relatively rare in the United States, develops after 1 to 10 years in 15% of untreated patients. Latent syphilis occurs when patients are asymptomatic but have a positive serologic test for syphilis. Early latent syphilis is when latent syphilis has been acquired within the last year. Late latent syphilis occurs after this. Tertiary infection may develop out of latent syphilis. Manifestations of tertiary infection include but are not limited to gummas and cardiac, ophthalmologic, and auditory abnormalities. Gummas are nonspecific, granulomatous lesions once common in late syphilis but rarely seen today. The skin gumma is a superfi-

cial nodule or deep granulomatous lesion that may develop punched-out ulcers. Superficial gummas respond dramatically to therapy. Gummas also may involve bone, liver, and the cardiovascular or central nervous system. Deep-seated gummas may have serious pathophysiologic consequences, and treatment often does not reverse organ dysfunction. Gradually progressive cardiovascular syphilis begins within 10 years in more than 10% of untreated patients and occurs most frequently in men. Patients develop aortitis with medial necrosis secondary to an obliterative endarteritis of the vasa vasorum. Central nervous system syphilis develops in 8% of untreated patients 5 to 35 years after primary infection and includes the following: meningovascular syphilis, tabes dorsalis, and general paresis (see Chapter 97). Late central nervous system syphilis may be asymptomatic despite cerebrospinal fluid (CSF) abnormalities indicating active inflammation.

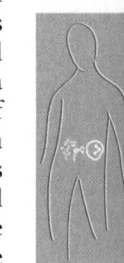

The natural history of syphilis may be altered by co-infection with HIV; such patients may develop signs and symptoms of secondary syphilis more rapidly, sometimes even before healing of the primary chancre (see Chapter 108).

Diagnosis

Serologic studies are the primary method for diagnosis of syphilis, but the diagnosis may also be made by darkfield examination or direct fluorescent antibody tests of clinical specimens. Spirochetes can be seen in darkfield preparations of chancres or moist lesions of secondary syphilis. Serologic diagnosis is considered in Table 107-2. The differential diagnosis of a primary chancre includes herpes simplex and three conditions that are relatively rare in the United States: chancroid, lymphogranuloma venereum (LGV), and granuloma inguinale. The characteristics of these diseases are presented in Table 107-1.

Treatment

The treatment of syphilis is considered in Table 107-3. In general, all stages and manifestations of syphilis can be treated with intramuscular benzathine penicillin; however, the presence of neurosyphilis requires modification of this standard therapy. For this reason, a lumbar puncture should be considered in all patients with latent syphilis or latent syphilis of unknown duration especially if HIV co-infected. An elevated CSF white blood cell count, elevated protein, and a positive result of a Venereal Disease Research Laboratory (VDRL) test on diluted samples of CSF establish the diagnosis of neurosyphilis. In absence of other CSF abnormalities, a patient with a persistently positive blood VDRL test result and a positive CSF VDRL test result should be considered to have neurosyphilis and treated accordingly. It should be noted, however, that the sensitivity of the CSF VDRL test in proven cases of neurosyphilis is only 40% to 50%. Therefore, in the absence of a positive CSF VDRL test result, treatment of neurosyphilis is still indicated in patients with a consistent neurologic syndrome, characteristic CSF changes, and a positive serum VDRL test result. Furthermore, because the VDRL test result may be negative in late syphilis, the presence of a positive serum fluorescent treponemal antibody absorption (FTA-abs) test in a patient with a neurologic syndrome consistent with syphilis is also a sufficient indication for treatment. Some experts recommend

Table 107-2 Serologic Studies in Syphilis

	VDRL	**FTA-abs**
Technique	Standard nontreponemal test; antibody to cardiolipin-lecithin	Standard treponemal test; antibody to Nichol strain of *Treponema pallidum* after absorption on nontreponemal spirochetes
Indications	Screening and assessing response to therapy; should be quantified by diluting serum	Confirmation of specificity of positive VDRL test; remains reactive longer than VDRL test; useful for late syphilis, particularly neurosyphilis
Percent Positive in Syphilis		
Primary	77%	86%
Secondary	98%	100%
Early latent	95%	99%
Late latent and late	73%	96%
False positives	Weakly reactive VDRL test is common (~30% of normals); if result of VDRL test is positive, test should be repeated; if positive result confirmed, FTA-abs performed; relative frequency of false positives determined by prevalence of syphilis in the population	Borderline positive is frequent (80%) in pregnancy; test should be repeated

FTA-abs, fluorescent treponemal antibody absorption; VDRL, Venereal Disease Research Laboratory.

Table 107-3 Treatment for Syphilis in the Nonimmunocompromised Patient

Clinical Category	Regimen of Choice	History of Penicillin Allergy
Primary Secondary Early latent Healthy contact*	Benzathine penicillin, 2.4 MU IM once	Penicillin desensitization or doxycycline, 100 mg PO twice daily, or tetracycline, 500 mg PO 4 times daily, both for 14 days; some experts recommend ceftriaxone or azithromycin
Late latent or latent syphilis of unknown duration	Benzathine penicillin, 2.4 MU IM per week for 3 wk	Penicillin desensitization, no regimen adequately evaluated; doxycycline, 100 mg PO twice daily, or tetracycline, 500 mg 4 times daily, both for 28 days
Neurosyphilis	Aqueous penicillin G, 20 MU IV daily for 10-14 days	Penicillin desensitization or ceftriaxone, 2g IV or IM daily for 10-14 days

*Contact of patient with active skin or mucous membrane lesions.
IM, intramuscularly; IV, intravenously; MU, million units; PO, orally.

performing an FTA-abs test on CSF to improve diagnostic accuracy in neurosyphilis. This test does, however, have a high false-positive rate in the CSF.

After initiation of treatment for syphilis, some patients may develop an acute febrile reaction called a *Jarisch-Herxheimer reaction*. This reaction is thought to represent a systemic response to penicillin-induced lysis of spirochetes, and manifestations include fever, myalgias, and headache within 24 hours of treatment. Antipyretics may be used. This reaction is especially important in neurosyphilis, as patients may display an acute worsening of original presenting symptoms and signs. Corticosteroid therapy may be administered for severe reactions.

Serologic studies for syphilis must be followed after treatment. With the recommended treatment schedules, 1% to 5% of patients with primary syphilis will develop relapse or be reinfected. In successfully treated primary syphilis, the VDRL test result should become negative by 2 years after therapy (usually by 6 to 12 months). The FTA-abs test result, however, often remains positive for life. In secondary syphilis, 75% of adequately treated patients will have a negative serum VDRL test result by 2 years. If the VDRL test result does not become negative or if a low fixed titer is not achieved, lumbar puncture should be performed to evaluate

the possibility of asymptomatic neurosyphilis, and the patient should be re-treated with penicillin. Of patients with central nervous system syphilis, 2% to 10% will experience relapse after treatment. However, asymptomatic patients rarely develop symptomatic disease after penicillin therapy. The only major exception is the patient infected with HIV, in whom meningovascular syphilis can develop within months of the standard treatment for primary syphilis. All patients who are treated for syphilis should become seronegative or *serofast* with a low fixed titer before cessation of follow-up. If this does not occur, therapy should be repeated.

Because of the documented progression to neurosyphilis in some individuals infected with HIV who have received treatment for primary syphilis, the following approach is suggested. All patients with syphilis should be tested for HIV infection. All individuals infected with HIV should be tested for syphilis. If dual infection is likely or documented, a lumbar puncture should be performed regardless of the stage or activity of the syphilis unless it is primary syphilis. Any CSF abnormality warrants a 10- to 14-day course of intravenous penicillin to treat neurosyphilis. If the CSF is unremarkable, treatment as described in Table 107-3 is appropriate. In any event, careful clinical and laboratory follow-up is essential.

Urethritis, Cervicitis, and Pelvic Inflammatory Disease

These syndromes can be considered broadly as gonococcal and nongonococcal in origin.

GONORRHEA

Neisseria gonorrhoeae is second only to *C. trachomatis* as the most common STI in the United States.

Epidemiologic Factors

It is estimated that 600,000 new infections with *N. gonorrhoeae* occur each year. Particular risk factors are urban location, low socioeconomic status, unmarried status, and large numbers of unprotected sexual contacts. Fifty percent of women having intercourse with a man with gonococcal urethritis will develop symptomatic infection. The risk for men is 20% after a single sexual contact with an infected woman. Orogenital contact and anal intercourse also transmit infection. Both men and women can have this infection and not have symptoms. In fact, asymptomatic infection of men is an important factor in transmission. Indeed, untreated patients may remain culture positive and capable of transmitting infection for periods of up to 6 months. Co-infection with *C. trachomatis* is observed in up to 30% to 40% of patients with gonorrhea. Higher rates of gonorrhea are being observed in MSM.

Pathogenesis

N. gonorrhoeae is a gram-negative, kidney bean–shaped diplococcus. Specialized projections from the organism, called *pili,* aid in attachment to mucosal surfaces, contribute to resistance to killing by neutrophils, and constitute an important virulence factor. In women, several factors alter susceptibility to infection. Group B blood type increases susceptibility, whereas vaginal colonization with normal flora, high immunoglobulin (Ig) A content of vaginal secretions, and high progesterone levels may be protective. Spread from the cervix to the upper genital tract is associated with menstruation as well as intrauterine contraceptive devices, and binding of gonococci to spermatozoa.

Clinical Presentation

Men with gonorrhea generally develop symptoms of urethritis including purulent discharge and severe dysuria. These symptoms develop 2 to 7 days after sexual contact with an infected partner. Prompt treatment usually follows, so more extensive genital involvement is uncommon.

In women, asymptomatic infection is common and is why screening of women is advocated so highly during routine gynecologic examination. For symptomatic infections, cervicitis is the most frequent manifestation and results in copious, yellow, vaginal discharge. Overall, 20% of women with gonococcal cervicitis develop PID, usually beginning at a time close to the onset of menstruation. PID manifests as endometritis (abnormal menses and midline abdominal pain), salpingitis (bilateral lower abdominal pain and tenderness), or pelvic peritonitis. Salpingitis can cause tubal occlusion and sterility. Gonococcal perihepatitis or Fitz-Hugh-Curtis syndrome may complicate PID. Women also may develop urethritis with dysuria and urinary frequency. In certain populations of sexually active women, 25% of those with urinary tract symptoms and 60% of those with symptoms but no bacteriuria have urethral cultures positive for *N. gonorrhoeae.*

Gonorrhea can infect sites other than the genitourinary tract. Anorectal gonorrhea occurs in both MSM and heterosexual women. In men, the resultant rectal pain, tenesmus, mucopurulent discharge, and bleeding may represent the only signs of infection. In women, however, asymptomatic anorectal involvement is a frequent complication of symptomatic genitourinary disease, occurring in up to 44%. This is possible even in the absence of anal intercourse. Isolated anorectal infection and acute or chronic proctitis are rare. Treatment failure is common and occurs in 7% to 35%. Pharyngeal gonorrhea may occur in MSM or heterosexual women after oral sex and is less frequent in heterosexual men. The pharynx is rarely the lone site of gonococcal infection, occurring in 5% to 8%. Because of the frequency of asymptomatic infection in each of the potential sites, patients with symptoms suggestive of gonococcal infection should have cultures from the urethra, cervix, anus, and, where applicable, pharynx.

Extragenital dissemination occurs in approximately 1% of men and 3% of women with gonorrhea. Strains of *N. gonorrhoeae* causing dissemination are generally more penicillin sensitive but resist the normal bactericidal activity of antibody and complement. This may result from binding of a naturally occurring blocking antibody by the gonococci. Complement deficiency states can predispose patients to disseminated gonorrhea. Dissemination of gonococcal infection may take several forms. First, it may manifest as an arthritis-dermatitis syndrome with 3 to 20 papular, petechial, pustular, necrotic, or hemorrhagic skin lesions, usually found on the extensor surfaces of the distal extremities. An associated finding is an asymmetrical polytenosynovitis, with or without arthritis, predominantly involving the wrists, fingers, knees, and ankles. Joint fluid cultures usually are negative in the arthritis-dermatitis syndrome, leading to speculation that circulating immune complexes, demonstrable in most patients, are important in its pathogenesis. However, synovial biopsies may yield positive cultures. Biopsy of skin lesions reveals gonococcal antigens by immunofluorescent antibody staining in two thirds of patients. Blood cultures are positive in 50% of patients. Septic arthritis is another manifestation of dissemination. Indeed, *N. gonorrhoeae* is the most frequent cause of septic arthritis in sexually active 16- to 50-year-old persons. The joint fluid cultures are positive in less than 50% of cases and generally not unless the leukocyte count in the joint fluid exceeds 80,000/μL. Blood cultures are positive in less than 25%. The diagnosis is most often confirmed by extra-articular cultures, usually at genital sites. Finally, gonococcemia may lead to endocarditis, meningitis, myopericarditis, or toxic hepatitis in rare cases.

Diagnosis

Gram stain and culture, nucleic acid hybridization tests, and nucleic acid amplification tests are available for the diagnosis of *N. gonorrhoeae* (and *C. trachomatis*). Culture and hybridization tests require a swab of the urethra or other potentially infected site. The amplification test can be performed on swabs or urine specimens. In men with symptomatic infection, Gram stain of the urethral discharge is sufficient to make the diagnosis of gonorrhea because typical intracellular diplococci are diagnostic (**Web Fig. 107-1**). Furthermore, the absence of gonococci on a smear of urethral discharge from a man virtually excludes the diagnosis. If, however, gram-negative diplococci are only seen extracellularly, this test is equivocal. In women, Gram staining of cervical exudates is insensitive (<60%) but relatively specific. Therefore further diagnostic modalities are necessary for women. Culture for *N. gonorrhoeae* is possible with a modified Thayer-Martin medium containing antibiotics that inhibit the growth of other organisms. This medium increases the yield of gonococci from samples likely to be contaminated. Thayer-Martin culture of normally sterile fluids, such as joint fluid, blood, and CSF, is not necessary; specimens from these sites should be cultured on chocolate agar. Other important considerations for isolating gonococci in culture include the following: (1) a synthetic swab must be used for specimen collection, as unsaturated fatty acids in cotton may be inhibitory; (2) a calcium alginate swab or a loop must be inserted 2 cm into the male urethra for adequate specimen sampling; (3) vaginal douching should be avoided for 12 hours and urination for 2 hours before specimen collection; and (4) vaginal speculum lubricants should not be used when cervical specimens are obtained. In all suggested cases of gonorrhea, the urethra, cervix, anus, and pharynx should be cultured. In women, 20% of cases in which initial cervical cultures were negative yield *N. gonorrhoeae* when cultures are repeated. Although hybridization and amplification tests are very attractive options for diagnosis of gonorrhea, the importance of culture should not be underestimated. Growing the organism in culture is currently the only means by which susceptibility testing can be performed, and with resistance to many antibiotic classes developing in *N. gonorrhoeae,* this becomes important.

Treatment

Gonococcal resistance to penicillin is increasing worldwide. The current recommendation for the treatment of uncomplicated gonorrhea is ceftriaxone, 125 mg given intramuscularly once, or cefixime, 400 mg orally once. Currently, the Centers for Disease Control and Prevention recommends this single class of antimicrobials for gonorrhea infection, given the high rate of resistance to other classes. Fluoroquinolones are no longer recommended for treatment of gonorrhea in the United States and in many other geographic areas. Treatment of gonorrhea should always be followed by a course of doxycycline, 100 mg orally twice daily for 7 days, or azithromycin, 1 g orally as a single dose, to treat possible concurrent chlamydial infection. In patients with severe β-lactam allergy, spectinomycin, 2 g intramuscularly once, can be used; however, this therapy is inadequate for pharyngeal infection. PID should be treated with cefoxitin, 2 g given intramuscularly once, with probenecid, 1 g orally once, followed by doxycycline, 100 mg orally twice daily for 14 days. Ceftriaxone, 250 mg intramuscularly once, may be substituted for cefoxitin plus probenecid. Metronidazole, 500 mg orally twice daily for 14 days, may be added as well. Seriously ill women with PID should be hospitalized.

Therapy with cefoxitin, 2 g intravenously every 8 hours, or cefotetan, 2 g intravenously every 12 hours, should be administered with doxycycline, 100 mg orally twice a day. Evaluation by ultrasonography for the presence of a pelvic abscess or peritonitis is warranted in this setting. Surgery or percutaneous drainage may be indicated if a tubo-ovarian or pelvic abscess is found.

Disseminated gonococcal infection should be treated with ceftriaxone, 1 g every 24 hours, until clinical symptoms and signs improve, generally in 24 to 48 hours. The treatment course can then be complete with cefixime, 400 mg twice a day orally to complete at least a week of therapy. In patients with severe β-lactam allergy, spectinomycin, 2 g intramuscularly twice a day for 7 to 10 days, is recommended.

Other considerations regarding the management and treatment of a patient with gonorrhea follow. A VDRL test should be performed in all patients with gonorrhea. If the result is negative, no further follow-up is necessary because ceftriaxone in the dosage used is probably effective in treating incubating syphilis. If alternative drugs are used, the VDRL test should be repeated after 4 weeks. Next, anal cultures for *N. gonorrhoeae* should be part of the routine follow-up of women because persistent anorectal carriage may be a source of relapse. Finally, postgonococcal urethritis occurs in 30% to 50% of men 2 to 3 weeks after treatment if doxycycline is not prescribed concomitantly. It usually is caused by *C. trachomatis* or *Ureaplasma urealyticum.*

NONGONOCOCCAL URETHRITIS, CERVICITIS, AND PELVIC INFLAMMATORY DISEASE

The diagnosis of nongonococcal urethritis (NGU) requires the exclusion of gonorrhea because considerable overlap exists in the clinical syndromes. In addition, infections frequently occur concurrently.

Epidemiologic Factors

Chlamydia is the most commonly reported infectious disease in the United States, and *C. trachomatis* is implicated in NGU 15% to 50% of the time. Other causative agents in NGU include: *U. urealyticum, Mycoplasma genitalium, Trichomonas vaginalis,* HSV, and adenovirus. Typically, NGU predominates in higher socioeconomic groups. NGU is less contagious than gonococcal infection, and the incubation period is 7 to 14 days.

Clinical Presentation

Men and women with chlamydial infections may be asymptomatic. However, in symptomatic infection, men generally report urethral discharge, itching, and dysuria, which are characteristic complaints indicating urethritis. It is important to note that the discharge is not spontaneous but becomes apparent after milking the urethra in the morning. The mucopurulent discharge consists of thin, cloudy fluid with purulent specks. These characteristics do not always allow clear distinction from gonococcal disease. *C. trachomatis* also is a common cause of epididymitis and prostatitis in men younger than 35 years of age and proctitis in men (or women) who practice receptive anal intercourse.

Symptomatic women most commonly report vaginal discharge. Two thirds of women with mucopurulent cervicitis have chlamydial infection. Similarly, many women with the acute onset of dysuria, urinary frequency, and pyuria, but sterile urine, have *C. trachomatis* infection. Untreated chlamydial infection in women may lead to PID, ectopic pregnancy, and infertility.

Diagnosis

Culture, direct immunofluorescence, enzyme immunoassay, and nucleic acid hybridization and amplification tests are available for identification of *C. trachomatis*. For diagnosis of cervicitis, nucleic acid amplification is the preferred method, as it is the most sensitive and specific test for *Chlamydia*. In addition, this test may be performed on cervical swabs or urine specimens, making it a convenient option in clinics. The exclusion of gonorrhea relies mainly on Gram-stained preparations of exudates and ultimately culture. However, a nucleic acid amplification test may be performed for this purpose as well. Screening for chlamydia at routine gynecologic examinations is now recommended for all women 25 years of age or younger.

Treatment

The patient and all sexual contacts should be treated with azithromycin, 1 g orally as a single dose, or doxycycline, 100 mg orally twice daily for 7 days. Recurrence may occur and requires longer duration of treatment (i.e., 2 to 3 weeks). In pregnancy, erythromycin base, 500 mg orally four times daily for 7 days, is an alternative regimen. Patients who fail to respond to doxycycline may be infected with *U. urealyticum*, given that 30% of strains are doxycycline resistant. Furthermore, patients who fail to respond to doxycycline

and azithromycin may have a syndrome of NGU caused by *T. vaginalis*, and consideration should be given to therapy with metronidazole.

Vaginitis

Table 107-4 considers salient features in the diagnosis and management of patients with vaginitis. The vaginal milieu is normally maintained by an intricate balance of microorganisms. This balance may be upset by a number of factors including administration of antibiotics, vaginal douching, or a new sexual partner. Disruption of the usual vaginal flora may lead to vaginitis. In this setting vulvovaginal candidiasis and bacterial vaginosis are two common conditions that contribute to the development of vaginitis. A third cause of vaginitis is trichomoniasis, which is sexually transmitted. Characteristic signs and symptoms of any vaginitis are vulvar irritation, pruritus, odor, and vaginal discharge. Diagnosis can now be made with rapid tests; however, the standard method for diagnosis remains evaluation of the vaginal pH, the whiff test, and microscopic examination of discharge collected during speculum examination. Treatment of vaginitis depends on the causative infection and may involve intravaginal application or oral administration of antimicrobials. See Table 107-4 for specific diagnostic and treatment modalities for the vulvovaginal candidiasis, bacterial vaginosis, and trichomoniasis. Of note, any woman with recurrent or refractory candidiasis should be tested for diabetes mellitus and HIV infection, as these conditions promote this infection.

Table 107-4 **Vaginitis**				
Disease	**Epidemiology and Pathogenesis**	**Clinical Findings**	**Diagnosis**	**Treatment**
Candidiasis (generally, *Candida albicans*)	Yeast is part of normal flora; overgrowth favored by broad-spectrum antibiotics, high estrogen levels (pregnancy, before menses, oral contraceptives), diabetes mellitus; may be early clue to HIV infection	Itching, occasional dysuria; little or no urethral discharge; labia pale or erythematous with satellite lesions; vaginal discharge thick, adherent, with white curds; balanitis in 10% of male contacts	Vaginal pH = 4.5 (normal); negative whiff test; yeast seen on wet mount in 50%; culture positive; rapid tests available	Miconazole, butoconazole, terconazole, clotrimazole, nystatin or tioconazole cream or suppository for 3-7 days; fluconazole, 150 mg PO once
Trichomonas vaginalis infection	STI; incubation 5-28 days; symptoms begin or exacerbate with menses	Soreness, irritation, mild dysuria, dyspareunia; copious loose discharge, one fifth yellow-green, one third bubbly	Elevated pH; wet mount shows large numbers of WBCs, trichomonads; positive whiff test (10% KOH causes fishy odor); rapid tests available	Metronidazole, 2 g PO once; tinidazole, 2 g PO once; treat sexual contacts
Bacterial vaginosis	Replacement of *Lactobacillus* species with *Gardnerella vaginalis*, *Mycoplasma hominis*, and anaerobes (*Mobiluncus* and *Prevotella* species); associated with multiple or new partners, douching	Vaginal odor, little inflammation; mild discharge, grayish, thin, homogeneous with small bubbles	Elevated pH; positive whiff test; wet prep contains clue cells (vaginal epithelial cells with intracellular coccobacilli), few WBCs; rapid tests available	Metronidazole, 500 mg PO twice daily for 7 days; metronidazole gel (0.75%), 5 g intravaginally once daily for 5 days, or clindamycin cream (2%), 5 g intravaginally daily at night for 7 days; do not treat contacts unless recurrent vaginitis

HIV, human immunodeficiency virus; KOH, potassium hydroxide; PO, orally; STI, sexually transmitted Trafection; WBCs, white blood cells.

Genital Warts and Other Human Papilloma Virus–Associated Diseases

HPV is the most important cause of genital warts as well as cervical dysplasia and cancer in women and anorectal dysplasia and cancer in MSM. Of importance, there is now a quadrivalent vaccine that protects against infection with HPV types 6, 11, 16, and 18, types most commonly implicated in genital warts and cervical cancer. Currently the three-vaccine series is recommended for 11- and 12-year-old girls, with catch-up vaccination offered to female patients aged 13 to 26 years.

EPIDEMIOLOGIC FACTORS

More than 100 types of HPV have been identified, and more than 30 can cause genital infection. Important types include HPV types 6 and 11, which cause the majority of genital warts, and HPV types 16, 18, 31, 33, and 35, which can lead to cervical, vaginal, or anal cancer. Patients infected with HPV can have more than one type of the HPV virus present simultaneously.

CLINICAL PRESENTATION

Genital warts are flat, papular, or pedunculated and are asymptomatic, in general. However, depending on size and location, warts can be painful, pruritic, and friable. The natural history of genital warts is benign, but recurrence is common. Immunocompromised patients such as those with HIV may have warts that are larger in size and number.

DIAGNOSIS

HPV infection may be diagnosed by detection of HPV DNA, RNA, or capsid proteins in cells. Identification of HPV infection is recommended as part of cervical cancer screening and is used in triage of women with atypical squamous cells of undetermined significance (ASC-US). Outside of cervical cancer screening, however, routine testing for HPV infection is not recommended. The diagnosis of genital warts is made by visual inspection and may be confirmed by biopsy. Biopsy should be performed in any case where the diagnosis is in question, if the warts do not respond or worsen during therapy, if the patient is immunocompromised, or if the warts have any red flag signs such as pigmentation, induration, friability, or ulceration. Specialized testing for HPV infection is generally unnecessary.

TREATMENT

Treatment for HPV is not indicated unless a patient has a cervical squamous intraepithelial lesion (SIL) or warts, as subclinical HPV infection frequently resolves spontaneously. Furthermore, untreated genital warts may also spontaneously resolve. Therefore the decision to initiate treatment for genital warts needs to be individualized. Consideration of the following should enter into the decision regarding whether to treat and what modality should be used: number, size, morphology, and location of the warts, patient preference, cost of therapy, convenience, adverse effects, and provider experience. If treatment is initiated, the goal is to remove visible warts. Removal of warts may induce a wart-free period but does not guarantee that the HPV virus has been eradicated or that HPV cannot continue to be transmitted. Response to therapy will depend on the immune status of the patient as well as adherence.

For external warts, treatment may be patient or provider applied. Patient-applied modalities include podofilox 0.5% solution or gel or imiquimod 5% cream. Podofilox is an antimitotic agent that destroys warts. Imiquimod stimulates an immune reaction to increase the production of interferon and cytokines, which in turn leads to destruction of the warts. These agents are applied once or twice daily for a defined period, and then several days of no therapy is allowed. This cycle may be repeated for several weeks. Mild to moderate irritation and inflammation occur with the application of these medications. Provider-applied modalities include cryotherapy, podophyllin resin 10% to 25%, trichloroacetic acid (TCA) or bichloroacetic acid (BCA) 80% to 90%. Cryotherapy with liquid nitrogen destroys warts by thermal-induced cytolysis. Pain and blistering are common after treatments. Podophyllin resin contains several compounds including antimitotic agents. Local irritation may occur if the agent spreads to areas surrounding the warts. TCA and BCA are caustic and destroy warts by chemical coagulation of proteins. Damage to adjacent areas of tissue may be encountered if the product is allowed to spread. A final treatment for eternal warts is surgical removal. Warts may be removed by scissor or shave excision, curettage, electrosurgery, or laser surgery. Surgery offers the advantage of treatment of warts in one visit and is most beneficial for those with a large number of genital warts or warts that cover a large area.

The presence of genital warts is not an indication to increase the frequency of cervical cancer screening or to perform cervical colposcopy. However, for cervical warts, underlying cervical dysplasia needs to be ruled out. Management should occur in conjunction with a specialist.

For vaginal or anal warts, cryotherapy or TCA or BCA is the recommended treatment modality. Surgery is also an option. For those with anal warts, a digital rectal examination and anoscopy should be performed to rule out the presence of warts on the rectal mucosa. Management of warts on the rectal mucosa should occur in conjunction with a specialist. Lastly, warts in the urethral meatus may be treated with cryotherapy or podophyllin. Surgical management may be required.

Proctocolitis in Men Who Have Sex with Men

Men who practice receptive anal intercourse may have proctitis or proctocolitis, causing anorectal pain, mucoid or bloody discharge, tenesmus, diarrhea, or abdominal pain. Sigmoidoscopy should be performed, with culture and Gram stain of the discharge. The potential causative organisms are diverse (**Web Table 107-1**), and 10% of patients harbor two or more pathogens. That being said, proctitis may occur without a definable pathogen in up to 42% of cases. LGV has been recognized as an important causative agent in this population. If not treated early, LGV may lead to chronic colorectal fistulas and strictures. Diarrheal syndromes are considered in Chapter 103, and diarrhea in the HIV-infected patient has an entirely different set of implications (see Chapter 108).

Prospectus for the Future

Effective treatment of sexually transmitted infections (STIs) will be increasingly important in worldwide efforts to counter the human immunodeficiency virus (HIV) epidemic. However, more extensive treatment of STIs may lead to increasing resistance of gonococci and other genital pathogens to currently available antimicrobial agents. Molecular-based diagnostic testing continues to be developed and will aid in rapid identification of pathogens. Treatment guidelines will necessarily evolve in response to the changing patterns of antimicrobial resistance.

References

Centers for Disease Control and Prevention (CDC): Trends in reportable sexually transmitted diseases in the United States, 2006. Available at: www.cdc.gov/std/stats/trends2006.htm.

Corey L, Handsfield HH: Genital herpes and public health. JAMA 283:791-794, 2000.

Naresh A, Beigi R, Woc-Colburn L, Salata RA: The bidirectional interactions of HIV-1 and sexually transmitted infections: A review. Infect Dis Clin Pract, in press.

Rein MF: Introduction to sexually transmitted diseases and common syndromes. In Goldman L, Ausiello D (eds): Cecil Textbook of Medicine, 22nd ed. Philadelphia, WB Saunders, 2004, pp 1914-1916.

Update to CDC'S Sexually Transmitted Diseases Treatment Guidelines, 2006: Fluoroquinolones no longer recommended for treatment of gonococcal infections. MMWR Morb Mortal Wkly Rep 56:332-336, 2007.

Workowski KA, Berman SM: Sexually transmitted diseases treatment guidelines, 2006. MMWR Recomm Rep 55:1-94, 2006.

Workowski KA, Levine WC: Sexually transmitted diseases treatment guidelines, 2002. MMWR Recomm Rep 51:1-80, 2002.

Human Immunodeficiency Virus Infection and Acquired Immunodeficiency Syndrome

Curt G. Beckwith, Edward J. Wing, Benigno Rodríguez, and Michael M. Lederman

Almost three decades after the acquired immunodeficiency syndrome (AIDS) was recognized as a new disease entity in 1981, more than 65 million individuals worldwide have been infected with the human immunodeficiency virus (HIV), the causative agent. The World Health Organization (WHO) estimates that by the end of 2007 there were 33 million persons living with HIV or AIDS in the world, and 2.7 million acquired HIV in the previous year alone. Of these, more than 90% live in the developing world, and the vast majority acquired the infection through heterosexual intercourse.

HIV type 1 (HIV-1) is responsible for the majority of infections worldwide. A second type of HIV (HIV-2) was identified in West Africa in the mid 1980s. HIV-2 infection also results in AIDS, but HIV-2 infection has a considerably longer clinically latent period than HIV-1. Although HIV-2 shares many biologic and genetic characteristics with HIV-1, each of the two viruses has regulatory and structural genes that are unique. Whereas HIV-1 is closely related to the simian immunodeficiency virus (SIV) isolated from a subspecies of chimpanzee (SIV_{cpz}), HIV-2 is more closely related to an SIV that is commonly found in the sooty mangabey (SIV_{sm}). The rare HIV-2 infections in the United States, Europe, and Asia to date have been of West African origin. Throughout the remainder of this chapter, the abbreviation *HIV* refers to HIV-1.

Epidemiology

Available data suggest that humans first became infected with HIV in the 1930s or 1940s, in the process of slaughtering chimpanzees for human consumption in the African bushmeat market. In retrospect, HIV infection had spread extensively in Central Africa by the early 1970s; the significant wasting of advanced HIV disease was then reflected by the descriptive eponym *slim disease,* which was applied to the unexplained illness that was occurring in large numbers of young adults in Uganda at that time.

AIDS was first recognized as a clinical entity in previously healthy men who had sex with men (MSM) who had serious infections caused by unusual opportunistic pathogens, most frequently *Pneumocystis jirovecii* pneumonia (PCP), an illness previously found only among patients with severe cellular immunodeficiency. Studies confirmed profound immunodeficiency in these individuals, leading to the name *acquired immunodeficiency syndrome,* or AIDS.

When similar opportunistic infections (OIs) were subsequently observed in injection drug users and in men with hemophilia and their female sexual partners, it became clear that this syndrome was caused by an agent transmitted either through sexual contact or through infusion of blood or blood products. HIV was identified in 1983 and confirmed in 1984 as the causative agent of AIDS.

Table 108-1 Opportunistic Infections Indicative of a Defect in Cellular Immune Function Associated with AIDS

Protozoan Infection

Toxoplasma gondii encephalitis
Cryptosporidium parvum enteritis (>1 mo)
Isospora belli enteritis (>1 mo)

Fungal Infection

Candida esophagitis
Cryptococcus neoformans meningitis
Disseminated histoplasmosis
Disseminated coccidioidomycosis
Pneumocystis jirovecii pneumonia (PCP)

Bacterial Infection

Disseminated *Mycobacterium avium-intracellulare*
Active *Mycobacterium tuberculosis* infection
Recurrent *Salmonella* septicemia
Recurrent bacterial pneumonia

Viral Infection

Chronic (>1 mo) mucocutaneous or esophageal herpes
  simplex virus infection
Cytomegalovirus retinitis, esophagitis, or colitis
Progressive multifocal leukoencephalopathy (JC virus)

Table 108-2 Other Conditions Fulfilling Clinical Criteria for AIDS

Neoplasms

Kaposi sarcoma
High-grade, B-cell non-Hodgkin lymphoma
Immunoblastic sarcoma
Primary brain lymphoma
Invasive carcinoma of the cervix

Systemic Illness

Human immunodeficiency virus (HIV) wasting syndrome
  (unintentional, unexplained loss of >10% of body weight)

Although the average lag period between initial infection by HIV and the clinical manifestations of severe immunodeficiency (AIDS) suggests that the introduction of the virus into North America may have occurred in the early 1970s, preserved specimens suggest that cases may have occurred in this part of the world as early as the 1960s.

The Centers for Disease Control and Prevention (CDC) surveillance criteria for the diagnosis of AIDS, as modified in 1987, included a large number of OIs (Table 108-1) indicative of defects in cellular and/or humoral immunity, as well as certain neoplasms and other conditions associated with severe immunodeficiency (Table 108-2). The occurrence of any one of these conditions in an HIV-infected individual with no other cause of immunosuppression constituted the diagnosis of AIDS. In 1992 the CDC broadened the surveillance definition of AIDS to include all HIV-infected persons with severely depressed levels of cell-mediated immunity as indicated by $CD4^+$ T-lymphocyte counts (CD4 counts) less than 200 cells/mm^3.

By 1993, AIDS had become the leading cause of death of American adults ages 25 to 44, a trend dramatically reversed by the introduction of highly active antiretroviral therapy (HAART) at the end of 1995 (Fig. 108-1). By the end of 2006, approximately 1.1 million persons in the United States were living with HIV and AIDS, and an estimated 56,300 persons became infected that year.

Retrospective analysis of stored serum has revealed that HIV infection had been present in parts of Central Africa for decades before recognition of the clinical syndrome of AIDS. Since the early 1980s, HIV infection has become a major worldwide pandemic. HIV infection continues to spread, albeit at strikingly different rates, throughout all continents. Since the late 1990s, exceptionally rapid transmission has occurred throughout India, Southeast Asia, Southern Africa, the former Soviet Union, and some parts of Eastern Europe.

Because of latency between HIV infection and the development of AIDS-associated illnesses, the clinically recognized epidemic of AIDS has lagged 6 to 8 years behind the spread of the virus into new populations. Although initially observed most frequently among homosexual men and intravenous drug users in the United States, heterosexual intercourse has been the dominant mode of HIV transmission throughout most of the world. The virus is present in semen and cervicovaginal secretions of infected individuals and can be transmitted by either partner during vaginal or anal intercourse. The concurrent presence of other sexually transmitted diseases (STDs), especially those associated with genital ulcerations, strongly facilitates sexual transmission of HIV-1 (see Chapter 107). In the United States, HIV infection has increased rapidly in women in the last decade; in several rural areas in the Southeast, women accounted for over one half of new cases in 2005. Over the past several years, there has also been a resurgence of HIV infection among young MSM.

A disproportionate number of North American men and women infected by HIV are African American or Hispanic. Transmission by injection drug use (IDU) has been a major factor in this imbalance, given that IDU transmission has occurred most commonly in impoverished inner-city areas, where intravenous drug abuse is most prevalent. Differences in regional patterns of IDU have been a major factor in the greater than 100-fold regional variation in prevalence of AIDS cases in the United States. Since 2003, IDU transmission has significantly declined in the United States, whereas heterosexual transmission has continued to increase (Fig. 108-2).

Vertical transmission of HIV from infected mother to child may occur in utero, during labor, or through breastfeeding. In the absence of antiretroviral treatment, HIV infects 25% to 30% of infants born to HIV-infected mothers. The rate of vertical transmission can be reduced to less than 2% by prenatal and perinatal treatment of the mother and postnatal treatment of the infant with effective antiretroviral drugs.

HIV is almost always detectable in the blood of infected persons in the absence of effective antiretroviral therapy (ART). Before the nationwide implementation of a blood screening test in late 1985, infection by means of transfused blood or blood products accounted for nearly 3% of AIDS cases in the United States. Since 1985, all blood products in North America have been screened for HIV antigens and antibodies to HIV. The risk of transfusion-acquired HIV infection in North America and Western Europe is now exceedingly small, but not absent.

HIV infection may occur after accidental parenteral exposures among health care workers. After injury by an

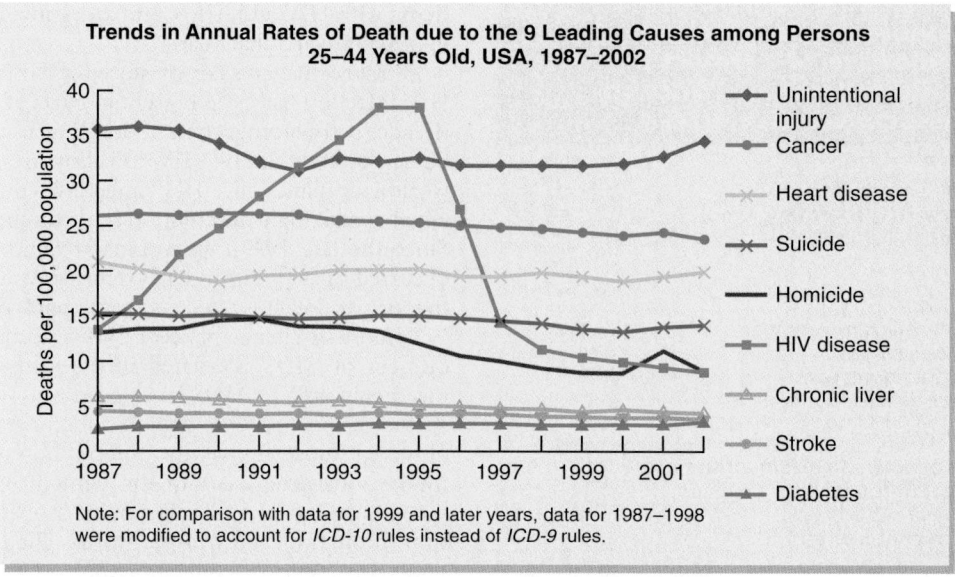

Figure 108-1 Trends in annual death rates in persons ages 25 to 44, United States, 1987-2004. In 1993, AIDS became the leading cause of death of Americans in this age group. Since the widespread adoption of effective combination antiretroviral therapy in 1996, AIDS-related death rates have fallen sharply. By 1998, AIDS ranked fifth among the causes of death in this age group. (Data courtesy of Centers for Disease Control and Prevention.)

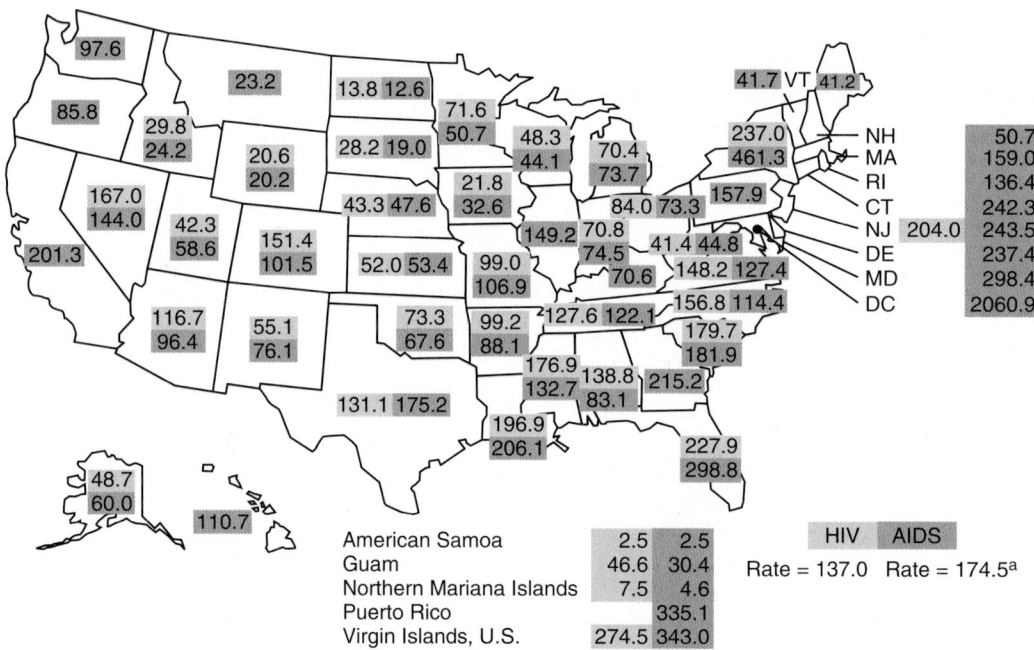

Figure 108-2 Estimated rates (per 100,000 population) for adults and adolescents living with HIV infection (not AIDS; 37 states and territories require confidential name-based HIV infection reporting) or with AIDS, United States and dependent areas (revised June 2007). AIDS rates show tremendous regional variation, from 2060 in the District of Columbia to 12 in Montana. (From Centers for Disease Control and Prevention: HIV/AIDS Surveillance Report, 2005. Vol 17, Rev ed. 2007.)

HIV-contaminated hollow needle, the risk of infection is approximately 0.3%. Observational data suggest that this risk can be reduced at least 10-fold by prompt postexposure prophylaxis.

Pathophysiology

HIV is a member of the lentivirus family of retroviruses, which includes the agents of visna, equine infectious anemia virus, and the SIVs. The core of HIV contains two single-stranded copies of the viral RNA genome, together with the virus-encoded enzymes reverse transcriptase, protease, and integrase (Fig. 108-3). Surrounding the structural (p24 and p18) proteins is a lipid bilayer derived from the host cell, through which protrude the transmembrane (gp41) and surface (gp120) envelope glycoproteins.

The HIV envelope glycoproteins have a high affinity for the CD4 molecule on the surface of T-helper lymphocytes and other cells of monocyte-macrophage lineage. After HIV

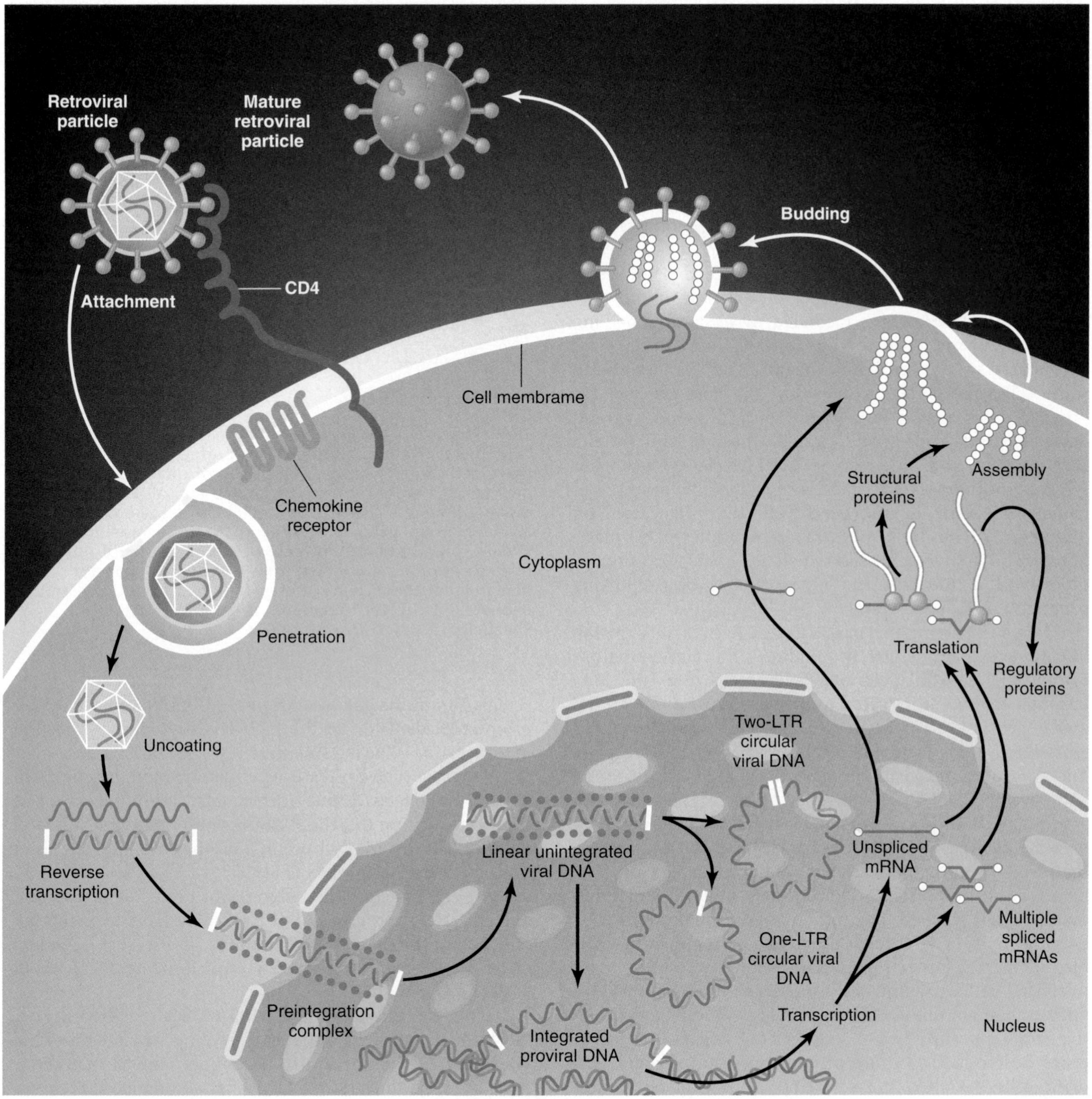

Figure 108-3 Essential steps in the life cycle of human immunodeficiency virus–1 (HIV-1). The first step is the attachment of the virus particle to the CD4 and chemokine (CCR5 or CXCR4) receptors on the surface of the lymphocyte (site of action of viral entry inhibitors; see text). The HIV-1 RNA genome then enters the cytoplasm as part of a nucleoprotein complex. The viral RNA genome is reverse-transcribed into a DNA duplex (site of action of reverse transcriptase inhibitors; see text). Once the viral DNA has been synthesized, the linear viral DNA molecule is incorporated into a preintegration complex that enters the nucleus. In the nucleus, unintegrated viral DNA is found in both linear and circular forms. The viral integrase (target for integrase inhibitors) catalyzes integration of the linear viral DNA into the host genome, where it remains for the life of the cell and serves as a template of viral transcription. Transcription of the integrated DNA template and alternative messenger RNA (mRNA) splicing creates spliced viral mRNA species encoding the viral accessory proteins, including Tat, Rev, and Nef, and the unspliced viral mRNA encoding the viral structural proteins, including the Gag-Pol precursor protein (cleaving of the precursor proteins is prevented by protease inhibitors; see text). A shift in the transcriptional pattern from the expression of predominantly multiply spliced viral mRNA to predominantly unspliced viral mRNA is indicative of active viral replication. All the viral transcripts are exported into the cytoplasm, where translation, assembly, and processing of the retroviral particle take place. The cycle is completed by the release of infectious retroviral particles from the cell. (Modified from Furtado MR, Callaway DS, Phair JP, et al: Persistence of HIV-1 transcription in patients receiving potent antiretroviral therapy. N Engl J Med 340:1614-1622, 1999, with permission.)

binds to CD4, the envelope undergoes a conformational change that facilitates binding to another cellular co-receptor (the most important of these are the chemokine receptors CCR5 and CXCR4). This second binding event promotes a major conformational change that causes approximation of the viral and cellular membranes; fusion of these membranes is mediated by insertion of the newly exposed fusion domain of the envelope gp41 into the host cell membrane. As a result, the HIV nucleoprotein complex enters the cytoplasm, where the RNA viral genome undergoes reverse transcription by the virally encoded reverse transcriptase. The resulting double-stranded viral DNA enters the nucleus, where proper localization of the viral preintegration complex is mediated by host proteins, and integration of the DNA provirus into the host chromosome is catalyzed by the retroviral integrase (see Fig. 108-3). In some cells, after integration within the host genome the provirus may remain in a latent state for years, without detectable transcription of RNA or synthesis of viral protein. Latently infected resting memory CD4 lymphocytes serve as reservoirs of persistent infection for the life of infected patients even in the presence of effective ART (see later discussion). The bulk of viral replication takes place, however, in activated T cells, which are both more susceptible to HIV infection and more capable of supporting productive HIV replication.

When a CD4 lymphocyte is activated (e.g., by recognition of antigenic peptides or by binding of proinflammatory cytokines), the viral promoter-enhancer region (the long terminal repeat) is activated to increase expression of HIV messenger RNA (mRNA). Virus-encoded regulatory proteins Tat and Rev facilitate mRNA expression and cytoplasmic transport, respectively. Core proteins, viral enzymes, and envelope proteins are encoded by the *gag*, *pol*, and *env* genes of HIV, respectively. *Gag*- and *pol*-encoded polyproteins are cleaved by viral proteases (see Fig. 108-3), whereas the envelope protein is cleaved and glycosylated by host proteases and glycosylases. Recent data indicate that more than 100 host proteins, in addition to the viral proteins, may be important for viral replication. Viral particles are assembled at the cell membrane, each containing two copies of unspliced mRNA within the core as the viral genome, and virions then are released from the cell by budding. Productive viral replication is lytic to infected T cells. A number of other host cells, including macrophages and certain dendritic cells, are also infected by HIV, but viral replication does not appear to be lytic to these cells.

IMMUNE DEFICIENCY IN HUMAN IMMUNODEFICIENCY VIRUS INFECTION

Following HIV infection, high-level viral multiplication occurs in mucosal lymphoid tissues of the gut and in other lymphatic sites, and plasma HIV RNA levels (plasma viral load [PVL]) often exceed 1 million copies per milliliter during the second to fourth weeks after infection. Almost all instances of acute HIV infection are caused by R5 tropic viruses, viruses that use the chemokine receptor CCR5 for cellular entry. CD4+ T cells that express CCR5 are typically memory cells that are concentrated in mucosal tissues. In the first few weeks of infection, the memory CD4+ T-cell

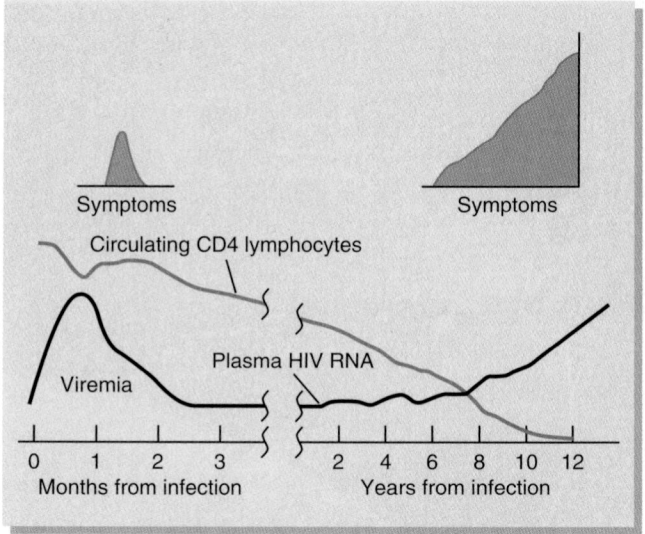

Figure 108-4 Natural history of HIV-1 infection in the untreated adult. Note the long period of clinical latency between the acute retroviral syndrome and AIDS-related disease. Note also the relative stability of the plasma HIV RNA level for several years after recovery from the initial burst of viremia, followed by an increase before the onset of AIDS-related symptoms. (Modified from Shaw GW: Biology of human immunodeficiency viruses. Modified from Goldman L, Bennett JC [eds]: Cecil Textbook of Medicine, 21st ed. Philadelphia, WB Saunders, 2000, p 1896.)

population in the gut-associated lymphoid tissue (GALT) is profoundly depleted by the high-level cytopathic infection in these tissues. During subsequent weeks the PVL decreases, often rapidly. The decrease in viremia results largely from a partially effective, but incomplete, immune response. After 6 to 12 months, the PVL generally stabilizes at a level often called the viral "set point," and may remain roughly at this level for several years (Fig. 108-4). The PVL at 6 to 12 months after infection is a significant predictor of the subsequent rate of progression of HIV disease but accounts for only half of the population variability in disease progression rates. Thus other factors likely contribute to the pace of disease progression.

During the initial burst of viral replication shortly after infection, the majority of patients develop an acute retroviral syndrome (see discussion of sequential clinical manifestations of HIV-1 infection, later). After spontaneous recovery from the acute retroviral syndrome, the patient may feel entirely well for several years. During this period of clinical latency, however, high-level viral multiplication continues in multiple tissues. In the asymptomatic infected individual, over 100 billion new virions may be produced daily, while an equal number are removed from circulation. Rapid production and turnover of circulating CD4+ T-helper cells (CD4 cells) also occurs throughout the course of HIV infection. Although a highly dynamic and complex equilibrium between HIV and CD4 cells may be maintained for several years, a progressive decline in circulating CD4 cells occurs in the great majority of individuals; as disease progresses, a more dramatic CD4 cell decline is observed, following a sharp rise in PVL (see Fig. 108-4). HIV replication, with its attendant cell lysis, accounts only partially for this progressive loss of CD4 cells. An ongoing state of cellular immune activation, not all of which can be attributed directly to HIV itself, appears to play a central role in this progressive immune deficiency.

An HIV-specific immune response contributes to the decrease in the rate of viral replication during the initial weeks after acute HIV infection. During the years of clinical latency, virions are present in large numbers in the follicular dendritic processes of the germinal centers of the lymph nodes, which undergo both hyperplasia and progressive fibrosis. As HIV disease progresses over several years, the lymphatic tissue atrophies, and plasma viremia intensifies. In later-stage HIV disease, there is often persistent high-level viremia (see Fig. 108-4).

The decline in the number of CD4 cells is accompanied by profound functional impairment of the remaining lymphocyte populations. Anergy may develop early in HIV infection and eventually occurs in virtually all persons with AIDS. With development of anergy, T-helper lymphocyte proliferation in response to antigenic stimuli is dramatically impaired. T-cell cytotoxic responses are diminished, and natural killer cell activity against virus-infected cells is greatly impaired, despite normal or increased numbers of these cells. Decrease in function as well as number of CD4 cells is central to the immune dysfunction, and this impairment partly underlies the failure of B-lymphocyte function, as measured by impaired capacity to synthesize antibody in response to new antigens. Profound impairment of multiple arms of the immune system underlies the enhanced risk of acquiring the OIs that are characteristic of AIDS.

INADEQUATE HOST DEFENSE MECHANISMS

HIV continues to replicate despite brisk antibody responses to many components of the virus and demonstrable cell-mediated immune responses to several HIV-derived proteins. There are several possible explanations for the inability of host responses to control HIV infection. The viral replication cycle allows integrated provirus to persist in the host genome in a transcriptionally latent state, in which it is not recognized by either humoral or cellular immune mechanisms (see Fig. 108-3). Conserved domains of the HIV envelope that are potential targets for neutralizing antibody are relatively inaccessible for generation of antibody responses, and extensive glycosylation of the viral envelope also hinders antibody formation and binding. Other conserved potential targets for antibody neutralization are typically unstable and manifest briefly only during the binding and fusion process. Envelope regions vary among different isolates, and although neutralizing antibody responses can be detected early after infection in most persons, mutational escape is readily and reproducibly demonstrable; errors in retroviral reverse transcription underlie this rapid escape from selection pressures and the resultant high degree of genetic variability among HIV isolates. Likewise, while CD8[+] T-cell responses are key to control of retroviral replication in established infection, there is evidence of both CD8[+] T-cell dysfunction and the emergence of escape mutations in sequences targeted by these cells. Preferential infection and deletion of HIV-specific CD4 T helper cells additionally hamper development of an effective anti-HIV immune response.

Diagnosis and Testing for Human Immunodeficiency Virus Infection

Because HIV transmission is preventable, ART is effective, and prophylaxis against the major OIs can prevent these life-threatening events, it is important that routine testing for HIV infection be applied effectively. Testing should *not* be confined only to individuals at recognized high risk. Although not fully implemented nationwide yet, the current recommendation from the CDC is that HIV testing be considered a part of routine medical care, and that it be offered to all patients at the time of contact with the health care system without requirements for written consent or formal pretest and posttest counseling. Confidential pretest discussion is important to ensure that persons appreciate the importance and consequences of the test results. All individuals, regardless of the reason for their interaction with the health care system, should be counseled regarding safer sexual practices. Injection drug users should strongly be advised not to share needles. Positive test results should be given in a face-to-face meeting, during which the patient is given assurance that with adherence to current therapy he or she may live asymptomatically with HIV infection for decades. Arrangements for continuing medical care should be made at this time. All patients should be encouraged to notify their sexual partners and persons with whom they have shared needles. This is often difficult; regional health authorities may be of great assistance in confidential notification of persons at risk. All pregnant women should routinely be offered HIV testing, because ART will dramatically reduce mother-to-child transmission.

Diagnosis of HIV infection is established by detection of antibodies to HIV in serum or in oral fluid and is confirmed by Western blot. These techniques are very sensitive in detecting HIV antibody, but individuals who have been infected recently may be antibody negative. During this "window period," typically 1 to 2 weeks, infected persons have detectable HIV RNA and core p24 antigen in plasma. For recently exposed persons whose initial enzyme-linked immunosorbent assay (ELISA) result is negative, repeat ELISAs at 6 weeks and 3 months are indicated. False-positive ELISA results do occur because the HIV ELISA has been calibrated to achieve maximum sensitivity; all positive ELISA results must therefore be confirmed by Western blot reactivity with at least two different HIV proteins. In a person at high risk for HIV exposure, an indeterminate Western blot reaction pattern often represents early seroconversion; in such cases a positive plasma HIV RNA (>10,000 copies/mL) is indicative of acute HIV infection.

Rapid and accessible testing methods play an increasingly important role in the diagnosis and confirmation of HIV infection. Oral fluid and/or urine testing are noninvasive approaches, and rapid test kits can provide tentative results within 30 minutes.

Table 108-3 Acute HIV Retroviral Syndrome: Common Signs and Symptoms

Sign or Symptom	Frequency (%)
Fever	98
Lymph node enlargement	75
Sore throat	70
Myalgia or arthralgia	60
Rash	50
Headache	35

Sequential Clinical Manifestations of Human Immunodeficiency Virus Type 1 Infection

ACUTE HUMAN IMMUNODEFICIENCY VIRUS INFECTION AND THE ACUTE RETROVIRAL SYNDROME

Over 50% of HIV-infected persons experience a mononucleosis-like syndrome (acute retroviral syndrome) 2 to 6 weeks after initial infection (see Fig. 108-4). Acute symptoms may include fever, sore throat, lymph node enlargement, rash, arthralgias, and headache and usually persist for several days to 3 weeks (Table 108-3). A maculopapular rash is common, is short-lived, and usually affects the trunk or face. Acute, self-limited aseptic meningitis, documented by cerebrospinal fluid (CSF) pleocytosis and isolation of HIV from CSF, is the most common clinical neurologic presentation and occurs in up to 10% of patients.

The acute retroviral syndrome is sufficiently severe that a large proportion of patients seek medical attention. In the absence of a high index of suspicion, these symptoms are often mislabeled as an "acute viral syndrome." This is especially unfortunate, because a very high plasma HIV RNA level during this period indicates a high likelihood of HIV transmission to sexual or needle-sharing partners, or from mother to infant.

During the acute retroviral syndrome, HIV antibody is often not detectable, but HIV infection can be demonstrated by detection of HIV RNA or the HIV core p24 antigen in plasma. Within 4 to 12 weeks after HIV infection, specific antibodies develop that are directed against the three main gene products of HIV: *gag*, *pol*, and *env*.

ASYMPTOMATIC PHASE

Untreated HIV infection usually results in a slow, nonlinear progression to severe immunodeficiency. Approximately 50% of untreated individuals develop AIDS within 10 years after HIV infection (see Fig. 108-4); an additional 30% have milder symptoms related to immunodeficiency, and less than 20% are entirely asymptomatic 10 years after infection. Progression of disease varies greatly among individuals. Adolescents with HIV progress to AIDS at a slower rate than older persons, and fewer than 30% develop AIDS within 10 years after HIV infection. The rate of progression of immunodeficiency is not influenced by the route of HIV transmission and, in the long term, does not appear to differ by gender, although typically women with HIV infection tend to experience more rapid disease progression with lower levels of HIV in plasma.

The majority of HIV-infected individuals are not diagnosed during the acute retroviral syndrome, are unaware of their infection, and are asymptomatic, often until their CD4 counts fall below 200 cells/mm³. Clinically recognized lymph node enlargement occurs in 35% to 40% of asymptomatic HIV-infected persons but is not significantly associated with either rate of progression of immunodeficiency or subsequent development of lymphoma. During early HIV infection, thrombocytopenia, probably caused by autoimmune platelet destruction, is common.

EARLY SYMPTOMATIC PHASE

Mucocutaneous lesions may be the first manifestations of immune dysfunction, especially polydermatomal varicella-zoster infection (shingles), recurrent genital herpes simplex virus (HSV) infections, oral or vaginal candidiasis, or oral hairy leukoplakia (OHL). Patients with only moderate immunodeficiency (CD4 counts between 200 and 500 cells/mm³) exhibit diminished antibody response to protein and polysaccharide antigens, as well as decreased cell-mediated immune function. These functional impairments are manifested clinically by a threefold to fourfold increase in incidence of bacteremic pneumonias caused by common pulmonary pathogens (especially *Streptococcus pneumoniae* and *Haemophilus influenzae*), as well as a marked increase in incidence of active pulmonary tuberculosis in endemic areas.

ADVANCED SYMPTOMATIC PHASE: OPPORTUNISTIC INFECTIONS

With advanced immunodeficiency, indicated by CD4 counts below 200 cells/mm³, patients are at high risk for developing OIs (Table 108-4). For example, in the late 1980s, in the absence of specific prophylaxis and before the availability of effective antiretroviral drugs, 60% of HIV-infected North American men developed PCP.

CD4 counts less than 50 cells/mm³ indicate profound immunosuppression and, in the absence of effective ART, are associated with a high mortality within the subsequent 12 to 24 months. Cytomegalovirus (CMV) retinitis, which can lead rapidly to blindness, and disseminated *Mycobacterium avium-intracellulare* (MAI) infections occur frequently. They respond adequately to specific therapy only when it is accompanied by effective control of viral replication.

SEX-SPECIFIC MANIFESTATIONS

Several sex-specific manifestations are relevant to the management of HIV infection in women. Recognition of these manifestations is especially important because they are responsive to specific therapy; each manifestation may serve as the signal for HIV testing in a person with no prior clinical manifestations of immunodeficiency.

- The earliest clinical manifestation of HIV infection in women may be frequent recurrence of *Candida* vaginitis in the absence of predisposing factors. Because recurrent

Table 108-4	**Relation of CD4 Lymphocyte Counts to the Onset of Certain HIV-Associated Infections and Neoplasms in North America**
CD4 Count (cells/mm³)*	**Opportunistic Infection or Neoplasm**
>500	Herpes zoster, polydermatomal
200-500	*Mycobacterium tuberculosis* infection Oral hairy leukoplakia *Candida* pharyngitis (thrush) Kaposi sarcoma, mucocutaneous (M) Bacterial pneumonia, recurrent Cervical neoplasia (F)
100-200	*Pneumocystis jirovecii* pneumonia *Histoplasmosis capsulatum* infection, disseminated Kaposi sarcoma, visceral (M) Progressive multifocal leukoencephalopathy Lymphoma, non-Hodgkin
<100	*Candida* esophagitis Cytomegalovirus retinitis *Mycobacterium avium-intracellulare*, disseminated *Toxoplasma gondii* encephalitis *Cryptosporidium parvum* enteritis *Cryptococcus neoformans* meningitis Herpes simplex virus, chronic, ulcerative Cytomegalovirus esophagitis or colitis Lymphoma, central nervous system

*CD4 count at which specific infections or neoplasms generally begin to appear. Each infection may recur or progress during the subsequent course of HIV disease.

F, exclusively in women; M, usually in men.

Table 108-5	**Management of Early HIV Disease**

Monitoring

Confirm positive HIV test result
Complete baseline history and physical examination: HIV-specific interval interview and examination every 3-4 mo

Laboratory Evaluation

Baseline plasma HIV RNA level and CD4 cell count with repeat every 3-4 mo
Baseline purified protein derivative (PPD)
Baseline *Toxoplasma* antibody, syphilis serology, hepatitis B and C antibodies, liver function tests, and chest radiograph*
Baseline genotypic resistance testing

Health Care Maintenance

Assessment for ongoing counseling needs and referral for significant psychiatric or social problems
Discussions regarding safer sex and avoidance of needle sharing
Pneumococcal vaccine, hepatitis A and B vaccine (if HAV, HBV seronegative)
Yearly influenza vaccine

*Many experts order a chest X-ray film only when clinically indicated.
   HAV, hepatitis A virus; HAV, hepatitis B virus.

Candida vaginitis may develop at a time of only moderate immunodeficiency (CD4 count above 200 cells/mm³), it may serve as a trigger to discuss HIV testing and lead to earlier diagnosis in otherwise asymptomatic women.

- Recurrent large painful genital, perianal, or perineal ulcers, caused by HSV-2, are more frequent in women than in men. Occurring at a time of more advanced immunodeficiency, such lesions should always prompt HIV testing, as well as specific antiviral therapy (see Chapter 107).
- A rare but potentially life-threatening complication may be development of cervical dysplasia or neoplasia. HIV-infected women show an increased prevalence of high-grade squamous intraepithelial lesions on Papanicolaou (Pap) smear. HIV-infected women should therefore undergo two Pap smears at a 6-month interval; if the initial two Pap smears are both normal, smears should be repeated once a year. Conversely, all women with high-grade squamous intraepithelial lesions on Pap smear should be encouraged to undergo testing for HIV infection.

Management of Human Immunodeficiency Virus Infection

Because patients are asymptomatic during most of the course of HIV-1 infection (see Fig. 107-4), and even seri-

ously immunocompromised individuals can function productively between bouts of OIs, the ambulatory management of persons with HIV infection deserves major emphasis.

INITIAL AMBULATORY EVALUATION

Once HIV infection is recognized, the physician should discuss, in an unhurried manner, the clinical course and treatment of HIV infection and the use of immunologic and virologic studies (e.g., CD4 counts, PVL assays) to guide therapy. The physician should emphasize that most patients, even without antiviral therapy, live for 10 to 12 years after acquiring HIV infection and are asymptomatic during most of that time. The physician should then emphasize that, with effective currently available ART, HIV disease progression can be prevented indefinitely.

Prevention of further transmission through unprotected sex or sharing of needles must be discussed not only at the first visit but also periodically thereafter. It is important to emphasize that these high-risk activities place both the "contact" and the patient at risk, as they may lead to transmission of new HIV strains to the patient, some of which may be resistant to current or future medications used in his or her treatment.

Initial evaluation should include both an HIV-oriented review of systems and a complete physical examination (Table 108-5). In particular, the skin must be examined for HIV-associated rashes and Kaposi sarcoma. Examination of the oral cavity may reveal thrush, gingivitis, hairy leukoplakia, superficial ulcers caused by HSV, aphthous ulcers, or lesions characteristic of Kaposi sarcoma. In persons with very advanced disease, the optic fundi may have hemorrhagic lesions characteristic of CMV retinitis. Lymph node enlargement, hepatomegaly, splenomegaly, and any genital lesions should all be carefully noted. Neurologic examination for both peripheral neuropathy and decreased global cognition deserves close attention. Pelvic examination with Pap smear should be routine for women.

Purified protein derivative (PPD) testing should be performed early in the course of HIV infection. Induration of 5 mm or more should be considered positive. Any patient with a positive PPD test result should be evaluated for the presence of active tuberculosis; if no active disease is present, the patient should receive 9 months of prophylaxis with isoniazid or combination drug therapy for a shorter time period (see Chapter 99). If active tuberculosis is identified, multidrug therapy should be initiated after careful consideration of possible interactions with antiretroviral medications.

Serologic testing for *Toxoplasma gondii* infection is important in the event that a person subsequently develops an intracerebral lesion (see later discussion). Serologic testing for syphilis should be followed by prompt treatment if patient is confirmed to be positive (see Chapter 107). Antibody responses to pneumococcal polysaccharides are better among patients with higher CD4 counts. The optimal timing of immunization is uncertain; however, if ART is indicated, some authorities will delay immunization for at least 3 to 4 months until HIV replication is better controlled and CD4 counts are increased.

The CD4 count and the PVL should be obtained at the first visit and repeated at intervals of 3 to 4 months. The patient should understand that the CD4 count and the PVL are rough guides to the degree of immunodeficiency and the rate of viral replication, respectively, and that modest fluctuations in these measurements may not indicate a change in clinical course. It is helpful for the physician to use graphic illustrations of the interaction between PVL and CD4 count as predictors of the course of illness in the absence of treatment, as well as a guide to the initiation and monitoring of ART (Table 108-6). Resistance testing should be performed on all patients at entry into clinical care and before initiation of ART (see later) if a considerable amount of time has elapsed between initial contact and therapy start. Transmitted resistance in some antiretroviral-naive populations is greater than 10%.

GOALS OF ANTIRETROVIRAL THERAPY

The goal of ART is to ensure that persons living with HIV infection lead symptom-free, productive lives. Currently available therapy makes achieving this goal possible in almost all individuals with early, asymptomatic HIV infection who have not acquired major resistance mutations as the result of earlier suboptimal ART. This circumstance is in stark contrast to the situation only 15 years ago, when progression to marked immunodeficiency was almost inevitable, and such devastating health consequences as blindness caused by CMV retinitis and crippling neurologic deficits as the result of *Toxoplasma* encephalitis were common preterminal events.

PRINCIPLES OF ANTIRETROVIRAL THERAPY

Treatment of HIV infection is exceptional among infectious diseases because specific therapy is not initiated as soon as the diagnosis has been established. Principles underlying this approach include the following:

- Antiretroviral treatment is not curative but suppressive; because HIV infection cannot be eradicated, treatment may be lifelong with currently available drugs.
- All effective treatment regimens may be associated with toxicities, some of which can be life threatening.
- There is a risk for the development of resistance to therapy that increases with the degree of nonadherence to therapy.
- Although damage to the host immune system occurs throughout the course of HIV infection, loss of protective immune response to the most serious OIs occurs only with advanced HIV disease.

ART should therefore be initiated at a time when the benefit of halting replication of the virus exceeds the risks and toxicities of prolonged treatment with available drugs.

WHEN TO INITIATE THERAPY

It is critical that initiation of therapy be based on a joint decision by the informed patient and the physician. Initiation of ART in an asymptomatic patient is seldom an urgent issue, and the physician should spend whatever time is necessary (e.g., three patient visits over a 12-week period) for the patient to understand both the potential benefits and the risks of the specific regimen that is to be undertaken. Graphs such as that shown in Figure 108-5 can be very effective in helping the patient to understand the importance of the CD4

Table 108-6	**Guidelines for the Initiation of Antiretroviral Therapy in the Chronically HIV-Infected Patient***	
Clinical Category	**CD4⁺ T-Cell Count and HIV RNA**	**Recommendation**
Symptomatic (e.g., AIDS, thrush)	Any value	Treat
Asymptomatic	CD4⁺ T cells <350/mm³	Treat
Asymptomatic	CD4⁺ T cells >350/mm³	Treatment may be considered in some cases, although benefit may be limited in this group of patients.
Asymptomatic with concomitant (a) pregnancy; (b) hepatitis B with an indication for treatment; or (c) HIV-associated nephropathy	Any value	Treat

*These general guidelines should be used only in conjunction with the text. There are no absolute laboratory thresholds on which the initiation of therapy can be based. This decision must always be made jointly by the informed patient and the physician.

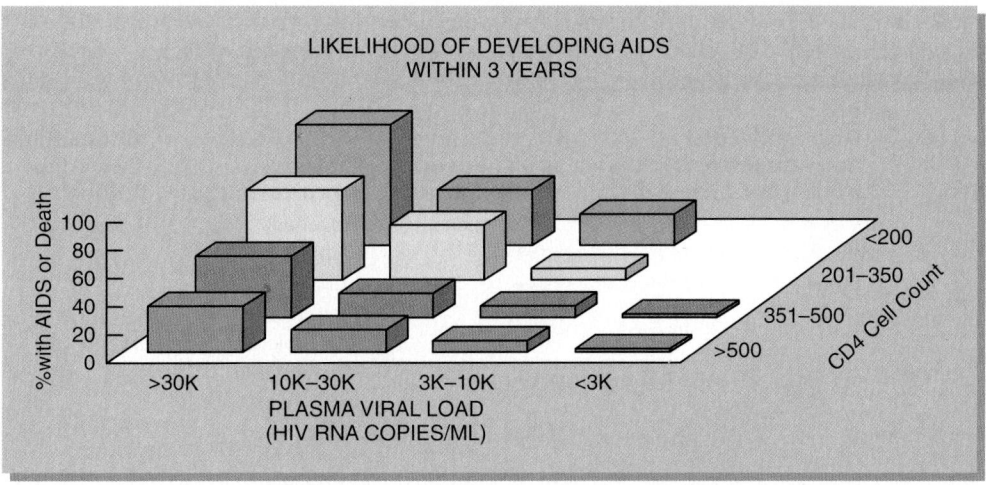

Figure 108-5 Likelihood of developing symptomatic AIDS-related illness or death within 3 years in the absence of treatment. Values in the yellow and red zones are considered indication for initiation of antiretroviral therapy. Values in the yellow zone indicate a 6% to 24% likelihood of progression in 3 years. Values in the purple zone suggest initiation of patient-physician discussion of antiretroviral therapy (see text). Values in the green zone indicate small likelihood of 3-year progression. (Data from Mellors JW, Muñoz A, Giorgi JV, et al: Plasma viral load and CD4+ lymphocytes as prognostic markers of HIV-1 infection. Ann Intern Med 126:946-954, 1997.)

count in providing the information essential to determining when to initiate therapy. Therapy should be individualized to the extent possible (e.g., a woman of reproductive age who uses contraceptive measures unreliably may be a poor candidate for a medication that is contraindicated during pregnancy). Because the patient may anticipate lifelong ART, and because inadequate adherence to any antiretroviral regimen will result, over time, in resistance to the antiretroviral drugs, it is essential that the patient have as full an understanding of the regimen as possible before initiating ART. The physician must emphasize to the patient the critical importance of consistent adherence with the treatment regimen once started because suboptimal drug levels both provide a selection pressure and permit viral replication. This selects for emergence of viruses with drug-resistant escape mutations that will remain with the patient for the rest of his or her life.

Symptomatic Patients

All patients with symptomatic AIDS (with active or past OIs) should receive ART. Without effective ART, patients with symptomatic AIDS have a high risk of death within 6 to 18 months.

Some experts recommend treatment of patients in whom the acute retroviral syndrome is recognized. There is suggestive evidence that initiation of effective ART at this early stage may lead to more effective restoration of immune function and less rapid subsequent progression of HIV disease, but the data are insufficient to support a definitive recommendation for treatment at this stage of infection.

Asymptomatic Patients

Treatment should be initiated before the patient becomes symptomatic. The CD4 count is the major determinant of when to start antiviral treatment. Although the optimal time to initiate therapy in a given asymptomatic patient cannot be precisely defined, it is currently recommended that all

patients should receive effective ART once the CD4 count falls below 350 cells/mm³ (see Table 108-6). For persons with CD4 counts greater than 350 cells/mm³, decisions about initiating treatment should be individualized by balancing the potential disadvantages of initiating ART (short- and long-term toxicities and development of antiretroviral resistance) against the potential benefits (prevention of progressive immunologic damage and resultant risk for comorbidities) in the context of what the patient is prepared and able to do. No uniform recommendation on treatment initiation can be made for this subset of patients.

In addition to CD4 count, certain clinical circumstances can modify the timing of initiation of ART. Pregnant women, patients with hepatitis B co-infection who require treatment for hepatitis B, and patients with HIV-associated nephropathy should all receive antiretroviral treatment regardless of CD4 count. Current guidelines for treatment initiation are summarized in Table 108-6.

ANTIRETROVIRAL DRUG REGIMENS

Clarification of the mechanisms of HIV replication has identified several potential sites at which retroviral replication might be limited or blocked (see Fig. 108-3). Drugs approved by the U.S. Food and Drug Administration for treatment of HIV infection include seven nucleoside analogues (NRTIs) and one nucleotide analogue that inhibit HIV reverse transcriptase; four non-nucleoside reverse transcriptase inhibitors (NNRTIs); nine HIV protease inhibitors (PIs); and one agent each belonging to the viral fusion inhibitor, chemokine coreceptor inhibitor, and integrase inhibitor classes (Table 108-7). Additional agents in each of these categories are currently in clinical trials; several will likely be approved soon.

The goal of ART is to ensure that the patient has the highest possible quality of life for as long as possible. In general, this requires therapy that durably suppresses the PVL below levels that are detectable by the most sensitive

Table 108-7	**Antiretroviral Drugs Approved for Use in Highly Active Antiretroviral Therapy Regimens for Treatment of HIV Infection**					
Nucleoside or Nucleotide Reverse Transcriptase Inhibitors (RTIs)	**Non-nucleoside Reverse Transcriptase Inhibitors (non-RTIs)**	**Viral Fusion Inhibitor**	**Protease Inhibitors (PIs)**	**Chemokine Receptor Inhibitor**	**Integrase Inhibitor**
Abacavir	Efavirenz	Enfuvirtide	Atazanavir	Maraviroc	Raltegravir
Didanosine	Nevirapine		Amprenavir		
Emtricitabine	Etravirine		Indinavir		
Lamivudine			Lopinavir		
Stavudine			Nelfinavir		
Zidovudine			Ritonavir		
Zalcitabine			Saquinavir		
Tenofovir*			Tipranavir		
			Fosamprenavir		
			Darunavir		

*Nucleotide RTI; other agents in the column are nucleoside RTIs.

available assays (<50 copies of HIV RNA per milliliter). Achievement of this objective currently demands that the patient take combination ART with a minimum of three antiretroviral drugs.

Currently recommended initial regimens that predictably provide profound and durable suppression of viral replication include a potent NNRTI plus two NRTIs or a potent PI plus two NRTIs (often in addition to a low dose of the PI ritonavir, which tends to inhibit the hepatic metabolism of other drugs in this group). In addition, combinations that include the newer classes of antiretrovirals (fusion inhibitors, integrase inhibitors, and chemokine receptor inhibitors) have been effective in highly experienced patients with viruses that have substantial levels of resistance to reverse transcriptase inhibitors and PIs. Each of these regimens can result in durable suppression of PVL, usually associated with gradual recovery of immunologic competence. Each regimen has specific advantages and potential toxicities of which the patient must be aware. For example, an efavirenz-based regimen has the advantage of simplicity of administration (once a day) but the disadvantage of a low genetic barrier to the acquisition of mutations that confer high-grade resistance to several NNRTIs if adherence is poor. Because the long-term effectiveness of any regimen is largely determined by the patient's ability to adhere closely to it, the choice of regimen should always be made jointly by the physician and the informed patient. Ease of administration and lack of adverse effects are critical to adherence, so each regimen must be tailored, as much as possible, to the individual patients. As more agents that can be given once a day are becoming available, once-a-day regimens may become regimens of choice, especially for patients with rigorous occupational schedules, or for patients receiving directly observed therapy. Most available regimens can be taken at twice-daily intervals (see Department of Health and Human Services HIV Treatment Guidelines at *www.aidsinfo.nih.gov/guidelines* for regularly updated treatment information). The recent development of a coformulation of efavirenz, tenofovir, and emtricitabine in a single tablet, taken once daily, represents a major step forward in providing an effective regimen that does not interfere with normal activities of daily living.

WHEN TO CHANGE THERAPY

When an effective antiretroviral regimen is initiated in an asymptomatic patient with no previous ART, the PVL should decrease sharply, generally by 10-fold in 4 weeks and to an undetectable level (<50 copies/mL) within 16 to 24 weeks. If reduction of this magnitude is not achieved, the physician should, with the patient, assess whether adherence has been adequate. If adherence has been nearly complete (>95%), the physician and patient should consider testing for resistance mutations and changing to another effective regimen. Whereas all patients should undergo resistance testing at the time of initial entry into care, minority viral subpopulations carrying resistance mutations may have been too infrequent to be detected at baseline, before exposure to antiretrovirals, but may rapidly overtake the sensitive virus once the selective pressure exerted by the medications is applied. Combination therapies permit suppression of viruses resistant to one drug. Incomplete adherence to treatment that permits drug levels to fall below those needed for complete suppression of viral replication permits the development of additional resistance mutations as viral replication is needed for new mutations to emerge; thus resistance mutations are promoted by a drug-induced selection pressure that is incompletely suppressive. Therefore, if an antiretroviral drug must be stopped for reasons of intolerance or toxicity, it is important to stop temporarily all antiretroviral drugs or alternatively to revise the regimen to sustain complete virologic suppression in order to prevent induction of resistance by an incompletely suppressive regimen. If a given regimen achieves a reduction of PVL below detectable limits and continuing adherence is achieved, the patient can anticipate effective viral suppression for many years and perhaps indefinitely. The PVL should be monitored at 3- to 4-month intervals throughout the course of therapy. If, after months or years of adequate viral suppression, the viral load again becomes detectable on two consecutive determinations, re-testing for resistance mutations and consideration of a change in therapy is indicated. Small viral load elevations on a single determination, however, are usually not significant. See regularly updated International AIDS Society–USA resistance guidelines at www.iasusa.org/guidelines/index.html.

Table 108-8 Prophylaxis Against Certain Opportunistic Infections (OIs) in HIV-Infected Adults*

Pathogen	Indication	First Choice	Alternatives
Pneumocystis jirovecii[†]	CD4 count <200, or history of thrush	TMP-SMZ, 1 tablet qd	Dapsone, 100 mg qd Atovaquone, 1500 mg qd Pentamidine, aerosolized, 300 mg q mo
Mycobacterium tuberculosis[†]			
Isoniazid-sensitive	TST reaction >5 mm, or prior positive TST result without treatment, or contact with case of active tuberculosis	Isoniazid, 300 mg PO, plus pyridoxine, 50 mg qd × 9 mo	Rifampin, 600 mg qd × 4 mo
Isoniazid-resistant	Same as above	Rifampin, 600 mg qd × 4 mo	Rifabutin, 300 mg qd × 4 mo
Toxoplasma gondii[†]	IgG antibody to Toxoplasma and CD4 count <100	TMP-SMZ, 1 double-strength tablet qd	Dapsone, 50 mg PO qd, plus pyrimethimine, 50 mg PO q wk
Mycobacterium avium-intracellulare[†]	CD4 count <50	Azithromycin, 1200 mg q wk	Clarithromycin, 500 mg PO bid

*Department of Health and Human Services recommendations for prophylaxis against OIs are updated regularly and are available at www.aidsinfo.nih.gov/guidelines.
[†]Strongly recommended as standard of care in all patients.
IgG, immunoglobulin G; PO, orally; TMP-SMZ, trimethoprim-sulfamethoxazole; TST, tuberculosis skin test.

Available data do not precisely define the threshold at which a change in therapy is indicated. Some experts recommend change as soon as the PVL is above detectable limits on two determinations. Others would not change until the viral load exceeds an arbitrary figure of 3000 to 5000 copies/mL. At this point, results of resistance testing should be used to define a second effective regimen. The most durable second regimen usually requires a change in at least two antiretroviral drugs.

After failure of a second antiretroviral regimen, change becomes more difficult because the remaining options are reduced. Antiviral resistance testing is even more critical in this setting because viral isolates will commonly demonstrate a significant number of resistance mutations, making the choice of the next regimen considerably more challenging. Many treated patients continue to do well clinically, with stable CD4 counts, for months to years after viral "escape" indicated by increasing PVL. In such patients, stopping ART generally results in clinical deterioration. The basis for continued clinical well-being, despite increasing PVL, during long-term ART is uncertain but may reflect diminished "pathogenicity" of viruses with antiretroviral drug resistance mutations and/or ongoing low-level antigenic stimulation in the setting of partially controlled viremia, potentially resulting in improved immunologic control of viral replication. Thus, many patients continue to receive clinical and immunologic benefit from continued ART despite loss of complete viral control. Continued administration of the ART maintains selection pressure, which results in drug-resistant viruses that tend to be less *fit* in terms of replicative capacity and possibly also less pathogenic. How long the clinical benefit will be sustained in such patients is unknown, but it is clear that these patients do not maintain CD4 cell numbers as well as do patients with more complete suppression of HIV replication. Moreover, HIV tends to accumulate further resistance mutations during periods of incomplete virologic suppression that could potentially compromise future options for salvage therapy;

hence, continuation of a partially suppressive regimen is reasonable only when no other options exist.

PROPHYLAXIS AGAINST OPPORTUNISTIC INFECTIONS

During the first 15 years of the HIV pandemic, the most effective medical interventions for HIV infection were prophylactic measures against OIs. The greatest success was the prevention of PCP in individuals with CD4 counts less than 200 cells/mm³; routine use of prophylaxis resulted in a greater than fourfold (from 60% to <15%) decrease in the frequency of PCP as the initial OI in North American men with HIV infection. Specific antimicrobial prophylaxis (Table 108-8) is also effective for prevention of *T. gondii* encephalitis in patients with anti-*Toxoplasma* antibodies with CD4 counts less than 100 cells/mm³, and for prevention of active tuberculosis in patients with positive tuberculin skin test results at any CD4 level (see Table 108-8). Prophylaxis against disseminated MAI infection is recommended at lower CD4 counts (<50 cells/mm³). Prophylaxis against CMV retinitis is moderately effective in patients with CD4 counts less than 50 cells/mm³, but prompt initiation of effective ART and early treatment of active disease are the currently preferred strategy. Prophylaxis is very effective against recurrent HSV-2 infection (acyclovir, famciclovir, or valacyclovir) and against recurrent *Candida* esophagitis (fluconazole) but should generally be reserved for those patients with recurrent symptomatic disease.

Management of Specific Clinical Manifestations of Immunodeficiency

In the course of HIV infection, OIs vary considerably in time of onset (see Table 108-4). For example, some patients may

Table 108-9 **Dermatologic Conditions Common in HIV Infection**		
Condition	**Description**	**Treatment**
Herpes simplex	Clear or crusted vesicles with an erythematous base; ulceration common when chronic; location: oral or genital mucous membranes, face, and hands	Acyclovir, 200 mg 5 times/day, or famciclovir, 250 mg tid, or valacyclovir, 1000 mg bid, each for 7-10 days
Herpes zoster (shingles)	Cluster of vesicles in a dermatomal distribution; may involve adjacent dermatomes or may disseminate	Acyclovir, 800 mg 5 times/day, or famciclovir, 500 mg tid, or valacyclovir, 1000 mg bid, each for 7 days; if disseminated or involvement of ophthalmic branch of trigeminal nerve, IV acyclovir, 10 mg/kg q8h
Staphylococcal folliculitis	Erythematous pustules on face, trunk, and groin, often pruritic	Dicloxacillin, 500 mg qid, or erythromycin, 500 mg qid for 1 wk
Bacillary angiomatosis	Friable vascular papules or subcutaneous nodules on skin; may involve liver, spleen, and lymph nodes	Clarithromycin, 500 mg bid, or doxycycline, 200 mg qd for 1 wk
Molluscum contagiosum	Chronic, flesh-colored papules, often umbilicated, on face or anogenital area	Cryotherapy and curettage
Seborrheic dermatitis	White scaling or erythematous patches on scalp, eyebrows, face, trunk, axilla, and groin	Hydrocortisone cream 2.5% and ketoconazole cream
Psoriasis	Scaling, marginated patches on elbows, knees, and lumbosacral areas	Triamcinolone acetonide cream 0.1%
Eosinophilic folliculitis	Recurrent pruritic follicular papules and rare pustules	Immune restoration with antiretroviral therapy, topical steroids
Candidal dermatitis	Urticarial scaling or erythematous patches on face, trunk, axilla, and groin	Hydrocortisone cream 1% and ketoconazole cream

IV, intravenous.

develop multidermatomal herpes zoster with CD4 counts greater than 500 cells/mm^3 and then have no other OIs until they develop PCP with CD4 counts less than 200 cells/mm^3. Conversely, some patients may remain entirely asymptomatic until their CD4 counts are below 50 cells/mm^3, at which time they may develop major life-threatening OIs, such as *T. gondii* encephalitis (see Table 108-4).

In general, OIs that occur with higher CD4 counts respond to routine therapy for the specific infection (e.g., appropriate β-lactam antibiotic for pneumococcal pneumonia, standard multidrug therapy for pulmonary tuberculosis), whereas OIs occurring with CD4 counts less than 200 cells/mm^3 require chronic suppressive therapy after treatment of acute infection (e.g., PCP pneumonia, CMV retinitis, or *Cryptococcus neoformans* meningitis).

Effective ART has had a dramatic impact on the incidence of OIs. Although the impact on specific OIs has varied, with decreases greater than 75% in CMV retinitis and PCP pneumonia, all recognized OIs have decreased dramatically in frequency in North America and Western Europe since 1996. Furthermore, after partial restoration of immunologic function in response to effective therapy, withdrawal of prophylaxis against specific OIs is reasonable. After initiation of effective ART and two consecutive CD4 counts at least 3 months apart that exceed 100 cells/mm^3 or 200 cells/mm^3, prophylaxis against CMV and MAI or PCP and *T. gondii*, respectively, may be withdrawn safely.

Because of the great reduction in OIs associated with effective ART, rates of hospitalization and mortality for AIDS-related illnesses have dropped sharply since 1996, with decreases of as much as 80% in major North American and Western European cities.

CONSTITUTIONAL SYMPTOMS

Nonspecific symptoms may be the initial clinical manifestations of severe immunodeficiency. Patients may develop unexplained fever, night sweats, anorexia, weight loss, or diarrhea. These symptoms may last for weeks or months before the development of identifiable OIs in patients who do not receive effective ART. These constitutional symptoms may represent manifestations of specific, but unidentified, OIs.

CUTANEOUS DISEASE

Cutaneous infections ultimately occur in most patients with untreated HIV disease. Most respond to specific therapy as outlined in Table 108-9.

MUCOSAL DISEASE

Oral *Candida* stomatitis, or thrush, is often the earliest recognized OI. Early thrush may be entirely asymptomatic; as infection becomes more extensive, it causes pain on eating. The characteristic cheesy white exudate on the mucous membranes can easily be scraped off, and the underlying mucosa may be normal or inflamed.

OHL is a white, lichenified, plaquelike lesion most commonly seen on the lateral surfaces of the tongue that is likely caused by Epstein-Barr virus (EBV). Unlike thrush, the lesions of OHL cannot be scraped off with a tongue depressor. OHL may also be an early manifestation of moderately severe immunodeficiency. OHL is painless, may remit and relapse spontaneously, and almost always responds to effective ART.

Patients may develop painful ulcers in the mouth. These may be caused by HSV but often represent aphthous lesions of uncertain cause. Small oral aphthous ulcers may respond to topical corticosteroids, whereas giant oral or esophageal ulcers require oral administration of thalidomide or corticosteroids. It is important to obtain cultures for HSV and CMV to exclude a viral origin before initiating corticosteroid or thalidomide therapy. Thalidomide should be used, if at all, only when birth control can be ensured in women with childbearing potential because of its well-documented adverse effects on fetal development.

Kaposi sarcoma has a predilection for the oral cavity and skin. Oral lesions may be purple, red, or blue and may be raised or flat. Usually painless, these lesions cause symptoms when they enlarge, bleed, or ulcerate. The incidence of Kaposi sarcoma has decreased dramatically in the United States, but the condition continues to be a major problem in Africa.

ESOPHAGEAL DISEASE

Symptomatic esophageal disease seldom occurs with CD4 counts greater than 100 cells/mm³. Pain on swallowing and substernal burning are common and most often indicate *Candida* esophagitis, particularly when oral thrush is present. Diagnostic esophagoscopy with biopsy, cytology, and culture should be performed if symptoms do not rapidly respond (within 3 to 5 days) to antifungal therapy. If esophagoscopy shows ulcerative lesions, they are usually caused by CMV (50%), aphthae (45%), or HSV (5%). Because each of these lesions is responsive to appropriate therapy, definitive etiologic diagnosis is essential (Table 108-10). CMV esophageal ulcers respond well to intravenous ganciclovir or foscarnet therapy for 2 to 3 weeks or until resolution is confirmed endoscopically. Esophageal ulcerations caused by HSV usually respond well to intravenous acyclovir (see Table 108-10).

GENITAL DISEASE

Recurrent genital ulcers are most often caused by HSV. Viral culture or specific immunofluorescence of ulcer scrapings confirms the diagnosis. Primary syphilis also occurs with increased frequency (see Chapter 107). Chancroid is unusual in North America.

Many genital inflammatory diseases increase the risk for acquisition of HIV infection; some, such as HSV infection, increase genital shedding of HIV, and persons with genital ulcer disease are at greater risk for transmitting HIV to their uninfected partners. These considerations make it imperative that genital mucosal infections be treated promptly and definitively.

Candida species, most often *Candida albicans,* can cause an irritating vulvovaginitis in women with HIV infection as well as in healthy HIV-seronegative women. A potassium hydroxide preparation of the cheesy white exudate will reveal budding yeast or pseudohyphae.

Bacterial vaginosis and trichomoniasis are common, and although both typically respond to specific treatment (e.g., metronidazole), bacterial vaginosis often recurs.

Infection with HPV is associated not only with development of genital warts in both men and women, but also with a greater frequency of cervical dysplasia in HIV-infected women and anal carcinoma in men. Pap smears indicative of cervical dysplasia should be followed by prompt colposcopy, biopsy when indicted, and appropriate treatment of any dysplastic lesions. With this approach, progression of cervical dysplasia to invasive cervical cancer is exceedingly rare. Some clinicians also recommend anal Pap testing for MSM with HIV infection, but the utility of routine screening in this setting has not been established.

NERVOUS SYSTEM DISEASES

Nervous system complications ultimately occur in the majority of untreated HIV-infected persons. They range from mild cognitive disturbances or peripheral neuropathy to severe dementia and life-threatening central nervous system (CNS) infections. As with other lentiviruses, HIV enters microglial cells of the CNS early in the course of HIV infection. This process may be associated with neuronal vacuolization, cell loss, and occasional lymphocytic infiltration. Both direct neuronal destruction and effects of viral proteins on neuronal cell function may contribute to nervous system disease in AIDS.

Cognitive Dysfunction

Intellectual impairment rarely occurs early in HIV infection, but subtle changes (decreased learning accuracy and learning speed) may be present in patients with only moderate immunodeficiency, and more striking changes often occur with advanced immunodeficiency. AIDS dementia complex (ADC) often begins insidiously and usually progresses over months to years (Table 108-11). ADC is characterized by poor concentration, diminished memory, slowing of thought processes, motor dysfunction, and occasionally behavioral abnormalities characterized by social withdrawal and apathy. Symptoms of clinical depression overlap with many of the characteristics of early ADC and must be considered carefully in differential diagnosis and therapy. Computed tomography (CT) of the head in ADC reveals only atrophy, with enlarged sulci and ventricles, but these findings do not reliably predict cognitive deficits. CSF is most often normal on examination.

Table 108-10 **HIV-Associated Esophagitis**		
Condition	**Characteristics**	**Treatment**
Candida infection	Thrush usual, esophageal plaques	Fluconazole, 400 mg/day
CMV infection	Large, shallow esophageal ulcers on endoscopy	Ganciclovir, 5 mg/kg IV bid
Herpes simplex	Deep ulceration on endoscopy	Acyclovir, 800 mg 5 times/day
Aphthae	Giant ulcers on endoscopy; no virus on biopsy	Prednisone, 40-60 mg/day, or thalidomide, 200 mg/day*

*Thalidomide must never be given during pregnancy or when pregnancy is possible.
CMV, cytomegalovirus.

Table 108-11	**Major Clinical Manifestations of AIDS Dementia Complex**	
	Early	**Late**
Cognition	Inattention, reduced concentration, forgetfulness, impaired memory	Global dementia
Motor performance	Slowed movements, clumsiness, ataxia	Paraplegia
Behavior	Apathy, altered personality, agitation	Mutism

Motor abnormalities may include a progressive gait ataxia. As the disease progresses, patients may develop focal neurologic complications characterized by spastic weakness of the lower extremities and incontinence secondary to vacuolar myelopathy.

Focal Lesions of the Central Nervous System

A large variety of neurologic problems may complicate the later stages of HIV infection. A neuroanatomic classification of these manifestations is presented in Table 108-12. Several of the more frequent or treatable problems are discussed here and in the next section.

Several opportunistic complications of HIV infection produce focal CNS lesions. Patients with focal neurologic signs, seizures of new onset, or recent onset of rapidly progressive cognitive impairment should undergo magnetic resonance imaging (MRI) and/or CT of the brain. Toxoplasmosis, CNS lymphoma, and progressive multifocal leukoencephalopathy (PML) are the most common causes of CNS focal lesions in this setting (Table 108-13).

In the absence of ART, *T. gondii* encephalitis occurs in up to one third of HIV-infected patients who have serologic evidence of *T. gondii* infection but is rare in individuals who have no such antibodies. Patients often have progressive headache and focal neurologic abnormalities, usually associated with fever. CT with contrast dye usually shows multiple ring-enhancing lesions. MRI is a more sensitive technique and often shows multiple small lesions not apparent on CT. Management of symptomatic, ring-enhancing brain lesions in persons with AIDS includes initiation of empirical therapy with pyrimethamine, sulfadiazine, and folinic acid. Brain biopsy should be reserved for patients with atypical presentations, those with no serum antibodies to *T. gondii*, or those whose lesions do not respond after 10 to 14 days of antiprotozoal treatment. After the initial response, patients must remain on chronic suppressive therapy until a sustained rise in CD4 count above 200 cells/mm^3 is achieved with effective ART.

Primary CNS lymphoma complicates advanced HIV infection in 3% to 6% of cases and is almost invariably associated with detectable EBV DNA in the CSF (see Table 108-13). Lesions may be single or multiple and are often weakly ring enhancing. Irradiation often provides remission, which may be sustained as immune function is restored by effective ART.

PML is a demyelinating disease caused by a papovavirus (JC virus). Presenting signs and symptoms may include progressive dementia, visual impairment, seizures, and/or

Table 108-12	**Neuroanatomic Classification of the Common Complications of HIV Infection**

Meningitis and Headache

Aseptic meningitis
Cryptococcal meningitis
Tuberculous meningitis

Diffuse Brain Diseases

With Preservation of Consciousness

AIDS dementia complex

With Concomitant Depression of Arousal

Toxoplasma encephalitis
Cytomegalovirus encephalitis

Focal Brain Diseases

Cerebral toxoplasmosis
Primary central nervous system lymphoma
Progressive multifocal leukoencephalopathy
Tuberculous brain abscess (*Mycobacterium tuberculosis*)

Myelopathies

Subacute or chronic progressive vacuolar myelopathy
Cytomegalovirus myelopathy

Peripheral Neuropathies

Predominantly sensory polyneuropathy
Toxic neuropathies (zalcitabine, didanosine, stavudine)
Autonomic neuropathy
Cytomegalovirus polyradiculopathy

Myopathies

Noninflammatory myopathy
Zidovudine myopathy

hemiparesis. MRI usually shows multiple lesions predominantly involving the white matter. These lesions are usually less visible on CT than on MRI and are not ring enhancing, which helps to distinguish PML from other mass lesions of the CNS. There is no effective specific treatment for PML; the disease often, but not always, regresses in response to effective ART.

Central Nervous System Diseases without Prominent Focal Signs

Evaluation of the HIV-infected patient with fever and headache is difficult because of the often subtle manifestations of serious CNS lesions in immunocompromised patients. Patients with bacterial meningitis (see Chapter 97) are managed as are noncompromised patients. Meningeal diseases in HIV-infected patients often, however, fall into the broad categories of aseptic meningitis, chronic meningitis, and meningoencephalitis.

Aseptic Meningitis

Patients with aseptic meningitis, which may be a manifestation of the acute retroviral syndrome, complain most often of headache; their sensorium is generally intact, and findings on neurologic examination are normal (see Chapter 97). In the person with established HIV infection, aseptic meningitis may result from several potentially treatable causes (see Chapters 97 and 107).

Chronic Meningitis

Patients with chronic meningitis characteristically have headache, fever, difficulty in concentrating, and/or changes

Table 108-13 Comparative Clinical and Radiologic Features of Cerebral Toxoplasmosis, Primary Central Nervous System Lymphoma, and Progressive Multifocal Leukoencephalopathy

	Clinical Onset			Neuroradiologic Features		
Condition	**Temporal Profile**	**Level of Alertness**	**Fever**	**Number of Lesions**	**Characteristics of Lesions**	**Location of Lesions**
Cerebral toxoplasmosis	Days	Reduced	Common	Usually multiple	Spheric, ring-enhancing on CT	Basal ganglia, cortex
Primary CNS lymphoma	Days to weeks	Variable	Absent	One or few	Irregular, weakly enhancing on CT	Periventricular
Progressive multifocal leukoencephalopathy	Weeks to months	Variable	Absent	Often multiple	Multiple lesions, visible on MRI	White matter

CNS, central nervous system; CT, computed tomography; MRI, magnetic resonance imaging.

in sensorium. CSF examination shows low glucose concentration, elevated protein level, and mild to modest lymphocytic pleocytosis. Cryptococcal meningitis is the most common type. The presence of cryptococcal antigen in serum or CSF or a positive CSF India ink preparation establishes the diagnosis (see Chapter 97). Treatment with amphotericin B for at least 2 weeks followed by high-dose fluconazole is usually effective. Serial lumbar punctures, with removal of CSF to decrease intracranial pressure, may be necessary in the early management of cryptococcal meningitis.

Mycobacterium tuberculosis is an eminently treatable cause of subacute or chronic meningitis in the HIV-infected patient, although rare in North America. Antituberculosis therapy should be considered in the setting of chronic meningitis if the cryptococcal antigen test is negative (see Chapter 97).

Coccidioides immitis or *Histoplasma capsulatum* may cause subacute or chronic meningitis in patients residing in, or with a travel history to, endemic regions (desert Southwest or Ohio and Mississippi River drainage areas, respectively) (see Chapter 97).

Meningoencephalitis

Patients with meningoencephalitis manifest alterations in sensorium varying from mild lethargy to coma. Patients are usually febrile, and neurologic examination often shows evidence of diffuse CNS involvement. CT or MRI may show only nonspecific abnormalities, whereas electroencephalography often is consistent with diffuse disease of the brain.

CMV encephalitis is rare and difficult to diagnose. Patients may demonstrate confusion, cranial nerve abnormalities, or long tract signs. CSF findings may resemble those of bacterial meningitis, with a modest polymorphonuclear leukocyte pleocytosis and depressed CSF glucose levels. CT scan or MRI may reveal periventricular abnormalities. Many patients have associated CMV retinitis. PCR detection of CMV DNA in CSF appears to be a sensitive and specific method for diagnosis of CMV encephalitis and polyradiculopathy.

Meningoencephalitis caused by HSV is unusual in HIV infection (see Chapter 97).

PULMONARY DISEASES

Pulmonary infections are common in persons living with HIV and range from nonspecific interstitial pneumonitis to life-threatening pneumonias (Table 108-14).

HIV-infected patients have a threefold to fourfold increased risk of bacterial pneumonia, generally caused by encapsulated bacteria, including *S. pneumoniae* and *H. influenzae*. The increased risk begins with modest degrees of immunodeficiency (CD4 counts of 200 to 500 cells/mm^3). The onset is often abrupt, and the response to prompt initiation of therapy is usually good; however, delay in appropriate antimicrobial therapy may result in a fulminant downhill course. Initial therapy is guided by the results of Gram stain of sputum (see Chapter 99).

Pneumonia caused by PCP remains a common life-threatening infection in North American persons with AIDS. Patients frequently complain of gradual onset of nonproductive cough, fever, and shortness of breath with exertion; a productive cough suggests another process. A substernal "catch" with inspiration is common and suggestive of PCP. In contrast to the acute onset of PCP in other immunocompromised patients, AIDS patients with PCP may have pulmonary symptoms for weeks before presentation to a physician. Arterial hypoxemia is usual and rapidly worsens with slight exertion, and oxygen desaturation with exercise as measured by pulse oximetry can be used to suggest the diagnosis. The chest radiograph often shows a subtle interstitial pattern but may be entirely normal. The patient often appears more sick than the radiograph would suggest. The presence of pleural effusions is suggestive of a cause other than PCP.

If PCP is suspected clinically, therapy should be started immediately; treatment for several days does not interfere with the ability to make a specific diagnosis. Confirmation of PCP is essential; delay in establishing a correct diagnosis of another treatable condition may be lethal. Some experienced centers, by Giemsa or direct fluorescent-antibody stain of induced sputum, may confirm the diagnosis, although many patients are unable to produce a specimen. Alternatively, bronchoalveolar lavage with silver or immunofluorescence staining is adequate to diagnose PCP in more than 95% of patients.

Treatment with high-dose trimethoprim-sulfamethoxazole for 3 weeks is effective therapy (see Table 108-14). Patients with advanced PCP and arterial hypoxemia (oxygen tension 75 mm on breathing of room air) benefit from administration of corticosteroids (40 mg of prednisone twice daily), with tapering of the drug over a 3-week period.

As with acute bacterial pneumonia, active pulmonary tuberculosis may develop at a time when the CD4 count

Table 108-14 Pulmonary Disease Associated with HIV Infection

Condition	Characteristic	Chest Radiograph	Diagnosis	Treatment
Pneumocystis jirovecii pneumonia	Subacute onset, dry cough, dyspnea	Interstitial infiltrate most common	Sputum or bronchoalveolar lavage for organism by stain	Trimethoprim-sulfamethoxazole, pentamidine, or atovaquone or primaquine + clindamycin
Bacterial (pneumococcus, *Haemophilus* most common)	Acute onset, productive cough, fever, chest pain	Lobar or localized infiltrate	Sputum Gram stain and culture, blood culture	Cefuroxime or alternative antibiotics
Mycobacterial (*Mycobacterium tuberculosis* or *Mycobacterium kansasii*)	Chronic cough, weight loss, fever	Localized infiltrate, lymphadenopathy	Sputum acid-fast stain and mycobacterial culture	Isoniazid, rifampin, pyrazinamide, ethambutol
Kaposi sarcoma	Asymptomatic or mild cough	Pulmonary nodules, pleural effusion	Open lung biopsy	Chemotherapy

remains well above 200 cells/mm³ (see Table 108-4). Chest radiographs in HIV-infected patients may show features of primary tuberculosis, including hilar adenopathy, lower or middle lobe infiltrates, miliary pattern, or pleural effusions, as well as classic patterns of reactivation. Extrapulmonary *M. tuberculosis* infection also occurs with increased frequency with advanced immunodeficiency.

Both pulmonary and extrapulmonary tuberculosis generally respond promptly to standard antituberculosis therapy. Treatment therefore should begin with four antituberculosis drugs (see Chapter 99).

Disseminated histoplasmosis and coccidioidomycosis occur with much greater frequency in persons with HIV infection. Either fungal infection may cause nodular infiltrates or a miliary pattern on chest radiograph. Histoplasmosis usually involves bone marrow as well as skin; bone marrow examination often shows the organism. Standard treatment of disseminated mycoses in AIDS patients is high-dose amphotericin. Because relapse is common, oral azole therapy (fluconazole for coccidioidomycosis, itraconazole for histoplasmosis) must be continued after resolution of signs and symptoms. In patients treated for histoplasmosis receiving suppressive ART for at least 6 months, this secondary prophylaxis may be discontinued after 1 year of therapy, provided that the CD4 count is 150 cells/μL, blood cultures are negative, and the serum *Histoplasma* antigen titers are low. Patients treated for systemic, meningeal, or diffuse pulmonary coccidioidomycosis have a greater risk of relapse and should likely continue indefinite suppressive therapy. In patients with localized pneumonia receiving successful ART and with sustained CD4 counts of 250 cells/mcL, on the other hand, cautious interruption of secondary prophylaxis after 1 year of treatment is a reasonable option.

GASTROINTESTINAL DISEASES

HIV affects the gastrointestinal tract early in infection, with profound depletion of memory CD4 T cells in GALT within the first few weeks of infection. Symptomatic disease of the gut is, however, unusual in the early stage of infection.

With advanced immunodeficiency (CD4 count <50 cells/mm³), gastrointestinal disease manifesting as dysphagia (see Table 108-10), diarrhea, or colitis is common. Each process may contribute to inadequate nutrition, compounding the weight loss associated with advanced HIV disease. Nausea and vomiting are often related to medications; these must be reviewed, and the likely offending drug (or drugs) withheld as a therapeutic trial. If symptoms of nausea and vomiting do not respond to empirical therapy with histamine-2 (H₂) antagonists or antiemetics, more extensive gastrointestinal evaluation is indicated.

Abnormalities of liver function tests are common in HIV disease and often are nonspecific. Elevations of serum alanine aminotransferase and aspartate aminotransferase often represent chronic active hepatitis B or C but may reflect hepatic inflammation caused by medications, including trimethoprim-sulfamethoxazole and/or antiretroviral agents. Marked elevations in serum alkaline phosphatase levels may reflect infiltrative disease of the liver (e.g., MAI or CMV) but also may occur in patients with acalculous cholecystitis, cryptosporidiosis, or AIDS-associated sclerosing cholangitis.

DIARRHEA

Diarrhea occurs, at least intermittently, in many persons with advanced immunodeficiency and may be caused by a variety of microorganisms (Table 108-15) as well as by certain antiretroviral therapies. In many instances, no clear cause is found. Stool specimens should be cultured for the common bacterial pathogens. *Salmonella*, *Campylobacter*, and *Yersinia* species are frequent causes; patients usually respond to standard antimicrobial therapy (see Chapter 103). Patients may also have recurrent episodes of diarrhea associated with *Clostridium difficile* toxin; this probably reflects the frequent use of broad-spectrum antibiotics.

In cases of persistent diarrhea, a fresh stool specimen should be examined for parasites, using a modified acid-fast stain for *Cryptosporidium parvum*, microsporidia, and *Isospora belli*, the most common enteric protozoal infections in

Table 108-15 **Diarrhea in Advanced HIV Infection**			
Cause	**Characteristics**	**Diagnosis**	**Treatment**
Frequent			
Cryptosporidium parvum	Varies from increased frequency to large-volume diarrhea	Acid-fast stain of stool	Nitazoxanide, 100 mg bid; antiretroviral therapy
Clostridium difficile	Abdominal pain, fever common	*C. difficile* toxin in stool or endoscopy	Metronidazole or vancomycin
Cytomegalovirus	Small bowel movements with blood or mucus (colitis)	Colonoscopy and biopsy	Ganciclovir
Mycobacterium avium-intracellulare	Abdominal pain, fever, retroperitoneal lymphadenopathy	Blood culture or endoscopy with biopsy	Multidrug regimen, including clarithromycin; ethambutol
Less Frequent			
Salmonella or *Campylobacter*	Sometimes with blood or mucus in bowel movements (colitis)	Stool culture	A fluoroquinolone (check sensitivities)
Microsporidia	Watery diarrhea	Calcofluor white or trichrome staining of stool; electron microscopy of biopsy material	Albendazole, antiretroviral therapy
Isospora belli	Watery diarrhea	Acid-fast stain of stool	Trimethoprim-sulfamethoxazole

AIDS patients. Microsporidium infection often requires biopsy with electron microscopy for diagnosis. Although cryptosporidiosis may be self-limited, massive diarrhea (up to 10 L/day) may occur. Isosporiasis responds to oral trimethoprim-sulfamethoxazole, and several microsporidial species to albendazole. Symptoms of both cryptosporidiosis and isosporiasis resolve in response to effective ART.

If stool diagnostic studies are negative and diarrhea persists, patients should undergo endoscopy (see Chapter 34). Biopsy of the duodenum or small bowel may show histologic evidence of cryptosporidial, microsporidial, MAI, or CMV infection. Biopsy of the colon may be indicative of HSV proctitis, CMV colitis, or MAI infection. For patients with refractory diarrhea, symptomatic treatment may improve the quality of life.

VIRAL HEPATITIS

Because of common routes of transmission, HIV-infected persons have a much greater prevalence of hepatitis B and hepatitis C infection than the general population. With improved survival as a result of effective ART, the consequences of liver disease from these viruses have become increasingly apparent. HIV co-infection alters the natural history of viral hepatitis, leading to more rapid progression to end-stage liver disease, greater infectiousness, and diminished response to specific treatments. Conversely, co-infection with hepatitis viruses may have deleterious consequences on the natural history of HIV disease and may compromise the effectiveness of ART. Thus, all HIV-infected patients should be screened for viral hepatitis co-infection, and immunized against those that are preventable by vaccination. Treatment of viral hepatitis and HIV co-infection is best done in consultation with an expert, as management of the combinations of drugs required in these circumstances is complex. It is especially important to screen for active hepatitis B co-infection before initiating antiretroviral therapies, as some agents (e.g., lamivudine, emtricitabine, tenofovir) are also active against hepatitis B virus and may select for resistance mutations when used injudiciously.

UNEXPLAINED FEVER

Most persistent fevers late in the course of HIV infection reflect a definable OI.

The most common cause of unexplained fever and anemia in patients with CD4 counts less than 50 cells/mm^3 is disseminated MAI infection. This may be diagnosed by bone marrow biopsy, but blood cultures in *Mycobacterium*-selective media are usually positive. Treatment (see Table 108-8) usually results in resolution of fever and weight gain.

Aggressive non-Hodgkin lymphoma may cause unexplained fever and weight loss. A rapidly enlarging spleen or asymmetrical lymph node enlargement may suggest the diagnosis. CT-guided biopsy of enlarged intra-abdominal nodes may provide the diagnosis.

WASTING

Cachexia may be prominent in advanced HIV disease. In some instances the wasting is caused by an intercurrent infectious process. Heightened production of tumor necrosis factor may contribute to fever, cachexia, and hypertriglyceridemia in advanced HIV disease.

If orthostatic hypotension occurs, especially if associated with hyperkalemia, the possibility of adrenal insufficiency, which rarely can result from CMV adrenalitis, should be investigated (see Chapter 67).

Most patients with AIDS-associated cachexia gain weight and achieve a sense of well-being after initiation of effective ART. In instances where cachexia is refractory, weight gain may be enhanced by administration of recombinant growth hormone, nonmethylated androgens, or megestrol, but definitive indications for these therapies have not been established.

ACQUIRED IMMUNODEFICIENCY SYNDROME–ASSOCIATED MALIGNANCIES

Among HIV-infected MSM, the frequency of Kaposi sarcoma fell from 40% at the outset of the epidemic to less than 15% in 1999. Human herpesvirus–8 is the causative agent. In many instances, lesions resolve after institution of effective ART. Systemic chemotherapy can cause remission in many patients with symptomatic visceral disease.

Non-Hodgkin lymphomas (largely B cell, with small non-cleaved or immunoblastic histology) occur 150 to 250 times more often in HIV-infected persons than in the general population. Up to 40% of AIDS-related systemic lymphomas, but virtually all of those in a primary CNS location, are related to EBV. Extranodal presentation of these tumors is the rule, with a high frequency of gastrointestinal or intracranial presentation. Chemotherapy for systemic disease or radiation therapy for CNS disease generally provides a clinical response, which may be maintained if accompanied by effective ART. Other malignancies, including Hodgkin disease, have increased incidence in untreated HIV-infected patients. More recently, and with more treated persons surviving with subclinical immune deficiency, an increasing incidence of a variety of non-AIDS–defining malignancies is being observed. The risk of these other cancers is greater in persons with lower CD4 counts, and incidence is expected to increase with time.

Renal Disorders

Renal insufficiency in AIDS patients may be a consequence of nephrotoxic drug administration, heroin injection, or HIV-associated nephropathy (HIVAN). Renal biopsy is indicated to establish a diagnosis, as certain histologic features such as focal and segmental glomerulosclerosis may distinguish HIVAN from renal failure associated with intravenous heroin use and from other causes of renal failure. In the United States, HIVAN is almost exclusively seen in African Americans and usually manifests as heavy proteinuria and progressive renal insufficiency. Without treatment, most patients develop end-stage renal disease within several months. Short-term, high-dose corticosteroid therapy may slow the progression of HIVAN, but treatment with combination antiretroviral therapies is indicated in this setting, irrespective of CD4 cell count, to arrest the course of this disease. The incidence of this complication has also been decreased by the availability of effective ART.

Rheumatologic Disorders

Musculoskeletal complaints are common; the relationship of circulating autoantibodies to these manifestations is not known. Muscle weakness, if localized, may be indicative of myelopathy-neuropathy (see Table 108-12). When weakness is proximal or is associated with myalgia and tenderness, myopathy should be suspected. The myopathy may be HIV associated or may, rarely, represent zidovudine toxicity. On muscle biopsy, inflammatory changes are more prominent in AIDS-associated myopathy, whereas mitochondrial abnormalities predominate in zidovudine-related myopathy. Arthralgias are common; both a Reiter-like syndrome and a Sjögren-like syndrome occur with increased frequency.

Prevention of Human Immunodeficiency Virus Infection

Three approaches—behavioral modification, treatment of STDs, and ART of seropositive pregnant women—can have a major impact on HIV transmission. In addition, the identification of HIV-infected individuals through HIV counseling and testing remains a cornerstone of prevention efforts.

In several communities at increased risk for HIV (e.g., homosexually active men in the United States and Western Europe, young adults in Uganda and Thailand), adoption of safer sexual practices, specifically the use of condoms during sexual activity, has been associated with a decrease in incidence of HIV infection. Sustaining these behavioral changes over long periods requires behavioral reinforcement.

Several recent controlled trials have demonstrated that male circumcision can decrease, by more than half, the risk of acquiring HIV infection.

Antiretroviral treatment of HIV-infected pregnant women and of their infants during the peripartum period has decreased maternal-child transmission from 25% to less than 4% in North America, without harm to the newborn children.

The use of universal blood and body fluid precautions during the care of all patients irrespective of known HIV status is routinely recommended to protect health care workers. Meticulous attention to use and disposal of sharp instruments is most important, because most nosocomial acquisition of HIV infection has occurred through accidental needlesticks. Prompt administration of antiretroviral drugs is thought to significantly decrease the risk of HIV infection after needlestick injuries. Current provisional recommendations by the U.S. Public Health Service for prophylaxis after high-risk occupational exposure include a combination regimen of three effective antiretroviral drugs, initiated as soon as possible after exposure and continuing for 4 weeks (see www.cdc.gov/mmwr/preview/mmwrhtml/rr5409a1.htm).

The development of an effective vaccine is the target of active research. Early clinical trials of vaccine candidates are ongoing but to date have proved disappointing. Induction of brisk T-cell responses to HIV antigens has neither protected against HIV acquisition nor decreased the magnitude of HIV replication among vaccinated subjects. A legitimate goal for vaccines, the induction of antibody responses that can broadly inhibit or neutralize the infectivity of diverse HIV strains, has to date eluded vaccine developers. Thus other strategies to prevent HIV acquisition are urgently needed. Several agents designed to be applied topically to the anogenital tract (commonly referred to as *microbicides*) are in development as preventive interventions that can be controlled by sexually active persons at the time of high-risk exposures. Some of these agents have proven highly effective in preclinical studies, and some are now being tested in humans. Likewise, preexposure prophylaxis (PREP) strategies with antiretroviral drugs are also being tested among persons at risk for HIV acquisition.

Prospectus for the Future

- Development of more well-tolerated antiretroviral therapies active against drug-resistant strains
- New treatment strategies targeting additional stages of the viral life cycle
- Increased understanding of the mechanisms of disease progression and CD4 depletion
- Heightened awareness of and improved treatment modalities for long-term toxicities of antiretroviral agents
- Increased focus on immunotherapeutic interventions

- Development of new prophylactic and therapeutic vaccine strategies
- Testing of strategies to eradicate reservoirs of HIV
- Tests of novel microbicides
- Continuing evaluation of the optimal timing for starting antiretroviral therapy
- Continued surveillance for and optimized management of risks for long-term complications of treated HIV infection such as cardiovascular and neoplastic events

References

Aberg JA, Gallant JE, Anderson J, et al: Primary care guidelines for the management of persons infected with human immunodeficiency virus: Recommendations of the HIV Medicine Association of the Infectious Diseases Society of America. Clin Infect Dis 39:609-629, 2004.

Castro KG, Ward JW, Slutsker L, et al: 1993 Revised classification system for HIV infection and expanded surveillance case definition for AIDS among adolescents and adults. Morbidity & Mortality Weekly Report Recomm Rep 41(RR-17):1-19, 1992.

DHHS Panel on Clinical Practices for Treatment of HIV Infection: Guidelines for the use of antiretroviral agents in HIV-infected adults and adolescents. Bethesda, Department of Health and Human Services, November 3, 2008, p. 139. Available at: http://aidsinfo.nih.gov/guidelines/.

Egger M, May M, Chene G, et al: Prognosis of HIV-1–infected patients starting highly active antiretroviral therapy: a collaborative analysis of prospective studies. Lancet 360:119-129, 2002.

Hammer SM, Eron JJ Jr, Reiss P, et al: Antiretroviral Treatment of Adult HIV Infection 2008: Recommendations of the International AIDS Society–USA Panel. JAMA 300:555-570, 2008.

Hirsch M, Brun-Vézinet F, D'Aquila RT, et al: Antiretroviral drug testing in adult HIV-1 infection. JAMA 283:2417-2426, 2000.

Lederman MM, Nicholson A, Cho M, Mosier D: Biology of CCR5 and its role in HIV infection and treatment. JAMA 296:815-26, 2006.

Masur H, Kaplan JE, Holmes KK, et al: Guidelines for preventing opportunistic infections among HIV-infected persons—2002: Recommendations of the U.S. Public Health Service and the Infectious Diseases Society of America. MMWR Recomm Rep 51:1-52, 2002.

Masur H, Kaplan JE, Holmes KK, et al: Guidelines for Prevention and Treatment of Opportunistic Infections in HIV-Infected Adults and Adolescents. National Institutes of Health, June 18, 2008, p 286. Available at: http://AIDSinfo.nih.gov.

Mellors J, Munoz AM, Giorgi VJ, et al: Plasma viral load and CD4 lymphocytes as prognostic markers of HIV-1 infection. Ann Intern Med 126:946-954, 1997.

Palella FJ, Delaney KM, Moorman AC, et al: Declining morbidity and mortality among patients with advanced human immunodeficiency virus infection. N Engl J Med 338:853-860, 1998.

Scheld WM: HIV and the acquired immunodeficiency syndrome. In Goldman L, Bennett JC (eds): Cecil Textbook of Medicine, 22nd ed. Philadelphia, Elsevier, 2004, pp 2136-2137.

Skiest DJ: Focal neurological disease in patients with acquired immunodeficiency syndrome. Clin Infect Dis 34:103-115, 2002.

Infections in the Immunocompromised Host

Tracy Lemonovich, David A. Bobak, and Robert A. Salata

Immunosuppression is an increasingly common byproduct of diseases and modern approaches to their treatment. The immunocompromised host has increased susceptibility to *opportunistic infection,* defined as infection caused by organisms of low virulence that constitute normal mucosal and skin flora or by pathogenic microbial agents that are usually maintained in a latent state. Compromised hosts include patients with congenital immunodeficiencies, those infected with human immunodeficiency virus (HIV), and those who are immunocompromised as a consequence of cancer and its treatment, bone marrow failure, or treatment with steroids, cytotoxic therapy, or other immunosuppressive agents.

Immunocompromise is not an all-or-nothing phenomenon. The extent of immunosuppression varies with the underlying cause and must exceed a threshold to predispose the individual to opportunistic infections. Analysis of the type of immunosuppression can help predict the spectrum and types of agents likely to cause infections in an individual patient. Accordingly, opportunistic infections are usually considered in categories that reflect the nature of the immune deficiency. An important point to remember, however, is that most patients have several interacting risk factors that may cause combinations of defects affecting several different aspects of host defense and immune function.

Disorders of Cell-Mediated Immunity

Cell-mediated immunity is the major host defense against facultative and some obligate intracellular pathogens (see also Chapter 92). A partial list of diseases and conditions that impair cell-mediated immunity is presented in Table 109-1. However, only a certain number of these conditions result in increased susceptibility to infection with intracellular pathogens. Several forms of congenital immunodeficiencies are associated with severe infections early in childhood (Table 109-2). Foremost among the acquired immunodeficiencies are HIV infection, Hodgkin disease and other lymphomas, hairy cell leukemia, and disseminated solid tumors. Severe malnutrition, as well as treatment with high-dose corticosteroids, cytotoxic drugs, or radiation therapy, can produce a similar predilection to infections. Patients with impaired cell-mediated immunity are especially susceptible to the types of organisms shown in Table 109-3 (**Web Figs. 109-1** to **109-8**).

The relative frequency of infection varies with the underlying disease (e.g., *Mycobacterium avium* complex is common in HIV infection, whereas *Listeria* is not), the geographic area (*Mycobacterium tuberculosis* is more common in developing countries than in developed countries), and the extent and type of immunosuppression (*M. tuberculosis* is an early, and *M. avium* complex a late, complication of HIV infection). Immunosuppressive medications vary greatly in their potency and mechanisms of action. In addition, the duration of immunosuppressive therapy is as important as the potency of the medication in assessing potential risk for opportunistic infection. For example, a patient receiving relatively high doses of corticosteroids for a short period (e.g., for an allergic reaction) is at much less risk for infection compared with a patient with an autoimmune disease receiving much lower doses of the same agent for a prolonged period.

Depression of cell-mediated immunity also permits organisms ordinarily constituting the normal flora, such as *Candida* species, to act as virulent opportunistic pathogens capable of causing aggressive infections. Latent viruses, fungi, mycobacteria, and parasites can reactivate to cause locally progressive or disseminated disease. In many instances the signs, symptoms, and laboratory abnormalities indicating an infection are subtle and nonspecific, an important

Table 109-1	**Conditions Causing Impaired Cell-Mediated Immunity**

Infectious Diseases

Measles
Chickenpox
Human immunodeficiency virus
Typhoid fever
Tuberculosis
Leprosy
Histoplasmosis

Malignant Diseases

Hodgkin disease
Lymphomas
Advanced solid tumors

Vaccinations

Measles
Mumps
Rubella

Drugs

Corticosteroids
Cytotoxic drugs
Antirejection drugs and antilymphocyte antibodies used for organ transplant patients
Monoclonal antibodies targeting tumor necrosis factor–α (e.g., infliximab, etanercept)

Miscellaneous

Congenital immunodeficiency states
Sarcoidosis
Uremia
Diabetes mellitus
Malnutrition

Table 109-2	**Examples of Congenital Immunodeficiency Syndromes**

Severe combined immunodeficiency (SCID)
  X-linked SCID
  Adenosine deaminase deficiency
  Purine-nucleosidase phosphorylase deficiency
  Zeta-associated protein (ZAP)-70 kinase deficiency
Wiskott-Aldrich syndrome
DiGeorge syndrome
Ataxia telangiectasia

Table 109-3	**Agents Commonly Causing Infections in Patients with Impaired Cell-Mediated Immunity**

Viruses

Varicella-zoster virus
Herpes simplex virus
Cytomegalovirus **(Web Fig. 109-8)**
Epstein-Barr virus
JC virus
Human herpesvirus 6
Human herpesvirus 8
Respiratory viruses (e.g., influenza, parainfluenza, adenovirus, respiratory syncytial virus)

Bacteria

Listeria monocytogenes
Salmonella species
Legionella species
Nocardia species
Mycobacterium tuberculosis
Nontuberculous mycobacteria

Fungi

Pathogenic: *Histoplasma, Coccidioides, Blastomyces* **(Web Fig. 109-4)**
Saprophytic: *Cryptococcus* **(Web Fig. 109-5)**, *Candida, Pneumocystis jirovecii* **(Web Fig. 109-6)**; less commonly, *Aspergillus* **(Web Fig. 109-1)**, *Zygomycetes* **(Web Fig. 109-2 and Web Fig. 109-3)**

Protozoa

Cryptosporidium parvum
Leishmania donovani
Toxoplasma gondii **(Web Fig. 109-7)**

Helminths

Strongyloides stercoralis

---

distinction to the clinical presentations commonly observed in immunocompetent patients.

In some instances, treatment of the underlying disease causing the immunodeficiency, or progression of the disease itself, produces an increased severe and generalized compromised state, one that predisposes the individual to infection by additional types of microorganisms. For example, during chemotherapy for lymphoma, bacterial infections initially predominate. Disease progression may also alter other factors that favor bacterial infections, such as mucosal breakdown and obstruction by tumor masses of the bronchi, the ureters, or the biliary tract. The result is a marked increase in severe bacterial infection and sepsis syndrome, often caused by multiple-resistant pathogens, late in the course of many diseases associated with impaired cell-mediated immunity.

Disorders of Humoral Immunity

The acquired disorders of antibody production associated with increased frequency of infection in adults are common variable immunodeficiency, chronic lymphocytic leukemia, lymphosarcoma, multiple myeloma, nephrotic syndrome, major burns, and protein-losing enteropathy. The paraproteinemic states belong in this category because of secondary decreases in levels of functioning antibody. Therapy with cytotoxic drugs may produce similar immunocompromised states.

Infections with pneumococci, *Haemophilus influenzae*, meningococci, streptococci, and staphylococci predominate early in the course of the humoral immunodeficiency. As the underlying disease itself progresses, infections with gram-negative bacilli become increasingly frequent. Treatment of the underlying condition with corticosteroids and cytotoxic drugs causes additional defects in cell-mediated immunity and provides susceptibility to infections with the group of pathogens presented in Table 109-3. Some agents predicted to alter humoral immunity may have unexpected effects. For example, the monoclonal antibody rituximab, used for treating certain types of lymphoma, profoundly depletes B lymphocytes but causes increased risk of hepatitis B reactivation, rather than increased risk of infection by the bacterial pathogens outlined previously.

In sickle cell anemia, heat-labile opsonic activity is diminished. Complement depletion by erythrocyte stroma impairs opsonization of pneumococci and *Salmonella* species and leads to frequent infections with these organisms. Impaired reticuloendothelial system function resulting from erythrophagocytosis and functional asplenia also predisposes patients with sickle cell disease to other serious bacterial infections. The predisposition to infection is related to age; once children with sickle cell disease develop antibodies to pneumococcal capsular polysaccharide, they lose their thousand-fold increased susceptibility to severe pneumococcal infection.

Splenectomy results in a loss of mechanisms for the clearing of opsonized organisms. Splenectomy therefore predisposes patients to fulminant infections caused by encapsulated bacteria. Over a period of years, the liver may partially compensate for certain aspects of splenic function. The splenic tissue also represents a major source of production of antibody, as well as other opsonic factors such as tuftsin, which opsonizes staphylococci. Splenectomized patients are also predisposed to severe and overwhelming infection with *Capnocytophaga* species (found in canine oral flora) and additionally have an increased risk for acquiring babesiosis. Pneumococcal, meningococcal, and possibly *H. influenzae* type b (Hib) vaccines should be administered to adult patients who will be undergoing splenectomy or who have diseases likely to produce functional asplenia. The newer protein conjugate forms of the pneumococcal and meningococcal vaccines may offer increased response rates for splenectomized or functionally asplenic patients. Although the 7-valent pneumococcal conjugate vaccine is currently recommended only for children, with the 23-valent polysaccharide vaccine used for high-risk adults and the elderly (including asplenic patients), the conjugate vaccine has been shown to decrease invasive pneumococcal disease in older adults by herd immunity. Conjugate meningococcal vaccine is recommended for asplenic adults <55 years of age. There is no specific recommendation for the conjugate Hib vaccine in this population, as efficacy is unknown, but the use of the vaccine should be considered. Fever in a patient with asplenia should immediately raise concern for possible underlying sepsis, and such a patient should be immediately treated with empirical antibiotics pending results of cultures and laboratory tests.

Impaired Neutrophil Function

Many types of inherited or acquired diseases impair neutrophil function. The defect may be extrinsic or intrinsic to the neutrophil itself. For example, impaired chemotaxis predisposes patients with inherited C3 and C5 deficiencies to frequent bacterial infections (see also Chapter 92). Corticosteroid therapy is generally associated with defective cell-mediated immunity (see previous discussion) but may also interfere with neutrophil chemotaxis. Even though circulating neutrophil counts are frequently normal or increased in patients receiving corticosteroids, these cells do not localize normally to the site of infection. Leukocyte adhesion deficiencies are caused by mutations in leukocyte integrins needed for binding to endothelial intercellular adhesion molecules, with resulting lack of neutrophils at sites of infection despite elevated serum neutrophil counts. Many other illnesses and conditions are associated with impaired neutrophil function, including myelodysplasia, paroxysmal nocturnal hemoglobinuria, radiation therapy, and cytotoxic drug therapy.

Inherited intrinsic defects in neutrophils are rare but have provided insights into understanding the microbicidal mechanisms of these cells. Neutrophils from patients with chronic granulomatous disease (CGD) cannot develop an oxidative burst. Catalase-negative organisms produce sufficient hydrogen peroxide to facilitate their own killing by CGD neutrophils via the myeloperoxidase pathway. Catalase-producing organisms such as staphylococci, *Serratia*, *Nocardia*, and *Aspergillus*, however, scavenge hydrogen peroxide. These organisms therefore cannot be killed effectively by neutrophils from patients with CGD, and serious recurrent infections can result.

The most severe intrinsic neutrophil defects occur in the Chédiak-Higashi syndrome. The neutrophils of patients with this syndrome have giant and abnormal granules and also exhibit defective microtubule assembly. These defects together cause impaired chemotaxis, abnormal phagolysosomal fusion, and delayed bacterial killing, predisposing patients to recurrent infections. Other phenotypic abnormalities often associated with this rare syndrome include partial albinism, depigmentation of the iris, peripheral neuropathies, and nystagmus.

Neutropenia

Neutropenia is one of the most common and most important risk factors for serious infection in the compromised host. Other alterations in host defense mechanisms frequently coexist with neutropenia, and these additional alterations often further increase the risk of infection. Most data regarding the incidence of fever and risk of infection associated with neutropenia come from studies of patients with leukemia undergoing cytotoxic chemotherapy. As the neutrophil count falls below 500/mcL, an exponential increase occurs in both the frequency and severity of associated infections. Neutrophil counts between 100 and 500/mcL are frequently associated with infections, whereas with neutrophil counts below 100/mcL, fever and some form of infection are almost universal. The duration of neutropenia is also important in determining the level of risk and types of infections in individual patients.

Chemotherapy-associated neutropenia in acute leukemia is usually profound and sustained and occurs in conjunction with other predisposing factors for infection such as mucositis and the presence of indwelling central venous catheters. These patients therefore become susceptible to organisms that are ubiquitous in the environment and are part of the normal flora (Table 109-4). In contrast, in patients with chronic or cyclic neutropenias, the susceptibility to infection varies inversely with the monocyte count because these cells help substitute for some of the antibacterial capacity of the missing neutrophils. This type of neutropenia may be either hereditary (often resulting from neutrophil elastase

Table 109-4 Agents That Frequently Cause Infections in Neutropenic Patients

Viruses

Cytomegalovirus (Web Fig. 109-8)
Herpesviruses

Bacteria

Pseudomonas aeruginosa
Serratia
Enterobacter
Escherichia coli
Klebsiella
Staphylococcus aureus (including methicillin-resistant staphylococci)
Coagulase-negative staphylococci
Corynebacterium group JK
Viridans group streptococci (e.g., *Streptococcus mitis*)
Enterococci (including vancomycin-resistant enterococci)

Fungi

Candida, including non-*albicans* species
Pneumocystis jirovecii (Web Fig. 109-6)
Aspergillus (Web Fig. 109-1)
Zygomycetes (Web Fig. 109-2 and Web Fig. 109-3)

mutations) or acquired. In contrast to patients with acute neutropenia caused by chemotherapy, patients with chronic or cyclic neutropenia rarely have life-threatening infection or bacteremia. Common manifestations are recurrent digital and oral ulcers, perineal infections, and relatively low baseline neutrophil counts with more profoundly low nadirs.

Diagnostic Problems in the Compromised Host

PULMONARY INFILTRATES

Pneumonia and bloodstream infections represent the most serious forms of infection for most immunocompromised patients. The immunocompromised patient with pulmonary infiltrates presents a particularly difficult diagnostic problem. Pulmonary infiltrates can represent infection, extension of underlying tumor, a complication of chemotherapy, fluid overload, pulmonary infarction, hemorrhage, or any combination of these conditions. Because of the seriousness of the condition and the variety of possible causes, obtaining a specific diagnosis is essential. Unfortunately, noninvasive serodiagnostic tests are rarely helpful in this setting, and accurate diagnosis can often be made only by direct sampling and examination of lung tissue by bronchoalveolar lavage and/or biopsy.

The clinical setting and radiographic appearance of pulmonary infiltrates will influence the decision about whether to proceed with lung biopsy. For example, in patients with leukemia, parenchymal infiltrates occurring before or within 3 days of initiation of chemotherapy are usually caused by infection from common bacterial pathogens. Major efforts should be directed first at collecting adequate sputum samples to stain and culture for bacterial, mycobacterial, and fungal pathogens. The course of pneumonitis after initial antibiotic therapy indicates whether to proceed with lung

biopsy. Pulmonary infiltrates after chemotherapy and prolonged neutropenia are frequently caused by *Aspergillus* species or mucormycoses.

In contrast, diffuse infiltrates occurring *after* treatment of leukemia are suggestive of infection by opportunistic microorganisms. *Pneumocystis jirovecii* (see Web Fig. 109-6), for example, is an important preventable, treatable cause of diffuse infiltrates and occurs most often after treatment of acute lymphocytic leukemia or in patients with an acquired deficiency of cell-mediated immunity (see Chapter 108). In these settings the diagnosis should be established by examination of induced sputum, by bronchoalveolar lavage, or by transbronchial biopsy. If these diagnostic approaches are not helpful, empirical therapy with trimethoprim-sulfamethoxazole may be initiated. It is important to note that the clinical presentation of *Pneumocystis* pneumonia (PCP) frequently differs in HIV-negative immunocompromised hosts compared with HIV-infected individuals. PCP in HIV-negative patients is often more acute, more severe, and more frequently associated with other concurrent pathogens. In addition, the diagnostic sensitivity of bronchoalveolar lavage for detecting *Pneumocystis* organisms is considerably reduced in HIV-negative patients, and lung biopsy may be needed to obtain the correct diagnosis.

The indication and timing for lung biopsy must be individualized. Delay in proceeding with biopsy may reduce the chances of favorably affecting the outcome of the infection, even if the biopsy shows a potentially treatable disease. Thrombocytopenia and/or coagulopathies frequently coexist in compromised patients with pulmonary infiltrates and need to be corrected to minimize bleeding risk of a biopsy. If a decision has been made to perform a biopsy, several technical options are available. Transbronchial biopsy by fiberoptic bronchoscopy will often provide adequate tissue samples for diagnosis, particularly in the evaluation of diffuse pulmonary lesions. Open-lung biopsy has an additional yield of 50% to 75% in the patient with a nondiagnostic transbronchial biopsy and should be performed without delay if progression of the patient's illness mandates immediate diagnosis. Early treatment of most pulmonary infections in immunocompromised hosts, even aspergillosis (Fig. 109-1), can be associated with an initially favorable outcome.

DISSEMINATED MYCOSES

Disseminated mycoses represent another major diagnostic problem in the immunocompromised host. Fungal infections, particularly in the lungs, are found postmortem in more than one half of patients with leukemia or lymphoma; usually the nature of the infection has not been established antemortem. Culture of a saprophytic organism such as *Candida* from superficial sites does not establish pathogenicity. Even in patients with widespread infection, detectable fungemia may be a late event.

How, then, can the diagnosis of fungal infection be established early, at a time when the infection is potentially curable? Lung biopsy (either transbronchial or open) can be definitive. The physician should search for superficial lesions accessible to scraping, aspiration, or biopsy (Fig. 109-2). Dissemination of *Candida tropicalis* frequently causes hyperpigmented macular or pustular skin lesions that show the organisms within blood vessel walls on punch skin biopsy.

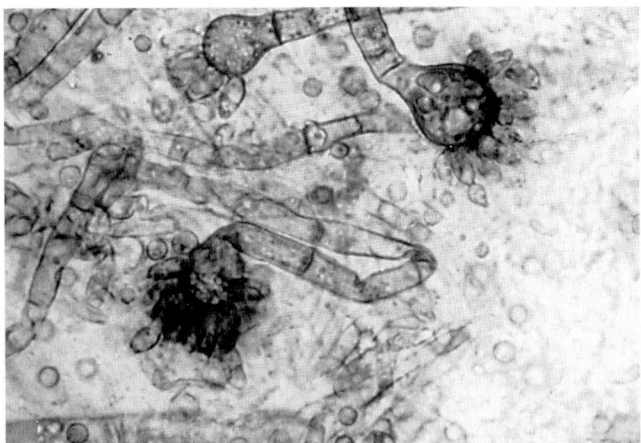

Figure 109-1 Fruiting head of *Aspergillus fumigatus* on a lung biopsy **(see Web Fig. 109-1).** Aspergillosis usually causes an expanding perihilar pulmonary infiltrate with a characteristic halo sign noted on a computed tomographic scan of the lungs. Prompt institution of potent antifungal therapy is essential in attempting to achieve a good clinical response.

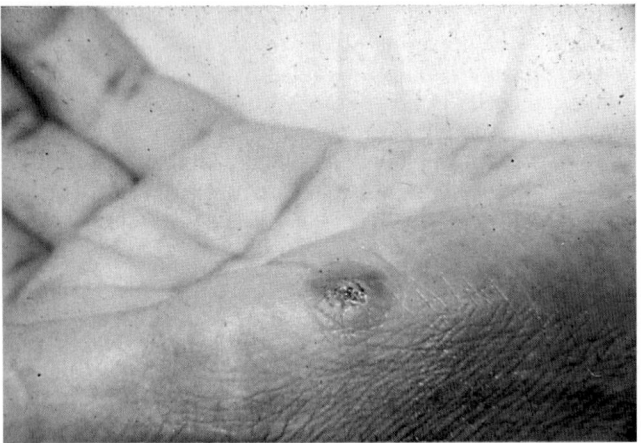

Figure 109-2 Skin lesion in a 76-year-old woman treated with corticosteroids and cytotoxic drugs for chronic lymphocytic leukemia and exhibiting nodular pulmonary infiltrates and lymphocytic meningitis. Fluid expressed from the lesion contained encapsulated yeast seen on India ink preparation and yielded *Cryptococcus neoformans* on culture **(see Web Fig. 109-5).**

Distinct skin lesions may also represent a disseminated mold infection such as *Fusarium* or *Aspergillus* species that may be diagnosed by biopsy. Hepatosplenic candidiasis is most frequently encountered in patients with fever after recovery from neutropenia. The presence of bull's-eye lesions on computed tomographic scans of the liver and spleen suggests hepatosplenic candidiasis and may be confirmed by biopsy. Cryptococcal polysaccharide antigen is usually present in the serum and/or cerebrospinal fluid of the patient with disseminated cryptococcosis **(see Web Fig. 109-5).** Specific antigen testing of serum and urine can also be performed for the endemic mycoses histoplasmosis, coccidioidomycosis, and blastomycosis for the diagnosis of both localized and disseminated infection. *Histoplasma* urine antigen testing, in particular, is a sensitive predictor of disseminated histoplasmosis. An assay for β-D-glucan, a cell wall component of many fungi, may become a valuable tool in the diagnosis of invasive fungal infections. This test appears to be useful in both exclusion of invasive fungal infections and early diagnosis in immunocompromised hosts, although it is nonspecific for type of fungal infection. In general, serologic diagnosis by antibody testing is rarely useful during a patient's initial clinical presentation.

Acute invasive pulmonary aspergillosis occurs most often in patients with prolonged, profound neutropenia who complain of fever and pleuritic chest pain during or after broad-spectrum antibacterial therapy. Accurate diagnosis of invasive disease caused by *Aspergillus* species usually requires examination of affected tissue obtained from a biopsy **(see Web Fig. 109-1).** The diagnosis of pneumonia caused by *Aspergillus,* or other molds, is also strongly suggested by the appearance of a distinctive halo sign visible on a computed tomographic scan of the lungs in at-risk patients.

In the absence of a definitive diagnosis, empirical use of antifungal drugs is generally indicated in the immunocompromised host with a moderate to high clinical suggestion of invasive fungal disease (e.g., in the febrile patient with neutropenia for more than 3 to 5 days despite empirical broad-spectrum antibacterial therapy). Several new antifungal agents have become available over the last few years (e.g., the echinocandins and newer azoles with broader activity such as posaconazole) and have widened our choices for immunocompromised patients with fungal infection. Current efforts focus on improved strategies for prophylaxis (see later discussion), as well as studying potential synergistic combinations of antifungal agents.

Prevention and Treatment of Infections in the Patient with Neutropenia

PREVENTION

Acute bacterial infections and sepsis caused by organisms comprising the gut flora occur frequently in patients with neutropenia and may have fever as their sole clinical sign. Prophylactic nonabsorbable antibiotics and protective isolation have generally failed to prevent such infection. Certain antibiotics, given prophylactically, may decrease the number of infections and bacteremic episodes in some patients with neutropenia. Prophylactic trimethoprim-sulfamethoxazole also decreases the risk of pneumonia caused by *P. jirovecii* (see Chapter 108). However, the bone marrow toxicity of this drug and selection of resistant organisms decrease the suitability for widespread prophylactic use in patients with neutropenia. Quinolones, such as ciprofloxacin, may be equally effective in preventing bacterial infections and generally have reduced toxicity. Quinolones have no activity against *P. jirovecii*, however, and have also been associated with an increased risk of severe streptococcal (including *Streptococcus viridans* group) infection in some patients. Prophylactic administration of agents to prevent systemic fungal infections is not routine for all patients with neutropenia but is generally used for patients with hematologic malignancies or those undergoing bone marrow or stem cell transplantation. Prophylactic antivirals such as acyclovir or valacyclovir are often given to prevent reactivation of latent viral infections such as herpes simplex virus and varicella-zoster virus in patients with neutropenia.

Adherence to strict hand-washing procedures by all hospital personnel remains the single best approach to preventing infection in patients with neutropenia.

TREATMENT

Empirical antibiotic therapy is indicated in febrile patients with granulocytopenia because at least two thirds have an underlying infection. Selection of two drugs with activity against gram-negative enteric bacilli and *Pseudomonas* is usually necessary (e.g., use of an antipseudomonal β-lactam and an aminoglycoside). Initial empirical therapy for staphylococci is indicated when clinical concern exists about infections of vascular catheters or of skin or soft tissue. Methicillin-resistant *Staphylococcus aureus* (MRSA) has become a major pathogen in this clinical situation. Antibiotic coverage for MRSA, though, is generally reserved for documented infection, given that empirical addition of an agent such as vancomycin does not affect short-term outcomes in neutropenic febrile patients without a documented source of infection. However, an empirical regimen containing vancomycin should be considered in patients with known MRSA colonization, those with positive blood cultures for gram-positive bacteria before further identification and susceptibility testing, those with evidence of central venous catheter infection, or those with hemodynamic instability. Despite the early use of empirical antibiotics, the clinical outcome of patients with both neutropenia and bacterial infections is poor unless the initial neutrophil count exceeds 500/mcL, the count rises during treatment, or the pathogen is a gram-positive organism. Adjunctive treatment with granulocyte colony-stimulating factors may result in shorter duration of neutropenia and fewer infectious complications in certain situations. Use of these biologics may also be beneficial in cases of documented or suggested invasive fungal disease (e.g., *Aspergillus* pneumonia) or refractory infection with gram-negative bacilli.

The appropriate duration of antimicrobial therapy of febrile patients with neutropenia is uncertain. If a specific diagnosis is made, narrowing antimicrobial coverage is sometimes appropriate to target the isolated organism, assuming that the neutrophil counts recover. If no causative agent is identified, many physicians continue to administer the empirical antibiotic regimen until the neutropenia resolves. The empirical addition of antifungal therapy is indicated in the patient with neutropenia who remains febrile for at least 3 days despite broad-spectrum antibacterial therapy. In this setting, the best approach is often to continue broad-spectrum antibiotics for the duration of the neutropenia unless the cause of the patient's fever can be clearly defined. In some centers, certain relatively low-risk patients with neutropenia and fever (e.g., highly dependable individuals with absolute neutrophil counts of 500/mcL) are initially managed at home using outpatient intravenous or oral combinations of highly active antibiotics.

With ever-increasing numbers of patients receiving a variety of potent and novel immunosuppressive agents, the number and variety of infections occurring in susceptible individuals can only be expected to increase. In addition to newly recognized pathogenic organisms, increases in antimicrobial resistance among known pathogens will also likely be observed. Newer strategies for dealing with infections in immunocompromised hosts include expanded use of targeted forms of prophylaxis, development of molecular assays permitting diagnosis at an earlier stage, and the evolution of combination therapies for particularly resistant organisms.

Prospectus for the Future

- The increasing use of immunosuppressive drugs with novel modes of action will predispose patients to infections by additional opportunistic pathogens.

- Increased use of prophylactic antimicrobials will lead to parallel increases in antibiotic resistance, increasing the demand for novel antimicrobial agents.

References

Giles JT, Bathon JM: Serious infections associated with anticytokine therapies in the rheumatic diseases. J Intensive Care Med 19:320-334, 2004.

Kotloff RM, Ahya VN, Crawford SW: Pulmonary complications of solid organ and hematopoietic stem cell transplantation. Am J Respir Crit Care Med 170:22-48, 2004.

Lexau CA, Lynfield R, Danila R, et al: Changing epidemiology of invasive pneumococcal disease among older adults in the era of pediatric pneumococcal conjugate vaccine. JAMA 294:2043-2051, 2005.

Odabasi A, Mattiuzzi G, Estey E, et al: Beta-D-glucan as a diagnostic adjunct for invasive fungal infections: validation, cutoff development, and performance in patients with acute myelogenous leukemia and myelodysplastic syndrome. Clin Infect Dis 39(2):199-205, 2004.

Pfeiffer CD, Fine JP, Safdar N: Diagnosis of invasive aspergillosis using a galactomannan assay: a meta-analysis. Clin Infect Dis 42:1417-1427, 2006.

Ramphal R: Changes in the etiology of bacteremia in febrile neutropenic patients and the susceptibilities of the currently isolated pathogens. Clin Infect Dis 39(Suppl 1):S32-S37, 2004.

Senn L, Robinson JO, Schmidt S, et al: 1,3-Beta-D-glucan antigenemia for early diagnosis of invasive fungal infections in neutropenic patients with acute leukemia. Clin Infect Dis 46:878-885, 2008.

Singh N, Paterson DL: *Aspergillus* infections in transplant recipients. Clin Microbiol Rev 18:44-69, 2005.

Sipsas NV, Bodey GP, Kontoyiannis DP: Perspectives for the management of febrile neutropenic patients with cancer in the 21st century. Cancer 103:1103-1113, 2005.

Wingard JR: The changing face of invasive fungal infections in hematopoietic cell transplant recipients. Curr Opin Oncol 17:89-92, 2005.

Infectious Diseases of Travelers: Protozoal and Helminthic Infections

Jessica K. Fairley, Keith B. Armitage, and Robert A. Salata

Medical advice for overseas travelers, some common clinical symptoms that may develop on their return, and the diagnosis and treatment of common parasitic diseases endemic in the United States and abroad are reviewed in this chapter.

Preparation of Travelers

More than 12 million Americans travel to developing countries each year. Major increases in international travel and the resurgence of malaria, dengue fever, and other infectious diseases worldwide bring the issues of prevention and management of health problems in travelers into the office of every physician.

Risks associated with international travel are dependent on the destination, duration of the trip, underlying health and age of the traveler, and activities while abroad. In general, destinations within the industrialized world require no specific health precautions. In contrast, travelers to developing areas, especially the tropics, can occasionally be exposed to life-threatening infections. Major issues to be addressed in the pretravel period include required and recommended immunizations, malaria prophylaxis, traveler's diarrhea, and other problems that can be avoided or prevented. Information about health risks in specific geographic areas, updated weekly, can be obtained from the Centers for Disease Control and Prevention (CDC) through its publications or by calling the International Travelers' Hotline (1-877-394-8747; website, www.cdc.gov/travel).

IMMUNIZATIONS

Only yellow fever vaccination may be required by law for international travel. Both polio and meningococcal meningitis vaccinations may be required during outbreak situations, and the meningococcal vaccine is required for religious pilgrimages (Hajj) to Saudi Arabia. Although some immunizations are not generally considered *travel* immunizations, many Americans have allowed routine diphtheria-tetanus immunizations to lapse or may not have been fully immunized against measles and polio. Finally, other immunizations are often strongly recommended, depending on the type and duration of travel. With a few exceptions, vaccines can be given simultaneously. Before immunization, a thorough history should be obtained to determine allergies to eggs or chick embryo cells. Pregnant women and individuals immunocompromised by human immunodeficiency virus (HIV), malignancy, or chemotherapy pose specific and important challenges; most live virus vaccines are contraindicated in these patients.

Hepatitis A

Hepatitis A is a major risk for travelers to areas of poor sanitation, affecting an estimated 1 in 500 to 1000 travelers per 2- to 3-week trip in some areas. Therefore, hepatitis A is the most frequent and important vaccine-preventable infection for travelers. Hepatitis A vaccine should be given at least 2 weeks before departure but remains effective if given up until the time of travel. A single dose provides protection for 1 to 2 years; a booster 6 to 18 months later is required for long-lasting immunity (>15 years).

Yellow Fever

Yellow fever is a live, attenuated virus vaccine that is highly effective and recommended for persons traveling to areas in South America and Africa where yellow fever is endemic. Vaccination is generally safe and lasts for 10 years, but it must be given at designated vaccination centers. Severe adverse events are rare and include yellow fever vaccine–

associated viscerotropic and neurologic disease, both more common in those with thymus disease. Benefits of the vaccine still far outweigh this small risk for most. However, because the adverse events occur more commonly in people over 60 years old, a careful assessment of risks and benefits for these travelers should be done before vaccination.

Cholera

Cholera is endemic in parts of Asia and Africa and has returned to South and Central America, where it is a major concern to travelers. The currently available vaccine is not highly effective and is not routinely recommended for travel into endemic areas. Health education on likely sources of transmission is far more effective in preventing disease than is vaccination.

Measles

Up to 20% of first-year college students have no serologic evidence of prior measles infection or immunization and must be presumed to be susceptible. Individuals born after 1956 with no physician-documented record of immunization are at greatest risk for measles. In addition, a single immunization with measles vaccine at 15 months of age may permit breakthrough infection as a young adult. A second measles vaccination after age 5 is now recommended; international travelers born after 1956 who have not received a booster after early childhood should have a one-time booster.

Diphtheria-Tetanus

Tetanus is a ubiquitous problem and is most prevalent in tropical countries. A booster within the previous 5 years is recommended. This precaution eliminates the need for a tetanus booster if the traveler sustains a tetanus-prone injury overseas. This recommendation is made primarily because of the uncertainty of obtaining sterile, disposable needles in many overseas locations. Given the resurgence of diphtheria in countries of the former Soviet Union and the occurrence of disease in travelers to these areas, diphtheria toxoid should be co-administered with tetanus toxoid. The current recommended booster for adults includes the acellular pertussis component as well.

Polio

Polio remains endemic in some regions of Asia and Africa, and small, geographically restricted, vaccine-associated outbreaks have occurred in the Western Hemisphere. Most young adults were immunized with at least four doses of trivalent oral poliovirus vaccine (OPV) before the elimination of this oral vaccine for use in all age groups in the United States. Many adults (>18 years of age) cannot remember, however, whether they received OPV; such individuals should be given inactivated poliovirus vaccine.

Meningococcal Meningitis

Meningococcal meningitis is a worldwide disease, but cases in international travelers are infrequent except with prolonged contact with the local population. Vaccination with the quadrivalent polysaccharide vaccine (A, C, Y, and W-135) is recommended for travelers to northern India, Nepal, and Saudi Arabia during the Hajj; certain parts of sub-Saharan Africa; and other locations for which travel advisories have been issued (www.cdc.gov/travel/). The newer quadrivalent A/C/Y/W-135 meningococcal protein-conjugated vaccine was licensed in the United States in 2005 for preferred use in persons 11 to 55 years of age.

Typhoid

American international travelers are at greatest risk for contracting typhoid in the Indian subcontinent, Central America, western South America, and sub-Saharan Africa. Vaccination is recommended for travel to endemic areas where exposure to contaminated food and water is likely. Vaccination is also strongly indicated for travelers with achlorhydria, immunosuppression, or sickle cell anemia and for those taking broad-spectrum antibiotics. Both an oral vaccine (four enteric-coated capsules given over 7 days) and an injectable vaccine (one dose) are available and are essentially equivalent in effectiveness, which ranges from 50% to 70%.

Influenza

Although influenza is not necessarily considered a travel-related illness, the influenza vaccine should be considered in the panel of vaccines offered to the traveler. Influenza seasons can occur at different times of the year than in North America. Therefore, if a traveler is planning a trip to the Southern Hemisphere from April to September or to the tropics at any time of the year, or is traveling in a group, vaccination should be offered if not done already in the fall or winter. Attention should be paid to vaccinating before the end of spring because vaccine supplies may be limited after that time. If a patient cannot be vaccinated or if there is concern regarding exposure to avian influenza, a course of the antiviral medication oseltamivir can be given to take at the first sign of a flulike illness. However, there are limited data to date on the effectiveness of oseltamivir for human cases of avian influenza, and resistance to neuraminidases in strains of seasonal influenza is increasing worldwide.

Other Vaccines

Some travelers, including missionaries, physicians, and anthropologists, need special consideration. These individuals live for prolonged periods in developing countries or are at special risk for contracting certain highly contagious diseases. Consideration should be given to immunization with hepatitis B, Japanese B encephalitis, plague, and rabies vaccines. In general, such travelers should be referred to a qualified travelers' clinic.

MALARIA PROPHYLAXIS

Malaria infection is associated with significant morbidity and mortality, particularly if caused by *Plasmodium falciparum*, especially in nonimmune travelers. Appropriate malaria prophylaxis should be prescribed and strictly adhered to. Malaria prophylaxis is a major problem for international travelers because of the high and increasing prevalence of drug resistance by the parasite. The need for, as well as the type of, prophylaxis is dependent on the exact itinerary within a given country because transmission risk is quite regional. Recommended chemoprophylactic regimens have changed frequently within the last few years. In general, travelers to areas where chloroquine-sensitive *P. falciparum* strains are exclusively found (parts of Central America, the

Caribbean, North Africa, and the Middle East) should take chloroquine phosphate (300-mg base or 500-mg salt) weekly starting 1 week before, continuing during, and for 4 weeks after leaving areas in which malaria is endemic. Travelers to areas where chloroquine-resistant *P. falciparum* is common may take mefloquine (Lariam), atovaquone-proguanil (Malarone), or doxycycline. These areas currently include Southeast Asia, sub-Saharan Africa, South America, and South Asia. Mefloquine, 250 mg/wk starting a week before travel, continuing during travel, and for 4 weeks after, is effective and convenient but may be associated with minor neurologic side effects (dizziness and vivid dreams) and, rarely, significant neuropsychiatric side effects. Some recommend starting mefloquine up to 2 to 4 weeks before travel to determine if there are any intolerable side effects. Mefloquine is not completely effective in Myanmar, rural Thailand, or some parts of East Africa, where resistance is a growing problem. Atovaquone-proguanil and doxycycline are effective in Southeast Asia and may be used in other areas of chloroquine resistance. Atovaquone-proguanil is well tolerated but must be taken every day and is relatively expensive. Doxycycline is inexpensive but must also be taken every day and is associated with photosensitivity and occasionally vaginal candidiasis. Although not yet approved by the U.S. Food and Drug Administration (FDA) for primary prophylaxis, primaquine has been used more frequently in travel to areas of higher *Plasmodium vivax* or *Plasmodium ovale* infections and has the advantage of both preventing acute infection from all malaria parasites, as well as preventing the later recurrent infections of *P. vivax* and *P. ovale*. However, it cannot be used in those with G6PD deficiency, and this needs to be screened for before administration. Although the sickle cell trait provides significant protection from death caused by *P. falciparum* malaria, this protection is not absolute and does not alter recommendations for prophylaxis. Emphasis must also be given to the use of mosquito netting, screens, and insect repellents with at least 30% DEET, as well as to the prompt diagnosis and treatment of any febrile episodes (temperature >102° F [39° C]) in malaria-endemic areas.

TRAVELER'S DIARRHEA

Between 20% and 50% of individuals traveling to developing countries will develop diarrhea during or shortly after their trip. Bacterial infections are most common, with enterotoxigenic *Escherichia coli* topping the list. Viruses and parasites can also be causes. The average duration of an episode of traveler's diarrhea is 3 to 6 days. Approximately 10% of episodes last longer than 1 week. The diarrhea may be accompanied by abdominal cramping, nausea, headache, low-grade fever, vomiting, or bloating. Fewer than 5% of persons have fever greater than 101° F (38° C), bloody stools, or both. Travelers with these symptoms may not have simple traveler's diarrhea and should see a physician at once (see Chapter 103).

Diarrheal illness (including cholera) can be avoided through precautions with food and beverages. All water should be presumed to be unsafe. Salads are often contaminated by protozoal cysts and, along with street vendor foods, are the most dangerous foods encountered by most travelers. Food should be well cooked, including meat, seafood, and vegetables. Dairy products should be avoided.

Diphenoxylate (Lomotil) and loperamide (Imodium) may give symptomatic relief of diarrhea but should be avoided if the diarrhea is severe, fever exists, or blood is present in the stool. First-line treatment includes one of the newer fluoroquinolones, which can be taken orally for 3 days to reduce the duration of symptoms and is effective against a wide variety of bacterial pathogens, including most *Shigella* and *Salmonella* species. In some countries, such as Thailand and Nepal, fluoroquinolone resistance, especially among *Campylobacter* species, has been on the rise; azithromycin is an alternative in these situations (CDC). Prophylactic antibiotics are not generally recommended. Bismuth subsalicylate (Pepto-Bismol) can be used as a prophylactic measure (two tablets 4 times a day) or used to treat acute bouts of diarrhea (1 oz every 30 minutes for eight doses).

AVIAN INFLUENZA

The highly pathogenic H5N1 strain of avian influenza is an emerging concern and public health threat in many Middle East and Southeast Asian countries. Although the avian influenza A viruses remain primarily avian pathogens, cases of human infection have occurred with direct contact with infected poultry. From 2003 to 2008, almost 400 human cases were reported, with a case fatality rate of over 60%. Although the majority of transmission has been from poultry to humans, there have been isolated cases of possible human to human transmission among close contacts. Signs and symptoms can range from conjunctivitis to influenza-like symptoms (fever, myalgias, sore throat) to severe pneumonia and respiratory failure. Occasionally vomiting, diarrhea, and neurologic symptoms can also be present. First-line treatment or prophylaxis for avian influenza is the antiviral medication oseltamivir, as the H5N1 virus is resistant to amantadine and rimantadine. Preventive measures for travelers include avoiding contact with live birds (poultry or wild), not visiting live animal markets, eating properly cooked food, and washing hands frequently. The routine influenza vaccine is not protective for avian influenza, but travel to areas endemic for avian influenza provides an ideal opportunity to discuss immunization against seasonal influenza when appropriate. Vaccination for seasonal influenza should decrease the risk for developing a febrile illness resulting from influenza A and B, which could be confused with avian influenza.

GENERAL HEALTH INFORMATION

Other potentially dangerous activities overseas include exposure to dogs and cats (rabies), swimming in fresh water (schistosomiasis or leptospirosis), walking barefoot (hookworm or strongyloidiasis), and insect bites. In addition to malaria, many diseases, including dengue, sleeping sickness, and yellow fever, are transmitted by insect bites, and avoidance measures should be stressed when applicable. Travelers should also be reminded to use seat belts.

SPECIAL PROBLEMS
Pregnant Women

Live virus vaccines are contraindicated in women during pregnancy, which greatly complicates pretravel preparations. Chloroquine probably can be used safely. Travel to areas of chloroquine-resistant malaria should be strongly discouraged. If a pregnant woman must travel, mefloquine has been used more frequently in pregnancy and appears to be safe, although data overall, and especially during the first trimester, are lacking. Ideally, if travel is to be undertaken at all, it should be postponed to the second trimester. No drug regimen to prevent or treat chloroquine-resistant malaria is known to be completely safe in pregnant women, and malaria during pregnancy is a medical emergency for both the mother and her fetus. If a pregnant woman must travel, her care should be managed by a travel clinic with experience in this area.

Acquired Immunodeficiency Syndrome

Many countries bar entry to patients with acquired immunodeficiency syndrome (AIDS). As of the fall of 2008, the United States ban was lifted. Several countries require HIV serologic testing for all travelers applying for more than a 3-month visa, which requires official documentation well in advance of travel. Patients with HIV infection need special preparation before travel to developing countries because of their increased susceptibility to certain illnesses (e.g., pneumococcal infection, tuberculosis).

Most international travelers are concerned about the risk of acquiring HIV infection while abroad. Most concerns center on untested blood or nonsterile needles, which might be used in an emergency. Issues of HIV infection and other sexually transmitted diseases should be discussed, especially with young, sexually active adults.

Returning Traveler

Fever

With the exception of skin testing for tuberculosis, asymptomatic returning travelers generally do not need screening tests. The clinical problems that most often arise in travelers soon after return are fever and diarrhea, whereas eosinophilia is the most common cause for later referral. Fever is most important because delay in the diagnosis of *P. falciparum* malaria is often fatal. Fever should always prompt consideration of malaria until proved otherwise in travelers returning from countries where malaria is endemic, even if they are still taking prophylactic drugs. Determining the malaria species with a blood film is important because this finding affects therapy. Chloroquine-sensitive *P. falciparum* is treated with 1 g of chloroquine given orally, followed by 500 mg at 6, 24, and 48 hours. For *P. vivax* and *P. ovale* (also generally chloroquine sensitive, although some resistance is emerging in certain areas), this regimen is followed by primaquine daily for 14 days to eradicate latent hepatic forms. Resistant *P. falciparum* is treated with atovaquone-proguanil, four full-strength pills a day for 3 days; or quinine sulfate, 650 mg given orally every 8 hours for 3 days, plus doxycycline, 100 mg orally twice daily for 7 days. Intravenous quinidine is used in patients with severe malaria. Artemisinin compounds are used in many parts of the world to treat chloroquine-resistant malaria but may be associated with a high rate of relapse. All patients with possible resistant malaria infection should be hospitalized, and if intravenous quinidine is warranted, than hospitalization in the intensive care unit with close monitoring of the QTc interval is necessary. If quinidine is not available or contraindicated,

parenteral artesunate is available as an investigational drug through the CDC. If fever is not caused by malaria, then dengue fever (the second most common cause of febrile illness in travelers after malaria), tuberculosis, typhoid fever, amebic liver abscess, leptospirosis, and rickettsial diseases, among other conditions, should be considered. Chikungunya virus, an arbovirus transmitted by mosquitoes, is an emerging pathogen related to several recent outbreaks and can also cause unexplained fever. Joint pains are common and can lead to chronic arthralgias. Evaluation of the febrile returned traveler should take into account the travel itinerary, exposures during the trip, immunization status, and host factors, such as immunosuppression.

Gastrointestinal Symptoms

Persistent traveler's diarrhea that is unresponsive to empiric antibiotics is often caused by *Giardia lamblia,* transmitted by contaminated water or food (fecal-oral route). Three stool specimens for ova and parasites and a stool culture are warranted (**Web Fig. 110-1**). Unfortunately, *G. lamblia* may be missed in up to one third of patients even after this workup. Assessment of stool *Giardia* antigen by enzyme-linked immunosorbent assay is more sensitive than culture. If clinical suggestion is high, an empiric course of metronidazole (500 mg orally three times a day for 7 days) is usually justified. Alternatives include tinidazole administered in one dose, or a 3-day course of nitazoxanide. Antibiotic-resistant bacteria, amebiasis, temporary lactose intolerance, bacterial overgrowth, and tropical sprue should also be considered.

Eosinophilia

Eosinophilia, often accompanied by persistent gastrointestinal symptoms, in a returning traveler usually manifests weeks or months after travel. It is usually caused by one of a wide variety of helminth infections. A stool specimen for ova and parasites is indicated but may be negative during the tissue-migrating phase of many intestinal worms or in tissue nematode infections, such as filariasis or onchocerciasis. Management of the more common parasitic infections encountered in travelers is included in the next section.

Respiratory Symptoms

Respiratory illnesses are common complaints in the returned traveler. Air travel has made the transmission and movement of respiratory microbes even easier, and the incubation period of many infections often exceeds travel time. Although many symptoms can be caused by common respiratory viruses not necessarily particular to the recent travel, there are some infections to consider. Respiratory symptoms, especially when accompanied by fever, may be indicative of influenza or possibly avian influenza if severe and associated with exposure to birds or poultry in a known endemic area. A new or undiagnosed pathogen, as was seen in the severe acute respiratory syndrome (SARS) outbreak, should also be considered in the differential diagnosis in severe, acute cases. Although the usual presentation is more chronic, tuberculosis is a consideration as well. Other infections that can cause respiratory symptoms include histoplasmosis, tularemia, plague, viral hemorrhagic fevers, coccidiomycosis, and Q fever. Helminth infections, such as schistosomiasis, strongyloidiasis, and ascariasis, can occasionally also cause pulmonary infections.

Rash

Skin lesions with or without fever can be a common complaint in the returning traveler. Overall, insect bites and cutaneous larva migrans, erythematous serpiginous pruritic lesions caused by migration of larvae, are the most common causes of skin lesions, with bacterial skin infections being the most common cause in those returning from sub-Saharan Africa. A black eschar in a patient returning from southern Africa is typical of African tick bite fever, a tick-borne rickettsial disease caused by *Rickettsia africae*. Ulcerative lesions can be indicative of cutaneous leishmaniasis (see later), and purpuric or petechial rashes may be signs of more serious illness such as viral hemorrhagic fevers, rickettsial diseases, and invasive meningococcal diseases, among others. Schistosomal dermatitis, which occurs after swimming in fresh water, is characterized by a transient maculopapular, pruritic eruption.

Protozoal and Helminthic Infections

PROTOZOAL INFECTIONS IN THE UNITED STATES

More than two billion people worldwide are infected with helminths. The incidence of protozoan parasitic infections is increasing in part because of the emergence of antimicrobial resistance (e.g., malaria) and an increasing number of susceptible hosts, especially those with HIV infection. Protozoal infections in the United States occur more frequently in immunocompromised hosts than in the general population (Table 110-1) (see Chapter 109). Babesiosis is very severe in asplenic individuals, and *Toxoplasma* encephalitis primarily affects patients with AIDS.

GIARDIASIS AND AMEBIASIS

Giardiasis, although endemic to the United States, is a common cause of persistent (longer than 2 to 3 weeks), nonbloody diarrhea in returning travelers. *G. lamblia* is prevalent throughout much of the developing world. Latin America is the most common site of *Giardia* acquisition by North American travelers. Men who have sex with men also have a high prevalence of infection because of specific sexual practices. Persons who work in day-care centers are also at increased risk for giardiasis because of its relatively high prevalence in young children. The diagnosis and treatment are described in the earlier section on returning travelers.

As with *Giardia, Entamoeba histolytica* is transmitted by the fecal-oral route; the vast majority of infected individuals are asymptomatic. When *E. histolytica* causes acute illness, it is generally identified by bloody diarrhea. In the United States, amebic dysentery is occasionally misdiagnosed as ulcerative colitis or Crohn disease, and the administration of corticosteroids may cause significant worsening and toxic megacolon. Stool examination for ova and parasites is generally diagnostic, but sigmoidoscopy may be required. Serologic testing is useful to exclude amebiasis in individuals from industrialized countries because the background antibody positivity is quite low. Treatment involves a 5- to 10-day course of metronidazole. Extraintestinal amebiasis generally manifests as hepatic liver abscess (see Chapter 102).

PROTOZOAL INFECTIONS COMMON IN TRAVELERS AND IMMIGRANTS

Leishmaniasis

Cutaneous and mucocutaneous leishmaniasis, transmitted by the sandfly (see Table 110-1), should be considered in any traveler returning from the Middle East or endemic areas of Latin America who has a persistent skin or mucous membrane lesion. Diagnosis is made by tissue biopsy. Visceral leishmaniasis should be anticipated in immigrants with fever and splenomegaly. Diagnosis is made by bone marrow biopsy and culture. Cutaneous leishmaniasis is generally self-limited. Other types are treated with sodium stibogluconate (Pentostam), 20 mg/kg/day for up to 20 days. Amphotericin B, paromomycin (for cutaneous infection), and pentamidine have been used in resistant cases.

African Trypanosomiasis

African trypanosomiasis is a protozoal infection, endemic in Africa, which causes sleeping sickness. Rarely imported into developed countries, it should be presumed in systemically ill patients from Africa who exhibit fever, headache, and development of encephalitic and neurologic signs and symptoms (see Table 110-1). Many patients will remember a painful chancre at the site of an insect bite (**Web Fig. 110-2**). Diagnosis is made by direct examination of the blood, lymph aspirate, or cerebrospinal fluid (**Web Figs. 110-3 and 110-4**). Treatment is highly toxic and should be supervised by an expert in the field.

Chagas Disease (American Trypanosomiasis)

Trypanosoma cruzi is the most common cause of heart failure in Brazil. Transmission is through contact with feces from infected reduviid bugs (kissing bugs) (**Web Fig. 110-5**), and cases of transfusion-associated *T. cruzi* infection have been recognized in the United States (see Table 110-1). Most patients are asymptomatic for decades and then exhibit cardiomegaly, megaesophagus, or megacolon. Diagnosis of acute disease is made by direct examination of the blood (**Web Fig. 110-6**). Serologic testing is also used but requires two to three different assays per patient to maximize sensitivity and specificity. As of 2007, the U.S. blood supply is screened for *T. cruzi* infection. Early diagnosis is critical because patients may respond to nitrofuran or nitroimidazole derivatives, available through the CDC. Treatment of chronic Chagas disease is largely supportive.

HELMINTHIC INFECTIONS COMMON IN THE UNITED STATES

Pinworm

Enterobiasis is common in the United States (Table 110-2), particularly among children. Perianal pruritus is the major clinical presentation. Infection is maintained by fecal-oral contamination. Diagnosis is made by the application of cellophane tape to the anus and subsequent microscopic examination for ova. Treatment is with mebendazole,

Table 110-1 Protozoal Infections

Protozoan	Setting	Vectors	Diagnosis	Special Considerations	Treatment
Endemic in the United States					
Babesia microti	New England	Ixodid ticks, transfusions	Thick or thin blood smear	Severe disease in asplenic persons	Quinine and clindamycin
Giardia lamblia	Mountain states	Humans, small mammals	Microscopic examination of stool or duodenal fluid	Common in homosexual men, travelers, children in day-care centers	Quinacrine, nitazoxanide, or metronidazole
Toxoplasma gondii	Ubiquitous	Domestic cats, raw meat	Clinical; serologic confirmation	Pregnant women, immunosuppressed host (AIDS)	Pyrimethamine and sulfadiazine
Entamoeba histolytica	Southeast	Human	Microscopic examination of stool or touch preparation from ulcer	Common in homosexual men, travelers, institutionalized persons	Metronidazole
Cryptosporidium species	Ubiquitous	Human	Acid-fast stain of stool	Severe in immunosuppressed hosts (AIDS)	Nitazoxanide
Trichomonas vaginalis	Ubiquitous	Human	Wet preparation of genital secretions	Common cause of vaginitis	Metronidazole
Primarily Seen in Travelers and Immigrants					
Plasmodium species	Africa, Asia, South America	Anopheles mosquito	Thick and thin blood smears	Consider in returning travelers with fever	Dependent on regional resistance pattern (see text)
Leishmania donovani	Middle East	Sandfly	Tissue biopsy	Consider in immigrants with fever and splenomegaly	Sodium stilbogluconate
Trypanosoma species	Africa, South America	Reduviid bugs, transfusion	Direct examination of blood or CSF	Very rare in travelers, transfusion associated	Dependent on species and stage of disease

AIDS, acquired immunodeficiency syndrome; CSF, cerebrospinal fluid.

100 mg given once. In heavy or recurrent infection, treating all family members is advisable.

Other Intestinal Nematodes

Ascaris (giant roundworm), *Ancylostoma duodenale* and *Necator americanus* (hookworm), and *Trichuris* (whipworms), still endemic in the United States, are extremely common in immigrants and are ubiquitous in the developing world, with co-infection with other helminths being very common (see Table 110-2). Most individuals are asymptomatic. Ascariasis and hookworm may cause transient pulmonary infiltrates with eosinophilia during the tissue migratory phase of infection. Heavy *Ascaris* infection may cause intestinal, biliary, or pancreatic obstruction. Hookworm infection can be associated with iron deficiency, and significant anemia in some cases. Diagnosis is made based on stool examination for ova and parasites (**Web Figs. 110-7 and 110-8**). Each of these worms can be eradicated with appropriate anthelmintic therapy such as mebendazole, 100 mg orally twice daily for 3 days.

HELMINTH INFECTIONS COMMON IN TRAVELERS AND IMMIGRANTS

Strongyloidosis

Strongyloides stercoralis is a common cause of eosinophilia in returning long-term travelers and immigrants, particularly those from Southeast Asia (see Table 110-2). Infection occurs when the parasite penetrates the skin, migrates to the lungs, and then is swallowed. Infection can persist for years; many men who served in the Pacific theater during World War II or in Vietnam still harbor infections. *S. stercoralis* is unique in its ability to complete its life cycle in the host and produce persistent infection. Although usually asymptomatic, infection can cause diarrhea, abdominal pain, and malabsorption. This helminth can cause life-threatening disseminated infection in individuals who are immunosuppressed from cancer chemotherapy, corticosteroids, or HIV infection. Diagnosis may be made by stool examination (**Web Fig. 110-9**), but this is not a very sensitive technique. Treatment with thiabendazole, 25 mg/kg (maximum 3 g/day) orally twice daily for 2 days, is curative in more than 90% of immunocompetent hosts. Ivermectin (200 mcg/kg/day) may be more effective than thiabendazole and is now the preferred drug for treatment of strongyloidosis, especially for immunocompromised hosts.

Schistosomiasis

Schistosoma mansoni (Africa, South America, and the Caribbean), *Schistosoma japonicum* (the Philippines, China, and Indonesia), and *Schistosoma mekongi* (Cambodia, Laos, and Vietnam) are the most common causes of hepatosplenic enlargement in the world (see Table 110-2). Chronic infection can lead to periportal hepatic fibrosis, obstruction of

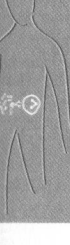

Table 110-2 **Helminthic Infections**

Helminth	Setting	Vectors	Diagnosis	Treatment
Endemic in the United States				
Pinworm (enterobiasis)	Ubiquitous	Human	Direct examination for ova	Mebendazole, albendazole
Ascaris lumbricoides	Southeast	Human	Stool examination for ova	Mebendazole, albendazole
Trichuris trichiura	Southeast	Human	Stool examination for ova	Mebendazole, albendazole
Hookworm	Southeast	Human	Stool examination for ova	Mebendazole, albendazole
Common in Travelers and Immigrants				
Strongyloides stercoralis	Developing world	Human	Stool examination for larvae	Thiabendazole, ivermectin
Schistosoma species	Developing world	Snails	Stool or urine examination for ova	Praziquantel
Wuchereria and *Brugia* species	Asia, some parts of Africa	Mosquitoes	Nocturnal blood examination	Ivermectin
Onchocerca volvulus	Africa, South and Central Americas	Black flies	Biopsy	Ivermectin
Loa loa	Africa	Tabanid flies	Blood examination, clinical setting	Diethylcarbamazine or Ivermectin
Clonorchis sinensis	Asia	Undercooked fish and snails	Stool examination for ova, radiology	Praziquantel
Echinococcus species	Worldwide	Canines and livestock	Radiology, serology, biopsy	Surgery, supportive therapy
Taenia solium (cysticercosis)	Developing world	Humans, pigs	Radiology, serology	Surgery, albendazole
T. solium, Taenia saginata, Diphyllobothrium latum (tapeworms)	Worldwide	Pigs, bovine, fish	Stool examination for ova or proglottids	Praziquantel

portal blood flow, and bleeding esophageal varices. Patients in the United States are often misdiagnosed as having hepatitis B or alcohol-induced liver disease. A clue to the correct diagnosis is that the liver is enlarged, in contrast to the small, shrunken liver of alcoholic cirrhosis. *Schistosoma haematobium* (Africa) commonly causes hematuria and leads to urinary obstruction. Diagnosis is made by examination of stool or urine for ova and parasites. Praziquantel is the drug of choice.

Lymphatic Filariasis

Wuchereria bancrofti and *Brugia malayi* cause elephantiasis throughout the tropics (see Table 110-2). Patients may exhibit acute lymphadenitis or asymptomatic eosinophilia. Some patients have pulmonary symptoms, infiltrates, and marked eosinophilia (tropical pulmonary eosinophilia). The diagnosis is made by finding microfilariae in blood specimens obtained at midnight. Treatment currently consists of a single oral dose of ivermectin, 100 to 400 mcg/kg.

Loa loa

Eyeworm is endemic in West and Central Africa (see Table 110-2). Patients exhibit transient pruritic subcutaneous swellings, and less commonly joint manifestations and neurologic symptoms. Eosinophilia is universal. In the United States, patients are often misdiagnosed for years as having chronic urticaria. In rare instances the adult worm can be visualized as it crosses the anterior chamber of the patient's eye, giving this worm its common name. Diagnosis

is generally suggested on clinical grounds and is confirmed by biopsy or presence of microfilaria on peripheral blood samples. Loasis can be treated with diethylcarbamazine or ivermectin.

River Blindness

Infection from *Onchocerca volvulus* occurs in West and Central Africa, as well as in South and Central America (see Table 110-2). Although the most severe manifestations occur in the eye, the most common clinical presentation in the United States is recurrent pruritic dermatitis. The diagnosis can be made by direct examination of skin snips for microfilariae; a specific serologic test is also available. Ivermectin, 150 mcg/kg orally for one dose, is the treatment of choice. Ivermectin should be repeated after 3 to 6 months to suppress cutaneous and ocular microfilariae.

Clonorchiasis

The Chinese liver fluke, *Clonorchis sinensis,* is important to diagnose in Asian immigrants. Symptoms may be confused with those of biliary tract disease. If untreated, infection can lead to cholangiocarcinoma. Praziquantel is curative.

Cysticercosis

The invasive larval form of pork tapeworm *(Taenia solium)* is the most common cause of seizures throughout the world, as well as in young adults in Los Angeles, chiefly among immigrants from Mexico. Typically, patients exhibit new onset of seizures or severe headache. Single or multiple ring-enhancing lesions are the characteristic finding on computed tomographic scan. The diagnosis may be confirmed by an immunoblot assay using peripheral blood. Treatment includes surgical removal when possible, and antiparasitic treatment in some cases, depending on the site of infection and clinical syndrome. Studies are ongoing for optimal treatment. Management must be individualized in each case. Praziquantel (50 mg/kg/day in three divided doses for 15 days) or albendazole (for 30 days, dosed by weight: >60 kg, 400 mg orally twice daily; <60 kg, 15 mg/kg/day in divided doses twice daily) can be curative in some cases but may precipitate focal cerebral edema and seizures by killing other cysticercariae within the central nervous system. An expert should be consulted before treatment.

Intestinal Tapeworms

Three intestinal tapeworms commonly infect humans: *Taenia saginata* from raw beef, *T. solium* from raw pork, and *Diphyllobothrium latum* from raw fish. Most individuals are asymptomatic, but *T. solium* can cause invasive disease (cys-ticercosis) if humans ingest ova of the adult worm. *D. latum* is associated with vitamin B$_{12}$ deficiency. All three infections are treated with praziquantel.

Hydatid Disease and Alveolar Cyst Disease

Hydatid disease, caused by the cestode *Echinococcus granulosus,* commonly produces a cystic liver mass in emigrants from sheep-raising parts of the world. Early diagnosis is important because rupture of the cyst can lead to dissemination. Diagnosis is often suggested from the appearance of the cyst (calcified wall and dependent hydatid *sand*) on abdominal computed tomographic scan. Serologic testing can be helpful but is occasionally negative if the cyst has not leaked. Currently, primary therapy is the surgical removal of the cyst without spillage of its contents, often with pretreatment with albendazole. *Echinococcus multilocularis,* endemic to more northern climates and far less common, causes alveolar cyst disease, a more severe disseminated syndrome with few treatment options and a worse prognosis.

Prospectus for the Future

- Treatment guidelines for malaria will continue to evolve in response to patterns of drug resistance.
- Increased international cooperative efforts, coupled with promising basic research advances, suggest that an effective malaria vaccine may become available over the next decade.
- Significant drug resistance in helminths has not been seen, but surveillance for the development of resistance is gaining support.

- Active research in helminth vaccines is ongoing, with the goal of better control of many of the neglected tropical diseases endemic to the developing world.
- Antimicrobial resistance among enteric pathogens may complicate the management of traveler's diarrhea.
- Changing patterns of established infections and new and emerging pathogens will continue to challenge travelers and health care providers.

References

Arguin P: Approach to the patient before and after travel. In Goldman L, Ausiello D (eds): Cecil Textbook of Medicine, 23rd ed. Philadelphia, WB Saunders, 2007, pp 2147-2150.

Arguin PM, Kozarsky PE, Reed C, Centers for Disease Control and Prevention: Health Information for International Travel 2008. Atlanta, Department of Health and Human Services, Public Health Service, 2007. Available at: www.cdc.gov/travel/yb/.

Bern, C, Montgomery SP, Herwaldt BL, et al: Evaluation and treatment of Chagas Disease in the United States. JAMA 298:2171-2181, 2007.

Boussinesq M: Loiasis. Ann Trop Med Parasitol 100:715-731, 2006.

Centers for Disease Control and Prevention: Human Infection with Avian Influenza A (H5N1) Virus: Advice for Travelers, 2008. Available at: www.cdc.gov/travel/contentAvianFluAsia.aspx.

Freedman DO: Malaria prevention in short-term travelers. N Engl J Med 359:603-612, 2008.

Gluckman SJ: Acute respiratory infections in a recently arrived traveler to your part of the world. Chest 134:163-171, 2008.

Greenwood BM, Bojang K, Whitty CJ, Targett GA: Malaria. Lancet 365:1487-1498, 2005.

Hill DR, Ericcson CD, Pearson RD, et al: The practice of travel medicine: Guidelines by the Infectious Diseases Society of America. Clin Infect Dis 43:1499-1539, 2006.

Hotez, PJ: Hookworm Infections. In Guerrant RL, Walker DH, Weller PF, eds. Tropical Infectious Diseases: Principles, Pathogens, and Practice. Philadelphia, Churchill Livingstone, 2006, pp 1265-1273.

Huang DB, White AC: An updated review on *Cryptosporidium* and *Giardia*. Gastroenterol Clin North Am 35:291-314, 2006.

King CH: Cestodes. In Mandell GL, Bennett JE, Dolin R, eds. Principles and Practices of Infectious Diseases, 6th ed. Philadelphia, Churchill Livingstone, 2005, pp 3285-3292.

Newman RD, Parise ME, Barber AM, Steketee RW: Malaria-related deaths among U.S. Travelers, 1963-2001. Ann Intern Med 141:547-558, 2004.

Pritt BS, Clark CG: Amebiasis. Mayo Clin Proc 83:1154-1164, 2008.

Santos DO, Coutinho CER, Madeira MF, et al: Leishmaniasis treatment—a challenge that remains: A review. Parasitol Res 103:1-10, 2008.

Siddiqui AA, Genta RM, Berk SL: Strongyloidiasis. In Guerrant RL, Walker DH, Weller PF (eds): Tropical Infectious Diseases: Principles, Pathogens, and Practice. Philadelphia, Churchill Livingstone, 2006, pp 1274-1285.

Speil C, Mushtaq A, Adamski A, Khardori N: Fever of unknown origin in the returning traveler. Infect Dis Clin North Am 21:1091-1113, 2007.

Udall DN: Recent updates on onchocerciasis: Diagnosis and treatment. Clin Infect Dis 44:53-60, 2007.

Section XVIII

Bioterrorism

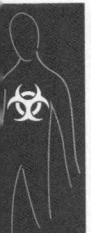

Bioterrorism

Robert W. Bradsher, Jr.

Bioterrorism returned to the consciousness of physicians in the days after the attacks on the World Trade Center and the Pentagon on September 11, 2001. Before a month had passed, the first case of inhalational anthrax in more than 50 years was diagnosed in the United States when a man was hospitalized and rapidly died in Florida. Soon thereafter, cases of cutaneous and inhalational anthrax were reported in New York; Washington, DC; New Jersey; Virginia; and Connecticut. The nation's attention was galvanized on the topics of anthrax, the U.S. Postal Service, gas masks, and antibiotic stockpiling, as well as other bioterrorism concerns. The Federal Bureau of Investigation reported 7 years later that it had concluded its case on the source of the outbreak with the suicide death of an anthrax researcher who worked at the U.S. Army Medical Research Institute of Infectious Diseases. Since September 11, 2001, bioterrorism has been a major topic of medical concern. The need to review bioterrorism is obvious; health professionals are unfamiliar with disease manifestations from these biologic agents used as weapons because they no longer occur or occur only rarely in nature. Those health care professionals on the frontline will likely be emergency department personnel, primary care physicians, pediatricians, and nurse practitioners rather than experts from the Centers for Disease Control and Prevention (CDC) or even traditional first responders, public health officers, or military officials. The purpose of this chapter is to highlight the recognition of these weapons, which are designed for use in terrorism.

Definition and Categorization

Bioterrorism is the intentional use of biologic agents to cause disease in humans or animals to provoke terror. The agents can cause disease either by specific infection or by action of a toxin produced by microorganisms. Depending on the microbe or toxin, resulting disease may or may not be contagious. The CDC has categorized bioterrorism agents into three categories (Table 111-1).

Category A includes agents that can be easily transmitted to humans and that can cause substantial mortality and morbidity. These agents have been most strongly considered as bioweapons and would lead to panic and social disruption. Category A agents have been the major focus for public health officials in preparation for bioterrorism episodes. These agents include anthrax, botulism, plague, smallpox, tularemia, and viral hemorrhagic fevers.

Category B agents (see Table 111-1) are moderately easy to transmit with moderate morbidity and mortality. These agents are not well known, and the CDC considers that increased awareness and surveillance are required. In addition, agents associated with water safety threats and food safety threats are included in category B.

Category C agents include emerging pathogens that could be engineered; they are included because of their availability and potential for having a major health impact.

Chemical weapons (see Table 111-1) are divided by the CDC into biotoxins, vesicants, blood agents, caustics, long-acting anticoagulants, metals, organic solvents, toxic alcohols, choking or pulmonary agents, and nerve agents, as well as vomiting, riot control, and incapacitating agents. Finally, the CDC website for bioterrorism provides links to radiation emergencies. This listing of potential biologic, chemical, and radiation weapons is likely to change substantially. Websites from federal agencies or universities will be the most likely sources for up-to-date information in the event of terrorist attacks, rather than textbooks or journal articles (Table 111-2 and **Web Table 111-1**).

History

Biologic weapons are part of the history of warfare. The Roman army is said by historians to have poisoned the wells of their enemies to shorten their military campaigns. The Tartar's siege of Kaffa in the Crimea in the Middle Ages included the use of cadavers who had died from plague being tossed over the walls of the city, presumably along with fleas that were the source of transmission of *Yersinia pestis.* In the

Table 111-1 **Biologic and Chemical Weapons**

Biologic Weapons

Category A	Category B	Category C
Anthrax (Bacillus anthracis)	Brucellosis (Brucella species)	Nipah virus
Botulism (Clostridium botulinum toxin)	Epsilon toxin—Clostridium perfringens	Hantavirus
Plague (Yersinia pestis)	Glanders (Burkholderia mallei)	
Smallpox (variola major)	Melioidosis (Burkholderia pseudomallei)	
Tularemia (Francisella tularensis)	Psittacosis (Chlamydia psittaci)	
Viral hemorrhagic fevers (Ebola, Marburg, Lassa, Machupo)	Q fever (Coxiella burnetii)	
	Ricin toxin—castor beans	
	Enterotoxin B—Staphylococcus aureus	
	Typhus fever (Rickettsia prowazekii)	
	Viral encephalitis (Venezuelan equine, Eastern equine, Western equine)	
	Water safety—Vibrio cholerae, Cryptosporidium parvum	
	Food safety—Salmonella, Escherichia coli 0157:H7, Shigella	

Chemical Weapons

Vesicants	Blood and Pulmonary Agents	Nerve Agents	Other
Distilled mustard	Arsine	G agents	Vomiting agent
Nitrogen mustard	Cyanide	Sarin (GB)	Riot-control agent
Lewisite	Nitrogen oxide	Soman (GD)	Incapacitating agent
Phosgene oxime	Chlorine	Tabun (GA)	
Ethyldichloroarsine	Phosgene	GF	Benzene
Methyldichloroarsine	Diphosgene	GE	Super warfarin
Phosgene oxime	Perfluoroisobutylene	V agents	Arsenic, barium, mercury, thallium
Phenyldichloroarsine	Red phosphorous	VX	
Sesqui mustard	Sulfur trioxide–chlorosulfonic acid	VM	
	Titanium tetrachloride	VE	
		VG	
		V-gas	

Data from the Centers for Disease Control and Prevention (CDC): Emergency Preparedness and Response website. Available at: www.bt.cdc.gov/Agent/Agentlist.asp.

twentieth century, German and Japanese troops investigated the distribution of biologic weapons before and during World Wars I and II. The United States began investigating biologic warfare at Fort Dietrich in 1942 and later at the Pine Bluff, Arkansas, arsenal before President Nixon ended all offensive efforts in biologic warfare in 1969 (microorganisms) and 1970 (toxins). After the termination of these investigative programs, the U.S. Army Medical Research Institute of Infectious Diseases (USAMRIID) was started to conduct research for medical defense against biologic weapons.

The former Soviet Union had multiple sites for the production of biologic weapons. Even after signing the 1972 treaty on prohibition of biologic weapon development, 55,000 employees in six separate sites were reported to be working on bioweapons under the name *Biopreparate*. An unintentional release of a relatively minute number of spores at the Sverdlovsk bioweapon production site caused anthrax to infect humans and animals over a 2-month period with at least 100 persons dying. Iraq is one of a number of nations considered to have a modern biologic warfare program. Between 1985 and the end of Operation

Desert Storm of the Persian Gulf War, Iraq developed anthrax, botulinum toxin, and aflatoxin for warfare use. In 1990, 200 bombs were produced, with one half containing botulinum toxin and one fourth containing anthrax. The more recent war in Iraq was started, in large part, because of the concern regarding the existence of weapons of mass destruction including bioweapons, although none were identified.

These biologic agents are clearly weapons of mass destruction. It has been estimated that 100 kg of anthrax would lead to the death of up to 3 million individuals if released near a major metropolitan area. Evans and associates estimate that 62,000 individuals would be killed with the release of 5 pounds of anthrax powder in St Louis. This amount compares with the 2 to 3 g of powder estimated to be used in terrorist mailings in 2001. Furthermore, it has been suggested that the release of 100 kg of anthrax spores would cause a number of deaths comparable to the number a hydrogen bomb would cause. However, the agents have also been dubbed "weapons of mass disruption." To illustrate this fact, in October through November 2001, when anthrax was delivered through the U.S. Postal Service, only

Table 111-2 **Websites Related to Biologic, Chemical, and Radiologic Weapons**

www.bt.cdc.gov—Centers for Disease Control and Prevention (CDC) Bioterrorism Preparedness and Response network

www.cidrap.umn.edu/cidrap/—University of Minnesota through the Center for Infectious Disease Research and Policy (CIDRAP)

bioterrorism.slu.edu/—Institute for Biosecurity; St Louis University, School of Public Health

www.usamriid.army.mil/—U.S. Army Medical Research Institute of Infectious Diseases Fort Detrick, Maryland

www.upmc-biosecurity.org/—Center for Biosecurity; University of Pittsburgh Medical Center

https://www.cbrniac.apgea.army.mil/Pages/default.aspx—Chemical, Biological, Radiological & Nuclear Defense Information Analysis Center (CBRNIAC)

www.state.gov/s/ct/—Office of the Coordinator for Counterterrorism, U.S. Department of State

www.idsociety.org/BT/ToC.htm—Infectious Diseases Society of America in collaboration with CIDRAP

www.acponline.org/clinical_information/resources/bioterrorism/—American College of Physicians bioterrorism resources

www.emergency.com/cntrterr.htm—"Counter-Terrorism Archive," Emergency Response and Research Institute (ERRI)

www.foodsafety.gov/~fsg/bioterr.html—Food safety information from the United States Department of Agriculture (USDA), the CDC, and the Canadian Food Inspection Agency

www.who.int/ipcs/en/—International Programme on Chemical Safety (IPCS)

www.emergency.cdc.gov/radiation/—Information from the Radiation Emergency section of CDC's Emergency Preparedness and Response network

www.who.int/ionizing_radiation/en/—World Health Organization (WHO) coordinates response to radiation emergencies, nuclear facility accidents, or weapons of mass destruction (WMD) incidents

22 confirmed or probable cases of infection were discovered, but the nation was almost paralyzed by the event. Holloway and colleagues have reported that the idea of infection caused by invisible agents is particularly frightening. Feelings of horror, anger, panic, magical thinking about microbes, fear of contagion, scapegoating and xenophobia, paranoia, social isolation, helplessness, and demoralization are considered to be results of terrorist acts such as the discovery of bioterrorism agents.

Biologic Agents

ANTHRAX

Anthrax, named for the appearance of the black eschar of the cutaneous lesions (Greek *anthrakos,* meaning coal), is primarily a disease of grazing animals. The organism exists in a spore form in soil as the reservoir. Humans become infected after contact either with soil or animal material infected with the organisms. The cutaneous form is the most common, accounting for approximately 95% of cases of anthrax. After 1 to 7 days of incubation, a small papule develops into an ulcer. Edema and erythema surround the ulcer, which develops a blackened eschar that will dry and fall off within 1 to 2 weeks (see **Web Table 111-1,** links 1, 3, 9, 10 for clinical photographs). This form is not as highly lethal as are other forms; response to antimicrobials is prompt. Gastrointestinal anthrax is very rare and follows the ingestion of contaminated meat. Progression to toxemia is thought to be common, with a high mortality rate. Inhalation anthrax follows respiratory inhalation of spores, although the incubation period may be significantly longer (up to 60 days) than in the cutaneous form. Symptoms include fever, malaise, myalgia, substernal pressure, and discomfort, with progression over days to high fever, dyspnea, cyanosis, progressive shock, and death. Hemorrhagic meningitis develops during this stage in approximately one half of patients. Hemorrhagic mediastinitis and pleural effusion are also common at this stage (see **Web Table 111-1,** links 1, 3, 9, 10 for clinical photographs).

The pathogenesis of anthrax involves ingestion of spores by macrophages, followed by sporulation to vegetative organisms in lymph nodes, which drains the initial site of infection. Toxins known as *lethal toxin* and *edema factor* lead to death. This toxin mediation of the disease explains why the mortality is high despite effective antimicrobial therapy.

Penicillin used to be the treatment of choice for anthrax infection; however, because of the production of β-lactamase by the organisms, either doxycycline or a quinolone (ciprofloxacin) is now the first-line treatment. The earlier the treatment is started, the more likely a response to the antimicrobial therapy will occur, because the late manifestations are caused by toxin rather than replication of the organism. Ciprofloxacin or doxycycline for a total of 60 days has been used as postexposure prophylaxis.

The only human vaccine for anthrax is the supernatant from culture of an attenuated strain and is not available for the general population. The U.S. military uses the vaccine for troops; however, some controversy has developed regarding the safety and efficacy of this immunization. It appears to protect against cutaneous disease and possibly inhalational anthrax. A very effective animal vaccine program is used in agricultural settings.

SMALLPOX

The smallpox virus is one of the most feared organisms that could be considered as a biologic weapon because of its 30% mortality rate (with a range toward 100% with certain forms of the disease) and because of its ability to spread person to person with a multiplier effect of 10 to 20. Another reason for the fear of smallpox relates to one of the greatest successes of the twentieth century. The organism was eliminated in the 1970s from natural infection after a worldwide public health vaccination effort. The elimination effort was successful because smallpox has a single, stable serotype, and only human hosts were infected (no animal reservoir). Other factors included the observation that prompt antibody response occurred with vaccination; even exposed individuals were protected if vaccinated early. The disease was easily recognized clinically, which enabled exposed persons to be immunized promptly, and no carrier or subclinical state was observed with smallpox. However, diagnosis of a patient may very likely be missed because smallpox has not been seen anywhere in the world since 1978. In the last decade, shortages of smallpox vaccine were reported; since the events of 2001, however, an adequate vaccine supply is available.

The virus of variola major and variola minor causes smallpox, named in the fifteenth century to differentiate it from the Great Pox, or syphilis. After an incubation of approximately 2 weeks, smallpox has a prodrome of fever, nausea, headache, and backache, followed by a transient erythematous rash. The typical exanthem then occurs, beginning on the head and upper extremities and spreading to the trunk and lower extremities. The number of lesions on the head and extremities remains greater than on the trunk for the duration of the rash (see **Web Table 111-1,** links 1, 3, 9, 10 for clinical photographs). The lesions begin as macules, which develop into vesicles and then pustules. The pustules dry and shrink in approximately 12 days with a hard crust or scab that then falls off, leaving a sunken scar. The variants of flat smallpox and hemorrhagic smallpox do not have the typical appearance and have a mortality rate approaching 100%. Except for the lesions on the skin and mucous membranes, other organs are not thought to be involved. Secondary bacterial infection is uncommon. Toxemia from the virus is considered to be the most likely cause of death. Complications include encephalitis and blindness from panophthalmitis and keratitis. Cough is not particularly prominent, but it is considered a key element in the transmission of the virus to others.

The differential diagnosis for smallpox includes a number of illnesses with rash. However, the most likely illness to be confused with smallpox is the primary varicella zoster viral infection (chickenpox), which produces crops of lesions, resulting in various stages of papule, vesicle, and pustule that can be observed at the same time in different areas of the body. In addition, chickenpox is more likely to be concentrated on the trunk than it is on the face and extremities as is smallpox.

Smallpox is spread by respiratory droplet nuclei or contaminated clothing or bedding material and is not transmitted during the incubation period but only during the initial fever and through the first week of the rash illness. Cough may transmit the virus in a widespread area. An example reviewed by Henderson is a patient admitted to a first-floor hospital room with subsequent transmission to individuals located on the third floor of the building.

Treatment of patients with smallpox centers on preventing transmission, with respiratory isolation and possibly institution of a quarantine in the setting of a large epidemic. Studies are underway to examine antiviral agents. Cidofovir is licensed for cytomegalovirus and has activity against smallpox; some benefit has been recognized in animals with monkeypox and vaccinia infection, but obviously no trials have been performed.

Prevention of infection with smallpox has been accomplished with vaccinia vaccination. The cutaneous inoculation of this modified virus (cowpox) leads to local infection (Fig. 111-1) with immunity, which should persist for at least a decade or longer. Even when given during the early incubation period, the vaccine can attenuate or abolish the manifestations of smallpox. The National Vaccination Program for the Smallpox Response Plan was ordered in December 2002; a total of 38,440 vaccinations were administered to civilian health care workers and first responders, and the

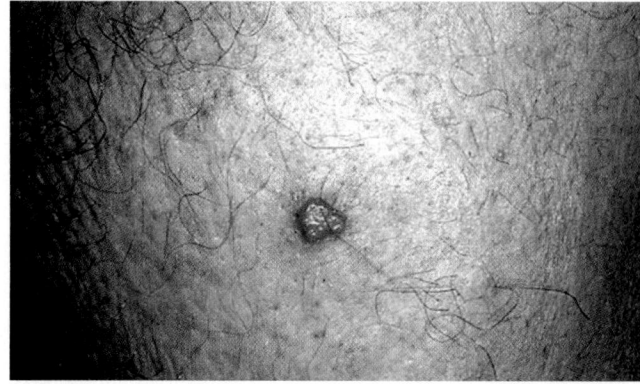
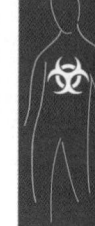

A

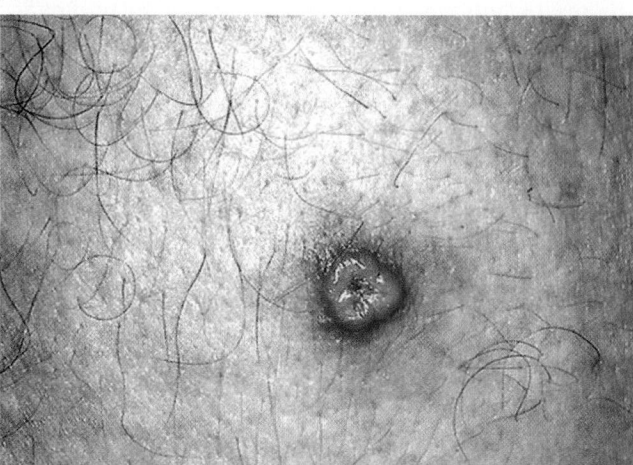

B

Figure 111-1 **A,** Vaccinia vaccination day 3. **B,** Vaccinia vaccination day 7.

number of adverse events was smaller than predicted. The complications of vaccine that occurred included skin lesions that ranged from accidental vaccination lesions to generalized vaccinia to eczema vaccinatum. These complications included 29 reports of generalized vaccinia, 3 patients with potential eczema vaccinatum, and 7 individuals with potential progressive vaccinia. The voluntary vaccination program was placed on hold after 21 cases of potential myocarditis or pericarditis were identified (see **Web Table 111-1,** link 1 for further discussion). Vaccinia immune globulin (VIG) can modify or ameliorate the complications. Pregnant women, those with eczema, and individuals who are immunosuppressed should not receive vaccinia vaccination.

PLAGUE

Y. pestis is the cause of plague, which occurs at a rate of 10 to 12 patients per year in the United States, predominantly in the western states. This organism was used by Japan in bioterrorism attempts in the 1940s but with infected fleas rather than airborne distribution. The infection occurs as either the bubonic form or the septicemic form, usually with pneumonia; unlike anthrax, this organism can be spread from person to person with the pneumonic form. The incubation period is from 2 to 8 days after inoculation, followed by the sudden onset of high fever, chills, generalized weakness, and tender regional lymphadenitis, known as *buboes*.

Inguinal, axillary, or cervical lymphadenopathy is most commonly found (see **Web Table 111-1,** links 1, 3, 9, 10 for clinical photographs). With late-stage disease, purpuric lesions develop and may be the source of the name *black plague* in the Middle Ages. The septicemic form can follow either cutaneous disease in a secondary manner or pneumonic infection as a primary disease. The systemic inflammatory response syndrome follows the severe endotoxemia with subsequent multiorgan dysfunction syndromes exhibited as acute respiratory distress syndrome (ARDS), disseminated intravascular coagulation (DIC), shock, and death. The pneumonic form has sudden onset with headache, malaise, fever, myalgia, and prominent cough, and the pneumonia progresses rapidly with pronounced dyspnea, cyanosis, and hemoptysis. Death results from either respiratory collapse or sepsis. Because secondary transmission is possible and likely, contact and droplet isolation precautions should be maintained for at least 48 hours after sputum cultures are negative or pneumonic plague is excluded. Antibiotic therapy with a quinolone, aminoglycoside, or doxycycline is warranted, as is supportive therapy. Prophylaxis with ciprofloxacin, doxycycline, or trimethoprim-sulfamethoxazole is used in contacts of patients with pneumonic plague. In the event of a bioterrorism event, federal authorities will give recommendations regarding the definition of the exposure that should prompt prophylaxis.

BOTULINUM TOXIN

Botulism is caused by toxin from *Clostridium botulinum,* which is a ubiquitous microorganism found in soil. The toxin types A, B, and E are most commonly associated with human disease, of which about 100 cases per year are reported in the United States. This toxin is the most potent lethal substance known to man, with a lethal dose of 1 ng/kg. No person-to-person transmission is observed with this toxin.

The clinical manifestations of botulism occur after an incubation of 18 to 36 hours in a dose-dependent fashion. The patient will be afebrile, alert, and oriented with normal sensory examination findings; the hallmark symptoms of the disease are cranial nerve abnormalities, such as ptosis, blurry or double vision, difficulty swallowing or talking, and decreased salivation. Progressive motor symptoms then develop, with bilateral descending flaccid paralysis and resultant respiratory paralysis (see **Web Table 111-1,** link 1 for clinical photographs). Death rates of 60% are documented in untreated patients, whereas fewer than 5% of patients who are treated die.

The treatment of botulism includes ventilatory assistance and supportive care. Botulinum antitoxin with the trivalent equine product against types A, B, and E, currently available only from the CDC, is recommended. It is most effective if administered early in the course of the illness. Antibiotic therapy with penicillin is used for infantile and wound botulism. The recovery period may be prolonged with supportive care, including mechanical ventilation, necessary for weeks to months. After antitoxin, no new nerve endings are affected, but recovery is dependent on the generation of new motor end plates at the neuromuscular junction. Vaccine for botulism is only investigational and is not available for clinical use.

VIRAL HEMORRHAGIC FEVERS

A number of viruses cause hemorrhagic fever. These include several different viral families of filoviruses (Ebola, Marburg), arenaviruses (Lassa, Junin, Machupo, Sabia, Guanarito), bunyaviruses (Rift Valley fever), and flaviviruses (yellow fever). Each of these has virus-dependent natural vectors of rodents, mosquitoes, or ticks. These viruses have no natural occurrence in the United States; consequently, identification of a patient with this illness will likely be a bioterrorism event.

Signs and symptoms of viral hemorrhagic fevers include fever, headache, malaise, dizziness, myalgias, nausea, and vomiting. Initial signs of infection would be flushing, conjunctival injection, and periorbital edema. A positive tourniquet test with petechiae is an indication of the bleeding propensity. Hypotension from blood loss and intraabdominal hemorrhage is a marker of the end stages of this infection. Progressive disease is also indicated by prostration; pharyngeal, chest, or abdominal pain or discomfort; mucous membrane bleeding; and skin ecchymosis. Shock and multiorgan dysfunction follow. Usually the patient is either improving or moribund within a week. Clinical bleeding, central nervous system involvement, and significant elevation of hepatic enzymes are indicators of a poor prognosis. The mortality rate is dependent on the infectious agent and ranges from 10% to 90%.

The viruses that cause hemorrhagic fevers are thought to be spread by contact with infected body fluids and not by aerosol or droplet transmission. Therefore standard infection control procedures will prevent the spread of infection to others. The patient should be in a private room with an adjoining anteroom, if available. Particular attention should be paid to strict adherence to hand washing, using an adequate facility with decontamination solution such as Betadine-containing or other hand-washing agents. Negative air pressure rooms should be used, although aerosol transmission is not believed to occur. Strict barrier precautions including protective eyewear and a face shield should be followed. Disposable equipment should be used, with "sharps" being disposed of in rigid containers with disinfectant stored inside and then autoclaved or incinerated. All body fluids should be disinfected because they are believed to be responsible for transmission.

Chemical Agents and Radiation

Chemical weapons are primarily either vesicants similar to nitrogen mustard or nerve agents, although terrorists could use vomiting agents and incapacitating agents such as mace as weapons. As would be expected, a substantial number of individuals would simultaneously exhibit the same symptoms and likely be from the same location. Individuals exposed to chemical warfare would exhibit ocular findings; upper airway symptoms such as rhinorrhea, wheezing, or dyspnea; skin complaints of itching to necrosis; and central nervous system findings from headache to confusion to seizures (see **Web Table 111-1,** links 1, 7, 13 for further discussion).

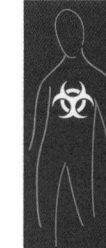

Illness caused by radiation exposure would initially manifest as acute radiation sickness. The severity and timing of the symptoms would depend on the dose of radiation. Bone marrow, gastrointestinal, vascular, neurologic, or cutaneous manifestations would be found, once again depending on the source and total dose. Suppression of blood elements might result in infection and sepsis. Gastrointestinal injury would result in diarrhea, gastrointestinal hemorrhage, and electrolyte abnormalities. Nervous system radiation might lead to ataxia, central nausea, or seizures. Other effects of blindness, pneumonitis, and cutaneous burns would be observed with acute radiation injury (see **Web Table 111-1,** links 1, 7, 13, 14 for further discussion).

The major difference in chemical weapons or intentional radiation injury from "dirty" bombs and biologic weapons is in the incubation time required for the latter. Illness caused by biologic warfare would not be seen until days to weeks after the release of the weapon. In contrast, chemical weapons would likely cause symptoms within minutes to hours in individuals located near the weapon and would likely be recognized by the traditional first responders. Likewise, radiation from a nuclear device would be immediately obvious. The CDC and other sites linked from the CDC website provide recognition and treatments for these conditions.

Prospectus for the Future

- Development of rapid detection systems for environmental monitoring for biologic, chemical, and radiologic weapons
- Development of newer vaccines and consideration of vaccine strategies to prevent bioterrorism outbreaks
- Construction of local, state, and federal plans to control and manage bioterrorism events

- Upgrading of the local, state, and federal public health infrastructures
- Reeducation of physicians in practice and in training regarding infectious diseases that are extremely rare or no longer occur but which might be used as biologic weapons

References

General

Doolan DL, Freilich DA, Brice GT, et al: The US Capitol bioterrorism anthrax exposures: Clinical epidemiological and immunological characteristics. J Infect Dis 195:174-184, 2007.

Evans RG, Crutcher JM, Shadel B, et al: Terrorism from a public health perspective. Am J Med Sci 323:291-298, 2002.

Greenfield RA, Brown BR, Hutchins JB, et al: Microbiological, biological, and chemical weapons of warfare and terrorism. Am J Med Sci 323:326-340, 2002.

Hogan DE, Kellison T: Nuclear terrorism. Am J Med Sci 323:341-349, 2002.

Holloway HC, Norwood AE, Fullerton CS, et al: The threat of biological weapons: Prophylaxis and mitigation of psychological and social consequences. JAMA 278:425-427, 1997.

Matheny J, Mair M, Smith B: Cost/success projections for US biodefense countermeasure development. Nat Biotechnol 26:981-983, 2008.

Vellozzi C, Lane JM, Averhoff G, et al: Generalized vaccinia, progressive vaccinia, and eczema vaccinatum are rare following smallpox (vaccinia) vaccination: United States surveillance, 2003. Clin Infect Dis 41:689-697, 2005.

Anthrax

Bartlett JG, Ingelsby TV Jr, Borio L: Management of anthrax. Clin Infect Dis 35:851-858, 2002.

Bush LM, Abrams BH, Beall A, Johnson CC: Index case of fatal inhalational anthrax due to bioterrorism in the United States. N Engl J Med 345:1607-1610, 2001.

Jernigan JA, Stephens DS, Ashford DA, et al: Bioterrorism related inhalational anthrax: The first 10 cases reported in the United States. Emerg Infect Dis 7:933-944, 2001.

Purcell BK, Worsham PL, Friedlander AM: Anthrax. In Dembek ZR (ed): Medical Aspects of Biological Warfare. Washington DC, Office of the Surgeon General, Borden Institute, Walter Reed Army Medical Center, 2007, pp 69-90.

Swartz MN: Recognition and management of anthrax. N Engl J Med 345:1621-1626, 2001.

Smallpox

Breman JG, Henderson DA: Current concepts: Diagnosis and management of smallpox. N Engl J Med 346:1300-1308, 2002.

Frey SE, Couch RB, Tacket CO, et al: Clinical responses to undiluted and diluted smallpox vaccine. N Engl J Med 346:1265-1274, 2002.

Henderson DA: Bioterrorism as a public health threat. Emerg Infect Dis 4:488-492, 1998.

Consensus Papers on Bioterrorism Agents

Arnon SS, Schechter R, Inglesby TV, et al: Botulinum toxin as a biological weapon: Medical and public health management. JAMA 285:1059-1070, 2001.

Borio L, Inglesby T, Peters CJ, et al: Hemorrhagic fever viruses as biological weapons: Medical and public health management. JAMA 287:2391-2405, 2002.

Dennis DT, Ingelsby TV, Henderson DA, et al: Tularemia as a biological weapon: Medical and public health management. JAMA 285:2763-2773, 2001.

Henderson DA, Inglesby TV, Bartlett JG, et al: Smallpox as a biological weapon: Medical and public health management. JAMA 281:2127-2137, 1999.

Inglesby TV, Dennis DT, Henderson DA, et al: Plague as a biological weapon: Medical and public health management. JAMA 283:2281-2290, 2000.

Inglesby TV, O'Toole T, Henderson DA, et al: Anthrax as a biological weapon, 2002: updated recommendations for management. JAMA 287:2236-2252, 2002.

Section XIX

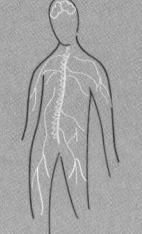

Neurologic Disease

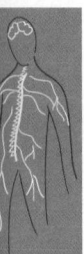

Neurologic Evaluation of the Patient

Frederick J. Marshall

To arrive at an accurate neurologic diagnosis, the clinician generates and tests hypotheses about the location and the mechanism of injury to the nervous system. Hypotheses are refined as the clinician progresses from the interview to the physical examination to the laboratory assessment of the patient. The focus is first placed on those entities that are common, serious, and treatable. Typical presentations of common diseases account for 80% of all cases, unusual presentations of common diseases account for 15%, typical presentations of rare diseases account for 5%, and unusual presentations of rare diseases account for less than 1%.

Taking a Neurologic History

The clinician must determine the location, quality, and timing of symptoms. He or she must avoid hearsay and ask the patient to report the progression of actual symptoms rather than a litany of diagnostic procedures and specialty evaluations. Establishing when the patient last felt perfectly normal is important. Ambiguous descriptors such as *dizzy* should be rejected in favor of evocative descriptors such as *light-headed* (which might implicate cardiovascular insufficiency) or *off balance* (which might implicate cerebellar or posterior column dysfunction).

Family members and other witnesses must corroborate historical information when appropriate. Historical information should include the medical and surgical histories; current medications; allergies; family history; review of systems; and social history, including the patient's level of education, work history, possible toxin exposures, substance use, sexual history, and current life circumstance.

Clues to localization are sought during the interview. For example, pain is generally caused by a lesion of the peripheral nervous system, whereas aphasia (disordered language

processing) indicates an abnormality of the central nervous system. Because sensory and motor functions are anatomically relatively distant in the cerebral cortex but progressively closer together as fibers converge in the brainstem, spinal cord, roots, and peripheral nerves, the co-existence of sensory loss and motor dysfunction in a limb implies either a large lesion at the level of the cortex or a smaller lesion lower down in the neuraxis. Small lesions in areas of *high traffic* such as the spinal cord or brainstem can result in widespread neurologic dysfunction, whereas small lesions elsewhere may be asymptomatic.

Table 112-1 lists the potential localizing values of common neurologic symptoms to help settle the issue of lesion localization. Tables 112-2 and 112-3 list symptoms that are commonly associated with lesions at specific locations in the nervous system. Some symptoms can result from a lesion at any of several levels of the nervous system. For example, double vision can result from a focal lesion in the brainstem, peripheral nerves (cranial nerve III, IV, or VI), neuromuscular junction, or extraocular muscles; or it can be nonfocal from an increase in intracranial pressure. Associated symptoms (or the lack thereof) may lead the interviewer to reject certain hypotheses that at first seemed most likely. Table 112-4 lists the most important types of neuropathologic conditions and provides examples of diseases in each category.

Some neuroanatomic locations point to a specific diagnosis or a limited number of diagnoses. For example, disease of the neuromuscular junction is usually caused by an autoimmune process—myasthenia gravis (common) or Eaton-Lambert myasthenic syndrome (uncommon). The exceptions—botulism and congenital myasthenic disorders—are rare. Alternatively, some areas of the nervous system (e.g., the cerebral hemispheres) are vulnerable to practically any of the categories of disease outlined in Table 112-4.

The pace and temporal order of symptoms are important. Degenerative diseases generally progress gradually, whereas vascular diseases (e.g., stroke, aneurysmal subarachnoid hemorrhage) progress rapidly. Certain symptoms such as double vision almost invariably develop abruptly, even if the underlying disorder has been developing gradually over days to weeks.

Neurologic Examination

Although the performance of the main elements of a general screening neurologic examination is imperative

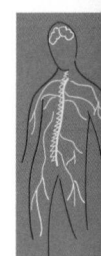

(Table 112-5), the examination should be tailored to confirm or disprove the clinical hypotheses generated from the patient's history. Unexpected signs must be explained (often with a return to the history for further clarification).

The examination is approached as if only one of two possible injuries has occurred: either the *final common pathway* to a structure is disrupted or the input to that pathway is disrupted (Fig. 112-1). In the case of the motor system, the *final common pathway* includes the anterior horn cells giving rise to axons in a nerve, the nerve itself, the neuromuscular junction, and the muscle. Injury to any of these structures will result in dysfunction of the muscle. Conversely, if these structures are intact, observing the muscle function may be possible under the right circumstances. If all modes of engaging the final common pathway fail to elicit a response, then the clinician can conclude that the lesion is located somewhere within the final common pathway.

For example, a man with paralysis of facial movement on one side that is caused by a lesion of cranial nerve VII cannot smile voluntarily, close his eye, or wrinkle his forehead on the affected side. Spontaneous laughter or smiling as an automatic response to a joke also fails to move the paretic side. If the problem is central, however, then facial movement with involuntary (spontaneous) smiling may be preserved or even increased. This observation is common in patients with facial weakness caused by a stroke.

Central input to a final common pathway in the nervous system is usually tonically inhibitory. Damage to this input typically results in overactivity of the involved muscle group. Signs of damage to central inhibitory systems include

Table 112-1 Potential Localizing Value of Common Neurologic Symptoms

Potential Localizing Value	Sign or Symptom
High	Focal weakness, sensory loss, or pain Focal visual loss Language disturbance Neglect or anosognosia
Medium	Vertigo Dysarthria Clumsiness
Low	Fatigue Headache Insomnia Dizziness Anxiety, confusion, or psychosis

Table 112-2 Use of Symptoms and Signs for Localization in the Central Nervous System

Sign or Symptom	Location
Cerebral Hemispheres	
Unilateral weakness or sensory complaints	Contralateral cerebral hemisphere
Language dysfunction	Left hemisphere (frontal and temporal)
Spatial disorientation	Right hemisphere (parietal and occipital)
Anosognosia (lack of insight into deficit)	Right hemisphere (parietal)
Hemivisual loss	Contralateral hemisphere (occipital, temporal, and parietal)
Flattening of affect or social disinhibition	Bihemispheric (frontal and limbic)
Alteration of consciousness	Bihemispheric (diffuse)
Alteration of memory	Bihemispheric (hippocampus, fornix, amygdala, and mammillary bodies)
Cerebellum	
Limb clumsiness	Ipsilateral cerebellar hemisphere
Unsteadiness of gait or posture	Midline cerebellar structures
Basal Ganglia	
Slowness of voluntary movement	Substantia nigra and striatum
Involuntary movement	Striatum, thalamus, and subthalamus
Brainstem	
Contralateral weakness or sensory complaints in the body with ipsilateral weakness or sensory complaints in the face	Midbrain, pons, and medulla
Double vision	Midbrain and pons
Vertigo	Pons and medulla
Alteration of consciousness	Midbrain, pons, medulla (reticular formation)
Spinal Cord	
Weakness and spasticity (ipsilateral) and anesthesia (contralateral) below a specified level	Corticospinal and spinothalamic tracts
Unsteadiness of gait	Posterior columns
Bilateral (can be asymmetrical) weakness and sensory complaints in multiple contiguous radicular distributions	Central cord

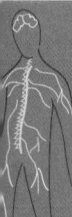

Table 112-3 Symptom Localization in the Motor Unit (Anterior Horn Cell and the Peripheral Nervous System)

Sign or Symptom	Location
Anterior Horn Cell	
Weakness and wasting with muscle twitching (fasciculation) but no sensory complaints	Anterior horn of spinal cord (diffuse or segmental)
Spinal Root	
Weakness and sensory loss confined to a known radicular distribution (pain, a common feature, may spread)	Cervical, thoracic, lumbar, and sacral
Plexus	
Pain, weakness, and sensory loss in a limb; not limited to a single radicular or peripheral nerve distribution	Brachial and lumbosacral (may also be caused by polyradiculopathy)
Nerve	
Pain, distal weakness, and/or sensory changes confined to a single peripheral nerve distribution	Peripheral nerves (mononeuropathy)
Pain, distal weakness, and/or sensory changes affecting both sides symmetrically (generally starting in feet)	Peripheral nerves (polyneuropathy)
Pain, distal weakness, and/or sensory changes affecting scattered single peripheral nerve distributions	Peripheral nerves (mononeuropathy multiplex)
Unilateral special sensory loss	Cranial nerves I, II, V, VII, VIII, and IX
Unilateral facial weakness involving entire one half of face	Cranial nerve VII (ipsilateral)
Neuromuscular Junction	
Progressive weakness with repeated use of a muscle; no sensory complaints	Ocular, pharyngeal, and skeletal
Muscle	
Proximal weakness; no sensory complaints	Diffuse and various patterns

Table 112-4 Categories of Neurologic Disease

Disease Category	Example
Genetic	
Autosomal dominant	Huntington disease
Autosomal recessive	Friedreich ataxia
Sex-linked recessive	Duchenne muscular dystrophy
Sporadic	Down syndrome
Neoplastic	
Intrinsic	Glioblastoma
Extrinsic	Metastatic melanoma
Paraneoplastic	Cerebellar degeneration
Vascular	
Stroke	Thrombotic, embolic, lacunar, hemorrhagic
Structural	Arteriovenous malformation
Inflammatory	Cranial arteritis
Infectious	
Bacterial	Meningococcal meningitis
Viral	Herpes encephalitis
Protozoal	Toxoplasmosis
Fungal	Cryptococcal meningitis
Helminthic	Cysticercosis
Prion	Creutzfeldt-Jakob disease
Degenerative	
Central	Parkinson disease
Central and peripheral	Amyotrophic lateral sclerosis
Autoimmune	
Central demyelinating	Multiple sclerosis
Peripheral demyelinating	Guillain-Barré syndrome
Neuromuscular junction	Myasthenia gravis
Toxic and Metabolic	
Endogenous	Uremic encephalopathy
Exogenous	Alcoholic neuropathy
Other Structural	
Trauma	Spinal cord injury
Hydrodynamic	Normal pressure hydrocephalus
Psychogenic	Hysterical paraparesis

(1) spasticity and hyperreflexia (motor cortex, subcortical white matter, or corticospinal pathways in the brainstem and spinal cord); (2) dystonia, rigidity, tremor, and tic (basal ganglia or extrapyramidal systems); and (3) ataxia and dysmetria (cerebellum). An exception is hypotonia caused by cerebellar disease.

Technologic Assessment

Laboratory investigations and special testing should be used to confirm a clinical suggestion and to finalize the diagnosis. Testing should be selectively performed because of expense, risk, and discomfort to the patient. Frequently helpful tests are discussed in this text; diagnostic tests should never be ordered without a specific differential diagnosis firmly in mind. Many neurodiagnostic tests disclose diagnoses unrelated to a patient's symptomatic disease process.

LUMBAR PUNCTURE

Investigation of the cerebrospinal fluid (CSF) is indicated in a small number of specific circumstances (usually meningitis and encephalitis) (Table 112-6). A CSF specimen should be routinely sent for laboratory testing to determine cell and differential counts, protein and glucose levels, and bacterial cultures. The CSF should also be examined for its color and clarity. Cloudy or discolored CSF should be centrifuged and examined for xanthochromia in comparison with water. Special studies may be supplemented as appropriate, including Gram stain; fungal, viral, and tuberculous cultures; cryptococcal and other antigens; tests for syphilis; Lyme titers; malignant cytologic patterns; or oligoclonal bands. Polymerase chain reaction for specific viruses holds promise for many conditions. Recording the opening and closing pressures is important. Tissue infection in the region of the puncture site is an absolute contraindication to lumbar puncture. Relative contraindications include known or

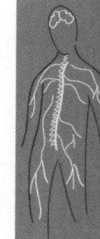

Table 112-5 Elements of a General Screening Neurologic Examination

General Systemic Physical Examination

Head (trauma, dysmorphism, and bruits)
Neck (tone, bruits, and thyromegaly)
Cardiovascular (heart rate, rhythm, and murmurs; peripheral pulses and jugular venous distention)
Pulmonary (breathing pattern and cyanosis)
Abdomen (hepatosplenomegaly)
Back and extremities (skeletal abnormalities, peripheral edema, and straight-leg raising)
Skin (neurocutaneous stigmata and hepatic stigmata)

Mental Status

Level of consciousness (awake, drowsy, and comatose)
Attention (coherent stream of thought, serial 7s)
Orientation (temporal and spatial)
Memory (short- and long-term)
Language (naming, repetition, comprehension, fluency, reading, and writing)
Visuospatial skills (clock drawing and figure copying)
Judgment, insight, thought content (psychotic)
Mood (depressed, manic, and anxious)

Cranial Nerves

Olfactory (smell in each nostril)
Optic (afferent pupillary function, funduscopic examination, visual acuity, visual fields, and structural eye findings)
Oculomotor, trochlear, and abducens (smooth pursuit and saccadic eye movements, nystagmus, efferent pupillary function, and eyelid opening)
Trigeminal (jaw jerk, facial sensation, afferent corneal reflex, and muscles of mastication)
Facial (efferent corneal reflex, facial expression, eyelid closure, nasolabial folds, and power and bulk)
Vestibulocochlear (nystagmus, speech discrimination, Weber test, and Rinne test)
Glossopharyngeal and vagus (afferent and efferent gag reflex and uvula position)
Spinal accessory (power and bulk of sternocleidomastoid and trapezii muscles)
Hypoglossal (position, bulk, and fasciculations of tongue)

Motor Examination

Pronator drift (subtle corticospinal lesion)
Tone and bulk of muscles (basal ganglia lesion yields rigidity, cerebellar lesion yields hypotonia, corticospinal lesion yields spasticity, nonspecific bihemispheric disease yields paratonia, hypertrophy indicates dystonia, pseudohypertrophy indicates muscle disease, and atrophy indicates lower motor neuron disease)
Adventitious movements (tremor, tic, dystonia, and chorea indicate disease of the basal ganglia; asterixis and myoclonus may indicate toxic metabolic process)
Power of major muscle groups (scale 0-5)
Upper extremities: deltoids, biceps, triceps, wrist extension and flexion, finger extension and flexion, and interossei
Lower extremities: hip flexion, extension, abduction, and adduction; knee extension and flexion; ankle dorsiflexion, plantar flexion, inversion, and eversion; toe extension and flexion

Sensory Examination

Light touch (posterior columns)
Pinprick (spinothalamic tract)
Temperature (spinothalamic tract)
Joint position sense (posterior columns)
Vibration (posterior columns)
Graphesthesia (cortical sensory)
Double simultaneous stimulation (cortical sensory)
Two-point discrimination (posterior columns and cortical sensory)

Table 112-5 Elements of a General Screening Neurologic Examination—Cont'd

Reflex Examination

Standard reflexes (grades 0-4)
Biceps
Triceps
Brachioradialis
Knee jerk
Ankle jerk
Pathologic reflexes
Babinski sign (if present)
Myerson sign (if present)
Snout (if present)
Jaw jerk (if brisk)
Palmomental (if present)
Hoffmann sign (if brisk)

Coordination and Gait

Finger-nose-finger (intention tremor suggesting cerebellar disease)
Rapid alternating movements (dysdiadochokinesia suggesting cerebellar disease)
Fine motor movements (slowness and small amplitude suggesting basal ganglia or corticospinal tract abnormalities)
Heel-to-shin (ataxia suggesting cerebellar disease)
Arising from chair with arms folded across chest (inability in advanced basal ganglia, cerebellar, corticospinal, or muscle disease)
Walking naturally (look for decreased arm swing, spasticity, broad base, festination, waddle, footdrop, start hesitation, and dystonia)
Tandem gait (look for ataxia)
Walking with feet everted or inverted (look for latent dystonia)
Hopping on each foot separately (look for latent dystonia)
Stand with feet together and eyes open, eyes closed (sensory ataxia and cerebellar disease)
Response to retropulsive stress (loss of postural righting mechanisms)

probable intracranial or spinal mass lesion, increased intracranial pressure as a result of mass lesions, coagulopathy caused by thrombocytopenia (usually correctable), anticoagulant therapy, or bleeding disorders. Rare but severe complications include transtentorial or foramen magnum herniation, spinal epidural hematoma, spinal abscess, herniated or infected disk, meningitis, and adverse reaction to a local anesthetic agent. More common and relatively benign complications include headache and backache.

TISSUE BIOPSIES

In select specialty centers, a diagnostic biopsy is performed on various tissues, including brain, peripheral nerve (see Chapter 130), muscle (see Chapter 131), and skin. On occasion, biopsy provides the only means of arriving at a definitive diagnosis.

ELECTROPHYSIOLOGIC STUDIES

Electrophysiologic studies include electroencephalography, electromyography, nerve conduction studies, and evoked potentials. These studies are helpful in situations in which the patient cannot be examined or interviewed adequately.

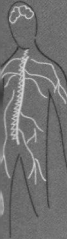

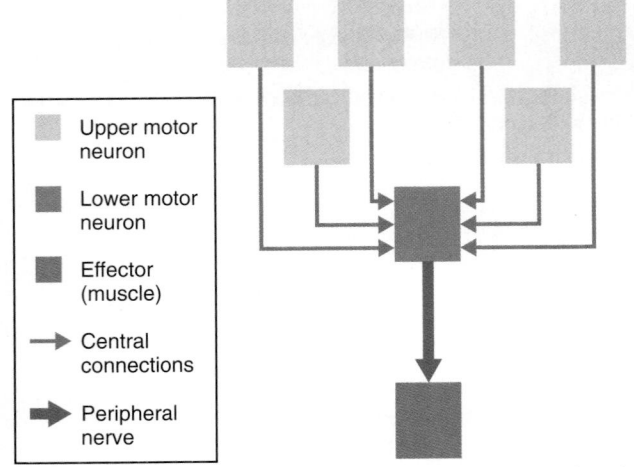

Upper motor neuron

Lower motor neuron

Effector (muscle)

Central connections

Peripheral nerve

Figure 112-1 The nervous system can be conceptually reduced to a series of higher-order inputs that converge on final common pathways. For example, upper motor neurons converge on lower motor neurons, whose axons form the final common pathway to an effector muscle.

Table 112-7	**Magnetic Resonance Imaging (MRI) versus Computed Tomography (CT)**
MRI	
Resolution 1-2 mm (higher with newer 3-Tesla magnets)	
Gadolinium contrast relatively safe (except in severe renal insufficiency)	
Unaffected by bone	
Multiple planes of imaging available	
Functional (physiologic) imaging capacity	
CT	
Resolution >5 mm	
Iodine contrast associated with anaphylaxis and rash	
Faster acquisition than MRI	
Metallic objects such as pacemaker or aneurysm clip preclude MRI	
Acute hemorrhage well visualized	
Better tolerated by patients who are severely ill or claustrophobic	

Table 112-6	**Indications for Lumbar Puncture**
Urgent (Do Not Wait for Brain Imaging)	
Acute central nervous system infection in the absence of focal neurologic signs	
Less Urgent (Wait for Brain Imaging)	
Vasculitis, subarachnoid hemorrhage, or cryptic process	
Increased intracranial pressure in the absence of mass lesion on magnetic resonance imaging or computed tomography	
Intrathecal therapy for fungal or carcinomatous meningitis	
Symptomatic treatment for headache from idiopathic intracranial hypertension or subarachnoid hemorrhage	

Electroencephalography is most often used to investigate seizures (see Chapter 126). It can document encephalopathy, in which case the background electrical activity of the brain is slowed, and it is also used in the evaluation of brain death.

Electromyography is useful in the differential diagnosis of muscle disease, neuromuscular junction disease, peripheral nerve disease, and anterior horn cell disease (see Chapters 130 and 131). Nerve conduction studies (see Chapters 130 and 131) may show decreased amplitude (characteristic of axonal neuropathy) or decreased velocity (characteristic of demyelinating neuropathy).

Visual-evoked potential studies are commonly used in the evaluation of possible multiple sclerosis (see Chapter 129). Asymmetrical slowing of the cortical response to visual pattern stimulation suggests demyelination in the optic nerve or central optic pathways. Brainstem auditory-evoked potential studies are useful in the diagnosis of diseases affecting cranial nerve VIII or its central projections. Lesions at the cerebellopontine angle and the brainstem cause abnormal delay in conduction. Brainstem auditory-evoked potentials are helpful in the diagnosis of deafness in infants. Somatosensory-evoked potentials are used to identify a slowing of central sensory conduction that results from demyelinating disease, compression, or metabolic derange-

ments. They are also used to evaluate spinal cord–mediated sensory abnormalities.

IMAGING STUDIES

Magnetic resonance imaging (MRI) and computed tomography (CT) are high-resolution imaging techniques that provide extraordinary diagnostic precision for central nervous system lesions. Most neurologic diseases, however, can have normal CT and MRI findings. Moreover, many abnormal findings on CT and MRI bear no relation to the diagnosis responsible for the patient's symptoms. Table 112-7 compares CT with MRI. MRI is used for most purposes, although CT has the advantage of wider accessibility, greater speed of acquisition, and better tolerability by the patient. CT detects acute hemorrhage and is preferred for emergencies. MRI provides more detail and simultaneously obtains images in the horizontal, vertical, and coronal planes. Contrast media for CT or MRI are useful in the diagnosis of tumors, abscesses, and other processes that derange the blood-brain barrier. MRI can now be used for functional imaging and spectroscopy; both techniques have great promise for the evaluation of cognitive and metabolic disorders, epilepsy, multiple sclerosis, and many other conditions.

Magnetic resonance angiography allows noninvasive visualization of the major vessels of the head and neck. Conventional angiography with an intra-arterial injection of contrast agent is used for evaluation of many intracranial vascular abnormalities, including small aneurysms and arteriovenous malformations and inflammation of small blood vessels.

Noninvasive ultrasonography of the carotid and vertebral arteries can define stenotic vessels and has been supplemented by transcranial Doppler technology, which allows characterization of blood flow in intracranial arteries.

Single-photon emission CT is useful for the evaluation of intracranial blood flow. Moreover, the development of new radioligands makes it possible to visualize the dopamine transporter on nigral-striatal dopaminergic projection neurons by using a ligand (β-CIT) to follow cell loss in patients with Parkinson disease. As the techniques of neural transplantation for Parkinson disease improve, it may be possible to image restoration of function.

Positron-emission tomography (PET) is a functional imaging technology that can demonstrate specific metabolic derangements. It remains a largely investigational method but is particularly useful for evaluating local abnormalities of glucose and oxygen metabolism. PET is of particular value in defining the site of origin of focal seizures. Customized ligands may be used to identify specific pathologic processes. An example is the thioflavin derivative known as Pittsburgh Compound B (PiB), which binds to the amyloid plaque of Alzheimer disease and may become useful as a clinical diagnostic test in the near future. The high cost of the cyclotron technology needed to generate the radioactive ligands limits the clinical use of PET to specialized centers.

GENETIC AND MOLECULAR TESTING

There are more neurologic diseases than diseases of all other systems combined. Recent discoveries have revolutionized the diagnostic approach to many of these diseases; new genetic tests are discovered every year. Table 112-8 outlines tests that are now commercially available. Genetic testing for a disorder requires that the clinician perform a thoughtful

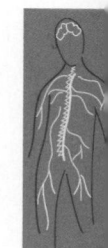

Table 112-8 Some Neurologic Conditions for Which Genetic Tests Are Available

Peripheral neuropathies (Charcot-Marie-Tooth 1A, Kennedy syndrome)

Neuromuscular diseases (myotonic dystrophy, Duchenne muscular dystrophy, Becker muscular dystrophy, spinal muscular atrophy, MELAS, MERRF, familial amyotrophic lateral sclerosis)

Movement disorders (spinocerebellar ataxia, multiple types; Friedreich ataxia; dystonia DYT1; Huntington disease)

Mental retardation (fragile X)

MELAS, mitochondrial encephalomyelopathy, lactic acidosis, and strokelike symptoms (syndrome); MERRF, myoclonus epilepsy with ragged red fibers (syndrome).

and caring evaluation of the patient, usually with input from and evaluation of the patient's family. Important ethical issues surround the use of genetic tests, including the ability to ensure privacy, to ensure adequate psychological and social support for patients who may be given devastating news, and to address adequately the appropriateness of prenatal screening or presymptomatic testing when no treatment is available.

Prospectus for the Future

Novel imaging techniques and molecular diagnostic studies are beginning to shed light on the pathogenesis of neurological conditions that have been identifiable only by clinical phenomenology. The dystonias, many degenerative diseases, the epilepsies, headache, and other conditions are not subject to specific diagnosis and disease localization. Despite these and foreseeable future advances, the clinical aspects of neurological disease remain of fundamental importance in understanding the impact of disease on patients and their families.

References

Hackney D: Radiologic imaging procedures. In Goldman L, Ausiello DA (eds): Cecil Textbook of Medicine, 23rd ed. Philadelphia, WB Saunders, 2007.

Samuels MA, Feske S (eds): Office Practice of Neurology, 2nd ed. New York, Churchill Livingstone, 2003.

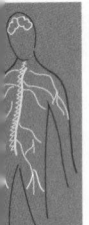

Disorders of Consciousness

Roger P. Simon

Coma is a sleeplike state in that the patient is unresponsive and the eyes are closed even with vigorous stimulation. A poorly responsive state in which the eyes are open, or an agitated confused state, or delirium, is not coma, but it may represent early stages of the same disease processes and should be investigated in the same manner.

Consciousness requires an intact and functioning brainstem reticular activating system and its cortical projections. The reticular formation begins in the midpons and ascends through the dorsal midbrain to synapse in the thalamus; it then innervates higher centers through thalamocortical connections. Knowledge of this anatomic substrate provides the short list of regions to be investigated in the search for a structural cause of coma: brainstem or bihemispheric dysfunction satisfies these anatomic requirements. Structural lesions elsewhere are not the cause of the patient's unconsciousness. In addition to structural lesions, meningeal inflammation, metabolic encephalopathy, and seizures diffusely affect the brain and complete the differential diagnosis for the patient in coma.

Pathophysiologic Factors

Meningeal irritation caused by infection or blood in the subarachnoid space is an essential early consideration in coma evaluation because its cause requires immediate attention (especially with purulent meningitis) and may not be diagnosed by computed tomography (CT).

Hemispheric mass lesions result in coma either by expanding across the midline laterally to compromise both cerebral hemispheres or by impinging on the brainstem to compress the rostral reticular formation. These processes—*lateral herniation* (lateral movement of the brain) and *transtentorial herniation* (vertical movement of the brain)—most commonly occur together. At the bedside, clinical signs of an expanding hemispheric mass evolve in a level-by-level, rostral-caudal manner (Fig. 113-1). Hemispheric lesions of adequate size to produce coma are readily seen on CT.

Brainstem mass lesions produce coma by directly affecting the reticular formation. Because the pathways for lateral eye movements (the pontine gaze center, medial longitudinal fasciculus, and oculomotor—third nerve—nucleus) traverse the reticular activating system, impairment of reflex eye movements is often the critical element of diagnosis of a brainstem lesion. A comatose patient without impaired reflex lateral eye movements does not have a mass lesion compromising brainstem structures in the posterior fossa. CT is not able to show some lesions in this region. Posterior fossa lesions may block the flow of cerebrospinal fluid from the lateral ventricles and result in the dangerous situation of *noncommunicating hydrocephalus.*

Metabolic abnormalities are caused by deficiency states (e.g., thiamine, glucose), by derangements of metabolism (e.g., hyponatremia), or by the presence of *exogenous toxins* (drugs) or *endogenous toxins* (organ system failure). Metabolic abnormalities result in diffuse dysfunction of the nervous system and therefore produce, with rare exceptions, no localized signs such as hemiparesis or unilateral pupillary dilation. The diagnosis of *metabolic encephalopathy* means that the examiner has found no focal anatomic features on examination or neuroimaging studies to explain coma, but it does not state that a specific metabolic cause has been established. Drugs have a predilection for affecting the reticular formation in the brainstem and for producing paralysis of reflex eye movement on examination. *Multifocal structural disorders* may simulate metabolic coma (Table 113-1).

In the late stages of status epilepticus, motor movements may be subtle even though *seizure activity* is continuing throughout the brain (nonconvulsive status epilepticus). Once seizures stop, the so-called *postictal state* can also cause unexplained coma.

Diagnostic Approach

The history and examination are essential in the diagnosis and are not replaced by brain imaging (Table 113-2). History of a premonitory headache supports a diagnosis of meningitis, encephalitis, or intracerebral or subarachnoid hemorrhage. A preceding period of intoxication, confusion, or delirium points to a diffuse process such as meningitis or endogenous or exogenous toxins. The sudden apoplectic onset of coma is particularly suggestive of ischemic or

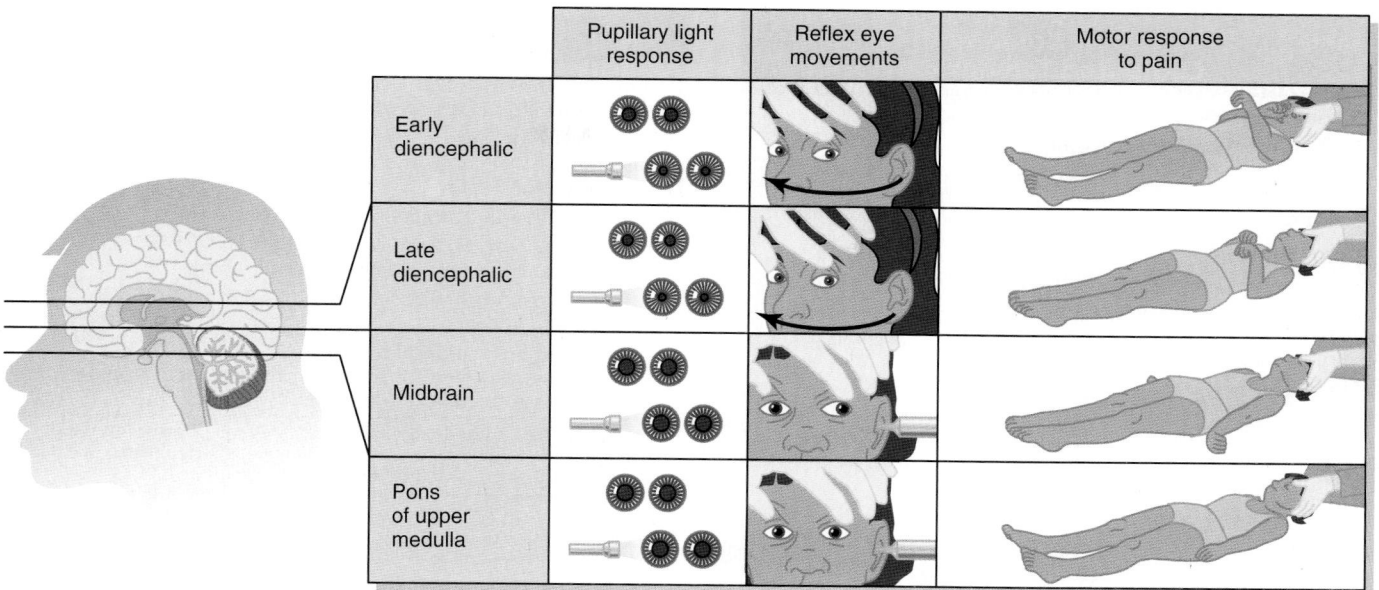

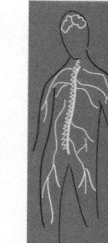

Figure 113-1 The evolution of neurologic signs in coma from a hemispheric mass lesion as the brain becomes functionally impaired in a rostral-caudal manner. *Early* and *late diencephalic* refer to levels of dysfunction just above (early) and just below (late) the thalamus. (From Aminoff MJ, Greenberg DA, Simon RP: Clinical Neurology. Stamford, CT, Appleton and Lange, 1996).

Table 113-1 **Multifocal Disorders Indicating Metabolic Coma**
Disseminated intravascular coagulopathy
Sepsis
Pancreatitis
Vasculitis
Thrombotic thrombocytopenic purpura
Fat emboli
Hypertensive encephalopathy
Diffuse micrometastases

hemorrhagic stroke affecting the brainstem or of subarachnoid hemorrhage or intracerebral hemorrhage with intraventricular rupture. Lateralized symptoms of hemiparesis or aphasia before coma occur in patients with hemispheric masses or infarctions.

The physical examination is critical, quickly accomplished, and diagnostic. The issues are three: (1) Does the patient have meningitis? (2) Are signs of a mass lesion present? (3) Is this condition a diffuse syndrome of exogenous or endogenous metabolic cause? Emergency management should then be instituted accordingly (Table 113-3).

IDENTIFICATION OF MENINGITIS

Although signs of meningeal irritation are not invariably present and have differing sensitivity with regard to cause (extremely common with acute pyogenic meningitis and subarachnoid hemorrhage, less common with indolent, fungal meningitis), the presence of these signs on examination is the central clue to the diagnosis. Missing these signs results in time-consuming additional tests such as brain imaging and the potential loss of a narrow window of opportunity for directed therapy. Passive neck flexion should be carried out (Fig. 113-2) in all comatose patients unless a history of head trauma exists. When the neck is passively flexed, by attempt-

ing to bring the chin within a few fingerbreadths of the chest, patients with irritated meninges reflexively flex one or both knees. This sign (*Brudzinski reflex*) is usually asymmetrical and not dramatic, but any evidence of knee flexion during passive neck flexion requires that the cerebrospinal fluid be examined. Is CT required before lumbar puncture in this setting? In the absence of lateralized signs (such as hemiparesis) supporting a superimposed mass lesion, a spinal puncture should be performed immediately. Although rare cases of herniation after lumbar puncture have been reported in children with bacterial meningitis, the urgency of diagnosis and treatment at the point of coma is paramount. The time needed for CT may result in a fatal therapeutic delay. An alternative approach involves obtaining blood cultures and immediately initiating antibiotic therapy with subsequent lumbar puncture; cerebrospinal fluid cell count, glucose determination, and protein content are unchanged, and Gram stain and culture often remain positive despite a short period of antibiotic treatment. Bacterial antigens in the cerebrospinal fluid or blood can also be detected.

SEPARATION OF STRUCTURAL FROM METABOLIC CAUSES OF COMA

The goal of this differential diagnosis is achieved by neurologic examination. Because the evaluation and potential treatments for structural and metabolic coma are widely divergent and the disease processes in both categories are often rapidly progressive, initiating the evaluation medically or surgically may be life saving. Identification of a structural versus a metabolic case is accomplished by focusing on three features of neurologic examination: the *motor response* to a painful stimulus, *pupillary function*, and *reflex eye movements*.

Motor Response

Asymmetrical or reflex function of the motor system provides the clearest indication of a mass lesion. Elicitation of a

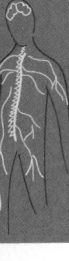

Table 113-2	**Causes of Coma with Normal Computed Tomography Scan**

Meningeal Disorders

Subarachnoid hemorrhage (uncommon)
Bacterial meningitis
Encephalitis
Subdural empyema

Exogenous Toxins

Sedative drugs and barbiturates
Anesthetics and γ-hydroxybutyrate*
Alcohols
Stimulants
Phencyclidine†
Cocaine and amphetamine‡
Psychotropic drugs
Cyclic antidepressants
Phenothiazines
Lithium
Anticonvulsants
Opioids
Clonidine§
Penicillins
Salicylates
Anticholinergics
Carbon monoxide, cyanide, and methemoglobinemia

Endogenous Toxins, Deficiencies, Derangements

Hypoxia and ischemia
Hypoglycemia
Hypercalcemia

Osmolar

Hyperglycemia
Hyponatremia
Hypernatremia

Organ system failure

Hepatic encephalopathy
Uremic encephalopathy
Pulmonary insufficiency (carbon dioxide narcosis)

Seizures

Prolonged postictal state
Spike-wave stupor

Hypothermia or hyperthermia

Brainstem ischemia

Basilar artery stroke

Pituitary apoplexy

Conversion or malingering

*General anesthetic, similar to γ-aminobutyric acid; recreational drug and body building aid. Rapid onset, rapid recovery often with myoclonic jerking and confusion. Deep coma (2-3 hr; Glasgow Coma Scale score = 3) with maintenance of vital signs.
†Coma associated with cholinergic signs: lacrimation, salivation, bronchorrhea, and hyperthermia.
‡Coma after seizures or status (i.e., a prolonged postictal state).
§An antihypertensive agent active through the opiate receptor system; frequent overdose when used to treat narcotic withdrawal.

Table 113-3	**Emergency Management**

Ensure airway adequacy.
Support ventilation and circulation.
Obtain blood for glucose, electrolytes, hepatic and renal function, prothrombin and partial thromboplastin times, complete blood count, and drug screen.
Administer 100 mg of thiamine intravenously (IV).
Administer 25 g of dextrose IV (typically 50 mL of 50% dextrose) to treat possible hypoglycemic coma.*
Treat opiate overdose with naloxone (0.4-1.2 mg IV).
The specific benzodiazepine antagonist flumazenil (0.2 mg IV repeated once and followed by 0.1 mg IV to 1-3 mg total) should be given for the reversal of benzodiazepine-induced coma or conscious sedation.†

*The glucose level is poorly correlated with the level of consciousness in hypoglycemia; stupor, coma, and confusion are reported with blood glucose concentrations ranging from 2 to 60 mg/dL.
†Not recommended in coma of unknown origin because seizures may be precipitated in patients with polydrug overdoses which include benzodiazepines with tricyclic antidepressants or cocaine.

spheric masses at their early stage (*early diencephalic*, i.e., compromising the brain above the thalamus) produce appropriate movement of one upper extremity, that is, movement toward the painful stimulus. The attenuated contralateral arm movement reflects a hemiparesis. This lateralized motor response in a comatose patient establishes the working diagnosis of a hemispheric mass. As the mass expands to involve the thalamus (*late diencephalic*), the response to pain becomes reflex arm flexion associated with extension and internal rotation of the legs (*decorticate posturing*); asymmetry of the response in the upper extremities is seen. With further brain compromise at the midbrain level, the reflex posturing changes in the arms such that both arms and legs respond by extension (*decerebrate posturing*); at this level, the asymmetry tends to be lost. At this point, the pupils become midposition in size, and the light reflex is lost, first unilaterally and then bilaterally. With further progression to the level of the pons, no response to painful stimulation is the most frequent finding, although spinal-mediated movements of leg flexion may occur. The classic postures illustrated in Figure 113-1, and particularly their asymmetry, strongly support the presence of a mass lesion. These motor movements, especially early in coma, are, however, most frequently seen as fragments of the fully developed, asymmetrical flexion or extension of the arms illustrated as decorticate and decerebrate postures in Figure 113-1. A small amount of asymmetrical flexion or extension of the arms in response to a painful stimulus carries the same implications as the full-blown postures of decortication or decerebration.

Metabolic lesions do not compromise the brain in a progressive, level-by-level manner as do hemispheric masses, and they rarely produce the asymmetrical motor signs typical of masses. Reflex posturing may be seen, but it lacks the asymmetry of decortication from a hemispheric mass and is not associated with the loss of pupillary reactivity at the stage of decerebration.

Pupillary Reactivity

In metabolic coma, one feature is central to the examination: Pupillary reactivity is present. This reactivity is seen both early in metabolic coma, when an appropriate motor

motor response requires that a painful stimulus be applied to which the patient will react. The patient's arms should be placed in a semiflexed posture, and a painful stimulus should be applied to the head or trunk. Strong pressure on the supraorbital ridge or pinching of the skin on the anterior chest or inner arm is the most useful method; finger nail bed pressure is also used, but it makes the interpretation of upper limb movement difficult.

The neurologic examination of a patient with an expanding hemispheric mass lesion is shown in Figure 113-1. Hemi-

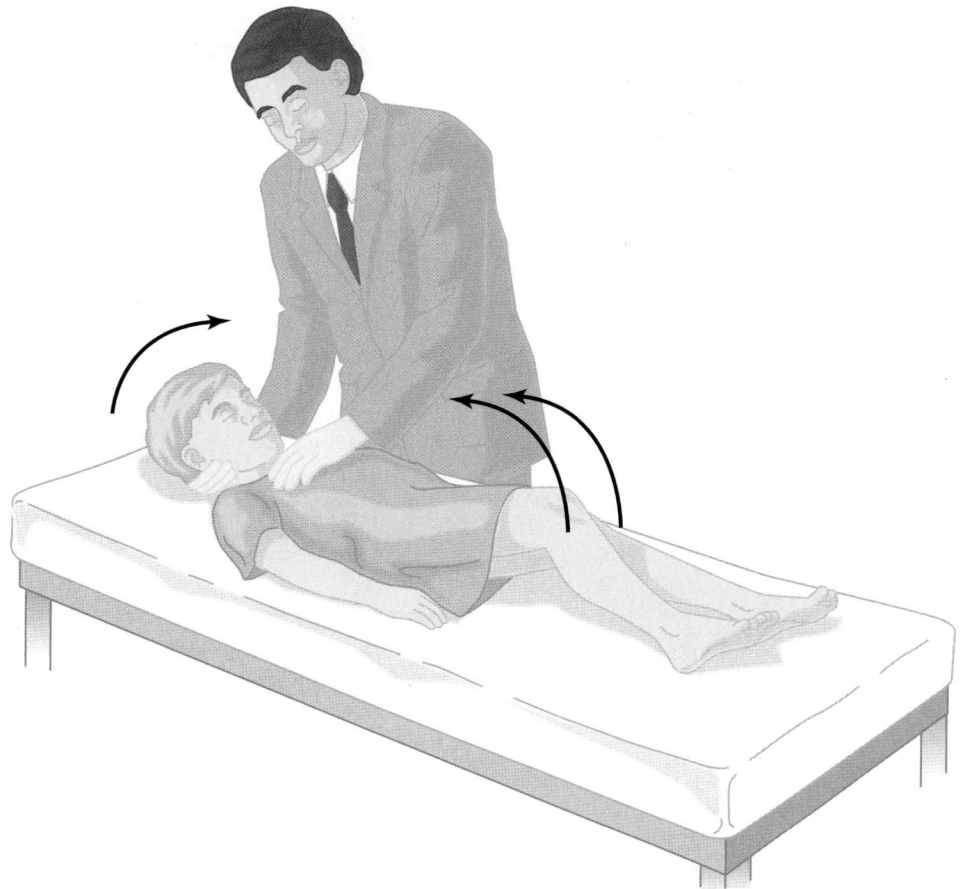

Figure 113-2 Elicitation of Brudzinski's sign of meningeal irritation as seen in infectious meningitis or subarachnoid hemorrhage. (From Aminoff MJ, Greenberg DA, Simon RP: Clinical Neurology. Stamford, CT, Appleton and Lange, 1996).

response to pain may be retained, and late in coma, when no motor responses can be elicited. The pupillary reaction in metabolic coma is lost only when coma is so deep that the patient requires ventilatory and blood pressure support.

Reflex Eye Movements

The presence of inducible lateral eye movements reflects the integrity of the pons and midbrain. These reflex eye movements (see Fig. 113-1) are brought about by passive head rotation to stimulate the semicircular canal input to the vestibular system (so-called *doll's eyes maneuver*) or by inhibiting the function of one semicircular canal by infusion of ice water against the tympanic membrane (caloric testing).

In metabolic coma, reflex eye movements may be lost or retained. Lack of inducible eye movements with the doll's eyes maneuver, in the setting of preserved pupillary reactivity, is virtually diagnostic of drug toxicity. With metabolic coma of non–drug-induced origin, such as organ system failure, electrolyte disorders, or osmolar disorders, reflex eye movements are preserved.

Brainstem mass lesions are most commonly caused by hemorrhage or infarction. Reflex lateral eye movements, the pathways for which traverse the pons and midbrain, are particularly affected, and the reflex postures of decortication and decerebration typical of brainstem injury are common. Lesions restricted to the midbrain (e.g., embolization from the heart to the top of the basilar artery) cause sluggish pupillary reflexes or their absence, with or without impaired medial eye movements (both are controlled by the third cranial nerve). With lesions restricted to the pons (e.g., intrapontine hypertensive hemorrhage), pupils are reactive but very small (pinpoint or pontine pupils), which reflects focal impairment of sympathetic innervation; pinpoint pupils are rare. Ocular bobbing (spontaneous symmetrical or asymmetrical rhythmic vertical ocular oscillations) is most often seen as a manifestation of a pontine lesion.

Seizures occurring in a patient with acute brain injury (e.g., that resulting from encephalitis, hypertensive encephalopathy, hyponatremia or hypernatremia, hypoglycemia or hyperglycemia) or chronic brain injury (e.g., dementia, mental retardation) often result in prolonged postictal coma. The examination shows reactive pupils and inducible eye movements (in the absence of overtreatment with anticonvulsants) and often up-going toes or focal signs (Todd paresis). Nonconvulsive seizures, particularly spike-wave stupor, may occur in a patient without a history of epilepsy. The diagnosis is made by electroencephalogram (see Chapter 126).

Prognosis in Coma

In coma after cardiac arrest, the prognosis for meaningful recovery can be assessed from clinical signs. Return of pupillary reactivity within 24 hours and purposeful motor

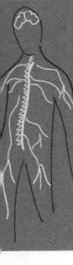

Table 113-4 **Percentage of Patients Recovering Independent Function from Coma After Cardiac Arrest (Predicted by Signs on Examination at 0, 1, 3, and 7 Days)**				
	Days After Cardiac Arrest			
Sign	0	1	3	7
No verbal response	13	8	5	6
No eye opening	11	6	4	0
Unreactive pupils	0	0	0	0
No spontaneous eye movements	6	5	2	0
No caloric response	5	6	6	0
Extensor posturing	18	0	0	0
Flexor posturing	14	3	0	0
No motor response (N = 210)	4	3	0	0
No eye opening to pain	31	8	0	0
Absent or reflex motor response	25	9	0	0
Unreactive pupils (N = 131)	17	7	0	0

Data from Levey DE, Caronna JJ, Singer BH: Predicting the outcome from hypoxic coma. JAMA 523:1420-1426, 1985; and from Edgren E, Hedstrand U, Kelsey S: Assessment of neurologic prognosis in comatose survivors of cardiac arrest. Lancet 343:1055-1059, 1994.

Table 113-5 **Locked-in Syndrome**
Clinical Features
Eye opening
Reactive pupils
Volitional vertical eye movements to command
Muteness
Quadriparesis
Sleep-wake cycles
Causes
Pontine vascular lesions (common)
Head injury, brainstem tumor, pontine myelinolysis (rare)
Recovery Possible
Onset 1-12 weeks (vascular)* *or*
Onset 4-6 months (nonvascular)*
Prognosis favorable
Normal CT scan*
Early recovery of lateral eye movements*

*Implications for care.
   CT, computed tomography.

Table 113-6 **Persistent Vegetative State: Common Causes***
Trauma (diffuse axonal injury)
Cardiac arrest and hypoperfusion (laminar necrosis of cortical mantle and/or thalamic necrosis)
Bihemispheric infarctions
Purulent meningitis or encephalitis (cortical injury)
Carbon monoxide
Prolonged hypoglycemic coma

*A vegetative state may not necessarily begin with coma but can also develop as the end stage of neurodegenerative diseases (e.g., Alzheimer disease) of adults or children and can accompany severe congenital developmental abnormalities of the brain such as anencephaly.

movements within the first 72 hours after cardiac arrest are highly correlated with a favorable outcome (Table 113-4). Rare late recoveries, however, have been reported.

Coma-like States

Locked-in patients are those in whom a lesion (usually a hemorrhage or an infarct) transects the brainstem at a point below the reticular formation (therefore sparing consciousness) but above the ventilatory nuclei of the medulla (therefore maintaining cardiopulmonary function) (Table 113-5). Such patients are awake, with eye opening and sleep-wake cycles, but the descending pathways through the brainstem necessary for volitional vocalization or limb movement have been transected. Voluntary eye movement, especially vertically, is preserved, and patients open and close their eyes or produce appropriate numbers of blinking movements in answer to questions. The electroencephalogram is usually normal, reflecting normal cortical function.

Psychogenic unresponsiveness is a diagnosis of exclusion. The neurologic examination shows reactive pupils and no reflex posturing in response to pain. Eye movements during the doll's eyes maneuver show volitional override rather than the smooth, uninhibited reflex lateral eye movements of coma. Ice water caloric testing either arouses the patient because of the discomfort produced or induces cortically mediated nystagmus rather than the tonic deviation typical of coma. Slow, conjugate roving eye movements of metabolic coma cannot be imitated and therefore rule out psychogenic unresponsiveness. In addition, the slow, often asymmetrical, and incomplete eye closure seen after passive eye opening of a comatose patient cannot be feigned. These signs therefore rule out psychogenic coma. In contrast, conscious patients usually exhibit some voluntary muscle tone in the eyelids during passive eye opening. The electroencephalogram in psychogenic unresponsiveness is that of normal wakefulness with reactive posterior rhythms on eye opening and eye closing. In patients with catatonic stupor, lorazepam administration may produce awakening.

In *persistent vegetative states* (PVSs), patients have awakened from coma but have not regained awareness. Wakefulness is exhibited by eye opening and sleep-wake cycles. The reticular activating system of the brainstem is intact to produce wakefulness, but the connections to the cortical mantle are interrupted, precluding awareness.

Clinical features do not differ by cause (Table 113-6). Patients in a PVS open their eyes diurnally and in response to loud sounds; blinking occurs with bright lights. Pupils react and eye movements occur both spontaneously and with the doll's eyes maneuver. Yawning, chewing, swallowing, and, uncommonly, guttural vocalizations and lacrimation may be preserved. Spontaneous roving eye movements (very slow, constant velocity) are particularly characteristic and distressing to the patient's visitors because the patient appears to be looking about the room. The brainstem origin of the eye movements is documented by their being readily redirected by the oculocephalic (doll's eyes) reflex. The limbs may move, but motor responses are only primitive; pain usually produces decorticate or decerebrate postures or fragments of these movements.

A vegetative state is termed *persistent* after 3 months if the brain injury was medical and after 12 months if the brain injury was traumatic. The determination as to when

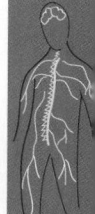

Table 113-7 **Criteria for Cessation of Brain Function***	
Anatomic Region Tested	**Confirmatory Sign**
Hemispheres	Unresponsive and unreceptive to sensory stimuli including pain[†]
Midbrain	Unreactive pupils[‡]
Pons	Absent reflex eye movements[§]
Medulla	Apnea[¶]

*Sequential testing is necessary for a clinical diagnosis of brain death; at least 6 hr for all cases and at least 24 hr in the setting of anoxic-ischemic brain injury.

[†]The patient does not rouse, groan, grimace, or withdraw limbs; purely spinal reflexes (deep tendon reflexes, plantar flexion reflex, plantar withdrawal, and tonic neck reflexes) may be maintained.

[‡]Most easily assessed by the bright light of an ophthalmoscope viewed through its magnifying lens when focused on the iris; unreactive pupils may be either midposition (as they will be in death) or dilated, as they often are in the setting of a dopamine infusion.

[§]No eye movement toward the side of irrigation of the tympanic membrane with 50 mL of ice water; the oculocephalic response (doll's eyes) will always be absent in the setting of absent oculovestibular testing.

[¶]No ventilatory movements in the setting of maximum CO_2 stimulation (≥60 mm Hg; with apnea, P_{CO_2} will passively rise 2-3 mm Hg/min); disconnect the ventilator from the endotracheal tube and insert cannula with 6 L of oxygen per minute.

CO_2, carbon dioxide; P_{CO_2}, partial pressure of carbon dioxide.

Table 113-8 **Exclusionary Criteria for Brain Death**
Seizures
Decorticate or decerebrate posturing
Sedative drugs
Hypothermia (<32.2° C)
Neuromuscular blockade
Shock

Table 113-9 **Confirmatory Tests for Brain Death**
EEG isoelectricity: Deep coma from sedative drugs or hypothermia (temperature below 20° C) can produce EEG flattening; patients clinically brain dead may have residual EEG activity for a significant number of days after a brain death diagnosis.
No cerebral blood flow at angiography (the most definitive confirmatory test).

EEG, electroencephalogram.

persistent equals *permanent* cannot be stated absolutely. Prediction of which patients early in the vegetative state will remain persistently vegetative is particularly difficult in trauma. Lesions of the corpus callosum and dorsolateral brainstem seen on magnetic resonance images 6 to 8 weeks after trauma correlated with persistence of the vegetative state at a year. In rare cases, patients show late improvement, but none of these patients returns to normal. Slight recovery to a minimally responsive state has also been described.

Brain imaging studies depict the sequelae of the causative injury but are not diagnostic of PVS. Magnetic resonance spectroscopy has shown a decrease in the neuronal marker of *N*-acetylaspartate. Positron-emission tomographic studies have shown decreased glucose usage and cerebral blood flow. Bilateral absence of somatosensory-evoked responses in the first week predicts death or vegetative state.

Brain death characterizes the *irreversible cessation* of brain function. Therefore death of the organism can be determined based on death of the brain. Although local laws may dictate some details, the standard definition permits a diagnosis of brain death based on documentation of irreversible cessation of all brain function, including function of the brainstem (Table 113-7).

Documentation of *irreversibility* requires that the cause of the coma be known, that the cause be adequate to explain the clinical findings of brain death, and that exclusionary criteria are absent (Table 113-8). Confirmatory tests are sometimes used but are not required for diagnosis (Table 113-9).

Brain death results in asystole, usually within days (mean, 4) even if ventilatory support is continued. Recovery after appropriate documentation of brain death has never been reported. Removal of the ventilator results in terminal rhythms (most often complete heart block without ventricular response), junctional rhythms, or ventricular tachycardia. Purely spinal motor movements may occur in the moments of terminal apnea (or during apnea testing in the absence of passive administration of oxygen): arching of the back, neck turning, stiffening of the legs, and upper extremity flexion.

Prospectus for the Future

Functional imaging (positron-emission tomography and functional magnetic resonance imaging) is now being employed for study of acute coma and stupor in emergency rooms and the intensive care units. These techniques will provide a better understanding of the metabolic derangements occurring in acute brain dysfunction. As specific ion channels of brain neurons are characterized, targeted molecular therapies will enter clinical trials.

References

Bernat JL: Chronic disorders of consciousness. Lancet 367:1181-1192, 2006.

Fins JJ, Master MG, Gerber LM, Giacino JT: The minimally conscious state: A diagnosis in search of an epidemiology. Arch Neurol 64:1400-1405, 2007.

Plum F, Posner JB: The Diagnosis of Stupor and Coma (Contemporary Neurology Series), vol 71, 4th ed. New York, Oxford University Press, 2007.

Quality Standards Subcommittee of the American Academy of Neurology: Practice parameters: Assessment and management of patients in the persistent vegetative state. Neurology 45:1015-1018, 1995.

Wijdicks EFM: Neurologic Complications of Critical Illness (Contemporary Neurology Series), vol 64, 2nd ed. New York, Oxford University Press, 2002.

Wijdicks EFM: The diagnosis of brain death. N Engl J Med 344:1215-1221, 2001.

Wijdicks EFM, Hijdra A, Young GB, et al: Practice parameter: Prediction of outcome in comatose survivors after cardiopulmonary resuscitation (an evidence-based review). Neurology 67:203-210, 2006.

Young GB, Ropper AH, Bolton CF: Coma and Impaired Consciousness: A Clinical Perspective. New York, McGraw-Hill, 1998.

Young GB: Neurologic prognosis after cardiac arrest. New Engl J Med 361:605-611, 2009.

Zandbergen EGJ, Hijdra A, Koelman JH, et al: Prediction of poor outcome within the first 3 days of postanoxic coma. Neurology 66:62-68, 2006.

Zeman A: Persistent vegetative state. Lancet 350:795-799, 1997.

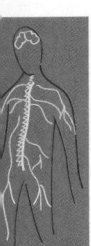

Disorders of Sleep

Lynn Liu

Neurobiology of Sleep

Sleep is essential for life. Rat models with complete sleep deprivation die within 10 to 30 days. Although the function of sleep is not clearly understood, there are demonstrable physiologic, psychological, and social consequences of chronic sleep deprivation. Recent advances in sleep medicine have enhanced recognition of sleep disorders, improved understanding of their pathophysiology, and resulted in development of new treatment strategies. The International Classification of Sleep Disorders (ICSD-2) divides sleep disorders into six major clinical categories.

Sleep and wakefulness include three states: wake, non–rapid eye movement (NREM) sleep, and rapid eye movement (REM) sleep. The entry and termination of each of these states are under active neurologic control. Wakefulness is maintained by activation of the cortex via the reticular activating system through the thalamus and the posterior hypothalamus. The ventrolateral preoptic nucleus (VLPO) of the anterior hypothalamus signals the onset of NREM sleep by descending inhibitory projections to the brainstem nuclei responsible for maintaining wakefulness, and the lateral dorsal tegmentum (LDT) and parapontine tegmentum (PPT) activate the transition into REM sleep.

Sleep stages can be differentiated by their physiologic characteristics and polysomnographic (PSG) criteria (Fig. 114-1). The transition from wake into sleep is cyclic. Each cycle takes approximately 90 to 120 minutes, and there are about four to six sleep cycles over the course of a nocturnal sleep period. These cycles can be graphically represented as a hypnogram. Sleep is entered through NREM stage 1 (N1), followed by a descent into deeper stages of sleep including stage 2 (N2), slow-wave sleep (N3), and then REM sleep (R). Physiologically, REM sleep represents a relatively activated state similar to waking and can be further subdivided into tonic stage, quiet periods of muscle atonia, and phasic stage, characterized by bursts of REM, small muscle twitches, penile erections, and labial engorgement. Of subjects awakened from REM sleep, 80% reported vivid dreaming, in comparison with only 20% of subjects awakened from NREM sleep.

Insomnia

ICSD-2 defines insomnia as difficulty initiating or maintaining sleep, early morning awakenings, or chronically nonrestorative or poor-quality sleep, despite adequate opportunity and circumstances for sleep, leading to daytime impairment. Insomnias can be categorized as acute or chronic and according to the timing of sleep disruption: sleep onset, sleep maintenance, or early awakening. In the National Sleep Poll 2005, 54% of U.S. respondents reported experiencing insomnia on a regular basis. Most can identify with *adjustment sleep disorder* (acute insomnia), which occurs in the setting of acute stressors such as death of a family member or work or social issues. Most acute insomnias resolve once the acute stressor has resolved. If the insomnia is severe, hypnotics are indicated for short-term use. Choice of hypnotic depends on matching the symptoms with the pharmacokinetic profile of the hypnotic; patients with sleep onset insomnia should use a short-acting medication, whereas those with sleep maintenance insomnia should use a longer-acting medication.

The most common chronic insomnia, *psychophysiologic insomnia*, is related to poor sleep hygiene (Table 114-1) and maladaptive sleep habits. Clinical characteristics include altered arousal threshold and rumination with precipitating and perpetuating factors. Treatment involves reeducating the patient about his or her attitudes and beliefs about sleep through cognitive behavioral therapy (CBT) by a trained sleep behaviorist. Sleep can also be disrupted by medical conditions, other sleep disorders, psychiatric disorders, and drugs.

Sleep-Related Breathing Disorders

At sleep onset the control of respiration changes from voluntary control to predominantly automatic control based on chemoreceptors and mechanoreceptor reflexes. Apnea is defined as a cessation of breathing lasting longer than 10

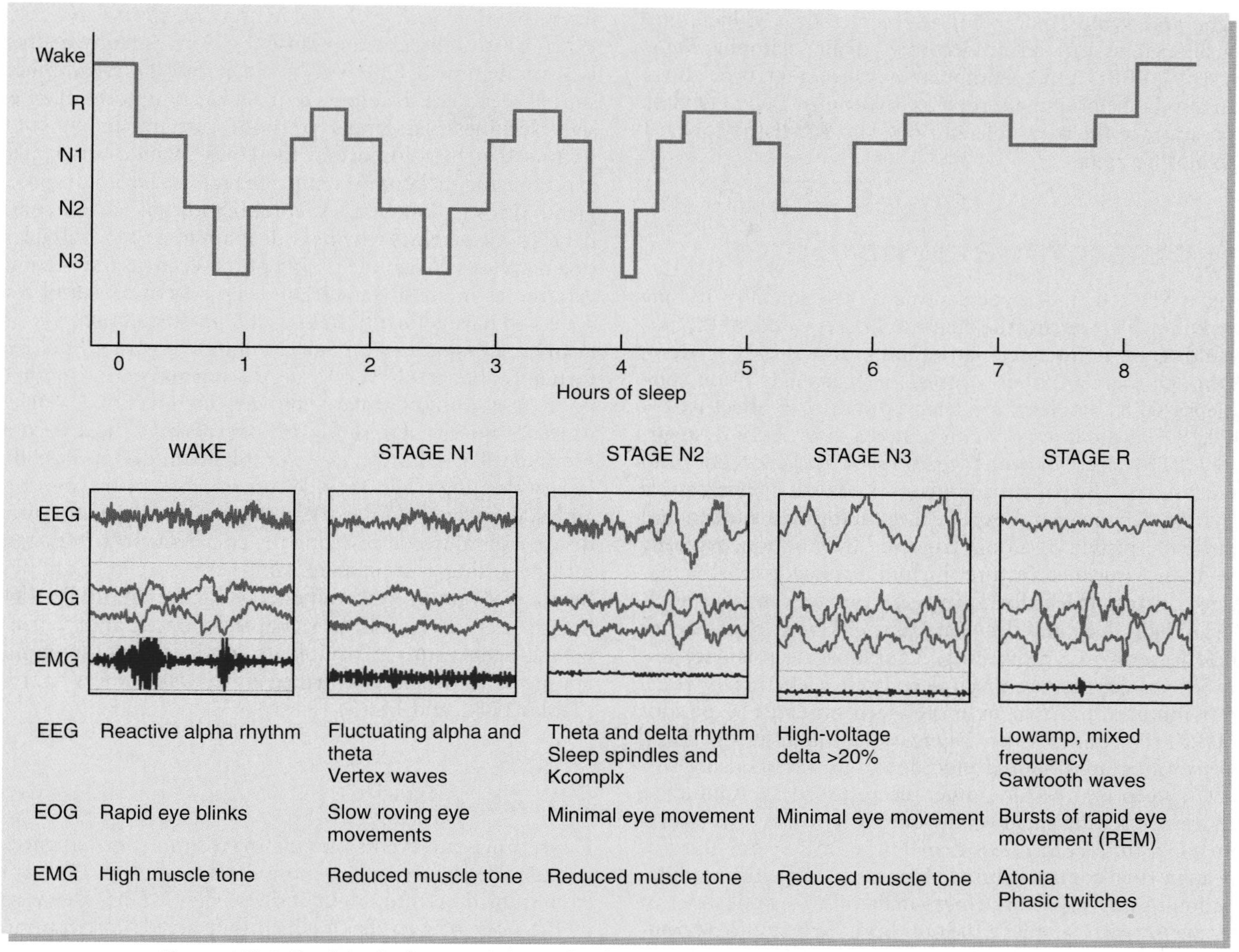

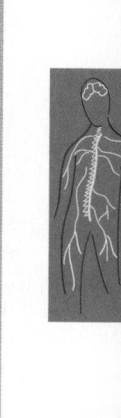

Figure 114-1 Physiologic characteristics and polysomnographic (PSG) criteria for stages of sleep.

The figure shows a hypnogram with axes labeled Wake, R, N1, N2, N3 against Hours of sleep (0 to 8), and below it five panels labeled WAKE, STAGE N1, STAGE N2, STAGE N3, STAGE R, each showing EEG, EOG, EMG traces with the following descriptions:

	WAKE	STAGE N1	STAGE N2	STAGE N3	STAGE R
EEG	Reactive alpha rhythm	Fluctuating alpha and theta Vertex waves	Theta and delta rhythm Sleep spindles and Kcomplx	High-voltage delta >20%	Lowamp, mixed frequency Sawtooth waves
EOG	Rapid eye blinks	Slow roving eye movements	Minimal eye movement	Minimal eye movement	Bursts of rapid eye movement (REM)
EMG	High muscle tone	Reduced muscle tone	Reduced muscle tone	Reduced muscle tone	Atonia Phasic twitches

Table 114-1 Sleep Hygiene

1. Maintain a regular schedule each day.
2. Wake at the same time each morning.
3. Exposure to natural light entrains the circadian rhythm.
4. Exercise in the morning or early afternoon; avoid vigorous exercise in the evening.
5. Avoid napping during the day, especially after 3 PM.
6. Avoid stimulants such as caffeine, nicotine, and alcohol too close to bedtime.
7. Avoid large meals close to bedtime.
8. Maintain regular and relaxing routines at bedtime.
9. Maintain a comfortable sleep environment.
10. Reserve the bed for sleep; avoid other activities (TV, radio, or reading).
11. Sleep only when sleepy.
12. Do not worry in bed, resolve issues before sleeping.
13. Get out of bed if not sleeping in 20 minutes.

seconds. There are three types of apnea: obstructive, central, and mixed. Obstruction of the upper airway results in a loss of airflow with maintained effort. Loss of a central signal to initiate a breath results in the loss of airflow signal and no signs of respiratory effort. Mixed apnea is the combination of these two types.

Obstructive sleep apnea syndrome is the most common sleep-related breathing disorder. It affects 2% to 5% of the adult population of the United States, as many as 20% of whom are not diagnosed. The typical patient with sleep apnea is an overweight middle-aged man, and its incidence increases with age; however, sleep apnea occurs in young children and people with a normal body mass index. Untreated sleep apnea increases the risk of cardiovascular disease, cerebrovascular disease, depression, and accidents. ICSD-2 criteria include complaints of unintentional sleep episodes during wakefulness, daytime sleepiness, unrefreshing sleep, fatigue or insomnia, or periods when the individual awakens with breath holding, gasping, or choking or the bed partner reports loud snoring or breathing interruptions. Polysomnography quantifies respiratory events per sleep hour, and a patient with more than five events per sleep hour with clinical complaints should receive treatment. Other factors that can exacerbate sleep apnea include crowding of the oropharyngeal space, oromaxillofacial disproportions, body position (supine position exacerbates airway patency), and sedatives that reduce the tone of the soft tissue. Treatment targets the opening of the airway. Weight loss is critical but difficult for most patients to achieve. Continuous positive airway pressure (CPAP) splints the airway, allowing uninterrupted respiration through the night and symptomatic improvement. Surgery including tonsillectomy and adenoidectomy, uvulopalatopharyngoplasty (UPPP), and mandibular advancement procedures can also be helpful in appropriate situations. Dental devices that advance the mandible and pull the soft tissue forward can also be used.

Hypersomnia Syndromes

The ICSD-2 defines hypersomnia as the inability to stay awake and alert during the major waking episodes of the day, resulting in unintended lapses into drowsiness or sleep. Although there are many causes, the classic condition, narcolepsy with cataplexy, has been estimated to affect 0.02% to 0.18% of the U.S. population. It is a disorder of dysregulated REM sleep in which features of REM intrude into wakefulness. The patient complains of almost daily excessive daytime sleepiness and experiences cataplexy, a sudden and transient episode of atonia triggered by emotion, typically laughter. Associated features include hypnagogic hallucinations, during which dream imagery intrudes into wakefulness or light sleep, and sleep paralysis, which is the persistence of REM atonia on awakening. A multiple sleep latency test (MSLT) to determine a mean sleep latency less than or equal to 8 minutes and two or more sleep onset REM periods (SOREMP) confirms the diagnosis, although an overnight polysomnography should precede the MSLT to ensure sufficient sleep and exclude other sleep disorders. Adjunctive laboratory testing includes hypocretin-1 levels in the cerebrospinal fluid (CSF) (less than 110 pg/mL or one third of mean normal control values). Hypocretin is a neuromodulator found in the posterior hypothalamus. In some cases of narcolepsy with cataplexy, the number of hypocretin neurons is reduced. Furthermore, human leukocyte antigen (HLA) subtype DQB1*0602 occurs at a higher frequency in these patients than in the general population.

Symptomatic treatment for narcolepsy minimizes daytime sleepiness and reduces cataplectic attacks. Scheduled naps are helpful because most patients find the naps to be refreshing and to help the patients continue to function. Stimulants, methylphenidate and amphetamines, improve daytime sleepiness, but patients may develop tolerance, weight loss, and jitteriness. Also of benefit is modafinil, a novel wakefulness-promoting agent that may enhance aminergic transmission in the anterior hypothalamus. It has a modest side effect profile that includes headache and nausea. The pontine inhibition of motor control during REM is thought to be under cholinergic control. Tricyclic antidepressants, specifically clomipramine, reduce the frequency of cataplectic attacks. Other antidepressants including selective serotonin reuptake inhibitors (SSRIs) have also been used. Sodium oxybate, a controlled substance, consolidates sleep and improves both the symptoms of excessive daytime sleepiness and cataplexy.

Circadian Rhythm Sleep Disorders

The circadian clock in the suprachiasmatic nucleus of the anterior hypothalamus maintains the appropriate timing for many physiological cycles including the sleep-wake cycle. When sleep is disrupted because the clock is faulty or there is a misalignment between the clock and the environment such as seen in shift workers or in jet lag, symptoms of excessive sleepiness, insomnia or both can impair function. Factors that help to entrain the clock include bright light exposure and melatonin, a hormone released from the pineal gland during darkness. A combination of genetics and behavior determines whether one is apt to be a morning lark or a night owl. When the timing of the sleep period becomes extreme as in some adolescents who stay awake until 3 to 4 AM and have difficulty waking at 8 AM to go to school, this *delayed sleep phase syndrome* can interfere with school performance, but if allowed to sleep a normal period until 12 noon, they would not have any sleep complaints. As society works 24 hours a day, *shift work sleep disorders* have become prevalent. For example, those on night shift often have difficulty sleeping when they get off of work in the morning and staying awake to work at night. Treatment for these disorders is aimed at resetting the circadian clock. Strategies include setting of strict sleep habits, exposure to bright light before periods of wakefulness, avoidance of bright light before sleep, melatonin to signal sleep onset, and pharmacologic agents such as stimulants, modafinil, and hypnotics appropriately timed to enhance either wakefulness or sleep (Tables 114-2 and 114-3).

Parasomnias

Parasomnias are events ranging from simple movements to complex behaviors without conscious awareness. They arise from transitions into or out of sleep. They can be categorized by the stage of sleep from which they arise. Most common childhood parasomnias arise from slow wave sleep and

Table 114-2 Hypnotics

	Dose Range	Half-Life
Benzodiazepines		
Estazolam (Prosom)	1-2 mg	10-24 hr
Flurazepam (Dalmane)	15-30 mg	2-3 hr
Quazepam (Doral)	7.5-30 mg	39 hr
Temazepam (Restoril)	7.5-30 mg	3.5-18.4 hr
Triazolam (Halcion)	0.125-0.15 mg	1.5-5.5 hr
Clonazepam (Klonopin)	0.25-2 mg	30-40 hr
Nonbenzodiazepines		
Zolpidem (Ambien, Ambien CR)	5-10 mg; CR: 6.25, 12.5 mg	2.5-2.8 hr
Zaleplon (Sonata)	5-20 mg	1 hr
Eszopiclone (Lunesta)	1-3 mg	6 hr
Ramelteon (Rozerem)	8 mg	1-2.6 hr

Table 114-3 Wakefulness Promoting Agents

Drug	Dose Range
Amphetamine (Dexedrine, Desoxyn, Adderall, Adderall XR)	5-40 mg
Methylphenidate (Ritalin, Metadate, Methylin, Concerta)	10-60 mg
Modafinil (Provigil)	200-400 mg

include *confusional arousals*, *sleepwalking*, and *sleep terrors*. Sleep terrors are episodes of intense autonomic arousal characterized by loud vocalization and fear with associated papillary dilation, diaphoresis, tachycardia, and tachypnea, all without recall. Although these events are thought of as childhood disorders, 2% to 5% of adults sleepwalk, and many have a family history. In contrast, events arising from REM sleep such as *nightmares* and *REM behavior disorders* (RBDs) typically involve vivid recall of dream content before arousal. During RBDs there is loss of the protective atonia of REM sleep, which inhibits dream enactment. This disorder tends to affect middle-aged or older men and may precede the diagnosis of a degenerative neurologic condition by a decade. Autopsy studies suggest that pontine lesions may be responsible for the release from motor inhibition. The physical behavioral response to the characteristically violent dream imagery can result in injuries to the patient or his or her bed partner. Treatment strategies are prevention of sleepwalkers from getting into dangerous situations such as by opening windows and doors. If the behaviors are persistent and affect daytime functioning, suppressing arousals with the use of a benzodiazepine can be particularly successful for RBDs.

Sleep-Related Movement Disorders

Sleep-related movement disorders involve abnormal movements that occur during sleep and result in an arousal or

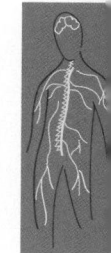

Table 114-4 **Dopamine Agonists**

Drug	Dose Range
Levodopa or carbidopa (Sinemet)	50-200 mg
Ropinirole (Requip)	0.25-4.0 mg
Pramipexole (Mirapex)	0.125-0.5 mg

disruption in the continuity of sleep. The clinical characteristics of *restless legs syndrome* (RLS), the most common sleep-related movement disorder, include the urge to move the legs because of an unpleasant sensation in the legs that tends to begin during periods of rest or inactivity, especially in the evening, and that is relieved by movement. Most cases are idiopathic, but some are familial and tend to have an earlier onset. Secondary causes include iron deficiency anemia, renal disorders, pregnancy, neurologic conditions such as peripheral neuropathies, radiculopathies, parkinsonian syndromes, rheumatoid arthritis, and fibromyalgia. Diagnosis is made by clinical history, although polysomnography can demonstrate increased periodic limb movements of sleep, repetitive movements of the lower extremities that result in arousals from sleep. The workup should exclude secondary causes including serum ferritin levels or iron saturations studies. The treatment for secondary causes entails iron replacement or symptomatic treatment of the underlying condition. For those with idiopathic RLS, the treatment of choice is a dopamine agonist such as levodopa, ropinirole, or pramipexole. Alternative medications include opioids, anticonvulsants for neuropathic pain, and hypnotics (Table 114-4).

Prospectus for the Future

Sleep medicine is a rapidly growing specialty bolstered by an increasing respect for the need to sleep well. As the basic science of how and why we sleep expands, pharmacologic management of certain sleep complaints will improve. Soon we will be able to target the pathophysiology in addition to the symptomatology of sleep disorders.

References

Basner RC: Continuous positive airway pressure for obstructive sleep apnea. N Engl J Med 356:1751-1758, 2007.

Dauvilliers Y, Arnulf I, Mignot E: Narcolepsy with cataplexy. Lancet 369:499-511, 2007.

Saper CB, Scammell TE, Lu J: Hypothalamic regulation of sleep and circadian rhythms. Nature 437:1257-1263, 2005.

Trenkwalder C: The restless legs syndrome. Lancet Neurol 4:465-475, 2005.

Wilson JF: In the clinic. Insomnia. Ann Int Med 148:ITC13-1–ITC13-16, 2008.

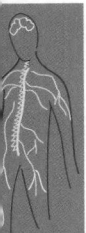

Cortical Syndromes

Sinéad M. Murphy and Timothy J. Counihan

Anatomy

The paired cerebral hemispheres are connected by a large band of white matter fibers, the *corpus callosum*. Each hemisphere consists of four anatomically and functionally distinct regions: frontal, temporal, parietal, and occipital lobes. The two cerebral hemispheres supplement each other functionally in a variety of behavioral and sensorimotor tasks; however, certain functions, particularly language, manual dexterity, and visuospatial perception, are strongly lateralized to one hemisphere. Language function, for instance, is lateralized to the left hemisphere in 95% of the population; although 15% of the population is left-handed, only a minority possesses a right hemisphere that is dominant for language. Visuospatial functions are largely subserved by the right (nondominant) hemisphere.

The Rolandic fissure separates the motor cortex (precentral gyrus) from the sensory cortex (postcentral gyrus). In these regions, cortical representations of the different parts of the body are arranged as the motor (in the frontal lobe) and sensory (in the parietal lobe) homunculi.

Regional Syndromes

Because many neurologic disorders affect the cerebral hemispheres in a regionally specific or focal manner, a careful history and clinical examination that includes the Mini-Mental State Examination are helpful not only in localizing brain lesions (Fig. 115-1), but also in establishing the cause. Tables 115-1 to 115-4 summarize some of the core clinical features involved with damage to individual hemispheres. The rate of onset of symptoms and the tempo of progression influence the extent of the clinical deficit. The homuncular arrangement of cortical motor and sensory representation may allow for more precise localization of a lesion. For instance, motor or sensory signs confined to the lower extremities may suggest a parasagittal lesion, whereas signs involving the face and upper limb may be found in laterally placed cortical lesions.

APHASIA

Aphasia or *dysphasia* refers to a loss or impairment of language function as a result of damage to the specific language centers of the dominant hemisphere. It is distinct from dysarthria, which is a disturbance in the articulation of speech. The principal types of aphasia are summarized in Table 115-5. A good bedside screening test for aphasia is to have the patient read and write a sentence; writing is almost invariably affected in patients with disturbances of language (Fig. 115-2). An exception to this occurs in the syndrome of *alexia without agraphia;* this syndrome results from a vascular lesion of the dominant hemisphere's posterior cerebral artery, in which the patient's language center is "disconnected" from the contralateral (unaffected) visual cortex. Such patients can write a sentence but are unable to read what they have written. Clinical assessment for aphasia requires testing of fluency, comprehension, repetition, naming, reading, calculation, and writing. *Anomia* (difficulty in recalling the names of objects) in isolation has little localizing value.

Broca aphasia is characterized by a severe disruption in the fluency of speech, with profound impairments in expression in both speech and writing. Comprehension may be mildly affected. The language disturbance is almost invariably accompanied by contralateral face and arm weakness as a result of the proximity of the motor homunculus to Broca's speech area.

Wernicke aphasia is characterized by an inability to comprehend spoken or written language. Affected patients speak fluently but the content is meaningless; they may use words that are close in meaning to the intended word (semantic paraphasias) or words that sound like the intended word (literal paraphasias). Some patients with Wernicke aphasia have an associated contralateral homonymous hemianopia.

Conduction aphasia is characterized by an inability to repeat a spoken phrase such as "no ifs, ands, or buts," although patients have normal comprehension. The responsible lesion lies in the arcuate fasciculus connecting Broca's and Wernicke's areas. *Global aphasia* results from large

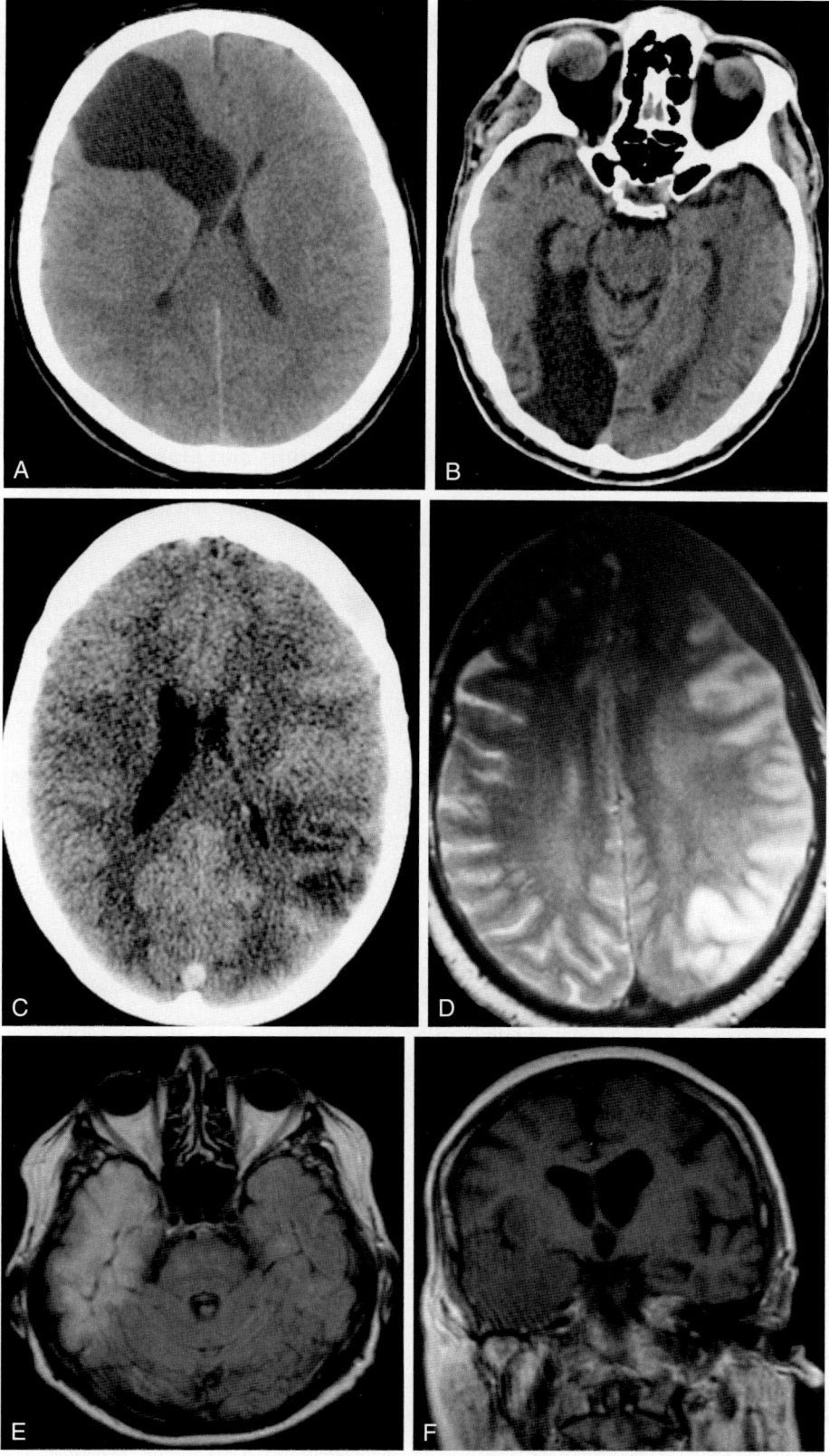

Figure 115-1 Computed tomography of the brain showing **(A)** large cystic lesion in right frontal lobe in a young man with seizures and a dysexecutive syndrome; **(B)** infarction in the right occipital lobe (posterior cerebral artery territory) in a man with a left homonymous hemianopia; and **(C)** hemorrhagic infarction in the left parietal lobe caused by venous sinus thrombosis (note thrombus in superior sagittal sinus) in a woman with headache and seizures. Magnetic resonance imaging of the brain showing **(D)** infarction in the left frontal and parietal lobes (middle cerebral artery territory) caused by internal carotid artery dissection in a man with right-sided neglect and hemiparesis; **(E)** high signal in the right temporal lobe in a patient with herpes simplex encephalitis; and **(F)** swollen right temporal lobe with mass effect in a woman with acute herpes simplex encephalitis.

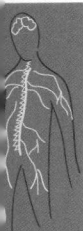

Table 115-1 Frontal Lobe Syndromes

Symptoms and Signs	Site of Lesion
Contralateral spastic weakness	Primary motor or premotor cortex
Broca aphasia	Dominant inferior frontal lobe
Forced eye deviation	Frontal eye fields
Executive dysfunction, poor sequencing	Dorsolateral prefrontal lobe
Akinetic mutism, urinary incontinence	Medial frontal cortex
Disinhibition, emotional lability	Orbitofrontal cortex

Table 115-3 Syndromes of Temporal Lobe Lesions

Symptoms and Signs	Site of Lesion
Anomic or sensory aphasia	Lateral temporal lobe (dominant)
Contralateral superior quadratic anopsia	Superior lateral temporal lobe
Amnesia	Hippocampus
Oral-exploratory behavior, passivity, hypersexuality (Klüver-Bucy syndrome)	Amygdala (bilateral)
Visual delusions (déjà vu, jamais vu), olfactory hallucinations	Inferomedial temporal lobe

Table 115-2 Parietal Lobe Syndromes

Symptoms and Signs	Site of Lesion
Contralateral sensory loss	Postcentral gyrus
Contralateral sensory neglect	Postcentral gyrus (nondominant)
Wernicke aphasia, apraxia	Inferior parietal or superior temporal cortex
Acalculia, finger agnosia, right-left confusion, agraphia (Gerstmann syndrome)	Angular gyrus

Table 115-4 Occipital Lobe Syndromes

Symptoms and Signs	Site of Lesion
Contralateral homonymous hemianopia	Striate cortex
Alexia without agraphia	Primary visual cortex (dominant) and splenium of corpus callosum
Visual agnosia, denial of blindness (Anton syndrome), visual hallucinations	Medial occipital lobe
Optic apraxia, absent optokinetic nystagmus	Lateral (visual association) cortex

Table 115-5 Principal Types of Aphasia

Type	Lesion Site	Fluency	Comprehension	Repetition	Naming	Other Signs
Broca	Inferior frontal lobe	↓	Good	↓	↓	Contralateral weakness
Wernicke	Posterior superior temporal lobe	Good	↓	↓	↓	Homonymous hemianopia
Conduction	Supramarginal gyrus	Good	Good	↓	↓	None
Global	Frontal lobe (large)	↓	↓	↓	↓	Hemiplegia

lesions of the frontal lobe, in which all aspects of language are affected. Lesions of the nondominant hemisphere language areas result in *dysprosody*. For instance, patients with lesions in the inferior frontal lobe of the nondominant (usually right) hemisphere, analogous to Broca's area, speak with a monotonous voice, losing the natural cadence of speech.

In *dysarthria*, language function is intact (which can be confirmed by having the patient write a sentence), but patients are unable to articulate speech. Dysarthria results from either supranuclear, nuclear, or peripheral lesions of the lower cranial nerves or from lesions of the bulbar musculature or neuromuscular junction.

AGNOSIA AND APRAXIA

Agnosia is the inability to recognize a specific sensory stimulus despite preserved sensory function. For instance, visual agnosia is the inability to recognize a visual stimulus despite normal visual acuity. Similar syndromes include the inability to recognize sounds (auditory agnosia), color (color agnosia), and familiar faces (prosopagnosia). Usually the responsible lesions are located in the occipitotemporal region.

Apraxia refers to an inability to perform learned motor tasks despite sufficient memory and sensorimotor function to understand the command (Fig. 115-3). The responsible lesions are usually in the dominant inferior parietal lobe. Lesions of the right parietal lobe often result in hemispatial neglect: The patient does not attend to stimuli in the left visual field or on the left side of the body. In a milder form of neglect, called *extinction*, patients can attend to stimuli contralateral to the side of the brain with the lesion (and the lesion is usually on the right side), but when presented with bilateral stimuli simultaneously, they respond only on the ipsilateral (right) side. Anosognosia, or the lack of awareness of one's deficit, frequently accompanies hemispatial neglect.

AMNESIA

Memory and mechanisms for recall are located in the hippocampus of the temporal lobe. The common memory disorders are summarized in Table 115-6. Degeneration of the hippocampus or its connections results in the inability to form new memories and is a central accompaniment of Alzheimer disease. Concussion injuries typically induce severe retrograde amnesia (the inability to recall events that

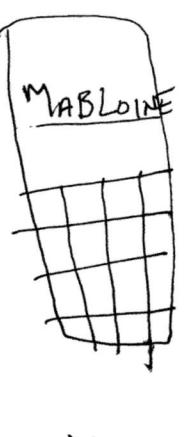

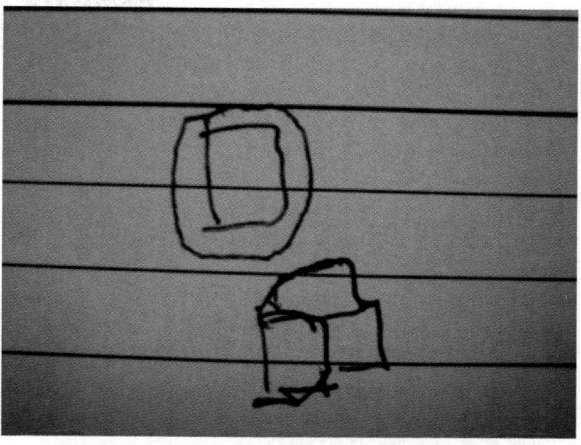

Figure 115-3 Attempts to draw a cube by a patient with a neurodegenerative disorder.

Figure 115-2 Neologisms written by a patient with aphasia attempting to name mobile phone, keys, camera, watch, pen, bag, boots.

occurred before the injury) and mild anterograde amnesia (the inability to recall events that occur after the injury).

Transient global amnesia typically affects persons older than 65 years and consists of abrupt onset of amnesia for time, place, and recent memory and lasts less than 12 hours. Patients are distressed and repeatedly require reorientation to their environment. They are, however, able to carry out complex, previously learned tasks such as driving. A number of precipitants have been identified, including extreme emotion, physical activity, sexual intercourse, and immersion in cold water. Recurrent episodes are rare.

Table 115-6 **Common Disorders of Memory**
Benign forgetfulness of aging
Alzheimer disease and other dementias
Head trauma
Transient global amnesia
Korsakoff syndrome (thiamine deficiency)
Encephalitis (herpes simplex)
Stroke (posterior cerebral artery)
Temporal lobe seizures
Psychogenic disorders

Korsakoff syndrome is the end result of untreated or partially treated Wernicke encephalopathy caused by thiamine deficiency. Patients (many of whom are alcoholic or malnourished) demonstrate confusion, gait ataxia, nystagmus, and ophthalmoparesis. The condition may be precipitated by the administration of glucose unless thiamine is given in advance. If the condition is untreated, a profound inability to form new memories results, with devastating consequences for the patient. In the chronic phase, patients confabulate freely in an attempt to fill the memory void.

Psychogenic amnesia often affects long-term memory as well as recent memory, and patients are occasionally unable to recall their own names. This is in contrast to most organic amnestic states, in which only short-term memory is affected and disorientation is greatest for time and place, but never for self.

Prospectus for the Future

There have been many recent advances in functional neuroimaging technology, which allows neuroscientists to study not only the functional anatomy of a particular brain structure, but also its metabolic activity. Functional magnetic resonance imaging (MRI) now permits mapping of the metabolic anatomy of subcortical gray and white matter structures, such as the basal ganglia, and their role in conditions such as dystonia. These imaging modalities are now able to study white matter tracts (tractography) in great detail, using a technique called *diffusion tensor imaging*. Similarly, modern MRI technology is now able to discriminate brain tissue that is infarcted from tissue that is ischemic (and therefore potentially still viable) in the setting of acute stroke. It is likely that such imaging techniques will become increasingly available in the acute hospital setting.

Reference

Preston DC, Shapiro BE: Neuroimaging in Neurology. An interactive CD. Philadelphia, WB Saunders, 2007.

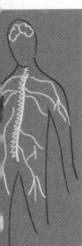

Dementia and Memory Disturbances

Frederick J. Marshall

Major Dementia Syndromes

Dementia is defined as the progressive loss of intellectual function. Memory loss is the central feature, and specific dementia syndromes characteristically cause particular forms of memory impairment. Dementia syndromes also produce specific abnormalities of cognition: language, spatial processing, *praxis* (learned motor behavior), and *executive function* (the ability to plan and sequence events). *Cortical dementia* and *subcortical dementia* subdivide the dementias (Table 116-1). Table 116-2 provides the differential diagnosis of neurodegenerative causes of dementia, and Table 116-3 outlines other causes of dementia. Neurodegeneration is the most common underlying cause of dementia and is seen in Alzheimer disease (AD), frontotemporal dementia, and diffuse Lewy body disease, among others. Most causes of dementias are currently untreatable. Potentially correctable causes account for less than 5% of all cases of dementia. Structural processes or infections must be considered, along with metabolic and nutritional diseases. Every patient with dementia should have tests of serum electrolytes and vitamin B$_{12}$, as well as assessments of liver, renal, and thyroid function; serologic studies for syphilis should be done if risk factors are identified. Chronic infections (see Chapter 128) and normal-pressure hydrocephalus should be considered. Brain imaging should be performed.

Neuropsychological testing characterizes the pattern of cognitive and memory impairments and is helpful in the differential diagnosis. The Mini-Mental State Examination (Table 116-4) is a standard test that can be used as a bedside or office screening tool for identifying patients with dementia. This examination emphasizes memory and language and is best at detecting cortical rather than subcortical dementia. In addition to the Mini-Mental State Examination, patients with dementia should have tests of visuospatial processing (clock drawing), praxis *(show how you would comb your hair; show how you would blow out a match),* and verbal fluency *(name as many animals as you can in 60 seconds).*

ALZHEIMER DISEASE

AD accounts for approximately 70% of all cases of dementia in older adults. Nearly 5 million persons in the United States are affected, and this number will double by 2020 as the population ages. AD places enormous burdens on the patient, on the family, and on society; annual direct and indirect expenditures are estimated to exceed $100 billion. The disease occurs in up to 30% of persons older than 85 years of age.

AD has many causes, but none are fully defined. All causes, however, produce similar clinical and pathologic findings. Pathologically, the disease is characterized by the progressive loss of cortical neurons and the formation of amyloid plaques and intraneuronal neurofibrillary tangles. β-amyloid (Aβ) is the major component of the plaques, whereas hyperphosphorylated tau protein is the major constituent of the neurofibrillary tangles. The process starts in the hippocampus and entorhinal cortex and spreads to involve diffuse areas of association cortex in the temporal, parietal, and frontal lobes. The relative deficiency of cortical acetylcholine (resulting from the loss of neurons in the nucleus basalis) provides the rationale for symptomatic treatment of the disease with centrally acting acetylcholinesterase inhibitors.

Pathogenesis

AD is often categorized into two forms: (1) a young-onset hereditary or familial form, which is extremely uncommon and for which three specific genetic abnormalities have been determined, and (2) a more common, sporadic form that typically occurs in persons older than 65 years of age (Table 116-5).

The autosomal-dominant, early-onset forms of AD have provided clues to the molecular pathogenesis of sporadic AD. Progressive dementia and pathologic changes characteristic of AD are almost universal in older patients with Down syndrome (trisomy 21). This observation suggested that chromosome 21 harbors a gene responsible for AD. Aβ is a

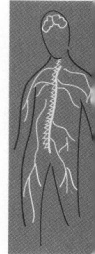

Table 116-1 Distinguishing Characteristics of Cortical and Subcortical Dementias

Cortical Dementia

Symptoms: major changes in memory, language deficits, perceptual deficits, praxis disturbances
Affected brain regions: temporal cortex (medial), parietal cortex, and frontal lobe cortex
Examples: Alzheimer disease, diffuse Lewy body disease, vascular dementia, frontotemporal dementias

Subcortical Dementia

Symptoms: behavioral changes, impaired affect and mood, motor slowing, executive dysfunction, less severe changes in memory
Affected brain regions: thalamus, striatum, midbrain, striatofrontal projections
Examples: Parkinson disease, progressive supranuclear palsy, normal-pressure hydrocephalus, Huntington disease, Creutzfeldt-Jakob disease, chronic meningitis

Table 116-2 Etiologic Diagnosis of Neurodegenerative Dementia in Adults

Alzheimer disease*
Parkinson disease*
Diffuse Lewy body disease*
Progressive supranuclear palsy
Corticobasal-ganglionic degeneration
Striatonigral degeneration
Olivopontocerebellar degeneration
Huntington disease
Frontotemporal dementias
Pick disease
Frontotemporal dementia without characteristic neuropathology
Frontotemporal dementia with motor neuron disease
Hallervorden-Spatz disease

*Denotes conditions for which symptomatic treatment is available.

Table 116-3 Other Causes of Progressive Dementia in Adults

Structural Disease or Trauma

Normal-pressure hydrocephalus*
Neoplasms*
Dementia pugilistica (multiple concussions in boxers)

Vascular Disease

Vascular dementia†
Vasculitis*

Heredometabolic Disease

Wilson disease*
Neuronal ceroid lipofuscinosis (Kufs disease)
Other late-onset lysosomal storage diseases

Demyelinating or Dysmyelinating Disease

Multiple sclerosis†
Metachromatic leukodystrophy

Infectious Disease

Human immunodeficiency virus, type 1*
Tertiary syphilis*
Creutzfeldt-Jakob disease
Progressive multifocal leukoencephalopathy
Whipple disease*
Chronic meningitis*
Cryptococcal meningitis*
Others

Metabolic or Nutritional Disease

Vitamin B_{12} deficiency*
Thyroid hormone deficiency or excess*
Thiamine deficiency* (Wernicke-Korsakoff syndrome)
Alcoholism†

Psychiatric Disease

Pseudodementia from depression*

*Denotes conditions for which preventive or corrective treatment is available.
†Denotes conditions for which symptomatic treatment is available.

Table 116-4 Elements of the Mini-Mental State Examination*

Cognitive Domain	Items	Score
Attention, concentration	Spell *world* backward (or perform *serial 7s* subtraction)	5
Memory and Orientation		
Temporal	Indicate year, season, month, day, date	5
Spatial	Indicate state, country, city, building, floor	5
Learning		
Immediate recall	Register three words (*apple, table, penny*)	3
Delayed recall	Recall three words (*apple, table, penny*)	3
Language		
Naming	Name two objects (*pen, watch*)	2
Repetition	Repeat phrase (*no ifs, ands, or buts*)	1
Comprehension	Follow three-step verbal command	3
	Follow one-step written command	1
Writing	Write original sentence	1
Visuospatial processing	Copy intersecting pentagons	1
	Total possible score	30

*Based on data from Folstein M, Folstein S, McHugh P: "Mini-mental state"—A practical method for grading the cognitive state of patients for the clinician. J Psychiatr Res 12:189-198, 1975.

cleavage product of the amyloid precursor protein, coded by a gene on chromosome 21. Abnormal processing of amyloid precursor protein into the amyloidogenic fragment $A\beta_{42}$ may be important in the pathogenesis of AD. The *apolipoprotein E (ApoE)* gene was found to be a susceptibility locus for sporadic AD in late-onset familial AD pedigrees. The gene is polymorphic (ε2/3/4), and persons who inherit one or both ε4 alleles are at increased risk for developing AD. ApoE-ε4 interacts selectively with Aβ and with tau protein, but how ApoE-ε4 increases the risk of AD is still unknown.

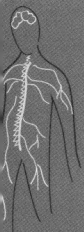

Table 116-5 **Familial versus Sporadic Alzheimer Disease**			
Chromosome or Gene	**Age at Onset (yr)**	**Percentage of All FAD Cases**	**Percentage of All AD Cases**
FAD: Early Onset, Autosomal Dominant			
1/presenilin 2	40-80	5-10	<0.5
14/presenilin 1	30-60	70	<1
21/amyloid precursor protein	35-65	5	<0.5
Sporadic AD: Late Onset, Possibly Polygenetic ± Possibly Environmental			
No single determinant gene*	Usually >60	—	98

*Apolipoprotein E-ε4 allele on chromosome 19 yields increased risk compared with ε2 or ε3 allele.
AD, Alzheimer disease; FAD, familial Alzheimer disease.

Table 116-6 **Diagnostic Criteria for Probable Alzheimer Disease**
Progressive functional decline and dementia established by clinical examination and mental status testing and confirmed by neuropsychological assessment
Cognitive deficits in two or more domains (including memory impairment)
Normal level of consciousness at presentation
Not developmentally acquired; onset between 40 and 90 years of age
Absence of other illnesses capable of causing dementia

Clinical Features

AD begins gradually and affects memory, orientation, language, visuospatial processing, praxis, judgment, and insight. Depression is frequent early in AD; frank psychosis with agitation and behavioral disinhibition often occur in advanced stages. Patients become dependent on others for all activities of daily living. The rate of progression of AD is variable, usually taking 5 to 15 years to progress from presentation to advanced illness. Diagnostic criteria are outlined in Table 116-6. Although a definitive diagnosis of AD requires biopsy (rarely done) or autopsy confirmation, these diagnostic criteria establish the diagnosis with more than 85% specificity in moderately demented patients. The positron emission tomography (PET) ligand Pittsburgh Compound B (PiB), which binds to amyloid, is currently being developed as a promising diagnostic and clinical marker of disease progression.

Treatment

Although their benefits are modest, the cholinesterase-inhibiting drugs tacrine (Cognex), donepezil (Aricept), rivastigmine (Exelon), and galantamine (Reminyl, Razadyne) represent important advances. Tacrine can be hepatotoxic and must be given 4 times a day; donepezil is given once a day and has fewer side effects than tacrine; rivastigmine may be given as a once-daily transdermal patch; and galantamine now has an extended release form that can also be given once a day. In clinical trials, cholinesterase inhibitors benefited fewer than 50% of patients. The glutamate antagonist memantine (Namenda) has been shown to prolong daily function in patients with moderate-to-advanced AD.

Nursing services provide oversight of hygiene, nutrition, and medication compliance. Antipsychotics, antidepressants, and anxiolytics are useful for patients with behavioral disturbances, which are the most common cause of nursing home placement. Acetylcholinesterase inhibition may also benefit the behavioral disorder. Patients and families can be referred to a local Alzheimer's Association chapter for further information on available community supports.

DIFFUSE LEWY BODY DISEASE

Lewy bodies are pathologic inclusions that are the hallmark of Parkinson disease when they are restricted to the brainstem (see Chapter 122). Patients with diffuse Lewy body disease have clinical parkinsonism (slow movement, rigidity, and balance problems) combined with early and prominent dementia. Pathologically, Lewy bodies are found in the brainstem, limbic system, and cortex. Visual hallucinations and cognitive fluctuations are common, and patients are unusually sensitive to the adverse effects of neuroleptic medication. Diffuse Lewy body disease may represent the second most common cause of dementia after AD. However, the common concurrence of the pathologic features of diffuse Lewy body disease with the classic neuritic plaques and neurofibrillary tangles of AD complicates the identification of the cause of dementia in a given patient.

VASCULAR DEMENTIA

Approximately 10% to 20% of older patients with dementia have radiographic evidence of focal stroke on magnetic resonance imaging (MRI) or computed tomography (CT), combined with focal signs on the neurologic examination. When the dementia syndrome begins with a stroke, and when the progression of the illness is stepwise (suggesting recurrent vascular events), the diagnosis of *vascular dementia* is likely. Patients typically develop early incontinence, gait disturbances, and flattening of affect. A subcortical dementing process attributed to small vessel disease in the periventricular white matter has been referred to as *Binswanger disease,* but it may merely be a radiographic finding rather than a true disease. Appropriate treatment of risk factors for vascular disease—blood pressure control, smoking cessation, diet modification, and anticoagulation (in select settings such as atrial fibrillation)—is clearly mandatory and may be of benefit.

FRONTOTEMPORAL DEMENTIAS

Unlike AD, in which the presenting symptom is typically memory loss, frontotemporal dementia often begins with significant behavioral disturbances. Patients with *Pick disease,* the classic form of frontotemporal dementia, are frequently irascible and socially disinhibited. As in AD, the illness progresses for years; no intervention slows the inevitable decline of these patients. Approximately 50% of patients have a family history of the disease; in some families, a mutation in the tau protein gene on chromosome 17 is the cause.

PARKINSON DISEASE

Nearly 50% of patients with Parkinson disease (see Chapter 122) become demented by the time they reach the age of 85 years. The dementia of Parkinson disease affects executive function out of proportion to its impact on language and visuospatial processing. Thought processes appear to slow down *(bradyphrenia),* analogous to the slowing of movement *(bradykinesia).* Because dementia occurs relatively late in the progression of Parkinson disease, most patients are taking drugs to improve their movement disorder by enhancing dopaminergic neurotransmission. These drugs can induce psychosis. Dose reductions should be attempted before the diagnosis of underlying dementia in these patients is made. Acetylcholinesterase inhibition has been shown to be helpful in patients with dementia caused by Parkinson disease.

NORMAL-PRESSURE HYDROCEPHALUS

The triad of dementia (typically subcortical), gait instability, and urinary incontinence suggests the possibility of *normal-pressure hydrocephalus.* These patients appear to walk with their feet stuck to the floor, without lifting up the knees and with a broad base. Symptoms evolve over the course of weeks to months, and brain imaging reveals ventricular enlargement out of proportion to the degree of cortical atrophy. Numerous diagnostic tests have been described, including radionuclide cisternography and MRI flow studies. The most important test remains the clinical response to removal of large volumes of cerebrospinal fluid, either through serial lumbar punctures or through the temporary placement of a lumbar drain, followed by examination of the patient's gait and cognitive function. Neurosurgical placement of a permanent ventriculoperitoneal shunt may correct the problem. Patients likely to benefit from shunt placement have a clear response to the removal of 30 to 40 mL of spinal fluid, with improved gait and alertness within minutes to hours of the procedure. The cause of normal-pressure hydrocephalus is a derangement of the cerebrospinal fluid hydrodynamics. Shunt placement is most likely to be effective if normal-pressure hydrocephalus occurs after severe head trauma or subarachnoid hemorrhage.

PRION INFECTION, CHRONIC MENINGITIS, DEMENTIA RELATED TO ACQUIRED IMMUNODEFICIENCY SYNDROME

Creutzfeldt-Jakob disease (CJD) is a subacute, dementing, transmissible illness with typical onset between 40 and 75 years of age and an incidence of 1 in 1,000,000 (see Chapter 128). The disease causes spongiform degeneration and gliosis in widespread areas of the cortex. Clinical variants of the disorder are differentiated by the relative predominance of cerebellar symptoms, extrapyramidal hyperkinesias, or visual agnosia and cortical blindness *(Heidenhain variant).* Ninety percent of patients with CJD have myoclonus, compared with 10% of patients with AD. Patients with all forms of the disease share a relentlessly progressive dementia and disruption of personality over weeks to months. The electroencephalogram develops characteristic abnormalities, including diffuse slowing and periodic sharp waves or spikes. The transmissible agent, a prion protein, is invulnerable to routine modes of antisepsis. Cerebrospinal fluid can be tested for the 14-3-3 protein, although this test is not 100% sensitive or specific for CJD (see Chapter 128). Diffusion-weighted MRI images show characteristic cortical ribbon changes.

Certain *infectious agents* can cause the subacute or chronic development of subcortical dementia. These chronic meningitides are discussed in Chapter 128.

Human immunodeficiency virus accesses the central nervous system through monocytes and the microglial system and causes associated neuronal cell loss, vacuolization, and lymphocytic infiltration. The dementia associated with this infection is characterized by bradyphrenia and bradykinesia. Patients have executive dysfunction, impaired memory, poor concentration, and apathy. Treatment of the underlying viral infection with protease inhibitors and reverse transcriptase inhibitors may slow the progression of the dementia (see Chapter 128).

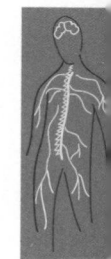

Other Memory Disturbances

STRUCTURE OF MEMORY

Memory function is divided into introspective processes (declarative, explicit, aware memories) and processes that are not accessible to introspection (nondeclarative, implicit, procedural memories). Short-term memory (e.g., for words on a list) is a form of *declarative memory.* Other forms include the conscious recall of episodes from personal experience *(episodic memory),* and factual knowledge *(semantic memory)* that can be consciously recalled and stated (declared). Declarative memories involve consciously *knowing that.* . . . Patients with amnesia resulting from lesions of the medial temporal lobes or midline diencephalic structures have deficits of declarative memory.

Nondeclarative memory encompasses several distinct and neuroanatomically less clearly localized functions related to the performance of specific learned motor, cognitive, or perceptual tasks. Nondeclarative (procedural) memories involve unconsciously *knowing how.* . . . Deficits in nondeclarative memory may involve various areas of association neocortex, depending on the nature of the task (e.g., parieto-temporal-occipital junction cortex for visual perceptual tasks, frontal association cortex for motor tasks). Patients with amnesia resulting from lesions of the medial temporal lobes tend to perform normally on tests of nondeclarative memory.

Anterograde amnesia refers to the inability to learn new information. It commonly occurs after brain injury or in association with dementia. The inability to recollect prior information is known as *retrograde amnesia*. Both types of amnesia usually occur together in brain injury syndromes, although the extent of one type or the other may vary. The degree of anterograde amnesia after head injury is correlated with the severity of the injury.

ISOLATED DISORDERS OF MEMORY FUNCTION

Memory can be impaired in relative isolation as a consequence of head injury, thiamine deficiency (Korsakoff syndrome), benign forgetfulness of aging, transient global amnesia, or psychogenic disease.

Head injury typically results in retrograde amnesia in excess of anterograde amnesia, with both forms stretching out in time away from the discrete event. As time passes, these disrupted memories generally gradually return, although rarely to the point at which the events immediately surrounding the trauma are recalled.

Korsakoff syndrome is characterized by the near-total inability to establish new memory. Patients often confabulate responses when they are asked to convey the details of their current circumstance or to relay the content of a recently presented story. Deficiency of thiamine and other nutritional deficiencies in the context of chronic alcoholism are the most common underlying causes. Thiamine is a necessary cofactor in the metabolism of glucose, and for this reason, thiamine must be replenished at the same time glucose is administered whenever a comatose patient is presented to the emergency department.

Aging is associated with mild loss of memory, exhibited by difficulty in recalling names and by forgetfulness for dates. Population-based assessments of neuropsychological function have demonstrated that poor performance on delayed-recall tasks is the most sensitive indicator of cognitive change with advancing age. Verbal fluency, in contrast, remains intact with advancing age, and vocabulary may increase with time, even into old age.

Transient global amnesia is a dramatic memory disturbance that affects older patients (>50 years of age). Patients usually have only one episode; occasionally, episodes recur over the course of several years. Patients have complete temporal and spatial disorientation; orientation for person is preserved. Near-total retrograde and anterograde amnesia persists for variable periods, typically 6 to 12 hours. Patients are often anxious and may repeat the same question over and over again. Transient global amnesia may be confused with psychogenic amnesia, fugue state, or partial complex status epilepticus. Transient global amnesia is thought to reflect underlying vascular insufficiency to the hippocampus or midline thalamic projections.

Unlike patients with organic memory disturbances, patients with *psychogenic amnesia* typically have inconsistent loss of recent and remote memory, relatively more loss of emotionally charged memory (rather than relatively less loss of such memory in organic disease), and an apparent indifference to their own plight—they ask few questions. Most characteristically, patients with psychogenic amnesia tend to express disorientation to person (asking, *Who am I?*), a phenomenon seldom seen in organic memory disturbance.

Patients with *severe depression* may exhibit *pseudodementia*. Vegetative signs, including changes in appetite, weight, and sleep pattern, are common, whereas signs of cortical impairment, such as aphasia, agnosia, and apraxia, are rare. Memory and bradyphrenia improve with antidepressant therapy. Depression often coexists with other causes of dementia: AD, Parkinson disease, and vascular dementia.

Prospectus for the Future

Molecular Genetics and the Future of the Diagnosis and Treatment of Dementia

Breakthroughs in the fields of proteomics, information processing of megadata sets, and messenger-RNA expression profiling promise to improve the diagnosis and treatment of dementia in the future. In all likelihood, Alzheimer disease (AD) will be subcategorized into more precise etiologic categories, and patients will be offered selective treatments based on their particular pharmacogenetic background. Drug development will be enhanced by emerging knowledge about the molecular mechanisms of Aβ deposition, synaptic loss, and tau protein hyperphosphorylation. Treatment strategies currently in clinical trials include decreasing Aβ peptide production by blocking α-secretase or β-secretase or upregulating cleavage of the amyloid precursor protein at the α-secretase site. In addition, studies of active and passive immunization designed to lower brain Aβ levels are ongoing. Although acetylcholinesterase inhibition has not been shown to be effective in the treatment of mild cognitive impairment (considered to be a precursor condition to AD), these novel molecular and immunologic approaches continue to hold promise for disease-modifying treatments in the future.

References

Bird T: Genetic aspects of Alzheimer disease. Gen Med 10:231-239, 2008.

Cummings JL, Doody R, Clark C: Disease-modifying therapies for Alzheimer disease: Challenges to early intervention. Neurology 69:1622-1634, 2007.

Knopman DS: Regional cerebral dysfunction: Higher mental functions. In Goldman L, Ausiello DA (eds): Cecil Textbook of Medicine, 23rd ed. Philadelphia, WB Saunders, 2007, pp 2662-2667.

McKeith I: Dementia with Lewy bodies and Parkinson's disease with dementia: Where two worlds collide. Pract Neurol 7:374-382, 2007.

Nordberg A: Amyloid imaging in Alzheimer's disease. Curr Opin Neurol 20:398-402, 2007.

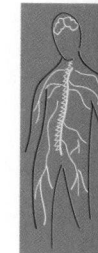

Major Disorders of Mood, Thoughts, and Behavior

Jeffrey M. Lyness

Introduction to and Classification of Mental Disorders

Mental (psychiatric) disorders are defined as alterations in mood, thoughts, and behavior that produce substantive subjective distress or affect the patient's functional status. Many mental disorders are caused by the direct effects of drugs, systemic disease, or neurologic disease on brain physiology. These may be broadly considered as secondary psychiatric disorders, as opposed to the primary or idiopathic psychiatric disorders. Table 117-1 shows the types of psychiatric disorders with an identified cause. The distinguishing feature of cognitive disorders is impairment in intellectual functions such as level of consciousness, orientation, attention, or memory; however, these disorders also often include disruption of mood, thoughts, and behaviors similar to that seen in other psychiatric syndromes. Cognitive disorders are the focus of Chapters 113 and 116.

The noncognitive secondary syndromes by definition cause psychiatric phenomenology similar to their idiopathic counterpart. Therefore, during the evaluation of any patient with new or worsened psychiatric symptoms, it is essential to conduct a thorough evaluation for specific "organic" causes, including at least a careful history and physical examination (with screening neurologic examination), often supplemented by laboratory evaluations. Table 117-2 outlines important causes of psychiatric syndromes. Although some conditions are more likely to produce certain psychiatric syndromes, many may manifest as any of several psychiatric syndromes. Conversely, a psychiatric syndrome may be caused by any of a wide range of conditions.

Because the cause of primary psychiatric disorders is not known, approaches to classification depend on reliable empirical observations of phenomenology, clustered into recognizable syndromes. Table 117-3 shows the most important psychiatric syndromes and the disorders in which they may manifest. Table 117-4 shows the major idiopathic disorders excluding substance use disorders (see Chapter 135).

Many psychiatric disorders can be present with multiple syndromes. For example, major depression with psychotic features, classified as a mood disorder, manifests with both a depressive syndrome and a psychotic syndrome. Therefore, in evaluating a patient with new or worsened psychiatric symptoms, one must construct a differential diagnosis based on syndromes alongside the differential diagnosis based on potential ("organic" or secondary) causes.

Mood Disorders

Mood disorders are characterized by idiopathic episodes of depression ("unipolar") or mania ("bipolar"). The core symptoms of depressive episodes include emotional symptoms (dysphoria, irritability, anhedonia, loss of interests), ideational symptoms (thought content of hopeless, worthless, guilty, or suicidal themes), and neurovegetative symptoms and signs (altered sleep, appetite, and weight; anergia; psychomotor slowing or agitation; decreased concentration). Major depressive disorder is defined by episodes of at least five such symptoms, including depressed mood or anhedonia or loss of interests, present most of the day for most days over at least 2 consecutive weeks, sufficient to cause significant distress and affect functional status. Other prominent symptoms may include associated anxiety, somatic worry or somatoform symptoms, and, in the most severe cases, psychotic symptoms including nihilistic or self-deprecatory ("mood-congruent") delusions. Major depression is common, with a point prevalence of 3% to 5% in men and 8% to 10% in women, and a lifetime prevalence approximately double the point prevalence. True disorder incidence is difficult to estimate in the population given the high recurrence rates, but new episodes have an annual incidence of approximately 3%. First onset may occur at any age but is most common in the third through fifth decades of life. Whereas most episodes of major depression fully remit spontaneously or with treatment, the lifetime risk of recurrence may be as high as 90%, and up to 20% of patients may experience chronic symptoms over many years. Major

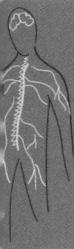

Table 117-1 Psychiatric Disorders (Syndromes) with an Identified Cause

Cognitive

Global (More than one realm of cognition affected; e.g., memory and language)

Delirium
Dementia

Specific (One realm of cognition affected: memory)

Amnestic disorder

Secondary

_____ caused by general medical condition
Substance-induced _____
where _____ may be any of the following:
    Mood disorder
    Anxiety disorder
    Psychotic disorder
    Sleep disorder
    Personality change
    Catatonic disorder

Based on data from *Diagnostic and Statistical Manual of Mental Disorders, Fourth Edition* (DSM-IV).

Table 117-2 Important Causes of Psychiatric Syndromes

Central Nervous System Conditions

Tumor
Toxins
Vascular disorders
Seizure
Infection
Genetic disorders
Congenital malformation
Demyelinating conditions
Degenerative conditions
Hydrocephalus

Systemic Diseases

Cardiovascular diseases
Pulmonary diseases
Cancer
Infection
Nutritional disorders
Endocrine disorders
Metabolic disorders

Drugs

Drug intoxication
Drug withdrawal

Table 117-3 Important Psychiatric Syndromes

Syndrome	Main Symptoms and Signs	Present in These Disorders
Cognitive	Impairment in intellectual functions (e.g., level of consciousness, orientation, attention, memory, language, praxis, visuospatial, executive functions)	Cognitive disorders Mental retardation (if onset in childhood)
Mood	Depressive: lowered mood, anhedonia, negativistic thoughts, neurovegetative symptoms Manic: elevated or irritable mood; grandiosity; goal-directed hyperactivity with increased energy; pressured speech; decreased sleep need	Cognitive disorders Mood disorders (primary or secondary) Psychotic disorders (schizoaffective disorder)
Anxiety	All include anxious mood and associated physiologic signs and symptoms (e.g., palpitations, tremors, diaphoresis). May include various types of dysfunctional thoughts (e.g., catastrophic fears, obsessions, flashbacks) and behaviors (e.g., compulsions, avoidance behaviors)	Cognitive disorders Mood disorders (primary or secondary) Psychotic disorders (primary or secondary) Anxiety disorders (primary or secondary)
Psychotic	Impairments in reality testing: hallucinations, thought process derailments	Cognitive disorders Mood disorders (primary or secondary) Psychotic disorders
Somatoform	Somatoform symptoms: physical symptoms from psychogenic causes	Mood disorders (primary or secondary) Anxiety disorders (primary or secondary) Somatoform disorders
Personality pathology	Dysfunctional enduring patterns of emotional regulation, thought patterns, interpersonal behaviors, impulse regulation	Cognitive disorders (dementia) Personality change from general medical condition Personality disorders

Based on data from *Diagnostic and Statistical Manual of Mental Disorders, Fourth Edition* (DSM-IV).

depression is a leading correlate of disability worldwide, is an important determinant of death by suicide, and is associated with increased risk of death from comorbid physical illnesses. Dysthymic disorder is a condition defined by chronic depressive symptoms of insufficient severity to meet criteria for major depression.

Depressive disorders are heterogeneous, with many potential pathogenic mechanisms. Genetic factors, such as polymorphisms of the serotonin transporter protein, affect vulnerability to depressive episodes in the face of psychosocial stressors. Depression is both polygenic and multifactorial, with genetic factors accounting for about 50% of the risk for depression onset. Alterations in the functioning of brain serotonergic and noradrenergic systems and of the hypothalamic-pituitary-adrenal axis are present in depression; neuroimaging studies show smaller hippocampal volumes and altered metabolic activity in several regions including the anterior cingulate cortex. However, at present such studies are not accurate in making the clinical diagnosis, which depends on identification of the clinical syndrome. Improvement in regional cerebral metabolic activity is seen with successful treatment of depression, with different

Table 117-4 Major Idiopathic ("Primary") Disorders of Mood, Thoughts, and Behavior

Mood Disorders

Unipolar

Major depressive disorder
Dysthymic disorder

Bipolar

Bipolar disorder
Cyclothymic disorder
Bipolar II disorder (bipolar disorder not otherwise specified)

Anxiety Disorders

Panic disorder (without or with agoraphobia)
Obsessive-compulsive disorder
Acute stress disorder or posttraumatic stress disorder
Generalized anxiety disorder
Social phobia
Specific phobia

Psychotic Disorders

Schizophrenia
Schizophreniform disorder
Brief psychotic disorder
Schizoaffective disorder
Delusional disorder

Somatoform Disorders

Conversion disorder
Pain disorder
Somatization disorder
Undifferentiated somatoform disorder
Body dysmorphic disorder
Hypochondriasis

Personality Disorders

Cluster A: Odd Eccentric

Schizoid personality disorder
Schizotypal personality disorder
Paranoid personality disorder

Cluster B: Dramatic/Emotional

Borderline personality disorder
Narcissistic personality disorder
Antisocial personality disorder
Histrionic personality disorder

Cluster C: Anxious/Fearful

Avoidant personality disorder
Dependent personality disorder
Obsessive-compulsive personality disorder

Based on data from *Diagnostic and Statistical Manual of Mental Disorders, Fourth Edition* (DSM-IV).

Table 117-5 Psychotherapies for Depression and Antidepressant Medications

Psychotherapy

Name	Approach
Cognitive psychotherapy	Identify and correct negativistic patterns of thinking
Interpersonal psychotherapy	Identify and work through role transitions or interpersonal losses, conflicts, or deficits
Problem-solving therapy	Identify and prioritize situational problems; plan and implement strategies to deal with top-priority problems

Commonly Used Antidepressants

Name	Mechanism of Action
SSRIs (selective serotonin reuptake inhibitors)	Inhibit presynaptic reuptake of serotonin
Citalopram and escitalopram	
Fluoxetine	
Paroxetine	
Sertraline	
SNRIs (serotonin and norepinephrine reuptake inhibitors)	Inhibit presynaptic reuptake of serotonin and norepinephrine
Duloxetine	
Venlafaxine and desvenlafaxine	
TCAs (tricyclic antidepressants)	Inhibit presynaptic reuptake of serotonin and norepinephrine (in varying proportions depending on the specific TCA)
Amitriptyline	
Desipramine	
Doxepin	
Imipramine	
Nortriptyline	
MAOIs (monoamine oxidase inhibitors)	Inhibit monoamine oxidase, the enzyme that catalyzes oxidative metabolism of monoamine neurotransmitters
Isocarboxazide	
Phenelzine	
Selegiline	Selective MAO-B inhibitor
Tranylcypromine	
Other	
Bupropion	Unknown, although it is weak inhibitor of presynaptic reuptake of norepinephrine and dopamine
Mirtazapine	Antagonist at α_2 and $5HT_2$ receptors
Trazodone	Inhibits presynaptic reuptake of serotonin; antagonist at $5HT_2$ and $5HT_3$ receptors

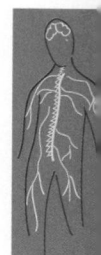

patterns of improvement visible on functional neuroimaging scans after psychotherapy versus pharmacotherapy. Dysfunctional negativistic patterns of thinking, impaired social relationships, and stressful life events also contribute to depression.

Mild to moderate forms of depression respond to focused psychotherapies or antidepressant medications (Table 117-5). Other psychosocial interventions, including exercise, also may produce benefit. More severe forms of depression will not respond to psychosocial interventions alone. Severe or refractory depression may be treated safely and effectively with electroconvulsive therapy. Other evidence-based somatic therapies include light therapy (for depression with a seasonal component) and possibly vagal nerve stimulation.

Bipolar disorder (bipolar I) is characterized by recurrent episodes of mania, usually with episodes of major depression as well. Manic episodes include elevated (euphoric) or irritable mood, goal-directed hyperactivity (often with poor judgment leading to substantial adverse consequences, e.g., sexual, spending, or gambling sprees), grandiose thought content, pressured speech, increased energy level with decreased need for sleep, and racing thoughts that may

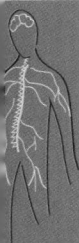

progress to objectively observable flight of ideas or more severe thought process derailments such as loose associations. Compared with unipolar depression, bipolar disorder has a lower point prevalence (approximately 1%), an approximately equal gender distribution, and a younger average age of onset (typically late teens to twenties). There are few data regarding incidence rates beyond studies of the peak years of disease onset, with wide variability also depending on other characteristics of the study sample. Most patients return to baseline functioning between acute mood episodes, but some have a deteriorating course; others have rapid cycling, defined as four episodes per year. Genetic factors play a greater role in the pathogenesis of bipolar disorder than in major depressive disorder; twin studies indicate that genetic factors again account for approximately 50% of the risk for bipolar disorder, representing a 50-fold increase over the population base rate (as compared with a fivefold to 10-fold increase for major depression). Bipolar disorder is polygenic and has been linked in individual families to different loci. The pathogenesis is unclear, but functional neuroimaging evidence suggests dysregulation of frontostriatal systems. Structural neuroimaging studies (computed tomography [CT] and magnetic resonance imaging [MRI] scans) show increased ventricular-brain ratios consistent with parenchymal agenesis or atrophy, similar to many other psychiatric disorders. Psychosocial stressors often play a role in precipitating episodes of both mania and depression. The mainstay of treatment for bipolar disorder is mood stabilizer medications (e.g., lithium, anticonvulsants such as valproic acid and carbamazepine) for both acute episodes and maintenance therapy. The anticonvulsant lamotrigine may be particularly useful for bipolar depression. Antipsychotic medications are useful for acute manic episodes and may have a role in maintenance therapy. Benzodiazepines may be used to treat acute agitation and aggression while waiting for more definitive antimanic therapies to take effect. Antidepressants have long been used for depressive episodes, although they may precipitate manic episodes and their efficacy for depression in bipolar patients is not established. Electroconvulsive therapy is effective for both refractory mania and depression. Psychosocial treatments alone do not effectively treat mania and may be less effective for bipolar depression, but psychoeducation and support to manage psychosocial stressors and encourage medication compliance improve longer-term outcomes.

A spectrum of less severe bipolar disorders includes conditions marked by episodes of hypomania (i.e., low-level manic symptoms without psychosis or significant impairment in functioning). These disorders include bipolar II disorder (bipolar disorder not otherwise specified [NOS]), characterized by episodes of hypomania and major depression, and cyclothymic disorder, characterized by hypomania and low-level depression not meeting criteria for major depression. Patients with bipolar II disorder are most likely to seek care during depressive episodes, so it is important to inquire about a prior history of manic symptoms to avoid precipitating mania with the use of antidepressant medications. Bipolar II appears to have heritability somewhat distinct from that of bipolar ("I") and major depressive disorders. The pathogeneses of these less severe mood disorders is unknown.

Table 117-6 **Common Somatic Symptoms of Anxiety**
Cardiorespiratory
Palpitations
Chest pain
Dyspnea or sensation of being smothered
Gastrointestinal
Sensation of choking
Dyspepsia
Nausea
Diarrhea
Abdominal bloating or pain
Genitourinary
Urinary frequency or urgency
Neurologic or Autonomic
Diaphoresis
Warm flushes
Dizziness or pre-syncope
Paresthesias
Tremor
Headache

Anxiety Disorders

The idiopathic anxiety disorders manifest with troublesome thoughts and somatic symptoms (Table 117-6) along with the emotional sensation of anxiety. A panic attack is a transient episode of crescendo anxiety, catastrophic thoughts (e.g., fears of dying, going insane, or losing self-control), and somatic symptoms. If panic attacks or other clinically significant anxiety symptoms occur only in predictable response to environmental stimuli, the anxiety disorder is known as a *phobia,* which may further be classified as agoraphobia (anxiety about being in places from which escape might be difficult or embarrassing, e.g., being alone, in crowds, in tunnels, or on bridges); social phobia (anxiety in interpersonal situations); and specific phobia (anxiety provoked by other situations or objects, e.g., blood, animals, heights). Panic disorder manifests with recurrent panic attacks of which at least some are unexpected and unpredictable, along with anticipatory anxiety (i.e., fears of having another attack) and avoidance behaviors (i.e., avoiding situations that might provoke a panic attack or in which having an attack is perceived to be embarrassing or dangerous).

Other anxiety disorders may not cause discrete panic attacks. Obsessive-compulsive disorder is characterized by recurrent obsessions (thoughts, impulses, or mental images that are anxiety-producing, perceived as intrusive and inappropriate, and resistant to attempts to suppress or neutralize them) and compulsions (repetitive behaviors or mental acts performed in response to obsessions or other rigid rules). Individuals exposed to severely stressful events (typically involving the actual or threatened loss of life or limb) may experience any of a wide variety of psychiatric sequelae. If the sequelae include symptoms of reexperiencing of the traumatic event (e.g., intrusive memories, nightmares, flashbacks), avoidance phenomena (e.g., avoiding reminders of the event, sense of foreshortened future), and hyperarousal symptoms (e.g., irritability, exaggerated startle response), the disorder is termed *acute stress disorder* (if the duration is up to 1 month) or *post-traumatic stress disorder* (if the duration is >1 month). Enduring anxiety symptoms that are not captured by these diagnoses (or by diagnoses of cognitive, mood, or psychotic disorders) may be diagnosed as generalized anxiety disorder. Anxiety disorders are common, with point prevalences of 1% to 2% each for panic disorder and obsessive-compulsive disorder and up to 10% for phobias. Although there are fewer data on long-term outcome than for mood disorders, many anxiety disorders tend to have a chronic waxing and waning course. There are few data that provide clear incidence rates, but it is clear that most anxiety disorders have first onset in the teens, 20s, and 30s; although new-onset anxiety is common in later life, the cause is only rarely a primary anxiety disorder (see Table 117-3).

The pathogeneses of most anxiety disorders may be understood as inappropriate activation of the stress response system involving a variety of neuroendocrine and autonomic outputs, coordinated by the central nucleus of the amygdala and other brain structures. The amygdala receives excitatory glutamatergic inputs from cortical sensory areas and the thalamus and has outputs to the major monoaminergic centers (e.g., noradrenergic neurons of the locus coeruleus, dopaminergic neurons of the ventral tegmental area, serotonergic neurons of the raphe nuclei) that in turn project to the many brain regions subserving the symptoms of anxiety. Unlike the other anxiety disorders, obsessive-compulsive disorder appears to be related more specifically to altered functioning of striatofrontal connections, leading to patterns of altered regional cerebral metabolism, visible on functional neuroimaging scans, that improve with successful psychotherapy or pharmacotherapy. The identification and correction of dysfunctional patterns of thinking ("cognitive therapy") and the extinction of pathologic behaviors and positive reinforcement of more functional behaviors ("behavior therapy") are evidence-based psychotherapies useful in most anxiety disorders. Such psychotherapies are the sole therapies for specific phobias and may be the sole or primary therapy for most other anxiety disorders. Antidepressant, anxiolytic, and other drug therapies are also used in treatment. Increasingly, antidepressant medications have replaced anxiolytics as the mainstay of pharmacotherapy for panic disorder, post-traumatic stress disorder, generalized social phobia, and generalized anxiety disorder. For obsessive-compulsive disorder, only antidepressant agents with pronounced activity on the serotonergic system (selective serotonin reuptake inhibitors [SSRIs; see Table 117-5], and also clomipramine) are efficacious.

Psychotic Disorders

Psychosis is defined as a loss of reality testing, manifested as hallucinations (false sensory perceptions), delusions (fixed false beliefs), and thought process derailments. Schizophrenia is the prototypic psychotic disorder; it includes acute episodes of psychosis ("positive" symptoms) and often declining overall functioning over time related to the presence of "negative symptoms" such as affective flattening, abulia, apathy, and social withdrawal. The point prevalence of schizophrenia is approximately 1%, and its chronic, debilitating course takes a considerable toll on patients, families, and society. Peak onset is in late adolescence to young

adulthood, slightly younger for males than females. The annual incidence is approximately 15 per 100,000, but with marked variability across study samples and populations. The pathogenesis of schizophrenia remains unknown, despite there being neurobiologic abnormalities. Twin studies show that the disease is multifactorial; genetic factors account for approximately 50% of the risk, and multiple gene loci appear to be involved. Studies of postmortem brains indicate a nongliotic neuropathologic process with subtle disruptions of cortical cytoarchitecture. It is likely that psychosocial factors and neurodevelopment interact with a nonlocalizable brain "lesion" either present at birth or acquired early in life. Dopaminergic mesocortical and mesolimbic pathways are important in the production of psychotic symptoms. Antipsychotic medications, often with adjunctive benzodiazepines, are used to treat acute psychotic episodes. Although maintenance antipsychotic medications help reduce the severity and frequency of acute psychotic episodes, comprehensive psychosocial rehabilitation programs are required to help patients manage interpersonal and other stressors and to improve overall clinical outcomes. In the past decade, second-generation ("atypical") antipsychotic medications have replaced first-generation antipsychotics because of their greater short-term tolerability and much lower rates of extrapyramidal side effects including tardive dyskinesia. However, there is concern that the second-generation drugs may contribute to the increase of obesity and metabolic syndrome among chronic schizophrenia patients.

Patients with single schizophrenia-like psychotic episodes of briefer duration, with subsequent return to asymptomatic baseline functioning, may be diagnosed with brief psychotic disorder (<1 month) or schizophreniform disorder (1 to 6 months). Schizoaffective disorder is a chronic recurrent disorder, with a prevalence slightly lower than that of schizophrenia, characterized by episodes of non-mood psychosis and also mood episodes (manic or depressed) with psychotic features. Its diagnosis therefore cannot be based on the patient's presentation at any one point in time, but requires knowledge of overall course. The outcomes of schizoaffective disorder are heterogeneous but on average are intermediate between schizophrenia and mood disorders. Treatment is symptomatic, using antipsychotic, mood stabilizing, and antidepressant medications to target specific psychotic and mood symptoms. Delusional disorder is characterized by potentially plausible ("nonbizarre") delusions such as marital infidelity, in the absence of thought process disorder, prominent hallucinations, or the negative symptoms of schizophrenia. Delusional disorder has a point prevalence of approximately 0.03% and a lifetime prevalence of 0.05% to 0.1%. It often is only partially responsive to antipsychotic medications, but patients' functioning may be largely unimpaired if they are able (with the aid of antipsychotics and psychotherapy) to not publically speak of or act on their delusions. The pathogeneses of the nonschizophrenic primary psychotic disorders remain largely unknown.

Somatoform Disorders

Somatoform symptoms, often broadly referred to as "somatization," resemble symptoms from systemic or neurologic

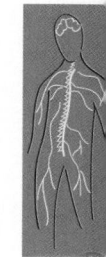

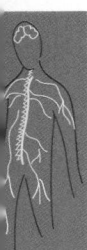

diseases but are thought to arise from unconscious psychogenic rather than identifiable physical causes. Somatization may range from normal human experiences (e.g., abdominal cramping in response to an acute stressor) to time-limited episodes to chronic, disabling conditions. The somatoform disorders are classified as pain disorder (pain); conversion disorder (other neurologic symptoms or signs, e.g., alteration in sensory functioning, motor functioning, coordination, or cognitive functioning); somatization disorder (Briquet syndrome: chronic recurrent somatoform symptoms of multiple organ systems); and undifferentiated somatoform disorder (somatoform symptoms not meeting criteria for the other disorders). The somatoform disorders also include hypochondriasis, manifested by inappropriate illness worry rather than somatoform symptoms per se, and body dysmorphic disorder, characterized by preoccupation with a perceived bodily defect ("imagined ugliness"), which may have more in common with the obsessions of obsessive-compulsive disorder than with the other somatoform disorders. The prevalence of somatoform disorders varies widely with both population being studied and the method of research diagnosis ascertainment. Somatization disorder may have a lifetime prevalence of 0.2% to 2% in females and <0.2% in males. Prevalence estimates for conversion disorder are as low as 0.01% in the general population but may be much higher (1% to 14%) in medical or surgical inpatient samples. Management of patients with somatoform disorders is often difficult, as physicians need to simultaneously maintain an appropriate level of vigilance for undiagnosed physical illness while avoiding unnecessary tools and therapies. Keys to ongoing care include maintaining an ongoing therapeutic alliance, setting regular office visits, conveying empathy for the patient's very real distress without colluding with the patient's belief in an identifiable physical disorder, and assertive treatment of depression, anxiety, or other comorbid psychopathology. Antidepressant medications may have some benefit in selected patient populations (e.g., some chronic pain syndromes) even in the absence of comorbid psychiatric disorders.

Somatoform symptoms and disorders should be distinguished from two conditions in which psychological factors lead to presentations resembling physical disorders. Factitious disorder (Munchausen syndrome) is a mental disorder in which patients consciously produce stigmata of disease (e.g., simulated or artificially induced fever or hypoglycemia) for the unconscious gain of assuming the sick role. Malingering is the conscious feigning of illness for conscious gain and therefore is not a mental disorder.

Personality Disorders

Personality is defined as the total repertoire of enduring patterns of thinking, feeling, and behaving, including affect and impulse regulation, defense and coping mechanisms, and interpersonal relatedness. Personality traits must be distinguished from time-limited states; for example, a patient who exhibits dependent features solely while acutely depressed does not have a dependent personality. A personality disorder is diagnosed when personality trait repertoires lead to enduring (if variable) subjective distress or dysfunction in social role performances. The major personality disorders are listed in Table 117-4. Personality and personality disorders are the result of complex interactions among genetic, environmental, and developmental factors. Approaches to patients with personality disorders will vary greatly depending on the specific type, but in most clinical circumstances other than longer-term psychotherapy, the realistic goal is not to alter fundamental personality structure but to help the patient maximize use of personality strengths (e.g., optimal defense mechanisms) while minimizing the harmful effects of emotional dysregulation, unhelpful defenses, and destructive behaviors. Although not the mainstay of most treatments for personality disorders, pharmacotherapy can be useful in selected patients (e.g., antipsychotics to target escalating paranoia in paranoid personality disorder; mood stabilizers; or antidepressants to target emotional dysregulation in borderline personality disorder). As well, patients with personality disorders are prone to mood, anxiety, eating, substance use, and other treatable psychiatric disorders.

Prospectus for the Future

Advances in neuroscience will lead to better pharmacologic or other somatic therapies. One example, deep brain stimulation, is currently under study for severe refractory mood and anxiety disorders. In the future, specifically tailored regimens for each individual may be based on genetic, pharmacogenomic, or proteomic profiles. These same advances may help identify patients for whom evidence-based psychotherapies or other psychosocial interventions are most likely to be effective. Identification of more specific and powerful risk markers may lead to the development of preventive interventions for at-risk individuals or groups. The current U.S. health care system, however, provides both barriers and disincentives that often prevent implementation of mental health treatments.

References

American Psychiatric Association: Diagnostic and Statistical Manual of Mental Disorders, 4th ed. Washington, DC, American Psychiatric Association, 1994.

Belmaker RH, Agam G: Major depressive disorder. N Engl J Med 358:55, 2008.

Freedman R: Schizophrenia. N Engl J Med 349:1738, 2003.

Sadock BJ, Sadock VA: Kaplan and Sadock's Comprehensive Textbook of Psychiatry, 8th ed. Philadelphia, Lippincott Williams & Wilkins, 2004.

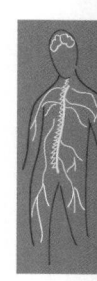

Disorders of Thermal Regulation

William P. Cheshire, Jr.

Core body temperature is tightly regulated to within half of one degree from its set point near 37° C (98.6° F). Serious and potentially fatal organ dysfunction ensues when temperatures depart from that range by more than a few degrees.

Hypothermia

Hypothermia is defined as a core body temperature <35° C (95° F) and may be therapeutic (induced for neuroprotective or cardioprotective purposes) or accidental. Prolonged environmental cold exposure leads to life-threatening hypothermia, particularly under conditions of impaired thermoregulation. At increased risk are neonates and elderly adults, whose ability to vasoconstrict and shiver is diminished; injured winter wilderness explorers; and the homeless, whose mobility is restricted. Water contact accelerates heat loss. Additional causes (Table 118-1) include drugs that depress the sensorium (alcohol abuse and sedative overdose), disorders that impair the anterior hypothalamus (Wernicke encephalopathy), and conditions that decrease the sympathetic thermoregulatory and shivering responses (hypoglycemia, hypothyroidism).

Initial signs of hypothermia consist of shivering, increased muscle tone, impaired judgment, slurred speech, and incoordination. With further temperature reduction, shivering ceases and hypometabolism leads to lethargy, stupor, and multisystem complications (Table 118-2). Atrial arrhythmias occur with moderate hypothermia, and ventricular arrhythmias with severe hypothermia. Even mild hypothermia can provoke cardiac arrhythmias in those with underlying cardiovascular disease. Severe cases can mimic death, as the skin is cold to the touch, the pupils dilate, and the pulse, respirations, and blood pressure may be barely detectable. For this reason, determination of death requires a core temperature <32.2° C (90° F). Hypothermic neurologic abnormalities are reversible with rewarming.

Treatment should be initiated promptly, beginning with passive external warming (blankets, reflective metalo-plastic sheets, heating lamps) for mild hypothermia. For moderate hypothermia, active surface (heated blankets, hot air circulators, hot tubs) and core warming methods (heated hemodialysis, hemodiafiltration, or peritoneal lavage) are recommended. Severe hypothermia with cardiac arrest may require cardiopulmonary bypass. Hypothermic patients are hypovolemic and require intravenous hydration.

Hyperthermia

Hyperthermia is defined as a core body temperature >40.5° C (105° F). It results from uncompensated body warming with or without exertion and manifests as heat exhaustion or heat stroke. The cause may be environmental, pharmacologic, metabolic, or neurologic. Unlike fever, which elevates the hypothalamic set point, hyperthermia does not subside when treated with cyclo-oxygenase inhibitors.

Heat exhaustion or heat stroke can occur during strenuous exertion in hot and/or humid climates, often occurring to healthy young athletes or military recruits. Lightheadedness, fatigue, and weakness can progress to confusion and coma as body temperature rapidly rises. Flushing and tachycardia are present. Profuse sweating in heat exhaustion may be followed by loss of sweating in heat stroke (Table 118-3). Predisposing factors include deficient thermoregulatory sweating (e.g., Ross syndrome, Sjögren syndrome, after bilateral sympathectomy). Also at risk are older adults during summer heat waves, particularly those unable to dissipate heat generated at rest because of drugs that inhibit sweating (tricyclic antidepressants, antihistamines, neuroleptics and other M3 anticholinergics; carbonic anhydrase inhibitors such as topiramate and zonisamide). Some drugs may cause hyperthermia via idiosyncratic reactions (drug fever), central dopamine antagonism (neuroleptic malignant syndrome), or dysregulation of skeletal muscle calcium transport in genetically susceptible patients given volatile anesthetic agents or succinylcholine (malignant hyperthermia). Drugs that enhance serotonin neurotransmission (serotonin syndrome) or sympathetic outflow

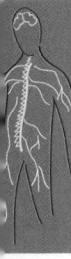

(psychomotor stimulant abuse) may also cause hyperthermia. Hyperthermia can complicate status epilepticus.

Neuroleptic malignant syndrome is a hypermetabolic state occurring in 0.2% of patients taking dopamine 2 receptor antagonists (e.g., haloperidol). CYP2D6 polymorphisms may determine vulnerability. Onset is over hours to days. Hyperthermia, rigidity, profuse sweating, tachycardia, labile blood pressure, delirium, tremors, dysphagia, and dysarthria can progress to coma. Creatine kinase is elevated. Treatment consists of reversing dopamine blockade by removing the offending drug. Although not FDA-approved for this purpose, effective treatment has been described using bromocriptine (2.5 to 10 mg three times daily) or, in severe cases, dantrolene (1 to 2.5 mg/kg intravenously [IV] every 6 hours until muscular relaxation occurs, followed by 4 to 8 mg/kg every 6 hours for 24 to 48 hours).

Malignant hyperthermia is an autosomal dominantly inherited syndrome in which exposure to volatile anesthetic agents (e.g., halothane) or succinylcholine provokes hyperthermia and muscle rigidity involving the limbs, trunk, and masseter muscles. The most frequent causal mutations involve the *RYR1* gene on chromosome 19q13.1. Onset is usually within 30 minutes but can be delayed by hours. Treatment consists of drug discontinuation and dantrolene (as described earlier).

Serotonin syndrome is a dose-related syndrome that occurs in patients taking serotonin-selective reuptake inhibitors (e.g., fluoxetine, sertraline) multiply or in combination with other medications (e.g., monoamine oxidase inhibitors, meperidine, tramadol, fentanyl) that enhance the availability of serotonin in the brain. Onset is within hours. Initial signs of agitation, tremor, and hyperreflexia can progress to hyperthermia, rigidity, sweating, and muscle and eye twitching. The offending drug should be promptly withdrawn.

Recreational abuse of psychomotor stimulants such as cocaine, amphetamine, 3,4-methylenedioxymethamphetamine (MDMA or "ecstasy"), and heroin can cause heat stroke via pathologic brain warming combined with peripheral vasoconstriction. Onset is within 1 hour. Chest pain, dilated pupils, or seizures can occur.

Hyperthermia in each of these conditions is a medical emergency, and rapid reduction of core temperature is mandatory. Evaporative cooling (tepid water sponging with fans) or cooling blankets are preferred for lowering core temperature to 38° to 39° C. Cold water immersion has occasionally been used for heat stroke. Benzodiazepines are useful to inhibit shivering.

Table 118-1 Causes of Hypothermia*

Alcohol abuse	43%
Wernicke encephalopathy	18%
Age >70	26%
Sepsis or shock	25%
Exposure without other causes	14%
Hypoglycemia	12%
Sedative overdose	10%
Hepatic encephalopathy, uremia	8%
Structural brain disorder, head trauma, hypothyroidism, diabetic ketoacidosis, renal failure, ethylene glycol poisoning	<5%

*N = 148: more than one factor occurred in 35 patients.
Data from Fischbeck KH, Simon RP: Neurological manifestations of accidental hypothermia. Ann Neurol 10:384-387, 1981.

Table 118-2 Effects of Hypothermia

	Mild (90°-95° F; 32°-35° C)	Moderate (82°-90° F; 28°-32° C)	Severe (<82° F; <28° C)
Cardiovascular	Tachycardia, increased blood pressure, PR and QT interval prolongation	Atrial fibrillation	Bradycardia, hypotension, ventricular arrhythmias, asystole at <20° C
Respiratory	Tachypnea	Hypopnea	Pulmonary edema, apnea at <24° C
Muscular	Shivering	Loss of shivering	Hypotonia
Neurologic	Impaired judgment, dysarthria, ataxia	Progressive lethargy, hallucinations, sluggish pupils	Stupor or coma, areflexia, dilated pupils, electroencephalographic silence at <26° C
Renal	Diuresis		Oliguria
Hematologic	Hemoconcentration, coagulopathy		
Gastrointestinal	Ileus, gastric stress ulcer, pancreatitis, hepatic dysfunction		
Metabolic	Declines by 5% for each 1° C		

Table 118-3 Effects of Hyperthermia

	Heat Stress (>100° F; >38° C)	Heat Exhaustion (>102° F; >39° C)	Heat Stroke (>104° F; >40° C)
Skin	Sweating, flushing	Profuse sweating, flushing	Anhidrosis,* flushing
Neurologic	Fatigue, postural syncope	Weakness, muscle cramps, paresthesia, headache, agitation, mild confusion	Encephalopathy, hallucinations, coma, seizures, focal deficits
Cardiovascular	Tachycardia	Tachycardia	Cardiac failure
Metabolic	Dehydration	Oliguria	Myoglobinuria, renal failure, acidosis, vomiting, coagulopathy

*Half of patients with heat stroke may sweat initially.

Prospectus for the Future

Accumulating evidence is showing that induction of mild hypothermia (32° to 35° C) improves neurologic outcome after cardiac arrest or anoxic brain injury. Perfection of this technique in the neurocritical care setting will broaden the clinical understanding of the relationship between brain function and temperature.

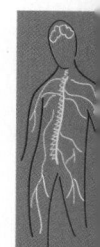

References

Cheshire WP, Fealey RD: Drug-induced hyperhidrosis and hypohidrosis: incidence, prevention and management. Drug Saf 31:109-126, 2008.

Cheshire WP, Low PA: Disorders of sweating and thermoregulation. Continuum Lifelong Learn Neurol 13:143-164, 2007.

Connolly E, Worthley LI: Induced and accidental hypothermia. Crit Care Resusc 2:22-29, 2000.

Kempainen RR, Brunette DD: The evaluation and management of accidental hypothermia. Respir Care 49:192-205, 2004.

Polderman KH: Induced hypothermia and fever control for prevention and treatment of neurological injuries. Lancet 371:1955-1969, 2008.

Smith JE: Cooling methods used in the treatment of exertional heat illness. Br J Sports Med 39:503-507, 2005.

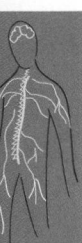

Headache, Neck Pain, and Other Painful Disorders

Timothy J. Counihan

Headache

PAIN-SENSITIVE INTRACRANIAL STRUCTURES

Headache is caused by irritation of pain-sensitive intracranial structures, including the dural sinuses; the intracranial portions of the trigeminal, glossopharyngeal, vagus, and upper cervical nerves; the large arteries; and the venous sinuses. Many structures are insensitive to pain, including the brain parenchyma, the ependymal lining of the ventricles, and the choroid plexuses. That the brain parenchyma itself is insensitive to pain accounts for the common clinical observation of patients who have large intracerebral lesions (such as intracerebral hematomas or malignant brain tumors) but little or no headache. Painful stimuli arising from brain tissue above the tentorium cerebelli are conveyed by means of the trigeminal nerve, whereas the glossopharyngeal, vagus, and first two cervical nerves convey impulses from the posterior fossa. The term "cervicogenic" headache is sometimes used to indicate that the source of headache (usually occipital in location) arises from an abnormality in the cervical spine.

EVALUATION OF THE PATIENT WITH HEADACHE

It is important to distinguish benign from ominous causes of headache. A detailed history (the quality, location, duration, and time course of the headache) helps in determination of which patients have a symptomatic structural intracranial lesion (Table 119-1). What exacerbates or relieves it? Pain intensity is not of much diagnostic value, except for the patient who complains of the acute onset of the worst headache of his or her life. This headache suggests subarachnoid hemorrhage (SAH). The quality of pain ("throbbing," "pressure," "jabbing") and the location may also be helpful, especially if the pain is of extracranial origin, such as temporal in temporal arteritis. Posterior fossa lesions cause occipitocervical pain, occasionally associated with unilateral retro-orbital pain. In general, multifocal pain

usually implies a benign cause. It is most important to clarify the acuity of onset of the headache; patients who describe the onset of pain as "like being hit on the head with a bat" should be suspected of having the sentinel headache of subarachnoid headache. Equally important is to establish the time course of the headache. Is this paroxysmal, nonprogressive headache (typical of migraine or tension-type headache)? Or is the headache daily persistent (such as in temporal arteritis) or progressive (suggesting the presence of a structural brain lesion)? Patients should be asked about any known triggers for the headache, such as menses, particular foods, caffeine, alcohol, or stress. Positional headache (headache that is maximal in the upright position and disappears rapidly on lying down) is characteristic of intracranial hypotension (low pressure headache). Diurnal variation in headache severity may give a clue to cause; morning headache or headache that awakens a patient from sleep may indicate raised intracranial pressure or sleep apnea as a cause. The presence of associated symptoms such as visual disturbances, nausea, or vomiting should be noted. The history should include inquiries about medications, especially use of analgesics and over-the-counter remedies. Information regarding the patient's past medical history as well as family history should also be taken into consideration. In the majority of patients with headache, the physical and neurologic examination findings are normal, although special attention may be directed toward examination of the eyes for papilledema, as well as the temporal arteries for a palpable nonpulsatile artery.

HEADACHE SYNDROMES

Headache is classified into primary and secondary headache syndromes (Table 119-2).

Migraine
Clinical Features
Migraine is an episodic headache disorder characterized by various combinations of neurologic, gastrointestinal, and autonomic changes. The diagnosis is based on the

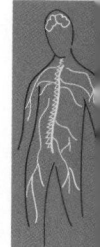

Table 119-1 Key Questions in the Assessment of Headache

1. For how long have you been having headaches?
2. What were they like when they first began? Were they intermittent, daily persistent, or progressive from the beginning?
3. What is the length of time from the start of the headache until its peak intensity?
4. Are there any warning symptoms (aura)?
5. Does the headache interfere significantly with normal activity (work, school, etc)?
6. What aggravates the headache (such as light, noise, odors)?
7. What do you do for relief from the headache (rest, move around, take medication)?
8. What time of day are the headaches most likely to occur? Do they regularly awaken you from sleep?
9. Are you aware of any specific triggers (foods, stress, lack of sleep, menstrual cycle)?
10. Does anyone else in the family have headaches?

Table 119-2 Classification of Headache Syndromes

Primary	Secondary
Migraine	Trauma
Tension-type	Stroke
Trigeminal autonomic cephalgias	Structural brain lesion
Other primary cephalgias	Substance use or withdrawal Infection Other secondary causes Skull and sinus disease

Table 119-3 Classification of Migraine

Migraine without aura (common migraine)
Migraine with aura (classic migraine)
Migraine variants
Hemiplegic migraine
Confusional migraine
Ophthalmoplegic migraine
Basilar migraine

of phosphenes that is characteristic of the migrainous aura. The pain of migraine is often pulsating, unilateral, and frontotemporal in distribution and often accompanied by anorexia, nausea, and, occasionally, vomiting. In characteristic attacks, patients are markedly intolerant of light (photophobia) and seek rest in a dark room. There may also be intolerance to sound (phonophobia) and occasionally to odors (osmophobia). The diagnosis of migraine requires the presence of at least one of these features, particularly in the absence of gastrointestinal symptoms. The presence of these symptoms results in a syndrome that is invariably disabling for the patient, to the extent that for the duration of the attack he or she is unable to function normally. In children, migraine is often associated with episodic abdominal pain, motion sickness, and sleep disturbances. Onset of typical migraine late in life (older than age 50) is rare, although recurrence of migraine that had been in remission is not uncommon. Recurrent migraine headache associated with transient hemiparesis or hemiplegia occurs rarely as a clearly genetically determined (Mendelian) disease (familial hemiplegic migraine).

Basilar migraine is unusual and occurs primarily in childhood. Severe episodic headache is preceded, or accompanied by, signs of bilateral occipital lobe, brainstem, or cerebellar dysfunction (e.g., diplopia, bilateral visual field abnormalities, ataxia, dysarthria, bilateral sensory or motor disturbances, other cranial nerve signs, and occasionally coma). *Vestibular migraine* or migrainous vertigo is characterized by symptoms of vertigo with or without the other typical migraine symptoms. The term *complicated migraine* refers to migraine attacks with major neurologic dysfunction (e.g., migraine with hemiplegia or coma) separate from the visual aura; in these cases, neurologic dysfunction outlasts the headache by hours to 1 or 2 days. Acute severe headache can reflect serious central nervous system disease (Table 119-4). Certain symptoms raise suspicion for a structural brain lesion (Table 119-5).

Causes

A migraine attack is the end result of the interaction of a number of factors of varying importance in different individuals. These factors include a genetic predisposition, a susceptibility of the central nervous system to certain stimuli, hormonal factors, and a sequence of neurovascular events. A positive family history is reported in 65% to 91% of cases. Familial hemiplegic migraine is associated with mutations in a gene for *P/Q* type calcium channel on chromosome 19 and a gene encoding a sodium-potassium ion pump on chromosome 1. Thus, mutations of diverse channels result in a common phenotype. The cause of migraine in the majority of patients remains uncertain.

headache's characteristics and associated symptoms. Results of the physical examination as well as the laboratory studies are usually normal.

The prevalence of migraine is up to 16% in women and 8% in men. It is estimated that 28 million Americans have disabling migraine headaches. All varieties of migraine may begin at any age from early childhood on, although peak ages at onset are adolescence and early adulthood.

Seven types of migraine are described (Table 119-3). The two most common are migraine without aura and migraine with aura; migraine without aura accounts for 80% of patients. Migraine auras are focal neurologic symptoms that precede, accompany, or, rarely, follow an attack. The aura usually develops over 5 to 20 minutes, lasts less than 60 minutes, and can involve visual, sensorimotor, language or brainstem disturbances. The most common aura is typified by positive visual phenomena (such as scintillating scotomata) that often precede the headache; they resemble the effect of being too close to a photographer with a flash camera *(phosphenes)*. The differential diagnosis of an aura includes a focal epileptic seizure arising from the visual cortex of the occipital lobe, or a transient ischemic attack (TIA). In the latter, there is no evolution of symptoms, and the symptoms themselves are typically "negative" (such as a hemianopia) rather than the "positive" visual phenomenon

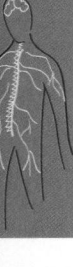

Table 119-4 Differential Diagnosis of Acute Headache—Major Causes

Migraine
Cluster headache
Stroke
   Subarachnoid hemorrhage
   Intracerebral hemorrhage
   Cerebral infarction
   Arterial dissection (carotid or vertebral)
Acute hydrocephalus
Meningitis or encephalitis
Giant cell arteritis (often chronic)
Tumor (usually chronic)
Trauma

Table 119-5 Clinical Features of Headaches Suggesting a Structural Brain Lesion

Symptoms

Worst of the patient's life
Progressive
Onset >50 years of age
Worse in early morning—awakens patient
Marked exacerbation with straining
Focal neurologic dysfunction

Signs

Nuchal rigidity
Fever
Papilledema
Pathologic reflexes or reflex asymmetry
Altered state of consciousness

The traditional view has been that the neurologic phenomena of migraine were caused by spasm of cerebral vessels and the pain was caused by subsequent dilation of extracranial arteries. There is good evidence that diminished cerebral blood flow accompanies the aura of the migraine attack. One of the key structures in the mechanism of pain in all migraine is the trigeminal vascular system. Stimulation of the trigeminal nerve or its ganglion can activate serotonin receptors and nerve endings on small dural arteries and result in a state of neurogenic inflammation. It is postulated that, in migraine, these processes in turn stimulate perivascular nerve endings, with resultant orthodromic stimulation of trigeminal nerve and pain referred to its *distribution*. The precise role of other factors such as female sex hormones, environmental triggers, and stress in the pathogenesis of migraine remains unclear.

Treatment

The goals of treatment are (1) making an accurate and confident diagnosis of migraine to reassure the patient that there is no more sinister cause for the headache; (2) relieving acute attacks; and (3) preventing pain and associated symptoms of recurrent headaches. The first step is to inform the patient that he or she has a migraine. The benign nature of the disorder and the patient's central role in the treatment plan should be emphasized. It is important that the patient keep a headache diary, which serves several functions: it helps identify covert headache triggers; it assists in monitoring headache frequency and response to treatment, and it actively involves the patient in the management of the condition.

Acute Migraine Attack

Acute attacks are alleviated with single agents or varying combinations of drugs (Fig. 119-1) as well as with behavioral modification therapy. Many attacks of migraine respond to simple analgesics, such as acetaminophen, aspirin, or nonsteroidal anti-inflammatory agents. Opioid drugs have a limited use in the migraine attack. Overuse of analgesics is particularly frequent in headache patients; one of the most important aspects of therapy of migraine patients, therefore, is the monitoring of amounts of analgesic used. In patients who are nauseated, it is often helpful to prescribe an antiemetic agent early in an attack. Phenothiazine drugs have antiemetic, prokinetic, and useful sedative properties, but they can produce involuntary movements as an acute adverse effect (acute dystonic reaction).

A number of *migraine-specific* serotonin agonist drugs have become available These agents, commonly referred to as "triptans," are useful in the acute treatment of migraine, having a rapid onset of action; sumatriptan, available as a subcutaneous preparation, results in a headache response rate of close to 70% (see Fig. 119-1). Although many are highly effective in alleviating migraine, patients must be carefully instructed in their appropriate use. Moreover, a response to these medications does not confirm a diagnosis of migraine.

Migraine Prevention

A number of agents have been used in the prevention of migraine (Table 119-6). The use of these agents should be restricted to patients who have frequent attacks (usually more than four per month) and who are willing to take daily medication. With any of the medications, an adequate trial period should be given, using adequate doses, before it is declared ineffective. Combination therapy is occasionally required but is not routinely prescribed. For a preventative drug to be considered successful, it should reduce the headache frequency rate by 50%. Magnesium supplementation, the plant extract feverfew, and high-dose riboflavin (vitamin B_2) have been effective in some patients.

The Future of Migraine Treatment

Given the increasing experimental evidence that neurogenic inflammation is the principal cause of migraine pain, there has been a predictable increase in the use of anticonvulsant medication (see Table 119-6) for prevention. Clinical trials using an antagonist to calcitonin gene–related peptide (CGRP) have shown some efficacy for the treatment of acute migraine.

Cluster Headache

Clinical Features

Cluster headache is the prototypic trigeminal autonomic cephalgia, consisting of a group of symptoms with a relatively specific temporal course. It is uncommon, occurring in less than 10% of all people with headache. Unlike migraine, it is much more common in men than in women, and its mean age at onset is later in life than migraine. Also, unlike migraine, cluster headache rarely begins in childhood,

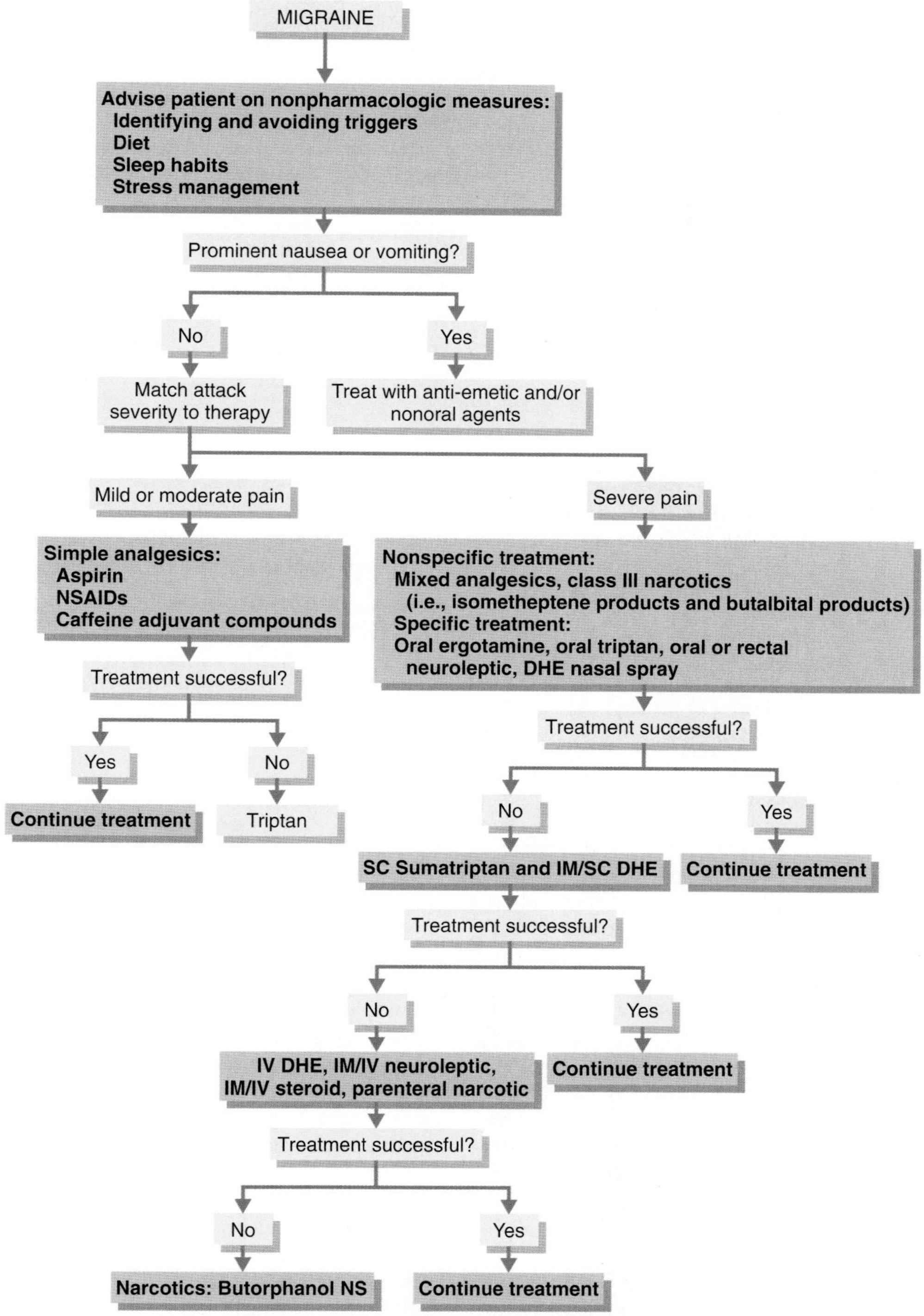

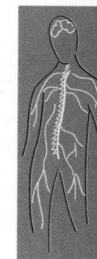

```
                        ┌──────────────┐
                        │   MIGRAINE   │
                        └──────┬───────┘
                               ↓
┌─────────────────────────────────────────────────────┐
│ Advise patient on nonpharmacologic measures:         │
│   Identifying and avoiding triggers                  │
│   Diet                                               │
│   Sleep habits                                       │
│   Stress management                                  │
└─────────────────────────┬───────────────────────────┘
                          ↓
              ┌──────────────────────────┐
              │ Prominent nausea or       │
              │ vomiting?                 │
              └───────┬──────────┬────────┘
                   No ↓          ↓ Yes
          ┌────────────────┐  ┌──────────────────────┐
          │ Match attack   │  │ Treat with anti-emetic│
          │ severity to    │  │ and/or nonoral agents │
          │ therapy        │  └──────────────────────┘
          └───┬────────┬───┘
              │        │
   ┌──────────────────┐  ┌────────────┐
   │ Mild or moderate │  │ Severe pain│
   │ pain             │  └────────────┘
   └──────────────────┘
```

Mild or moderate pain

Simple analgesics:
  Aspirin
  NSAIDs
  Caffeine adjuvant compounds

Treatment successful?
  Yes → **Continue treatment**
  No → Triptan

Severe pain

Nonspecific treatment:
  Mixed analgesics, class III narcotics
   (i.e., isometheptene products and butalbital products)
Specific treatment:
  Oral ergotamine, oral triptan, oral or rectal
   neuroleptic, DHE nasal spray

Treatment successful?
  No → **SC Sumatriptan and IM/SC DHE**
  Yes → **Continue treatment**

Treatment successful?
  No → **IV DHE, IM/IV neuroleptic, IM/IV steroid, parenteral narcotic**
  Yes → **Continue treatment**

Treatment successful?
  No → **Narcotics: Butorphanol NS**
  Yes → **Continue treatment**

Figure 119-1 Algorithm for the treatment of migraine. DHE, dihydroergotamine; IM, intramuscular; IV, intravenous; NS, normal saline; NSAIDs, nonsteroidal anti-inflammatory drugs; SC, subcutaneous. (From Silberstein SD, Young WB, Lipton RB: Migraine and cluster headaches. In Johnson RT, Griffin JW [eds]: Current Therapy in Neurologic Disease, 5th ed. St Louis, Mosby, 1997, p 88).

and there is less often a family history. The pain in cluster headache is of extreme intensity, is unilateral, and is associated with congestion of the nasal mucosa and injection of the conjunctiva on the side of the pain. Increased sweating of the ipsilateral side of the forehead and face may occur. There may be associated ocular signs of Horner syndrome: miosis, ptosis, and the additional feature of eyelid edema. The pain is usually steady, nonthrobbing, and invariably localized retro-orbitally on one side of the head; it may occasionally spread to the ipsilateral side of the face or neck. Attacks often awaken patients, usually 2 to 3 hours after the onset of sleep ("alarm-clock headache"). In contrast to migraineurs, the pain is not relieved by resting in a dark, quiet area; on the contrary, patients sometimes seek some activity that can distract them. The duration of headache is usually around 1 hour, although it may recur several times in a day, recurring paroxysmally (in *clusters*) for several weeks.

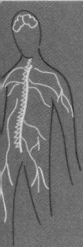

Table 119-6 Preventive Therapy for Migraine

Drug Class	Agent	Dose	Adverse Effects
β-adrenergic receptor blockers	Propranolol Nadolol	40-160 mg/day 40-160 mg/day	Contraindicated in asthma; nightmares, fatigue, syncope
Tricyclic antidepressants	Amitriptyline	10-75 mg qhs	Dry mouth, confusion, palpitations
Serotonin reuptake inhibitors	Paroxetine Sertraline	10-50 mg/day 50-200 mg/day	Insomnia, somnolence, sexual dysfunction
Calcium-channel blockers	Verapamil Flunarizine*	120-900 mg/day 5 mg/day	Constipation, edema, hypotension Parkinsonism
Serotonin antagonists	Methysergide Pizotifen*	2-8 mg/day 0.5-1.5 mg/day	Prolonged use associated with fibrotic reactions
Anticonvulsants	Divalproex sodium Gabapentin Topiramate	500-1000 mg/day 300-900 mg/day 50-200 mg/day	Weight gain, tremor Somnolence Renal calculi

*Not licensed in United States.

Table 119-7 Clinical Features Distinguishing Migraine from Tension Headache

	Migraine with Aura	Migraine without Aura	Tension Headache
Aura	Focal neurologic deficit (visual, sensory, language) Onset over 4 min Lasts <60 min	No focal neurologic deficit	No focal neurologic deficit
Headache	Unilateral Throbbing or pulsating Aggravated by activity Inhibits or prohibits activity Onset within 60 min of aura	Unilateral Throbbing or pulsating Aggravated by activity Inhibits or prohibits activity	Bilateral Nonpulsating ("pressure") Not aggravated by activity May inhibit but not prohibit activity
Associated symptoms	Nausea ± vomiting Photophobia Phonophobia	Nausea ± vomiting Photophobia Phonophobia	No nausea or vomiting Minimal photophobia

These periods of frequent headaches are separated by headache-free periods of varying duration, often several months or years. Attacks have a striking tendency to be precipitated by even small amounts of alcohol. There are rare variants of cluster headache: a "chronic variety" in which remissions are brief (less than 14 days); *"chronic paroxysmal hemicrania,"* in which attacks are shorter and strikingly more prevalent in women; and *"hemicrania continua,"* in which there is continuous, moderately severe, unilateral headache. The cause of all these syndromes is unknown, although the distribution of the pain suggests dysfunction of the trigeminal nerve.

Treatment
Therapy for cluster headache may be abortive for acute headache or prophylactic to prevent headache. Acute headache may respond to oxygen by mask (7 to 10 L/min for 15 minutes), which is effective within several minutes in 70% of patients. Sumatriptan and dihydroergotamine are also effective. Preventive medications include lithium, divalproex sodium, verapamil, methysergide, and corticosteroids. Paroxysmal hemicrania and related syndromes are often strikingly sensitive to indomethacin.

Tension-Type Headache
In contrast to migraine, tension-type headache is featureless (Table 119-7). The pain is usually not throbbing but rather steady and often described as a "pressure feeling" or a "vise-like" sensation. It is usually not unilateral and may be frontal,

occipital, or generalized. There is frequently pain in the neck area, unlike in migraine. Pain commonly lasts for long periods of time (e.g., days) and does not rapidly appear and disappear in attacks. There is no "aura." Photophobia and phonophobia are usually absent (see Table 119-2). Although tension-type headache may be related by the patient to occur or be exacerbated at times of particular emotional stress, the pathophysiology may relate to sustained craniocervical muscle contraction; hence, a more appropriate term for this syndrome is *muscle-contraction headache.*

A careful evaluation should be made of the patient's psychosocial milieu and the presence of anxiety or depression. The tricyclic antidepressant drugs in low doses have proven the most useful for prevention of tension-type headache; although the best documented is amitriptyline, newer agents with fewer side effects may be equally effective. Nonpharmacologic therapies such as relaxation therapy, massage, physiotherapy, or acupuncture may be useful in refractory cases. Intramuscular botulinum toxin injections have been used both in migraine and tension-type headache but are not of established benefit.

Other Defined Primary Headache Syndromes
Several acute short-lasting headache syndromes need to be differentiated from migraine, cluster, or tension headache. These include "thunderclap" headache, *primary stabbing headache, primary exertional headache,* "ice cream" headache, and coital headache. The latter may be indistinguish-

able from the headache of SAH and requires computed tomography (CT) and lumbar puncture to exclude SAH. All of these headache syndromes are more common in migraineurs. Two additional rare short-lasting headache syndromes deserve mention: short-lasting unilateral neuralgiform headache with conjunctival tearing (SUNCT); and *hypnic* headache. The latter refers to multiple episodes of very brief headache that awaken the patient (typically an older woman) from sleep. The syndrome of SUNCT causes multiple very brief (seconds to minutes) episodes of cluster-like headache and autonomic disturbance.

Chronic daily headache is defined arbitrarily as headache lasting for more than 4 hours on more than 15 days in the month for more than 3 months. In clinical practice this means that the patient has a headache more often than not. In these cases it is important to establish whether the headache syndrome began as an episodic disorder (as in migraine or tension-type headache) or whether it consists of new daily persistent headaches.

New Daily Persistent Headache

New daily persistent headache needs to be distinguished from both tension-type and migraine headaches that have transformed into chronic daily headache; new daily persistent headaches need investigation to exclude a secondary cause.

Headache may be a manifestation of underlying structural brain disease (Table 119-8). Headache can be seen in all forms of cerebrovascular disease: infarction, TIAs, and intracerebral hemorrhage and SAH. The headache in SAH is usually extremely severe and often described by the patient as "the worst headache of my life." Nuchal rigidity, third nerve palsy (usually involving the pupil), and retinal, pre-retinal, or subconjunctival hemorrhages may be found. CT

of the head usually shows subarachnoid, intraventricular, or other intracranial blood.

The patient with headache and fever presents a common diagnostic problem in the emergency department. Neck stiffness is a common symptom. Meningismus is confirmed by eliciting Brudzinski and Kernig signs. Vomiting occurs in about 50% of patients. Suspicion for meningitis should prompt further investigation, including a lumbar puncture. If the patient shows focal signs, papilledema, or profound alteration in level of consciousness, CT of the head before lumbar puncture is required to rule out focal disease such as an abscess or subdural empyema. These lesions, however, are rare.

Acute Sinusitis

Head and face pain is the most prominent feature of sinusitis. Malaise and low-grade fever are usually present. The pain is dull, aching, and nonpulsatile; is exacerbated by movement, coughing, or straining; and is improved with nasal decongestants. The pain is most pronounced on awakening or after any prolonged recumbency and is diminished with maintenance of an upright posture.

The location of the pain depends on the sinus involved. Maxillary sinusitis provokes ipsilateral malar, ear, and dental pain with significant overlying facial tenderness. Frontal sinusitis produces frontal headache that may radiate behind the eyes and to the vertex of the skull. Tenderness to frontal palpation may be present with point tenderness on the undersurface of the medial aspect of the superior orbital rim. In ethmoidal sinusitis, the pain is between or behind the eyes with radiation to the temporal area. The eyes and orbit are often tender to palpation, and, in fact, eye movements themselves may accentuate the pain. Sphenoidal sinusitis causes pain in the orbit and at the vertex of the skull and occasionally in the frontal or occipital regions. Given that the trigeminal nerve mediates pain perception from the sinuses, many patients who complain of "sinus headaches" are probably suffering from the trigeminovascular disturbance of migraine, rather than sinusitis. Chronic sinusitis is seldom a cause of headache.

Brain Tumors

Posterior fossa tumors (particularly of the cerebellum) frequently produce headache, especially if hydrocephalus occurs because cerebrospinal fluid (CSF) flow is partially obstructed. Supratentorial tumors, however, are less likely to cause headache and are more frequently heralded by altered mental status, focal deficits, or seizures. Although increased intracranial pressure is often associated with headache, it is usually not the primary mechanism, because uniform pressure elevations do not usually produce distortions of pain-sensitive structures.

Idiopathic Intracranial Hypertension

Idiopathic intracranial hypertension (IIH), also called *benign intracranial hypertension,* is defined as a syndrome of elevated intracranial pressure without evidence of focal lesions, hydrocephalus, or frank brain edema. It occurs usually between the ages of 15 and 45 and is more frequent in obese women. The disorder is characterized by headache with features of raised intracranial pressure. The headache is usually insidious in onset, is typically generalized, is relatively mild

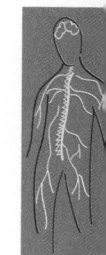

Table 119-8 **Headache Secondary to Underlying Brain Disease**
Cerebrovascular Disease
Ischemic stroke
Intracerebral hemorrhage
Subarachnoid hemorrhage
Inflammatory Disease
Cranial arteritis
Isolated central nervous system vasculitis
Tolosa-Hunt syndrome
Systemic lupus erythematosus
Infectious Disease
Meningitis
Abscess
Encephalitis
Sinusitis
Post-Traumatic Disorder
Subdural hematoma
Empyema
Neoplastic Disease
Malignant brain tumor
Benign brain tumor
Metastasis
Other
Idiopathic intracranial hypertension

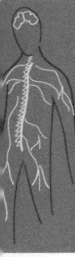

in severity, and is often worse in the morning or after exertion (e.g., straining or coughing).

At times, patients have visual disturbances, such as restricted peripheral visual fields, enlarged blind spots, slight visual blurring, or diplopia secondary to abducens nerve palsies. Funduscopic examination shows papilledema, which is often more impressive than the clinical picture. IIH is usually a benign and self-limited disorder, but it may lead to visual loss, including blindness.

The condition has been associated with drugs—vitamin A intoxication, nalidixic acid, danazol (Danocrine), and isotretinoin (Accutane)—as well as corticosteroid withdrawal and systemic disorders such as hypoparathyroidism and lupus.

CT scans are usually normal but can show small ventricles and an "empty sella" in some cases. CSF opening pressure is elevated, usually in the range of 250 to 450 mm of water, with the pressure fluctuating markedly when monitoring occurs over a prolonged period. There is increasing evidence that some cases of IIH are caused by cerebral venous sinus occlusion. These cases can occur in hypercoagulable states, including peripartum, in association with the combined oral contraceptive pill, and in association with antiphospholipid antibody syndrome.

Treatment

After secondary causes of IIH have been eliminated, the patient should have dietary counseling for weight loss. Carbonic anhydrase inhibitors (acetazolamide) and corticosteroids have proved useful in headache control. As a second-line agent, furosemide also acts to lower CSF production. Serial lumbar punctures are understandably unpopular with patients even though transient headache relief is obtained. CSF shunting procedures (ventriculoperitoneal shunt) are occasionally necessary. For patients with progressive visual loss, optic nerve sheath fenestration has been shown to preserve or restore vision in 80% to 90% and provide headache relief in a majority. Intracranial hypotension (usually secondary to a CSF leak after trauma or lumbar puncture) may also cause headache, exacerbated by standing.

Idiopathic Intracranial Hypotension

Also known as *low pressure headache*, idiopathic intracranial hypotension is commonly encountered as a sequela of lumbar puncture, resulting from leakage of CSF through the dural sac. Low pressure headaches may also occur spontaneously as a result of rupture of subarachnoid cysts. The headache is initially characteristically positional, being severe on standing but relieved rapidly on lying down. Occasionally the headache is associated with focal or "false localizing" signs, especially abducens nerve palsies.

Post-Traumatic Headache

Headache in individuals who have experienced trauma has no specific quality and is associated with irritability, concentration impairment, insomnia, memory disturbance, and light-headedness. Anxiety and depression are present to variable degrees. Multiple treatment options are available, and amitriptyline and nonsteroidal anti-inflammatory agents are useful. Occasionally, muscle relaxants and anxiolytics are beneficial.

Giant Cell Arteritis

Headache occurs in 60% of patients with giant cell arteritis, a granulomatous vasculitis of medium and large arteries. More than 95% of patients are 50 years of age or older. Malaise, fever, weight loss, and jaw claudication occur early, in addition to headache. Polymyalgia rheumatica, a syndrome of painful stiffness of the neck, shoulders, and pelvis, is found in half the patients. Visual impairment secondary to ischemic optic neuritis may occur. The headache is usually described as aching and is exacerbated at night and after exposure to cold. The superficial temporal artery is frequently swollen and very tender, and may be pulseless. The erythrocyte sedimentation rate is usually elevated; the mean is 100 mm/hr. Anemia is frequently present. Temporal artery biopsy usually confirms the diagnosis, but, because the arteritis is segmental, large or multiple sections may be required. Prednisone therapy is often dramatically effective and must be given promptly to preserve vision on the affected side.

HEADACHE ASSESSMENT IN THE EMERGENCY ROOM

Assessment of the patient with acute nontraumatic headache in the emergency room can be challenging; it is essential to establish how the headache evolved. Acute-onset severe headache should prompt investigation to exclude SAH, intracranial hemorrhage, acute obstructive hydrocephalus, and meningitis. Appropriate initial investigations should include brain imaging with CT or magnetic resonance imaging (MRI). Patients with suspected meningitis without focal neurologic signs or impaired consciousness should not have their lumbar puncture delayed unnecessarily before imaging. All patients should have standard blood tests including blood cultures if bacterial meningitis is suspected.

HEADACHE IN SYSTEMIC DISEASE

A wide variety of systemic diseases have headache as a prominent symptom; some of the more prevalent disorders are summarized in Table 119-9.

Table 119-9 **Headache Secondary to Systemic Disease**
Endocrine or Metabolic
Malignant hypertension (e.g., pheochromocytoma)
Acromegaly
Cushing disease
Carcinoid
Hyperparathyroidism
Paget disease
Pulmonary
Hypercapnea
Sleep apnea
Pharmacologic
Alcohol
Nitrates
Caffeine withdrawal
Analgesic withdrawal ("rebound") headache
Others: dipyridamole, cyclosporine, tacrolimus, calcium channel antagonists

Cranial Neuralgias

Neuralgias are differentiated from other head pains by the brevity of the attacks (usually 1 to 2 seconds or less) and by the distribution of the pain.

Trigeminal Neuralgia

In trigeminal neuralgia (tic douloureux), stabbing, spasmodic pain occurs unilaterally in one of the divisions of the trigeminal nerve. It lasts seconds, but it may occur many times a day for weeks at a time. It is characteristically induced by even the lightest touch to particular areas of the face, such as the lips or gums. Trigeminal neuralgia is the most frequent neuralgia of the elderly and is thought to be caused by compression of the trigeminal nerve root in the pons by an aberrant arterial loop. A very small minority of cases are caused by multiple sclerosis, cerebellopontine angle tumors, aneurysms, or arteriovenous malformations, although in these cases (unlike "true" trigeminal neuralgia) there are usually objective signs of neurologic deficit, such as areas of diminished sensation. In these cases of "symptomatic" neuralgia, the pain is often atypical. MRI is indicated in patients who have sensory loss, those who are under 40, and those with bilateral or atypical symptoms. Trigeminal neuralgia may be life threatening when it interferes with eating. Neuralgic pain is often responsive to treatment with standard doses of an anticonvulsant such as phenytoin, carbamazepine, gabapentin, pregabalin, and, occasionally, baclofen. Antidepressant drugs such as amitriptyline and, more recently, duloxetine may also be useful in this setting. Combination therapy including an antidepressant, anticonvulsant, and opiate analgesic has been shown to have synergistic effects.

If medical treatments are unsuccessful, a variety of surgical procedures are used, including microvascular decompression and radiofrequency lesioning of the sensory portion of the trigeminal nerve.

Glossopharyngeal Neuralgia

Glossopharyngeal neuralgia is much less common than trigeminal neuralgia. Brief paroxysms of severe, stabbing, unilateral pain radiate from the throat to the ear or vice versa and are frequently initiated by stimulation of specific "trigger zones" (e.g., tonsillar fossa or pharyngeal wall). Swallowing often provokes an attack; yawning, talking, and coughing are other potential triggers. Microvascular decompression is necessary if medical treatment is ineffective.

Postherpetic Neuralgia

Herpes zoster produces head pain by cranial nerve involvement in one third of cases. In some cases a persistent intense burning pain follows the initial acute illness. The discomfort may subside after several weeks or persist (particularly in the elderly) for months or years. The pain is localized over the distribution of the affected nerve and associated with exquisite tenderness to even the lightest touch. The first division of the trigeminal nerve is the most frequent cranial nerve involved (ophthalmic herpes) and is occasionally associated with keratoconjunctivitis. When the seventh nerve is affected ("geniculate herpes"), the pain involves the external auditory meatus and pinna. Occasionally, concomitant facial paralysis may occur (Ramsay Hunt syndrome).

Occipital Neuralgia

Occipital neuralgia is a syndrome that includes occipital pain starting at the base of the skull and often provoked by neck extension. Physical examination shows tenderness in the region of the occipital nerves and altered sensation in the C2 dermatome. Treatment includes the use of a soft collar, muscle relaxants, physical therapy, and local injections of analgesics and anti-inflammatory agents.

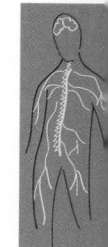

Complex Regional Pain Syndrome

Complex regional pain syndrome (CRPS), formerly known as *reflex sympathetic dystrophy*, is a syndrome that consists of pain and hyperesthesia and autonomic changes. Almost any type of injury can lead to CRPS, including blunt trauma, lacerations, and burns. Patients often suffer from coexisting emotional disturbances, which may contribute to as well as result from the pain.

Neck and Back Pain

Most patients with acute neck or back pain have a musculoskeletal disorder that is self-limiting and does not require specific therapy. The pain may originate from a number of sources, including the vertebrae and intervertebral disks, facet joints, and muscles and ligaments of the vertebral column.

Because the thoracic spine is designed for rigidity rather than mobility, thoracic disk rupture is exceedingly rare. Acute-onset pain in the thoracic region may be a result of dissection of the aorta or anterior spinal artery thrombosis.

CERVICAL SPONDYLOSIS

Cervical spondylosis is a degenerative disorder of the cervical intervertebral disks leading to osteophyte formation and hypertrophy of adjacent facet joints and ligaments. In contrast to the lumbar spine, herniation of cervical intervertebral disks (nucleus pulposus) accounts for only 20% to 25% of cervical root irritation. Cervical spondylosis is probably the most common pathology seen in office practice of neurologists and is present radiographically in over 90% of the population older than 60. For unknown reasons, the degree of anatomic abnormality is not directly correlated with the clinical signs and symptoms. Clinical disease may represent a combination of normal, age-related, degenerative changes in the cervical spine and a congenital or developmental stenosis of the cervical canal; the process may be aggravated by trauma. It may manifest as a painful stiff neck, with or without symptoms or signs of cervical root irritation or spinal cord compression. Patients with root irritation (cervical radiculopathy) complain of pain and paresthesias radiating down the arm roughly in the dermatomal distribution of the affected nerve root. More typically, the pain radiates in a myotomal pattern, whereas numbness and paresthesias follow a dermatomal distribution. Discrete sensory loss is uncommon and certainly less prominent than symptoms (Table 119-10). For relief, patients often adopt a position

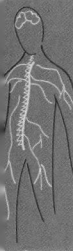

Table 119-10 Common Root Syndromes of Intervertebral Disk Disease

Disk Space	Root Affected	Muscles Affected	Distribution of Pain	Distribution of Sensory Symptoms	Reflex Affected
C4-5	C5	Deltoid, biceps	Medial scapula; shoulder	Shoulder	Biceps
C5-6	C6	Wrist extensors	Lateral forearm	Thumb; index finger	Triceps
C6-7	C7	Triceps	Medial scapula	Middle finger	Brachioradialis
C7-T1	C8	Hand intrinsics	Medial forearm	Fourth and fifth fingers	Finger flexion
L3-4	L4	Quadriceps	Anterior thigh	Across knee joint	Knee jerk
L4-5	L5	Peronei	Great toe, dorsum of foot	Great toe	
L5-S1	S1	Gastrocnemius, glutei	Calf	Lateral sole of foot	Ankle jerk

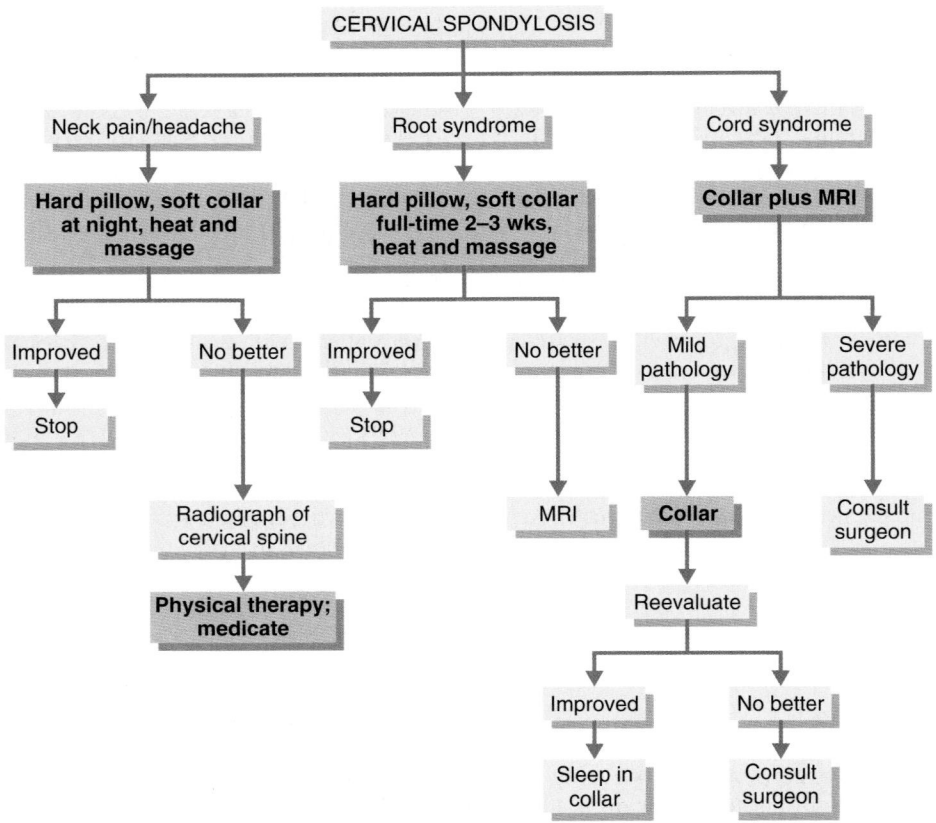

Figure 119-2 Algorithm for the treatment of cervical spondylosis. MRI, magnetic resonance imaging. (From Ronthal M, Rachlin JR: Cervical spondylosis. In Johnson RT, Griffin JW [eds]: Current Therapy in Neurologic Disease, 5th ed. St Louis, Mosby, 1997, p 77).

with the arm elevated and flexed behind the head. Pain is exacerbated by turning the head, ear down, to the side of the pain (Spurling maneuver). Objective neurologic findings may be limited to reflex asymmetry because weakness may be obscured by pain. Patients who have some degree of spinal cord compression demonstrate gait and bladder disturbances and evidence of spasticity on examination of the lower extremities. These patients require investigation with an imaging study, ideally MRI or CT myelography. Plain radiographs of the cervical spine add little information except in patients with rheumatoid arthritis in whom basilar invagination or atlantoaxial subluxation is suspected.

Cervical spondylosis is so common in the general population that it may be present coincidentally in a patient with another disease of the spinal cord. Among other diseases that may mimic cervical spondylosis are multiple sclerosis, amy-otrophic lateral sclerosis, and, rarely, subacute combined system disease (vitamin B_{12} deficiency). Conservative treatment includes the use of anti-inflammatory medication, cervical immobilization, and physical therapy for isometric strengthening of neck muscles once pain has subsided (Fig. 119-2). Surgery should be considered if there is progression of the neurologic deficit, especially the emergence of signs of cervical cord compression.

ACUTE LOW BACK PAIN

Low back pain without sciatica (radiating radicular pain) is common, with a reported point prevalence of up to 33%. Acute low back pain lasting several weeks is usually self-limiting, with a low risk for serious permanent disability. Risk factors for prolonged disability include psychological

Table 119-11	**Clinical Features of Low Back Pain Suggestive of Structural Pathology**

Vertebral Column Pathology

Pain maximal at rest or at night
Worsening pain over time
Constitutional symptoms
Focal vertebral tenderness
History of recent trauma
History of cancer (especially breast, bronchial, renal cell, prostate, myeloma)

Nerve Root Pathology

Radicular pain (sciatica)
Dermatomal sensory loss
Absent or asymmetrical reflexes
Positive result on straight leg raise test (S1 root compression)
Urinary or bowel incontinence
Perineal sensory loss } Cauda equina syndrome

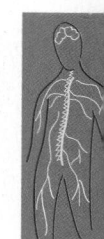

distress, compensation conflict over work-related injury, and other coexistent pain syndromes. The evaluation of patients with acute low back pain should center around distinguishing pain of mechanical origin from neurogenic pain caused by nerve root irritation (Table 119-11). The same pathologic changes that affect the cervical spine may also affect the lumbar spine. Because the spinal cord ends at the level of the first lumbar vertebra, lumbar canal stenosis from intervertebral disk disease and degenerative spondylosis will affect the roots of the cauda equina. The most common levels for lumbar degenerative disk disease are at L4 to L5 and L5 to S1, resulting in the common complaint of sciatica caused by irritation of the lower lumbar roots. Pain tends to improve with sitting or lying down, in contrast to the pain from spinal or vertebral tumors, which is aggravated by prolonged recumbency. Examination shows loss of the normal lumbar lordosis, paraspinal muscle spasm, and exacerbation of pain with straight leg raising, owing to stretching of the lower lumbar roots. About 10% of disk herniations occur lateral to the spinal canal, in which case the more rostral root is compressed. Percussion of the spine may cause focal tenderness of one of the vertebrae, suggesting bony infiltration by infection or tumor.

Spinal stenosis of the lumbar region may manifest as "neurogenic claudication," which is usually described as unilateral or bilateral buttock pain that is worse on standing or walking and relieved by rest or flexion at the waist. Patients may have pain that is worse when walking downhill, in contrast to patients with vascular claudication, whose pain is maximal when walking up an incline.

MRI in many patients with isolated low back pain shows nonspecific findings; MRI early in the course of an episode of low back pain does not improve clinical outcome. MRI should be performed in patients with back pain who have associated neurologic symptoms or signs, especially new onset disturbances of bladder or bowel continence or perineal sensory symptoms suggestive of a *cauda equina syndrome*. Patients with risk factors for malignancy, infection, or osteoporosis, as well as those with pain maximal at rest (or nocturnal pain) require imaging (see Table 119-11).

Treatment strategies for lumbar pain are similar to those for cervical pain, with surgery reserved for patients with neurologic signs and clear pathologic processes seen on imaging studies. Most cases of acute low back pain, even with rupture of an intervertebral disk, can be treated conservatively with a short period of rest, muscle relaxants, and analgesics. Prolonged bed rest is no longer recommended except for patients in severe pain. Patient education regarding proper posture and appropriate back exercises is helpful, as is a formal physical therapy program. Chiropractic manipulation should be reserved for patients who have no evidence of neurologic injury or spine instability.

Prospectus for the Future

A number of novel therapeutic approaches hold promise for the treatment of medically refractory headache. Electrical stimulation of the occipital nerve has been effective in some patients with severe cluster headache, as has deep brain stimulation of the hypothalamic region. Some patients with chronic daily headache respond to local intramuscular botulinum toxin injection. The association between patent foramen ovale (PFO) and migraine headache has prompted treatment trials of PFO closure. Thus far there is inadequate evidence to support this approach. Nonetheless the association merits further investigation.

References

Detsky ME, McDonald MR, Baerlocher MO, et al: Does this patient with headache have migraine or need neuroimaging? JAMA 296:1274-1283, 2006.

Gronseth G, Cruccu G, Alksne J, et al: Practice parameter: The diagnostic evaluation and treatment of trigeminal neuralgia (an evidence-based review): Report of the Quality Standards Subcommittee of the American Academy of Neurology and the European Federation of Neurological Societies. Neurology 71:1183-1190, 2008.

Headache Classification Subcommittee of the International Headache Society: The International Classification of Headache Disorders: 2nd edition. Cephalalgia 24(Suppl 1):9-160, 2004.

Ho TW, Mannix LK, Fan X, et al: Randomized controlled Trial of an oral CGRP receptor antagonist MK0974 in acute treatment of migraine. Neurology 70:1304-1312, 2008.

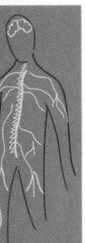

Disorders of Vision and Hearing

Allan McCarthy and Timothy J. Counihan

Disorders of Vision and Eye Movements

EXAMINATION OF THE VISUAL SYSTEM

Acuity

The clinical examination of visual function should begin with the testing of visual acuity. The patient should wear corrective lenses if they are available, and, if possible, testing should be performed with a Snellen chart at a distance of 20 feet to minimize the influence of pupil size and lens accommodation on visual acuity. When errors of refraction are responsible for decreased visual acuity, vision may be improved by having the patient look through a pinhole. Corrected vision in one eye of less than 20/40 suggests damage to the lens (cataract) or retina or a disorder of the anterior visual (prechiasmal) pathway. Color vision in each eye should also be tested; even when visual acuity is normal, patients with lesions of the optic nerve may complain that colors appear "washed out" in the affected eye.

Visual Fields

Thorough examination of the visual fields (Fig. 120-1) can often localize lesions interrupting the afferent (sensory) visual system. Visual fields in all four quadrants should be tested by comparing the patient's field with that of the examiner (confrontation). The examiner's head should be level with that of the patient's, and a white pin used to map peripheral visual fields and a red pin to assess for the presence of a scotoma. Asking the patient to count the number of the examiner's extended fingers is more sensitive than presenting moving objects in detecting visual field deficits. The field should be tested first unilaterally and then bilaterally because uncovering a defect (particularly in the left hemifield) with bilateral testing only (extinction) suggests a lesion in the contralateral parietal lobe.

Partial or complete visual loss in one eye only implies damage to the retina or optic nerve anterior to the optic chiasm, whereas a visual field abnormality involving both eyes implies a defect at or posterior to the optic chiasm. Scotomas are areas of partial or complete visual loss and may be central or peripheral; central scotomas reduce visual acuity as a result of damage to macular fibers. A scotoma impairing half of a visual field is known as a *hemianopia*. A homonymous hemianopia implies a postchiasmal lesion. Quadrantanopias are smaller defects in the visual field and may be superior (which suggests a temporal lobe lesion) or inferior (which suggests a parietal lobe lesion). Bitemporal hemianopia implies a lesion at the chiasm, such as a pituitary tumor. An altitudinal hemianopia occurs with vascular damage to the retina. Scintillating scotomas are hallucinations of flashing lights. If they are monocular, they may be caused by retinal detachment; binocular scintillations suggest occipital oligemia (as in migraine) or seizure. Any suspicious findings on bedside confrontation testing warrant formal visual field testing using perimetry.

Pupils

Pupil constriction results from stimulation of parasympathetic system of the oculomotor (third cranial) nerve, whereas dilation is mediated by the sympathetic system. If the balance of these systems is upset, pupillary inequality (anisocoria) results. The pupils should be examined in both dim and bright light; if the anisocoria increases going from dim to bright light, a lesion of the parasympathetic system is likely (Fig. 120-2). *Physiologic anisocoria* is characterized by a difference in pupil size that appears less in bright light and has no associated pathologic findings.

Both the direct and consensual light responses should be noted for each eye; in the latter, when the light is shone in one eye, both pupils should constrict. This is best tested using the "swinging light test," in which the light is moved quickly from one eye to the other. If there is dilation of one

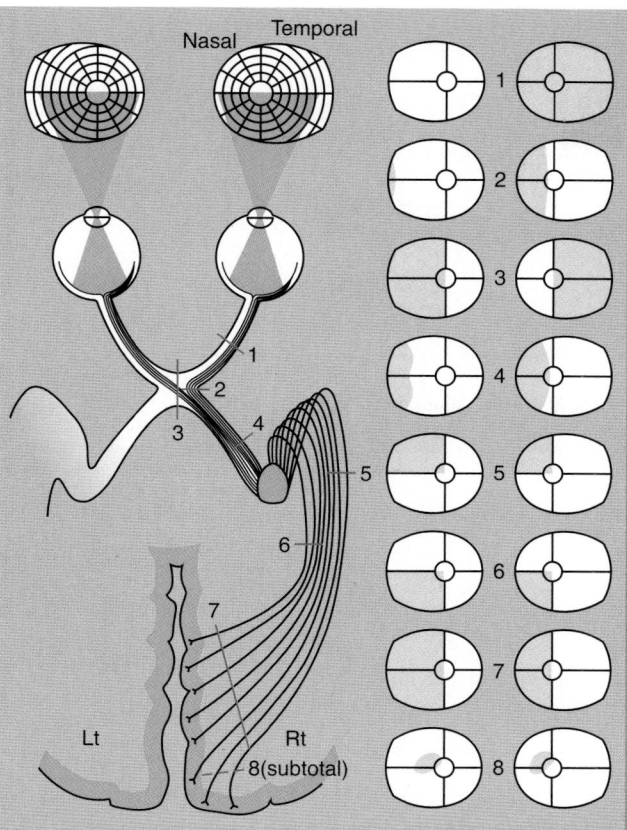

Figure 120-1 Visual fields that accompany damage to the visual pathways: *1,* Optic nerve: unilateral amaurosis. *2,* Lateral optic chiasm: grossly incongruous, incomplete (contralateral) homonymous hemianopia. *3,* Central optic chiasm: bitemporal hemianopia. *4,* Optic tract: incongruous, incomplete homonymous hemianopia. *5,* Temporal (Meyer) loop of optic radiation: congruous partial or complete (contralateral) homonymous superior quadrantanopia. *6,* Parietal (superior) projection of the optic radiation: congruous partial or complete homonymous inferior quadrantanopia. *7,* Complete parieto-occipital interruption of optic radiation: complete congruous homonymous hemianopia with psychophysical shift of foveal point often sparing central vision, giving "macular sparing." *8,* Incomplete damage to visual cortex: congruous homonymous scotomas, usually encroaching at least acutely on central vision. (From Baloh RW: Neuro-ophthalmology. In Goldman L, Bennett JC [eds]: Cecil Textbook of Medicine, 21st ed. Philadelphia, WB Saunders, 1998, p 2236).

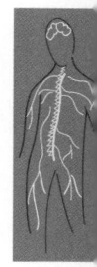

pupil as the light is moved to it from the other side, an abnormality of the optic nerve in that eye should be suspected. This abnormality is referred to as an *afferent pupillary defect.* The accommodative pupillary response is tested by asking the patient to look first in the distance and then at the examiner's finger, held 12 inches away. The pupils should constrict symmetrically and rapidly.

The presence of ptosis should be noted. A large, unreactive pupil with ptosis indicates a lesion of the oculomotor nerve *(third cranial nerve palsy)* interrupting the parasympathetic nerve supply to the pupil. The associated paralysis of the medial and inferior rectus and inferior oblique muscles (see later discussion) results in distortion of the eye (inferolaterally, "down and out") and a subjective complaint of diplopia by the patient. Common causes of a third nerve palsy include compression by an aneurysm of the posterior

communicating artery, by transtentorial herniation, or from ischemia, usually in the setting of diabetes or vasculitis. A third nerve palsy caused by ischemia often spares the pupil but results in complete paralysis of the oculomotor and eyelid levator muscles. An acute painful third nerve palsy should be treated as an emergency, with the need to investigate for an intracranial aneurysm.

A small, poorly reactive pupil with associated ptosis is known as *Horner syndrome* and results from damage to the sympathetic fibers to the pupil. There may be associated unilateral anhidrosis resulting from damage to sympathetic fibers. Horner syndrome may result from lesions of the hypothalamus, brainstem, cervical spinal cord, or sympathetic fibers to the pupil. Horner syndrome from sympathetic fiber involvement may be the first sign of an apical lung tumor (Pancoast) or may occur in diseases affecting the carotid artery.

Argyll-Robertson pupils are small, irregular pupils that constrict to near vision but not in response to light. They are associated with neurosyphilis, diabetes, and other disorders. This so-called *light-near dissociation* may also occur in rostral dorsal midbrain lesions, in which there are abnormalities of vertical gaze, eyelid retraction, and convergence retraction nystagmus. This uncommon constellation of clinical findings is frequently secondary to a pineal lesion.

Tonic (Adie) pupils constrict slowly and incompletely in response to light; this is usually an incidental finding on examination but may be associated with areflexia (Adie syndrome). Reaction to accommodation is preserved, and it has been suggested that the disorder is a result of parasympathetic denervation. *Hippus* refers to pupillary unrest with synchronous oscillation of the pupil size; it is considered a normal phenomenon.

Eye Movements

The history helps in evaluating the patient with diplopia. Is the diplopia primarily horizontal or vertical, or is it greater looking to the right or to the left? Double vision that varies during the day suggests myasthenia gravis. Is the diplopia maximal with near or distant vision? Greater difficulty with near vision suggests impairment of the medial rectus, oculomotor nerve, or convergence system, whereas abducens nerve weakness results in horizontal diplopia when objects are viewed at a distance. Diplopia that worsens on going down stairs may suggest a fourth nerve lesion. Monocular diplopia is usually caused by diseases of the retina or lens and is corrected by having the patient look through a pinhole, unless the cause is psychogenic.

The examination should begin by determining the position of the head and eyes with the eyes in primary gaze. Both smooth pursuit and (voluntary) saccadic eye movements in horizontal and vertical directions are checked to determine whether the movements are conjugate or disconjugate. Disconjugate eye movements suggest a disorder of the brainstem (at the level of the ocular motor nuclei or their connections), the peripheral nerves (cranial nerves III, IV, or VI), individual eye muscles (ocular myopathy), or the neuromuscular junction (myasthenia gravis or botulism). A large deficit in the range of eye movements may provide sufficient diagnostic information. However, in many cases, although the patient complains of diplopia, no clear misalignment is visible on testing eye movements. The corneal

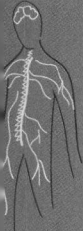

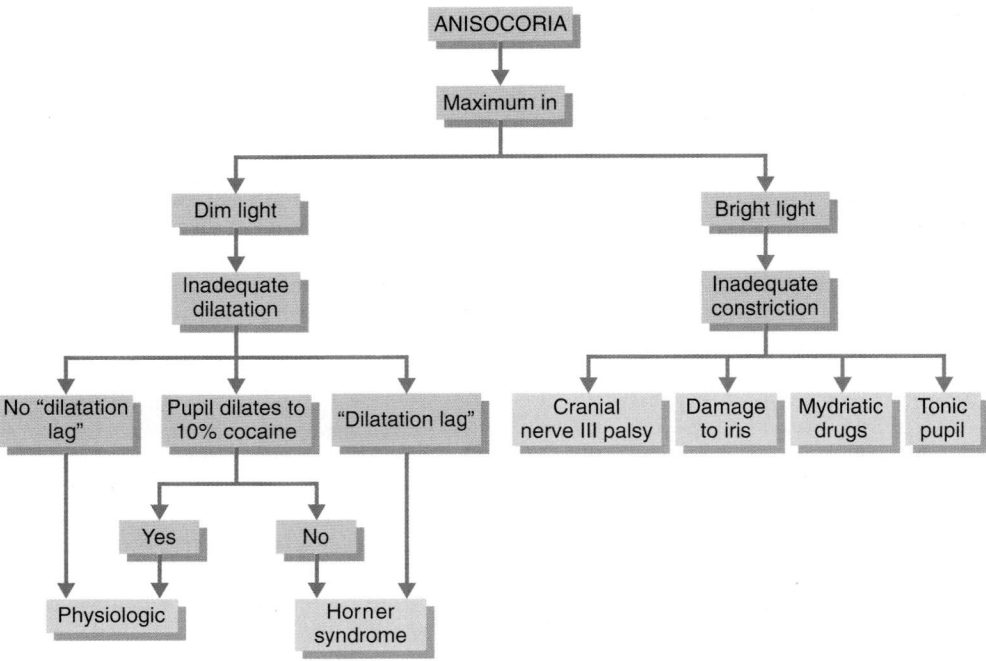

Figure 120-2 Algorithm for the approach to unequal pupils (anisocoria).

reflection test may help identify misalignment in these cases. The patient is instructed to look at a light shining directly at the eyes. If the eyes are normally aligned, the light reflection will be about 1 mm nasal to the center of the cornea. If one eye is deviated medially, the reflection will be displaced outward; the reflection will be displaced inward if the eye is deviated outward.

The abducens (sixth cranial) nerve supplies the lateral rectus muscle. The trochlear (fourth cranial) nerve subserves the superior oblique muscle, which intorts the eye as well as depresses the eye in adduction (such as when a patient tries to look downstairs). All other muscles are supplied by the oculomotor nerve. Abnormalities of the cranial nerves in the brainstem are usually accompanied by other signs, such as weakness, ataxia, or dysarthria. The abducens nerve has a long ascending course through the posterior fossa, where it is prone to compression at multiple sites and as a result of raised intracranial pressure; hence, a sixth nerve palsy may be a false localizing sign. Table 120-1 lists the major causes of acute ophthalmoplegia.

Conjugate eye movement is regulated by supranuclear pathways from the cerebral hemisphere to the medial longitudinal fasciculus in the brainstem. A lesion in the cerebral hemisphere resulting from hemorrhage, infarction, or tumor disrupts conjugate gaze to the contralateral side, so that the eyes "look away" from the hemiplegia. Lesions of the brainstem cause conjugate paralysis to the ipsilateral side (eyes looking toward the side of the hemiplegia). Lesions of the medial longitudinal fasciculus, which connects the nuclei of the oculomotor and abducens nerves, leads to *internuclear ophthalmoplegia*. In this case, horizontal gaze results in failure of adduction in one eye and nystagmus in the abducting eye. The lesion is on the side of failed adduction; bilateral lesions are frequently seen in multiple sclerosis.

Table 120-1 Major Causes of Acute Ophthalmoplegia

Condition	Diagnostic Features
Bilateral	
Botulism	Contaminated food; high-altitude cooking; pupils involved
Myasthenia gravis	Fluctuating degree of paralysis; responds to edrophonium chloride (Tensilon) IV
Wernicke encephalopathy	Nutritional deficiency; responds to thiamine IV
Acute cranial polyneuropathy	Antecedent respiratory infection; elevated CSF protein level
Brainstem stroke	Other brainstem signs
Unilateral	
P Comm aneurysm	Third cranial nerve, pupil involved
Diabetic-idiopathic	Third or sixth cranial nerve, pupil spared
Myasthenia gravis	As above
Brainstem stroke	As above

CSF, cerebrospinal fluid; IV, intravenous; P Comm, posterior communicating artery.

Funduscopy

The retina should be carefully examined in each patient by direct ophthalmoscopy, which provides a magnified view of the fundus without the necessity for dilation of the pupil.

UNILATERAL VISUAL LOSS

Loss of vision in one eye may be caused by lesions of the cornea, lens, vitreous, retina, or optic nerve. Careful funduscopic examination will usually reveal ocular and retinal lesions, but acute lesions of the optic nerve (optic neuritis) may not be associated with abnormalities of the optic nerve head. *Optic neuritis* is a condition characterized by inflammation of the optic nerve accompanied by non-homonymous defects in vision. The term *papillitis* refers to ophthalmoscopically observable changes in the optic nerve; *retrobulbar neuritis* refers to this condition without observable changes in the funduscopic examination findings.

The patient with optic neuritis complains of difficulty with vision in the affected eye. Loss of vision may be insidious and recognized only when the unaffected eye is accidentally occluded. Patients often complain of periorbital pain on eye movement on presentation. The evolution of visual loss is highly variable, progressing over a period ranging from less than a day to several weeks, although most patients will have reached their maximal visual deficit in 3 to 7 days. Patients may describe their vision as blurred or dim, and colors may appear less bright than usual or "gray." Red desaturation may occur with optic neuritis and may be detected using Ishihara color plates. At the time the patient is first examined, visual acuity may range from almost 20/20 to the extreme of total blindness. Examination of the visual field shows defects within the central 25 degrees, with central and paracentral scotomas being the most common types. An afferent pupillary defect is frequently present. The funduscopic examination is abnormal in only about one half of the cases. The disc may appear hyperemic with blurred margins, and hemorrhages, when present, are few and found only on the disc or in the area immediately surrounding the disc. Optic neuritis should be treated acutely with high-dose intravenous corticosteroids, as this is proven to shorten time to recovery. The most common cause of optic neuritis is multiple sclerosis. Bilateral optic neuritis is much less common and may coincide with cervical spine demyelinating disease, or *acute tranverse myelitis*. The combination of optic nerve disease and transverse myelitis is known as *neuromyelitis optica* (NMO) or *Devic disease*. The recent discovery of antibodies directed toward aquaporin 4 (a water channel present on astrocytes and vascular endothelial cells), associated with NMO, has identified this as a separate disease entity, with a different treatment regimen emerging for it. The NMO antibody is the first sensitive and specific biomarker associated with a central demyelinating disorder.

Ischemic optic neuropathy occurs in two forms. The *atherosclerotic* variety occurs mostly between the ages of 50 and 70, and no evidence of systemic disease is present. The *arteritic* form is usually a manifestation of giant cell arteritis; there may be systemic manifestations of the disease, including headache, scalp tenderness, and generalized myalgias. Laboratory evaluation shows anemia and elevated erythrocyte sedimentation rate in almost every case. Patients with arteritis should be treated with high doses of corticosteroids to prevent permanent loss of vision.

The optic nerve may be compressed by tumors that originate in the nerve itself or in the region of the optic chiasm. Pathologic processes that appear acutely as optic disc edema frequently result in a secondary optic atrophy, including papilledema, optic neuritis, and ischemic optic neuropathy. Glaucoma is responsible for more cases of optic atrophy in the adult population than any other cause. In young patients with inherited optic atrophy, Leber hereditary optic

neuropathy is often the cause; it is usually bilateral. *Foster-Kennedy* syndrome is optic atrophy in one eye with papilledema in the other eye, secondary to a tumor compressing the atrophied optic nerve and causing raised intracranial pressure to produce papilledema in the opposite eye.

Acute transient monocular blindness is usually the result of embolization to the central retinal artery from an atheromatous plaque in the carotid artery *(amaurosis fugax)*. Any complaint of transient visual loss constitutes an emergency, and steps must be taken to prevent permanent loss of vision by making a prompt diagnosis and initiating appropriate therapy. Examples of sight-saving procedures include corticosteroid therapy for cranial arteritis, reduction of intraocular pressure for acute glaucoma, and carotid surgery, anticoagulation, or antiplatelet therapy for embolic cerebrovascular disease.

BILATERAL VISUAL LOSS

Gradual bilateral visual loss caused by optic nerve lesions is rare. Causes include Leber hereditary optic neuropathy and a toxic-nutritional deficiency state. Acute transient bilateral visual loss (visual obscuration) may be a symptom of raised intracranial pressure caused by a brain tumor or idiopathic intracranial hypertension (IIH); papilledema is often severe. IIH, formerly known as *pseudotumor cerebri*, requires prompt investigation and treatment to prevent potential bilateral visual failure. It occurs most often in overweight women in their second or third decade of life. Vitamin A and tetracycline ingestion have been associated with the condition. Unilateral or bilateral lateral rectus palsy may be present. It is one of the few situations in which, after imaging, performance of a lumbar puncture is safe in the setting of marked bilateral papilledema. Cerebral venous sinus thrombosis may mimic IIH and should be screened for with neuroimaging.

Lesions of the optic chiasm or postchiasmal optic pathways lead to specific patterns of partial visual loss, as summarized in Figure 120-1. Bilateral damage to the optic radiations or visual cortex results in cortical blindness. The pupillary light reflex is normal, as are the funduscopic examination findings, and the patient may occasionally be unaware that he or she is blind (Anton syndrome). Patients are often misdiagnosed as having a conversion reaction. Transient cortical blindness occurs most often in basilar artery insufficiency but is also seen in hypertensive encephalopathy. Positive visual phenomena (e.g., phosphenes, scintillating scotomas) are characteristic of migrainous aura and probably reflect oligemia to the occipital lobes from vasoconstriction. Arteriovenous malformations, tumors, and seizures may produce similar symptoms and should be distinguished from migraine with aura by a careful history and examination as well as by imaging in appropriate cases.

Visual hallucinations are visual sensations independent of external light stimulation; they may be either simple or complex, may be localized or generalized, and may occur in patients with a clear or clouded sensorium. Visual illusions are alterations of a perceived external stimulus in which some features are distorted. The simplest visual phenomena consist of flashes of light (photopsias), blue lights (phosphenes), or scintillating zigzag lines, which last a fraction of

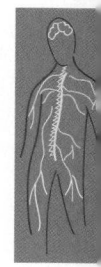

a second and recur frequently or which appear to be in constant motion. These can arise from dysfunction within the optic pathways at any point from the eye to the cortex. Glaucoma, incipient retinal detachment, retinal ischemia, or macular degeneration can cause simple visual hallucinations based on dysfunction in the eye. Lesions of the occipital lobe are often associated with simple hallucinations; classic migraine is by far the most common condition of this type. Complex visual hallucinations such as seeing objects as people, animals, landscapes, or various indescribable scenes occur most frequently with temporal lobe lesions or parieto-occipital association areas. Visual hallucinations of epileptogenic origin are typically stereotyped.

Hearing and Its Impairments

SYMPTOMS OF AUDITORY DYSFUNCTION

The main symptoms of lesions within the auditory system are hearing loss and tinnitus. Hearing loss can be classified as conductive, sensorineural, mixed, or central, based on the anatomic site of pathology (Fig. 120-3). Tinnitus can be either subjective or objective. Conductive hearing loss results from lesions involving the external or middle ear. Patients with a conductive hearing loss can hear speech in a noisy background as well as in a quiet background, because they can understand loud speech as well as anyone. The ear often feels full, as if it is blocked. The Weber test localizes to the deaf ear, if the deafness is unilateral.

Sensorineural hearing loss usually results from lesions of the cochlea or the auditory division of the vestibulocochlear (eighth cranial) nerve (Table 120-2). Patients with sensorineural hearing loss often have difficulty hearing speech that is mixed with background noise and may be annoyed by loud speech. They usually hear low tones better than high-frequency ones. Distortion of sounds is

common with sensorineural hearing loss. Central ("retrocochlear") hearing disorders are rare and result from bilateral lesions of the central auditory pathways, including the cochlear and dorsal olivary nuclear complexes, inferior colliculi, medial geniculate bodies, and auditory cortex in the temporal lobes. Damage to both auditory cortices may result in pure word deafness, in which patients are selectively unable to discriminate language but may be able to hear nonverbal sounds.

Tinnitus is the perception of a noise or ringing in the ear that is usually audible only to the patient (subjective), although, rarely, an examiner can hear the sound as well. The latter, so-called *objective tinnitus,* can be heard when the examining physician places a stethoscope against the patient's external auditory canal. Tinnitus that is pulsatory and synchronous with the heartbeat suggests a vascular abnormality within the head or neck (Fig. 120-4). Aneurysms, arteriovenous malformations, and vascular tumors can produce this type of tinnitus.

Subjective tinnitus, heard only by the patient, can result from lesions involving the external ear canal, tympanic membrane, ossicles, cochlea, auditory nerve, brainstem, and

Table 120-2 **Cause of Acute Unilateral Sensorineural Deafness**
Cochlear
Idiopathic (85%)
Trauma
Ménière disease
Lyme disease
Syphilis
Autoimmune disease
Retrocochlear
Demyelination
Vestibular schwannoma (usually gradual onset)
Stroke

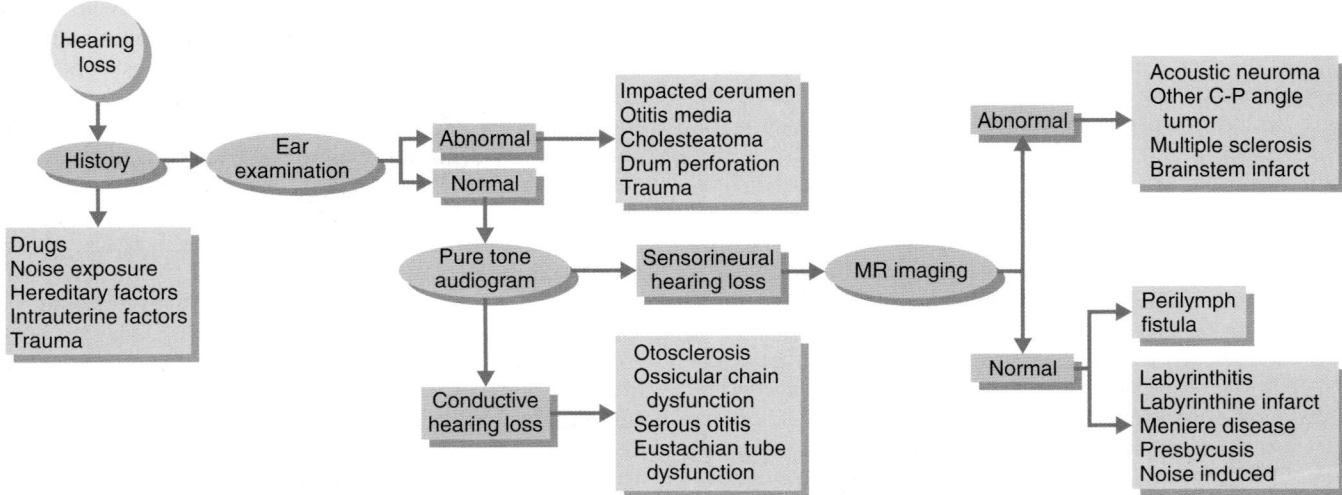

Figure 120-3 Evaluation of deafness (unilateral and bilateral). C-P, cerebellopontine; MR, magnetic resonance. (Modified from Baloh RW: Hearing and equilibrium. In Goldman L, Bennett JC [eds]: Cecil Textbook of Medicine, 21st ed. Philadelphia, WB Saunders, 1998, p 2250).

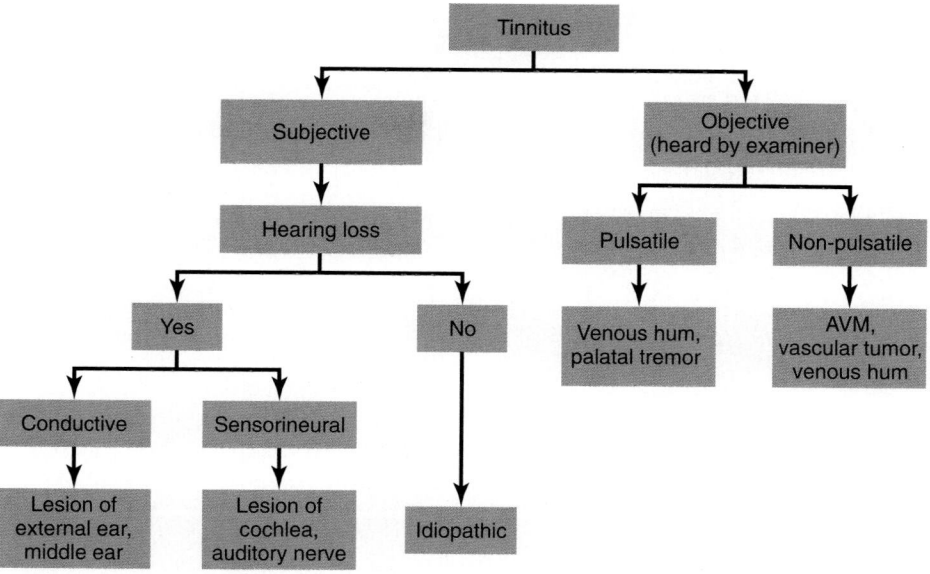

Figure 120-4 Algorithm for the approach to the patient with tinnitus. AVM, arteriovenous malformation; CNS, central nervous system.

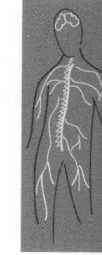

cortex. The character of the tinnitus does not usually aid in determining the site of the disturbance. For this, one must rely on associated symptoms and signs. When tinnitus results from a lesion of the external or middle ear, it is usually accompanied by a conductive hearing loss. The patient may complain that his or her voice sounds hollow and that other sounds are muffled. Because the masking effect of ambient noise is lost, the patient may be disturbed by normal muscular sounds such as chewing, tight closure of the eyes, or clenching of the jaws. The characteristic tinnitus associated with Ménière syndrome is low pitched and continuous, although fluctuating in intensity. Often the tinnitus becomes very loud immediately preceding an acute attack of vertigo and then may disappear after the attack. Tinnitus resulting from lesions within the central nervous system is usually not associated with hearing loss but is nearly always associated with other neurologic symptoms and signs. High-dose salicylates frequently result in tinnitus.

EXAMINATION OF THE AUDITORY SYSTEM

A quick test for hearing loss in the speech range is to observe the response to spoken commands at different intensities (whisper, conversation, and shouting). The examiner must be careful to prevent the patient from reading his or her lip movement. A high-frequency stimulus such as a watch tick should also be used, because sensorineural disorders often involve only the higher frequencies. Tuning fork tests permit a rough assessment of the hearing level for pure tones of known frequency. The Rinne test compares the patient's hearing by air conduction with that by bone conduction. A 512-cps tuning fork is first held against the mastoid process until the sound fades. It is then placed 1 inch from the ear. Normal subjects can hear the fork about twice as long by air conduction as by bone conduction. If hearing by bone con-

duction is longer than by air conduction, a conductive hearing loss is suggested. The Weber test compares the patient's hearing by bone conduction in the two ears. The fork is placed at the center of the forehead, and the patient is asked where he or she hears the tone. Normal subjects hear it in the center of the head, patients with unilateral conductive loss hear it on the affected side, and patients with unilateral sensorineural loss hear it on the side opposite the loss. Otoscopic examination may reveal impacted cerumen as a cause of conductive hearing loss.

CAUSES OF HEARING LOSS

The bilateral hearing loss commonly associated with advancing age is called *presbycusis*. Presbycusis is not a distinct disease entity but rather represents multiple effects of aging on the auditory system. Presbycusis may include conductive and central dysfunction, although the most consistent effect of aging is on the sensory cells and neurons of the cochlea; as a result, higher tones are lost early.

Otosclerosis is a disease of the bony labyrinth that usually manifests itself by immobilizing the stapes and thereby producing a conductive hearing loss. Seventy percent of patients with clinical otosclerosis notice hearing loss between the ages of 11 and 30. There is a family history of otosclerosis in approximately 50% of cases. *Stapedectomy*, a procedure in which the stapes is replaced with a prosthesis, is effective in correcting the conductive component of hearing loss.

A lesion of the cerebellopontine angle, such as a vestibular schwannoma (Fig. 120-5), often causes unilateral hearing loss that progresses slowly; symptoms are caused by compression of the nerve in the narrow confines of the canal. The most common symptoms associated with vestibular schwannomas are slowly progressive hearing loss and tinnitus from compression of the cochlear nerve. Vertigo occurs in fewer than 20% of patients, but approximately 50% complain of imbalance or disequilibrium. Next to the

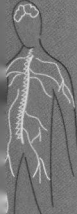

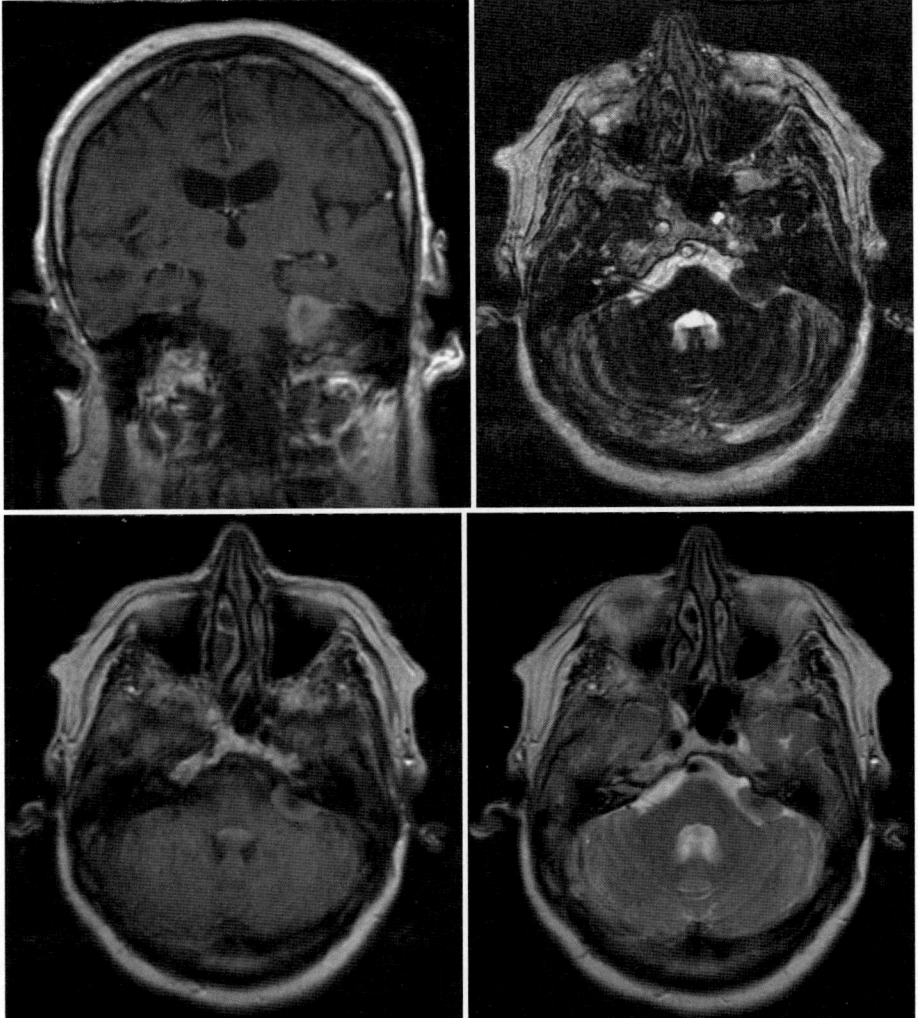

Figure 120-5 Magnetic resonance imaging scan of the brain showing coronal and axial views of a tumor of the left cerebellopontine angle, consistent with a schwannoma.

auditory nerve, the cranial nerves most commonly involved by compression are the seventh (facial weakness) and fifth (sensory loss). Loss of the corneal reflex on the affected side is often the first clinical sign. Treatment in most cases is surgical removal.

Ménière syndrome (endolymphatic hydrops) is characterized by fluctuating hearing loss and tinnitus, episodic vertigo, and a sensation of fullness or pressure in the ear. Typically the patient develops a sensation of fullness and pressure, along with decreased hearing and tinnitus in one ear. Vertigo rapidly follows, reaching a maximum intensity within minutes and then slowly subsiding over the next several hours. The patient is usually left with a sense of unsteadiness and dizziness for days after the acute vertiginous episode. In the early stages the hearing loss is completely reversible, but in later stages a residual hearing loss remains. Up to 50% of patients with idiopathic Ménière syndrome frequently have a positive family history, suggesting genetic predisposing factors. The key to the diagnosis of Ménière syndrome is to document fluctuating hearing levels in a patient with the characteristic clinical history. Medical therapy for endolymphatic hydrops includes dietary sodium restriction and oral diuretics.

Acute unilateral deafness usually results from damage to the cochlea and may be caused by viral or bacterial labyrinthitis or vascular occlusion in the territory of the anterior inferior cerebellar artery. Perilymphatic fistulas may also cause abrupt unilateral deafness, usually in association with tinnitus and vertigo.

Drugs that cause acute irreversible bilateral hearing loss include aminoglycosides, cisplatin, and furosemide. Salicylates may cause reversible hearing loss and tinnitus.

TREATMENT OF HEARING LOSS

The best treatment is prevention, particularly by the appropriate use of earplugs for those working in a noisy environment. Hearing aids help patients with conductive hearing loss, and developments with cochlear implants may help patients with sensorineural hearing loss.

Prospectus for the Future

There has been accumulating evidence that a substantial minority of patients with symptoms of idiopathic intracranial hypertension (IIH) have underlying anatomic abnormalities of cerebral venous sinuses. In patients who have demonstrable abnormalities on cerebral venography, endoluminal venous sinus stenting has been reported as effective. This approach is receiving further study. In patients with sudden idiopathic sensorineural hearing loss who do not respond to oral corticosteroid therapy, intratympanic steroid injection has emerged as a potential therapeutic option. Aminoglycoside antibiotics are known to be associated with ototoxicity; a small study has found that co-administration of aspirin appears to attenuate the ototoxic potential of gentamicin, possibly through an antioxidant effect. This finding, if substantiated in larger studies, may have implications for parts of the world where appropriate monitoring facilities for aminoglycoside levels are not readily available.

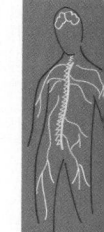

References

Plant GT: Optic neuritis and multiple sclerosis. Curr Opin Neurol 21:16-21, 2008.

Rauch SD: Clinical practice. Idiopathic sudden sensorineural hearing loss. N Engl J Med 359:833-840, 2008.

Sajjadi H, Paparella MM: Ménière's disease. Lancet 372:406-414, 2008.

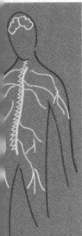

Dizziness and Vertigo

Kevin A. Kerber

Vestibular System

Understanding the vestibular system and common peripheral vestibular disorders is of central importance in the evaluation of patients with dizziness. This is because the dilemma is often discriminating a benign peripheral vestibular disorder from a small focal brain lesion. The vestibular system is a common source of confusion. Many clinicians assume a "peripheral" cause in the absence of motor, sensory, or language deficits, but this approach is flawed. A more effective approach is to aim to "rule in" a *specific* peripheral vestibular disorder. When a specific peripheral vestibular disorder does not fit, then a workup for a central nervous system lesion is usually warranted. The three common peripheral vestibular disorders all have highly characteristic history and examination features, thus enabling this approach.

BASIC VESTIBULAR SYSTEM CONCEPTS

The peripheral vestibular system maintains a balanced tonic input to the brain. The input represents the circuitry that links the inner ear to eye movements, the vestibulo-ocular reflex (VOR). A normal functioning VOR is important for balance and maintaining clear vision when moving. When an imbalance is caused by a lesion or aberrant stimulation, then vertigo ensues. A characteristic sign of vestibular system imbalance is nystagmus: rhythmic slow and fast movements of the eyes in opposite directions. The location of pathology determines the pattern of nystagmus (Table 121-1). Dysfunction at the semicircular canal level leads to nystagmus in the plane of the affected canal. Therefore problems in the vertical canals (i.e., posterior and anterior canals) lead to vertical and torsional nystagmus, whereas problems in the horizontal canal lead to horizontal nystagmus. At the vestibular nerve level a mixed horizontal-torsional nystagmus is generated because input from all the semicircular canals converge at this level and the signals from the vertical canals mostly cancel each other out. The pathways and thus the patterns of eye movements become less predictable with lesions of the central vestibular pathways, although some general rules apply. Pure vertical (downbeat or upbeat) spontaneous nystagmus, bidirectional gaze-evoked nystagmus (look left, beats left; look right, beats right) (**Web Video 121-1**), and persistent downbeating positional nystagmus are signs of central dysfunction (see Table 121-1).

Another characteristic sign of vestibular disturbance is a positive head-thrust test (**Web Video 121-2**). A subject with an intact VOR will maintain gaze on a stationary, straight-ahead target after a brief, small-amplitude, high-acceleration movement of the head to one side. A subject with vestibular impairment on one side loses this reflex on the ipsilateral side and therefore, after the quick head movement, will need to make a re-fixation voluntary eye movement (i.e., a "saccade") back to the target because the eyes moved with the head. This so-called "catch-up" or "corrective" saccade is easily appreciated at the bedside and indicates vestibular deafferentation.

PERIPHERAL VESTIBULAR DISORDERS

There are three common peripheral vestibular disorders: vestibular neuritis, Ménière disease, and benign paroxysmal positional vertigo (BPPV). An understanding of these three disorders is important because each one is the primary consideration for the cause of one of the three common dizziness presentation categories (Table 121-2). In addition, these disorders are the prototypes for most pathology that involves the peripheral vestibular system.

Vestibular neuritis manifests with the abrupt onset of severe vertigo, nausea, and imbalance without other neurologic symptoms. The disorder is caused by a viral disturbance of the vestibular nerve, analogous to Bell palsy. On examination, the acute peripheral vestibular pattern of nystagmus is seen (see Table 121-2) (**Web Video 121-3**). A positive head-thrust test in the direction of the affected ear (but in the direction opposite the fast phase of nystagmus) further supports a vestibular nerve localization. If the nystagmus changes direction with gaze (i.e., look left, beat left; then look right, beat right), then vestibular neuritis is not the diagnosis because these findings localize to the central nervous system. Small strokes of the cerebellum or brainstem can closely mimic vestibular neuritis. Symptoms may

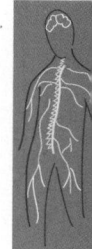

Table 121-1 Common Types and Patterns of Nystagmus

Types	Patterns	Localization	Principal Causes
Spontaneous	Unidirectional horizontal >> torsional	Vestibular nerve, or rarely the brainstem	Vestibular neuritis, or rarely stroke
	Downbeat, upbeat, or pure torsional	Brain	Stroke
Gaze-evoked	Unidirectional	Vestibular nerve	Vestibular neuritis (recovery pattern)
	Bidirectional	Brain	Stroke, cerebellar syndrome, medication side effect*
Positional	Burst of upbeat torsional with DH	Posterior SCC	BPPV
	Horizontal with supine positional testing	Horizontal SCC or rarely the brainstem	BPPV, brainstem lesion
	Persistent downbeat	Brain	Chiari malformation, cerebellar degeneration

*Most common with antiepileptic drugs.
   BPPV, benign paroxysmal positional vertigo; DH, Dix-Hallpike positional test; SCC, semicircular canal; >>, greater than.

Table 121-2 Common Categories of Dizziness Presentations

	Acute Severe Dizziness	Recurrent Spontaneous Attacks	Recurrent Positional Attacks
Primary consideration	Vestibular neuritis	Ménière disease	BPPV
Key features	Constant vertigo, unidirectional horizontal nystagmus,* positive head-thrust test†	Vertigo lasting hours, unilateral auditory symptoms	Positionally triggered, brief (<1 min) attacks Upbeat-torsional burst of nystagmus in DH position, cured by Epley maneuver‡
Red flags	Other CNS features, other patterns of nystagmus, imbalance as the principal symptom, chest pain, cardiovascular risk factors	Other CNS features, CNS patterns of nystagmus, imbalance as the principal symptom, attacks lasting only minutes, chest pain, cardiovascular risk factors, recent onset and crescendo pattern	Other CNS features, CNS patterns of nystagmus
Other considerations	Stroke, myocardial infarction, metabolic disturbances, demyelinating attack	TIA, cardiac arrhythmia, migraine, panic attacks	Horizontal or anterior canal BPPV, migraine, Chiari malformation, posterior fossa tumor, orthostatic hypotension

*This nystagmus never changes direction. Gaze in the direction of the fast phase will increase the velocity of the nystagmus, whereas gaze in the opposite direction will decrease the velocity of the nystagmus.
   †The head-thrust test will be positive in the direction of the affected ear, which is opposite the direction of the fast phase of nystagmus.
   ‡These features apply to BPPV stemming from the posterior canal.
   BPPV, benign paroxysmal positional vertigo; CNS, central nervous system; DH, Dix-Hallpike; TIA, transient ischemic attack.

respond to a short course of corticosteroids and vestibular rehabilitation.

Ménière disease is characterized by recurrent episodes of vertigo, nausea, and imbalance typically lasting hours; prominent auditory features must be present to make the diagnosis. Early in the course, auditory symptoms fluctuate along with vertigo attacks, but later they become a fixed symptom. The auditory symptoms are nearly always unilateral at the onset and consist of hearing loss, roaring tinnitus, or severe fullness in one ear. If attacks are brief (i.e., minutes rather than hours), then transient ischemic attacks should be considered. The dizziness of migraine can also closely mimic Ménière disease. The initial treatment of Ménière disease is a low-salt diet or a diuretic. However, neither of these treatments is of established efficacy. Ablative surgical procedures are appropriate in refractory vertigo cases.

Patients with BPPV report very brief episodes (<1 minute) of vertigo triggered by head movement—most often tilting the head back to look up, getting in or out of bed, or rolling over in bed. Dizziness from any cause may worsen after certain movements, but the dizziness of BPPV is *triggered* by certain movements. The most common form of BPPV

occurs when otoliths enter the posterior canal. Posterior canal BPPV is identified at the bedside using the Dix-Hallpike test (Fig. 121-1). In response to the Dix-Hallpike test, otoliths move in the canal and lead to a burst of upbeat-torsional nystagmus lasting about 20 to 30 seconds (**Web Video 121-4**). This disorder is cured in minutes by using the repositioning maneuver described by Epley. BPPV is less commonly caused by otoliths in the horizontal canal and very rarely the anterior canal. When the otoliths are in one of these other canals, the pattern of nystagmus is different from that of posterior canal BPPV, as are the repositioning maneuvers. Positional vertigo and nystagmus are common in patients with migraine. If a persistent downbeating nystagmus is seen during the Dix-Hallpike test, then a central nervous system cause (e.g., Chiari malformation, cerebellar tumor, or cerebellar degeneration) should be considered.

Approach to the Patient

"Dizziness" means different things to different people, so first start by defining the symptom. Is it true vertigo (i.e.,

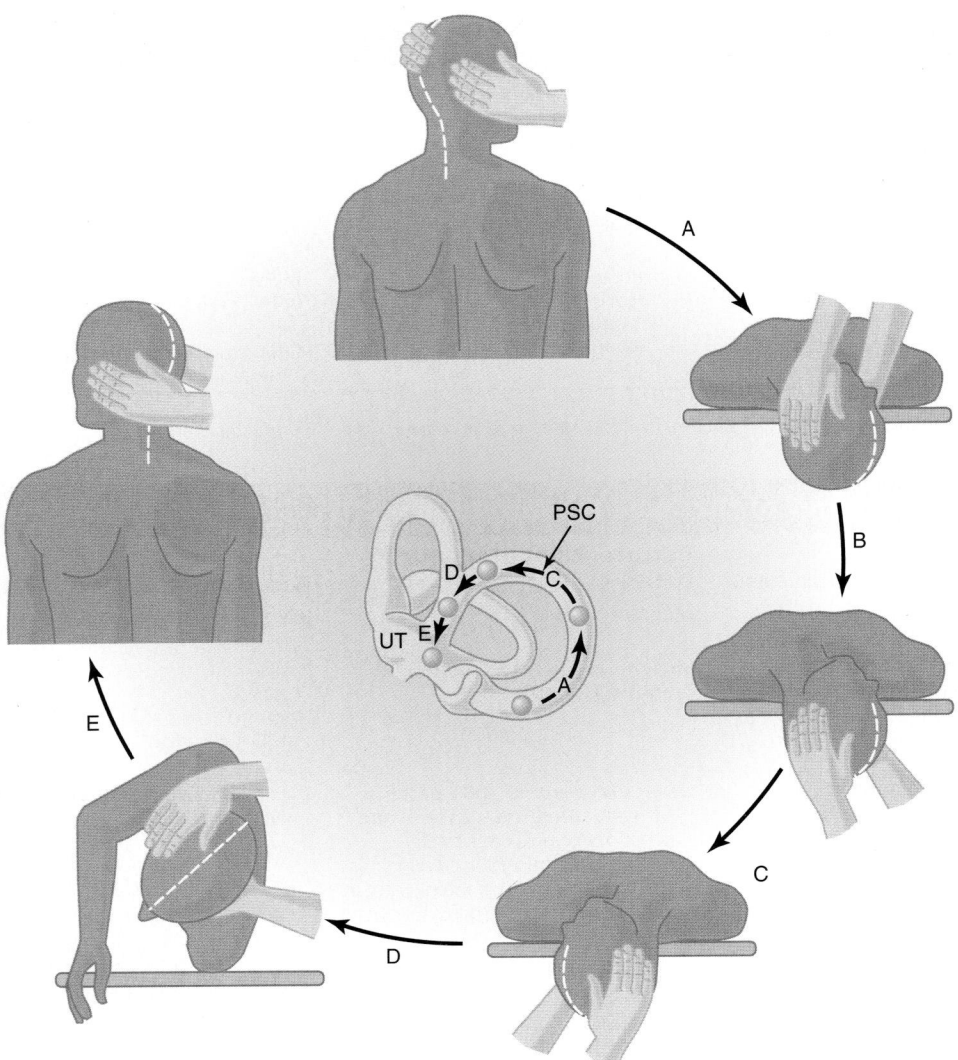

Figure 121-1 Repositioning treatment for benign positional vertigo designed to move endolymphatic debris out of the posterior semicircular canal (PSC) of the right ear and into the utricle (UT). The patient is seated, and the patient's head is turned 45 degrees to the right **(A)**. The head is then lowered rapidly to below the horizontal **(B)**. The examiner shifts hand positions **(C)**, and the patient's head is rotated rapidly 90 degrees in the opposite direction, so it now points 45 degrees to the left, where it remains for 30 seconds **(D)**. The patient then rolls onto the left side without turning the head in relation to the body and maintains this position for another 30 seconds **(E)** before sitting up. The treatment is repeated until nystagmus is abolished. The procedure is reversed for treating the left ear. The patient must avoid the supine position for 2 days. (Adapted from Foster CA, Baloh RW: Episodic vertigo. In Rakel RE [ed]: Conn's Current Therapy. Philadelphia, WB Saunders, 1995).

visualized spinning of the environment), lightheadedness, imbalance, or some other symptom? The next step is to define the characteristics of the symptom. When did it start? Is it constant or episodic? If episodic, what are the duration and frequency of the episodes, and are there any triggers? This information helps categorize the patient's presentation (see Table 121-2). Next, ask about aggravating or alleviating factors and about accompanying symptoms. The patient's past medical history may identify a risk for certain disorders. The list of medications should be carefully scrutinized, because dizziness is a common medication side effect. The family history may reveal a familial pattern of similar symptoms. Whenever possible it is always preferable to examine the patient with dizziness at the time of active symptoms. Hearing should be tested one ear at a time with either tuning

forks or finger rub. If the general examination is unrevealing, then the focus should shift to the ocular motor examination to search for signs of vestibular or brain dysfunction. Does the patient have nystagmus? If so, what type and pattern? Is the head-thrust test result positive? Instruct the patient to follow your finger back and forth and assess whether the eyes move smoothly. This is a test of the smooth pursuit system, and pathologically impaired smooth pursuit is a central nervous system sign. If the patient reports that symptoms are triggered by head or body turns, then positional testing should be performed.

True vertigo suggests a disturbance of the vestibular system but does not discriminate a peripheral from a central vestibular localization. If the patient's features do not fit with a common peripheral vestibular disorder then central nervous system causes should be considered. If the patient reports imbalance as the principal symptom and has a gait disorder, then the following causes should be considered: stroke (if the onset was acute), a musculoskeletal disorder, peripheral neuropathy, bilateral vestibulopathy, or a neuro-degenerative disorder involving the cerebellum. When the dizziness is described as lightheadedness, wooziness, or a similar symptom, and the neurologic examination findings are normal, then general medical causes should be considered. Dizziness can be a prominent symptom of anxiety and panic disorders. Migraine should be on the differential diagnosis of any dizziness presentation. When none of these seem to fit, the examination findings are normal, and the symptom has been present for more than several months,

then the patient likely has chronic dizziness—typically considered a benign hypersensitivity disorder.

Treating Dizziness

Unless a specific disorder can be identified, symptomatic treatment is usually needed: meclizine, a benzodiazepine, or an antiemetic. However, these are not appropriate long-term treatment regimens. Patients with chronic dizziness may benefit from lifestyle modifications (e.g., exercise, optimizing sleep and diet, and stress management). Migraine prophylactic agents are reasonable to try, but their effectiveness for dizziness has not been established.

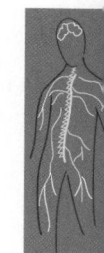

Prospectus for the Future

To optimize patient care and health care system usage, we need rigorous research to better define the clinical utility of diagnostic tests in dizziness—with a focus on defining which patients will benefit from having which test. Understanding the underlying mechanisms of migraine dizziness would be a major breakthrough.

References

Baloh RW, Honrubia V: Clinical Neurophysiology of the Vestibular System, 3rd ed. New York, Oxford University Press, 2001.

Fife TD, Iverson DJ, Lempert T, et al: Practice parameter: Therapies for benign paroxysmal positional vertigo (an evidence-based review): Report of the Quality Standards Subcommittee of the American Academy of Neurology. Neurology 70:2067-2074, 2008 (and accompanying video clips accessible at www.aan.com/go/practice/guidelines).

Disorders of the Motor System

Frederick J. Marshall

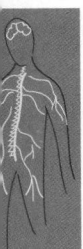

The voluntary motor system originates in the motor areas of the frontal lobe cortex that send their output caudally in the corticospinal tract. The basal ganglia and cerebellum have additional integrating, postural, and coordinating influences (Fig. 122-1). Descending influences from the red nuclei, vestibular nuclei, and brainstem reticular formation converge with descending corticospinal pathways on bulbospinal motor neurons to activate functionally automatic motor programs. At every level, afferent feedback provides input from muscle, nerves, spinal segment, brainstem, cerebellum, basal ganglia, and cortex to guide the efferent messages from the motor cortex. Figures 122-2 and 122-3 indicate the corticobasal ganglia connections and corticocerebellar loops that unconsciously precede movement.

Disease can selectively affect every level of the motor system from brain to muscle. Table 122-1 lists the anatomic locations of diseases affecting the motor system.

Symptoms and Signs of Motor System Disease

The patient with motor system disease usually complains of difficulty with accomplishing specific tasks. Patients with central nervous system (CNS) disorders (see Table 122-1) typically have difficulty with coordination, balance, and rapid movements. Muscle strength is frequently normal, and muscle atrophy (wasting) is usually lacking. Muscle tone is usually increased, characterized by spasticity or rigidity. Patients with peripheral nervous system (PNS) disorders (see Table 122-1) usually complain of difficulty with tasks; if weakness is proximal, there is impairment in climbing or descending stairs, rising from a chair, or lifting heavy objects above the head. If weakness is distal, then the patient complains of stumbling and tripping or of having problems fastening buttons or opening locks or doors with the hands.

The patient with weakness of gradual onset may not recognize it, emphasizing the useful axiom that "signs of muscle weakness precede symptoms of weakness." A patient with weakness who is unfamiliar with what is taking place may use words such as *numbness, deadness, tiredness,* or *fatigue.* In contrast, when a patient complains of *weakness,* it often results from systemic rather than neurologic disease. In such patients, strength is often normal or only mildly reduced because the complaint is usually a loss of stamina and endurance. The patient with a complaint of fatigue should be asked to distinguish between true weakness and the less specific symptoms of lassitude and asthenia. If the patient is unable to perform a specific normal activity, then true weakness is suggested. Objective evidence of weakness is established if symptoms exceed the boundaries of normal variation (e.g., double vision, drooping eyelids, difficulty swallowing, repeated aspiration of food or liquids into the airway), as opposed to the more subjective complaints of inability to lift, carry, or push an object.

CNS motor disorders (see Table 122-1) can result from focal brain or spinal cord diseases such as those that occur with stroke, tumor, or inflammatory or demyelinating disease, each of which is covered in specific chapters elsewhere in this text. CNS motor disorders can also be the result of a widespread, nonfocal *system* degeneration, which is considered in this chapter. Focal brain disease usually produces abnormalities on neuroimaging procedures. System degeneration, in contrast, seldom produces detectable abnormalities on neuroimaging and other neurodiagnostic tests until long after patients first report symptoms and have signs of abnormal function on examination.

Corticospinal diseases from system degeneration are uncommon and are characterized by upper motor neuron signs (spasticity and hyperreflexia). The most common is amyotrophic lateral sclerosis, which differs from other CNS motor diseases by the prominent involvement of both the CNS and PNS. The hereditary spastic paraplegias are rare diseases with only upper motor neuron signs.

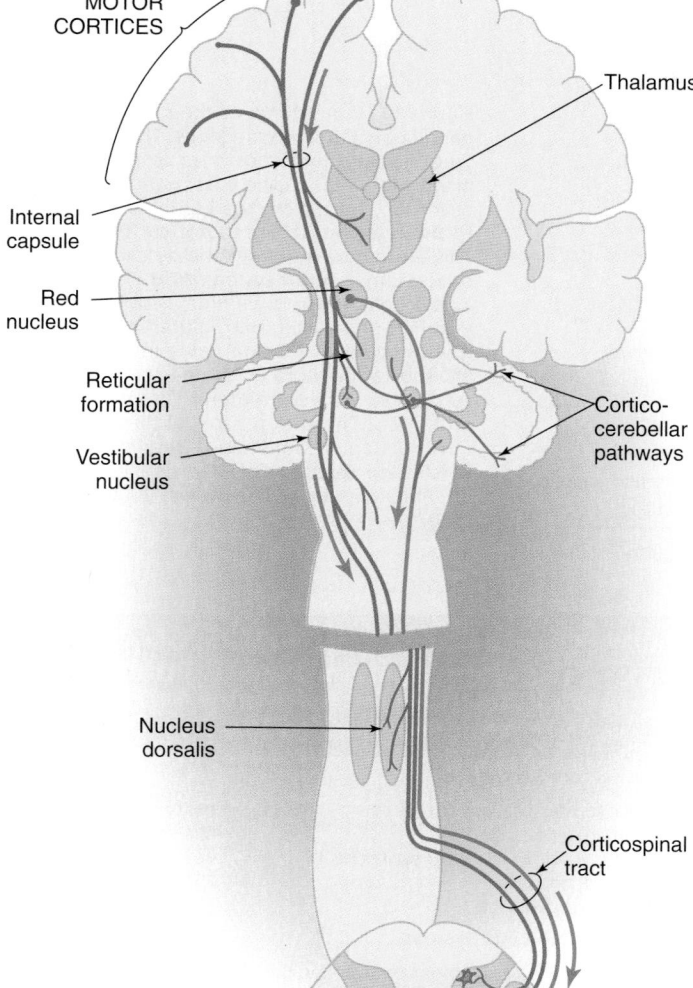

Figure 122-1 Normal human voluntary motor system.

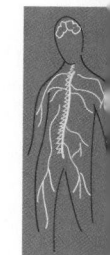

Movement Disorders and Ataxia

Central motor systems are divided into three constituents: pyramidal, extrapyramidal, and cerebellar. The pyramidal system (named for the pyramidal cross-section of fiber tracts in the medulla) is the major outflow from motor cortex to spinal cord. Lesions of the pyramidal system cause motor weakness (paresis), spasticity, and hyperreflexia. Although lesions of this system disturb motor function, they are not considered *movement disorders*. Movement disorders are caused by extrapyramidal or cerebellar dysfunction. The term *extrapyramidal* refers to the basal ganglia and their projections. The main components of the extrapyramidal system are noted in Table 122-2, and their major interconnections are depicted in Figure 122-4.

The basal ganglia receive input from the cortex and give feedback to the cortex through projections from the thalamus. Multiple neurotransmitters are involved in complex feedback loops. The basal ganglia modulate not only motor cortical activity but also the activity of association cortex, particularly in the frontal lobes. Many movement disorders therefore involve complex neurobehavioral symptoms (e.g., dementia in Huntington disease, attentional deficits and obsessive-compulsive behavior in Tourette disorder, depression in Parkinson disease). Clinicoanatomic correlations between lesions in a component of the system and development of a characteristic movement disorder or neurobehavioral syndrome remain elusive. An exception is hemiballismus, a dramatic flailing movement of the extremities on one side of the body usually caused by a lesion of the contralateral subthalamic nucleus. Neurosurgical interventions designed to ablate or stimulate specific nuclei, and neuropharmacologic treatments designed to modulate selective receptor systems are increasingly widespread.

Movement disorders entail either too little movement (hypokinesia) or too much movement (hyperkinesia). Table 122-3 outlines the hypokinetic disorders in the differential diagnosis of akinetic-rigid syndrome. The disorders listed in Table 122-3 cause progressive immobility. *Rigidity* refers to increased muscular tone throughout the range of motion. It does not vary with passive acceleration of the limb by the examiner. Lead-pipe rigidity connotes the ductile quality of metal being passively bent. Cogwheel rigidity is the superimposition of tremor on underlying rigidity. Paratonic rigidity or paratonia is a velocity-dependent resistance to passive movement. Such resistance increases as the speed of passive limb displacement increases. Patients with paratonic rigidity demonstrate *gegenhalten,* an inability to fully relax a limb for passive range-of-motion testing. This group of patients also demonstrates *mitgehen,* the tendency to *help out* as the examiner attempts to move the limb passively. Paratonia is clinically nonspecific; it is common in patients with diminished cerebral function resulting from a variety of causes. True rigidity always implies basal ganglia dysfunction on the contralateral side.

Many different hyperkinetic movements may be exhibited (Table 122-4). Accurate identification of these movements is required for proper diagnosis and treatment of extrapyramidal diseases. For example, chorea occurring in successive generations is most likely caused by Huntington disease (hereditary chorea). Parkinson disease is most likely the cause of resting tremor in an older patient with rigidity and bradykinesia (slow movement). Essential tremor (a common, often inherited disorder) is most likely the cause of action tremor in a patient without rigidity or bradykinesia).

Table 122-5 outlines a number of signs commonly associated with lesions of the cerebellar system. Disorders of proprioceptive function may result in *sensory* ataxia caused by impairment of the spinocerebellar inputs.

Hypokinetic Movement Disorders

IDIOPATHIC PARKINSON DISEASE

James Parkinson, an English physician, first described the clinical triad of tremor, bradykinesia, and muscular rigidity in 1817. Later, physicians recognized that postural instability

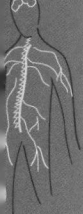

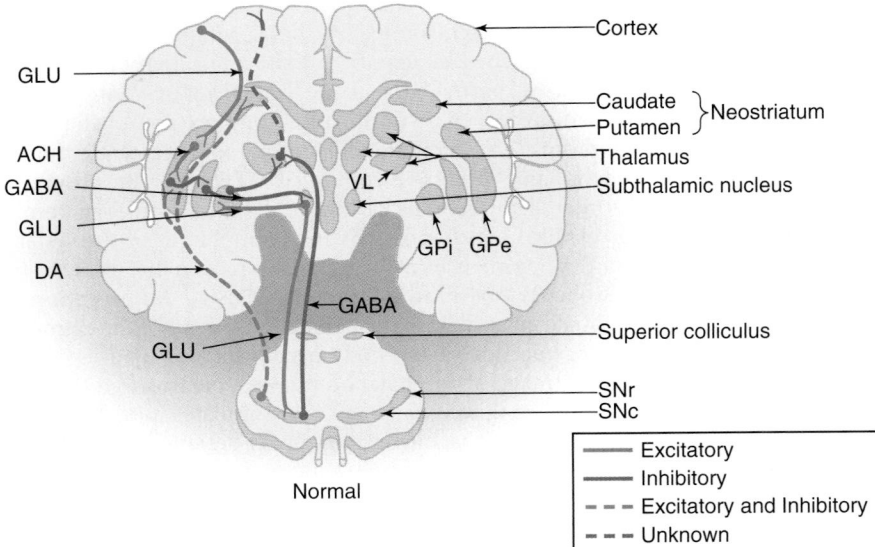

Normal

Excitatory
Inhibitory
Excitatory and Inhibitory
Unknown

Figure 122-2 Anatomy of the basal ganglia and their connections. The feedback loop proceeds from cerebral prefrontal areas to the basal ganglia and eventually back from the basal ganglia to the thalamus to the motor cortex. This ultimately regulates the descending corticospinal motor system. ACH, acetylcholine; DA, dopamine; GABA, γ-aminobutyric acid; GLU, glutamate; GP, globus pallidum (e, external; i, internal); SN, substantia nigra (c, compacta; r, reticulate); VL, ventrolateral. (From Jankovic J: The extrapyramidal disorders: Introduction. In Goldman L, Bennett JC [eds]: Cecil Textbook of Medicine, 21st ed. Philadelphia, WB Saunders, 2000, p 2078).

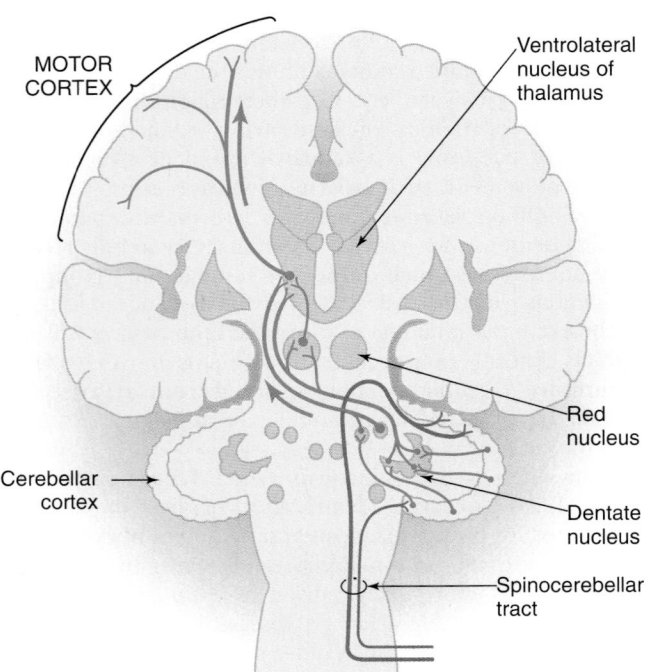

Figure 122-3 Corticocerebellar loop. The major cerebellar input is from the spinocerebellar tract. Outflow is to the motor cortex via the mesencephalon and thalamus.

Table 122-1 Anatomic Classification of Motor System Disease: Principal Disorders of the Motor System from Proximal to Distal

Central Nervous System

Corticospinal diseases (disorders of the upper motor neuron)
Extrapyramidal movement disorders
Cerebellar ataxias
Spinal cord diseases

Peripheral Nervous System

Radiculopathies and lower motor neuron diseases
Peripheral nerve disorders
  Polyneuropathy
  Focal neuropathy
Neuromuscular junction
  Myasthenia
  Lambert-Eaton myasthenic syndrome
  Botulism
Muscular disorders

Table 122-2 Major Components of the Basal Ganglia and Extrapyramidal Nervous System

Substantia nigra
  Pars reticulata
  Pars compacta
Striatum
  Caudate
  Putamen
Globus pallidus
  Pars medialis
  Pars lateralis
Subthalamus
Thalamus
  Ventroanterior
  Ventrolateral

was also a fundamental aspect of the illness. These four signs remain the diagnostic criteria for Parkinson disease. Parkinson disease affects 500,000 to 750,000 people in the United States and is a leading cause of neurologic disease in individuals older than 65 years of age. Premature death of pigmented dopaminergic neurons in the pars compacta of the substantia nigra is the underlying basis of the disease, but the cause remains unclear. Neuronal loss occurs in the substantia nigra, with characteristic eosinophilic hyaline intraneuronal inclusions called Lewy bodies. Dopamine-containing neurons with cell bodies in the substantia nigra

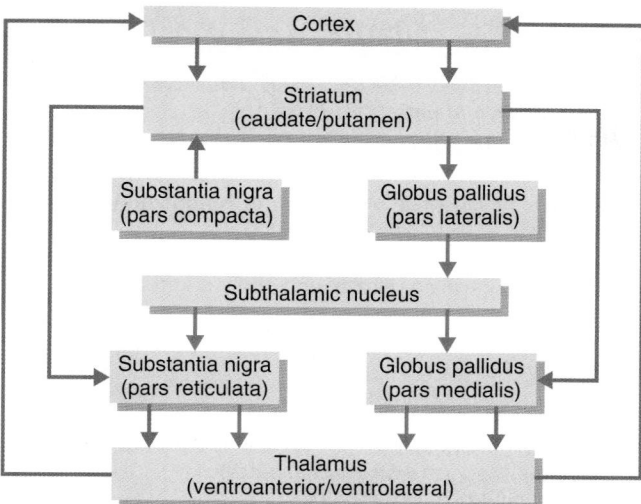

Figure 122-4 In this simplified version of the basal ganglia wiring diagram, information flows in one of two ways, either facilitating motor output by means of the direct pathway *(red lines)* or inhibiting motor output by means of the indirect pathway *(blue lines).* In Parkinson disease, loss of neurons in the pars compacta of the substantia nigra shifts the balance away from the direct pathway and toward the indirect pathway, resulting in hypokinesia. Conversely, in Huntington disease, loss of select neurons in the striatum shifts the balance away from the indirect pathway and toward the direct pathway, resulting in hyperkinesia.

Table 122-4 **Descriptive Terms of the Hyperkinesias**	
Asterixis	Transitory loss of motor tone resulting in rapid movement of a joint (the conceptual opposite of myoclonus) **(Web Video 122-2)**
Athetosis	Slow writhing movement
Ballism	Flailing movement (typically unilateral—hemiballism)
Chorea	Irregular flicking, dancelike movement **(Web Video 122-3)**
Choreoathetosis	The combination of chorea and athetosis
Dyskinesia	Nonspecific term for hyperkinesia (generally chorea, athetosis, and dystonia, alone or in combination)
Dystonia	Sustained contortion resulting from excess muscular activity across a joint: generalized, segmental, or focal **(Web Video 122-4)**
Myoclonus	Rapid jerking muscular movement: multifocal or segmental, rhythmic or irregular **(Web Video 122-5)**
Tic	Semi-suppressible motor or vocal gestural movement (may be simple, such as eye blinking or throat clearing, or complex, such as hopping or swearing)
Tremor	Rhythmic oscillating movement: predominantly at rest or with action

Table 122-3 **Differential Diagnosis of the Akinetic-Rigid Syndrome**
Idiopathic Parkinson disease
Drug-induced parkinsonism
Diffuse Lewy body disease
Progressive supranuclear palsy
Corticobasal-ganglionic degeneration
Multisystem atrophy: parkinsonian type, cerebellar type, mixed type
Vascular parkinsonism
Other hereditary neurodegenerative disorders: Huntington disease; Hallervorden-Spatz disease
Toxic parkinsonism: carbon monoxide; manganese; MPTP
Catatonia (psychosis)

MPTP, methyl-phenyl-tetrahydropyridine.

Table 122-5 **Signs of Cerebellar System Impairment**	
Ataxia	Poorly coordinated, broad-based, lurching gait
Ataxic dysarthria	Abnormal modulation of speech velocity and volume
Dysmetria	Irregular placement of voluntary limb or ocular movement
Hypometria	Movement falling short of the intended target
Hypermetria	Movement overshooting the intended target
Dysdiadochokinesis	Breakdown in precision and completeness of rapid alternating movements (as with a pronation-supination task)
Dysrhythmokinesis	Irregularity of the rhythm of rapid alternating movements or planned movement sequences
Dyssynergia	Inability to perform movement as a coordinated temporal sequence
Hypotonia	Decreased resistance to passive muscular extension (seen immediately after injury to the lateral cerebellum)
Intention tremor	Tremor orthogonal to the direction of intended movement (tends to increase in amplitude as the target is approached)
Titubation	Rhythmic rocking tremor of the trunk and head

project to the striatum (caudate and putamen), where they synapse on a variety of cell types. Early in the course of the disease, dopamine receptors in the striatum are upregulated in response to decreased dopaminergic input from the substantia nigra. This compensatory ability of the striatum is eventually overwhelmed, and progressive clinical dysfunction ensues.

In the past decade a number of monogenic causes have been identified, including the following causative genes: α-synuclein *(SNCA),* parkin, PTEN-induced kinase 1 *(PINK1), DJ-1,* and leucine-rich repeat kinase 2 *(LRRK2).* However, altogether, these gene defects likely account for only 2% to 3% of all cases of classic parkinsonism. Characterization of the encoded proteins suggests a pathogenic role

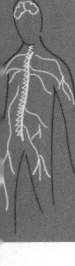

Table 122-6 Clinical Features of Parkinson Disease

Primary Features

Bradykinesia, rest tremor, rigidity, postural instability, therapeutic response to levodopa

Secondary Features

Masked facies (facial hypomimia)

Dysphagia; hypophonia or palilalia, micrographia, stooped posture, festinating gait, start hesitation, dystonic cramps

Autonomic dysfunction: orthostatic hypotension, urinary incontinence, constipation

Behavioral alterations: depression, dementia, sleep disorders including restless legs syndrome

Sensory complaints: aching, numbness, tingling

Table 122-7 Medications for Parkinson Disease

Anticholinergic Agents

Trihexyphenidyl (Artane)
Benztropine (Cogentin)

Dopamine Precursors (Combined with Peripheral Aromatic Amino Acid Decarboxylase Inhibitors)

Carbidopa-levodopa (Sinemet, Sinemet-CR, Parcopa) (regular, controlled-release, and orally disintegrating forms)
Benserazide-levodopa (Madopar) (marketed in Europe)

Dopamine Agonists

Apomorphine (Apokyn) (injectable short acting), bromocriptine (Parlodel)
Pramipexole (Mirapex)
Rotigotine (Neupro) (transdermal patch)
Ropinirole (Requip, Requip XR)

Monoamine Oxidase Type B (MAO-B) Inhibitors

Selegiline (deprenyl) (Carbex, Eldepryl, Zelapar)
Rasagiline (Azilect)

Catechol-*O*-Methyltransferase (COMT) Inhibitors

Tolcapone (Tasmar)
Entacapone (Comtan)

Catechol-*O*-Methyltransferase (COMT) Inhibitors Combined with Carbidopa-Levodopa

Entacapone-carbidopa-levodopa (Stalevo)

in the process of protein degradation and in mitochondrial function.

Symptoms and signs of Parkinson disease are listed in Table 122-6. The patient notes unilateral symptoms initially: characteristically, hand tremor, decreased arm swing, foot dragging, or micrographia. Symptoms and signs subsequently spread to involve both sides. Gradually worsening postural instability ultimately results in wheelchair confinement. Symmetrical onset of symptoms and early falls caused by postural instability are atypical of idiopathic Parkinson disease, whereas they are common in other causes of the akinetic-rigid syndrome (see Table 122-3). Tremor may be a prominent feature of idiopathic Parkinson disease, but it is not usually a prominent feature of other akinetic-rigid disease states (**Web Video 122-1**).

Treatment of Parkinson disease is outlined in Table 122-7. Carbidopa-levodopa (Sinemet) remains the mainstay of treatment for advanced Parkinson disease. Failure of bradykinesia and rigidity to improve in response to a trial of levodopa treatment raises the possibility of another disease (see Table 122-3) because these diseases typically involve primary pathologic deterioration at the level of the striatum rather than the substantia nigra.

Levodopa requires enzymatic conversion to dopamine within substantia nigra neurons. Unlike levodopa, the dopamine agonists do not compete with other amino acids to cross the blood-brain barrier; they require no enzymatic conversion and act directly at the level of the striatum, bypassing the substantia nigra. Concern has been expressed that treatment with levodopa may eventually provoke motor complications, such as *on-off* fluctuations and dyskinesias. Initiating therapy with dopamine agonists allows the physician to reserve levodopa treatment for later stages of the illness. The co-administration of a dopamine agonist in the later stages of illness may reduce the amount of levodopa required.

Selegiline delays the need for levodopa treatment in patients with early Parkinson disease. Selegiline inhibits monoamine oxidase type B, an enzyme that breaks down dopamine. Toxic free radicals generated in the normal catabolism of dopamine may damage dopaminergic neurons in the substantia nigra, which may cause Parkinson disease in patients who are vulnerable as a result of a combination of inherited risk and as yet undetermined environmental exposures. It has been postulated that selegiline may act as a neuroprotective agent if the formation of free radicals is

inhibited. Rasagiline is a second generation selective monoamine oxidase type B inhibitor. Patients may tolerate it better because it is not metabolized to amphetamine. Alternatively, selegiline is now available as an orally disintegrating tablet, which decreases production of amphetamine from first-pass hepatic metabolism.

The aromatic amino acid decarboxylase inhibitor carbidopa and the catechol-*O*-methyltransferase (COMT) inhibitors entacapone and tolcapone block the breakdown of levodopa. Co-administration of levodopa with carbidopa and a COMT inhibitor suppresses levodopa's peripheral catabolism, maximizing the amount available to cross the blood-brain barrier and prolonging its effective half-life. Tolcapone has been associated with rare but potentially lethal liver toxicity; the hepatic function of patients undergoing treatment with this drug must be monitored closely. Entacapone has no adverse effect on liver function and is now in widespread use.

Because enhancing dopaminergic neurotransmission is the underlying rationale of drug treatments for Parkinson disease, most antiparkinsonian drugs have unwanted dopaminergic side effects. These include nausea, orthostatic hypotension, hallucinations, psychosis, and dyskinesia (i.e., abnormal involuntary hyperkinetic movements such as chorea and dystonia). Management of progressive Parkinson disease requires a careful balance between the potential beneficial effects of medication and these potential side effects.

In the past decade, great advances have been made in the surgical treatment of Parkinson disease. Most centers of excellence in the care of Parkinson disease now offer deep-brain stimulation (DBS) of the subthalamic nuclei (STN) as a treatment option. This procedure is performed with the

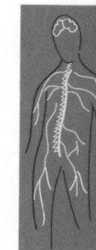

patient awake, using the combined expertise of the stereo-tactic neurosurgeon and an electrophysiologist and clinical neurologic assessment. Parameters such as the pulse frequency, pulse width, amplitude, and electrical port can be modulated to achieve dynamic suppression of output from the STN to the thalamus. This procedure can be performed bilaterally. Documented benefits in rigidity, tremor, and bradykinesia can occur; gait and postural instability are relatively refractory to treatment. Although dyskinesia increases initially, overall dyskinesia is reduced in a majority of patients with DBS by improvement of other symptoms and consequently reduction in the levodopa and dopamine agonist doses. The ideal patient is young, free of dementia or neuropsychiatric complications, and highly responsive to medications for Parkinson disease. Patients with a poor response to levodopa are less likely to benefit from DBS surgery.

DRUG-INDUCED PARKINSONISM

The most common cause of drug-induced parkinsonism is treatment with neuroleptic medication. A number of other agents may provoke a bradykinetic-rigid syndrome (Table 122-8).

DIFFUSE LEWY BODY DISEASE

Lewy body disease may be classified into three types based on the pathologic distribution of underlying Lewy bodies: brainstem, transitional, and diffuse. Restriction of Lewy bodies to the brainstem defines *Parkinson disease*. In the *transitional phase*, Lewy bodies spread to involve the limbic system. In *diffuse Lewy body disease*, clinical parkinsonism combined with prominent dementia occurs. Visual hallucinations are common, patients may be extremely sensitive to the adverse effects of neuroleptic medication, and cognitive fluctuations occur (see Chapter 116).

PROGRESSIVE SUPRANUCLEAR PALSY

In the early 1960s Steele, Richardson, and Olszewski described a series of patients who exhibited gait disturbance, falls, bradykinesia, and rigidity. Unlike patients with idiopathic Parkinson disease, patients with progressive supranuclear palsy typically do not have tremor. A progressive loss of voluntary eye movements occurs with the preservation of oculocephalic reflex eye movements (the hallmark of a supranuclear eye movement abnormality). Patients develop

Table 122-8 **Drugs Causing Bradykinesia or Rigidity**
Established
Neuroleptics (virtually all phenothiazines, butyrophenones, others)
Metoclopramide
Tetrabenazine
Reserpine
Reported
Lithium
Phenytoin
Angiotensin-converting enzyme inhibitors

dementia, pseudobulbar affect (i.e., affective lability without correlative underlying emotional content), and frontal release signs. Progression is faster than it is in patients with idiopathic Parkinson disease, and symptomatic response to dopaminergic agents is limited. The cause of progressive supranuclear palsy remains unknown. Tau-containing neurofibrillary tangles develop, with neuronal loss and gliosis involving the globus pallidus, subthalamic nucleus, substantia nigra, pons, oculomotor complex, medulla, and dentate nucleus of the cerebellum.

CORTICOBASAL-GANGLIONIC DEGENERATION

Like progressive supranuclear palsy, corticobasal-ganglionic degeneration is also a tauopathy involving neurofibrillary tangles, neuronal loss, and gliosis. Classically the disease manifests with marked asymmetry of motor dysfunction characterized by bradykinesia, rigidity, and apraxia (failure of learned motor movements) on one side of the body or in a single limb. The "alien hand" syndrome can be a hallmark of the disorder; the limb adopts seemingly deliberate movements that are not under the direct voluntary control of the patient. As the disease progresses, a combination of cortical dementia (aphasia, agnosia, apraxia) and basal-ganglia dysfunction (bradykinesia, rigidity, and postural instability, with or without tremor) becomes increasingly disabling. Asymmetry persists late into the course.

MULTISYSTEM ATROPHY

Three entities are included under the term *multisystem atrophy* (see Table 122-3). Abnormal glial cytoplasmic inclusions containing α-synuclein are the pathologic hallmark of the disorder, with progressive loss of neurons—in particular, brain nuclei—determining the particular clinical presentation. All eventually progress to a profoundly akinetic-rigid state. In olivopontocerebellar atrophy, the predominant early manifestations are cerebellar dysmetria and ataxia, with abnormalities of vocal modulation, appendicular coordination, and smooth pursuit eye movements. A dramatic and progressive loss of neurons occurs in the olivary nucleus of the medulla, pons, and cerebellum, giving rise to characteristic atrophy of these regions on computed tomography (CT) or magnetic resonance imaging (MRI). In striatonigral degeneration, predominant bradykinesia, symmetrical rigidity, and postural instability develop relatively early, typically without prominent resting tremor. These signs are relatively refractory to levodopa treatment, differentiating these from similar signs caused by idiopathic Parkinson disease. In Shy-Drager syndrome, bradykinesia, rigidity, and postural instability are combined with early and prominent loss of autonomic function. Severe orthostatic hypotension results in syncopal events. Cardiac arrhythmias, urinary incontinence, constipation, diarrhea, sudomotor instability, and disordered central temperature regulation may occur. Recently, a reclassification of multisystem atrophy has been proposed, outlining predominantly cerebellar, parkinsonian, or mixed cerebellar-parkinsonian subtypes—all of which have prominent dysautonomia as a core feature. Multisystem atrophy is a sporadic disease in which dementia, if it occurs, is a late-stage finding. A positive family history for

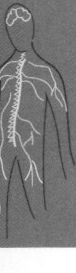

a similar disorder should suggest an alternative diagnosis such as a dominant spinocerebellar degeneration.

VASCULAR PARKINSONISM

Vascular parkinsonism is a controversial entity because its findings are varied and its pathogenesis is ill defined. Patients have signs of Parkinson disease and have microangiopathic changes in the basal ganglia that cause periventricular high T2-weighted signals on MRI. However, such changes are commonly seen on MRI in older individuals, regardless of whether they have bradykinesia and rigidity. Vascular parkinsonism is often diagnosed whenever vascular risk factors are known and periventricular white matter lesions that are evident on MRI accompany clinical evidence of parkinsonism. A lack of improvement with levodopa therapy or the overt evidence of stroke involving the basal ganglia supports this diagnosis.

TOXIC PARKINSONISM

Carbon monoxide intoxication may cause bilateral necrosis of the basal ganglia, leading to an akinetic-rigid state. Chronic exposure to manganese has also been associated with the development of parkinsonism. An intriguing clue to a possible toxic basis for idiopathic Parkinson disease was discovered in the 1970s with the report of a series of formerly asymptomatic individuals who developed bradykinesia, postural instability, tremor, and rigidity after exposure to the designer street drug 1-methyl-4-phenyl-1,2,3,6-tetrahydropyridine (MPTP). Selective uptake of this agent into pigmented cells of the substantia nigra, with conversion by monoamine oxidase type B to the toxic free radical MPP(+), accounts for selective cell death of dopaminergic neurons. MPTP has been widely studied in animal models of Parkinson disease.

Hyperkinetic Movement Disorders

ESSENTIAL TREMOR

The most common cause of tremor is *essential tremor*. This condition is inherited and ranges in severity from cosmetic to disabling. Unlike the tremor of Parkinson disease, essential tremor typically affects both sides of the body symmetrically and is more prominent with action than it is at rest. The frequency of the tremor oscillation is relatively constant, but the amplitude may vary. As with all forms of tremor, stress, sleep deprivation, and stimulants (e.g., caffeine) make the condition worse. Alcohol often relieves essential tremor. When essential tremor occurs in the context of a dominant family history, it is called *familial tremor*. Essential tremor starts somewhat earlier than it does with Parkinson disease and may affect the neck and head muscles and the voice, as well as the arms and hands. The most useful medications for essential tremor include propranolol (Inderal), primidone (Mysoline), and topiramate (Topamax). DBS surgery with electrode placement in the ventral intermediolateral nucleus of the thalamus is highly effective but should

be reserved for patients whose condition is refractory to pharmacotherapies.

OTHER CAUSES OF TREMOR

Parkinson disease tremor is worse at rest, is often slower than essential tremor, and responds best to anticholinergic treatment rather than to medications for essential tremor. Cerebellar tremor has a more irregular rhythm, is coarser than either essential tremor or the tremor of Parkinson disease, and is more pronounced as the limb approaches a target (action tremor). So-called *rubral tremor* is an extremely coarse tremor with significant intention dysmetria that occurs with lesions in the area of the red nucleus in the mesencephalon. Numerous drugs can provoke tremor, including stimulants (e.g., theophylline, methylphenidate), dopamine receptor–blocking drugs, lithium, tricyclic antidepressants, anticonvulsants (e.g., valproate, phenytoin, carbamazepine), cardiac agents (e.g., amiodarone, calcium channel blockers, procainamide), and immunosuppressive agents (e.g., cyclosporin A, corticosteroids).

DYSTONIA

Dystonia consists of sustained muscle contractions that result in abnormal postures and contortions. It may occur as a primary process or as a secondary symptom of an underlying neurologic disease (e.g., Wilson disease, Huntington disease, cerebral anoxia). Derangements in the physiologic makeup of the dopamine synapse may lead to acute drug-induced dystonic reactions. Such reactions can be life threatening if respiratory function is compromised, but they generally respond to emergent treatment with anticholinergic medication. Metoclopramide (Reglan), commonly prescribed for nausea and vomiting, may induce dystonia. DBS with implantable electrodes has been used experimentally for dystonia.

Although the primary dystonias presumably involve basal ganglia dysfunction, no underlying pathologic structure has been convincingly documented. Mutations of the *DYT* gene on chromosome 9 have been defined in some families with generalized dystonia. Five percent to 10% of patients with primary generalized dystonia are responsive to treatment with levodopa (i.e., dopa-responsive dystonia as a result of mutations of the GTP-cyclohydrolase gene), and all patients with symptoms of generalized dystonia should receive a therapeutic trial of levodopa.

A large number of common focal dystonias were once considered emotional disorders: writer's cramp, spasmodic dysphonia, and torticollis (Table 122-9). Intramuscular injection of botulinum toxin is the treatment of choice for symptomatic control of focal dystonia.

WILSON DISEASE

Wilson disease is a rare (approximately 1 per 40,000 births) but treatable autosomal recessive disorder that is debilitating and eventually fatal if left untreated. It should be considered in the differential diagnosis of new-onset hyperkinesia or parkinsonism in the young adult. Wilson disease almost never develops after the age of 50 years. Wilson disease may also exhibit neuropsychiatric manifestations. Psychosis is

Table 122-9 **Features of the Primary Dystonias**	
Feature	**Description**
Generalized (Usually Childhood Onset, Autosomal Dominant with Variable Penetrance)	
Idiopathic torsion dystonia	Intorsion of a foot, followed by progressive spread of dystonia to involve the muscles of the limbs, trunk, neck, and face
Dopa-responsive dystonia	As above, with bradykinesia and rigidity common and hyperreflexia in 25%. Dramatic response to low-dose levodopa (50-200 mg)
Focal (Usually Adult Onset, Sporadic)	
Spasmodic torticollis	Involuntary contraction of neck musculature resulting in various combinations of twisting, tilting, extension, or flexion
Meige syndrome	Lower facial or mandibular dystonia with dyskinetic movements of the tongue and lips
Blepharospasm	Involuntary forced eyelid closure
Spasmodic dysphonia	Dystonic vocal cord contraction resulting in hoarse or breathy whisper
Writer's cramp	Task-specific contortion of the hand or forearm during attempts to write

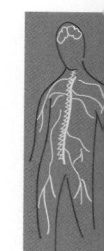

common. The disease is a systemic disorder of copper metabolism. In addition to the neurologic signs and symptoms, hepatic dysfunction (including death from fulminant hepatic failure) occurs in variable degrees. All young adult patients with a movement disorder should be screened for Wilson disease by means of a ceruloplasmin level. In patients with suspected Wilson disease, slit-lamp examination for Kayser-Fleischer rings (i.e., characteristic depositions of copper pigment in the limbus of the iris), 24-hour urine collection for copper, determination of serum copper level, and hepatic biopsy are indicated. Treatment with copper chelation and zinc can arrest further neurologic decline and can occasionally improve neurologic deficits. Mobilization of copper from liver stores can result in neurologic worsening during initial treatment with standard chelation regimens. Patients should be referred to experienced centers for initiation of treatment.

HUNTINGTON DISEASE

Huntington disease is an inexorably progressive autosomal dominant neurodegenerative disorder affecting motor function, cognition, and behavior. The mean age at onset is 40 (10% of cases begin in childhood), and the mean duration of illness is 20 years. In the adult-onset form, chorea affects the limbs and trunk. Other movement abnormalities commonly occur, including dystonia, rigidity, postural instability, and myoclonus. Bradykinesia and rigidity predominate in the juvenile-onset form. Eye movements are often abnormal early in the disease, with slowing of saccadic initiation and velocity and eventual breakdown of smooth pursuit movements. The disease involves premature death of specific neurons in the caudate and putamen.

An abnormal expansion in the number of trinucleotide CAG repeat sequences occurs in a *350-kD* gene on chromosome 4, coding for the protein huntingtin. Excessive CAG sequences encode an overly expanded number of polyglutamine repeats in the protein. CAG expansion in excess of 37 repeats is diagnostic of the disease. On average, the higher the CAG-repeat expansion, the earlier the age at onset. Despite this inverse correlation between CAG expansion length and age at onset, the variability in age at onset for a given CAG expansion is too high to enable precise prognostication regarding onset for individual patients. No treatment currently exists that slows the progression of Huntington disease. Downregulation of dopaminergic neurotransmission by means of neuroleptic agents may suppress chorea but often worsens underlying postural instability and rigidity. The U.S. Food and Drug Administration (FDA) has recently approved the vesicular monoamine transport (VMAT) inhibitor tetrabenazine for treatment of chorea associated with Huntington disease. This drug, widely available in Europe for several years, functions by depleting dopamine from the presynaptic neuron. The therapeutic window for tetrabenazine can be low, however, because it also has the potential to deplete serotonin and norepinephrine and can increase depression, parkinsonism, and akathisia (a restless hyperkinetic movement disorder). Treating depression and psychosis may enhance the patient's quality of life. Use of antenatal diagnosis and presymptomatic genetic testing of adult patients at risk for the disease raises ethical and personal questions. Presymptomatic testing of at-risk children is not indicated.

OTHER CAUSES OF CHOREA

Sydenham chorea occurs in childhood as a postinfectious complication of group A β-hemolytic streptococcal pharyngitis. The illness is usually self-limited, but prolonged chorea may occur, as may other neuropsychiatric symptoms. The caudate and STN are affected, presumably on an autoimmune basis. Some patients respond to a short course of corticosteroids. Treatment with intravenous immunoglobulin is also an option.

A number of drugs occasionally cause chorea, including isoniazid, lithium, oral contraceptives, and reserpine. Metabolic causes include thyrotoxicosis, hypoparathyroidism, and hypomagnesemia. Hemichorea may result from stroke or tumor, and autoimmune or vascular mechanisms may underlie the chorea sometimes observed in patients with lupus erythematosus.

MYOCLONUS

Myoclonus occurs in many neurologic disorders, but it may also occur in isolation. *Physiologic (hypnagogic) myoclonus* occurs in healthy individuals as they fall asleep. *Essential myoclonus* is a nonprogressive, generalized disorder that can occur as an autosomal dominant trait. Patients experience multifocal, large-amplitude lightning jerks that are provoked by action and are disabling, or they may have mild, small-amplitude jerks that do not disrupt their function. Patients with essential myoclonus almost always also have some degree of underlying dystonia. Myoclonus also occurs in generalized epilepsy syndromes that are not inherently progressive (e.g., benign myoclonus of infancy, juvenile myoclonic epilepsy) or in tonic-clonic epilepsy and progressive encephalopathy (e.g., progressive myoclonic encephalopathy). Static myoclonic encephalopathy occurs most commonly as a consequence of severe anoxia (Lance-Adams syndrome) or head trauma and may be spontaneous or action induced, multifocal, or generalized. Secondary causes of focal or multifocal myoclonus include underlying structural lesions of the nervous system (e.g., stroke, arteriovenous malformation, demyelinating disease, tumor, abscess, other infectious processes) or toxic-metabolic conditions (e.g., hypoxia, uremia, hepatic encephalopathy, sepsis, electrolyte disturbances, hormonal abnormalities). Treatment should be directed to the underlying cause. Valproate or clonazepam are commonly prescribed for symptomatic treatment of myoclonus.

TOURETTE DISORDER

In 1885, Gilles de la Tourette described a series of patients with motor and vocal tics, some of whom had coprolalia (foul language). For most of the ensuing century, Tourette disorder was considered a rare curiosity, existing on the border zone of neurology and psychiatry. Although coprolalia is an uncommon manifestation, Tourette disorder and its related primary tic disorders (e.g., chronic motor tics, chronic vocal tics, transient tic disorder) have been increasingly recognized in the past decade as common entities. A substantial proportion of children with learning disorders have Tourette disorder.

Transitory tics are a normal part of child development. Tourette disorder is defined as the history of both motor and vocal tics (for more than 1 year) with onset before the age 18 years. The tics are associated with obsessions and compulsive behavior in 50% of patients and are accompanied by attention-deficit disorder in 50% of patients. Tourette disorder is probably an autosomal dominant condition with variable penetrance.

Treatment focuses on the most functionally incapacitating aspect of the disorder (not necessarily the tics), and patients and families should be reassured that the disorder is not progressive or fatal. Approximately two thirds of patients outgrow their tics (but not necessarily the other neuropsychiatric manifestations of the illness) by adulthood. Useful medications are outlined in Table 122-10. Strategies to reduce stress on the patient, including education of parents, peers, and teachers, are frequently preferable. Treatment of attention deficit with stimulants may exacerbate tics; treatment of tics with neuroleptic drugs may blunt affect, disrupt learning, provoke depression, and lead to unwanted weight gain.

OTHER CAUSES OF TICS

Tics may be drug induced (i.e., stimulants or neuroleptic medications causing tardive tics), or they may be sympto-

Table 122-10 **Medications Used in the Management of Incapacitating Tourette Disorder**
Tics
Neuroleptics (haloperidol, pimozide, others)
Clonidine (oral or transdermal patch)
Calcium channel blockers (diltiazem, verapamil)
Benzodiazepines (clonazepam, others)
Guanfacine
Obsessive-Compulsive Behavior
Selective serotonin reuptake inhibitors (fluoxetine, sertraline, others)
Clomipramine
Attention-Deficit Disorder
Stimulants (methylphenidate, pemoline)
Clonidine
Selegiline
Tricyclic antidepressants

matic of developmental, degenerative, toxic-metabolic, or infectious neurologic disorders. Patients with chromosomal abnormalities (e.g., Down and fragile X syndromes) frequently have tics, as do those with pervasive developmental delay, anoxic encephalopathy, and autism. Tics occasionally occur in patients with Huntington disease, progressive supranuclear palsy, Creutzfeldt-Jakob disease, and encephalitis, as well as those with sequelae of carbon monoxide poisoning or hypoglycemia.

Cerebellar Ataxias

The cerebellum receives input from the spinal cord (spinocerebellar tracts), from the vestibular nuclei in the brainstem, and from pontine relays, carrying information from the motor and premotor cortex. The cerebellar cortex is made up of four main neuronal types. Granule cells input onto Purkinje cells, whose axons form the sole output of the cerebellar cortex, terminating in cerebellar nuclei or select brainstem nuclei. Golgi cells and stellate-basket cells function as inhibitory interneurons within the cerebellar cortex. The cerebellar cortex is organized into three main sagittal zones. The most medial (vermal) zone projects to the fastigial nuclei, which in turn project to the vestibulospinal and reticulospinal tracts. Injuries to this zone or its projections lead to abnormal stance and gait, truncal titubation, and disturbances of extraocular movement. The intermediate (paravermal) zone projects to the interposed nuclei, which in turn project to the red nucleus and the thalamus. Isolated injuries to this zone are rare, and clinical manifestations generally overlap with medial or lateral cerebellar syndromes. The lateral zone projects to the dentate nuclei, which in turn project to the thalamus and cerebral cortex. Injuries to this zone or its projections result in abnormal stance and gait, appendicular dysmetria, eye movement dysmetria, dysdiadochokinesia, dysrhythmokinesia, intention tremor, ataxic dysarthria, and hypotonia.

NONHEREDITARY ATAXIAS

Lesions of the cerebellum, its inflow tracts, or its outflow tracts may all be associated with ataxia. The rapid onset

Table 122-11 Hereditary Ataxias

Disease	Onset	Associated Signs
Autosomal Recessive Inheritance		
Ataxia-telangiectasia	Childhood	Telangiectasia, recurrent sinus and pulmonary infections, choreoathetosis, mental retardation in 30%, neoplasms (lymphoma, lymphocytic leukemia)
Abetalipoproteinemia (Bassen Kornzweig syndrome or acanthocytosis)	Childhood	Absent serum apolipoprotein B leads to fat malabsorption with decreased vitamins A, E, and K; retinitis pigmentosa; nystagmus
Friedreich ataxia	Childhood	Scoliosis, cardiomyopathy, dysarthria, areflexia, Babinski signs, loss of joint position and vibration sense in legs, dysmetria
Autosomal Dominant Inheritance		
Spinocerebellar ataxia types 1-8, 10-23, and 25-27	Adulthood	Variable combinations of long-tract signs, parkinsonism, dementia
Dentatorubral-pallidoluysian atrophy		Sensory loss, myoclonus, chorea
Other forms of olivopontocerebellar atrophy		Dystonia and seizures

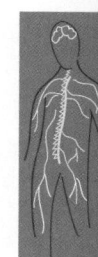

of ataxia suggests an underlying structural condition, an immune-mediated process, drug intoxication, or conversion disorder. Structural lesions of the cerebellum or its connecting tracts include tumors, demyelinating plaques, abscesses, and vascular events such as vertebrobasilar occlusion, cerebellar parenchymal hemorrhage, traumatic hematoma, and arteriovenous malformation. Immune-mediated processes include acute postinfectious cerebellitis or myoclonic encephalopathy with neuroblastoma in children, and paraneoplastic cerebellar degeneration in adults. Migraine headaches, particularly in childhood, may be accompanied by ataxia. Radiographic studies, drug screening, and cerebrospinal fluid analysis will clarify the diagnosis in most patients with acute-onset ataxia.

Chronic or progressive ataxia may result from slow-growing brain tumors (e.g., cerebellar astrocytoma, hemangioblastoma, ependymoma, medulloblastoma, supratentorial tumors), congenital malformations (e.g., basilar impression, Dandy-Walker malformation, Chiari malformation), drug effects (e.g., alcoholic cerebellar vermian degeneration, chronic phenytoin toxicity), or hereditary ataxias.

HEREDITARY ATAXIAS

Progressive ataxia is a feature of numerous hereditary neurologic diseases (Table 122-11). Determining which hereditary disease is responsible depends on a thorough assessment of the familial pattern of inheritance and knowledge of the typical age at onset and progression of symptoms and signs associated with these conditions.

Molecular tests for a number of specific hereditary ataxias have become available within the past decade, but caution should be used to ensure adequate informed consent, support services, and follow-up before such tests are used to determine a potentially fatal diagnosis, especially in presymptomatic individuals. Genetic test results have immediate implications for the risk status of extended family members. Definitive therapies are generally lacking, genetic testing is expensive, and few mechanisms can ensure against genetic testing results being used by insurers or employers to the disadvantage of the patient or family.

Similar to Huntington disease, several of the autosomal dominant spinocerebellar ataxias are caused by abnormal expansions in the number of repeated CAG codons within unique genes. These diseases display the phenomenon of *anticipation:* the age at onset is progressively younger in successive generations of a family. This phenomenon occurs because the CAG repeat length of the abnormal genes is upwardly unstable during gametogenesis, and higher CAG repeat burden results in younger age at onset. Other dominant spinocerebellar ataxias are caused by noncoding regions, through mRNA mechanisms like those elucidated in myotonic dystrophy (see Chapter 131), or through conventional mutations.

Prospectus for the Future

Advances in molecular genetics, gene profiling, stem cell research, and fetal tissue transplant techniques are all proceeding rapidly and promise to improve the diagnosis and therapy of many movement disorders in the coming decade. Initial studies of fetal nigral tissue transplantation in patients with Parkinson disease have been controversial. A number of patients developed disabling dyskinesias after receiving fetal nigral grafts. Nonetheless, the fact that these grafts survived, developed connections to target structures in the striatum, and had a functional impact on patients' parkinsonian symptoms is encouraging. More work will need to be done in animal models of parkinsonism in which dyskinesia develops. Great interest exists in developing gene therapy for Parkinson disease because creating viral vectors with relative tropism for the striatum, specifically targeting the molecular biochemistry of dopamine production and metabolism, is possible. Experimental gene therapy in animal models (e.g., rodents, primates) is promising, and early trials of gene transfection using adeno-associated virus are underway in humans. Studies of co-affected siblings with Parkinson disease have revealed new genetic loci of interest. Similar approaches hold promise in most other motor system disorders.

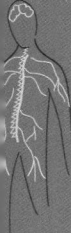

References

Klein C, Lohmann-Hedrich K: Impact of recent genetic findings in Parkinson's disease. Curr Opin Neurol 20:453-464, 2007.

Lang A: Other movement disorders. In Goldman L, Ausiello DA (eds): Cecil Textbook of Medicine, 23 ed. Philadelphia, WB Saunders, 2007.

Pahwa R, Factor S, Lyons K, et al: Practice parameter: Treatment of Parkinson disease with motor fluctuations and dyskinesia (an evidence-based review): Report of the Quality Standards Subcommittee of the American Academy of Neurology. Neurology 66:983-995, 2006.

Soong B-W, Paulson HL: Spinocerebellar ataxias: An update. Curr Opin Neurol 20:438-446, 2007.

Suchowersky O, Gronseth G, Perlmutter J, et al: Practice parameter: Neuroprotective strategies and alternative therapies for Parkinson disease (an evidence-based review): Report of the Quality Standards Subcommittee of the American Academy of Neurology. Neurology 66:976-982, 2006.

Suchowersky O, Reich S, Perlmutter J, et al: Practice parameter: Diagnosis and prognosis of new onset Parkinson disease (an evidence-based review): Report of the Quality Standards Subcommittee of the American Academy of Neurology. Neurology 66:968-975, 2006.

Vulkmann J: Update on surgery for Parkinson's disease. Curr Opinion Neurol 20:465-469, 2007.

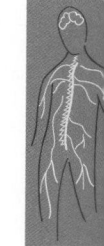

Developmental and Neurocutaneous Disorders

Emily C. de los Reyes and E. Steve Roach

Advances in magnetic resonance imaging and genetic microarray technology have improved our understanding of neurodevelopmental disorders. High-resolution neuroimaging now detects congenital and developmental abnormalities that were previously unrecognized. Moreover, neurodevelopmental disorders in one group are now being diagnosed with alarming frequency: the autistic spectrum disorders. Although the exact cause of these disorders is unclear, this chapter will discuss the various syndromes associated with autistic spectrum disorders.

Neural Tube Defects

Neural tube defects are developmental defects associated with failure of the anterior and posterior neuropore to close during the 24th to 26th days of gestation. Disturbances of neural tube closure manifest with a spectrum of abnormalities including anencephaly, encephalocele, and myelomeningocele with Chiari II malformation. Genetic factors may play a role, because there is a higher incidence in trisomy syndromes. However, folic acid affects cell division, and folic acid supplementation during pregnancy has been advocated in pregnancies as a preventive measure.

Chiari malformation is the displacement of the hindbrain (cerebellar) tonsils more than 5 mm below the foramen magnum. Chiari I malformation is frequently asymptomatic, but some individuals develop headaches or lower cranial neuropathies. Additional signs include syringomyelia or scoliosis. Surgical decompression may be necessary when the symptoms are severe.

Chiari II malformations are characterized by displacement of the cerebellum and lower brainstem through the foramen magnum. These malformations typically occur in conjunction with a myelomeningocele and hydrocephalus, so seizures, cognitive delay, paraplegia, and sphincter dysfunction are common. Treatment is surgical repair of the myelomeningocele with subsequent shunting of the hydrocephalus. Bladder dysfunction may necessitate intermittent catheterization and treatment of urinary tract infections and genitourinary reflux.

Spinal Malformations

Developmental anomalies of the vertebral bodies are common and cause pain and neurologic symptoms when they cause scoliosis or accelerated degenerative changes of the spine. Neurologic disability is likely when cord anomalies are present or when they compress neural structures or alter cerebrospinal fluid flow.

Tethered Spinal Cord

A tethered spinal cord results from an anomalous filum terminale that causes either lack of normal ascent of the conus medullaris to the L1 vertebral level or an ischemic or metabolic disturbance of the caudal spinal cord. Associated spinal anomalies are common: diastematomyelia (split cord), spinal lipomas, dermal sinuses, and fibrolipomas of the filum terminale. Affected individuals exhibit bladder and sexual dysfunction and leg extremity weakness or spasticity. Symptoms develop more often in childhood or adolescence. Cutaneous hypertrichosis, hemangiomas, and/or dimpling often occurs in the lumbar area. Treatment involves surgical release of the tethered cord.

Syringomyelia

Syringomyelia is a cystic cavitation of the central portion of the spinal cord, whereas hydromyelia is the dilatation of the central canal. Both are usually located in the cervical cord but may extend in to the medullary region (syringobulbia) or toward the thoracic cord. A syringomyelia may develop in association with Chiari malformations, trauma, tumor, or a tethered cord. The classic presentation is a dissociated sensory loss (pain and temperature loss with preservation of light touch and proprioception) in the neck, arms, or legs. A cervical lesion produces a capelike dissociated sensory loss of the arms and shoulder, along with atrophy of the hands and arms with increased tone and hyperreflexia in the legs. Extension into the medulla may cause lower cranial neuropathies. Diagnosis is confirmed by magnetic resonance imaging. If the cause is associated with Chiari II malformation, then posterior fossa decompression and shunting of the hydrocephalus may improve the symptoms. Rarely, a large syrinx unassociated with a Chiari malformation may require shunting

Brain Malformations

Malformations of cortical development can be identified with accuracy through neuroimaging procedures. Most such lesions develop during the first trimester. Disorders of ventral induction include holoprosencephaly, agenesis of the corpus callosum, and septo-optic dysplasia. Holoprosencephaly is the failure of the prosencephalon to divide into two separate structures. The disorder is heterogeneous with a spectrum of abnormalities ranging from alobar holoprosencephaly (cortex with a single ventricle) to lobar holoprosencephaly (cerebral hemispheres are mostly separated except for the frontal lobes).

Migrational abnormalities occurring during the second to the fourth month of gestation include lissencephaly, schizencephaly, and polygyria and pachygyria. Diagnosis is established by magnetic resonance imaging. Symptoms include cognitive delay, spasticity, and seizures. Intractable seizures may require resection of the focal cortical dysplasias. These disorders may be caused by congenital intrauterine infections, gene mutations, or teratogenic agents. The identification of various gene mutations (Table 123-1) has allowed genetic counseling for families of affected children. X-linked gene mutation is milder in women because of X inactivation.

Autism and Autism Spectrum Disorders

Autism spectrum disorders are characterized by impaired social communication, delayed expressive and receptive language, and repetitive, stereotypic behavior. Although these disorders are increasingly diagnosed, their cause remains unclear. Autism is clearly genetic in individuals with tuberous sclerosis complex (TSC), Rett syndrome, and fragile X syndrome. The treatment that has shown the most promise is intensive behavioral intervention. Speech therapy is helpful. Alternative medicine is popular but has not been studied in a well-designed manner. Genetic syndromes that have a high risk of autistic spectrum disorders are discussed in the following paragraphs.

RETT SYNDROME

Rett syndrome is an X-linked dominant disorder caused by a mutation of the methyl-cytosine binding protein (MeCP2) that functions as a transcriptional repressor. The identification of this gene has permitted characterization of the phenotypic spectrum of Rett syndrome. Patients with Rett syndrome develop normally until the first year of life, when they manifest loss of communication skills and deceleration of head growth. A classic feature is loss of hand function and stereotypic hand wringing. Seizures are common. Diagnosis is confirmed by DNA testing. Treatment is currently limited to treatment of seizures and spasticity.

FRAGILE X SYNDROME

Next to Down syndrome, fragile X syndrome is the most common genetic cause of mental retardation and is caused by expanded CGG triplet repeats (>200 CGG repeats) in the first exon of the fragile X mental retardation gene (*FMR1*). Symptomatic females have a milder mental

---

Table 123-1 Malformations of Central Nervous System Cortical Development Recognized on Magnetic Resonance Imaging

Malformation	Locus	Gene(s)	Clinical Manifestations
Holoprosencephaly	7q36,13q32 2p21 Trisomy 13 or 18	SHH, ZIC2 SIX3	Dysmorphic features Mental retardation Pituitary dysfunction
Lissencephaly	17p13.3	LIS-1	Mental retardation Epilepsy Motor disability
Lissencephaly with agenesis of corpus callosum	Xq22.3	RELN	
Band heterotopia	Xq22.3	DCX	Epilepsy
Polymicrogyria	Xq28 11p13	Unknown PAX6	Epilepsy Cognitive delay
Schizencephaly	10q26		Mental retardation Spasticity Epilepsy
Periventricular nodular	Xq28 20q13.13	FLNA ARFGEF2	Normal vs heterotopia Severe epilepsy

ARFGEF2, ADP-ribosylation factor guanine nucleotide–exchange factor 2, brefeldin A–inhibited; *DCX*, doublecortin; *FLNA*, both filamin 1 gene and filamin A, alpha; *LIS*, lissencephaly; *PAX6*, paired box; *RELN*, reelin; *SHH*, sonic hedgehog gene; *SIX3*, homolog of *Drosophila so*; *ZIC2*, homolog of *Drosophila* odd-paired or *opa*.

deficiency compared with their male counterparts. Children have a distinctive appearance: macrocephaly with a long narrow face, and prominent ears, pubertal macroorchidism, and joint laxity. Neurobehavioral features include autism and attention deficit disorder. Some individuals with 55 to 200 CGG repeats develop ataxia and tremor and cognitive dysfunction beginning in adulthood, which may mimic parkinsonism.

Neurocutaneous Disorders

Neurocutaneous disorders are congenital, often hereditary disorders characterized by pathognomonic cutaneous and central nervous system lesions that uniquely distinguish each disease. The most important of these syndromes are neurofibromatosis (types 1 and 2), TSC, Sturge-Weber syndrome, and von Hippel-Lindau disease. There is considerable variability in the spectrum of clinical manifestations.

NEUROFIBROMATOSIS TYPE 1

Neurofibromatosis type 1 (NF1) is an autosomal dominant disorder with a prevalence of 1 in 3000 births. Almost half of the cases are sporadic mutations. The *NF1* gene on chromosome 17q expresses neurofibromin, a tumor-suppressor protein. In NF1, there is loss of expression of neurofibromin, leading to dysregulated cell growth and differentiation. Mutations in the *NF1* gene are identified in approximately 75% of patients, but no correlation exists between a particular genotype and phenotype. Many manifestations of NF1 appear during childhood and adult life. The criteria for the diagnosis include two or more of the following: (1) six or more café-au-lait macules larger than 5 mm in prepubertal patients or more than 15 mm in postpubertal individuals, (2) two or more neurofibromas of any type or one plexiform neurofibroma, (3) axillary or inguinal freckling, (4) sphenoid bone dysplasia, (5) optic nerve glioma, (6) Lisch nodules, and (7) a family history of NF1. Diagnosis is based on clinical criteria, supplemented by neuroimaging findings, or by DNA testing. Other manifestations include learning disabilities, attention deficit disorder, macrocephaly, and epilepsy. Important complications include scoliosis, gastrointestinal neurofibromas, pheochromocytomas, and renal artery stenosis. Most individuals with NF1 do not require treatment. Painful subcutaneous neurofibromas can be excised. Intraspinal and intracranial tumors are typically benign and treated surgically. Genetic counseling should be provided to all patients and families. New mutations occasionally occur in the germline of an unaffected parent and can be transmitted to more than one offspring.

NEUROFIBROMATOSIS TYPE 2

Neurofibromatosis type 2 (NF2) is an autosomal-dominant disease that occurs less frequently than NF1 (approximately 1 in 50,000 individuals). The *NF2* gene is located on chromosome 22q. The gene product (merlin) is a cytoskeletal protein. Most NF2 patients have bilateral VIII nerve schwannomas. However, multiple meningiomas and multiple other tumors are common. Skin lesions are present in a minority of patients with NF2, and the diagnosis is based on the following criteria: (1) bilateral VIII nerve tumors detected by magnetic resonance imaging, (2) a family member with either NF2 or unilateral VIII nerve schwannoma, and (3) juvenile posterior subcapsular lens opacities. Symptoms of NF2 begin in the second to fourth decades. Removal of the schwannomas and other tumors is often usually indicated, and early recognition is important for successful treatment of VIII nerve tumors.

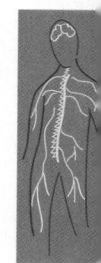

TUBEROUS SCLEROSIS COMPLEX

TSC causes hamartomatous lesions involving multiple organs at different stages in the course of the disease. Transmission is autosomal dominant, but sporadic cases are frequent because of spontaneous mutations. The incidence is 1 in 6000. The *TSC* gene loci are at chromosome 9p34 for *TSC1* and chromosome 16p for *TSC2*. The gene product for *TSC1* is hamartin and for *TSC2*, tuberin. Both gene products interact with the mammalian target of rapamycin (mTOR), which is essential in cell growth, proliferation, and angiogenesis. Hereditary cases not linked to these two loci also occur.

The most significant organs affected include the brain (cortical tubers, subependymal giant cell astrocytomas), heart (cardiac rhabdomyomas), skin (facial angiofibromas, hypomelanotic skin macules or "ash leaf spot," shagreen patches, and subungual fibromas), kidney (renal angiomyolipoma), eye (retinal hamartoma), and lung (pulmonary lymphangioleiomyomatosis).

Seizures, most commonly infantile spasms, are the usual early clinical presentation. Treatment is directed toward the epilepsy, especially for infantile spasms. A surgical approach may be necessary for intractable epilepsy. Subependymal nodules may enlarge and cause hydrocephalus. The lesions enlarge especially during adolescence. Renal angiomyolipomas are prone to hemorrhage. Pulmonary lymphangioleiomyomatosis may be life threatening, especially in females. Cognitive disability may require special education.

STURGE-WEBER SYNDROME

Sturge-Weber syndrome is variably characterized by an upper facial vascular nevus (port-wine stain), a leptomeningeal angioma, and ocular abnormalities (glaucoma and choroidal hemangioma). The disorder occurs sporadically in less than 1 in 20,000 births. Clinical features include focal epilepsy, cognitive impairment, and, less frequently, hemiparesis, hemianopia, or glaucoma. If antiepileptic drugs do not control seizures, surgical excision of epileptogenic areas may be indicated.

The diagnosis is usually made by the port-wine stain and neuroimaging confirmation of the intracranial abnormality. Magnetic resonance imaging is a more reliable tool for diagnosis because calcifications on computed tomographic scans are classic but unnecessary for the diagnosis. However, 80% of people with a facial port-wine stain have no associated brain involvement. Laser treatment of the port-wine stain is of cosmetic benefit.

VON HIPPEL–LINDAU DISEASE (CENTRAL NERVOUS SYSTEM ANGIOMATOSIS)

Von Hippel–Lindau disease is an autosomal-dominant disorder caused by a defective tumor suppressor gene (*VHL* gene) on chromosome 3p25-p26. It is variably associated with retinal angiomas, brain and spinal cord hemangioblastomas, renal cell carcinomas, pheochromocytomas, angiomas of the liver and kidney, and cysts of the pancreas, kidney, liver, and epididymis. The diagnosis is established if patients have more than one central nervous system hemangioblastoma, one hemangioblastoma with a visceral manifestation of the disease, or one manifestation of the disease and a known family history.

Symptoms typically begin during the third or fourth decade. Retinal inflammation with exudates, hemorrhage, and retinal detachment may antedate cerebellar symptoms (headache, vertigo, and vomiting) or signs (incoordination, dysmetria, and ataxia).

Retinal detachments and tumors are treated by laser therapy. Brain tumors, renal cell carcinomas, pheochromocytomas, and epididymal tumors are treated surgically. Early evaluation and repeated imaging studies are indicated once the diagnosis has been made, and genetically at-risk individuals should also be evaluated.

Prospectus for the Future

Understanding of the neurocutaneous disorders associated with tumor development is increasing. As the molecular signals causing tumors are clarified, novel genetic treatment strategies will become feasible. Improved imaging and surgical techniques are already making it possible to treat some aspects of the neurocutaneous disorders.

References

Barkovich AJ, Kuzniecky RI, Jackson GD, et al: A developmental and genetic classification for malformations of cortical development. Neurology 65:1873-1887, 2005.

Brega AG, Goodrich G, Bennett RE, et al: The primary cognitive deficit among males with fragile X-associated tremor/ataxia syndrome (FXTAS) is a dysexecutive syndrome. J Clin Exp Neuropsychol 15:1-17, 2008.

Guerrini R, Marini C: Genetic malformations of cortical development. Exp Brain Res 173:3, 2003.

Hankinson TC, Klimo P, Feldstein N: Chiari malformations, syringohydromyelia and scoliosis. Neurosurg Clin North Am 18:549-568, 2007.

Nass R, Crino P: Tuberous sclerosis complex: A tale of two genes, Neurology 70:904-905, 2008.

Roach ES, Miller VS: Neurocutaneous Disorders. New York, Cambridge University Press, 2004.

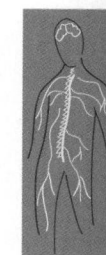

Cerebrovascular Disease

Sinéad M. Murphy and Timothy J. Counihan

The term *cerebrovascular disease* refers to disorders of the arterial or venous circulatory systems of the central nervous system. Stroke is a clinical syndrome defined by the World Health Organization as "rapidly developing clinical signs of focal or global disturbance lasting 24 hours or longer or leading to death with no apparent cause other than of vascular origin." Approximately 80% of strokes are ischemic in origin. *Focal* ischemic stroke is caused by either thrombotic or embolic occlusion of a major artery, whereas *global* ischemia usually results from inadequate cerebral perfusion such as that occurring after cardiac arrest or ventricular fibrillation. Rarely is isolated cerebral hypoxia (such as occurs in carbon monoxide poisoning or asphyxiation) a cause of stroke.

Epidemiology

Stroke remains the third leading medical cause of death and the leading cause of acquired physical disability in developed countries. Since 1990 the incidence of stroke in the United States has declined, with an annual incidence of approximately 250 per 100,000 population, accounting for about 1 in every 16 deaths. Mortality from stroke has also declined with advances in medical care. Rates of stroke among men and women are similar. The incidence and rate of mortality from stroke are higher in blacks than whites. Although the reasons for the decline in the incidence of stroke remain unclear, a greater understanding of the importance of controlling risk factors in stroke prevention may be in part responsible. This decrease in incidence is coincident with the decline of cardiovascular deaths and better control of hypertension and other risk factors (Table 124-1). In addition, the increasing public awareness of the warning symptoms of stroke as constituting a *brain attack* (analogous to chest pain as a warning of a *heart attack*) is beginning to result in earlier presentation and therefore access to acute stroke treatments.

Anatomy

Two pairs of major arteries, the carotid (anterior circulation) and vertebral (posterior circulation) arteries, supply the brain (Fig. 124-1).

ANTERIOR CIRCULATION

The common carotid artery bifurcates into an internal and an external branch at the level of the thyroid cartilage in the neck. The internal carotid artery (ICA) gives off no branches within the neck, enters the skull through the carotid canal in the petrous part of the temporal bone, and passes through the cavernous sinus as the carotid siphon. Within the cavernous sinus the ICA is in close proximity to the oculomotor, trochlear, and abducens nerves (cranial nerves III, IV, and VI) as well as the ophthalmic and maxillary branches of the trigeminal nerve (cranial nerve V). Small branches are given off to supply the adjacent meninges and posterior lobe of the hypophysis before the ICA pierces the dura. The ICA then gives off the ophthalmic, posterior communicating, and anterior choroidal arteries before bifurcating into the anterior cerebral artery (ACA) and middle cerebral artery (MCA). The ACA supplies the medial surfaces of the cerebral hemispheres, and the MCA supplies the lateral surface (convexity), in addition to much of the basal ganglia and subcortical white matter.

POSTERIOR CIRCULATION

The vertebral arteries (VAs) arise from the subclavian arteries and course upward within the transverse processes of the cervical vertebrae. The extracranial VA gives off a branch to form the anterior spinal artery. The first intracranial branch of the VA is the posterior inferior cerebellar artery (PICA), which supplies the posterolateral medulla, inferior vermis, choroid plexus of the fourth ventricle, and inferior cerebellum. The two VAs unite to form the basilar artery (BA) at

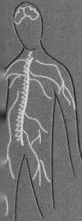

Table 124-1 **Risk Factors for Ischemic Stroke**
Diabetes
Hypertension
Smoking
Family history of premature vascular disease
Hyperlipidemia
Atrial fibrillation
History of transient ischemic attack
History of recent myocardial infarction
History of congestive heart failure (left ventricular ejection fraction <25%)
Drugs (sympathomimetics, oral contraceptive pill, cocaine)

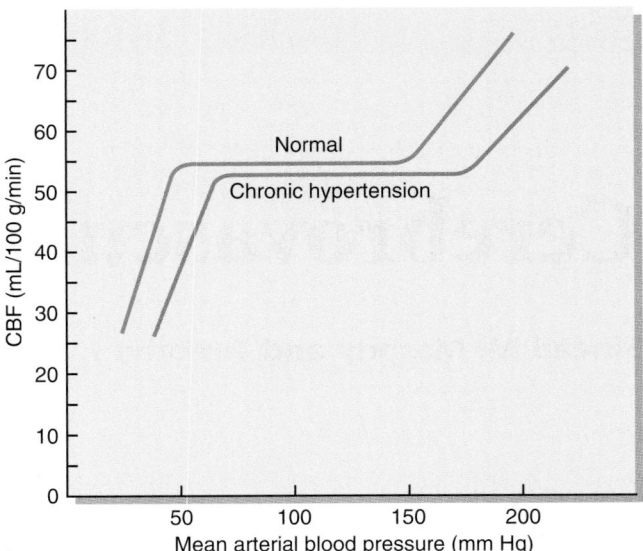

Figure 124-2 Autoregulatory cerebral blood flow (CBF) response to changes in mean arterial pressure in normotensive and chronically hypertensive persons. Note the shift of the curve toward higher mean pressures with chronic hypertension. (From Pulsinelli WA: Cerebrovascular diseases-principles. In Goldman L, Bennett JC [eds]: Cecil Textbook of Medicine, 21st ed. Philadelphia, WB Saunders, 2000, p 2097).

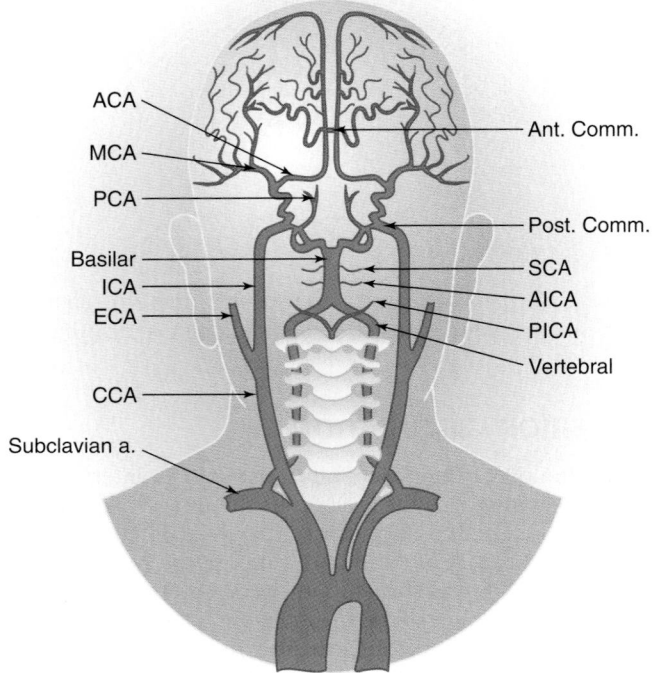

Figure 124-1 Coronal view of the extracranial and intracranial arterial supply to the brain. Vessels forming the circle of Willis are highlighted. A, artery; ACA, anterior cerebral artery; AICA, anterior inferior cerebellar artery; Ant Comm, anterior communicating artery; CCA, common carotid artery; ECA, external carotid artery; ICA, internal carotid artery; MCA, middle cerebral artery; PCA, posterior cerebral artery; PICA, posterior inferior cerebellar artery; Post Comm, posterior communicating artery; SCA, superior cerebellar artery. (Modified from Lord R: Surgery of Occlusive Cerebrovascular Disease. St Louis, Mosby, 1986).

the pontomedullary junction. The BA supplies the remainder of the cerebellum via the anterior inferior cerebellar artery (AICA) and superior cerebellar artery (SCA). The BA also supplies the pons via the paramedian, long and short circumferential branches before bifurcating into the posterior cerebral arteries (PCAs) at the level of the pontomesencephalic junction.

CIRCLE OF WILLIS

The circle of Willis is formed at the base of the brain by the union of both ACAs via the anterior communicating artery

and the union of the ICA with the PCA via the posterior communicating artery (see Fig. 124-1). Hence communication exists between both anterior circulations, as well as between the posterior and anterior circulations on each side. Congenital anomalies of the circle are frequent; they include hypoplasia or atresia of a PCA or ACA, which may reduce collateral blood supply if an adjacent vessel becomes occluded.

CEREBRAL VENOUS CIRCULATION

Superficial veins drain into the transverse, superior sagittal, and cavernous sinuses. The deep venous drainage is via the great vein of Galen, which drains into the straight sinus, which in turn drains into the torcula along with the sagittal sinus. Blood drains from the torcula to the transverse sinus, then to the sigmoid sinus, and thereafter the jugular vein. Anterior venous drainage is via the cavernous sinus, which communicates with the contralateral cavernous sinus, the transverse sinus via the superior petrosal sinus, and the inferior petrosal sinus, which drains directly into the jugular bulb.

Physiologic Factors

Unlike other body tissues, the brain has few energy stores but relies on a sizable and reliable cerebral blood flow (CBF) to meet its energy demands. CBF averages 50 mL/100 g of brain tissue per minute. A complex system of neural pathways regulates CBF in a process known as *autoregulation*, which maintains CBF at a constant level despite wide fluctuations in cerebral perfusion pressure (CPP) (Fig. 124-2). CBF remains relatively constant when the mean arterial pressure (MAP) remains between 50 and 150 mm Hg. In the case of chronic systemic hypertension, however, both the upper and lower levels of autoregulation are raised, which indicates a higher tolerance of hypertension but a greater susceptibility to the effects of hypotension. CPP is the difference between MAP and intracranial pressure (ICP). CPP is usually approximately 80 mm Hg. When CPP falls below 50 mm Hg there is evidence of ischemia and reduced cellular channel activity.

Ischemic Stroke

PATHOGENESIS

Cerebral ischemia may result from thrombotic or embolic occlusion of a major vessel that reduces blood flow within the involved vascular territory, or it may be a consequence of diminished systemic perfusion. Prolonged brain ischemia results in infarction, characterized histologically by necrosis of neurons, glia, and endothelial cells. Cerebral infarcts are classified as either *pale* (anemic) or *hemorrhagic* (in areas of endothelial necrosis). In transitional zones between normally perfused tissue and the infarcted central core is a rim of moderately ischemic tissue known as the *ischemic penumbra*, which is the target area for treatment trials of neuroprotective agents.

Global cerebral ischemia usually results from cardiac arrest or ventricular fibrillation. Some neuronal populations are selectively vulnerable to transient global ischemia, particularly neurons of the hippocampus, cerebellar Purkinje cells, and the deeper layers of the cerebral cortex (inducing so-called *laminar necrosis*). Pure hypoxia causes cerebral dysfunction (exhibited clinically as lethargy and confusion) but rarely produces irreversible brain injury unless accompanied by other factors such as hypoglycemia.

When CBF falls to 20 mL/100 mg of brain per minute, neuronal function is affected and electrical activity of cortical cells ceases. The critical threshold for irreversible cell damage is about 10 mL/100 g of brain per minute. At this level of hypoperfusion mitochondrial metabolism is inhibited and anaerobic metabolism of glucose occurs, causing a rise in lactate and thus acidosis. Intracellular membranes are no longer able to control ion fluxes. Potassium leaks out of cells; sodium, water, and calcium enter cells, causing cytotoxic edema (see later). Activation of membrane lipases further compromises cell membrane integrity and leads to release of excitatory neurotransmitters, which in turn may further exacerbate tissue injury. For a short period of time the cells may remain viable if perfusion is restored.

CEREBRAL EDEMA

Cerebral edema may be intracellular (cytotoxic) or interstitial (vasogenic). Intracellular edema develops rapidly in ischemic neurons as energy-dependent ion-channel pumps fail, whereas vasogenic edema occurs as a result of damage to endothelial cells, disrupting the blood-brain barrier and allowing macromolecules such as plasma proteins to enter the interstitial space. Fluid accumulates over 3 to 5 days after an ischemic stroke and can increase brain water content by as much as 10%; such large volume increases can lead to transtentorial herniation and death.

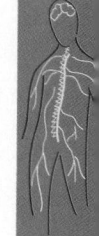

Table 124-2 **Causes of Cerebral Ischemia**
Focal
Large artery atherothrombotic
• In-situ thrombosis
• Artery-to-artery embolism
Cardioembolism
• Atrial fibrillation
• Intracardiac thrombus
• Cardiomyopathy
• Atrial myxoma
• Valvular vegetations
• Paradoxical embolism via patent foramen ovale
Small vessel disease
Other determined cause
• Fibromuscular dysplasia, moyamoya disease
• Vasculitis
• Dissection (spontaneous, traumatic)
• Vasospasm (migraine, subarachnoid hemorrhage)
• Drugs (cocaine, sympathomimetics, oral contraceptive pill)
• Fat or air embolism
• Sickle cell disease
• Hypercoagulable state
• Homocystinuria
• Antiphospholipid syndrome (lupus anticoagulant, anticardiolipin antibodies)
• Protein C or protein S deficiency
• Paraneoplastic disorder
Undetermined or cryptogenic
Global
Hypoperfusion
Cardiac arrest
Ventricular fibrillation

ETIOLOGIC FACTORS

Table 124-2 lists the major causes of acute cerebral ischemia. The TOAST classification system is often used for classification of stroke mechanism. This includes large artery atherosclerosis, which accounts for approximately one quarter of strokes, either through embolization of plaque to distal vessels (artery-to-artery embolus) or by in situ thrombosis. Certain sites of the cerebral vasculature are more prone to the development of atheromatous plaques (Fig. 124-3). Cardioembolism makes up 20% to 30% of ischemic strokes, arising most commonly as a result of atrial fibrillation. Mural thrombi, valvular vegetations, and atrial myxomas are also potential sources of embolus, as are *paradoxical emboli* (emboli of venous origin passing through a patent foramen ovale [PFO]). Small vessel disease accounts for another 20% to 30% of strokes, with a small proportion having other causes, including arterial dissection, vasculitis, and illicit drug use such as cocaine; in 20% to 30% of stroke patients the mechanism remains unclear (*cryptogenic* stroke).

Certain conditions predispose younger patients to stroke (Table 124-3).

TRANSIENT ISCHEMIC ATTACK VERSUS STROKE

A transient ischemic attack (TIA) is a brief episode of neurologic dysfunction caused by focal brain or retinal ischemia, with clinical symptoms typically lasting less than 1 hour. The previous 24-hour time window has largely been abandoned; some patients with only transient symptoms may have

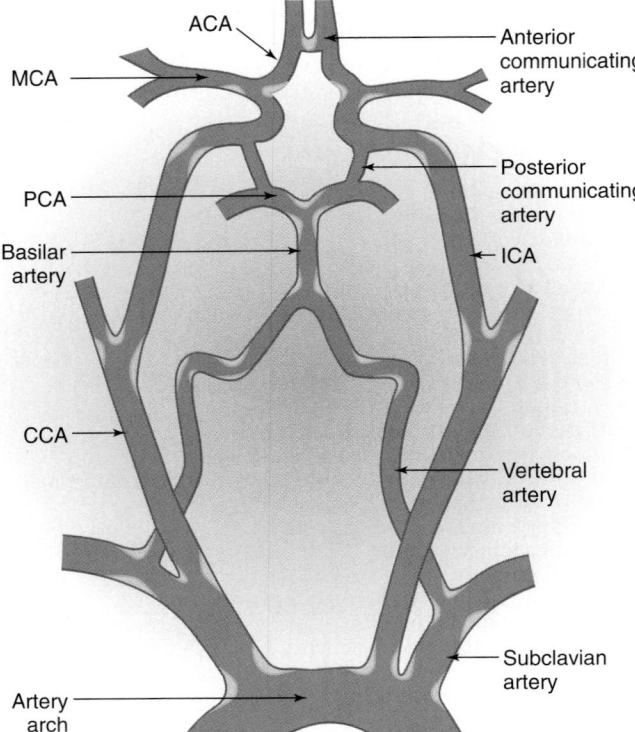

Figure 124-3 Sites of predilection for atheromatous plaque. ACA, anterior cerebral artery; CCA, common carotid artery; ICA, internal carotid artery; MCA, middle cerebral artery; PCA, posterior cerebral artery. (From Caplan LR: Stroke—A Clinical Approach. Boston, Butterworth-Heinemann, 1993).

Table 124-3 **Causes of Stroke in Young Adults**
Migraine
Arterial dissection
Drugs (cocaine, heroin, oral contraceptive pill)
Premature atherosclerosis (homocystinuria, hyperlipidemia)
Postpartum angiopathy
Cardiac Factors
Atrial septal defect
Patent foramen ovale
Mitral valve prolapse
Endocarditis
Hematologic Factors
Deficiency states (antithrombin III, protein S, protein C)
Disseminated intravascular coagulation
Thrombotic thrombocytopenic purpura
Inflammatory Factors
Systemic lupus erythematosus
Polyarteritis nodosa
Neurosyphilis
Cryoglobulinemia
Other Factors
Fibromuscular dysplasia
Moyamoya disease

imaging evidence of established infarction. In most instances the maximal clinical deficit occurs at the onset of symptoms, with subsequent recovery. Several factors may contribute to symptom progression (often referred to as a *stroke in evolution*), including propagation of a thrombus or progression of cerebral edema or hemorrhage into an infarcted area. Coexistent medical conditions such as systemic hypotension, fever, hyperglycemia, or hypoxemia may further adversely affect the outcome.

LACUNAR STROKE

A *cerebral lacuna* is a small, deep infarction involving a penetrating branch of a large cerebral artery. Lacunae are usually associated with chronic hypertension, although they are occasionally found in normotensive patients, presumably as a result of microatheroma of penetrating arteries, especially of the basal ganglia, thalamus, and white matter of the internal capsule and pons.

Probably the most common clinical syndrome caused by a lacunar stroke is *pure motor hemiparesis,* resulting from a lesion in the internal capsule. Another common lacunar syndrome is *ataxic hemiparesis* with both unilateral weakness and ataxia; the responsible lesion is usually in the internal capsule or pons. Other lacunar syndromes include *pure sensory stroke* and *dysarthria–clumsy hand* syndromes. The clinical pattern of weakness in lacunar syndromes is typically that of face-arm-leg paresis affected in equal proportion.

BRAINSTEM SYNDROMES

A number of brainstem syndromes have been described, with a combination of contralateral hemiplegia and cranial nerve dysfunction. *Weber syndrome,* caused by a midbrain lesion, is associated with an ipsilateral cranial nerve III palsy and contralateral weakness; *Claude syndrome,* caused by a lesion in the red nucleus, consists of a cranial nerve III palsy with a contralateral *rubral* tremor. *Millard-Gubler syndrome* results from a lesion of the ventral pons, manifesting with a contralateral hemiplegia and ipsilateral cranial nerve VI and VII palsies. *Raymond syndrome,* also caused by a ventral pontine lesion, causes an ipsilateral sixth nerve palsy with a contralateral hemiplegia. In the lateral medulla, a syndrome involving cranial nerves IX and X, Horner syndrome, cerebellar ataxia, and crossed hemibody pain and temperature loss is known as *Wallenberg syndrome.* This syndrome is most often the result of occlusion of the ipsilateral VA with resulting ischemia in the territory of the PICA.

Major Stroke Syndromes

The clinical manifestations of ischemic stroke are summarized in Table 124-4.

INTERNAL CAROTID ARTERY

TIAs that occur in the anterior circulation affect either the retinal artery or MCA distribution most frequently. Symptoms of retinal artery involvement consist of several seconds of a *graying out* of vision in one eye or monocular blindness *(amaurosis fugax),* often described as being like a curtain coming down over the affected eye. An important finding on retinoscopy is the presence of refractile arterial lesions, which represent cholesterol crystals *(Hollenhorst plaques)*

Table 124-4 Clinical Manifestations of Ischemic Stroke

Occluded Vessel	Clinical Signs
ICA	Ipsilateral blindness (variable) MCA syndrome
MCA	Contralateral hemiparesis, hemisensory loss (face or arm more than leg) Aphasia (dominant) or anosognosia (nondominant) Homonymous hemianopsia (variable)
ACA	Contralateral hemiparesis, hemisensory loss (leg more than arm) Abulia (especially if bilateral)
VA or PICA	Ipsilateral facial sensory loss, hemiataxia, nystagmus, Horner syndrome Contralateral loss of temperature or pain sensation Dysphagia
SCA	Gait ataxia, nausea, vertigo, dysarthria
BA	Quadriparesis, dysarthria, dysphagia, diplopia, somnolence, amnesia
PCA	Contralateral homonymous hemianopsia, amnesia, sensory loss

ACA, anterior cerebral artery; BA, basilar artery; ICA, internal carotid artery; MCA, middle cerebral artery; PCA, posterior cerebral artery; PICA, posterior inferior cerebellar artery; SCA, superior cerebellar artery; VA, vertebral artery.

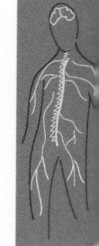

that have become detached from a more proximal cholesterol plaque. Most anterior circulation TIAs occur in the setting of significant stenosis or ulceration of the ICA (>75%); cardiogenic embolism accounts for some of the remainder. Other causes to consider include traumatic or spontaneous arterial dissection.

Acute occlusion of a previously widely patent ICA usually results in contralateral hemiplegia and hemisensory loss, reflecting ischemia in the MCA territory. Headache frequently accompanies ICA occlusion. The extent of the deficit depends on the availability of collateral circulation; in the case of occlusion of a previously severely stenotic ICA, little or no clinical deficit may be apparent, because of extensive collateral circulation. Severe bilateral ICA stenosis may occasionally cause *border zone (watershed)* ischemia (between the ACA and MCA) in the setting of systemic hypotension; this results in a well-recognized clinical syndrome consisting of bilateral proximal limb weakness (*man-in-a-barrel* syndrome). The clinical recognition of ICA stenosis or occlusion may be unreliable because although the presence of a bruit in the region of the angle of the jaw suggests significant extracranial vascular disease, it does not distinguish the external carotid artery from the ICA.

ANTERIOR CEREBRAL ARTERY

Occlusion of the ACA distal to the anterior communicating artery causes weakness and sensory loss in the contralateral leg. Other clinical manifestations include urinary incontinence and *abulia*, a state of akinetic mutism reflecting bilateral frontal lobe dysfunction.

MIDDLE CEREBRAL ARTERY

Embolism accounts for the majority of MCA occlusions. Emboli may be either cardiogenic or artery to artery from the ICA. Occlusion of the main MCA trunk results in contralateral hemiplegia, hemianesthesia, and homonymous hemianopsia with a gaze preference away from the side of the hemiplegia. The hemiplegia usually affects the face and arm more than the leg. A global aphasia occurs with dominant hemisphere lesions, and anosognosia occurs with nondominant hemisphere involvement. Occasionally, selective occlusion of the lenticulostriate branches from the proximal MCA causes capsular infarction without evidence of cortical infarction, as a result of collateral filling of the distal MCA. Occlusion of the superior division of the MCA causes faciobrachial weakness; an expressive (Broca) aphasia results from dominant hemisphere lesions, or a motor neglect (characterized by motor impersistence and spatial disorientation) results from lesions in the nondominant side. Inferior division occlusion usually produces impairment of sensory perception (astereognosis) and occasionally a visual field disturbance. Dominant hemisphere lesions result in a fluent (Wernicke) aphasia.

VERTEBROBASILAR ISCHEMIA

Vertebrobasilar ischemia produces various combinations of symptoms such as dizziness (vertigo), diplopia, ataxia, bilateral sensory or motor symptoms, and fluctuating episodes of drowsiness. Scintillations or transient visual field deficits may indicate ischemia in the PCA distribution. Distinguishing the vertigo of vertebrobasilar ischemia from labyrinthine vertigo can be difficult, although isolated positional vertigo is more likely to be of labyrinthine origin.

VERTEBROBASILAR OCCLUSION

Occlusion of the vertebral or basilar arteries or their branches (PICAs, AICA, and SCA) results in discrete syndromes (see Table 124-4). Acute infarction of the cerebellum from occlusion of any of its three supplying vessels may result in its swelling within the posterior fossa, causing obstruction of the fourth ventricle, and obstructive hydrocephalus. Such patients require close monitoring and occasionally neurosurgical intervention.

BA occlusion produces massive brainstem dysfunction and is often fatal. If the medulla is spared, a number of syndromes can occur, including the *locked-in syndrome*, in which patients are fully awake yet quadriplegic and can communicate only by means of vertical eye movements and blinking.

POSTERIOR CEREBRAL ARTERY OCCLUSION

Proximal PCA occlusions cause contralateral hemiparesis (from damage to the cerebral peduncle), hemisensory loss (thalamus), amnesia (medial temporal lobe), and hemianopsia. Macular (central) vision may be spared because of collateral vessels from the MCA. Dominant thalamic involvement may cause aphasia and thus simulate an anterior circulation stroke.

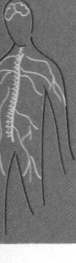

Table 124-5 **Causes of Cerebral Venous Sinus Thrombosis**
Hematoloic conditions
Paroxysmal nocturnal hemoglobinuria
Thrombotic thrombocytopenic purpura
Sickle cell disease
Polycythemia
Protein C or S deficiency
Antithrombin III deficiency
Lupus anticoagulant
Factor V Leiden deficiency
Prothrombin gene mutation
Malignancy
Pregnancy
Inflammatory bowel disease
Collagen vascular conditions
Systemic lupus erythematosus
Wegener granulomatosis
Behçet syndrome
Drugs (oral contraceptive pill, steroids)
Nephrotic syndrome
Dehydration

CEREBRAL VENOUS THROMBOSIS

Occlusion of the cerebral venous sinuses may occur in several settings, often in association with a hyperviscosity or hypercoagulable state (Table 124-5). The condition is associated with pregnancy. The clinical picture varies: patients may have headache, seizures, or focal neurologic symptoms; they often have papilledema on examination. The diagnosis frequently rests on imaging findings: bilateral hemorrhagic infarctions in a parasagittal distribution are common, as are areas of extensive white matter edema. Contrast-enhanced computed tomography (CT) may demonstrate the *empty delta* sign, suggesting a filling defect in the sagittal sinus. Magnetic resonance venography (MRV) or formal cerebral angiography should confirm the sinus filling defect.

Diagnosis

Evaluation of the patient with a suspected stroke should seek to answer three questions: Is it a stroke? Where is the lesion? And what is the mechanism? Some useful bedside pointers that may be elicited from the history and help define the stroke mechanism include the time of symptom onset and the temporal course and progression of symptoms. The type of activity preceding symptom onset and the presence of accompanying symptoms (such as headache, vomiting, or syncope) are also useful, as is the presence or absence of stroke risk factors.

The physical examination determines lesion localization and identifies clues to pathogenesis. A thorough cardiovascular examination, including blood pressure and cardiac rhythm, is essential. Palpation of the facial artery occasionally discloses reversal of flow, which suggests ICA occlusion. Ophthalmoscopy can detect platelet and cholesterol emboli, as well as giving information about the chronicity and sever-

ity of systemic hypertension. Papilledema may accompany cerebral venous thrombosis.

Ancillary blood tests include a complete blood count, sedimentation rate, glucose, coagulation screen, and fasting lipid profile. Toxicology screen (e.g., for cocaine) may be useful in young patients with unexplained stroke, especially in the setting of intracerebral hemorrhage (ICH). In young patients and those with unexplained venous sinus thrombosis, a search for a hypercoagulable state is necessary (see Tables 124-3 and 124-5).

Brain imaging with CT is the most reliable test for differentiating ischemic stroke from hemorrhage. With advances in technology it is now possible to detect early infarct signs on CT within the first 6 hours after symptom onset. These include hyperdense MCA sign, attenuation of the lentiform nucleus, loss of the insular ribbon, and sulcal effacement (Fig. 124-4). Magnetic resonance imaging (MRI) may be used to verify infarction if the diagnosis remains in doubt, and can be useful in determination of stroke mechanism (Fig. 124-5).

The extracranial carotid arteries can be assessed with duplex ultrasonography or magnetic resonance angiography (MRA). Cerebral angiography is reserved for such indications as cerebral vasculitis and cerebral aneurysms.

Differential Diagnosis

TIAs need to be distinguished from other paroxysmal events affecting the nervous system. In rare cases, patients with migraine headache have weakness contralateral to the side of the headache *(hemiplegic migraine)*. Some partial-onset seizures are followed by a transient hemiparesis *(Todd paralysis)*. Metabolic conditions such as hyponatremia, hypoglycemia, and hyperglycemia can all cause focal neurologic disturbance, which may be mistaken for stroke; however, in such cases routine blood tests should make the diagnosis clear.

The acute onset of a stroke generally distinguishes it from other brain lesions, although hemorrhage into a primary or metastatic tumor may simulate stroke. Strokes and seizures may coexist, and 10% of strokes are associated with seizure at the time of onset. As a general rule, a single, unilateral stroke rarely produces an alteration of consciousness.

Primary Stroke Prevention

The identification and reduction of stroke risk factors (see Table 124-1), including therapy for hypertension, cessation of smoking, and treatment of diabetes and hyperlipidemia, as well as treatment with antiplatelet agents for individuals with vascular risk factors have led to a decline in the incidence of stroke.

ATRIAL FIBRILLATION

Atrial fibrillation occurs in approximately 10% of people over the age of 80. The most devastating complication of atrial fibrillation is thromboembolic stroke. Twenty percent

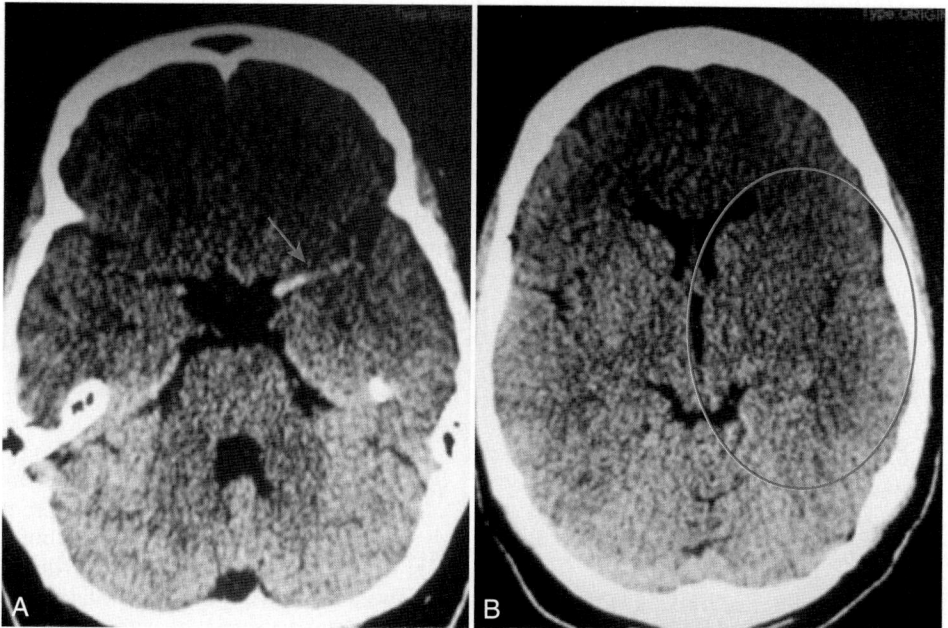

Figure 124-4 Early signs of infarction on computed tomography of the brain. **A,** Hyperdense middle cerebral artery sign *(red arrow)* and **B,** hypoattenuation of the left caudate and lentiform nuclei, loss of the insular ribbon, and sulcal effacement *(outlined in red).*

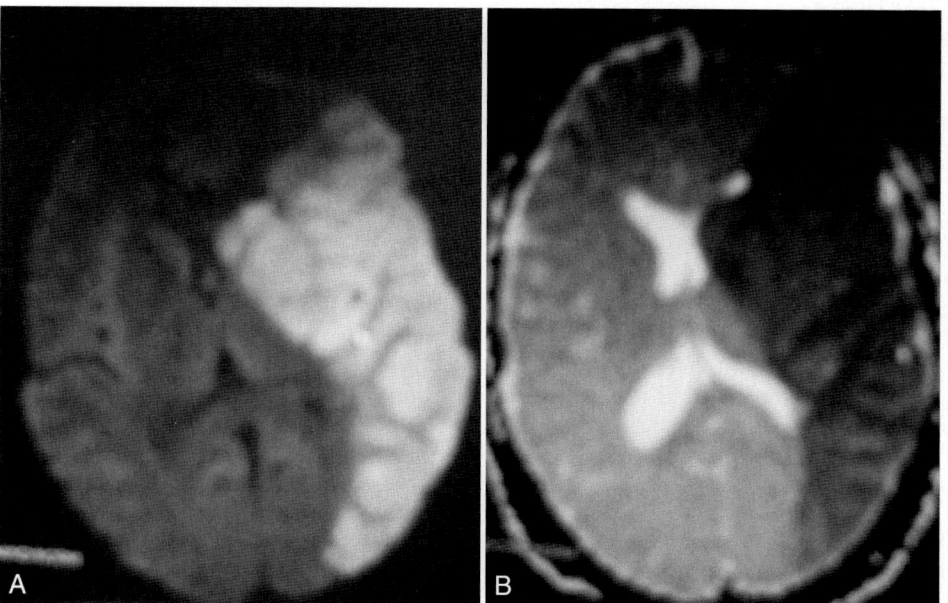

Figure 124-5 Magnetic resonance imaging scan of the brain of the same patient shown in Figure 124-4. **A,** Diffusion-weighted image (DWI) shows bright signal in the left middle cerebral artery territory. **B,** Apparent diffusion coefficient (ADC) shows dark signal in the same area, confirming acute infarction.

to 30% of ischemic strokes are cardioembolic in origin. The risk of stroke in patients with atrial fibrillation depends on a wide variety of risk factors, including age, sex, and the presence of comorbid conditions. All patients with atrial fibrillation require investigation with electrocardiography, thyroid function tests, and transthoracic echocardiography. In general, the presence of valvular heart disease increases the annual risk of stroke 17-fold. For these patients, anticoagulation with warfarin to an international normalized ratio (INR) of 2 to 3 is recommended. Patients with prosthetic heart valves require long-term anticoagulation. Patients with

paroxysmal (self-terminating) atrial fibrillation have the same risk of stroke as patients in permanent atrial fibrillation. Patients with an episode lasting less than 48 hours may be candidates for electrical cardioversion without the need for anticoagulation. The CHADS score is used to estimate the risk of stroke in patients with nonvalvular atrial fibrillation. The presence of congestive cardiac failure (C), hypertension (H), age >75 years (A), and diabetes (D) each scores one point, and a history of prior stroke or TIA (S) scores two points. A CHADS score of two or more is associated with an annual risk of stroke of over 4%. International treatment

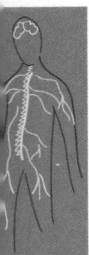

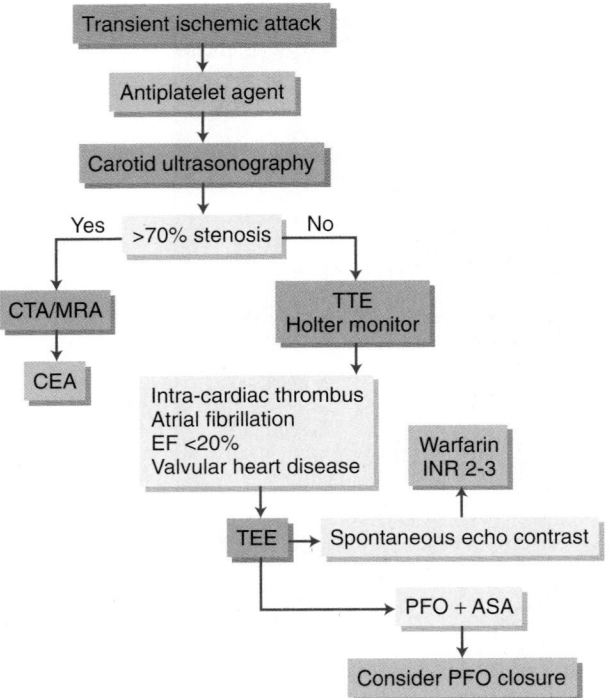

Figure 124-6 Algorithm for the treatment of transient ischemic attacks (TIAs). ASA, atrial septal aneurysm; CTA, computed tomography angiography; EF, ejection fraction; INR, international normalized ratio; MRA, magnetic resonance angiography; PFO, patent foramen ovale; TEE, transesophageal echocardiography; TTE, transthoracic echocardiography.

recommendations are aspirin 325 mg/day for those with a CHADS score of 0; for those with a CHADS score of 1, aspirin or warfarin may be used depending on patient preference. Patients with a CHADS score of 2 or more should be anticoagulated unless there is a specific contraindication. Patients with bacterial endocarditis should not receive warfarin because of the risk of cerebral hemorrhage from septic embolization. New direct thrombin inhibitors such as dabigatran are being evaluated as possible oral alternatives to warfarin for the future.

TRANSIENT ISCHEMIC ATTACK

The occurrence of a TIA or stroke is a significant risk factor for recurrent stroke, with an average 5% risk per year, although the annual risk of stroke after an episode of amaurosis fugax is only 1% to 2%.

Hospital admission is advisable for new-onset and recurrent TIAs unless a confident diagnosis of the cause of the event can be made. Imaging studies (carotid Doppler ultrasound or MRA of the neck) and cardiac investigations should be performed and a decision made promptly to treat the patient as appropriate (Fig. 124-6).

Antiplatelet therapy with aspirin, with or without dipyridamole, or clopidogrel has been shown to reduce the risk of recurrent events. Patients with a significant risk for cardiogenic thromboembolism should be treated with warfarin.

CAROTID STENOSIS

For patients with extracranial ICA stenoses of more than 70% (with or without symptoms of ischemia in that vascular

distribution), *carotid endarterectomy* reduces the risk of stroke. In high-risk patients, carotid artery stenting has emerged as an alternative to endarterectomy. For patients with moderate (60% to 70%) asymptomatic carotid stenosis, evidence that early endarterectomy is superior to deferred surgery is increasing, but only if the surgical center has a very low complication rate. In patients with an asymptomatic bruit or extracranial carotid stenosis of less than 60%, treatment with antiplatelet therapy may be effective.

Management of Acute Ischemic Stroke

GENERAL MEASURES

Specific medical and nursing measures should be initiated in cases of acute stroke, with particular emphasis on reducing the risk of complications from immobility, such as pneumonia, deep venous thrombosis, and urinary tract infection. The early introduction of physical, occupational, and speech therapy and a thorough evaluation of swallowing ability reduce morbidity. Judicious treatment of hypertension and hyperglycemia and correction of dehydration should be instituted. Prevention and prompt treatment of hyperthermia with antipyretics may reduce the extent of the deficit. Early awareness of poststroke depressive symptoms is especially important in preparing patients for rehabilitation.

USE OF ANTICOAGULANTS

No evidence has been found to support the use of anticoagulation (heparin) in the management of acute stroke. Although heparin might reduce the risk of early recurrent stroke, any benefit is offset by the increased risk of intracranial hemorrhage. Antiplatelet therapy remains the treatment of choice to prevent recurrent thromboembolism in the majority of patients with stroke. Anticoagulation may be appropriate in selected patients with cervical artery dissection, basilar thrombus, or suspected propagation of thrombus or stroke in evolution. Cranial CT is necessary before institution of heparin to confirm or rule out intracerebral or subarachnoid hemorrhage. Baseline prothrombin time, partial thromboplastin time, and platelet count, as well as tests for hypercoagulable states, should be obtained before initiation of therapy. A history of active peptic ulceration or uncontrolled hypertension (systolic blood pressure consistently >200 mm Hg) precludes the use of anticoagulants, unless the benefits clearly outweigh the risks.

THROMBOLYSIS

Patients who are within 3 hours of the onset of ischemic stroke should be considered for intravenous recombinant tissue-type plasminogen activator (rt-PA). A thorough clinical evaluation is essential to determine whether the patient is an appropriate candidate for the treatment (Fig. 124-7). The risks (6% risk of symptomatic intracranial hemorrhage) and benefits (50% chance of little or no disability at 3 months, compared with 38% chance without rt-PA) must be fully explained to the patient and family so that an informed decision can be made rapidly. The odds for a favorable outcome at 3 months improve the earlier the

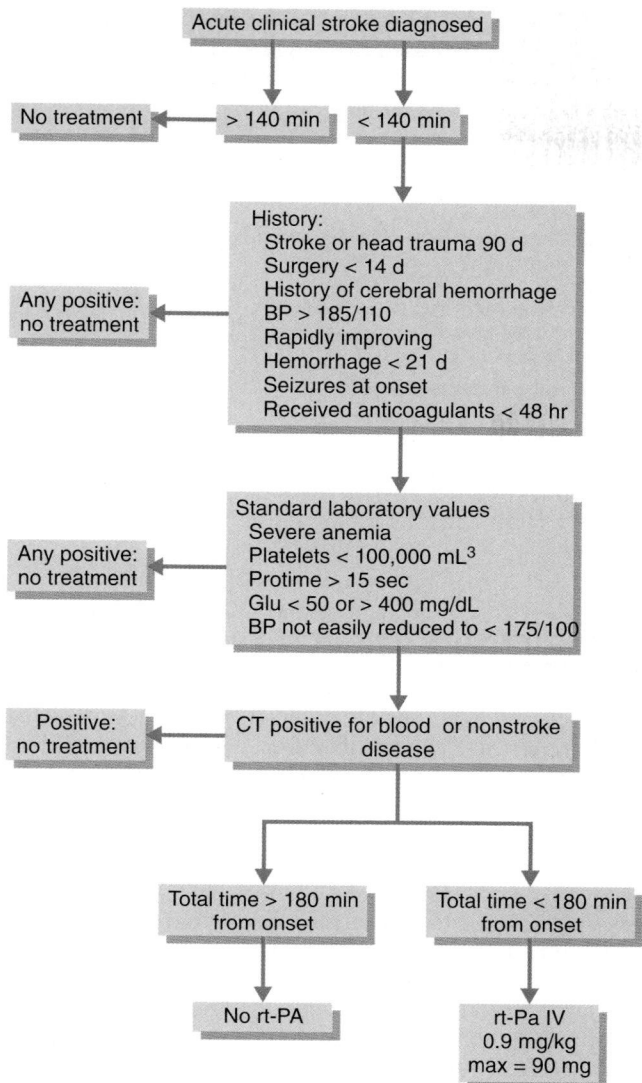

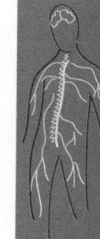

Figure 124-7 Evaluating acute stroke for safe recombinant tissue-type plasminogen activator (rt-PA) therapy. BP, blood pressure; CT, computed tomography; Glu, glucose; IV, intravenous. (Data from National Institute of Neurological Disorders and Stroke rt-PA Stroke Study Group: Tissue plasminogen activator for acute ischemic stroke. N Engl J Med 333:1581-1587, 1996.)

treatment is administered within the 3-hour window. There is increasing evidence that the benefit of thrombolysis exists up to 4.5 hours after symptom onset. Careful monitoring of blood pressure and avoidance of anticoagulants and antiplatelet agents are required for 24 hours after rt-PA administration.

There is increasing evidence that intra-arterial thrombolysis is effective for acute stroke treatment up to 6 hours after stroke onset. A potential future development of thrombolytic therapy may be combination therapy with neuroprotective agents (such as glutamate antagonists and magnesium), which may extend the therapeutic time window beyond 3 hours. Use of platelet glycoprotein IIb/IIIa complex antagonists is also under study.

MANAGEMENT OF HYPERTENSION

In the setting of an acute stroke, care must be taken regarding blood pressure control. Antihypertensive therapy is instituted if the blood pressure persistently exceeds 220 mm Hg systolic or 120 mm Hg diastolic (except in patients undergoing thrombolysis, in whom more stringent guidelines apply). Less marked elevations of blood pressure should not be treated acutely. Ideally an agent with a short half-life that can be easily titrated, such as intravenous labetalol, is used in the acute setting when necessary.

MANAGEMENT OF CEREBRAL EDEMA

Only in large hemispheric infarction is ischemic cerebral edema sufficient to cause brain shift and transtentorial herniation. This is termed *malignant MCA syndrome* and usually results from infarction of the entire MCA territory in younger patients. If signs of herniation appear, airway intubation and mechanical hyperventilation produce transient cerebral vasoconstriction and may reduce ICP. Mannitol acts by reducing the volume of the surrounding unaffected brain, but its effects are also transient. Corticosteroids are of no benefit in cytotoxic edema.

Decompressive hemicraniectomy has been shown to reduce mortality and increases the number of patients with a favorable functional outcome in patients with malignant MCA syndrome.

HYPERTENSIVE ENCEPHALOPATHY

The term *hypertensive encephalopathy* refers to the diffuse cerebral effects of severe hypertension that are not caused by infarction or hemorrhage and that are potentially reversible with control of blood pressure. Patients experience headache, visual blurring (obscurations), confusion, and drowsiness. Seizures may develop. The blood pressure is typically very high (250/150 mm Hg), and papilledema and retinal hemorrhages are usually apparent on funduscopic examination. CT and MRI show diffuse cerebral edema with a predilection for the occipital lobes. A related disorder, *reversible posterior leukoencephalopathy syndrome*, has been described in hypertensive patients taking cyclosporin, tacrolimus, and erythropoietin.

Hypertensive encephalopathy is a medical emergency. Treatment should be directed to the prompt but controlled lowering of blood pressure (e.g. with sodium nitroprusside), with care taken to avoid hypotension. The condition is clinically and pathophysiologically analogous to eclampsia.

REHABILITATION

The majority of stroke-related deaths result from medical complications (e.g., pneumonia, myocardial infarction, sepsis) rather than the neurologic deficit. Admission to a specialist stroke unit improves functional outcome and reduces medical complications that follow stroke.

TREATMENT OF CEREBRAL VENOUS SINUS THROMBOSIS

Acute anticoagulation with heparin is indicated for treatment of cerebral venous sinus thrombosis, even in the presence of hemorrhage. Interventional therapy with intra-sinus rt-PA has been used in situations where the patient does not respond to anticoagulation. Warfarin is indicated

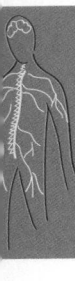

for prevention of recurrent cerebral venous sinus thrombosis; patients are usually treated for a minimum of 6 months.

SECONDARY PREVENTION OF ISCHEMIC STROKE

Recent multicenter clinical trials have shown that aggressive control of stroke risk factors reduces the rate of recurrence. The use of cholesterol-lowering agents and angiotensin-converting enzyme inhibitors reduces the rate of stroke recurrence, even in normotensive patients.

Antiplatelet Therapy

Prophylactic therapy with aspirin, with or without dipyridamole, or clopidogrel prevents recurrent events. Aspirin inhibits platelet aggregation by blocking platelet cyclooxygenase and thus prevents formation of thromboxane. Dipyridamole is a phosphodiesterase inhibitor that blocks uptake and metabolism of adenosine by vascular endothelial cells as well as potentiating the antiaggregating effects of prostacyclin. Clopidogrel inhibits ADP-induced platelet aggregation. All may be used for secondary stroke prevention. The addition of aspirin to clopidogrel does not confer added benefit for stroke prevention, as there is a significantly increased risk of hemorrhage.

Anticoagulation

Warfarin is indicated for secondary stroke prevention in the setting of atrial fibrillation, in patients with severely reduced ejection fraction, and in those with valvular heart disease. Warfarin has not yet been proven any more effective than aspirin for secondary prevention of stroke in patients with PFO or intracranial ICA stenosis, although trials are ongoing.

Hypertension

Hypertension is a well-recognized risk factor for ischemic and hemorrhagic stroke. A target blood pressure of less than 140/90 mm Hg is appropriate. Studies have indicated that the use of angiotensin-converting enzyme inhibitors in combination with a thiazide diuretic reduces the risk of stroke recurrence, even in normotensive patients.

Lipid-Lowering Agents

There is evidence that treatment with 3-hydroxy-3-methylglutaryl-coenzyme A (HMG-CoA) reductase inhibitors ("statins") reduces stroke recurrence. This seems to be independent of their cholesterol-lowering effects and may result in part from upregulation of endothelial nitric oxide synthase and anti-inflammatory properties. All patients with TIA or stroke should be treated with a statin regardless of cholesterol level.

Intracerebral Hemorrhage

ICH may be diffuse (subarachnoid hemorrhage) or focal (intraparenchymal) and accounts for 20% of all strokes. Table 124-6 lists the causes of spontaneous ICH. The acute rise in ICP from arterial rupture frequently results in loss of consciousness at the outset; some patients die from herniation.

Table 124-6 **Causes of Spontaneous Intracerebral Hemorrhage**
Intraparenchymal Hemorrhage
Hypertension
Amyloid (congophilic) angiopathy
Arteriovenous malformation
Bleeding diathesis
Drugs (amphetamines, cocaine, anticoagulants, thrombolytics)
Tumors
Cerebral venous sinus thrombosis
Hemorrhagic transformation of ischemic stroke
Cerebral vasculitis
Subarachnoid Hemorrhage
Congenital saccular aneurysm (85%)
Mycotic aneurysm
Arteriovenous malformation
Unknown (10%)

HYPERTENSIVE INTRACEREBRAL HEMORRHAGE

Hypertensive ICH often occurs at the same sites that are affected in lacunar infarction. Pathologically, microaneurysms known as *Charcot-Bouchard aneurysms* have been identified in some patients. The most common sites for hypertensive hemorrhage are the putamen (40%), thalamus (12%), lobar white matter (15% to 20%), caudate (8%), pons (8%), and cerebellum (8%). Although CT readily identifies the hemorrhage, several clinical findings may help localize the site (Table 124-7). In general, severity of headache correlates with the size of the lesion. Diminished level of alertness is caused by mass effect, increased ICP, or direct involvement of the brainstem reticular-activating system. Seizures are slightly more frequent during the acute phase in ICH than in ischemic stroke. Both basal ganglia and thalamic hemorrhages may rupture into the adjacent ventricle and result in secondary hydrocephalus; cerebellar hemorrhage may cause obstructive hydrocephalus as a result of compression of the fourth ventricle.

With intracerebral hematoma, the patient's level of consciousness often deteriorates during the first 24 to 48 hours after the initial symptoms, usually because of the development of edema around the lesion or expansion of the hematoma. Edema that is sufficient to cause significant brain shift results in herniation of brain tissue. In addition to causing direct pressure on vital brainstem structures, herniation may cause compression of adjacent blood vessels (particularly the PCAs and ACAs), resulting in infarction.

LOBAR HEMORRHAGE

Lobar hemorrhages occur in a peripheral distribution of the cerebral cortex. They are usually smaller than hypertensive ICHs and have a more benign prognosis. In young persons, lobar hemorrhages may be secondary to arteriovenous malformations or ingestion of sympathomimetic drugs. In elderly persons, they may occur because of congophilic amyloid angiopathy (CAA). The diagnosis of CAA is suggested by the finding of multiple *microbleeds* on gradient

Table 124-7 Clinical Manifestations Related to Site of Intracerebral Hemorrhage

Site			Manifestation		
	Headache	**Pupils**	**Eye Movements**	**Sensorimotor Signs**	**Other**
Basal ganglia	Severe	Normal	Normal	Hemiparesis	Confusion, aphasia
Thalamus	Moderate	Small, poorly reactive to light	Hyperconvergence Absent vertical gaze	Hemisensory > motor loss	Hypersomnolence
Pons	Severe	Small, reactive	Horizontal gaze paresis	Quadriplegia	Coma
Cerebellum	Severe, occipital	Normal	Normal	Ataxia	Early vomiting

echo MRI. Patients with CAA often have associated dementia and seizures.

DIAGNOSIS, MANAGEMENT, AND PROGNOSIS

CT remains the diagnostic test of choice in the diagnosis of acute ICH, showing a hyperintense area with mass effect and (later) hypointense surrounding edema. MRI is less sensitive than CT for detecting hemorrhage in the early stages. The management of ICH depends on the size and location of the lesion. In the acute phase, the mass effect of a cerebral hematoma is far greater than in a large cerebral infarction, with a greater risk of herniation and death. In the chronic phase, however, the prognosis for recovery in patients who survive is much better for those with hemorrhage than for those with ischemic stroke. Therefore therapy for acute hemorrhage is directed at reducing mass effect either by medical decompression with controlled hyperventilation or mannitol or, in rare cases, by surgical decompression. This latter option should be considered urgently in cases of cerebellar hemorrhage in which patients are especially at risk of sudden deterioration either because of acute obstructive hydrocephalus (from compression of the fourth ventricle) or as a result of direct pressure on the caudal brainstem.

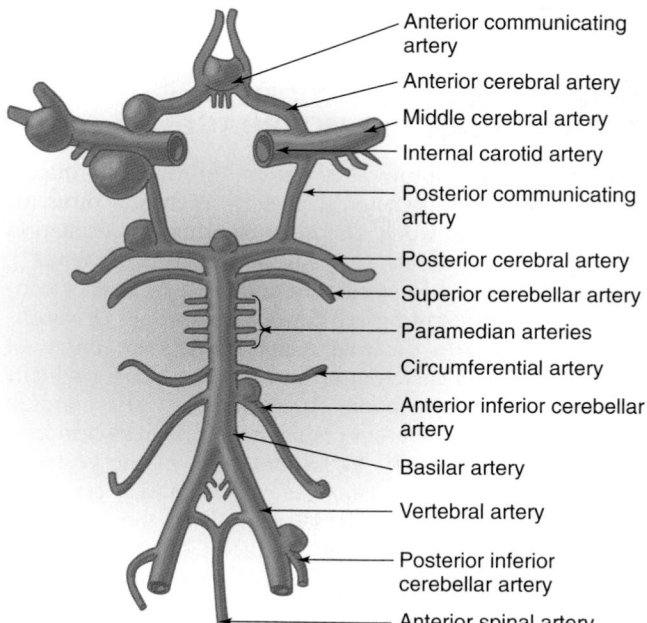

Figure 124-8 The more common sites of berry aneurysms. The diagrammatic size of the aneurysm at the various sites is directly proportional to its frequency at that locus.

- Anterior communicating artery
- Anterior cerebral artery
- Middle cerebral artery
- Internal carotid artery
- Posterior communicating artery
- Posterior cerebral artery
- Superior cerebellar artery
- Paramedian arteries
- Circumferential artery
- Anterior inferior cerebellar artery
- Basilar artery
- Vertebral artery
- Posterior inferior cerebellar artery
- Anterior spinal artery

Intracranial Aneurysms

Intracranial aneurysms occur in three forms: fusiform, mycotic, and saccular (congenital *berry*) aneurysms.

Fusiform aneurysms represent ectatic dilations of large arteries, usually the basilar or intracranial carotid arteries. They rarely rupture but may compress adjacent brain tissue or cranial nerves and cause local neurologic dysfunction. Fusiform aneurysms are rarely accessible to surgical repair.

Mycotic aneurysms occur in the context of bacterial endocarditis when septic emboli lodge in a peripheral vessel (see Chapter 100). They are often multiple and located distally in the arterial tree, and thus they are accessible to surgical repair should they fail to respond to antibiotic therapy.

Saccular aneurysms form at arterial bifurcations (Fig. 124-8); 80% are located in the anterior circulation. They are thought to arise from a combination of a congenital defect in the arterial media and elastic lamina and gradual

deterioration from hemodynamic stress. Their incidence is higher in patients with polycystic kidney disease and Marfan syndrome.

Approximately 6% of the population harbors an unruptured saccular aneurysm; 25% of patients have multiple aneurysms. Fortunately, the annual incidence of rupture is only approximately 10 per 100,000. The risk of rupture is 1% per year. Of individuals with aneurysms that do rupture, 33% die before reaching a hospital, and another 20% die in the hospital. Overall, only 30% of patients recover without significant disability.

Incidental aneurysms of the anterior circulation smaller than 7 mm have a very low risk of rupture (<0.05% per year); the risk of rupture rises with increasing size of aneurysm and location within the posterior circulation. Within families, aneurysms tend to be at the same site and to rupture during the same decade. The risk of an unruptured aneurysm in a first-degree relative of a patient with subarachnoid hemorrhage is 4% to 5% with one affected relative and 8% to 10% with two or more affected relatives. The natural history of

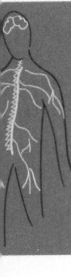

aneurysms is unknown. Whether they pose an early high risk after formation or whether a constant risk of rupture exists over time is unknown.

Treatment of Unruptured Intracranial Aneurysms

Treatment of asymptomatic aneurysms remains controversial. Aneurysms may be treated by open surgical clipping or by endovascular coiling. The latter procedure has emerged as the treatment of choice in the majority of patients and has a low morbidity and mortality. The risk-benefit ratio of treatment depends on life expectancy. In older persons the risk of rupture over their remaining lifetime may be very low and not warrant intervention.

CLINICAL MANIFESTATIONS OF SUBARACHNOID HEMORRHAGE

Aneurysms may rupture at any time but especially during periods of strenuous activity, such as exercise, coitus, or strenuous physical work. The most common manifestation is sudden severe headache ("the worst headache of my life"), often accompanied by neck pain and rigidity. Loss of consciousness and vomiting are common sequelae. Occasionally, with so-called *sentinel hemorrhages,* the onset of symptoms is less cataclysmic, and the headache gradually resolves over 24 to 48 hours. Aneurysms may also manifest by compression of adjacent cranial nerves, such as compression of cranial nerve III by an aneurysm of the posterior communicating artery. *Giant aneurysms* (>2.5 cm) may compress cranial nerves III, IV, and VI in the cavernous sinus. Aneurysms occasionally produce a TIA as a result of embolization from a thrombus within an aneurysm.

DIAGNOSIS

CT of the brain shows subarachnoid hemorrhage in nearly all patients, and its location may suggest a site of rupture. A normal CT scan may not totally exclude subarachnoid hemorrhage and mandates a lumbar puncture in patients with suggestive symptoms. Care must be taken to centrifuge cerebrospinal fluid to detect true xanthochromia, the yellow coloration that develops by 6 hours after subarachnoid hemorrhage. Contrast CT or MRI identifies aneurysms larger than 5 mm as well as arteriovenous malformations. Cerebral angiography remains the *gold standard* for diagnosing intracranial aneurysms, and it is usually performed when surgery is being contemplated and deferred in severe cases in which significant risk of vasospasm exists. A small group of patients with predominantly peri-mesencephalic hemorrhage on CT have normal cerebral angiograms and a more benign outcome. The electrocardiogram may show deep, symmetrical T-wave inversion. Once the diagnosis of subarachnoid hemorrhage has been made (or if clinical suspicion persists, even with inconclusive testing), the patient should be managed under the guidance of a neurosurgical team.

Table 124-8 **Complications of Subarachnoid Hemorrhage**
Hypertension (systemic and intracranial)
Vasospasm
Hemorrhage (rebleeding)
Hydrocephalus
Hyponatremia (syndrome of inappropriate antidiuretic hormone; cerebral salt wasting)

MANAGEMENT AND PROGNOSIS

An essential part of management of patients with subarachnoid hemorrhage is to prevent its complications (Table 124-8). To reduce the risk of rebleeding, patients are placed on bed rest with analgesics for pain relief, mild sedation, and the use of laxatives to reduce straining. Management of hypertension requires balancing the need to maintain a steady CPP in the context of raised ICP and possible vasospasm and, in contrast, the risk of rebleeding. Most rebleeding occurs within the first 3 days after rupture. The peak timing for vasospasm is between 5 and 9 days after the hemorrhage, and it may be accompanied by an alteration in the neurologic status. Oral nimodipine, a calcium channel blocker, should be given for 21 days after subarachnoid hemorrhage to prevent vasospasm.

Vascular Malformations

Vascular malformations of the brain and spinal cord are grouped according to vessel size and composition. *Venous angiomas* are the most common and tend to lie close to the brain surface. Malformations composed of capillaries are called *capillary telangiectases* and are typically located within the brainstem. *Cavernous angiomas* are composed of dilated sinusoidal channels, are readily detectable on CT, and rarely bleed.

Arteriovenous malformations are composed of tangles of arteries connected directly to veins without intervening capillaries. They may produce headache, seizures, or hemorrhage, accounting for 1% of all strokes. The initial hemorrhage typically occurs before the fourth decade, with a 7% risk of rebleeding within the first year afterward. Hemorrhage may occur into the brain parenchyma, subarachnoid space, or intraventricular space.

Treatment of arteriovenous malformations is guided by individual factors, such as the age of the patient, location and composition of the lesion, and manifestations. As the natural history of unruptured arteriovenous malformations is unknown, treatment of asymptomatic patients is controversial. In general, arteriovenous malformations in older patients (>55 years) are treated conservatively, whereas younger patients are treated by surgical excision, embolization, or, less commonly, if small, by irradiation.

Prospectus for the Future

The risk of both ischemic and hemorrhagic strokes can be reduced by vascular risk factor modification. Additional progress can be expected in this area, particularly in defining genetic factors that may increase stroke susceptibility. Important clinical trials are ongoing in the areas of treatment of PFO, warfarin in heart failure, and alternatives to warfarin for anticoagulation. Improved public recognition of stroke symptoms and better access to acute stroke units should result in greater use of thrombolysis and reduced morbidity from stroke. Trials of neuroprotective agents have been disappointing to date, although animal models were promising; research in this area is ongoing. Hemorrhagic stroke has been somewhat neglected in the past. The natural history of unruptured aneurysms and arteriovenous malformations is unknown, which makes treatment decisions difficult. These areas require further study.

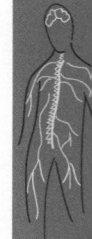

References

Adams HP, del Zoppo G, Alberts MJ, et al: Guidelines for the early management of adults with ischemic stroke. Stroke 38:1655-1711, 2007.

Friedlander RM: Arteriovenous malformations of the brain. N Engl J Med 356:2704-2712, 2007.

Mant J, Hobbs F, Fletcher K, et al: Warfarin versus aspirin for stroke prevention in an elderly community population with atrial fibrillation (the Birmingham Atrial Fibrillation Treatment of the Aged Study, BAFTA): A randomised controlled trial. Lancet 370:493-503, 2007.

Wahlgren N, Ahmed N, Davalos A, et al: Thrombolysis with alteplase for acute ischaemic stroke in the Safe Implementation of Thrombolysis in Stroke-Monitoring Study (SITS-MOST): An observational study. Lancet 369:275-282, 2007.

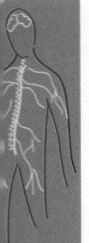

Traumatic Brain Injury and Spinal Cord Injury

Geoffrey S. F. Ling

Traumatic brain injury (TBI) and traumatic spinal cord injury (TSCI) are leading causes of traumatic death and disability. Over 8 million patients undergo TBI each year, with approximately 52,000 patients in the United States dying as a direct consequence. An additional 11,000 patients are severely disabled by TSCI. The majority of TBIs and TSCIs are a result of falls, motor vehicle accidents, sports-related occurrences, and assaults. Among the almost 5.5 million TBI and TSCI survivors, most require prolonged rehabilitation.

Types of Traumatic Brain Injury

Certain lesions necessitate neurosurgical intervention, whereas others do not. TBI conditions for which emergency neurosurgery is needed are penetrating wounds, intracerebral hemorrhage with mass effect including subdural and epidural blood, bony injury such as displaced fracture, and vertebral subluxation. However, focal, hypoxic-anoxic, diffuse axonal, and diffuse microvascular injuries typically do not necessitate surgery.

Traumatic Brain Injury Management

The initial goals in TBI care are the ABCs of airway, breathing, and circulation. Next is D for disability (neurologic). Every patient should undergo a detailed neurologic examination to ascertain the level of neurologic disability. An initial Glasgow Coma Score (GCS) should be assigned to each patient. The GCS (Table 125-1) categorizes TBI patients and provides a quantifiable measure of impairment.

Patients with mild or moderate TBI typically recover quickly and fully. In the early stage of management, it is important to determine the duration of amnesia or loss of consciousness a patient may have experienced. The American Academy of Neurology Guideline uses a grading scale for concussion that is based primarily on the length of these intervals (Table 125-2). Longer periods of abnormal sensorium are associated with higher grades. Higher grades necessitate longer periods of convalescence. Other clinical guides that are used include the Cantu Grading System and the Colorado Medical Society Guidelines.

In general, patients with mild or moderate TBI will not require major medical intervention, and almost all will do well after adequate convalescence. It is essential that patients have adequate recovery even from mild TBI. A subsequent head injury before full recovery may be catastrophic as it could result in "second impact syndrome" (SIS), which leads to worse clinical outcome including death.

Severe TBI is defined as an injury that results in a GCS score of eight or less. This is a serious condition so to optimize outcome, medical management should adhere to currently accepted clinical guidelines such as the Brain Trauma Foundation "Clinical Guidelines for Severe TBI." An important early intervention is airway protection, usually by endotracheal intubation. If elevated intracranial pressure (ICP) is suspected or if GCS < 8, the ICP should be monitored. Options for ICP monitoring are epidural fiberoptic catheter, subdural bolt, intraparenchymal fiberoptic catheter, or intraventricular catheter (IVC). All of these devices require drilling a small burr hole through the skull. The fiberoptic catheters are closed system devices and thus are associated with very low infection rates. However, measurements can drift after 5 days of use. As they cannot be zeroed, fiberoptic monitors are usually changed at this time. The subdural bolt can be zeroed but is associated with a slightly higher incidence of infection. The IVC or external drainage device is the most invasive as it requires inserting a catheter through brain parenchyma into a lateral cerebral ventricle. It can be zeroed and has the highest incidence of infection. The greatest benefit of the IVC is that it provides a therapeutic option in that CSF can be drained, which helps reduce intracranial volume and thus ICP.

If there is elevated ICP, the patient's head should be elevated to 30 degrees and kept midline, with a rigid neck collar used (until the cervical spine can be evaluated for stability). Mannitol should be given intravenously at a dose of 0.5 to 1.0 g/kg. Hyperventilation may also be used, with a goal of P_{CO_2} of 34 to 36 mm Hg. ICP should be kept less than 20 mm Hg, with the cerebral perfusion pressure (CPP) greater than 60 mm Hg. CPP is the mathematical difference between mean arterial pressure (MAP) and ICP. Thus, CPP represents the arterial pressure that globally perfuses the brain. A head CT without contrast should be done as soon as possible both to identify lesions that will require surgery and to determine the extent of injury.

If ICP remains poorly controlled, one can consider administering an intravenous bolus of 23% hypertonic saline (30 ml) followed by continuous infusion of 2% or 3% hypertonic saline (75 to 125 ml/hr) through a central venous catheter. If these interventions are unsuccessful, pharmacologic coma or surgical decompression should be considered. Pharmacologic coma can be induced with pentobarbital. This is given as a loading dose of 5 mg/kg, intravenously.

followed by an infusion of 1 to 3 mg/kg/hr. Alternatively, propofol can be administered as a loading dose of 2 mg/kg intravenously, followed by an infusion of up to 200 µg/kg/min. Continuous electroencephalographic (EEG) monitoring is helpful, as the limit of drug-induced coma is achieving ICP control or cerebral electrical burst-suppression. Persistently elevated ICP after all these efforts is ominous. Consideration should be made regarding frontal or temporal lobe decompression and hemicraniectomy.

To meet CPP goals, patients must first be adequately hydrated. The goal of TBI fluid management is to increase the osmolar gradient between systemic vasculature and brain, not dehydration. For this purpose, hyperosmolar intravenous solutions, such as normal saline, are used. Other options are hypertonic saline (e.g., 3% sodium solutions). If meeting CPP goals is difficult with intravenous fluids alone, vasoactive pharmacologic agents such as norepinephrine and phenylephrine can be administered. These two agents are preferred because they are considered to have the least effect on cerebral vasomotor tone. Barbiturates and propofol are myocardial depressants, and therefore aggressive cardiovascular management entailing close cardiac monitoring and maintenance of euvolemia with appropriate fluid hydration and vasopressors as needed to maintain CPP will probably be necessary in the event of pharmacologic coma.

Agitation can be treated with lorazepam or haloperidol. If these are inadequate, then infusions of midazolam or propofol may be used. Pain should be treated adequately. Acetaminophen and nonsteroidal anti-inflammatory agents may be adequate, but for moderate to severe pain, a narcotic analgesic such as fentanyl or morphine should be used. A benefit of opioids is that they can be reversed by naloxone, which allows reassessment of neurologic status.

Hypoxia, seizures, and fever must be avoided. Maintaining P_{O_2} at approximately 100 mm Hg is sufficient. Phenytoin is administered for the first 7 days after injury, as it reduces early onset seizures. After 7 days, this medication should be stopped. It can be restarted if late-onset seizures occur. Fever should be reduced with antipyretics such as acetaminophen, with cooling blankets used as needed. Other important

Table 125-1 Glasgow Coma Score

Best Eye Response	Best Verbal Response	Best Motor Response
1 = No eye opening	1 = No verbal response	1 = No motor response
2 = Eye opening to pain	2 = Incomprehensible sounds	2 = Extension to pain
3 = Eye opening to verbal command	3 = Inappropriate words	3 = Flexion to pain
4 = Eyes open spontaneously	4 = Confused	4 = Withdrawal from pain
	5 = Oriented	5 = Localizing pain
		6 = Obeys commands

Score = Eye Response + Verbal Response + Motor Response.

Table 125-2 American Academy of Neurology Concussion Management

Grade 1 (Mild)	Grade 2 (Moderate)	Grade 3 (Severe)
Remove from duty, work, or play	Remove from duty for the rest of the day	Take to emergency department
Examine immediately and at 5-min intervals	Examine frequently for signs of CNS deterioration	Neurologic evaluation, including appropriate neuroimaging
May return to duty or work if clear within 15 min	Physician's neurologic examination ASAP (within 24 hr)	Consider hospital admission
	Return to duty after 1 full asymptomatic week (after being cleared by physician)	

Grade of Concussion	Return to Play or Work
Grade 1 (first injury)	15 minutes
Grade 1 (second injury)	1 week
Grade 2 (first injury)	1 week
Grade 2 (second injury)	2 weeks
Grade 3 (first injury) (brief LOC)	1 week
Grade 3 (first injury) (long LOC)	2 weeks
Grade 3 (second injury)	1 month
Grade 3 (third injury)	Consult a neurologist

ASAP, as soon as possible; CNS, central nervous system; LOC, loss of consciousness.

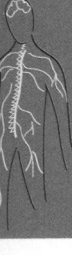

management considerations include prevention of gastric stress ulcers, deep vein thrombosis (DVT), and decubitus ulcer. Nutrition should be maintained, ideally with enteral feeds. However, if hyperosmolar therapy is used, then one should use concentrated enteral feeds that minimize free water content.

After the first few hours have elapsed, efforts should be made to reduce hyperventilation. This therapy should be reserved only for initial emergency management. If the therapy is continued over 12 hours, metabolic compensation negates the ameliorative effects of respiratory alkalosis caused by a hypocapnic state.

Regular neurologic examinations and continuous ICP and CPP measurements should be made. Generally, the peak period of cerebral edema is from 48 to 96 hours after TBI. Thereafter, this spontaneously resolves and clinical improvement should follow.

A complication of TBI is "postconcussive syndrome." The most common symptoms are headache, difficulty concentrating, appetite changes, sleep abnormalities, and irritability. Depending on the patient and the severity of TBI, postconcussive syndrome has a variable presentation and duration. In general, this condition lasts only a few weeks after injury. However, uncommonly, it can persist beyond a year or more. Therapies are focused on managing symptoms. For headache, nonsteroidal anti-inflammatory agents, migraine drugs, and biofeedback can be effective. For cognitive dysfunction, neuropsychologic testing may be helpful in determining appropriate intervention.

Traumatic Spinal Cord Injury Management

The emergency management of traumatic injury to the spinal cord has improved with the measures recommended by the "Guidelines for the Management of Cervical Spine and Spinal Cord Injuries" from the American Association of Neurological Surgeons. As with TBI, therapy begins with the ABCs of airway, breathing, and circulation. For patients with high cervical lesions, spontaneous ventilation will be lost. Lesions lower than C5 may also be associated with insufficient ventilatory capability. If there is any concern that the airway or if ventilatory efforts are compromised, then emergency intubation is required. In a patient in whom the cervical spine has not been adequately imaged, the preferred method is nasotracheal intubation using fiberoptic guidance. Other approaches are nasotracheal (blind) or orotracheal intubation, but traction must be applied to maintain spinal column alignment.

Maintaining adequate intravascular volume is of particular importance in the spinal cord–injured patient. Hypotension may result from either neurogenic shock or hypovolemia. For neurogenic shock, vasopressive pharmacologic agents such as phenylephrine may be needed. If tachycardia is present, then hypovolemia is the more likely cause, and fluid administration is the appropriate initial management. As with TBI, normal saline is the preferred fluid.

After these issues have been addressed, a neurologic assessment should be made. An accompanying TBI needs to be considered. Up to 50% of TSCI patients have an associated

TBI. History with complete neurologic examination is the best method for diagnosis. Neuroimaging is often indicated for diagnostic evaluation, but not all patients need radiographic study. Normal neurologic history and examination findings in patients with a clear sensorium obviates the need for imaging studies. However, complaints of pain over the spine or of numbness, tingling, or weakness should raise the suspicion of spinal cord injury. In particular, a complaint of burning hands suggests cervical spinal cord injury. As accurately as possible, the time of injury should be recorded. A detailed neurologic examination is needed to identify the level of the injury and the completeness of any deficits and to document the degree of neurologic dysfunction at the earliest time possible. The level of the injury is the lowest spinal cord segment with intact motor and sensory function. The prognosis for neurologic improvement is better if the lesion is incomplete than if it is complete. During this acute period, serial examinations must be made frequently.

If spinal cord injury is suspected, the patient should be immediately and appropriately immobilized, that is, with a rigid collar or back board or both. Radiologic evaluation should begin with plain x-ray films of the bony spine. Abnormalities on x-ray films should lead to further neuroimaging. Bony vertebrae should be examined with computed tomography (CT), and the spinal cord with magnetic resonance imaging (MRI). Intervertebral and paravertebral soft tissue are best studied with MRI. A chest radiograph should also be obtained in order to visualize the lower cervical and thoracic vertebrae. Presence of a pleural effusion in the setting of a possible thoracic spine injury suggests a hemothorax.

If the C-spine radiograph is normal but the patient complains of neck pain, then ligamentous injury may be present. Ligamentous injury is evaluated by flexion-extension C-spine x-ray studies. However, in the acute period, pain may prevent an adequate study. Such patients should be kept in a rigid cervical collar for at least 24 to 48 hours until the pain and neck muscle spasm resolve. At that time, the study may be performed. If abnormal, the patient will need surgical evaluation.

If spinal cord injury is identified, methylprednisolone should be given at an initial dose of 30 mg/kg intravenous bolus followed by a continuous infusion of 5.4 mg/kg/hr. The infusion should be for 23 hours if it is started within 3 hours of injury. If beyond 3 hours but still within 8 hours, then methylprednisolone should be given for 48 hours. The efficacy of methylprednisolone in TSCI from penetrating causes has not been demonstrated, so this therapy is reserved only for closed compartment injury. This is the only indication for steroid use in TSCI. At this time, the decision for surgical intervention should be made, based on the stability of the vertebral column.

SPINAL CORD SYNDROMES

There are three main spinal cord syndromes: Brown-Séquard (hemisection), central cord, and anterior cord. Anterior cord syndrome is associated with deficits referable to bilateral anterior and lateral spinal cord columns. There is loss of touch, pain, and temperature sensations and motor function below the level of the lesion. The posterior column functions of proprioception and vibratory sensation remain intact. In Brown-Séquard syndrome, the deficits are caused by injury to a lateral half of the cord. There is functional loss of ipsilateral motor function, touch, proprioception, and vibration sensations, and contralateral pain and temperature sensations. Central cord or "man in a barrel" syndrome manifests as motor paralysis of both upper extremities while the lower extremities are spared. Weakness is greater proximally than distally. Pain and temperature sensations are generally reduced, but proprioception and vibration are spared.

SPINAL SHOCK

After acute injury, spinal shock may occur, causing a temporary loss of spinal reflexes below the level of injury. Neurologic examination will reveal loss of deep tendon reflexes, bulbocavernosus reflex, and the anal wink. In high cervical injuries, the lower reflexes (bulbocavernosus and anal wink) may be preserved. There may also be the "Schiff-Sherrington" phenomenon, in which reflexes are affected above the level of injury. In addition, there will likely be loss of autonomic reflexes, leading to neurogenic shock, bowel ileus, and urinary retention.

OTHER TRAUMATIC SPINAL CORD INJURY MANAGEMENT ISSUES

In the intensive care unit, the patient will need continued treatment. Once methylprednisolone therapy has been completed, there is no need for further steroid use. TSCI patients require close cardiovascular and ventilatory care. Other issues are genitourinary, bowel, infectious disease, nutrition, skin and prophylaxis against skin ulcers, and DVT formation.

Patients with spinal cord injury are at risk for neurogenic shock and dysautonomia, which lead to peripheral vasodilation and hypotension. If the lesion is at T3 or above, then sympathetic tone to the heart is compromised. In this setting, hypotension is accompanied by bradycardia: the classic neurogenic shock triad of bradycardia, hypotension, and peripheral vasodilation.

Therapy for dysautonomia begins by ensuring adequate circulating volume. The goal is to administer fluids to restore a euvolemic state. Blood should be transfused if the patient is anemic—that is, if the hematocrit is less than 30. If blood is not required, then either colloid (e.g., albumin solutions) or crystalloid (e.g., normal saline) may be used to maintain a central venous pressure (CVP) of 4 to 6 mm Hg. Hypervolemia should be avoided, as this will exacerbate peripheral edema. Once an adequate circulating volume has been achieved, a vasopressive agent such as phenylephrine, norepinephrine, or dopamine can be used. The goal MAP is 85 mm Hg or greater. Symptomatic bradycardia can be treated with atropine.

Spinal cord patients are at risk for ventilatory compromise. Patients whose injuries are at C5 or higher typically require mechanical ventilation with an appropriate tidal volume (6 to 10 ml/kg) and F_{IO_2} and mandatory machine-driven rate. The F_{IO_2} should be set at a value that gives a P_{O_2} of 80 to 100 mm Hg. The rate should be set to give a P_{CO_2} of 40 mm Hg. Positive end-expiratory pressure (PEEP) should also be used to minimize atelectasis. If the patient does not show signs of ventilatory recovery within 2 weeks of intubation, a tracheostomy should be considered.

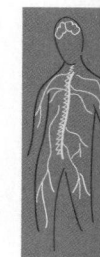

Lesions below C5 may also be associated with inadequate spontaneous ventilation. Midcervical lesions may be associated with intact but compromised diaphragm function. If suspected, a "sniff" test under fluoroscopy can be performed to determine if both hemidiaphragms are functioning properly. If not, intubation and tracheostomy with volume-controlled ventilation may be needed. If function is intact, then pressure support (PS) ventilation may be sufficient. The amount of PS to administer is dependent on patient requirements and should be sufficient to lead to an appropriate tidal volume. F_{IO_2} and PEEP should be set as described previously.

Patients with cervical lesions at C6 and below, including the thoracic cord, are generally not mechanical ventilator–dependent. However, their ventilatory effort may be inadequate, as the thoracic cord innervates intercostal muscles, which are accessory muscles of respiration. Such patients have decreased cough and inability to increase ventilation when needed. This leads to atelectasis and comprised ability to clear secretions, which may lead to pneumonia. These patients may benefit from chest physical therapy.

Thromboembolic disease often complicates TSCI and is a leading cause of morbidity and mortality in these patients, as up to 80% will develop DVT without proper prophylaxis. Therefore all patients with TSCI should receive both anticoagulation and leg mechanical compression devices. As soon as possible, sequential compression devices (SCDs) or compression stockings should be placed on patients. Then, as soon as hemostasis is ensured, low–molecular-weight heparin (LMWH) should be initiated. Unfractionated heparin may also be used in conjunction with SCD, but LMWH is preferred. An inferior vena cava filter may be placed in those patients in whom anticoagulation therapy is contraindicated but should not be the primary means of preventing DVT.

Mid to low thoracic spinal cord injury can lead to ileus. A nasogastric tube should be placed to decompress the stomach. Parenteral nutrition should be started as soon as possible. Enteral feeding should be delayed until gastrointestinal motility returns. This normally takes about 2 to 3 weeks. The pharmacologic agents metoclopramide, erythromycin, and cisapride may promote gastrointestinal motility.

Gastric ulcer prophylaxis needs to be administered: H_2-receptor antagonists, proton pump inhibitors, antacids, or sucralfate. Pancreatitis and trauma-related perforated bowel are potential problems. Loss of abdominal muscle tone and visceral sensation may mask clinical signs such as pain, guarding, or rigidity. Bladder tone may be lost because of spinal shock. A Foley catheter should be placed and maintained for a minimum of 5 to 7 days to help drain the bladder and to evaluate circulatory volume and renal function. After spinal shock has resolved, autonomic dysreflexia may occur from bladder distention. Clinical signs such as sweating, skin flushing, and hypertension may be present. Clinical examination using palpation and percussion will reveal a distended bladder, which can be treated with bladder training or intermittent catheterization. Phenoxybenzamine may be helpful in this condition.

Until enteral feeding can begin, parenteral nutrition should be used. A caloric level of 80% of the Harris-Benedict prediction, which approximates a patient's total daily energy expenditures, should be used for quadriplegic patients. This is an approximation of a patient's total daily energy expenditure and is based on the patient's basal metabolic rate and activity level. The full Harris-Benedict predicted amount should be used for patients with thoracic spine injuries and below.

There is a propensity for decubitus ulcers from pressure to develop in patients with TSCI. Mechanical kinetic beds, regular log rolling (every 2 hours), and padded orthotics are all useful in minimizing this complication.

Orthotics, physical therapy, and occupational therapy (for cervical cord injury) are also important. Therapy should begin as soon as the spine is stabilized. This will serve to minimize contractures and to begin the rehabilitation process. It should be remembered that once therapy begins, energy expenditures will increase, and consequently additional nutrition will be needed. Also, as intermittent compression devices will need to be removed during therapy, the heparin dose may need to be increased.

Prognosis

TRAUMATIC BRAIN INJURY

The most useful prognostic indicator after TBI is the neurologic examination at presentation. Clearly, the better the neurologic examination findings, the higher the likelihood of improved recovery. The initial GCS is a very reliable

Table 125-3 American Spinal Injury Association Impairment Scale

Grade	Injury Type	Definition
A	Complete	No motor or sensory function below the lesion
B	Incomplete	Sensory but no motor function
C	Incomplete	Some motor strength (<3)
D	Incomplete	Motor strength >3
E	None	Sensory and motor function normal

prognostic indicator. The lower the initial GCS, the less likely a patient will have meaningful neurologic or functional recovery.

TRAUMATIC SPINAL CORD INJURY

For TSCI, the completeness of the injury is the most useful prognosticator. The American Spine Injury Association Impairment Scale grades spinal cord injury on the basis of completeness (Table 125-3). A grade A or complete motor and sensory deficit below the lesion is associated with the most ominous prognosis. If this status persists for longer than 24 hours, there is little reasonable likelihood of meaningful recovery. On the other hand, partial injuries, even severe, have substantial probability of recovery.

Prospectus for the Future

Traumatic brain injury (TBI) and traumatic spinal cord injury (TSCI) prevention remains the most effective way of reducing the incidence of these disorders. Practice guidelines have contributed to improved outcome after TBI and TSCI. However, morbidity remains high. Medical management is largely confined to supportive efforts primarily directed toward minimizing secondary injury, optimizing perfusion and oxygenation, and preventing nonneurologic morbidity. Surgical intervention helps restore structural stability, minimize further injury, and reduce lesion size. However, neither medicine nor surgical treatment reverses neuronal death nor fully prevents secondary injury processes. Research is needed to improve our understanding of the pathogenesis of these injuries and find ways to mitigate it. As new pharmacologic, medical, and surgical approaches are introduced, there will be increasing opportunities to improve the still-poor prognosis of many patients.

References

Belanger E, Levi AD: The acute and chronic management of spinal cord injury. J Am Coll Surg 190:603-618, 2000.

Brain Trauma Foundation, American Association of Neurological Surgeons, Congress of Neurological Surgeons: Guidelines for the management of severe traumatic brain injury. J Neurotrauma 24 (Suppl 1): S1-S106, 2007.

Quality Standards Subcommittee, American Academy of Neurology: Practice parameter: The management of concussion in sports (summary statement). Neurology 48:581-585, 1997.

Cushman JG, Agarwal N, Fabian TC, et al: Practice management guidelines for the management of mild traumatic brain injury: The EAST practice management guidelines work group. J Trauma 51:1016-1026, 2001.

Hadley MN, Walters BC, Grabb PA, et al: Guidelines for the management of acute cervical spine and spinal cord injuries. Clin Neurosurg 49:407-498, 2002.

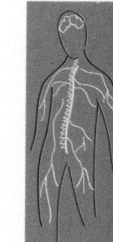

Epilepsy

Michel J. Berg

Definition

Epileptic (or *electrical*) *seizures* are caused by abnormal highly synchronous discharges of neurons. They are a common sign of brain dysfunction. A wide variety of symptoms can occur depending on the location in the brain affected, including involuntary movements, sensations, and impaired consciousness.

Seizures often occur during the course of medical or neurologic illnesses in which brain function is temporarily deranged (symptomatic seizures) (Table 126-1). The most common secondary causes are childhood febrile seizures, metabolic derangements (such as hypoglycemia or hyponatremia), intoxications (alcohol, cocaine), acute head traumas, and hypoxic-ischemic conditions (syncope, embolic stroke). Symptomatic seizures are usually self-limited, and recurrent seizures do not occur after the underlying disorder has been corrected. Therefore symptomatic seizures do not indicate epilepsy.

Epilepsy is a chronic disorder defined as a condition with recurrent seizures not produced directly by a secondary cause. There are many different epileptic syndromes (the epilepsies). Classification of the epilepsy syndrome depends on a number of factors including the seizure type, cause, genetic factors, neuroimaging, and response to therapy. The phrase *seizure disorder* is synonymous with the word *epilepsy*.

A single seizure may occur as an unprovoked event with no discoverable reason. By definition, two separate seizures are required to make the diagnosis of epilepsy; that is, a single seizure does not constitute epilepsy.

Individuals with epilepsy have increased seizure susceptibility (lowered seizure threshold). Genetic factors and prior brain injury (from a multitude of causes) are the major contributors to such susceptibility.

Most seizures in someone with epilepsy occur in an unpredictable fashion. It is this unpredictable timing that results in the major negative impact on quality of life. If functionally impairing seizures occur during waking hours (*diurnal seizures)*, then activity restrictions are required including restriction from driving, operating heavy machinery, heights, and unobserved swimming or bathing (showering with a good drain is recommended). These activity restrictions lead to loss of independence. The psychological impact of having intermittent involuntary loss of body control and the dependant status imposed by the activity restrictions are major contributors to the substantial increased incidence of comorbid depression in people with epilepsy (up to 50%).

In many people with epilepsy there is a higher seizure frequency during sleep because of increased synchronization of neuronal activity. Seizures that occur exclusively in sleep constitute *nocturnal epilepsy.* In women with epilepsy (WWE), seizures sometimes occur more often during the week around menses or at ovulation (*catamenial epilepsy).* Sleep deprivation, alcohol consumption, infectious illness, certain medications, and severe emotional stressors can further lower the seizure threshold and are associated with more seizures in people with epilepsy (see Table 126-1).

Incidence and Etiology

Seizures can occur at any time. Ten percent of people in developed countries have a seizure at some time during their lives. In contrast, 0.7% to 1% have current epilepsy (prevalence), and 3% to 4% have epilepsy at some time during their lives (lifetime prevalence). In the United States, there are approximately 125,000 new cases of epilepsy diagnosed each year (incidence). The incidence and prevalence are biphasic, with epilepsy being more common in childhood (primarily resulting from perinatal injury, infections, and genetic factors) and in old age (from stroke, tumors, and dementia) (Fig. 126-1). In developing countries the frequency of epilepsy is higher because of a variety of factors including increased brain infections with organisms such as cysticercosis.

Before the 1990s, in most people with epilepsy the cause was not determined. The advent of magnetic resonance imaging (MRI) and, more recently, genetic analysis has substantially improved our ability to identify the underlying cause of many types of epilepsy. About 70% of adults and

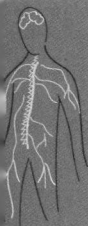

Table 126-1 Causes of Symptomatic Seizures*

Acute electrolyte/metabolic disorders
  Acute hyponatremia (<120 mEq/L)
  Acute hypernatremia (>155 mEq/L)
  Hyperosmolality (>310 mOsm/L)
  Hypocalcemia (<7 mg/dL)
  Hypoglycemia (<30 mg/dL)
Drugs
  Quinolone antibiotics, isoniazid, penicillins (in renal insufficiency)
  Theophylline, aminophylline, ephedrine, phenylpropanolamine, terbutaline
  Tramadol, lidocaine, meperidine (in renal insufficiency)
  Tricyclic antidepressants
  Cyclosporine
  Cocaine (crack), phencyclidine, amphetamines
  Alcohol and benzodiazephine withdrawal
Central nervous system disease
  Hypertensive encephalopathy, eclampsia
  Hepatic and uremic encephalopathy
  Sickle cell disease, thrombotic thrombocytopenic purpura
  Systemic lupus erythematosus
  Meningitis, encephalitis, brain abscess
  Acute head trauma, stroke, brain tumor

*The metabolic derangements and drugs listed in Table 126-1 also lower the seizure threshold in people with epilepsy.

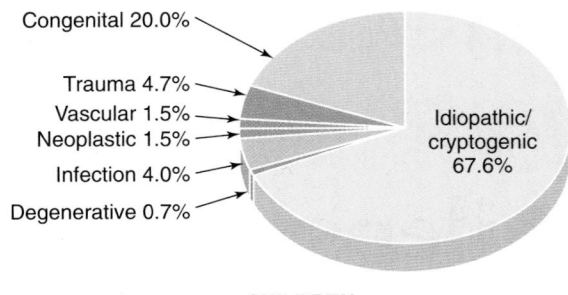

CHILDREN

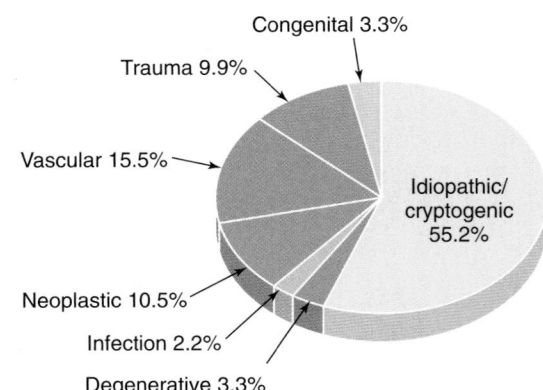

ADULTS

Figure 126-1 Causes of epilepsy according to age in all newly diagnosed cases in Rochester, Minnesota, 1935 to 1984. (Modified from Hauser WA, Annegers JF, Kurland LT: Incidence of epilepsy and unprovoked seizures in Rochester, Minnesota: 1935-1984. Epilepsia 1994;34:453.)

40% of children with new-onset epilepsy have partial (focal) seizures. In many it is not possible to identify a specific cause, although focal seizures imply a cerebral injury or lesion. The most common specific lesions are hippocampal sclerosis, neuronal and glial tumors, vascular malformations, neuronal migration disorders (e.g., cortical dysplasia), hamartomas, encephalitis, cerebral trauma, embolic stroke, and hemorrhage. Not all patients with cerebral lesions develop epilepsy; how or why a particular lesion becomes epileptogenic is poorly understood.

Hereditary influences have long been associated with epilepsy. During the past decade, a number of gene mutations have been associated with specific epilepsy syndromes.

At least 10 of the genetic epilepsies are known to be channelopathies; that is, a specific channel in a population of neurons, such as one isoform of the sodium channel, is mutated. Although still rare, new channelopathies are being identified, and it is likely that channel dysfunction will contribute to many of the epilepsies. An example of a channelopathy is *Dravet syndrome*, also known as *severe myoclonic epilepsy of infancy* (SMEI). Dravet syndrome is caused by a complete loss of function mutation in the voltage-gated sodium channel gene, *SCN1A*. Dravet syndrome typically manifests at about 6 months of age with prolonged hemiclonic seizures associated with fever. Most cases of supposed vaccine (DPT)–associated encephalopathy are now known to result from Dravet syndrome first manifesting with the minor febrile reaction to the pertussis vaccine. Adults with Dravet syndrome are typically mentally retarded with spasticity or ataxia, gait dysfunction, and occasion nocturnal clonic seizures as well as other seizure types. Dravet syndrome is a more common cause of mental retardation with epilepsy than previously appreciated. Recognition of Dravet

syndrome is important because certain antiepileptic drugs (AEDs) worsen it (lamotrigine, phenytoin), whereas others are particularly beneficial (topiramate, levetiracetam, valproate, benzodiazepines).

Neuronal migration disorders (see Chapter 123) identified by MRI are another cause of epilepsy that is being increasingly recognized.

Classification and Clinical Manifestations

Seizures are classified by their clinical symptoms and signs. The manifestations of a seizure depend on whether its onset involves most or only a part of the cerebral cortex, on the functions of the cortical areas, and on the subsequent pattern of spread within the brain. Seizures are of two broad types: (1) those with onset limited to part of the cerebral hemisphere (*partial* or *focal seizures*) and (2) those with onset that involves the cerebral cortex diffusely (*generalized seizures*). Seizures are dynamic and evolve; a patient's seizure pattern varies depending on the extent and manner of spread of the electrical discharge. Thus simple partial seizures (SPSs) can evolve into complex partial seizures (CPSs), and partial seizures can evolve into secondarily generalized tonic-clonic (GTC) seizures.

In an individual, seizures are typically stereotyped, although a person can have more than one seizure type and a specific seizure type can have varying intensities. The behaviors that occur during the seizure are termed the *semiology*. The seizure itself is referred to as the *ictus,* and the period of time during which the seizure occurs is termed the *ictal phase.* The time after the seizure, until the patient is fully recovered, is the *postictal phase,* and the time between seizures (which can be years) is the *interictal phase.*

The epileptic syndromes can be divided into three major categories: *partial epilepsy, primary (idiopathic) generalized epilepsy,* and *symptomatic generalized epilepsy.* This classification is based on the widely used scheme of the International League against Epilepsy. Specific seizure types occur in each of these groups.

PARTIAL SEIZURES

Simple Partial Seizures

In *partial seizures* (also known as *localization-related* or *focal seizures*), a localized region of the brain has abnormal neurons that intermittently fire hypersynchronously, recruiting the surrounding, otherwise normal neurons, generating a seizure. If the abnormal neuronal firing is confined, there may be no clinical manifestation, and the event, which can be detected only with electroencephalography (EEG), is termed a *subclinical or electrical seizure.* If the electrical discharge involves a slightly larger area, an SPS occurs and manifests as a symptom *without* impairment of consciousness. The symptom may be a sensation, autonomic function (e.g., nausea or another epigastric sensation), abnormal thought (e.g., fear, déjà vu), or involuntary movement. An SPS is commonly called an *aura* and can serve as a warning that a more intense seizure is about to occur. Auras occur in about 60% of patients with partial epilepsy.

During an SPS the patient can interact normally with the environment except for limitations imposed by the seizure itself on specific localized brain functions. SPSs are divided into *SPS without impairment,* which do not interfere with function (e.g., just an internal sensation) and *SPSs with impairment,* which can interfere with function (e.g., a jerking limb that would disrupt the ability to drive safely).

SPSs with motor signs manifest as *clonic* (rhythmic jerking) or *tonic* (stiffening) movements of a discrete body part. When the seizure begins in the primary motor cortex and spreads to involve adjacent areas of the precentral gyrus, clonic movements progress in an orderly sequence *(Jacksonian march)* that reflects the motor cortex homunculus topographic organization (e.g., mouth to hand to arm to leg).

Complex Partial Seizures

A CPS is a focal-onset seizure *with* impairment of consciousness. The degree of consciousness impairment spans from minimal to complete unresponsiveness. Almost always the patient's eyes are open during the ictus, indicating an awake state (albeit impaired). The eyes may close after the seizure ends, and the patient typically experiences some degree of postictal confusion, fatigue, and sometimes headache (with the head pain usually ipsilateral to the seizure focus). A CPS typically lasts 1 to 3 minutes, with a postictal state of a few minutes to hours.

The specific signs and symptoms that occur during a partial seizure characteristically reflect the location of seizure

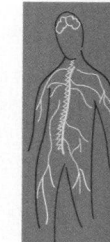

Table 126-2	**Ictal Manifestations: Localization of Seizures by Signs and Symptoms**
Locus	**Manifestation**
Temporal lobe	
Uncus or amygdala	Foul odor
Middle or inferior temporal gyrus	Visual changes: micropsia, macropsia
Parahippocampal-hippocampal area	Déjà vu; jamais vu
Parahippocampal-septal area	Fear, pleasure, anger, dreamy sensation
Auditory association cortex	Voices, music
Insular, anterior temporal cortex	Lip smacking, drooling, abdominal symptoms, cardiac arrhythmia
Frontal lobe	
Motor cortex	Contralateral clonic movements of face, fingers, hand, foot
Premotor cortex	Contralateral arm extension; fencing posture
Language areas	Speech arrest, aphasia
Lateral cortex	Contralateral eye deviation
Bifrontal	Absence-like
Parietal lobe	Sensory symptoms
Occipital lobe	Visual hallucinations (often in color), teichopsias, metamorphopsias

onset (Table 126-2). The location of the focus is important as it predicts the nature of the pathology and directs diagnostic testing. Both medical and surgical treatments are determined, in part, by focus location.

Psychomotor, temporal lobe, and *limbic seizures* are all terms that have been used in the past to describe a variety of the ictal behaviors now classified as CPSs, but they are not synonymous. Not all CPSs arise from the temporal lobe, nor do all involve the limbic system. Similarly, certain temporal lobe and limbic phenomena may not be associated with the alteration in awareness that is required to designate it a CPS.

Medial temporal lobe seizures involve the hippocampal and amygdalar areas. An epigastric sensation or a vague cephalic sensation is the most common aura symptom. Less frequently, the classical symptom of a foul smell, déjà vu, or other odd thinking occurs. Olfactory auras are referred to as *uncinate seizures* because of their origin in or near the uncus of the medial temporal lobe. In lateral temporal seizures (neocortical), language impairment (dominant hemisphere) or formed visual or auditory hallucinations occur. As a temporal lobe seizure spreads to involve the dominant temporal lobe or bilateral temporal lobe structures including the limbic system, the seizure becomes complex. A blank stare is often described by witnesses. Automatic motor behaviors, termed *automatisms,* are common in seizures that involve the limbic system (usually in the temporal lobe). Automatisms include oroalimentary signs (e.g., lip-smacking, repetitive swallowing) and repetitive hand movements (manual automatisms). Other temporal lobe seizure signs include speech arrest (dominant hemisphere), recurring vocalizations (nondominant hemisphere), and eye blinking.

Frontal lobe seizures have at least four different semiologic patterns, as follows:

1. *Supplementary motor seizures* (superior frontal gyri, posterior aspect) consist of contraversive posturing of the head and arms such that a fencing posture is assumed; the contralateral arm is extended, the head is turned strongly to that side, and the ipsilateral arm is flexed and held either up above the head or across the chest.
2. *Lateral frontal seizures* manifest as contralateral head and eye deviation.
3. *Hypermotor seizures* (frontal, poorly localized) can be dramatic, consist of wild asynchronous movements, and are often confused with psychogenic non-epileptic attacks (PNEAs); thus they are sometimes termed *pseudo-pseudoseizures*. Almost all hypermotor seizures last less than 40 seconds and typically occur one to five times a night during sleep and less often during waking. Obscene verbal explicatives are commonly uttered loudly during hypermotor seizures.
4. *Frontal absence seizures* are rare and caused by diffuse, bisynchronous epileptic activity. These consist of staring and mimic typical or atypical absence seizures (see later).

Parietal lobe seizures consist of somatosensory sensations or higher cognitive function disruption. The somatosensory sensations can have a "Jacksonian march." *Occipital lobe seizures* involve unformed or poorly formed visual hallucinations that are often in color (in contrast to the visual aura of migraine, which is black, gray, and white). Forced eye deviation can occur with occipital seizures. Occipital seizures can have a prolonged discharge lasting tens of minutes that is subclinical or minimally clinical before propagating. Parietal and occipital seizures do not become complex until propagating to the temporal lobes or limbic system.

Reflex seizures are precipitated by a specific stimulus, such as touch, a musical tune, a particular movement, reading, stroboscopic lights, or certain complex visual images. Reflex seizures arise in the parietal or occipital lobes, as these mediate sensory functions. Reflex seizures are uncommon, with the exception of the photosensitive response in juvenile myoclonic epilepsy (JME).

Secondarily Generalized Convulsive Seizures

A focal-onset seizure that spreads throughout the brain results in a *secondarily generalized seizure*. Typically there is a tonic phase that consists of extensor posturing lasting 20 to 60 seconds, followed by progressively longer periods of inhibition manifesting as a clonic phase that lasts up to another minute—hence the descriptive name *generalized tonic-clonic* seizure. The terms *convulsion, generalized tonic-clonic, grand-mal,* and *major-motor seizure* are often used interchangeably, although *generalized tonic-clonic* is a specific phenomenologic description of the behavior. In some patients, a few clonic jerks precede the tonic-clonic sequence; in others, only a tonic or clonic phase is present.

As a partial seizure transitions into a secondarily generalized convulsion, the arm contralateral to the seizure focus may extend first while the ipsilateral arm is flexed at the elbow. This is termed the *"figure-4 sign"* and is useful for lateralizing the seizure focus. A loud, *"tonic cry"* may occur at the onset of a convulsion as air is forcibly expelled through tightly contracted vocal cords. The eyes are open and commonly described to roll back. During a convulsion, breathing does not occur and cyanosis becomes evident. Foaming at the mouth may be present. Oral trauma, especially involving the tongue, is typical. Urinary incontinence is common. Fecal incontinence is rare. First aid involves turning the patient onto a side as the seizure ends to allow the saliva to drool from the mouth, decreasing the likelihood of aspiration. Witnesses commonly describe a GTC as lasting 5 to 10 minutes or longer; however, the GTC phase rarely lasts longer than 2 minutes.

The postictal phase is marked by transient deep stupor, followed in 15 to 30 minutes by a lethargic, confused state, sometimes with automatic behaviors. As recovery progresses, many patients complain of headache, muscle soreness, mental dulling, lack of energy, or mood changes lasting for hours to days.

Convulsions result in a number of striking but transient physiologic changes, including hypoxemia, lactic acidosis, elevated catecholamine levels, and increased serum concentrations of creatine kinase, prolactin, corticotropin, and cortisol. Complications include oral trauma, vertebral compression fractures, shoulder dislocation, aspiration pneumonia, and very rarely sudden death, which may be related to acute pulmonary edema, cardiac arrhythmia, or suffocation.

Partial seizures (of all intensities) may be followed by a transient neurologic abnormality reflecting postictal depression of the epileptogenic cortical area. Therefore focal weakness may follow a partial motor seizure, or numbness a sensory seizure. These reversible neurologic deficits are referred to as *Todd paralysis* and last minutes to hours, rarely more than 48 hours. Examination of a patient immediately after a seizure may show transient focal abnormalities that indicate the site or at least the side of seizure origin.

PARTIAL EPILEPSY

The classification of the epilepsy syndromes closely follows the classification of the seizures, but epilepsy is the condition with recurrent seizures. *Partial* (localization-related, focal) *epilepsy* is characterized by recurrent partial seizures. It is divided into two main groups, idiopathic and symptomatic.

Idiopathic Partial Epilepsy

The idiopathic partial epilepsies are thought to result from a subtle genetic developmental abnormality. The most common type is *benign epilepsy with central midtemporal spikes* (BECTS), also known as *benign rolandic epilepsy* (BRE). This common epilepsy syndrome of childhood represents about 15% of all pediatric epilepsies. Seizures usually begin between the ages of 3 and 13 years in an otherwise normal child. The seizures consist of brief simple partial hemifacial motor or sensory events. There is typically twitching of one side of the face, speech arrest, drooling, and paresthesias of the face, gums, tongue, or inner cheeks. These signs may be so minor that they escape notice, although the affected child often points to his face and goes to a parent and holds on until it is over; the child then quickly resumes normal activity. Seizures may progress to include hemiclonic movements or hemitonic posturing. Secondarily GTC seizures occasionally occur, usually during sleep. The parents may report only the convulsions; the focal signature can be

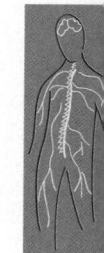

missed unless the child is carefully questioned. The electroencephalogram reveals distinctive, stereotyped epileptiform discharges over the central and midtemporal regions that are dramatically activated by sleep with a normal underlying background. Prognosis is invariably good; the seizures disappear and the electroencephalogram normalizes by mid to late adolescence. Outcome is not affected by treatment, but AEDs prevent recurrent attacks.

Symptomatic Partial Epilepsy

The symptomatic partial epilepsies are the most common type of epilepsy and are classified based on the cerebral lobe involved during the initial phase of the seizure. Temporal lobe epilepsy (TLE) is the most frequent, followed by frontal, with rarer cases of parietal and occipital. Although often not identified in life, all cases of symptomatic partial epilepsy have an underlying focal abnormality in the cerebral cortex such as a scar, malformation, growth, or abnormal gene expression. An individual patient with symptomatic partial epilepsy usually has a single focus. However, the focus can involve a large, multilobar circuit. Some patients have multiple foci, each with different seizure manifestations.

TLE is the most common epilepsy syndrome of adults, accounting for at least 40% of epilepsy cases. Habitual seizures begin in late childhood or adolescence. There is often a history of childhood febrile seizures. Virtually all patients have CPSs, some of which secondarily generalize. Most TLE arises from medial temporal limbic structures, typically associated with gliosis in the hippocampus (*hippocampal sclerosis; mesial temporal sclerosis*). In a quarter of cases, TLE is caused by another structural lesion such as a cavernous malformation, hamartoma, cortical dysplasia, glial tumor, or scar related to previous head injury or encephalitis. When a lesion is present in addition to hippocampal sclerosis, the condition is termed *dual pathology*.

Post-Traumatic Epilepsy

The likelihood of developing post-traumatic epilepsy relates directly to the severity of the head injury. The relative risk for developing epilepsy after a penetrating wound to the brain (e.g., bullet or shrapnel) is up to 600 times that in the general population; such wounds lead to epilepsy in most cases. Severe closed head injuries result in epilepsy 20% of the time. Severe closed head injuries are defined by the presence of an intracranial hemorrhage (subdural, epidural, subarachnoid, or cerebral contusion), unconsciousness or amnesia lasting more than 24 hours, or persistent abnormalities on neurologic examination, such as hemiparesis or aphasia. Although the majority of the patients with a severe head injury who develop seizures do so within 1 to 2 years, new-onset epilepsy may appear after 20 years or longer. Mild closed head injuries (uncomplicated brief loss of consciousness, no skull fracture, absence of focal neurologic signs, and no contusion or hematoma) may minimally increase the risk of seizures. Post-traumatic epilepsy is always partial, although only convulsions may be clinically evident, especially with multifocal injury. Early seizures within a week of the head injury do not necessarily signify future epilepsy.

PRIMARY GENERALIZED SEIZURES

Primary generalized seizures begin diffusely and involve both cerebral hemispheres simultaneously from the outset. They lack focal clinical and electroencephalographic features. Primary generalized seizures must be distinguished from partial seizures; in some cases they have similar clinical features.

Absence seizures (petit mal) occur mainly in children and are characterized by sudden, momentary lapses in awareness with staring. Sometimes rhythmic blinking occurs with a slight loss of neck tone. Most absence seizures last less than 10 seconds. If the absence lasts longer than 20 seconds, automatisms (see earlier) are usually present. The electroencephalogram has a characteristic pattern of three-per-second spike and slow waves (Figure 126-2) during an absence seizure. Behavior and awareness return to normal immediately after the seizure ends, although brief confusion may be present if the surroundings changed during the seizure.

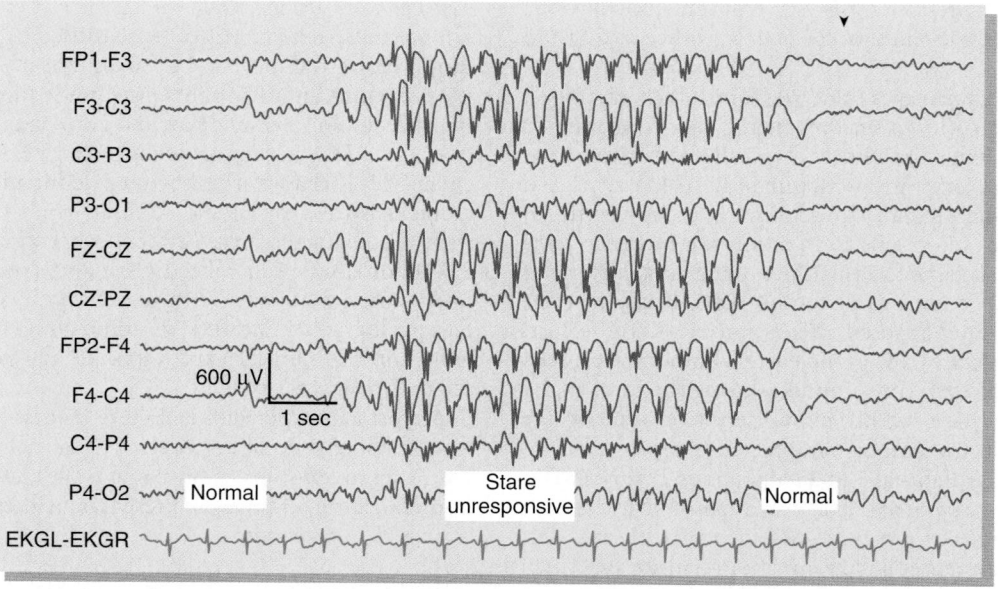

Figure 126-2 Absence (petit mal) epilepsy. The electroencephalogram shows the typical pattern of generalized 3-Hz spike-wave complexes associated with a clinical absence seizure.

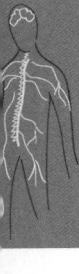

There is no postictal period and usually no recollection that a seizure occurred.

Myoclonic seizures manifest as rapid, recurrent, brief muscle jerks that can occur bilaterally, synchronously or asynchronously, or unilaterally without loss of consciousness. The myoclonic jerks range from small movements of the face or hands to massive bilateral spasms that simultaneously affect the head, limbs, and trunk. Repeated myoclonic seizures may crescendo and evolve to a GTC seizure. Although they can occur at any time, myoclonic seizures often cluster shortly after waking.

Primary GTC seizures may begin with a few myoclonic jerks or abruptly with a tonic phase lasting 20 to 60 seconds, followed by up to 1 minute of a clonic phase, followed by a postictal state (as described earlier). Although there are usually no focal features, sometimes head turning occurs; this movement does not suggest a specific localization.

IDIOPATHIC (PRIMARY) GENERALIZED EPILEPSY

The idiopathic generalized epilepsies (IGEs) are likely polygenic, resulting from a combination of mutations and polymorphisms in genes involved in thalamocortical circuitry. Different members of the same family may have dissimilar phenotypes. However, no specific IGE genes have been identified. A person with IGE has a 10% chance of passing the condition to a child. Most people with IGE have normal intelligence.

Childhood absence epilepsy (CAE; pyknolepsy, petit mal epilepsy) is the most common type of childhood epilepsy. It begins at 3 to 12 years of age with a peak at 7 years. Children with CAE have frequent absences (often hundreds per day) and are sometimes initially thought to have attention problems or to be daydreamers. Parents tend to report more absences at mealtimes, but that is because of closer observation; the absences are usually present throughout the day. One half of children with CAE have occasional GTC seizures. CAE is self-limited, and seizures and the electroencephalographic abnormalities resolve by young adulthood. The absence seizures of CAE are typically provoked by hyperventilation, a useful procedure in the office setting and during EEG.

JME begins between ages 8 and 20 years. It is characterized by clusters of myoclonic seizures in the morning, starting shortly after waking. The clusters typically persist for 10 to 30 minutes. The jerks are predominantly in the arms and last less than one second. Consciousness is preserved. An affected teenager often fails to mention the morning jerks unless specifically asked. Sometimes there is a history of throwing breakfast utensils or toothbrushes because of the jerks. JME is often diagnosed after a morning GTC seizure. In JME, GTC seizures are particularly common after sleep deprivation or alcohol consumption during the prior night. People with JME are usually photic sensitive—that is, the seizures and electroencephalographic discharges are activated by flickering lights at 5 to 20 Hz (*photic-paroxysmal* or *photic-convulsive* response). This is a type of reflex seizure (see earlier). Some people with JME also have absence seizures. The electroencephalogram is similar to that seen in CAE, but the generalized spike and slow wave discharges are slightly faster (3 to 4 Hz) nd often have polyspike components. In contrast to CAE, the seizures in JME persist

into adulthood and can be lifelong, although they lessen with age.

Less common IGE phenotypes include *juvenile absence epilepsy* (JAE) and *GTC seizures alone* (GTCA). In JAE the predominant seizure type is absence and, like JME, the condition persists into adulthood. In GTCA the predominant seizure type is a convulsion, sometimes with a predilection for the morning. Less frequent absences or myoclonic seizures can occur in GTCA. Although onset of JME, JAE, and GTCA is typically during the teen years, cases of IGE with onset in elder age have been reported.

SYMPTOMATIC SECONDARY GENERALIZED EPILEPSY

Symptomatic generalized epilepsy occurs in people with multifocal or diffuse brain dysfunction from early in life. There is usually an associated encephalopathy with some degree of mental retardation. In addition to all of the seizure types that occur in partial epilepsy and IGE, people with symptomatic generalized epilepsies have tonic and atonic drop seizures and atypical absence seizures.

Drop seizures can be tonic and/or atonic. "Drop" implies that if the patient is upright, he or she falls, with no protective reflexes. Patients with drop seizures often experience head injuries and should wear a helmet except when they are directly attended by a care provider, in a secure chair, or lying down. During a *tonic seizure,* the arms abruptly thrust forward at a 90-degree angle to the body and the entire body stiffens. Classically the fall is backward. During an *atonic seizure,* tone is abruptly lost in the postural muscles and the patient falls forward.

Atypical absence seizures manifest as staring or mental slowing associated with a slow generalized spike and slow wave discharge (2.5 Hz or less) on the electroencephalogram. They may last minutes or even hours. Fluctuating levels of awareness and gradual onset and offset are described with atypical absences.

Lennox-Gastaut Syndrome

The *Lennox-Gastaut syndrome* (LGS) is a common form of symptomatic generalized epilepsy caused by diffuse or multifocal brain dysfunction. LGS manifests at 2 to 10 years of age. Sixty percent of patients have preexisting encephalopathy and developmental delay, and 20% had infantile spasms (see later). LGS is responsible for 5% to 10% of childhood epilepsy. It is characterized by the combination of tonic and atonic seizures, myoclonic seizures, and atypical absences with the characteristic electroencephalographic pattern of 2.5 Hz or slower generalized spike and slow waves. During sleep there are bursts of diffuse fast rhythms on the electroencephalogram indicative of tonic-atonic seizures, often with minimal clinical expression. Tonic-clonic and partial seizures may also occur.

Almost all people with LGS have mental retardation with associated behavioral disorders. LGS is a chronic condition requiring supervision; many patients ultimately live in group homes. If drop seizures are present, a helmet should be prescribed for protection.

Infantile Spasms

Infantile spasms are often a precursor of LGS, although not formally classified as a symptomatic generalized epilepsy. By definition, infantile spasms begin during the first year of life. They affect approximately 1 in 5000 children. The epileptic spasms manifest as flexor or extensor tonus, myoclonus, or a mixed pattern. The spasms last 1 to 20 seconds each and occur in clusters for up to 20 minutes. *West syndrome* is the combination of epileptic spasms, hypsarrhythmia (a chaotic, disorganized epileptiform electroencephalographic pattern), and mental retardation. It is common for the term *infantile spasms* to be used synonymously with *West syndrome*. Infantile spasms have a poor prognosis, with over 90% of patients developing mental retardation and most progressing to symptomatic generalized epilepsy; only a small percent of patients with cryptogenic cases recover. There are many causes of infantile spasms, including perinatal insults, cerebral malformations, central nervous system (CNS) infections, tuberous sclerosis, and inborn errors of metabolism.

OTHER SEIZURE CONDITIONS

Febrile Seizures

Febrile seizures affect between 3% and 5% of children younger than the age of 6 years. About 30% of children have more than one attack; the likelihood of recurrence is greater if the first seizure occurs before 1 year of age or there is a family history of febrile seizures. Although most affected children have no long-term consequences, febrile seizures increase the risk of developing epilepsy later in life. This risk is low for most children (2% to 3%) but is 10% to 15% in those who had prolonged or focal febrile seizures, a family history of nonfebrile seizures, or neurologic abnormalities before the first febrile seizure.

Diagnosis

Accurate diagnosis is the cornerstone of epilepsy treatment. The diagnostic evaluation has three objectives: (1) to determine that the events are epileptic seizures; (2) to identify a specific underlying cause; and (3) to establish if the seizures are symptomatic and isolated or if epilepsy is present and, if so, to determine the specific epilepsy syndrome.

HISTORY AND EXAMINATION

The patient's and witnesses' descriptions of the events are central to making the diagnosis. Extra attention should be given to exploring details of the behavior during the seizure. The setting of the seizure can suggest acute causes such as drug withdrawal, CNS infection, trauma, or stroke. A history of recent-onset seizures in an adult suggests a new intracranial lesion, and a more chronically sustained or remote history of attacks suggests chronic epilepsy. Any focal feature before, during, or after the seizure suggests a structural brain lesion requiring appropriate investigation. The pattern of the seizures and the patient's age are often important clues to the seizure and epilepsy type.

The physical examination findings are normal in most patients with epilepsy. Physical findings that should be sought include overt or subtle focal neurologic signs, including slight unilateral lower facial paresis, clumsy fine finger movements, and mild hyperreflexia, as these can be present in partial epilepsy with a contralateral seizure focus. Careful skin examination is indicated to detect features of neurocu-

taneous syndromes such as a facial port-wine stain involving the upper eyelid in Sturge-Weber syndrome; hypopigmented macules (ash-leaf spots), shagreen patch, and facial angiofibromas in tuberous sclerosis; and café-au-lait spots and axillary freckling in neurofibromatosis. Asymmetry in the size of the hands, feet, or face signifies a long-standing abnormality of the cerebral hemisphere contralateral to the smaller side. Absence seizures can be triggered in untreated children with hyperventilation for 2 to 3 minutes.

LABORATORY TESTS

EEG is the most important diagnostic test for seizures and epilepsy. Electroencephalographic findings are useful and sometimes essential for establishing the diagnosis, classifying the seizures correctly, identifying the epilepsy syndrome, and making therapeutic decisions. In combination with suitable clinical findings, *epileptiform* electroencephalographic discharges, termed *spikes* or *sharp waves,* strongly support a diagnosis of epilepsy.

In patients with recurrent seizures, focal epileptiform discharges are consistent with focal epilepsy, whereas generalized epileptiform activity usually indicates a generalized form of epilepsy. However, most electroencephalograms are obtained between seizures, and interictal abnormalities alone cannot prove or disprove a diagnosis of epilepsy.

Forty percent to 50% of patients with epilepsy show epileptiform abnormalities on the initial electroencephalogram. The chance of capturing epileptiform activity is enhanced by sleep deprivation the night before the test so that the patient sleeps during a portion of the electroencephalographic recording. Serial electroencephalograms increase the yield of positive tracings. A small proportion of patients with epilepsy have normal interictal electroencephalograms despite all efforts to record an abnormality.

The interpretation of the interictal electroencephalogram is confounded by two factors. One is that epileptiform discharges occur in about 2% of normal people; many of these are thought to be asymptomatic markers of a genetic trait, especially in children. Second is that the interpretation of the electroencephalogram is subjective and there are normal benign variant waveforms and artifacts that can be misinterpreted as epileptiform activity and erroneously considered to be evidence of seizure susceptibility.

Epilepsy can be definitively established by recording a characteristic ictal discharge during a representative clinical attack. This is uncommon during routine electroencephalographic recordings but can be accomplished with *inpatient video-EEG long-term monitoring* (LTM) performed at many epilepsy centers throughout the world. Inpatient video-EEG monitoring is indicated in people who have ongoing seizures despite being treated with appropriate AEDs. About one third of patients admitted for LTM are found to not have epilepsy; the majority of these patients have PNEAs (see later). In the 25% to 30% of people with partial epilepsy who continue to have disabling seizures despite trials with multiple AEDs, inpatient video-EEG monitoring is a critical test for determining candidacy for resective epilepsy surgery.

NEUROIMAGING

Brain MRI complements electroencephalographic findings by identifying structural pathology that may be causally

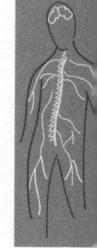

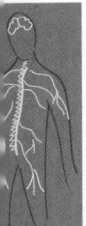

related to the development of epilepsy. MRI is the best test to detect epileptogenic cerebral lesions including hippocampal sclerosis, neuronal migration disorders, tumors, focal atrophy, arteriovenous malformations, and cavernous malformations. It is important to obtain a complete imaging study that includes T1-weighted, T2-weighted, and inversion-recovery sequences in coronal and axial planes with and without contrast. Imaging in the coronal plane perpendicular to the long axis of the hippocampus has improved detection of hippocampal atrophy and hippocampal high T2 signal, findings that correlate with the pathologic finding of mesial temporal sclerosis and an epileptogenic temporal lobe. Additional sequences that should be routine include T2-weighted gradient-echo (GRE), to detect hemosiderin indicating old hemorrhage associated with vascular malformations or trauma, and diffusion-weighted images (DWI) for cytotoxic edema present with acute cerebral injury including the effects from prolonged seizures.

An MRI should be obtained in all patients suspected of having epilepsy except those with definite benign epilepsy with centro-temporal spikes (BRE) or definite IGE (e.g., CAE and JME). Computed tomography (CT) scan with contrast is an alternate study for those who cannot have MRI but is not as good at detecting small lesions. CT scan can complement MRI because it is better for detecting calcium and a more practical test for acute bleeding. Any patient with seizures and abnormal neurologic findings or focal slow-wave abnormalities on EEG should have neuroimaging. If there is an unexplained change in seizure pattern, repeat neuroimaging should be considered, to evaluate for a new lesion.

Positron emission tomography (PET) and single-photon emission computed tomography (SPECT) provide information about brain function. These techniques use physiologically active, radiolabeled tracers to image the brain's metabolic activity (PET) or blood flow (SPECT). Typically these studies are reserved for select patients undergoing evaluation for epilepsy surgery. About 70% to 85% of patients with TLE have temporal lobe hypometabolism on interictal PET corresponding to the seizure focus. SPECT is most useful when an ictal and interictal study are combined to identify an extratemporal seizure focus. Abnormalities on PET or SPECT are often present even when brain structure on MRI is normal.

OTHER TESTS

Routine blood tests rarely offer diagnostic assistance in otherwise healthy patients with epilepsy. Serum electrolytes, liver function tests, and complete blood count are useful as baseline studies before AED therapy is started. Blood tests are necessary in older patients with acute or chronic systemic disease. Adolescents and young adults with unexplained seizures should be screened for substance abuse (especially cocaine) with blood or urine studies.

Lumbar puncture is indicated only if there is a suspicion of meningitis, encephalitis, or a CNS glucose transporter abnormality; it is otherwise unnecessary. Repeated generalized seizures and status epilepticus can increase cerebrospinal fluid protein content slightly and produce a pleocytosis for 24 to 48 hours; cerebrospinal fluid pleocytosis should be

Table 126-3 **Non-Epileptic Episodic Disorders That May Resemble Seizures**
Movement disorders: myoclonus, paroxysmal choreoathetosis, episodic ataxias, hyperexplexia (startle disease)
Migraine: confusional, vertebrobasilar, visual auras
Syncope
Behavioral and psychiatric: psychogenic non-epileptic attacks (pseudoseizures), hyperventilation syndrome, panic or anxiety disorder, dissociative states
Cataplexy (usually associated with narcolepsy)
Transient ischemic attack
Alcoholic blackouts
Hypoglycemia

attributed to seizures only in retrospect after an intracranial inflammatory process has been excluded.

An electrocardiogram (ECG) should be obtained in any young person with a first generalized seizure if there is a family history of arrhythmia, sudden unexplained death, or episodic unconsciousness. An ECG should also be obtained in any patient with a personal history of cardiac arrhythmia or valvular disease.

Differential Diagnosis

Not every paroxysmal event is a seizure, and misidentification of other conditions as epilepsy leads to ineffective, unnecessary, and potentially harmful treatment. Misdiagnosis accounts for a substantial portion of patients who have not responded to AED treatment. A variety of conditions can be confused with epilepsy, depending on the age of the patient and the nature and circumstances of the attacks (Table 126-3). Non-epileptic paroxysmal disorders that are confused with epileptic seizures have sudden, discrete abnormal behaviors, variable responsiveness, changes in muscle tone, and various postures or movements.

PNEAs (*pseudoseizures, psychogenic non-electrical attacks*) frequently cause intractable "epilepsy" in adults. PNEAs result when the unconscious mind converts emotional conflicts or stressors into a physical state that mimics a seizure (see Chapter 117). Some patients with psychogenic seizures also have epilepsy. Definitive diagnosis requires video-EEG documentation, although a history of atypical and non-stereotyped attacks, emotional or psychological precipitants, psychiatric illness, lack of response to AEDs, and repeatedly normal interictal electroencephalograms suggests the possibility of psychogenic attacks. About 80% of patients with PNEA have been the victims of physical or sexual abuse. PNEAs are more common in females.

Panic attacks (anxiety attacks) with hyperventilation can superficially resemble partial seizures with affective, autonomic, or special sensory symptoms. Hyperventilation typically causes perioral and finger tingling. Prolonged hyperventilation results in muscle twitching or spasms (tetany); affected patients may faint.

Syncope (see Chapter 121) refers to the symptom complex that results when there is a transient, global reduction in cerebral perfusion. Loss of consciousness lasts only a few seconds, uncommonly a minute or more, and recovery is usually rapid. If the cerebral ischemia is sufficiently severe, the syncopal episode may include tonic posturing of the trunk or clonic jerks of the arms and legs and incontinence (*convulsive syncope*).

Some forms of *migraine* can be mistaken for seizures, especially if the headache is atypical or mild. The visual aura, present in some migraineurs, is typically black, gray, and white; a color aura almost always indicates an epileptic seizure. Basilar artery migraine, a variant noted most often in children and young adults, can include lethargy, mood changes, confusion, disorientation, vertigo, bilateral visual disturbances, and loss of consciousness.

Treatment

If the cause of symptomatic seizures is corrected, AEDs are usually not necessary. Adults with a single, unprovoked seizure and normal clinical and laboratory findings frequently do not have subsequent seizures; antiepileptic treatment is usually not indicated if only one seizure has occurred. However, patients with focal neurologic findings on clinical, radiologic, or electroencephalographic examinations are more likely to have repeated seizures. In individual patients, social considerations may dictate treatment after a single seizure.

If seizures are recurrent, the goal of treatment is complete seizure freedom. There is no perfect AED. They all have potential toxic side-effects and idiosyncratic reactions. For more than half of people with epilepsy, any of the appropriate AEDs for their particular type of seizures can be completely effective and well tolerated. However, for about one quarter of people with epilepsy, no AED or combination of AEDs is completely effective. Once the seizure type and epilepsy syndrome have been determined an initial and, if needed, subsequent AED should be chosen based on both the anticipated efficacy and toxicity profile. All AEDs can cause sedation, cognitive dysfunction, and incoordination in some patients, especially at high levels. Various rare, sometimes life-threatening reactions may occur with all of the AEDs. Commonly encountered situations are as follows:

1. IGE (CAE, JME, others)
   a. In all IGEs, valproate or lamotrigine is the first line agent and results in complete control in 85% to 90% of patients.
      i. Valproate tends to cause weight gain and has been associated with the development of polycystic ovary syndrome, particularly in adolescent girls. It results in hair loss in about 5%. It has an increased risk of teratogenicity.
      ii. Lamotrigine has a small but significant risk of a severe rash (toxic epidermal necrolysis—Stevens-Johnson syndrome) for about the first 2 months after the medication is started. A slow dose escalation substantially reduces this risk. Lamotrigine metabolism is dramatically inhibited by valproate, so in combination, much lower doses of lamotrigine are required. Occasionally lamotrigine worsens myoclonus, but it is effective in most cases of JME.

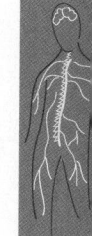

   b. Second-line options include topiramate, levetiracetam, and zonisamide.
   c. In CAE with exclusively absence seizures, ethosuximide is an appropriate first choice. If any convulsions have occurred, valproate or lamotrigine should be used.
   d. If there is a history of more than 5 minutes of crescendo in absences or myoclonus (often described as a "foggy" state) culminating in a convulsion, then oral benzodiazepines (lorazepam or diazepam) can abort the absence cluster and prevent a convulsion.
   e. Absences and myoclonus can be exacerbated by carbamazepine, oxcarbazepine, and GABAergic compounds including gabapentin, pregabalin, and tiagabine. These AEDs should be avoided in IGE.
2. Partial epilepsy
   a. Almost all of the AEDs (except ethosuximide) can be effective in partial epilepsy. The choice of the first AED should be guided by side effect concerns and pharmacokinetics.
   b. Phenytoin is the most commonly used AED in partial epilepsy in developed countries. It is typically loaded in the emergency room after the initial seizures and subsequently continued. However, phenytoin has substantial short- and long-term toxicity, and its levels are difficult to regulate because of saturation kinetics and multiple drug interactions. Its toxicities include hirsutism, coarsening of features, and gingival hyperplasia, especially in children and adolescents. Long-term toxicities include osteomalacia, peripheral neuropathy, and cerebellar degeneration with permanent incoordination. Peak level toxicities include nystagmus, gait instability, ataxia, and, if the level rises above 50, acute cerebellar degeneration and cardiac arrhythmias.
   c. Carbamazepine, oxcarbazepine, topiramate, levetiracetam, lamotrigine, and zonisamide are currently used as first-line therapy for partial seizures. Carbamazepine and oxcarbazepine can cause hyponatremia. Topiramate can lead to weight loss (often desired) but has cognitive side effects. Levetiracetam can cause severe mood changes and marked sedation but is usually well tolerated. Lamotrigine needs to be titrated slowly because of the rash risk. Zonisamide has a long half-life (48 to 72 hours), so it is a good option for intermittently noncompliant patients.
   d. Patients with Asian ancestry should be tested for the HLA-B*1502 allele before treatment with carbamazepine is initiated. Patients with this allele (which is present only in the Asian population) are at substantial risk for Stevens-Johnson syndrome and toxic epidermal necrolysis when exposed to carbamazepine.
   e. Adjunctive treatment for partial seizures includes valproate, pregabalin, lacosamide, gabapentin, tiagabine, and primidone. The proportion of gabapentin absorbed decreases with increasing dose, which limits its effectiveness. For most patients, pregabalin is a better choice. Primidone is rapidly converted to phenobarbital by some people, limiting its use.
   f. Phenobarbital is the most widely used AED in the world because of its low cost. However, it causes sedation and cognitive impairment and it should be

avoided except in difficult-to-control epilepsy. The exception is neonatal seizures, for which it is the most commonly accepted AED.

3. Symptomatic generalized epilepsy (LGS, others)
   a. All AEDs have a role in the treatment of symptomatic generalized epilepsy, but seizure freedom is rarely achieved. At a minimum, control of the more severe seizures including drop seizures and convulsions should be the target of therapy. Polytherapy is usually required.
   b. Valproate is commonly the initial medication instituted.
   c. Added efficacy can be achieved with lamotrigine, topiramate, levetiracetam, and zonisamide.
   d. Felbamate may be effective, but its use should be limited to epileptologists because of the significant risk of fatal aplastic anemia and liver failure.
   e. The vagus nerve stimulator (VNS; see later) has a specific role in reducing the severity of seizures in this condition.
   f. Dravet syndrome and possibly the related syndrome of generalized epilepsy with febrile seizures plus (GEFS+) respond best to topiramate, levetiracetam, and benzodiazepines. Some drugs, including lamotrigine and probably phenytoin, worsen Dravet syndrome.

Determining the dose of AEDs must be done with care. Only a few of the AEDs are safe to load or start at a full therapeutic dose. Most should be started with a gradual dose escalation. Management guidelines are as follows:

1. The type of seizures and epilepsy should be defined, and the preferred medication should be given in usual doses and then increased until seizure control is complete or side effects occur (Table 126-4).
2. If seizures persist at toxic levels, or if major side effects occur, another agent should be tried.
3. Do not stop one agent until another has been added. Otherwise, status epilepticus may result.

4. If seizures persist after two agents have been given to toxic levels, consider referral to a specialized epilepsy center for complex combination therapy and video-EEG LTM.
5. Toxic levels of some AEDs (particularly phenytoin and carbamazepine) can cause seizures.
6. Extended-release and longer-acting AEDs are preferred for most patients.
7. Patients should be counseled repeatedly to adhere to the medication regimen. Pill boxes should be encouraged. Medication noncompliance is the leading cause of breakthrough seizures.

EPILEPSY SURGERY

In the majority of patients, epilepsy is controlled with medication. When seizures cannot be controlled by adequate trials of two appropriate single agents or by the combination of two agents, the epilepsy is termed *medically intractable* (or *refractory*), a situation encountered in approximately 25% of patients with symptomatic partial epilepsy. Such patients are at risk for the consequences of seizures: inability to drive; stigmatization by schools, employers, and families; and threats to personal educational and occupational goals. In appropriately selected cases, epilepsy surgery can abolish seizures with restoration of normal neurologic function. The accurate localization of a small, resectable seizure focus requires intensive investigation at a specialized center.

KETOGENIC DIET

The ketogenic diet is a very high-fat diet with restricted carbohydrates and protein carefully designed to cause a ketotic state mimicking starvation, but supplying adequate nutrition. It is mainly used in children with severe symptomatic generalized epilepsy. The ketogenic diet can be effective in this most refractory form of epilepsy, resulting in seizure freedom in 15% to 20%. However, the diet is hard to maintain and requires a dedicated, cooperative caregiver (usually the patient's mother) and a specially trained dietician.

Table 126-4 **Frequently Prescribed Antiepileptic Drugs**

Drug	Adult Total Dose per day	Dose Frequency (hr)	"Therapeutic" Concentrations
Carbamazepine	400-1600 mg	6-8 (12 for sustained release)	6-12 µg/mL
Ethosuximide	500-1500 mg	8-12	40-100 µg/mL
Gabapentin	900-3600 mg	6-8	Uncertain
Lacosamide	200-400 mg	12	Uncertain
Lamotrigine*	100-800 mg	12	2-15 µg/mL
Levetiracetam	500-3000 mg	12	15-40 µg/mL
Oxcarbazepine	600-2400 mg	8-12	15-40 µg/mL
Phenobarbital	60-240 mg	24	15-40 µg/mL
Phenytoin	200-400 mg	24	10-20 µg/mL
Pregabalin	100-600 mg	8-12	Uncertain
Rufinamide	1600-3200 mg	8-12	Uncertain
Topiramate	100-600 mg	12	2-20 µg/mL
Valproate	500-6000 mg	8	50-120 µg/mL
Zonisamide	100-600 mg	24	Uncertain

*Slow initial dose titration mandatory for lamotrigine *and often indicated for other agents.*

VAGUS NERVE STIMULATOR (VNS)

The VNS is an implanted device similar in appearance to a cardiac pacemaker. It is placed into contact with the left vagus nerve in the neck. Typically it is programmed to stimulate the nerve for 30 seconds every 3 to 5 minutes, although there are many other options. Swiping a magnet over the device can give an extra stimulation and sometimes abort a seizure. In up to two thirds of patients, partial seizures are reduced by 50% or more and seizure intensity decreases. The VNS rarely results in seizure freedom. The VNS may have a role in symptomatic generalized epilepsy, improving drop seizures and overall seizure severity. Once a VNS has been implanted, the patient cannot have an MRI of the neck and certain other body regions. MRIs of the head with standard field strengths are permitted, but not with higher field strengths, above 2 Tesla.

STATUS EPILEPTICUS

Status epilepticus can occur with partial or generalized epilepsy and is defined as prolonged or rapidly recurring seizures without full intervening recovery. Various durations have been specified including longer than the patient's typical seizures or seizures ongoing for more than 10 to 30 minutes. *Acute repetitive seizures* are defined as a cluster of seizures over minutes to hours with intervening recovery.

Convulsive status epilepticus (grand mal, major-motor) is a medical emergency. Continuous generalized epileptic activity can damage the brain permanently. The most frequent cause is abrupt withdrawal of AEDs (e.g., noncompliance) in a person with known epilepsy. Other precipitants include withdrawal from alcohol or drugs in a habitual user, cerebral infection, trauma, hemorrhage, and brain tumor.

Complex partial status epilepticus manifests as a sustained state of confusion often associated with motor and autonomic automatisms. Some attacks produce bizarre behavior, whereas others are marked by a stuporous state. Patients may resist assistance because of their abnormal state, which can last for hours or even days. The electroencephalogram usually shows nearly continuous discharging activity predominating in one or both temporal regions.

Absence status epilepticus (petit mal status) resembles complex partial status and consists of a confused state with some automatic behaviors. The electroencephalogram is characteristic, with continuous runs of generalized 3- to 4-Hz spike and slow wave activity. The condition occurs in children to young adults with known absence epilepsy. Rarely, absence status occurs as the first manifestation of epilepsy in older persons with no history of seizures. *Atypical absence status* with fluctuating confusion lasting for hours or longer occurs in patients with symptomatic generalized epilepsy (e.g., LGS) and is accompanied by a generalized spike–slow wave pattern of 2.5 Hz or slower on the electroencephalogram.

Partial motor status, also known as *epilepsy partialis continua,* ranges from highly focal, clonic movements of the face or hand to jerks that involve most of the limb or half the body. The clonus frequency can vary from one every 3 seconds to 3 per second. It is relatively uncommon. Its causes include stroke, trauma, neoplasms, and encephalitis; sometimes the cause never becomes clear. Epilepsy partialis continua often resists all efforts at treatment, and neurosurgical removal of the causative lesion is sometimes required.

Physicians infrequently witness seizures; most of the time they learn about the semiology while taking the history. Merely observing a patient in the midst of a seizure does not indicate that the patient should be treated for status epilepticus. However, once status epilepticus is diagnosed, the need for treatment is urgent.

The longer status epilepticus lasts, the more difficult it is to terminate and the more likely it is to cause brain damage. Aggressive therapy is mandatory for convulsive status epilepticus (Table 126-5). If initial therapy is not rapidly effective, anesthetic agents requiring intubation and ventilation should be used within an hour of onset. Complex partial status can also result in permanent neuronal injury and should similarly be treated aggressively, although therapeutic decisions are often made to try to stop complex partial status with agents that do not cause respiratory suppression to avoid intubation. Absence status is unlikely to result in permanent sequelae and usually responds promptly to benzodiazepine treatment.

Investigation of the cause of the status epilepticus should be undertaken during the treatment and continued after the seizures stop. Severe hyperglycemia can produce refractory partial motor and complex partial status; seizures stop once hyperglycemia is corrected.

Postanoxic status myoclonus, although it can last for weeks and is accompanied by generalized polyspike epileptiform discharges on the electroencephalogram, is usually not treated as status epilepticus. It typically indicates an irreversible condition caused by severe brain injury with a very poor prognosis.

Genetic Counseling and Pregnancy

HEREDITY

Patients with epilepsy should be advised about the hereditary risks for their offspring, although in most people with epilepsy it does not influence their decision about having children. The idiopathic epilepsies have complex inheritance, with about 10% of children of an affected parent developing seizures. There are over 200 Mendelian-inherited syndromes with epilepsy, but these are all rare.

TERATOGENICITY

Children of mothers taking antiepileptic medication have a birth defect rate of 6% to 9%, which is 2 to 3 times that of the general population. Convulsions, however, pose a substantial risk to the mother and fetus. Therefore AEDs should not be stopped during pregnancy. Two AEDs, valproate and carbamazepine, have been incriminated in neural tube closure defects. Because the neural tube closes by 28 days of fetal development, this defect will develop before the mother is aware she is pregnant. Phenytoin, phenobarbital, and primidone have been associated with a spectrum of neurodevelopmental abnormalities. All five of these older AEDs are classified as pregnancy category D by the U.S. Food and Drug Administration (FDA) and should be avoided if

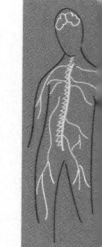

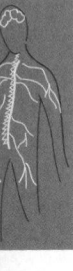

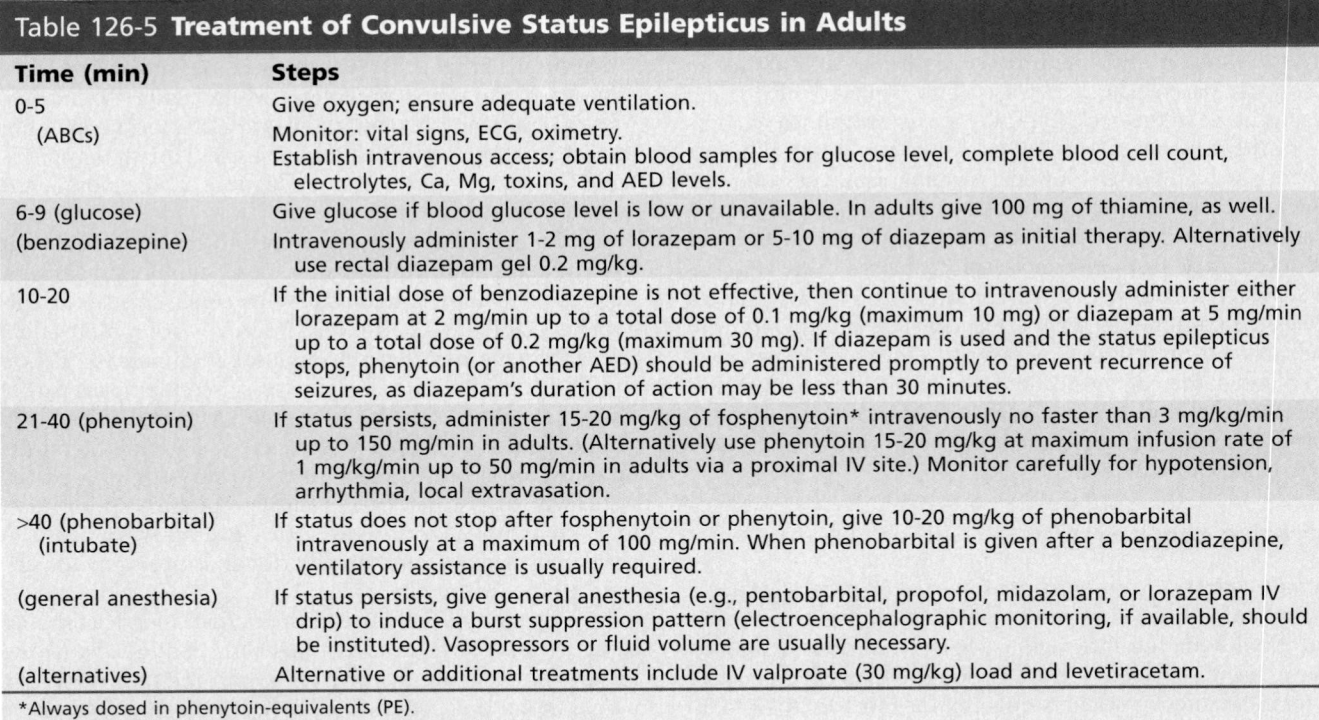

Table 126-5 Treatment of Convulsive Status Epilepticus in Adults

Time (min)	Steps
0-5 (ABCs)	Give oxygen; ensure adequate ventilation.
	Monitor: vital signs, ECG, oximetry.
	Establish intravenous access; obtain blood samples for glucose level, complete blood cell count, electrolytes, Ca, Mg, toxins, and AED levels.
6-9 (glucose) (benzodiazepine)	Give glucose if blood glucose level is low or unavailable. In adults give 100 mg of thiamine, as well.
	Intravenously administer 1-2 mg of lorazepam or 5-10 mg of diazepam as initial therapy. Alternatively use rectal diazepam gel 0.2 mg/kg.
10-20	If the initial dose of benzodiazepine is not effective, then continue to intravenously administer either lorazepam at 2 mg/min up to a total dose of 0.1 mg/kg (maximum 10 mg) or diazepam at 5 mg/min up to a total dose of 0.2 mg/kg (maximum 30 mg). If diazepam is used and the status epilepticus stops, phenytoin (or another AED) should be administered promptly to prevent recurrence of seizures, as diazepam's duration of action may be less than 30 minutes.
21-40 (phenytoin)	If status persists, administer 15-20 mg/kg of fosphenytoin* intravenously no faster than 3 mg/kg/min up to 150 mg/min in adults. (Alternatively use phenytoin 15-20 mg/kg at maximum infusion rate of 1 mg/kg/min up to 50 mg/min in adults via a proximal IV site.) Monitor carefully for hypotension, arrhythmia, local extravasation.
>40 (phenobarbital) (intubate)	If status does not stop after fosphenytoin or phenytoin, give 10-20 mg/kg of phenobarbital intravenously at a maximum of 100 mg/min. When phenobarbital is given after a benzodiazepine, ventilatory assistance is usually required.
(general anesthesia)	If status persists, give general anesthesia (e.g., pentobarbital, propofol, midazolam, or lorazepam IV drip) to induce a burst suppression pattern (electroencephalographic monitoring, if available, should be instituted). Vasopressors or fluid volume are usually necessary.
(alternatives)	Alternative or additional treatments include IV valproate (30 mg/kg) load and levetiracetam.

*Always dosed in phenytoin-equivalents (PE).
AED, antiepileptic drug; ECG, electrocardiogram; IV, intravenous.

possible. Large registries suggest that the newer AEDs have less teratogenicity, but the data are incomplete. Use of two or more AEDs (polytherapy) increases the teratogenic risk.

Pregnancies in WWE should be planned. During the year before conception, an attempt should be made to minimize the teratogenic potential of the AEDs by changing to a newer AED, changing to monotherapy from polytherapy, or tapering off the AEDs, but only if there are clear reasons to believe that seizures will not recur (see later). The lowest effective dose of the AEDs should be used, but this must be balanced with the risk of a breakthrough seizure.

Folic acid deficiency is a well-established factor in neural tube closure defects in the general population. There is little evidence that additional folic acid in a well-nourished woman with epilepsy decreases the AED effects on neural tube closure. However, it is common practice to place WWE of childbearing age on supplemental folic acid (1 mg) as prophylaxis against a neural tube closure defect. Once pregnancy is planned or recognized, the dose of folic acid is commonly increased to 4 mg per day.

MANAGEMENT DURING AND AFTER PREGNANCY

WWE have a 1.5- to 3-fold increased rate of complications of pregnancy, including bleeding, toxemia, abruptio placentae, and premature labor. They should be managed as having high-risk pregnancies. High-quality (focused or type 2) ultrasound, maternal serum alpha-fetoprotein level (elevated in neural tube closure defects), and amniocentesis for chromosomal analysis are used to identify fetal malformations.

During pregnancy, AED concentrations decrease because of increased hepatic and renal clearance and increased plasma volume. The free fraction of highly protein-bound AEDs (e.g., phenytoin and valproate) increase because of decreased albumin concentration and increased competition

for binding sites by sex steroids. Therefore it is essential to monitor drug levels (free levels for highly protein-bound AEDs) before conception and at regular intervals throughout pregnancy. Hepatic induction of glucuronidation can dramatically reduce lamotrigine levels, sometimes requiring doubling or tripling of the lamotrigine dose to maintain pre-pregnancy levels. Lamotrigine levels should be measured at least every month throughout pregnancy. Similarly, oxcarbazepine levels fall by about a third beginning in the first trimester, and thus the dose should be increased and followed at least each trimester.

Emesis, a common problem during early pregnancy, can result in missed and partial doses of AEDs. The expectant mother should have specific instructions to retake a full or partial dose of her AEDs if vomiting occurs shortly after medications have been taken.

After the child is born, the dose of AEDs should be tapered to the pre-pregnancy amount within days to weeks. The AED levels can be checked 1 to 2 weeks after the taper is completed, to confirm they are at the patient's baseline.

In general, breastfeeding is not contraindicated in women taking AEDs.

During the postpartum period the mother with epilepsy may be at increased risk for seizures, especially if her seizures are activated by lack of sleep. To decrease this risk, a support person should perform at least one of the nighttime feedings. Patients whose seizure semiology would put the infant at risk (e.g., dropping or excessively clutching the baby) may require child care modification or supervision.

Psychosocial Concerns

Ongoing epileptic seizures often result in major emotional consequences for the patient and family. Comorbid depression is present in up to 50% of patients with refractory

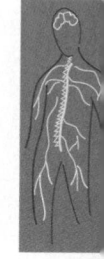

epilepsy and 20% of patients with controlled epilepsy. Anxiety disorders are similarly common. Both are often unrecognized and untreated. In people with epilepsy, quality-of-life impairment is better correlated with depression than seizure frequency. The unpredictable nature of seizures and the necessary activity restrictions cause dependence, decreased self-worth, embarrassment, underemployment, and helplessness. Reduced libido and hyposexuality are common in patients with epilepsy and often unrecognized.

Family dynamics are often disrupted by the presence of epilepsy. Both families and patients often fear seizures (seizure phobia). It is common for family members to perceive that their loved one is dying when he or she has a convulsion, especially for the first time.

Patients with epilepsy are helped most by complete seizure control, but reassurance and optimistic social guidance aid immeasurably. Once seizure control has been achieved, affected persons should be encouraged to live a normal life, using common sense as their guide. Although activity restrictions may eventually be lifted, patients with past epilepsy should be advised to avoid head-contact sports, high alpine climbing, scuba diving, and professions requiring work at heights, large amounts of driving, or weapon use (with the exception of CAE or BECTS, which may completely remit).

All states grant automobile driver's licenses to patients with epilepsy, provided that no seizures have occurred for specified periods. Life-and-health insurance policies can generally be obtained. The Epilepsy Foundation of America and local social service organizations can assist with patients' social-vocational considerations.

Prognosis

Sixty percent to 70% of people with epilepsy achieve a 5-year remission of seizures within 10 years of diagnosis. About half of these patients are eventually seizure-free without AEDs. Factors favoring remission include an idiopathic form of epilepsy, a normal neurologic examination, and onset in early to middle childhood (excluding neonatal seizures).

Approximately 30% of patients continue to have seizures and never achieve a permanent remission with medications. In the United States, the prevalence of intractable epilepsy

cases is 1 to 2 per 1000 population. Such patients should be evaluated at an epilepsy center.

Injuries resulting from seizures are common. Advising patients not to cook, or to use back burners or microwave ovens, can prevent some serious burns. A helmet is advisable for those with drop seizures.

Sudden unexplained death in epilepsy (SUDEP) occurs in 1 per 1000 patients per year, taking all forms of epilepsy together. In the most refractory epilepsies, the SUDEP rate is greater than 1 per 200 patients per year. SUDEP is believed to result from excessive autonomic nervous system sympathetic tone during an unwitnessed seizure with resultant cardiac arrhythmia or pulmonary edema. Suffocation can occur after an unwitnessed convulsion if the patient ends up face down in a pillow. Accidental deaths related to seizures (e.g., motor vehicle collisions) further increase the death rate. Aspiration with convulsions is common but can be prevented by turning the head to one side as the convulsion ends.

Discontinuing Antiepileptic Drugs

Many patients with epilepsy become seizure-free on medication for an extended period of time. Some patients can discontinue AEDs without a relapse. Successful drug withdrawal is most likely if initial seizure control was readily achieved using monotherapy, there were relatively few seizures before remission, and the electroencephalogram and neurologic examination findings are normal just before drugs are tapered off. A seizure-free interval of at least 2 years is important to reduce the likelihood of relapse; some advocate that seizure freedom should be for at least 5 years unless the epilepsy syndrome is known to remit (e.g., CAE or BECTS). Conversely, risk of relapse is high if seizure control was difficult to establish and required polytherapy, if there were frequent convulsions before control was achieved, if a focal abnormality is present on neurologic examination, or if the electroencephalogram demonstrates focal disturbances of background activity or epileptiform activity at the time drug withdrawal is considered.

Prospectus for the Future

- For the past eight decades, new drugs have been developed for epilepsy. This trend should continue, and one to three new AEDs with differing mechanisms of action should become available every 5 years.
- The molecular pathogenesis of some genetic epilepsies has been defined. These still rare disorders will provide insights and targets for novel antiepileptic treatments that correct neuronal dysfunction. The molecular causes of the common epilepsies will be defined.

- Improved imaging techniques will further facilitate cortical localization and selective ablation of the epileptic focus, resulting in more patients becoming seizure-free and returning to normal life.
- Chronically implanted electrodes located at the seizure foci attached to implanted computers will allow direct monitoring of seizures, and treatments (e.g., electrical stimulation, drugs, cooling) delivered directly to the seizure focus without the need for removal of a portion of the brain.

References

Bleck TP. Refractory status epilepticus. Curr Opin Crit Care 11:117-120, 2005.

French JA, Pedley TA. Initial management of epilepsy. N Engl J Med 359:166-176, 2008.

Hirtz D, Berg AT, Bettis D, et al. Practice parameter: Treatment of the child with a first unprovoked seizure. Report of the Quality Standards Subcommittee of the American Academy of Neurology and the Practice Committee of the Child Neurology Society. Neurology 60:166-175, 2003.

Krumholz A, et al. Practice parameter: Evaluating an apparent unprovoked first seizure in adults (an evidence-based review). Report of the Quality Standards Subcommittee of the American Academy of Neurology and the American Epilepsy Society. Neurology 69:1996-2007, 2007.

Lowenstein D, Messing R. Epilepsy genetics: yet more exciting news. Ann Neurol 62:549-551, 2007.

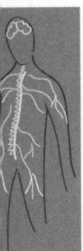

Central Nervous System Tumors

Lisa R. Rogers and Jennifer J. Griggs

Central nervous system (CNS) tumors can produce devastating effects and are often associated with high mortality rates. Even histologically benign tumors may be unresectable and thus incurable because of their location. Some benign tumors transform into higher grade (malignant) tumors over time. Malignant tumors in the brain or spinal cord have the potential for rapid recurrence.

Brain tumors are the second most common cancers in children. The incidence of brain tumors is low in young adults but increases with advancing age and reaches a plateau between the ages of 65 and 79 years. There may be a recent rise in the incidence of primary brain tumors among elderly patients, but such an increase may reflect better detection rather than increasing incidence. The incidence of primary CNS lymphoma is increasing in all age groups, accounted for only in part by lymphoma that occurs in the acquired immunodeficiency syndrome (AIDS).

The cause of most CNS tumors is unknown. With the exception of gliomas associated with vinyl chloride and tumors that occur after CNS irradiation, no environmental agents are known to be causative. There is no definite evidence supporting a viral origin of CNS tumors. Hereditary syndromes associated with an increased risk of CNS tumors, including von Hippel-Lindau disease, tuberous sclerosis, Li-Fraumeni syndrome, and neurofibromatosis, account for less than 1% of primary CNS tumors. Although the chromosomal abnormality associated with many of these syndromes is known, the specific mechanisms leading to CNS neoplasia have not been defined.

Classification

The World Health Organization has classified primary CNS tumors on the basis of cell of origin. Most primary CNS tumors are of neuroepithelial origin and result from neoplastic transformation of astrocytes, ependymocytes, or oligodendrocytes. Astrocytomas are the most common. Overall, brain metastases occurring from a systemic cancer are the most common CNS tumor, but these tumors are often not resected and are thus under-represented in incidence figures that rely on surgical pathology registries. In a patient with a known systemic malignant disease, metastasis to the CNS is more likely than a primary CNS tumor.

Clinical Manifestations

In general, symptoms caused by intracranial tumors result from one or more of the following: compression of the brain by tumor, vasogenic edema associated with the tumor or tumor cell infiltration, and destruction of brain parenchyma. Because of the uncompromising rigidity of the cranial vault, both histologically benign and malignant tumors may cause symptoms even when they are small. Symptoms caused by primary brain tumors tend to be slowly progressive rather than acute. In contrast, metastatic tumors are more likely to produce acute symptoms because they grow more rapidly and are associated with more edema. Moreover, hemorrhage into metastatic tumors, particularly renal cell cancer, melanoma, lung tumors, and choriocarcinomas, may cause acute neurologic symptoms.

The majority of pediatric brain tumors arise in the posterior fossa, whereas the majority of adult brain tumors arise in the cerebral hemispheres. Therefore the symptoms of brain tumors are very different in these patient populations. Patients with cerebral hemisphere or posterior fossa tumors may have generalized symptoms that arise from increased intracranial pressure or with focal symptoms resulting from specific areas of compromise. Headache is a common generalized neurologic sign of brain tumor and occurs in up to two thirds of patients as a presenting sign. There are no characteristics unique to the headache resulting from a brain tumor, but useful clinical clues are the new onset of headache, a progressively worsening headache, a headache of a different characteristic from prior chronic headaches, or a headache accompanied by new neurologic symptoms or signs. The pain may localize to the side of the tumor in patients with supratentorial tumors; patients with infratentorial tumors frequently describe pain in the retro-orbital,

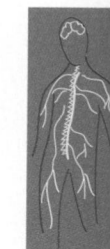

retroauricular, or occipital region. Other generalized symptoms include changes in mood or personality, a decrease in appetite, and nausea. Projectile vomiting, common in children, is rare in adults. The frequency of seizures depends on the type and location of brain tumor, and seizures occur in 20% to 80% of patients. The occurrence of the first seizure in an adult should prompt an evaluation for a brain tumor.

A careful history and neurologic examination helps in localizing the site of a suspected brain tumor. The focal symptoms depend on the location of the tumor. *Tumors of the frontal lobe* may grow to a massive proportion before symptoms prompt the patient or the patient's family to seek medical help. Progressive difficulty with concentration and memory, personality changes, hemiparesis, and lack of spontaneity may also occur with a frontal lobe tumor. Aphasia (language disturbance) may occur from involvement of the dominant frontal lobe. Urinary incontinence and gait disorder may also appear if the tumor involves both frontal lobes, such as the "butterfly glioma," which crosses the corpus callosum, or multicentric tumors such as lymphoma, or multiple brain metastases. Neurologic examination may show speech, cognitive, or motor abnormalities, and primitive reflexes may be present.

Involvement of the *temporal lobes* by tumor can lead to memory loss, personality changes, auditory hallucinations, and upper quadrantanopia. Speech may also be affected if the involved temporal lobe is in the dominant hemisphere. If tumors are large enough, they can cause herniation of the uncus through the tentorial notch *(uncal herniation).*

Parietal lobe tumors may cause subtle signs or more dramatic findings such as hemianesthesia and hemianopia, typically upper quadrantic. Tumors of the right parietal lobe may also manifest with spatial disorientation. *Occipital lobe* tumors may cause a homonymous hemianopia.

Tumors that arise in the posterior *fossa,* such as pediatric medulloblastoma, ependymoma, brainstem glioma, or cerebellar astrocytoma, can cause gait ataxia and cranial nerve dysfunction.

Metastatic spread of primary CNS tumors to sites outside the CNS is exceedingly rare. Spread along the neuraxis to the meninges and spinal cord; however, can occur with a variety of malignant CNS tumors.

Evaluation of the Patient

RADIOGRAPHIC EVALUATION

All patients suspected of having a brain tumor should undergo a contrast-enhanced computed tomography (CT) scan or magnetic resonance imaging (MRI) brain scan. Brain MRI is the preferred test because it is more useful in imaging the temporal and posterior fossae and because it is more sensitive in detecting the extent of parenchymal involvement by tumor. It is important to obtain both fluid-attenuated inversion recovery (FLAIR) and contrast-enhanced MRI sequences. CT scans done without contrast enhancement are not adequate for evaluation of either primary or metastatic tumors. Although there are exceptions, most low-grade brain tumors do not demonstrate enhancement after intravenous contrast injection. Vasogenic edema can accompany any type of brain tumor and is easily visible on FLAIR MRI

sequences. Cerebral angiography is indicated only when an understanding of tumor blood supply is deemed necessary before surgical resection, for example, in patients with a highly vascularized meningioma. 2-fluoro-2-deoxy-D-glucose positron emission tomography (FDG-PET), scanning reveals regions of increased glucose metabolism in many malignant tumors. PET scans are also useful in assessing response to treatment and in distinguishing recurrent tumor from radiation necrosis in tumors treated with brain radiation. Research is currently being conducted with advanced MRI sequences, including magnetic resonance spectroscopy and diffusion-weighted MRI, for the diagnosis and monitoring of brain tumors.

HISTOLOGIC DIAGNOSIS

Biopsy, or removal when possible, of a suspected brain tumor is essential in making an accurate tumor histologic diagnosis or in detecting non-neoplastic disease that can mimic a brain tumor, such as a brain abscess. Exceptions to tissue diagnosis include brainstem tumors that show MRI characteristics of a glioma, because there is significant risk associated with biopsy of the brainstem. Tumor tissue may be obtained by open craniotomy or with MRI- or CT-guided stereotactic techniques. Because the histologic features of the tumor may be mixed, small biopsy specimens can be misleading. When the suspicion of a primary brain tumor is high, the tissue diagnosis can be made at the time of surgical resection. This approach yields the greatest amount of tissue for pathologic examination. In up to 10% of patients with brain metastatic tumors, the primary systemic tumor site is not evident and brain biopsy or resection can be helpful in identifying the most likely primary site.

OTHER DIAGNOSTIC TESTS

Lumbar puncture for CSF examination is helpful if the patient is suspected of having leptomeningeal involvement with tumor, as can occur in patients harboring a lymphoma or medulloblastoma. CSF examination may also be indicated if the diagnosis of a brain tumor is in doubt and CNS infection or another condition needs to be excluded. Lumbar puncture is contraindicated when there is significant mass effect from an intracranial lesion, because removing fluid may lead to brain herniation. Electroencephalography is not routinely performed in patients with brain tumors, even if seizures are part of the clinical presentation.

Treatment

SURGICAL RESECTION

Surgical resection is attempted in most patients with primary brain tumors and in many patients with a single brain metastasis. Even when a surgical cure is unlikely, resection of a large portion of the tumor may relieve symptoms. Such "debulking" of primary and metastatic brain tumors also leads to improvement in survival. Extensive tumor resection is not possible in most patients with tumors arising in areas that are critical for neurologic function, such as the brainstem, language or sensorimotor cortex, basal ganglia, or

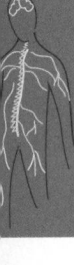

corpus callosum because of the risk of permanent and debilitating neurologic dysfunction. Newer methods of mapping cortical areas of language, sensory, and motor function during surgery have improved the results of radical resection in some patients. Surgical resection is not recommended for primary CNS lymphoma because these tumors are often multifocal.

ACUTE TREATMENT OF INCREASED INTRACRANIAL PRESSURE

Most patients with parenchymal CNS tumors have vasogenic edema caused by disruption of the blood-brain barrier. This disruption is a result of the invasion of brain vessels by the tumor or to tumor angiogenesis, the vessels of which are embryonic and lack a tight barrier. Such patients usually benefit from the use of glucocorticoids, which reduce edema possibly by stabilization of this barrier. Dexamethasone is the preferred glucocorticoid because of its long half-life. Patients with symptoms related to vasogenic edema often improve within 48 hours of dexamethasone administration. Doses used for treatment of tumor-related edema are typically 4 to 24 mg per day given in divided doses (2 to 4 times daily). Dexamethasone can be given orally because it is well absorbed from the gastrointestinal tract. Because steroids can be associated with a variety of adverse effects, the lowest dose and duration of administration should be sought.

In patients with severe neurologic signs related to brain edema, an intravenous bolus of 10 to 20 mg dexamethasone should be considered. If the neurologic signs are life threatening, including signs of brain herniation, mannitol should be given at a dose of 0.5 to 2.0 g/kg intravenously to reduce intracranial pressure, and dexamethasone should be given concurrently. Neurosurgical consultation should be obtained to determine if emergency surgery is indicated.

ANTICONVULSANTS

Brain tumors can result in focal or generalized seizures at any time in the clinical course. It is routine to administer anticonvulsants to patients before they undergo biopsy or resection of a brain tumor. Aside from the immediate preoperative and postoperative periods, however, prophylactic anticonvulsants are not indicated for those patients who do not have seizures. Chronic administration of anticonvulsants is indicated in any brain tumor patient suspected or proven to have a seizure. There are important interactions between anticonvulsants and other medications often used by brain tumor patients, such as steroids and chemotherapy, and these interactions must be considered when selecting an anticonvulsant.

RADIATION THERAPY

Brain radiation therapy is commonly delivered by one of three methods: external beam (conventional) radiation therapy, brachytherapy, or radiosurgery. *External beam radiation therapy* uses x-ray beams directed either at the whole brain or to the focal area involved by tumor. Such treatments are typically given over 2 to 6 weeks, depending on the type of tumor. *Brachytherapy* involves the implantation of either permanent or temporary radiation seeds within the tumor.

This approach allows higher than standard doses of radiation therapy to be delivered to the tumor while the surrounding normal tissue is protected. The third approach, *radiosurgery,* involves convergence of multiple radiation beams on a small, well-defined target, the brain tumor. With radiosurgery the dose of radiation to normal brain is minimal. Radiosurgery is typically used for treating small tumors that are not surgically accessible and is ideal for acoustic neuromas and other small tumors that arise adjacent to critical brain structures.

CHEMOTHERAPY

Chemotherapy is rarely used as the sole therapy for primary CNS neoplasms. Exceptions are primary CNS lymphoma, for which high-dose chemotherapy has recently been proven to be very effective, and brain tumors in very young children, in whom chemotherapy is given and brain and spinal radiation is delayed or not given. In other tumors, chemotherapy is typically administered during or after CNS radiation. The major obstacle to the effective use of chemotherapy in most tumors is the blood-brain barrier, which limits the passage of many drugs. Although the barrier is often disrupted by the tumor, the surrounding intact barrier, which often harbors microscopic tumor, limits penetration of the chemotherapy. This leads to tumor regrowth at the margins of the tumor. Attempts to overcome the blood-brain barrier by giving intra-arterial chemotherapy have not shown an advantage over standard intravenous administration. In addition, CNS tumors can be drug resistant, limiting the effectiveness of chemotherapy. Temozolomide, an oral agent, has been shown to be effective in patients with malignant gliomas and is well tolerated. Anaplastic oligodendrogliomas, an uncommon type of malignant glioma, are often unusually sensitive to chemotherapy.

Specific Tumors
MALIGNANT GLIOMA

The term *malignant glioma* refers to a group of heterogenous tumors and includes glioblastoma multiforme, anaplastic astrocytoma, and anaplastic oligodendroglioma. Some gliomas have histologic features of both astrocytoma and oligodendroglioma (mixed glioma). Of the malignant gliomas, *glioblastoma multiforme* has the worst prognosis; survival beyond 2 years is unusual. Surgical resection, radiation therapy, and chemotherapy are combined to improve symptoms and quality of life. A number of clinical factors, including patient age, the degree of surgical resection, and performance status affect survival. When disease relapse occurs, additional surgical resection, a change of chemotherapy, or use of molecularly targeted agents may be of short-term benefit.

In contrast, *anaplastic astrocytomas* and *anaplastic oligodendrogliomas* are associated with more favorable median survival times. Patients with anaplastic oligodendrogliomas typically benefit the most from chemotherapy or radiation. An important biologic correlate in the anaplastic oligodendroglioma is the status of the 1p and 19q chromosomes within the tumor tissue.

LOW-GRADE GLIOMA

Low-grade gliomas include *astrocytoma, oligodendroglioma,* and *ependymoma.* These tumors are more common in young patients, and the outcome is more favorable than in the malignant gliomas.

PRIMITIVE NEUROECTODERMAL TUMOR

Medulloblastoma is the most common form of a primitive neuroectodermal tumor. It typically arises in the midline of the cerebellum in children. It can be difficult to diagnose on clinical grounds because a child cannot describe the symptoms resulting from posterior fossa mass effect. Treatment involves surgical resection, radiation, and chemotherapy.

MENINGIOMA

Meningiomas arise from the meningeal lining surrounding the brain or spinal cord and generally grow slowly; they may also be found incidentally during the evaluation of unrelated neurologic symptoms. They often arise along the dorsal surface of the brain, falx cerebri, sphenoid ridge, or base of the skull or within the lateral ventricles. Most meningiomas are histologically benign.

Complete resection of meningiomas should be attempted, as the risk of recurrent disease is proportionate to the extent of resection. For example, the risk of recurrent disease in the subsequent two decades is close to 20% in patients who do not have complete resection or coagulation of dural attachments. In these patients, and in those who have only partial resection of the tumor itself, postoperative radiation therapy may be considered. In the patient with malignant meningioma, radiation therapy should be recommended regardless of the extent of resection. There is no definitive role for chemotherapy in the treatment of meningiomas.

CENTRAL NERVOUS SYSTEM LYMPHOMA

Primary CNS lymphomas are increasing in incidence among both immunocompromised and immunocompetent people. By definition, a patient with primary CNS lymphoma has no evidence of lymphoma outside the CNS. These tumors most often arise deep within the brain and are therefore less likely to manifest with seizures than are other primary or metastatic CNS neoplasms. Headache, personality changes, and focal symptoms corresponding to the location of the tumor are the usual presenting complaints. Lymphoma is multifocal at the time of diagnosis in 40% of immunocompetent patients and close to 100% of patients with AIDS. Many patients have neoplastic involvement of the leptomeninges, but such involvement is rarely symptomatic. Up to 20% of patients will also have lymphomatous involvement of the eye, and a small percentage of these patients develop eye involvement before the diagnosis of the brain tumor.

Treatment of primary CNS lymphomas requires first that the correct diagnosis be made. Because the disease is often multifocal, it may be confused with metastatic disease from a solid tumor. Symptoms often improve with corticosteroids because of the cytotoxic effects of steroids on lymphoma cells. However, administration of steroids before brain biopsy should be discouraged, as the prompt resolution of tumor reduces the yield of tissue biopsy. Surgical biopsy, but not resection, is the recommended method for diagnosis. The treatment for this tumor is currently evolving as new treatments emerge. It responds well to whole brain radiation as well as to high-dose chemotherapy, in particular methotrexate. Specific treatment should be based on patient age, performance status, and other variables.

METASTATIC TUMORS TO THE BRAIN

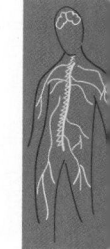

Most brain tumors are metastatic from cancer elsewhere in the body; typically those arising in the lung, breast, colon, or skin (melanoma), but nearly any solid tumor can metastasize to the CNS. Patients have headache, seizures, and focal symptoms reflecting the areas of involvement. Brain metastases are usually multiple. Single lesions are termed *solitary* if there is no other site of active disease in the body.

Treatment of metastases usually begins with corticosteroids to reduce edema and thus improve neurologic symptoms. Surgical resection is indicated for selected patients with a single brain metastasis when it is resectable, when the systemic cancer is well controlled, and when the patient is functioning well physically. In addition, resection or at least biopsy is indicated if there is no known site of systemic cancer and a brain metastasis is suspected. Most surgical patients are also treated with whole brain radiation therapy, as are those patients with multiple brain metastases. Because most chemotherapeutic agents do not cross the blood-brain barrier, the CNS is considered a sanctuary site for the development of metastasis when systemic cancer is treated. When CNS metastases grow and disrupt the blood-brain barrier, however, the chemotherapy may be more effective, and a variety of agents are currently being studied. Stereotactic radiosurgery is also an option for some patients with a limited number of brain metastases.

SPINAL CORD TUMORS

Much less common than tumors of the brain, spinal cord tumors are described as *extradural* (outside of the dural sac) or *intradural.* Most extradural tumors result from extension of vertebral metastasis from other sites, typically lung, breast, and prostate cancers. Intradural tumors are further described as either *extramedullary* (arising outside the spinal cord) or *intramedullary* (arising within the spinal cord). Examples of intradural extramedullary tumors are schwannomas and meningiomas. Ependymomas and astrocytomas are the most common intramedullary tumors. The most common location for spinal tumors is the thoracic region.

Patients with extradural or intradural extramedullary spinal cord tumors develop symptoms as a result of compression of normal structures by the tumor or impairment of the vascular supply, rather than by tumor invasion of the spinal cord parenchyma. Back pain and distal paresthesias in the legs are among the earliest symptoms, followed by loss of sensation and weakness below the level of the tumor and loss of bowel and bladder control.

MRI is the most useful test to evaluate the patient with suspected spinal cord tumor. Unless there is a contraindication to MRI, it has replaced myelography in most cases.

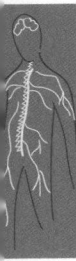

In patients with progressing deficits, urgent evaluation and treatment are indicated. High doses of intravenous corticosteroids are indicated to reduce spinal cord edema. Surgical resection of extradural tumor followed by local radiation therapy or radiation therapy alone are the treatments of choice, depending on a variety of clinical factors. Surgery for biopsy is indicated if there is no known cancer.

Treatment of intradural intramedullary or extramedullary primary spinal tumors is with surgical resection, when possible. In many patients, however, resection carries an unacceptable risk of neurologic damage, and biopsy alone is performed to establish the diagnosis. Most patients require spinal radiation for definitive treatment.

Prospectus for the Future

For patients with high-grade gliomas, such as glioblastoma, there is recent promising evidence that agents that target tumor growth factors, such as vascular endothelial growth factor, may play an important role in therapy. Clinical trials of these agents with standard radiation and chemotherapy are ongoing. In many cancers, including brain tumors, a molecular "signature" can now be obtained from the tumor tissue resected at surgery (Cancer Genome Atlas project). This signature predicts which therapies, including chemotherapies and agents targeting growth factors, will be most effective.

An exciting new concept in our understanding of cancer is that a population of tumor stem cells may be responsible for tumor initiation and self-renewal. These cells are typically not damaged by radiation or chemotherapy. Research is ongoing to determine if these tumor stem cells underlie the failure to eradicate tumors with current therapies. The pathways underlying tumor stem cell growth have been identified in high-grade gliomas and in medulloblastomas. Drugs targeting the tumor stem cell population in these tumors are in early clinical trials.

References

Batchelor TT, Byrne TN: Neurological complications of primary brain tumors. In Schiff D, Kesari S, Wen PY (eds): Cancer Neurology in Clinical Practice. Totowa, NJ, Humana Press, 2008.

Eichler AF, Loeffler JS: Multidisciplinary management of brain metastases. Oncologist 12: 884-898, 2007.

Wen PY, Kesari S: Malignant gliomas in adults. N Engl J Med 359:492-507, 2008.

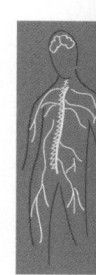

Infectious Diseases of the Nervous System

Avindra Nath

This chapter focuses on central nervous system (CNS) infections that manifest as abscesses within the parenchyma itself or as parameningeal infections. A category of infections with clinical signs confined to the brain and spinal cord—prion diseases—is also discussed.

Brain Abscess

Brain abscesses produce symptoms and findings similar to those of other space-occupying lesions, such as brain tumors, but often progress more rapidly and affect meningeal structures more frequently than tumors. They originate or extend from extracerebral locations, resulting from (1) blood-borne metastases from unknown sources, lungs, or heart, and (2) direct extension from parameningeal sites of infection (otitis, cranial osteomyelitis, and sinusitis), sites of recent or remote head trauma or neurosurgical procedures, and infections associated with cyanotic congenital heart disease. Commonly isolated pathogens are aerobic and microaerobic streptococci and gram-negative anaerobes, such as *Bacteroides* and *Prevotella*. Less common are gram-negative aerobes and *Staphylococcus*. *Actinomyces*, *Nocardia*, and *Candida* are less frequently found. Infection may be polymicrobial. Culture-negative abscesses from surgical specimens occur in 30% of antibiotic-treated patients and in 5% of patients undergoing surgery before antibiotic administration.

DIAGNOSIS

The classical clinical picture is composed of a triad of elements: those reflecting the infectious nature of the lesion (e.g., fever), those related to focal brain involvement, and those caused by increasing intracranial mass effect. Elements of one or two categories are often absent in a given case, particularly early in the course. For example, nearly one half of patients may not have a fever or leukocytosis. Recent onset of a headache is the most common symptom; headache may increase in severity and may be associated with

focal signs related to the location of the abscess (e.g., hemiparesis or aphasia, followed by obtundation and coma). Seizures precede diagnosis in 30%. Toxoplasma abscesses are often associated with movement disorders because of their propensity for the basal ganglia. The period of evolution may be as brief as hours or as long as days to weeks with more indolent organisms. Cerebrospinal fluid (CSF) examination should be avoided. It is seldom diagnostic, and CSF can be normal. Lumbar puncture in the setting of a mass lesion carries the risk of aggravating an impending transtentorial herniation.

Magnetic resonance imaging (MRI) provides better soft tissue contrast than computed tomography (CT) and is particularly useful for detecting multiple and posterior fossa abscesses, with intravenous gadolinium contrast, or for demonstrating cerebritis, the extent of mass effect, associated venous thrombosis, and the response to therapy. In the early cerebritis stage, although CT scans may be normal, the fluid-attenuated inversion recovery (FLAIR) sequence of MRI is very sensitive for visualization of brain edema. On T1-weighted images, the area of cerebritis is seen initially as a low–signal intensity, ill-defined area. Later stages of infection are noted by the formation of a rim of slightly high signal intensity on T1-weighted images and central necrosis. This area of central necrosis appears bright on diffusion-weighted images (DWI) and dark on apparent diffusion coefficient (ADC) images, which helps differentiate it from tumors, which show the opposite features (Fig. 128-1). That distinction (i.e., brain abscess from tumor) is important for the stereotactic approach to ring-enhancing lesions before biopsy or surgical excision. An abscess is best drained centrally, whereas a tumor is best biopsied along its rim. Other neuroimaging techniques, such as perfusion imaging, MR spectroscopy, and positron emission tomography have limited use in differentiation of brain abscesses from tumors.

TREATMENT

A suspected brain abscess requires urgent intervention. Unless the surgical procedure poses a substantial risk,

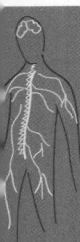

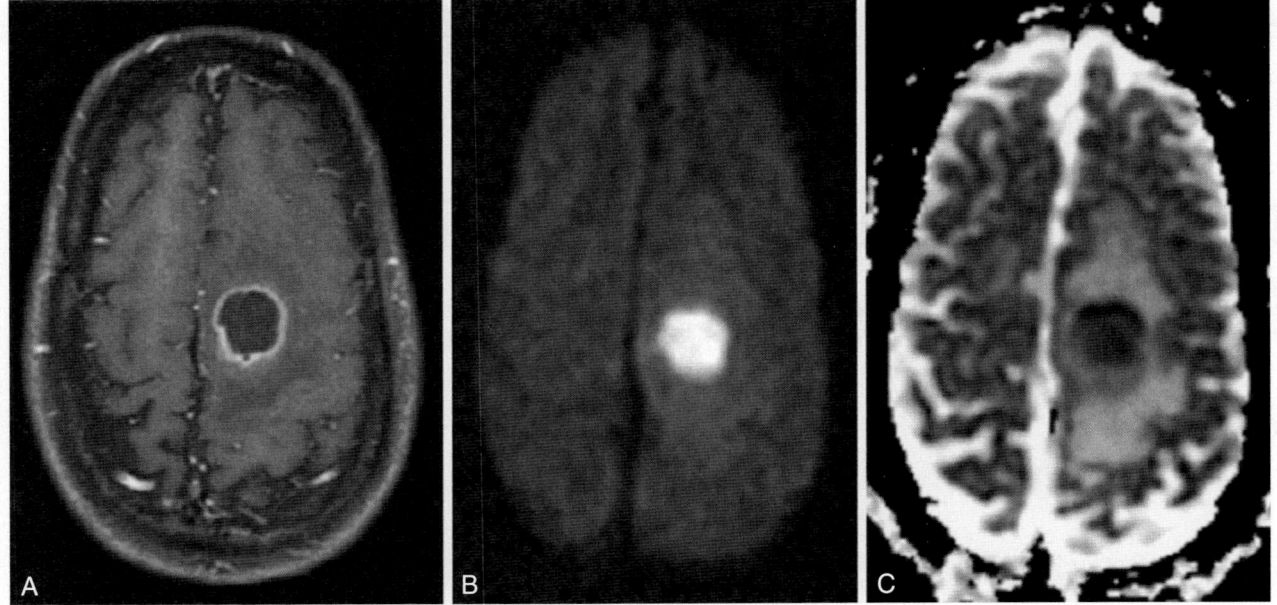

Figure 128-1 Magnetic resonance imaging features of a brain abscess. **A,** Contrast-enhanced scan shows ring-enhancing lesion in the left frontal lobe. **B,** The diffusion-weighted image shows restricted diffusion in the cavity resulting from viscous pus and cellular material. **C,** Corresponding apparent diffusion coefficient map shows dark viscous material in the cavity and surrounding edema.

aspiration of the lesion is needed for microbial diagnosis. If antiedema measures are necessary, intravenous dexamethasone in high dosages may be used (16 to 24 mg/day in four divided dosages) for short periods of time until surgical intervention is possible, because it may retard the formation of the capsule and also cause immunosuppression. Proper control of seizures is critical because the tonic phase of a generalized seizure may increase intracranial pressure. In a patient with a large abscess, seizures may trigger a brain herniation. Therefore seizure prophylaxis should be initiated in all patients with cortical or temporal lobe abscesses. Anticonvulsants that can be administered intravenously are the drugs of choice.

Successful antibiotic management of brain abscess is based on knowledge of proved or suspected pathogens together with familiarity with the properties of the antibiotic armamentarium. CNS drug penetration capabilities as well as antibiotic spectrum of activity are important considerations. Empirical antibiotic therapy without surgical intervention may be used if the primary source of infection outside of the CNS is identified or in patients with cerebritis without capsule formation and those with multiple small abscesses or abscesses in basal ganglia or brainstem. If the organism is unknown, empirical therapy may include vancomycin, metronidazole, and a third-generation cephalosporin. In brainstem abscesses, the possibility of *Listeria* infection should be considered and treatment should include intravenous ampicillin. In human immunodeficiency virus (HIV)–infected patients with multiple ring-enhancing lesions, empirical therapy for toxoplasmosis should be initiated even if the patient is seronegative for toxoplasma. Whenever empirical therapy is undertaken, the patient needs to be followed by repeat CT or MRI scanning. Those patients who fail to respond should undergo surgical intervention. An important aspect of the management strategy is the

eradication of the predisposing condition or cause of the brain abscess such as an oral, ear, cardiac, or pulmonary infection.

Parameningeal infections include those that produce suppuration in potential spaces covering the brain and spinal cord (epidural abscess and subdural empyema) and those that produce occlusion of the contiguous venous sinuses and cerebral veins (cerebral venous sinus thrombosis).

Subdural Empyema

Subdural empyema refers to infection in the space separating the dura and arachnoid. Two thirds of subdural empyemas originate from the frontal or ethmoid sinuses, 20% from inner ear infections, and the rest from trauma or neurosurgical procedures. The empyema results from direct or indirect extension from infected paranasal sinuses through a retrograde thrombophlebitis. Unilateral empyema is most common because the falx prevents passage across the midline, but bilateral or multiple empyemas can occur. Cortical venous thrombosis or brain abscess develops in about one fourth of patients. In some patients the subdural empyema may be associated with an epidural abscess or meningitis. These infections occur more often in children than in adults.

Initial symptoms are caused by chronic otitis or sinusitis, on which lateralized headache, fever, and obtundation become superimposed. Vomiting, meningeal signs, and focal neurologic abnormalities (hemiparesis or seizures) follow. If untreated, obtundation progresses and the septic mass and swollen underlying brain lead to venous thrombosis or death from herniation. The major differential diagnosis is that of meningitis. Nuchal rigidity and obtundation occur in both, but papilledema and lateralizing deficits are

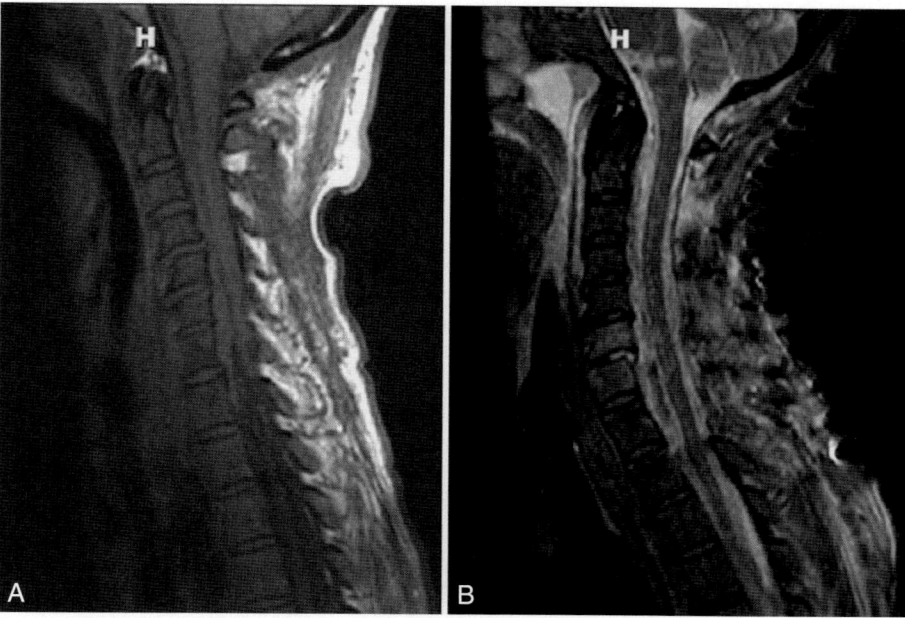

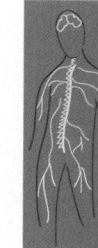

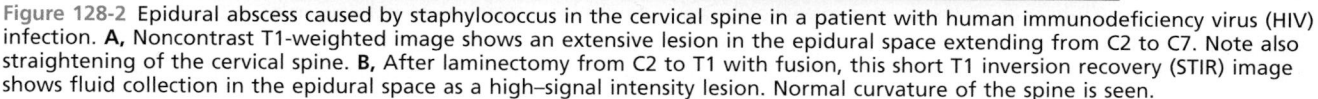

Figure 128-2 Epidural abscess caused by staphylococcus in the cervical spine in a patient with human immunodeficiency virus (HIV) infection. **A,** Noncontrast T1-weighted image shows an extensive lesion in the epidural space extending from C2 to C7. Note also straightening of the cervical spine. **B,** After laminectomy from C2 to T1 with fusion, this short T1 inversion recovery (STIR) image shows fluid collection in the epidural space as a high–signal intensity lesion. Normal curvature of the spine is seen.

more common in empyema. Lumbar puncture should be avoided in patients with subdural empyema to prevent cerebral herniation. Contrast-enhanced CT or MRI can be diagnostic of empyema, showing an extra-axial, crescent-shaped mass with an enhancing rim lying just below the inner table of the skull over the cerebral convexities or in the interhemispheric fissures. On MRI, subdural empyemas have decreased signal on T1-weighted imaging and increased signal on T2-weighted scans. Similar to brain abscess, subdural empyema has a high signal intensity on DWI and a low signal intensity on ADC maps. Treatment requires both prompt surgical drainage of the empyema cavity and high-dose intravenous antibiotics directed toward organisms found at the time of craniotomy.

Malignant External Otitis

Malignant (necrotizing) external otitis occurs commonly in older patients with diabetes or in any immunosuppressed patient. It is often caused by *Pseudomonas aeruginosa*. It progresses rapidly, with ear pain, facial swelling, osteomyelitis of the base of the skull, dural sinus thrombosis, and purulent meningitis. Multiple cranial nerve palsies, most often facial and auditory, occur because of their proximity to the external ear canal. CT scan may identify bony erosion, and MRI scan shows soft tissue changes and dural enhancement. Urgent treatment is essential: an antipseudomonal penicillin or a third-generation cephalosporin combined with an aminoglycoside or ciprofloxacin, as well as surgical débridement and drainage. If the condition is untreated, the mortality rate is high. Patients with an inadequate response to antibiotic therapy should undergo biopsy for investigation of possible malignancy.

Spinal Epidural Abscess

Infection within the epidural space around the spinal cord can cause paralysis and death. Its incidence is 0.5 to 1.0 per 10,000 hospital admissions in the United States; the frequency is increased in intravenous drug users. The classical triad of fever, spinal pain, and neurologic deficits may not be present in all patients, leading to a delay in diagnosis. Patients are usually febrile and have acute or subacute neck or back pain, with focal percussion tenderness being a prominent sign; stiff neck and headache are common. The pain can be mistaken for sciatica, a visceral abdominal process, chest wall pain, or cervical disk disease. If the infection goes unrecognized at this stage, the symptoms can rapidly evolve, over a few hours to a few days, to produce weakness and finally paralysis distal to the spinal level of the infection. In this clinical setting, spinal epidural abscess should be assumed, systemic antibiotics begun, and urgent neuroradiologic imaging pursued. The differential diagnosis includes compressive and inflammatory processes involving the spinal cord (transverse myelitis, intervertebral disk herniation, epidural hemorrhage, and metastatic tumor), which can usually be detected by MRI (Fig. 128-2). Epidural abscess may be accompanied by diskitis or osteomyelitis of the vertebral bodies.

PATHOPHYSIOLOGIC FACTORS

Infections of the epidural space originate from contiguous spread or through hematogenous routes from a distant source. Cutaneous infection is the most common remote source, especially in intravenous drug users. Abdominal, respiratory tract, and urinary sources are also common. As the use of epidural catheters is increasing for pain management, epidural abscess and hematoma are also being increasingly reported. The anatomy of the epidural space dictates the location of the abscess. Because the size of the intravertebral canal remains relatively constant whereas the circumference of the spinal cord changes, abscess formation is maximal in the thoracic and lumbar regions and minimal at the cervical spine enlargement.

BACTERIOLOGIC FACTORS

Causative organisms can be identified by culture or Gram stain from pus obtained at exploration (90% of patients), blood cultures (60% to 90% of patients), or CSF (20% of patients). *Staphylococcus aureus* is most common, followed by streptococci and gram-negative anaerobes. Tuberculous abscesses represent as many as 25% of patients in high-risk populations.

TREATMENT

Unless culture and sensitivities dictate otherwise, penicillinase-resistant penicillin should be started empirically as antistaphylococcal treatment for presumed bacterial infection. If methicillin resistance is suspected, vancomycin should be used. Considering the severity of the disease, additional gram-negative coverage with a third-generation cephalosporin or a quinolone may be needed. Surgical decompression was considered mandatory; now, early diagnosis by MRI allows for effective medical therapy alone if started before the occurrence of neurologic complications. Affected patients should be monitored closely; if signs of neurologic deterioration emerge, surgical intervention may be necessary.

Septic Cavernous Sinus Thrombosis

Septic cavernous sinus thrombosis usually occurs as a result of spread of infection from facial structures via facial veins or from the sphenoid or ethmoid sinuses. Symptoms include headache or lateralized facial pain, followed in a few days to weeks by fever and involvement of the orbit, which produces proptosis and chemosis secondary to obstruction of the ophthalmic vein. Paralysis of oculomotor nerves follows rapidly. In some instances, sensory dysfunction occurs in the first and second divisions of the trigeminal nerve and a decrease develops in the corneal reflex. Further involvement of the contiguous orbital contents follows, with mild papilledema and decreased visual acuity, sometimes progressing to blindness. Extension to the opposite cavernous sinus or to other intracranial sinuses with cerebral infarction or increased intracranial pressure secondary to impaired venous drainage can result in stupor, coma, and death. The CSF is abnormal if there is accompanying meningitis or parameningeal infection. The most common causative organism is *S. aureus,* followed by streptococci and pneumococci; anaerobic infection may occur. Diagnosis of cavernous sinus thrombosis is usually made with MRI scan with venogram. Radiologic evaluation includes imaging of the sphenoidal and ethmoidal sinuses, which if infected may require drainage. Empirical antimicrobial therapy should

include an antistaphylococcal agent. Empirical combination therapy with parenteral metronidazole, vancomycin, and ceftriaxone will achieve reasonable CSF and brain penetration and is likely to be active against *S. aureus* as well as the usual sinus pathogens. Parenteral flucloxacillin or dicloxacillin can be added if *S. aureus* infection is strongly suspected, as penicillins have better bactericidal effects than vancomycin for methicillin-susceptible strains of *S. aureus.*

Lateral Sinus Thrombosis

Septic thrombosis of the lateral sinus results from acute or chronic infections of the middle ear and spreads via emissary veins that connect the mastoid with the lateral venous sinus. It may spread to involve the sigmoid sinus. The symptoms include ear pain followed over several weeks by fever, headache, nausea, vomiting, and vertigo. Mastoid swelling may be seen. Sixth cranial nerve palsies and papilledema can occur, but other focal neurologic signs are rare. The diagnosis can be established by MR angiography. Treatment includes empirical broad-spectrum intravenous antibiotics to cover staphylococci and anaerobes (nafcillin or oxacillin with penicillin or metronidazole), but surgical drainage (mastoidectomy) may be required.

Septic Sagittal Sinus Thrombosis

Septic sagittal sinus thrombosis is uncommon and occurs as a consequence of purulent meningitis, infections of the ethmoidal or maxillary sinuses spreading through venous channels, infected compound skull fractures, or, rarely, neurosurgical wound infections. Symptoms include manifestations of elevated intracranial pressure (headache, nausea, and vomiting) that evolve rapidly to stupor and coma. Diagnosis and treatment are similar to those for lateral venous sinus thrombosis, described earlier.

Neurologic Complications of Infectious Endocarditis

Neurologic complications occur in one third of patients with bacterial endocarditis and triple the mortality rate of the disease. Most of these complications derive from valvular vegetations. Cerebral (but not systemic) emboli are increasingly common from mitral valve endocarditis. Most emboli, regardless of the bacterial cause of the infection, occur before or early in the course of treatment. By 2 weeks of therapy, the risk of embolization decreases dramatically. Cerebral emboli are distributed in the brain in proportion to cerebral blood flow. Therefore most emboli lodge in the branches of the middle cerebral artery peripherally, with resultant hemiparesis. Focal seizures may result.

Mycotic aneurysms complicate endocarditis in 2% to 10% of patients and are more common in acute than subacute disease. The middle cerebral artery is most commonly involved, with the aneurysms being located distally in the vessel, differentiating them from congenital berry aneurysms. Multidetector CT angiography may be necessary

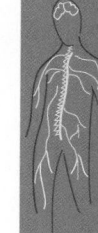

to diagnose these aneurysms. Small brain abscesses may complicate the course of endocarditis, but macroscopic abscesses are rare, with most occurring in the setting of acute, rather than subacute, endocarditis. Multiple micro-abscesses, however, can result in a diffuse encephalopathy similar to that seen in sepsis. Such lesions may escape detection on CT scan and are not amenable to surgical drainage. Antibiotic treatment of the primary disease is indicated. The CSF is abnormal in 70% of patients and simulates that seen in purulent meningitis (polymorphonuclear predominance, elevated protein level, and low glucose level) or a parameningeal infection (lymphocytic predominance, modest protein elevation, and normal glucose level). Endovascular treatment of infectious aneurysms is possible, but endovascular coiling may not prevent hemorrhage associated with panvasculitic rupture of a new aneurysm. Patients with infectious endocarditis who do not respond to conservative medical therapy can have prompt valve surgery after endovascular treatment despite the presence of intracerebral hemorrhage.

Prion Diseases

Several human diseases have been attributed to a unique infectious protein—the prion. The infectious form of prion protein is rich in beta-sheets and is detergent-insoluble, multimeric, and resistant to proteinase K treatment. Prion illnesses (transmissible spongiform encephalopathies) can be classified as sporadic, hereditary, or acquired. The most common form is sporadic Creutzfeldt-Jakob disease (CJD). Familial forms include Gerstmann-Sträussler-Scheinker syndrome, and familial fatal insomnia. Acquired forms are caused by the transmission of abnormal prion protein (PrP) from human to human or from cattle to human. Accidental transmission of CJD from human to human appears to have occurred with cadaveric dura mater grafts, corneal transplantation, receipt of human growth hormone or pituitary gonadotropin, contaminated electroencephalogram (EEG) electrodes, and contaminated surgical instruments. The appearance of variant CJD in Great Britain, in association with the outbreak of bovine spongiform encephalopathy and the contamination of beef, has greatly increased interest in this group of illnesses. Kuru is another transmissible spongiform encephalopathy that was spread in New Guinea by cannibalism, the practice of which ceased in the 1950s. This disease is now nearly extinct.

SPORADIC CREUTZFELDT-JAKOB DISEASE

Illness from CJD is seen worldwide, with an incidence of 0.5 to 1.0 cases per 1 million population per year. CJD is frequently diagnosed incorrectly initially. Prodromal symptoms include altered sleep patterns and appetite, weight loss, changes in sexual drive, and impaired memory and concentration. Disorientation, hallucinations, depression, and emotional lability are early signs, followed by a rapidly progressive dementia associated with myoclonus (approximately 90% of patients). Myoclonus is generally provoked by tactile, auditory, or visual startle stimuli. CJD has an abrupt onset in 10% to 15% of patients. Other distinctive presentations include seizures, autonomic dysfunction, and lower motor neuron disease suggesting amyotrophic lateral sclerosis. Cerebellar ataxia occurs in one third of patients. Atypical presentations, such as with pure ataxia or visual phenomena (the so-called Heidenhain variant), may go initially undiagnosed.

The clinical tetrad supporting the diagnosis of CJD consists of a subacute progressive dementia, myoclonus, typical periodic complexes on EEG, and normal CSF. FLAIR imaging sequences on MRI show extensive curvilinear

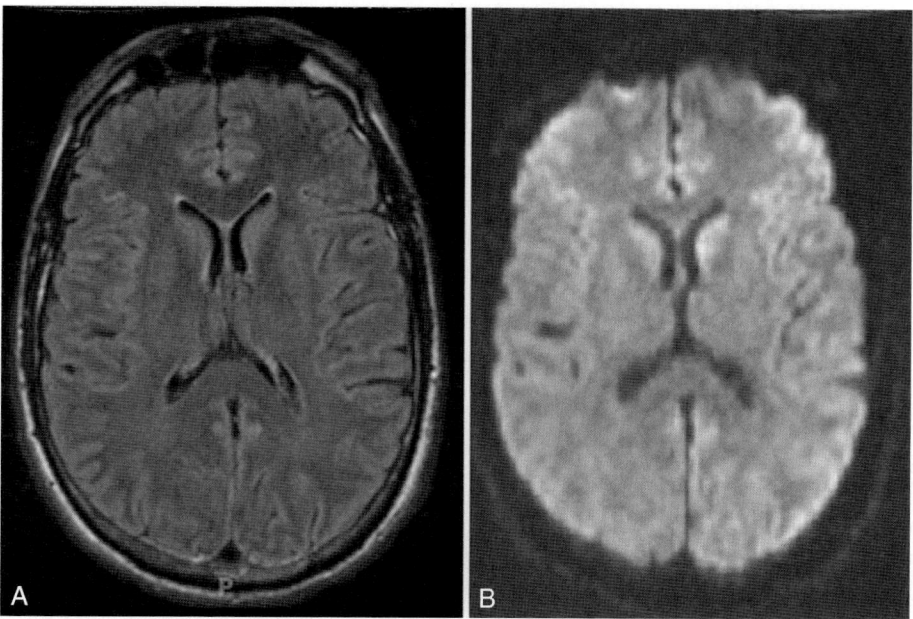

Figure 128-3 Magnetic resonance imaging (MRI) scan of a patient with pathologically proven Creutzfeldt-Jakob disease. **A,** An axial fluid-attenuated inversion recovery (FLAIR) image is relatively normal, but corresponding **(B)** diffusion-weighted scan shows high signal intensity in the cortical ribbon, most prominent in the frontal regions as well as the caudate nucleus.

hyperintensity along the neocortex, termed *cortical ribbon-ing*, affecting frontal, parietal, and temporal lobes, in decreasing order of frequency. Nearly 90% of CJD FLAIR sequences show cortical ribboning to some extent, with a clear majority of cases also showing involvement of the limbic cortex, striatum, and thalamus. The pattern of extensive increased neocortical and/or striatal FLAIR signal and DWI abnormality has a diagnostic accuracy for CJD approaching 95% (Fig. 128-3). A characteristic "pulvinar sign" has been described, denoting a "hockey stick" distribution of hyperintensity in the posteromedial thalamus. Bilateral presence of this sign reliably allows diagnosis of vCJD. Routine CSF study is generally normal. A CSF test for the protein 14-3-3, in the appropriate clinical context, is highly specific and sensitive for CJD. No effective therapy has been developed. The disease is inexorably progressive. The median time to death from onset is 5 months, and 90% of patients with sporadic CJD die within 1 year. The pathogenic isoform of prion protein can be demonstrated in brain by immunocytochemical staining and by Western-blot analysis.

Although the illness is not communicable in the conventional sense, a risk exists in handling materials contaminated with the prion protein. Gloves should be worn during handling of blood, CSF, and other body fluids. Instruments must be disinfected by steam autoclaving for 1 hour at 132° C, by steam autoclaving for 4.5 hours at 121° C (1.5 psi), or by immersion in 1 N sodium hydroxide for 1 hour at room temperature.

Prospectus for the Future

Major progress continues to be made in magnetic resonance imaging with seven tesla magnets now being available for human imaging and new sequence techniques that are capable of differentiating between blood, necrosis, and pyogenic lesions with great precision and sensitivity. These techniques are expected to greatly advance the diagnosis of CNS infections and the monitoring of treatment. Molecular biological techniques currently lack the sensitivity in detection of non-viral pathogens in CSF. Hence, further research is needed to advance these diagnostic methods. Advances in surgical techniques, such as minimally invasive laparoscopic techniques are expected to help in evacuation of deep-seated abscesses. However, substantial effort is necessary to develop new antimicrobial agents that penetrate the CNS. Similarly, there are no available drugs for treatment of many viral pathogens and prions, which requires investment of resources for drug development.

References

Carfrae MJ, Kesser BW: Malignant otitis externa. Otolaryngol Clin North Am 41:537-549, 2008.
Johnson RT: Prion diseases. Lancet Neurol 4:635-642, 2005.

Nath A: Brain abscess and parameningeal infections. In Goldman L, Ausiello DA (eds): Cecil Textbook of Medicine, 23rd ed. Philadelphia, WB Saunders, 2007.
Tsai YD, Chang WN, Shen CC, et al: Intracranial suppuration: A clinical comparison of subdural empyemas and epidural abscesses. Surg Neurol 59:191-196, 2003.

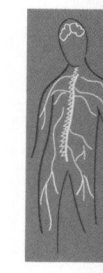

Demyelinating and Inflammatory Disorders

Joanne Lynn

Demyelination is a process of injury to myelin of the central nervous system (CNS) or the peripheral nervous system. Diseases of peripheral nervous system myelin are discussed in Chapter 130. Demyelinating diseases of the CNS include acquired and hereditary (referred to as *dysmyelinating*) disorders. The acquired inflammatory demyelinating disorders of the CNS include multiple sclerosis (MS), neuromyelitis optica (NMO), transverse myelitis (TM), optic neuritis, and acute disseminated encephalomyelitis. Table 129-1 lists common disorders of CNS myelin.

Multiple Sclerosis

MS is the most common acquired inflammatory demyelinating disease of the CNS and affects 2.5 million people worldwide with a predominance in women (female:male ratio is 2:1). The prevalence generally increases with distance from the equator and varies from 5 to 119 per 100,000 people in the United States. Onset commonly occurs from age 15 to 50 years. The course is highly variable but for 85% of patients begins with discrete episodes of neurologic dysfunction termed *relapses* that are initially largely reversible and separated by periods of stability or remission. This course is termed *relapsing-remitting*. In many patients the course eventually advances to a steady irreversible progression termed *secondary progressive MS*. Approximately 10% to 15% of patients have a *primary progressive* course, with progressive myelopathy or ataxia without discrete relapses (PPMS). Patients who experience a single episode of CNS demyelination are said to have a clinically isolated syndrome (CIS), and a subset at particularly high risk to subsequently develop MS may be identified by the presence of asymptomatic white matter lesions on brain magnetic resonance imaging (MRI).

ETIOLOGY

The cause remains unknown. Although evidence suggests that MS is an autoimmune disease triggered by environmental factors, a specific auto-antigen has not been identified. Genetic risk factors have been implicated by familial aggregation and high prevalence in some ethnic populations. MS is a complex genetic disease, with the interaction of genetic and environmental factors contributing to susceptibility and expression. Latitude-based differences in prevalence suggest that the disorder may be the result of a variety of possible factors including immune dysregulation incited by a regional pathogen in a susceptible population, relative lack of sunlight, or decreased vitamin D.

PATHOLOGY

Demyelination in MS occurs in perivenular extensions preferentially in the periventricular areas, termed "Dawson's fingers." Entry of immune cells from the vasculature into the brain is facilitated by the specific interaction of lymphocytic molecule VLA-4 with its vascular endothelium ligand, VCAM. After diapedesis through the endothelium and dissolution of the basement membrane, these mononuclear cells migrate to the brain parenchyma. The majority of cells are macrophages and resident microglia, but there are also T, B, and natural killer (NK) cells. T cells, particularly Th1 and Th17 lymphocytes and their cytokines, are considered pivotal in the induction of inflammation that precedes all acute exacerbations of MS and causes demyelination and irreversible axonal injury. After repeated attacks, loss of brain parenchyma and brain atrophy occur. CD8 cells are present in MS lesions, but their role in mediating injury is only beginning to be understood. B cells present in well-formed lymphoid follicles in the brain and meninges secrete immunoglobulins, which may be important in antibody- and complement-mediated injury and are also responsible for the presence of the oligoclonal bands in the CSF. Th2 cells are anti-inflammatory and probably abrogate inflammation and induce clinical remissions. Accordingly, immunomodulatory therapies attempt to modify the immune response from a Th1 state to the more desirable Th2 state.

Table 129-1 **Demyelinating Disorders**
Multiple sclerosis (MS)
Neuromyelitis optica (Devic disease, NMO)
Clinically isolated syndromes
Optic neuritis
Acute transverse myelitis (TM)
Brainstem demyelination
Acute disseminated encephalomyelitis
Viral infections
Human immunodeficiency virus 1 (HIV-1)–associated myelopathy
Progressive multifocal leukoencephalopathy
Subacute sclerosing panencephalitis
Toxic demyelination
Chemotherapy-related leukoencephalopathy
Radiation leukoencephalopathy
Nutritional or metabolic disorders
Subacute combined degeneration (vitamin B_{12} deficiency)
Demyelination of the corpus callosum (Marchiafava-Bignami disease)
Central pontine myelinolysis
Vascular or ischemic disorders
Leukodystrophies

Table 129-2 **Common Symptoms and Signs of Multiple Sclerosis**
Symptoms
Numbness, paresthesias
Weakness
Muscle spasms and tightness
Fatigue
Monocular visual impairment
Diplopia
Decreased balance
Vertigo
Urinary dysfunction
Depression
Cognitive impairment
Signs
Sensory deficits
Spasticity
Extensor plantar responses
Optic atrophy
Deafferent papillary defect
Visual field defects
Internuclear ophthalmoplegia
Nystagmus
Tremor
Abnormal affect
Absent abdominal reflexes
Sensory deficits, paresthesias
Weakness
Monocular central scotoma, optic atrophy, afferent papillary defect
Lhermitte phenomenon
Eye movements: diplopia, internuclear ophthalmoplegia, nystagmus
Vertigo
Ataxia, dysmetria or intention tremor, dysarthria
Fatigue
Neurogenic bladder and bowel dysfunction
Sexual dysfunction
Depression
Cognitive impairment
Uhthoff phenomenon: neurologic deficits worsened by fever, heat neuropathic pain

CLINICAL AND LABORATORY DIAGNOSIS

Relapses are manifested as the subacute development of one or often multiple symptoms or signs of neurologic dysfunction referable to the CNS (Table 129-2). The diagnosis is based on the demonstration of dissemination of disease in time (multiple clinical events) and space (multiple sites of involvement) and the exclusion of other neurologic disorders. The 2005 revision of the McDonald Criteria (Table 129-3) for diagnosis of relapsing-remitting MS uses the clinical history, neurologic examination, MRI, evoked responses, and abnormalities in the cerebrospinal fluid to establish the occurrence of lesions in the brain disseminated in time and space.

Magnetic Resonance Imaging

MRI generates image contrast based on the spin resonance properties of protons and is the single best laboratory technique to demonstrate demyelination in the CNS because of its ability to show the contrast between normal myelin and MS lesions. The most abundant source of protons in the brain is water, and water content of an area of demyelination is always higher than that of normal myelin, which is hydrophobic because of its high lipid content.

Lesions of MS are best seen on T2 and T2-FLAIR (fluid-attenuated inversion recovery) sequences. Lesions often assume an ovoid shape and preferentially occur at right angles to the lateral walls of the lateral ventricles and the corpus callosum. Although T1 sequences detect fewer lesions than T2, the presence of hypointensities on T1 images ("black holes") indicates underlying axonal loss and greater severity of disease. Enhancement after intravenous administration of gadolinium is helpful in detection of lesions where a breach of the blood-brain barrier has occurred within the previous 6 weeks because of active disease (Fig. 129-1).

Cerebrospinal Fluid

Cerebrospinal fluid cell count, total protein, and glucose are usually normal. A slight mononuclear pleocytosis or elevation in protein may occur rarely during exacerbations. The typical CSF abnormality in MS is evidence of increased intrathecal synthesis of immunoglobulin G (IgG), indicated by an elevated IgG index (calculated from CSF and serum IgG and albumin) or the presence of oligoclonal IgG bands on isoelectric focusing (Fig. 129-2).

Visual Evoked Potentials

Evoked potentials have been useful in detecting subclinical demyelination in the brainstem using auditory stimuli (auditory evoked potential) or the spinal cord and brain using sensory stimuli (somatosensory evoked potential). The visual evoked potential (VEP) is the most sensitive and the only evoked potential used by the McDonald criteria for diagnosis of MS.

The differential diagnosis of MS is broad and includes diseases that can mimic discreet attacks and gradual progression of neurologic deficits (Table 129-4).

Table 129-3 McDonald Multiple Sclerosis Diagnostic Criteria*

Clinical (Attacks)	Objective Lesions	Additional Requirements to Make Diagnosis
2 or more	2 or more	None Clinical evidence alone will suffice Additional evidence desirable but must be consistent with MS
2 or more	1	Dissemination in space by MRI *or* two or more MRI lesions consistent with MS plus positive CSF *or* await further clinical attack implicating other site
1	2 or more	Dissemination in time by MRI or second clinical attack
1	1	Dissemination in space by MRI *or* two or more MRI lesions consistent with MS plus positive CSF *and* dissemination in time by MRI or second clinical attack
0 (progression from onset)	1 or more	Disease progression for 1 yr (retrospective or prospective) *and* two out of three of the following: • Positive brain MRI (nine T2 lesions *or* four or more T2 lesions with positive VEP) • Positive spinal cord MRI (two or more focal T2 lesions) • Positive CSF
Paraclinical Evidence in MS Diagnosis		
What is a positive MRI?		Three out of four of the following: • 1 Gd-enhancing brain or cord lesion or 9 T2 hyperintense brain and/or cord lesions if there is no Gd-enhancing lesion • 1 or more brain infratentorial or cord lesions • 1 or more juxtacortical lesions • 3 or more periventricular lesions
What provides MRI evidence of dissemination in time?		• A Gd-enhanced lesion detected in scan at least 3 months after onset of initial clinical event at a site different from initial event • A new T2 lesion detected in a scan done at any time compared with a reference scan done at least 30 days after initial clinical event
What is positive CSF?		Oligoclonal IgG bands in CSF (and not serum) or elevated IgG index
What is positive VEP?		Delayed but well-preserved wave form

Individual cord lesions can contribute, along with individual brain lesions, to reaching required number of T2 lesions.

*These diagnostic criteria were developed through the consensus of the International Panel on the Diagnosis of MS and data from Polman CH, Reingold SC, Edan G, et al: Diagnostic criteria for multiple sclerosis: 2005 revisions to the "McDonald Criteria". Ann Neurol 58:840-846, 2005; Barkhof F, Filippi M, Miller DH, et al: Comparison of MRI criteria at first presentation to predict conversion to clinically definite multiple sclerosis. Brain 120:2059-2069, 1997; and Tintoré M, Rovira A, Martínez MJ, et al: Isolated demyelinating syndromes: comparison of different MR imaging criteria to predict conversion to clinically definite multiple sclerosis. AJNR Am J Neuroradiol 21:702-706, 2000.

CSF, cerebrospinal fluid; Gd, gadolinium; IgG, immunoglobulin G; MRI, magnetic resonance imaging; MS, multiple sclerosis; VEP, visual evoked potential.

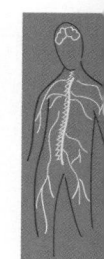

TREATMENT

The treatment of patients with MS consists of management of acute relapses, disease-modifying therapies (DMTs) aimed at reduction of the severity and frequency of acute relapses or slowing of progressive disease, and symptomatic therapies (Table 129-5). Treatment for a major relapse is intravenous (IV) methylprednisolone at a dose of 500 to 1000 mg daily for 3 to 5 days, sometimes followed by a taper of oral prednisone. A small randomized study demonstrated efficacy for plasmapheresis for steroid-refractory fulminant attacks of demyelination.

Various DMTs are available for MS, and selection is dependent on disease course and severity, drug efficacy, and patient comorbidities and preferences. Studies have shown that early treatment of patients with CIS at high risk for the development of MS with interferon-β or glatiramer acetate (GA) can delay progression to clinically definite MS. The six currently approved DMTs for relapsing-remitting MS are interferon-β-1b (Betaseron), two forms of interferon-β-1a (Avonex and Rebif), and GA (Copaxone), as well as second-line agents natalizumab (Tysabri) and mitoxantrone (Novantrone). Three formulations of interferon-β have been approved for treatment of relapsing forms of MS. Binding of interferon-β to its receptor induces multiple immuno-modulatory effects including enhancement of Th2 activity, downregulation of antigen presentation, reduction of inflammatory cytokines, and decreased lymphocyte trafficking into the CNS. Adverse events include injection site reactions for subcutaneous formulations, flulike symptoms, and headache. GA is a synthetic polypeptide designed to simulate myelin basic protein and is administered as a daily subcutaneous injection. The exact mechanism of action is not completely understood, but GA competes with myelin-derived antigens for binding with MHC molecules and causes a shift in GA-reactive lymphocyte populations from a Th1 to a Th2 state. GA therapy is well tolerated; adverse events include local injection site reactions and a sporadic postinjection transient reaction of flushing and dyspnea.

Natalizumab is a humanized monoclonal antibody that binds α_4 integrins present on leukocytes and blocks their interaction with vascular endothelial cell adhesions molecules, thereby inhibiting the migration of leukocytes across the blood-brain barrier. It is administered by monthly IV infusion and causes a potent reduction in relapse rate and new and enhancing MRI lesions. Treatment with natalizumab has been associated with the development of progressive multifocal leukoencephalopathy. Mitoxantrone is an anthracenedione chemotherapeutic agent that is U.S. Food

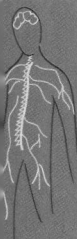

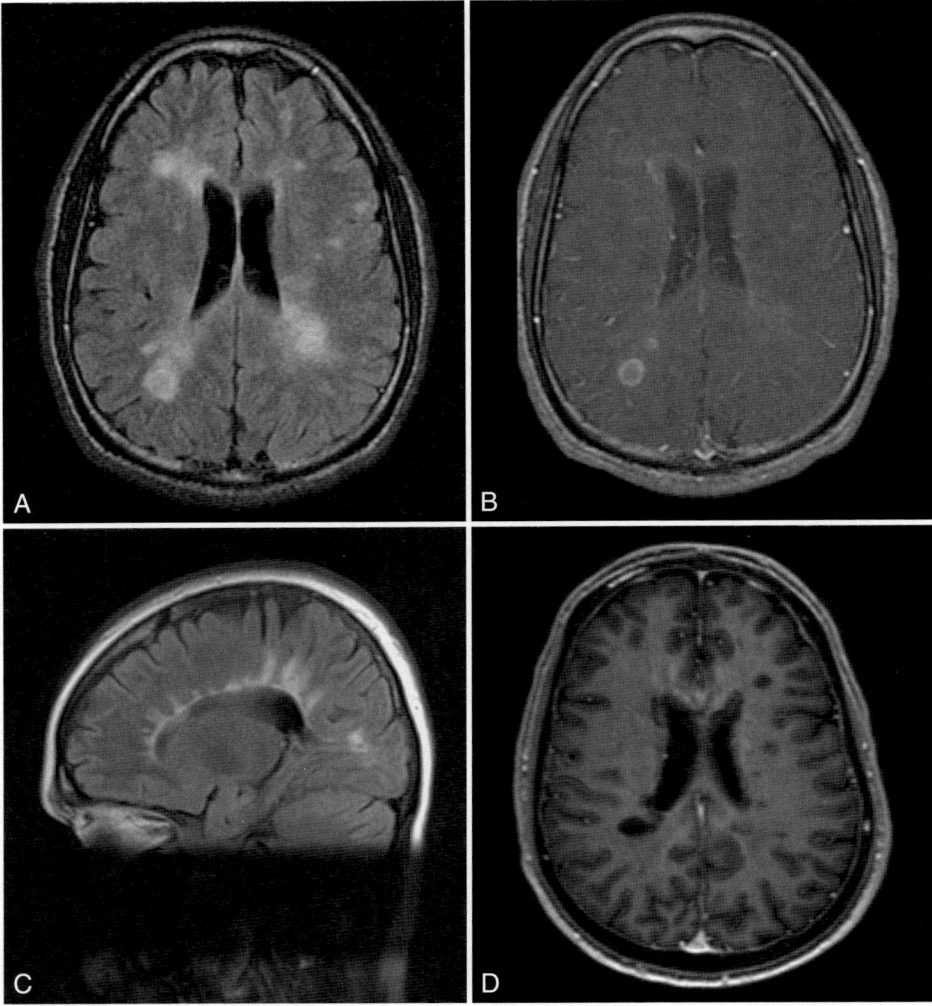

Figure 129-1 **A,** Axial fluid-attenuated inversion recovery (FLAIR) image of the brain from a patient with MS revealing classical multiple periventricular and deep white matter high-signal lesions. **B,** Axial T1-weighted image with gadolinium contrast from the same patient shows that two of the lesions are actively inflamed and enhanced with contrast. **C,** Sagittal FLAIR image of the brain from a patient with MS demonstrating classical periventricular lesions radiating outward from the ventricles. **D,** Axial T1-weighted image showing areas of T1 low signal ("black holes").

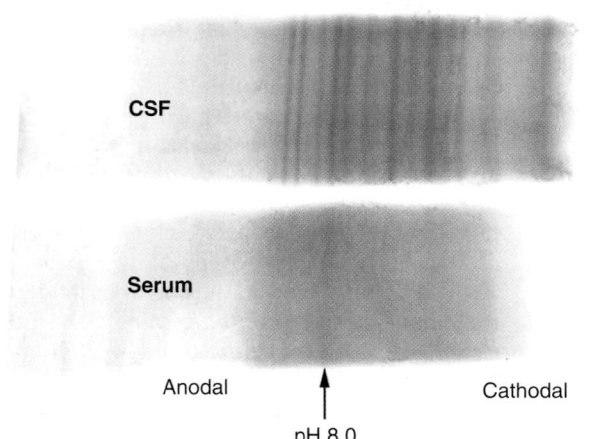

Figure 129-2 Isoelectric focusing gel of cerebrospinal fluid (CSF) and serum of a patient with multiple sclerosis. The CSF *(upper lane)* shows oligoclonal bands cathodal to (to the right of) pH 8.0, which are not seen in the serum *(lower lane).*

Table 129-4 Differential Diagnosis of Multiple Sclerosis

Relapsing-Remitting

Vascular disease: strokes, vasculitis, CADASIL
Inflammatory: neuromyelitis optica, acute TM, acute disseminated encephalomyelitis, paraneoplastic syndromes
Rheumatologic disease: systemic lupus erythematosus, Sjögren syndrome, sarcoidosis, Behçet syndrome, antiphospholipid antibody syndrome
Spinal cord disease: compression, abscess, spinal arteriovenous malformation

Progressive Syndromes

Degenerative: spinocerebellar ataxias, spine disease, hereditary spastic paraparesis, syrinx
Infections: HTLV-1, HIV-related, epidural abscess
Neoplastic: epidural tumor, lymphoma
Metabolic: adrenomyeloleukodystrophy; vitamin B_{12}, vitamin E, or copper deficiency
Vascular: spinal arteriovenous malformation; dural venous fistula

CADASIL, cerebral autosomal dominant arteriopathy with subcortical infarcts and leukoencephalopathy; HIV, human immunodeficiency virus; HTLV-1, human T-cell lymphotropic virus type 1; TM, transverse myelitis.

Table 129-5 Treatment of Multiple Sclerosis

Acute Exacerbations

Intravenous methylprednisolone, 500-1000 mg/day for 3-5 days, variably followed by oral prednisone taper
Plasma exchange (very severe exacerbations)

Disease-Modifying Therapies

Interferon-β-1a
Interferon-β-1b (two formulations)
Glatiramer acetate
Natalizumab
Mitoxantrone

Symptomatic Therapies

Weakness: physical therapy, assistive devices, exercise
Spasticity: stretching, baclofen (oral and intrathecal), tizanidine, benzodiazepines, dantrolene, botulinum toxin
Fatigue: amantadine, modafinil, energy conservation strategies
Neuropathic pain: carbamazepine, gabapentin, pregabalin, amitriptyline, narcotics
Bladder dysfunction: anticholinergic medications for failure to store, intermittent self-catheterization or chronic catheterization, sacral neuromodulation therapy
Depression: antidepressants, psychotherapy
Antipyretics for intercurrent infection

and Drug Administration (FDA) approved for treatment of aggressive relapsing and secondary progressive disease. It is administered intravenously every 3 months as the most common dosing interval. The cumulative dosage is limited to 140 mg/m^2 because of dose-related cardiotoxicity; there is also a risk of treatment-related acute leukemia. Various other immunosuppressive agents such as cyclophosphamide are in wide use as well. At the present time, there are no FDA-approved therapies available for PPMS.

Neuromyelitis Optica (Devic Disease)

Once regarded as a variant of MS, NMO is now recognized as a distinct relapsing, inflammatory demyelinating disease that preferentially affects the spinal cord and optic nerves. Brain MRI is typically normal early on, but nonspecific white matter abnormalities often develop that do not meet MS radiologic diagnostic criteria. A role for humoral immunopathogenesis is supported by the presence of the NMO-IgG autoantibody, which binds to aquaporin-4, a water transport protein in the CNS. Multiple clinical features distinguish NMO from MS. Whereas MS preferentially affects persons of Northern European white ancestry, NMO accounts for a substantial proportion of CNS demyelinating disease in nonwhite populations including Asians, Hispanics, and African Americans. NMO-associated myelitis differs from MS myelitis in that the clinical impairment is often more severe and MRI typically reveals a longitudinally extensive involvement of the cord (extending three or more vertebral segments, whereas MS lesions rarely exceed one or two segments in length). CSF may show pleocytosis with a predominance of neutrophils. Oligoclonal bands are found in the CSF in only 20% to 30% of NMO cases. NMO attacks are initially treated with IV methylprednisolone but often fail to respond. Plasmapheresis has been shown to be helpful in some cases as a rescue therapy. Maintenance immunosuppressive therapy is generally recommended to decrease the frequency of relapses. Anecdotal reports suggest benefit from azathioprine, rituximab, and other agents; however, optimal treatment regimens are yet to be defined, as no controlled treatment trials have been conducted.

Optic Neuritis

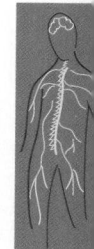

Optic neuritis is an inflammation of the optic nerve that may occur in isolation or in association with a variety of autoimmune disorders including MS and NMO. The clinical presentation consists of visual loss that is more often monocular than binocular, diminished perception of colors, especially red hues, and pain on eye movement. Symptoms progress over a period of hours to 1 week. Examination reveals variable impairments of visual acuity and color vision, visual field loss, and an afferent papillary defect. The optic disc appears normal in the approximately two thirds of patients who have retrobulbar optic neuritis affecting the posterior two thirds of the optic nerve. Papillitis or swelling of the optic disc may be present in patients with inflammation in the anterior portion of the optic nerve. Visual function usually improves to some degree. The differential diagnosis includes optic neuropathy from anterior ischemic optic neuropathy, tobacco-nutritional amblyopia, vasculitis, optic nerve compression, pernicious anemia, Leber hereditary optic neuropathy, infections, and systemic autoimmune inflammatory diseases such as systemic lupus erythematosus (SLE) and Behçet disease. Treatment with intravenous methylprednisolone (500 to 1000 mg) for 3 days followed by a short prednisone taper hastens recovery and is generally administered for moderately severe or bilateral visual loss; however, a significant benefit to long-term visual outcome has not been demonstrated.

Gadolinium-enhanced MRI of the brain should be performed to assess the risk of subsequent development of MS in patients with isolated optic neuritis and other forms of CIS (TM, brainstem syndromes). Patients with characteristic but asymptomatic brain demyelinating lesions are at high risk for eventual development of clinically definite MS; benefit has been shown for initiation of MS DMTs for this subgroup with CIS.

Acute Transverse Myelitis

Acute TM is a focal inflammatory disorder of the spinal cord manifested as sensory, motor, and/or autonomic dysfunction that develops over hours to 3 weeks. Other causes of acute myelopathy including compression, infarction, and infection must be ruled out by clinical presentation, MRI, and other investigations. Acute TM occurs with a yearly incidence of one to four new cases per million people. Severity and recovery are variable. The potential causes of this syndrome include TM; MS; NMO; and post-infectious, postvaccinal, and other systemic inflammatory disorders, such as SLE, sarcoid, Behçet disease, and Sjögren syndrome. Many cases are idiopathic. Inflammation within the cord should be demonstrated as abnormal signal on MRI or be suggested by CSF pleocytosis or elevated IgG index. Treatment of the acute presentation is 1000 mg methylprednisolone daily for 5 days. Cases secondary to inflammatory conditions require consideration of chronic immunosuppression.

Acute Disseminated Encephalomyelitis

Acute disseminated encephalomyelitis (ADEM) is typically a monophasic immune-mediated inflammatory demyelinating disorder that primarily affects the brain and spinal cord. It occurs more commonly in children but can occur at any age. Symptoms typically begin 2 days to 6 weeks after an antigenic challenge such as a vaccination or antecedent infection; however, there are many cases without history of either. Prodromal features of fever, headache, myalgias, and malaise are followed by the rapid development of meningeal signs, declining mental status, weakness, ataxia, cranial nerve palsies, visual loss and seizures. MRI shows multiple large and asymmetrical white matter lesions with variable gadolinium enhancement. Oligoclonal bands may be present transiently in approximately one third of cases. There may be occasional relapsing courses that render differentiation from MS difficult. Acute hemorrhagic leukoencephalitis is a rare, rapidly progressive and fulminant variant of ADEM that is usually triggered by an upper respiratory tract infection and is often fatal. Treatment of ADEM with intravenous methylprednisolone often hastens recovery.

Prospectus for the Future

The cause of multiple sclerosis (MS) remains unknown. However, recent progress in the understanding of its pathogenesis is stimulating the development of many therapeutic strategies.

The development of treatments that reduce central nervous system injury in MS without compromising patient safety is the current challenge.

References

Balcer LJ: Optic neuritis. N Engl J Med 354:1273-1280, 2006.

Frohman EM, Racke MK, Raine CS: Multiple sclerosis—The plaque and its pathogenesis. N Engl J Med 354:942-955, 2006.

Goodin DS, Frohman EM, Garmany GP Jr, et al: Disease modifying therapies in multiple sclerosis: Report of the Therapeutics and Technology Assessment Subcommittee of the American Academy of Neurology and the MS Council for Clinical Practice Guidelines. Neurology 58:169-178, 2002.

Polman CH, Reingold SC, Edan G, et al: Diagnostic criteria for multiple sclerosis: 2005 revisions to the "McDonald Criteria." Ann Neurol 58:840-846, 2005.

Wingerchuck DM, Lennon VA, Lucchinetti CF, et al: The spectrum of neuromyelitis optica. Lancet Neurol 6:805-815, 2007.

Neuromuscular Diseases: Disorders of the Motor Neuron and Plexus and Peripheral Nerve Disease

Carlayne E. Jackson

Neuromuscular diseases are classified into four groups, according to which portion of the motor unit is involved (Table 130-1). Motor neuron and peripheral nerve diseases are considered in this chapter; myopathies are considered in Chapter 131, and neuromuscular junction diseases are considered in Chapter 132. The symptoms and signs of the neuromuscular diseases are at times indistinguishable. However, some useful general rules apply to assist with localization based on the distribution of weakness, presence or absence of sensory symptoms, reflex abnormalities, and specific associated clinical features (Table 130-2).

Electromyography and Nerve Conduction Studies

Electromyography (EMG) and nerve conduction studies can also be useful diagnostic tools in localizing the lesion in a patient with a suspected neuromuscular disease. The measurement of electrical activity arising from muscle fibers is performed by inserting a needle electrode percutaneously into a muscle. Normal muscle is electrically silent at rest. Spontaneous activity during complete relaxation occurs in myotonic disorders, in inflammatory myopathies, and in denervated muscles. Spontaneous activity of a single muscle fiber is called a *fibrillation*, and such activity of part of or an entire motor unit is called a *fasciculation*. In myotonia, repeated muscle depolarization and contraction occur despite voluntary relaxation. Abnormalities in motor unit potentials occur during the course of denervation; with the development of reinnervation, the remaining motor units increase in amplitude and become longer in duration and

polyphasic (**Web Figure 130-1**). Conversely, in muscle diseases such as the muscular dystrophies and other diseases that destroy scattered fibers within a motor unit, the motor unit action potentials are of lower amplitude and shorter duration and are polyphasic. A reduced recruitment (interference) pattern from maximum voluntary effort occurs in denervation. Conversely, in patients with primary muscle disease, submaximal voluntary effort produces a full recruitment pattern despite marked weakness.

Nerve conduction is studied by stimulating a peripheral nerve (e.g., the ulnar) with surface electrodes placed over the nerve. The resulting action potential is recorded by electrodes placed over the nerve more proximally in the case of large sensory nerve fibers and over the muscle distally in the case of motor nerve fibers in a mixed motor sensory nerve. For sensory nerves, the sensory nerve action potential (SNAP) is quantitated, and for motor nerves, the compound muscle action potential (CMAP) is quantitated.

Diseases of the Motor Neuron (Anterior Horn Cell)

AMYOTROPHIC LATERAL SCLEROSIS

The most common *acquired* motor neuron disease, amyotrophic lateral sclerosis (ALS), is a progressive, typically fatal disorder resulting from degeneration of the cortical motor neurons originating in layer five of the motor cortex and descending via the pyramidal tract (resulting in upper motor neuron signs and symptoms) and from degeneration of the anterior horn cells in the spinal cord and their brainstem homologues innervating bulbar muscles (resulting in lower motor neuron signs and symptoms) (Table 130-3). The incidence is approximately 2 per 100,000 population, and there is a slight male predominance. The peak age of onset is in the sixth decade, although the disease can occur at any time throughout adulthood. Epidemiologic studies have incriminated risk factors for ALS including exposure to insecticides, smoking, participation in varsity athletics, and military service in the Gulf War. Mean survival from onset of symptoms is 2 to 5 years, with 10% of patients surviving beyond 10 years. The majority of deaths are related to respiratory muscle failure and aspiration pneumonia. The cause of ALS is largely unknown, with 95% of cases considered "sporadic," and 5% related to an autosomal dominant disease (familial ALS [FALS]). FALS is an adult-onset disease that is clinically and pathologically indistinguishable from sporadic ALS. FALS is caused by missense mutations in the superoxide dismutase gene *(SOD1)* in 20% of patients. Other genetic causes are also being identified (see **Web Table 130-1**).

Clinical symptoms relating to the upper motor neuron degeneration include loss of dexterity, slowed movements, muscle weakness, stiffness, and emotional lability. Signs on neurologic examination that confirm an upper motor neuron lesion include pathologic hyperreflexia, spasticity, and extensor plantar responses (Babinski sign). Lower motor neuron signs and symptoms caused by anterior horn cell degeneration include weakness, muscle atrophy, fasciculations, and cramps. Fasciculations in the absence of associated muscle atrophy or weakness are usually benign and may be aggravated by sleep deprivation, stress, and excessive caffeine ingestion. Muscle weakness in patients with ALS usually begins distally and asymmetrically and may manifest as a monoparesis, hemiparesis, paraparesis, or quadriparesis. It may also be limited initially to the bulbar region, resulting in difficulty with chewing, swallowing, speech, and movements of the face and tongue. For unclear reasons, ocular motility is spared until the very late stages of the illness. Bowel and bladder function and sensation remain spared throughout the course of the disease. Degeneration of the corticobulbar projections innervating the brainstem can lead to involuntary emotional expression disorder (IEED), causing difficulty controlling laughter and/or tearfulness (also called *pseudobulbar affect*). Up to 50% of patients with ALS may also have a component of frontotemporal dementia characterized by executive dysfunction, poor insight, personality changes (disinhibition, impulsivity, apathy), abnormal eating habits, poor hygiene, and language dysfunction.

The diagnosis of ALS remains one of "exclusion," in which other potential causes must be ruled out through a variety of neuroimaging, laboratory, and electrodiagnostic investigations (**Web Table 130-2**). For example, compression of the cervical spinal cord or cervicomedullary junction from tumors or cervical spondylosis can produce weakness, atrophy, and fasciculations in the upper extremities and spasticity in the lower extremities, closely resembling ALS.

The only current U.S. Food and Drug Administration (FDA)–approved therapy for ALS is riluzole 50 mg twice per day, which in clinical trials prolonged survival by 2 to 3 months. The mechanism of this effect is not known with certainty; however, riluzole may reduce excitotoxicity by diminishing presynaptic glutamate release. Initiation of

Table 130-1 Classification of Neuromuscular Diseases

Site of Involvement	Typical Examples
Anterior Horn Cell	

Without upper motor neuron involvement	Spinal muscular atrophy
	  Progressive muscular atrophy
	  Bulbospinal muscular atrophy
	  Poliomyelitis
	  West Nile virus

With upper motor neuron involvement	Amyotrophic lateral sclerosis Primary lateral sclerosis
Peripheral Nerve	
Mononeuropathy	Carpal tunnel syndrome Ulnar palsy Meralgia paresthetica
Multiple mononeuropathies	Mononeuritis multiplex (e.g., polyarteritis nodosa), leprosy, sarcoidosis, amyloidosis

Polyneuropathies	Diabetic neuropathy
	  Charcot-Marie-Tooth disease
	  Guillain-Barré syndrome

Neuromuscular Junction	
	Myasthenia gravis Eaton-Lambert syndrome
Muscle	
	Duchenne muscular dystrophy Dermatomyositis

Table 130-2 Clinical Features of the Neuromuscular Diseases

Clinical Feature	Anterior Horn Cell	Peripheral Nerve	Neuromuscular Junction	Muscle
Distribution of weakness	Asymmetrical limb or bulbar	Symmetrical, usually distal	Extraocular, bulbar, proximal limb	Symmetrical, proximal limb
Atrophy	Marked and early	Mild, distal	None (or very late)	Slight early; marked later
Sensory Involvement	None	Dysesthesias, loss of sensation	None	None
Reflexes	Variable (depending on degree of upper motor neuron involvement)	Decreased out of proportion to weakness	Normal in myasthenia gravis, depressed in Lambert-Eaton syndrome	Decreased in proportion to weakness
Characteristic features	Fasciculations, cramps	Combined sensory and motor abnormalities	Fatigability	Usually painless

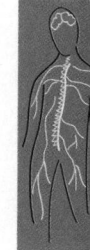

Table 130-3	**Symptoms and Signs Associated with Amyotrophic Lateral Sclerosis**

Symptoms	Signs
Upper Motor Neuron Degeneration	
Loss of dexterity	Pathologic hyperreflexia
Slowed movements	Babinski response
Weakness	Hoffman response
Stiffness	Jaw jerk
Emotional lability	Spasticity
Lower Motor Neuron Degeneration	
Weakness	Muscle atrophy
Fasciculations	Fibrillation potentials on electromyography
Cramps	Neurogenic atrophy on muscle biopsy

Table 130-4	**Symptom Management for Motor Neuron Diseases**

Respiratory Insufficiency
Noninvasive positive pressure ventilation
Cough assist devices

Dysarthria
Augmentative speech device

Dysphagia
Percutaneous endoscopic gastrostomy placement
Suction machine

Sialorrhea
Amitriptyline 25-75 mg qhs
Glycopyrrolate 1-2 mg q8h

Spasticity
Baclofen 10-20 mg qid
Dantrium 25-100 mg qid

Emotional Lability
Serotonin reuptake inhibitors
Amitriptyline 25-75 mg qhs

Weakness
Ankle foot orthosis
Wheelchair
Elevated toilet seat

noninvasive positive pressure ventilation (NPPV) on a spontaneous timed mode has also been shown to prolong survival up to 20 months and to improve quality of life. NPPV should be initiated when the forced vital capacity (FVC) is less than 50% or when patients report symptoms that suggest nocturnal hypoventilation (daytime fatigue, frequent arousals, supine dyspnea, morning headaches). A cough-assist device can be used to assist with clearing upper airway secretions and has been shown to minimize the risk of pneumonia in clinical trials. A percutaneous gastrostomy (PEG) tube should be recommended before the FVC drops below 50% or when patients are unable to maintain weight with oral intake alone. Symptomatic therapy for spasticity, emotional lability, muscle cramping, and drooling is also essential in maintaining patient dignity and quality of life (Table 130-4). Augmentative speech devices can be prescribed to assist patients with communication and computer access.

OTHER ACQUIRED MOTOR NEURON DISEASES

Other motor neuron diseases involve only particular subsets of motor neurons (Table 130-5). Progressive muscular atrophy (PMA) is a pure lower motor neuron disease that accounts for 8% to 10% of patients with motor neuron disease. Weakness is typically distal and asymmetrical, and bulbar involvement is rare. Patients with PMA generally have a better prognosis than those with ALS, with a survival of 3 to 14 years. Primary lateral sclerosis (PLS) is a pure upper motor neuron syndrome in which patients demonstrate either a slowly progressive spastic paralysis or dysarthria. This is a rare disorder, accounting for 2% of all motor neuron cases. Survival is generally years to decades.

SPINAL MUSCULAR ATROPHY

Spinal muscular atrophy (SMA) is a hereditary form of motor neuron disease in which only the lower motor neuron is affected. The SMAs may begin in utero, in infancy, in childhood, or in adult life and represent the first class of neurologic disorders in which a developmental defect in neuronal apoptosis most likely produces the disease. Two genes are involved in SMA types 1 to 3: the neuronal

Table 130-5	**Clinical Spectrum of Motor Neuron Diseases***

Upper and Lower Motor Neuron Involvement
Sporadic amyotrophic lateral sclerosis
Familial amyotrophic lateral sclerosis

Upper Motor Neuron Involvement
Primary lateral sclerosis
Familial spastic paraparesis

Lower Motor Neuron Involvement
Motor neuronopathy related to malignancy or paraproteinemia
Poliomyelitis
West Nile virus
Postpolio syndrome
Hexosaminidase deficiency
Progressive muscular atrophy
Spinal muscular atrophy
    Type I: Infantile onset (Werdnig-Hoffmann disease)
    Type II: Late infantile onset
    Type III: Juvenile onset (Kugelberg-Welander disease)

*Italicized disorders are hereditary.

apoptosis inhibitor protein *(NAIP)* and survival motor neuron *(SMN)* genes.

Bulbospinal muscular atrophy (BSMA) or Kennedy disease is an X-linked recessive disorder in which the mean age at onset is 30 years; the range is from 15 to 60 years. BSMA is a trinucleotide repeat disorder with a CAG expansion encoding for a polyglutamine tract in the first exon of the androgen receptor gene, on chromosome Xq11-12. The mechanism by which disruption of the androgen receptor gene alters the function of bulbar and spinal motor neurons is not known. An inverse correlation exists between the number of CAG repeats and the age of onset of the disease. Affected individuals exhibit chin fasciculations, midline furrowing and atrophy of the tongue, and proximal weakness. Dysphagia and dysarthria are common, and up to 90% of patients demonstrate gynecomastia and infertility. Two findings distinguishing this disorder from ALS are the absence of upper motor neuron signs and in some patients the presence of a subtle sensory neuropathy.

Disorders of the Brachial and Lumbosacral Plexus

The roots within the cervical, lumbar, and sacral regions organize into the cervical, lumbar, and sacral plexuses before giving rise to individual peripheral nerves. Diseases of these plexuses (plexopathies) tend to be *focal* in symptoms and signs, whereas many diseases of the peripheral nerves and muscles are *generalized.*

BRACHIAL PLEXOPATHY

The brachial plexus is constituted by mixed nerve roots from C5 to T1 that fuse into upper, middle, and lower trunks above the level of the clavicle and redistribute into lateral, posterior, and medial cords below that landmark **(Web Fig. 130-2)**. Symptoms include weakness, pain, and sensory loss in the shoulders or arms. Upper trunk lesions may be due to trauma and idiopathic brachial plexitis (see later). Lower trunk lesions may result from malignant tumor invasion, thoracic outlet syndrome, or as a complication of sternotomy. If the entire plexus is involved, radiation injury, trauma, and late metastatic disease are the most common causes.

ACUTE AUTOIMMUNE BRACHIAL NEURITIS

Acute autoimmune brachial neuritis is characterized by the abrupt onset of severe pain, usually over the lateral shoulder, but at times extending into the neck or entire arm. The acute pain generally subsides after a few days to a week; by this time, weakness of the proximal arm becomes apparent. The serratus anterior, deltoid, and supraspinatus are the most commonly affected muscles, but other muscles of the shoulder girdle may also be affected. In rare cases, most of the patient's arm and even the ipsilateral diaphragm are involved. Sensory loss is usually slight and generally involves the axillary nerve distribution. Weakness may last weeks to months and be accompanied by severe atrophy of the shoulder girdle. No therapy has been shown to alter or shorten the clinical course, although steroids and analgesics may reduce pain. Most patients recover within several months to 3 years. The disorder frequently follows an upper respiratory infection or an immunization, but in many instances no antecedent illness occurs. It is bilateral in one third of cases but is always asymmetrical; it may recur in 5% of patients. Recurrent brachial plexopathies that are painless may be related to an autosomal dominant disorder, hereditary neuropathy with liability to pressure palsies (HNPP), caused by a deletion or point mutation of PMP-22 protein (chromosome 17p).

LUMBOSACRAL PLEXOPATHY

The lumbosacral plexus is formed from the ventral rami of spinal nerves T12 to S4. These divide within the plexus into ventral and dorsal branches that form the femoral, sciatic, and obturator nerves. The plexus is located within the substance of the psoas major muscle. Clinical features include proximal pain and weakness in anterior thigh muscles (femoral) or posterior thigh muscles and the buttocks. Bowel and bladder dysfunction may also occur. Diabetes, malignant invasion, radiation therapy, infection (herpes zoster), psoas abscess, trauma, and retroperitoneal hemorrhage are common causes. An autoimmune form is much less frequent than brachial neuritis.

Disorders of the Peripheral Nerves

Peripheral neuropathy refers to a large group of disorders that can produce focal (mononeuropathy or multiple mononeuropathies) or generalized nerve dysfunction (polyneuropathies) (Table 130-6). Peripheral neuropathies are among the most prevalent neurologic conditions, affecting 2% to 8% of adults, with the incidence increasing with age. They range in severity from mild sensory abnormalities, found in up to 70% of patients with long-standing diabetes, to fulminant, life-threatening paralytic disorders such as Guillain-Barré syndrome (GBS).

MONONEUROPATHY AND MULTIPLE MONONEUROPATHIES

Mononeuropathies are disorders in which only a single peripheral nerve is affected. The most common cause is

Table 130-6 **Classification and Causes of Peripheral Neuropathy**	
Type of Neuropathy	**Examples**
Mononeuropathies	
Compressive	Carpal tunnel syndrome, ulnar palsy
Hereditary	Hereditary neuropathy with predisposition to pressure palsies
Inflammatory	Bell palsy
Multiple mononeuropathies	Vasculitis (mononeuritis multiplex), diabetes, leprosy, sarcoidosis, amyloidosis
Polyneuropathies	
Hereditary	Charcot-Marie-Tooth disease
Endocrine	Diabetes, hypothyroidism
Metabolic	Uremia, liver failure
Infections	Leprosy, diphtheria, human immunodeficiency virus, Lyme disease
Immune-mediated	Guillain-Barré syndrome, chronic inflammatory demyelinating polyneuropathy
Toxic	Lead-, arsenic-, alcohol-, drug-induced
Paraneoplastic	Lung cancer

Table 130-7 Common Mononeuropathies

	Precipitating Factors	Motor Signs and Symptoms	Sensory Signs and Symptoms	Treatment
Median Nerve				
Entrapment at the wrist (carpal tunnel syndrome)	Repetitive wrist flexion or sleep	Weakness in thenar muscle; inability to make a circle with the thumb and index fingers	Numbness, tingling, and/or pain in thumb, index finger, middle finger, and medial half of ring finger. Tinel and Phalen signs	Neutral wrist splint, carpal tunnel injections or surgery
Ulnar Nerve				
Entrapment at the elbow	External compression in condylar groove, fracture of humerus	Weakness or atrophy of the interossei and thumb adductor	Sensory loss in the little finger and contiguous half of the ring finger	Elbow pads; ulnar nerve transposition or decompression of cubital tunnel
Radial Nerve				
Entrapment at the spiral groove	Prolonged sleeping on arm after drinking excessive amounts of alcohol: "Saturday night palsy"	Wrist drop with sparing of elbow extension; weakness of finger and thumb extensors	Sensory loss on dorsum of hand	Spontaneous recovery; wrist splint
Femoral Nerve				
	Abdominal hysterectomy, hematoma, prolonged lithotomy position, diabetes	Weakness and atrophy of quadriceps	Sensory loss in anterior thigh and medial calf	Physical therapy
Lateral Femoral Cutaneous Nerve				
Meralgia paresthetica	Obesity, pregnancy, diabetes, constrictive belts	None	Sensory loss, pain, or tingling over anterolateral thigh	Weight loss; spontaneous recovery
Peroneal Nerve				
Entrapment at the fibular head	Habitual leg crossing, knee casts, prolonged squatting, profound weight loss	Weakness of ankle dorsiflexors or evertors and toe extensors	Sensory loss in anterolateral leg and dorsum of foot	Ankle-foot orthosis; remove source of compression
Sciatic Nerve				
	Injection injury, fracture or dislocation of hip	Weakness of hamstrings, ankle plantar flexors or dorsiflexors	Sensory loss in buttock, lateral calf and foot	Ankle-foot orthosis; physical therapy
Tibial Nerve				
Entrapment in tarsal tunnel	External compression from tight shoes, trauma, tenosynovitis	None	Sensory loss and tingling in sole of foot	Tarsal tunnel injection, eliminate source of compression, medial arch support

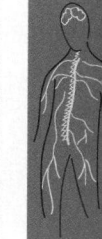

nerve entrapment such as median nerve compression resulting in carpal tunnel syndrome or peroneal nerve injury causing foot drop (Table 130-7). When more than one peripheral nerve is involved, the term *mononeuropathy multiplex* or *multiple mononeuropathies* is often used. Multiple mononeuropathies are most commonly seen in diabetes mellitus and vasculitis but have also been reported in leprosy, sarcoidosis, hereditary neuropathy with predisposition to pressure palsies, and amyloidosis.

Polyneuropathies

Polyneuropathy refers to a group of disorders affecting the motor, sensory, and autonomic nerves. These disorders may predominantly affect the nerve axon (axonal neuropa-

thies), myelin sheath (demyelinating neuropathies), or the small- to medium-sized blood vessels supplying the nerves (vasculitic neuropathies). The clinical features of the polyneuropathies reflect the pathology of the underlying process.

AXONAL NEUROPATHIES

In the symmetrical polyneuropathies, the underlying pathology is usually a slowly evolving type of axonal degeneration that involves the ends of long nerve fibers first and preferentially. With time, the degenerative process involves more proximal regions of long fibers, and shorter fibers are affected. This pattern of distal axonal degeneration or *dying back* of nerve fibers results from a wide variety of metabolic, toxic, and endocrinologic causes. The resulting clinical picture of an axonal polyneuropathy includes early loss of muscle stretch reflexes at the ankle and weakness that initially involves the intrinsic muscles of the feet, the extensors of the toes, and the dorsiflexors at the ankle. The motor signs are usually mild in contrast to the sensory abnormalities, which may include numbness, tingling, and burning sensations (dysesthesias). The sensory symptoms usually begin symmetrically in the toes and feet and then ascend proximally to the legs in a "stocking" distribution. When the sensory abnormalities reach the level of the knees, the symptoms begin in the hands, in a "glove" distribution. Truncal and abdominal dysesthesias may develop once the sensory abnormalities ascend to the level of the elbows. Peripheral neuropathies caused by axonal degeneration are generally progressive unless the underlying cause can be identified and treated. Recovery from axonal degeneration requires nerve regeneration, a process that often requires 2 to 3 years.

DEMYELINATING NEUROPATHIES

Demyelination of a peripheral nerve at even a single site can block conduction, resulting in a functional deficit identical to that seen after axonal degeneration. In contrast to repair by regeneration, however, repair by remyelination can be rapid. Autoimmune attack on the myelin sheath occurs in the inflammatory demyelinating neuropathies (GBS and chronic inflammatory demyelinating polyneuropathy [CIDP]) and some neuropathies associated with paraproteinemias (see later). Inherited disorders of myelin such as Charcot-Marie-Tooth (CMT) disease comprise the other major category of demyelinating neuropathies. Other causes include toxic, mechanical, and physical injuries to nerves. Although these examples have nearly pure demyelination, many neuropathies have both axonal degeneration and demyelination. This mixed pathologic abnormality reflects the mutual interdependency of the axons and the myelin-forming Schwann cells. The prominent clinical feature of an acquired demyelinating polyneuropathy is weakness that affects not only the distal muscles, but also the proximal and facial muscles. Unlike in an axonal neuropathy, sensory loss is rarely the presenting symptom. Patients generally have diffuse hyporeflexia or areflexia.

VASCULITIC NEUROPATHIES

Vasculitic neuropathies occur as a result of disease of the small or medium-sized blood vessels that leads to ischemia and infarction of isolated peripheral nerves. The term *mononeuritis multiplex* is also used to describe this clinical situation, in which there is multifocal involvement of individual nerves leading to asymmetrical, predominantly distal weakness and sensory loss associated with severe pain. Causes include systemic vasculitis (rheumatoid arthritis, systemic lupus erythematosus, Wegener granulomatosis, Churg-Strauss syndrome, polyarteritis nodosa) and primary peripheral system vasculitis (25% of cases). Therapy with corticosteroids in addition to a cytotoxic agent can stabilize and in some cases improve the neuropathy.

Etiology of Neuropathies

Neuropathic disorders can be broadly divided into those that are acquired and those that are hereditary (Table 130-8). Acquired disorders are the more common and have many causes: metabolic or endocrine disorders (diabetes mellitus, renal failure, porphyria); immune-mediated disorders (GBS, CIDP, multifocal motor neuropathy, anti-myelin-associated glycoprotein neuropathy); infectious causes (human immunodeficiency virus [HIV], Lyme disease, cytomegalovirus [CMV], syphilis, leprosy, diphtheria); medications (HIV drugs, chemotherapies); environmental toxins (heavy metals); or paraneoplastic processes. Diabetes mellitus and alcoholism are the most common causes of polyneuropathy in developed countries. As many as one third of acquired neuropathies are idiopathic.

Clinical Approach to the Patient with Suspected Polyneuropathy

Because of the many causes, it is important to approach the patient with neuropathy systematically, beginning with the patient's history and physical examination. It is essential to determine which nerves are involved (motor, sensory, or autonomic) and in what specific combination (Table 130-9). Small-fiber neuropathies often manifest with unpleasant or abnormal sensations such as a burning pain, electric shock–like sensations, cramping, tingling, pins and needles, or prickly feelings such as the limb "feeling asleep." Large-fiber neuropathies can manifest as numbness,

Table 130-8 Hereditary Neuropathic Disorders

	Inheritance Pattern	Genetic Defect	Clinical Features
Hereditary sensorimotor neuropathies	AR, AD, or X-linked	See **Web Table 130-4**	Pes cavus, distal atrophy and weakness, hammer toes
Familial amyloid polyneuropathy	AD	Transthyretin Gelsolin Apolipoprotein AI	Pain, autonomic dysfunction
Fabry disease	X-linked	α-Galactosidase	Cardiac ischemia, renal disease, stroke, cutaneous angiokeratomas
Tangier disease	AR	Apolipoprotein A	Low HDL levels, orange tonsils
Refsum disease	AR	Phytanic acid oxidase	Retinitis pigmentosa, cardiomyopathy, deafness, ichthyosis

AD, autosomal dominant; AR, autosomal recessive; HDL, high-density lipoprotein.

Table 130-9 **Differential Diagnosis of Neuropathic Disorders Based on Symptoms**		
Motor Symptoms Only	**Sensory Symptoms Only**	**Autonomic Symptoms**
Porphyria	Cryptogenic sensory polyneuropathy	Amyloid neuropathy
Charcot-Marie-Tooth	Metabolic, drug-related, or toxic neuropathy	Diabetic neuropathy
Chronic inflammatory demyelinating polyneuropathy	Paraneoplastic sensory neuropathy	Fabry disease
Guillain-Barré syndrome		Guillain-Barré syndrome
Lead neuropathy		Hereditary sensory or autonomic neuropathy
Motor neuron disease		Porphyria

Table 130-10 **Neuropathies Associated with Pain**
Alcoholic neuropathy
Amyloidosis
Cryptogenic sensorimotor neuropathy
Diabetic neuropathy
Fabry disease
Guillain-Barré syndrome
Heavy metal toxicity (arsenic, thallium)
Hereditary sensory or autonomic neuropathy
HIV sensorimotor neuropathy
Radiculopathy or plexopathy
Syphilis
Vasculitis
HIV, human immunodeficiency virus.

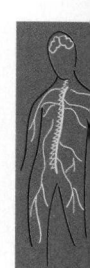

tingling, or as gait ataxia. Symptoms suggesting motor nerve involvement include muscle weakness that typically involves the distal foot muscles. Autonomic nerve involvement is suggested by symptoms of orthostatic hypotension, impotence, cardiac arrhythmia, or bladder dysfunction.

The distribution of muscle weakness is important. In axonal neuropathies the weakness predominantly involves the distal lower extremity muscles, and in demyelinating neuropathies the weakness can involve both proximal and distal muscles as well as facial muscles. Most neuropathies result in *symmetrical* weakness. If asymmetry is present, motor neuron disease, radiculopathy, plexopathy, compressive mononeuropathies, or mononeuritis multiplex should be considered. The intensity and distribution of painful dysesthesias can be informative. Although many axonal neuropathies are associated with a burning sensation in the feet, pain as the chief complaint suggests specific causes of neuropathy (Table 130-10). A neuropathy that manifests with acute, asymmetrical weakness and severe pain suggests vasculitis.

In patients with severe, asymmetrical proprioceptive deficits, with sparing of motor function, the site of the lesion is usually the sensory neuron. This specific syndrome has a relatively limited differential diagnosis, including paraneoplastic process, Sjögren syndrome, cisplatinum toxicity, vitamin B6 toxicity, and HIV infection.

Most neuropathies are relatively insidious in onset, particularly those associated with metabolic or endocrine disorders. Acute neuropathies may be caused by a vasculitic process, toxin exposure, porphyria, or GBS. GBS is commonly preceded by a viral illness, immunization, or a surgical procedure. The neurologic history must thoroughly explore potential toxic exposures such as prior medications and alcohol use (**Web Table 130-3**).

Because many neuropathies are hereditary, it is essential to obtain a detailed family history, specifically inquiring about a history of gait instability, use of adaptive equipment, or skeletal deformities of the feet. Hereditary neuropathies may be autosomal recessive, autosomal dominant, or X-linked. In some situations it may be helpful to actually examine family members because the severity of disease may vary considerably from one generation to the next. The most common hereditary neuropathy is CMT disease (see later).

A complete neurologic examination should always be performed in a patient complaining of numbness. If the patient shows evidence of upper motor neuron involvement in addition to the sensory loss, vitamin B12 or copper deficiency should be considered, even in the absence of apparent anemia. An elevated methylmalonic acid or homocystine level can also help confirm this diagnosis in patients with borderline B12 levels. The presence of weakness and upper motor neuron signs without associated sensory loss suggests ALS.

If the neuropathy is associated with mental status abnormalities, then pyridoxine intoxication or deficiencies of thiamine, niacin ("dementia, diarrhea, dermatitis"), and vitamin B12 should be considered in the differential diagnosis. Lyme disease (see Chapter 97) may result in both peripheral nervous system symptoms (facial nerve palsies, paresthesias, weakness) and central nervous system symptoms (dementia, headache). Acquired immunodeficiency syndrome (AIDS) can also affect both the central and the peripheral nervous systems. GBS and CIDP usually occur at the time of HIV seroconversion, whereas sensory neuropathy, mononeuritis multiplex, and CMV polyradiculopathy generally occur in the context of low CD4 counts in the terminal stages of the disease.

Laboratory Approach to the Patient with Suspected Neuropathy

Once a preliminary differential diagnosis is developed based on the history and neurologic examination findings, laboratory studies can confirm the diagnosis. Laboratory tests to identify potentially treatable causes of neuropathy are included in Table 130-11. Additional studies can be ordered based on the suspected diagnosis. An impaired glucose tolerance test is found in more than half of patients with idiopathic sensory neuropathy and is more sensitive than tests

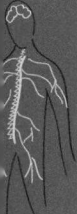

Table 130-11 **Peripheral Neuropathy Laboratory Studies**	
Standard Tests	**Tests Indicated in Selected Cases**
B$_{12}$	Anti-Hu antibody
Complete blood count (CBC)	ESR, ANA, RF, SS-A, SS-B
Glucose tolerance test	Genetic studies for Charcot-Marie-Tooth
RPR	Human immunodeficiency virus (HIV)
Sequential multi-channel analysis (SMA) 20	Lyme antibody
Serum protein electrophoresis (SPEP) and immunofixation electrophoresis (IFE)	Phytanic acid
Thyroid function tests	24-hr urine for heavy metals
Nerve conduction studies or electromyogram (EMG)	Quantitative sensory testing Lumbar puncture Nerve biopsy Skin biopsy Tilt table testing

Table 130-12 **Symptomatic Treatment for Neuropathic Pain**
Tricyclic Antidepressants
Amitriptyline 10-150 mg qhs
Nortriptyline 10-150 mg qhs
Imipramine 10-150 mg qhs
Desipramine 10-150 mg qhs
Anticonvulsants
Lamotrigine 200-400 mg qd
Gabapentin 300-1200 mg tid
Carbamazepine 100-200 mg tid
Topiramate 150-200 mg bid
Oxcarbazepine 1200-2400 mg qd
Pregabalin 150-600 mg qd
Alternative Treatments
Tramadol 50-100 mg qid
Mexiletine 150 mg bid-tid
Lidoderm patches
Capsaicin cream
Transcutaneous nerve stimulation
Acupuncture

of fasting glucose or hemoglobin A$_{1c}$ (HbA$_{1c}$). In a patient with acute, asymmetrical weakness and sensory loss, screening for an inflammatory process (ESR, ANA, RA, SS-A, SS-B) is appropriate. In addition, genetic testing is now available for most patients with CMT disease. If a monoclonal protein is identified on serum protein electrophoresis, a skeletal survey, urine immunofixation electrophoresis, and bone marrow biopsy should be ordered to rule out an underlying lymphoproliferative disorder. If the patient has a monoclonal protein associated with autonomic dysfunction, congestive heart failure, or renal insufficiency, a biopsy (rectal, abdominal fat, or sural nerve) is essential to exclude a diagnosis of amyloidosis. CIDP can be associated with a monoclonal gammopathy, and in this situation patients should be treated with immunosuppressive therapy. Monoclonal gammopathies observed in patients with an axonal peripheral neuropathy are frequently benign (monoclonal gammopathy of unknown significance) and do not necessarily warrant therapy.

A lumbar puncture is indicated only if an acquired demyelinating neuropathy such as GBS or CIDP is being considered. In these cases one would expect to find an "albuminocytologic dissociation" with an elevation in cerebrospinal fluid (CSF) protein and a relatively normal white blood cell (WBC) count. If the CSF WBC count is >50, Lyme disease, HIV-associated disease, or a paraneoplastic process must be considered.

Electrodiagnostic studies consisting of nerve conduction testing and EMG can be a helpful extension of the physical examination. These studies are useful in defining whether the neuropathic process is caused by a primarily axonal or demyelinating process. In general, axonal degeneration decreases the amplitude of the CMAP out of proportion to the degree of reduction in peripheral nerve conduction velocity, whereas demyelination produces prominent reduction in conduction velocities. Nerve conduction testing can help determine, in the case of a demyelinating neuropathy, whether the process has an acquired or hereditary cause.

A uniform slowing of nerve conduction usually suggests a hereditary cause. Electrodiagnostic studies can identify subclinical neuropathy (in patients receiving potentially neurotoxic medications) and can quantitate the extent of axon loss. Finally, these studies can localize the lesion in the case of radiculopathies, plexopathies, and multiple mononeuropathies.

Sensory nerve biopsies are necessary in the diagnosis of a vasculitic neuropathy because treatment involves potentially toxic medications. Performing a muscle biopsy in addition to the nerve biopsy may improve the diagnostic yield and should be considered because the inflammation is random and focal and easily missed. Nerve biopsies are not indicated in "cryptogenic" neuropathies, diabetic neuropathy, or motor neuron disease.

Treatment Strategies in Peripheral Neuropathy

Despite a very thorough history, examination, and laboratory studies, as many as one third of patients remain undiagnosed. In this situation, the focus of management is pain control. Patients with neuropathy frequently report a burning, searing, and aching sensation in their feet and hands that interferes with sleep. Neuropathic pain is difficult to treat but may respond to various medications having different mechanisms of action (Table 130-12). It is important to "start low and taper slow" and to treat for a minimum of 4 weeks before concluding that an agent is ineffective.

Common Mononeuropathies

(see Table 130-7)

CARPAL TUNNEL SYNDROME

Carpal tunnel syndrome results from compression of the median nerve at the wrist as it passes beneath the flexor

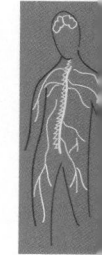

retinaculum. Symptoms usually begin in the dominant hand but commonly involve both hands over time. Patients typically report numbness, tingling, and burning sensations in the palm and in the fingers supplied by the median nerve: the thumb, index finger, middle finger, and medial one half of the ring finger. Some patients report that all fingers become numb. Pain and paresthesias are most prominent at night and often interrupt sleep. The pain is prominent at the wrist but may radiate to the forearm and occasionally to the shoulder. Shaking the hand relieves both pain and paresthesias. Percussion of the median nerve at the wrist provokes paresthesias in a median nerve distribution in 60% of patients (Tinel sign), and flexion of the wrist for 30 to 60 seconds provokes pain or paresthesias in 75% of cases (Phalen sign). Precipitating factors include activities that require repetitive wrist movements: mechanical work, gardening, house painting, and typing. Predisposing causes include pregnancy, diabetes, acromegaly, rheumatoid arthritis, chronic renal failure, thyroid disorders, and primary amyloidosis.

The diagnosis is based on clinical symptoms and signs. Electrodiagnostic studies may demonstrate prolongation of the sensory or motor latencies across the wrist in up to 85% of patients. In more severe cases, EMG may demonstrate evidence of denervation in the abductor pollicis brevis. Treatment initially includes avoidance of repetitive wrist activities and the use of a neutral wrist splint. If these conservative measures fail, injections of lidocaine and methylprednisolone can be given into the carpal tunnel or surgical treatment by section of the transverse carpal ligament can effectively decompress the nerve. Indicators that have been shown to predict failure with conservative management include age >50, disease duration >10 months, constant paresthesias, and a positive Phalen sign in <10 seconds.

ULNAR PALSY

The ulnar nerve may become entrapped at the elbow because of external compression in the condylar groove. Injury may also occur years after a malunited supracondylar fracture of the humerus with bony overgrowth. Contrary to the findings in carpal tunnel syndrome, muscle weakness and atrophy characteristically predominate over sensory symptoms and signs. Patients notice atrophy of the first dorsal interosseous muscle and difficulty performing fine manipulations of the fingers. Numbness of the little finger, the contiguous one half of the ring finger, and the ulnar border of the hand may be present. Ulnar nerve compression can be confirmed with electrodiagnostic studies demonstrating slowed motor conduction velocity across the elbow. Treatment includes the use of elbow pads to avoid compression or surgical procedures including transposition of the ulnar nerve or decompression of the cubital tunnel.

PERONEAL NEUROPATHY

The peroneal nerve can become compressed as it wraps around the fibular head and passes into the fibular tunnel between the peroneus longus muscle and the fibula. Compression may occur as a result of habitual leg crossing, prolonged bed rest, knee casts, prolonged squatting, anesthesia, or profound weight loss. The nerve can also be compressed as a result of Baker cysts, fibular fractures, blunt trauma, tumors, or hematomas at the knee. Symptoms include "foot drop" with selective weakness of the ankle dorsiflexors and evertors as well as the toe extensors. Reflexes remain normal, and sensory loss generally involves the anterolateral leg and dorsum of the foot. Electrodiagnostic studies demonstrate slowing of the peroneal conduction velocity across the fibular head and may demonstrate denervation if axonal injury is present. Compressive injuries usually resolve spontaneously within weeks to months. Magnetic resonance imaging (MRI) and surgical exploration should be considered if symptoms are progressive.

Specific Acquired Polyneuropathies

GUILLAIN-BARRÉ SYNDROME: ACUTE INFLAMMATORY DEMYELINATING POLYNEUROPATHY

Since the advent of polio vaccination, GBS has become the most frequent cause of acute flaccid paralysis throughout the world. GBS is an immune-mediated disorder that follows an identifiable infectious disorder in approximately 60% of patients. The best-documented antecedents include infection with *Campylobacter jejuni,* infectious mononucleosis, CMV, herpesvirus, and mycoplasma. *C. jejuni* is often associated with more severe axonal cases.

The initial symptoms of GBS often consist of tingling and pins-and-needles sensations in the feet and may be associated with dull low-back pain. By the time of presentation, which occurs hours to 1 to 2 days after the first symptoms, weakness has usually developed. The weakness is usually most prominent in the legs, but the arms or cranial musculature may be involved first. Muscle stretch reflexes are lost early, even in regions where strength is retained. Cutaneous sensory deficits (loss of pain and temperature) are relatively mild; however, large fiber function (vibration and proprioception) are more severely impaired. Other clinical features include pain (20%), paresthesias (50%), autonomic symptoms (20%), facial weakness (50%), ophthalmoparesis (9%), bulbar weakness, and respiratory failure (25%). Symptoms associated with GBS typically evolve over a 2- to 4-week period, with approximately 90% of patients showing no evidence of progression beyond 4 weeks. For this reason, patients who are seen within several weeks from onset continue to require hospitalization for close observation. Respiratory muscle strength should be monitored with bedside measurements of the FVC. Intubation should be initiated when the FVC falls below 15 mL/kg.

Treatment may include either intravenous gammaglobulin (0.4 g/kg/day × 5 days) or plasmapheresis—the exchange of the patient's plasma for albumin (200 mL/kg over 7 to 10 days). Clinical studies have confirmed equal efficacy between these two therapies, with no additional benefit conferred with combination therapy. Corticosteroids are not effective in GBS. Indications for therapy include inability to ambulate independently, impaired respiratory function, or rapidly progressive weakness. Clinical features predicting a poor prognosis or prolonged recovery time include rapidly progressive weakness, need for mechanical ventilation, and low-amplitude CMAPs. The mortality rate remains 5% to 10%, usually because of respiratory complications, cardiac arrhythmia, or pulmonary embolism. With appropriate supportive care and rehabilitation, 80% to 90% of patients recover with little or no disability.

CHRONIC INFLAMMATORY DEMYELINATING POLYNEUROPATHY

CIDP has been considered the "chronic form" of GBS, because by definition the symptoms must progress for at least 8 weeks. The clinical features include proximal and distal weakness, areflexia, and distal sensory loss. Autonomic dysfunction, respiratory insufficiency, and cranial nerve involvement can occur but are much less common than in GBS. Treatment for CIDP includes the use of oral immunosuppressive agents such as prednisone, cyclosporine, mycophenolate mofetil, and azathioprine. Intravenous immune globulin and plasmapheresis are also indicated for severe or refractory cases.

DIABETIC NEUROPATHY

Diabetes mellitus is the most frequent cause of peripheral neuropathy worldwide. The diabetic neuropathies take many clinical forms, including symmetrical polyneuropathies and a wide variety of individual plexus or nerve disorders.

Diabetes mellitus often causes a slowly progressive, distal, symmetrical sensorimotor polyneuropathy (DSPN). DSPN is uncommon at the time of diagnosis of diabetes, but its prevalence increases with duration of diabetes with a lifetime prevalence of 55% for type 1 and 45% for type 2. The precise pathogenesis is not defined, but, similar to the ocular and renal complications, diabetic neuropathy can be reduced in incidence and in severity by maintaining blood glucose levels close to normal. Initial symptoms may consist of numbness, tingling, burning, or prickling sensations affecting the feet and toes. Mild distal weakness and gait instability may subsequently develop. The sensory symptoms can then chronically progress to involve a "stocking-glove pattern." The small-fiber dysfunction often produces spontaneous neuropathic pain in which unpleasant sensations can be evoked by normally innocuous stimuli, such as the bed sheets on the toes at night. Continuous burning or throbbing pain may occur, and prolonged walking is often distressing. In severe cases, patients may develop foot ulcers in insensitive areas that necessitate amputation. Autonomic dysfunction is also frequently associated with DSPN including impotence, nocturnal diarrhea, sweating abnormalities, orthostatic hypotension, and gastroparesis.

Other less common neuropathies associated with diabetes include cranial neuropathies (the sixth, third, and rarely fourth nerves), mononeuropathies, mononeuropathy multiplex, radiculopathies, and plexopathies. Diabetic amyotrophy (also known as *diabetic lumbosacral polyradiculopathy*) is a distinctive disorder characterized by severe thigh pain followed by proximal>distal lower extremity weakness that progresses over a period of months. The onset is invariably unilateral, but the condition may progress to involve both lower extremities. Physical therapy and effective pain management are essential; treatment with immune modulators is controversial.

TOXIC-INDUCED NEUROPATHIES

Toxic neuropathies constitute a large number of disorders caused by alcohol, drugs, heavy metals, and environmental substances (**Web Table 130-3**). The majority of toxic neuropathies manifest as a distal sensorimotor axonal neuropathy that chronically progresses over time unless the offending agent is eliminated. Clinical evaluation should focus on the temporal relationship between exposure and the onset of sensory or motor symptoms as well as symptoms of systemic toxicity.

CRITICAL ILLNESS POLYNEUROPATHY

Critical illness polyneuropathy (CIP) is a common cause of failure to wean from a ventilator in a patient with associated sepsis and multi-organ failure. Clinical features include generalized or distal flaccid paralysis, especially involving the lower extremities, depressed or absent reflexes, and distal sensory loss with relative sparing of cranial nerve function. The diagnosis can be confirmed with nerve conduction studies showing evidence of a severe, generalized axonal neuropathy. CSF protein should be normal and, in addition to conduction studies, distinguishes CIP from GBS.

Specific Hereditary Polyneuropathies

CHARCOT-MARIE-TOOTH DISEASE

The eponym Charcot-Marie-Tooth (CMT) identifies a group of heritable disorders of peripheral nerves that share clinical features but differ in their pathologic mechanisms and the specific genetic abnormalities (**Web Table 130-4**). CMT is the most common heritable neuromuscular disorder, with an incidence of 17 to 40 cases per 100,000.

CMT disease usually manifests during the first to second decades with symptoms related to insidious foot drop: frequent tripping and inability to jump well or run as fast as other children. Over time, distal upper extremity weakness develops, resulting in difficulty with buttoning, handling keys, and opening jars. Examination reveals distal weakness and wasting of the intrinsic muscles of the feet, the peroneal muscles, the anterior tibial muscles, and the calves (inverted champagne bottle legs). A variable degree of impaired large-fiber sensory function is reflected in reduced vibratory sensation at the toes. Muscle stretch reflexes are lost, first at the ankles. Typically, a foot deformity exists, with high arches (pes cavus) and hammer toes, reflecting long-standing muscle imbalance in the feet. Most patients with CMT disease have nearly normal occupational and daily activities, and they have a normal life span. Although no specific treatment has been developed, the foot drop can be treated by appropriate bracing of the ankle with ankle-foot orthoses. Genetic counseling and education of affected patients and their families are important, both for reassurance and to preclude unnecessary diagnostic evaluation of affected members in future generations.

Demyelinating forms of CMT are classified as CMT1 and axonal forms as CMT2. CMT is usually transmitted as an autosomal dominant trait; however, X-linked dominant transmission is responsible for approximately 10% of cases. Rare autosomal recessive forms are designated CMT4, and these patients tend to have an earlier onset and more severe phenotype. CMT1A is the most common form and accounts for 90% of CMT1 and 50% of all CMT cases. CMT1A is associated with the 17p11.2-p12 duplication in the *PMP22* gene expressed by Schwann cells. A deletion or a point mutation of the *PMP22* gene produces a different phenotype—HNPP, which is characterized by recurrent episodes of focal entrapment with attacks of weakness and numbness in the peroneal, ulnar, radial, and median nerves (in descending order of frequency) or in a brachial plexus distribution. Commercial testing for the *PMP22* duplication or deletion is now widely available.

Familial Amyloid Neuropathies

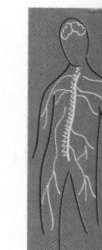

Amyloid neuropathy is an autosomal dominant disorder caused by extracellular deposition of the fibrillary protein amyloid in peripheral nerve and sensory and autonomic ganglia, as well as around blood vessels in nerves and other tissues. The age of onset varies from 18 to 83 years. In all forms of amyloidosis, the initial and major abnormalities affect the small sensory and autonomic fibers. Involvement of small fibers responsible for pain and temperature sensibilities leads to loss of the ability to perceive mechanical and thermal injuries and to an increased risk of tissue damage. As a result, painless injuries present a major hazard of this disorder; in advanced stages, they can lead to chronic infections or osteomyelitis of the feet or hands and the necessity for amputation. Amyloid deposition in the heart can lead to cardiomyopathy. Mutations in transthyretin, apolipoprotein A1, or gelsolin are responsible. Early recognition is essential, as liver transplantation has been shown to halt disease progression.

Prospectus for the Future

The discovery of the cause of some cases of familial amyotrophic lateral sclerosis (ALS) has not yet translated into treatment strategies, nor has it shed light on potential treatments for the more common, clinically identical sporadic syndrome. Genetic and environmental factors that might alter a patient's predisposition of developing sporadic ALS are also being sought, and with this knowledge comes the hope that novel treatments will soon be developed. In the meantime, many innovative clinical trials are being conducted. The identification of the molecular cause of many of the hereditary peripheral neuropathies has opened the prospect of genetic approaches to treatment. For the acquired neuropathies, symptomatic treatments continue to be developed and improved.

References

Dyck PJ, Thomas PK (eds): Peripheral Neuropathy, 4th ed. Philadelphia, WB Saunders, 2005.

Feldman EL: Amyotrophic lateral sclerosis and other motor neuron diseases. In Goldman L, Ausiello DA (eds): Cecil Textbook of Medicine, 23rd ed. Philadelphia, WB Saunders, 2007.

Griggs RC: Neuromuscular diseases: Disorders of the motor neuron and plexus and peripheral nerve disease. In Goldman L, Ausiello DA (eds): Cecil Textbook of Medicine, 23rd ed. Philadelphia, WB Saunders, 2007.

Shy M: Peripheral neuropathies. In Goldman L, Ausiello DA (eds): Cecil Textbook of Medicine, 23rd ed. Philadelphia, WB Saunders, 2007.

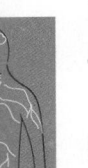

Muscle Diseases

Robert C. Griggs

Skeletal muscle diseases (myopathies) are disorders in which a primary structural or functional impairment of muscle occurs. Myopathies can be broadly classified into hereditary and acquired disorders. The hereditary disorders include the muscular dystrophies, congenital myopathies, channelopathies, metabolic disorders, and mitochondrial disorders. The acquired include inflammatory disorders, metabolic disorders, endocrine disorders, disorders associated with systemic illness, and drug-induced or toxic disorders.

Organization and Structure of Muscle

Muscle consists of many motor units. The number of muscle fibers innervated by a single motor unit varies from muscle to muscle. Muscles subserving finely coordinated movements, such as an ocular muscle, can have fewer than 10 muscle fibers in a motor unit. Powerful proximal limb muscles have large motor units with 1000 to 2000 fibers innervated by a single motor neuron.

The muscle fibers consist of thick and thin filaments (myofibrils). The myofibrils are surrounded by the sarcolemmal membrane and basal lamina. A large number of muscular dystrophies are now known to be caused by genetic defects in this region (Fig. 131-1). The sarcolemmal components are known as the *dystrophin-glycoprotein complex* (DGC). The DGC is a trans-sarcolemmal complex of proteins and glycoproteins that links the subsarcolemmal cytoskeleton to the extracellular matrix. Dystrophin was the first well-characterized protein in the DGC. Other DGC components include the dystroglycan complex (α and β), the sarcoglycan complex (α, β, γ, and δ), and the syntrophin complex (α, $\beta1$, and $\beta2$). Closely adherent to the extracellular portion of the sarcolemma is the basal lamina, components of which are known as *laminins*.

Assessment

The most important aspect of evaluating a patient with a myopathy is the history. The most common symptom of a patient with muscle disease is a loss of function caused by weakness. If the weakness is in the legs, then patients report difficulty climbing stairs and rising from a low chair or toilet or from the floor. When the arms are involved, patients notice trouble lifting objects (especially over their heads) and washing or brushing their hair. These symptoms point to proximal weakness, the most common site of weakness in a myopathy. In less common distal myopathies, patients first complain of poor hand grip (difficulty opening jar tops and turning door knobs) or tripping as a result of ankle weakness from muscle weakness. Rarely they may exhibit a change in speech or swallowing, droopy eyelids, and double vision from weakness of cranial nerve–innervated muscles.

The tempo of the disease course is important. Weakness may be present all of the time (fixed) or intermittently (episodic). Myopathies can produce either fixed or episodic symptoms. Muscle disorders can be *acute* (<4 weeks), *subacute* (4 to 8 weeks), or *chronic* (>8 weeks). Examples include (1) acute or subacute inflammatory myopathies (dermatomyositis [DM] and polymyositis [PM]), (2) chronic slow progression over years (most muscular dystrophies), or (3) fixed weakness with little change over decades (congenital myopathies). Patients with channelopathies or metabolic myopathies have recurrent attacks over many years, whereas a patient with acute muscle destruction caused by a toxin such as cocaine may have a single acute episode.

Patients who report a generalized global *weakness* or *fatigue* seldom have a myopathy, particularly if the neurologic examination findings are normal. Fatigue is a complaint of the patient with myasthenia gravis but otherwise is usually a nonspecific symptom. Muscle pain (myalgia) is also a nonspecific complaint that infrequently accompanies some myopathies. Myalgias may be episodic (e.g., metabolic myopathies) or nearly constant (e.g., occasional inflammatory myopathies). However, muscle pain is surprisingly uncommon in most muscle diseases, and limb pain is more likely to be caused by bone or joint disorders. Rarely is a muscle disease responsible for vague aches and discomfort in muscle if strength is normal. The involuntary muscle cramp is localized to a single muscle and lasts from seconds to minutes. In most instances, cramps are benign and normal; they do not reflect myopathy. Cramps occur with dehydration, hyponatremia, azotemia, and myxedema and

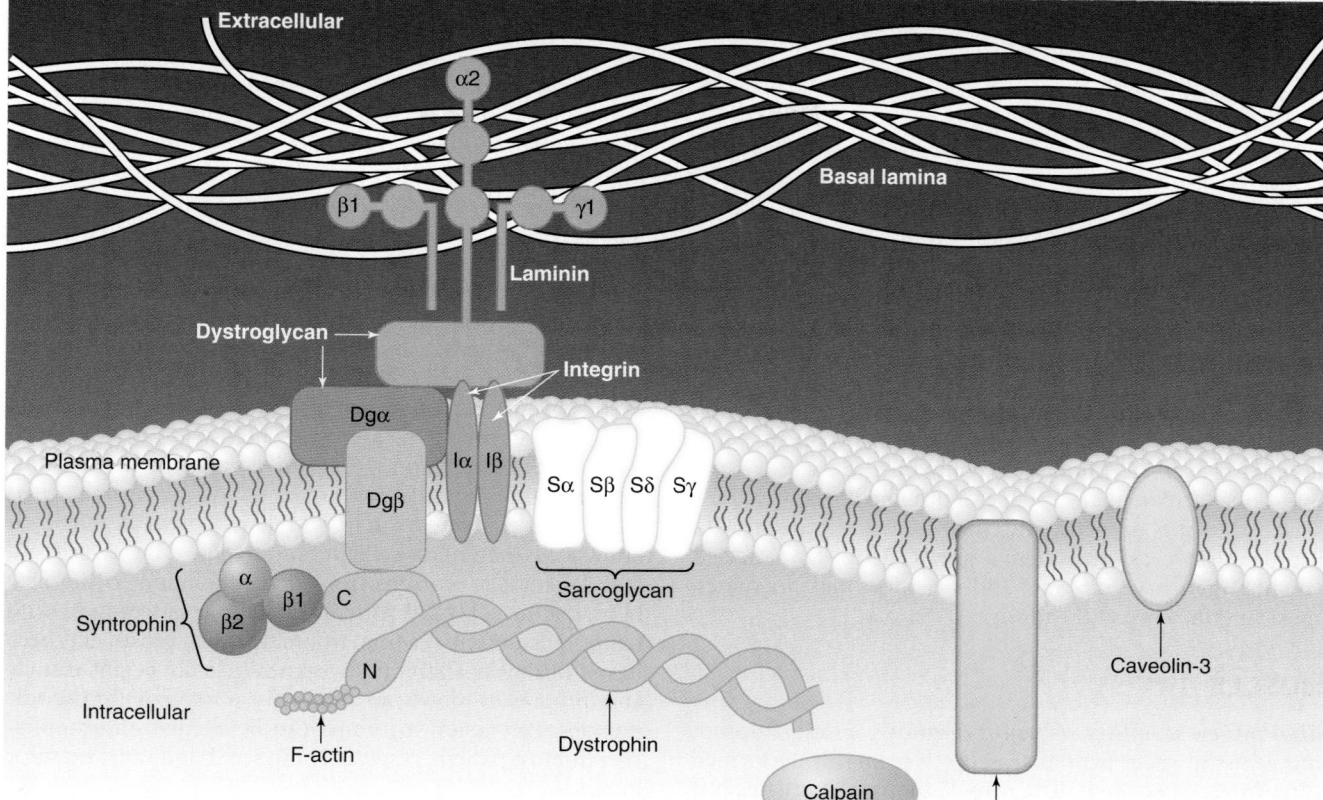

Figure 131-1 The dystrophin-glycoprotein complex and related proteins.

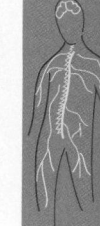

in nerve disease such as amyotrophic lateral sclerosis. Muscle contractures are rare and resemble a cramp. They last longer than cramps and occur with exercise in glycolytic enzyme defects. On electromyographic (EMG) examination, contractures are electrically silent, whereas cramps have rapidly firing motor unit discharges. Muscle contracture should not be confused with fixed tendon contracture. Myotonia is the phenomenon of impaired relaxation of muscle after forceful voluntary contraction. Patients report muscle stiffness or persistent contraction in almost any muscle group but particularly the hands. Exercise-induced weakness and myalgias may be accompanied by dark or red urine (myoglobinuria). Myoglobinuria follows rapid muscle destruction.

EXAMINATION

Specific muscle function should be tested. Muscle strength is quantitated by the Medical Research Council of Great Britain (MRC) grading scale of 0 to 5:

5: Normal power
4: Active movement against gravity and resistance
3: Active movement against gravity
2: Active movement only with gravity eliminated
1: Trace contraction
0: No contraction

Muscles should be inspected for atrophy or hypertrophy. Atrophy of proximal limb muscles is usual in longstanding myopathies. Muscles can also become diffusely hypertrophic in dystrophic or myotonic conditions. In Duchenne and Becker dystrophies, the calves enlarge as a result of pseudohypertrophy from replacement with connective tissue and fat. The sensory examination findings should be normal in muscle disease. Reflexes are preserved early in the disease process, but when muscles become extremely weak, reflexes become hypoactive or unelicitable. Evidence of upper motor neuron damage (e.g., spasticity, Babinski signs, clonus) is present in myopathies only if coincidental central nervous system disease exists.

PATTERNS OF WEAKNESS

Six broad patterns of muscle weakness occur in myopathies:

1. The most common is in proximal muscles of the arms and legs: a limb-girdle distribution. Neck flexor and extensor muscles can also be affected. The reason why most myopathies begin in proximal muscles is unknown.
2. Distal weakness may begin in the upper or lower extremities. Such distal weakness is often a feature of neuropathies.
3. Scapuloperoneal weakness includes weakness of the periscapular muscles and distal lower extremity weakness of the anterior compartment. The scapular muscle weakness is usually accompanied by scapular winging.
4. Distal upper extremity weakness in the distal forearm muscles (wrist and finger flexors), and proximal lower extremity weakness involving the knee extensors

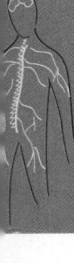

(quadriceps) may occur. This pattern is typical of inclusion body myositis (IBM) and frequent in myotonic dystrophy.

5. Involvement of ocular or pharyngeal muscles may be predominant.

6. Neck extensor weakness (the *dropped head syndrome*) may be prominent.

These six patterns of myopathy are useful in differential diagnosis, but neuromuscular diseases other than myopathies can also exhibit one of these weakness patterns. For example, whereas proximal greater than distal weakness is characteristic of myopathies, patients with acquired demyelinating neuropathies (Guillain-Barré syndrome and chronic inflammatory demyelinating polyneuropathy) often have proximal as well as distal muscle involvement. Such neuropathies are additionally accompanied by sensory and reflex loss. Ocular, pharyngeal, and proximal limb weakness is characteristic of neuromuscular junction transmission disorders such as myasthenia gravis. However, affected patients often have diplopia and weakness that fluctuates, suggesting the correct diagnosis.

MUSCLE BIOPSY

Fixed muscle is of little value for diagnosis. Examination of muscle tissue under light microscopy is primarily performed using frozen specimens. The muscle biopsy can establish if either a neuropathic or a myopathic disorder is present; it can also suggest a specific diagnosis of many hereditary and acquired myopathies.

Muscular Dystrophies

Muscular dystrophies are inherited myopathies characterized by progressive muscle weakness and degeneration and subsequent replacement by fibrous and fatty connective tissue. Historically, muscular dystrophies were categorized by their distribution of weakness, age at onset, and inheritance pattern. Advances in the molecular understanding of the muscular dystrophies have defined the genetic mutation and abnormal gene product for most of these disorders (Table 131-1).

Dystrophinopathies are X-linked disorders resulting from mutations of the large dystrophin gene located at Xp21. Dystrophin is a large subsarcolemmal cytoskeletal protein that, along with the other components of the DGC, provides support to the muscle membrane during contraction. Mutations disrupting the translational reading frame of the gene result in near-total loss of dystrophin (Duchenne dystrophy), whereas in-frame mutations result in the translation of semifunctional dystrophin of abnormal size or amount (Becker dystrophy). The incidence of Duchenne dystrophy is 1 in 3500 male births; one third of the cases result from a new mutation. Duchenne dystrophy manifests as early as age 2 to 3 years as delays in motor milestones and difficulty running. The proximal muscles are the most severely affected, and the course is relentlessly progressive. Patients begin to fall frequently by age 5 to 6, have difficulty climbing stairs by age 8 years, and are usually confined to a wheelchair by age 12. Most patients die of respiratory complications in

their 20s. Congestive heart failure and arrhythmias can occur late in the disease. The smooth muscle of the gastrointestinal tract is involved and may cause intestinal pseudo-obstruction. The average IQ of boys with Duchenne dystrophy is low, reflecting central nervous system involvement. Becker dystrophy is a milder form of dystrophinopathy and varies in severity depending on the gene lesion. It is less common than the Duchenne form, with an incidence of 5 per 100,000.

Myotonic dystrophy occurs in two forms: DM-1 and DM-2. Both dystrophies are autosomal-dominant multisystem disorders that affect skeletal, cardiac, and smooth muscle and other organs, including the eyes, the endocrine system, and the brain. DM-1 is the most prevalent muscular dystrophy, with an incidence of 13.5 per 100,000 live births. DM-1 can occur at any age, with the usual onset of symptoms in the late second or third decade. However, some affected individuals may remain symptom-free their entire lives. A severe form of DM-1 with onset in infancy is known as *congenital myotonic dystrophy*. The severity of DM-1 generally worsens from one generation to the next (anticipation). Typical patients exhibit facial weakness with temporalis muscle wasting, frontal balding, ptosis, and neck flexor weakness. Extremity weakness usually begins distally and progresses slowly to affect the proximal limb-girdle muscles. Percussion myotonia can be elicited on examination in most patients, especially in thenar and wrist extensor muscles.

Associated manifestations in DM-1 include cataracts, testicular atrophy and impotence, intellectual impairment, and hypersomnia associated with both central and obstructive sleep apnea. Respiratory muscle weakness may be severe, with impairment of ventilatory drive. Cardiac conduction defects are common and can produce sudden death. Pacemakers may be necessary, and annual electrocardiographic examinations are recommended. Chronic hypoxia can lead to cor pulmonale. The molecular defect of myotonic dystrophy (DM-1) is an abnormal expansion of CTG repeats in chromosome 19q13.2. The second myotonic dystrophy (DM-2) is caused by an abnormal expansion of a tetranucleotide repeat on chromosome 3q. The precise pathomechanisms of DM-1 and DM-2 are unknown but probably relate to abnormal RNA transcribed by the pathologic repeats. DM-2 resembles DM-1. However, weakness is often proximal; patients may complain of myotonia and myalgias. Patients with DM-2 may have less severe cardiac and other organ involvement than those with DM-1.

Congenital Myopathies

Congenital myopathies are defined by their appearance on biopsy (Table 131-2). They are usually present at birth with hypotonia and subsequent delayed motor development. Most congenital myopathies are relatively nonprogressive and may not be diagnosed until the second or third decade. Clinical findings common in the congenital myopathies are reduced muscle bulk, slender body build, a long, narrow face, skeletal abnormalities (high-arched palate, pectus excavatum, kyphoscoliosis, dislocated hips, and pes cavus), and absent or reduced muscle stretch reflexes. The molecular

Table 131-1 **Major Muscular Dystrophies**

Disease	Mode of Inheritance	Gene Mutation Location	Gene Defect or Protein
X-Linked MD			
Duchenne, Becker	XR	Xp21	Dystrophin
Emery-Dreifuss	XR	Xq28	Emerin
Limb-Girdle MD			
LGMD 1A	AD	5q22-34	Myotilin
LGMD 1B	AD	1q11-21	Lamin A/C
LGMD 1C	AD	3p25	Caveolin-3
LGMD 2A	AR	15q15	Calpain-3
LGMD 2B*	AR	2p12	Dysferlin
LGMD 2C	AR	13q12	γ-sarcoglycan
LGMD 2D	AR	17q12	α-sarcoglycan
LGMD 2E	AR	4q12	β-sarcoglycan
LGMD 2F	AR	5q33	δ-sarcoglycan
LGMD 2G	AR	17q11	Telethonin
LGMD 2H	AR	9q31	E3-ubiquitin-ligase
LGMD 2I	AR	19q13.3	Fukutin-related protein 1
LGMD 2J	AR	2q31	Titin
Congenital MD With CNS Involvement			
Fukuyama CMD	AR	9q31-33	Fukutin
Walker-Warburg CMD	AR	9q31-33	Fukutin
Muscle-eye-brain CMD	AR	1p	Glycosyltransferase
Without CNS Involvement			
Merosin-deficient classic type	AR	6q2	Laminin-2 (merosin)
Merosin-positive classic type	AR	Unknown	Not known
Integrin-deficient CMD	AR	12q13	Integrin α7
Rigid spine syndrome	AR	1p3	Selenoprotein N
Distal MD			
Late adult-onset 1A (Welander)	AD	2p15	Unknown
Late adult-onset 1B (Udd)	AD	2q31	Titin
Early adult-onset 1A (Nonaka)	AR	9p1-q1	GNE
Early adult-onset 1B (Miyoshi)†	AR	2q12-14	Dysferlin
Early adult-onset 1C (Laing)	AD	14	MYH7
Other MD			
Facioscapulohumeral	AD	4q35	Deleted chromatin
Oculopharyngeal	AD	14q11	Poly(A) binding protein 2
Myotonic dystrophy type 1	AD	19q13	RNA accumulation
Myotonic dystrophy type 2	AD	3q	RNA accumulation
Myofibrillar myopathy	AD	11q21-23	β-crystallin
Myofibrillar myopathy	AD	2q35	Desmin
Bethlem myopathy	AD	21q22	Collagen VI

*Probably the same condition as Miyoshi distal MD.
†Probably the same condition as LGMD 2B.
 AD, autosomal dominant; AR, autosomal recessive; CMD, congenital muscular dystrophy; CNS, central nervous system; GNE, UDP-*N*-acetylglucosamine 2-epimerase/*N*-acetylmannosamine kinase; LGMD, limb-girdle muscular dystrophy; MD, muscular dystrophy; XR, X-linked recessive; MYH7, myosin heavy chain 7.

Table 131-2 **Major Morphologically Distinct Congenital Myopathies**

Central core
Nemaline
Centronuclear (myotubular)
Congenital fiber type disproportion
Sarcotubular
Reducing body
Myofibrillar

genetic defects of most congenital myopathies are now known, and these disorders, as well as the muscular dystrophies, are being reclassified.

Metabolic Myopathies

Metabolic myopathies (Table 131-3) include (1) glucose and glycogen metabolism disorders, (2) lipid metabolism disorders, and (3) mitochondrial disorders.

GLUCOSE AND GLYCOGEN METABOLISM DISORDERS

Glucose, and its storage form glycogen, is essential for the short-term, predominantly anaerobic energy requirements of muscle. Disorders of glucose and glycogen metabolism (called *glycogenoses*) have two distinct syndromes: (1) dynamic symptoms of exercise intolerance, pain, cramps, and myoglobinuria; and (2) static symptoms of fixed weakness without exercise intolerance or myoglobinuria. Of the

11 glycogenoses, only glucose 6-phosphate (type I) and liver phosphorylase (type VI) deficiencies spare muscle.

Glycogenoses with Exercise Intolerance (Myoglobinuria)

Exercise intolerance (Table 131-4) begins in childhood with exertional muscle pain, cramps, and myoglobinuria appearing in the second or third decade. Many patients note a *second wind* phenomenon after a period of brief rest so that they can continue the exercise at the previous level of activity. Muscle pain is caused by electrically silent contractures. Strength, blood creatine kinase (CK) levels, and EMG findings between attacks are usually normal early in the disease, but they may become abnormal with advancing age. After episodes of severe myoglobinuria, EMG shows myopathic units and fibrillations. EMG performed during a contracture shows electrical silence. In the forearm exercise test, the venous lactate level fails to rise in myophosphorylase, phosphofructokinase, and phosphoglycerate kinase deficiencies and rises subnormally in phosphorylase β kinase, phosphoglucomutase, and lactate dehydrogenase deficiencies. Diagnosis is made by muscle biopsy study of the enzymes or by defining specific genetic mutations.

Glycogenoses with Fixed Weakness and No Exercise Intolerance

Glycogenoses with fixed weakness and no exercise intolerance (see Table 131-3) produce a syndrome of progressive proximal weakness. Diagnosis requires muscle biopsy or genetic mutation definition. Acid maltase deficiency can now be treated with enzyme replacement.

DISORDERS OF FATTY ACID METABOLISM

Lipids are essential for the aerobic energy needs of muscle during sustained exercise. Serum long-chain fatty acids are the primary lipid fuel for muscle metabolism. They are transported into the mitochondria as carnitine esters and

---

Table 131-3 Metabolic and Mitochondrial Myopathies

Glycogen Metabolism Deficiencies

Type II	$\alpha_{1,4}$-glucosidase (acid maltase)
Type III	Debranching enzyme
Type IV	Branching enzyme
Type V	Phosphorylase* (McArdle disease)
Type VII	Phosphofructokinase* (Tarui disease)
Type VIII	Phosphorylase β kinase*
Type IX	Phosphoglycerate kinase*
Type X	Phosphoglycerate mutase*
Type XI	Lactate dehydrogenase*

Lipid Metabolism Deficiencies

Carnitine palmitoyl transferase*
Primary systemic or muscle carnitine deficiency
Secondary carnitine deficiency

Mitochondrial Myopathies

Pyruvate dehydrogenase complex deficiencies
Progressive external ophthalmoplegia (PEO)
Autosomal dominant with multiple mitochondrial DNA deletions
Adenine nucleotide translocator 1 (ANT1)
Twinkle (mitochondrial protein)
Polymerase gamma
Kearns-Sayre syndrome
Myoclonic epilepsy and ragged-red fibers (MERRF)
Mitochondrial encephalopathy with lactic acidosis and strokelike episodes (MELAS)
Mitochondrial neurogastrointestinal encephalomyopathy (MNGIE)
Mitochondrial depletion syndrome
Leigh disease and neuropathy, ataxia, retinitis pigmentosa (NARP)
Succinate dehydrogenase deficiency*

*Deficiency can produce exercise intolerance and myoglobinuria.

Table 131-4 Channelopathies and Related Disorders

Disorder	Clinical Features	Inheritance	Chromosome	Gene
Chloride Channelopathies				
Myotonia congenita				
Thomsen disease	Myotonia	Autosomal dominant	7q35	*CLC-1*
Becker disease	Myotonia and weakness	Autosomal recessive	7q35	*CLC-1*
Sodium Channelopathies				
Paramyotonia congenita	Paramyotonia	Autosomal dominant	17q13.1-13.3	*SCNA4A*
Hyperkalemic periodic paralysis	Periodic paralysis, myotonia, and paramyotonia	Autosomal dominant	17q13.1-13.3	*SCNA4A*
Hypokalemic periodic paralysis (<10% of cases)	Periodic paralysis	Autosomal dominant	17q13.1-13.3	*SCNA4A*
Calcium Channelopathies				
Hypokalemic periodic paralysis	Periodic paralysis (most cases)	Autosomal dominant	1q31-32	Dihydropyridine receptor
Malignant hyperthermia (some cases)	Anesthetic-induced delayed relaxation	Autosomal dominant	19q13.1	Ryanodine receptor
Potassium channelopathy (Andersen-Tawil syndrome)	Periodic paralysis, cardiac arrhythmia, skeletal abnormalities	Autosomal dominant	17q23	*KCNJ2*
Rippling muscle disease (Web video 131-1)	Muscle mounding or stiffness	Autosomal dominant	1q41	Caveolin-3

are metabolized by means of beta-oxidation. Carnitine palmitoyl transferase (CPT) I converts cytoplasmic acyl coenzyme A (CoA) to acylcarnitine, which is then transported into the mitochondria by carnitine acyltransferase in exchange for carnitine. CPT II on the inner mitochondrial membrane reconstitutes acyl CoA. A deficiency of carnitine, CPT, or the enzymes of beta-oxidation can lead to impaired muscle lipid metabolism.

As with glycogen pathway defects, abnormal fatty acid metabolism causes exercise intolerance with myoglobinuria or static weakness with a lipid storage myopathy. In addition, some disorders of lipid metabolism can produce multiorgan metabolic crises, with hepatic failure and altered mental status. Most lipid disorders are believed to be autosomal recessive (see Table 131-3).

MITOCHONDRIAL MYOPATHIES

Mitochondrial myopathies (see Table 131-3) produce slowly progressive weakness of proximal limbs or external ocular and other cranial muscles and abnormal fatigability on sustained exertion. Some of these myopathies affect multiple organs or systems, in addition to muscle. In mitochondrial myopathies, some muscle fibers contain abnormal mitochondria. These fibers appear *ragged red* on biopsy stains (trichrome) and may fail to react for cytochrome *c* oxidase. Serum lactic acid levels are often elevated at rest in mitochondrial myopathy. Mitochondrial diseases are caused by mutations in either nuclear or mitochondrial DNA. During fertilization, all of the mitochondria are contributed by the mother; thus all mutations of mitochondrial DNA are either maternally transmitted or arise de novo in the maternal ovum or in early embryonic life. However, because the majority of mitochondrial proteins (95%) are encoded from nuclear genes, mitochondrial disorders can also have autosomal-dominant or X-linked heredity. Mitochondrial disorders produce biochemical defects proximal to the respiratory chain (involving substrate transport and usage) or within the respiratory chain.

SPECIFIC MITOCHONDRIAL DISORDERS AFFECTING MUSCLE

Progressive External Ophthalmoplegia

Severe ptosis and progressive external ophthalmoplegia (PEO) are clinical hallmarks of mitochondrial disease. Ptosis is often the presenting symptom and can be noted in childhood. Patients and their physicians often overlook both ptosis and PEO (lack of eye movements). Patients often do not complain of double vision. Slight proximal weakness may occur. PEO caused by mitochondrial disease is associated with single or multiple mitochondrial DNA deletions. Patients with single mitochondrial deletions have Kearns-Sayre syndrome, which manifests before age 20 years and includes a wide variety of multisystem abnormalities: retinitis pigmentosa, heart block, hearing loss, short stature, ataxia, delayed puberty, peripheral neuropathy, and impaired ventilatory drive. Kearns-Sayre syndrome is caused by single large mitochondrial deletions; it is sporadic with no family history of the disorder. Patients with PEO who have multiple mitochondrial deletions have an autosomal-dominant

inheritance pattern. Many of the responsible genes have been identified (see Table 131-3).

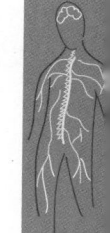

Myoclonic Epilepsy and Ragged Red Fibers

Patients with myoclonic epilepsy and ragged red fibers (MERRF) have varying symptoms of myoclonus, generalized seizures, ataxia, dementia, sensorineural hearing loss, and optic atrophy, as well as limb-girdle weakness. Some patients also have peripheral neuropathy, cardiomyopathy, and cutaneous lipomas. Ptosis and PEO are usually not present.

Mitochondrial Encephalomyopathy with Lactic Acidosis and Strokelike Episodes

Patients with mitochondrial encephalomyopathy with lactic acidosis and strokelike episodes (MELAS) have normal early development, experience migraine-like headaches and strokes before age 40 years, and have chronic lactic acidosis. Other features can include dementia, hearing loss, and episodic vomiting, ataxia, and coma, as well as diabetes. Ptosis and PEO are uncommon.

Channelopathies (Nondystrophic Myotonias and Periodic Paralyses)

The myotonias are categorized into dystrophic and nondystrophic disorders. The nondystrophic myotonias and the periodic paralyses are caused by mutations of various ion channels in muscle (see Table 131-4). The term *channelopathies* is often used to describe this group of disorders.

CHLORIDE CHANNELOPATHIES

Myotonia congenita is caused by point mutations in the muscle chloride channel gene. Autosomal-dominant and autosomal-recessive forms are allelic. The autosomal-dominant form (Thomsen disease) and the autosomal-recessive form (Becker myotonia congenita) are both benign and are associated with muscle hypertrophy and action, percussion, and electrical myotonia. Cold increases the myotonia, and exercise improves it. The heart or other organs are not involved. Patients with Thomsen disease are not weak, but patients with Becker myotonia congenita have fluctuations in strength and may develop persistent limb-girdle weakness. Many patients do not require treatment, but drugs such as quinine, procainamide, phenytoin, and mexiletine reduce myotonia and may improve strength.

SODIUM CHANNELOPATHIES

Several autosomal-dominant disorders are caused by point mutations in the voltage-dependent sodium channel gene. All of these disorders have symptoms beginning in the first decade. Paramyotonia congenita has paradoxical myotonia in that myotonia *increases* with exercise. Myotonia is worsened by cold temperature. The myotonia can be treated with sodium channel blockers such as mexiletine.

In hyperkalemic periodic paralysis, attacks of weakness last 1 to 2 hours and are precipitated by fasting, by rest after exercise, or by ingesting potassium-rich foods. During attacks, patients are hyporeflexic with normal sensation, and no ocular or respiratory muscle weakness is present. The serum potassium level may be normal during the attack, and therefore a more appropriate term may be *potassium-sensitive periodic paralysis*. Episodes of weakness rarely necessitate acute therapy; oral carbohydrates or glucose improves weakness. Treatments to prevent attacks include thiazide diuretics, β-agonists, and a low-potassium, high-carbohydrate diet, with avoidance of fasting, strenuous activity, and cold.

In a small proportion of patients, hypokalemic periodic paralysis results from mutations in the sodium channel (see **Web video 131-2**).

CALCIUM CHANNELOPATHIES

The majority of cases of hypokalemic periodic paralysis are caused by mutations in the muscle calcium channel. Attacks begin by adolescence and are triggered by exercise, sleep, stress, or meals rich in carbohydrates and sodium. Attacks last from 3 to 24 hours. A vague prodrome of stiffness or heaviness in the legs can occur, and if the patient performs mild exercise, then a full-blown attack may be aborted. Ocular, bulbar, and respiratory muscles are rarely involved. Early in the disease, patients have relatively normal interattack examinations except for eyelid myotonia (approximately 50%). Later, many patients have proximal weakness. Preventive measures include a low-carbohydrate, low-sodium diet and carbonic anhydrase inhibitors. Acute attacks are treated with oral potassium. Patients with hypokalemic periodic paralysis and mutations in the sodium channel are often worsened by carbonic anhydrase inhibitors.

Thyrotoxic periodic paralysis resembles hypokalemic periodic paralysis and is common in male Asian young adults; β-adrenergic blocking agents reduce the frequency and severity of attacks, but the ultimate treatment is directed against the thyrotoxicosis. A channel defect has not yet been identified.

Malignant hyperthermia is characterized by severe muscle rigidity, fever, tachycardia precipitated by depolarizing muscle relaxants, and inhalational anesthetic agents such as halothane. The symptoms usually occur during surgery but can first be noticed in the postoperative period. Patients may have had previous anesthesia without symptoms. During attacks, the CK level is markedly elevated, and myoglobinuria develops. The disorder is caused by excessive calcium release by the sarcoplasmic reticulum calcium channel, the ryanodine receptor. Some patients have mutations in the ryanodine receptor gene on chromosome 19q13, which is the same gene mutated in central core disease. The symptoms are treated with dantrolene, and at-risk patients should not be given known provocative anesthetic agents. The occurrence of malignant hyperthermia in one member of a family should prompt consideration as to whether other family members might also be at risk.

OTHER FORMS OF MUSCLE STIFFNESS

Neuroleptic malignant syndrome with muscular rigidity, altered mental status, and hyperthermia is caused by central dopaminergic blockade from neuroleptics. The muscle rigidity can produce myoglobinuria.

Stiff-person syndrome is an acquired autoimmune condition that produces severe muscle stiffness of proximal, and especially paraspinous, muscles. Excess motor unit activity caused by autoantibodies to glutamic acid decarboxylase is present, which is a major enzyme in the synthesis of δ-aminobutyric acid, and this circumstance results in disinhibition in the central nervous system. Some patients also have antibodies to islet cells and develop diabetes mellitus. Symptomatic treatment consists of diazepam; immunosuppressive treatment can improve the condition.

Inflammatory Myopathies

Inflammatory myopathies are acquired, nonhereditary disorders (Table 131-5) that are characterized by muscle weakness and inflammation on muscle biopsy. Most are associated with elevated CK levels, myopathic EMG findings, and a limb-girdle distribution of weakness. Occasionally, inflammatory myopathies have distal, focal, or other selective involvement of particular muscles.

IDIOPATHIC INFLAMMATORY MYOPATHY

The three major categories of idiopathic inflammatory myopathy are DM, PM, and IBM (Table 131-6). PM and DM are both characterized by the onset of symmetrical weakness subacutely over weeks or several months. Myalgias can occur, but muscle pain and tenderness are rarely chief complaints. Patients complaining of myalgia who do not have demonstrable weakness are more likely to have polymyalgia rheumatica or fibromyalgia than PM. Esophageal muscles are affected in up to 30% of both PM and DM cases, leading to dysphagia.

The rash of DM may accompany or precede the onset of muscle weakness. This rash can be a heliotrope rash (purplish discoloration of the eyelids often associated with

---

Table 131-5 Major Inflammatory Myopathies

Idiopathic

Polymyositis
Dermatomyositis
Inclusion body myositis
Overlap syndromes with other connective tissue disease (e.g., systemic lupus erythematosus)
Sarcoidosis
Inflammatory myopathies with eosinophilia
Eosinophilic polymyositis
Diffuse fasciitis with eosinophilia
Myositis ossificans

Infections

Bacterial (e.g., *Staphylococcus*, *Streptococcus*, gas gangrene, *Clostridium welchii*)
Viral: acute myositis after influenza or other viral infections; retrovirus-related myopathies (HIV, HTLV-1)
Parasitic: toxoplasmosis, trypanosomiasis, cysticercosis, trichinosis
Fungal

HIV, human immunodeficiency virus; HTLV-1, human T-cell leukemia virus type 1.

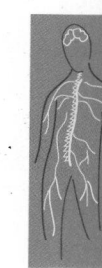

Neuromuscular Junction Disease

Emma Ciafaloni

Disorders of the neuromuscular junction interfere with the transmission of electrical impulses from peripheral nerve to muscle. They can be acquired or inherited and are associated with weakness and fatigability on exertion (Table 132-1). In each disorder the safety margin of neuromuscular transmission is compromised by one or more specific defects: acetylcholine (ACh) synthesis or packaging of ACh quanta into synaptic vesicles, the release of ACh quanta from the nerve terminal by nerve impulses, and the efficiency of the released ACh quanta to generate a postsynaptic depolarization.

Myasthenia Gravis

Myasthenia gravis (MG) is an acquired autoimmune disorder. Pathogenic autoantibodies induce acetylcholine receptor (AChR) deficiency at the motor end plate. Circulating AChR antibodies are present in 70% to 80% of cases, and immunoglobulin G and complement components are deposited on the postsynaptic membrane. AChR deficiency results from lysis of the junctional folds and destruction of AChRs cross-linked by antibodies that block the binding of ACh to AChR. The incidence is 2 to 5 per year per 1 million population, and the prevalence 13 to 64 per million. The female-to-male ratio is 6:4. The disease may manifest at any age, but the incidence in women peaks in the third decade and that in men in the sixth or seventh decade.

CLINICAL FEATURES

MG can involve either the external ocular muscles selectively (ocular MG) or the general voluntary muscle system (generalized MG). The symptoms usually fluctuate, tending to be worse later in the day (diurnal fluctuation). They are provoked or worsened by exertion, intercurrent infections, menses, and excitement. Ocular muscle involvement is usually bilateral and asymmetrical, and typically is associated with ptosis and diplopia. Weakness of other muscles innervated by cranial nerves results in loss of facial expression, a smile that resembles a snarl, nasal regurgitation of liquids, choking on foods and secretions, and slurred, nasal speech. Abnormal fatigability of the limb muscles causes difficulty in combing the hair, lifting objects repeatedly, climbing stairs, walking, and running. On examination, fatigue is most reliably demonstrated in the eyes: the *curtain sign* of worsening ptosis with upgaze or asymmetrical nystagmus on extremes of lateral and medial gaze. Proximal limb muscles are affected more than distal ones, but in advanced cases weakness is widespread. Initially, the symptoms are ocular in 40%, are generalized in 40%, involve only the extremities in 10%, and involve only the bulbar or bulbar and eye muscles in another 10%. Ocular muscles are affected in nearly all patients after a year of disease. The symptoms remain ocular in only 15%. When the disease becomes generalized, usually it does so within the first year of onset. Two thirds of patients with MG have thymic hyperplasia, and 10% to 15% have thymoma. In about 10% the MG is associated with another autoimmune disease. Circulating AChR antibodies can be detected in most infants born to myasthenic mothers, but only 12% of such children develop transient neonatal MG, usually during the first few hours of life. The disease is caused by the transfer of AChR antibodies and is self-limited.

DIAGNOSIS

Anticholinesterase Tests (Tensilon Test)

Edrophonium given intravenously acts within a few seconds and lasts for a few minutes. Two milligrams of the drug are injected intravenously over 15 seconds. If no response occurs in 30 to 45 seconds, an additional 8 mg is injected. The evaluation of the response requires objective assessment of one or more signs not easily influenced by motivation, such as degree of ptosis and range of ocular movements. Possible cholinergic side effects of the drug include fasciculations, flushing, lacrimation, abdominal cramps, nausea, vomiting, and diarrhea. The drug must be given cautiously to patients with cardiac disease because it may cause sinus bradycardia,

Table 132-1 **Disorders of the Neuromuscular Junction**
Autoimmune
Myasthenia gravis
Lambert-Eaton myasthenic syndrome
Congenital
Presynaptic defects in ACh resynthesis, packaging, or release
Synaptic defect: congenital end plate AChE deficiency
Postsynaptic defects: slow-channel syndromes
Postsynaptic defects: decreased response to ACh
Fast-channel syndromes
AChR deficiency without kinetic abnormality
Familial limb-girdle myasthenia
Toxic
Botulism
Drug-induced disorders
Organophosphate intoxication
Ach, acetylcholine; AChE, acetylcholinesterase; AChR, acetylcholine receptor.

atrioventricular block, and, rarely, cardiac arrest. Atropine should be available during the test. Edrophonium should not be given to patients having respiratory difficulty.

Diagnostic Testing

Repetitive Nerve Stimulation

Supramaximal stimulation of a motor nerve at 2 or 3 Hz results in a 10% or greater decrement of the amplitude of the evoked compound muscle action potential from the first to the fifth response. The test is positive in about 75% with generalized MG, provided that two or more distal and two or more proximal muscles are examined. It is less frequently abnormal (approximately 50%) in purely ocular MG.

Single Fiber Electromyography

Single fiber electromyography (SFEMG) is currently the most sensitive method for diagnosis of MG and reveals increased jitter and blocking in 99% of patients with generalized MG and in 97% of those with purely ocular MG when a weak muscle is tested. SFEMG is usually available only in specialized EMG laboratories.

Blood Tests and Radiography

The AChR antibody test measures the binding of antibody to AChR labeled with radioactive α bungarotoxin. The antibody-binding test result is positive in nearly all adults with moderately severe or severe MG, in 80% with mild generalized MG, and in 50% with ocular MG. Some patients without AChR have abnormal antibodies to MuSK, a muscle-specific tyrosine kinase with a role in aggregation of AChR and the end plate. Striated muscle antibodies also occur in MG patients. Their role is unknown, but they are often associated with thymoma. Because of the frequency of thymomas, chest x-ray studies and chest computed tomography (CT) scanning are indicated.

TREATMENT

Anticholinesterases, thymectomy, alternate-day prednisone, azathioprine, cyclosporine, plasmapheresis, and intravenous immunoglobulin are used to treat MG. Anticholinesterases

are useful in all forms of the disease. Pyridostigmine bromide (60-mg tablets) acts for 3 to 4 hours, and neostigmine bromide, 15 mg, acts for 2 to 3 hours. Pyridostigmine bromide has fewer muscarinic side effects and is therefore more widely used. One-half to two tablets are given every 4 hours in the daytime. This medication is also available in 180-mg "time-span" tablets for use at bedtime and as a syrup for children and patients requiring nasogastric feeding. In critically ill patients or postoperatively, neostigmine can be used intramuscularly (1.5 mg is equivalent to 60 mg pyridostigmine) or intravenously (0.5 mg is equivalent to 60 mg of pyridostigmine). Patients who have difficulty with respiration, feeding, or handling secretions and who are not responding to relatively high doses of anticholinesterases are best treated by anticholinesterase withdrawal, tracheal intubation, and ventilator support.

In patients with generalized disease not responding adequately to anticholinesterases, other forms of therapy must be used. Thymectomy has been believed to improve the clinical course of MG, but a controlled clinical trial of the procedure is now in progress. On the other hand, thymoma is an indication for thymectomy because the tumor is often locally invasive. Alternate-day prednisone treatment induces remission or improves the disease in more than half the patients. Azathioprine in doses of 2 to 3 mg/kg/day also induces remissions or improvement in more than half of patients treated. The time required for improvement is 12 to 15 months. Surveillance for side effects (pancytopenia, leukopenia, and hepatocellular injury) must be maintained during therapy. Azathioprine as an adjunct to alternate-day prednisone reduces the maintenance dose of prednisone and is associated with fewer corticosteroid side effects. Mycophenolate mofetil, cyclosporine, and other immunosuppressants are also used. Plasmapheresis is helpful in patients with sudden worsening of MG and is indicated in severe generalized MG refractory to other forms of treatment. A course of five exchanges of 2 L of plasma on alternate days often results in objective improvement and lowers the AChR antibody titer in a few days. Plasmapheresis is expensive and not usually suitable for long-term treatment. Intravenous immunoglobulin, 2 g/kg divided over 2 to 5 days, also improves severe MG and may be more widely available. The mean duration of the response is 9 weeks in patients who are also treated with corticosteroids and 5 weeks in those who are not.

Lambert-Eaton Myasthenic Syndrome

Lambert-Eaton myasthenic syndrome (LEMS) is a presynaptic neuromuscular junction disorder in which pathogenic autoantibodies against the voltage-sensitive calcium channels at the motor nerve terminal cause a decreased release of acetylcholine. Among patients older than age 40 years, 70% of men and 30% of women have an associated carcinoma, usually a small cell carcinoma of the lung. LEMS may predate tumor detection by up to 3 years. SOX antibodies in patients with LEMS predict the presence of small cell lung cancer. Non-neoplastic LEMS has an association with other autoimmune disorders, HLA-B8 and Drw3 antigens, and organ-specific autoantibodies. Patients with LEMS have weakness and fatigability of proximal limb and trunk muscles with relative sparing of extraocular and bulbar muscles. The lower limbs are more severely involved than the upper ones. On maximal voluntary contraction, the force produced by a weak muscle increases for a few seconds and then again decreases. Tendon reflexes are usually hypoactive or absent and reappear after short activation of the muscles. Autonomic manifestations (dry mouth, impotence, decreased sweating, orthostatic hypotension, and altered pupillary reflexes) occur in 50% of patients. Nerve conduction studies are always abnormal and show a small compound muscle action potential that facilitates more than 100% after short activation of the muscle. Repetitive stimulation at 2 to 3 Hz induces a further decrement, but stimulation at frequencies higher than 10 Hz or voluntary exercise for a brief period facilitates the response to normal amplitude. Treatment strategies include pyridostigmine, corticosteroids, azathioprine, and intravenous immune globulin. 3, 4-Diaminopyridine is an effective treatment but is not widely available in the United States; it can cause seizures and other side effects.

Botulism

Botulism is a paralytic illness caused by the neurotoxin produced by the anaerobic bacterium *Clostridium botulinum*. Botulinum toxin binds irreversibly to the presynaptic nerve endings, where it inhibits the release of acetylcholine. Types of the disease include foodborne botulism, most commonly caused by home-canned food; wound botulism, with most cases occurring among heroin users; and infant botulism, occurring most commonly in the second month of life because of intestinal colonization. Botulism should be suspected in any infant with poor feeding, constipation, poor sucking and crying, muscle weakness, and respiratory distress. The disease is characterized by symmetrical descending flaccid paralysis starting with blurred vision, dysphagia, and dysarthria. Prompt recognition and treatment with mechanical ventilatory support and early administration of antitoxin are crucial to reduce mortality. Health Department and Centers for Disease Control and Prevention (CDC) laboratories can confirm the diagnosis by detecting the toxin in serum or stool specimens and can provide the antitoxin. Nerve conduction studies and repetitive nerve stimulation testing can also confirm the diagnosis. Recovery of muscle strength may take several months.

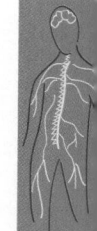

Drug-Induced Myasthenic Syndromes

Aminoglycoside antibiotics, antiarrhythmic agents (procainamide and quinidine), β-adrenergic blockers (propranolol and timolol), phenothiazines, lithium, trimethaphan, methoxyflurane, and magnesium given parenterally or in cathartics reduce the safety margin of neuromuscular transmission. However, overt myasthenic symptoms do not usually appear unless an overdose of the drug is administered or the renal or hepatic elimination of the drug is impaired. The drugs may worsen MG or LEMS.

Succinylcholine, a depolarizing blocking drug, is used to induce muscle relaxation during anesthesia. A single dose of the drug sufficient to cause transient apnea is eliminated by plasma pseudocholinesterase in 10 to 20 minutes. In approximately 1 in 2500 patients receiving the drug, prolonged apnea occurs and persists up to several hours. Most of these patients have an autosomal recessive abnormality of the plasma pseudocholinesterase. Curare and related agents used during surgery and in critically ill patients to induce muscle relaxation produce blockade of the neuromuscular junction. Their use in patients with MG and other myasthenias is associated with profound and prolonged weakness.

Organophosphate insecticides irreversibly inhibit cholinesterases. Ingestion is associated with alterations in sensorium, convulsions, coma, severe muscarinic side effects, cramps, fasciculations, and muscle weakness from a depolarization block.

Prospectus for the Future

A multicenter, randomized, controlled trial of thymectomy in MG began in early 2006. This trial may provide long-needed answers about the value of this procedure. Randomized, controlled trials of other treatments (e.g., mycophenolate mofetil) are also in progress.

References

Engel AG: Acquired autoimmune myasthenia gravis. In Engel AG, Franzini-Armstrong C (eds): Myology, 3rd ed. New York, McGraw-Hill, 2004.

Engel AG: Disorders of neuromuscular transmission. In Goldman L, Ausiello DA (eds): Cecil Textbook of Medicine, 23rd ed. Philadelphia, Saunders, 2007.

Engel AG: Myasthenic syndromes. In Engel AG, Franzini-Armstrong C (eds): Myology, 3rd ed. New York, McGraw-Hill, 2004.

Gronseth GS, Barohn RJ: Practice parameter: Thymectomy for autoimmune myasthenia gravis (an evidence-based review). Report of the Quality Standards Subcommittee of the American Academy of Neurology. Neurology 55:7-15, 2000.

Sabater L, Titulaer M, Saiz A, et al: SOX1 antibodies are markers of paraneoplastic Lambert-Eaton myasthenic syndrome. Neurology 70:924-928, 2008.

Shapiro RL, Hatheway C, Swerdlow DL: Botulism in the United States: A clinical and epidemiologic review. Ann Intern Med 129:221-228, 1998.

Section XX

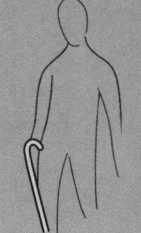

The Aging Patient

The Aging Patient

Mitchell T. Heflin and Harvey Jay Cohen

Over the last century, the number of Americans over the age of 65 years increased from 3 million to over 35 million. During the same period the population over age 85 grew most rapidly, expanding from 100,000 in 1900 to over 4 million by the end of the 20th century. By 2030, the number of adults over age 65 will likely reach 70 million, or just over 20% of the total population. Ten million of those people will be over age 85 (Fig. 133-1). A 2007 report from the National Institute on Aging and the U.S. State Department points out that this phenomenon is not isolated to the United States. Around the globe, the percentage of the population over 65 years of age will increase by 25% to 50% over the next 25 years and by 140% in developing nations.

The aging of the world's population will compel virtually all health care providers to gain competency in geriatrics, the clinical science of assessment, prevention, and treatment of illness in older adults. A basic grasp of geriatrics requires understanding at epidemiologic, biologic, and clinical levels. The provider must appreciate the impact of aging on presentation of and predisposition to certain conditions, identification of goals of care, and selection of treatment strategies. Moreover, care of older adults demands a multi-faceted approach, accounting for individual, family, and community resources for caregiving. Finally, the practice of geriatrics requires an appreciation for systems of care that include interprofessional teams working in a variety of settings ranging from home to hospital to long-term care. This chapter will provide an introduction to geriatrics and the essentials of caring for older adults.

Epidemiology of Aging

Most experts believe that the rapid growth of the population of older adults reflects the many health care successes of the twentieth century. Fries, in his landmark paper, attributes the extension of the human life span to "the elimination of premature death, particularly neonatal mortality." Improvements in other aspects of public health, including adequate nutrition and housing, safe drinking water, immunizations, and antibiotics, have led to lower rates of mortality throughout childhood and early adulthood, affording an opportunity for more people to survive to late life. Examination of survival curves across the twentieth century demonstrates a marked change in the shape of the overall graph from nearly linear in 1900 to rectangular in the 1990s, with much of the mortality compressed into late life (Fig. 133-2). Although the life expectancy at birth over the same period has risen dramatically from 47 years to nearly 77 years, the maximum life span has remained remarkably stable.

The Biology of Aging

The relatively static nature of the maximum life span reflects the human body's limits at the cellular, tissue, and organ level in dealing with the stresses of aging. Across cell types and organ systems, certain consistent age-related alterations in function exist. Variability in tissue and organ function decreases, as evidenced by less fluctuation in heart rate or hormone secretion. Organ systems also exhibit predictable declines in function over time. These changes are most evident at times of stress, and ultimately these systems are slower to react and recover. The overall result is an impaired ability to deal with any demands beyond a narrow range outside the normal. This progressive narrowing in reserve, often termed "homeostenosis," can be depicted as a steady tapering in the reserve available in multiple organ systems as time progresses (Fig. 133-3). In this situation an individual may function within the normal range in the absence of crisis, but stress such as acute illness may exceed his or her capacity to restore function and recover health. The result at best may be a decline in health and ability, and at worst, death.

THEORIES OF AGING

Scientific research provides a number of plausible theories of aging, which can be grouped into two major categories. *Error* or *damage theories* propose that aging occurs because

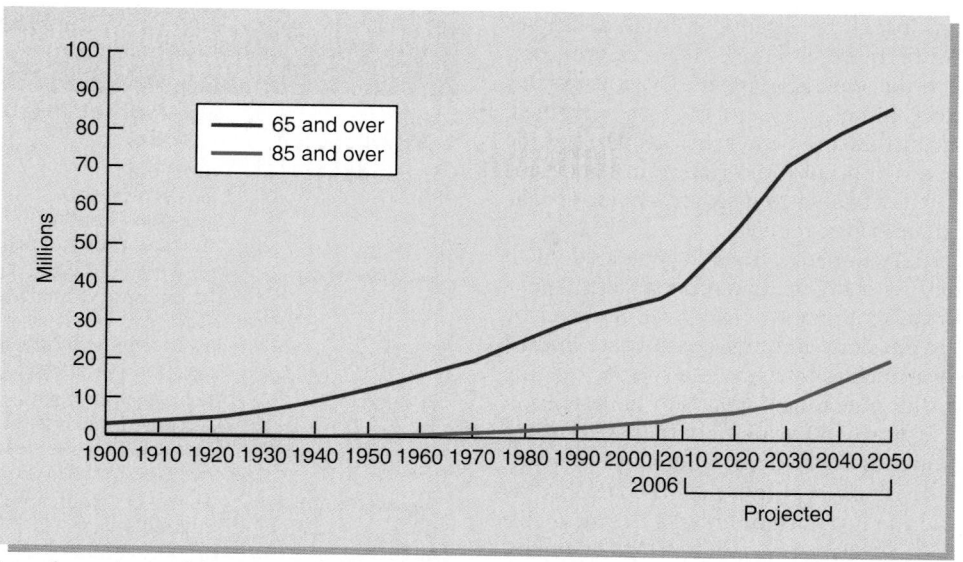

Figure 133-1 Number of people aged 65 years and older, by age group, for selected years 1900 to 2006 and projected years 2010 to 2050. (From Federal Interagency Forum on Aging-Related Statistics: Older Americans 2008: Key Indicators of Well-Being. Federal Interagency Forum on Aging-Related Statistics. Washington, DC, U.S. Government Printing Office, March 2008.)

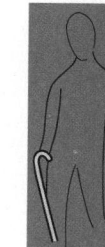

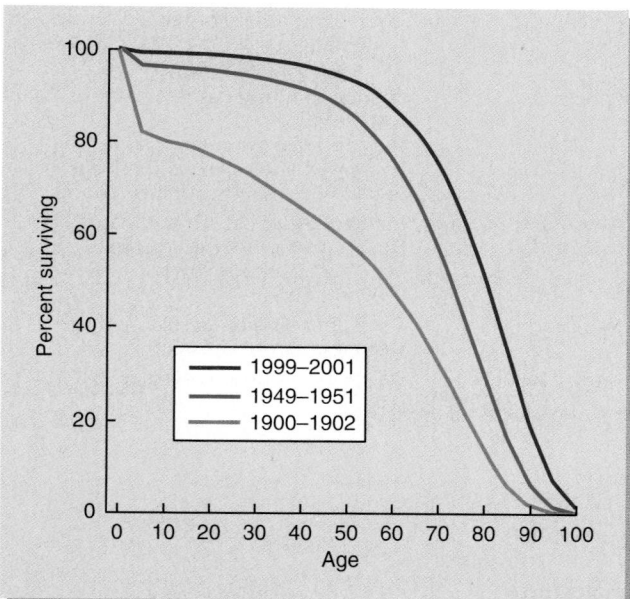

Figure 133-2 Percent surviving by age. Death registration by states, 1900 to 1902, and in the United States, 1949 to 1951 and 1999 to 2001. (From U.S. Decennial Life Tables for 1999-2001, United States Life Tables. Natl Vital Stat Rep 57:1-10, 2008.)

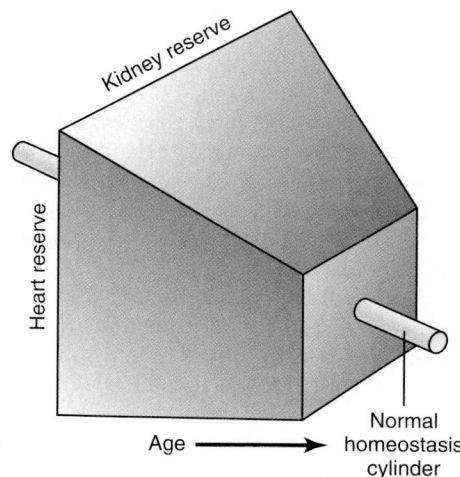

Figure 133-3 Schematic representation of decreased homeostatic reserve or "homeostenosis." (From Fries J, Crapo LM: Vitality and aging: Implications of the rectangular curve. San Francisco, WH Freeman, 1981.)

of persistent threats from damaging agents and an ever-declining ability to respond to or repair this damage. *Program theories* postulate that genetic and developmental factors most significantly determine the biologic life course and the maximal age of the organism. In actuality, biologic aging may reflect a complex combination of many types of events.

The free radical theory of aging proposes that oxidative metabolism results in an excess of highly reactive byproducts, called *oxygen free radicals,* which damage proteins, DNA, and lipids. Molecular injury leads to cell dysfunction and ultimately to tissue and organ disrepair. Proponents of this hypothesis may argue that organisms with higher

metabolic rates live shorter lives (presumably because of a more rapid accumulation of byproducts). Although the latter portion of the theory has been called into question, many still contend that limiting the production of oxidants can improve health and possibly extend life. A second theory asserts that the accumulation of glucose-related molecules on proteins contributes to their dysfunction and degradation. These "glycosylated" molecules become more abundant over time and lead to impaired function at the tissue and organ level. Theory proponents point to the many chronic problems that routinely arise in patients with diabetes mellitus as proof of the significance of this phenomenon.

A different line of reasoning asserts that the human life span and aging result from genetic based timing mechanisms. Older theories suggest that evolutionary pressures are biased for traits that promote health and reproduction in early adulthood, possibly at the expense of health and function in late life. Furthermore, little selective pressure exists against negative traits that emerge in late life, leaving humans prone to the ill effects of aging. Geneticists have identified, among species of fruit flies and certain nematodes, specific genes that result in a significant prolongation in the organism's life span. Work is ongoing to discover similar genetic sequences among mammalian models.

Study of the enzyme telomerase has also generated much interest among theorists on aging. In a process called apoptosis, cells undergo programmed death to be replaced by younger cells. These divisions and replacements are limited by the number of generations intrinsic to a specific cell line (the so-called "Hayflick phenomenon"). With the extension of life expectancy to nearly 80 years over the last century, some scientists postulate that people are outliving their allotted number of cell divisions (replicative aging). DNA in the telomeres at the end of chromosomes marks the inevitable loss of chromosomal material with replication. As telomeres shorten, cell aging and demise eventually occur. The enzyme telomerase prevents telomere shortening and may increase a cell's number of allotted replications and thereby extend the life span of the organ. Of course, this advantage must be weighed against the price of "immortality," namely the increased risk of malignancy.

The most recent development in the biology of aging goes beyond theory to application. Caloric restriction, or the purposeful reduction of food intake, is the only intervention that has been shown to reproducibly extend the maximal life span. In rats, life span increases an average of 20 months with a 40% reduction in calories. Rhesus monkeys enrolled in a trial of caloric restriction appear to have a lower disease burden and mortality than controls after 15 years. The mechanism is not well understood but may be metabolically mediated. In observational studies in humans, those with lower average body temperature, lower insulin levels, and higher dehydroepiandrosterone sulfate (DHEAS) levels (all changes found in calorically restricted monkeys) appeared to survive longer. Current research is focused on reproducing this phenomenon in human subjects and discovering chemical agents that mimic these metabolic effects.

To understand the changes in the individual's ability to cope with physiologic stress with age, one must also examine the changes at the level of the organ system. Table 133-1 provides an overview of these changes by system. As will be evident, although normal aging is not itself a diagnosis, it is, indeed, fertile ground for disease and disability.

THE FRAILTY PHENOTYPE

The concept of "homeostenosis" bridges the biologic changes of aging and the increased vulnerability of humans to illness and functional decline in late life—a state commonly referred to as "frailty." Recent research has established a definition of frailty that moves beyond traditional components of chronologic age, comorbidity, and disability to identify a unique clinical entity with independent predictive capacity. The "cycle of frailty" ties together the individual system-specific changes and identifies key events or clinical presentations that create a specific phenotype (Fig. 133-4). Five key elements form the core of this cycle, including the following:

Table 133-1 Changes in Physiologic Function with Age

Organ System	Age-Related Decline in Function
Special senses	Presbyopia Lens opacification Decreased hearing Decreased taste, smell
Cardiovascular	Impaired intrinsic contractile function Decreased conductivity Decreased ventricular filling Increased systolic blood pressure Impaired baroreceptor function
Respiratory	Decreased lung elasticity Decreased maximal breathing capacity Decreased mucus clearance Decreased arterial PO_2
Gastrointestinal	Decreased esophageal and colonic motility
Renal	Decreased glomerular filtration rate
Immune	Decreased cell-mediated immunity Decreased T-cell number Increased T-suppressor cells Decreased T-helper cells Loss of memory cells Decline in antibody titers to known antigens Increased autoimmunity
Endocrine	Decreased hormonal responses to stimulation Impaired glucose tolerance Decreased androgens and estrogens Impaired norepinephrine responses
Autonomic nervous	Impaired response to fluid deprivation Decline in baroreceptor reflex Increased susceptibility to hypothermia
Neurologic	Decreased vibratory sense Decreased proprioception
Musculoskeletal	Decreased muscle mass

PO_2, partial pressure of oxygen.

1. Weight loss
2. Weakness
3. Poor endurance
4. Slowness
5. Inactivity

Frailty is defined as the presence of three or more of these conditions. By this definition, frailty independently predicts falls, declines in mobility, loss of ability to perform activities of daily living (ADLs), hospitalization, and death. This definition seems to provide a defined link between aging-related disease and disability and, perhaps, a target for interventions to prevent the onset of functional decline—that is, a means of further compressing comorbidity and disability in late life.

Clinical Care of Older Adults

Caring for older adults requires a strong foundation in the basics of internal medicine integrated with an appreciation for the complexity and heterogeneity of the impact of aging

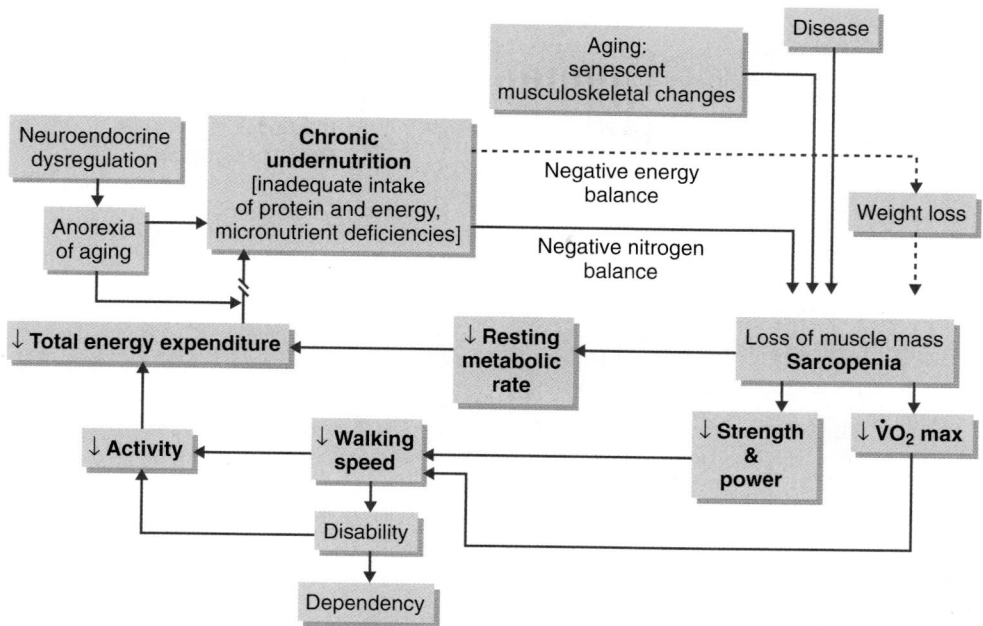
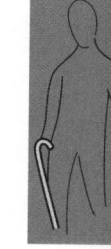

Figure 133-4 Cycle of frailty hypothesized as consistent with demonstrated pairwise associations and clinical signs and symptoms of frailty. (From Fried LP, Walston J: Frailty and failure to thrive. In Hazzard WR, Blass JP, Ettinger WH Jr, et al (eds). Principles of Geriatric Medicine and Gerontology, 4th ed. New York, McGraw-Hill, 1998, pp 1387-1402.)

on health and well-being. The clinician must possess strong diagnostic skills, given that older adults may have atypical presentations or multiple comorbid conditions and functional decline. In addition, he or she must monitor for a number of nonspecific conditions, such as problems with mobility, mood, or mentation, that affect self-care capacity and safety. Treatment strategies present unique challenges as well, often requiring a balance of pharmacologic and non-pharmacologic interventions with careful consideration of the individual's goals for care. This section presents the core components of the comprehensive assessment of the older patient.

COMORBID CONDITIONS, FUNCTION, AND LIFE EXPECTANCY

With advancing age and declines in reserve, older adults experience high rates of chronic illness and related functional decline. Eighty percent of those over age 65 years have at least one chronic illness, and 50% have two or more comorbid conditions. Some of these conditions contribute directly to increased rates of mortality, including the leading causes of death among older adults—heart disease, cancer, and stroke. Many common diseases, however, primarily threaten function and result in disability and institutionalization. Arthritis, dementia, hearing loss, and vision impairment are all important problems in this respect. The presence of multiple comorbid conditions may compound the disabling effects of individual diseases and further complicate management. In the era of evidence and guidelines, a provider caring for a patient with several common chronic conditions, such as diabetes mellitus, coronary artery disease, and osteoporosis, may feel compelled to prescribe six or seven medications to remain in compliance with current recommendations. This practice can result in significant cost to the patient and with limited accounting for risks, benefits,

and individual preferences. In addition to considering the discrete management of individual diseases, care of the older adult requires assessment of the overall impact of treatment on symptoms, function, and life expectancy.

Function, defined formally, is "a person's ability to perform tasks and fulfill social roles across a broad range of complexity"—more succinctly, self-care capacity. Assessing this ability provides the clinician with a means of understanding the impact of illness, assessing quality of life, identifying care needs, and estimating progress and prognosis. Comprehensive assessment of function should include questions about self-care capacity as well as objective measures of cognition and mobility. (The latter two are detailed in separate sections later.) Self-care capacity is most often divided into basic, instrumental, and advanced ADLs. Basic ADLs include those actions that maintain personal health and hygiene, including transferring, bathing, toileting, dressing, and eating. Instrumental ADLs (IADLs) include activities necessary for living independently, specifically driving, cooking, shopping, managing medications and finances, using the telephone (or other communication device), and doing housework. Advanced ADLs include social or occupational functions associated with activities such as hobbies, employment, or caregiving. Approximately 28% of adults over age 65 and 78% of those over age 85 have difficulty with IADLs or one or more basic ADLs. Predictably, as the incidence of disability rises, so does the rate of dependence and nursing home residence. Long-term care in skilled facilities increases from 1.4% among those age 65 to 74 to 20% among those older than age 85. Impairment in ADLs is also associated with an increased risk of falls, depression, and death in the affected elder. Among older adults the assessment of self-care capacity provides key health status information independent of age and comorbid conditions.

For clinicians, navigating the myriad options for management of multiple chronic conditions requires individualized

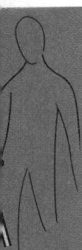

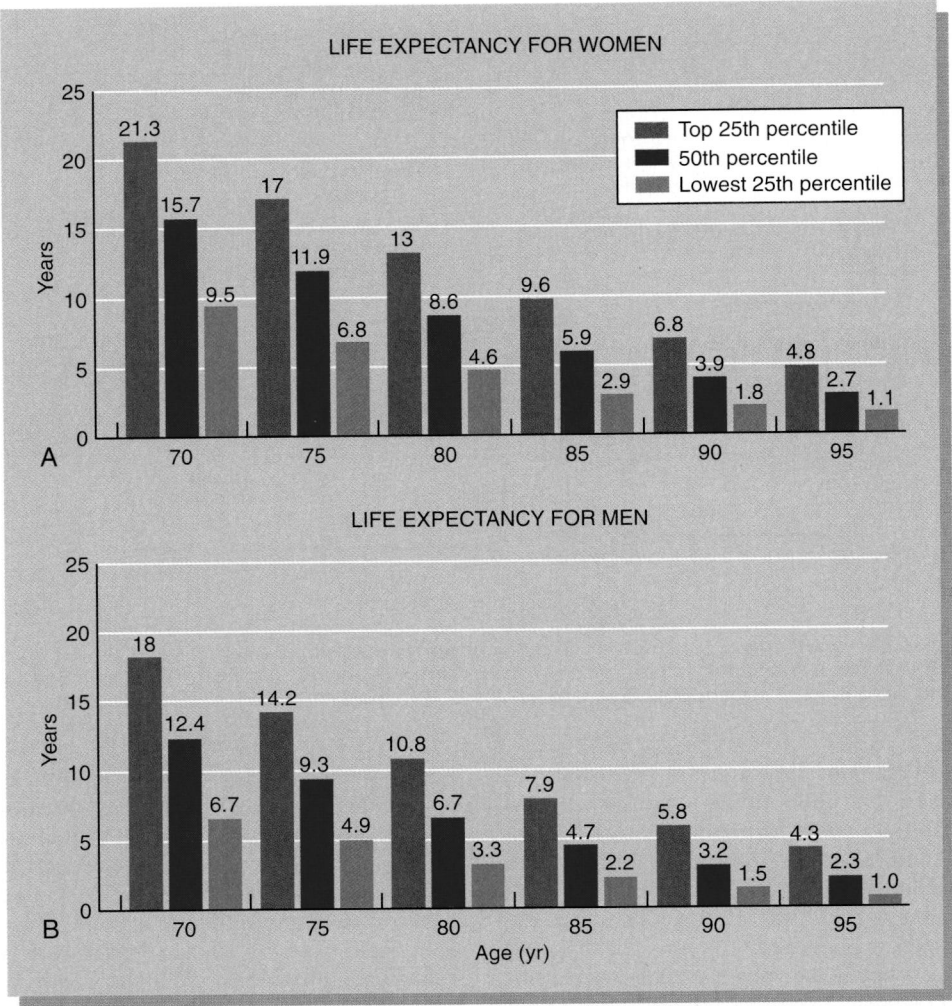

Figure 133-5 Upper, middle, and lower quartiles of life expectancy for women and men at selected ages. (From Walter LC, Covinsky KE: Cancer screening in elderly patients—a framework for individualized decision making. JAMA 285:2750, 2001.)

assessment of risks, benefits, and specific goals of various therapies. Estimates of life expectancy, integrating the impact of age, comorbid illness, and function, have been generated to assist in medical decision making. These estimates assist providers in predicting median survival and thus can help in estimating the potential life remaining in which one might benefit from a given procedure or therapy (Fig. 133-5). For example, the options offered to a frail 85-year-old man with less than 3 years left to live may be quite different from those presented to his healthy counterpart of the same age with a median life expectancy of 5 to 7 years. In addition, any decision should take into account the individual patient's goals and preferences.

ALTERED PRESENTATION OF DISEASE

Competent care of the frail older adult starts with recognition of disease, even in the absence of typical signs and symptoms. Presentation of disease among the elderly may differ dramatically from that expected; manifestations of distress may be subtle or nonspecific, and improvement is less obvious and slower. This phenomenon occurs for a number of reasons. As noted previously, older adults experience high rates of comorbid illness, which may confound the clini-

cian's ability to diagnose a problem accurately. For example, a patient with heart disease and chronic obstructive pulmonary disease who visits the office because of dyspnea may be experiencing a flare of his pulmonary disease or an atypical presentation of ischemic heart disease or both. Reporting of symptoms may also be affected by psychosocial factors, including limited access to the health care system, cognitive problems, or minimization of symptoms as "normal aging." Likewise, health care providers may minimize complaints by older adults with complex medical illness or frail health.

The alert clinician may anticipate atypical presentations for certain conditions (Table 133-2). Hyperthyroidism can manifest with apathy, malaise, depression, and fatigue, while lacking classic symptoms of tremor, tachycardia, or sweating. It can also manifest with heart failure and is highly prevalent among older adults with new-onset atrial fibrillation. Likewise, older patients with hypothyroidism may atypically demonstrate failure to thrive, weight loss, cognitive decline, or depression. In the presence of infection, older adults may not reliably mount fever or experience localized symptoms. Studies have demonstrated that lowering the threshold definition of fever can improve the diagnostic utility of body temperature as a sign of bacterial infection. Although chest pain remains the most common and important symptom of

Table 133-2 **Atypical Disease Presentations in Older Adults**	
Diagnosis	**Potential Presenting Symptoms and Signs**
Myocardial infarction	Altered mental status Fatigue Fever Functional decline
Infection	Altered mental status Functional decline Hypothermia
Hyperthyroidism	Altered mental status Anorexia Atrial fibrillation Chest pain Constipation Fatigue Weight gain
Depression	Cognitive impairment Failure to thrive Functional decline
Electrolyte disturbance	Altered mental status Falls Fatigue Personality changes
Malignancy	Altered mental status Fever Pathologic fracture
Pulmonary embolus	Altered mental status Fatigue Fever Syncope
Vitamin deficiency	Altered mental status Ataxia Dementia Fatigue
Fecal impaction	Altered mental status Chest pain Diarrhea Urinary incontinence
Aortic stenosis	Altered mental status Fatigue

Note: This table represents only a limited list of select disease processes and presentations; it is not meant to serve as an exhaustive reference for use during patient care activities.

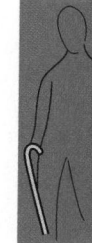

average, three to five medications. Although medications may be indicated for specific medical conditions, use of multiple medications increases the risk for drug-drug interactions and associated adverse drug events. Altered pharmacokinetics and pharmacodynamics contribute to adverse drug events, which are a common cause of hospitalization and morbidity in the elderly. Common changes in pharmacokinetics include changes in body composition, with increased fat stores and decreased body water. Fat-soluble medications, such as benzodiazepines, have a prolonged duration of effect because of this phenomenon. Age-related declines in glomerular filtration rates result in decreased clearance of many medications, including such drugs as atenolol, digoxin, and lithium. Accurate calculations of creatinine clearance will inform drug choice and dosing and improve prescribing safety. Pharmacodynamic changes include decreased sensitivity to certain commonly prescribed drugs, such as β blockers, and increased sensitivity to other agents, such as narcotics and warfarin.

Given the risks of medication use in older adults, health care providers and systems should employ strategies to improve both the effectiveness and safety of prescribing. Evidence-based recommendations include the following:

- Maintain an up-to-date medication list, including over-the counter medications and herbal supplements.
- Comprehensively review medications at least once annually (if not at every visit) and, in particular, at the time of transitions between care settings (e.g., after hospitalization). A clear indication for each medication, and documentation of response to therapy (particularly for chronic conditions), should be included.
- Assess for duplication and drug-drug or drug-disease interactions. Using a drug information database will help with this process.
- Assess adherence and affordability and inquire about the patient's system for administering medications (e.g., a pillbox).
- Assess for specific classes of medications commonly associated with adverse events: warfarin, analgesics (particularly narcotics and nonsteroidal anti-inflammatory drugs [NSAIDs]), antihypertensives (particularly angiotensin-converting enzyme [ACE] inhibitors and diuretics), insulin and hypoglycemic agents, and psychotropics.
- Minimize or avoid use of anticholinergic medications, which present specific risks.

A clear and rational approach to prescribing and ongoing management of medications that accounts for indication, interactions, and adherence may reduce the risk of common adverse events.

ischemic heart disease, dyspnea in the absence of chest pain is a commonly reported symptom, particularly in older adults and those with multiple comorbidities.

In truth, any medical illness may manifest nonspecifically among older adults, particularly those in frail health. Nonspecific symptoms related to an underlying illness include changes in mentation, difficulty with balance and falls, new urinary incontinence (UI), and a general change in functional ability. A lack of understanding of the phenomenon of altered presentation of disease can lead to delays in diagnosis and treatment and result in worse outcomes for older adults. Research indicates that altered presentation predicts not only suboptimal care, but future functional decline and increased mortality.

MEDICATIONS

Medication-related problems are very common in older adults. In the United States, outpatients over age 65 take, on

COGNITION

Dementia

The prevalence of dementia increases with age, with estimates ranging from 20% to 50% after age 85. The most common forms of dementia include Alzheimer disease, Lewy body dementia, and vascular dementia. The latter is commonly present in combination with Alzheimer disease in a condition termed *mixed etiology dementia*. Dementia is most often characterized by impairment in one or more cognitive domains severe enough to disrupt function or occupation. Mild cognitive impairment (MCI) is present when an individual has discernible cognitive limitations without apparent functional impact. Patients with MCI develop dementia at a rate of approximately 15% per year. In general, a diagnosis of dementia is associated with a higher risk of falls, functional impairment, institutionalization, and death. Caregivers of demented individuals also face increased rates of stress and health problems. Clinicians diagnose dementia through symptom and functional history (often including the input of caregivers), cognitive assessment, and physical examination. A number of instruments, including the Mini Mental Status Examination (MMSE), clock-drawing test (CDT), and the Mini-Cog, are validated screening tools. The time-tested MMSE offers an assessment of multiple cognitive domains but does not provide adequate measure of executive function and is prone to lack of sensitivity in individuals with high premorbid intelligence and lack of specificity in those with low levels of education. Validated assessments of executive function include the CDT, verbal fluency test, or the Trail B test. Instruments also exist for collecting data regarding patient function from a relative or caregiver. In patients suspected of having dementia, assessments of personal safety with respect to firearms, driving, and the home environment should be performed. A careful medication review and physical examination, including vital signs, complete neurologic assessment, and evaluations of gait and balance, are, of course, essential in dementia to reveal specific findings that point to a specific cause (see Chapter 116).

Delirium

The differential diagnosis for cognitive problems other than dementia is broad and includes delirium, mood disturbance, and drug effects. The differentiation of dementia and delirium may present the most significant challenge, particularly in the hospitalized elderly (Table 133-3). Delirium is characterized by its acuity and alteration in global cognitive function, whereas dementia is chronic and affects specific cognitive domains. Delirium affects more than 2 million hospitalized persons each year. Its incidence is variably estimated at 25% to 60% among patients in acute care settings and results in extra hospital days and related expenditures. Delirium is also associated with prolonged hospital stay, increased costs, increased readmission rate to the hospital (12% to 65% at 6 months), and higher in-hospital and 1-year mortality. The Confusion Assessment Method (CAM) offers a validated tool to diagnose delirium. Per the CAM, delirium is likely present if the patient has both an acute onset of confusion with fluctuating course and inattention and either disorganized thinking or altered level of consciousness. Key risk factors for delirium include older age, cognitive impairment, comorbid illness, and functional decline. Precipitating factors related to acute illness include hypoxia, electrolyte abnormalities, dehydration, and malnutrition as well as medications and alcohol withdrawal. Although treatment of delirium is difficult and revolves around the underlying medical issues, controlled trials have demonstrated that a multi-modal intervention may be effective in preventing delirium in high-risk patients. The evidence demonstrates that the use of restraints in combative or confused older adults leads to increased morbidity and mortality. Nonpharmacologic management strategies include reorientation and preservation of sleep patterns, family or caregiver presence at the bedside, and early mobilization. The use of pharmacologic agents, specifically neuroleptics or sedative hypnotics such as benzodiazepines, should be reserved for cases in which nonpharmacologic strategies do not help and the patient presents a risk of harm to himself or herself or others.

MOOD

Older adults commonly experience depressive symptoms, with prevalence estimates as high as 15% to 19% among those over age 75. The presence of comorbid illness and grief often confound the presentation of depression. As a result, it can remain undetected despite its significant adverse impact on quality of life, morbidity, and mortality. Suicide rates are almost twice as high in the elderly when compared with the general population, with the rate highest for white men over 85 years of age. Among older adults, depression can manifest atypically with cognitive, functional, or sleep problems as well as complaints of fatigue or low energy. Several instruments have been developed and validated for screening for depression in the elderly. Asking two simple questions about mood and anhedonia ("Over the past 2 weeks have you felt down, depressed, or hopeless?" and "Over the past 2 weeks have you felt little interest or pleasure in doing things?") may be as effective as using longer instruments. Any positive screening test result should trigger a full diagnostic interview. When screening for depression in the elderly, it is particularly important to have systems in place to provide feedback of screening results, a readily accessible means of making an accurate diagnosis, and a mechanism for providing treatment and careful follow-up. Recent trials indicate that the addition of counseling to pharmacologic therapy confers additional benefit for older, frail patients with depression. Anxiety, like depression, is also common among older adults and may similarly result in physical and cognitive symptoms, insomnia, agitation, psychosis, and isolation. Clinicians should consider a diagnosis of generalized

Table 133-3	**Features of Delirium versus Dementia**	
Feature	**Delirium**	**Dementia**
Onset	Acute	Insidious
Course	Fluctuating, lucid at times	Generally stable
Duration	Hours to weeks	Months to years
Alertness	Abnormally low or high	Usually normal
Perception	Illusions and hallucinations common	Usually normal
Memory	Immediate and recent impaired	Recent and remote impaired
Thought	Disorganized	Impoverished
Speech	Incoherent, slow or rapid	Word-finding difficulty
Physical illness or medication causative	Frequently	Usually absent

anxiety, panic, or agoraphobia in older adult patients with any of these symptoms.

MOBILITY

Problems with mobility are particularly common in the elderly. Among those over age 65, 20% of men and 32% of women report difficulty with one or more of five specific physical activities (stooping or kneeling, reaching overhead, writing, lifting 10 pounds, or walking two to three blocks). Among these, respondents cite problems with walking most commonly. Difficulties with balance and gait present significant risks for older adults. Approximately 30% of community-dwelling elders fall each year. The annual incidence of falls approaches 50% in patients over 80 years of age. Five percent of falls in older adults result in fracture or hospitalization. Risk factors for falls include a history of falls, fear of falling, decreased vision, cognitive impairment, medications (particularly anticholinergic, psychotropic, and cardiovascular medications), diseases causing problems with strength and coordination, and environmental factors. Effective interventions for people with a history of falls or who are at risk for falling involve addressing multiple contributing factors. Providers should regularly inquire about recent falls or a fear of falling in older patients. For patients who report falling, the assessment should include review of circumstances of the fall(s), measure of orthostatic vital signs, visual acuity testing, cognitive evaluation, and gait and balance assessment. A brief physical examination maneuver called the "timed get up and go" has the patient arise from a sitting position, walk 10 feet, turn, and return to the chair to sit. A time of more than 16 seconds to complete the process, or observation of postural instability or gait impairment, suggests an increased risk of falling. Gait speed, an additional measure of mobility, has recently received much attention for its predictive ability in older adults. Gait speed is measured over a 10-meter span with the patient walking at a comfortable pace. A speed of less than 0.8 m/sec predicts difficulty navigating outside the home, and a speed of less than 0.6 m/sec predicts a high risk of falls and functional decline. For those found to be at risk for falls, providers should also review all medications for possible causative agents and inquire about home safety. High-risk patients should be evaluated for assistive devices and a supervised exercise program (Table 133-4).

HEARING AND VISION

Problems with vision and hearing are very common among older adults and frequently complicate the management of comorbid conditions and accelerate functional decline. Significant vision loss occurs in 16% to 18% of adults over age 65. Common causes include glaucoma, cataracts, age-related macular degeneration, and retinopathy from hypertension and diabetes. Decreased visual acuity increases fall risk and has been associated with all-cause mortality. Such problems may be detectable with regular testing via bedside tools such as the Snellen or Jaeger eye chart. Given the implications of vision loss for function and safety, a general ophthalmologic examination every 1 to 2 years is recommended for all older adults. Furthermore, ophthalmologic centers have recognized the multifaceted challenges faced by older adults with

vision impairment and have developed specialized low vision clinics offering evaluation by optometrists, occupational therapists, and social workers with a focus on improving quality of life and maintaining independence.

Hearing loss is the third most common ailment in older adults (behind hypertension and arthritis), affecting an estimated 40% to 66% of those over age 75. It is associated with depression, social isolation, poor self-esteem, and functional disability. Pure tone audiometry is the reference standard for screening for hearing loss, but a simple whispered voice test is also highly sensitive and specific. Ideally all older adults would undergo annual hearing screen by questionnaire and handheld audiometry. Unfortunately, the lack of reimbursement for hearings aids under most insurance plans, including Medicare, presents a major barrier for many older adults.

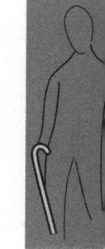

CONTINENCE

UI affects up to 30% of community-dwelling older adults and at least half of those residing in skilled nursing facilities (SNFs). It occurs more frequently in women, but this gender disparity narrows as the rate of UI in men increases after age 85. The impact of UI on health ranges from increased risk of skin irritation, pressure wounds, and falls to social isolation, functional decline, and depression. For caregivers of older adults, UI complicates physical care and can contribute to decisions for placement in SNFs. Common comorbid conditions include diabetes mellitus, heart failure, arthritis, and dementia.

A systematic approach to the investigation of UI can often reveal a cause and potential solution. It is important to first determine if the incontinence is acute or chronic in nature. Acute causes of incontinence are often attributable to specific medical problems, including infection, metabolic disturbance, or medication effects. The pneumonic DIAPERS recalls the various potential acute causes of UI (D, delirium; I, infection; A, atrophic vaginitis; P, pharmaceuticals; E, excess urine output from congestive heart failure (CHF) or hyperglycemia; R, restricted mobility; and S, stool impaction). If the UI is chronic, then further history can characterize the nature of the symptom from among four types. Urge incontinence from detrusor overactivity is the most common type. Patients with this problem will complain of urinary frequency, nocturia, and a sudden onset of urge to void. Stress incontinence occurs with incompetence of pelvic musculature or urethral sphincter and is characterized by small amounts of leakage with laughing, sneezing, coughing, or even standing. Overflow incontinence results from urinary retention, often related to prostatic hyperplasia in men or bladder atony in patients with diabetes or spinal cord injury. Patients often have constant dribbling or leakage without a true sense of needing to void. Finally, functional incontinence results from comorbid conditions that limit a patient's ability to act on or interpret the need to void, mobility problems such as arthritis, and weakness or cognitive problems. Table 133-5 describes the various types of incontinence and suggested approaches. Of course, older adults with multiple comorbid conditions often have incontinence that results from a combination of chronic and/or acute causes.

Continence problems are frequently treatable but are often not raised by patients as a concern. A targeted history

Table 133-4 Recommended Components of Clinical Assessment and Management for Older Persons Living in the Community Who Are at Risk for Falling

Assessment and Risk Factor	Management
Circumstances of previous falls*	Change in environment and activity to reduce the likelihood of recurrent falls
Medication use • High-risk medications (e.g., benzodiazepines, other sleep medications, neuroleptics, antidepressants, anticonvulsives, or class IA antiarrhythmics)*†‡ • Four or more medications‡	Review and reduction of medications
Vision* • Acuity <20/60 • Decreased depth perception • Decreased contrast sensitivity • Cataracts	Ample lighting without glare; avoidance of multifocal glasses while walking; referral to an ophthalmologist
Postural blood pressure (after ≥5 min in a supine position, immediately after standing, and 2 min after standing)‡ • ≥20 mm Hg (or ≥20%) drop in systolic pressure, with or without symptoms, either immediately or after 2 min of standing	Diagnosis and treatment of underlying cause, if possible; review and reduction of medications; modification of salt restriction; adequate hydration; compensatory strategies (e.g., elevating head of bed, rising slowly, or performing dorsiflexion exercises); pressure stockings; pharmacologic therapy if the above strategies fail
Balance and gait†‡ • Patient's report or observation of unsteadiness • Impairment on brief assessment (e.g., the "get up and go" test or performance-oriented assessment of mobility)	Diagnosis and treatment of underlying cause, if possible; reduction of medications that impair balance; environmental interventions; referral to physical therapist for assistive devices and for gait, balance, and strength training
Targeted neurologic examinations • Impaired proprioception* • Impaired cognition* • Decreased muscle strength†‡	Diagnosis and treatment of underlying cause, if possible; increase in proprioceptive input (with an assistive device or appropriate footwear that encases the foot and has a low heel and thin sole); reduction of medications that impair cognition; awareness on the part of caregivers of cognitive deficits; reduction of environmental risk factors; referral to physical therapist for gait, balance, and strength training
Targeted musculoskeletal examinations of legs (joints and range of motion) and examination of feet*	Diagnosis and treatment of underlying cause, if possible; referral to physical therapist for strength, range-of-motion, and gait and balance training, and for assistive devices; use of appropriate footwear; referral to podiatrist
Targeted cardiovascular examination† • Syncope • Arrhythmia (if there is known cardiac disease, abnormal electrocardiogram, and syncope	Referral to cardiologist; carotid-sinus massage (in case of syncope)
Home-hazard evaluations after hospital discharge†‡	Removal of loose rugs and use of nightlights, nonslip bathmats, and stair rails; other interventions as necessary

*Recommendation of this assessment is based on observations that the finding is associated with an increased risk of falling.
†Recommendation of this assessment is based on one or more randomized controlled trials of a single intervention.
‡Recommendation of this assessment is based on one or more randomized controlled trials of a multifactorial intervention strategy that included this component.
From Tinetti ME. Preventing falls in elderly persons. N Engl J Med 348:42-49, 2003.

Table 133-5 Causes, Types, and Treatment of Urinary Incontinence

Type	Definition	Cause	Treatment
Stress	Leakage associated with increased intra-abdominal pressure (coughing, sneezing)	Hypermobility of the bladder base, frequently caused by lax perineal muscles	Pelvic muscle exercise, timed voiding, α-adrenergic drugs, estrogens, surgery
Urge	Leakage associated with a precipitous urge to void	Detrusor hyperactivity (outflow obstruction, bladder tumor, detrusor instability), idiopathic (poor bladder), compliance (radiation cystitis), hypersensitive bladder	Bladder training, pelvic muscle exercise, bladder-relaxant drugs (anticholinergics, oxybutynin, tolterodine, imipramine)
Overflow	Leakage from a mechanically distended bladder	Outflow obstruction, enlarged prostate, stricture, prolapsed cystocele, acontractile bladder (idiopathic, neurologic [spinal cord injury, stroke, diabetes])	Surgical correction of obstruction, intermittent catheter drainage
Functional	Inability or unwillingness to void	Cognitive impairment, physical impairment, environmental barriers (physical restraints, inaccessible toilets), psychological problems (depression, anger, hostility)	Prompted voiding, garment and padding, external collection devices

and physical examination can often identify the cause of UI and lead to appropriate intervention. We recommend asking about and documenting the presence or absence of UI biannually and determining whether the UI, if present, is bothersome to the patient or caregiver. In addition to a history of acute and chronic causes, a targeted physical examination should include an assessment for fluid overload, genital and rectal examination, and neurologic evaluation. Urine and blood tests are indicated to evaluate for infection, metabolic causes, and renal dysfunction. In addition, in patients suspected of having urinary retention, catheterization or ultrasound can help define the postvoid residual and determine the need for catheter placement and further urologic evaluation. Many institutions now offer more specialized evaluation and care through incontinence clinics, which offer multidisciplinary approaches to management addressing both pharmacologic and nonpharmacologic options. Effective nonpharmacologic options include scheduled toileting, bladder training, and biofeedback. Use of these strategies may avoid the use of medications with common adverse effects, such as anticholinergic medications for detrusor overactivity.

NUTRITION

Older adults experience high rates of malnutrition related to various causes, including medical illness, dental problems, or access issues related to limited mobility, cost, or cognitive problems. Approximately 15% of older outpatients and half of the hospitalized elderly are malnourished and have clearly associated increases in morbidity and mortality. The utility of general laboratory testing is limited, but a combination of serial weight measurements and inquiries about changing appetite can reveal problems with nutritional status in the elderly. Vulnerable elders with an involuntary weight loss of 10% or more in 1 year or less should undergo further evaluation for undernutrition, including assessment of medical or medication-related causes, dental status, problems with acquiring or preparing food, appetite and intake, swallowing ability, and previous directions for dietary restrictions.

Social and Legal Issues

The geriatric social history includes assessments of resources for direct caregiving and financial support available to a patient. These issues become particularly important for frail older adults, given their physical and economic vulnerability.

CAREGIVING

The clinician should always inquire about who is providing care for the older patient. This includes both personal care with ADLs and help with IADLs such as transportation, medications, food preparation, finances, and housekeeping. This list should include both formal caregivers, such as home health professionals or hired aides, and informal caregivers, such as family members, neighbors, or friends. The majority of care provided in the United States is delivered by informal caregivers. Over 34 million people in the United States provide informal care for older adults and, of these, 8.9

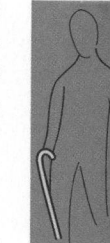

million are caring for persons suffering from dementia. The majority of informal caregivers are women and elderly themselves, with an average age of 63 years. The stress and strain of providing daily care can have serious deleterious effects on the caregiver's health. Studies have demonstrated adverse effects on blood pressure and immune function and increased rates of cardiovascular disease and death. In addition, caregivers have alarmingly high rates of psychological illness, with symptoms of depression reported in up to 50%. This problem is particularly prevalent in those providing care for patients with dementia or other cognitive problems. The presence of mental illness further raises the risk of verbal or physical abuse or neglect of the patient. The clinician must recognize caregiver problems early and consider referral to a social worker, patient resource manager, or, when available, a geriatric assessment team. Key risk factors for stress include (1) a frail family caregiver; (2) a patient with cognitive impairment, emotional disturbance, substance abuse, sleep disruption, or behavioral problems; (3) low income or financial strain; and (4) acute illness or hospitalization. Providers should recognize the overt signs and symptoms of physical or mental strain and regularly inquire about caregiver burden with an offer to talk apart from the patient if need be.

A number of resources exist to support caregivers and provide strategies for problem solving and self-care. Community-based programs provide assistance with meals, transportation, or respite care options through volunteer organizations or subsidized programs. Counseling on both the physical and emotional aspects of care has been demonstrated to reduce health risks to the caregiver and delay institutionalization. This includes in-home or institutional respite stays to provide caregivers with precious time off. Studies consistently demonstrate that such services are underused by caregivers.

MISTREATMENT

All too often, caregiver stress and social isolation increase the risk of abuse or neglect of older adults. Elder mistreatment has been reported in 3% to 8% of the older adult population in the United States. A variety of forms of neglect or physical abuse can result in adverse health outcomes for older victims. Victims themselves are unlikely to report instances of abuse, making it difficult to address issues in the clinical setting. Older adults who are noted to have contusions, burns, bite marks, genital or rectal trauma, pressure ulcers, or unexplained weight loss without clinical explanation should be asked about mistreatment or referred to social work services.

FINANCES

The older adult population in the United States varies widely in measures of wealth. Although the overall rate of poverty among adults over age 65 has declined over the last 50 years, 10% of older adults still live at or below the poverty line, and the percentage is higher among African Americans (24%) and Hispanics (21%). Providers should screen for problems with financial resources, as these issues have direct implications for health status and well-being. Older adults with limited means may be more prone to have problems affording medications, meals, and basic amenities. Referrals to community resource networks can help identify options for help with basic needs, including housing options and congregate meals. Information on agencies and services in specific locales can be identified at www.eldercarelocator.org.

ADVANCE DIRECTIVES

Older patients may experience periods of altered sensorium or cognitive impairment and become unable to participate in their financial or health care decisions. In such situations a surrogate must intervene on behalf of the patient. Powers of attorney, living wills, advance directives, and guardianship documents become important in these situations. A power of attorney lists a surrogate who is authorized to manage a patient's financial affairs. Trust in this representative is important because the surrogate has the right to spend the patient's money and incur debt in the patient's name. A health care power of attorney designates a representative to make health care choices for the patient. For patients who have not created a health care power of attorney, typically the spouse or other first-degree relative is the default surrogate decision maker. The patient's preferences are sometimes detailed in a living will or other more detailed advance directive. This document often addresses situations in which the patient has a terminal illness, persistent vegetative state or progressive neurologic condition and can include explicit directions for care management including withdrawal or withholding of specific measures, including artificial nutrition and hydration. If no surrogate is designated and no next of kin is available, guardianship may be obtained. Guardianship is a legal proceeding whereby the court appoints a surrogate decision maker. For more information on legal issues and the elderly the reader is referred to the National Academy of Elder Law Attorneys at www.naela.org.

High-Risk Circumstances

THE HOSPITALIZED PATIENT

Millions of older adults are hospitalized in the United States each year for a variety of acute illnesses and elective procedures. Fortunately, in the United States, Medicare Part A covers nearly all the costs associated with acute care, including the costs of hospitalization and follow-up rehabilitation. While in the hospital, however, older adults are vulnerable to myriad complications related to both their compromised health state and problems inherent to the acute care environment itself. As noted previously, delirium plagues the hospitalized elderly at a very high rate and increases their risk of prolonged hospital stays, nursing home admission, and death. Hospitalized older adults also experience the effects of immobilization, with loss of muscle strength and deconditioning. Acutely, these factors increase the risk of falls and impair function and ability to provide self-care. In addition, poor oral intake may result in malnutrition, and illness-related fluid losses cause dehydration. As a result, hypotension and protein-calorie malnutrition are common problems. Immobility and malnutrition both predispose the acutely ill patient to the development of pressure wounds, which, in

the right circumstance, can develop in under 2 hours. All these problems worsen in the presence of delirium or depressed mood. Environmental factors also contribute to problems, including tethers such as catheters and intravenous lines, which increase risk of falls, and noisy wards, frequent tests, and procedures that further disrupt diurnal rhythms and sleep. Up to a third of hospitalized older adults experience a decline in their ability to perform ADLs in the course of their hospitalization. Patients who experience declines in function during hospitalization have higher rates of rehospitalization, prolonged institutionalization, and mortality after discharge, and many (41%) never return to their preadmission level of function. To combat these problems, some hospitals have created specialized inpatient geriatric care units, often termed *acute care for elders (ACE) units*. These units incorporate adaptations in the physical environment and specially trained staff to provide safe, patient-centered care designed to maximize restoration of function and prevent common complications of hospitalization. Likewise, geriatric evaluation and management (GEM) units (described later) offer specialized, team-based postacute care with an emphasis on rehabilitation and return to prior level of function.

CARE TRANSITIONS

As noted previously, older adults experience high rates of complications during acute illness and require prolonged periods of time to recover. For this reason, management in the postacute period represents a critical and complex time in their care. Specifically, older adults with acute illness often find themselves transferred between different care settings and providers. Nearly a quarter of hospitalized older adults are discharged to SNFs, and another 12% are discharged with home health care. Of those discharged to skilled facilities, 19% will return to the hospital within 30 days. Transitions in care represent high-risk episodes, and evidence shows that patients and caregivers frequently experience miscommunication, medication errors, and missed essential laboratory tests or appointments during this period of time. Recent trials have demonstrated a reduction in rehospitalization through a structured discharge and transition plan that includes medication reconciliation before and after discharge, careful planning for laboratory and appointment follow-up, communication with patients and caregivers about expectations and preferences, and specific coaching for caregivers in symptom management and care. More information on care management in transitions is available at www.caretransitions.org.

Systems of Care

AMBULATORY AND HOME CARE

The majority of care for older adults occurs in the outpatient clinic. Much of the cost of this care, including visit fees, laboratory tests, x-ray studies, and vaccinations, is covered under Medicare Part B, for which patients pay a monthly premium. Outpatient visits may occur with the physician, physician's assistant, nurse practitioner, or clinical nurse specialists, depending on the nature of the problem and the structure of the clinic. Other key members of the care team include social workers, pharmacists, psychologists, and physical and occupational therapists. Most assessments discussed in this chapter can be performed in the clinic, including functional assessments, cognitive and mood screening, gait and balance assessment, medication review, eye and ear examinations and continence evaluations. Interview of a caregiver can augment the information collected. Care in this setting can be complicated, though, by problems with transportation and ineffective or inefficient communication among multiple providers, particularly for patients with multiple specialists.

Over the last several years, home care has re-emerged as a very effective means of providing health care for older adults. As with the outpatient clinic, Medicare Part B will reimburse providers in part for services rendered in the home. In addition, if a rehabilitative or skilled service is needed, Medicare Part A provides coverage. Patients receiving services in the home must be "homebound," implying that they are significantly functionally impaired and travel with assistance out of the home infrequently and usually for medical purposes. Services rendered in the home include a full range of evaluations by teams of providers from a variety of health professions depending on needs. Social workers often lead these visits and perform case management, assessing financial and other resource needs. Nurses, clinical nurse specialists, and/or nurse practitioners provide skilled services when necessary, including health education, symptom monitoring, or wound care. Physical and occupational therapy can assess mobility and home safety and greatly enhance function and independence. Furthermore, examination of a person's home environment can reveal much about his or her nutritional habits and can facilitate education or intervention in this area. Physicians may serve as medical directors of such programs but may also perform visits themselves to learn more about a given patient's health status. If significant concerns exist about a patient's safety, particularly in the setting of cognitive impairment, a home visit may provide information about the need for more urgent interventions, including referrals to Adult Protective Services. Research has demonstrated that coordinated home care programs can improve management of chronic disease, including dementia, diabetes mellitus, and CHF, and can reduce rehospitalization in CHF.

LONG-TERM CARE

The phrase *long-term care* describes the array of services available to provide care for patients with disability from chronic and acute conditions. This definition includes the services offered in the outpatient and home settings described previously. Most associate the term, however, with the system of living facilities providing personal and medical care for disabled adults of all ages. SNFs provide long-term care for those with permanent disabilities from chronic illness or short rehabilitative stays after acute illness (e.g., stroke) or procedures (e.g., joint replacement). The scope of services may also include end-of-life care in conjunction with a hospice care team. Facility staff includes licensed nurses who give 24-hour supervision, with much of the personal care provided by certified nursing assistants (CNAs). Each facility also has a medical director overseeing various

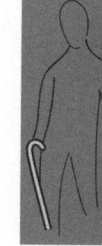

aspects of medical care. An attending physician, who may or may not be the medical director, performs patient visits every 30 to 60 days. Most SNFs also employ physical, occupational, and speech therapists for rehabilitation care, dietitians, social workers, and recreational therapists. Patients with moderate or severe dementia constitute approximately 60% of patients living in SNFs. Although Medicare Part A provides payment for rehabilitative stays of 100 days or less (with a co-payment for days 21 to 100), it does not finance long-term stays. Patients of this type pay out of pocket, through long-term care insurance, or through Medicaid, a joint federal and state assistance program. Medicaid constitutes 47% of all payment sources for SNF care.

For patients with less complex care needs, assisted living facilities or domiciliary care homes provide an alternative arrangement for long-term care. Although these facilities vary dramatically in their size and structure, most provide nonskilled care for patients who need some assistance with ADLs. Licensed nurses may be present during discrete periods of time, and other professions may visit the facility intermittently to provide specific services such as physical therapy. Facilities do not have medical directors, and patients normally continue to see a primary care provider in the outpatient clinic. Unlicensed staff, including nursing aides, provides most of the personal care and assistance. Medicaid provides some reimbursement for this type of care, but the majority of residents pay out of pocket or through other assistance programs, such as social security.

PACE

In the 1970s a group providing care for older adults in San Francisco developed a model of long-term care centered in the community. Proponents of this model, entitled the Program of All-inclusive Care for the Elderly (PACE), believed that the community (rather than the institution) provided a better location to meet the chronic care needs of older adults. From its start as a community-based effort in California, the PACE model has grown with the support of foundations and now Medicare and Medicaid and offers services for seniors at 42 locations in 22 states. Participants must be over 55 and certified by the state to be eligible for nursing home care. The PACE program then uses resources otherwise slated to pay for the individual's long-term care to provide care in the community—much of it coordinated through senior centers offering an array of resources and services, including the following:

- Adult day care, offering nursing; physical, occupational, and recreational therapies; meals; nutritional counseling; social work; and personal care
- Medical care provided by a PACE physician familiar with the history, needs, and preferences of each participant
- Home health care and personal care
- All necessary prescription drugs
- Social services
- Medical specialists such as audiology, dentistry, optometry, podiatry, and speech therapy
- Respite care*

*Information from the National PACE Association website at www. npaonline.org.

When necessary, PACE participants are admitted to the hospital or nursing home. These services are provided under the auspices of the PACE program as part of the care package. The benefits of care for older adults, particularly those of limited means, appear to be substantial; questions about cost, generalizability, and sustainability remain.

GERIATRIC CARE

In caring for frail older adults with complex care needs, consultation with a geriatrician or geriatrics-focused team can often provide highly useful information. The geriatrician can assist in the assessment and management of the specific conditions or situations described earlier. He or she can help with difficult decisions regarding treatment options in the context of multiple comorbidities and limited life expectancy and offer advice on appropriate level or setting of care for an older adult. Geriatricians complete a minimum of 1 year of fellowship after residency training in internal medicine or family practice. After training they are eligible for board certification and qualified to work in a number of different settings, including the hospital, long-term care, home care, or outpatient clinics. Comprehensive assessment by a geriatrician or geriatrics team includes components detailed previously, including evaluation of the patient's medical condition, function, and social support. Normally the consultant will work with an interdisciplinary team (IDT) that may include a nurse case manager, physician's assistant, social worker, physical or occupation therapist, pharmacist, psychologist, or others. The outcome of the geriatric assessment is a comprehensive plan for safely restoring the patient to optimal function with mutually agreeable and realistic goals of care.

In the setting of acute illness, geriatricians also provide important services. As described earlier, acute-care-for-elders (ACE) units can improve patient care and prevent iatrogenic complications. Similarly, once patients are medically stable, transfer to a specialized geriatrics care unit, often termed a geriatric evaluation and management (or GEM) unit, may be possible, to provide a comprehensive medical assessment and plan for transition of care. Early consultation with a geriatrician and an IDT in the acute care setting can help in the management of complex medical illness and with communication with patients and caregivers about posthospitalization options. Subsequent to hospitalization, locating facilities or services that offer comprehensive care by a geriatrician and IDT would be ideal, including a coordinated approach that uses specific strategies to manage transitions of care.

Prospectus for the Future

Over the last quarter century, our understanding of the biology of human aging and chronic disease has expanded dramatically and allowed us to begin to develop novel strategies for more effective prevention and management of the medical ailments of late life. Concurrently with these scientific advances, however, we have also seen an increase in the population of older adults that has outpaced the resources available for care. In facing this challenge, the current generation of physicians and physicians-in-training must recognize the unique principles of care for the older patient and gain competence, if not mastery, in this area. These principles include (1) age-related changes in biology and physiology that make older adults more vulnerable to chronic illness and disability; (2) the presence of comorbid illness and functional decline, which predict health outcomes and life expectancy independent of age; (3) that older adults manifest illness in a number of nonspecific ways, including impairments in mobility, mentation, and mood; (4) effective and optimal care, which includes careful assessment of health status and social circumstances, in identifying preferred treatment strategies; and 5) novel systems of care that incorporate interprofessional teams providing care across the spectrum of settings. Indeed, it is this last point that most accurately foretells the future of geriatric medicine. In recent years, randomized controlled trials of multifaceted, interdisciplinary interventions accounting for both host and environmental factors have proven highly effective in management of a variety of conditions. Examples include home-based interventions for congestive heart failure, dementia, and depression and specific protocols for prevention and management of falls and delirium in hospitals and nursing homes. In order to continue to meet the challenge of providing care for the oldest members of society, we must support the development and dissemination of these measures that adopt a holistic view of the individual patient's experience across providers and settings.

References

Boyd CM, Darer J, Boult C, Fried LP, et al: Clinical practice guidelines and quality of care for older patients with multiple comorbid diseases: Implications for pay for performance. JAMA 294:716-724, 2005.
Cohen HJ, Feussner JR, Weinberger M, et al: A controlled trial of inpatient and outpatient geriatric evaluation and management. N Engl J Med 346: 905-912, 2002.
Coleman E: Improving the quality of transitional care for persons with complex care needs. J Am Geriatr Soc 51:556-557, 2003.
Creditor MC: Hazards of hospitalization of the elderly. Ann Intern Med 118:219-223, 1993.
Cristafolo VJ, Tresini M, Francis MK, Volker C: Biological theories of senescence. In Bengston VL, Schaie W (eds): Handbook of Theories of Aging. New York, Springer, 1999.
Federal Interagency Forum on Aging-Related Statistics: Older Americans 2008: Key indicators of well-being. Washington, DC, U.S. Government Printing Office, March 2008.
Fried LP, Tangen CM, Walston J: Frailty in older adults: Evidence for a phenotype. J Gerontol Med Sci 56:146-156, 2001.
Fries JF: Aging, natural death, and the compression of morbidity. N Engl J Med 303:130-135, 1980.

Ganz DA, Bao Y, Shekelle PG, Rubenstein LZ: Will my patient fall? JAMA 297:77, 2007.
Holsinger T, Deveau J, Boustani M, Williams JW: Does this patient have dementia? JAMA 297:2391, 2007.
Inouye SK: Delirium in older persons. N Engl J Med 354:1157-1165, 2006.
Jarrett PG, Rockwood K, Carver D, et al: Illness presentation in elderly patients. Arch Intern Med 155:1060-1064, 1995.
Li RM, Iadarola AC, Maisano CC (eds): Why Population Aging Matters: A Global Perspective. A booklet prepared in follow-up to the 2007 Summit on Global Aging hosted by the U.S. State Department and the National Institute on Aging. National Institute on Aging and the National Institutes of Health, March 2007.
National Alliance for Caregiving and AARP: Caregiving in the U.S. Bethesda, National Alliance for Caregiving, and Washington, DC, AARP, 2004.
Ouslander JG: Management of overactive bladder. N Engl J Med 350:786-799, 2004.
Shrank WH, Polinski JM, Avorn J: Quality indicators for medication use in vulnerable elders. J Am Geriatr Soc 55(Suppl 2):S373, 2007.
Tinetti ME: Preventing falls in elderly persons. N Engl J Med 348:42-49, 2003.
Tinetti ME, Bogardus ST, Agostini JV: Potential pitfalls of disease-specific guidelines for patients with multiple conditions. N Engl J Med 351:2870-2874, 2004.
Walter LC, Covinsky KE: Cancer screening in elderly patients—a framework for individualized decision making. JAMA 285:2750, 2001.

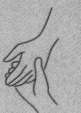

Section XXI

Palliative Care

Palliative Care

Robert G. Holloway and Timothy E. Quill

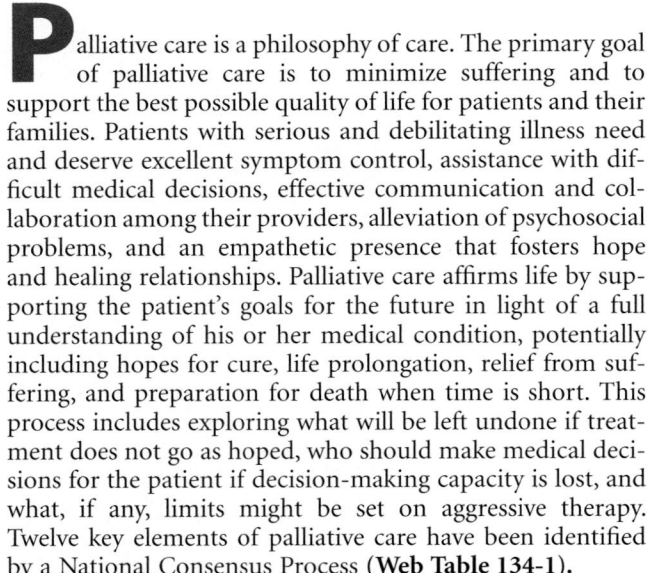

Palliative care is a philosophy of care. The primary goal of palliative care is to minimize suffering and to support the best possible quality of life for patients and their families. Patients with serious and debilitating illness need and deserve excellent symptom control, assistance with difficult medical decisions, effective communication and collaboration among their providers, alleviation of psychosocial problems, and an empathetic presence that fosters hope and healing relationships. Palliative care affirms life by supporting the patient's goals for the future in light of a full understanding of his or her medical condition, potentially including hopes for cure, life prolongation, relief from suffering, and preparation for death when time is short. This process includes exploring what will be left undone if treatment does not go as hoped, who should make medical decisions for the patient if decision-making capacity is lost, and what, if any, limits might be set on aggressive therapy. Twelve key elements of palliative care have been identified by a National Consensus Process (**Web Table 134-1**).

Palliative care provides an organized, highly structured system for delivering care by an interdisciplinary team, including physicians, nurses, social workers, chaplains, counselors, and other health care professionals. Palliative care should be integrated within various health care settings including the hospital, emergency department, nursing home, home care setting, assisted living facilities, and outpatient settings. Palliative care remains very unevenly available, so many patients and families needlessly suffer, having no, limited, or delayed access to appropriate palliative care.

The integration of palliative care into the experiences of patients and families is designed to meet four objectives. First, to ensure that pain and symptom control, psychosocial distress, spiritual issues, and practical needs are addressed throughout the continuum of care. Second, to make certain that patients and families obtain the information they need in an ongoing and comprehensible manner to understand their prognosis and treatment options. This process incorporates their values and preferences and is sensitive to changes in the patient's condition over time. Third, palliative care seeks to provide seamless care coordination across settings with high-quality communication among providers.

Finally, for those patients who are not going to recover, to the extent possible palliative care prepares patients and families for the dying process and for death, including providing options for hospice care, opportunities for personal growth, and bereavement support.

Common Illness Trajectories and Palliative Care

There are distinct trajectories of functional decline before dying (**Web Fig. 134-1**). These four trajectories have major implications for palliative care and health care delivery. Patients and families likely have different physical, psychological, social, and spiritual needs depending on the trajectory of their illness before they die. Being aware of these trajectories can help providers deliver appropriate care that integrates both disease-directed and palliative treatments.

TRAJECTORY 1: SHORT PERIOD OF EVIDENT DECLINE BEFORE DEATH

Cancer typifies trajectory 1. Function is preserved until rather late, followed by a predictable and precipitous decline over weeks to months. The onset of decline usually suggests metastatic tumor. A more predictable decline in function can assist in anticipating care needs, transitioning away from curative treatments toward a more exclusive emphasis on palliation, and eventually into hospice care. Not all malignancies follow this trajectory (e.g., prostate, breast), and some nonmalignant conditions may follow this course.

TRAJECTORY 2: CHRONIC ILLNESS WITH EXACERBATIONS AND SUDDEN DYING

Congestive heart failure (CHF), chronic obstructive pulmonary disease (COPD), end-stage liver disease, and acquired immunodeficiency syndrome (AIDS) typify trajectory 2.

These organ system diseases represent chronic illnesses with occasional, acute exacerbations (e.g., physiologic stress that overwhelms the body's reserves), often requiring hospital admission. Patients can have a return of function after an exacerbation, but often not to the level of their baseline. They also may die suddenly during an exacerbation, but it is difficult to predict in advance. Prognosticating is very challenging in this trajectory. For example, patients with heart failure who die suddenly also have a 50% chance of living 6 months or longer 1 week before their sudden death. When patients choose to forego or stop aggressive life support, planning for aggressive symptom relief during a future exacerbation is essential.

TRAJECTORY 3: PROLONGED DWINDLING

Dementia and frailty typify trajectory 3. Affected patients have a prolonged course of physical and cognitive decline and slowly dwindle away. Additional diagnoses include other neurodegenerative conditions (e.g., Parkinson's disease, amyotrophic lateral sclerosis) and patients with multiple moderate to severe comorbidities (e.g., arthritis, visual impairment, past mild strokes, diabetes with neuropathy). Gradual decline in function, weight loss, fatigue, and low levels of activity are core features. Caregiver demands are usually immense. Prognosticating survival is difficult, and complications such as pneumonia and fractures may be terminal events. The benefits and burdens of artificial nutrition must be balanced in the late stages.

TRAJECTORY 4: SUDDEN, SEVERE NEUROLOGIC INJURY

Sudden impairment trajectories are those that stem from sudden neurologic injury that can lead to profound cognitive and functional impairment. These include stroke, hypoxic ischemic encephalopathy, and traumatic brain injury. The vast majority of deaths occur either early after the event when treatments are withheld or withdrawn or in the chronic stage in survivors who have accumulating

debility (these events represent the leading cause of adult disability). At the extremes of impairment are persistent vegetative states, minimally conscious states, and locked-in syndrome. But there is a vast spectrum of severe impairments short of these extremes that raise questions about how to manage potentially severe debility with little chance of improvement. This trajectory requires a health system responsive to negotiating goals of treatment with patients and surrogates who may consider these future health states "worse than death."

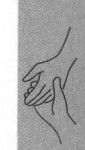

Communication Skills and Negotiating Goals of Treatment

Excellent communication skills are central to palliative care: communication with patients, family, other physicians, nurses, and other members of the health care team. The overarching aim is to assist the patient and family in establishing the goals of current and future treatment in a process of shared decision making. When negotiating goals of treatment in palliative care, the focus is often to assist with the following decisions: to help decide types and aggressiveness of disease-directed therapies, to ensure optimum palliation of symptoms, to assist in hospice determinations, to discuss withholding or withdrawing therapies, and to facilitate advance care planning and to initiate surrogate decision making if patient lacks capacity. These discussions occur at various time points in the course of advancing illness when new and important information is learned and needs to be communicated to the patient and family. The need to renegotiate goals should also be anticipated when triggers of advancing disease suggest limited life expectancy or excessive suffering. These discussions are almost always variants of "bad news" discussions.

The overall approach to communication and negotiating goals of care in each of these scenarios is similar (Table 134-1). This includes running an effective family meeting with or without the patient present. Initial elements include

Table 134-1	**General Strategy for Communicating and Negotiating Goals of Care in Common Palliative Care Settings**
Step	**Goals of Care**
1	Prepare and establish setting Do not have a rigid preset agenda
2	Ask patient and family what they know and understand Provide sufficient time for patients and families to "tell their story" Use active listening skills
3	Find out how much patient and family want to know Acknowledge and explore emotions
4	Discuss prognosis and benefits and burdens of treatment options Be mindful of optimistic and pessimistic predictions Be prepared to make recommendations
5	Respond to emotions and empathetic response Convey honesty, and reframe hope Use "I wish" statements
6	Summarize, establish, and implement plan, follow-up Possible time-limited trial

establishing the proper setting, identifying key stakeholders, and "doing your homework" (i.e., discussing potential plans with people from all relevant subspecialties who may have communicated with the patient and families). When the meeting begins, first find out what the patient and family understand about the medical condition, and ask about what added information they want. Keeping an open mind and trying to hold back on a fixed agenda (e.g., to "get the DNR" or to "stop futile care") helps clinicians allow patients and families sufficient time to "tell their stories" and provides the context within which effective decision making can occur. In general, the more patients and families speak in the early parts of such meetings, the better.

The provider then needs to share prognostic information and discuss the benefits and burdens of the available treatment options. Alerting the patient or family of impending bad news ("I am afraid I have some difficult news to share with you") is a useful initial communication strategy. The amount of information should be paced with frequent pauses to allow time for emotional responses. Comprehension should be frequently checked, and questions should be encouraged. The skilled clinician can flexibly assess, probe, and pace the content and depth of the discussions and negotiations in an emotionally responsive (acknowledge, explore, empathize, and legitimize) and culturally competent manner. This includes the ability to understand and respect diverse religious practices and differing preferences about degree of truth telling. When appropriate, the clinician should make recommendations based on scientific knowledge as well as awareness of a patient's values and preferences and should be prepared to help resolve conflicts among patient, family members, and providers. Finally, providers need to develop strategies to preserve and potentially reframe hope, including ways to "hope for the best" while simultaneously "preparing for the worst." Commitments to minimize suffering and to not abandon the patient and family are essential. At the end of the discussions, the provider should summarize key aspects of what was reviewed and establish a follow-up plan for future communications and treatments.

Estimating and Communicating Prognosis

A core component of information shared in the palliative care setting is prognosis. Understanding prognosis is central to making decisions about aggressive treatment as well as hospice. Prognosis is a prediction of possible future outcomes of a disease (survival, symptoms, function, quality of life, family impact, and financial considerations) with or without treatment. Most patients and families want to know prognosis; they both hate it and crave it at the same time. Because there are some patients and families who may not want to know prognosis or may want it communicated in a particular way, it is essential to begin by finding out what the patient and family know and want to know.

Inaccurate predictions may lead to poor decision making. Indeed, physicians tend to overestimate survival in patients with advanced cancer by about 30%, and the bias is more pronounced the longer the physician-patient relationship.

Overly optimistic predictions can lead to overuse of ineffective or unwanted disease-directed treatment, delay in hospice referrals, false expectations, unnecessary tests and procedures, and poor symptom control. Therefore accurately estimating and communicating prognosis is central to optimal decision making in advanced illness and at the end of life.

In advanced illnesses, common factors found to be predictive of short-term survival (i.e., less than 3 to 6 months) include performance status, anorexia-cachexia syndrome, delirium, and dyspnea. In addition to physicians' subjective predictions of survival, there exist models to assist with prognostic estimates, including generic models for particular populations (e.g., hospice enrollees) as well as disease-specific models (e.g., cancers, heart failure, liver disease, stroke, AIDS, spinal cord compression). Hospice eligibility criteria also exist for different diseases. Although not uniformly reliable, they can be useful in formulating estimates when prognosis might be 6 months or less if the disease were allowed to run its natural course (a prognostic criterion for hospice referral).

For an individual patient, however, prognostic uncertainty remains the rule. Therefore it is important to integrate both evidence and experience-based medicine and present the information in formats tailored to the particular patient (verbal descriptions, numerics, frequencies, or graphics). Prognostic estimates should be bounded with ranges to convey realistic uncertainty, being sure to allow for exceptions in both directions. For example, "in my experience, patients with your condition live on average a few weeks to a few months. It could be longer if you are lucky, but it could also be shorter." For survival-predominant prognoses (e.g., "How long do I have?"), be mindful of overly optimistic prognoses, remembering to think of and convey the lower bound (e.g., "some may live longer, but others may unfortunately live shorter"). For outcome-predominant prognoses (e.g., "What will life be like?"), be mindful of overly pessimistic predictions, remembering the power of adaptation and engendering hope by helping patients and families find new meaning.

Suffering and Symptom Management

In addition to establishing and facilitating goals of treatment, palliative care aims to relieve suffering, defined as severe distress related to events that threaten the stability of personhood or how the physical, psychological, spiritual, and social aspects of self are interconnected. Beginning with simple, open-ended screening questions such as "In what ways are you suffering most?" and then following with more domain-related screening questions (physical, psychological, spiritual, social) may allow for more probing and multidimensional inquiries to better understand the various sources of and contributions to an individual's suffering.

One of the first steps in the care of any seriously ill patient is to control pain and other forms of physical suffering. There are striking similarities between the burden of symptoms experienced in patients dying of cancer and the symptoms experienced in noncancerous conditions. Although the profile of symptoms may differ, each disease carries with it troubling symptoms that can potentially be addressed and managed.

PHYSICAL SYMPTOMS

Pain

Uncontrolled pain dominates all other experiences, and most pain can be relieved using basic pain management strategies. These include a detailed history and physical examination, categorizing the likely type(s) (i.e., somatic, visceral, neuropathic) and severity (rated on a 0 to 10 scale) of pain, knowledge about proper opioid dosing strategies, and judicious use of consultations and invasive interventions (e.g., nerve blocks, epidural analgesia). The overarching three-tiered approach is to use nonopioids (e.g., acetaminophen, nonsteroidal anti-inflammatory drugs) for mild pain, weak opioids (e.g., hydrocodone or codeine) for mild to moderate pain, and strong opioids (e.g., morphine, hydromorphone, fentanyl, methadone) for moderate to severe pain.

Most patients with chronic moderate to severe pain should be initially started on around-the-clock administration of a short-acting opioid. Table 134-2 shows the equianalgesic dosing, usual starting doses, half-life, duration, and relative costs for the commonly available opioid agents. Once the total daily dosage has been determined (sum of all scheduled and "as needed" doses), the patient may be switched to a long-acting opioid to cover the baseline requirements. As-needed opioids for breakthrough pain should be approximately 10% of the total daily dose every 1 to 2 hours orally or every 30 to 60 minutes subcutaneously or intravenously. Continuous intravenous (IV) or subcutaneous (SC) infusions of opioids may be needed for rapid control of severe pain. Methadone is useful in palliative care because of its excellent oral bioavailability, lack of active metabolites in renal impairment, low cost, flexible route of administration (oral [PO], IV, SC), and possible effect on both neuropathic and somatic pain. However, it does have a dose-dependent, progressively long half-life and arrhythmogenic potential.

Constipation occurs with all opioids, and it should be anticipated and treated. Other predictable but less common side effects include nausea, myoclonus, urinary retention, pruritus, and delirium. Some of these side effects are time-limited with initiation (e.g., nausea), whereas others can be managed by dose reduction or opioid rotation (e.g., myoclonus, delirium). Major respiratory depression is extremely rare if the opioid dose is appropriate and proportionate to the severity of symptoms. In the absence of a prior history of drug and alcohol abuse, addiction is rare, but physical dependence (i.e., withdrawal symptoms on abrupt cessation) and tolerance (i.e., a decrease in drug effect over time) should be expected. Naloxone should be rarely used unless a clear overdose is suspected or if life-threatening complications occur. Special caution is needed about opioid prescribing in elderly and debilitated patients, and recommended starting doses should be reduced by approximately 50%. There are additional opioid selection recommendations for patients with renal insufficiency (avoid morphine and codeine; use hydromorphone and oxycodone with caution; methadone and fentanyl optimal) and hepatic insufficiency (cautiously use fentanyl, hydromorphone, oxycodone, or methadone; avoid or decrease dose of morphine).

Other Symptoms

There are numerous physical symptoms not related to pain that can dominate and overwhelm the clinical picture in any given patient. These include dyspnea, nausea and vomiting, constipation, anorexia-cachexia, fatigue, bleeding, agitation, apathy, myoclonus, pruritus, and specific functional deficits. Each symptom requires a structured approach to the history and physical examination, with a full exploration of the potential causes and treatment options, and informed by the prognosis and preferences of the patient and family.

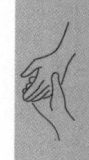

Psychological Pain

Depression, anxiety, and delirium are all common in the palliative care setting. They are frequently underrecognized and under-treated. Appropriate diagnosis and treatment can improve quality of life.

Nearly all patients in palliative care and their families experience sadness, preparatory grief, and transient anxiety as illness advances. Grief or normal sadness is often experienced in waves with retained capacity for pleasure. Depression is more enduring, persistent, and intense and may be associated with hopelessness, helplessness, worthlessness, and guilt. Two screening question assessing depressed mood and anhedonia include "Are you depressed?" and "Do you have much interest and pleasure in doing things?" One should be cautious using somatic symptoms to diagnose depression (e.g., fatigue, anorexia, sleep disturbance), as they frequently overlap with physiologic changes associated with advanced disease. For depression and anxiety, consider and rule out contributions from physical symptoms (e.g., uncontrolled pain), medical causes (e.g., hypothyroidism, hyperthyroidism), and medications. Effective pharmacologic and nonpharmacologic treatments exist for both depression and anxiety, although treatment selection depends on symptom intensity, patient prognosis, and treatment benefits and burdens. Other members of the interdisciplinary team (social worker, chaplain, and psychologist) often play a critical role in assessment and ongoing management.

Delirium, an acquired and fluctuating disorder of consciousness and cognition, occurs commonly in the palliative care setting. The level of psychomotor activity can vary from hyperactive ("agitated" delirium) to hypoactive ("quiet" delirium). Nearly 80% of the delirium in the palliative care setting is the hypoactive variant. As a result, it is often underdiagnosed, or misdiagnosed as depression and fatigue. The most common causes of delirium in palliative care include medications (e.g., opioids), metabolic disorders caused by progressive organ failure, and infection. Meticulous attention to the history from collateral sources (nurses, caregiver) and a detailed medication history are essential for an accurate diagnosis. Although delirium may reverse if an obvious cause is identified and removed, frequently it represents an important marker of progressive illness, so cognitive improvements may be transient and incomplete. In addition to cause-specific treatment (e.g., change or stop medications, treat infection, administer oxygen, ensure adequate hydration, administer bisphosphonates), environmental interventions are recommended for all patients (e.g., quiet reassurance, gentle reorientation, optimization of sensory

Table 134-2 Equianalgesic Table for Adults with Moderate to Severe Pain

Medication	Equianalgesic Dose (for chronic administration) IM/IV onset 15-30 min	Equianalgesic Dose (for chronic administration) PO onset 30-60 min	Usual Starting Doses Adult > 50 kg; For opioid naive patients (♦1/2 dose for elderly, or severe renal or liver disease) Parenteral	Usual Starting Doses Adult > 50 kg; For opioid naive patients PO	Comments
Morphine	10 mg	30 mg	2.5-5 mg IV q3-4h (♦1.25-2.5 mg)	5-15 mg q3-4h (IR or oral solution) (♦2.5-7.5 mg)	IR tablets (15, 30 mg) oral sol. (2 mg/ml, 4 mg/ml) Conc solution (20 mg/ml) can give buccally Morphine ER tables (15, 30, 60, 100, 200 mg) q 8-12h Kadian ER pellets (10, 20, 30, 50, 60, 60, 100, 200 mg) q 12-24h Avinza ER pellets (30, 60, 90, 120 mg) q 24h Rectal suppositories (5, 10, 20, 30 mg) Not recommended in renal failure
Oxycodone	Not available	20 mg	Not available	5-10 mg q3-4h (♦2.5 mg)	OxyIR capsule (5 mg); IR tablet (5, 10, 15, 20, 30 mg); conc solution (20 mg/ml) Oxycontin (10, 15, 30, 40, 60, 80 mg) – due to high cost and potential for abuse, use only if failure or contraindication to morphine ER Not enough literature regarding dosing in renal failure; use caution
Hydromorphone	1.5 mg	7.5 mg	0.2-0.6 mg IV q 2-3h (♦0.2 mg)	1-2 mg q3-4h (♦0.5-1 mg)	Tablet (2, 4, 8); oral liquid (1 mg/ml) Use carefully in renal failure
Methadone*	½ oral dose 2 mg PO methadone = 1 mg parenteral methadone	Oral morphine: Methadone ratio — 24 hr. oral morphine: <30 mg → 2:1; 31-99 mg → 4:1; 100-299 mg → 8:1; 300-499 mg → 12:1; 500-999 mg → 15:1; 1000-1200 mg → 20:1; >1200 mg → Consider consult	1.25-2.5 mg q 8h (♦1.25 mg)	2.5-5 mg q 8h (♦1.25-2.5 mg)	Table (5,10 mg); sol (1 mg/ml, 2 mg/ml & concentrated 10 mg/ml) Usually q 12h or q 8h; long variable T ½ Acceptable with renal disease Small dose change makes big difference in blood level Tends to accumulate with higher doses, always advise "hold for sedation" Because of long half life, do not use methadone prn When converting from oral to parenteral, cut dose in half for safety When converting parenteral to oral, keep dose the same
Fentanyl*	100 mcg (single dose) (T1/2 and duration of parenteral doses variable)	24 hr oral MS dose : Initial patch — 30-59 mg → 12.5 mcg/hr; 60-134 mg → 25 mcg/hr; 135-224 mg → 50 mcg/hr; 315-404 mg → 100 mcg/hr	25-50 mcg IM/IV q 1-3h (♦12.5-25 mcg)	Transderm patch 12.5 mcg/hr q72h (Use with caution in opioid naive and in unstable patients because of 12 hour delay in onset and offset)	Transdermal patch (12.5, 25, 50, 75, 100 mcg); N.B. Incomplete cross-tolerance already accounted for in conversion to fentanyl; when converting to other opioids from fentanyl, generally reduce the equianalgesic amount by 50% Acceptable with renal disease, monitor carefully if using long term IV: Very short acting; associate with chest wall rigidity Oral lozenge (200 mcg start) and buccal tablet (100 mcg start)—indicated for breakthrough cancer pain only (see PDR and package insert)

*Parenteral methadone and fentanyl are not integrated into the equianalgesic table. See Quill, 2010 for more detail on dosing and prescribing.

input, minimization of night disruptions). Pharmacologic management should be used sparingly and cautiously and may include antipsychotic medications, benzodiazepines, and psychostimulants (for the hypoactive variant).

Spiritual and Existential Pain

Spiritual and existential distress is prevalent in patients and families with serious illness, especially at the end of life. Spirituality is about one's relationship with and responses to transcendent questions that confront one as a human being (i.e., search for meaning and purpose in life). Religion is a set of texts, practices, and beliefs about the transcendence shared by a community. Spirituality is broader than religion. The spiritual issues of seriously ill and dying patients often center on questions of meaning, value, and relationships. Dying patients want to be assured of their value in the face of actual or perceived threats to their intactness as a human being (physical or cognitive declines, altered appearances). Spirituality helps people find hope in despair and can help restore purpose.

One of the goals of palliative care is to relieve spiritual and existential distress. Patients and families often welcome such discussions. Examples of open-ended questions to facilitate this dialogue include "Are you at peace with all of this?" and "Is faith (religion, spirituality) important to you?" Acknowledgment and empathetic listening are the most important responses for most clinicians, not "correct answers."

Other strategies for fostering hope and meaning include developing caring relationships, setting attainable goals, involving the patient in the decision-making process, affirming the patient's worth, using lighthearted humor (when appropriate), and reminiscing with life review. It is important, however, to know one's professional boundaries and to refer to other members of the care team as appropriate ("Would you like to explore religious matters with someone?").

The Role and Use of Diagnostic Tests and Invasive Procedures

Several questions should be considered in determining the appropriateness of aggressive medical or palliative interventions near the end of life. What is the goal or expected outcome of the proposed intervention? What is the probable efficacy of the intervention? What are the patient's baseline levels of function and life expectancy? What are the potential side effects and burdens of the intervention? What are the patient's and family's wishes?

The range of medical and palliative options available is huge, so the challenge is to determine what makes sense to enhance the well-being of this patient at this particular stage of illness. Palliative interventions range from simple laboratory tests to more invasive options such as chemotherapy, radiotherapy, surgical or endoscopic interventions, stenting procedures, thoracentesis, paracentesis, pericardiocentesis, home inotropic therapy, noninvasive ventilation, antibiotics, and transfusions. The challenge is to individualize, so that patients can take full advantage of treatments that will

help them meet their goals while not having their experience dominated by near-futile invasive interventions.

The Role of Hospice

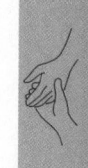

Hospice care is a specialized form of palliative care aimed at patients in the terminal stages of illness and their families. In 2007, 1.3 million patients were served by hospice programs in the United States. In order for a patient to qualify for the Medicare Hospice Benefit, two physicians must sign a statement certifying that the patient's prognosis for survival, if the disease were to run its natural course, is more likely than not to be 6 months or less. In addition, patients and families must agree to the hospice philosophy of care, aimed primarily at comfort, and forgo insurance coverage for disease-directed therapies. Hospice criteria exist to assist in making these determinations for most common medical conditions. Hospice care can be delivered in hospitals, patient's homes, nursing homes, or dedicated "hospice houses." The Medicare Hospice Benefit covers most costs related to terminal care without a deductible, which includes palliative medications, nursing oversight, supplies, and bereavement care. Hospice also covers up to 4 hours of custodial caregiver services per day, but family and/or friends have to provide the remaining care and support if a patient is to stay at home.

Cancer continues to be the most common diagnosis for patients dying in hospice programs. However, the prevalence of noncancer diagnoses is increasing, and patients with noncancerous conditions now represent more than 50% of all hospice admissions. Discussing hospice with patients and families can be challenging. First, it is often initially viewed as a "bad news" discussion, given that patients and families need to confront the fact that disease-directed treatment is no longer effective and that prognosis is likely to be 6 months or less. Second, given the reimbursement restrictions, patients may also need to forgo particular types of treatment that are important to them (e.g., acute hospital or intensive care unit [ICU]–level care, dialysis, chemotherapy, milrinone for heart failure).

Request for Hastened Death—Last Resort Options

The prevalence of suicidal ideation and suicide attempts is higher in patients with advanced life-limiting illness compared with those without serious disease. The prevalence of patients requesting a health care professional to help hasten death is not precisely known, but the situation is not uncommon. The motivation behind such requests may relate to relentless physical suffering, disfigurement, hopelessness, loss of dignity, fear of being a burden, or a "cry for help." Most enduring requests from patients with progressive medical illnesses, however, arise not from inadequate symptom control, but from a patient's belief about dignity, meaning, and control over the circumstances of death. Although some providers might be uncomfortable with exploring such requests, they need to be approached systematically with a diligent search to understand the root causes before a response is given.

A careful evaluation includes a precise clarification and exploration of exactly what the patient is asking and why. Is the request based on transient thoughts about ending life (common) or a serious appeal for assistance (relatively rare)? Does the request occur in the context of intense physical suffering, psychological despair, an existential crisis, or a combination of factors? Does the patient have full decision-making capacity, and is the request proportionate to the level of suffering? Evaluating such requests can be emotionally fatiguing and conflicting, and clinicians need self-awareness in distinguishing their emotions from the patient's, including tending to one's own support.

Responding to such a request should first include intensification of potentially reversible contributions to suffering. This will often include treating physical and psychological symptoms, aggressive attempts to foster hope, consulting psychiatrists or spiritual counselors, and creative brainstorming with trusted colleagues and team members. Some requests for hastened death persist despite optimal palliative care. In such circumstances, the clinicians should seek out a second opinion and confront the possibilities. These possibilities include withdrawal of life-sustaining interventions, palliative sedation, voluntary cessation of oral intake, and assisted suicide (illegal in the United States except for the states of Oregon and Washington). Although it is important to support the patient, clinicians must balance this desire with integrity and nonabandonment. This may include drawing specific boundaries regarding what the clinician can and cannot do, while still searching in earnest for a mutually acceptable solution.

Common Ethical Challenges in Palliative Care

INADEQUATE TREATMENT OF PAIN AND THE MYTH THAT PAIN MEDICATION HASTENS DEATH

Evidence abounds that pain is undertreated in many medical settings, including in those patients who are severely and even terminally ill (especially women, the elderly, minorities, and those who are cognitively impaired). Some undertreatment stems from fears about addiction as well as concerns about the possibility of hastening death. When patients with prior addiction problems are excluded, the incidence of new addictive behavior when opioids are used to treat pain in those with well-defined serious illness is probably less than 1%. Similarly, data suggesting that properly prescribed opioids hasten death are virtually nonexistent. In fact, there is some suggestion that opioids might even prolong life in these settings, and they certainly enhance quality of life in those with advanced illness and major pain or dyspnea.

WHEN PATIENTS AND FAMILIES WANT NEAR-FUTILE TREATMENT

The patient autonomy movement in medicine has led to patients and families taking an active role in their own medical decision making. This is generally a positive development except in two circumstances: (1) when physicians stop taking an active role and using their expertise to guide patients in their decision making, thereby abdicating their professional responsibility of advocating for the best possible treatment based on the patient's medical condition and personal values, and (2) when patients or their families want and even demand near-futile treatment toward the end of life despite physicians' advice that treatment will cause much more burden than benefit. Physicians might try to respond to patients who want "everything" by suggesting that they might want to try everything that is "more likely to help than harm," but avoid any treatment that is most likely to "do more harm than good." But some patients and families will accept no limits on treatment no matter what the burden and the improbability of success. Of course, truly futile treatment should not be offered or provided on request, but absolute futility has been difficult to define in many cases.

FEEDING TUBE QUESTIONS WHEN PATIENTS STOP EATING AND DRINKING

Many patients gradually stop eating and drinking as a natural part of the dying process, but this can be very hard for patients and families to accept in light of fears about "starving to death" and in view of seemingly simple technologies that can potentially combat and even reverse the problem. In fact, with few exceptions, feeding tubes have not been shown to prolong life in most advanced illnesses such as metastatic cancer or advanced Alzheimer disease. It is important to know about the exceptions (e.g., esophageal and oropharyngeal cancers, amyotrophic lateral sclerosis, and perhaps acute stroke) but also to have an open and frank discussion about the naturalness of eating and drinking less and less as many illnesses progress. If there is uncertainty about whether a particular patient might benefit from a feeding tube, and patient and family are clear about wanting to give it a try, the clinician can frame the decision as a "time-limited trial" to see how the patient tolerates tube feeding psychologically as well as physiologically in a specified timeframe. A nasogastric tube has a built-in time limit of about a month before a percutaneous endoscopic gastrostomy (PEG) tube needs to be inserted; this provides a potential framework for such a trial. Explaining to patients and families about the positive aspects of natural feeding, even in small amounts, of real food (smell, taste, enjoyment) may help focus the decision on important quality-of-life issues that may otherwise be ignored, rather than on more technical, physiologic issues.

Last Hours and Days of Living

An integral aspect of palliative care is preparing and guiding the patient and caregivers through the dying process. When prognosis is measured in hours to days, there are typical signs and symptoms that occur. Patients become weak and fatigued and gradually lose mobility. There is also a gradual and predictable decrease in food and fluid intake. Most patients do not experience hunger and thirst, and the associated mouth dryness that occurs is easily palliated with small sips or sponges of cold water. Caregivers will frequently ask about IV hydration. In rare instances, IV or SC fluids may temporarily improve mental status and energy in the final days of life. Most of the time, however, the benefits are difficult to discern, and the excessive fluids may contribute to end-of-life physiologic conditions (edema, ascites, effusions, and pulmonary secretions) that do not improve longevity and may worsen comfort.

As patients become weaker, there is a predictable decrease in the level of consciousness with increasing periods of somnolence eventually giving way to a comatose state. Education about this process should include associated changes in respiratory patterns and anticipation of progressive periods of apnea, interspersed with episodes of hyperpnea and deep breathing (Cheyne-Stokes respirations). During this process caregivers often feel they are on "a roller-coaster ride," and gentle guidance on what to expect can allay concerns. As consciousness wanes, swallowing slows and the cough reflex weakens. As a result, saliva pools in the oropharynx and can result in noisy respiration ("death rattle"), which can usually

be palliated with transdermal scopolamine, glycopyrrolate (given via oral [PO], IV, or SC route), or sublingual atropine ophthalmic drops. Families should be reminded that these symptoms are a natural part of the dying process, and that persistent shortness of breath is relatively uncommon but can be treated with opiates and benzodiazepines if needed.

As death approaches, reduced perfusion causes cooling and cyanosis of the extremities and a decrease in and darkening of the urine. Most deaths are relatively peaceful, but a few can be preceded by periods of intense agitation and restlessness (hyperactive terminal delirium). Antipsychotic medications and conventional doses of benzodiazepines can usually treat terminal delirium. Before and when death occurs, families should be encouraged to carry out cultural or religious rituals that are important to them. Providers should express condolences, be available for questions, and be responsive to intense emotional reactions that sometimes occur. A short condolence card or letter is almost always appreciated. If possible, efforts should be made to follow up with family members and caregivers deemed at risk for complicated bereavement and grief.

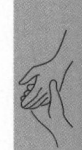

Prospectus for the Future

Palliative care became an officially recognized subspecialty in the United States in 2006. Physicians from 10 specialties can be board certified in hospice and palliative medicine, including family medicine, internal medicine, emergency medicine, pediatrics, physical medicine and rehabilitation, anesthesiology, psychiatry, neurology, radiology, and surgery. As patients live longer with chronic illness, there will be an increasing need to fully integrate palliative care providers and programs within hospitals, in nursing homes, and in the outpatient setting. There is a compelling need for research to better define the optimal timing, setting, and delivery of palliative care to improve the quality of life and lessen the suffering of patients and families with advanced illness.

References

Gazelle G: Understanding hospice—An underutilized option for life's final chapter. N Engl J Med 357:321-324, 2007.

Hudson P, Quinn K, O'Hanlon B, Aranda S: Family meetings in palliative care: Multidisciplinary clinical practice guidelines. BMC Palliat Care 7:12, 2008.

Moryl N, Coyle N, Foley KM: Managing an acute pain crisis in a patient with advanced cancer: "This is as much of a crisis as a code." JAMA 299:1457-1467, 2008.

Quill TE, Holloway RG, Shah MS, et al: Primer of Palliative Care, 5th ed. Glenview, Ill, American Academy of Hospice and Palliative Medicine, 2007.

Walsh D, Caraceni AT, Fainsinger R, et al (eds): Palliative Medicine. Philadelphia, WB Saunders, 2009.

Section XXII

Substance Abuse

Alcohol and Substance Abuse

Richard A. Lange and L. David Hillis

Alcohol Dependence and Abuse

Alcohol dependence and abuse are major public health problems. Seventeen million adults in the United States, about 1 in every 12, abuse alcohol or are alcohol-dependent, and 58 million have participated in binge drinking within the past month. In the United States, alcohol use is the third leading preventable cause of death—exceeded only by cigarette smoking and obesity—and claims over 85,000 lives annually. Alcohol-related liver disease, which affects more than 2 million Americans, is responsible for approximately 13,000 deaths per year. Alcohol use contributes to roughly 30% of all fatalities caused by motor vehicle accidents, or approximately 13,000 vehicular deaths annually, and is a major contributor to risky sexual behavior, domestic violence, homicide, and suicide. For the year 1998, the economic cost of alcohol abuse was estimated to be $185 billion.

Definitions of Alcohol Abuse and Dependence

The American Psychiatric Association has specific criteria for the diagnoses of *alcohol abuse* and *alcohol dependence;* these criteria are described in the *Diagnostic and Statistical Manual of Mental Disorders,* fourth edition, and are listed in Table 135-1. A person can be diagnosed with abuse only if he or she does not fit the criteria for dependence, and a person who meets the criteria for both abuse and dependence is diagnosed with dependence. The so-called *binge drinker* is defined as one who typically consumes five or more drinks on a single occasion. The terms *tolerance* and *dependence* are used to describe a continuum in the adaptation of the central nervous system (CNS) to drug usage. Tolerance may enable the alcoholic to maintain sobriety even in the setting of markedly elevated blood alcohol concentrations. Alcohol dependence is present when the individual has tolerance, withdrawal symptoms, and an uncontrollable urge to consume alcohol (see Table 135-1).

Epidemiologic Factors

Among individuals aged 12 or older, whites are more likely to report current alcohol use than other racial groups (Fig. 135-1), and men are more likely than women to be drinkers (57% versus 46%, respectively). Surveys indicate that approximately 40% of high school seniors and 65% of college students currently use alcohol (Fig. 135-2), and more than one half of all college students admit to heavy episodic drinking. Although the prevalence of ethanol use is highest in individuals younger than 30 years of age, survey data suggest that about two thirds of persons over age 30 consume ethanol.

Pharmacologic and Metabolic Factors

After oral ingestion, alcohol is absorbed predominantly in the small intestine, and its rate of intestinal absorption is accelerated by the simultaneous ingestion of carbohydrates and carbonated beverages. Prolonged retention of alcohol in the stomach, as occurs when food is consumed before drinking, delays alcohol absorption, because absorption in the stomach is considerably slower than in the duodenum. Once in the blood, alcohol equilibrates rapidly across all membranes, including the blood-brain barrier, thereby accounting for the prompt onset of its euphoric effects. Maximal blood alcohol concentrations are reached 45 to 75 minutes after alcohol is ingested.

The liver metabolizes approximately 90% of ethanol to acetaldehyde via the alcohol dehydrogenase pathway; subsequently, acetaldehyde is converted by aldehyde dehydrogenase to acetate, which enters the Krebs cycle. At low or moderate serum concentrations of ethanol, the alcohol dehydrogenase pathway functions almost exclusively in metabolizing ethanol. At high concentrations, the microsomal ethanol oxidizing system contributes to metabolism. Less than 10% of ethanol is excreted unchanged through the skin, kidneys, and lungs. Variability among individuals in

Table 135-1	Criteria for the Diagnosis of Alcohol Abuse and Dependence in a 12-Month Period	
Alcohol Abuse (One or More of the Following)	**Alcohol Dependence (Three or More of the Following)**	
Failure to meet obligations at home, school, or work	Alcohol tolerance: increased consumption as a result of decreased effects of alcohol	
Inappropriate or recurrent use of alcohol in harmful or hazardous situations	Symptoms or signs of alcohol withdrawal	
Evidence of legal problems	Alcohol consumption increases for long periods	
Concerns related to alcohol consumption are ignored or minimized	Attempts to quit typically fail	
	More time is diverted to obtain, use, and recover from use of alcohol	
	Withdrawal from customary social, occupational, and recreational contacts	
	Alcohol abuse continues despite knowledge of psychophysical dependence	

Adapted from the American Psychiatric Association: *Diagnostic and Statistical Manual of Mental Disorders,* 4th ed. Washington, DC, American Psychiatric Press, 2000.

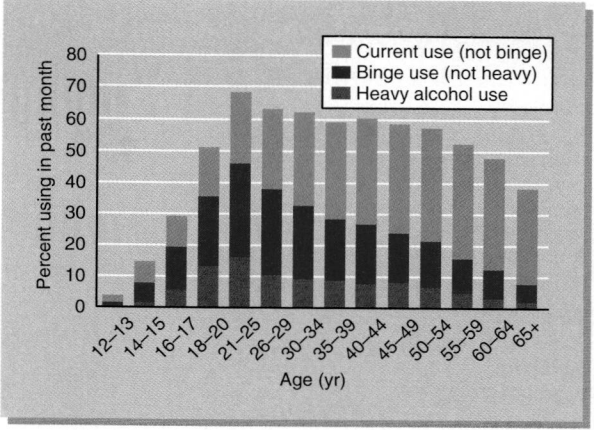

Figure 135-2 Current, binge, and heavy alcohol use among persons aged 12 or older, by age, according to the National Survey on Drug Use and Health (2007). *Binge* drinking is defined as having five or more drinks on a single occasion. *Heavy* alcohol use is defined as having had five or more drinks on the same occasion on each of five or more days in the previous 30 days. (From Substance Abuse and Mental Health Services Administration, Office of Applied Studies: Results from the 2007 National Survey on Drug Use and Health: National Findings. NSDUH Series H-34, DHHS Publication No. SMA 08-4343. Rockville, Md, 2008.)

oxidation of ethanol (in cases of more active alcohol dehydrogenase variants) or slower acetaldehyde oxidation (in cases of less active aldehyde dehydrogenase variants). Acetaldehyde is a toxic substance, the accumulation of which leads to a highly aversive reaction that includes facial flushing, nausea, and tachycardia.

Mechanisms of Alcohol-Induced Organ Damage

The major organs that are susceptible to damage by alcohol are the liver, pancreas, heart, brain, and bone (Table 135-2). Several alcohol-related medical disorders are caused by various nutritional deficiencies; ethanol is deficient in proteins, minerals, and vitamins. Therefore the initial management of the alcoholic must attend to suggested dietary deficiencies (e.g., thiamine) and electrolyte imbalances, including potassium, magnesium, calcium, and zinc.

Alcohol-related liver disease is the leading preventable cause of hepatic failure in the industrialized world. Genetic factors are thought to play a role in susceptibility to this disorder because alcoholic liver disease is more prevalent in whites than in other ethnic groups, despite a similar magnitude of ethanol consumption. The histopathologic features of alcoholic liver disease include fatty infiltration, hepatitis, fibrosis, and end-stage cirrhosis.

Clinical Manifestations of Alcohol Ingestion

ACUTE ALCOHOL INTOXICATION

Mild ethanol intoxication produces slurred speech, ataxia, irregular eye movements, and poor coordination. Signs of

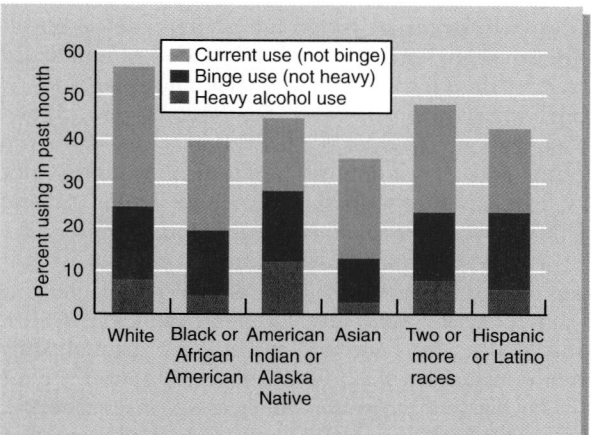

Figure 135-1 Current, binge, and heavy alcohol use among persons aged 12 or older, by race and ethnicity, according to the National Survey on Drug Use and Health (2007). *Binge* drinking is defined as having five or more drinks on a single occasion. *Heavy* alcohol use is defined as having had five or more drinks on the same occasion on each of five or more days in the previous 30 days. (From Substance Abuse and Mental Health Services Administration, Office of Applied Studies: Results from the 2007 National Survey on Drug Use and Health: National Findings. NSDUH Series H-34, DHHS Publication No. SMA 08-4343. Rockville, Md, 2008.)

the efficiency of the alcohol and aldehyde dehydrogenase systems has been observed. These variations have been shown to influence a person's risk of developing alcohol abuse or dependence. The mechanism is thought to involve elevated acetaldehyde levels, resulting from a more rapid

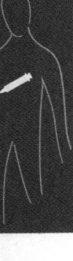

Table 135-2 **Medical Complications of Alcohol Abuse**

Neurologic

Encephalopathy (Wernicke, with oculomotor dysfunction; gait ataxia)
Cognitive dysfunction
Amnesia (i.e., Korsakoff syndrome)
Dementia
Cerebellar degeneration
Peripheral neuropathy

Hematologic

Anemia (often with macrocytosis)
Leukopenia
Thrombocytopenia

Gastrointestinal

Esophagitis
Esophageal varices
Gastritis
Gastrointestinal bleeding
Pancreatitis
Hepatitis
Cirrhosis
Splenomegaly

Cardiovascular

Hypertension
Cardiomyopathy
Stroke
Arrhythmias (especially atrial fibrillation)

Electrolyte or Nutritional

Thiamine deficiency
Hypokalemia
Hypomagnesemia
Ketoacidosis
Hypoglycemia
Hypertriglyceridemia
Malnutrition

Endocrine

Diabetes mellitus
Gynecomastia

Musculoskeletal

Myopathy
Osteoporosis
Testicular atrophy
Amenorrhea
Infertility

Miscellaneous

Spontaneous abortion
Fetal alcohol syndrome
Increased risk of cancer (breast, oropharyngeal, esophageal, hepatocellular)
Accidents, trauma, violence, suicide

CNS depression and associated cerebellar or vestibular dysfunction include dysarthria, ataxia, and nystagmus. Although blood alcohol concentrations are not precisely correlated with the degree of intoxication and the clinical effect of ethanol widely varies among individuals, stupor and coma usually develop at blood concentrations approaching 400 mg/dL, and blood levels of 500 mg/dL often are fatal. However, it is important to understand that death may occur even when the blood alcohol concentration is as low as 300 mg/dL.

WITHDRAWAL SYNDROME (CONVULSIONS)

Alcohol withdrawal occurs in three stages. The signs of minor withdrawal usually appear 6 to 12 hours after the discontinuation of ethanol and are caused by central adrenergic hyperexcitability; they consist of anxiety, tremors, sweating, tachycardia, diarrhea, and insomnia. Additional evidence of autonomic nervous system hyperactivity often appears within 12 to 24 hours and includes increased startle response, nightmares, and visual hallucinations. Alcohol withdrawal seizures (so-called *rum fits*) are generalized clonic-tonic convulsions that occur 12 to 48 hours after the discontinuation of ethanol and are estimated to occur in 2% to 5% of alcoholics.

DELIRIUM TREMENS

Delirium tremens (DTs) is characterized by delirium (a confused state with varying levels of consciousness), hallucinations, tremor (caused by marked autonomic nervous system overactivity), and agitation. It occurs in approximately 5% of alcoholics, most often in chronic heavy abusers with underlying neurologic damage. If unrecognized and untreated, the in-hospital mortality rate of DTs approaches 25%.

Management and Treatment

Intervention strategies in alcohol abusers are designed to modify the individual's attitudes, knowledge, and skills to prevent alcohol misuse. In the outpatient setting, increased frequency of contact between the primary care physician and the patient increases the likelihood of detection, intervention, and prevention of heavy alcohol consumption. All scheduled office visits should include alcohol screening, assessment, and possible brief attempts at intervention (one or more discussions lasting 10 to 15 minutes), as studies show that this approach decreases alcohol intake and its consequences. Behavioral or pharmacologic treatment should be considered, because two thirds of treated patients have a reduction in the amount of consumption (by more than 50%) as well as the consequences of consumption (e.g., alcohol-related injury or job loss). A year after treatment, one third of patients are either abstinent or drink moderately without consequences.

SCREENING AND INTERVENTION STRATEGIES

The National Institute on Alcohol Abuse and Alcoholism (NIAAA) provides several web-based guidelines for alcohol screening during routine health examination (see www.niaaa.nih.gov). A four-step plan exists with which physicians can (1) screen patients for alcohol use, (2) assess for the presence of alcohol-related problems, (3) provide advice concerning appropriate action, and (4) monitor the patient's progress. For the current drinker the physician should inquire about the number of drinks consumed per day,

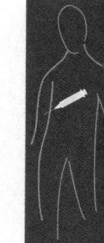

Table 135-3 **CAGE: An Alcoholism Screening Test**
1. Have you ever felt you should *cut* down on your drinking?
2. Have people *annoyed* you by criticizing your drinking?
3. Have you felt *guilty* about your drinking?
4. Have you ever had a drink first thing in the morning to steady your nerves or to get rid of a hangover (i.e., as an *eye-opener*)?

number of days per week on which ethanol is consumed, and total number of drinks consumed per month. Alcohol consumption that exceeds 14 drinks per week or three drinks per day should trigger an in-depth assessment of alcohol-related problems. The physician should ascertain if the individual is at risk for alcohol-related problems, has an existing problem, or may be alcohol-dependent.

The CAGE questionnaire (each of the letters in the acronym refers to one of the questions) (Table 135-3) is a useful screening tool for identifying alcohol-dependent individuals. A positive response to two or more of the four questions is indicative of a potential alcohol problem and should prompt questions regarding the quantity and frequency of consumption. Difficulties with work-related, interpersonal, and family relationships and/or evidence of high-risk behavior despite self-reported low-risk consumption indicate that the individual is at risk for alcohol dependence. To assess for alcohol dependence, the individual should be queried about morning drinking, blackouts, depression, abdominal pain, hypertension, sexual dysfunction, and problems with sleep. If drinking has been associated with legal problems, impaired behavior, feelings of guilt, or trauma, alcohol dependence should be suspected. The patient with alcohol dependence exhibits a compulsion (e.g., a preoccupation) to drink, lack of control once drinking has started, symptoms of withdrawal, drinking to relieve symptoms, and increased tolerance to alcohol. On physical examination, evidence of alcoholic liver disease may be exhibited as jaundice, hepatomegaly, palmar erythema, male gynecomastia, spider angiomata, and ascites. The serum γ-glutamyltransferase concentration typically is elevated in individuals who drink excessively.

LOW-RISK DRINKING

A standard drink contains 12 g of alcohol, an amount similar to that found in one 12-oz bottle of beer or wine cooler, one 5-oz glass of wine, or 1.5 oz of distilled (e.g., 80 proof) spirits. In men older than age 64 and in women, the limit for moderate drinking is one drink per day. For younger men, moderate drinking is defined as no more than two drinks per day. For the same amount of ingested ethanol, women and older adult men achieve a higher blood-ethanol concentration than younger men owing to their smaller volume of body water. A reasonable blood alcohol level should not exceed 50 mg/dL.

A blood-alcohol level as low as 80 mg/dL may exceed the legal definition for driving under the influence (DUI) or driving while intoxicated (DWI). In national surveys the strategy of the *designated driver* appears to be effective at preventing unsafe driving by drinkers at risk for DWI. Complete abstinence is recommended for people with a history of alcohol dependence, other serious medical conditions (e.g., liver disease), and pregnancy.

NONPHARMACOLOGIC THERAPIES

For the foreseeable future, pharmacologic agents will remain complementary and adjunctive to the traditional approaches of abstinence, group therapy, coping mechanisms, and behavior modification. The most widely employed behavioral approach is the 12-step program administered by Alcoholics Anonymous (AA), with which the recovering alcoholic moves through 12 specific steps aided by his or her attendance at regular meetings within a self-help peer group. Cognitive behavioral therapy is based on the principle that the alcoholic first must identify the internal and external cues to drinking so that he or she can develop effective countermeasures for drinking behavior. Motivation enhancement therapy is a four-session, brief-contact intervention program that encourages self awareness and behavioral changes in the alcoholic. These therapies provide similar efficacy.

CONSIDERATIONS FOR DRUG INTERVENTIONS

If desired, medications can be administered in conjunction with behavioral modification. Disulfiram, naltrexone, and acamprosate have been approved by the U.S. Food and Drug Administration (FDA) for adjunctive therapy.

Disulfiram (Antabuse) inhibits aldehyde dehydrogenase (i.e., the enzyme that converts acetaldehyde to acetate), resulting in a 5- to 10-fold increase in serum acetaldehyde concentrations when alcohol is consumed. This produces uncomfortable symptoms (e.g., facial flushing, tachycardia, nausea, vomiting, and headache), which act to deter alcohol consumption. Because of low medication compliance and limited efficacy, disulfiram is rarely prescribed.

Naltrexone, an opioid antagonist used for the treatment of opiate addiction, is the first medication to be approved by the FDA for the treatment of alcoholism in over 50 years. In clinical trials a combination of naltrexone and psychosocial intervention reduced the number of drinking days, induced a longer period of abstinence from ethanol, and decreased the relapse rate in heavy drinkers when compared with psychosocial intervention alone. Naltrexone is administered in a dose of 50 mg daily for 12 weeks, although larger doses (i.e., 100 to 150 mg daily) and a longer duration of administration may improve its success in preventing relapse. Some recovering alcoholics develop nausea when it is initiated. Because hepatic toxicity may occur at high doses (300 mg), periodic testing of liver function is recommended. Naltrexone is contraindicated in patients receiving opioids, given that opiate withdrawal is an unintended adverse effect of the drug.

Nalmefene, an opiate antagonist, has a mechanism of action similar to that of naltrexone, but the FDA has yet to approve nalmefene for the treatment of alcohol abuse. In placebo-controlled trials, nalmefene was substantially better than placebo at reducing the rate of relapse in heavy drinkers. In comparison with naltrexone, hepatotoxicity occurs less often.

Acamprosate (Campral) is a structural analog of γ-aminobutyric acid (GABA). It decreases excitatory glutaminergic neurotransmission during alcohol withdrawal. The recommended dosage of Campral is 666 to 1000 mg 3 times a day, and its most common side effects are diarrhea and intestinal cramping. In placebo-controlled trials involving more than 4600 alcoholic patients, acamprosate reduced relapse rates and increased abstinence from ethanol. In comparative trials it did not appear to be as efficacious as naltrexone. Because the liver does not metabolize acamprosate, it is safe in persons with alcoholic liver disease.

Several other drugs have been associated with a reduction in alcohol consumption, including ondansetron (a selective serotonin reuptake inhibitor), topiramate (an anticonvulsant), baclofen (a GABA agonist), and varenicline (a nicotinic acetylcholine-receptor and dopamine partial agonist), but they are not yet approved by the FDA for treatment of alcohol dependence.

FETAL ALCOHOL SPECTRUM DISORDERS

Alcohol freely crosses the placenta and is teratogenic. It is a leading preventable cause of birth defects with mental deficiency, with up to 1 in 100 children in the United States being born with fetal alcohol spectrum disorders (FASDs). The scope of disabilities and malformations varies and depends on the amount of alcohol consumed, the frequency of exposure, the stage of fetal development when alcohol is present, maternal parity, nutrition, and individual variation in maternal and fetal alcohol metabolism.

The term *fetal alcohol spectrum disorders* is used to characterize the full range of prenatal alcohol damage varying from mild to severe and encompassing a broad array of physical defects and cognitive, behavioral, and emotional deficits. It includes conditions such as fetal alcohol syndrome (FAS), alcohol-related neurodevelopmental disorder (ARND), and alcohol-related birth defects (ARBDs).

FAS, the most severe form of FASD, is characterized by growth retardation, neurodevelopmental abnormalities (i.e., microcephaly, hyperactivity, irritability, altered motor skills, learning disabilities, seizure disorders, and mental retardation), and dysmorphic facial features, including short palpebral fissures, flat midface, short nose, smooth philtrum, and a thin upper lip. Children with typical dysmorphic facial features who lack the other features have partial FAS. Children with ARBDs have typical facies associated with FAS and anomalies in other organs (i.e., cardiac, renal, skeletal, auditory) but no growth retardation or neurodevelopmental abnormalities. Children with ARND exhibit behavioral or cognitive abnormalities in the absence of dysmorphic facial features.

Although the damage from prenatal exposure to alcohol cannot be reversed, children with FASDs benefit from early diagnosis and aggressive intervention with physical, occupational, speech and language, and educational therapies Early recognition can also benefit the impaired mother, resulting in access to alcohol treatment and a better social situation for the entire family.

The diagnosis of FASD is important, but prevention is the answer. Given that no safely established level of alcohol consumption in pregnancy exists, recommendations suggest that pregnant women maintain abstinence. In addition, women who are considering pregnancy or are already pregnant must be counseled about the effects of alcohol on the fetus.

MEDICAL MANAGEMENT OF ALCOHOL WITHDRAWAL AND DELIRIUM TREMENS

For the patient with probable alcohol withdrawal, comorbid conditions that may coexist or mimic the symptoms of withdrawal (e.g., infection, trauma, hepatic encephalopathy, meningitis, drug overdose, metabolic derangements) should be excluded. Once these conditions have been excluded, the patient should be placed in a quiet and protective environment and should receive parenteral thiamine and multivitamins to decrease the risk of Wernicke encephalopathy or Korsakoff amnestic syndrome. Benzodiazepines are the only medications proved to ameliorate symptoms and to decrease the risk of seizures and DTs in patients with alcohol withdrawal. Typically, diazepam (5 to 20 mg), chlordiazepoxide (50 to 100 mg), or lorazepam (1 to 2 mg) is administered intravenously every 5 to 10 minutes until symptoms subside, with the last of these medications preferred in patients with advanced cirrhosis, considering that the liver minimally metabolizes it. Continued administration of a benzodiazepine with a fixed-interval approach (i.e., administered even if symptoms are absent) or a symptom-driven approach typically continues for 24 to 72 hours. All benzodiazepines appear to be similarly efficacious in treating alcohol withdrawal, but long-acting agents may be more effective in preventing withdrawal seizures and are associated with fewer rebound symptoms. Conversely, short-acting agents may offer a lower risk of oversedation. For the patient who is resistant to benzodiazepines, intravenous phenobarbital (130 to 260 mg administered intravenously every 15 minutes) may be given.

Prescription Drug Abuse

According to the National Survey on Drug Use and Health, an estimated 19.9 million Americans aged 12 years or older were current illicit drug users in 2007, meaning they had used prescription drugs for nonmedical purposes or illicit drugs within 1 month of the survey interview (Fig. 135-3). This estimate of current illicit drug users represents 8% of the population aged 12 years or older. Marijuana was the most commonly used illicit drug: 53% of illicit drug users used marijuana only, 27% used drugs other than marijuana (including sedatives, hypnotics, stimulants, hallucinogens, and inhalants), and 19% used both.

SEDATIVES AND HYPNOTICS

Benzodiazepines and barbiturates are the major sedative-hypnotic drugs among the commonly abused drugs that are listed in Table 135-4. The patient with sedative-hypnotic intoxication may have slurred speech, incoordination,

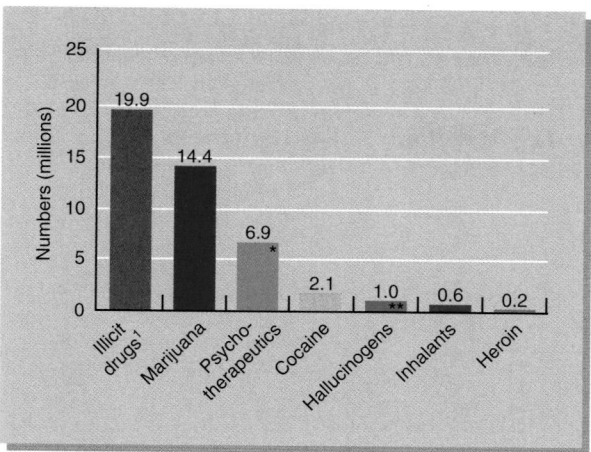

Figure 135-3 Past-month illicit drug use among persons aged 12 or older, according to the National Survey on Drug Use and Health (2007). (From Substance Abuse and Mental Health Services Administration, Office of Applied Studies: Results from the 2007 National Survey on Drug Use and Health: National Findings. NSDUH Series H-34, DHHS Publication No. SMA 08-4343. Rockville, Md, 2008.)

unsteady gait, impaired attention or memory, stupor, and coma. The psychiatric manifestations of intoxication include inappropriate behavior, labile mood, and impaired judgment and social functioning. On physical examination the person may have respiratory depression or even arrest, nystagmus, and hyperreflexia. Although benzodiazepines rarely depress respiration to the extent that barbiturates do (and, as a result, have a much wider margin of safety), the effects of these drugs are additive with those of other CNS depressants, such as ethanol. Chronic use may produce physical and psychological dependence and a potentially dangerous withdrawal syndrome.

Benzodiazepines potentiate the effects of GABA, which inhibits neurotransmission. They are available as short-acting agents (temazepam [Restoril] and triazolam [Halcion]), intermediate-acting agents (alprazolam [Xanax], chlordiazepoxide [Librium], estazolam [ProSom], lorazepam [Ativan], and oxazepam [Serax]), and long-acting agents (clorazepate [Tranxene], clonazepam [Klonopin], diazepam [Valium], flurazepam [Dalmane], halazepam [Paxipam], Prazepam [Centrax], and quazepam [Doral]).

Table 135-4 Commonly Abused Drugs

Substance: Category and Name	Examples of Commercial and Street Names	How Administered*	Intoxication Effects and Potential Health Consequences
Cannabinoids			Euphoria, slowed thinking and reaction time, drowsiness, inattention, confusion, impaired balance and coordination, enhanced perception; cough, frequent respiratory infections; impaired memory and learning; increased heart rate, anxiety; panic attacks; tolerance, addiction
Hashish	Boom, chronic, gangster, hash, hash oil, hemp	Smoked, swallowed	
Marijuana	Blunt, dope, ganja, grass, herb, joints, Mary Jane, pot, reefer, sinsemilla, skunk, weed	Swallowed, smoked	
Sedative-Hypnotics (CNS Depressants)			Reduced pain and anxiety, feeling of well-being, lowered inhibitions, labile mood, impaired judgment, poor concentration, fatigue, confusion, impaired coordination and memory, respiratory depression and arrest, addiction
Benzodiazepines (other than flunitrazepam)	Restoril, Halcion, Xanax, Librium, ProSom, Ativan, Serax, Tranxene, Klonopin, Valium, Dalmane, Doral; candy, downers, sleeping pills, tranks	Swallowed	Sedation, drowsiness, dizziness

Continued

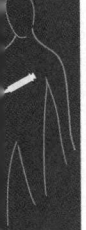

Table 135-4 Commonly Abused Drugs—Cont'd

Substance: Category and Name	Examples of Commercial and Street Names	How Administered	Intoxication Effects and Potential Health Consequences
Flunitrazepam[†]	Rohypnol; forget-me pill, Mexican Valium, R2, Roche, roofies, roofinol, rope, rophies	Swallowed, snorted	Visual and gastrointestinal disturbances, urinary retention, amnesia while under drug's effects
Barbiturates	Amytal, Nembutal, Seconal, phenobarbital; barbs, reds, red birds, phennies, tooies, yellows, yellow jackets	Injected, swallowed	Sedation, drowsiness, depression, unusual excitement, fever, irritability, poor judgment, slurred speech, dizziness
GHB[†]	γ-hydroxybutyrate; G, Georgia home boy, grievous bodily harm, liquid ecstasy	Swallowed	Drowsiness, dizziness, nausea and vomiting, headache, loss of consciousness, hallucinations, peripheral vision loss, nystagmus, loss of reflexes, seizures, coma, death
Dissociative Anesthetics			Increased heart rate and blood pressure; impaired function, memory motor loss, numbness, nausea and vomiting
PCP and analogues	Phencyclidine; angel dust, boat, hog, love boat, peace pill	Injected, swallowed, smoked	Possible decrease in blood pressure and heart rate; panic, aggression, violence, suicidal ideation; loss of appetite, depression
Ketamine*	Ketalar SV; cat Valiums, K, Special K, vitamin K	Injected, snorted, smoked	At high doses: delirium, depression, respiratory depression and arrest, amnesia while under drug's effects
Hallucinogens			Altered states of perception and feeling, nausea, chronic mental disorders, persisting perception disorder (flashbacks)
LSD	Lysergic acid diethylamide; acid, blotter, boomers, cubes, microdot, yellow sunshines	Swallowed, absorbed through mouth tissues	Also, for LSD and mescaline: increased body temperature, heart rate, blood pressure; loss of appetite; sleeplessness, numbness, weakness, tremors
Mescaline	Buttons, cactus, mesc, peyote	Swallowed, smoked	
Opioids and Morphine Derivatives			Pain relief, euphoria, drowsiness, respiratory depression and arrest, pinpoint pupils, nausea, confusion, constipation, sedation, unconsciousness, seizures, coma, tolerance, addiction
Codeine or oxycodone	Empirin with Codeine, Fiorinal with Codeine, Robitussin A-C, Tylenol with Codeine, OxyContin, Roxicodone, Vicodin; Captain Cody, Cody, schoolboy (with glutethimide), doors and fours, loads, pancakes and syrup	Injected, swallowed	Less analgesia, sedation, and respiratory depression than morphine

Table 135-4 **Commonly Abused Drugs—Cont'd**

Substance: Category and Name	Examples of Commercial and Street Names	How Administered	Intoxication Effects and Potential Health Consequences
Fentanyl	Actiq, Duragesic, Sublimaze; Apache, China girl, China white, dance fever, friend, goodfella, jackpot, murder 8, TNT, Tango and Cash	Injected, smoked, snorted	
Heroin	Diacetylmorphine; brown sugar, dope, H, horse, junk, skag, skunk, smack, white horse	Injected, smoked, snorted	Staggering gait
Morphine or meperidine	Roxanol, Duramorph, Demerol; M, Miss Emma, monkey, white stuff	Injected, swallowed, smoked	
Opium	Laudanum, paregoric; big O, black stuff, block, gum, hop	Swallowed, smoked	
Stimulants			Increased heart rate, blood pressure, metabolism; feelings of exhilaration, energy, increased mental alertness, rapid or irregular heart beat; reduced appetite, weight loss, heart failure, seizures, coma
Amphetamine	Adderall, Biphetamine, Dexedrine; bennies, black beauties, crosses, hearts, LA turnaround, speed, truck drivers, uppers	Injected, swallowed, smoked, snorted	Rapid breathing, paranoia, hallucinations, tremors, loss of coordination, irritability, anxiety, restlessness, delirium, panic, impulsive behavior, aggressiveness, Parkinson disease, tolerance, addiction
Methamphetamine	Desoxyn; chalk, crank, crystal, fire, glass, go fast, ice, meth, speed	Injected, smoked, snorted	Aggression, violence, psychotic behavior, memory loss, cardiac and neurologic damage, impaired memory and learning, tolerance, addiction
Methylphenidate	Ritalin; JIF, MPH, R-ball, Skippy, the smart drug, vitamin R	Injected, swallowed, snorted	Increase or decrease in blood pressure, psychotic episodes, digestive problems, loss of appetite, weight loss
Cocaine	Cocaine hydrochloride; blow, bump, C, candy, Charlie, coke, crack, flake, rock, snow, toot	Injected, smoked, snorted	Increased temperature, chest pain, respiratory failure, nausea, abdominal pain, stroke, seizures, malnutrition
MDMA† (methylenedioxymethamphetamine)	DOB, DOM, MBDB, MDA; Adam, clarity, ecstasy, Eve, lover's speed, peace, Methyl-J, Eden, STP, X, XTC	Swallowed	Mild hallucinogenic effects, hallucinations, paranoia, increased tactile sensitivity, empathic feelings, nystagmus, ataxia, tremor, hyperthermia, impaired memory and learning

Continued

Table 135-4 **Commonly Abused Drugs—Cont'd**			
Substance: Category and Name	**Examples of Commercial and Street Names**	**How Administered**	**Intoxication Effects and Potential Health Consequences**
Other Compounds			Stimulation, loss of inhibition, headache, nausea or vomiting, slurred speech, loss of motor coordination, wheezing, unconsciousness, cramps, weight loss, muscle weakness, depression, memory impairment, damage to cardiovascular and nervous systems, sudden death
Inhalants	Solvents (paint thinners, gasoline), glues, gases (butane, propane, aerosol propellants, nitrous oxide), nitrites (isoamyl, isobutyl, cyclohexyl); laughing gas, poppers, snappers, whippets	Inhaled through nose or mouth	

*Taking drugs by injection can increase the risk of infection through needle contamination with staphylococci, human immunodeficiency virus, hepatitis, and other organisms.
†Associated with sexual assaults (e.g., *date rapes*).
CNS, central nervous system.

Flunitrazepam (Rohypnol, also known as *roach, roofies, circles, Mexican valium,* or *rope*) is a popularly abused benzodiazepine that is not legally available in the United States but is often smuggled here from other countries. Flunitrazepam has been implicated in cases of *date rape* and is known as a *club drug* because adolescents and young adults often use it at nightclubs and bars or during all-night dance parties called *raves.*

In persons with an acute benzodiazepine overdose, respiratory depression is the major danger. Flumazenil (Romazicon), a competitive antagonist of benzodiazepines, can be given intravenously for acute overdose. Although it reverses the sedative effects of benzodiazepines, flumazenil may not completely reverse respiratory depression, and it may cause seizures in patients with physical dependence or concurrent tricyclic antidepressant poisoning.

Benzodiazepine cessation may precipitate withdrawal symptoms, depending on the half-life of the benzodiazepine, the duration of use, and the dose. Such withdrawal is characterized by intense anxiety, insomnia, irritability, perceptual changes, hypersensitivity to light and sound, psychosis, hallucinations, palpitations, hyperthermia, tachypnea, diarrhea, muscle spasms, tremors, and seizures. Withdrawal symptoms usually peak 2 to 4 days after the discontinuation of a short-acting agent and 5 to 6 days after discontinuation of a longer-acting one; however, panic attacks and nightmares may recur for months. In general, agents with shorter half-lives produce more intense withdrawal symptoms compared with agents with longer half-lives. Detoxification requires a change to a longer-acting benzodiazepine (e.g., clonazepam, diazepam) or phenobarbital and a tapering regimen of 7 to 10 days for short-acting agents or 10 to 14

days for longer-acting ones. For hemodynamically unstable patients who require very rapid medication titration to control withdrawal symptoms and for those with severe hepatic failure, short-acting medications are indicated in lieu of phenobarbital. Propranolol can be given to decrease tachycardia, hypertension, and anxiety.

Barbiturates may be short acting (pentobarbital and secobarbital), intermediate acting (amobarbital, aprobarbital, and butabarbital), or long acting (mephobarbital and phenobarbital). The symptoms of acute intoxication with and withdrawal from barbiturates are similar to those of benzodiazepines. For acute barbiturate overdose, oral charcoal and alkalinization of the urine (to a pH >7.5) with forced diuresis are effective in lowering the blood concentration. For patients with hemodynamic compromise refractory to aggressive supportive therapy, barbiturate elimination can be increased by hemodialysis or charcoal hemoperfusion. The effective treatment of withdrawal symptoms requires estimating the daily dose of the abused drug and substituting an equivalent phenobarbital dose to stabilize the patient, after which the dose of phenobarbital is tapered over 4 to 14 days, depending on the half-life of the abused drug. Benzodiazepines may also be used for detoxification, and propranolol and clonidine may help reduce symptoms.

Abuse of γ-hydroxybutyrate (GHB) has increased substantially over the last decade in the United States. This drug is abused for its sedative, euphoric, and bodybuilding effects. GHB is a metabolite of the neurotransmitter GABA, and it also influences the dopaminergic system. It potentiates the effects of endogenous or exogenous opiates. The ingestion of GHB results in immediate drowsiness and dizziness, with the feeling of a *high.* These effects can be potentiated by the concomitant use of alcohol or benzodiazepines. Similar to flunitrazepam and ketamine, GHB is a popular club drug, and it has been implicated in cases of date rape. Its street names include *G, liquid E, liquid X, fantasy, Georgia home boy, and grievous bodily harm.* Adverse effects that may occur within 15 to 60 minutes of its ingestion include headache, nausea, vomiting, hallucinations, loss of peripheral vision, nystagmus, hypoventilation, cardiac dysrhythmias, seizures, and coma. In rare instances these adverse effects have led to death. The withdrawal from GHB becomes clinically apparent within 12 hours and may last up to 12 days.

OPIOIDS

Opioids include the natural and semisynthetic alkaloid derivatives of opium, as well as the purely synthetic drugs that mimic heroin. They bind to opioid receptors in the brain, spinal cord, and gastrointestinal tract; in addition, they act on several other CNS neurotransmitter systems, including dopamine, GABA, and glutamate, to produce analgesia, CNS depression, and euphoria. With continued opioid use, tolerance and physical dependence develop. As a result, the user must use larger amounts of the drug to obtain the desired effect, and withdrawal symptoms may occur if use is discontinued. The commonly abused opioids include heroin, morphine, codeine, oxycodone (OxyContin or Roxicodone), meperidine (Demerol), propoxyphene (Darvon), hydrocodone (Vicodin), hydromorphone (Dilaudid), buprenorphine (Temgesic) and fentanyl (Sublimaze). Intravenous heroin use, particularly when combined with cocaine (a so-called *speedball*), is increasing in the United States. The controlled-release pain reliever OxyContin was made available for use in 1995. By 2001, OxyContin was the most prescribed brand-name narcotic and was frequently diverted for illicit use, in which it was ingested orally, inhaled, or dissolved in water and administered intravenously to obtain an immediate high. In 2002, buprenorphine (Subutex) was made available in the United States for use in opiate addiction therapy. Unlike methadone, which must be dispensed from a clinic, buprenorphine can simply be prescribed by a physician. As a result, its illicit use has increased substantially.

Acute opioid overdose produces pulmonary congestion, with resultant cyanosis and respiratory distress, and changes in mental status that may progress to coma. Other manifestations include fever, pinpoint pupils, and seizures. Unsterile intravenous practices can lead to skin abscesses, cellulitis, thrombophlebitis, wound botulism, meningitis, rhabdomyolysis, endocarditis, hepatitis, or human immunodeficiency virus (HIV) infection. Neurologic complications from intravenous heroin use include transverse myelitis, inflammatory polyneuropathy, and peripheral nerve lesions.

For acute opioid overdose, the patient's respiratory status must be assessed and supported. Naloxone should be administered intravenously and repeated at 2- to 3-minute intervals, often in escalating doses. The patient should respond within minutes with increases in pupil size, respiratory rate, and level of alertness. If no response occurs, opioid overdose is excluded, and other causes of somnolence and respiratory depression must be considered. Naloxone should be titrated carefully because it may precipitate acute withdrawal symptoms in opioid-dependent patients.

Withdrawal symptoms may appear as early as 6 to 10 hours after the last injection of heroin. Initially the individual often has feelings of drug craving, anxiety, restlessness, irritability, rhinorrhea, lacrimation, diaphoresis, and yawning; these signs are followed by dilated pupils, piloerection, anorexia, nausea, vomiting, diarrhea, abdominal cramps, bone pain, myalgias, tremors, muscle spasms, and, in rare cases, seizures. These symptoms and signs peak at 36 to 48 hours and then subside over 5 to 10 days, if untreated. A protracted abstinence syndrome characterized by bradycardia, hypotension, mild anxiety, sleep disturbance, and decreased responsiveness may occur for up to 5 months.

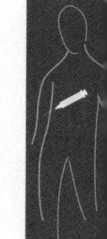

Withdrawal from opioids can be managed with methadone, a long-acting synthetic agonist drug; withdrawal symptoms of methadone develop more slowly and are less severe than those caused by heroin. Methadone can be given twice daily and tapered over 7 to 10 days. Alternatively, levo-α-acetylmethadol (LAAM), a long-acting agonist, or buprenorphine, a partial agonist, can be given. The latter is combined with naloxone in a formulation (Suboxone) developed to decrease the potential for abuse. Clonidine reduces autonomic hyperactivity and is particularly effective if combined with a benzodiazepine.

Patients with repeated relapses can be maintained on methadone or LAAM. Buprenorphine may also be used as maintenance therapy. Naltrexone is a long-acting opioid antagonist that blocks impulsive opioid use. It can be given daily or two to three times weekly, but only after the patient is thoroughly detoxified because it may precipitate withdrawal. Pharmacotherapy must be combined with psychotherapy and structured rehabilitation to achieve an optimal outcome.

AMPHETAMINES

Amphetamines have been used therapeutically for weight reduction and treatment of attention-deficit disorder and narcolepsy. Similar to cocaine, they cause a release of monoamine neurotransmitters (dopamine, norepinephrine, and serotonin) from presynaptic neurons. In addition, however, they have neurotoxic effects on dopaminergic and serotonergic neurons. Their euphoric and reinforcing effects are mediated through dopamine and the mesolimbic system, whereas their cardiovascular effects are caused by the release of norepinephrine. Chronic use leads to neuronal degeneration in dopamine-rich areas of the brain, which may increase the risk for the eventual development of Parkinson disease.

Amphetamines can be abused orally, intranasally, intravenously, or by smoking. The most frequently used drugs are dextroamphetamine (Dexedrine), methamphetamine (Desoxyn), and methylphenidate (Ritalin). Methamphetamine is known on the street as *ice, crank, meth, crystal, tina, glass, and yaa baa.* Recently the illicit use of amphetamines has increased substantially, in part because (1) it is easily and quickly synthesized from ephedrine or pseudoephedrine (Fig. 135-4), and (2) its psychotropic effects persist for up to 24 hours. The anorexiants phenmetrazine and phentermine, which are structurally and pharmacologically similar to amphetamine, also have been used illicitly.

Tolerance to the stimulant effects of amphetamines develops rapidly, and toxic effects can occur with higher doses. Acute amphetamine toxicity is characterized by excessive

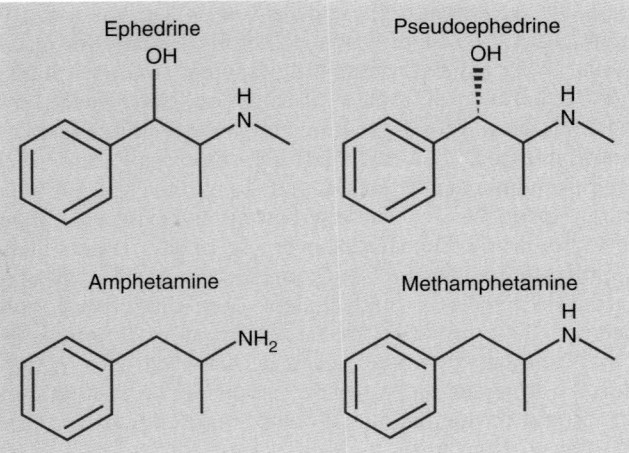

Figure 135-4 The chemical structures of amphetamine and methamphetamine, which can be easily manufactured from ephedrine or pseudoephedrine given that they are structurally similar and widely available.

sympathomimetic effects, including tachycardia, hypertension, hyperthermia, cardiac arrhythmias, tremors, seizures, and coma. The patient may experience irritability, hypervigilance, paranoia, stereotyped compulsive behavior, and tactile, visual, or auditory hallucinations. The clinical picture may simulate an acute schizophrenic psychosis. The symptoms of withdrawal are similar to those seen with cocaine (described in the next section), but the acute psychosis and paranoia are often significantly pronounced.

The treatment of amphetamine abuse centers on a quiet environment, benzodiazepines for anxiety, and sodium nitroprusside for severe hypertension. Antipsychotics, such as haloperidol, can reduce the agitation and psychosis by blocking dopamine's effects on the CNS receptor. Urine acidification with ammonium chloride accelerates amphetamine excretion.

Illicit Drug Abuse

COCAINE

Cocaine use has increased dramatically among adolescents and young adults. Among individuals 12 years old or older in 2007, 2.1 million had used cocaine within the previous month and 906,000 had used it for the first time within the previous 12 months, which averages to about 2500 initiates per day. It is a frequent cause of drug-related visits to emergency rooms. Cocaine can be taken orally or intravenously; alternatively, because it is well absorbed through all mucous membranes, abusers may achieve a high blood concentration after intranasal, sublingual, vaginal, or rectal administration. Its freebase form—called *crack* because of the popping sound it makes when heated—is heat stable so that it can be smoked. Crack cocaine is considered to be the most potent and addictive form of the drug. Euphoria occurs within seconds after crack cocaine is smoked and is short lived. Compared with smoking of crack cocaine or the intravenous injection of the drug, mucosal administration results in a slower onset of action, a later peak effect, and a longer duration of action. The blood half-life is approximately

1 hour. The drug's major metabolite is benzoylecgonine, which can be detected in the urine for 2 to 3 days after a single dose.

An intense, pleasurable reaction lasting 20 to 30 minutes occurs after cocaine use, after which rebound depression, agitation, insomnia, and anorexia occur, which are then followed by fatigue, hypersomnolence, and hyperphagia (the *crash*). This crash usually lasts 9 to 12 hours but occasionally may last up to 4 days. Users often ingest the drug repetitively at relatively short intervals to recapture the euphoric state and to avoid the crash. On occasion, sedatives or alcohol are ingested concomitantly to reduce the intensity of anxiety and irritability associated with the crash. The combination of cocaine and intravenously administered heroin (so-called *speedball, snowball, Belushi,* or *dynamite*) is frequently used so that the abuser can experience the cocaine-induced euphoria and then *float* down on the opiate. Unfortunately, this combination has been reported to cause sudden death. People who use cocaine in temporal proximity to the ingestion of ethanol produce the metabolite cocaethylene, which has also been implicated in cocaine-related deaths.

Cocaine blocks the presynaptic reuptake of norepinephrine and dopamine, producing an excess of these neurotransmitters at the site of the postsynaptic receptor. Thus cocaine acts as a powerful sympathomimetic agent, resulting in tachycardia, hypertension, tachypnea, hyperthermia, agitation, pupillary dilation, peripheral vasoconstriction, and seizures. Cocaine causes potent vasoconstriction of cerebral arteries and therefore may result in a stroke. It is associated with myocardial ischemia and arrhythmias and, in rare cases, with myocardial infarction in young persons with normal or nearly normal coronary arteries. The principal mechanisms of ischemia and infarction are coronary arterial vasoconstriction, thrombosis, platelet aggregation, tissue plasminogen activator inhibition, increased myocardial oxygen demand, and accelerated atherosclerosis (Fig. 135-5).

For patients with cocaine-induced hypertension or tachycardia, labetalol and benzodiazepines are usually effective in lowering systemic arterial pressure and heart rate. Patients with acute myocardial infarction should receive aspirin, heparin, nitroglycerin, and, if indicated, reperfusion therapy (with a thrombolytic agent or primary coronary intervention). The use of β-adrenergic blockers should be avoided because ischemia may be worsened by unopposed α-adrenergically mediated coronary arterial vasoconstriction. Patients with a normal electrocardiogram or nonspecific changes can be managed safely with observation.

The immediate treatment of acute cocaine intoxication includes obtaining vascular and airway access, if needed, and careful electrocardiographic monitoring. Benzodiazepines can be given to control CNS agitation, and haloperidol or risperidone can be used in the severely agitated patient. A supportive environment is needed, but detoxification is not required, given that few physical signs of true dependence are present.

Most chronic cocaine abusers have psychological dependence and an intense craving for cocaine. Personal and group therapies are important adjuncts to pharmacologic treatment, but relapse is common and is difficult to manage. Although no medication is FDA approved for treatment of cocaine addiction, disulfiram, modafinil, anticonvulsants

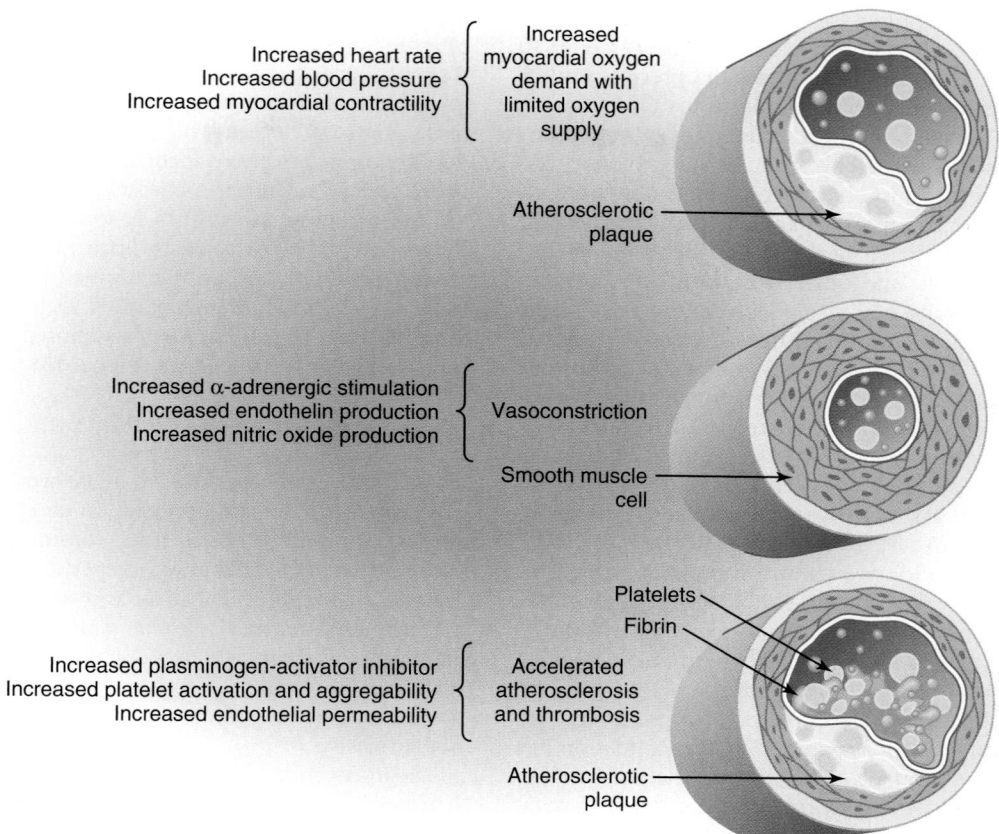

Figure 135-5 The mechanisms by which cocaine may induce myocardial ischemia or infarction. Cocaine may cause increases in the determinants of myocardial oxygen demand when oxygen supply is limited *(top)*, when intense vasoconstriction of the coronary arteries occurs *(middle)*, or when accelerated atherosclerosis and thrombosis are present *(bottom)*.

(e.g., topiramate and tiagabine), serotonin reuptake inhibitors (e.g., citalopram), serotonin receptor antagonists (e.g., ondansetron), and GABA receptor agonists (e.g., baclofen) have shown some promise in promoting cocaine abstinence. More recent research is focused on so-called *vaccine strategies*, whereby protein-conjugated analogues of cocaine would be administered to produce anti-cocaine antibodies that bind cocaine, thereby preventing its passage across the blood-brain barrier.

CANNABIS

The cannabinoid drugs include marijuana (the dried flowering tops and stems of the hemp plant) and hashish (a resinous extract of the hemp plant). Marijuana is the illicit drug with the highest rate of dependence or abuse. Of the 6.9 million persons in the United States with dependence on or abuse of illicit drugs in 2007, 3.9 million were dependent on or abused marijuana or hashish (representing 1.6% of the total population aged 12 years old or older). Marijuana and hashish are among the drugs most commonly used by adolescents, with approximately one half of 12th graders admitting use at least once and 20% reporting that they are current users. Most of their pharmacologic effects come from metabolites of δ-9-tetrahydrocannabinol, which bind to specific cannabinoid receptors located in the CNS, spinal cord, and peripheral nervous system. The primary mode of use is smoking, with mood-altering

and intoxicating effects noted within 3 minutes and peak effects in approximately 1 hour. The acute physiologic effects are dose related and often include increased heart rate, conjunctival congestion, dry mouth, fine tremor, muscle weakness, and ataxia. Psychoactive effects include euphoria, enhanced perception of colors and sounds, drowsiness, inattentiveness, and inability to learn new facts. Tolerance and physical dependence occur, and chronic users may experience mild withdrawal symptoms of irritability, restlessness, anorexia, insomnia, or mild hyperthermia. Rarely, acute psychosis with panic reactions occurs. The treatment of withdrawal is supportive and includes reassurance; benzodiazepines may be used in severely agitated patients. Cannabinoids have been used as antiemetic agents in patients with cancer receiving chemotherapy, for weight stimulation (in patients with cancer or HIV infection), and in the treatment of glaucoma.

HALLUCINOGENS AND DISSOCIATIVE DRUGS

Hallucinogens (drugs that cause hallucinations) include lysergic acid diethylamide (LSD), mescaline, psilocybin, and ibogaine. *Dissociative drugs* distort perceptions of sight and sound and produce feelings of detachment—dissociation—without causing hallucinations. They include phencyclidine (PCP), ketamine, and dextromethorphan (a widely available cough suppressant).

LSD is the most potent of the hallucinogenic drugs. Although it is known to interact with serotonin receptors in the cerebral cortex and *locus ceruleus,* the precise psychoactive mechanism is unknown. Within 30 minutes of its oral ingestion, sympathomimetic effects appear, including mydriasis, hyperthermia, tachycardia, elevated blood pressure, diaphoresis, dry mouth, increased alertness, tremors, and nausea. Within 2 hours, the psychoactive effects become apparent, with heightened perceptions (highly intensified colors, smells, sounds, and other sensations), body distortions, mood variations, and visual hallucinations. An acute panic reaction may occur, sometimes leading to self-injury or suicide. After approximately 12 hours, the syndrome begins to subside, but fatigue and tension may persist for another day. Flashbacks (brief recurrences of the hallucinations) may occur days or even weeks after the last dose but tend to disappear without treatment. Acute panic reactions are best treated in a supportive environment; benzodiazepines can be given to severely agitated patients.

PCP is a potent addictive hallucinogen that produces a prompt stimulant effect similar to that of amphetamines, with feelings of euphoria, power, and invincibility. Patients may have hypertension, tachycardia, hyperthermia, bidirectional nystagmus, slurred speech, ataxia, hallucinations, extreme agitation, and rhabdomyolysis. With more severe reactions, patients may be brought to medical attention in a coma-like state, with open eyes and pupils that are partially dilated, a decreased pain response, brief periods of excitation, and muscle rigidity. On occasion, patients may have hypertensive urgency, seizures, and bizarre (often violent) behavior, which lead to suicide or extreme violence toward others. Tolerance and mild withdrawal symptoms have been seen in daily users, but the major problem is drug craving. Treatment entails a quiet environment, sedation with benzodiazepines, hydration, haloperidol for terrifying hallucinations, and suicide precautions. Continuous gastric suction and acidification of the urine with intravenous ammonium chloride or ascorbic acid may aid in the drug's excretion, but acidification may increase the risk of renal failure if rhabdomyolysis is present.

Ketamine is a rapidly acting general anesthetic; unlike most anesthetics, it produces only mild respiratory depression and appears to stimulate the cardiovascular system. Adverse effects, including delirium and hallucinations, limit the use of ketamine as a general anesthetic in humans. Similar to PCP, ketamine is a dissociative anesthetic. In addition, it has both analgesic and amnestic properties and is associated with less confusion, irrationality, and violent behavior than PCP. Ketamine is one of the club drugs that has been implicated in date rape.

INHALANTS

The inhalants may be classified as (1) *organic solvents,* including toluene (airplane glue and spray paint), paint thinners, kerosene, gasoline, carbon tetrachloride, shoe polish, acetone (nail polish removers and Liquid Paper), xylene (permanent markers), and degreasers (dry cleaning fluids); (2) *gases,* such as butane, propane, aerosol propellants, and anesthetics (ether, chloroform, halothane, and nitrous oxide); and (3) *nitrites,* such as cyclohexyl nitrite, amyl nitrite, and butyl nitrite (room deodorizer). These drugs are most often inhaled by children or young adolescents, after which they produce dizziness and intoxication within minutes. Prolonged exposure or daily use may lead to hearing loss, bone marrow depression, cardiac arrhythmias, cerebral degeneration, peripheral neuropathies, and damage to the liver, kidneys, or lungs. A characteristic "glue sniffer's rash" around the nose and mouth is sometimes seen after prolonged use. In rare instances death may occur, most likely from hypoxemia, cardiac arrhythmias, pneumonia, or aspiration of vomit while unconscious. Detoxification is rarely required for the patient who has abused these substances, but psychiatric treatment may be needed to prevent relapse.

DESIGNER DRUGS

The term *designer drugs* refers to illicit synthetic drugs, many of which have increased potency in comparison with their parent compounds. The most common designer drugs include analogs of fentanyl, meperidine, piperazine, and methamphetamines. The best-known fentanyl derivatives are α-methyl fentanyl *(China white),* parafluorofentanyl, and 3-methyl fentanyl. Because these drugs are approximately 1000 times as potent as heroin, the fact that fatal overdoses from respiratory depression have been reported is not surprising.

The major meperidine derivatives are 1-methyl-4-phenyl-4-propionoxypiperidene (MPPP) and 1-methyl-4-phenyl-1,2,3,6-tetrahydropyridine (MPTP). These drugs produce euphoria similar to that caused by heroin. In some users, MPTP causes neuronal degeneration in the substantia nigra, which produces an irreversible form of Parkinson disease.

Piperazines, a new class of designer drugs of abuse, are commonly sold as party pills in the form of tablets, capsules, or powders on the drug black market and in so-called "head shops" or over the internet. 1-Benzylpiperazine (BZP) is the most prevalent of these compounds. Aside from BZP and 1-(3,4-methylenedioxybenzyl)piperazine (MDBP), the phenylpiperazine derivatives 1-(3-trifluoromethylphenyl) piperazine (TFMPP), 1-(3-chloro phenyl) piperazine (mCPP), and 1-(4-methoxyphenyl)piperazine (MeOPP) are often abused. Because piperazines and amphetamines cause similar pharmacologic symptoms, piperazine poisoning can easily be wrongly diagnosed as amphetamine poisoning. Furthermore, piperazines are not detected by routinely used immunochemical screening procedures for drugs of abuse, but they require an appropriate toxicologic analysis (e.g., by gas chromatography–mass spectrometry). The methylenedioxy synthetic derivatives of amphetamine and methamphetamine are generally referred to as *ecstasy* and include 3,4-methylenedioxy methamphetamine (MDMA, also known as *Adam*); 3,4-methylenedioxyethylamphetamine (MDEA, also known as *Eve*); and N-methyl-1-(3,4-methylenedioxyphenyl)-2-butanamine (MBDB, also known as *Methyl-J* or *Eden*). These drugs have CNS stimulant and hallucinogenic properties. They produce elevated mood and increased self-esteem and may cause acute panic, anxiety, paranoia, hallucinations, tachycardia, nystagmus, ataxia, and tremor. Deaths in some users have been attributed to cardiac arrhythmias, hyperthermia with seizures, and intracranial hemorrhage.

Prospectus for the Future

The elucidation of ligands to psychotropic drugs is being used to provide molecular clues for the derivation of structural analogs that have therapeutic benefits. For example, recent studies have identified the receptors to which tetrahydrocannabinoid binds to mediate its effects. In the brain, activation of the cannabinoid-1 receptor causes the psychotropic effects associated with marijuana use. Cannabinoid-1 receptors also are found in adipose tissue and the gastrointestinal tract, where they regulate food intake and glycemic control. A cannabinoid-1 receptor antagonist, rimonabant, has been shown to be effective in suppressing the reinforcing and rewarding properties of different agents that are often abused (e.g., cocaine, nicotine, alcohol) and reducing food intake and body weight. This agent appears to be effective in treating drug addiction and obesity-related disorders, although its high rate of adverse psychiatric effects (i.e., depression, anxiety, and suicidal ideation) have halted its clinical development. The identification of other receptors and signaling pathways may permit the development of other agonists or antagonists that will serve as effective pharmacotherapeutic agents.

References

Anton RF: Naltrexone for the management of alcohol dependence. N Engl J Med 359:715-721, 2008.

Anton RF, O'Malley SS, Ciraulo DA, et al: Combined pharmacotherapies and behavioral interventions for alcohol dependence: The COMBINE study: A randomized controlled trial. JAMA 295:2003-2017, 2006.

Dick DM, Agrawal A: The genetics of alcohol and other drug dependence. Alcohol Res Health 31:111-118, 2008.

Edenberg HJ: The Genetics of Alcohol Metabolism: Role of Alcohol Dehydrogenase and Aldehyde Dehydrogenase Variants. Available at: http://pubs.niaaa.nih.gov/publications/arh301/5-13.htm.

Ferri MMF, Amato L, Davoli M: Alcoholics Anonymous and other 12-step programmes for alcohol dependence. Cochrane Database Syst Rev 4:1-26, 2008.

Heilig M, Mark E: Pharmacological treatment of alcohol dependence: Target symptoms and target mechanisms. Pharmacol Ther 111:855-876, 2006.

Lopez-Moreno JA, Gonzalez-Cuevas G, Moreno G, Navarro M: The pharmacology of the endocannabinoid system: Functional and structural interactions with other neurotransmitter systems and their repercussions in behavioral addiction. Addict Biol 13:160-182, 2008.

Preti A: New developments in the pharmacotherapy of cocaine abuse. Addict Biol 12:133-151, 2007.

Saitz R: Unhealthy alcohol use. N Engl J Med 352:596-607, 2005.

Staack RF: Piperazine designer drugs of abuse. Lancet 369:1411-1413, 2007.

Substance Abuse and Mental Health Services Administration: Results from the 2007 National Survey on Drug Use and Health: National Findings (Office of Applied Studies, NSDUH Series H-34, DHHS Publication No. SMA 08-4343). Rockville, Md, 2008. Available at: http://oas.samhsa.gov.

Index

Page numbers followed by f indicate figures; t, tables.

A

A_{1c} (glycosylated hemoglobin), 698, 703-704, 704t, 706
Abatacept, for rheumatoid arthritis, 827, 827t
Abciximab, 109-110, 582
Abdominal pain, 382-385, 383t, 384f
  in acute intermittent porphyria, 655-656
  gastrointestinal bleeding with, 387
  in pancreatic carcinoma, 453
  in pancreatitis
    acute, 447-448
    chronic, 451-452
Abdominal pain syndrome, functional, 385
Abortion, septic, acute kidney injury secondary to, 367-368
Abscess(es)
  antimicrobial therapy for, 905
  brain, 1159-1160, 1160f
    infective endocarditis with, 962, 1162-1163
    parasitic, 942, 943f
    subdural empyema leading to, 1160
  fever of unknown origin and, 921
  hepatic, 921, 975-976, 976t
  infective endocarditis with, 961-963, 1162-1163
    surgery for, 966
  intra-abdominal, 975-977, 976t
    fever associated with, 921, 975
  lung, 248, 256
  pancreatic, 976t, 977
  paravertebral, in mycobacterial osteomyelitis, 988
  pelvic, 976t, 977
  perinephric, 976t, 990-991
  peritonsillar, 949
  pharyngeal space, 949-950
  prostatic, 757, 922, 991
  renal, 922, 962
  retroperitoneal, 976t, 977
  retropharyngeal space, 949-950
  spinal epidural, 987, 1161-1162, 1161f
  staphylococcal, 886-887
  subcutaneous, 969
Absence epilepsy
  childhood, 1146, 1149-1150
  juvenile, 1146
Absence seizures, 1145-1146, 1145f
  atypical, 1146
  frontal, 1144
  hyperventilation and, 1147
Absence status epilepticus, 1151
Absolute risk reduction, 18
Abuse. See Domestic violence; Elder abuse.
Acamprosate, for alcoholism, 1224
Acanthocytes, 529
Acarbose, 710t-713t, 712
Accessory pathways, 129
  catheter ablation of, 142-143
  concealed, 129
ACE. See Angiotensin-converting enzyme (ACE).
ACE inhibitors. See Angiotensin-converting enzyme (ACE) inhibitors.
Acetaminophen
  for osteoarthritis pain, 872
  overdose of, 264t, 472, 477
Acetazolamide, mechanism of action, 307-308, 308t
Acetylcholine, neuromuscular junction disease and, 1191-1193
Acetylcholinesterase inhibitors, for dementia symptoms
  in Alzheimer disease, 1072, 1074
  in Parkinson disease, 1075
N-Acetylcysteine
  for acetaminophen overdose, 472
  contrast media–associated nephropathy and, 365-366, 371-372
  for idiopathic pulmonary fibrosis, 230
  in Wilson disease, 652
Achalasia, 411, 412f, 412t
Achilles tendinitis, 875

Acid-base balance, 294-295, 316-319, 317f
Acid-base disorders, 316-319. See also Acidosis; Alkalosis.
  adaptive responses to, 317, 318t
  systematic assessment of, 317, 317t
Acidosis
  as ketoacidosis, 318-319
    diabetic, 698, 715-716, 715t
  metabolic. See Metabolic acidosis.
  renal tubular, 319, 319f-320f, 319t
    urinary pH in, 299-300, 320
  respiratory, 321-322
Acquired cystic kidney disease, 339
Acquired immunodeficiency syndrome (AIDS), 884.
    See also Human immunodeficiency virus (HIV) infection.
  antiretroviral therapy for, initiation of, 1016t, 1017
  chest infections in, 194
  cholecystitis in, acalculous, 492
  diagnostic criteria for, 1009, 1009t
  enteric protozoal infections in, 1024-1025
  epidemiology of, 1008-1010, 1010f
  malignancies in, 1009t, 1026. See also Kaposi sarcoma.
    non-Hodgkin lymphoma, 553, 1025-1026
    primary CNS lymphoma, 1026, 1154, 1157
  nervous system disease in, 1021-1023, 1022t-1023t, 1177
  progression to, 1012f, 1013-1014, 1017f
  travel by patients with, 1037
  travelers' risk of acquiring, 1037
Acromegaly, 662-663, 662t-663t
  hyperphosphatemia in, 791-792
  musculoskeletal manifestations of, 881t
Acropachy, thyroid, 882
ACTH. See Adrenocorticotropic hormone (ACTH).
Actin, of myocytes, 25, 25f-26f
Actinomyces, 887-888
Actinomycetales, 887-888
Actinomycin D, mechanism of action, 4
Action potentials
  cardiac, 118, 119f
  hyperkalemia and, 312
Action tremor, 1114
Activated protein C, 561. See also Protein C.
  for sepsis syndrome, 930-932, 931t
  for septic shock, 262
Activated protein C resistance, 582-583, 582t, 587
Activities of daily living (ADLs), 1198-1199, 1205-1207
Acute chest syndrome, in sickle cell disease, 530
Acute coronary syndromes, 106-112. See also Myocardial infarction; Unstable angina.
  glycoprotein IIb/IIIa inhibitors in, 582
  plaque disruption and, 95
  secondary prevention of, 116-117
  treatment algorithm for, 109f
Acute intermittent porphyria, 655-656, 655f, 656t
Acute kidney injury (AKI), 359-368. See also Acute tubular necrosis (ATN) ; Renal failure, acute.
  causes of, 359, 360f
    aortic dissection as, 349-350
    endogenous nephrotoxins, 367-368
    exogenous nephrotoxins, 365-366, 365t
  in chronic kidney disease, 372, 372t, 372t
  vs. chronic kidney disease, 362, 363t, 369
  clinical importance of, 359, 360t
  definition of, 359
  diagnostic criteria for, 359, 359b
  future prospects for, 368b
  in hospitalized patients, 360
    with chronic kidney disease, 372
    diagnostic approach to, 360-361, 361t-362t
  hyperkalemia in, 364
  in outpatients, 362-363, 363t
  of pregnancy, 367-368
Acute limb ischemia, 166-167

Acute lung injury, 262
  in idiopathic pulmonary fibrosis, 230
Acute phase reactants, in rheumatic disease, 821, 826
Acute respiratory distress syndrome. See Adult respiratory distress syndrome (ARDS).
Acute stress disorder, 1080-1081
Acute tubular necrosis (ATN), 359, 360f. See also Acute kidney injury (AKI).
  clinical presentation of, 363
  complications of, 363-364, 364t
  in hospitalized patients, 360-362, 362t
  outcome and prognosis in, 364
  pathogenesis of, 365
  in pregnancy, 368
  prevention of, 364-365
  in sepsis syndrome, 929
Adalimumab
  for Crohn disease, 437
  for rheumatoid arthritis, 827, 827t
  for spondyloarthropathies, 832
ADAMTS-13, 558
  therapeutic preparations of, 587
  in thrombotic thrombocytopenic purpura, 331-332, 586-587
  von Willebrand disease and, 575
Addison disease, 680-681, 683
Addisonian crisis, hypercalcemia in, 786-787
Adenocarcinoma
  breast, 610
  esophagus, 410, 439, 606
  gastric, 440-441
  kidney, 612
  lung, 266-267, 269, 603
  of unknown primary, 615
Adenoma-to-carcinoma sequence, 596, 596f
Adenosine
  as antiarrhythmic agent, 139
  coronary blood flow and, 28-29
Adenosine deaminase deficiency, gene therapy for, 13
Adenosine diphosphate (ADP) inhibitors, 581-582, 581t. See also Clopidogrel.
Adenosine stress testing, 55
  with myocardial perfusion imaging, 57-58
Adenosine triphosphate (ATP)
  coronary blood flow and, 28-29
  myocardial contraction and, 25, 26f
Adhesive capsulitis, in diabetics, 881
Adie pupils, 1097
Adipocytokines, 631
Adipose tissue, secretory products of, 631
Adjuvant chemotherapy, 624
ADLs. See Activities of daily living (ADLs).
Adolescent women's health, 734-736
Adrenal glands, 679-690
  anatomy of, 679, 679f
  future prospects for, 690b
  physiology of
    cortical, 679-680, 680f
    medullary, 689
Adrenal hyperplasia
  congenital, 683-684
  primary aldosteronism secondary to, 177-178
Adrenal insufficiency, 680-683, 682t
  ACTH levels and, 664-665
  in HIV-infected patients, 1025
  hypoglycemia in, 724-725
  in sepsis, 930-932
Adrenal medullary hyperfunction, 689-690. See also Pheochromocytoma.
Adrenal tumors
  adenoma
    aldosterone-producing, 177-178, 689
    cortisol-secreting, 688
  carcinoma, 690
  incidentaloma, 690
α_2-Adrenergic agonists, perioperative, with noncardiac surgery, 279